For Instructors

Instructor's Electronic Resource

ISBN: 1-4160-2569-3

This helpful Instructor's CD provides the necessary tools for the instructor to quickly and consistently prepare for class. Key features include:

- A full Instructor's Resource Manual in the most common word processing formats.
- A comprehensive Test Bank using the ExamView test generator platform.
- PowerPoint lecture slides on the CD.
- An image collection in a variety of downloadable formats. Images can also be imported into the PowerPoint lecture slides of your choice.
- Also available online in Evolve Resources.

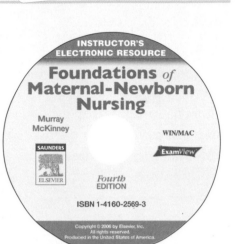

INSTRUCTOR'S ELECTRONIC RESOURCE

Foundations *of* **Maternal-Newborn Nursing**

Murray
McKinney

WIN/MAC

SAUNDERS
ELSEVIER

ExamView

Fourth EDITION

ISBN 1-4160-2569-3

Copyright © 2006 by Elsevier, Inc.
All rights reserved.
Produced in the United States of America

Evolve Course Management System

evolve http://evolve.elsevier.com/Murray/foundations/

Evolve is an interactive learning environment that works in coordination with *Foundations of Maternal-Newborn Nursing,* fourth edition, providing Internet-based course content that reinforces and expands on the concepts that instructors deliver in class. Instructors are able to access all of the resources available to students. Instructors can use Evolve to:

- Publish class syllabi, outlines, and lecture notes.
- Set up "virtual office hours" and e-mail communication.
- Share important dates and information through the online class Calendar.
- Encourage student participation through Chat Rooms and Discussion Boards.

Instructors are encouraged to contact their sales representative for more information about integrating Evolve into their curricula.

Brief Table of Contents

Fourth
EDITION

Foundations *of* Maternal–Newborn Nursing

Sharon Smith Murray, MSN, RN, C

Professor, Health Professions
Golden West College
Huntington Beach, California

Emily Slone McKinney, MSN, RN, C

Baylor Healthcare System
Dallas, Texas

With 400 Illustrations

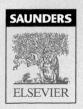

SAUNDERS

ELSEVIER

SAUNDERS
ELSEVIER

11830 Westline Industrial Drive
St. Louis, Missouri 63146

Notice

Knowledge and best practice in this field are constantly changing. As new research and experience broaden our knowledge, changes in practice, treatment and drug therapy may become necessary or appropriate. Readers are advised to check the most current information provided (i) on procedures featured or (ii) by the manufacturer of each product to be administered, to verify the recommended dose or formula, the method and duration of administration, and contraindications. It is the responsibility of the practitioner, relying on their own experience and knowledge of the patient, to make diagnoses, to determine dosages and the best treatment for each individual patient, and to take all appropriate safety precautions. To the fullest extent of the law, neither the Publisher nor the Authors assume any liability for any injury and/or damage to persons or property arising out or related to any use of the material contained in this book.

The Publisher

Executive Editor: Michael S. Ledbetter
Acquisitions Editor: Catherine Albright Jackson
Senior Developmental Editor: Lisa P. Newton
Publishing Services Manager: Jeff Patterson
Project Manager: Anne Konopka
Design Manager: Teresa McBryan

Printed in the United States of America.

Last digit is the print number: 9   8   7   6   5   4   3   2

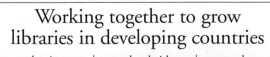

Working together to grow
libraries in developing countries

www.elsevier.com | www.bookaid.org | www.sabre.org

ELSEVIER   BOOK AID International   Sabre Foundation

Reviewers

Jessica Lynn Alexander, MN

Assistant Professor
Mississippi University
Columbus, Mississippi

Darlene Del Prato, MS, RN, C

Faculty
St. Joseph's Hospital
Syracuse, New York

Jill Janke, RNC, ANP, DNSc

Professor
University of Alaska Anchorage
School of Nursing
Anchorage, Alaska

Debra Migues, RN, MSN, ICCE

Associate Professor of Nursing
Louisiana College
Division of Nursing
Pineville, Louisiana

Virginia Bradford Pearson, RN, MSN

Instructor
University of Southern Mississippi
School of Nursing
Hattiesburg, Mississippi

For Skip, whose love and support make it all possible.
For my daughters, Vicki, Holly, and Shannon, who make me proud.
For Marina, Nicholas, and Giovanni, who provide such joy.
And to my mother, Clare, who has always shown the way.
S.S.M.

For Michael, the love of my life.
For the blessings of our daughters, Cathy and Amy.
And to the love of my late parents, Juanita and Charles Slone.
E.S.M.

For the nursing students who have challenged us to learn something new each day.
For the clients who make our caring as a nurse worthwhile.
S.S.M and **E.S.M.**

Preface

Our challenge as nursing educators is to keep up with the rapid changes in health care while preparing students to stay focused on the *care* of nursing. In clinical rotations that seem to grow shorter each year, the nursing faculty must teach the student ways to use the nursing process, drugs, and technology that are beneficial while imparting the values of client-centered care. Our text tries to help the student learn to balance "high-touch" care with "high-tech," often life-saving, care.

Although health care delivery has changed dramatically, with greater emphasis now on outcome management and use of clinical pathways to decrease the length of stay in the birth facility, the family's need for education and support during the childbearing period does not lessen. Nurses have responded to families' needs by developing alternative means of education that use every possible moment before admission and during their stay in the birth facility. A student's clinical experience often includes the home and a variety of community clinics.

An effective textbook must present comprehensive content that can be read with ease, because nursing students differ in learning abilities, experience, and primary language. Our objective for the fourth edition of *Foundations of Maternal-Newborn Nursing* continues to be the presentation of complex material as simply and clearly as possible. We again provide step-by-step instruction in assessments and interventions so that students can function quickly in the clinical area at a beginning level. To this end, proven learning aids, such as summaries, illustrations, tables, and highlights are used generously throughout the book.

CONTENT

Maternity nurses must be flexible to accommodate families from different cultures and who communicate in different languages and hold different health beliefs. Nurses must use critical thinking skills to devise culture-specific care that includes providing necessary education and support. The six elements we consider most important are a scientific base of information, nursing process, communication, client teaching, critical thinking, and cultural diversity.

Scientific Base

Effective nursing care depends on having a sound understanding of the bases for medical treatments and nursing actions. Although anatomy and physiology courses are part of every curriculum, students often need a review, particularly of the specific content related to childbearing. Because of

this, we have incorporated principles of physiology and pathophysiology throughout the book. We have presented these scientific concepts in a clear and understandable manner so that the reader can comprehend the forces underlying both health and dysfunction. We have included research evidence that supports specific nursing care methods when available.

Chapters 4, 5, and 6 provide general information about reproductive physiology, genetics, and the process of conception and fetal development. Chapters 7, 12, 17, and 19 explain physiologic adaptation during pregnancy, birth, and the postpartum period and in the newborn. Part V, Families at Risk during the Childbearing Period, describes the pathophysiological, psychological, and social bases of complications in the mother and in the newborn.

The Nursing Process

The nursing process is the accepted framework for client assessment and analysis of client needs. It is used to plan and provide nursing care and evaluate the client's response to care. Client needs often are a mixture of those for which nurses have the primary accountability and those for which another discipline provides definitive therapy yet for which nurses have some responsibility. Therefore for analyzing client needs we have chosen either a *nursing diagnosis* or a *collaborative problem,* depending on whether nurses are primarily responsible for helping the client meet those needs. All nursing diagnoses are drawn from the most recent list of those approved by the North American Nursing Diagnosis Association (NANDA).

The nursing process is treated two ways in our text: in a narrative format and in nursing care plans. In each method we lead the reader through the five steps of the nursing process. In the narrative format, basic information about the condition is presented and general nursing care follows, organized by the steps of the nursing process. Interventions are general rather than client specific and are explained by rationales. Because nursing students often have difficulty transferring general information to the care of a specific client, we have created nursing care plans based on scenarios of client situations most often encountered in maternity nursing.

Communication

Although they seldom are included as core content in maternal-newborn nursing texts, communication skills are essential to provide adequate care for a childbearing family. We reinforce the student's previous learning and give practical examples of ways in which communication skills can be used in the maternity setting.

Guidelines and examples of effective communication and potential blocks are reviewed in Chapter 2. Color-highlighted *communication cues* in the text give tips on how to interact with families. Tips include ways to avoid potentially embarrassing situations, role modeling of effective communication styles, and reading nonverbal signals.

In addition, dialogues throughout the text present realistic possible nurse-client interactions. As the interaction develops, we identify communication techniques and explain their rationale. Because no one is perfect, we occasionally insert communication blocks, identify them, and suggest alternate responses.

Client Teaching

Childbearing families are entitled to comprehensive information about how to achieve the best pregnancy outcome and how to best care for the mother and baby after birth. Women of all ages need current information about maintaining their health, including when they are not pregnant. Nurses are their primary instructors in most areas of maternal-newborn nursing, and they must be well prepared and well organized to be effective. We present client teaching in three ways:

- Teaching-learning principles are discussed in Chapter 2.
- Chapters are organized to highlight key content so that the student can gather information and translate it into client teaching. For example, Chapter 22, Infant Feeding, lays a foundation of basic information, discusses some common problems, identifies relevant assessments, and presents nursing interventions devoted to teaching parents ways to feed their infant successfully.
- Client teaching guidelines are highlighted in *Want to Know* features, which give ideas on ways to answer the most common client questions on a topic. These features are constructed to show students ways to present information in everyday language rather than in professional language so that the family will better understand the teaching. For instance, the feature "When to Go to the Hospital or Birth Center" (p. 267, Chapter 13) addresses the concern of many expectant parents that they will not recognize the onset of labor.

Critical Thinking

Nurses must learn critical thinking skills to overcome habits or impulses that can lead to poor clinical decisions. Chapter 2 discusses steps in critical thinking and describes how critical thinking is used in each step of the nursing process. In addition, critical thinking exercises are presented in two ways. First, exercises based on clinical scenarios of common situations with questions to stimulate critical thinking are placed throughout the text. Answers to the questions follow each exercise to provide reinforcement for student learning. Second, client-specific nursing care plans (described earlier) contain critical thinking exercises that require participation by the student. This makes the care plans interactive and reinforces the concept of critical thinking in clinical practice.

Cultural Diversity

Cultural values are among the most significant factors that influence a woman's perception of childbirth, and effective nursing care must be culture specific. This requires nurses to consider their own cultural values and examine how these values may create conflict with those whose values are different.

Chapter 1 offers an overview of Western cultural values and identifies some areas such as communication and health beliefs that may be sources of conflict. Because many different cultural groups exist in the United States and Canada, emphasis is placed on ways to do a cultural assessment. Plans for care then can show how understanding a family's culture helps nurses provide care that shows respect for cultural differences and traditional healing practices.

New information is integrated throughout the book in all areas, such as the antepartum period, nutrition, birth, the postpartum period, and care of the newborn. Chapter 33, Women's Health Care, includes information about cardiovascular disease in women, physical inactivity, and weight control issues that have increased in recent years.

The Internet is often used by lay people and professionals as a source of health information. We provide the addresses for many websites throughout our text that contain reliable, current information relevant to maternal, newborn, and women's health nursing. Examples of these sites are the March of Dimes, Centers for Disease Control and Prevention, National Institutes of Health, and American Cancer Society. Websites for professional associations are included when appropriate.

ORGANIZATION

The fourth edition of *Foundations of Maternal-Newborn Nursing* is divided into six parts. Part I, Foundations for Nursing Care of Childbearing Families, presents an overview of contemporary maternity care including ethical, social, and legal aspects. A review of reproductive anatomy and physiology and the hereditary and environmental factors that affect care are also presented. This material is especially important for students who have not recently completed a full anatomy and physiology course.

Part II, The Family Before Birth, begins with conception and fetal development. These chapters also cover the physiologic and psychosocial adaptations to pregnancy and include a thorough explanation of recommended nutrition during pregnancy and after childbirth.

Part III, The Family during Birth, addresses the physiologic processes of birth and nursing care during labor and birth. These chapters include intrapartum fetal monitoring, pain management, and obstetric procedures such as cesarean birth.

Part IV, The Family Following Birth, describes care of the new mother and infant. Alternative methods for continuing care, such as home visits and telephone follow-up, also are covered. Separate chapters address infant feeding and home care of the infant.

Part V, Families at Risk during the Childbearing Period, includes a chapter on the family with special needs such as age-related concerns, childbearing in a substance-abusing or violent environment, birth of an infant with congenital anomalies, and responses to fetal or neonatal death. Additional chapters describe the most common complications of pregnancy, childbirth, and the postpartum and neonatal periods. Prematurity is a major health concern in the United States. Measures to reduce prematurity's rate, severity, and long-term effects on the child and family are discussed in several chapters.

Part VI, Other Reproductive Issues, focuses on family planning, care of the infertile couple, and women's health care.

FEATURES

- *Visual Appeal.* The book is visually appealing, with numerous up-to-date full-color illustrations and photographs that clarify concepts and reinforce learning. Beautiful color pictures also illustrate a childbirth story and cesarean birth.
- *Objectives and Definitions.* Each chapter begins with a list of objectives that spells out the purposes of the chapter. A list of key terms with their definitions follows the objectives. A glossary at the back of the book contains key terms from all chapters and other terms related to this course.
- *Check Your Reading.* Questions to help students monitor their understanding of the material presented are placed at intervals throughout each chapter. Answers to questions are placed in Appendix D so that students can have immediate feedback.
- *Critical Thinking Exercises.* Clinical situations are boxed and set apart to stimulate critical thinking. We believe strongly that immediate feedback is a powerful learning tool, so answers to critical thinking exercises in the text appear at the end of every chapter.
- *Critical to Remember.* Condensed summaries of the essential facts to remember are boxed and set apart to reinforce critical information.
- *Want to Know.* This feature can be used by students who must begin teaching very early in their clinical rotations. These include answers to the most common questions asked by women and parents, often phrased in laymen's terms or as the nurse would actually answer a client.
- *Procedures.* Illustrated procedures that are specific to maternity and women's health nursing, such as assessment of the uterine fundus, are presented in a step-by-step format with rationales for each step.
- *Drug Guides.* Guides for medications often administered in maternity nursing and women's health care are available in appropriate chapters. Information about additional drugs may be given in tables or in the narrative.
- *Complementary and Alternative Therapies.* We have included content about these therapies when appropriate throughout the text, and it is highlighted with a special heading. Several herbal and botanical preparations have been added to Appendix B, Use of Drugs and Botanical Preparations during Pregnancy and Breastfeeding.
- *Summary Concepts.* A concise review of content is provided at the end of each chapter. In addition, tables and flow charts are frequently used to summarize complex material.
- *Keys to Clinical Practice.* A description of how to prepare for clinical experience is presented in Appendix C. This feature provides care guides for assessments and interventions for the woman in labor, the woman after childbirth, and the infant. It also provides teaching on key topics such as assisting the inexperienced mother to breastfeed. This feature is designed to help students through their earliest clinical experiences before they have had much theory.

ANCILLARIES

Materials that complement *Foundations of Maternal-Newborn Nursing* include:

- The *Foundations of Maternal-Newborn Nursing Companion CD*: This interactive CD-ROM is included with the text. The CD includes New Maternity videos, NCLEX-style review questions; nursing skills outlines, case studies, neonatal video clips with learning exercises, and a glossary with definitions and sound pronunciations.
- *Instructor's Electronic Resource:* Four separate teacher support programs are available on a single CD-ROM or from this book's Evolve website: (a) a full instructor's manual in the most common word processing formats; (b) a computerized test bank using the Exam View program; (c) PowerPoint lecture slides, and (d) an image collection in a variety of downloadable formats.
- *Virtual Clinical Excursions workbook/CD-ROM package:* A groundbreaking learning tool guides the student through a computer-generated virtual clinical environment and helps the student apply textbook content to "virtual clients" in that environment. The clinical simulations and workbook represent the next generation of research-based learning tools that promote critical thinking and meaningful learning.
- *Study Guide for Foundations of Maternal-Newborn Nursing:* This manual presents a variety of additional activities designed to help students master content and become more proficient in the clinical area. Review questions at various levels of difficulty are included.
- *Clinical Companion for Foundations of Maternal-Newborn Nursing:* This portable reference book can be easily carried to the clinical area, where information that relates to hands-on practice is most useful. The primary focus of the companion is on nursing assessments and interventions.

EVOLVE LEARNING RESOURCES

Weblinks for both instructors and students allows access to information and resources based on topics covered in this edition of *Foundations of Maternal-Newborn Nursing* at http://evolve.elsevier.com/Murray/foundations/.

The *Instructor's Electronic Resource* includes the Instructor's Resource Manual, Test Bank, Image Collection, and Power Point Lecture slides.

Evolve Course Management System (CMS):

- The CMS is available to instructors on adoption of the fourth edition of *Foundations of Maternal-Newborn Nursing.*
- Instructors and students will have **full access** to a comprehensive suite of communication and organization tools, including discussion boards, e-mail, chat rooms, calendars, address books, task organizers, and more.
- Instructors will have **exclusive access** to the course management tools that allow them to customize their course content, build online tests, create assignments, enter grades, post announcements, manage student groups, and much more.

ACKNOWLEDGMENTS

We give special thanks to Lisa Newton, Senior Developmental Editor in Editorial, who helped organize the project and guide it to completion. Anne Konopka in Book Production helped us refine and clarify our writing with her suggestions and critiques. We also thank Teresa McBryan, Design Manager, for the beautiful cover and the clear and attractive page layouts.

We thank Michael Ledbetter, Executive Editor, Nursing Division for helping us plan the fourth edition of our text. Although our book had a successful framework in place, Michael helped us consider changes and additions that improve it for students and teachers.

Finally, we want to thank Trula Myers Gorrie, our co-author on the first two editions of this textbook. Tru has continued to be our colleague, mentor, and coach as we have continued with the fourth edition. Most of all, Tru is a great friend to us. Although we miss her company as our co-author, we wish Tru only the best as she enjoys a well-earned retirement.

Special Features

Objectives and **Definitions** with glossary-style definitions at the beginning of each chapter set the stage for student learning.

Illustrated procedures that are specific to maternity and women's health nursing are presented in a step-by-step format with rationales for each step.

Critical to Remember boxes provide condensed summaries of the essential facts to remember and are set apart to reinforce critical information.

CHAPTER

33 Women's Health Care

OBJECTIVES

After studying this chapter, you should be able to:

1. Explain examinations and screening procedures recommended to maintain the health of women.
2. Explain benign disorders of the breast, relate them to usual age of onset, and describe the diagnostic procedures used to rule out cancer of the breast.
3. Describe the incidence, risks, pathophysiology, management, and nursing considerations related to malignant breast tumors.
4. Discuss cardiovascular disease in women, including risk factors, signs and symptoms, and prevention measures.
5. Discuss common menstrual cycle disorders.
6. Explain premenstrual syndrome, management options, and nursing considerations.
7. Discuss medical termination of pregnancy in terms of procedures, possible complications, and follow-up care.
8. Describe the physical and psychological changes associated with menopause and options to alleviate uncomfortable changes.
9. Discuss measures to reduce severity of osteoporosis.
10. Describe the major disorders associated with pelvic relaxation in terms of cause, treatment, and nursing considerations.
11. Discuss the most common benign and malignant disorders of signs and symptoms, management, and nursing con
12. Describe care of the woman with an infectious disorder sexually transmissible diseases, pelvic inflammatory dis

Go to your Student CD-ROM for

DEFINITIONS

Adjuvant Therapy Additional treatment that increases or enhances the action of the primary treatment.

Adnexa Accessory parts or organs, such as the fallopian tubes and ovaries associated with the uterus.

Amenorrhea Absence of menstruation. Primary amenorrhea is a delay of the first menstruation. Secondary amenorrhea is cessation of menstruation after its initiation.

Angina Pectoris Myocardial pain usually brought on by physical activity or stress; usually called simply *angina*.

Atrophic Vaginitis Inflammation that occurs when the vagina becomes dry and fragile, usually as a result of estrogen deficit after menopause.

878

---

554   PART IV The Family Following Birth

NIPPLE CONFUSION

Nipple confusion (or nipple preference) may occur when an infant who has been fed by bottle confuses the tongue movements necessary for bottle feeding with the suckling of breastfeeding. Some infants develop a preference for bottle feeding and refuse to breastfeed. Others use bottle feeding tongue movements that impede breastfeeding.

Movements of the mouth and tongue are different in breastfeeding and bottle feeding. To feed from a bottle, infants must push the tongue over the nipple to slow the flow of milk and prevent choking (Figure 22-9). This can be demonstrated by noting the steady drip of milk when a bottle is held upside down. In bottle feeding, the infant's lips are relaxed because the infant does not need to hold the nipple in place. If the infant uses the same thrusting tongue motion and relaxed lips while nursing, the breast may be pushed out of the mouth.

During breastfeeding, the infant uses suction to hold the nipple in place near the soft palate. The tongue cups around the nipple and areola with the tip over the lower gum. With each compression of the lower jaw, the tongue presses

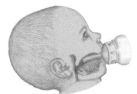

Tongue thrusts forward
to control milk flow

Figure 22-9 ■ During bottle feeding, infants must push the tongue over the nipple to slow the rapid flow of milk.

CRITICAL TO REMEMBER

Infant Signs of Breastfeeding Problems

Falling asleep after feeding less than 5 minutes
Refusal to breastfeed
Tongue thrusting
Smacking or clicking sounds
Dimpling of the cheeks
Failure to open the mouth widely at latch-on
Lower lip turned in
Short, choppy motions of the jaw
No audible swallowing
Use of formula

sess suckling. The peristaltic motion of the tongue should be felt as the infant sucks. The infant who is thrusting the tongue may have become confused by the use of latex nipples, which should be avoided until the problem is resolved. If the infant tends to place the tongue on top of the nipple, inserting a finger in the mouth and pressing the infant's tongue down just before latch-on may be effective. The tongue should be cupped under the breast and should cover the lower gum. Helping the infant open the mouth widely before attachment may improve suckling. More complicated suckling problems may require assistance from a lactation educator or consultant.

CHECK YOUR READING

11. What wake-up techniques should the nurse teach the mother of a sleepy infant?
12. How does sucking from a bottle differ from suckling from the breast?

INFANT COMPLICATIONS

Infant complications may be minor and cause minimal interference with breastfeeding or may prevent the infant from breastfeeding for a long period.

JAUNDICE. Jaundice (hyperbilirubinemia) need not interfere with breastfeeding or may prevent the infant from breastfeeding for a long period. Even when infants receive phototherapy, they usually can be removed from the lights for feedings. Concern about adequate intake may be more prevalent in caring for the infant with jaundice. Insensible water loss from the skin is increased as a result of the heat and lights used in treatment and could lead to dehydration.

---

280   PART III The Family during Birth

PROCEDURE

13-1 Leopold's Maneuvers

PURPOSE: To determine presentation and position of the fetus and aid in location of fetal heart sounds

1. Explain the procedure to the woman and the rationale for each step as it is performed. Tell her what is found at each step. *Gives information, teaches the woman, and reassures her when the assessment findings are normal.*
2. Ask the woman to empty her bladder if she has not done so recently. Have her lie on her back with her knees flexed slightly. Place a small pillow or folded towel under one hip. *Decreases discomfort of a full bladder during palpation and improves ability to feel fetal parts in the suprapubic area. Knee flexion helps the woman relax her abdominal muscles to enhance palpation. Uterine displacement prevents aortocaval compression, which could reduce blood flow to the placenta.*
3. Wash your hands with warm water. Wear gloves if contact with secretions is likely. *Warm hands are more comfortable during palpation and prevent tensing of abdominal muscles.*
4. Stand beside the woman, facing her head, with your dominant hand nearest her. *The first three maneuvers are most easily performed in this position.*

5. Palpate the uterine fundus. The breech (buttocks) is softer and more irregular in shape than the head. Moving the breech also moves the fetal trunk. The head is harder and has a round, uniform shape. The head can be moved without moving the entire fetal trunk. *Distinguishes between a cephalic and breech presentation. If the fetus is in a cephalic presentation, the breech is felt in the fundus. If the presentation is breech, the head is felt in the fundus.*

SECOND MANEUVER

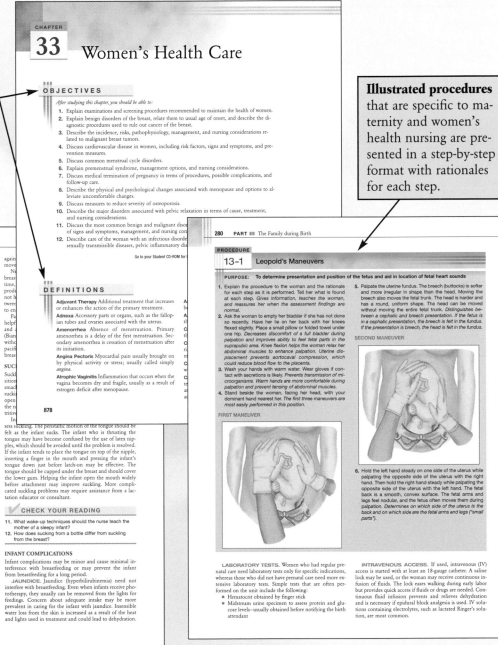

6. Hold the left hand steady on one side of the uterus while palpating the opposite side of the uterus with the right hand. Then hold the right hand steady while palpating the opposite side of the uterus with the left hand. The fetal back is a smooth, convex surface. The fetal arms and legs feel nodular, and the fetus often moves them during palpation. *Determines on which side of the uterus is the back and on which side are the fetal arms and legs ("small parts").*

FIRST MANEUVER

LABORATORY TESTS. Women who had regular prenatal care need laboratory tests only for specific indications, whereas those who did not have prenatal care need more extensive laboratory tests. Simple tests that are often performed on the unit include the following:

■ Hematocrit obtained by finger stick
■ Midstream urine specimen to assess protein and glucose levels—usually obtained before notifying the birth attendant

INTRAVENOUS ACCESS. If used, intravenous (IV) access is started with at least an 18-gauge catheter. A saline lock may be used, or the woman may receive continuous infusion of fluids. The lock eases walking during early labor but provides quick access if fluids or drugs are needed. Continuous fluid infusion prevents and relieves dehydration and is necessary if epidural block analgesia is used. IV solutions containing electrolytes, such as lactated Ringer's solution, are most common.

Want to Know Boxes can be used by students who must begin teaching very early in their clinical rotations. These include answers to the most common questions asked by women and parents, often phrased in laymen's terms or as the nurse would actually answer a client.

Critical Thinking Exercises presented in real-life clinical situations challenge students to determine what to do and why.

Therapeutic Communications shows actual client-nurse dialogues to illustrate interactions.

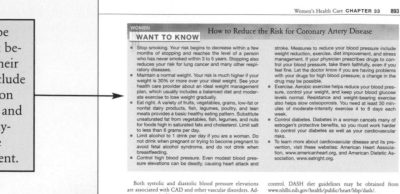

WOMEN
WANT TO KNOW
How to Reduce the Risk for Coronary Artery Disease

- Stop smoking. Your risk begins to decrease within a few months of stopping and reaches the level of a person who has never smoked within 3 to 5 years. Stopping also reduces your risk for lung cancer and many other respiratory diseases.
- Maintain a normal weight. Your risk is much higher if your weight is 30% or more over your ideal weight. See your health care provider about an ideal weight management plan, which usually includes a balanced diet and moderate exercise to lose weight gradually.
- Eat right. A variety of fruits, vegetables, grains, low-fat or nonfat dairy products, fish, legumes, poultry, and lean meats provides a basic healthy eating pattern. Substitute unsaturated fat from vegetables, fish, legumes, and nuts for foods high in saturated fats and cholesterol. Limit salt to less than 6 grams per day.
- Limit alcohol to 1 drink per day if you are a woman. Do not drink when pregnant or trying to become pregnant to avoid fetal alcohol syndrome, and do not drink when breastfeeding.
- Control high blood pressure. Even modest blood pressure elevations can be deadly, causing heart attack and

stroke. Measures to reduce your blood pressure include weight management, exercise, diet improvement, and stress management. If your physician prescribes drugs to control your blood pressure, take them faithfully, even if you feel fine. Let the doctor know if you are having problems with your drugs for high blood pressure; a change in the drug may be possible.
- Exercise. Aerobic exercise helps reduce your blood pressure, control your weight, and keep your blood glucose levels normal. Resistance and weight-bearing exercise also helps slow osteoporosis. You need at least 30 minutes of moderate-intensity exercise 4 to 6 days each week.
- Control diabetes. Diabetes in a woman cancels many of estrogen's protective benefits, so you must work harder to control your diabetes as well as your cardiovascular risks.
- To learn more about cardiovascular disease and its prevention, visit these websites: American Heart Association, www.americanheart.org, and American Dietetic Association, www.eatright.org.

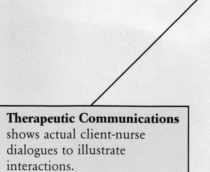

ules are chaotic for a while, the infant's behavior is generally more predictable by 12 to 16 weeks of age.
- Encourage open expression of feelings between parents as a first step in coping with stress.
- Remind parents of the need for healthy nutrition and recreation. Fatigue and tension easily can overwhelm the anticipated joys of parenting if no respite is available from constant care.
- Suggest that new parents enlist grandparents, other relatives, and friends to help with meal preparation and shopping.

HELPING THE FATHER CO-PARENT. Fathers often later remember the early interactions with their infants as being significant events in their lives (de Montigny & Lacharite, 2004). Help the father become involved with his infant by including him in teaching and providing opportunities for him to participate in diapering, comforting activities, and feeding the infant or helping the mother breastfeed. Offer frequent encouragement and praise.

PROVIDING WAYS TO REDUCE SIBLING RIVALRY. Suggest that parents plan time alone with older children. Frequent praise and expressions of love and affection help reassure older children of their places in the family. Suggest that visitors and relatives avoid focusing exclusively on the infant and include older children in their gift giving and exclamations about the newborn.

Emphasize the importance of responding calmly and with understanding when a child regresses to more infantile behaviors or expresses hostility toward the infant. Acknowledging the child's feelings and offering prompt reassurance of continued love are the most valuable actions.

Some children, particularly those older than 3 years of age, enjoy being a big brother or sister and respond well when they are included in infant care. This participation may not be possible with younger children, and setting aside separate time to participate in a favorite activity may be more worthwhile for the parents.

IDENTIFYING RESOURCES. In many homes women assume the major responsibilities of day-to-day homemaking. With the birth of an infant, this task becomes more difficult. A division of labor must be negotiated to prevent undue stress and fatigue. This division of labor is particularly important when there are other children whose needs for time, attention, and comfort must also be met.

Although the mother's primary support often is the father of the baby, extended family members, particularly grandmothers and sisters, also provide valuable support. Community resources such as daycare centers, parenting classes, and breastfeeding support are available in many areas. In addition, close friends and neighbors often share solutions to specific problems. Remind the mother that resources are available when she begins to feel isolated and exhausted.

Evaluation
A prompt, gentle response to infant crying and fussing indicates...

CRITICAL THINKING EXERCISE 18-1

Carol, a 35-year-old primipara, had an infant daughter by cesarean birth after failure to progress in labor. Carol is very tired, although she is relatively comfortable. Her husband was present during the labor and birth and is excited about being a father. He has no experience with children, and his job requires almost constant travel. Carol has never taken care of a newborn.

On the day of delivery, Carol readily accepts assistance with hygiene. She passively follows the nurse's requests to turn, cough, and breathe deeply. She discusses the details of her labor and wonders why the physician did not perform a cesarean birth earlier. She examines her baby girl closely and touches the face and hands gently with her fingertips. She remarks that she plans to breastfeed and is surprised that the infant sleeps so much.

Questions
1. What are Carol's priority needs at this time?
2. What phase of recovery is she manifesting? Why does she "fingertip" the infant?

The first postoperative day, Carol's indwelling catheter is removed and intravenous (IV) fluids are discontinued. Carol ambulates with minimal assistance and is pleased to be able to urinate without difficulty. She asks about bowel function and requests the prescribed stool softener. She spends a great deal of time getting the baby to breastfeed. She is very frustrated that the infant does not breastfeed well and asks for assistance from the lactation educator.

Questions
3. What are Carol's priority needs now?
4. How have her behaviors changed?

Before discharge, Carol is breastfeeding well. The infant latches on and nurses for 10 to 15 minutes on each breast, and Carol's nipples are free of tenderness or signs of trauma. Carol has no relatives in the area, and her husband is home for the weekend only. She states that she will just have to get along by herself after that.

Questions
5. What anticipatory guidance should Carol receive before she goes home?
6. What further nursing interventions would be most helpful to her and the baby?

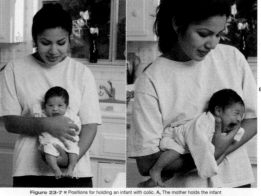

THERAPEUTIC COMMUNICATIONS
Coping with Crying

Shannon Gray tells the nurse, Mark Winston, about her daughter, Marina, who has been having crying spells every day lasting 4 hours or longer. Shannon looks tired and worried. Marina, age 4 weeks, eats well, shows good weight gain, and is developing appropriately for her age.

Shannon: It seems like all I do is try to stop Marina's crying. I can't get anything else done.
Mark: You spend a lot of time trying to find ways to comfort her. (Paraphrasing to encourage the mother to continue.)
Shannon: I've tried everything! I rock her, walk with her, feed and change her. We go for car rides and put her in her swing, but nothing works for long. She just starts crying again.
Mark: It's so frustrating when nothing seems to work! (Reflecting mother's feelings shows that the nurse is trying to understand them.)

Shannon: Sometimes I wonder if I was cut out to be a mother. I never thought it would be like this.
Mark: Being a mother is so much harder than you expected that sometimes you aren't sure you made the right choice. (Reflecting the content of what the mother said helps her focus and shows acceptance.)
Shannon: But I really do love her. I just don't know how to help her. I must be a terrible mother. (becomes teary.)
Mark: Parents often feel guilty when they can't find a way to help an upset baby. And yet, we really don't know all the reasons why babies cry. You've tried very hard to help Marina. Maybe we can work together to think of some other techniques to use. (Gives reassurance that what the mother is feeling is normal, then offers information and further help.)
Shannon: I'd love that. It worries me to have Marina so unhappy. What else can I do for her?

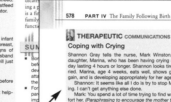

Figure 23-7 Positions for holding an infant with colic. A, The mother holds the infant facing forward. One hand creates slight pressure against the abdomen, while the other flexes the legs. This position may help the infant expel flatus. B, The prone hold is also effective for some infants. The mother holds the infant in a horizontal position along her arm.

Contents

CHAPTER 13

Nursing Care during Labor and Birth, 266

CHAPTER 14

Intrapartum Fetal Surveillance, 306

CHAPTER 15

Pain Management during Childbirth, 335

PART V

Families at Risk during the Childbearing Period

CHAPTER 24

The Childbearing Family with Special Needs, 589

CHAPTER 25

Complications of Pregnancy, 622

PART VI

Other Reproductive Issues

CHAPTER 31
Family Planning, 832

CHAPTER 32
Infertility, 856

CHAPTER 33
Women's Health Care, 878

APPENDIXES

GLOSSARY, 969

Maternity Care Today

Go to your Student CD-ROM for Review Questions keyed to these Objectives.

OBJECTIVES

After studying this chapter, you should be able to:

1. Describe changes in maternity care, from home birth with lay midwives to the emergence of medical management.
2. Compare current settings for childbirth both within and outside the hospital setting.
3. Identify trends that led to the development of family-centered maternity care.
4. Describe current trends that affect perinatal nursing, such as cost containment, outcomes management, evidence-based practice, community-based perinatal care, advances in technology, and increased use of complementary and alternative medicine.
5. Explain changes in family structure and their impact on family functioning.
6. Compare Western cultural values with those of differing cultural groups.
7. Describe the effect of cultural diversity on nursing practice.
8. Discuss the downward trends in infant and maternal mortality rates, and compare current infant mortality rates among specific racial groups and nations.

DEFINITIONS

Antepartum Pertaining to the time during pregnancy before the onset of labor.

Complementary and Alternative Medicine Nonmainstream or unconventional health care treatments and practices that are generally not used in hospitals and often not reimbursed by insurance companies.

Culture Sum of values, beliefs, and practices of a group of people that is transmitted from one generation to the next.

Ethnic Pertaining to religious, racial, national, or cultural group characteristics, especially speech patterns, social customs, and physical characteristics.

Ethnicity Condition of belonging to a particular ethnic group; also refers to ethnic pride.

Ethnocentrism Opinion that the beliefs and customs of one's own ethnic group are superior.

Infant Mortality Rate Number of deaths per 1000 live births that occurs within the first 12 months of life.

Intrapartum Pertaining to the time of labor and childbirth.

Lactation Secretion of milk from the breasts; also describes the period during which a child is breastfed.

Maternal Mortality Rate Number of maternal deaths from births and complications of pregnancy, childbirth, and puerperium (the first 42 days after the pregnancy ends) per 100,000 live births.

Neonatal Mortality Rate Number of deaths per 1000 live births occurring at birth or within the first 28 days of life.

Postpartum Pertaining to the first 6 weeks after childbirth.

Major changes in maternity care occurred in the first half of the twentieth century as childbirth moved from the home to a hospital setting. Change continues and confusion abounds as health care providers and payers attempt to control the increasing cost of care and the rapid growth of expensive technology. Despite these challenges, health care professionals try to maintain the quality of care.

Alterations in family structure and function and differing cultural beliefs and customs also affect nursing care. Although improvements in health care have resulted in a significant decline in maternal and infant mortality rates in the United States, statistics show a wide disparity between outcomes for whites and those for nonwhites.

HISTORICAL PERSPECTIVES ON CHILDBEARING

Granny Midwives

Before the twentieth century, childbirth occurred most often in the home with the assistance of a "granny" midwife, whose training was obtained through an apprenticeship with a more experienced granny, or lay, midwife. Women who were charity cases might give birth in a hospital in which medical students learned. The preferred attendant for wealthy women was a midwife, who attended at a home birth. The midwife continued to care for the mother and newborn after birth.

Many women and infants fared well when a lay midwife assisted with birth in the home, but maternal and infant death rates from childbearing were high for both hospital and home births. The primary causes of maternal death were postpartum hemorrhage, postpartum infection (also known as *puerperal sepsis,* or "childbed fever"), and toxemia, now known as *preeclampsia.* The primary causes of infant death were prematurity, dehydration from diarrhea, and contagious diseases.

Emergence of Medical Management

In the late nineteenth century, developments available to physicians but not always midwives led to a decline in home births and an increase in physician-assisted hospital births. Significant discoveries that set the stage for a change in maternity care included the following:

- The discovery by Semmelweis that puerperal infection could be prevented by hygienic practices
- The development of forceps to facilitate birth
- The discovery of chloroform, used to control pain during childbirth and available only to physicians
- The use of drugs to start or induce labor and increase uterine contractions (augmentation of labor)
- Advances in operative procedures such as cesarean birth

With good intentions to prevent infections, hospitals hurried to develop policies and procedures to meet the needs of physicians and take advantage of technology. By 1960, 90% of all births in the United States occurred in hospitals.

Maternity care became highly regimented. Physicians managed all antepartum, intrapartum, and postpartum care. Lay midwifery became illegal in many areas, and nurse-midwifery was not well established. The woman's role in childbirth was seen as passive: the physician "delivered" her infant. The primary functions of nurses were to assist the physician and follow prescribed medical orders after childbirth. Teaching and counseling were not valued nursing functions at that time.

Unlike home births, hospital births hindered bonding between parents and infants. During labor the woman received medication such as "twilight sleep," a combination of a narcotic and scopolamine that provided pain relief but left her disoriented, confused, and heavily sedated. Because of this practice and the lack of knowledge regarding the importance of early contact between parent and child, the mother often did not see her infant for several hours after the delivery. The father was sent to a waiting area and was not allowed to see the mother until some time after the birth of the infant.

Despite technologic advances and the move from home to hospital, maternal and infant mortality rates declined slowly. The slow decline primarily resulted from problems that could have been prevented, such as poor maternal nutrition, infectious diseases, and inadequate prenatal care. These stubborn problems remained because of inequalities in health care delivery. Affluent families could afford comprehensive medical care early in the pregnancy, but poor families had very limited access to prenatal care or information about childbearing. Two concurrent trends, federal involvement and consumer demands, led to additional changes in maternity care.

Government Involvement in Maternal-Infant Care

The high rates of maternal and infant mortality among poor women provided the impetus for federal involvement in maternity care. The Sheppard-Towner Act of 1921, the first federally sponsored program, provided funds for state-managed programs for mothers and children. Although the Sheppard-Towner Act was later repealed, it set the stage for future allocation of federal funds. Today the federal government supports several programs to improve the health of mothers, infants, and young children (Table 1-1). Although government funds partially solved the problem of maternal and infant mortality, the distribution of health care remains inequitable. Most physicians practice in urban or suburban areas in which more people have insurance through their work and can afford to pay for medical services. Women in rural or inner city areas have difficulty obtaining care because they are poor or because work-related health coverage is unavailable or too expensive.

The ongoing problem of providing health care for poor women and children left the door open for nurses to expand their roles, and advanced educational programs prepared nurses as certified nurse-midwives (CNMs), nurse practitioners, and clinical specialists (see Chapter 2).

TABLE 1-1 Federal Projects for Maternal Child Care

Program	Purpose
Title V of Social Security Act	Provides funds for maternal-child health programs
National Institute of Health and Human Development	Supports research and education of personnel needed for maternal and child health programs
Title V Amendment of Public Health Service Act	Established the Maternal and Infant Care (MIC) projects to provide comprehensive prenatal and infant care in public clinics
Title XIX of Medicaid	Provides funds to facilitate access to care by pregnant women and young children
Head Start	Provides educational opportunities for low-income children of preschool age
Women, Infants, and Children (WIC) Program	Provides supplemental food and nutrition information
Temporary Assistance to Needy Families (TANF)	Provides temporary money for basic living costs of poor children and their families, with eligibility requirements and time limits varying among states; tribal programs available for Native Americans; replaced the Aid to Families with Dependent Children (AFDC) program
National Center for Family Planning	A clearinghouse for contraceptive information
Healthy Start	Enhances community development of culturally appropriate strategies designed to decrease infant mortality and causes of low birth weight

Effects of Consumer Demands on Health Care

In the early 1950s consumers began to insist on their right to be involved in their own health care. Pregnant women were no longer willing to accept only what was offered. They wanted information about planning and spacing their children, and they wanted to know what to expect during pregnancy. Fathers, siblings, and grandparents wanted to be part of the extraordinary time of pregnancy and childbirth. Parents wanted more "say" in the way their child was born.

Early in the 1950s, Dr. Grantly Dick-Read proposed a method of childbirth that allowed the mother to control her fear and therefore to control her pain during labor, allowing for birth without pharmacologic intervention. Methods such as Lamaze and Bradley also gained favor (see Chapter 11). A growing consensus among child psychologists and nurse researchers affirmed that early parent-newborn contact outweighed risks of infection. Knowledgeable parents insisted that their infants remain with them at all times. The practice of separating the infant from the family was abandoned when infections did not increase in nurseries, and family-centered maternity care became the standard.

Development of Family-Centered Maternity Care

The term *family-centered maternity care* describes safe, high-quality care that recognizes and adapts to both the physical and the psychosocial needs of the family, including the newborn. The goal is to foster family unity while maintaining physical safety.

The basic principles of family-centered care are as follows:
- Childbirth is usually a normal, healthy event in the life of a family.
- Childbirth affects the entire family, and family relationships will need to be restructured.
- Families are capable of making decisions about care if they are given adequate information and professional support.

Family-centered care greatly increased the responsibilities of nurses. Nurses do not only provide physical care and as-

sist physicians; they also now assume a major role in teaching, counseling, and supporting families in their decisions. (See Chapter 2 for additional information regarding the nurse's role in maternity care.)

CURRENT SETTINGS FOR CHILDBIRTH

Traditional Hospital Setting

In traditional hospital childbirth settings of the past, labor took place in a functional labor room, similar to a small hospital or an emergency department room. The mother was moved to a delivery area similar to an operating room when birth was imminent. The mother was transferred to a recovery area for 1 to 2 hours of observation after birth and then taken to the postpartum unit, which resembled a standard hospital room. The infant was usually moved to the newborn nursery when the mother was transferred to the recovery area. Mother and infant were reunited when the mother was settled in the postpartum unit. The nurse who cared for the mother in the postpartum unit was rarely the same nurse who cared for her baby. Beginning in the 1970s the father or another significant support person could usually remain with the mother throughout labor, birth, and recovery in this setting.

Although birth in a traditional hospital setting was safe, the setting was impersonal, and the multiple moves were uncomfortable for the mother. The move from the labor room to the delivery room just before the birth of the baby was particularly difficult for the mother. Furthermore, each move disrupted the family's time together and often separated the parents and infant. Because of these disadvantages, hospitals began to devise settings that were more comfortable and facilitated family participation.

Labor, Delivery, and Recovery Rooms

Today the most common location for vaginal birth is the labor, delivery, and recovery (LDR) room. In an LDR room, normal labor, birth, and recovery from birth take place in one setting (Figure 1-1). LDR rooms are homelike, often with refrigerators, entertainment media, and soothing light-

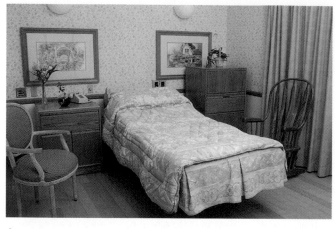

A

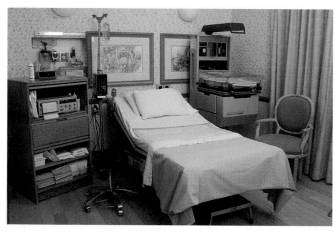

B

Figure 1-1 ■ A typical labor, delivery, and recovery room. Homelike furnishings **(A)** can be adapted quickly to expose the necessary technical equipment **(B)**.

ing. The furniture can quickly be transformed, turning the LDR into a birthing room when needed. Decorative items are moved to expose suction and oxygen apparatus, ceiling spotlights are activated, and wood chests open to reveal fetal monitors and equipment for the birth. Because childbearing families now expect technology such as computer charting, intravenous pumps, and fetal monitoring, the concealing of equipment is often less common than when use of LDR rooms started.

During labor the woman's significant others are allowed to remain with her. These people may include relatives, friends, and her other children, depending on the policies of the agency and the mother's desires. After she has given birth, the mother typically remains in the LDR room for 1 to 2 hours, after which she is transferred to her postpartum room for the remainder of her hospital stay. The healthy infant may remain with the mother throughout her stay in the LDR room. When the mother is transferred to her postpartum room, the infant may be transferred to the nursery for assessment or may remain with the mother in a mother-baby postpartum room while being assessed.

The major advantages of LDR rooms are that the setting is more comfortable and homelike and the family can remain with the mother throughout her stay. However, if the family prefers a low-intervention birth, they may regard technologic components of the LDR room as disadvantages.

Labor, Delivery, Recovery, and Postpartum Rooms

Some hospitals offer rooms similar to LDR rooms in layout and function, with the exception that the mother is not transferred to a postpartum unit after recovery. She and the infant remain in the labor, delivery, recovery, and postpartum (LDRP) room until discharge. The father or the woman's primary support person is encouraged to stay with the mother and infant, and sleeping equipment may be provided.

Birth Centers

Freestanding birth centers are designed to provide maternity care to low-risk women outside a hospital setting. Many centers also provide gynecologic services, such as annual checkups and contraceptive counseling. The mother usually attends classes at the birth center or elsewhere to prepare for childbirth, breastfeeding, and infant care. Both the mother and the infant continue to receive follow-up care during the first 6 weeks after birth. This may include help with breastfeeding problems, a postpartum examination at 4 to 6 weeks, family planning information, and examination of the newborn. Birth is often assisted by CNMs who have provided care for the woman throughout her pregnancy and will continue to provide primary care for the mother and infant.

Birth centers are less expensive than traditional hospitals, which provide advanced technology that may be unnecessary for low-risk clients. Moreover, women who want a safe, homelike birth in a familiar setting with personnel they have known throughout their pregnancies often express satisfaction.

The major disadvantage is that most independent birth centers are not equipped for major obstetric emergencies. If unforeseen difficulties develop during labor, the woman must be transferred by ambulance to a nearby hospital to the care of a back-up physician who has agreed to perform this duty. Although procedures have been designed for these situations, a sudden transfer is frightening for the family. Liability issues also affect the CNM's decision to transfer the woman, possibly sooner than might have occurred in the recent past.

Home Births

In the United States only a small number of women give birth at home. Because malpractice insurance for midwives who attend home births is expensive and difficult to obtain, only a small number of CNMs offer this service. Many CNMs have moved their practices to hospitals or birth centers. Mothers who once sought home births have found that they can have many of the advantages of family-centered care in the safe environment of a hospital or birth center, yet retain the nurse-midwife's care and low-intervention approach that they prefer.

Home birth provides the advantage of keeping the family together in its own familiar environment throughout the childbirth experience. When all goes well, birth at home can be a growth-enhancing experience for every family member. Young siblings are not separated from their mothers and are able to establish positive relationships with the new baby immediately after birth. Bonding with the infant is unimpeded by hospital routines, and breastfeeding is highly encouraged and supported. Women who have their babies at home maintain a feeling of control because they actively plan and prepare for each detail of the birth.

Giving birth at home also has disadvantages. Women who plan a home birth must be screened carefully to make sure that they have a very low risk for complications. If transfer to a nearby hospital becomes necessary, the time required may be too long in an emergency. Other problems associated with home birth include the need for the parents to provide a setting and adequate supplies for the birth. Moreover, the mother must take care of herself and the infant without the immediate help she would have in a hospital or birth center setting.

CHECK YOUR READING

1. What led to federal involvement in the health care of women and infants? Is health care equal among poor and more affluent women now?
2. How does family-centered maternity care differ from maternity care during the first half of the nineteenth century?
3. How do LDR and LDRP rooms differ from birth centers and home births in their advantages and disadvantages?

CURRENT TRENDS IN MATERNITY CARE

Recently the government, insurance companies, hospitals, and health care providers made a concerted effort to control the increasing cost of health care in the United States. Reform has involved a change in the ways and in which settings money is spent. In the past, most of the health care budget was spent in acute-care settings, in which the facility charged for services after they were provided. Because the facility was paid for any services billed, hospitals had no incentive to be efficient or cost conscious.

Cost Containment

One way in which health care payers have attempted to control costs is with a prospective form of payment; that is, they will no longer pay whatever a hospital charges for a service. Instead, the facility and payers agree in advance on a fixed amount of money for necessary services for specifically diagnosed conditions. An example of this approach is diagnosis-related groups (DRGs).

DIAGNOSIS-RELATED GROUPS

DRGs classify related medical diagnoses based on the type or complexity of services generally required by a client with that condition. This method became a stan-

dard in 1987 when the federal government set the amount of money that Medicare would pay for each DRG. If a client requires more services than that DRG will pay or if the services are more costly, the hospital must absorb the costs. Conversely, if the hospital delivers the care at a lower cost than the payment for that DRG, the hospital keeps the remaining money. Hospitals benefit financially if they can reduce the client's length of stay (LOS) in the facility and thereby reduce the costs for service. Although the DRG system originally applied only to Medicare clients, most states have adopted the system for Medicaid payments, and most insurance companies use a similar system.

MANAGED CARE

Health insurance companies also examined the cost of health care and instituted a health care delivery system that has been called *managed care.* Examples of managed care organizations are health maintenance organizations (HMOs), point of service plans (POSs), and preferred provider organizations (PPOs). HMOs provide relatively comprehensive health services for persons enrolled in the organization for a set fee or premium. However, HMOs usually have limited referral to specialists within the HMO, and care outside the HMO group may not be covered. POS plans provide more flexibility in that the primary care physician within the POS organization can make referrals to specialists not in the network. Similarly, PPOs are groups of health care providers who agree to provide health services to a specific group of clients at a discounted cost. When the client needs medical treatment, managed care includes strategies such as payment arrangements and preadmission or pretreatment authorization to control costs. Co-payments for non-network providers are often higher.

CAPITATED CARE

Capitation may be incorporated into any type of managed care plan. In a pure capitated care plan, the payer of the health insurance (usually the employer or the government) pays a set amount of money each year to a network of primary care providers (PCPs). The contracted amount paid to the PCP may be adjusted for the age and gender of the client group. The PCPs include physicians and often include advanced practice nurses in community clinics or private practices with physicians. In exchange for access to a guaranteed client base, the PCP agrees to provide general health care to each client under contract and to pay for all other covered services such as laboratory work, specialist visits, and hospital care.

Capitated plans are of interest to employers and the government because the plans allow payers of health care to predictably budget for health care for a plan year. Health care consumers do not have unexpected financial burdens from illness. The disadvantage for consumers is that they lose most of their freedom of choice regarding their health care providers. PCPs can lose money if they refer too many clients to specialists, who may have no restrictions on their fees, or if they order too many diagnostic tests. Many providers and consumers fear that this method of cost containment will inevitably affect treatment decisions.

EFFECTS OF COST CONTAINMENT ON MATERNITY CARE

Prospective payment plans have had major effects on maternity care, primarily with regard to LOS. Mothers who have a normal vaginal birth are typically discharged from the hospital at 48 hours, and mothers who give birth by cesarean section leave at 96 hours. Many mothers and infants developed problems with shorter lengths of stay, often called *drive-through deliveries*, that were mandated under early prospective pay arrangements. The problems might require disruptive readmission and more expensive treatment than needed with earlier identification of the problem. As a result, many states passed legislation requiring a minimum 48-hour LOS for vaginal births and 4 days (96 hours) for cesarean births, unless the woman and her health care provider choose an earlier discharge time. Some insurance plans use a compromise, in which the woman who elects to leave 24 hours after vaginal birth is provided one or more home visits by a nurse to check on her status and that of her baby.

Unfortunately, 48 hours is still a short time to accomplish the teaching needed before discharge, particularly when the new mother is tired and uncomfortable from the birth. She may or may not have had prenatal classes to prepare her for the care she and her infant will need, and she may not have had prenatal care at all.

Reduced lengths of stay have also affected caregivers, particularly nurses. Since the mid 1990s nurses have become increasingly concerned with meeting the needs of families who leave the hospital a short time after the birth of an infant. Nurses find it especially difficult to provide adequate information about self-care and infant care when the mother is still recovering from childbirth.

CASE MANAGEMENT. *Case management* is a practice model that uses a systematic approach to identify specific clients and to manage care collaboratively to ensure optimal outcomes through access to the best available resources (Alfaro-LeFevre, 2004). In this model a case manager or case coordinator, who focuses on both quality and cost outcomes, coordinates the services needed by the client and family. Inherent to case management is the coordination of care by all members of the health care team. The guidelines established in 1995 by the Joint Commission on Accreditation of Healthcare Organizations (JCAHO) require an interdisciplinary, collaborative approach to client care. This concept is at the core of case management. Nurses who provide case management evaluate client needs, establish needs documentation to support reimbursement, and may be part of long-term care planning in the home or a rehabilitation facility.

OUTCOMES MANAGEMENT. Regardless of how health care costs may be controlled, the determination to lower health care costs while maintaining the quality of care has led to a clinical practice model called *outcomes management.* This is a systematic method to identify client outcomes and to focus care on interventions that will accomplish the stated outcomes for specific case types, such as the woman who has just given birth. The planning tools used by the health care team to identify and meet stated outcomes are *clinical pathways.* Other names for clinical pathways include *critical* or *clinical paths, care paths, care maps, collaborative plans of care, anticipated recovery paths,* and *multidisciplinary action plans.*

Clinical Pathways. Clinical pathways are standardized, interdisciplinary plans of care devised for clients with a specific health problem. Clinical pathways identify client outcomes, specify timelines for achievement of those outcomes, direct appropriate interventions and sequencing of interventions, include interventions from a variety of disciplines, promote collaboration, and involve a comprehensive approach to care. Although the concept of clinical pathways is not new, it has only recently been widely accepted as the use of case management has become widespread in various health care settings. The purpose, as in managed care and case management, is to provide high-quality care while controlling costs.

Facilities differ in how they use clinical pathways. For instance, they may be used for change-of-shift reports to indicate information about LOS, individual needs, and priorities of the shift for each client. They may also be used for documentation of the client's nursing care plan and his or her progress in meeting the desired outcomes. Many pathways are particularly helpful in identification of families that need follow-up care. Computer-based systems are replacing many printed pathways. (See Figure 1-2 for an example of a clinical pathway.)

Variances. Deviations, often called *variances,* may occur, either in the time line or in the expected outcomes. A variance is the difference between what was expected and what actually happened. A variance may be positive or negative. A positive variance occurs when a client progresses faster than expected and is discharged sooner than planned. A negative variance occurs when progress is slower than expected, outcomes are not met within the designated time frame, and the LOS is prolonged.

Students' Use of Clinical Pathways. Clinical pathways are guidelines for care. Although a pathway provides insight into the scheduling of assessments and care, it is not meant to teach nursing skills and procedures. One purpose of this book is to provide ample information so that students can *use* clinical pathways in a clinical setting. This involves teaching *why and how to perform assessments* and interpreting the significance of the data obtained. Moreover, the book emphasizes ways of providing information, care, and comfort for clients and their families as they progress along a clinical pathway.

Evidence-Based Practice

Closely related to outcomes management is a change in focus referred to as *evidence-based* or *research-based* clinical practice guidelines to provide safe and effective care. Nurses and other professionals cannot perform assessments and care solely because "we've always done it that way." They rely on research data rather than tradition or habit to determine care measures that improve both quality and outcomes of client care to achieve *best practice* outcomes. Nurses must carefully study evidence-based practices to determine if the research was done reliably and whether guidelines based on the research are appropriate for their clinical area. Poor reliability in the guidelines can lead to more expensive care because of harm to patients, ineffective interventions, or use of scarce resources without benefit. Poorly researched or inadequate practice guidelines are likely to result in frustration among nurses and patients. Nurses may need to adapt evidence-based practice guidelines for best local use (Graham et al., 2002).

The Agency for Healthcare Research and Quality (AHRQ) actively sponsors research in health issues facing women to guide best practice. From research generated through this agency and organizations such as the Association of Women's Health, Obstetric and Neonatal Nurses (AWHONN), American College of Obstetricians and Gynecologists (ACOG), and American Academy of Pediatrics (AAP), evidence to guide the best clinical practices grows (AHRQ, 2001, 2002). Examples of guidelines for pregnancy and infants' and women's health include the following:

- Folic acid prevention of neural tube defects
- Management of preterm labor
- Regional anesthesia and analgesia in labor
- Breast cancer screening
- Cardiovascular disease prevention
- Perinatal care at the threshold of fetal viability
- Shoulder dystocia of the newborn
- Circumcision
- Immunization for preterm and low-birth-weight infants

Another resource for evidence-based practice in perinatal nursing is the Cochrane Collaboration, which provides coordination of research results by an international network of individuals and institutions. The results in the Cochrane database do not prescribe policies, procedures, or protocols that a facility should take. However, the evaluations of research identify and distill results from available research so that the best practices may be incorporated into the facility practices. The Internet address for the Cochrane Collaboration is www.cochrane.org.

Community-Based Perinatal Nursing

Because an acute-care setting is the most expensive for delivery of health care services, community-based care has increased in perinatal nursing. Advances in portable technology and wireless transmission allow nurses in many practice areas to perform procedures in the home that were once limited to the hospital. Additionally, women and their families are taught to manage less-severe pregnancy complications at home under the supervision of a nurse, entering the hospital only for possible worsening of the complication. Consumers often prefer home care because of decreased stress on the family when a woman or newborn does not need to be separated from the family support system for hospitalization.

Ample evidence shows that the health care system of the future will be community oriented and involve care for greater numbers of clients in the home and through community agencies. Because home care is a growing part of maternity care, community-based or home care nursing is discussed for specific conditions throughout the text. Public health agencies have existed for many years, and many women obtain all antepartum, postpartum, and neonatal care in these clinics. Other community facilities such as neighborhood health centers, shelters for women and children, school age mothers' programs, and nurse-managed postpartum centers also provide care to a variety of clients.

Nurses need a broad array of skills to function effectively in community-based care, whether that care takes place in individuals' homes or large clinics. They must understand the communities in which they practice and the diversity within those communities. Nurses need skills to work with a multidisciplinary team. They are often responsible for assisting clients through high-technology choices and therefore need to be proficient in communication and teaching skills.

Perinatal nursing services delivered in a community setting encompass antepartum, postpartum, and neonatal care. Because care is given in an environment that is physically separated from an acute-care institution, nurses must be able to function independently and have superior clinical and critical thinking skills. They should be proficient in interviewing, counseling, and teaching. They assume a leadership role in the coordination of the services a family may require in a complex case, and they frequently supervise the work of other care providers.

COMMON TYPES OF PERINATAL HOME CARE

ANTEPARTUM HOME CARE. Most preconceptional and low-risk antepartum care takes place in private offices or public clinics. High-risk conditions that may be seen in home-based perinatal nursing include preterm labor, hyperemesis gravidarum (intractable vomiting during pregnancy), bleeding problems, preterm premature rupture of membranes, hypertension, and diabetes during pregnancy.

POSTPARTUM AND NEONATAL HOME CARE. Even with legislation to limit discharge requirements of managed care agencies, providing the necessary education to new mothers in their own self-care, basic care of their infants, and signs of problems they should report after discharge is a challenge for health care professionals. Before the woman is discharged, hospitals may offer classes, closed circuit television programs, written materials (often in multiple languages), and individual teaching and demonstration.

After the woman is discharged, various services are offered for home care. These services may include telephone

Text continued on p. 12

YORK HEALTH SYSTEM
YORK, PENNSYLVANIA
CLINICAL PATHWAY
VAGINAL DELIVERY

CLINICAL PATH DAY		EXPECTED PATIENT/ FAMILY OUTCOMES	INTERDISCIPLINARY ASSESSMENT	TESTS	CONSULT
Pre-Natal	DATE	☐ Prenatal test results available [4] ☐ 8 or more prenatal visits complete [4] ☐ Attended baby care and post-partum classes [3] ☐ Risk assessment complete and referral(s) to appropriate agency made as needed.[5] ☐ Low risk pregnancy or monitored high risk pregnancy [4] ☐ _____ ☐ _____	Each visit-maternal weight; BP; urine dipstick-sugar, protein ketones; FHT S/S of pregnancy complication Perinatal risk assessment Social support Knowledge of self and newborn care Knowledge of warning signs of complications Knowledge of signs of labor	Type and Rh Antibody Screen H and H Sickle cell Rubella RPR HBSAG Trutol or 3h GTT GC, Chlamydia Triple Screen Group B Strep	☐ Perinatologist ☐ Diabetic Educator ☐ Behavioral Health ☐ Social Service ☐ _____ ☐ _____ ☐ _____
Admission		☐ Demonstrates knowledge of pain management options [1, 2, 3] ☐ Support person present [2] ☐ Referral made for identified risk factors ☐ Admission procedures completed [4] ☐ _____	Admission assessment Patient needs/desires for pain relief in labor Support system _____ _____	WCBC Type and Rh prn Tube to hold US scan prn _____	☐ Perinatologist ☐ Behavioral Health ☐ Social Service ☐ Neonatology ☐ _____
Labor First Stage		☐☐ Achieves desired level of pain relief [1, 2, 3] ☐☐ Support person present [2] ☐☐ Referral made for identified maternal/fetal risk during labor ☐☐ Mother demonstrates normal physiologic parameters [4] ☐☐ Fetus demonstrates normal physiologic parameters [4] ☐☐ _____	FHR q 30 min UC q 30-60 min P, R, BP q 2h T q 4° (q2 if ROM) Support system Progress of labor Level of comfort _____	_____ _____	☐ Neonatology ☐ _____
Labor Second Stage		☐ Pushing effectively [4] ☐ Support person present {2} ☐ Referral made for identified maternal/fetal risk during labor [4] ☐ Mother demonstrates normal physiological parameters [4] ☐ Fetus demonstrates normal physiological parameters [4] ☐ _____	FHR q 5 min BP q 30 min Vaginal exam prn _____	_____ _____	☐ Neonatology ☐ _____
NAME			INITIALS	NAME	INITIALS

Figure 1-2 ■ Clinical pathway for vaginal delivery. (Courtesy Women and Children Services of the York Health System, York, PA.)

DOCUMENTATION CODES
Initial=Meets Standard
★=Exception on pathway identified
C=Chronic problems
N=Not applicable

PARENT/FAMILY PROBLEMS
1. Pain r/t childbirth
2. Anxiety r/t childbirth and/or parenting
3. Knowledge deficit r/t childbirth and/or parenting
4. Potential alteration maternal/fetal homeostasis

5. Potential for ineffective parenting
6. _____
7. _____

INTERVENTIONS/ACTIVITIES	MEDS	NUTRITION	EDUCATION AND DC PLANNING
_____ _____	Prenatal vitamin, Fe as per order _____ _____	Regular diet _____ _____	Childbirth preparation class Baby care class Breastfeeding class when appropriate Prenatal education
Bed rest with fetal monitor x 30 minutes _____	IV/mini cath _____	NPO with ice chips _____	☐ Orient pt/SO/family to L and D area ☐ Reinforce breathing and relaxation techniques ☐ _____
Insertion of scalp electrode and IUPC as appropriate Warm/cold compress, massage, position change, ambulates and warm showers prn Encourage to void q 1-2° EFM as ordered Vaginal exam prn Catheterize prn _____ _____	IV as ordered Analgesia prn as ordered Epidural as ordered Induction/augmentation of labor as ordered _____ _____	NPO with ice chips _____	☐☐☐ Reinforce breathing and relaxation technique ☐☐☐ Review options for pain management ☐☐☐ Encourage support person involvement ☐☐☐ Provide explanation of labor progress prn
Position for comfort Catheterize prn Warm/cold compress, massage, position change and void prn _____ _____	IV as ordered Continue epidural as ordered Augmentation of labor as ordered _____ _____	NPO with ice chips _____	☐ Assist with pushing ☐ Encourage support person involvement ☐ _____ ☐ _____

NAME	INITIALS	NAME	INITIALS

Figure 1-2 ■ *Continued*

Continued

CLINICAL PATH DAY		EXPECTED PATIENT/ FAMILY OUTCOMES	INTERDISCIPLINARY ASSESSMENT	TESTS	CONSULT
Delivery	DATE _____ TIME _____	☐ Deliver live newborn vaginally [4] ☐ Support person present [2] ☐ Mother demonstrates normal physiologic parameters ☐ _____	Fundus, bleeding _____ _____	Cord blood Rh studies when indicated Placenta to pathology as ordered _____	_____ _____
Early Recovery	DATE _____	☐ Postpartum parameters stable [4] ☐ Achieves desired level of pain relief [1] ☐ _____ ☐ _____	Temp X 1 P, R, BP, fundus, lochia, bladder, episiotomy q 15 min x 4, and q 30 min x 2 Level of comfort _____	_____ _____	_____ _____
2-24 Hours	DATE _____	☐☐☐ Achieves desired level of pain relief [1] ☐☐☐ Cares for self and infant [3] ☐☐☐ Postpartum parameters stable ☐☐☐ Voiding qs [4] ☐☐☐ Adequate home support system identified [5] ☐☐☐ _____ ☐☐☐ _____	T, P, R, BP, Breasts, fundus, lochia, bladder, episiotomy q 4h Readiness to learn Knowledge of self and newborn care Level of comfort Home support system _____	_____ _____	_____ _____
24-48 Hours	DATE _____	☐☐☐ Achieves desired level of pain relief [1] ☐☐☐ Postpartum parameters stable [4] ☐☐☐ Referral made for potential or identified risk (physical/psychosocial) ☐ Cares for self and infant [3] ☐☐☐ _____	T, P, R, BP, bid Breasts, fundus, lochia, bladder, episiotomy q shift WA Level of comfort Readiness to learn Knowledge of self and newborn care _____	WCBC _____ _____	_____ _____
Day of Discharge	DATE _____	☐☐☐ Achieves desired level of pain relief [1] ☐☐☐ Postpartum physiological parameters within D/C guidelines [4] ☐ Patient/SO/family verbalization of D/C instructions [3] ☐ Postpartum Home Visit not needed based on Interqual Criteria ☐ Discharge within 2 days after delivery ☐ _____ ☐ _____	T, P, R, BP, bid Breasts, fundus, lochia, bladder, episiotomy bid Level of comfort Readiness to learn Pt/SO/family knowledge of self and newborn care _____ _____	_____ _____	_____ _____

NAME	INITIALS	NAME	INITIALS

NOTE: EACH PATIENT REQUIRES AN INDIVIDUAL ASSESSMENT AND TREATMENT PLAN. THIS CLINICAL PATH IS A RECOMMENDATION FOR THE AVERAGE PATIENT WHICH REQUIRES MODIFICATION WHEN NECESSARY BY THE PROFESSIONAL STAFF.

Figure 1-2, *cont'd* ▪ Clinical pathway for vaginal delivery.

INTERVENTIONS/ACTIVITIES	MEDS	NUTRITION	EDUCATION AND DC PLANNING
Catheterize prn Continue IV Continue epidural or local anesthetic _____ _____	Oxytocin after placenta delivered as ordered ☐ _____ ☐ _____	NPO _____ _____	☐ Support parent/infant bonding ☐ _____ ☐ _____
OOB with assist first time Perineal ice pack q 30 min prn Cath prn Shower _____	Analgesia prn Continue epidural if PPTL Continue IV oxytocin as ordered D/C IV or cap IV ☐ _____ ☐ _____	Reg diet as tolerated _____ _____	☐ Support parent/infant bonding ☐ Teach pericare ☐ _____ ☐ _____
OOB with assist first time, then OOB ad lib Catheterize per protocol Epifoam, Tucks prn Ice pack prn Sitz bath 12° after delivery prn _____	Analgesia prn _____ _____	Adv to reg diet as tolerated _____ _____	☐☐☐ Initiate and continue maternal/newborn education record, D/C instructions ☐☐☐ _____ _____ ☐☐☐ _____
OOB ad lib Epifoam, Tucks prn Sitz bath prn _____	Analgesia prn _____ _____	Regular diet _____ _____	☐☐☐ Continue maternal newborn education record ☐☐☐ _____ _____ ☐☐☐ _____

OOB ad lib
Epifoam, Tucks prn
Sitz bath prn
_____
_____
	Analgesia prn
	☐ RhoGAM, when indicated
	☐ Rubella, when indicated
	_____
	_____
		Regular diet
		_____
		_____
			☐ Completion of maternal newborn education record
			☐ Physician discharge instructions
			☐ Support services in community:
			  ☐ Breastfeeding Support Services
			  ☐ Perinatal Coaching
			  ☐ City/State Health
			  ☐ Other
			☐ D/C after Pt./family review instructions

DISCHARGE DATE	DISCHARGE TIME	DISCHARGED TO	ACCOMPANIED BY ☐ W/C ☐ AMBULATE

Figure 1-2 ■ Continued

calls, home visits, information lines, and lactation consultations. At the time of discharge, some hospitals provide parents with videotapes of infant care to supplement written materials for later reference. In addition, nurse-managed outpatient clinics provide care for mothers and infants in some areas. (See Chapters 18 and 23 for additional information about home care for mothers and infants.)

HOME CARE FOR HIGH-RISK NEONATES. Neonatal home care nurses may provide care for infants who are discharged from the acute-care facility with serious medical conditions. Parents of preterm or low-birth-weight infants require a great deal of information and support. Infants with congenital anomalies such as cleft palate may require care adapted to their conditions. Moreover, increasing numbers of technology-dependent infants, such as those who require ventilator assistance, total parenteral nutrition, intravenous medications, and apnea monitoring, are now cared for at home.

The coordination of care for the high-risk newborn is a major challenge for home care nurses. The involvement of multiple specialty providers, such as physicians, nurses, respiratory therapists, and equipment vendors, may result in duplication or fragmentation of services. Duplication of services results in unnecessary costs, and fragmentation of services can result in dangerous gaps in care. (See Chapters 29 and 30 for home care for high-risk infants.)

STANDARDS OF PRACTICE FOR PERINATAL NURSING

Both community-based and acute-care perinatal services must meet guidelines for practice established by the agency itself, appropriate specialty practice organizations, and accrediting agencies.

AGENCY STANDARDS. Health care agencies are required to have policies, procedures, and protocols to define and guide all elements of care. These standards, which must comply with established national standards, must be kept current and accessible to the nursing personnel. Manuals for these agency standards are often available online within the agency for easier access. Updates and periodic reviews are required to maintain validity of care guidelines.

ORGANIZATIONAL STANDARDS. Organizational standards provide broader guidelines that are nationally recognized. AWHONN is recognized as the national professional organization for perinatal nursing services, publishing standards, education guides, monographs, professional issues, and nursing practice guidelines. Standards set by other professional organizations such as the ACOG, AAP, and the National Association of Home Care, may influence standards for perinatal nurses.

LEGAL STANDARDS. Nurses who practice in any health care delivery system must understand the definition of nursing practice and the rules and regulations that govern its practice in their work settings. Nurses must also be aware of their scope of practice in varying locations as defined by state nurse practice acts. (Chapter 3 gives additional information on legal aspects of nursing.)

Other regulatory bodies, such as the Occupational Safety and Health Administration (OSHA), Food and Drug Administration (FDA), and Centers for Disease Control and Prevention (CDC), also provide guidelines for practice in those areas. Accrediting agencies such as the JCAHO and Community Health Accreditation Program (CHAP) give their approval after visiting facilities and observing whether standards are being met in practice. Approval from these accrediting agencies affects reimbursement and funding decisions as well.

Advances in Technology

As with other areas of health care, perinatal care must keep pace with technologic advances. Health care professionals and clients have online access to information from a variety of databases that are frequently updated and many that have provided data used throughout our book. Today's nurse must be as much at ease with a keyboard, mouse, and pointer as yesterday's nurse was with pen and paper. Fetal monitoring data may be stored on electronic media rather than on paper. Video and digital imaging methods are used to preserve and recall crisp images and allow image overlay and computerized comparison, often at distant locations. Personal computer systems are linked to share information about staffing, scheduling, communication, and employee benefits. Today's nursing student routinely communicates with instructors by electronic mail (e-mail) and receives grades and completes tests and assignments over the Internet. Laptop computers are often common ways to take notes in class or at a meeting. The personal digital assistant (PDA), often with security features, can be used to support nurses with drug information, send and receive wireless e-mail, maintain contacts, and download journal articles from publications such as *Journal of Obstetric, Gynecologic, and Neonatal Health* and *AWHONN Lifelines.* Maintaining security is essential to ensure appropriate privacy for personal and professional information.

Complementary and Alternative Medicine

Complementary and alternative medicine (CAM) is common, and its use is not restricted to recent immigrants to North America, although some techniques originated thousands of years ago in Eastern cultures. CAM can be defined as those systems, practices, interventions, modalities, professions, therapies, applications, theories, and claims that are currently not an integral part of the conventional medical system in North America (ACOG, 2001). The therapies may be used alone (alternative therapy), combined with other therapies, or used in addition to conventional medical therapy (complementary therapy) (Bostwick & Raines, 2003). Table 1-2 gives examples of therapies for complementary or alternative care.

In 2002 almost 75% of the population surveyed by the National Center for Health Statistics used at least one CAM measure. At 69%, women were more likely than men to use

TABLE 1-2 Complementary and Alternative Medicine Categories

Category	Examples
Mind-body interventions: Behavioral, psychologic, social, and spiritual approaches to health	Yoga, relaxation response techniques, meditation, tai chi, hypnotherapy, spirituality, and biofeedback; some, such as support groups and cognitive-behavioral therapy, are now mainstream
Manipulative and body-based methods: Based on manipulation or movement of one or more parts of the body	Chiropractic or osteopathic manipulation, massage
Alternative medical systems: Systems developed outside the Western biomedical approach or that evolved apart from the early conventional medical approach in the United States	Examples of systems developed within Western cultures include homeopathy, naturopathic, and chiropractic medicine; non-Western approaches include traditional Chinese medicine, ayurveda, Native American medicine, and acupuncture
Biologically based therapies: Use of substances found in nature such as herbs, foods, and vitamins	Dietary supplements, herbal products or medicinal plants such as ginkgo biloba, ginseng, echinacea, saw palmetto, witch hazel, bilberry, aloe vera, feverfew, and green tea

Energy therapies: Two types involve the energy fields
  Biofield therapies: Presumed to affect energy fields that surround the body
  Bioelectromagnetic-based therapies: Unconventional use of electromagnetic fields
	Biofield therapies have not been scientifically proved; examples include qi gong, reiki, and therapeutic touch
	Examples of bioelectromagnetic-based therapies include pulsed fields, magnetic fields, and alternating-current or direct-current fields

CAM. Major reasons for using CAM cited by both men and women surveyed were as follows (Barnes, 2004):

- CAM combined with conventional medical therapy would help.
- Use of CAM might be interesting to try.
- CAM was suggested by a conventional medical professional.
- Conventional medical treatments would not help.
- Conventional medical therapy was expensive.

Safety is a major concern in the use of CAM. Many people who use these techniques or substances are self-referred. They may delay necessary care from a conventional physician or nurse-midwife, or they may ingest herbal remedies or other substances that are harmful during pregnancy or lactation. Some CAM therapies are harmful if combined with conventional medications or when taken in excess. Additionally, because herbs and vitamins are classified as foods rather than medications, they are not heavily regulated, if at all. People may take in variable amounts of active ingredients from these substances. Laypeople often do not consider CAM to be medicine and may not report the use of such therapies to their conventional health care providers, which sets the stage for an interaction between conventional medications and CAM therapies that have pharmacologic properties. Also, many people may not consider some therapies to be alternative because they are considered mainstream in their cultures, in which Western medicine is considered alternative. (See "Cultural Perspectives in Childbearing" on page 15 for more information on health practices used in specific cultures.)

Nurses may find that their professional values do not conflict with many of the CAM therapies. As a profession, nursing supports a self-care and preventive approach to health care in which individuals bear much of the responsibility for their health. Nursing practice has traditionally emphasized a holistic, or body-mind-spirit, model of health that fits with CAM. Nurses may already widely practice some CAM therapies such as therapeutic touch. The rising interest in CAM provides opportunities for nurses to participate in research related to the legitimacy of these treatment modalities.

The National Institutes of Health has a web page (www.nih.gov) for the National Center for Complementary and Alternative Medicine to answer questions people may have about CAM. This web page provides information to both laypeople and professionals about CAM.

✔ CHECK YOUR READING

4. How do cost-containment strategies affect maternal-newborn nursing?
5. What are the functions of clinical pathways?
6. How do standards guide community-based perinatal care?
7. What are possible dangers in the use of complementary and alternative medicine?

THE FAMILY

Families are sometimes categorized into three groups: traditional, nontraditional, and high risk. In theory, traditional families require care that differs from that needed by nontraditional or high-risk families.

Traditional Families

Traditional families, or nuclear families, are headed by a father and mother who view parenting as the major priority in their lives and whose energies are not depleted by stressful conditions such as poverty, illness, or substance abuse. Generally, traditional families are motivated to learn all they can about pregnancy, childbirth, and parenting. These families are best served by providing information as the need arises. Traditional families can be single or dual income. Today, the family structure that is composed of two married parents and their children represents 69% of families with children, down from 87% in 1970 (Fields & Casper, 2001).

SINGLE-INCOME FAMILIES

Single-income families in which one parent, usually the father, is the sole provider constitute a minority among households in the United States. Most two-parent families depend on two incomes, either to make ends meet or to provide nonessentials that they could not afford on one income. One or both parents must often travel as a work responsibility. Dependence on two incomes has created greater stress on parents, subjecting them to many of the same problems that single-parent families face. For instance, reliable, competent child care is an issue and that has increased the stress and financial burdens many families experience. A high consumer debt load gives them less cushion for financial setbacks such as job loss. It may be difficult for parents in these families to have the time and flexibility to attend to the requirements of both their careers and their children.

Nontraditional Families

Nontraditional families are defined by their unique structure and may be single parent, blended, or extended. As with traditional families, nontraditional families require information. They often benefit from referrals to meet specific needs such as single-parenting classes, classes for parents of multiples, and group classes for adoptive families.

SINGLE-PARENT FAMILIES

Millions of families are now headed by a single parent, most often the mother, who must function as a homemaker and caregiver and is often the major financial provider for the family's needs. Divorce is the most common cause of single-parent families, although childbirth among unmarried women is also a major factor. Widowhood of the parent sometimes occurs as well. The proportion of families with children that are headed by a single mother is now 26%, and single-father families, once rare, now make up 5% of this group.

Single-parent families headed by women are more likely to have an income below the poverty level (32%) than those headed by men (16%) (Fields, 2004). Single parents may feel overwhelmed by the prospect of assuming all child-rearing responsibilities and may be less prepared for illness or loss of a job than two-parent families.

Nurses can support and encourage single-parent families with a focus on the unique problems of each specific family. Nurses are often the primary source of information about health care for many of these families and are often instrumental in the initiation of the necessary referrals to social and governmental agencies.

BLENDED FAMILIES

Blended families are formed when divorced or widowed parents remarry and bring children from a previous marriage into the new relationship. In many situations the members of the couple desire children with each other, which creates a contemporary family structure commonly described as "yours, mine, and ours." These families may have difficulty forming a cohesive family unit unless they can overcome differences in parenting styles and values. Differing expectations of children's behavior and development and differing beliefs about discipline often cause family conflict. Financial hardships may occur in the blended family when a parent must pay child support from a previous relationship.

EXTENDED FAMILIES

The extended family includes members from at least three generations living under one roof. This family structure is becoming increasingly common in the United States and has given rise to the term *boomerang families*. Elderly parents may live with their adult children, or single or married adults with children of their own return to their parents' homes because they either are unable to support their families or want the additional support that grandparents provide for grandchildren. Extended families are vulnerable to generational conflicts and may require education and referral to prevent disintegration of the family unit. However, extended families can also provide a great deal of support for all members.

Grandparents or other older family members, because of the inability of the parents to care for the children, now head a growing number of households with children. The strain of raising children a second time may cause tremendous physical, financial, and emotional stress.

SAME-SEX PARENT FAMILIES

Although families headed by same-sex parents are relatively uncommon, they are recognized increasingly in the United States. Children in these families may be from previous heterosexual unions, adopted, or conceived by an artificial reproductive technique such as in vitro fertilization. These families may face a great many challenges from a community that is unaccustomed to alternative lifestyles. The children's adaptation depends on the parents' psychologic adjustment, the degree of participation and support of the absent biologic parent, and community acceptance and support.

ADOPTIVE FAMILIES

People who adopt a child may have problems that biologic parents do not face. Biologic parents have the long period of gestation and the gradual changes of pregnancy to help them adjust emotionally and socially to the birth of a child. An adoptive family, both parents and siblings, is expected to make the same adjustments suddenly when the adopted child arrives, possibly from another country. Adoptive parents add pressure to themselves if they have an unrealistically high standard for themselves. Additional issues with adoptive families may include the following:

- Lack of knowledge of the child's health history
- Difficulty assimilating if the child is adopted from another country
- Unknown developmental or growth delays in the child
- The decision of when and how to tell the child about being adopted

Adoptive parents as well as biologic parents need information, support, and guidance to prepare them to care for the infant or child and to maintain their own relationship.

Adoptive parents may be older when the adoption is finalized. Friends in their age group may have children who are much older than the newly adopted child, particularly if the parents adopt an infant. This difference may make adoptive parents feel somewhat out of step with their peers, who are attending soccer and drill team practice while the adoptive parents are changing diapers and doing night feedings.

High-Risk Families

High-risk families include those below the poverty level, those headed by a single teenage parent, and those with unanticipated stress, such as an infant who is preterm, ill, or handicapped. In addition, families with lifestyle problems such as alcoholism, use of illicit drugs, and family violence are considered at high risk for problems in providing adequate care for the infant.

Many high-risk families require specialized services. In such cases the major responsibility of nurses is to refer these families to agencies that can provide comprehensive care. The most common referrals are to social service agencies for financial assistance, crisis intervention, home visits, and drug rehabilitation programs (see Chapter 24).

Characteristics of a Healthy Family

In general, healthy families are able to adapt to changes that occur in the family unit. Pregnancy and childbirth create some of the most powerful changes in a family. The relationship between adults must change to include the care of a helpless infant. Children must learn to share the attention of parents with a new sibling. The healthy, viable family is able to adapt to these changes without undue stress, but the family that is unprepared for change may suffer conflict.

Healthy families exhibit some common characteristics that provide a framework the nurse can use to assess the way all families function. These characteristics include the following:

- Members of healthy families communicate openly with each other to express the concerns and needs of each family member.
- Healthy families remain flexible in role assignment so that if one person is unable to complete the assigned tasks, another member offers assistance.
- Adults in healthy families agree on the basic principles of parenting so that discord about such things as discipline and sleep schedules is minimal.
- Healthy families are adaptable and not overwhelmed by changes that occur in the home and relationships as a result of childbirth. For instance, adaptable families can tolerate less-than-perfect housekeeping, an irregular schedule of meals, and interrupted sleep, all of which are common when an infant is added to the family structure.
- Members of healthy families volunteer assistance without waiting to be asked. Some young parents feel guilty if they must ask for help with the tasks of parenting but are relieved when assistance is offered.

Factors That Interfere with Family Functioning

Nurses need to recognize factors that interfere with the family's ability to provide for the individual needs of family members. These factors include lack of financial resources, absence of adequate family support, birth of an infant who requires specialized care, unhealthy habits such as smoking or substance abuse, and inability to make mature decisions that are necessary to provide care for an infant.

✔ **CHECK YOUR READING**

8. How do structures of traditional and nontraditional families differ?
9. What are four reasons families might be identified as high risk?
10. What are the characteristics of a healthy family?
11. What factors interfere with family functioning?

CULTURAL PERSPECTIVES IN CHILDBEARING

Culture is the sum of the beliefs and values that are learned, shared, and transmitted from generation to generation by a particular group. Cultural values guide the thinking, decisions, and actions of a group, particularly in pivotal events such as childbearing. Ethnicity is the condition of belonging to a particular group that shares race, language and dialect, religious faiths, traditions, values, and symbols, as well as food preferences, literature, and folklore. Cultural beliefs and values vary among different groups, and nurses must be aware that individuals often believe their cultural values and patterns of behavior are superior. This belief, termed *ethnocentrism*, forms the basis for many conflicts that occur when persons from different cultural groups have frequent contact.

Nurses must be aware that culture has visible and invisible layers that could be said to resemble an iceberg (Figure 1-3). Observable behaviors can be compared with the visible part—the tip of the iceberg. The history, beliefs, values, and religion

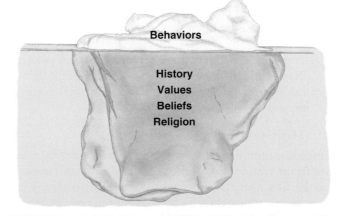

FIGURE 1-3 ■ Visible and hidden layers of culture are like the visible and submerged parts of an iceberg. Many cultural differences are hidden below the surface.

are not observed, but they are the hidden foundation on which behaviors are based and can be likened to the large submerged part of the iceberg. A full comprehension of cultural behavior includes knowledge of the hidden beliefs expressed by behaviors.

Implications of Cultural Diversity for Perinatal Nurses

Many immigrants and refugees are of childbearing age, which means that perinatal nurses in most localities will provide care for culturally diverse families. To provide effective care, nurses must be aware that culture is among the most significant factors that influence a woman's perception of childbirth.

WESTERN CULTURAL BELIEFS

Nursing practice in the United States is based largely on Western beliefs. Nurses must recognize that these beliefs may differ significantly from those of other societies and that the differences may cause a great deal of conflict.

Leininger (1978) identified seven dominant Western cultural values. These values, described in the following list, greatly influence the thinking and action of nurses in the United States but may not be shared by their clients.

1. Democracy is a cultural value not shared by families that believe decisions are made by elders or other higher authorities in the group. Fatalism, or a belief that events and results are predestined, may also affect health care decisions.
2. Individualism conflicts with the values of many cultural groups in which individual goals are subordinated to the greater good of the group.
3. Cleanliness is an American "obsession" that many others view with amazement.
4. Preoccupation with time, which is measured by health care professionals in minutes and hours, is a major source of conflict with those who mark time by different standards such as seasons and body needs.
5. Reliance on machines and equipment may intimidate families who have not reached even minimal comfort with technology.
6. The belief that optimal health is a right is in direct conflict with beliefs in many cultures in the world in which health is not a major emphasis or even an expectation.
7. Admiration of self-sufficiency and financial success may conflict with beliefs of other societies that place less value on wealth and more value on less-tangible principles such as spirituality.

COMMUNICATION

Communication may also be a source of conflict between "dominant culture" and "other culture" health care professionals. This is particularly true for Southeast Asians, Latinos, African-Americans, and Middle Eastern immigrants.

SOUTHEAST ASIANS. Language is the greatest barrier to health care for families who have recently immigrated to North America, including people from Southeast Asia (Mattson, 1995; Ottani, 2002). Women of childbearing age were often born in the United States or Canada, but elders in families may not have learned English. Besides the national languages of Vietnam, Cambodia, and Laos, tribal languages may be familiar to the family. People from Southeast Asia also speak softly and avoid prolonged eye contact, which they consider rude, in contrast to the Western belief that eye contact denotes honesty and forthrightness. They invariably show respect to the elderly, priests, and physicians. When medication or therapy is recommended, they seldom say "no." They may accept the prescription or medication sample but not take the medicine, or they may agree to undergo a procedure but not keep the appointment.

HISPANICS. Hispanics, also called Latinos, include those whose origin is Mexico, Central and South America, and Puerto Rico. The background of approximately 67% of Hispanics in the United States is Mexican. Most Hispanics of Mexican background reside in southern or western states, whereas Puerto Ricans often live in the northeast United States and those from Cuba tend to reside in the south. Hispanics are part of a rapidly growing population in the United States. Education and unstable employment are often problems in the Hispanic population. Two in five Hispanics have not graduated from high school. Lower pay and unemployment, which accompany incomplete education, are also more likely (Ramirez & de la Cruz, 2003).

Men usually serve as head of household and are considered strong ("macho"). Women are the homemakers. Hispanics usually have a close extended family and place a high value on children.

Hispanics tend to be polite and gracious in conversation. Preliminary social interaction is important, and Hispanics may be insulted if a problem is addressed directly without taking time for "small talk." This is counter to the value of "getting to the point" for many white people in the United States and may cause frustration for the client as well as for the health care worker.

There exists a strong association between religion and health. The *curandero*, a folk healer, may be consulted for health care before a U.S. health care worker is consulted.

AFRICAN-AMERICANS. African-Americans constitute 13% of the U.S. population, and the population of African-Americans has increased faster than the overall population in the United States (McKinnon, 2003). African-Americans are often part of a close extended family, although many heads of household are single women. They have a sense of loyalty to their people and community but sometimes distrust the majority group. African-Americans sometimes use a communication style that may cause conflict when they seek health care. They may use idioms, colloquial expressions, or speech patterns that are unfamiliar to many health care workers. Nurses must often clarify what is being said so that misunderstandings can be avoided and teaching can be effective. The black minister is influential, and religious rituals such as prayer may be used in coping with illness.

NATIVE AMERICANS. Native Americans include American Indians and Alaska Natives. This group makes up 1.5% of the total U.S. population. Many who consider themselves Native Americans are of mixed race. The largest American Indian tribal groups include Cherokee, Navajo, Latin American Indian, Choctaw, Sioux, and Chippewa. The largest tribe among Alaska Natives is the Eskimos (Ogunwole, 2002).

Native Americans may consider a willful child to be strong and a docile child to be weak. They have close family relationships, and respect for their elders is the norm. Native Americans may consider health to be a state of harmony with nature and may believe that supernatural influences have a great impact on health and illness. Native Americans may highly respect a medicine man, whom they believe to be given power by supernatural forces. The use of herbs and rituals is part of the medicine man's curative practice.

MIDDLE EASTERNERS. Middle Eastern immigrants come from a variety of countries, including Lebanon, Syria, Arabia, Egypt, Turkey, Iran, and Palestine. Islam is the dominant, and often the official, religion in these countries; its followers are known as *Muslims.* Obtaining health care information may be difficult, because Islam dictates that family affairs should be kept within the family. Personal information is shared only with personal friends, and health assessment must be done gradually. Decisions are usually made by the male head of household. Interpreters should be from the same country and religion as the client, if possible, because of regional differences and hostilities.

Islam requires believers to kneel and pray five times a day: at dawn, noon, afternoon, after sunset, and after nightfall. Muslims do not eat pork and do not use alcohol. Many are vegetarians.

Cross-Cultural Health Beliefs

More than 100 different ethnocultural groups exist in the United States, and numerous traditional health beliefs are observed among these groups. Culturally based definitions of health are common. Women of Asian origin may view health as the balance between "yin" and "yang." Those of African or Haitian origin may define health as "harmony with nature." People from Mexico, Central and South America, and Puerto Rico often see health as a balance between "hot" and "cold."

TRADITIONAL METHODS TO PREVENT ILLNESS

The traditional methods of illness prevention rely on the causes of a given illness as ascribed by a person's culture. These causes may include the following:

- Agents such as hexes, spells, or the "evil eye," which may strike a person (often a child) and cause injury, illness, or misfortune
- Phenomena such as soul loss or accidental provocation of envy, jealousy, or hatred of a friend or an acquaintance
- Environmental factors such as bad air and natural events such as solar eclipses

Practices to prevent illness developed from beliefs regarding the cause of illness. A believer must avoid those persons known to transmit hexes and spells. Elaborate methods are used to prevent inciting envy or jealousy of others and to avoid the evil eye. Protective or religious objects such as amulets with magic powers or consecrated religious objects (such as talismans) are frequently worn or carried to prevent illness. Also, numerous food taboos and traditional combinations are prescribed in traditional belief systems to prevent illness. For instance, people from many ethnic backgrounds eat raw garlic to prevent illness. Those of African origin may consume nonfood substances (pica) such as starch to facilitate labor.

TRADITIONAL PRACTICES TO MAINTAIN HEALTH

Several traditional practices are used to maintain health. Proper clothing such as scarves may prevent drafts and thus maintain the health of a woman who is pregnant and believes she must avoid cool air. Another example is a proper diet. Women of Asian origin eat rice daily. Mental and spiritual health are maintained by activities such as silence, meditation, and prayer. Many people view illness as punishment for breaking a religious code and adhere strictly to religious morals and practices to maintain health.

TRADITIONAL PRACTICES TO RESTORE HEALTH

Traditional practices to restore health often conflict with Western medical practice. Some of the most common practices include the use of natural substances such as herbs and plants to treat illness. Religious charms, holy words, and traditional healers may be tried before a medical opinion is sought. Religious medals, prayer cards, and sacrifices may also be used to treat illness.

A variety of substances may be ingested for the treatment of illnesses. The nurse should make an effort to identify the substance and determine whether its active ingredient may alter the effects of prescribed medication.

Dermabrasion, which is the rubbing or irritation of the skin to relieve discomfort, is a common health care practice in cultures such as those of Vietnam and Cambodia. The most popular form is coining, in which an area is covered with an ointment and the edge of a coin is rubbed over the area. All dermabrasion methods leave marks resembling bruises or burns on the skin and may be mistaken for signs of physical abuse (D'Avanzo & Geissler, 2003; Mattson, 1995).

Cultural Assessment

All health care professionals must develop skills in performing a cultural assessment so that they can understand the meaning of childbirth in different cultural groups. The following questions might be considered in making such an assessment:

- What is the family's ethnic affiliation?
- Is childbearing viewed as a normal process, a time of vulnerability, or a state of illness?

- What are the prescribed practices, customs, and rituals related to diet, activity, and behavior during pregnancy and childbirth?
- What maternal restrictions or precautions are considered necessary during pregnancy and childbirth? Are women exempted from any religious expectations at this time?
- Who provides support during pregnancy, childbirth, and beyond?
- What are the prescribed practices and restrictions related to care of the newborn?
- Who in the family hierarchy makes health care decisions?
- How is time marked—by minutes and hours, or by seasons and body needs?
- What are the views of life and death, including predestination and fatalism?
- How can health care professionals be most helpful?

After such an assessment, plans for care should show respect for cultural differences and traditional healing practices. (Additional information is presented throughout this book relating to culture-specific areas such as nutrition, pregnancy, birth, and the postpartum period.)

✔ CHECK YOUR READING

12. Why is it important for nurses to examine their own cultural values and beliefs?
13. How might communication be a source of conflict?
14. How is culture comparable to an iceberg?

STATISTICS ON MATERNAL AND INFANT HEALTH

Statistics is the science of collecting and interpreting numeric data. In health and medical science, data often focus on mortality rates within a given population. Mortality rates indicate the number of deaths that occur each year by different categories. They are important sources of information about the health of groups of people within a country. They may also be an indication of the value a society places on health care and the kind of health care available to the people. The newest statistics about maternal and infant health can be obtained from the National Center for Health Statistics (www.cdc.gov/nchs).

Maternal and Infant Mortality

Throughout history the number of deaths of women and infants has been high, especially around the time of childbirth. Infant and maternal mortality rates began to fall with the improved health of the general population, application of basic principles of sanitation, and increase in medical knowledge. Improvements in health care, including widely available antibiotics, public health facilities, and increased prenatal care further reduced infant mortality. Today, mothers seldom die in childbirth and infant mortality rates continue a downward trend. However, this downward trend is greater for whites than for nonwhites.

MATERNAL MORTALITY

In 2002 the maternal mortality rate was 8.9 per 100,000 live births for all women in the United States. African-American women are more likely to die from birth-related causes than white women. The maternal mortality rate for African-American women is 24.9, whereas for white women it is 6.0 (National Center for Health Statistics, 2004). The rate is higher if compared with that in previous years because deaths whose cause was aggravated by pregnancy are now included, even if the death occurs more than 42 days after the end of pregnancy.

INFANT MORTALITY

Between 1950 and 1990, infant mortality dropped from 29.2 to 9.2 deaths per 1000 live births. In 2002 the infant mortality rate (death before the age of 1 year) was 7.0 per 1000 live births, slightly higher than the 2001 infant mortality rate of 6.8 per 1000 live births in the United States. Moreover, the neonatal mortality rate (death before 28 days of life) was 4.7 deaths per 1000 live births, also slightly higher than the 2001 rate. The fall in infant mortality is attributed to better neonatal care and public awareness campaigns such as the "Back to Sleep" campaign to reduce the occurrence of sudden infant death syndrome (SIDS) (National Center for Health Statistics, 2004; Martin et al., 2003). Early and more consistent prenatal care, including at public clinics, reduces pregnancy complications and allows early identification of problems. However, women do not consistently receive the best care, because they may not enter prenatal care until their pregnancy nears term.

Although infant mortality rates in the United States have declined overall, rates have declined faster for whites than for non-Hispanic African-American infants. The mortality rate in 2002 for white infants was 5.8. For infants of non-Hispanic African-American mothers the rate was 14.4 (National Center for Health Statistics, 2004). Figure 1-4 compares the rates of infant mortality for all races and for whites and African-Americans since 1950.

Disparity across Racial Groups

The disparity in maternal and infant mortality rates is most obvious between whites and African-Americans, who constitute the largest minority group. The discrepancy is primarily because of greater numbers of premature and low-birth-weight (below 2500 g) infants among African-Americans. Premature and low-birth-weight infants have a greater risk for short-term and long-term health problems, such as respiratory disorders, developmental delay, or SIDS (Office of Minority Health, 2004).

Poverty, not race, is the important factor. The rate of poverty is higher for nonwhites than for whites in the United States. People who live below the poverty level are unlikely to be in good health, be well nourished, have ade-

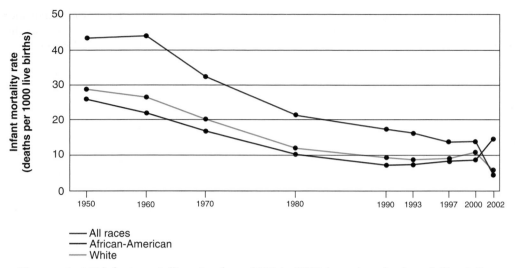

Figure 1-4 ■ Infant mortality rates from 1950 to 2002 based on final mortality statistics. (From Martin, J.A., et al. [2003]. Births: Final data for 2002. *National Vital Statistics Reports*, *52*(10). Retrieved August 9, 2004, from www.cdc.gov/nchs/data/nvsr52/nvsr52_10.pdf; and National Center for Health Statistics [2004]. Health, United States, 2004: *Chartbook on trends in the health of Americans.* Hyattsville, MD. Author.)

quate housing, and obtain adequate preventive health care. Obtaining care becomes vital during pregnancy and infancy, and lack of care is reflected in the high mortality rates in all categories.

The following *Healthy People 2010* objectives relate to infant mortality in the United States (United States Department of Health and Human Services, 2004):

- Reduce infant mortality from the 1998 rate of 7.2 per 1000 live births to 4.5 per 1000 live births in 2010
- Reduce neonatal mortality from the 1998 rate of 4.8 per 1000 live births to 2.9 per 1000 live births in 2010
- Reduce the percentage of low-birth-weight infants from 7.6 to 5
- Reduce the percentage of very-low-birth-weight infants from 1.4 to 0.9

Infant Mortality across Nations

A country such as the United States, which has one of the highest gross national products in the world, is expected to have one of the lowest infant mortality rates. Yet in 2000, the most recent year for which comparative data among countries are available, the mortality rate in the United States ranked 27th among developed nations (Table 1-3).

The major reasons for this poor showing are (1) unequal access to health care for women of all socioeconomic levels and (2) low birth weight and complications of prematurity that contribute to infant mortality. Congenital anomalies, SIDS, newborn problems after pregnancy complications, and respiratory distress syndrome are also leading causes of infant mortality.

TABLE 1-3 Infant Mortality Rates for Selected Countries (Based on 2000 Data)

Country	Infant Mortality (per 1000 Live Births)
Singapore	2.5
Greece	3.0
Japan	3.2
Sweden	3.4
Finland, Norway	3.8
Spain	3.9
Czech Republic	4.1
Germany	4.4
Italy	4.5
France	4.6
Austria, Belgium	4.8
Switzerland	4.9
Netherlands, Northern Ireland	5.1
Australia	5.2
Canada, Denmark	5.3
Israel	5.4
Portugal	5.5
England and Wales	5.6
Scotland	5.7
Greece	6.1
Ireland	6.2
New Zealand	6.3
United States	6.9

From National Center for Health Statistics. (2004). *Health, United States, 2004: Chartbook on Trends in the Health of Americans.* Hyattsville, MD.

✔ **CHECK YOUR READING**

15. Why is the infant mortality rate so much lower today than at the beginning of the twentieth century?
16. Why are African-American women and infants more likely to die than white women and children?
17. How does the infant mortality rate in the United States compare with the rates in other countries?

Adolescent Pregnancy

United States adolescent birth rates fell to a historic low in 2002. The rate decreased from 62.1 per 1000 teenagers aged 15 to 17 in 1991 to 23 per 1000 in 2001. Births to non-Hispanic black teenagers 15 to 17 years old fell from 86.1 per 1000 (1991) to 41 per 1000 (in 2002). The birth rate to the youngest mothers of all races, age 10 to 14 years, is now the lowest ever, 0.7 per 1000 mothers (Martin et al., 2003). These rates are nearing the *Healthy People 2010* target rates for girls 15 to 17 years old of 43 per 1000 (U.S. Department of Health and Human Services, 2004).

SUMMARY CONCEPTS

- Changes in maternity care in the United States came about as a result of technologic advances, increased knowledge, government involvement, and consumer demands.
- Alternative settings for childbirth are now available in hospitals and freestanding birth centers. Home birth is less frequently selected as an alternative.
- Family-centered maternity care, which is based on the principle that families can make decisions about health care if they have adequate information, has greatly enhanced the role of nurses.
- "Drive-through deliveries," or very short lengths of stay mandated by prospective payment plans, resulted in costly maternal and infant problems. Many states passed laws requiring a minimum stay of 48 hours after vaginal birth or 96 hours after cesarean birth. The woman and her care provider have the right to choose an earlier discharge time.
- Reduced lengths of stay make it more difficult for the nurse to provide information regarding self-care and infant care to the woman who is recovering from the fatigue and discomfort of birth.
- Clinical pathways are interdisciplinary guidelines for assessments and interventions that will accomplish the identified outcomes in the shortest time. A variance is a deviation in either the timeline or expected outcomes of the pathway and may indicate either faster or delayed progression.
- Students must learn the reason for and the way to perform assessments and interventions so that they can use clinical pathways to determine whether clients are achieving identified outcomes.
- Social trends such as poverty, early unplanned pregnancy, and the increased rate of divorce have altered family structure and function and have increased the need for information and support provided by nurses.

- To provide care for culturally diverse clients, nurses must examine their own beliefs and become familiar with different cultural values and customs encountered in their practice settings.
- Infant and maternal mortality rates have declined dramatically in the last 50 years. However, the United States continues to have a higher infant mortality rate than many other developed nations, and variation in mortality rates across ethnic groups is still wide.

REFERENCES & READINGS

Agency for Healthcare Research and Quality (AHRQ). (2001). AHRQ Publication No. 012-PO12: *Program brief: Women's health highlights.* Rockville, MD: Author. Retrieved August 10, 2004, from www.ahcpr.gov/research/womenh1.htm.

Agency for Healthcare Research and Quality (AHRQ). (2002). AHRQ Publication No. 02-MO17: *Health care for women.* Rockville, MD: Author. Retrieved August 10, 2004, from www.ahcpr.gov/news/focus/focwomen.htm.

Agency for Healthcare Research and Quality (AHRQ) (2004). *Clinical practice guidelines.* Retrieved August 10, 2004, from www.ahrq.gov.

Alfaro-LeFevre, R. (2004). *Critical thinking and clinical judgment: A practical approach* (3rd ed.). Philadelphia: Saunders.

American Academy of Pediatrics (AAP) & American College of Obstetricians and Gynecologists (ACOG). (2002). *Guidelines for perinatal care* (5th ed.). Elk Grove Village, IL: Author.

American College of Obstetricians & Gynecologists (ACOG). (2001). *Use of botanicals for management of menopausal symptoms* (ACOG Practice Bulletin No. 28). Washington, DC: Author. Retrieved September 14, 2004, from www.acog.org/from_home/publications/misc/pb028.htm.

Amour, K. (2004). PDAs in nursing: Here's why and how to use this emerging clinical tool. *AWHONN Lifelines, 8*(3), 241-247.

Association of Women's Health, Obstetric, and Neonatal Nurses (AWHONN). (2003). *Standards for professional nursing practice in the care of women and newborns,* (6th ed.). Washington, DC: Author.

Barnes, P.M., Powell-Griner, E., McFann, K., & Nahan, R.L. (2004). Complementary and alternative medicine use among adults: United States, 2002. *Advance data from vital and health statistics,* #343. Hyattsville, MD: National Center for Health Statistics.

Bostwick, D., & Raines, D.A. (2003). Complementary and alternative therapies during the perinatal period. In S.M. Levasseur & D.A. Raines (Eds.), *Perinatal nursing secrets* (pp. 209-216). Philadelphia: Hanley & Belfus.

Callister, L.C. (2001). Culturally competent care of women and newborns: Knowledge, attitude, and skills. *Journal of Obstetric, Gynecologic, and Neonatal Nursing, 30*(2), 209-215.

Cesario, S., Morin, K., & Santa-Donato, A. (2002). Evaluating the level of evidence of qualitative research. *Journal of Obstetric, Gynecologic, and Neonatal Nursing, 31*(6), 708-714.

D'Avanzo, C.E., & Geissler, E.M. (2003). *Mosby's pocket guide to cultural assessment* (3rd ed.). St. Louis: Mosby.

Dossey, B.M. (2000). *Florence Nightingale: Mystic, visionary, healer.* Springhouse, PA: Springhouse.

Fields, J. (2004). America's families and living arrangements: 2003. Current population reports p. 20-553. Washington, DC: U.S. Census Bureau. Retrieved December 31, 2004, from www.census.gov/prod/2004pubs/p20-553.pdf.

Fontaine, K.L. (2005). *Healing practices: Alternative therapies for nursing.* Upper Saddle River, NJ: Pearson.

Gennaro, S., Hodnett, E., & Kearney, M. (2001). Making evidence-based practice a reality in your institution: Evaluating the evidence and using the evidence to change clinical practice. *MCN: American Journal of Maternal-Child Nursing, 26*(5), 236-244.

Giger, J.N., & Davidhizar, R.E. (2004). *Transcultural nursing: Assessment & intervention* (4th ed.). St. Louis: Mosby.

Graham, I.D., Harrison, M.D., Browers, M., Davies, B.L. & Dunn, S. (2002). Facilitating the use of evidence in practice: Evaluating and adapting clinical practice guidelines for local use by health care organizations. *Journal of Obstetric, Gynecologic, and Neonatal Nursing, 31*(5), 599-611.

Leininger, M. (1978). *Transcultural nursing: Concepts, theories, practices.* New York: John Wiley & Sons.

Levine, M.A., Anderson, L., & McCullough, N. (2004). Hmong birthing. *AWHONN Lifelines, 8*(2), 147-149.

Lowe, N.K. (2004). Maternal mortality in the global village [Editorial]. *Journal of Obstetric, Gynecologic, and Neonatal Nursing, 33*(2), 153.

Kronenberg, F., Murphy, P.A., & Wade, C. (2003). Select populations: Women. In J.W. Spencer & J.J. Jacobs (Eds.), *Complementary and alternative medicine: An evidence-based approach.* St. Louis: Mosby.

Martell, L.K. (2000). The hospital and the postpartum experience: A historical analysis. *Journal of Obstetric, Gynecologic, and Neonatal Nursing, 29*(1), 65-72.

Martin, J.A., Hamilton, B.E., Sutton, P.D., Ventura, S.J., Menacker, F., & Munson, M.L. (2003). Births: Final data for 2002. *National Vital Statistics Reports, 52*(10). Retrieved August 9, 2004, from www.cdc.gov/nchs/data/nvsr52/nvsr52_10.pdf.

Mattson, S. (2002). Caring for Latino women: This population is surging throughout the U.S.–not just the big cities. *AWHONN Lifelines, 7*(3): 258-260.

Mattson, S. (1995). Culturally sensitive perinatal care for Southeast Asians. *Journal of Obstetric, Gynecologic, and Neonatal Nursing, 24*(4), 335-342.

Mattson, S. (2000a). Providing culturally competent care: Strategies and approaches for perinatal clients. *AWHONN Lifelines, 4*(5), 37-39.

Mattson, S. (2000b). Striving for cultural competence: Providing care for the changing face of the U.S. *AWHONN Lifelines, 4*(3), 48-52.

Mattson, S. (2000c). Working toward cultural competence: Making the first steps through cultural assessment. *AWHONN Lifelines, 4*(4), 41-43.

McKinnon, J. (2003). *The black population in the United States: Current population reports.* Retrieved August 23, 2004, from www.census.gov/prod/2003pubs/p20-541.pdf

National Center for Complementary and Alternative Medicine. (2004). What is complementary and alternative medicine (CAM)? Bethesda, MD: National Institutes of Health. Retrieved September 14, 2004, from nccam.nih.gov/health/whatiscam/.

National Center for Health Statistics. (2004). Health, United States, 2004 with chartbook on trends in the health of Americans. Hyattsville, MD.

Nichols, F.H. (2000). History of the women's health movement in the 20th century. *Journal of Obstetric, Gynecologic, and Neonatal Nursing, 29*(1), 56-64.

O'Connor, A.M., Jacobsen, M.J., & Stacey, D. (2002). An evidence-based approach to managing women's decisional conflict. *Journal of Obstetric, Gynecologic, and Neonatal Nursing, 31*(5), 570-581.

Office of Minority Health, Centers for Disease Control & Prevention. (2004). Eliminate disparities in infant health. Retrieved August 25, 2004, from www.cdc.gov/omh/AMH/factsheets/infant.htm.

Ogunwole, S.U. (2002). *The American Indian and Alaska Native population: Census 2000 brief.* Washington, DC: U.S. Census Bureau. Retrieved August 24, 2004, from www.census.gov/prod/2002pub/c2kbr01-15.pdf.

Ondeck, M. (2000). Historical development. In F.H. Nichols & S.S. Humenick (Eds.), *Childbirth education: Practice, research, and theory* (2nd ed., pp. 18-31). Philadelphia: Saunders.

Ottani, P.A. (2002). Embracing global similarities: A framework for cross-cultural obstetric care. *Journal of Obstetric, Gynecologic, and Neonatal Nursing, 31*(1), (33-38).

Petersen, M.F., Cohen, J., & Parsons, V. (2004). Family-centered care: Do we practice what we preach? *Journal of Obstetric, Gynecologic, and Neonatal Nursing, 33*(4), 421-427.

Ramirez, R.R., & de la Cruz, G.P. (2003). Current Population Reports P20-545. *The Hispanic population in the United States: March 2002.* Washington, DC: U.S. Census Bureau. Retrieved August 24, 2004, from www.census.gov/prod/2003pubs/p20-545.pdf.

U.S. Department of Health and Human Services. *Healthy People 2010.* Retrieved August 9, 2004, from www.healthypeople.gov/document/.

U.S. Department of Health and Human Services. (2003). *Health, United States, 2003, with chartbook on trends in the health of Americans.* Hyattsville, MD: Department of Health and Human Services.

U.S. Department of Health and Human Services, Administration for Children and Families. (2004). Fact sheet: Temporary Assistance for Needy Families (TANF). Retrieved August 26, 2004, from www.acf.dhhs.gov/news/facts/tanf.html.

West, Z. (2002). *Acupuncture in pregnancy and childbirth.* Edinburgh: Churchill Livingstone.

Yankowitz, J. (2003). Drugs in pregnancy. In J.R. Scott, R.S. Gibbs, B.Y. Karlan, & A.F. Haney (Eds.), *Danforth's obstetrics and gynecology* (9th ed, pp. 129-142). Philadelphia: Lippincott Williams & Wilkins.

The Nurse's Role in Maternity and Women's Health Care

OBJECTIVES

After studying this chapter, you should be able to:

1. Explain the roles of nurses with advanced preparation in maternal-newborn or women's health nursing, including the roles of nurse-midwives, nurse practitioners, and clinical specialists.
2. Discuss the roles for nurses in maternity and women's health care.
3. Explain the importance of critical thinking in nursing practice, and describe how it may be refined.
4. Relate the five steps of the nursing process to maternal-newborn and women's health nursing.
5. Explain how the nursing process relates to critical thinking.
6. Discuss the importance of nursing research in clinical practice.

Go to your Student CD-ROM for Review Questions keyed to these Objectives.

DEFINITIONS

Ambiguity (Ambiguous) Lack of clarity or certainty; having more than one meaning.

Assumptions Beliefs taken for granted without examination.

Baseline Data Information that describes the status of the client before treatment begins.

Bias A prejudice that sways the mind.

Cesarean Birth Surgical birth of the fetus through an incision in the abdominal wall and uterus.

Delegated Nursing Interventions Physician-prescribed nursing actions that require nursing judgment because nurses are accountable for correct implementation; also called *interdependent nursing interventions*. (See also *independent nursing interventions*.)

Fetus The developing baby from 9 weeks after conception until birth; term used in everyday practice to describe a developing baby during pregnancy, regardless of age.

Independent Nursing Interventions Nurse-prescribed actions used in both nursing diagnoses and collaborative problems. (See also *delegated nursing interventions*.)

Inference The act of drawing a conclusion or making a deduction.

Judgment An opinion.

Reflection Meditation, attentive consideration.

Skepticism Doubt in the absence of conclusive evidence.

Suspend To delay or bring to a stop temporarily.

Validate To make certain that the information collected during assessment is accurate.

As maternity care changed from regimented care of the mother and newborn to a family-centered approach, maternity nursing evolved to a new level of independence. Women's health has evolved from nursing that did not focus on the care of women from the early years of adolescence to late life. For the best care during the years preceding childbearing through the time after reproductive years, nurses must communicate and teach effectively. They must be able to think critically and use the nursing process to develop a plan of care that meets the unique needs of each family. Nurses are expected to base practice on valid and current research and to collaborate with other health care providers. Moreover, many nurses complete advanced programs of education that allow them to provide primary care to girls and women before, during, and after their childbearing years.

ADVANCED PREPARATION FOR MATERNAL-NEWBORN NURSES

Greater complexity of care and the need to contain costs have increased the need for nurses with various types of advanced preparation. Advanced practice nurses may practice as certified nurse-midwives (CNMs), nurse practitioners, nurse educators, and nurse researchers. Preparation for advanced practice involves obtaining a master's or doctoral degree. Nurses working in midlevel or higher management are often required to have a master's degree in health care administration or the specialty that they lead.

Certified Nurse-Midwives

CNMs are registered nurses who have completed an extensive program of study and clinical experience. They must pass a certification test administered by the American College of Nurse-Midwives. CNMs are qualified to take complete health histories and perform physical examinations. They can provide complete care during pregnancy, childbirth, and the postpartum period. They attend the mother and infant as long as the mother's progress is normal. CNMs are committed to providing information to prevent problems during pregnancy and preparation for normal pregnancy and childbirth. They spend a great deal of time counseling and supporting the childbearing family. The CNM also provides gynecologic services and family-planning information and counseling. The practice approach of the CNM to childbirth is noninterventionist and supportive, and pregnancy and birth are regarded as normal processes.

The effectiveness of care provided by nurse-midwives has a long history that continues to be validated. In the 1930s the Maternity Center Association, founded to provide care for indigent women, began to educate public health nurses in midwifery. Around the same time, Mary Breckinridge, a nurse-midwife from England, founded the Frontier Nursing Service to provide primary care (including midwifery services) for poor families in the remote mountains of Kentucky.

Despite the proved effectiveness of care, physicians opposed the widespread use of nurse-midwives. For many years the scope and locations of their practices were restricted. In 1970, however, many restrictions were removed when the American College of Obstetricians and Gynecologists and the Nurses' Association of the American College of Obstetricians and Gynecologists (NAACOG)—now known as the Association of Women's Health, Obstetric and Neonatal Nurses (AWHONN)—issued a joint statement that admitted CNMs as part of the health care team. In 1981 Congress authorized Medicaid payments for the services of CNMs. This measure has resulted in increased use of nurse-midwives, particularly in health maintenance organizations, birth centers, and some hospitals.

Nurse Practitioners

Nurse practitioners are registered nurses with advanced preparation that allows them to provide primary care for specific groups of clients. They can take a complete health history, perform physical examinations, order and interpret laboratory and other diagnostic studies, and provide primary care for health maintenance and health promotion. Most nurse practitioners collaborate with physicians for treatments and medications, but, depending on their scope of practice and the board of nursing mandates for their practice in the state, they may work independently and prescribe some medications. Nurse practitioners now specialize in many areas of practice, including women's health. Nurse practitioner programs in all specialties are a popular track for master's degree nursing preparation.

The women's health nurse practitioner (WHNP) provides wellness-focused, primary, reproductive, and gynecologic care over the life span, beginning during adolescence. Common responsibilities include performing well-woman examinations, screening for sexually transmitted diseases, and providing family planning services. Hospitals may employ WHNPs to assess and screen women who arrive at obstetric triage units; many of these women have nonobstetric problems during pregnancy.

Family nurse practitioners (FNPs) are prepared to provide preventive, holistic care for young and old family members. They care for women during uncomplicated pregnancies and provide follow-up care for mothers and infants after childbirth. Unlike CNMs, FNPs do not assist with childbirth.

Pediatric nurse practitioners (PNPs) provide health maintenance care for infants and children that do not require the services of physicians. They may see infants at well-baby visits and for common illnesses.

Clinical Nurse Specialists

Maternity, or perinatal, clinical specialists are registered nurses who, through study and supervised practice at the graduate level (master's or doctorate), have become expert in the care of childbearing women with complex problems. Four major subroles have been identified for clinical nurse specialists: expert practitioner, educator, researcher, and consultant. These professionals often function as clinical leaders, role models, client advocates, and change agents. They also act as consultants to assist other nurses in planning care for difficult problems encountered in the maternity unit. Unlike nurse practitioners, clinical nurse specialists do not provide primary care.

IMPLICATIONS OF CHANGING ROLES FOR NURSES

Nurses now work in a variety of highly specialized areas, such as fetal diagnostic centers, infertility clinics, and facilities offering genetic counseling, as well as in acute care settings. Home-based care is an option for some perinatal conditions, such as risk for preterm birth. Nurses also assume primary responsibility for independent functions such as teaching, counseling, and intervening for a wide variety of nonmedical problems that affect the childbearing family.

Because of the added responsibilities of teaching and counseling, all nurses must develop and maintain additional interpersonal skills. These skills include communication, effective teaching, critical thinking, and the use of the nursing process to identify and intervene for a variety of problems.

Therapeutic Communication

Unlike social communication, therapeutic communication is purposeful, goal directed, and focused. Although it may seem simple, therapeutic communication requires conscious effort and considerable practice. Therapeutic communication is a vital part of nursing. Communication is emphasized throughout this book for three reasons: (1) to review the process, (2) to emphasize the importance of communication in women's health and maternal-newborn nursing, and (3) to provide examples for using therapeutic communication with childbearing families.

GUIDELINES FOR THERAPEUTIC COMMUNICATION

Therapeutic communication requires great flexibility and cannot depend on a specific set of learned techniques. However, the following guidelines may prove helpful:

1. A restful setting that provides privacy, reduces distractions, and minimizes interruptions is ideal.
2. Interactions should begin with introductions and clarification of the nurse's role: "My name is Claudia Lyall; I am here to complete the discharge teaching that was started yesterday." This introduction acknowledges the nurse's purpose and sets the scene to discuss concerns about the family's discharge from the hospital.
3. Therapeutic communication should be focused and directed toward meeting the needs expressed by the family. One method of focusing the interaction is to begin with an open-ended question: "How do you feel about going home today?" Redirection of the conversation may also be necessary: "Thanks for showing me the beautiful pictures of the baby. I understand you're having some trouble getting him to nurse?"
4. Nonverbal behaviors may communicate more powerful messages than the spoken word. For example, facial expressions and eye movements can confirm or contradict what the woman says. Repetitive hand gestures, such as finger tapping and twirling a lock of hair, may indicate frustration, irritation, or boredom. Body posture, stance, and gait can convey energy, depression, or discomfort. Voice tone, pitch, rate, and volume may indicate joy, anger, or fear. Grooming also conveys messages about the way the woman feels about herself. If she is tired or depressed, she may neglect her own grooming, although she may not verbalize a problem.
5. Active listening requires that the nurse "attend" to the words being said and to nonverbal clues. Attending behaviors that convey the nurse's interest and a sincere desire to understand include the following:
   - Eye contact, which signals a readiness to interact
   - Relaxed but erect posture, with the upper portion of the body inclined toward the client
   - Minimal cues and leads such as nodding, leaning closer, and smiling. Verbal cues include "Uh-huh, go on," "Tell me about that," and "Can you give me an example?"
   - Touch, which can be a powerful response when words would break a mood or fail to convey the depth of feeling experienced between the woman and nurse
6. Cultural differences influence communication. In some cultures, such as certain Asian cultures, prolonged eye contact is perceived as confrontational and initiates a great deal of concern. People from some cultures, such as Middle Eastern or Native American, may be uncomfortable with touch and would be disturbed by unsolicited touching.
7. Clarifying communication involves a unique process in which the listener receives the message as the sender intended. The nurse may need to ask questions to clarify a statement. For instance, the nurse may say, "I'm not sure I understand," or "So you are undecided about breastfeeding?"
8. Emotions are part of communication, and nurses must often reflect feelings that are expressed verbally or nonverbally: "It sounds as if you were looking forward to delivery in a birth center and are disappointed that you needed a cesarean birth."

THERAPEUTIC COMMUNICATION TECHNIQUES

Therapeutic communication involves responding and listening, and nurses must learn to use responses that facilitate rather than block communication. These facilitative responses, often called *communication techniques*, focus on both the content of the message and the feeling accompanying the message. The techniques are useful at many ages and for those who are significant in the client's life. Communication techniques include clarifying, reflecting, maintaining silence, questioning, and directing (Table 2-1). In addition, nurses must be aware of blocks to communication (Table 2-2).

✔ CHECK YOUR READING

1. How does therapeutic communication differ from social communication?
2. What are the major communication techniques?
3. What are the major blocks to communication?

TABLE 2-1 Communication Techniques

Definition	Examples
Clarifying Clearing up or following up to understand both content and feelings expressed, to check the accuracy of how the nurse perceives the message.	"I'm confused about your plans. Could you explain?" "Tell me what you mean when you say you don't feel like yourself." "Are you saying that _____?" "Tell me more about _____?"
Paraphrasing Restating in words other than those used by the client what the client seems to express; a form of clarification.	**Example No. 1** Client: "My boyfriend won't even come into the room for the birth. I'm furious with him." Nurse: "You want him with you and you're angry because he won't be here?" **Example No. 2** Client: "My baby cries all the time. We aren't getting any sleep." Nurse: "You say that you're exhausted and it seems like your baby cries a great deal? What is a typical day like?"
Reflecting Verbalizing comprehension of what the client said and what the client seems to be feeling. It is important to link content and feeling and to reflect the client as a mirror reflects a person. The opinion, values, and personality of the nurse should not be in the reflected image.	**Example No. 1** Client: "I don't know what to do. My husband doesn't think a cesarean is needed, but the doctor says the baby is showing some stress." Nurse: "You're confused and frightened because they don't agree?" **Example No. 2** Client (woman in early labor): "It was my husband's idea to have a baby. I wasn't too excited about it at first." Nurse: "I'll bet the dad will be a pushover as a father." The nurse's statement reflects the nurse's opinion and fails to acknowledge the mother's statement. A better response might be: "Your husband was more excited early in the pregnancy than you were?"
Silence Waiting and allowing time for the client to continue. Verbal communication need not be constant.	The nurse waits quietly for the client to continue.
Structuring Creating guidelines or setting priorities.	"You said you don't know how to take care of the baby and also that you're afraid of getting pregnant again. What should we talk about first?"
Pinpointing Calling attention to differences or inconsistencies in statements.	Nurse talking to an 8-year-old child: "You said you didn't want your mother to spend the night with you, but you cry every night after she leaves. It can be scary being alone. I'll sit with you and we can talk about asking your mother to stay tomorrow night."
Questioning Eliciting information directly; using open-ended questions to avoid "yes" or "no" answers and to prevent controlling the answers.	"How do you feel about being pregnant?" instead of "Are you happy to be pregnant?" "How do you feel about your brother being very sick?" instead of "Are you frightened because your brother is very sick?"
Directing Using nonverbal responses or succinct comments to encourage the client to continue.	Nodding. "Um-mm." "You were saying?" "Please go on."
Summarizing Reviewing the main themes or issues that were discussed	"You had two major concerns today." "We have talked about breastfeeding and how to bathe the baby today."

The Nurse's Role in Teaching and Learning

Nurses are significant teachers on the health care team because of their relationships with clients. Clients often perceive nurses as less threatening than physicians and may expect nurses to have time to respond to concerns that a physician may find trivial. Nurses teach in several settings, including one-on-one interactions, formal classes, and group discussions (Figure 2-1). To teach effectively, nurses must be familiar with the basic principles of teaching and learning.

TABLE 2-2 Behaviors That Block Communication

Behavior	Example	Alternative
Conveying lack of interest	Looking away, fidgeting	Attending behaviors such as eye contact, nodding
Conveying sense of haste	Checking the time, standing near the door	Sitting at bedside
Closed posture	Arms crossed over chest, holding clipboard in front of body	Leaning forward with arms relaxed
Interrupting, finishing sentences	Woman: "I'm not sure how to…." Nurse: "We'll have a bath demonstration later."	"Go on, _____." "You were saying _____."
Providing false reassurance	"You're going to be okay."	"I sense you are concerned about how to care for the baby. I will help you give the bath today."
Inappropriate self-disclosure	To woman in labor: "I was in labor 12 hours, then had a cesarean."	"What concerns you most about labor?"
Giving advice	"You should _____." "If I were you, I would _____."	"How do you feel about that?" "What do you think is most important?"
Failure to acknowledge comments or feelings	Woman: "Being a parent is hard work. I never have time for myself." Nurse: "It's going to get worse before it gets better. Parenting is hard work."	"Parenting is hard work. Let's talk about some ways that you might get a break."

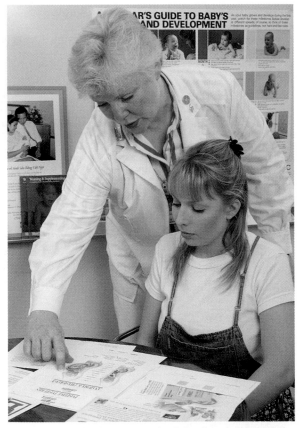

Figure 2-1 ■ In the prenatal clinic the nurse teaches a woman in a one-on-one setting.

PRINCIPLES OF TEACHING AND LEARNING

Application of the following principles helps nurses become effective teachers in the childbearing setting:

- Real learning depends on the readiness of the family to learn and the relevance of the content. Many childbearing families are highly motivated to learn. The parents want to be effective, and any content relevant to the health of either mother or child is eagerly sought.
- Active participation increases learning. Whenever possible, the learner should be involved in the educational process and not act as a passive listener or viewer. Therefore learning is enhanced when the family and nurse mutually develop goals and when time for questions and explanations is ample. A discussion format, in which all can participate, stimulates more learning than a straight lecture.
- Repetition of a skill increases retention and feelings of competence. For example, parents experience real learning when they are allowed to bathe, feed, and diaper the infant more than once. This learning often begins during infant care classes presented during the prenatal period and may continue during home or clinic visits after the mother and infant leave the birth facility.
- Praise and positive feedback are powerful motivators for learning and are particularly important when the family is trying to master a frustrating task such as breastfeeding an unresponsive infant.
- Role modeling is an effective method to demonstrate behavior. Parents benefit greatly from watching a competent nurse respond to their infant. Nurses must be aware that their behaviors are scrutinized carefully at all times and may be copied later.
- Conflicts and frustration impede learning, and they should be recognized and resolved for learning to progress. For instance, couples sometimes do not agree about the way the infant should be fed (breastfeeding versus formula feeding). This issue and the feelings it generates must be acknowledged before teaching about breastfeeding can be effective.
- Learning is enhanced when teaching is structured to present simple tasks before more complex material. For instance, the nurse should teach umbilical cord

care, which is simple, before teaching how to bathe and shampoo the infant, which is more difficult.

- A variety of teaching methods is necessary to maintain interest and illustrate concepts. Posters, videos, and printed materials supplement lectures and discussion. Models may be especially useful for teaching family planning or the processes of labor.
- Retention is greater when material is presented in small segments over time. Brief hospital stays do not promote this practice, making follow-up care particularly important.

FACTORS THAT INFLUENCE LEARNING

Many factors influence learning, including the developmental level of the family, their primary language, their cultural orientation, and their previous experiences.

DEVELOPMENTAL LEVEL. Not surprisingly, teenage parents have different concerns than older parents do. Also, younger people usually learn better in different ways than parents in their thirties. For example, very young parents often do not benefit from printed material to the same degree as older parents. However, teenagers often learn well from videos, computer-based lessons, and group discussions with those who share similar concerns. To be effective, the nurse must acknowledge this difference and structure teaching-learning sessions to meet the family's primary concerns.

LANGUAGE. Understanding the language used determines how well the family learns from the nurse's teaching. Those from countries other than the United States may learn two or more languages, including English, even if they are most comfortable with their country's main language. They may learn multiple languages because family members are from several countries. Newly arrived immigrants might speak English well, but they may not understand the idioms, nuances, medical words, or slang terms that are frequently used. The nurse must create a climate in which families feel free to ask questions when they do not understand.

One helpful method is to ask those who speak a different language to describe what they have learned and how they will use the information. The nurse may also want to determine whether the new information conflicts with the information the parents learned previously.

CULTURE. Background and culture influence learning. People tend to forget content with which they disagree. For instance, if the family is from a culture that believes the mother should eat certain foods after childbirth, family members may disregard other foods recommended by the nurse. Also, if the recommendations of the family's elders and the teachings of the nurse or physicians conflict, young parents often follow the advice of the elders. Therefore the nurse should determine the cultural beliefs and attempt to reach an understanding about what information will be useful before beginning to teach.

PREVIOUS EXPERIENCES. Parents who already have children have unique concerns. These families may not need instruction in newborn care, but they may be very concerned about how older children will accept a new infant. They may need advice in checking used toys and equipment to ensure the infant's safety.

PHYSICAL ENVIRONMENT. The physical environment also influences learning. The hospital room is generally suitable for individual teaching. If group instruction is planned, the instructor should arrange comfortable chairs in a circle so that all persons can hear and participate in face-to-face communication.

ORGANIZATION AND SKILL OF THE INSTRUCTOR. The instructor must determine the objectives of the class, develop a plan for meeting the objectives, and gather all material before the teaching session begins. If the objective is that participants will observe a bath demonstration, the nurse must decide how to demonstrate the bath, when to present care of the umbilical cord and circumcision, and which major principles should be addressed.

A summary of the major principles discussed is helpful after the teaching session. For example, after a bath demonstration, the nurse might conclude with "The important points to remember are to prevent the baby from becoming chilled; to be sure the infant doesn't fall; to start at the face, which is the cleanest area; and to bathe the baby's bottom, which is the dirtiest area, last."

EFFECTS OF EARLY DISCHARGE

Although the principles of teaching and learning should be used whenever possible, early discharge of the mother and infant often requires modifications (Figure 2-2). Rarely is there enough time for repetition and return demonstrations of infant care. Many families leave the hospital before they have attained much comfort with infant care. Self-care after birth and infant teaching often begins during prenatal care or on admission for birth.

Innovative methods have been developed to provide a safety net for families and make them feel more secure. These include follow-up telephone calls, home visits, information lines, videos on infant care, and mother-infant out-

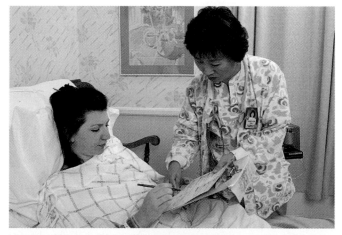

Figure 2-2 ■ Often the nurse must condense teaching by using a "check-off" sheet because mothers and infants leave the birth facility within a short time after birth.

patient clinics. Teaching self-care and infant care during the prenatal period is emphasized. This information must be reviewed before the mother and infant leave the birth facility, but review is generally less time consuming than the initial presentation. Printed materials are provided to parents at discharge in addition to the verbal teaching.

The Nurse's Role as Collaborator

Nurses collaborate with other members of the health care team, often coordinating and managing a client's care. Care is improved by an interdisciplinary approach as nurses work together with dietitians, social workers, physicians, and others.

Managing the transition from an acute care setting to the home involves discharge planning and collaboration with other health care professionals. The nurse must be knowledgeable about community and financial resources to promote a smooth transition. Cooperation and communication are essential to best encourage clients to participate in their care and meet the needs of newborns.

The Nurse's Role as Researcher

Nurses contribute to their profession's knowledge base by systematically investigating theoretic or practice-related issues in nursing. Nursing does not merely "borrow" scientific knowledge from medicine and basic sciences. Nursing generates and answers its own questions based on research of its unique subject matter. The responsibility for research within nursing is not limited to nurses with graduate degrees. It is important that all nurses apply valid research findings to their practices, rather than basing care decisions merely on intuition or tradition. Evidence-based practice is no longer just an ideal but an expectation of nursing practice. Nurses can contribute to the body of professional knowledge by demonstrating an awareness of the value of nursing research and assisting in problem identification and data collection. Nurses should keep their knowledge current by networking and sharing research findings at conferences, by publishing, and by reading research in professional journals.

The Nurse's Role as Advocate

An advocate is one who speaks on behalf of another. As the health care environment becomes increasingly complex, care can become impersonal. As the health professional who is closest to the client, the nurse is in an ideal position to humanize care and to intercede on the client's behalf. As an advocate the nurse considers the family's wishes in planning and implementing care. The nurse provides information to women and their families to ensure that they are involved in decisions and activities related to the care of the newborn. Nurses must be advocates for health promotion of vulnerable groups such as victims of domestic violence.

The Nurse's Role as Manager

As a result of the brief stay in the birth facility and cost-containment strategies, the role of nurses has changed from that of primary caregiver to that of manager and teacher. Nurses may provide less direct patient care and delegate tasks such as ambulation or taking vital signs to others. As a

result, nurses spend more time teaching families, supervising unlicensed personnel, planning and coordinating care, and collaborating with other professionals and agencies. Nurses are expected to understand the financial "squeeze" resulting from cost-containment strategies and to contribute to their institutions' economic viability. At the same time they must continue to act as patient advocates and maintain standards of care (see Chapter 3).

✔ CHECK YOUR READING

4. What are the major principles of teaching and learning?
5. What factors affect learning?
6. Why is nursing becoming more active in application of research?

CRITICAL THINKING

In recent years critical thinking has received widespread attention in nursing. Clearly, nurses must be concerned with developing critical thinking skills, needed not only to pass the National Council Licensure Examination but also to function clinically. Nurses must be concerned with learning and refining the critical thinking skills needed to function in the rapidly changing clinical arena. Critical thinking is controlled rather than undirected and directed toward finding solutions or forming opinions. People think critically in their everyday lives as they make decisions about, for example, when to pay a bill in relation to its due date and their payday, determining ways to make their grocery dollars go farther, and choosing a car with features that are necessary rather than simply desirable.

For effective critical thinking, nurses must gain insight into their own thought processes and analyze their own thinking by taking it apart for examination and criticism. Critical thinking includes recognizing and acknowledging specific habits and responses that can interfere with productive thinking.

Critical thinking is based on reason rather than preference or prejudice. It also seeks to examine feelings to understand how emotions affect thinking. Finally, critical thinking requires the suspension of judgment until evidence is adequate to support inferences or conclusions.

Purpose

The purpose of critical thinking is to help nurses make the best clinical judgments. The process begins when nurses realize that accumulating a fund of knowledge from texts and lectures is not enough. They must also be able to apply this knowledge to specific clinical situations and thus reach conclusions that provide the most effective care in each situation.

In addition, nurses must honestly examine their own thought processes for flaws that can lead to inaccurate conclusions or poor judgments. Although this examination requires self-analysis, a series of steps makes the process easier. Critical thinking exercises are presented throughout the book to help students develop skills in critical thinking and application of knowledge.

Steps

A series of steps may help clarify the way critical thinking is learned. These steps may be called the *ABCDEs of critical thinking*. They include recognition of assumptions, examination of personal biases, analysis of the amount of pressure for closure, examination of how data are collected and analyzed, and evaluation of how emotions may interfere with critical thinking.

RECOGNIZING ASSUMPTIONS

Assumptions are ideas, beliefs, or values that are taken for granted without basis in fact or reason. Such assumptions may lead to unexamined thoughts or unsound actions. For instance, the following assumptions can have negative consequences: "Anyone who wants a job can get one"; "Teenagers don't listen"; "Every woman wants a baby."

A list of everything known about a specific situation may help in the identification of assumptions. Each item on the list should be analyzed to determine whether it is true, whether it could be true, and whether it is untrue or evidence is insufficient to determine its truth.

EXAMINING BIASES

Biases are prejudices that sway the mind toward a particular conclusion or course of action on the basis of personal theories or stereotypes. Biases are based on unexamined beliefs, and many are widespread—for instance, "Fat people are lazy"; "Women are bad drivers"; "Men are insensitive."

People may be biased against those of different races, religions, or lifestyles. When faced with a predisposition to judge a person or a group of persons, it may be wise to ask oneself or a co-worker a series of questions:
- "Why do you think that?"
- "What if this was a different client?"
- "What if there were different circumstances?"
- "What might someone who disagrees say?"
- "What is influencing my thinking?"

DETERMINING THE NEED FOR CLOSURE

Many persons look for immediate answers and experience a great deal of anxiety until a solution is found for any problem. In other words, they have little tolerance for doubt or uncertainty, which is sometimes called *ambiguity.* As a result, they feel pressure to come to a decision or to reach closure as early as possible. This is one of the most important aspects of critical thinking, because those who feel pressure to come to an early decision or find a quick solution often do so with insufficient data.

To overcome pressure to reach an early conclusion, a conscious effort must be made to suspend judgment. This is sometimes called *reflective skepticism.* The first step is to acknowledge the anxiety created by postponed decisions. The next step involves deliberately waiting to make a decision. One method is to follow the example of judges who take information "under advisement" and announce they will "render a decision" at a later date.

Persons who jump to conclusions often stop with one answer. To overcome this tendency, they should always look for a second "right" answer. They could also imagine the problem from the perspective of someone else. They might ask a series of questions:
- "What alternatives do we have?"
- "What else might work?"
- "What information supports this?"
- "What effect would that have?"
- "Is there good evidence to support that decision?"
- "Is there reason to doubt that evidence?"

On the other hand, some persons can tolerate a great deal of doubt and uncertainty. They are comfortable with data collection and analysis but feel uncomfortable making decisions. They may procrastinate or postpone the decision for as long as possible. This procrastination may be of little consequence in some situations. For instance, a family might collect information about getting a pet for a considerable time, and the decision may be of slight importance.

Failure to make a decision in the clinical area may have serious consequences for clients and their families. Several questions may help overcome the tendency to postpone coming to a decision:
- "What signs indicate something is wrong?"
- "Do I need to do something about it?"
- "How much time do I have?"
- "What happens if I don't do something about this?"
- "What should I do first?"
- "What resources can help me?"

This step might also be called *priority setting*, and it is one of the most important aspects of critical thinking in nursing.

BECOMING SKILLFUL IN DATA MANAGEMENT

Expertise in collecting, organizing, and analyzing data involves developing an attitude of inquiry and learning to live with questions such as "Why?" "What if?" "What else?" "Is this relevant?" "How does it relate to that?" "How can I organize the data?" "Do the data form patterns?" "What can I infer from those patterns?"

COLLECTING DATA. To obtain complete data, nurses must develop skill in verbal communication. Open-ended questions elicit more information than questions that require only a one-word answer. Follow-up questions are often needed to clarify information or pursue a particular thought.

VALIDATING DATA. Unclear or incomplete information should be validated. This process may involve rechecking physical signs, collecting additional information, or determining whether a perception is accurate. For instance, the comment "you seem uncomfortable" may result in the client's denial or acknowledgment of discomfort.

ORGANIZING AND ANALYZING DATA. Data are more useful when organized into patterns or clusters. The first step is to separate the relevant data from data that may be interesting but are unrelated to the current situation. For example, the fact that her neighbor is pregnant with twins has little bearing on how a new mother breastfeeds her infant.

The next step is to compare data with expected norms to determine what is within the expected range (normal) and what is not (abnormal). Abnormal results provide cues that can be grouped or clustered so that conclusions can be made. For example, all data that may indicate excessive bleeding, such as pulse rate, blood pressure, amount of vaginal bleeding, and skin color, may seem more meaningful when grouped. Organizing data into clusters often reveals that additional data are needed before a decision can be reached.

ACKNOWLEDGING EMOTIONS AND ENVIRONMENTAL FACTORS

Several emotions and environmental factors can influence critical thinking. For instance, the clinical area is often a noisy, fast-paced, and hectic environment with time limitations and distractions that make calm reflection and reasoning difficult. Fatigue also reduces the ability to concentrate during a 12-hour shift. Inexperienced nurses and students may lack confidence in their knowledge and often feel anxious, which can reduce the ability to think critically.

Many nurses, both experienced and inexperienced, have a strong need to protect their self-image. As a result, they become defensive when they have said or done something wrong. This response is a serious barrier to critical thinking, which requires that all health care professionals learn to acknowledge mistakes and become comfortable with constructive criticism.

Extreme emotions such as anger and frustration impede critical thinking by narrowing the focus to only data that support the intense feeling. For example, persons who are extremely frustrated may often repeat the perceived cause of their frustration and may be unable to move on to other information to address the problem.

The first step is to recognize and acknowledge factors or emotions that impede thinking. For example, nurses may find it necessary to say, "I feel flustered by all the activity and need to find a quiet spot for a few minutes of concentration." To develop critical thinking skills, the nurse must learn to admit mistakes and become comfortable saying, "I was wrong." Asking for assistance, verification, or validation is wise when fatigue is a problem or when lack of confidence creates anxiety.

The person who experiences intense frustration or anger must recognize these emotions and their influence on rational thought. A trusted colleague may be asked to point out signs of these emotions such as repetitive vehement comments. Some persons use other methods of control such as visualizations, breathing exercises, and brief, self-imposed "time-outs" from the precipitating situation, if possible.

✔ CHECK YOUR READING

7. What is the purpose of critical thinking?
8. What steps may be helpful in refining critical thinking?
9. What is meant by *reflective skepticism?*

Application of the Nursing Process
Maternal-Newborn Nursing

The nursing process forms the basis for maternal-newborn and women's health nursing, as for all nursing. The nursing process consists of five distinct steps: (1) assessment, (2) analysis, (3) planning, (4) implementation, and (5) evaluation. In maternal-newborn nursing the nursing process applies to a population that is generally healthy and experiencing a life event that holds the potential for both growth and problems. Nursing activity in the maternal-newborn and women's health settings is devoted to the assessment and diagnosis of client strengths and healthy functioning to achieve a higher or more satisfying level of wellness. This focus often differs from that of providing care for clients who are ill.

The nursing process is written in the text as a linear, step-by-step process. However, with knowledge and experience, the nurse applies the nursing process in the clinical setting dynamically. For example, the nurse may discover that the woman has a full bladder early in a postpartum assessment. The nurse skips to an intervention and helps the woman to the restroom to urinate before completing the assessment to prevent client discomfort and possible excessive bleeding caused by a full bladder. In another example, the nurse goes to the woman's room to give her an injection of RhoGAM and discovers the woman nursing her baby, who is eagerly suckling for the first time in several hours. Based on critical thinking, the nurse delays the injection (an intervention), which would require that the woman change her position. The nurse realizes that the few minutes required for the infant to complete the feeding are more important than the short delay in giving the injection.

Assessment

Nursing assessment should be accomplished systematically and deliberately and include physiologic data and information related to psychologic, social, and cultural considerations. Although the woman or infant may be the primary client, nurses must assess the belief systems, available support, perceptions, and plans of other family members to provide the best nursing care. Two levels of nursing assessment are used to collect comprehensive data: (1) screening assessments and (2) focus assessments.

SCREENING ASSESSMENT

The screening, or database, assessment is usually performed at the first contact with the client. Its purpose is to gather information about all aspects of the client's health. This information, called *baseline data,* describes the client's health status before interventions begin. It forms the basis for the identification of both strengths and problems.

A variety of methods may be used to organize the assessment. For example, information may be grouped according to body systems. Assessment can also be organized around nursing theory models, such as Roy's adaptation to stress theory, Gordon's Functional Health Patterns, the Human Response Patterns of the North American Nursing Diagnosis Association (NANDA), or Orem's self-care deficit theory.

FOCUSED ASSESSMENT

A focused assessment is used to gather information specifically related to an actual health problem or a problem that the client or family is at risk for acquiring. A focused assessment is often performed at the beginning of a shift and centers on areas relevant to childbearing. For instance, in care of the mother and infant after birth the nurse should assess the breasts and nipples because the mother is at risk for problems if she does not have adequate information about breastfeeding or care of the nipples. A focused assessment may also reveal strengths that nursing care will enhance.

Analysis

The data gathered during assessment must be analyzed to identify existing or potential strengths or problems and their causes. Data are validated and grouped in a process of critical thinking to determine cues and inferences. Health needs that nurses can treat independently and for which they are legally accountable are termed *nursing diagnoses*. At present, more than 160 nursing diagnoses have been identified by NANDA.

Nursing Diagnosis

Each nursing diagnosis identified by NANDA consists of the following components:

1. The title, which offers a broad description of the health problem, although a few wellness diagnoses focus on positive client responses.
2. Defining characteristics, which refer to a cluster of signs and symptoms or cues often seen with that particular diagnosis.
3. Etiologic and related factors, which are factors that can cause or contribute to the problem. The etiology may be pathophysiologic, situational, or maturational. Although the majority of nursing diagnoses address actual or potential health problems, wellness diagnoses are often appropriate for the maternal, newborn, and women's health areas. An example of a wellness NANDA nursing diagnosis is "Breastfeeding, Effective."

Diagnoses may be actual, risk, or wellness nursing diagnoses (Table 2-3). Actual nursing diagnoses indicate that the diagnosis exists at the time of assessment and can be validated by the presence of defining characteristics. Risk nursing diagnoses are appropriate when the diagnosis does not exist but the individual or family is at risk to develop it based on contributing factors. Wellness nursing diagnoses are appropriate when the individual or family is moving from a specific level of wellness to greater wellness. Any nursing diagnosis may occur in maternal-newborn or women's health clients, although some diagnostic categories are common.

Planning

The third step in the nursing process involves planning care for problems that were identified during assessment and reflected in the nursing diagnoses. During this step, nurses set priorities, develop goals or outcomes, and plan interventions to accomplish these goals.

SETTING PRIORITIES

Setting priorities includes (1) determining what problems need immediate attention (life-threatening problems) and taking immediate action; (2) determining whether potential problems call for a physician's orders for diagnosis, monitoring, or treatment; and (3) identifying actual nursing diagnoses that take precedence over risk nursing diagnoses.

ESTABLISHING GOALS AND EXPECTED OUTCOMES

Although the terms *goals* and *expected outcomes* are sometimes used interchangeably, they are different. Generally, broad goals do not state the specific outcome criteria and are less measurable than outcome statements. Broad goals should be linked with more specific and measurable outcome criteria. For example, if the goal is that the parents will demonstrate effective parenting by discharge, expected outcomes that serve as evidence might include prompt, consistent responses to infant signals and competence in bathing, feeding, and comforting the infant.

TABLE 2-3 Examples of Actual and Risk Nursing Diagnosis

Actual Nursing Diagnoses		
Problem	**Etiology**	**Signs and Symptoms**
Imbalanced Nutrition: Less Than Body Requirements	Lack of knowledge about nutritional needs during lactation	Weight loss of 5 kg and daily caloric intake <1500 calories
Ineffective Breastfeeding	Nipple trauma	Cracked nipples and reports of discomfort during nursing

Risk Nursing Diagnoses	
Problem	**Risk Factors**
Risk for Imbalanced Nutrition: Less Than Body Requirements	Knowledge deficit of nutritional needs during lactation
Risk for Ineffective Breastfeeding	Lack of knowledge of correct positioning of infant and appropriate breast care

Certain rules apply to written expected outcomes:

- Outcomes should be stated in client-oriented terms, identifying who is expected to achieve the goal. This is usually the woman, infant, or family.
- Measurable verbs must be used. For example, *identify, demonstrate, express, walk, relate,* and *list* are observable and measurable verbs. Examples of verbs that are difficult to measure are *understand, appreciate, feel, accept, know,* and *experience.* For instance, "Ms. Brown will experience less anxiety about assuming care of her infant" poses a problem because determining whether she experiences less anxiety is difficult. This outcome can be reworded as "Ms. Brown will state that she feels less anxious about assuming care of her infant and will participate in infant care (umbilical cord, circumcision, bathing) before discharge."
- A time frame is necessary. When is the person expected to perform the action? By the first postpartum day? After teaching? By discharge? Within the second trimester?
- Goals and expected outcomes must be realistic and attainable. For instance, if a nursing diagnosis of "pain related to lack of knowledge about pain control" is chosen, a realistic expected outcome might be "The woman will state that her pain during labor is manageable using techniques taught by the nurse." A goal such as "will remain free of pain throughout labor" is not attainable by nursing interventions only and is not realistic.
- Goals and expected outcomes are worked out with the client and family to ensure their participation in the plan of care.

DEVELOPING NURSING INTERVENTIONS

After the goals and expected outcomes are developed, nurses write nursing interventions that will help the client meet the established outcomes.

INTERVENTIONS FOR ACTUAL NURSING DIAGNOSES. Nursing interventions for actual nursing diagnoses are aimed at reducing or eliminating the causes or related factors. For instance, the nursing diagnosis is "Impaired parenting related to interruption of bonding process secondary to illness of infant as manifested by absences of attachment behaviors (eye contact, holding)." The desired outcome might be that the parents will demonstrate progressive attachment behaviors such as touching, palming, eye contact, and participation in infant care within 1 week. Nursing interventions focus on increasing contact between parents and the infant and facilitating attachment behaviors.

INTERVENTIONS FOR RISK NURSING DIAGNOSES. Interventions are aimed at (1) monitoring for onset of the problem, (2) minimizing risk factors, and (3) preventing the problem. For example, the nursing diagnosis for an infant is "Risk for Impaired Skin Integrity related to frequent, loose stools." The planned outcome is that the skin remains intact. Nursing interventions include monitoring the condition of the skin at prescribed intervals for signs of skin impairment and initiating measures to keep the skin clean and dry to reduce the risk of skin impairment.

INTERVENTIONS FOR WELLNESS NURSING DIAGNOSES. Interventions focus on health enhancement for wellness nursing diagnoses. Nursing care seeks to promote client success through the teaching of self-care measures. Examples of wellness interventions include teaching related to weight reduction, exercise to lower high blood pressure, or reconditioning the body after birth.

Implementing Interventions

Implementing nursing interventions may be a problem if written interventions are not specific. Nursing interventions should be as specific as physician's orders and may be formulated with computerized care plans. If a physician orders "hydrocodone with acetaminophen, 5 mg/500 mg, 1 tablet PO every 6 hours prn for pain," the order specifies the combination drug to be given, the dose to be given, the route of administration, the time, and the reason. A well-written nursing intervention is equally specific: "Teach woman not to break, chew, or crush the drug tablet."

Conversely, poorly written interventions, such as "Assist with breastfeeding," provide generalizations rather than specific steps. Specific methods that the nurse should use to assist breastfeeding are more effective. For example, "Demonstrate correct positioning in cradle and football hold at first attempt to breastfeed. Teach mother to elicit rooting reflex by stroking infant's lips with nipple. Demonstrate how to latch infant to nipple, and request a return demonstration before mother is discharged."

Evaluation

The evaluation determines the effectiveness of the plan and its goals or expected outcomes. The nurse must assess the status of the client and compare the current status with the goals or outcome criteria developed during the planning step. The nurse then judges the client's progression toward goal achievement and makes a decision: Should the plan be continued? Modified? Abandoned? Are the problems resolved or the causes diminished? Is another nursing diagnosis more relevant?

The nursing process is dynamic, and evaluation frequently results in expanded assessment and additional or modified nursing diagnoses and interventions. Nurses are cautioned not to view lack of goal achievement as a failure but as a signal to reassess and begin the process anew.

Individualized Nursing Care Plans

Nurses are responsible for documenting nursing diagnoses, expected outcomes, and interventions for each problem. This information is often communicated to colleagues through a written plan of care. Many institutions have standards of care for groups of clients, such as those who have had normal spontaneous vaginal births. However, individual nursing care plans may be necessary on the basis of needs or problems identified during the assessment step of

---

BOX 2-1   Developing Individualized Nursing Care Through the Nursing Process

Although the nursing process is the foundation for nursing, initially it is a challenging process to apply in the clinical area. It requires proficiency in focused assessments of the new mother and infant and the ability to analyze data and plan nursing care for individual clients and families. Asking questions at each step of the nursing process may be helpful.

Assessment
1. Did some data not fit within normal limits or expected parameters? For example, the client states that she feels "dizzy" when she tries to ambulate.
2. If so, what else should be assessed? (What else should I look for? What might be related to this symptom? How do my assessments compare with previous assessments?) For example, what are the blood pressure, pulse, skin color, temperature, and amount of lochia if the client feels dizzy? Is my assessment similar to earlier ones, or has there been a change?
3. Did the assessment identify the cause of the abnormal data? What are the lab values for her hemoglobin and hematocrit value? What was her estimated blood loss at childbirth? Did she lose excessive blood during the hours and days after birth?
4. Are other factors present? Did she receive medication during labor? What kind of medication? Did she receive an anesthetic for labor pain? When? What medication is the client now taking? How long has it been since she has eaten? Is the environment a related factor (crowded, warm, unfamiliar)? Is she reluctant to ask for assistance?

Analysis
1. Are adequate data available to reach a conclusion? What else is needed? (What do you wish you had assessed? What would you look for next time?)
2. What is the major concern? (On the basis of the data, what are you worried about?) The client who is dizzy may fall as she ambulates to the bathroom, particularly if she does not ask for help.
3. What might happen if no action is taken? (What might happen to the client if you do nothing?) She may suffer an injury or a complication.
4. Is there a NANDA-approved diagnostic category that reflects your major concern? How is it defined? Suppose that during analysis you decide the major concern is that the patient will faint and suffer an injury. What diagnostic category most closely reflects this concern? "Risk for Injury"? Definition: The state in which an individual is at risk for harm because of a perceptual or physiologic deficit, a lack of awareness of hazards, or maturational age.

5. Does this diagnostic category "fit" this client? Is she at greater risk for a problem than others in a similar situation? Why? What are the additional risk factors?
6. Is this a problem that nurses can manage independently? Are medical interventions also necessary?
7. If the problem can be managed by nurses, is it an actual problem (defining characteristics present) or a risk problem (risk factors present)?

Planning
1. What expected outcomes are desired? That the client will remain free of injury during the hospital stay? That she will demonstrate position changes that reduce the episodes of vertigo?
2. Would the outcomes be clear, specific, and measurable to anyone reading them?
3. What nursing interventions should be initiated and carried out to accomplish these goals or outcomes?
4. Are your written interventions specific and clear? Are action verbs used (assess, teach, assist)? After you have written the interventions, look them over. Do they define exactly what is to be done (when, what, how far, how often)? Will they prevent the client from suffering an injury?
5. Are the interventions based on sound rationale? For instance, dehydration possible during labor causes weakness that may result in falls; loss of blood during delivery often exceeds 500 ml, which results in hypotension that is aggravated when the client stands suddenly. A woman who has recently delivered with an epidural block may have lingering effects from this form of labor pain relief.

Implementing Nursing Interventions
1. What are the expected effects of the prescribed intervention? Are adverse effects possible? What are they?
2. Are the interventions acceptable to the client and family?
3. Are the interventions clearly written so that they can be carefully followed?

Evaluation
1. What is the status of the client right now?
2. What were the goals and outcomes? Were they specific and measurable or should they be clarified?
3. Compare the current status of the client with the stated goals and outcomes.
4. What should be done now?

NANDA, North American Nursing Diagnosis Association.

---

the nursing process. When nurses write individualized plans of care, they implement the plans through interventions that direct the care (Box 2-1).

The Nursing Process Related to Critical Thinking

Although the nursing process and critical thinking are similar and overlap in many respects, major differences exist (Figure 2-3). The five steps of the nursing process provide a logical method for problem solving. Problem solving begins with a specific problem and ends with a solution. Conversely, critical thinking is open-ended; it goes before and beyond problem solving. Critical thinking may be triggered by a problem, a positive event, or an opportunity to improve. It focuses on appraisal of the way the individual

thinks, and it emphasizes reflective skepticism. Critical thinking is used throughout each step of the nursing process (Table 2-4).

✔ **CHECK YOUR READING**

10. How does screening assessment differ from focused assessment?
11. How do actual nursing diagnoses differ from risk nursing diagnoses?
12. How should goals and expected outcome criteria be stated?
13. Why are interventions sometimes difficult to implement? How can this difficulty be overcome?

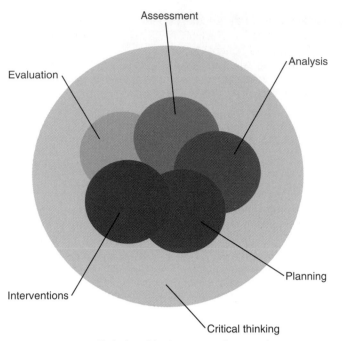

Figure 2-3 ■ Relationship between the nursing process and critical thinking.

TABLE 2-4 Use of Critical Thinking in The Nursing Process

Nursing Process	Critical Thinking Skills
Assessment	Collecting complete data, validating data Clustering data (normal versus abnormal, important versus unimportant, relevant versus irrelevant) Identifying emotions
Analysis	Identifying cues and making inferences Reflecting and suspending judgment Examining thought processes for biases and assumptions Identifying alternatives Determining priorities
Planning	Examining need for closure Searching for alternative solutions Validating plan with client or co-worker Communicating plan Acknowledging defensive behavior
Implementation	Applying knowledge Testing plan Carrying out plan
Evaluation	Examining insights gained Recognizing new ways of thinking or acting Examining options and criteria for action Appraising self and others in the situation

COLLABORATIVE PROBLEMS

In addition to nursing diagnoses, which describe problems that respond to independent nursing actions, nurses must also deal with problems beyond the scope of independent nursing practice. These are sometimes termed *collaborative problems,* which are physiologic complications that usually occur in association with a specific pathologic condition or treatment. Collaborative problems represent situations with both independent nursing as well as physician-prescribed as-

pects. The nurse often adapts care prescribed by the physician or advanced practice nurse, such as a CNM or nurse practitioner, to the individual client, observing for pathologic changes (Carpenito-Moyet, 2004; Murray & Atkinson, 2000).

An example of a collaborative problem is a woman's risk for preterm birth because her membranes ruptured at 30 weeks of gestation. The nurse assesses the woman regularly for signs of infection and subtle signs that suggest possible onset of labor well before term. If signs suggesting a complication occur, such as more frequent or painful contractions, the physician would be notified for further interventions.

Planning

Client goals and expected outcomes are not made for collaborative problems because the nurse's accountability is to detect early changes and manage these problems in conjunction with physicians or advanced practice nurses. Nursing diagnoses have client goals and expected outcomes that reflect the nurse's accountability to achieve or maintain a favorable status after nursing care (Carpenito-Moyet, 2004).

Collaborative problems should reflect the nurse's responsibility in situations that require delegated nursing interventions. Examples of nursing interventions in collaborative problems include the following:
- Observing for signs that suggest complications
- Implementing standing orders and protocols to minimize the severity of a complication
- Contacting physicians or advanced practice nurses if signs of complications are identified and interventions are started

Interventions

Interventions for collaborative problems include (1) performing assessments to monitor the status of the client and detect signs and symptoms of complications, (2) communicating with the physician when signs and symptoms of complications are noted, (3) performing delegated interventions to prevent or correct the complication, and (4) performing nursing interventions described in the standards of care or policy and procedure manuals.

Evaluation

Although client-centered goals or outcomes are not developed for collaborative problems, the nurse collects and compares data with established norms and judges whether data are within normal limits. If data are not within normal limits, the nurse communicates with the physician or advanced practice nurse for additional direction and implements delegated nursing and independent nursing interventions.

✓ CHECK YOUR READING

14. How do nursing diagnoses differ from collaborative problems?
15. Why are client-centered goals or expected outcomes inappropriate for collaborative problems?

NURSING RESEARCH

As maternal-newborn nursing and the health care system change, nurses are challenged to demonstrate that their work improves client outcomes and is cost effective. To meet this challenge, nurses must generate, participate in, and use research. With the establishment of the National Institute of Nursing Research (NINR) in the National Institutes of Health (www.nih.gov/ninr), nurses now have an infrastructure to ensure the support of nursing research and the education of well-prepared nurse researchers. The NINR seeks to establish a scientific basis for nursing care of clients throughout life. The translation of scientific advances into cost-effective, quality care is inherent to the mission of the NINR.

Clinically based nursing research is increasingly conducted, as nurse researchers strive to develop an independent body of knowledge that demonstrates the value of nursing interventions. However, a gap exists between knowledge acquired by the research team and its application to care of the client in the clinical setting.

Students and inexperienced nurses may not initiate research projects, but they may participate in nursing research planned by experts and use updated knowledge from research. Refereed professional journals such as *Lifelines; Journal of Obstetric, Gynecologic, and Neonatal Nursing; Nursing Research; Journal of Perinatal and Neonatal Nursing;* and *Journal of Neonatal Nursing* are sources of verified information about maternal, newborn, and women's health nursing that help validate nursing actions and remove measures that have not proved valid.

The Association of Women's Health, Obstetric and Neonatal Nurses (AWHONN) has created several research-based practice programs for nursing care of women and newborns (www.awhonn.org). Examples of AWHONN research projects to improve nursing care include the following:

- Transition of the preterm infant to an open crib
- Management of women in the second stage of labor
- Continence for women
- Neonatal skin care
- Cyclic pelvic pain and discomfort management
- Setting universal cessation counseling and screening standards: nursing care for pregnant women who smoke

SUMMARY CONCEPTS

- Registered nurses with advanced education are prepared to provide primary care for women and children as certified nurse-midwives and nurse practitioners.
- Clinical nurse specialists function as expert practitioners, educators, researchers, and consultants to provide in-depth interventions for many problems encountered in maternity care.
- Nurses must be adept at communication techniques and communication blocks to meet their responsibilities as educators and counselors.
- A major nursing responsibility covered in this book is to provide information on women's health issues and for childbearing families. Nurses must use the principles of teaching and learning to fulfill the role of educator.
- Nurses must refine their critical thinking abilities by examining their own thought processes for flaws that can lead to inaccurate conclusions or poor clinical judgments.
- The nursing process begins with assessment and includes analysis of data that may result in nursing diagnoses. Nurses are legally accountable for identifying and managing these problems independently.
- Collaborative problems are usually physiologic complications that require both delegated, or physician-prescribed, and independent, or nurse-prescribed, interventions.
- Nurses must base their practices on the evidence generated by research. Professional journals are the best sources for the latest research.

REFERENCES & READINGS

Alfaro-LeFevre, R. (2004). *Critical thinking in nursing: A practical approach* (3rd ed.). Philadelphia: Saunders.

Arnold, E., & Boggs, K. (1999). *Interpersonal relationships: Professional communication skills for nurses* (3rd ed.). Philadelphia: Saunders.

Breslin, E.T., & Lucas, V.A. (2003). *Women's health nursing: Toward evidence based practice*. Philadelphia: Saunders.

Capitulo, K.L. (1998). The rise, fall, and rise of nurse midwifery in America. *Maternal/Child Nursing Journal, 23*(6), 314-321.

Carpenito-Moyet, L.J. (2004). *Handbook of nursing diagnosis* (10th ed.). Philadelphia: Lippincott Williams & Wilkins.

Curran, L. (2003). The women's health nurse practitioner: Evolution of a powerful role. *AWHONN Lifelines, 6*(4), 332-337.

Davies, B.L. (2002). Sources and models for moving nursing research into clinical practice. *Journal of Obstetric, Gynecologic, and Neonatal Nursing, 31*(5), 558-562.

Katz, A. (2003). Words, powerful words: How our communication affects patient wellness and so much more. *AWHONN Lifelines, 7*(3), 205-207.

McRae, M. (2003). Men in obstetrical nursing: Perceptions of the role. *MCN: American Journal of Maternal-Child Nursing, 28*(3), 167-173.

Murray, M.E., & Atkinson, L.D. (2000). *Understanding the nursing process in a changing care environment* (6th ed.). New York: McGraw-Hill.

Redman, B.K. (2001). *The practice of patient education* (9th ed.). St. Louis: Mosby.

Riley, J.B. (2004). *Communication in nursing* (5th ed.). St. Louis: Mosby.

Tabone, S. (2004). Data suggest nurse fatigue threatens patient safety: Is prescribing the nurse's work hours the only answer? *Texas Nursing, 78*(2), 4-7.

Trossman, S. (2004). Increased hours, more errors. *The American Nurse, 36*(4), 1; 3-4.

Ethical, Social, and Legal Issues

After studying this chapter, you should be able to:

1. Apply theories and principles of ethics to ethical dilemmas.
2. Describe how the steps of the nursing process can be applied to ethical decision making.
3. Discuss ethical conflicts related to reproductive issues such as elective abortion, forced contraception, and infertility therapy.
4. Discuss the maintenance of client, institutional, and colleague confidentiality when using electronic communication.
5. Relate how major social issues such as poverty and access to health care affect maternal-newborn nursing.
6. Describe the legal basis for nursing practice.
7. Identify measures to prevent or defend malpractice claims.
8. Describe the nursing implications of current trends in health care.

Go to your Student CD-ROM for Review Questions keyed to these Objectives.

DEFINITIONS

Bioethics Rules or principles that govern right conduct, specifically those that relate to health care.

Deontologic Theory Ethical theory holding that the right course of action is the one dictated by ethical principles and moral rules.

Emancipated Minor An adolescent younger than the age of majority (usually 18 years) who is considered developmentally competent to make certain medical decisions independent of a parent or guardian.

Ethical Dilemma A situation in which no solution seems completely satisfactory.

Ethics Rules or principles that govern right conduct and distinctions between right and wrong.

Malpractice Negligence by a professional person.

Mutual Recognition Model A model of nurse licensure that allows nurses to hold licenses in their states

of residence and practice in other states that also recognize the home state's license; also known as a *multistate licensure compact.*

Negligence Failure to act in the way a reasonable, prudent person of similar background would act in similar circumstances.

Nurse Practice Acts Laws that determine the scope of nursing practice in each state.

Standard of Care Level of care that can be expected of a professional as determined by laws, professional organizations, and health care agencies.

Standard Procedures Procedures determined by nurses, physicians, and administrators that allow nurses to perform duties usually part of the medical practice.

Utilitarian Theory Ethical theory stating that the right course of action is the one that produces the greatest good.

Nurses often grapple with ethical and social dilemmas that affect individuals and families for whom they provide care. Nurses must know the way to approach these issues in a knowledgeable and systematic way. Some ethical and social issues result in the passage of laws that regulate reproductive practice. The nurse must understand the legal basis for his or her scope of practice to reduce vulnerability to malpractice claims.

ETHICS AND BIOETHICS

Ethics involves determining the best course of action in a certain situation. Ethical reasoning is the analysis of what is morally right and reasonable. Bioethics is the application of ethics to health care. Ethical behavior for nurses is discussed in codes such as the American Nurses Association Code for Nurses. Ethical issues have become more complex as technology has created more options in health care. These issues are controversial because agreement over what is right or best does not exist and because moral support is possible for more than one course of action.

Ethical Dilemmas

An ethical dilemma is a situation in which no solution seems completely satisfactory. Opposing courses of action may seem equally desirable, or all possible solutions may seem undesirable. Ethical dilemmas are among the most difficult situations in nursing practice. To find solutions, nurses must apply ethical theories and principles and determine the burdens and benefits of any course of action.

ETHICAL THEORIES

Two major theories guide ethical decision making: deontologic and utilitarian. Few people use one theory exclusively. Instead, they make decisions by examining both theories and determining which is most appropriate for the circumstances.

DEONTOLOGIC THEORY. The deontologic approach determines what is right by applying ethical principles and moral rules. It does not vary the solution according to individual situations. One example is the rule, "Life must be maintained at all costs and in all circumstances." Strictly used, the deontologic approach would not consider the quality of life or weigh the use of scarce resources against the likelihood that the life maintained would be near normal.

UTILITARIAN THEORY. The utilitarian theory approaches ethical dilemmas by analyzing the benefits and burdens of any course of action to find one that will result in the greatest amount of good. With this theory, appropriate actions may vary according to the situation. This practical approach is concerned more with the consequences of actions than the actions themselves. In its simplest form the utilitarian approach is "The end justifies the means." If the outcome is positive, the method of arriving at that outcome is less important.

BOX 3-1 Ethical Principles

Beneficence—People are required to do or promote good for others.
Nonmaleficence—People must avoid risking or causing harm to others.
Autonomy—People have the right to self-determination. This includes the right to respect, privacy, and information necessary to make decisions.
Justice—All people should be treated equally and fairly regardless of disease or social or economic status.

ETHICAL PRINCIPLES

Ethical principles are also important for solving ethical dilemmas. Four of the most important principles are beneficence, nonmaleficence, respect for autonomy, and justice (Box 3-1). Other important ethical rules, such as accountability and confidentiality, are derived from these four basic principles. These principles guide decision making, but in some situations the application of one principle conflicts with another principle. In such cases, one principle may outweigh another in importance.

Treatments designed to do good may also cause harm. For example, a cesarean birth may prevent permanent harm to a fetus in jeopardy. However, the surgery that saves the fetus also harms the mother, causing pain, temporary disability, and possible financial hardship. Both mother and health care providers may decide that the principle of beneficence outweighs the principle of nonmaleficence. If the mother does not want surgery, the principles of autonomy and justice also must be considered. Is the mother's right to determine what happens to her body more or less important than the right of the fetus to fair and equal treatment?

USING ETHICAL THEORIES AND PRINCIPLES TO SOLVE DILEMMAS

Nurses are often involved in supporting parents when tragedy strikes at birth. They must be knowledgeable regarding the disease process and the appropriate nursing care in these situations and the support families need when ethical dilemmas arise.

CRITICAL THINKING EXERCISE 3-1

The parents of an infant with anencephaly state that they would like to donate the organs from their dying infant to another infant who might live as a result. They believe that in this way their own infant will live on as a part of another baby. Although such transplants have been performed in the past, they are not currently practiced because of ethical concerns.

Questions
1. What is the deontologic view of this decision?
2. How would the utilitarian view differ?
3. What ethical principles are involved? If such transplants become routine, what problems might arise?

BOX 3-2 Applying the Nursing Process to Solve Ethical Dilemmas

Assessment—Gather data to clearly identify the problem and the decisions necessary. Obtain viewpoints from all who will be affected by the decision and applicable legal, agency policy, and common practice standards.
Analysis—Decide whether an ethical dilemma exists. Analyze the situation using ethical theories and principles. Determine whether and how these conflict.
Planning—Identify as many options as possible, their advantages and disadvantages, and which are most realistic. Predict what is likely to happen if each option is followed. Include the option of doing nothing. Choose the solution.
Implementation—Carry out the solution. Determine who will implement the solution and how. Identify all interventions necessary and what support is needed.
Evaluation—Analyze the results. Determine whether further interventions are necessary.

Many approaches can be used to solve ethical dilemmas. Although an approach does not guarantee a right decision, it provides a logical, systematic method for decision making. Because the nursing process is also a method of problem solving, nurses can use a similar approach when faced with ethical dilemmas (Box 3-2).

Decision making in ethical dilemmas may seem straightforward, but it rarely results in answers agreeable to everyone. Many agencies therefore have bioethics committees to formulate policies for ethical situations, provide education, and help make decisions in specific cases. The committees include a variety of professionals such as nurses, physicians, social workers, ethicists, and clergy members. The family members most closely affected by the decision also participate if possible. A satisfactory solution to ethical dilemmas is more likely to occur when people work together.

✔ CHECK YOUR READING

1. What is the difference between ethics and bioethics?
2. How does the deontologic theory differ from the utilitarian theory?
3. When might two ethical principles conflict?
4. How do the steps of the nursing process relate to ethical decision making?

Ethical Issues in Reproduction

Reproductive issues often involve conflicts in which a woman behaves in a way that may cause harm to her fetus or is disapproved of by some or most members of society. Conflicts between a mother and fetus occur when the mother's needs, behavior, or wishes may injure the fetus. The most obvious instances involve abortion, substance abuse, and a mother's refusal to follow the advice of caregivers. Health care workers and society may respond to such a woman with anger rather than support. However, the rights of both mother and fetus must be examined.

ELECTIVE ABORTION

Abortion was a volatile legal, social, and political issue even before the *Roe v. Wade* decision by the United States Supreme Court in 1973. Before that time, states could outlaw abortion within their boundaries. In *Roe v. Wade* the Supreme Court stated that abortion was legal in the United States and that existing state laws prohibiting abortion were unconstitutional because they interfered with the mother's constitutional right to privacy. This decision stipulated that (1) a woman could obtain an abortion at any time during the first trimester, (2) the state could regulate abortions during the second trimester only to protect the woman's health, and (3) the state could regulate or prohibit abortion during the third trimester, except when the mother's life might be jeopardized by continuing the pregnancy.

For many people the woman's constitutional right to privacy conflicts with the fetus' right to life. However, the Supreme Court did not rule on when life begins. This omission provokes debate between those who believe life begins at conception and those who believe life begins when the fetus is viable, or capable of living outside the uterus. Those who believe life begins at conception may be opposed to abortion at any time during pregnancy. Those who believe life begins when the fetus is viable (20 to 24 weeks of gestation) may oppose abortion after that time. Nurses need to understand abortion laws and the conflicting beliefs that divide society on this issue.

CONFLICTING BELIEFS ABOUT ABORTION. Some people believe abortion should be illegal at any time because it deprives the fetus of life. In contrast, others believe that women have the right to control their reproductive functions and that political discussion of reproductive rights is an invasion of a woman's most private decisions.

Belief That Abortion Is a Private Choice. Central to political action to keep abortion legal is the conviction that women have the right to make decisions about their reproductive functions on the basis of their own ethical and moral beliefs and that the government has no place in these decisions. Many women who support this view state that they would not choose abortion for themselves. Still, they support the right of each woman to make her own decision and view government action as interference in a very private part of women's lives. Many people who support the legality of abortion prefer to call themselves *pro-choice* rather than *pro-abortion* because they believe that *choice* more accurately expresses their philosophic and political position.

Each year more than 800,000 legal abortions are performed in the United States. In 2000, the latest year for which statistics are available, the rate was 24.5 abortions for every 100 live births. However, the abortion rate has steadily fallen since 1990, although the rate remains highest for minors under 15 years (National Center for Health Statistics, 2004). Advocates of the legal right to abortion point out that the performance of abortion, either legal or illegal, has always been a reality of life and will continue regardless of legislation or judicial rulings. Advocates also express concern regarding the unsafe conditions associated with illegal abortion, citing the deaths that resulted from illegal abortions performed before the *Roe v. Wade* decision.

Belief That Abortion Is Taking a Life. Many people believe that legalized abortion condones taking a life and feel morally bound to protect the lives of fetuses. This position is called *pro-life*. The term has become emotionally charged, and some believe it polarizes opinion and implies that those who do not agree with the anti-abortion position are not concerned about life or are "anti-life."

Persons opposed to abortion have demonstrated their commitment by organizing as a potent political force. They have willingly been arrested for civil disobedience during attempts to prevent admissions to clinics that perform abortions.

LEGAL ASPECTS OF ROE V. WADE. Abortion has been a complex legal issue, and the Supreme Court has made major decisions that affect abortion law since 1973. Some decisions have strengthened the original *Roe v. Wade* ruling, and others have weakened it (Box 3-3). Legislation introduced in 1995 that banned late-term abortions received a presidential veto because it did not provide an exception when the mother's health is at risk. Other versions of this bill will probably be introduced and, if passed, may come before the Supreme Court.

POLITICAL ASPECTS OF ABORTION. The abortion question is one of the primary issues confronting political candidates, who are often asked to explain their stand on abortion. Abortion-rights advocates emphasize that their message is to keep government out of the daily lives of citizens and that abridging women's right to abortion is unconstitutional. Anti-abortion leaders will probably continue a confrontational strategy to bring attention to their point of view. In addition, they will continue to try to pass legislation that would hinder abortion by any means possible.

IMPLICATIONS FOR NURSES. Nurses have several responsibilities that cannot be ignored in the conflict about abortion. First, they must be informed about the complexity of the abortion issue from a legal and an ethical standpoint and know the regulations and laws in their state. Second, they must realize that for many people, abortion is an ethical dilemma that results in confusion, ambivalence, and personal distress. Next, they must also recognize that for many others, the issue is not a dilemma but a fundamental violation of the personal or religious views that give meaning to their lives. Finally, nurses must acknowledge the sincere convictions and strong emotions of those on all sides of the issue.

Personal Values. Nurses respond to abortion issues in ways that illustrate the complexity of the issue and the ambivalence it often produces. For instance, some nurses have no objection to participation in abortions. Others do not assist with abortions but may care for women after the procedure. Some nurses will assist with a first-trimester abortion but may object to later abortions. Many nurses are com-

BOX **3-3** Supreme Court Decisions on Abortion Since *Roe v. Wade*

1976—States cannot give a husband veto power over his spouse's decision to have an abortion.
1977—States do not have an obligation to pay for abortions as part of government-funded health care programs. (This is considered by abortion rights advocates to be unfair discrimination against poor women who are unable to pay for an abortion.)
1979—Physicians have broad discretion in determining fetal viability, and states have leeway to restrict abortions of viable fetuses.
1979—States may require parental consent for minors seeking abortions if an alternative (such as judge's approval) is also available.
1989—Upheld a Missouri law barring abortions performed in public hospitals and clinics or performed by public employees. Also, required physicians to conduct tests for fetal viability at 20 weeks of gestation.
1990—States may require notification of both parents before a person under the age of 18 years has an abortion. A judge can authorize the abortion without parental consent.
1992—Validated a Pennsylvania law imposing restrictions on abortions. The restrictions upheld include the following:
• A woman must be told about fetal development and alternatives to abortion.
• She must wait at least 24 hours after this explanation before having an abortion.
• Unmarried women under the age of 18 must obtain consent from their parents or a judge.
• Physicians must keep detailed records of each abortion, subject to public disclosure.
• Struck down only one requirement of the Pennsylvania law: that a married woman must inform her husband before having an abortion.
1993—Rescinded the so-called "gag rule," which restricted counseling that health care professionals (with the exception of physicians) could provide at federally funded family planning clinics.
1995—Upheld a ruling that states cannot withhold state funds for abortions in cases of pregnancies resulting from rape or incest or when the mother's life is in danger.
2003—Bill that bans late-term abortions signed by president, George W. Bush.

fortable assisting with abortion if the fetus has severe anomalies but are uncomfortable in other circumstances. Some nurses feel that they could not provide care before, during, or after an abortion but that they are bound by conscience to try to dissuade a woman from the decision to end the pregnancy.

Professional Obligations. Nurses have no obligation to support a position with which they disagree. The nursing practice acts of many states allow nurses to refuse to assist with the procedure if it violates their ethical, moral, or religious beliefs. However, nurses are obligated to disclose this information before they are employed in an institution that performs abortions. For a nurse to withhold this information until assigned to care for a woman having an abortion and then refuse to provide care is unethical. As always, nurses must respect the decisions of women who look to nurses for care. If nurses believe they are not able to provide compassionate care because of personal convictions, they must inform a supervisor so that appropriate care can be arranged.

5. How did the *Roe v. Wade* ruling affect state laws related to abortion in the United States?
6. What are the major conflicting beliefs about abortion?
7. What are some Supreme Court decisions that have modified the *Roe v. Wade* ruling?
8. What are nurses' responsibilities if they are morally opposed to abortion?

MANDATED CONTRACEPTION

The availability of contraception that does not require taking a regular oral dose, such as using a hormone-releasing patch or having hormone injections, has led to speculation about whether certain women should be forced to use this method of birth control. Requiring contraception has been used as a condition of probation, allowing women accused of child abuse to avoid jail terms.

Some people believe that mandated contraception is a reasonable way to prevent additional births to women who are considered unsuitable parents and decrease government expenses for dependent children. A punitive approach to social problems does not provide long-term solutions. Requiring poor women to use contraception to limit the money spent supporting them is legally and ethically questionable and does not address the obligations of the children's father. Such a practice interferes with a woman's constitutional rights to privacy, reproduction, refusal of medical treatment, and freedom from cruel and unusual punishment. In addition, medication may pose health risks to the woman. Surgical sterilization (tubal ligation) also carries risks and must be considered permanent. Access to free or low-cost information on family planning would be more appropriate and ethical.

FETAL INJURY

If a mother's actions cause injury to her fetus, the question of whether she should be restrained or prosecuted has legal and ethical implications. In some instances courts have issued jail sentences to women who have caused or who may cause injury to the fetus. This response punishes the woman and places her in a situation in which she cannot further harm the fetus. In other cases, women have been forced to undergo cesarean births against their will when physicians have testified that such a procedure was necessary to prevent injury to the fetus.

The state has an interest in protecting children, and the Supreme Court has ruled that a child has the right to begin life with a sound mind and body. Many state laws require that evidence of prenatal drug exposure be reported. Women have been charged with negligence, involuntary manslaughter, delivery of drugs to a minor, and child endangerment.

However, forcing a woman to behave in a certain way because she is pregnant violates the principles of autonomy, self-determination of competent adults, bodily integrity, and personal freedom. Because of fear of prosecution, this practice could impede, not advance, health care during pregnancy.

The punitive approach to fetal injury also raises the question of how much control the government should have over a pregnant woman. Laws could be passed to mandate maternal human immunodeficiency virus (HIV) testing, fetal testing, intrauterine surgery, or even the foods the woman eats during pregnancy. The decision of just how much control should be allowed in the interests of fetal safety is difficult.

FETAL THERAPY

Fetal therapy is becoming more common as techniques improve and knowledge grows. Although intrauterine blood transfusions are relatively standard practice in some areas, fetal surgery is still relatively uncommon.

The risks and benefits of surgery for major fetal anomalies must be considered in every case. Even when surgery is successful, the fetus may not survive, may have other serious problems, or may be born preterm. The mother may require weeks of bed rest and a cesarean birth. Yet despite the risks, successful fetal surgery may result in birth of an infant who could not otherwise have survived.

Parents need help to balance the potential risks to the mother and the best interests of the fetus. They might feel pressured to have surgery or other fetal treatment they do not understand. As with any situation involving informed consent, women need adequate information before making a decision. They should understand whether procedures are still experimental, what the chances of success are, and what alternatives are available.

ISSUES IN INFERTILITY

INFERTILITY TREATMENT. Perinatal technology has found ways for some previously infertile couples to bear children (see Chapter 32). Many techniques are more successful, but ethical concerns include the high cost and overall low success of some infertility treatments. Because many of these costs are not covered by insurance, their use is limited to the affluent. Techniques may benefit only a small percentage of infertile couples. Despite treatment, many couples never give birth, regardless of the costs or invasiveness of therapy. Successful treatment may lead to multiple gestations, usually twins, and complications related to maternal age. See Chapter 32 for trends and issues associated with infertility therapy.

Other ethical concerns focus on the fate of unused embryos. Should they be frozen for later use by the woman or someone else or used in genetic research? What if the parents divorce or die? Who should make these decisions? In multiple pregnancies with more fetuses than can be expected to survive intact, reduction surgery may be used to destroy one or more fetuses for the benefit of those remaining. The ethical and long-term psychologic implications of this procedure are also controversial.

Assisted reproductive techniques now allow post-menopausal women to become pregnant. What are the ethical implications of conceiving and giving birth to children whose mother is several decades older than their friends' mothers and is more likely to die when the children are relatively young? Should the age and health of the parents be a factor in determining whether this treatment is offered? Should a consideration be the risk these women face for complications that might result in unhealthy infants? Should average life expectancy enter the decision?

SURROGATE PARENTING. In surrogate parenting a woman agrees to bear an infant for another woman. Conception may take place outside the body using ova and sperm from the couple who wish to become parents. These so-called "test-tube babies" are then implanted into the surrogate mother, or the surrogate mother may be inseminated artificially with sperm from the intended father.

Cases in which the surrogate mother has wanted to keep the child have created controversy. No standard regulations govern these cases, which are decided individually. Ethical concerns involve who should be a surrogate mother, what her role should be after birth, and who should make these decisions. Screening of parents and surrogates is necessary to determine whether they are suited for their roles. Who should perform the screening? Should it be left to the private interests of those involved, or should the government become involved? Answers to these questions are not definite at this time.

An issue closely related to surrogate parenting is the use of donor gametes. Will the use of donor gametes violate religious or moral beliefs of the parents? Does the child thus conceived have a right to know the identity of the biologic parents? What are the rights of the biologic parents? What about the ethics involved in the selling of gametes?

✔ CHECK YOUR READING

9. What dangers are involved in punitive approaches to ethical and social problems?
10. What problems are involved in the use of advanced reproductive techniques?

PRIVACY ISSUES

Many people are concerned about the possible misuse of their health information. They may fear that health information in the wrong hands, whether that information is accurate or not, may cost them a job, promotion, loan, or something equally valuable.

GOVERNMENT REGULATIONS

The Health Insurance Portability and Accountability Act (HIPAA) of 1996 was designed to reduce fraud in the insurance industry and make it simpler for people to remain insured if they move from one job to another. Also within the HIPAA's provisions was the mandate that Congress pass a law to protect the privacy of personal medical information by August 1999. Congress failed to do so, and the U.S. Department of Health and Human Services (HHS) Secretary proposed interim regulations in October 1999 to protect personal medical privacy as required by HIPAA. The HHS regulations provide consumers with significant new power over their records, including the right to see and correct their records, the application of civil and criminal penalties for violations of privacy standards, and protection against deliberate or inadvertent misuse or disclosure (HHS, 2001a).

ONLINE COMMUNICATIONS. Client health data are being converted to various computerized formats. One example involves the computerized storage of electronic fetal monitoring data, including background information, interventions, and graphics. Although this allows nearly instantaneous exchange of data among providers in an emergency situation, it also carries the potential for greater violation of privacy than data maintained on paper. Terminals may be placed conveniently in hallways or client rooms to facilitate entry and retrieval of information for staff. The nurse must remember that this information may also be easily accessed by a computer-savvy person despite the use of passcodes and other security measures.

Nurses must take care to avoid violating client confidentiality when using electronic client data formats. For example, nurses must log off terminals when finished so that unauthorized people cannot gain access to the system. Security codes should remain secret and committed to memory and should not be words or combinations that another person can easily guess. Suspected loss of a password should be promptly reported to the system administrator. Most systems require regular changes of security codes. Random codes may be issued by the computer network itself, based on an employee's clearance, to limit what others know about the individual's security code. Having a single code to be used for applications appropriate to a specific caregiver, such as charting, monitoring, e-mail, policies, and procedures for nurses and physicians, can reduce the likelihood that the employee will write down the many codes often required by different applications.

Internet discussion lists allow nurses to exchange information and nursing care tips that can improve practice. These forums also have the potential to allow lapses of client or institutional confidentiality because their communications cannot be considered private. When participating in discussion lists or using e-mail, nurses must respect the confidentiality of clients, colleagues, and institutions. Institutional documents such as chart forms, policies, and procedures should not be shared without the facility's approval. A personal message should not be forwarded without the original sender's permission.

SOCIAL ISSUES

Nurses are exposed to many social issues that influence health care and often have ethical implications. Some issues that affect maternity care include poverty, homelessness, access to care, allocation of health care resources, and care versus cure.

Poverty

Although the poverty rate for the United States is lower than during the 1990s, poverty remains an underlying factor in problems such as homelessness and inadequate access to health care. In general, 10.8% of families lived in poverty during 2003, but families headed by a female had a rate of 28% during the same year. Newer racial divisions within the census use three racial subdivisions for white people: white alone, white alone or in combination with another race, and white alone but not Hispanic. The poverty rate for non-Hispanic white families was 8.2% in 2002, whereas the rate was 22.5% for Hispanic families and 11.8% for Asian families (DeNavas-Walt, Proctor, & Mills, 2004). Because of adverse living conditions, poor health care, and poor nutrition, infants born to low-income women are more likely to begin life with problems such as low birth weight.

Poverty tends to breed poverty. In poor families, children may leave the educational system early, making them less likely to learn skills necessary to obtain good jobs. Childbearing at an early age is common and further interferes with education and the ability to work. The cycle of poverty may continue from one generation to the next as a result of hopelessness and apathy (Figure 3-1).

Even people with incomes above the poverty level may not be able to pay for health care because of rising costs. The working poor have jobs but receive wages that barely meet their day-to-day needs. These jobs often do not offer health insurance, or high health insurance premiums may be the only option. The working poor have little opportunity to save for emergencies such as serious illness. Nationwide in 2003, 16.1% of the population under age 65 years had no health insurance (Cohen & Ni, 2004; Fried et al., 2003). Millions of other people have limited insurance and would not be able to survive financially in the event of serious illness. People without insurance seek care only when absolutely necessary. Health maintenance and illness prevention may seem costly and unnecessary to them. Some receive no health care during pregnancy until they arrive at the hospital for birth.

Various government programs are available to help the poor. One such program is Temporary Assistance to Needy Families (TANF), which provides money for basic living costs of indigent children and their families. Created by the Welfare Reform Law of 1996, this replaced the Aid to Families with Dependent Children (AFDC) program of the older welfare system. TANF imposes time limits on the aid given to the family, unlike AFDC. Eligibility requirements, income limits, allowances for homelessness, and time limitations vary among states.

Homelessness

Families, many of which are composed of single women and their children, constitute the largest group of homeless people, and many are African-American or Hispanic. Homeless people often wait until health problems are severe because of feelings of shame for their homeless state and the inability to pay for services. Malnutrition, substance abuse, and mental health

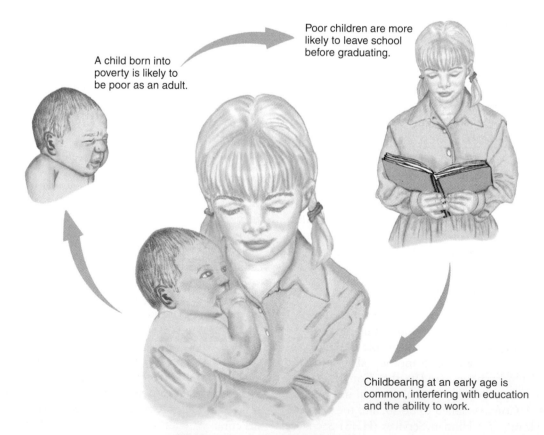

A child born into poverty is likely to be poor as an adult.

Poor children are more likely to leave school before graduating.

Childbearing at an early age is common, interfering with education and the ability to work.

Figure 3-1 ■ The cycle of poverty.

disorders are major problems among members of this group. Tuberculosis, skin infections, diarrhea, urinary tract infections, dental problems, and trauma are also common. Infants born to homeless women are subject to a lower birth weight and greater likelihood of neonatal mortality (Upvall, 2003).

Birth to a young teenager is a contributing cause and effect of homelessness. Pregnancy interferes with one's ability to work and may decrease income to the point at which housing is unattainable. Prostitution to earn money may result in pregnancy and add to its problems with factors such as infections, violence, and inadequate health care. Homeless teens are more likely to have poor eating habits, smoke, and have greater risks for preterm labor, anemia, or hypertension during pregnancy and to deliver a low-birth-weight infant. More than 3 million have one or more sexually transmitted diseases (STDs) that can damage mother or child, such as chlamydia, syphilis, and HIV (March of Dimes, 2004).

Access to Health Care

The United States ranks 27th in infant mortality compared with other developed countries (see Chapter 1). Data for 2002 showed that for every 1000 live births in the United States, seven infants died before their first birthday (National Center for Health Statistics). Many of these deaths are related to low birth weight, prematurity, and other prenatal factors.

PRENATAL CARE IN THE UNITED STATES

Prenatal care is widely accepted as an important element in a good pregnancy outcome. In 2002 almost 84% of mothers received care during the first trimester of pregnancy, and almost 4% had no prenatal care or started it during the last trimester. Late prenatal care among black, Hispanic, and Native American women was 5% (Martin et al., 2004). Prenatal care is often poor because health care, particularly that supported by programs such as Medicaid, is not easily available. Lack of access to prenatal care adds to the infant mortality rate and the large number of low-birth-weight infants born each year in the United States. Because preterm infants are the largest category of those needing intensive care, millions of dollars could be saved each year by ensuring adequate prenatal care and good maternal nutrition. Even a small improvement in an infant's birth weight or gestational age reduces complications and hospital time.

Box 3-4 summarizes factors that interfere with access to care. Many factors overlap; for example, poverty is often associated with the other characteristics listed. In the United States, minority women are more likely to be indigent, less

---

BOX 3-4 Factors Related to Lack of Access to Health Care

Poverty
Unemployment
Lack of medical insurance
Adolescence
Minority group membership
Inner city residence
Rural residence
Unmarried mother status
Less than high school education
Inability to speak English

---

likely to obtain adequate prenatal care, and more likely to die in childbirth when compared with white women.

Adolescent pregnancy is also associated with many factors listed in Box 3-4. In the United States adolescent pregnancy rates have fallen but remain high at approximately 11% of U.S. births. The 2002 birth rate for teenagers declined to 43 births per 1000 women aged 15 to 19 years. Approximately 17% of teens give birth to their second infant within 3 years of the first (March of Dimes, 2004). Teen mothers are less likely to complete their education and more likely to be poor than adult mothers.

In some situations women can obtain prenatal care but choose not to do so. These women may not understand the importance of the care or may deny they are pregnant. Some have had unsatisfactory past experiences with the health care system, avoiding care for as long as possible. Others want to hide substance use or other habits from disapproving health care workers. When women have major life problems, prenatal care is not a priority for them. Language and cultural differences also play a part in whether a woman seeks prenatal care. Although these are not access issues as such, they must be addressed to improve health care.

GOVERNMENT PROGRAMS FOR HEALTH CARE

MEDICAID. More than 45% of all money spent on health care in 2002 was publicly funded (National Center for Health Statistics). One government program that increases access to health care is Medicaid, which has existed since 1965. Medicaid provides health care for indigent persons, older adults, and persons with disabilities. Pregnant women and young children are especially targeted. Medicaid is funded by both the federal and the state governments. The states administer the program and determine which services are offered. Although the qualifying level of poverty varies among states, all women whose income is below 133% of the current federal poverty level are eligible for perinatal care.

Medicaid has a number of problems. Determination of a client's eligibility often takes weeks. The woman must fill out lengthy, complicated forms; provide documentation of income; and then wait for determination of eligibility. If a woman is not already enrolled at the beginning of pregnancy, she is unlikely to finish the process in time to receive the early prenatal care so beneficial to a good pregnancy outcome.

Some physicians are unwilling to care for Medicaid clients who may be at higher risk. Many are especially unwilling if reimbursement for physicians and hospitals is slow and less than that paid by other insurers. Physicians may be less inclined to accept high-risk, lower-paying clients because of the continual concern about malpractice suits.

Women who do not have private insurance may receive prenatal care at public clinics. However, such clinics are often understaffed and have large numbers of clients. Clinics may be located in areas not easily accessible to pregnant women who have transportation problems. Long waits for appointments may require time off from work, resulting in loss of pay for an hourly worker. A mother may not be able to find child care for older children while she visits the clinic. These problems decrease the chance that women will take steps to obtain care.

SHELTERS AND HEALTH CARE FOR THE HOMELESS. Federal funding has assisted homeless people with shelter and health care. However, as do other indigent people, the homeless have difficulties in obtaining health care because of lack of transportation, inconvenient hours, and poor continuity of care.

Quality and quantity of care in clinics may be poor because of inadequate funding. Nurses have been instrumental in opening shelters, clinics, and outreach services for the homeless, with nurse practitioners often playing a major role. Clinics headed by nurse-practitioners are often opened in underserved rural areas. Nurses also help inform the public and legislatures about the needs of the homeless and others with few health care options.

INNOVATIVE PROGRAMS. Innovative programs to ensure that all women receive good prenatal care are necessary to improve pregnancy outcomes. Some outreach programs are designed to improve health in women who traditionally do not seek prenatal care. Bilingual health care workers and bilingual educational classes are part of some programs. Programs may be located in schools, shopping centers, churches, workplaces, and neighborhoods that are easily accessible to clients. Mobile vans outfitted with basic equipment bring prenatal care to women who are unable or unwilling to attend care at fixed locations or in more distant neighborhoods. (Such vans often provide neighborhoods with additional programs such as dental care, immunizations, well-child care, women's health care and screening mammography.) The number of such neighborhood programs is insufficient to make adequate health care for women and children a reality.

Allocation of Health Care Resources

In 2002 the United States spent $1.5 trillion, or 14.9% of its gross domestic product, on health care (National Center for Health Statistics, 2004). Expenditures for health care continue to rise. Areas that must be addressed include ways to provide care for indigent persons, the uninsured or underinsured, and those with long-term care needs. Distribution of the limited funds available for health care among all these areas is a major concern.

The 1997 Balanced Budget Act has had a major impact on health care facilities, including those that provide maternal-newborn care. The act sought to limit Medicare fraud, extend the life of Medicare funds, and improve the benefits for staying healthy. The act also included changes in the Medicaid policies and the institution of a State Children's Health Insurance Program (SCHIP). Because the health care for a large percentage of any facility's clients is likely to be publicly funded by Medicare and Medicaid, the impact of the Balanced Budget Act cannot be ignored by nurses. This act has further limited income to hospitals and community agencies from the public sector, requiring that nurses work with even fewer financial resources than they did just a few years ago. However, the act's emphasis on preventive care also provides an opportunity for nurses to become innovators in such programs.

Health Care Rationing

Modern technology has greatly influenced health care rationing. Some argue that such rationing does not exist, but it occurs whenever some people have no access to care and money is insufficient for all people to equally share the available technology. Advanced medical care often benefits only a small number of people but at great cost. Health care is also rationed when it is more freely given to those who have money to pay for it than to those who do not.

Many questions will need answers as the costs of health care increase faster than the funds available. Is health care a fundamental right? Should a certain level of care be guaranteed to all citizens? What should that care entail? Should the cost of treatment and its effectiveness be considered when the amount covered by government or third-party payers is decided? Nurses will be instrumental in finding solutions to these vital questions.

Care versus Cure

One problem to be addressed is whether the focus of health care should be on preventive and caring measures or cures for disease. Medicine has traditionally centered more on treatment and cure than prevention and care. Yet prevention avoids suffering and is less expensive than treating diseases after diagnosis.

The focus on cure has resulted in technologic advances that have enabled some people to live longer, healthier lives. However, financial resources are limited, and the costs of expensive technology must be balanced against the benefits obtained. Indeed, the cost of one organ transplant would pay for prenatal care for many low-income mothers.

Although low-birth-weight infants constitute a small percentage of all newborns, they require a large percentage of total hospital expenditures. The expenses of one preterm infant for a single day in an intensive care nursery are more than enough to pay for care of the mother throughout her pregnancy and birth. Yet if the mother had received prenatal care early and regularly, the infant might have avoided intensive care.

In addition, quality-of-life issues are important with regard to technology. Neonatal nurseries are able to keep alive very-low-birth-weight babies because of advances in knowledge. Some of these infants go on to lead normal or near-normal lives. Others gain time but not quality of life. Families and health care professionals face difficult decisions about when to treat, when to end treatment, and how to recognize that the suffering outweighs the benefits.

✔ **CHECK YOUR READING**

11. How do poverty and inadequate prenatal care affect infant mortality and morbidity?
12. How has the Balanced Budget Act of 1997 affected nursing practice?
13. How does a decision to spend money on technology sometimes conflict with issues of disease prevention?

LEGAL ISSUES

The legal foundation for the practice of nursing provides safeguards for clients and sets standards by which nurses can be evaluated. Nurses need to understand how the law applies specifically to them. When nurses do not meet the standards expected, they may be held legally accountable.

Safeguards for Health Care

Three categories of safeguards determine the law's view of nursing practice: (1) nurse practice acts, (2) standards of care set by professional organizations, and (3) rules and policies set by the institution employing the nurse.

NURSE PRACTICE ACTS

Every state has a nurse practice act that determines the scope of practice of registered nurses in that state. Nurse practice acts define what the nurse is allowed to do when caring for clients. The acts also specify what the nurse is expected to do when providing care. Some parts of the law may be very specific. Others are stated broadly to allow flexible interpretation of the role of nurses. Nurse practice acts vary among states, and nurses must understand these laws wherever they practice. Nurses should have a copy of the nurse practice act for their state and refer to it for questions about their scope of practice. Most state nurse practice acts are also available on the Internet. The website of the National Council of State Boards of Nursing (NCSBN) (www.ncsbn.org) has information on nurse practice acts for all states, all territories, and the District of Columbia, as well as other information related to licensing and practice.

Laws relating to nursing practice also delineate methods, called *standardized procedures,* by which nurses may assume certain duties commonly considered part of medical practice. The procedures are written by committees of nurses, physicians, and administrators. They specify the nursing qualifications required for practicing the procedures, define the appropriate situations, and list the education required. Standardized procedures allow the role of the nurse to change to meet the needs of the community and expanding knowledge.

A number of states have adopted a mutual recognition model, or a multistate licensure compact, for nursing licensure proposed by the NCSBN. States involved in the compact, available at the NCSBN website, agree to recognize an unrestricted license to practice nursing issued by another state in the compact. This gives the license holder the authority to practice in the state in which the license was issued and those states that recognize the license. The nurse must abide by the rules and regulations in each state. Some advantages include reduced duplication and more cost-effective interstate practice.

Concerns have been raised about the NCSBN interstate compact model by the Association of Women's Health, Obstetric, and Neonatal Nurses (AWHONN), the major organization for maternal-newborn and women's health nurses (AWHONN, 1999). This organization recognizes that nursing practice must change to facilitate telehealth, transport nursing, and greater mobility of nurses. However, AWHONN opposes the proposed compact model for several reasons, including concerns about constitutionality; licensure changes from the state of practice to the state of residence, possibly making it more difficult for consumers to file complaints; and confidentiality of malpractice or complaint data filed against nurses in a centralized database maintained by NCSBN. Additional concerns include increased costs if a claim must be defended in multiple jurisdictions.

STANDARDS OF CARE

Court decisions have generally held that nurses must practice according to established standards and health agency policies in addition to nurse practice acts. Standards of care are set by professional associations and describe the level of care that can be expected from practitioners. For example, perinatal nurses are held to the national standards published by AWHONN, which are based on research and the agreement of experts. AWHONN also publishes practice resources, position statements, and other guidelines for nurses. Nurses should be familiar with the latest standards of care that cover their own practices.

AGENCY POLICIES

Each health care agency sets specific policies, procedures, and protocols that govern nursing care. All nurses should be familiar with those that apply in the agencies in which they work. Nurses are frequently involved in writing and revising nursing policies and procedures. In the event of a malpractice claim, the applicable policy, procedure, or protocol is likely to be used as evidence. The case of the professionals is strengthened if all agency policies were followed properly. These policies should be revised and updated regularly.

Malpractice

Negligence is the failure to perform as a reasonable, prudent person of similar background would act in a similar situation. Negligence may consist of doing something that should not be done or failing to do something that should be done.

Malpractice is negligence by professionals, such as nurses and physicians, in the performance of their duties. Nurses may be accused of malpractice if they do not perform according to established standards of care and in the manner of a reasonable, prudent nurse with similar education and

---

CRITICAL TO REMEMBER

Elements of Negligence

Duty—The nurse must have a duty to act or give care to the client. It must be part of the nurse's responsibility.

Breach of duty—A violation of that duty must occur. The nurse fails to conform to established standards in performing that duty.

Damage—An actual injury or harm to the client as a result of the nurse's breach of duty must occur.

Proximate cause—The nurse's breach of duty must be proved to be the cause of harm to the client.

experience in a similar situation. Four elements must be present to prove negligence: duty, breach of duty, damage, and proximate cause.

Prevention of Malpractice Claims

Malpractice claims continue to be a major cost in health care. As a result of awards from such claims, the cost of malpractice insurance has risen for all health care workers. In addition, more health care workers practice defensively and accumulate evidence that their actions are in the client's best interest. For example, nurses must be careful to include detailed data on charts. This responsibility is especially important in perinatal nursing, because most suits occur in this area.

Many reasons exist for perinatal malpractice claims. Complications are usually unexpected, because parents view pregnancy and birth as normal. The birth of a child with a problem is a tragic surprise, and they may look for someone to blame. Although very small preterm infants may survive, some have long-term disabilities that require expensive care. Statutes of limitations vary among different states, but plaintiffs often have more than 20 years for lawsuits that involve a newborn. Therefore the period during which a malpractice suit may be filed is longer.

Health care agencies and individual nurses must work together to prevent malpractice claims. Nurses are responsible and accountable for their own actions. Therefore they must be aware of the limits of their knowledge and scope of practice, and they must practice within those limits.

Prevention of claims is sometimes referred to as *risk management* or *quality assurance*. Although prevention of all malpractice claims is impossible, nurses can help prevent malpractice judgments against themselves by following guidelines for informed consent, refusal of care, and documentation; acting as a client advocate; and maintaining their levels of expertise.

INFORMED CONSENT

When clients receive adequate information, they are less likely to file malpractice suits. Informed consent is an ethical concept that has been enacted into law. Clients have the right to decide whether to accept or reject treatment options as part of their right to function autonomously. To make wise decisions, they need full information about treatments offered.

COMPETENCE. Certain requirements must be met before consent is considered informed. First, the client must be competent, or able to think through a situation and

CRITICAL TO REMEMBER

Requirements of Informed Consent

Client's competence to consent
Full disclosure of information needed
Client's understanding of information
Client's voluntary consent

make rational decisions. Infants, children, and clients who are comatose or severely mentally retarded are incapable of making such decisions. A client who has received drugs that impair the ability to think is temporarily incompetent. In these cases another person is appointed to make decisions for the client.

In most states the age of majority (the age at which a person can give consent to medical treatment) is 18 years. However, in some states, younger adolescents can consent independently to some treatments, such as those for mental illness, abortions, contraceptives, drug abuse, and STDs. Pregnant adolescents may be considered emancipated minors in some states as well. Nurses must be familiar with laws governing age of consent in their jurisdiction.

Another exception to the usual requirement of informed consent is in emergency circumstances, because in such situations consent is considered to be implied (Cady, 2000b). Treatment may proceed if evidence that the client does not want the treatment is lacking. *Emergency* may be specifically defined by state law and is usually restricted to unforeseen conditions that, if uncorrected, would result in severe disability or death. Emergency consent applies only for the emergency condition and does not extend to any other nonemergency problem that coexists with the emergency condition.

FULL DISCLOSURE. The second requirement is full disclosure of information, including details of what the treatment entails, the expected results, and the meaning of those results. The risks, side effects, benefits, and other treatment options must be explained to clients. The client also must be informed about the consequences if no treatment is chosen.

UNDERSTANDING OF INFORMATION. The third requirement is that the client must comprehend information about proposed treatment. Health professionals must explain the facts in terms the person can understand. If a client does not speak English, an interpreter is required. A hearing-impaired client must have a sign-language interpreter of the appropriate level to sign all explanations before consent is given. If the information to be provided or obtained is sensitive, foreign language or sign language interpreters should not be family or friends, because these people may interpret selectively rather than objectively. Additionally, client confidentiality is compromised when nonprofessional interpreters are used for sensitive information. Nurses must be client advocates when they find a client does not fully understand or has questions about a treatment. If it is a minor point, the nurse may be able to explain it. Otherwise the nurse must inform the physician that the client's misconceptions need to be clarified.

VOLUNTARY CONSENT. The fourth requirement is that clients must be allowed to make choices voluntarily without undue influence or coercion from others. Although others can give information, the client alone makes the decision. Clients should not feel pressured to choose in a certain way, and they should not believe that their future care depends on their decision.

REFUSAL OF CARE

Sometimes clients decline treatment offered by health care workers. Clients refuse treatment when they believe that the benefits of treatment are insufficient to balance the burdens of the treatment or their quality of life after treatment. Clients have the right to refuse care, and they can withdraw agreement to treatment at any time. When a person makes this decision, a number of steps should be taken.

First, the physician or nurse should establish that the client understands the treatment and consequences of refusal. If the physician is unaware of the client's decision, the nurse should notify that physician accordingly. The nurse documents the refusal, explanations given to the client, and notification of the physician on the chart. If the treatment is considered vital to the client's well-being, the physician discusses the need with the client and documents the results. Opinions by other physicians may be offered to the client as well.

Clients may be asked to sign forms indicating that they understand the possible results of rejection of treatment. This measure is to defend against any subsequent lawsuit in which a client claims lack of knowledge of the possible results of a decision. If no ethical dilemma exists, the client's decision stands.

In cases of an ethical dilemma a referral may be made to the hospital ethics committee. In rare situations the physician may seek a court ruling to force treatment. For example, if a woman refuses a cesarean birth, her decision may gravely harm the fetus. This situation is the only legal instance in which a person is forced to undergo surgery for the health of another. Indigent or minority women are more likely to have a court-ordered cesarean birth (Lindgren, 1996). However, court action is avoided if possible because it places the woman and her caregiver in adversarial positions. In addition, it invades the woman's privacy and interferes with her autonomy and right to informed consent. If legally mandated surgery were to become widespread and cause women to avoid health care during pregnancy, the resulting harm would affect more women and infants than would be protected by the surgery.

Coercion is illegal and unethical in obtaining consent. Even though the nurse may strongly believe that the client should receive the treatment, the client should not feel forced to submit to unwanted procedures. Nurses must be sure that personal feelings do not adversely affect the quality of their care. Clients have the right to good nursing care, regardless of their decisions to accept or reject treatment.

DOCUMENTATION

Documentation is the best evidence that a standard of care has been maintained. It includes nurses' notes, fetal monitoring strips, electronic data, flow sheets, care paths, consent forms, and any other data recorded on the chart. In many instances notations in hospital records are the only proof that care has been given. Unfortunately, accurate and thorough documentation is the most common area lacking in malpractice cases (Simpson & Chez, 2001). When documentation is not present, juries often assume that care was not given.

Documentation must be specific and complete in perinatal nursing. This careful step is critical because of the long statute of limitations when a newborn is involved. Nurses are unlikely to remember situations that happened years in the past and, if sued, must rely on their documentation to explain their care. Documentation must show that nurses assessed the client appropriately, continually monitored for problems, identified problems and instituted correct interventions, and reported changes in the client's condition to the primary care provider.

DOCUMENTING FETAL MONITORING. Fetal monitor paper strips or stored electronic data are important sources of information about the mother and fetus during labor and birth. Nurses record a great deal of information about nursing care on the monitor strip. Sometimes the client requires the nurse's full attention, and completion of other charting must be delayed temporarily. In this situation the nurse's notes on the monitor strip provide the basis for later charting.

Although monitor strips are a legal part of the chart, paper strips may become lost or separated from the chart, and electronic media may be erased. These risks increase the importance of nurses' recording of summaries about the fetal condition in the flowsheets at appropriate intervals. Complete, detailed charting ensures that the nurse's actions will be apparent many years later in a court, even without the monitor strip.

DOCUMENTING DISCHARGE TEACHING. Discharge teaching is important to ensure that clients know how to take care of themselves and their infants after they leave the facility. To prevent or defend against lawsuits, nurses must document the teaching they perform and the client's understanding of that teaching. Various documentation forms verify teaching and the degree of understanding about important topics. The nurse should also note the need for reinforcement and the method of providing that reinforcement.

DOCUMENTING INCIDENTS. Another form of documentation used in risk management is the incident report, sometimes called a *quality assurance report* or *variance report*. The nurse completes a report when something occurs that might result in legal action, such as injury to a client, visitor, or staff member. The report warns the agency's legal department that a problem may exist. It also identifies situations that might endanger clients in the future. Incident reports are not a part of the client's chart and should not be referred to on the chart. When an incident occurs, documentation on the chart should include the same type of factual information about the client's condition that would be recorded in any other situation.

CAMERAS IN THE BIRTHING ROOM

Another issue is that of cameras (primarily videocameras) in the birthing or operating room. Although the videos are a precious memento of the birth for families, health care providers (and especially their insurers) are concerned that the videotapes or photos may be used as evidence in any malpractice action against providers. Some institutions have prohibited photography altogether in the birth setting, and others limit photography to before and immediately after birth but not during the birth itself. Many facilities require clients to sign forms stating that the photos or videotapes cannot be used in legal action and placing other restrictions on photography. However, videotapes and photographs can help defend the providers in a malpractice case by showing that the standard of care was met.

The nurse must determine the woman's wishes regarding photography so that friends or family do not unintentionally photograph her against her wishes. The woman and her partner should be made aware of any facility policies about photography during pregnancy so that they are aware of restrictions before the birth. The labor record should note that a video recording was made, by whom the recording was made, and who will maintain possession of the video. This note makes the video discoverable evidence by the facility in a future legal action (Cesario, 1998). Staff must be careful of their speech and facial expressions when they are being videotaped and avoid any conversations that could sound unprofessional if taken out of context or facial expressions that do not match what the charted notes say.

THE NURSE AS CLIENT ADVOCATE

The plaintiff may win a malpractice suit if the nurse fails in the role of client advocate. Nurses are ethically and legally bound to act as the client's advocate. When nurses feel that the client's best interests are not being served, they are obligated to seek help from appropriate sources. This usually involves taking the problem through the facility's chain of command. The nurse consults a supervisor and the client's physician. If the results are not satisfactory, the nurse continues through administrative channels to the director of nurses, hospital administrator, and chief of the medical staff if necessary. All nurses should know the chain-of-command process for their workplaces.

Nurses must document their efforts to seek help for clients. For example, when postpartum clients are experiencing excessive bleeding, nurses document the methods used to control the bleeding. They also document each time they call the physician, the information given to the physician, and the response received. When nurses cannot contact the physician or do not receive adequate instructions, they should document their efforts to seek instruction from others such as the supervisor. They should also complete an incident report. Nurses must continue their efforts until the client receives the care needed.

MAINTAINING EXPERTISE

The nurse can also reduce malpractice liability by maintaining expertise. To ensure that nurses maintain their expertise in provision of safe care, most states require proof of continuing education for renewal of nursing licenses. Nursing knowledge grows and changes rapidly, and all nurses must keep current. New information from classes, conferences, and professional publications can help nurses perform as would a reasonably prudent peer. Nurses should analyze research articles to determine whether changes in client care are indicated by the research evidence.

Employers often provide continuing education classes for their nurses through conferences, satellite television systems, computer networks, and other means. Membership in professional organizations, such as state branches of the American Nurses Association or specialty organizations like AWHONN, gives nurses access to new information through publications, nursing conferences, and other educational offerings. Continuing nursing education is also widely available on the Internet.

Expertise is a concern when nurses are "floated" or required to work with clients whose needs differ from those of the nurses' usual clients. A nurse may be floated from one maternal-newborn setting to another or to a nonmaternity setting. In these situations nurses need cross-training, which includes orientation and education to perform care safely in new areas. The employer must provide appropriate cross-training for nurses who float. Nurses who work outside their usual area of expertise must assess their own skills and avoid performing tasks or taking responsibilities in areas until they have been educated to be competent in those areas.

✔ CHECK YOUR READING

14. How do state boards of nursing safeguard clients?
15. How do standards of care and agency policies influence judgments about malpractice?
16. How can standards of care be used to help defend malpractice claims against nurses?

COST CONTAINMENT AND DOWNSIZING

Measures to lower health care costs continue to directly and indirectly affect nurses' work. Two measures of special concern are the use of unlicensed assistive personnel and brief length of stay (LOS) for clients.

Delegation to Unlicensed Assistive Personnel

In an effort to reduce health care costs, facilities have increased the use of unlicensed assistive personnel to perform direct client care and have decreased the number of supervising nurses. An unlicensed person may be trained to do everything from housekeeping tasks to drawing blood and performing other diagnostic testing to giving medications, all in the same day. This practice raises concerns about the quality of care that clients receive when the nurse becomes responsible for the care of more clients but must rely on unlicensed persons to perform much of this care.

Nurses must be aware that they remain legally responsible for client assessments and must make the critical judgments necessary to ensure client safety when delegating tasks to unlicensed personnel. Nurses must know the capabilities of each unlicensed person who is caring for clients and must supervise them sufficiently to ensure their competence. The

American Nurses Association, AWHONN, and state boards of nursing have issued statements to help nurses understand their roles in working with unlicensed assistive personnel (American Nurses Association, 1997; AWHONN, 2000).

Early Discharge

Regardless of the client's diagnosis, the time from admission to discharge is as short as possible to keep costs in check. Because birth is considered a normal event that does not require a long LOS, care of new mothers and infants requires teaching from the earliest encounters. When discharge within 24 hours of vaginal birth or 48 hours of cesarean birth was mandated by many third-party payers, health care professionals were apprehensive about client safety.

In 1996 federal legislation was passed to require insurance companies to allow the option of a 48-hour hospital LOS after vaginal birth and a 4-day LOS after cesarean birth. Discharge may be earlier if deemed appropriate after discussion between the physician and client. Although it is not required by federal law, many states mandate prompt follow-up for early discharge in the client's home, an office, or a clinic. Some third-party payers voluntarily cover home visits for mothers who opt for earlier discharge because of the lower total cost for the home visit plus a short hospital LOS.

CONCERNS ABOUT EARLY DISCHARGE

Health care professionals are concerned about women's ability to care for themselves and their infants so soon after birth. Women may be exhausted from a long labor or illness and unable to absorb all the information nurses attempt to teach before discharge. Once home, many women must also care for other children, often without the assistance of family members or friends.

While mothers and infants are in the birth facility, nurses may detect early signs of maternal or infant complications that may not be evident to parents. Mothers at home may not recognize development of serious maternal or neonatal infection or jaundice, and care may be delayed until the illness is severe. The ethical and legal implications of sending a mother home before she is ready to adequately care for herself and her newborn are very real concerns for nurses who must balance cost constraints with client needs.

METHODS TO DEAL WITH SHORT LENGTHS OF STAY

Early discharge is both a challenge and an opportunity for nurses. More teaching must occur during pregnancy when the mother's physical needs do not interfere with her ability to comprehend the new knowledge. In the birth facility, careful documentation and notification of the primary care provider is essential so that clients are not discharged inappropriately if abnormal findings develop. Self- and infant-care discharge instructions should be explained to the woman and support person. A printed form, signed by both the client and nurse, is placed in the chart with a copy given to the woman for later reference. Other methods for follow-up, such as home visits, phone calls, and return visits to the birth facility for nursing assessments after discharge may

identify complications early when they can be dealt with most effectively.

Nursing follow-up by phone calls, sometimes called *phone triage*, is the least expensive of postdischarge methods. However, the nurse does not see or physically examine the client or her infant, and specific protocols and procedures should be in place for the triage call and for nursing actions that should be taken if a potential problem is identified during the call. Documentation should be kept on a form developed for follow-up phone calls. Any instructions given to the client (recommended actions if problems arise, if a minor problem does not improve, or if a problem worsens during phone triage) must be documented.

✓ CHECK YOUR READING

17. What concerns do nurses have about unlicensed personnel?
18. Why is early discharge a concern for nurses?
19. What are important points in phone-call triage?

SUMMARY CONCEPTS

- Ethical dilemmas are a difficult area of practice and are best solved by applying ethical theories and principles and the steps of the nursing process.
- When ethical principles of beneficence, nonmaleficence, autonomy, and justice result in ethical dilemmas, the nursing process may be used to guide ethical decision making.
- Elective abortion is a controversial issue that generates strong feelings in two opposing factions in the United States. Decisions by the Supreme Court have limited or upheld the right of states to impose restrictions on abortion.
- Nurses must examine their beliefs and come to personal decisions about abortion before they are faced with the situation in their own practices.
- When using online communications to transmit data about clients, colleagues, or facilities, nurses must be careful not to violate confidentiality and to maintain ethical conduct.
- Punitive approaches to ethical and social problems may prevent women from seeking adequate prenatal care.
- Issues in fetal therapy include weighing of the risks and benefits for the mother versus those for the fetus and determination of whose rights should prevail.
- Issues in infertility concern the high cost and low success rate of some treatments, the fate of unused embryos and multiple fetuses, and the rights of surrogate parents.
- Poverty is a major social issue that underlies adequacy of health care resources, access to prenatal care, government programs to increase health care to indigent women and children, and health care rationing.
- Nurses are expected to perform in accordance with nurse practice acts, standards of care, and agency policies. Doing so provides the best prevention of or defense against malpractice claims.
- Nurses can help defend malpractice claims by following guidelines for informed consent, refusal of care, and documentation and by maintaining their levels of expertise.

- To give informed consent, the client must be competent, receive full information, understand that information, and consent voluntarily.

- Complete documentation is the best evidence that the standard of care received by a client was met. Therefore nurses must ensure their documentation accurately reflects the care given.

- Continuing pressures on optimal nursing practice include use of unlicensed assistive personnel and short lengths of stay.

ANSWERS TO CRITICAL THINKING EXERCISE, p. 37

1. The deontologic view is that taking organs necessary for life from one human being to give to another is wrong, even when the donor cannot survive. This view disapproves of aggressive treatment necessary to maintain perfusion to the organs until a recipient is located because treatment does not help the dying infant and may increase suffering. This concern invokes the principle of nonmaleficence.

2. The utilitarian view is that anencephalic infants cannot survive, but that their organs could provide benefit to other infants (beneficence). Because this family feels strongly that helping other infants allows good to come from their own tragedy, the greatest good would be for an organ transplant.

3. Potential problems include the possibility that transplants might someday be required, even against the parents' will, which might deny them autonomy in making decisions for their child's benefit. A woman might be forced to carry a pregnancy to term so that the organs could be harvested, even if the parents would rather end the pregnancy. If anencephalic infants are used for organ donation, people with profound mental retardation or persistent vegetative states might be placed in the same situation. Choosing infants to benefit would also be a concern, involving principles of justice. An overriding concern would be determining who would make the decisions necessary.

REFERENCES & READINGS

Alfaro-LeFevre, R. (2004). *Critical thinking and clinical judgment: A practical approach.* Philadelphia: Saunders.

American Nurses Association. (1997). Registered professional nurses and unlicensed assistive personnel. Washington, DC: Author.

Association of Women's Health, Obstetric and Neonatal Nurses (AWHONN). (1999). Position statement: Issue: Interstate compact for mutual recognition of state licensure. Washington, DC: Author.

AWHONN. (2000). Position statement: Issue: The role of unlicensed assistive personnel in the nursing care for women and newborns. Washington, DC: Author.

Bloom, K., Bednarzyk, M.S., Devitt, D.L., Renault, R.A., Teaman, V., & Van Loock, D.M. (2004). Barriers to prenatal care for homeless pregnant women. *Journal of Obstetric, Gynecologic, and Neonatal Nursing,* 33(4), 428-435.

Brent, N.J. (2001). Reproductive and family concerns. In N.J. Brent (Ed.), *Nurses and the law: A guide to principles and applications* (2nd ed., pp. 181-204). Philadelphia: Saunders.

Cady, R. (2000a). Informed consent for adult patients, part 1. A review of basic principles. *MCN: The American Journal of Maternal/Child Nursing,* 25(2), 106.

Cady, R. (2000b). Informed consent for adult patients, part 2. *MCN: The American Journal of Maternal/Child Nursing,* 25(3), 164.

Centers for Medicare and Medicaid Services. (2004). Medicaid eligibility. Retrieved September 21, 2004, from www.cms.hhs.gov/medicaid/eligibility/criteria.asp.

Cesario, S.K. (1998). Should cameras be allowed in the delivery room? *MCN: The American Journal of Maternal/Child Nursing,* 23(2), 87-91.

Cohen, R.A., & Ni, H. (2004). National health insurance coverage estimates from the National Health Institute Survey, January-June 2003. Retrieved September 19, 2004, from www.cdc.gov/nchs/nhis.htm.

DeNavas-Walt, C., Proctor, B.P., & Mills, R.J. (2004). U.S. Census Bureau, Current Population Reports, p. 60-226. *Income, Poverty, and Health Insurance Coverage in the United States, 2003.* Washington, DC: US Government Printing Office. Retrieved January 1, 2005, from www.census.gov/prod/2004pubs/p60-226.pdf.

Douglas, M.R. (2001). Ethics and nursing practice. In N.J. Brent (Ed.), *Nurses and the law: A guide to principles and application* (2nd ed., pp. 31-52). Philadelphia: Saunders.

Driscoll, K.M., & Sudia-Robinson, T. (2003). Legal and ethical issues of neonatal care. In C. Kenner & J.W. Lott (Eds.), *Comprehensive neonatal nursing: A physiologic perspective* (3rd ed., pp. 43-107). Philadelphia: Saunders.

Foley, E.M. (2002). Drug screening and criminal prosecution of pregnant women. *Journal of Obstetric, Gynecologic, and Neonatal Nurses,* 31(2), 133-137.

Lindgren, K. (1996). Maternal-fetal conflict: Court-ordered cesarean section. *Journal of Obstetric, Gynecologic, and Neonatal Nursing,* 25(8), 653-656.

Lucas, V.A. (2003). The business of women's health care. In E.T. Breslin & V.A. Lucas (Eds.), *Women's health nursing: Toward evidence-based practice* (pp. 761-795). Philadelphia: Saunders.

March of Dimes Birth Defects Foundation. (2004). Teenage pregnancy. Retrieved September 19, 2004, from www.modimes.com.

Martin, J.A., Hamilton, B.E., Sutton, P.D., Ventura, S.J., Menacker, F., & Munson, M.L. (2004). *Births: Final data for 2002. National Vital Statistics Reports,* 52(10). Hyattsville, MD: National Center for Health Statistics. Retrieved September 21, 2004, from www.cdc.gov/nchs/data/nvsr52_10.pdf.

National Center for Health Statistics. (2004). Health, United States, 2004, with Chartbook on Trends in the Health of Americans. Hyattsville, MD.

Office of Public Affairs. (2004). Fact sheet: Office of Family Assistance (TANF). Washington, DC: U.S. Department of Health and Human Services. Retrieved September 19, 2004, from www.acf.hhs.gov/opa/fact_sheets/tanf_factsheets.html.

Simpson, K.R., & Chez, B.F. (2001). Professional and legal issues. In K.R. Simpson & P.A. Creehan (Eds.), *AWHONN perinatal nursing* (2nd ed., 21-49). Philadelphia: Lippincott.

Teschendorf, M. (2003). Women during the reproductive years. In E.T. Breslin and V.A. Lucas (Eds.), *Women's health nursing: Toward evidence-based practice* (pp. 553-627). Philadelphia: Saunders.

United States Department of Health and Human Services. (2001a). Health Insurance Portability and Accountability Act of 1996: Privacy rule: Provisions relevant to public health practice. Retrieved September 18, 2004, from www.cdc.gov/ncidod/HIP/NNIS/members/HIPAA_privacy.pdf.

United States Department of Health and Human Services. (2003). Fact sheet: Administrative simplification under HIPAA: National standards for transactions, privacy, and security. Retrieved October 26, 2004, from www.hhs.gov/news/2002pres/hipaa.html.

Upvall, M.J. (2003). Women and culture. In E.T. Breslin & V.A. Lucas (Eds.), Women's health nursing: Toward evidence-based practice. Philadelphia: Saunders.

Reproductive Anatomy and Physiology

OBJECTIVES

After studying this chapter, you should be able to:

1. Explain female and male sexual development from prenatal life through sexual maturity.
2. Describe the normal anatomy of the female and male reproductive systems.
3. Explain the normal function of the female and male reproductive systems.
4. Explain the normal structure and function of the female breast.

Go to your Student CD-ROM for Review Questions keyed to these Objectives.

DEFINITIONS

Amenorrhea Absence of menstruation. Primary amenorrhea is a delay of the first menstruation, and secondary amenorrhea is cessation of menstruation after its initiation.

Cilia Hairlike processes on the surface of a cell that beat rhythmically to move the cell or to move fluid or other substances over the cell surface.

Climacteric Endocrine, body, and psychic changes occurring at the end of a woman's reproductive period. Also informally called *menopause,* although this term does not encompass all changes.

Coitus Sexual union between a male and a female.

Fornix (Pl. *fornices*) An arch or pouchlike structure at the upper end of the vagina. Also called a *cul-de-sac.*

Gamete Reproductive cell; in the female an ovum and in the male a spermatozoon.

Genetic Sex Sex determined at conception by union of two X chromosomes (female) or an X and a Y chromosome (male) (also called *chromosomal sex*).

Gonad Reproductive (sex) gland that produces gametes and sex hormones. The female gonads are ovaries and the male gonads are testes.

Gonadotropic Hormones Secretions of the anterior pituitary gland that stimulate the gonads, specifically follicle-stimulating hormone and luteinizing hormone. Chorionic gonadotropin is secreted by the placenta during pregnancy.

Graafian Follicle A small sac within the ovary that contains the maturing ovum.

Menarche Onset of menstruation.

Menopause Permanent cessation of menstruation during the climacteric.

Puberty Period of sexual maturation accompanied by the development of secondary sex characteristics and the capacity to reproduce.

Ruga (Pl. *rugae*) Ridge or fold of tissue, as on the male's scrotum and in the female's vagina.

Secondary Sex Characteristics Physical differences between mature males and females that are not directly related to reproduction.

Somatic Sex Gender assignment as male or female on the basis of form and structure of the external genitalia.

Spermatogenesis Formation of male gametes (sperm) in the testes.

Spinnbarkeit Clear, slippery, stretchy quality of cervical mucus during ovulation.

An understanding of the structure and function of the reproductive organs is necessary for effective nursing care of women during and after their reproductive years and for couples that require family planning or infertility care. This chapter reviews basic prenatal development, sexual maturation, and the structure and function of the female and male reproductive systems. Because of its emphasis in this book, the female reproductive system is discussed most extensively.

SEXUAL DEVELOPMENT

Sexual development begins at conception when the genetic sex is determined by the union of an ovum and a sperm. During childhood the sex organs are inactive. They become active during puberty as the person begins sexual maturation.

Prenatal Development

The mother's ovum carries a single X chromosome. Each of the father's spermatozoa carries either an X chromosome or a Y chromosome. If an X-bearing spermatozoon fertilizes the ovum, the offspring's genetic sex is female. If a Y-bearing spermatozoon fertilizes the ovum, a genetic male offspring results.

Although genetic sex is determined at conception, the reproductive system of males and females is similar, or sexually undifferentiated, for the first 6 weeks of prenatal life. During the seventh week, differences between males and females appear in the internal structures. The external genitalia continue to look similar until the ninth week, when these outer structures begin to change. Differentiation of the external sexual organs is complete at about 12 weeks' gestational age.

The basic trend for prenatal sexual development is to have female structures. Presence of only a small part of the Y chromosome (the short arm) changes this trend and directs the early (primitive) sex cells to become testes. Absence of the critical part of the Y chromosome allows the primitive sex cells to continue on their course of becoming ovaries (see Chapter 6).

During fetal life, both ovaries and testes secrete their primary hormones, which are estrogen and testosterone, respectively. Testosterone causes development of male sex organs and external genitalia, and its absence results in development of female sex characteristics. Although estrogen is secreted by the fetal ovary, the hormone is not required to initiate development of female sex structures.

Childhood

The sex glands of girls and boys are inactive during infancy and childhood. At sexual maturity the hypothalamus stimulates the anterior pituitary gland to produce hormones, which in turn stimulate sex hormone production by the gonads.

Sexual Maturation

Puberty refers to the time during which the reproductive organs become fully functional. It is not a single event but a series of changes that occurs over several years during late

TABLE 4-1 Comparison of Secondary Sex Characteristics in Females and Males

Females	Males
Development of glandular and ductal systems in the breast; deposition of fat selectively in the breast, buttocks, and thighs, resulting in a rounded figure	Muscle mass 50% greater
Wide, round pelvis	Narrow, upright, and heavier pelvis
Pubic and axillary hair	Pubic and axillary hair; facial and chest hair; increased amount of hair on the upper back in some males; male pattern baldness, beginning on the top of the head
Soft, smooth skin texture	Coarser skin
Higher-pitched voice	Deeper voice

childhood and early adolescence. Primary sex characteristics relate to the maturation of those organs directly responsible for reproduction. Examples of primary sex characteristics are maturation of ova in the ovaries and production of sperm in the testes. Secondary sex characteristics are changes in other systems that differentiate females and males but do not directly relate to reproduction (Table 4-1).

INITIATION OF SEXUAL MATURATION

Not all factors that initiate sexual maturation are known. Secretions of the hypothalamus, anterior pituitary, and gonads all play a part. The hypothalamus can secrete gonadotropin-releasing hormone (GnRH) to initiate puberty during infancy and early childhood, but it does not do so in significant amounts until late childhood. Production of even tiny quantities of sex hormones by the young child's ovaries or testes inhibits secretions of the hypothalamus, preventing premature onset of puberty. Maturation of another brain area, as yet unknown, probably triggers the hypothalamus to initiate puberty (Guyton & Hall, 2000).

The maturing child's hypothalamus gradually increases production of GnRH beginning at age 9 to 12 years (Blackburn, 2003; Guyton & Hall, 2000; Jones & DeCherney, 2003b,c). The level of GnRH increases slowly until it reaches a level adequate to stimulate the anterior pituitary to increase its production of follicle-stimulating hormone (FSH) and luteinizing hormone (LH). The ovaries and testes increase production of sex hormones and begin maturing gametes in response to higher levels of FSH and LH. The sex hormones also induce development of secondary sex characteristics. (Table 4-2 lists the major hormones that play a role in reproduction.)

The age at which changes of puberty begin and the time required to complete these changes vary among individuals. The hormonal changes of puberty begin about 6 months to 1 year earlier in girls than in boys. The growth spurt that occurs with puberty also begins earlier for girls than for boys. The obvious changes of puberty in girls, such as breast de-

TABLE 4-2 Major Hormones in Reproduction

Produced by	Target Organs	Action in Female	Action in Male
Gonadotropin-Releasing Hormone			
Hypothalamus	Anterior pituitary	Stimulates release of FSH and LH, initiating puberty and sustaining female reproductive cycles; release is pulsatile	Stimulates release of FSH and LH, initiating puberty; release is pulsatile
Follicle-Stimulating Hormone			
Anterior pituitary	Ovaries (female) Testes (male)	1. Stimulates final maturation of follicle 2. Stimulates growth and maturation of graafian follicles before ovulation	Stimulates Leydig cells of testes to secrete testosterone
Luteinizing Hormone			
Anterior pituitary	Ovaries (female) Testes (male)	1. Stimulates final maturation of follicle 2. Surge of LH about 14 days before next menstrual period causes ovulation 3. Stimulates transformation of graafian follicle into corpus luteum, which continues secretion of estrogens and progesterone for about 12 days if ovum is not fertilized, if fertilization occurs, placenta gradually assumes this function	Stimulates Leydig cells of testes to secrete testosterone
Estrogens			
1. Ovaries and corpus luteum (female) 2. Placenta (pregnancy) 3. Formed in small quantities from testosterone in Sertoli cells of testes (male); other tissues, especially the liver, produce estrogen in the male	Internal and external reproductive organs Breasts (female) Testes (male)	1. Reproductive organs a. Maturation at puberty b. Stimulation of endometrium before ovulation 2. Breasts: induce growth of glandular and ductal tissue; initiate deposition of fat at puberty 3. Stimulate growth of long bones but cause closure of epiphyses, limiting mature height 4. Pregnancy: stimulate growth of uterus, breast tissue; inhibit active milk production; relax pelvic ligaments	Necessary for normal sperm formation
Progesterone			
Ovary, corpus luteum, placenta	Uterus, female breasts	1. Stimulates secretion of endometrial glands; causes endometrial vessels to become dilated and tortuous in preparation for possible embryo implantation 2. Pregnancy: induces growth of cells of fallopian tubes and uterine lining to nourish embryo; decreases contractions of uterus; prepares breasts for lactation but inhibits prolactin secretion	Not applicable
Prolactin			
Anterior pituitary	Female breasts	Stimulates secretion of milk (lactogenesis); estrogen and progesterone from placenta have an inhibiting effect on milk production until after placenta is expelled at birth; sucking of newborn stimulates prolactin secretion to maintain milk production	Not applicable
Oxytocin			
Posterior pituitary	Uterus, female breasts	1. Uterus: stimulates contractions during birth and stimulates postpartum contractions to compress uterine vessels and control bleeding 2. Stimulates let-down, or milk-ejection reflex, during breastfeeding	Not applicable
Testosterone			
Adrenal glands (female) Ovaries (female)	Sexual organs (male) Male body conformation after puberty	Small quantities of androgenic (masculinizing) hormones from adrenal glands cause growth of pubic and axillary hair at puberty; most androgens, such as testosterone, are converted to estrogen	1. Induces development of male sex organs in fetus 2. Induces growth and division of the cells that mature sperm 3. Induces development of male secondary sex characteristics

FSH, Follicle-stimulating hormone; GnRH, gonadotropin-releasing hormone; LH, luteinizing hormone.

velopment, begin an average of 2 years before changes in boys. Changes of puberty occur in an orderly sequence in both genders. Increases in height and weight are dramatic during puberty but slow after puberty until mature heights and weights are attained. The nutritional state can also influence the start of puberty, with earlier onset occurring in well-nourished children.

FEMALE PUBERTY CHANGES

As girls mature, the anterior pituitary gland secretes increasing amounts of FSH and LH in response to the hypothalamic secretion of GnRH. These two pituitary secretions stimulate secretion of estrogens and progesterone by the ovary, resulting in maturation of the reproductive organs and breasts and development of secondary sex characteristics. The first noticeable change of puberty in girls, development of the breasts, begins at about 8 to 13 years of age. Menstruation occurs about 2 to 2.5 years after breast development, with an average age range of 9 to 16 years (Needlman, 2004).

BREAST CHANGES. Initially, the nipple enlarges and protrudes. The areola surrounding the nipple enlarges and becomes somewhat protuberant, although less so than the nipple. These changes are followed by growth of the glandular and ductal tissue. Fat is deposited in the breasts to give them the characteristic rounded female appearance. During puberty a girl's breasts often develop at different rates, resulting in a lopsided appearance until one breast catches up with the other.

BODY CONTOURS. The pelvis widens and assumes a rounded, basinlike shape that favors passage of the fetus during childbirth. Fat is deposited selectively in the hips, giving them a rounder appearance than that of the male.

BODY HAIR. Pubic hair first appears downy and becomes thicker as puberty progresses. Axillary hair appears near the time of menarche. The texture and quantity of pubic and axillary hair vary among women and ethnic groups. Women of African descent usually have body hair that is coarser and curlier than that of white women. Asian women often have sparser body hair than women of other racial groups.

SKELETAL GROWTH. Girls grow taller for several years during early puberty in response to estrogen stimulation. The growth spurt begins about 1 year after breast development begins. Estrogen's other powerful effect on the skeleton is to cause the epiphyses (growth areas of the bone) to unite with the shaft of the bones, which eventually stops growth in height.

REPRODUCTIVE ORGANS. The girl's external genitalia enlarge as fat is deposited in the mons pubis, labia majora, and labia minora. The vagina, uterus, fallopian tubes, and ovaries grow larger. In addition, the vaginal mucosa changes, becoming more resistant to trauma and infection in preparation for sexual activity. Cyclic changes in the reproductive organs occur during each female reproductive cycle.

MENARCHE. Approximately 2 to 2.5 years after the beginning of breast development, girls experience their menarche, or first menstrual period. Early menstrual periods are often irregular and scant. These early menstrual cycles are not usually fertile because ovulation occurs inconsistently. Fertile reproductive cycles require preparation of the uterine lining precisely timed with ovulation. However, ovulation may occur during any female reproductive cycle, including the first. The sexually active girl can conceive even before her first menstrual period.

Delayed onset of menstruation is called *primary amenorrhea* if the girl's periods have not begun within 2 years after the onset of breast development or by age 16 or if the girl is more than 1 year older than her mother or sisters were when their menarche occurred. *Secondary amenorrhea* describes absence of menstruation for at least three cycles after regular cycles have been established or for 6 months (Kim, 2000). Both primary and secondary amenorrhea are more common in females who are thin. Women who are competitive athletes or ballet dancers or suffer from eating disorders (such as anorexia nervosa or bulimia) may have too little fat to produce enough sex hormones to stimulate ovulation and menstruation. Pregnancy is also a common cause of secondary amenorrhea. Both primary and secondary amenorrhea may result from inadequate pituitary stimulation of the ovary or failure of the ovary to respond to pituitary stimulation. Amenorrhea also may be caused by excessive androgenic hormones from the adrenal glands, which have a masculinizing effect.

MALE PUBERTY CHANGES

Secretion of GnRH by the hypothalamus stimulates secretion of LH and FSH from the anterior pituitary. LH and FSH then stimulate secretion of testosterone and eventually cause spermatogenesis in the maturing adolescent. Testosterone stimulates development of a boy's reproductive organs and secondary sex characteristics. The first outward sign of puberty is growth of the testes, which may begin as early as 9.5 years of age. Initial penile development extends from 9.2 to 13.7 years of age, with an average of 10.5 years. Final male sexual maturation is complete at approximately 16.5 years of age (Blackburn, 2003; Needlman, 2004). The skin of the scrotum thins and darkens as the sexual organs mature.

NOCTURNAL EMISSIONS. Often called *wet dreams,* nocturnal emissions commonly occur during the teenage years. The boy experiences a spontaneous ejaculation of seminal fluid during sleep, often accompanied by dreams with sexual content. Boys should be prepared for this normal occurrence so that they do not feel abnormal or ashamed or fear that they have an infection or other problem.

BODY HAIR. Pubic hair growth begins at the base of the penis. Gradually, the hair coarsens and grows upward and in the midline of the abdomen. About 2 years later, axillary hair appears. Facial hair begins as a fine, downy mustache and progresses to the characteristic beard of the adult male. In most boys, chest hair develops, and some boys have hair on their upper backs. The amount and character of body hair vary among men of different racial groups, with Asian and Native American men often having less than white or African men. The quantity and character of body hair among men of the same racial group also vary.

BODY COMPOSITION. Because of the influence of testosterone, men develop a greater average muscle mass than women. At maturity a man's muscle mass exceeds the woman's by an average of 50%, explaining the biologic advantage of men in tasks requiring muscle strength.

SKELETAL GROWTH. Testosterone causes boys to undergo a rapid growth spurt, especially in height. A boy's linear growth begins about 1 year later than a girl's and may continue into his twenties. Testosterone eventually causes union of the epiphysis with the shaft of long bones, as estrogen does in girls. The height-limiting effect of testosterone is not as strong as that of estrogen in females, with the result that boys grow in stature for several years longer than girls. The male's greater average height at maturity is the combined result of beginning the growth spurt at a slightly later age and continuing it for a longer time.

A boy's shoulders broaden as his height increases. His pelvis assumes a more upright shape, with narrower diameters and heavier composition than the female's. A man's pelvis is structurally suited for tasks requiring load bearing.

VOICE CHANGES. Hypertrophy of the laryngeal mucosa and enlargement of the larynx cause the male's voice to deepen. Before reaching their lower tones at maturity, many boys experience embarrassing "cracking" or "squeaking" of their voices when they speak.

Decline in Fertility

The climacteric is a transitional period starting as female fertility declines and extends through menopause and the postmenopausal period. In most women the climacteric occurs between ages 40 and 50. Maturation of ova and production of ovarian hormones gradually decline. The external and internal reproductive organs atrophy somewhat as well. *Menopause* is the term used to describe the final menstrual period. However, *menopause* and *climacteric* are often used interchangeably to describe the entire gradual process of change. Perimenopause is the time from onset of changes associated with the climacteric, continuing for approximately 2 to 5 years after the last menstrual period (Blackburn, 2003; Guyton & Hall, 2000). (See Chapter 33 for more information about the woman's needs during this phase of her life.)

Men do not experience a distinct marker event like menopause. Production of testosterone and sperm gradually declines, and sexual function decreases in the late 40s and 50s.

CHECK YOUR READING

1. What are the first noticeable changes of puberty in girls and boys?
2. What are common differences in body hair characteristics among women and men of different races?
3. What are basic differences between the mature male and female pelves?
4. Why do males generally attain greater mature height than females?
5. What are common male and female secondary sex characteristics?

FEMALE REPRODUCTIVE ANATOMY

The nurse needs a basic knowledge of the structure and function of the external and internal reproductive organs to understand their roles in pregnancy and childbirth (Table 4-3).

External Female Reproductive Organs

Collectively, the external female reproductive organs are called the *vulva*. These structures include the mons pubis, labia majora and minora, clitoris, structures of the vestibule, and perineum (Figure 4-1).

MONS PUBIS

The mons pubis is the rounded, fleshy prominence over the symphysis pubis that forms the anterior border of the external reproductive organs. It is covered with varying amounts of pubic hair.

LABIA MAJOR AND MINORA

The labia majora are two rounded, fleshy folds of tissue that extend from the mons pubis to the perineum. They have a slightly deeper pigmentation than surrounding skin and are covered with pubic hair. The labia majora protect the more fragile tissues of the external genitalia.

The labia minora run parallel to and within the labia majora. The labia minora extend from the clitoris anteriorly and merge posteriorly to form the fourchette, which is the posterior rim of the vaginal introitus, or vaginal opening. The labia minora do not have pubic hair. They are highly vascular and respond to stimulation by becoming engorged with blood.

CLITORIS

The clitoris is a small projection at the anterior junction of the two labia minora. This structure is composed of highly sensitive erectile tissue similar to that of the penis. The labia majora merge to form a prepuce over the clitoris.

TABLE 4-3 Functions of Female Reproductive and Accessory Organs

Organ	Function
Vagina	1. Provides the passageway for the menstrual flow 2. Is the female organ for coitus; receives the male penis during coitus 3. Provides the passageway for the fetus during birth
Uterus	Houses and nourishes the fetus to sufficient maturity to function outside the mother's body; propels fetus to outside
Fallopian tube	1. Provides passageway for ovum as it travels from ovary to uterus 2. Is the site of fertilization
Ovaries	1. Secrete estrogens and progesterone 2. Contain ova within follicles for maturation during the woman's reproductive life
Breasts Alveoli	Secrete milk after childbirth (acinar cells within alveoli)
Lactiferous ducts and sinuses	Collect milk from alveoli and conduct it to the outside

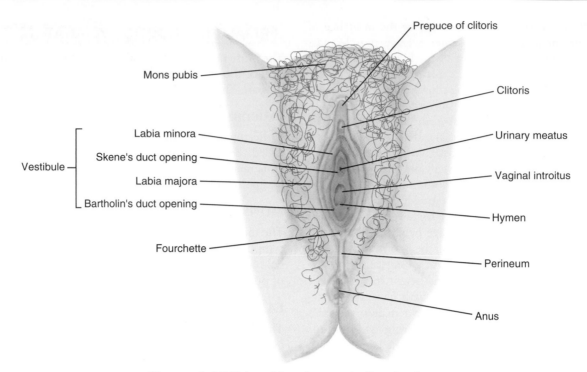

Figure 4-1 ■ External female reproductive structures.

VESTIBULE

The *vestibule* refers to structures enclosed by the labia minora. The urinary meatus, vaginal introitus, and ducts of Skene's and Bartholin's glands lie within the vestibule. Skene's, or periurethral, glands provide lubrication for the urethra. Bartholin's glands provide lubrication for the vaginal introitus, particularly during sexual arousal.

The vaginal introitus is surrounded by erectile tissue. During sexual stimulation, blood flows into the erectile tissue, allowing the introitus to tighten around the penis. This adds a massaging feeling that heightens the male's sexual sensations and encourages ejaculation.

The hymen is a thin fold of mucosa that partially separates the vagina and vestibule. The intactness or lack thereof of the hymen is not a criterion of virginity. The hymen may be broken by injury, tampon use, intercourse, or childbirth.

PERINEUM

The perineum is the most posterior part of the external female reproductive organs. The perineum extends from the fourchette anteriorly to the anus posteriorly. It is composed of fibrous and muscular tissues that provide support for pelvic structures. The perineum may be lacerated during childbirth, or it may be incised to enlarge the vaginal opening in a procedure called an *episiotomy.*

Internal Female Reproductive Organs

The internal reproductive structures are the vagina, uterus, fallopian tubes, and ovaries (Figures 4-2 and 4-3). These organs are supported and contained within the bony pelvis.

VAGINA

The vagina is a tube of muscular and membranous tissue about 8 to 10 cm long that lies between the bladder anteriorly and the rectum posteriorly. The vagina connects the uterus above with the vestibule below. The vaginal lining has multiple folds, or rugae, and a muscular layer capable of marked distention during childbirth. The vagina is lubricated by secretions of the cervix (the lowermost part of the uterus) and Bartholin's glands.

The vagina does not end abruptly at the uterine opening but arches to form a pouchlike structure called the *vaginal fornix.* Each fornix is described by its location: anterior, posterior, and lateral.

The vagina has three major functions: (1) it allows discharge of the menstrual flow; (2) it is the female organ of coitus; and (3) it allows passage of the fetus from the uterus to outside the mother's body during childbirth.

UTERUS

The uterus is a hollow, thick-walled, muscular organ shaped like a flat, upside-down pear. The uterus houses and nourishes the fetus until birth and then contracts rhythmically during labor to expel the fetus. Each month the uterus is prepared for a pregnancy, regardless of whether conception occurs.

The uterus measures about $7.5 \times 5 \times 2.5$ cm and is larger in women who have borne children. It is suspended above the bladder and is anterior to the rectum. Its normal position is anteverted (rotated forward over the bladder) and slightly anteflexed (flexed forward).

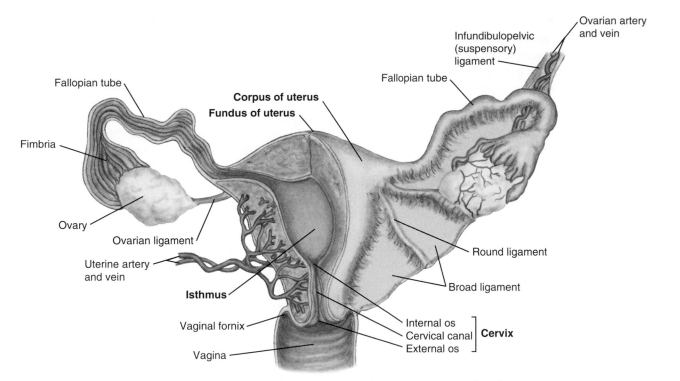

Fallopian tube

Fimbria

Ovary

Ovarian ligament

Uterine artery
and vein

Isthmus

Vaginal fornix

Vagina

Corpus of uterus

Fundus of uterus

Fallopian tube

Infundibulopelvic
(suspensory)
ligament

Ovarian artery
and vein

Round ligament

Broad ligament

Internal os
Cervical canal $\Big]$ **Cervix**
External os

Figure 4-2 ■ Internal female reproductive structures, anterior view.

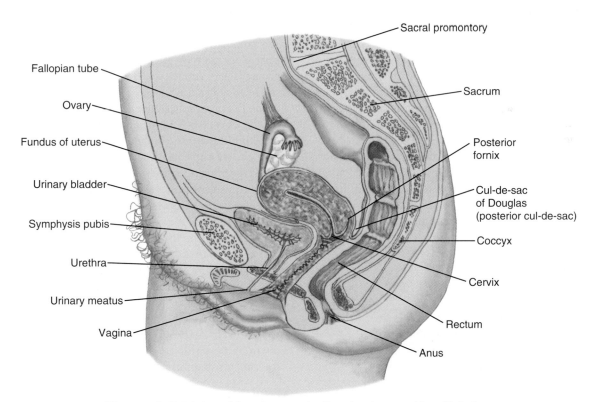

Fallopian tube

Ovary

Fundus of uterus

Urinary bladder

Symphysis pubis

Urethra

Urinary meatus

Vagina

Sacral promontory

Sacrum

Posterior
fornix

Cul-de-sac
of Douglas
(posterior cul-de-sac)

Coccyx

Cervix

Rectum

Anus

Figure 4-3 ■ Internal female reproductive structures, midsagittal view.

DIVISIONS OF THE UTERUS. The uterus has three divisions: the corpus, isthmus, and cervix.

Corpus. The corpus, or body, is the upper division of the uterus. The uppermost part of the uterine corpus, above the area where the fallopian tubes enter the uterus, is the fundus of the uterus.

Isthmus. A narrower transition zone, the isthmus, is located between the corpus of the uterus and cervix. During late pregnancy the isthmus elongates and is known as the *lower uterine segment.*

Cervix. The cervix is the tubular "neck" of the lower uterus and is about 2 to 3 cm in length. During labor the cervix effaces (thins) and dilates (opens) to allow passage of the fetus. The os is the opening in the cervix between the uterus and vagina. The upper and lower cervix are marked by the internal and external os, respectively. The external os of a childless woman is round and smooth. After vaginal birth the external os has an irregular, slitlike shape and may have tags of scar tissue.

LAYERS OF THE UTERUS. The uterus has three layers: the perimetrium, myometrium, and endometrium.

Perimetrium. The perimetrium is the outer peritoneal layer of serous membrane that covers most of the uterus. Laterally the perimetrium is continuous with the broad ligaments on both sides of the uterus.

Myometrium. The myometrium is the middle layer of thick muscle. Most muscle fibers are concentrated in the upper uterus, and their number diminishes progressively toward the cervix. The myometrium contains three types of smooth muscle fiber, each suited to specific functions in childbearing (Figure 4-4):

1. Longitudinal fibers are found mostly in the fundus and are designed to expel the fetus efficiently toward the pelvic outlet during birth.
2. Interlacing figure-8 fibers constitute the middle layer. These fibers contract after birth to compress blood vessels that pass between them to limit blood loss.
3. Circular fibers form constrictions where the fallopian tubes enter the uterus and surround the internal cervical os. Circular fibers prevent reflux of menstrual

blood and tissue into the fallopian tubes, promote normal implantation of the fertilized ovum by controlling its entry into the uterus, and retain the fetus until the appropriate time of birth.

Endometrium. The endometrium is the inner layer of the uterus. It responds to the cyclic variations of estrogen and progesterone during the female reproductive cycle (see p. 60). The endometrium has two layers:

1. The basal layer is the area nearest the myometrium that regenerates the functional layer of the endometrium after each menstrual period and after childbirth.
2. The functional layer lies above the basal layer. Endometrial arteries, veins, and glands extend into the functional layer and are shed during each menstrual period and after childbirth in the lochia.

FALLOPIAN TUBES

The fallopian tubes, also called *oviducts,* are 8 to 14 cm long and quite narrow (2 to 3 mm at their narrowest and 5 to 8 mm at their widest). They form a pathway for the ovum between the ovary and uterus. Fertilization occurs in the fallopian tubes. Each fallopian tube enters the upper uterus at the cornu, or horn, of the uterus.

The fallopian tubes are lined with folded epithelium containing cilia that beat rhythmically toward the uterine cavity to propel the ovum through the tube. The rough, folded surface of its lining and small diameter make the fallopian tube vulnerable to blockage from infection or scar tissue. Tubal blockage may result in sterility or a tubal pregnancy, because the fertilized ovum cannot enter the uterus for proper implantation.

The fallopian tubes have the following four divisions:

1. The interstitial portion runs into the uterine cavity and lies within the uterine wall.
2. The isthmus is the narrow part adjacent to the uterus.
3. The ampulla is the wider area of the tube lateral to the isthmus, where fertilization occurs.
4. The infundibulum is the wide, funnel-shaped terminal end of the tube. Fimbria are fingerlike processes that surround the infundibulum.

The fallopian tubes are not directly connected to the ovary. The ovum is expelled into the abdominal cavity near the fimbria at ovulation. Wavelike motions of the fimbria draw the ovum into the tube. However, the tubal isthmus remains contracted until 3 days after conception to allow the fertilized ovum to develop within the tube. Initial growth of the fertilized ovum within the fallopian tube promotes its normal implantation in the upper uterus.

OVARIES

The ovaries are the female gonads, or sex glands. They have two functions: (1) sex hormone production and (2) maturation of an ovum during each reproductive cycle.

The ovaries secrete estrogen and progesterone in varying amounts during a woman's reproductive cycle to prepare the uterine lining for pregnancy. Ovarian hormone secretion gradually declines to very low levels during the climacteric.

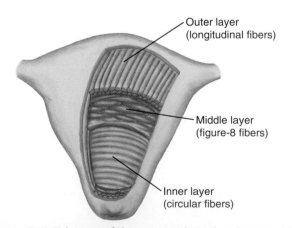

Outer layer
(longitudinal fibers)

Middle layer
(figure-8 fibers)

Inner layer
(circular fibers)

Figure 4-4 ■ Layers of the myometrium showing the three types of smooth muscle fiber.

At birth the ovary contains all the ova it will ever have. About 2 million immature ova are present at birth. Many of these degenerate during childhood, and at puberty 200,000 to 400,000 viable ova remain. Many ova begin the maturation process during each reproductive cycle, but most never reach maturity. During a woman's reproductive life, only about 400 of the ova ever mature enough to be released and fertilized. By the time a woman reaches the climacteric, almost all her ova have been released during ovulation or have regressed. The few remaining ova are unresponsive to stimulating hormones and do not mature (Blackburn, 2003; Moore & Persaud, 2003).

✓ CHECK YOUR READING

6. What is the vulva? Describe the location of each of these external female organs: labia majora and minora, clitoris, urinary meatus, vaginal introitus, hymen, and perineum.
7. What are the three divisions of the uterus? Where is the fundus located?
8. Describe the three myometrial layers of the uterus. What is the function of each layer?
9. How do the fallopian tubes conduct the ovum from the ovary to the uterus? Why does the fertilized ovum first grow within the fallopian tube?
10. What are the two functions of the ovaries?

Support Structures

The bony pelvis supports and protects the lower abdominal and internal reproductive organs. Muscles and ligaments provide added support for the internal organs of the pelvis against the downward force of gravity and increases in intraabdominal pressure.

PELVIS

The bony pelvis is a basin-shaped structure at the lower end of the spine (Figure 4-5). Its posterior wall is formed by the sacrum. The side and anterior pelvic walls are composed of three fused bones: the ilium, ischium, and pubis.

The linea terminalis, also called the *pelvic brim* or *ileopectineal line*, is an imaginary line that divides the upper, or false, pelvis from the lower, or true, pelvis. The false pelvis provides support for the internal organs and the upper part of the body. The true pelvis is most important during childbirth (see Chapter 12).

MUSCLES

Paired muscles enclose the lower pelvis and provide support for internal reproductive, urinary, and bowel structures (Figure 4-6). In addition, a fibromuscular sheet, the pelvic fascia, provides support for the pelvic organs. Vaginal and urethral openings are located in the pelvic fascia.

The levator ani is a collection of three pairs of muscles: the pubococcygeus, which is also called the *pubovaginal muscle* in the female; the puborectal; and the iliococcygeus. These muscles support internal pelvic structures and resist increases in the intraabdominal pressure.

The ischiocavernosus muscle extends from the clitoris to the ischial tuberosities on each side of the lower bony pelvis. The two transverse perineal muscles extend from fibrous tissue of the perineum to the two ischial tuberosities, stabilizing the center of the perineum.

LIGAMENTS

Seven pairs of ligaments maintain the internal reproductive organs and their nerve and blood supplies in their proper positions within the pelvis (see Figure 4-2).

LATERAL SUPPORT. Paired ligaments stabilize the uterus and ovaries laterally and keep them in the midline of the pelvis. The broad ligament is a sheet of tissue extending from each side of the uterus to the lateral pelvic wall. The round ligament and fallopian tube mark the upper border of the broad ligament, and the lower edge is bounded by the uterine blood vessels. Within the two broad ligaments are the ovarian ligaments, blood vessels, and lymphatics.

The right and left cardinal ligaments provide support to the lower uterus and vagina. They extend from the lateral walls of the cervix and vagina to the side walls of the pelvis.

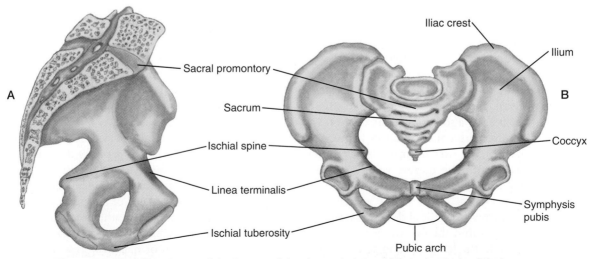

Figure 4-5 ■ Structures of the bony pelvis, shown in lateral **(A)** and anterior **(B)** views.

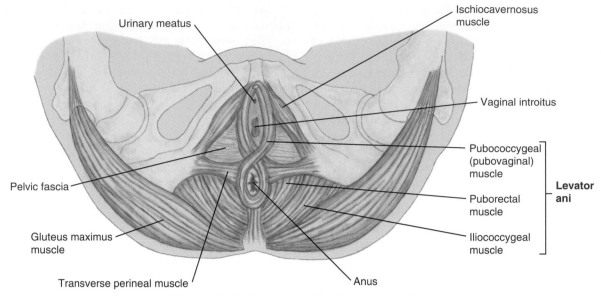

Figure 4-6 ■ Muscles of the female pelvic floor.

The two ovarian ligaments connect the ovaries to the lateral uterine walls. The infundibulopelvic (suspensory) ligaments connect the lateral ovary and distal fallopian tubes to the pelvic side walls. The infundibulopelvic ligament also carries the blood vessel and nerve supply for the ovary.

ANTERIOR SUPPORT. Two pairs of ligaments provide anterior support for the internal reproductive organs. The round ligaments connect the upper uterus to the connective tissue of the labia majora. These ligaments maintain the uterus in its normal anteflexed position and help direct the fetal presenting part against the cervix during labor.

The pubocervical ligaments support the cervix anteriorly. They connect the cervix and interior surface of the symphysis pubis.

POSTERIOR SUPPORT. The uterosacral ligaments provide posterior support, extending from the lower posterior uterus to the sacrum. These ligaments also contain sympathetic and parasympathetic nerves of the autonomic nervous system.

BLOOD SUPPLY

The uterine blood supply is carried by the uterine arteries, which are branches of the internal iliac artery. These vessels enter the uterus at the lower border of the broad ligament near the isthmus of the uterus. The vessels branch downward to supply the cervix and vagina and upward to supply the uterus. The upper branch also supplies the ovaries and fallopian tubes. The vessels are coiled to allow for elongation as the uterus enlarges and rises from the pelvis during pregnancy. Blood drains into the uterine veins and from there into the internal iliac veins.

Additional ovarian and tubal blood supply is carried by the ovarian artery, which arises from the abdominal aorta. The ovarian blood supply drains into the two ovarian veins. The left ovarian vein drains into the left renal vein, and the right ovarian vein drains directly into the inferior vena cava.

NERVE SUPPLY

Most functions of the reproductive system are under involuntary, or unconscious, control. Nerves of the autonomic nervous system from the uterovaginal plexus and inferior hypogastric plexus control automatic functions of the reproductive system.

Sensory and motor nerves that innervate the reproductive organs enter the spinal cord at the T12 through L2 levels. These nerves are important for pain management during childbearing (see Chapter 15).

✔ CHECK YOUR READING

11. Where is the true pelvis located?
12. What are the purposes of the muscles of the pelvis? What are the purposes of the ligaments?

FEMALE REPRODUCTIVE CYCLE

The term *female reproductive cycle* refers to the regular and recurrent changes in the anterior pituitary secretions, ovaries, and uterine endometrium that are designed to prepare the body for pregnancy (Figure 4-7). Associated changes in the cervical mucus promote fertilization during each cycle. The female reproductive cycle is often called the *menstrual cycle* because menstruation provides a marker for each cycle's beginning and end if pregnancy does not occur.

The female reproductive cycle is driven by a feedback loop between the anterior pituitary and ovaries. A feedback loop is a change in the level of one secretion in response to a change in the level of another secretion. The feedback loop may be positive, in which rising levels of one secretion cause another to rise, or negative, in which rising levels of one secretion cause another to fall.

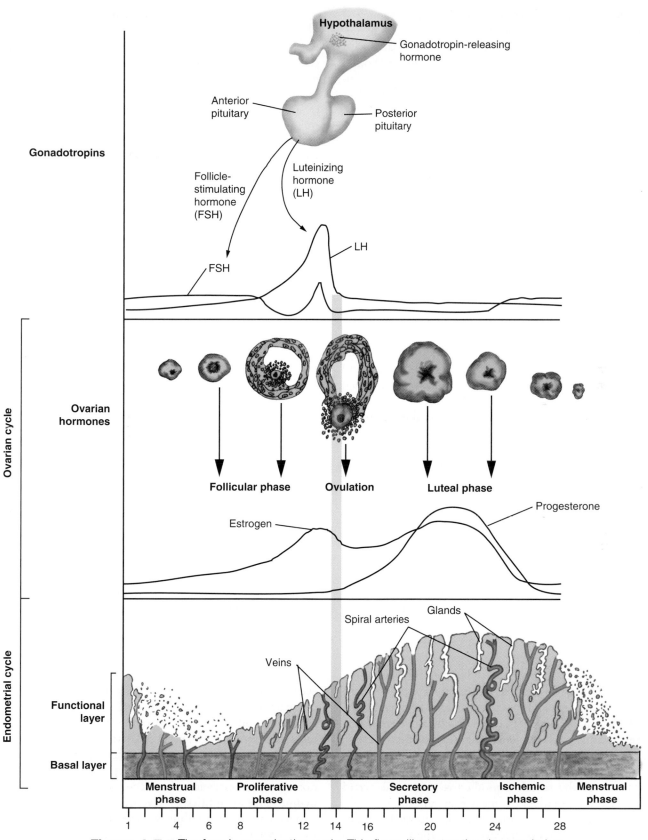

Figure 4-7 ■ The female reproductive cycle. This figure illustrates the changes in hormone secretion from the anterior pituitary and interrelated changes in the ovary and uterine endometrium.

The duration of the cycle is about 28 days, although it may range from 20 to 45 days (Guyton & Hall, 2000). Significant deviations from the 28-day cycle are associated with reduced fertility. The first day of the menstrual period is counted as day 1 of the woman's cycle. The female reproductive cycle is further divided into two cycles that reflect changes in the ovaries and uterine endometrium.

Ovarian Cycle

In response to GnRH from the woman's hypothalamus, the anterior pituitary secretes FSH and LH. These secretions stimulate the ovaries to mature and release an ovum and secrete additional hormones that will prepare the endometrium for implantation of a fertilized ovum. The ovarian cycle consists of three phases: the follicular, ovulatory, and luteal.

FOLLICULAR PHASE

The follicular phase is the period during which an ovum matures. It begins with the first day of menstruation and ends about 14 days later in a 28-day cycle. The length of this phase varies more among different women than do the lengths of the other two phases. The fall in estrogen and progesterone secretion by the ovary just before menstruation stimulates secretion of FSH and LH by the anterior pituitary. As the FSH and LH levels rise slightly, 6 to 12 graafian follicles, each containing an immature ovum, begin to grow. Each follicle secretes fluid containing high levels of estrogen, which accelerates maturation by making the follicle more sensitive to the effects of FSH. Eventually, one follicle outgrows the others to reach maturity. The mature follicle secretes large amounts of estrogen, which depresses FSH secretion. The dip in FSH secretion just before ovulation blocks further maturation of the less-developed follicles. Occasionally, more than one follicle matures and releases its ovum, which can lead to a multifetal pregnancy. Women who take fertility drugs may mature and release multiple ova that are used for assisted reproductive techniques (see Chapter 32).

OVULATORY PHASE

Near the middle of a 28-day reproductive cycle and about 2 days before ovulation, LH secretion rises markedly. Secretion of FSH also rises but to a lesser extent than that of LH. These surges in LH and FSH cause a slight fall in follicular estrogen production and a rise in progesterone secretion, which stimulates final maturation of a single follicle and release of its ovum. Ovulation marks the beginning of the luteal phase of the female reproductive cycle and occurs about 14 days before the next menstrual period.

The mature follicle is a mass of cells with a fluid-filled chamber. A smaller mass of cells houses the ovum within this chamber. At ovulation a blisterlike projection called a *stigma* forms on the wall of the follicle, the follicle ruptures, and the ovum with its surrounding cells is released from the surface of the ovary, where it is picked up by the fimbriated end of the fallopian tube for transport to the uterus.

LUTEAL PHASE

After ovulation and under the influence of LH, the remaining cells of the old follicle persist for about 12 days as a corpus luteum. The corpus luteum secretes estrogen and large amounts of progesterone to prepare the endometrium for a fertilized ovum. During this phase, levels of FSH and LH decrease in response to higher levels of estrogen and progesterone. If the ovum is fertilized, it secretes a hormone (chorionic gonadotropin) that causes persistence of the corpus luteum to maintain an early pregnancy. If the ovum is not fertilized, FSH and LH fall to low levels and the corpus luteum regresses. Decline of estrogen and progesterone with corpus luteum regression results in menstruation as the uterine lining breaks down.

The loss of estrogen and progesterone from the corpus luteum at the end of one cycle stimulates the anterior pituitary to again secrete more FSH and LH, initiating a new female reproductive cycle. The old corpus luteum is replaced by fibrous tissue called the *corpus albicans*.

Endometrial Cycle

The uterine endometrium responds to ovarian hormone stimulation with cyclic changes. Three phases mark the changes in the endometrium: the proliferative, secretory, and menstrual.

PROLIFERATIVE PHASE

The proliferative phase occurs as the ovum matures and is released during the first half of the ovarian cycle. After completion of a menstrual period the endometrium is very thin. The basal layer of endometrial cells remains after menstruation. These cells multiply to form new endometrial epithelium and endometrial glands under the stimulation of estrogen secreted by the maturing ovarian follicles. Endometrial spiral arteries and endometrial veins elongate to accompany thickening of the functional endometrial layer and nourish the proliferating cells. As ovulation approaches, the endometrial glands secrete thin, stringy mucus that aids entry of sperm into the uterus.

SECRETORY PHASE

The secretory phase occurs during the last half of the ovarian cycle as the uterus is prepared to receive a fertilized ovum. The endometrium continues to thicken under the influence of estrogen and progesterone from the corpus luteum, reaching its maximum thickness of 5 to 6 mm. The blood vessels and endometrial glands become twisted and dilated.

Progesterone from the corpus luteum causes the thick endometrium to secrete substances to nourish a fertilized ovum. Large quantities of glycogen, proteins, lipids, and minerals are stored within the endometrium, awaiting arrival of the ovum.

MENSTRUAL PHASE

If fertilization does not occur, the corpus luteum regresses and its production of estrogen and progesterone falls. About 2 days before the onset of menstruation, vasospasm of the endometrial blood vessels causes the endometrium to become ischemic and necrotic. The necrotic areas of endometrium separate from the basal layers, resulting in the menstrual flow. The duration of the menstrual phase is about 5 days.

During a menstrual period, women lose about 40 ml of blood. Because of the recurrent loss of blood, many women are mildly anemic during their reproductive years, especially if their diets are low in iron.

Changes in Cervical Mucus

During most of the female reproductive cycle, the mucus of the cervix is scant, thick, and sticky. Just before ovulation, cervical mucus becomes thin, clear, and elastic to promote passage of sperm into the uterus and fallopian tube, where they can fertilize the ovum. *Spinnbarkeit* refers to the elasticity of cervical mucus. A woman may assess the elasticity of her cervical mucus to either avoid or promote conception (see Procedure 33-1).

✔ CHECK YOUR READING

13. Which ovarian structures secrete estrogen and progesterone during the female reproductive cycle?
14. What three ovarian phases occur during each female reproductive cycle?
15. How does the uterine endometrium change during a woman's reproductive cycle?
16. Why does the cervical mucus become thin, clear, and elastic around the time of ovulation?

THE FEMALE BREAST

Structure

The breasts, or mammary glands, are not directly functional in reproduction, but they secrete milk after childbirth to nourish the infant. The small, raised nipple is located at the center of each breast (Figure 4-8). The nipple is composed of sensitive erectile tissue and may respond to sexual stimulation. A larger circular areola surrounds the nipple. Both the nipple and areola are darker than surrounding skin. Montgomery's tubercles are sebaceous glands in the areola. They are inactive and not obvious except during pregnancy and lactation, when they enlarge and secrete a substance that keeps the nipple soft.

Within each breast are lobes of glandular tissue that secrete milk. These lobes are arranged in a pattern similar to spokes of a wheel around the hub. Between 15 and 20 of these lobes are arranged around and behind the nipple and areola. Fibrous tissue and fat in the breast support the glandular tissue, blood vessels, lymphatics, and nerves.

Alveoli are small sacs that contain acinar cells to secrete milk. The acinar cells extract the necessary substances from the mammary blood supply to manufacture milk when the breasts are properly stimulated by the anterior pituitary gland. Myoepithelial cells surround the alveoli to contract and eject the milk into the ductal system when signaled by secretion of the hormone oxytocin from the posterior pituitary gland.

The alveoli drain into lactiferous ducts, which connect to drain milk from all areas of the breast. The lactiferous ducts

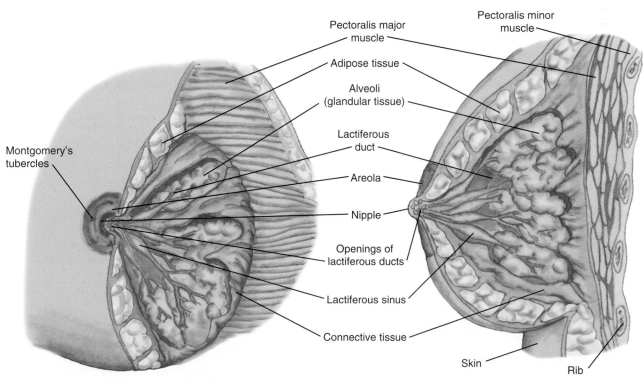

Figure 4-8 ■ Structures of the female breast.

become wider under the areola and are called *lactiferous sinuses* in this area. The lactiferous sinuses narrow again as they open to the outside in the nipple.

Function

The breasts are inactive until puberty, when rising estrogen levels stimulate growth of the glandular tissue. In addition, fat is deposited in the breasts, resulting in the mature female contour. The amount of fat is the major determinant of breast size; the amount of glandular tissue is similar for all mature women. Therefore breast size is unrelated to the amount of milk a woman can produce during lactation.

During pregnancy, high levels of estrogen and progesterone produced by the placenta stimulate growth of the alveoli and ductal system to prepare them for lactation. Prolactin secretion by the anterior pituitary gland stimulates milk production during pregnancy, but this effect is inhibited by estrogen and progesterone produced by the placenta. Inhibiting effects of estrogen and progesterone stop when the placenta is expelled after birth, and active milk production occurs in response to the infant's suckling while breastfeeding.

✓ CHECK YOUR READING

17. What is the function of Montgomery's tubercles?
18. How is a woman's breast size related to the amount of milk she can produce?
19. Why is milk not actively secreted during pregnancy?

MALE REPRODUCTIVE ANATOMY AND PHYSIOLOGY

External Male Reproductive Organs

The male has two external organs of reproduction: the penis and scrotum (Figure 4-9).

PENIS

The penis has two functions. As part of the urinary tract, it carries urine from the bladder to the exterior during urination. As a reproductive organ, the penis deposits semen into the female vagina during coitus.

The penis is composed mostly of erectile tissue, which is spongy tissue with many small spaces inside. The three areas of erectile tissue are the corpus spongiosum, which surrounds the urethra, and two columns of the corpus cavernosum on each side of the penis.

The penis is flaccid most of the time because the small spaces within the erectile tissue are collapsed. During sexual stimulation, arteries within the penis dilate and veins are partly occluded, trapping blood in the spongy tissue. Entrapment of blood within the penis causes erection and enables the man to penetrate the vagina during sexual intercourse.

The glans is the distal end of the penis. The urinary meatus is centered in the end of the glans. The loose skin of the prepuce, or foreskin, covers the glans. The prepuce may be removed during circumcision, a surgical procedure usually

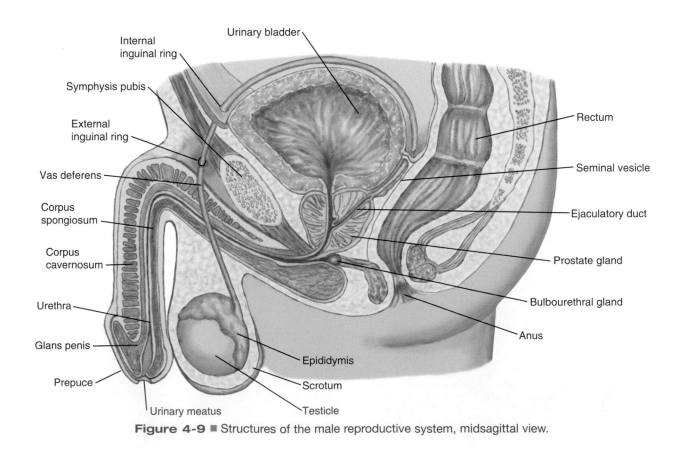

Figure 4-9 ■ Structures of the male reproductive system, midsagittal view.

performed during the newborn period, although it may be performed later. The glans is very sensitive to tactile stimulation, which adds to a man's sensation during coitus.

SCROTUM

The scrotum is a pouch of thin skin and muscle suspended behind the penis. The skin of the scrotum is somewhat darker than the surrounding skin and is covered with small ridges called *rugae*. The scrotum is divided internally by a septum. One of the male gonads (testicle) is contained within each pocket of the scrotum.

The scrotum's main purpose is to keep the testes cooler than the core body temperature. Formation of normal male sperm requires that the testes not be too warm. A cremaster muscle is attached to each testicle to either draw them closer to the body for warming or relax them, allowing them to move away from the body for cooling.

Internal Male Reproductive Organs

The functions of the male external and internal organs are summarized in Table 4-4.

TESTES

The male gonads, or testes, have two functions: (1) they serve as endocrine glands and (2) they produce male gametes, or sperm, also called *spermatozoa*. Androgens (male sex hormones) are the primary endocrine secretions of the testes. Androgens are produced by Leydig cells of the testes. The primary androgen produced by the testes is testosterone.

Unlike the female, who experiences a cyclic pattern of hormone secretion, the male secretes testosterone in a relatively even pattern. A feedback loop with the hypothalamus

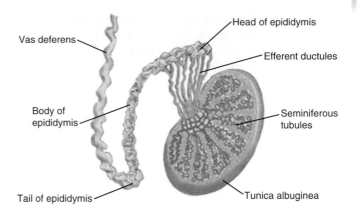

Figure 4-10 ■ Internal structures of the testis. Initial production of sperm begins within the tiny, coiled seminiferous tubules. Immature sperm pass from the seminiferous tubules to the epididymis and then to the vas deferens. During their passage through these structures, the sperm mature and acquire the ability to propel themselves after ejaculation.

and anterior pituitary stabilizes testosterone levels. A small amount of testosterone is converted to estrogen in the male and is necessary for sperm formation.

Spermatogenesis occurs within tiny coiled tubes, the seminiferous tubules of the testes (Figure 4-10). Leydig cells are interstitial cells that support the seminiferous tubules and secrete testosterone, which is necessary to form new cells that will mature into sperm. Sertoli cells within the seminiferous tubules respond to FSH secretion by nourishing and supporting sperm as they mature. Unlike the female, who has a lifetime supply of ova in her gonads at birth, the male does not begin producing sperm until puberty. The normal male produces new sperm throughout life, although production declines with age.

At ejaculation, about 40 to 250 million sperm are deposited in the vagina (Blackburn, 2003). This large number is needed for normal fertility, although a single sperm fertilizes the ovum. Only a few sperm ever reach the fallopian tube, where an ovum may be available for fertilization. When the first sperm penetrates the ovum, changes within the ovum prevent other sperm from also fertilizing it (see Chapter 6).

ACCESSORY DUCTS AND GLANDS

From the seminiferous tubules, sperm pass into the epididymis within the scrotum for storage and final maturation. In the epididymis, sperm develop the ability to be motile, although secretions within the epididymis inhibit actual motility until ejaculation occurs.

The epididymis empties into the vas deferens, where larger numbers of sperm are stored. The vas deferens then leads upward into the pelvis, then downward toward the penis through the internal and external inguinal rings. Within the pelvis the vas deferens joins the ejaculatory duct before connecting to the urethra.

Three glands—the seminal vesicles, prostate, and bulbourethral gland—secrete seminal fluids that carry sperm

TABLE 4-4 Functions of Male Reproductive and Accessory Organs

Organ	Function
Penis	1. Conduit for urine from bladder 2. Male organ of sexual intercourse
Scrotum	Housing of testes and maintenance of their temperature at a level cooler than the trunk of the body, thus promoting normal sperm formation
Testes	1. Endocrine glands that secrete the primary male hormone (testosterone) 2. Sperm formation
Seminiferous tubules	• Location of spermatogenesis within the testes
Epididymis	• Storage of some sperm • Final sperm maturation • The location where sperm develop the ability to be motile
Vas deferens	• Storage of sperm • Conduction of sperm from the epididymis to the urethra
Seminal vesicles, prostate, and bulbourethral glands	Secretion of seminal fluids that carry sperm and provide for the following: 1. Nourishment of sperm 2. Protection of sperm from the hostile acidic environment of the vagina 3. Enhancement of the motility of sperm 4. Washing of all sperm from the urethra

into the vagina during intercourse. The seminal fluid has four functions: (1) nourish the sperm, (2) protect the sperm from the hostile pH (acidic) environment of the vagina, (3) enhance the motility of the sperm, and (4) wash the sperm from the urethra so that the maximum number are deposited in the vagina.

✔ CHECK YOUR READING

20. What are the two functions of the penis?
21. What two types of erectile tissue are in the penis? What is their function?
22. Why is it important for the testes to be contained within the scrotum?
23. What are the two functions of the testes?

SUMMARY CONCEPTS

- Initial prenatal development of the reproductive organs is similar for both males and females. If a critical part of the Y chromosome is not present at conception, female reproductive structures will develop.
- During puberty the reproductive organs become fully functional, and secondary sex characteristics develop.
- Puberty begins about 6 months to 1 year earlier in girls than in boys, although the early growth spurt in girls makes it seem that they begin puberty much earlier than boys.
- Females are generally shorter than males at the completion of puberty because they begin their growth spurt at an earlier age and complete it more quickly than boys.
- Girls often do not ovulate in early menstrual cycles, although they can ovulate even before the first cycle. Therefore a girl can become pregnant before her first menstrual period if she is sexually active.
- The onset of puberty is more subtle in boys than in girls, beginning with growth of the testes and penis.
- Boys may have nocturnal emissions of seminal fluid, which may be distressing if the boy has not been educated that these events are normal and expected.
- At birth a girl has all the ova she will ever have. New ova are not formed after birth; almost all are depleted when the woman reaches the climacteric.
- The female reproductive cycle is often called the *menstrual cycle.* It includes changes in the anterior pituitary gland, ovaries, and uterine endometrium to prepare for a fertilized ovum. The character of cervical mucus also changes to encourage fertilization.
- Breast size is unrelated to glandular tissue or the quantity or quality of milk a woman can produce for her infant after childbirth. Breast size is primarily related to the amount of fat present.

- For normal sperm formation, a man's testes must be cooler than his core body temperature.
- Seminal fluids secreted by the seminal vesicles, prostate, and bulbourethral glands nourish and protect the sperm, enhance their motility, and ensure that most sperm are deposited in the vagina during sexual intercourse.

REFERENCES & READINGS

Blackburn, S.T. (2003). *Maternal, fetal, and neonatal physiology* (2nd ed.). Philadelphia: Saunders.

Carlson, B.M. (2004). *Human embryology and developmental biology* (3rd ed.). St. Louis: Mosby.

Cunningham, F.G., Gant, N.F., Leveno, K.J., Gilstrap, L.C., Hauth, J.C., & Wenstrom, K.D. (2001). *Williams obstetrics* (21st ed.). New York: McGraw-Hill.

Georges, J.M. (2000). Female genital and reproductive function. In L.C. Copstead & J. Banasik (Eds.), *Pathophysiology: Biological and behavioral perspectives* (2nd ed., pp. 648-666). Philadelphia: Saunders.

Guyton, A.C., & Hall, J.E. (2000). *Textbook of medical physiology* (10th ed.). Philadelphia: Saunders.

Jones, E.E., & DeCherney, A.H. (2003a). Fertilization, pregnancy, and lactation. In W.F. Boron & E.L. Boulpaep (Eds.), *Medical physiology: A cellular and molecular approach* (pp. 1167-1189). Philadelphia: Saunders.

Jones, E.E., & DeCherney, A.H. (2003b). The female reproductive system. In W.F. Boron & E.L. Boulpaep (Eds.), *Medical physiology: A cellular and molecular approach* (pp. 1141-1165). Philadelphia: Saunders.

Jones, E.E., & DeCherney, A.H. (2003c). The male reproductive system. In W.F. Boron & E.L. Boulpaep (Eds.), *Medical physiology: A cellular and molecular approach* (pp. 1122-1140). Philadelphia: Saunders.

Kim, M.H. (2000). Secondary amenorrhea. In F.P. Zuspan & E.J. Quilligan (Eds.), *Current therapy in obstetrics and gynecology* (5th ed., pp. 146-150). Philadelphia: Saunders.

Mikkelsen, D., & Cagle, C.S. (2000). Male genital and reproductive function. In L.C. Copstead & J. Banasik (Eds.), *Pathophysiology: Biological and behavioral perspectives* (2nd ed., pp. 708-725). Philadelphia: Saunders.

Moore, K.L., & Persaud, T.V.N. (2003). *The developing human* (7th ed.). Philadelphia: Saunders.

Needlman, R.D. (2004). Growth and development: Adolescence. In R.E. Behrman, R.M. Kliegman, & H.B. Jenson (Eds.), *Nelson textbook of pediatrics* (17th ed., pp. 53-58). Philadelphia: Saunders.

Riddick, D.H. (2000). Primary amenorrhea. In F.P. Zuspan & E.J. Quilligan (Eds.), *Current therapy in obstetrics and gynecology* (5th ed., pp. 143-146). Philadelphia: Saunders.

Toot, P.J., & Lu, J.K.H. (2004). Female reproductive physiology. In N.F. Hacker, J.G. Moore, & J.C. Gambone (Eds.), *Essentials of obstetrics and gynecology* (4th ed., pp. 33-45). Philadelphia: Saunders.

CHAPTER 5

Hereditary and Environmental Influences on Childbearing

OBJECTIVES

After studying this chapter, you should be able to:

1. Describe the structure and function of normal human genes and chromosomes.
2. Give examples of ways to study genes and chromosomes.
3. Explain some of the benefits and ethical implications of the Human Genome Project.
4. Describe the characteristics of single gene traits and their transmission from parent to child.
5. Relate chromosomal abnormalities to spontaneous abortion and birth defects in the infant.
6. Explain characteristics of multifactorial birth defects.
7. Identify environmental factors that can interfere with prenatal development and ways to prevent or reduce their effects.
8. Describe the process of genetic counseling.
9. Explain the role of the nurse in caring for individuals or families with concerns about birth defects.

Go to your Student CD-ROM for Review Questions keyed to these Objectives.

DEFINITIONS

Allele An alternate form of a gene.

Autosome Any of the 22 pairs of chromosomes other than the sex chromosomes.

Birth Defect An abnormality of structure, function, or body metabolism present at birth that results in physical or mental disability or is fatal (March of Dimes Birth Defects Foundation, 2004a).

Chromosomes Organization of DNA of specific genes into strings within the cell nucleus.

Congenital Present at birth.

Diploid Having a pair of chromosomes that represents one copy of every chromosome from each parent; the number of chromosomes (46 in humans) normally present in body cells other than gametes.

Familial Presence of a trait or condition in a family more often than would be expected by chance alone.

Gamete Reproductive cell or germ cell; in the female an ovum and in the male a spermatozoon.

Gene Segment of DNA that directs the production of a specific product needed for body structure or function.

Genetic Pertaining to the genes or chromosomes.

Genotype Genetic makeup of an individual.

Haploid Having one copy of a chromosome from each pair (23 in humans, or half the diploid number); normal for gametes.

Heterozygous Having two different alleles for a genetic trait.

Homologous Chromosomes that pair during meiosis, one received from the person's mother and one from the father.

Homozygous Having two identical alleles for a genetic trait.

Karyotype A display of a cell's chromosomes, arranged from largest to smallest pairs.

Monosomy Presence of only one of a chromosome pair in every body cell.

Mutation Alteration in DNA sequence in a gene, usually one that adversely affects its function.

Pedigree A graphic representation of a family's medical and hereditary history and the relationships among the family members (also called a *genogram*).

D E F I N I T I O N S—cont'd

Phenotype The outward expression of a person's genetic makeup; observed characteristics produced by the interaction of genes and environment.

Polymorphism Alternate form of a gene found in the population at a frequency greater than 1%.

Polyploidy Having additional full sets of chromosomes, such as 69 (triploidy) or 92 (tetraploidy).

Sex Chromosome The X or Y chromosome; females have two X chromosomes and males have one X and one Y chromosome.

Somatic Cells Body cells other than the gametes, or germ cells.

Teratogen An environmental agent that can cause defects in a developing baby during pregnancy.

Translocation Exchange of genetic material between nonhomologous chromosomes.

Trisomy Presence of three copies of a chromosome in each body cell.

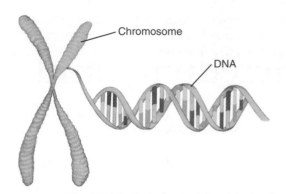

Figure 5-1 ■ The DNA helix is the building block of genes and chromosomes.

Hereditary and environmental forces shape a person's development from before conception until death. As people learn more about genes and their influences on the body's function, they are discovering that genes have more influence on health and disease than was previously thought. The nurse needs a basic knowledge of these forces to better understand disorders evident at birth and those that develop later in life. This chapter reviews the basics of hereditary influences on development and the impact of environmental factors in causing birth defects. The nursing role in relation to genetic knowledge is also discussed.

HEREDITARY INFLUENCES

Hereditary influences on development result from the directions for cellular functions provided by genes that constitute the 46 chromosomes in every somatic cell. Disorders can result if too much or too little genetic material is present in the cells and if one or more genes are abnormal and provide incorrect directions.

Structure of Genes and Chromosomes

A review of the structure of genes and chromosomes aids in understanding the reasons for the occurrence of disorders. Chromosomes are composed of genes that in turn are composed of deoxyribonucleic acid, or DNA (Figure 5-1).

DEOXYRIBONUCLEIC ACID

DNA is the building block of genes and chromosomes. Its three units are (1) a sugar (deoxyribose), (2) a phosphate group, and (3) one of four nitrogen bases (adenine, thymine, guanine, and cytosine).

DNA resembles a spiral ladder, with a sugar and a phosphate group forming each side of the ladder and a pair of nitrogen bases forming each rung. The four bases of the DNA molecule pair in a fixed way, allowing the DNA to be accurately duplicated during each cell division.

■ Adenine pairs with thymine.
■ Guanine pairs with cytosine.

The DNA also directs manufacture of proteins needed for cell function. The sequence of bases within the DNA determines which amino acids will be assembled to form a protein and the order in which they will be assembled for cell processes. Some proteins form the structure of body cells, whereas others are enzymes that control metabolic processes within the cell. If the sequence of nitrogen bases in the DNA is incorrect or some bases are missing or added in critical places, a defect in body structure or function may result.

Bases are arranged in groups of three called *codons* for translation into a specific amino acid in the cell. For example, a triplet base codon may consist of the bases GCC (guanine, cytosine, cytosine), which tells the cell to produce the amino acid alanine. Other codons, known as *stop codons*, signal the end of a gene sequence.

GENES

A gene is a segment of DNA that directs the production of a specific product needed for body structure or function. Humans have between 30,000 and 40,000 genes, fewer than previous estimates ranging from 50,000 to 140,000 (Guyton & Hall, 2000; March of Dimes, 2004a; National Human Genome Research Institute, 2004). Some genes are active only during prenatal life; others become functional at various times after birth.

Genes that code for the same trait often have two or more alternate forms, or alleles. Familiar examples of alleles are the ABO blood types. Normal alleles provide genetic variation and sometimes a biologic advantage. If an allele occurs at least 1% of the time in the population, it is called a *polymorphism*.

Some changed gene forms, or mutations, may be harmless, but many are harmful, such as those that cause the production of abnormal hemoglobin in sickle cell disease. Mutations may cause harm by the following actions:

- Substituting incorrect bases for the normal bases
- Interrupting the normal gene sequence or stopping it prematurely
- Duplicating some bases or entire gene sequences
- Adding or subtracting some bases within those making up a gene's sequence of bases, which will alter the amino acids it causes to be assembled

A mutation may occur in gametes or somatic cells. If the mutation occurs in a gamete, the mutation can be transmitted from one generation to the next. Mutations occurring in somatic cells are often associated with malignant change, but they are not transmitted from generation to generation.

Genes are too small to be seen under a microscope, but they can be studied in several ways:

- By measuring the products that they direct cells to produce, such as an enzyme or other substance
- By directly studying the gene's DNA
- By analyzing the gene's close association (linkage) with another gene that can be studied in one of the previous two ways

The tissue used for study of a gene depends on where the gene product is present in the body and the available technology. These tissues may include blood, skin cells, hair follicles, and fetal cells from the amniotic fluid or chorionic villi.

Genes that can be identified by direct analysis of DNA can be studied in any cells containing a nucleus, even if the gene product is not present in that tissue. Although not always used, DNA analysis of the blastomere (eight-cell stage of prenatal development) can be used to select embryos to be implanted in the uterus after in vitro fertilization. This prevents implantation of embryos with a specific gene defect or common chromosome defects.

The Human Genome Project is an international effort begun in 1990 to identify all genes contained in the 46 human chromosomes. The full sequence of human genes was completed in April, 2003 (National Human Genome Research Institute, 2004). Information gained from this project may allow advances such as the following:

- Performing genetic testing to determine the risk for a disorder or the actual or probable presence of the disorder
- Basing reproductive decisions on more accurate and specific information than has previously been available
- Identifying genetic susceptibility to a disorder so that interventions to reduce risk can be instituted
- Using gene therapy to modify a defective gene
- Modifying therapy such as medication based on an individual's genetic code or the genetic makeup of tumor cells

The explosion of knowledge about the genetic basis for many diseases raises many legal and ethical issues for which we

TABLE 5-1 Ethical Issues Created by Greater Genetic Knowledge

- Should testing be offered for a genetic disease for which no treatment is available? What if the disease is fatal? Should testing be required if a person may carry a diagnosable disorder that they might pass on to their children, even if they do not want the test?

  Huntington's disease is an example of a genetic disease that can be diagnosed. It has serious effects, with a fatal outcome during midlife. Should testing be offered? Should it be required before the person is allowed to reproduce?

- Who should own and control genetic information? Does an insurer have the right to a person's genetic information to assess risk and therefore set more accurate rates? Or is this information private? Should this information be disregarded for everyone when insurance rates are set?

  Geneticists may have the ability to identify conditions that a person will develop in the future even if the problem is not present. Examples include hypertension, diabetes, and heart disease. If an insurance company knows that the person will develop this disorder, rates would be higher or coverage would be denied. If an employer has this information, the person might not be hired to avoid raising insurance costs for the company. Yet the reverse could be true. Genetic testing might prove that a person *would not* develop a disorder, thereby gaining them lower rates. If genetic testing before being insured is not permitted, is it right that all persons insured by a company subsidize those who develop disorders that could have been determined before being insured by paying higher rates?

- How should issues of racial or ethnic identification be handled? What if a person's parentage is not what he or she has always thought?

  Discoveries in the process of genetic analysis may determine that a person is not of the racial identity previously thought, or a person might discover that a parent is not the biologic parent. What should be done if information of this nature is uncovered? What are possible implications for self-image and identity? How might other members of the family be involved in the unexpected discovery?

do not yet have answers (Table 5-1). As our knowledge base grows, new issues such as the following are likely to emerge:

- Genetic information has implications for others in the person's family, raising privacy issues.
- Knowledge about a genetic disorder often precedes knowledge about treatment of the disorder.
- Identification of genetic problems could lead to poor self-esteem, guilt, and excessive caution, or, conversely, a reckless lifestyle.
- Presymptomatic identification of genetically influenced illness would be a source of long-term anxiety.
- Genetic knowledge could affect one's choice of a partner.
- Discrimination may occur, such as the imposition of high insurance rates, the denial of insurance coverage, or the decision by an employer not to hire a qualified person who has a greater chance of genetically influenced illness.

CHROMOSOMES

Genes are organized in 46 paired chromosomes in the nucleus of somatic cells. A gene can be likened to a single bead; a chromosome is like a string of beads. Each chromosome is composed of varying numbers, often several thousand, genes. A total of 22 chromosome pairs are autosomes, and the twenty-third pairs are composed of the sex chromosomes. Added, missing, and structurally abnormal chromosomes are usually harmful.

Mature gametes have half the chromosomes (23) of other body cells. One chromosome from each pair is distributed randomly in the gametes, allowing variation of genetic traits among people. When the ovum and sperm unite at conception, the total is restored to 46 paired chromosomes.

Cells for chromosomal analysis must have a nucleus and be living. Chromosomes can be studied using any of several types of cells: white blood cells, skin fibroblasts, bone marrow cells, and fetal cells from the chorionic villi of the placenta or suspended in amniotic fluid.

Unlike genes, chromosomes can be seen under the microscope but only during cell division. Specimens must be obtained and preserved carefully to provide enough living cells for chromosomal analysis. Temperature extremes, blood clotting, and the addition of improper preservatives can kill the cells and render them useless for analysis.

Chromosomes look jumbled before they are arranged into a karyotype (Figure 5-2). Systematic study is possible using photography or computer imaging of prepared chromosomes and then arranging them into a karyotype (Figure 5-3). In a karyotype, autosomal pairs are arranged from largest to smallest. Letters describe groups of similar size and appearance. Sex chromosomes usually are arranged in a separate group.

A person's karyotype is abbreviated by a combination of numbers and letters. A number describes the total number of chromosomes, followed by either an XX to indicate the sex chromosomes are female or XY to indicate they are male. Therefore the chromosome complement is abbreviated 46,XX for a normal female and 46,XY for a normal male. If the chromosome number is abnormal, such as that in Down syndrome, which has an extra 21 chromosome, an added abbreviation indicates the abnormality: 47 (total number of chromosomes), XY (male), +21 (the number of the extra chromosome). Other abbreviations describe karyotypes with missing or structurally altered chromosomes.

Finer chromosome analysis makes use of fluorescent-labeled DNA probes that attach to specific chromosomes. This technique is called *fluorescent in-situ hybridization* (FISH) and permits testing for added, missing, or rearranged chromosome material that otherwise may not be visible microscopically. FISH analysis can be done rapidly because

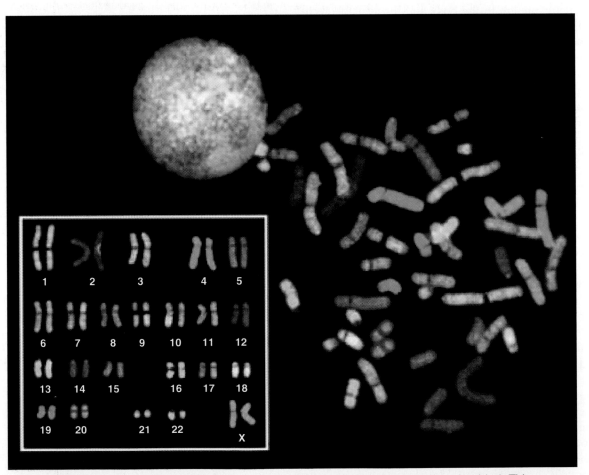

Figure 5-2 ■ Before arrangement in a karyotype, chromosomes appear jumbled. This photo is a spectral karyotype from a normal female. (From National Human Genome Research Institute. [2002]. Retrieved July 24, 2004, from www.genome.gov/Pages/Hyperion/DIR/VIP/Glossary/Illustration/Pdf/sky.pdf.)

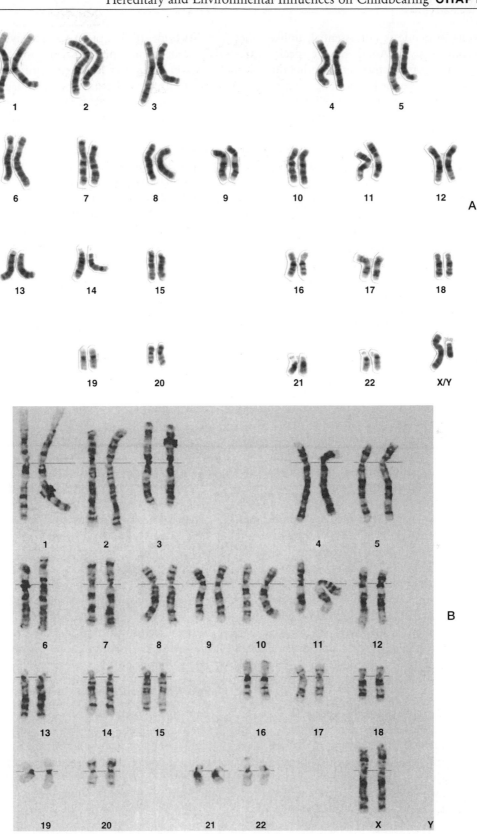

A

B

Figure 5-3 ■ Karyotypes of chromosomes that were stained, creating bands to distinguish each chromosome and identify missing or duplicated chromosome material. **A,** Normal male karyotype: 46,XY. **B,** Normal female karyotype: 46,XX. (**A** from National Human Genome Research Institute. [2002]. *Fact sheet: Karyotype.* Retrieved July 19, 2003, from www.genome.gov; **B** from Jorde, L.B., Carey, J.C., Bamshad, M.J., & White, R.L. [2003]. *Medical genetics* [3rd ed., p. 108]. St. Louis: Mosby.)

stimulation of cells to divide is not essential, unlike other types of chromosome analysis. Another more specific chromosome analysis is the comparative genomic hybridization used to identify losses or duplications of specific chromosome regions, which often occur in tumor cells (Jorde, Carey, Bamshad, & White, 2003). Spectral karyotyping colors or "paints" each chromosome differently to identify rearrangements, losses, or gains of chromosome material (Jorde, et al., 2003; National Human Genome Research Institute, 2004).

✔ CHECK YOUR READING

1. What is the relationship among DNA, genes, and chromosomes?
2. Can genes be studied by examining them under a microscope? Why or why not? What methods are used to study them?
3. Why do cell specimens for chromosomal analysis have to be alive, regardless of the tissue used?
4. What do each of these abbreviations mean: 46,XY and 46,XX? How are chromosome abnormalities described?

Transmission of Traits by Single Genes

Inherited characteristics are passed from parent to child by the genes in each chromosome. These traits are classified according to whether they are dominant (strong) or recessive (weak) and whether the gene is located on one of the autosome pairs or on the sex chromosomes. Both normal and abnormal hereditary characteristics are transmitted by these mechanisms.

Because humans have pairs of matched chromosomes, excepting the sex chromosomes in the male, they have one allele for a gene at the same location on each member of the chromosome pair. The paired alleles may be identical (homozygous) or different (heterozygous).

Some genes, both normal and abnormal, occur more frequently in certain groups than in the population as a whole. For example, the gene that causes Tay-Sachs disease is carried by approximately 1 of every 30 (3.3%) U.S. Jews, a rate approximately 100 times its occurrence in the general population. Persons of French-Canadian ancestry and members of the Cajun population in Louisiana are similarly at risk (March of Dimes, 2004d). Because the abnormal gene occurs more frequently in these groups, their incidence of Tay-Sachs disease is also higher. Other disorders that are more common in certain ethnic groups are cystic fibrosis, which occurs primarily in whites of northern European descent, and sickle cell disease, which occurs more frequently in people of African descent.

DOMINANCE

Dominance describes the way a person's genetic composition is translated into the phenotype, or observable characteristics. In the case of a dominant gene, one copy is enough to cause the trait to be expressed. For example, in the ABO blood system, genes for types A and B are dominant. Therefore a single copy of either of these genes is enough for it to be expressed in the person's blood type.

Two identical copies of a recessive gene are required for the trait to be expressed. The gene for blood type O is recessive. Laboratory testing identifies a person's blood type as O only if that person receives a gene for blood type O from both parents. If the person receives a gene for type O from one parent and type A from the other parent, blood type A is expressed in laboratory blood typing.

On the basis of dominant and recessive forms of a gene, a person with type A blood can have one of two possible combinations of gene alleles:

- Two type A alleles
- One type A allele and one type O allele

Other alleles are equally dominant. The person who receives a gene for blood type A from one parent and type B from the other will have type AB blood because both alleles are equally dominant and expressed in blood typing.

Dominance and recessiveness are relative qualities for many genes. Some people with a single copy of an abnormal recessive gene (carriers) may have a lower than normal level of the gene product (for example, an enzyme) that can be detected by biochemical methods. These people often do not have overt disease because the normal copy of the gene produces enough of the required product to allow normal or near-normal function.

CHROMOSOME LOCATION

Genes located on autosomes are either autosomal dominant or autosomal recessive, depending on the number of identical copies of the gene needed to produce the trait. However, genes located on the X chromosome are paired only in females, because males have one X and one Y chromosome.

A female with an abnormal recessive gene on one of her X chromosomes usually has a normal gene on the other X chromosome that compensates and maintains relatively normal function. However, the male is at a disadvantage if his only X chromosome has an abnormal gene. The male has no compensating normal gene because his other sex chromosome is a Y. The abnormal gene is expressed in the male because it is unopposed by a normal gene.

Patterns of Single Gene Inheritance

Three major patterns of single gene inheritance are (1) autosomal dominant, (2) autosomal recessive, and (3) X-linked (Table 5-2). Few genes are found on the Y chromosome, primarily the one that causes the embryo to differentiate into a male. Because very few Y-linked traits have been identified, these will not be discussed.

Although the word *pedigree* is widely used among genetic professionals, the nurse may need to interpret it for the client. Be cautious when referring to the illustration of a family's genetic history as a *pedigree,* because some associate the word only with animals. For example, when taking a genetic family history, the nurse might say, "I'm going to use several symbols to depict your family tree and its members' health histories. This diagram is called a *genogram,* but it's also often called a *pedigree.*"

TABLE 5-2 Single-Gene Traits

Genogram (Pedigree) Symbols

A genogram symbolically represents a family's medical history and the relationships of its members to one another. It helps identify patterns of inheritance that may help distinguish one type of disorder from another.

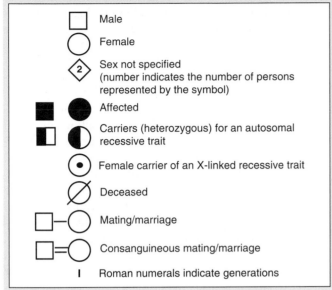

- ☐ Male
- ○ Female
- ◇ Sex not specified (number indicates the number of persons represented by the symbol)
- ■ ● Affected
- ◨ ◐ Carriers (heterozygous) for an autosomal recessive trait
- ⊙ Female carrier of an X-linked recessive trait
- ⊘ Deceased
- ☐—○ Mating/marriage
- ☐=○ Consanguineous mating/marriage
- I Roman numerals indicate generations

Autosomal Recessive

Characteristics

Two autosomal recessive genes are required to produce the trait.
Males and females are equally likely to have the trait.
There is often no prior family history of the disorder before the first affected child.
If more than one family member is affected, they are usually full siblings.
Consanguinity (close blood relationship) of the parents increases the risk for the disorder.
Disorders are more likely to occur in groups isolated by geography, culture, religion, or other factors.
Some autosomal recessive disorders are more common in specific ethnic groups.

Transmission of Trait from Parent to Child

Unaffected parents are carriers of the abnormal autosomal recessive trait.
Children of carriers have a 25% (1 in 4) chance for receiving both copies of the defective gene and thus having the disorder.
Children of carriers have a 50% (1 in 2) chance of receiving one copy of the gene and being carriers like the parents.
Children of carriers have a 25% (1 in 4) chance of receiving both copies of the normal gene. They are neither carriers nor affected.

Examples

Normal traits: Blood group O; Rh-negative blood factor.
Abnormal traits: Tay-Sachs disease; sickle cell disease; cystic fibrosis.

Genogram

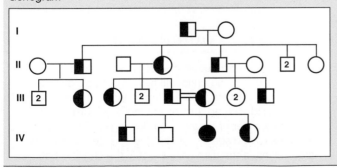

Autosomal Dominant

Characteristics

A single copy of the gene is enough to produce the trait.
Males and females are equally likely to have the trait.
Often appears in every generation of a family, although family members having the trait may have widely varying manifestations of it.
May have multiple and seemingly unrelated effects on body structure and function.

Transmission of Trait from Parent to Child

A parent with the trait has a 50% (1 in 2) chance of passing the trait to the child.
The trait may arise as a new mutation from an unaffected parent. The child who receives the mutated gene can then transmit it to future generations.

Examples

Normal traits: Blood groups A and B; Rh-positive blood factor.
Abnormal traits: Huntington's disease; neurofibromatosis.

Genogram

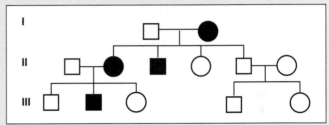

X-Linked Recessive

Characteristics

Although recessive, only one copy of the gene is needed to cause the disorder in the male, who does not have a compensating X without the trait.
Males are affected, with rare exceptions.
Females are carriers of the trait but not usually adversely affected.
Affected males are related to one another through carrier females.
Affected males do not transmit the trait to their sons.

Transmission of Trait from Parent to Child

Males who have the disorder transmit the gene to 100% of their daughters and none of their sons.
Sons of carrier females have a 50% (1 in 2) chance of being affected. They also have a 50% chance of being unaffected.
Daughters of carrier females have a 50% (1 in 2) chance of being carriers like their mothers. They also have a 50% chance of being neither affected nor carriers.
A new X-linked recessive gene also may arise by mutation.

Examples

Colorblindness; Duchenne muscular dystrophy; hemophilia A.

Genogram

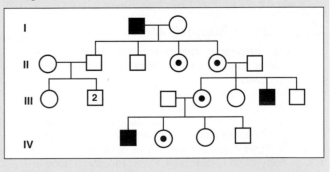

Single gene traits have mathematically predictable and fixed rates of occurrence. For example, if a couple has a child with an autosomal recessive disorder, the risk that future children will have the same disorder is one in four (25%) at every conception. The risk is the same at every conception, regardless of how many of a couple's children have been affected.

AUTOSOMAL DOMINANT TRAITS

An autosomal dominant trait is produced by a dominant gene on a nonsex chromosome. The expression of abnormal autosomal dominant genes may result in multiple and seemingly unrelated effects in the person. The gene's effects also may vary substantially in severity, leading a family to believe incorrectly that a trait skips a generation. A careful physical examination may reveal subtle evidence of the trait in each generation. In other cases some people may carry the dominant gene but have no apparent expression of it in their physical makeup.

In some autosomal dominant disorders, such as Huntington's disease, those with the gene will always have the disease if they live to the age at which the disorder becomes apparent. In other disorders, only a portion of those carrying the gene ever exhibit the disease.

New mutations account for the introduction of abnormal autosomal dominant traits into a family that has no history of the disorder. In this case parents of the child are normal because their body cells do not have the altered gene. Men over age 40 who father children are more likely to have offspring with a new autosomal dominant mutation (Jorde, et al., 2003; Nussbaum, McInnes, & Willard, 2004).

The person who is affected with an autosomal dominant disorder is usually heterozygous for the gene; that is, the person has a normal gene on one chromosome and an abnormal gene on the other chromosome of the pair. Occasionally a person receives two copies of the same abnormal autosomal dominant gene. Such an individual is usually much more severely affected than someone with only one copy.

AUTOSOMAL RECESSIVE TRAITS

An autosomal recessive trait occurs if a person receives two copies of a recessive gene carried on an autosome. Everyone is estimated to carry abnormal autosomal recessive genes

without manifesting the disorder because they have a compensating normal gene (Hoyme, 2004a; Jorde, et al., 2003; Kenner, 2003; Simpson & Elias, 2003). Because the probability that two unrelated people share even one of the same abnormal genes is low, the incidence of autosomal recessive diseases is relatively low in the general population.

Situations that increase the likelihood that two parents share the same abnormal autosomal recessive gene are the following:

- Consanguinity (blood relationship of the parents)—Blood relatives have more genes in common, including abnormal ones.
- Groups that are isolated by culture, geography, religion, or other factors—The isolation allows abnormal genes to become concentrated over the years and occur at a greater frequency than in more diverse groups.

Many autosomal recessive disorders are severe, and affected persons may not live long enough to reproduce. Two notable exceptions are phenylketonuria (PKU) and cystic fibrosis. Improved care of people with these disorders has allowed them to live into the reproductive years. If one member of the couple has the autosomal recessive disorder, all their children will be carriers. Their risk for having similarly affected children is also higher, depending on the prevalence of the abnormal gene in the general population and the likelihood that their mate is a carrier.

X-LINKED TRAITS

X-linked recessive traits are more common than X-linked dominant traits and are the only X-linked pattern discussed in this chapter. Gender differences in the occurrence of X-linked recessive traits and the relationship of affected males to one another are important factors that distinguish these disorders from autosomal dominant and recessive disorders. In general, males are the only ones to show full effects of an X-linked recessive disorder because their only X chromosome has the abnormal gene on it. Females can show the full disorder in two uncommon circumstances:

- If a female has a single X chromosome (Turner's syndrome)
- If a female child is born to an affected father and a carrier mother

X-linked recessive disorders can be relatively mild, such as colorblindness, or they may be severe, such as hemophilia. In addition, those having the disorder may be affected with varying degrees of severity.

CRITICAL TO REMEMBER

Single Gene Abnormalities

- A person affected with an autosomal dominant disorder has a 50% chance of transmitting the disorder to each biologic child.
- Two healthy parents who carry the same abnormal autosomal recessive gene have a 25% chance of having a child affected with the disorder caused by this gene.
- Parental consanguinity increases the risk for having a child with an autosomal recessive disorder.
- One copy of an abnormal X-linked recessive gene is enough to produce the disorder in a male.
- Abnormal genes can arise as new mutations. If these mutations are in the gametes, they are transmitted to future generations.

CHECK YOUR READING

5. If a parent has an autosomal dominant disorder, what is the chance that the child will have the same disorder?
6. Why would parents who are first cousins be more likely to have a child with an autosomal recessive disorder?
7. If each member of a couple carries a gene for an autosomal recessive disorder, what is the chance that the children will have the disorder? What is the chance that the children will be carriers? What is the chance that the children will not receive the abnormal gene from either parent?

8. Why are males more often affected with X-linked recessive disorders? If a female carries an X-linked recessive disorder such as hemophilia, what are the chances that her sons will have the disorder? What is the chance that her daughters will be carriers?

Chromosomal Abnormalities

Chromosomal abnormalities can be numerical or structural. They are quite common (50% or more) in the embryo or fetus that is spontaneously aborted (miscarried). Chromosomal abnormalities often cause major defects because they involve deletion or duplication of many genes.

NUMERICAL ABNORMALITIES

Numerical chromosomal abnormalities involve added or missing single chromosomes or multiple sets of chromosomes. Trisomy and monosomy are numerical abnormalities of single chromosomes. The term *polyploidy* refers to abnormalities involving full sets of chromosomes.

TRISOMY. A trisomy exists when each body cell contains an extra copy of one chromosome, bringing the total number to 47 (Figure 5-4). Each chromosome is normal, but there are too many in each somatic cell. The most common trisomy is Down syndrome, or trisomy 21, in which three

copies of chromosome 21 are in each somatic cell. Trisomies of chromosomes 13 and 18 are less common and have more severe effects. The incidence of bearing children with trisomies increases with maternal age, so most women who are 35 years old or older and become pregnant are offered prenatal diagnosis to determine whether the fetus has Down syndrome or another trisomy.

CRITICAL TO REMEMBER

Chromosome Abnormalities

Chromosome abnormalities are either numerical or structural.

Numerical	Structural
Entire single chromosome added (trisomy)	Part of a chromosome missing or added
Entire single chromosome missing (monosomy)	Rearrangements of material within chromosome(s)
One or more added sets of chromosomes, resulting in cells containing 69 (triploidy) or 92 (tetraploidy) chromosomes	Two chromosomes that adhere to each other
	Fragility of a specific site, such as on the X chromosome ("fragile X syndrome")

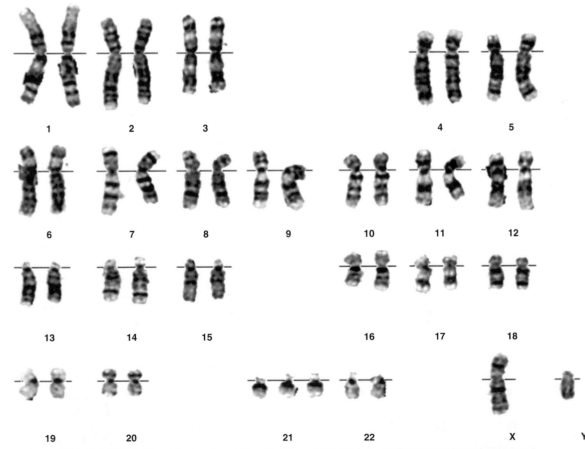

Figure 5-4 ■ Karyotype of a male with trisomy 21 (Down syndrome: 47,XY, +21). (From Jorde, L.B., Carey, J.C., Bamshad, M.J., & White, R.L. [2003]. *Medical genetics* [3rd ed., p. 114]. St. Louis: Mosby.)

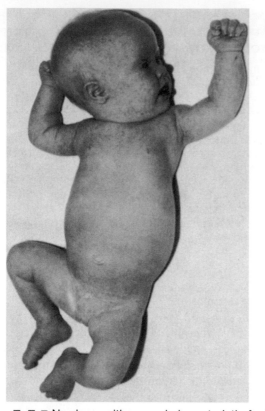

Figure 5-5 ■ Newborn with several characteristic features of Down syndrome. Note that the infant has less flexion of her extremities and a flat face and occiput. (From Jones, K.L. [1997]. *Smith's recognizable patterns of human malformation* [5th ed., p. 11]. Philadelphia: Saunders.)

Infants with Down syndrome have characteristic features that are usually noticed at birth (Figure 5-5). Chromosomal analysis is performed during the neonatal period to confirm the diagnosis and determine whether Down syndrome is caused by trisomy 21 or a rarer chromosomal anomaly that involves a structural rather than a numerical abnormality of chromosome 21.

Children with Down syndrome reach developmental milestones more slowly than normal children. They are mentally retarded, although the severity varies, just as intelligence varies in the general population. Early intervention programs and regular medical care help these children reach their full ability and manage the physical problems associated with Down syndrome.

MONOSOMY. A monosomy exists when each body cell has a missing chromosome, with a total number of 45. The only monosomy compatible with postnatal life is Turner's syndrome, or monosomy X (Figure 5-6). Over 99% of conceptions with the 45, XO karyotype are lost in spontaneous abortion (Jorde, et al., 2003). The person with Turner's syndrome has a single X chromosome and is always female.

Large cystic masses on either side of the neck (cystic hygromas) may be found on routine ultrasound exam and lead to the diagnosis. Liveborn infants have excess skin around the neck left from the hygromas and edema that is most noticeable in the hands and feet during infancy. If Turner's syndrome is not identified and treated during infancy or childhood, an affected girl will remain very short and will not have menstrual periods or develop secondary sex characteristics. Children with Turner's syndrome usually have

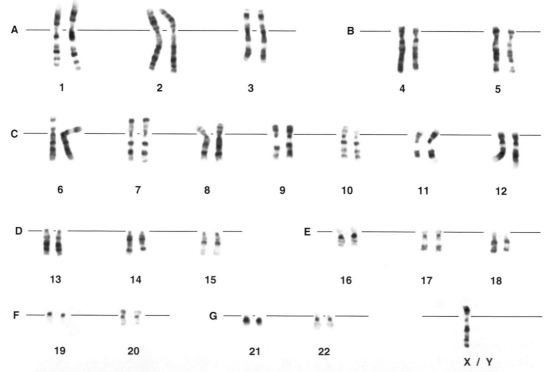

Figure 5-6 ■ Karyotype of a female with monosomy X (Turner's syndrome: 45,X). (Courtesy Dr. Mary Jo Harrod, University of Texas Southwestern Medical Center.)

normal intelligence, although they may have difficulty with spatial relationships or the solving of visual problems such as reading a map. The girl may have a broad, shieldlike chest with widely spaced nipples. Her kidneys may be joined at their upper poles (horseshoe kidney), and coarctation of the aorta may require corrective surgery.

POLYPLOIDY. Polyploidy may occur when gametes do not halve their chromosome number during meiosis and retain both members of each pair or when two sperm fertilize an ovum simultaneously. The result is an embryo with one or more extra sets of chromosomes. The total number of chromosomes is a multiple of the haploid number of 23 (69 or 92 total chromosomes). Polyploidy usually results in an early spontaneous abortion but may occasionally be seen in a liveborn infant. This abnormality may be found in chorionic villus sampling (see Chapter 10) and may reflect an abnormality of the chorionic villi rather than the fetus.

Structural Abnormalities

Chromosomal abnormalities may involve the structure of one or more chromosomes. Part of a chromosome may be missing or added, or DNA within the chromosome may be rearranged. Some of these rearrangements are common harmless variations. Others are harmful because important

genetic material is lost or duplicated in the structural abnormality or the position of the genes in relation to other genes is altered so that normal function is not possible.

Another structural abnormality occurs when all or part of a chromosome is attached to another (translocation) (Figure 5-7). Many people with a translocation chromosomal abnormality are clinically normal because the total of their genetic material is normal or balanced. If a parent has a balanced translocation, the offspring may have completely normal chromosomes or a balanced translocation, as the parent has. However, the offspring may receive too much or too little chromosomal material and be spontaneously aborted or have birth defects.

Balanced translocations are often discovered when amniocentesis reveals a translocation in the fetus or during infertility evaluations if a history of recurrent spontaneous abortions is reported. Either balanced or unbalanced chromosomal translocations may occur spontaneously in the offspring of parents who have no translocation.

Fragile X syndrome is an X-linked chromosomal abnormality. The syndrome was so named because a site on the X chromosome demonstrates breaks and gaps when the cells are grown in a medium deficient in folic acid. The syndrome is now usually diagnosed by molecular DNA studies.

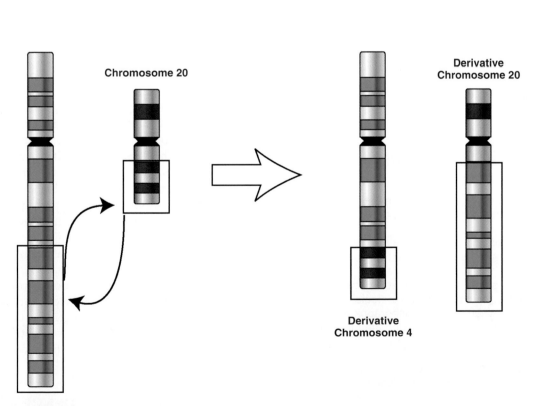

Before translocation

After translocation

Chromosome 20

Derivative Chromosome 20

Derivative Chromosome 4

Chromosome 4

Figure 5-7 ■ Illustration of a translocation of chromosome material between chromosomes 4 and 20. (From National Human Genome Research Institute [2003]. *Fact sheet: Translocation.* Retrieved July 19, 2003, from www.genome.gov/glossary.cfm.)

As in other X-linked traits, males are more severely affected than females, who have a compensating X chromosome that is usually normal. Fragile X syndrome is the most common inherited form of male mental retardation (Hall, 2004a).

✔ **CHECK YOUR READING**

9. What is a chromosomal trisomy? Describe a common trisomy.
10. What is a chromosomal monosomy? Which monosomy is compatible with life?
11. Why are structural chromosomal abnormalities often harmful?
12. What are the possible outcomes of the offspring of a parent who has a balanced chromosomal translocation?

MULTIFACTORIAL DISORDERS

Multifactorial disorders result from an interaction of genetic and environmental factors. The genetic tendency toward the disorder is modified by the environment. These interactions may either positively or negatively influence prenatal and postnatal development. For example, two embryos may have an equal genetic susceptibility for the development of a disorder such as spina bifida (open spine). However, the disorder will not occur unless an environment that favors its development, such as deficient maternal intake of folic acid, also exists.

Characteristics

Multifactorial birth defects are typically (1) present and detectable at birth and (2) isolated defects rather than defects that occur with unrelated abnormalities. However, a multifactorial defect may cause a secondary defect. For example, infants with spina bifida often have hydrocephalus (abnormal

⨆ **CRITICAL TO REMEMBER**

Multifactorial Birth Defects

Multifactorial defects are some of the most common birth defects encountered in maternity and pediatric nursing practice.

They are a result of interaction between a person's genetic susceptibility and environmental factors during prenatal development.

These are usually single, isolated defects, although the primary defect may cause secondary defects.

Some occur more often in certain geographic areas.

A greater risk of occurrence exists with the following:

• Several close relatives have the defect, whether mild or severe.
• One close relative has a severe form of the defect.
• The defect occurs in a child of the less frequently affected gender.

Infants who have several major or minor defects that are not directly related probably do not have a multifactorial defect but have another syndrome, such as a chromosomal abnormality.

collection of spinal fluid within the brain) as well. The hydrocephalus is not a separate defect but one that occurs because the primary defect—abnormal development of the spine and spinal cord—disrupts spinal fluid circulation, allowing the fluid to build up within the brain's ventricular system.

However, the infant who has defects other than those known to be associated with spina bifida probably does not have a multifactorial disorder. In this case the spina bifida is more likely to be part of a syndrome, such as a chromosome defect, that may pose a different risk for recurrence in a future child.

Multifactorial disorders are some of the most common birth defects that a maternal-child nurse encounters. Examples include the following:

■ Many heart defects
■ Neural tube defects such as anencephaly (absence of most of the brain and skull) and spina bifida
■ Cleft lip and cleft palate
■ Pyloric stenosis

Risk for Occurrence

Unlike single gene traits, multifactorial disorders are not associated with a fixed risk of occurrence or recurrence in a family. The risks are an average rather than a constant percentage. Factors that may affect the risk are as follows:

1. Number of affected close relatives—Risk increases as the number of affected close relatives (parent, full sibling, or child) increases.
2. Severity of the disorder in affected family members—For example, bilateral cleft lip is associated with a higher risk for recurrence in a close relative than is a unilateral cleft lip.
3. Sex of the affected person(s)—For example, pyloric stenosis occurs five times as often in males as in females. The couple who has a daughter with pyloric stenosis faces a higher risk for recurrence with future children because the genetic influence for development of the defect is greater if a female develops it.
4. Geographic location—The risk for some disorders, such as neural tube defects, is higher in some locations than others. Neural tube disorders have shown greater prevalence in some areas such as the Rio Grande Valley area in Texas.
5. Seasonal variations—Seasonal variations are noted with some multifactorial disorders.

If multifactorial disorders had no environmental component, the risk for occurrence and recurrence would be a precise percentage rather than a range. However, if no genetic component exists (if the disorder were totally related to environment), the ability to predict the risk for occurrence or recurrence would be minimal.

ENVIRONMENTAL INFLUENCES

Environment may positively influence prenatal development, such as good nutrition that supplies all necessary raw materials for fetal growth. However, some environmental influences are harmful, such as teratogens and mechanical forces that disrupt development.

Environmental influences on childbearing are those that are not known to have a genetic component. At one time the placenta was thought to be a shield against harmful agents within a pregnant woman's body. Now the fact that most agents can cross the placenta and affect the developing fetus is recognized.

Teratogens

Teratogens are agents in the fetal environment that either cause or increase the likelihood that a birth defect will occur. Some drugs have been definitely established as safe or harmful. With most agents, however, their potential for harming the fetus is not clear. Several factors make it difficult to establish the teratogenic potential of an agent:

1. Retrospective study—Investigators must rely on the mother's memory about substances she ingested or was exposed to during pregnancy. The conclusion that a specific agent is harmful and the ways in which it harms the fetus is possible only when many cases are collected in which the exposure history is similar and the birth defects are also similar.
2. Timing of exposure—Agents may be harmful at one stage of prenatal development but not at another. Exposure may be harmful but may vary with the prenatal development stage.
3. Different susceptibility of organ systems—Some agents affect only one fetal organ system, or they affect one system at one stage of development and another at a different stage of development.
4. Uncontrolled fetal exposure—Exposures cannot be controlled to eliminate extraneous agents or ensure a consistent dose. Interactions with other agents may reduce or compound the fetal effects. An agent that is toxic at one dose may have no apparent effect at another.
5. Placental transfer—Agents vary in their ability to cross the placenta.
6. Individual variations—Fetuses show varying susceptibility to harmful agents.
7. Nontransferability of animal studies—Results of animal studies cannot always be applied to humans. Agents that do not harm animal fetuses may damage the human embryo or fetus.
8. Risk for damage from an uncontrolled maternal disorder—Some maternal disorders, such as epilepsy or hypertension, may cause fetal damage if not controlled. A poorly controlled maternal disorder raises a question of whether the disorder itself or medication expected to control the disorder harms the fetus.

Teratogens typically cause more than one defect, which distinguishes teratogenic defects from multifactorial disorders. However, children affected by single gene and chromosome defects are also likely to have multiple defects. Therefore clinicians consider single gene disorders, chromosomal abnormalities, and effects of teratogenic agents when trying to diagnose an infant born with multiple anomalies.

BOX 5-1 Selected Environmental Substances Known or Thought to Harm the Fetus*

Alcohol
Aminoglycosides
Anticonvulsant agents
Antihyperlipidemic agents (statins)
Antineoplastic agents
Antithyroid drugs
Cocaine
Diethylstilbestrol (DES)
Folic acid antagonists
Infections
- Cytomegalovirus
- Herpes simplex virus
- Human immunodeficiency virus
- Rubella
- Syphilis
- Toxoplasmosis
- Varicella
Lithium
Mercury
Retinoic acid
Tetracycline
Tobacco
Warfarin

*Risks related to other drugs or additional substances are noted in Appendix B. The nurse should observe for new information about adverse fetal effects from these or other drugs that may be given during pregnancy.

Hundreds of individual agents are either known or suspected teratogens (Box 5-1). Types of teratogens include the following:

- Maternal infectious agents (for example, viruses, bacteria) that cross the placenta
- Drugs and other substances used by the woman (for example, therapeutic agents, illicit drugs, tobacco, alcohol)
- Pollutants, chemicals, and other substances to which the mother is exposed in her daily life
- Ionizing radiation
- Maternal hyperthermia
- Effects of maternal disorders such as diabetes mellitus and PKU

Theoretically, all or some of the risk to the developing fetus can be eliminated by avoiding exposure to the agent or changing the fetal environment in some way.

PREVENTING FETAL EXPOSURE

Ideally, prevention of exposure to harmful influences begins before conception because all major organ systems develop early in pregnancy, often before a woman realizes that she is pregnant. To avoid some agents such as alcohol and illicit drugs, some pregnant women must be committed to making substantial lifestyle changes.

INFECTIONS. Rubella immunization 28 days (1 month) before pregnancy virtually eliminates the risk that the mother will contract this infection, which can damage the fetus severely. If a woman becomes pregnant within 28 days after immunization, fetal risk is considered unlikely (American Academy of Pediatrics & American College of Obstetricians and Gynecologists, 2002; March of Dimes, 2002).

For infections that cannot be prevented by immunization, the nurse can counsel the woman to avoid situations in which acquiring the disease is more likely (see Chapters 26 and 30).

DRUGS AND OTHER SUBSTANCES. The United States Food and Drug Administration has established pregnancy categories for therapeutic drugs based on their potential to harm the fetus. The categories range from A through D and X. Class A drugs have no demonstrated fetal risk in well-controlled studies. At the opposite end, pregnancy category X drugs are well established as being harmful. The physician must balance the woman's need for the drug's therapeutic effects against the fetal need to avoid exposure to it (see Appendix B).

Establishing whether an illicit drug can cause prenatal damage is difficult because women who use illegal drugs often have other problems that complicate analysis of fetal effects. For example, these women may use multiple drugs and may have poor nutritional status, untreated sexually transmitted diseases, inadequate prenatal care, and stressful lives. In addition, illicit drugs are unlikely to be pure, and substances used to dilute them may themselves be harmful.

Drugs are often metabolized and excreted in urine, including drugs in the fetal system. Fetal blood levels of drug often remain high because the fetus swallows amniotic fluid that contains excreted drug products, even after the drug is eliminated by the mother.

The best action is for the woman to eliminate use of nontherapeutic drugs and substances such as alcohol. If she takes therapeutic drugs, the physician may be able to prescribe an alternative drug with a lower risk to the fetus or may eliminate nonessential therapeutic drugs such as acne medications.

The pregnant woman who abuses drugs presents a complicated picture because maintenance of her drug habit usually takes priority over her health needs. She often has late or no prenatal care, increasing the likelihood that fetal damage occurred long before she encountered health care professionals.

IONIZING RADIATION. Nonurgent radiologic procedures may be done during the first 2 weeks after the menstrual period begins, before ovulation occurs. For urgent procedures during pregnancy, the lower abdomen should be shielded with a lead apron if possible. The radiation dose is kept as low as possible to reduce fetal exposure.

MATERNAL HYPERTHERMIA. An important teratogen is maternal hyperthermia. The mother's temperature may rise unavoidably during illness. Nurses should caution pregnant women to avoid deliberate exposure to heat sources such as saunas and hot tubs. Temperatures vary widely among public hot tubs, and a specific guideline for duration of exposure is difficult. The important factor is how high the woman's body temperature rises and for how long, not just the sauna or hot tub temperature.

MANIPULATING THE FETAL ENVIRONMENT

Appropriate medical therapy can help a woman prevent fetal damage that could result from her illness. For example, a woman who has diabetes should try to keep her blood glucose levels normal and stable before and during pregnancy for the best possible fetal outcomes. A woman with PKU should return to her special phenylalanine-free diet before conception to prevent high levels of phenylalanine in her body that will damage the fetus.

All women of childbearing age should take at least 0.4 mg (400 mcg) of folic acid daily before conception because this has been found to reduce the incidence of neural tube defects by 50% to 70%. The recommended increase during later pregnancy is 0.6 mg (600 mcg). Women who have had a child with a neural tube defect need a higher amount of folic acid, 4 mg (4000 mcg) after consulting with their health care providers. In January 1999 the Centers for Disease Control and Prevention, March of Dimes Birth Defects Foundation, and National Council on Folic Acid began a national campaign to educate women about the importance of consuming adequate folic acid every day. A 2003 Gallup poll showed that more women of childbearing age now take a vitamin with folic acid, but that the total remains low at 32% (March of Dimes, 2004b). The neural tube closes during the fourth week after conception, often before the woman knows she is pregnant. Nurses can help make women aware of their need for a supplement of folic acid before conception to help reduce this serious birth defect.

Mechanical Disruptions to Fetal Development

Mechanical forces that interfere with normal prenatal development include oligohydramnios and fibrous amniotic bands.

Oligohydramnios, an abnormally small volume of amniotic fluid, reduces the cushion surrounding the fetus and may result in deformations such as clubfoot. Prolonged oligohydramnios can interfere with fetal lung development by interfering with normal branching and development of the alveoli. Oligohydramnios may not be the primary fetal problem; rather, it may be related to other fetal anomalies. Oligohydramnios may also be a sign of reduced placental blood flow that may occur in certain complications of pregnancy.

Fibrous amniotic bands may result from tears in the inner sac (amnion) of the fetal membranes and can result in fetal deformations or intrauterine limb amputation. Fibrous bands are usually sporadic and unlikely to recur. Because these bands can cause multiple defects, they may be confused with birth defects from other causes such as chromosome and single gene abnormalities.

✔ **CHECK YOUR READING**

13. What are the usual characteristics of multifactorial disorders?
14. What factors can vary the likelihood that a multifactorial disorder will occur or recur?
15. How can a woman avoid exposing her fetus to teratogens?
16. Why should a woman with PKU adhere to a low-phenylalanine diet before and during pregnancy?
17. Why is adequate folic acid intake before conception important?

GENETIC COUNSELING

Genetic counseling provides services to help people understand the genetic disorder about which they are concerned and the risk of its occurrence in their family. Those concerned about multifactorial or environmental hazards can receive up-to-date information at most centers as well.

Availability

Genetic counseling is often available through facilities that provide maternal-fetal medicine services. State departments of mental health, mental retardation, and rehabilitation services also may provide counseling services. Local chapters of the March of Dimes are an important source of information about birth defects and counseling services. Fact sheets and other information about birth defects and their prevention are available at the March of Dimes website, www.marchofdimes.com. Organizations that focus on specific birth defects provide valuable support and assistance in obtaining needed services for individuals and families affected by the disorder.

Focus on the Family

Genetic counseling focuses on the family rather than only the affected individual. One family member may have a birth defect, but study of the entire family is often needed for accurate counseling. This may involve obtaining medical records and performing physical examinations and laboratory studies on numerous family members. Counseling is impaired if family members are unwilling to provide medical records and agree to examinations and laboratory studies. In addition, those who seek counseling may be unwilling to request cooperation from other family members or share newly acquired genetic information.

Process of Genetic Counseling

Genetic counseling may be a slow process that is not always straightforward. Several visits spread over months may be needed. Multiple family members may be part of the process. Tests for rare disorders may be performed at only one or a few laboratories in the world, and several weeks may be needed to complete them. Despite a comprehensive evaluation, a diagnosis may never be established. An accurate diagnosis is crucial to provide families with the best information about the risks for a specific birth defect, prognosis for the person affected, and options available to prevent or manage the disorder (Box 5-2). Even if the counseling does not provide clear information, expanding knowledge may allow a definitive diagnosis later, and families are encouraged to contact the center for updates.

Individuals or families may request genetic counseling before or during pregnancy or after a child has been born with a defect. A genetic evaluation may include many factors:

- A complete medical history of the affected person, including prenatal and perinatal history
- The medical history of other family members
- Laboratory, imaging, and other studies

BOX 5-2 Diagnostic Methods that May be Used in Genetic Counseling

Preconception Screening
Family history to identify hereditary patterns of disease or birth defects
Examination of family photographs
Physical examination for obvious or subtle signs of birth defects
Carrier testing
   Persons from ethnic groups with a higher incidence of some disorders
   Persons with a family history suggesting that they may carry a gene for a specific disorder
Chromosomal analysis
Deoxyribonucleic acid (DNA) analysis

Prenatal Diagnosis for Fetal Abnormalities
Maternal tests to screen for abnormalities
Chorionic villus sampling
Amniocentesis
Ultrasonography
Percutaneous umbilical blood sampling

Postnatal Diagnosis for an Infant with a Birth Defect
Physical examination and measurements
Imaging procedures (such as ultrasonography, radiography, echocardiography)
Chromosomal analysis
DNA analysis
Tests for metabolic disorders (phenylketonuria, cystic fibrosis)
Hemoglobin analysis for disorders such as sickle cell disease
Immunologic testing for infections
Autopsy

- Physical assessment of a child with the birth defect and other family members as needed
- Examination of photographs, particularly for family members who are deceased or unavailable
- Construction of a genogram, or pedigree, to identify relationships among family members and their relevant medical history

If a diagnosis is established, genetic counseling educates the family about the following:

- What is known about the cause of the disorder
- The natural course of the disorder
- The likelihood that the disorder will occur or recur in other family members
- Availability of prenatal diagnosis for the disorder
- The ways a couple may be able to avoid having an affected child
- Availability of treatment and services for the person with the disorder

Genetic counseling is nondirective; that is, the counselor does not tell the individual or parents what decision to make but educates them about options for dealing with the disorder. However, families often subjectively interpret the counseling. Some parents may regard a 50% risk of occurrence or recurrence as low, whereas others may think that a 1% risk is unacceptably high. Also, the family's values and beliefs influence whether they seek counseling and what they do with the information provided.

When risks and probabilities are discussed, these numbers must be stated in terms the individual or parents can understand, and their understanding must be verified. A 1 in 100 risk may sound higher to many people than a 1 in 5 risk. However, when the same numbers are framed in terms of percentages, the 1% risk is obviously much lower than the 20% risk.

Supplemental Services

Comprehensive genetic counseling includes services of professionals from many disciplines, such as biology, medicine, nursing, social work, and education. These professionals provide family support and referrals to parent support groups, grief counseling, and intervention for problems that accompany the birth of a child with a birth defect, such as socioeconomic and family dysfunction.

NURSING CARE OF FAMILIES CONCERNED ABOUT BIRTH DEFECTS

Nurses have an important role in helping families that are concerned about birth defects. Some nurses work directly with family members who are undergoing genetic counseling. Many more nurses are generalists who bring their knowledge about birth defects and their prevention to those they encounter in everyday practice.

Nurses as Part of a Genetic Counseling Team

Many genetic counseling teams include nurses. Genetic nursing may include the following:

- Providing counseling after additional education in this area
- Guiding a woman or couple through prenatal diagnosis
- Supporting parents as they make decisions after receiving abnormal prenatal diagnostic results
- Helping the family deal with the emotional impact of a birth defect
- Assisting parents who have had a child with a birth defect to locate needed services and support
- Coordinating services of other professionals, such as social workers, physical and occupational therapists, psychologists, and dietitians
- Helping families find appropriate support groups to help them cope with the daily stresses associated with a child who has a birth defect

Nurses in General Practice

Nurses who work in women's health care and those who work in antepartum, intrapartum, newborn, or pediatric settings often encounter families who are concerned about

---

How can this birth defect be genetic? No one else in our family has ever had anything like it.

Autosomal recessive disorders are carried by parents who themselves are unaffected. The abnormal gene may have been passed down through many generations, but the risk for an affected child is nonexistent until two carrier parents mate.

Isn't the chance that this birth defect will happen to another of our children only one in a million?

Autosomal recessive disorders have a 25% (1 in 4) chance of recurring in children of the same parents. Autosomal dominant disorders may pose a 50% risk for recurrence unless they resulted from a new mutation in the parental germ cells.

Isn't this birth defect very likely to recur? We'd better not have any more children.

Some birth defects are associated with a relatively high risk of recurrence; others have a low risk. Prenatal diagnosis may offer parents a way to avoid having an affected child, or some disorders may be treated before birth. New genetic knowledge may provide therapies not available just a short time ago. Parents' values and perceptions of risks of recurrence affect the final decision.

Because we've already had a child with this birth defect (an autosomal recessive defect), will the next three be normal?

If both parents are carriers for an autosomal recessive disorder, there is a 25% (1 in 4) risk for their child to be affected that is constant with each conception. The chance

that their child will be neither affected nor a carrier is constant with each conception. Each child has a 25% (1 in 4) chance of receiving both copies of the normal gene (unaffected and not a carrier) and a 50% (2 in 4) chance of receiving a single abnormal gene from one parent (a carrier but not affected with the disorder).

If I undergo amniocentesis or another prenatal diagnostic test, can the test detect all birth defects?

Although many disorders can be prenatally diagnosed, not all can be diagnosed in the same fetus. Testing is offered for one or more specific disorders after a careful family history is taken to determine appropriate tests.

If the prenatal test results are normal, will my baby be normal?

Normal results from prenatal testing exclude those specifically tested disorders. Every healthy couple has about a 5% risk of having a child with a birth defect, some of which are not obvious at birth. This baseline risk remains, even if all prenatal test results are normal.

Will I have to have an abortion if my prenatal tests show that my baby is abnormal?

Abortion may be an option for parents whose fetus is affected with a birth defect, but most parents are reassured by normal test results. If results are abnormal, some parents appreciate the time to prepare for a child with special needs. Better medical management can be planned for a newborn who is expected to have problems. Prenatal diagnosis gives many parents the confidence to have children despite their increased risk for having a child with a birth defect.

birth defects. These families may include a member with a birth defect. Other families may believe that they have an increased risk for having a child with a birth defect. Generalist nurses provide care and support that complements that given by nurses who work on a genetic counseling team.

WOMEN'S HEALTH NURSES

The nurse who provides care in women's health may encounter families who should be referred for genetic counseling. The ideal time to provide counseling is before conception so that the childbearing couple has more options if risks are identified. Personal and family histories are taken and updated during primary care visits, and the nurse may identify factors that could affect a future child before conception.

For example, the nurse may identify a woman who belongs to a group in which the sickle cell gene is more frequent and arrange for testing to determine her carrier status. If testing reveals that she is a carrier for the gene, the woman can be advised that she could conceive a child with sickle cell disease if her partner is also a carrier. If her partner has not been tested, the nurse can arrange for his testing.

ANTEPARTUM NURSES

Antepartum nurses often identify those who may benefit from genetic counseling. The antepartum nurse also assists families with decision making, teaching, and emotional support. An added nursing role in the genetic counseling area is to help those who must deal with abnormal test results.

IDENTIFYING FAMILIES FOR REFERRAL. Nurses in antepartum settings often identify a woman or family for whom referral for genetic counseling is appropriate (Box 5-3). The personal and family history of the woman and her partner may reveal factors that increase their risks for having a child with a birth defect. In addition to the usual medical history about disorders such as hypertension and diabetes, the woman should be questioned about a family history of birth defects, diseases that seem to "run in the family," mental retardation, and developmental delay.

■ Some people are reluctant to disclose that they have a family member with mental retardation or a birth defect. The nurse can gently probe for sensitive information by asking questions about whether any family members have learning problems or are "slow." The use of words that are lay oriented and caring often elicits more information than clinical terms that may seem harsh, such as "low IQ."

HELPING THE FAMILY DECIDE ABOUT GENETIC COUNSELING. If genetic counseling is appropriate, the physician or nurse-midwife discusses it with the woman and refers the family to an appropriate center. However, the final decision rests with the family. The nurse can help the family weigh issues that are important to them as they decide.

Genetic counseling can raise issues that are uncomfortable, such as whether to undergo prenatal diagnosis, what to do if a condition cannot be prenatally diagnosed, and what options are acceptable if prenatal diagnosis shows abnormal results. Counseling may open family conflicts if information from other family members is needed or if family values differ on issues such as abortion of an abnormal fetus. In addition, the tests can show unexpected results (Box 5-4).

TEACHING ABOUT LIFESTYLE. Nurses can teach a pregnant woman about harmful factors in her lifestyle that can be modified to reduce the risk of defects to offspring. The nurse can support the woman in making lifestyle changes that may be difficult, such as stopping alcohol consumption, reducing or eliminating smoking, and improving her diet. Use of liberal praise can motivate a woman to continue her efforts to promote an optimal outcome. However, a negative attitude from nurses or other professionals may make her feel like a failure, and she may abandon her efforts to create a healthier lifestyle.

PROVIDING EMOTIONAL SUPPORT. Until they know that prenatal test results are normal, possibly a time

---

BOX 5-3 Reasons for Referral to a Genetic Counselor

Pregnant women who will be 35 years of age or older when the infant is born
Men who father children after age 40
Members of a group with an increased incidence of a specific disorder
Carriers of autosomal recessive disorders
Women who are carriers of X-linked disorders
Couples related by blood (consanguineous relationship)
Family history of birth defect or mental retardation
Family history of unexplained stillbirth
Women who experience multiple spontaneous abortions
Pregnant women exposed to known or suspected teratogens or other harmful agents either before or during pregnancy
Pregnant women with abnormal prenatal screening results, such as multiple-marker screen or suspicious ultrasound findings

---

BOX 5-4 Examples of Problems in Genetic Counseling and Prenatal Diagnosis

Inadequate medical records
Family members' refusal to share information
Records that are incomplete, vague, or uninformative
Inconclusive testing
Too few family members available when family studies are needed
Inadequate number of live fetal cells obtained during amniocentesis
Failure of fetal cells to grow in culture if other testing techniques are not useful
Ambiguous prenatal test results that are neither clearly normal nor clearly abnormal
Unexpected results from prenatal diagnosis
Finding an abnormality other than the one for which the person was tested
Nonpaternity revealed
Inability to determine the severity of a prenatally diagnosed disorder
Inability to rule out all birth defects
Client misunderstanding of the mathematical risk as it is presented

THERAPEUTIC COMMUNICATIONS

Assisting a Woman Who May Benefit from Genetic Counseling

Paula Crandall is a 41-year-old white woman who is 8 weeks pregnant with her first child after more than 10 years of infertility. Barbara Glenn is a nurse who works with Paula's obstetrician.

Paula: I know all about the risks at my age. I'm not so much worried about my own health but the baby's.

Barbara: You seem to be concerned that the baby might not be all right. *(Clarifying)*

Paula: Sure, what woman wouldn't be? I know I'm more likely to have a baby with Down syndrome at my age.

Barbara: Yes, the risks of having an infant with a chromosomal abnormality increase after the mother is 35 years old. Do you want prenatal diagnosis to see if the fetus has this kind of problem? *(Paraphrasing and giving information. Barbara also uses a closed-end question that tends to block communication because it is usually answered with a simple "yes" or "no.")*

Paula: Oh, yes. I know what's available from surfing the Internet. When we waited so long to have children, I just assumed that I'd have whatever tests were recommended. I just don't know....

Barbara: You're reconsidering prenatal testing now? *(Reflecting)*

Paula: Well, not exactly reconsidering.... It's just that I've waited so long for a baby, and this may be our only one.

Barbara: [Waiting quietly but attentively because Paula seems to be thinking.] *(Using silence)*

Paula: I'm just worried about testing. I know prenatal tests have a low risk, but what if I lose a normal baby? It took me so long to finally get pregnant, and I'm running out of time. I might not get another chance.

Barbara: It must be a very difficult decision. *(Reflecting)*

Paula: It is. Even if I have testing and the baby has Down syndrome, I'm not so sure I'd have an abortion. The outlook for people with Down syndrome is much better than it used to be. Why have testing if I wouldn't do anything about an abnormal baby?

Barbara: You certainly have some valid concerns. How does your husband feel about testing? *(Questioning using an open-ended question)*

Paula: Oh, Bill is all for it. He keeps reminding me that the baby is probably normal and that I probably won't have a miscarriage if I have testing. His cousin had a child with Down syndrome, and Bill doesn't think we should knowingly bring a child with a serious birth defect into the world. What would you do if you were in my place?

Barbara: I can't answer that question because I'm not in your place. Let's review some of the issues so you can make the best decision for yourself and your family. First, you know you have an increased risk for having a baby with a chromosomal defect such as Down syndrome because of your age. Second, the odds that the baby will be normal are higher than the risk that the baby will be abnormal. Third, amniocentesis poses a small but real risk of causing a miscarriage. Fourth, you are undecided about whether you would terminate a pregnancy if the fetus were abnormal. Other issues to consider are time limitations and the option of screening with a sample of your blood. The maternal serum alpha-fetoprotein test is done 8 to 10 weeks from now, but it does not require a sample from inside the uterus. An amniocentesis may be done slightly earlier but requires an amniotic fluid sample from your uterus to test. *(Summarizing)*

Paula: I know. I'm running out of time in more ways than one.

Barbara: If you like, I can set up an appointment with a genetic counselor. The counselor can provide you with the most accurate assessment of your risk for having a child with a birth defect and also the risks of any indicated prenatal diagnosis procedure. Then you can decide whether or not to have testing.

Paula: I think I'd like that, as long as I don't have to be committed to a particular decision before I go.

---

period spanning several days or weeks, many women delay telling friends or family about their pregnancy or investing in it emotionally. When results are abnormal, women face more difficult decisions about whether to terminate or continue the pregnancy.

HELPING THE FAMILY DEAL WITH ABNORMAL RESULTS. Because prenatal diagnostic tests are performed to detect disorders involving serious physical and often mental defects, the woman whose test results are abnormal must confront painful decisions. For many of these disorders, no effective prenatal or postnatal treatment exists. Only two choices may be available: to continue or terminate the pregnancy. In addition, the decision to terminate a pregnancy must be made in a short time. Making no decision is effectively a decision to continue the pregnancy. Although the physician or genetic counselor discusses abnormal results and available options, the nurse reinforces the information given to these anxious families and supports them.

When test results are abnormal, nurses can expect the couple to grieve. Even if a pregnancy was unplanned, the woman who reaches the time of prenatal diagnosis has already made the initial decision to continue the pregnancy. If results are abnormal, she must decide again if she will continue or end the pregnancy. Women who continue their pregnancies grieve over losing the expected normal infant.

INTRAPARTUM AND NEONATAL NURSES

Nurses working in intrapartum and neonatal settings encounter families who have given birth to an infant with a birth defect that may have been unexpected. Stillborn infants sometimes have birth defects that contributed to their intrauterine death. In addition to the loss of their baby, these parents face pain because of the associated abnormality. An autopsy may be performed to document all anomalies and to establish the most accurate diagnosis of the birth defect for future counseling. Nursing care for families that experience a perinatal loss, whether a result of the infant's death or the loss of the expected normal infant, is addressed in Chapter 24.

Nurses who care for these families in the intrapartum and neonatal settings will find the parents anxious, depressed, and sometimes hostile because of the unexpected event. The family's usual coping mechanisms may be inadequate for the situation, or new coping mechanisms may not have been developed. Diagnostic studies are often recommended soon after the birth of an abnormal infant to establish a diagnosis and give parents accurate information about the disorder and their options. However, a high anxiety level reduces the ability to understand the often massive amount of information received. The nurse is in the best position to evaluate the family's perception of the problem, help them understand the diagnostic tests, reinforce correct information, and correct misunderstandings. In addition, the nurse is often most therapeutic by simply being an available, active listener, helping to ease the family's pain over the event.

Nurses should encourage families to contact lay support groups, which are significant sources of support because members fully understand the daily problems encountered in the care of a child with a birth defect. Such groups can help the parents deal with the stress and chronic grief associated with prolonged care of these children. Support groups also can help the parents see the positive aspects and victories when caring for their special-needs child. Internet sites regarding specific birth defects are often available to offer parent education and support.

PEDIATRIC NURSES

Children with birth defects typically have numerous recurrent medical problems. They usually are hospitalized more often and for longer periods than children without birth defects. They may have to travel to specialized hospitals for care, adding to the family's stress. Their families often have substantial expenses for medical care and equipment that are not covered by insurance or public assistance programs. Income may be lost because one parent, usually the mother, stops working to care for the child.

Family dysfunction is common, and the strain of having a child with a serious birth defect may lead to divorce. Siblings often feel left out of their parents' attention because the needs of this child demand so much of their time.

The pediatric nurse can reduce the family's stress by helping them locate appropriate support services. The nurse can contact social services departments to help the family find financial and other resources needed to care for the child. If parents have not connected with a lay support group, the pediatric nurse can encourage them to do so.

SUMMARY CONCEPTS

- The 46 human chromosomes are long strands of deoxyribonucleic acid (DNA), each containing up to several thousand individual genes.

- With the exception of those genes located on the X and Y chromosomes in males, genes are inherited in pairs that may be identical or different. Some genes are dominant, and some are recessive.
- Many genes can be analyzed by the products they produce, their DNA, or their close association with another gene that is more easily analyzed.
- Cells for chromosome analysis must be living. Specimens must be handled carefully to preserve viability if analysis of dividing cells in the metaphase of cell division is necessary. Other techniques, such as fluorescent in situ hybridization, permit study of cells without requiring active cell division, allowing rapid test results.
- Chromosome abnormalities are either numerical, with the addition or deletion of an entire chromosome or chromosomes, or structural, with deletion, addition, rearrangement, or fragility of the chromosome material.
- Single gene disorders are associated with a fixed risk of occurrence or recurrence. The type of single gene abnormality (autosomal dominant, autosomal recessive, or X-linked) determines the risk.
- Multifactorial disorders occur because of a genetic predisposition combined with environmental factors.
- The risk for occurrence or recurrence of multifactorial disorders is not fixed but varies according to the number of close relatives that are affected, severity of the defect in affected persons, gender of the affected person, and geographic locale. Seasonal variations may affect the risk for some disorders.
- Relatively few agents that can enter the fetal environment are known to be definitely teratogenic or definitely safe.
- The risk for fetal damage from environmental agents can be decreased by reducing exposure to the agent or manipulating the fetal environment.
- The purpose of genetic counseling is to educate individuals or families with accurate information so that they can make informed decisions about reproduction and appropriate care for affected members.
- The nurse cares for people with concerns about birth defects by identifying those needing referral, teaching, coordinating services, and offering emotional support.

REFERENCES & READINGS

American Academy of Pediatrics & American College of Obstetricians and Gynecologists (ACOG). (2002). *Guidelines for perinatal care* (5th ed.). Washington, DC: Author.

American College of Obstetricians and Gynecologists. (2003). Immunization during pregnancy. *ACOG Committee Opinion number 282.* Author.

American College of Obstetricians and Gynecologists. (2000). Maternal phenylketonuria. *ACOG Committee Opinion number 230.* Author.

Andres, R.L. (2004). Effects of therapeutic, diagnostic, and environmental agents and exposure to social and illicit drugs. In R.K. Creasy, R. Resniki, & J.D. Iams (Eds.), *Maternal-fetal medicine: Principles and practice* (5th ed, pp. 281-314). Philadelphia: Saunders.

Banasik, J.L. (2000a). Genetics and developmental disorders. In L.C. Copstead & J.L. Banasik (Eds.), *Pathophysiology: Biological and behavioral perspectives* (2nd ed., pp. 110-133). Philadelphia: Saunders.

Banasik, J.L. (2000b). Molecular genetics and tissue differentiation. In L.C. Copstead & J.L. Banasik (Eds.), *Pathophysiology: Biological and behavioral perspectives* (2nd ed., pp. 62-109). Philadelphia, Saunders.

Centers for Disease Control. (2004). National Immunization Program: Guidelines for vaccinating pregnant women. Retrieved July 21, 2004, from www.cdc.gov/nip/publications/preg_guide.htm#rubella.

Cook, S.S. (2003). Deconstructing DNA: Understanding genetic implications on nursing care. *AWHONN Lifelines, 7*(2), 140-144.

Elias, S. (2004). The human gynome [sic] Presidential address. *American Journal of Obstetrics and Gynecology, 190*(6), 1528-1533.

Guyton, A.C., & Hall, J.E. (2000). *Textbook of medical physiology* (10th ed.). Philadelphia: Saunders.

Hall, J.G. (2004a). Chromosomal clinical abnormalities. In R.E. Behrman, R.M. Kliegman, & H.B. Jenson (Eds.), *Nelson textbook of pediatrics* (17th ed., pp. 382-391). Philadelphia: Saunders.

Hall, J.G. (2004b). Genetic counseling. In R.E. Behrman, R.M. Kliegman, & H.B. Jenson (Eds.), *Nelson textbook of pediatrics* (17th ed., pp. 395-396). Philadelphia: Saunders.

Hamilton, B.A., & Wynshaw-Boris, A. (2004). Basic genetics and patterns of inheritance. In R.K. Creasy, R. Resnik, & J.D. Iams (Eds.), *Maternal-fetal medicine: Principles and practice* (5th ed, pp. 3-36). Philadelphia: Saunders.

Hasenau, S.M., & Covington, C. (2002). Neural tube defects: Prevention and folic acid. *MCN: American Journal of Maternal/Child Nursing, 27*(2), 87-91.

Hoyme, H.E. (2004a). Patterns of inheritance. In R.E. Behrman, R.M. Kliegman, & H.B. Jenson (Eds.), *Nelson textbook of pediatrics* (17th ed., pp. 376-382). Philadelphia: Saunders.

Hoyme, H.E. (2004b). Molecular basis of genetic disorders. In R.E. Behrman, R.M. Kliegman, & H.B. Jenson (Eds.), *Nelson textbook of pediatrics* (17th ed., pp. 367-371). Philadelphia: Saunders.

Hoyme, H.E. (2004c). Molecular diagnosis of genetic diseases. In R.E. Behrman, R.M. Kliegman, & H.B. Jenson (Eds.), *Nelson textbook of pediatrics* (17th ed., pp. 371-376). Philadelphia: Saunders.

Jenkins, T.M., & Wapner, R.J. (2004). Prenatal diagnosis of congenital disorders. In R.K. Creasy, R. Resnik, & J.D. Iams (Eds.), *Maternal-fetal medicine: Principles and practice* (5th ed., pp. 235-280). Philadelphia: Saunders.

Jones, K.L. (1997). *Smith's recognizable patterns of human malformation* (5th ed.). Philadelphia: Saunders.

Jones, S.L., & Fallon, L.A. (2002). Reproductive options for individuals at risk for transmission of a genetic disorder. *Journal of Obstetric, Gynecologic, and Neonatal Nursing, 31*(2), 193-199.

Jorde, L.B., Carey, J.C., Bamshad, M.J., & White, R.L. (2003). *Medical genetics* (3rd ed). St. Louis: Mosby.

Kay, M.A. (2004). Gene therapy. In R.E. Behrman, R.M. Kliegman, & H.B. Jenson (Eds.), *Nelson textbook of pediatrics* (17th ed., pp. 333-341). Philadelphia: Saunders.

Kenner, C. (2003). Human genetics and implications for neonatal care. In C. Kenner & J.W. Lott (Eds.), *Comprehensive neonatal nursing: A physiologic perspective* (3rd ed., pp. 132-150). Philadelphia: Saunders.

March of Dimes Birth Defects Foundation. (2002). *Fact sheet: Rubella.* Retrieved July 22, 2004, from www.modimes.com//professionals/681_1225.asp.

March of Dimes Birth Defects Foundation. (2004a). *Fact sheet: Birth defects.* Retrieved July 18, 2004, from www.marchofdimes.com/professionals/681_1206.asp.

March of Dimes Birth Defects Foundation. (2004b). *Fact sheet: Folic acid.* Retrieved July 18, 2004, from www.marchofdimes.com//professionals/681_1151.asp.

March of Dimes Birth Defects Foundation. (2004c). *Fact sheet: Sickle cell disease.* Retrieved July 18, 2004, from www.marchofdimes.com/professionals/681_1221.asp.

March of Dimes Birth Defects Foundation. (2004d). *Fact sheet: Tay Sachs disease.* Retrieved July 18, 2004, from www.marchofdimes.com/professionals/681_1227.asp.

Moore, K.L. & Persaud, T.V.N. (2003). *Before we are born: Essentials of embryology and birth defects* (6th ed.). Philadelphia: Saunders.

National Human Genome Research Institute. (2004). *All about the Human Genome Project.* Retrieved July 20, 2004, from www.genome.gov/10001772.

Nussbaum, R.L., McInnes, R.R., & Willard, H.F. (2004). *Thompson & Thompson genetics in medicine* (6th rev. ed.). Philadelphia: Saunders.

Postlethwaite, D. (2003). Preconception health counseling for women exposed to teratogens: The role of the nurse. *Journal of Obstetric, Gynecologic, and Neonatal Nursing, 32*(4), 523-532.

Simpson, J.L., & Elias, S. (2003). *Genetics in obstetrics and gynecology* (3rd ed.). Philadelphia: Saunders.

Tinkle, M.B., & Cheek, D.J. (2002). Human genomics: Challenges and opportunities. *Journal of Obstetric, Gynecologic, and Neonatal Nursing, 31*(2), 178-187.

Ward, K. (2003). Genetics and prenatal diagnosis. In J.R. Scott, R.S. Gibbs, B.Y Karlan, & A.F. Haney (Eds.), *Danforth's obstetrics and gynecology* (9th ed., pp. 173-195). Philadelphia: Lippincott Williams and Wilkins.

Conception and Prenatal Development

After studying this chapter, you should be able to:

1. Describe formation of the female and male gametes.
2. Relate ovulation and ejaculation to the process of human conception.
3. Explain implantation and nourishment of the embryo before development of the placenta.
4. Describe normal prenatal development from conception through birth.
5. Explain structure and function of the placenta, umbilical cord, and fetal membranes.
6. Describe the occurrence of common deviations from normal conception and prenatal development.
7. Describe prenatal circulation and the circulatory changes after birth.
8. Explain the mechanisms and trends in multifetal pregnancies.

Go to your Student CD-ROM for Review Questions keyed to these Objectives.

Autosome Any of the 22 pairs of chromosomes other than the sex chromosomes.

Conceptus Cells and membranes resulting from fertilization of the ovum at any stage of prenatal development.

Corpus Luteum Graafian follicle cells remaining after ovulation that produce estrogen and progesterone.

Diploid The number of chromosomes (46 in humans) normally present in body cells other than gametes that represents one copy of every chromosome from each parent.

Ejaculation Expulsion of semen from the penis.

Embryo The developing baby from the beginning of the third week through the eighth week after conception.

Endometrium Lining of the uterus.

Fertilization Age Prenatal age of the developing baby, calculated from the date of conception. (Also called *postconceptional age.*)

Fetus The developing baby from 9 weeks after conception until birth; used in everyday practice to describe a developing baby during pregnancy, regardless of age.

Gamete Reproductive cell; in the female an ovum and in the male a spermatozoon.

Gestational Age Prenatal age of the developing baby (measured in weeks) calculated from the first day of the woman's last menstrual period; approximately 2 weeks longer than the fertilization age. (Also called *menstrual age.*)

Graafian Follicle A small sac within the ovary that contains the maturing ovum.

Haploid Normal number of chromosomes in male or female gamete; refers to one copy of a chromosome from each pair (23 in humans, or half the diploid number).

Meiosis Reduction cell division in gametes that halves the number of chromosomes in each cell.

Mitosis Cell division in body cells other than the gametes.

Nidation Implantation of the fertilized ovum (zygote) in the uterine endometrium.

Oogenesis Formation of gametes (ova) in the female.

Ovulation Release of the mature ovum from the ovary.

Placenta Fetal structure that provides nourishment and removes wastes from the developing baby and secretes hormones necessary for the continuation of pregnancy.

DEFINITIONS—cont'd

Sex Chromosome The X or Y chromosome. Females have two X chromosomes; males have one X and one Y chromosome.

Somatic Cells Body cells other than the gametes, or germ cells.

Spermatogenesis Formation of male gametes (sperm) in the testes.

Teratogen An agent that can cause defects in a developing baby during pregnancy.

Zygote The developing baby from conception through the first week of prenatal life.

A basic understanding of conception and prenatal development helps the nurse provide care to parents during normal childbearing and better understand problems such as infertility and birth defects. This chapter addresses formation of the gametes, the process of conception, prenatal development, and important auxiliary structures that support normal prenatal development. The reason for the occurrence of multifetal pregnancy (for example, twinning) is also discussed.

GAMETOGENESIS

Gametogenesis is the development of ova in the woman and sperm in the man (Table 6-1). Production of gametes requires a different process than formation of somatic cells. Somatic cells reproduce by a process called *mitosis*. Each somatic cell has 46 paired chromosomes: 22 pairs of autosomes and one pair of sex chromosomes. During mitosis the cell divides into two new cells, each having 46 chromosomes like the parent cell.

Gametogenesis requires a special reduction division called *meiosis*. Unlike mitosis, in which the diploid number of chromosomes is retained in the new cells, meiosis halves the number of chromosomes to arrive at the haploid number. Only one of each chromosome pair (22 autosomes and one sex chromosome) is directed to the gamete. Also, with the exception of the X and Y chromosomes in the male, each chromosome exchanges some material with its mate so that the new chromosome in the gamete contains some material from the mother and some from the father. This process, which is called *crossing over*, allows variation in genetic material while keeping constant the total amount of chromosome material from generation to generation. When the sperm and ovum unite at conception, the "halves" form a new cell and restore the chromosome number to 46.

Oogenesis

Oogenesis is the formation of female gametes (Figure 6-1, *A*) within the ovary. Oogenesis begins during prenatal life when primitive ova (oogonia), like all other cells, multiply by mitosis. Each oogonium contains 46 chromosomes, as do other body cells. Before birth these oogonia enlarge to form primary oocytes, each surrounded by a layer of follicular cells. These are called *primary follicles*. The primary oogonium begins its first meiotic division during fetal life but does not complete the process until puberty. The primary follicle and its oogonium, which still contains 46 chromosomes, remain dormant throughout childhood.

The female fetus has all the ova she will ever have by the thirtieth week of gestation. Many of these ova regress during childhood. When a girl's reproductive cycles begin at puberty, some of the primary follicles present at birth begin maturing. The process of gamete maturation continues

TABLE 6-1 Comparison of Female and Male Gametogenesis

	Oogenesis	Spermatogenesis
Time during which primary germ cells are produced	Fetal life; no others develop after about 30 weeks of gestation	Continuously after puberty
Hormones that control the process	GnRH FSH LH Estrogen	GnRH FSH LH Testosterone Estrogen (small amounts converted from testosterone) Growth hormone
Number of mature germ cells that develop from each primary cell	One	Four
Quantity	One during each reproductive cycle of about 28 days	40-250 million released with each ejaculation
Size	Large; visible to naked eye; abundant cytoplasm to nourish embryo until implantation	Tiny compared with ovum; little cytoplasm; head is almost all nuclear material (chromosomes)
Motility	Relatively nonmotile; carried along by action of cilia and currents within fallopian tubes	Independently motile by means of whiplike tail; mitochondria in middle piece provide energy for motility
Chromosome complement	23 total: 22 autosomes plus one X sex chromosome	23 total: 22 autosomes, plus either an X or a Y sex chromosome

GnRH, Gonadotropin-releasing hormone; *FSH,* follicle-stimulating hormone; *LH,* luteinizing hormone.

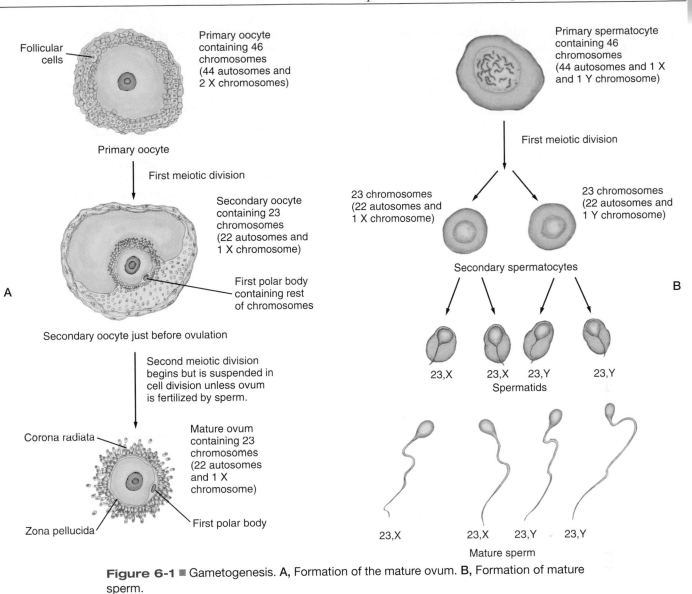

Figure 6-1 ■ Gametogenesis. **A,** Formation of the mature ovum. **B,** Formation of mature sperm.

throughout her reproductive years until the climacteric, which is sometimes called the *change of life.*

When the oocyte matures, two meiotic divisions reduce the chromosome number from 46 paired to 23 unpaired chromosomes: 22 autosomes and one X chromosome. Shortly before ovulation, the primary oocyte completes its *first meiotic division*, which began during fetal life. The result is a secondary oocyte that now contains 23 chromosomes. The primary cell's cytoplasm is divided unequally with this division, and most of it is retained by the secondary oocyte. The remainder of cytoplasm plus the other half of the chromosomes go into a tiny, nonfunctional polar body that soon degenerates.

At ovulation, the secondary oocyte begins to form a mature ovum (*second meiotic division*). Each of the 23 chromosomes divides without replication of the deoxyribonucleic acid (DNA). The second meiotic division is prolonged, and the mature ovum remains suspended in metaphase, the middle part of cell division. If fertilization occurs, the second meiotic division is completed, resulting in a mature ovum that also contains 23 chromosomes and a second tiny polar body containing the 23 discarded chromosomes that degenerates. If the ovum is not fertilized, it does not complete the second meiotic division and degenerates. In oogenesis, one primary oocyte results in a single mature ovum.

When the mature ovum is released from the ovary, it is surrounded by two layers: the zona pellucida and the cells of the corona radiata. These layers protect the ovum and prevent fertilization by more than one sperm. For fertilization to occur, the sperm must penetrate these two layers to reach the ovum's cell nucleus.

Spermatogenesis

Spermatogenesis (Figure 6-1, *B*) begins during puberty in the male and requires approximately 70 days to complete. Primitive sperm cells, or spermatogonia, develop during the prenatal period and begin multiplying by mitosis during puberty. Unlike the female, the male continues to produce new spermatogonia that can mature into sperm throughout his lifetime. Although male fertility gradually declines with age, men can father children in their 50s, 60s, and beyond.

Each spermatogonium contains 46 paired chromosomes, like other body cells. In the mature male a spermatogonium enlarges to become a primary spermatocyte that still contains all 46 chromosomes. The first meiotic division forms two secondary spermatocytes and reduces the number to 23 unpaired chromosomes in each gamete: 22 autosomes and one X or Y sex chromosome in each spermatocyte. Each chromosome of the secondary spermatocyte divides to retain 23 chromosomes in the second meiotic division, forming two spermatids. Therefore 50% of the four spermatids that result from the two meiotic divisions of the spermatogonium carry an X chromosome and 50% carry a Y chromosome. The spermatids gradually evolve into mature sperm.

The gamete from a male determines the gender of the new baby because the ovum carries only an X chromosome. Each mature sperm contains 23 chromosomes: 22 autosomes and either an X or a Y chromosome. If an X-bearing spermatozoon fertilizes the ovum, the baby is a girl. If a Y-bearing spermatozoon fertilizes the ovum, the baby is a boy.

The mature sperm has three major sections: a head, middle portion, and tail (Figure 6-2). The head is almost entirely a cell nucleus and contains the male chromosomes that join the chromosomes of the ovum. The middle portion supplies energy for the tail's whiplike action. The movement of the tail propels the sperm toward the ovum.

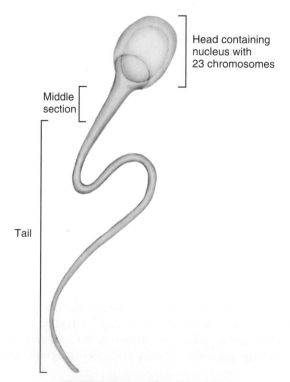

Head containing nucleus with 23 chromosomes

Middle section

Tail

Figure 6-2 ■ Mature sperm.

✓ CHECK YOUR READING

1. What is the purpose of meiosis in the gametes?
2. How many mature ova can be produced by each oogonium? When does meiosis occur in the female?
3. How many mature spermatozoa can be produced by each spermatogonium? When does meiosis occur in the male?

CONCEPTION

Natural conception is the interaction of many factors, including correct timing between release of a mature ovum at ovulation and ejaculation of enough healthy, mature, motile sperm into the vagina. Although exact viability is unknown, the ovum may survive no longer than 24 hours after its release at ovulation. Most sperm survive no more than 24 hours in the female reproductive tract, although a few may remain fertile in the woman's reproductive tract for as long as 5 days (Guyton & Hall, 2000).

Preparation for Conception in the Female

Before ovulation, several oocytes begin to mature under the influence of follicle-stimulating hormone (FSH) and luteinizing hormone (LH) from the woman's anterior pituitary gland. Each maturing oocyte is contained within a sac called the *graafian follicle*, which produces estrogen and progesterone to prepare the endometrium for a possible pregnancy. Eventually, one follicle outgrows the others. The less mature oocytes permanently regress.

RELEASE OF THE OVUM

Ovulation occurs approximately 14 days before a woman's next menstrual period would begin. The follicle develops a weak spot on the surface of the ovary and ruptures, releasing the mature ovum with its surrounding cells onto the surface of the ovary. The collapsed follicle is transformed into the corpus luteum, which maintains high estrogen and progesterone secretion necessary to make final preparation of the uterine lining for a fertilized ovum.

OVUM TRANSPORT

The mature ovum is released on the surface of the ovary, where it is picked up by the fimbriated (fringed) ends of the fallopian tube. The ovum is transported through the tube by the muscular action of the tube and movement of cilia within the tube. Fertilization normally occurs in the distal third of the fallopian tube (ampulla) near the ovary. The ovum, fertilized or not, enters the uterus approximately 3 days after its release from the ovary.

Preparation for Conception in the Male

The male preparation for fertilizing the ovum consists of ejaculation, movement of the sperm in the female reproductive tract, and preparation of the sperm for actual fertilization.

EJACULATION

When a male ejaculates during sexual intercourse, 40 to 250 million sperm, 50% to 90% of which are morphologically normal, are deposited in the upper vagina and over the cervix. The sperm are suspended in 2 to 5 ml of seminal fluid, which nourishes and protects the sperm from the acidic environment of the vagina (Blackburn, 2003; Toot & Lu, 2004). Many sperm are lost as the ejaculate drips from the vaginal introitus. Other sperm are inactivated by acidic vaginal secretions or digested by vaginal enzymes and phagocytes. The seminal fluid coagulates slightly after ejaculation to hold the semen deeply in the vagina. Many sperm are relatively immobile for approximately 15 to 30 minutes until other seminal enzymes dissolve the coagulated fluid and allow the sperm to begin moving upward through the cervix.

TRANSPORT OF SPERM IN THE FEMALE REPRODUCTIVE TRACT

The whiplike movement of the tails of spermatozoa propels them through the cervix, uterus, and fallopian tubes. Uterine contractions induced by prostaglandins in the seminal fluid enhance movement of the sperm toward the ovum. Only sperm cells enter the cervix. The seminal fluid remains in the vagina.

Many sperm are lost along the way. Some are digested by enzymes and phagocytes in the female reproductive tract, whereas others simply lose their direction, moving into the wrong tube or past the ovum and out into the peritoneal cavity. Fewer than 200 reach the fallopian tube where the ovum waits (Toot & Lu, 2004).

PREPARATION OF SPERM FOR FERTILIZATION

Sperm are not immediately ready to fertilize the ovum when they are ejaculated. During the trip to the ovum, the sperm undergo changes that enable one of them to penetrate the protective layers surrounding the ovum, a process called *capacitation*. During capacitation a glycoprotein coat and seminal proteins are removed from the acrosome, which is the tip of the sperm head. After capacitation the sperm look the same but are more active and can better penetrate the corona radiata and zona pellucida surrounding the ovum.

Sperm must also undergo an acrosome reaction to further prepare them to fertilize the ovum. The sperm that reach the ovum release hyaluronidase and acrosin to digest a pathway through the corona radiata and zona pellucida. Their tails beat harder to propel them toward the center of the ovum. Eventually, one spermatozoon penetrates the ovum.

Fertilization

Fertilization occurs when one spermatozoon enters the ovum and the two nuclei containing the parents' chromosomes merge (Figure 6-3).

ENTRY OF ONE SPERMATOZOON INTO THE OVUM

Entry of a spermatozoon into the ovum has three results. First is the zona reaction, in which changes in the zona pellucida surrounding the ovum prevent other sperm from entering. Second, the cell membranes of the ovum and sperm fuse and break down, allowing the contents of the sperm head to enter the cytoplasm of the ovum. Third, the ovum, which has been suspended in the middle of its second meiotic division since just before ovulation, completes meiosis. This results in a nucleus with 23 chromosomes and the expulsion of a second nonfunctional polar body. The mature ovum now contains 23 unpaired chromosomes (22 autosomes and one X chromosome) in its nucleus.

FUSION OF THE NUCLEI OF SPERM AND OVUM

Once a spermatozoon has penetrated the ovum, fusion of their nuclei begins. The sperm head enlarges and the tail degenerates. The nuclei of the gametes move toward the center of the ovum, where the membranes surrounding their nuclei touch and dissolve. The 23 chromosomes from the sperm mingle with the 23 from the ovum, restoring the diploid number to 46. Fertilization is complete, and cell division can begin when the nuclei of the sperm and ovum unite.

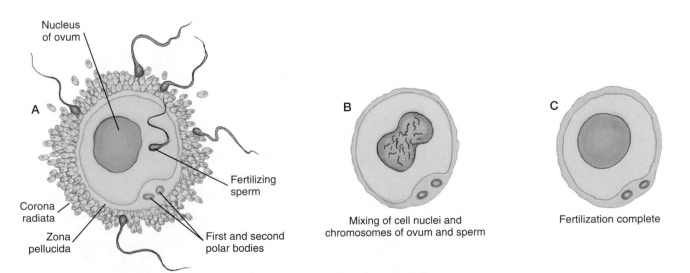

Nucleus of ovum

A

Corona radiata

Zona pellucida

Fertilizing sperm

First and second polar bodies

B

Mixing of cell nuclei and chromosomes of ovum and sperm

C

Fertilization complete

Figure 6-3 ■ Process of fertilization. **A,** A sperm enters the ovum. **B,** The 23 chromosomes from the sperm mingle with the 23 chromosomes from the ovum, restoring the diploid number to 46. **C,** The fertilized ovum is now called a *zygote* and is ready for the first mitotic cell division.

4. Where does fertilization usually occur?
5. What are the purposes of the seminal fluid?
6. What occurs when a spermatozoon penetrates the ovum?
7. When is fertilization complete and a new human conceived?

PREEMBRYONIC PERIOD

The preembryonic period is the first 2 weeks after conception (Figure 6-4). Around the fourth day after conception, the fertilized ovum, now called a *zygote*, enters the uterus.

Initiation of Cell Division

The zygote divides into 2, then 4, then 8 cells, and so on. Until the 16-cell stage, the cells become tightly compacted with each division so that they occupy approximately the same amount of space as the original zygote. When the conceptus is a solid ball of 12 to 16 cells, it is called a *morula* because it resembles a mulberry.

The outer cells of the morula secrete fluid, forming a blastocyst, a sac of cells with an inner cell mass placed off center within the sac. The inner cell mass develops into the fetus. Part of the outer layer of cells develops as the placenta and fetal membranes.

Entry of the Zygote into the Uterus

When the blastocyst contains approximately 100 cells, it enters the uterus. It lingers in the uterus another 2 to 4 days before beginning implantation. The endometrium, now called the *decidua*, is in the secretory phase of the reproductive cycle, 1½ weeks before the woman would otherwise begin her menstrual period. The endometrial glands are secreting at their maximum, providing rich fluids to nourish the conceptus before placental circulation is established. The endometrial spiral arteries are well developed in the secretory phase, providing easy access for development of the placental blood supply.

Implantation in the Decidua

The conceptus carries a small supply of nutrients for early cell division. However, implantation at the proper time and location in the uterus is critical for continued development. Implantation, or nidation, is a gradual process that occurs between the sixth and tenth days after conception. During the relatively long process of implantation, embryonic structures continue to develop.

Maintaining the Decidua

Implantation and survival of the conceptus require a continuing supply of estrogen and progesterone to maintain the decidua in the secretory phase. The zygote secretes human chorionic gonadotropin (hCG) to signal the woman's body that a pregnancy has begun. Production of hCG by the conceptus causes the corpus luteum to persist and continue secretion of estrogen and progesterone until the placenta takes over this function.

Location of Implantation

The conceptus must be in the right place at the right time for normal implantation to occur. The site of implantation is important because that is where the placenta develops. Normal implantation occurs in the upper uterus, slightly more often on the posterior wall than the anterior wall (Moore &

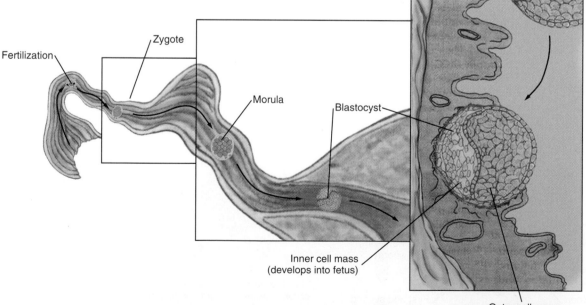

Fertilization

Zygote

Morula

Blastocyst

Inner cell mass
(develops into fetus)

Outer cell mass
(develops into placenta
and membranes)

Figure 6-4 ■ Prenatal development from fertilization through implantation of the blastocyst. Implantation gradually occurs from the sixth through the tenth day. Implantation is complete on the tenth day.

Persaud, 2003a). The upper uterus is the best area for implantation and placental development for three reasons:

- The upper uterus is richly supplied with blood for optimal fetal gas exchange and nutrition.
- The uterine lining is thick in the upper uterus, preventing the placenta from attaching too deeply into the uterine muscle and facilitating easy expulsion of the placenta after full-term birth.
- Implantation in the upper uterus limits blood loss after birth because strong interlacing muscle fibers in this area compress open endometrial vessels after the placenta detaches.

Mechanism of Implantation

Enzymes produced by the conceptus erode the decidua, tapping maternal sources of nutrition. Primary chorionic villi are tiny projections on the surface of the conceptus extending into the endometrium, now called the decidua basalis, that lies between the conceptus and the wall of the uterus. The chorionic villi eventually form the fetal side of the placenta. The decidua basalis forms the maternal side of the placenta (see p. 100, Figure 6-7, *A*).

At this early stage, nutritive fluid passes to the embryo by diffusion (the passive movement across a cell membrane from an area of higher concentration to one of lower con-

centration) because the circulatory system is not yet established. The conceptus is fully embedded within the mother's uterine decidua by 10 days, and the site of implantation is almost invisible.

As the conceptus implants, usually near the time of the next expected menstrual period, a small amount of bleeding ("spotting") may occur at the site. Implantation bleeding may be confused with a normal menstrual period, particularly if the woman's menstrual periods are usually light.

CHECK YOUR READING

8. When does implantation occur?
9. What are the advantages of implantation in the upper uterus?
10. How is the embryo nourished before the placenta develops?

EMBRYONIC PERIOD

The embryonic period of development extends from the beginning of the third week through the eighth week after conception (Figure 6-5). Basic structures of all major body organs are completed during the embryonic period (Table 6-2).

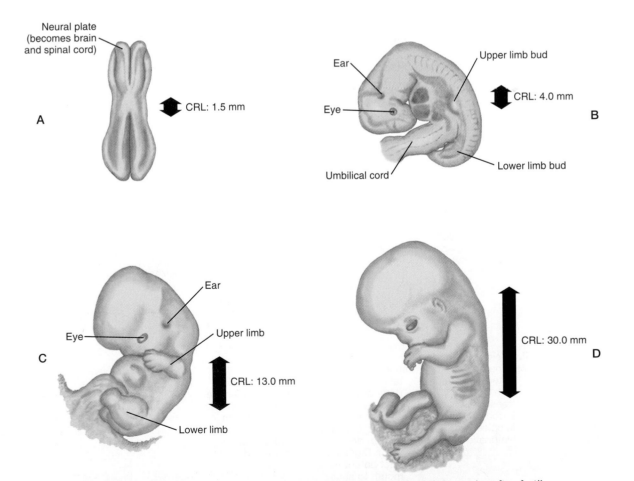

Figure 6-5 ■ Embryonic development from the third through eighth weeks after fertilization. **A**, Week 3. **B**, Week 4. **C**, Week 6. **D**, Week 8. (*CRL,* Crown-rump length.)

TABLE 6-2 Timetable of Prenatal Development Based on Fertilization Age*

Nervous and Sensory System	Cardiorespiratory System	Digestive System	Genitourinary System	Musculoskeletal System	Integumentary System
3 Weeks: 1.5 mm CRL					
Flat neural plate begins closing to form neural tube. Neural tube still open at each end.	Heart consists of two parallel tubes that fuse into a single tube. Contractions of heart tube begin. Chorionic villi of early placenta connect with heart.	Endoderm (inner germ layer) will become digestive tract.		Paired, cube-shaped swellings (somites) appear and will form most of the head and trunk skeleton. Muscle, bone, and cartilage develop from mesoderm.	Epidermis (outer skin layer) will develop from ectoderm (outer germ layer). Dermis (deep skin layer) and connective tissue will develop from mesoderm (middle germ layer).
4 Weeks: 4 mm CRL					
Neural tube closed at each end. Cranial end of neural tube will form brain; caudal end will form spinal cord. Eye development begins as an outgrowth of forebrain. Nose development begins as two pits. Inner ear begins developing from hind brain.	Heart begins partitioning into four chambers and begins beating. Blood circulating through embryonic vessels and chorionic villi. Tracheal development begins as a bud on the upper gut and branches into two bronchial buds.	Development of primitive gut as embryo folds laterally. Stomach begins as a widening of the tube-shaped primitive gut. Liver, gallbladder, and biliary ducts begin as a bud from primitive gut.	Primordial germ (reproductive) cells are present on embryonic yolk sac.	Upper limb buds are present and look like flippers. Lower limb buds appear.	Mammary ridges that will develop into mammary glands appear.
6 Weeks: 13 mm CRL					
Development of pituitary gland and cranial nerves. Head sharply flexed because of rapid brain growth. Eyelid development beginning. External ear development begins in neck region as six swellings.	Blood formation primarily in liver. Three right and two left lung lobes develop as outgrowths of the right and left bronchi. Completion of partitioning of the heart into four chambers.	Most intestines are contained within the umbilical cord because the liver and kidneys occupy most of the abdominal cavity. Stomach nearing final form. Development of upper and lower jaws.	Kidneys are near bladder in the pelvis. Kidneys occupy much of the abdominal cavity. Primordial germ cells incorporated into developing gonads. Male and female gonads are identical in appearance.	Arms paddle-shaped, fingers webbed. Feet and toes develop similarly, but a few days later than arms and hands. Bones cartilaginous, but ossification of skull begins.	Mammary glands begin development. Tooth buds for primary (deciduous) teeth begin developing.
8 Weeks: 30 mm CRL					
Spinal cord stops at end of vertebral column. Taste buds begin developing. Eyelids fuse. Ears have final form but are low-set.	Heart partitioned into four chambers. Heart beat detectable with ultrasound. Additional branching of bronchi.	Stomach has reached final form. Lips are fused. Intestines remain in umbilical cord.	Testes begin developing under influence of Y chromosome. Ovaries will develop if a Y chromosome is not present. External genitalia begin to differentiate but still appear quite similar.	Fingers and toes still webbed, but distinct by end of eighth week. Bones begin to ossify. Joints resemble those of adults.	Auricles of ear low-set but beginning to assume final shape.
10 Weeks: 61 mm CRL; Weight, 14 g					
Head flexion remains, but less. Eyelids closed and fused. Top of external ear slightly below eye level.	May be possible to detect heartbeat with Doppler transducer. Blood produced in spleen and lymphatic tissue.	Intestines contained within abdominal cavity as growth of this cavity catches up with digestive system development. Digestive tract patent from mouth to anus.	Kidneys in their adult position. Male and female external genitalia have different appearance but are still easily confused.	Toes distinct; soles face each other.	Fingernails begin developing. Tooth buds for permanent teeth begin developing below those for primary teeth.

CRL, Crown-rump length.
*Fertilization age is about 2 weeks less than gestational age.

TABLE 6-2 Timetable of Prenatal Development Based on Fertilization Age*—cont'd

Nervous and Sensory System	Cardiorespiratory System	Digestive System	Genitourinary System	Musculoskeletal System	Integumentary System
12 Weeks: 87 mm CRL; Weight, 45 g					
Surface of brain is smooth, without sulci (grooves) or gyri (convolutions). Nasal septum and palate complete development.	Heartbeat should be detected with Doppler transducer.	Sucking reflex present. Bile formed by liver.	Kidneys begin producing urine. Male and female external genitalia can be distinguished by appearance.	Limbs are long and thin. Involuntary muscles of viscera develop.	Downy lanugo begins developing at end of this week.
16 Weeks: 140 mm CRL; Weight, 200 g					
Face is human looking because eyes face forward rather than to side.	Pulmonary vascular system developing rapidly.	Fetus swallows amniotic fluid and produces meconium (bowel contents).	Urine excreted into amniotic fluid.	Lower limbs reach final relative length, longer than upper limbs. A woman who has been pregnant before may begin to feel fetal movements.	External ears have enough cartilage to stand away from head somewhat. Blood vessels easily visible through the delicate skin. Fingerprints developing.
20 Weeks: 160 mm CRL; Weight, 460 g					
Myelination of nerves begins and continues through first year of postnatal life.	Heartbeat should be detectable with regular fetoscope.	Peristalsis well developed.	Over 40% of nephrons are mature and functioning. Testes contained in abdomen but begin descent toward scrotum. Primordial follicles of ovary reach peak of 5 to 7 million and then gradually decline.	Fetal movements felt by mother and may be palpable by an experienced examiner.	Skin is thin and covered with vernix caseosa. Brown fat production complete. Nipples begin development.
24 Weeks: 230 mm CRL; Weight, 820 G					
Spinal cord ends at level of first sacral vertebra because of more rapid growth of vertebral canal.	Primitive thin-walled alveoli (air sacs) have developed and are surrounded by capillary network. Surfactant production begins in lungs. Respiration possible, but many fetuses die if born at this time.		Testes descending toward inguinal rings.	Fetus is active. Fetal movements become progressively more noticeable to both mother and examiner.	Body appearance lean. Skin wrinkled and red. Fingerprints and footprints developed. Fingernails present. Eyebrows and lashes present.
28 Weeks: 270 mm CRL; Weight, 1300 g					
Major sulci and gyri are present. Eyelids no longer fused after 26 weeks. Responds to bitter substances on tongue.	Erythrocyte formation completely in bone marrow. Sufficient alveoli, surfactant, and capillary network to allow respiratory function, although respiratory distress syndrome is common. Many infants born at this time survive with intensive care.		Testes descended through inguinal canal into scrotum by end of 26th week.		Skin slightly wrinkled but smoothing out as subcutaneous fat is deposited under it.

Continued

TABLE 6-2 Timetable of Prenatal Development Based on Fertilization Age*—cont'd

Nervous and Sensory System	Cardiorespiratory System	Digestive System	Genitourinary System	Musculoskeletal System	Integumentary System
32 Weeks: 300 mm CRL; Weight, 2100 g					
Maturation of parasympathetic nervous system nears that of sympathetic nervous system, resulting in greater fetal heart rate variability on electronic fetal monitor tracing.	Surfactant production nears mature levels. Respiratory distress still possible if born at 32 weeks.				Skin smooth and pigmented. Large vessels visible beneath skin. Fingernails reach fingertips. Lanugo disappearing.
38 Weeks: 360 mm CRL; Weight, 3400 g					
Sulci and gyri developed. Visual acuity about 20/600 at birth.	Newborn infant has about one eighth to one sixth the number of alveoli of an adult. Well-developed ability to exchange gas.		Both testes usually palpable in scrotum at birth. The newborn girl's ovaries contain about 1 million follicles. No new ones are formed after birth; their numbers continue to decline after birth.		Fetus plump, and skin smooth. Vernix caseosa present in major body creases. Lanugo present on shoulders and upper back only. Fingernails extend beyond the fingertips. Ear cartilage firm.

Differentiation of Cells

The embryo progresses from undifferentiated cells with essentially identical functions to differentiated, or specialized, body cells. By the end of the eighth week, all major organ systems are in place and many are functioning, although in a simple way.

Development of the specialized structures is controlled by three factors: (1) genetic information in the chromosomes received from the parents, (2) interaction between adjacent tissues, and (3) timing. Although basic instructions are carried within the chromosomes, one tissue may induce change toward greater specialization in another, but only if a signal between the two tissues occurs at a specific time during development. In this way, structures develop with appropriate sizes and relationships to each other.

During the embryonic period, structures are vulnerable to damage from teratogens because they are developing rapidly. Normal development of one structure often requires normal and properly timed development of another structure. Unfortunately, a woman may not realize she is pregnant during this sensitive time. For this reason the possibility of pregnancy should be explored with her before the prescription of drugs or administration of diagnostic procedures such as radiography. Some agents may be damaging at one time during pregnancy but not at another. Others may be damaging at any time during pregnancy (see Appendix B).

Weekly Developments

Development occurs simultaneously in all embryonic organ systems. Development of the embryo and fetus proceeds in a cephalocaudal (head-to-toe) and central-to-peripheral direction. The earliest cells are simple, are linked to no specific body system, and progress to complex cells that perform specialized functions. Generalized to specific development continues with refinement of organs, such as development of bones, joints, muscles, and tendons of the arm and hand beginning as a simple limb bud. This developmental pattern continues after birth.

Full term ranges from 36 to 40 weeks of fertilization age, or 38 to 42 weeks of gestational age (after last menstrual period). Because conception occurs approximately 2 weeks after the first day of the last menstrual period in most women who have 4-week cycles, the fertilization age, used in this chapter, is approximately 2 weeks shorter than the gestational age. However, gestational age is most commonly used in practice because the last menstrual period provides a known marker, whereas most women do not know exactly when they conceived.

WEEK 2

Implantation is complete by the end of the second week after fertilization. The most growth occurs in the outer cells, or trophoblast, which eventually becomes the fetal part of the placenta. The inner cell mass that will develop into the baby becomes flattened into the embryonic disk. Cells that eventually form part of the fetal membranes develop.

WEEK 3

Many women miss their first menstrual period during the third week after conception. The embryonic disk develops three layers called *germ layers* that in turn give rise to major organ systems of the body (Table 6-3). The three germ layers are the ectoderm, mesoderm, and endoderm.

The central nervous system begins developing during the third week. A thickened flat neural plate appears, extending to-

TABLE 6-3 Derivatives of the Three Germ Layers

Ectoderm	Mesoderm	Endoderm
Brain and spinal cord	Cartilage	Lining of gastrointestinal and respiratory tracts
Peripheral nervous system	Bone	Tonsils
Pituitary gland	Connective tissue	Thyroid
Sensory epithelium of the eye, ear, and nose	Muscle tissue	Parathyroid
Epidermis	Heart	Thymus
Hair	Blood vessels	Liver
Nails	Blood cells	Pancreas
Subcutaneous glands	Lymphatic system	Lining of urinary bladder and urethra
Mammary glands	Spleen	Lining of ear canal
Tooth enamel	Kidneys	
	Adrenal cortex	
	Ovaries	
	Testes	
	Reproductive system	
	Lining membranes (pericardial, pleural, and peritoneal)	

ward the end of the embryonic disk that will become the head. The neural plate develops a longitudinal groove that folds to form the neural tube. At the end of the third week the neural tube is fused in the middle but still open at each end.

Early heart development consists of a pair of parallel heart tubes that run and then fuse longitudinally. The primitive, or tubular, heart begins beating at 22 to 23 days, resulting in a wavelike flow of blood. By the end of the fourth week, coordinated contractions result in the unidirectional flow of blood that characterizes the mature heart. Vessels developing in the chorionic villi and membranes join the heart tube. Primitive blood cells arise from the endoderm lining the distal blood vessels.

WEEK 4

The shape of the embryo changes during the fourth week after conception. It folds at the head and tail end and laterally, resembling a C-shaped cylinder. A "tail" is apparent during the embryonic period because the brain and spinal cord develop more rapidly than other systems. The tail disappears as the rest of the body catches up with growth of the central nervous system. The neural tube closes during the fourth week. If the neural tube does not close, defects such as anencephaly and spina bifida result.

Formation of the face and upper respiratory tract begins. Beginnings of the internal ear and the eye are apparent. The upper extremities appear as buds on the lateral body walls. Because the embryo is sharply flexed anteriorly, the heart is near the embryo's mouth. Partitioning of the heart into four chambers begins during the fourth week and is completed by the end of the sixth week.

The lower respiratory tract begins growth as a branch of the upper digestive tract, which is a simple tube at this time. Gradually, the esophagus and trachea complete separation. The trachea branches to form the right and left bronchi. These bronchi in turn branch to form the three lobes of the right lung and two lobes of the left lung. Continued branching of the bronchi eventually forms the terminal air sacs, or alveoli. The alveoli proliferate and become surrounded by a rich capillary network that enables oxygen and carbon dioxide exchange at birth.

WEEK 5

The head is very large because the brain grows rapidly during the fifth week after fertilization. The heart is beating and developing four chambers. Upper limb buds are paddle shaped with obvious notches between the fingers. Lower limbs form slightly later than upper ones. Lower limbs are also paddle shaped, but the area between the toes is not as well defined as the division between the fingers.

WEEK 6

The rapidly developing head is bent over the chest. The heart reaches its final four-chambered form. Upper and lower extremities continue to become more defined.

The eyes continue to develop, and the beginnings of the external ears appear as six small bumps on both sides of the neck. Facial development begins with eyes, ears, and nasal pits that are widely separated and aligned with the body walls. Gradually the embryo grows so that the face comes together in the midline and the external ears assume their proper position on the sides of the head.

WEEK 7

General growth and refinement of all systems occur seven weeks after conception. The face becomes more human looking. The eyelids begin to grow, and the extremities become longer and better defined. The trunk elongates and straightens, although a C-shaped spinal curve remains in the newborn at birth.

The intestines have been growing faster than the abdominal cavity during the embryonic period. The relatively large liver and kidneys also occupy much of the abdominal cavity. Therefore most of the intestines are contained within the umbilical cord while the abdominal cavity grows to accommodate them. The abdomen is large enough to contain all its normal contents by 10 weeks.

WEEK 8

The embryo has a definite human form, and refinements to all systems continue. The ears are low set but approaching their final location. The eyes are pigmented but not yet fully covered by eyelids. Fingers and toes are stubby but well defined. The external genitalia begin to differentiate, but male and female characteristics are not distinct until 10 weeks after conception, or 12 weeks after the woman's last menstrual period.

✔ CHECK YOUR READING

11. Why is the embryo particularly susceptible to damage from teratogens?
12. How does the lower respiratory tract develop?
13. Why are the intestines mostly contained within the umbilical cord until the tenth week?

FETAL PERIOD

The fetal period is the longest part of prenatal development. It begins 9 weeks after conception and ends with birth. All major systems are present in their basic form. Dramatic growth and refinement in the structure and function of all organ systems occur during the fetal period (Figure 6-6). Teratogens may damage already formed structures but are less likely to cause major structural alterations. The central nervous system is vulnerable to damaging agents through the entire pregnancy. (In this discussion, *weeks of gestation* refer to weeks after conception. Add 2 weeks to obtain the approximate number of weeks from the woman's last menstrual period.)

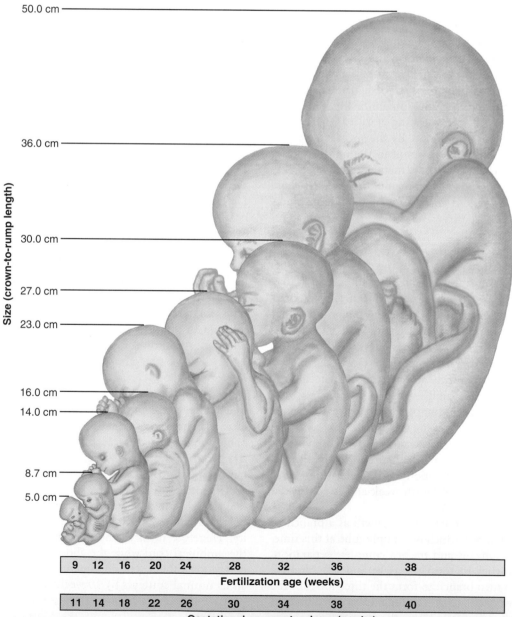

Figure 6-6 ■ Fetal development from 9 weeks through 38 weeks of fertilization age. The gestational age, measured from the first day of the last menstrual period, is approximately 2 weeks longer than the fertilization age.

Weeks 9 through 12

The head is approximately half the total length of the fetus at the beginning of this period. The body begins growing faster than the head, changing the proportions. The extremities approach their final relative lengths, although the legs remain proportionately shorter than the arms. The first fetal movements begin but are too slight for the mother to detect.

The face is broad with a wide nose and widely spaced eyes. The eyes close at 9 weeks and reopen at 26 weeks. The ears appear low set because the mandible is still small.

The intestinal contents that were partly contained within the umbilical cord enter the abdomen by 11 weeks as the capacity of the abdominal cavity catches up with them in size. Blood formation occurs primarily in the liver during the ninth week but shifts to the spleen by the end of the twelfth week. The fetus begins producing urine during this period and excretes it into the amniotic fluid.

Internal differences in males and females begin to be apparent in the seventh week. External genitalia look similar until the end of the ninth week. By the end of the twelfth week, the fetal gender can be determined by the appearance of the external genitalia.

Weeks 13 through 16

The fetus grows rapidly in length, so the head becomes smaller in proportion to the total length. Movements strengthen, and some women, particularly those who have been pregnant before, are able to detect them. This phenomenon is referred to as *quickening*. The face looks human because the eyes face fully forward. The ears near their final position at the sides of the head and in line with the eyes.

Weeks 17 through 20

Fetal movements feel like fluttering or "butterflies." Some women may not recognize these subtle sensations.

Changes in the skin and hair are evident. Vernix caseosa, a fatty, cheeselike secretion of the fetal sebaceous glands, covers the skin to protect it from constant exposure to amniotic fluid. Lanugo is fine, downy hair that covers the fetal body and helps the vernix adhere to the skin. Both vernix and lanugo diminish as the fetus reaches term. Eyebrows and head hair appear.

Brown fat is a special heat-producing fat deposited during this period that helps the newborn maintain temperature stability after birth. It is located on the back of the neck, behind the sternum, and around the kidneys.

Weeks 21 through 24

While continuing to grow and gain weight, the fetus still appears thin because of minimal subcutaneous fat. The skin is translucent and red because the capillaries are close to its fragile surface.

The lungs begin to produce surfactant, a surface-active lipid substance that facilitates lung expansion and makes it easier for the baby to breathe after birth. Surfactant reduces surface tension in the lung alveoli and prevents them from collapsing with each breath. Production of surfactant begins at approximately 20 weeks but does not reach levels that permit easy survival outside the uterus until 26 to 28 weeks after conception. Surfactant production increases during late pregnancy, particularly during the last 2 weeks (Moore & Persaud, 2003a). To reduce respiratory distress of prematurity, artificial surfactant may be given to infants who are at risk for a deficiency because of their immaturity. Maternal corticosteroids such as betamethasone may be given before birth to accelerate surfactant production in the preterm fetus likely to be born before completion of 34 weeks gestation (see Chapter 27 for discussion of preterm labor care).

The capillary network surrounding the alveoli is increasing but still very immature, although some gas exchange is possible. A fetus born at this gestation is less likely to survive, because of inadequate gas exchange. Other systems are extremely immature as well, such as blood vessels in the brain that may bleed.

Weeks 25 through 28

The fetus is more likely to survive if born during this period because of maturation of the lungs, pulmonary capillaries, and central nervous system. The fetus becomes plumper with smoother skin as subcutaneous fat is deposited under the skin. The skin gradually becomes less red. The eyes, which were closed during the ninth week, reopen. Head hair is abundant. Blood formation shifts from the spleen to the bone marrow.

During early pregnancy the fetus floats freely within the amniotic sac. However, the fetus usually assumes a head-down position during this time for two reasons:

- The uterus is shaped like an inverted egg. The overall shape of the fetus in flexion is similar, with the head being the small pole of the egg shape and the buttocks, flexed legs, and feet being the larger pole.
- The fetal head is heavier than the feet, and gravity causes the head to drift downward in the pool of amniotic fluid.

The head-down position is also most favorable for normal birth.

Weeks 29 through 32

The skin is pigmented according to race and is smooth. Larger vessels are visible over the abdomen, but small capillaries cannot be seen. Toenails are present, and fingernails extend to the fingertips. The fetus has more subcutaneous fat, which rounds the body contours. If the fetus is born during this period, chances of survival are good.

Weeks 33 through 38

Growth of all body systems continues until birth, but the rate of growth slows as full term approaches. The fetus is mainly gaining weight. The pulmonary system matures to enable efficient and unlabored breathing after birth.

The well-nourished term fetus is rotund with abundant subcutaneous fat. At birth, boys are slightly heavier than girls. The skin is pink to brownish pink, depending on race. Lanugo may be present over the forehead, upper back, and upper arms. Vernix often remains in major creases such as the groin and axillae.

The testes are in the scrotum. Breasts of both male and female infants are enlarged, and breast tissue is palpable beneath the areola and nipple.

✔ CHECK YOUR READING

14. What is the difference between fertilization age and gestational age? Which term is more commonly used and why?
15. Why does the fetus usually assume a head-down position in the uterus?
16. What is the purpose of each of these fetal structures or substances: Vernix caseosa? Lanugo? Brown fat? Surfactant?

AUXILIARY STRUCTURES

Three auxiliary structures sustain the pregnancy and permit normal prenatal development: the placenta, umbilical cord, and fetal membranes. These structures develop simultaneously with the baby's development.

Placenta

The placenta is a thick, disk-shaped organ. The placenta has two components: maternal and fetal (Figure 6-7). It is involved in (1) metabolic functions, (2) transfer functions, and (3) endocrine functions. The fetal side is smooth, with branching vessels covering the membrane-covered surface. The maternal side is rough where it attaches to the uterus (see Figure 12-14, *A* and *B*).

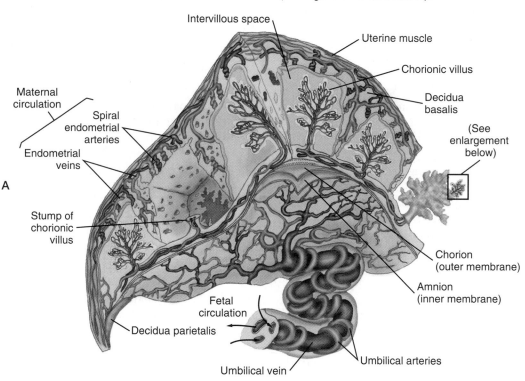

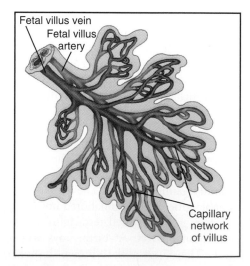

Figure 6-7 ■ A, Placental structure showing relationship of placenta, fetal membranes, and uterus. Arrows indicate the direction of blood flow between the fetus and placenta through the umbilical arteries and vein. Blood from the woman bathes the fetal chorionic villi within the intervillous spaces to allow exchange of oxygen, nutrients, and waste products without gross mixing of maternal and fetal blood. **B,** Structure of a chorionic villus; its fetal capillary network is illustrated.

The umbilical cord is normally inserted on the fetal side of the placenta, near the center. However, it may insert off center or even out on the fetal membranes (Figure 6-8).

During early pregnancy the placenta is larger than the embryo or fetus. However, the fetus grows faster than the placenta, so the placenta is approximately one sixth the weight of the fetus at the end of a full-term pregnancy.

MATERNAL COMPONENT

DEVELOPMENT. When conception occurs, cells of the endometrium undergo changes that promote early nutrition of the embryo and enable most of the uterine lining to be shed after birth. These changes convert endometrial cells into the decidua. In addition to providing nourishment for the embryo, the decidua may protect the mother from uncontrolled invasion of fetal placental tissue into the uterine wall.

The three decidual layers are (1) the decidua basalis, which underlies the developing embryo and forms the maternal side of the placenta; (2) the decidua capsularis, which overlies the embryo and bulges into the uterine cavity as the embryo and fetus grow; and (3) the decidua parietalis, which lines the rest of the uterine cavity. By approximately 22 weeks of gestation, the decidua capsularis fuses with the decidua parietalis, filling the uterine cavity.

CIRCULATION IN THE MATERNAL SIDE. Maternal and fetal blood normally do not mix in the placenta, although they flow very close to each other. Exchange of substances between mother and fetus occurs within the intervillous spaces of the placenta. While in the intervillous space, the mother's blood is briefly outside her circulatory system. Approximately 150 ml of maternal blood is contained within the intervillous space. Blood in the intervillous space is changed approximately three to four times per minute, requiring circulation of 450 to 750 ml per minute for placental perfusion.

Maternal blood spurts into the intervillous spaces through 80 to 100 spiral arteries in the decidua. After the

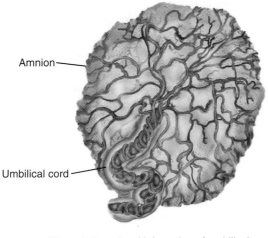

Amnion

Umbilical cord

Normal placenta with insertion of umbilical cord near center and branching of fetal umbilical vessels over the surface

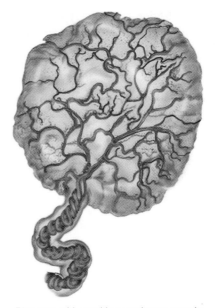

Placenta with cord inserted near margin of placenta

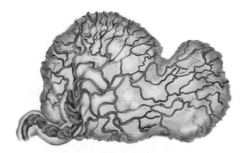

Placenta with a small accessory lobe

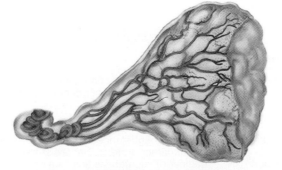

Velamentous insertion of umbilical cord. Cord vessels branch far out on membranes. When membranes rupture, fetal umbilical vessels may be torn and the fetus can hemorrhage.

Figure 6-8 ■ Placental variations.

oxygenated and nutrient-bearing maternal blood washes over the chorionic villi containing the fetal vessels, it returns to the maternal circulation through the endometrial veins for elimination of fetal waste products.

FETAL COMPONENT

DEVELOPMENT. The fetal side of the placenta develops from the outer cell layer (trophoblast) of the blastocyst at the same time the inner cell mass develops into the embryo and fetus. The primary chorionic villi are the initial structures that eventually form the fetal side of the placenta.

CIRCULATION IN THE FETAL SIDE. The umbilical cord contains the umbilical arteries and vein to transport blood between the fetus and placenta. Chorionic villi are bathed by oxygen- and nutrient-rich maternal blood in the maternal intervillous spaces. Each chorionic villus is supplied by a tiny fetal artery carrying deoxygenated blood and waste products from the fetus. The vein of the chorionic villus returns oxygenated blood and nutrients to the embryo and fetus.

Capillaries in the chorionic villi are separated from actual contact with the mother's blood by the membranes of each villus. This arrangement allows contact close enough for exchange and prevents mixing of maternal and fetal blood. The closed fetal circulation is important because the blood types of mother and fetus may not be compatible.

The placental arteries and veins converge in the blood vessels of the umbilical cord. Two umbilical arteries and one umbilical vein transport blood between the fetus and the fetal side of the placenta. Blood is circulated to and from the fetal side of the placenta by the fetal heart.

METABOLIC FUNCTIONS

The placenta produces some nutrients needed by the embryo and for placental functions. Substances synthesized include glycogen, cholesterol, and fatty acids (Moore & Persaud, 2003a,b).

TRANSFER FUNCTIONS

Exchange of oxygen, nutrients, and waste products across the chorionic villi occurs through several methods (Table 6-4). Placental transfer of harmful substances also may occur.

Most substances that enter the mother's bloodstream can enter the fetal circulation, and many agents enter it almost immediately.

GAS EXCHANGE. Respiration is a key function of the placenta. Oxygen and carbon dioxide pass through the placental membrane by simple diffusion. The average oxygen-partial pressure (PO_2) of maternal blood in the intervillous space is 50 mm Hg. The average blood PO_2 in the umbilical vein (after oxygenation) is approximately 30 mm Hg (Guyton & Hall, 2000; Jones & DeCherney, 2003).

The fetus can thrive in this low-oxygen environment for three reasons:

- Fetal hemoglobin can carry 20% to 50% more oxygen than adult hemoglobin.
- The fetus has a higher oxygen-carrying capacity because of a higher average hemoglobin (14.5 to 22.5 g/dl) and hematocrit value (approximately 48% to 69%).
- Hemoglobin can carry more oxygen at low carbon dioxide-partial pressure (PCO_2) levels than it can at high ones (Bohr effect). Blood entering the placenta from the fetus has a high PCO_2, but carbon dioxide diffuses quickly to the mother's blood, where the PCO_2 is lower, reversing the levels of carbon dioxide in the maternal and the fetal blood. Therefore the fetal blood becomes more alkaline and the maternal blood becomes more acidic. This allows the mother's blood to give up oxygen and the fetal blood to combine with oxygen readily.

Fetal PCO_2 is only about 2 to 3 mm Hg higher than the PCO_2 of maternal blood. However, carbon dioxide is very soluble, allowing it to pass across the placental membrane into maternal blood at this low pressure gradient.

NUTRIENT TRANSFER. The growing fetus requires a constant supply of nutrients from the pregnant woman. Glucose, fatty acids, vitamins, and electrolytes pass readily across the placenta. Glucose is the major energy source for fetal growth and metabolic activities.

WASTE REMOVAL. In addition to carbon dioxide, urea, uric acid, and bilirubin are readily transferred from fetus to mother for disposal. Because the normal placenta removes wastes for the fetus, metabolic defects such as phenylketonuria are usually not evident until after birth.

TABLE 6-4 Mechanisms of Placental Transfer

Mechanism	Description	Examples of Substances Transferred
Simple diffusion	Passive movement of substances across a cell membrane from an area of higher concentration to one of lower concentration	Oxygen and carbon dioxide Carbon monoxide Water Urea and uric acid Most drugs and their metabolites
Facilitated diffusion	Passage of substances across a cell membrane by binding with carrier proteins that assist transfer	Glucose
Active transport	Transfer of substances across a cell membrane against a pressure or electrical gradient, or from an area of lower concentration to one of higher concentration	Amino acids Water-soluble vitamins Minerals: Calcium, iron, iodine
Pinocytosis	Movement of large molecules by ingestion within cells	Maternal IgG class antibodies Some passage of maternal IgA antibodies

IgA, Immunoglobulin A; *IgG,* immunoglobulin G.

ANTIBODY TRANSFER. Many of the immunoglobulin G (IgG) class of antibodies are passed from mother to fetus through the placenta. This confers passive (temporary) immunity to the fetus against diseases such as measles if the mother is immune to them. Passage of antibodies against disease is beneficial because the newborn does not produce antibodies for several months after birth. The preterm or small-for-gestational age infant has little protection from maternal antibodies because they are transferred during late pregnancy and are poorly transferred if placental function is inadequate.

Passage of antibodies from expectant mother to fetus is not always beneficial. If maternal and fetal blood types are not compatible, the mother may already have or may produce antibodies against fetal erythrocytes. The mother's antibodies may then destroy the fetal erythrocytes, causing fetal anemia or even death. This situation may occur if the mother is Rh-negative and the fetus is Rh-positive.

TRANSFER OF MATERNAL HORMONES. Most maternal protein hormones do not reach the fetus in significant amounts. The female fetus exposed to androgenic hormones may have masculinization of her genitalia, and her true gender may be difficult to determine at birth.

ENDOCRINE FUNCTIONS

The placenta produces several hormones necessary for normal pregnancy. hCG causes the corpus luteum to persist for the first 6 to 8 weeks of pregnancy and secrete estrogens and progesterone. As the placenta develops further, it takes over estrogen and progesterone production and the corpus luteum regresses. When a Y chromosome is present in the male fetus, hCG also causes the fetal testes to secrete testosterone, necessary for normal development of male reproductive structures.

Human placental lactogen, also called *human chorionic somatomammotropin*, promotes normal nutrition and growth of the fetus and maternal breast development for lactation. This placental hormone decreases maternal insulin sensitivity and glucose use, making more glucose available for fetal nutrition.

Steroid hormones secreted by the placenta include estrogens and progesterone. Estrogens cause enlargement of the woman's uterus, enlargement of the breasts, growth of the ductal system of the breasts, and enlargement of the external genitalia. Estriol is the most plentiful estrogen produced during pregnancy.

Progesterone is essential for normal continuation of the pregnancy. Functions of progesterone include the following:
- Causes secretory changes in the endometrium, providing nourishment as the conceptus enters the uterus
- Causes the changes in endometrial cells that convert them into the larger and thicker cells of the decidua, which characterize pregnancy
- Reduces muscle contractions of the uterus to prevent spontaneous abortion
- May induce some immune tolerance in the mother's body for the conceptus

- Acts with estrogens and other hormones to cause growth of the breasts, budding of the alveoli that will secrete milk, and development of secretory characteristics in the alveolar cells

Other hormones produced by the placenta include human chorionic thyrotropin and human chorionic adrenocorticotropin.

CHECK YOUR READING

17. Which structure takes over the functions of the corpus luteum?
18. What is the purpose of the intervillous spaces of the placenta?
19. Why should fetal and maternal blood not actually mix?
20. What factors enable the fetus to thrive in a low-oxygen environment?
21. What are the purposes of these placental hormones: hCG? Human placental lactogen? Estrogen? Progesterone?

Fetal Membranes and Amniotic Fluid

The two fetal membranes are the amnion (inner membrane) and the chorion (outer membrane). The two membranes are so close as to be one (the "bag of waters"), but they can be separated. If the membranes rupture in labor, amnion and chorion usually rupture together, releasing the amniotic fluid within the sac.

The amnion is continuous with the surface of the umbilical cord, joining the epithelium of the fetus' abdominal skin. Chorionic villi proliferate over the entire surface of the gestational sac for the first 8 weeks after conception. A conceptus observed at this time looks like a shaggy sphere with the embryo suspended inside. As the embryo grows, it bulges into the uterine cavity. The villi on the outer surface gradually atrophy and form the smooth-surfaced chorion. The remaining villi continue to branch and enlarge to form the fetal side of the placenta.

Amniotic fluid protects the growing fetus and promotes normal prenatal development. Amniotic fluid protects the fetus by the following actions:
- Cushioning against impacts to the maternal abdomen
- Maintaining a stable temperature

Amniotic fluid promotes normal prenatal development by the following actions:
- Allowing symmetric development as the major body surfaces fold toward the midline
- Preventing the membranes from adhering to developing fetal parts
- Allowing room and buoyancy for fetal movement

Amniotic fluid is derived from two sources: (1) fetal urine and (2) fluid transported from the maternal blood across the amnion. Castoff fetal epithelial cells and vernix are suspended in the amniotic fluid. The water of the amniotic fluid changes by absorption across the amnion, returning to the mother. The fetus also swallows amniotic fluid and absorbs it in the digestive tract. Waste products are returned to the placenta through the umbilical arteries.

The volume of amniotic fluid increases during pregnancy and is approximately 700 to 800 ml at 40 weeks. An abnormally small quantity of fluid (less than 50% of the amount expected for gestation, or under 400 ml at term) is called *oligohydramnios* and may be associated with the following (Blackburn, 2003; Guyton & Hall, 2000; Toot & Lu, 2004):

- Poor placental blood flow
- Preterm membrane rupture
- Failure of fetal kidney development
- Blocked urinary excretion

Poor fetal lung development (pulmonary hypoplasia) and malformations such as skeletal abnormalities may result from compression of fetal parts.

Hydramnios (also called *polyhydramnios*) is the opposite situation, in which the quantity may exceed 2000 ml. Hydramnios may be associated with the following (Blackburn, 2003):

- Imbalanced water exchange among mother, fetus, and amniotic fluid that has no known cause
- Poorly controlled maternal diabetes mellitus that results in large quantities of fetal urine excretion having an elevated glucose level

- Malformations of the central nervous system, cardiovascular system, or gastrointestinal tract that interfere with normal fluid ingestion, metabolism, and excretion

FETAL CIRCULATION

The course of fetal blood circulation is from the fetal heart, to the placenta for exchange of oxygen, nutrients, and waste products, and back to the fetus for delivery to fetal tissues (Figure 6-9, *A*).

Umbilical Cord

The fetal umbilical cord is the lifeline between the fetus and placenta. It has two arteries that carry deoxygenated blood and waste products away from the fetus to the placenta, where these substances are transferred to the mother's circulation. The umbilical vein carries freshly oxygenated and nutrient-laden blood from the placenta back to the fetus. The umbilical arteries and vein are coiled within the cord to allow them to stretch and prevent obstruction of blood flow through them. The entire cord is cushioned by a soft sub-

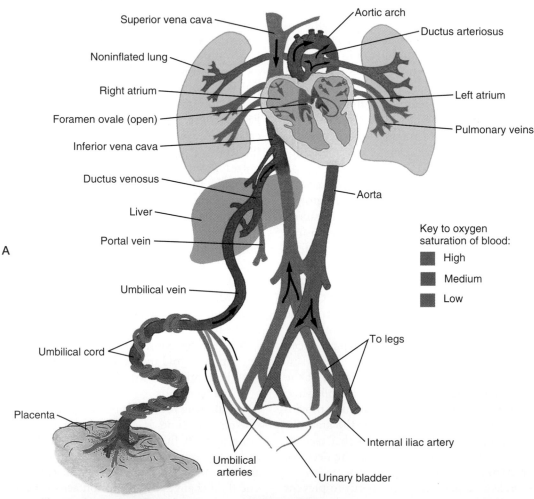

Fetal circulation

Figure 6-9 ■ **A**, Fetal circulation. Three shunts allow most blood from the placenta to bypass the fetal lungs and liver, ductus venosus, ductus arteriosus, and foramen ovale.

stance called *Wharton's jelly* to prevent obstruction resulting from pressure.

Fetal Circulatory Circuit

Because the fetus does not breathe air, several alterations of the postnatal circulatory route are needed (see Figure 6-9, *A*). Also, the fetal liver does not have the metabolic functions that it will have after birth, because the mother's body performs these functions. Three shunts in the fetal circulatory system allow blood with the highest oxygen content to be sent to the fetal heart and brain: the ductus venosus, foramen ovale, and ductus arteriosus. At birth the infant's lungs oxygenate the blood, the placenta is removed from the circulatory path, and the liver must perform its metabolic functions.

Oxygenated blood from the placenta enters the fetal body through the umbilical vein. About two thirds of the blood goes through the liver, and the rest bypasses the liver and enters the inferior vena cava through the first shunt, the ductus venosus. The blood then enters the right atrium and joins with deoxygenated blood from the lower body and head. Most of the blood passes directly into the left atrium through the second shunt, the foramen ovale, where it mixes with the small amount of blood returning from the lungs. Blood is pumped from the left ventricle into the aorta to nourish the body. A small amount of blood from the right ventricle is circulated to the lungs to nourish the lung tissue. The rest of the blood from the right ventricle joins oxygenated blood in the aorta through the third shunt, the ductus arteriosus. The head and upper body receive the greatest amount of oxygenated blood.

The wall of the right ventricle of the fetal heart is thicker than that of the left because resistance to blood flow through the uninflated lungs is high, similar to the resistance in other parts of the fetal body. When the infant begins breathing after birth, resistance to pulmonary blood flow from the right ventricle falls, while resistance to systemic flow from the left ventricle rises. Thickness of the wall of the left ventricle increases to meet greater resistance to systemic outflow. Thickness of the right ventricle has little change. As cardiac growth progresses throughout child-

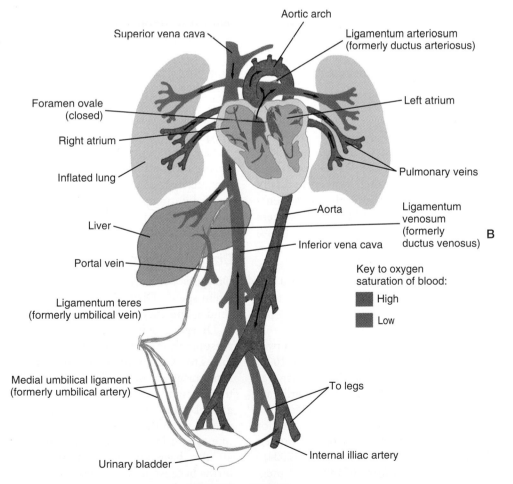

Circulation after birth

Figure 6-9 ■ **B,** Circulation after birth. Note that the fetal shunts have closed. The umbilical vessels (ductus venosus and ductus arteriosus) will be converted to ligaments.

hood, the thickness of the left ventricle remains greater than that of the right ventricle (Blackburn, 2003; Moore & Persaud, 2003b).

Changes in Blood Circulation after Birth

Fetal circulatory shunts are not needed after birth because the infant oxygenates blood in the lungs and is not circulating blood to the placenta (Figure 6-9, *B*). As the infant breathes, blood flow to the lungs increases, pressure in the right side of the heart falls, and the foramen ovale closes. The ductus arteriosus constricts as the arterial oxygen level rises. Persistent hypoxia may cause the ductus arteriosus to remain open for a prolonged period. The ductus venosus constricts when flow of blood from the umbilical cord stops.

Transition to the postnatal circulatory pattern is gradual. Functional closure begins when the infant breathes and the cord is cut, removing the placenta from the circulation. The foramen ovale and ductus venosus are permanently closed as tissue proliferates in these structures. The ductus venosus becomes a ligament, as do the umbilical vein and arteries (see Table 19-1, p. 453).

✓ CHECK YOUR READING

22. What are the purposes of the fetal membranes and amniotic fluid?
23. Trace the path of fetal circulation from the placenta through the fetal body and back to the placenta.

MULTIFETAL PREGNANCY

The incidence of multifetal pregnancy (multiple gestation) is increasing in the United States. Much of the increase is a result of a rise in maternal age, when women naturally are more likely to have twins, and infertility treatments that induce multiple ovulation. Twin births in 2002 were 3% higher than in 2001, at 31.1 per 1000 live births (3.2% of all births). The greatest rise in twin births has been among women aged 30 years and older. Triplet and higher-order multiple births rose from 37 to 193.5 per 100,000 live births between 1980 and 1998. Since 1998, the rate of high multiple births has declined slightly and was 184 per 100,000 live births in 2002 (Martin et al., 2003).

United States data for 2002 showed a 4% increase in twin births for non-Hispanic white women, to 34.8 per 1000, whereas the rate increase for non-Hispanic black women was 2%, or 34.7 per 1000 live births. The Hispanic twin birth rate remains lower at 20.7 per 1000 live births in 2002 (Martin et al., 2003). Asian women have a considerably lower rate for spontaneous twinning—about 1 in 150 for Japanese women and 1 in 300 for Chinese women (Stoll & Kliegman, 2004).

Twinning is the most common form of multifetal pregnancy. The same processes that occur in twin pregnancies also may occur in higher-order multiple gestations. Twins are often called *identical* or *fraternal* by lay people but are

more accurately described by their zygosity, or the number of ova and sperm involved. The two types of twins are monozygotic and dizygotic (Figure 6-10).

Monozygotic Twinning

Monozygotic twins are conceived by the union of a single ovum and spermatozoon, with later division of the conceptus into two. Monozygotic twins have identical genetic complements and are the same gender. However, they may not always look identical at birth because one twin may have grown much larger than the other or one may have a birth defect such as a cleft lip. Monozygotic twinning occurs essentially at random (about 3 to 5 per 1000 pregnancies), and a hereditary or racial component is not well established (Stoll & Kliegman, 2004).

Monozygotic twinning occurs when a single conceptus divides early in gestation. The blastocyst in most monozygotic twins is formed with two inner cell masses instead of one. If this occurs, usually in 70% of monozygotic twin pregnancies, the fetuses usually have two amnions (inner membranes) but a single chorion (outer membrane) (Blackburn, 2003).

If the conceptus divides earlier, two separate but identical morulas (and then blastocysts) develop and implant separately. These monozygotic twins have two amnions and two chorions. Although the placentas develop separately, they may fuse and appear as one at birth. The chorions also may fuse during prenatal development. Examination of the placenta and membranes after birth may not identify whether twins are monozygotic or dizygotic. Tests such as DNA analysis or detailed blood typing may be needed to determine whether twins are monozygotic or dizygotic.

Late separation of the inner cell mass may result in twins having a single amnion and a single chorion. These twins are more likely to die because their umbilical cords become entangled during pregnancy. Incomplete separation of the inner cell mass may result in conjoined (formerly called "Siamese") twins.

Dizygotic Twinning

Dizygotic twins arise from two ova that are fertilized by different sperm. Dizygotic twins may be the same or different gender, and they may not have similar physical traits.

Dizygotic twinning may be hereditary in some families, presumably because of an inherited tendency of the females to release more than one ovum per cycle. Women of some races are more likely to have dizygotic twins. Infertility therapy increases the incidence of twins, usually dizygotic, because induction of ovulation usually results in the release of multiple ova, with implantation of more than one zygote in the uterus. Women who conceive after age 40 also have an increased incidence of dizygotic twin births because multiple ova are more likely to be released near the climacteric.

Because dizygotic twins arise from two separate zygotes, their membranes and placentas are separate. The mem-

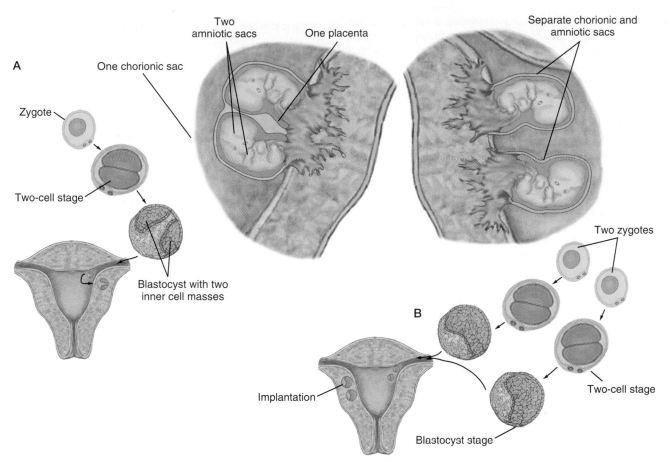

Figure 6-10 ▪ A, Monozygotic twinning. The single inner cell mass divides into two inner cell masses during the blastocyst stage. These twins have a single placenta and chorion, but each twin develops in its own amnion. **B,** Dizygotic twinning. Two ova are released during ovulation, and each is fertilized by a separate spermatozoon. The ova may implant near each other in the uterus, or they may be far apart.

branes, the placentas, or both may fuse during development if they implant closely. Dizygotic twins are not conjoined because they do not involve division of a single cell mass into two but arise from two separate conceptions.

High Multifetal Gestations

Pregnancies resulting in triplets or higher may arise from a single zygote or a combination of a single and multiple zygotes, or each may arise from a separate zygote. High multifetal pregnancies pose greater hazards to both mother and her fetuses. The incidence of long-term handicaps is higher as the number of fetuses increases.

✔ CHECK YOUR READING

24. How do monozygotic twins occur?
25. Why can examination of the placenta and membranes in a multifetal pregnancy not always establish whether they are monozygotic or dizygotic?
26. Why are dizygotic twins often of different genders?

SUMMARY CONCEPTS

- The purpose of gametogenesis is to produce ova and sperm that have half the full number of chromosomes, or 23 unpaired chromosomes. When an ovum and sperm unite at conception, the number is restored to 46 paired chromosomes.
- The female has all the ova she will ever have at 30 weeks of prenatal gestation. No other ova are formed after this time.
- One primary oocyte can mature into one mature ovum that contains 23 unpaired chromosomes (22 autosomes and one X chromosome).
- A male can continuously produce new sperm from puberty through the rest of his life, although fertility gradually declines after age 40.
- One primary spermatocyte can result in production of four mature sperm. Two of the mature sperm have 22 autosomes and one X sex chromosome. Two have 22 autosomes and one Y sex chromosome.
- The male determines the baby's gender because only sperm carry either an X or Y sex chromosome. The female contributes only an X chromosome to the baby.

- The basic structure of all organ systems is established during the first 8 weeks of pregnancy. Teratogens during this period may cause major structural and functional damage to the developing organs.
- The fetal period is one of growth and refinement of already established organ systems. Teratogens are less likely to cause major structural damage to the fetus but may cause major functional damage.
- The placenta is an embryonic or a fetal organ with metabolic, respiratory, and endocrine functions.
- Transfer of substances between mother and embryo or fetus occurs by four mechanisms: simple diffusion, facilitated diffusion, active transport, and pinocytosis.
- Most substances in the maternal blood can be transferred to the fetus.
- The fetal membranes contain the amniotic fluid, which cushions the fetus, allows normal prenatal development, and maintains a stable temperature.
- The umbilical cord is the lifeline between the fetus and the placenta. Two umbilical arteries carry deoxygenated blood and waste products to the placenta for transfer to the mother's blood. One umbilical vein carries oxygenated and nutrient-rich blood to the fetus. Coiling of the vessels and enclosure in Wharton's jelly reduce the risk of obstruction of the umbilical vessels.
- Three fetal circulatory shunts are needed to partially bypass the fetal liver and lungs: the ductus venosus, foramen ovale, and ductus arteriosus. These structures close functionally after birth but are not closed permanently until several weeks or months later.
- Multifetal pregnancy may be monozygotic or dizygotic. Twins are the most common form of multifetal pregnancy.
- Examination of the placenta and membranes alone cannot conclusively establish whether multiple fetuses are monozygotic or dizygotic.
- Dizygotic twins are more likely to occur in certain families and racial groups and especially in mothers older than 40 years and women who take fertility treatments to induce ovulation.

REFERENCES & READINGS

Benirschke, K. (2004). Multiple gestation: The biology of twinning. In R.K. Creasy, R. Resnik, & J.D. Iams (Eds.), *Maternal-fetal medicine: Principles and practice* (5th ed., pp. 55-67). Philadelphia: Saunders.

Benirschke, K. (2004). Normal early development. In R.K. Creasy, R. Resnik, & J.D. Iams (Eds.), *Maternal-fetal medicine: Principles and practice* (5th ed., pp. 37-44). Philadelphia: Saunders.

Bernstein, D. (2004). Developmental biology of the cardiovascular system. In R.E. Behrman, R.M. Kliegman, & H.B. Jenson (Eds.), *Nelson textbook of pediatrics* (17th ed., pp. 1475-1481). Philadelphia: Saunders.

Blackburn, S.T. (2003). *Maternal, fetal, and neonatal physiology: A clinical perspective.* Philadelphia: Saunders.

Callahan, L. (2004). Fetal and placental development and functioning. In S. Mattson & J.E. Smith (Eds.), *Core curriculum for maternal-newborn nursing* (3rd ed., pp. 41-72). Philadelphia: Saunders.

Carlson, B.M. (2004). *Human embryology and developmental biology,* 3rd ed. St. Louis: Mosby.

Carsten, M.E., & Lu, M.C. (2004). Endocrinology of pregnancy and parturition. In N.F. Hacker, J.G. Moore, & J.C. Gambone (Eds.), *Essentials of obstetrics and gynecology* (4th ed., pp. 57-64). Philadelphia: Saunders.

Guyton, A.C., & Hall, J.E. (2000). *Textbook of medical physiology* (10th ed.). Philadelphia: Saunders.

Jones, E.E., & DeCherney, A.H. (2003). Fertilization, pregnancy, and lactation. In W.F. Boron & E.L. Boulpaep (Eds.), *Medical physiology: A cellular and molecular approach.* Philadelphia: Saunders.

Malone, F.D., & D'Alton, M.E. (2004). Multiple gestation: Clinical inheritance and management. In R.K. Creasy, R. Resnik, & J.D. Iams (Eds.), *Maternal-fetal medicine: Principles and practice* (5th ed., pp. 281-314). Philadelphia: Saunders.

Martin, J.A., Hamilton, B.E., Sutton, P.D., Ventura, S.J., Menacker, F., & Munson, M.L. (2003). Births: Final data for 2002. *National Vital Statistics Reports, 53*(10). Hyattsville, MD: National Center for Health Statistics. Retrieved August 8, 2004, from www.cdc.gov/nchs/pressrooms/03facts/teenbirth.htm.

Moore, K.L., & Persaud, T.V.N. (2003a). *Before we are born: Essentials of embryology and birth defects* (6th ed.). Philadelphia: Saunders.

Moore, K.L., & Persaud, T.V.N. (2003b). *The developing human: Clinically oriented embryology* (7th ed.). Philadelphia: Saunders.

Stoll, B.J., & Kliegman, R.M. (2004). The high-risk infant. In R.E. Behrman, R.M. Kliegman, & H.B. Jenson (Eds.), *Nelson textbook of pediatrics* (17th ed., pp. 547-561). Philadelphia: Saunders.

Toot, P.J., & Lu, J.K.H. (2004). Female reproductive physiology. In N.F. Hacker, J.G. Moore, & J.C. Gambone (Eds.), *Essentials of obstetrics and gynecology* (4th ed., pp. 33-45). Philadelphia: Saunders.

Physiologic Adaptations to Pregnancy

After studying this chapter, you should be able to:

1. Describe the physiologic changes that occur during pregnancy.
2. Differentiate presumptive, probable, and positive signs of pregnancy.
3. Compute gravida, para, and estimated date of delivery.
4. Describe initial antepartum assessments in terms of history, physical examination, and risk assessment.
5. Identify subsequent antepartum assessments.
6. Discuss maternal adaptation to multifetal pregnancy.
7. Describe the common discomforts of pregnancy in terms of causes and measures that prevent or relieve them.
8. Use nursing process and critical thinking skills to develop plans of nursing care for the most common problems and discomforts of pregnancy.

Go to your Student CD-ROM for Review Questions keyed to these Objectives.

DEFINITIONS

Abortion Spontaneous or elective termination of pregnancy before the twentieth week of gestation based on the date of the last menstrual period. Spontaneous abortion is frequently called *miscarriage.*

Amenorrhea Absence of menstruation; either a delay of the first menstruation (primary amenorrhea) or cessation of menstruation after its initiation.

Braxton Hicks Contractions Irregular, usually mild uterine contractions that occur throughout pregnancy and become stronger in the last trimester.

Chadwick's Sign Bluish purple discoloration of the cervix, vagina, and labia during pregnancy as a result of increased vascular congestion.

Colostrum Breast fluid secreted during pregnancy and the first week after childbirth.

Diastasis Recti Separation of the longitudinal muscles of the abdomen (rectus abdominis) during pregnancy.

Goodell's Sign Softening of the cervix during pregnancy.

Gravida A woman who is or has been pregnant, regardless of the duration or outcome of the pregnancy.

Hegar's Sign Softening of the lower uterine segment that allows it to be easily compressed by the sixth week of pregnancy.

Hyperemia Excess blood in an area of the body.

Melasma Brownish pigmentation of the face during pregnancy; also called chloasma and "mask of pregnancy."

Multigravida A woman who has been pregnant more than once.

Multipara A woman who has given birth two or more times at 20 or more weeks of gestation.

Nullipara A woman who has never completed a pregnancy beyond a spontaneous or elective abortion.

Para Number of pregnancies that have progressed to 20 or more weeks at delivery, whether the fetus was born alive or stillborn; refers to the number of pregnancies, not the number of fetuses.

Physiologic Anemia of Pregnancy Decrease in hemoglobin and hematocrit values caused by dilution of erythrocytes by expanded plasma volume rather than by an actual decrease in erythrocytes or hemoglobin.

From the moment of conception, changes occur in the pregnant woman's body that are necessary to support and nourish the fetus, prepare the woman for childbirth and lactation, and maintain the woman's health. Pregnant women are often puzzled by the physical changes and unprepared for associated discomforts. Many pregnant women rely on nurses to provide accurate information and compassionate guidance throughout their pregnancy. To respond effectively, nurses must understand not only the physiologic changes but also how these changes affect the daily lives of expectant mothers.

CHANGES IN BODY SYSTEMS

Although pregnancy challenges each body system to adapt to increasing demands of the fetus, the most obvious changes are in the reproductive system.

Reproductive System

UTERUS

GROWTH. Perhaps the most dramatic change during pregnancy occurs in the uterus, which before conception is a small, pear-shaped organ entirely contained in the pelvic cavity. Before pregnancy the uterus weighs about 50 to 70 g (1.8 to 2.5 oz) and has a capacity of about 10 ml (one third of an ounce). By 36 weeks of gestation the uterus weighs 800 to 1200 g (1.8 to 2.6 lb) and has a capacity of 5000 ml (Blackburn, 2003).

Uterine growth occurs as the result of hyperplasia and hypertrophy. During the first trimester, growth is mainly caused by hyperplasia resulting from stimulation by estrogen and growth factors and stretching as the embryo grows. During the second and third trimesters, uterine growth results from hyperplasia and hypertrophy as the muscle fibers stretch in all directions to accommodate the growing fetus. In addition to muscle growth, fibrous tissue accumulates in the outer muscle layer of the uterus and the amount of elastic tissue increases. These changes greatly increase the strength of the muscle wall.

Muscle fibers in the myometrium increase in both length and width. Although the uterine wall thickens during early pregnancy, by the third trimester the wall of the uterus thins to about 1.5 cm (0.6 in) and the fetus can be easily palpated through the abdominal wall (Bond, 2004). As the uterus expands into the abdominal cavity at about 12 weeks of gestation, it displaces the intestines upward and laterally. It gradually rotates to the right as a result of pressure of the rectosigmoid colon on the left side of the pelvis.

PATTERN OF UTERINE GROWTH. The uterus grows in a predictable pattern that provides information about fetal growth and helps to confirm the estimated date of delivery (EDD), sometimes called the *estimated date of birth* (EDB) (Figure 7-1). For instance, by 12 weeks of gestation the uterus extends out of the maternal pelvis and can be palpated above the symphysis pubis. At 16 weeks the fundus reaches midway between the symphysis pubis and the umbilicus. At 20 weeks the fundus is located approximately at the umbilicus.

By 36 weeks the fundus reaches its highest level at the xiphoid process. It pushes against the diaphragm, and the expectant mother may experience shortness of breath, even during rest. By 40 weeks the fetal head descends into the pelvic cavity, and the uterus sinks to a lower level. This descent of the fetal head is called *lightening*, because it reduces pressure on the diaphragm and makes breathing easier.

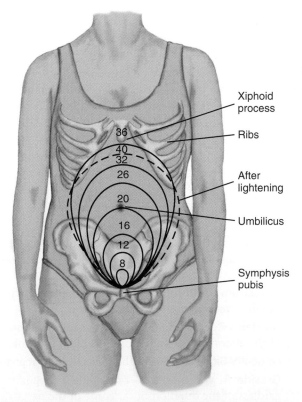

Figure 7-1 ■ Uterine growth pattern during pregnancy.

CONTRACTILITY. Throughout pregnancy the uterus undergoes irregular contractions called *Braxton Hicks contractions*. During the contractions the uterus temporarily tightens and becomes firm. It then returns to its original relaxed state. During the first two trimesters the contractions are infrequent and usually not felt by the woman. Contractions occur more frequently during the third trimester and may cause some discomfort. These are termed *false labor* when they are mistaken for the onset of early labor.

UTERINE BLOOD FLOW. As the uterus enlarges, an increase in the size and number of blood vessels expands blood flow dramatically. In early pregnancy, when the uterus and placenta are relatively small, most blood flow is to the myometrium and endometrium. As pregnancy continues, the delivery of materials needed for fetal growth and the removal of metabolic wastes depends on adequate perfusion of the placental intervillous spaces. During late pregnancy blood flow to the uterus and placenta reaches 450 to 650 ml/min (Cunningham et al., 2005). Maternal blood carried by the myometrial arteries enters the intervillous spaces, where oxygen and nutrients are transferred to the chorionic villi and hence to the fetus. Metabolic wastes from the fetus diffuse into venous structures of the mother (see Chapter 6).

Late in pregnancy, the uterine souffle, a soft, blowing sound, may be auscultated over the uterus. This is the sound of blood circulation through the placenta, and it corresponds to the maternal pulse. Therefore, to identify uterine souffle, the rate of the maternal pulse must be checked simultaneously with listening to the souffle. Uterine souffle differs from funic souffle, the soft, purring sound heard over the umbilical cord that corresponds to the fetal heart rate.

CERVIX

The cervix also undergoes significant changes after conception. The most obvious changes occur in color and consistency. In response to increasing levels of estrogen the cervix becomes congested with blood (hyperemic), resulting in the characteristic bluish purple color that extends to include the vagina and labia. This discoloration, referred to as *Chadwick's sign*, is one of the earliest signs of pregnancy.

The cervix is largely composed of connective tissue that softens when the collagen fibers decrease in concentration. Before pregnancy the cervix has a consistency similar to that of the tip of the nose. After conception the cervix feels more like the lobe of the ear. The cervical softening is referred to as *Goodell's sign*.

A less obvious change occurs as the cervical glands proliferate during pregnancy and the glandular walls become thin and widely separated. As a result, the endocervical tissue resembles a honeycomb that fills with mucus secreted by the cervical glands. The mucus forms a plug in the cervical canal. This plug blocks the ascent of bacteria from the vagina into the uterus during pregnancy and protects the fetus and membranes from infection (Figure 7-2). The mucous plug remains in place until the onset of labor

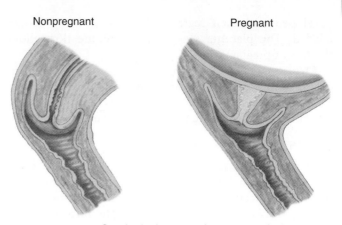

Nonpregnant

Pregnant

Figure 7-2 ■ Cervical changes that occur during pregnancy. Note enlargement of spaces in the cervical mucosa, which are filled with a thick mucous plug.

when the cervix begins to thin and dilate, allowing the mucous plug to be expelled. One of the earliest signs of labor may be "bloody show," which consists of the mucous plug and a small amount of blood produced by disruption of the cervical capillaries as the mucous plug is dislodged.

VAGINA AND VULVA

Changes of the vagina result from increased vascularity and are somewhat similar to those of the cervix. Softening of the abundant connective tissue allows the vagina to distend during childbirth. Because of hyperemia, the vaginal walls, like the cervix, appear blue or purple. The vaginal mucosa thickens, and vaginal rugae (folds) become very prominent.

Vaginal cells contain increasing amounts of glycogen, which causes rapid sloughing and increased thick, white, vaginal discharge. The pH of the vaginal discharge is acidic (3.5 to 6) because of the increased production of lactic acid that results from the action of Lactobacillus acidophilus on glycogen in the vaginal epithelium (Cunningham et al., 2005). The acidic condition helps to prevent growth of harmful bacteria found in the vagina. However, the glycogen-rich environment favors the growth of *Candida albicans*, and persistent yeast infections (candidiasis) are common during pregnancy.

Increased vascularity, edema, and connective tissue changes make the tissues of the vulva and perineum more pliable. Pelvic congestion during pregnancy can lead to heightened sexual interest and increased orgasmic experiences.

OVARIES

Once conception occurs, the major function of the ovaries is to secrete progesterone for the first 6 to 7 weeks of pregnancy. Progesterone, often called the "hormone of pregnancy," must be present in adequate amounts from the earliest stages to maintain pregnancy. Progesterone helps suppress contractions of the uterus and may also help prevent tissue rejection of the fetus (Liu, 2004). The corpus luteum secretes progesterone until the placenta is developed and then regresses because it is no longer needed. The placenta secretes progesterone throughout the rest of pregnancy.

Ovulation ceases during pregnancy because the high circulating levels of estrogen and progesterone inhibit the release of follicle-stimulating hormone (FSH) and luteinizing hormone (LH), which are necessary for ovulation.

BREASTS

During pregnancy the breasts change in both size and appearance (Figure 7-3). Estrogen stimulates the growth of mammary ductal tissue, and progesterone promotes the growth of lobes, lobules, and alveoli. The breasts become highly vascular, with a delicate network of veins often visible just beneath the surface of the skin. If the increase in breast size is extensive, striations ("stretch marks") similar to those that occur on the abdomen may develop.

Characteristic changes in the nipples and areolae occur during pregnancy. The nipples increase in size and become more erect, and the areolae become larger and more pigmented. The degree of pigmentation varies with the complexion of the expectant mother. Women with very light complexions exhibit less change in pigmentation than those with darker skin. Sebaceous glands called *tubercles of Montgomery* become more prominent during pregnancy and secrete a substance that lubricates the nipples. In addition, a thick, yellowish breast fluid, or colostrum, is present beginning in the second trimester and can readily be expressed by the third trimester.

✔ CHECK YOUR READING

1. What is the expected uterine growth at 16 weeks, 20 weeks, and 36 weeks of gestation?
2. How does uterine blood flow change during pregnancy?
3. What is the purpose of the cervical mucous plug?
4. What is the major purpose of progesterone?
5. How do the breasts change in size and appearance during pregnancy?

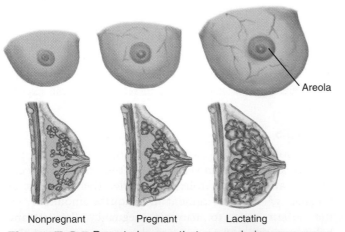

Nonpregnant   Pregnant   Lactating

Figure 7-3 ■ Breast changes that occur during pregnancy. The breasts increase in size and become more vascular, the areolae become darker, and the nipples become more erect.

Cardiovascular System

During pregnancy, alterations occur in heart size and position, blood volume, blood flow, and blood components.

HEART

HEART SIZE AND POSITION. Cardiac changes are minor and reverse soon after childbirth. The muscles of the heart (myocardium) enlarge slightly because of the increased workload during pregnancy. The heart is pushed upward and toward the left as the uterus elevates the diaphragm during the third trimester. As a result of the change in position, the locations for auscultation of heart sounds may be shifted upward and laterally in late pregnancy.

HEART SOUNDS. During pregnancy, some heart sounds may be so altered that they would be considered abnormal in a nonpregnant state. The changes are first heard between 12 and 20 weeks of gestation and continue for 2 to 4 weeks after childbirth. The most common variations in heart sounds include splitting of the first heart sound and a systolic murmur that is found in 90% of pregnant women (Cunningham et al., 2001). The murmur is best heard at the left sternal border. Although the second heart sound remains normal, many women have a third heart sound because of rapid filling during diastole (Gordon, 2002).

BLOOD VOLUME

Total blood volume is a combination of plasma and other components such as red blood cells (RBCs; erythrocytes), white blood cells (WBCs; leukocytes), and platelets (thrombocytes). Total blood volume increases about 40% to 50% during pregnancy (Bond, 2004).

PLASMA VOLUME

Plasma volume begins to increase at 6 to 8 weeks of gestation and peaks at 4700 to 5200 ml at 32 weeks. This is about 50% (1200 to 1300 ml) above nonpregnant values (Gordon, 2002). The increase is higher in multifetal pregnancies. The reason for the increase in plasma volume is unclear, but it may be related to vasodilation from nitric oxide, estrogen, progesterone, and prostaglandin stimulation of the renin-angiotensin-aldosterone system, which causes sodium and water retention (Blackburn, 2003; Monga, 2004).

Although the cause of plasma volume expansion is poorly understood, the increased volume is clearly needed for two reasons: (1) to transport nutrients and oxygen to the placenta, where they become available for the growing fetus, and (2) to meet the demands of the expanded maternal tissue in the uterus and breasts. An additional benefit of hypervolemia is that it provides a reserve to protect the pregnant woman from the adverse effects of blood loss that occurs during childbirth.

RED BLOOD CELL MASS. RBC mass increases by 250 to 450 ml, about 25% to 33% above prepregnancy values (Blackburn, 2003). Although both RBC volume and plasma volume expand, the increase in plasma volume is more pronounced and occurs earlier. The resulting dilution of RBC mass causes a decline in maternal hematocrit. This condition is frequently called *physiologic anemia,* or *pseudoanemia of pregnancy,* because it reflects dilution of RBCs in greatly expanded plasma volume rather than an actual decline of RBCs and does not indicate true anemia.

Physiologic anemia should not be dismissed as unimportant, however. Frequent laboratory examinations may be needed to distinguish between physiologic and true anemia. Generally, iron deficiency anemia occurs when the hemoglobin is less than 11 g/dl in the first and third trimesters or less than 10.5 g in the second trimester (Cunningham et al., 2005). Iron supplementation is often prescribed for all pregnant women by the second trimester to prevent anemia.

Dilution of RBCs by plasma may have a protective function. By decreasing blood viscosity, dilution may counter the tendency to form clots (thrombi) that can obstruct blood vessels and cause serious complications (see Chapter 28).

CARDIAC OUTPUT

A major consequence of the expanded blood volume of pregnancy is an increase in cardiac output. Cardiac output is the amount of blood discharged from the heart each minute. It is based on stroke volume (the amount of blood pumped from the heart with each contraction) and heart rate (the number of times the heart beats each minute). Cardiac output rises rapidly during the first trimester and increases 30% to 50% by the third trimester. The increase in cardiac output is primarily the result of a gain in stroke volume, but the heart rate also rises 10 to 20 beats per minute (bpm) by 32 weeks of gestation (Blackburn, 2003; Monga, 2004). Cardiac output is highest when the woman is lying on her side and lower in the sitting, standing, or supine position (Gordon, 2002).

PERIPHERAL VASCULAR RESISTANCE

Peripheral vascular resistance falls during pregnancy. This change is likely because of (1) smooth muscle relaxation in vessel walls resulting from the effects of progesterone; (2) the addition of the uteroplacental unit, which provides a greater area for circulation; (3) fetal heat production, which may produce vasodilation; (4) synthesis of prostaglandins that cause resistance to circulating vasoconstrictors such as angiotensin II and norepinephrine; and (5) increased nitric oxide levels that cause vasodilation.

BLOOD PRESSURE

The effect of decreased peripheral vascular resistance is that blood pressure (BP) remains stable during pregnancy despite the increase in blood volume. Systolic pressure remains largely unchanged or decreases slightly if it is measured when the woman is sitting or standing. Diastolic pressure shows a decrease (about 10 to 15 mm Hg) that is greatest at 24 to 32 weeks of gestation. BP returns to usual levels by term (Blackburn, 2003).

If the BP is measured with the woman lying on her left side, systolic pressure decreases 5 to 10 mm Hg and diastolic pressure decreases 10 to 15 mm Hg, especially from 24 to 32 weeks of gestation; then both systolic and diastolic pressure rise to nonpregnant levels by the end of pregnancy (Monga, 2004).

CONSISTENCY OF MEASUREMENT. Because the BP is affected by position during pregnancy, agencies should standardize the way BP is taken. The woman's position and pressure should be recorded so that the method of evaluation remains consistent.

Consistency is important throughout the antepartum, intrapartum, and postpartum periods regarding use of Korotkoff's fourth (muffling) phase or fifth phase (disappearance of sound) in recording diastolic BPs. Use of Korotkoff's fourth phase gives a higher diastolic reading than use of Korotkoff's fifth phase. Korotkoff's fifth phase is used most often because the fourth phase is not always identifiable. Consistency helps identify gradual changes accurately. BPs of 140/90 and above may indicate preeclampsia and require additional evaluation.

SUPINE HYPOTENSION. When the pregnant woman is in the supine position, particularly in the second and third trimesters, the weight of the gravid (pregnant) uterus partially occludes the vena cava and the aorta (Figure 7-4). The occlusion impedes return of blood from the lower extremities and consequently reduces cardiac return. Cardiac output may be reduced 25% to 30% (Monga, 2004).

Collateral circulation developed in pregnancy generally allows blood flow from the legs and pelvis to return to the heart when the woman is in a supine position (Blackburn, 2003). Some women develop a drop in BP known as *supine hypotensive syndrome,* with symptoms of faintness, lightheadedness, dizziness, and agitation. Some may experience syncope, a brief lapse in consciousness. Blood flow through the placenta is also decreased if the woman remains in the supine position for a prolonged time, which could result in fetal hypoxia.

A lateral recumbent position alleviates the pressure on the blood vessels and quickly corrects supine hypotension. Women should be advised to rest in a side-lying position to prevent or correct the occurrence of supine hypotension. If they must lie in a supine position for fetal surveillance testing, a wedge or pillow under the right hip may be effective in decreasing supine hypotension.

BLOOD FLOW

The following major changes in blood flow occur during pregnancy:

1. Blood flow is altered to include the uteroplacental unit. About 500 to 800 ml/min is required to perfuse the uterus and placenta (Monga, 2004).
2. About 50% more blood must circulate through the maternal kidneys to remove the increased metabolic wastes generated by the mother and the fetus (Monga, 2004).

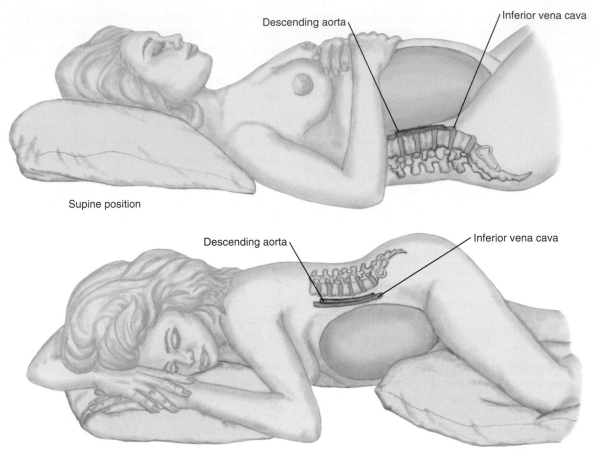

Descending aorta   Inferior vena cava

Supine position

Descending aorta   Inferior vena cava

Right lateral position

Figure 7-4 ■ Supine hypotensive syndrome. When the pregnant woman is in the supine position, the weight of the uterus partially occludes the vena cava and the descending aorta. A side-lying position corrects supine hypotension.

3. The woman's skin requires increased circulation to dissipate heat generated by increased metabolism during pregnancy.

4. Blood flow to the breasts is increased two to three times by the end of pregnancy, resulting in engorgement and dilated veins (Koos, Nuwayhid, & Moore, 2004).

5. The weight of the expanding uterus on the inferior vena cava and iliac veins partially obstructs blood return from veins in the legs, and blood pools in the deep and superficial veins of the legs. The resulting stasis of blood exerts pressure on the veins and causes them to become distended. Prolonged engorgement of the veins of the lower legs may lead to varicose veins of the legs, vulva, or rectum (hemorrhoids).

BLOOD COMPONENTS

Erythrocytes, leukocytes, and clotting factors increase during pregnancy. Erythrocytes increase by 25% to 33%, reflecting accelerated production of erythrocytes rather than prolonged red cell life. The gain in erythrocytes greatly increases the maternal demand for iron, which is necessary for hemoglobin formation.

Although iron absorption and iron-binding power are increased during pregnancy, sufficient iron is not always supplied by the woman's diet. Iron supplementation is necessary to promote hemoglobin synthesis and thus ensure sufficient erythrocyte production to prevent the development of iron-deficiency anemia (see Chapter 26).

Leukocytes increase during pregnancy, up to 12,000 cells/mm^3. Leukocytes increase further during labor and the early postpartum period, reaching levels as high as 25,000 cells/mm^3 (Cunningham et al., 2005).

Pregnancy is a hypercoagulable state in which changes in clotting factors cause an increased ability to form clots. Plasma fibrinogen (factor I) rises about 50%, and plasma fibrin increases about 40% (Bond, 2004). Levels of factors II, VII, VIII, X, and XII are also increased. Fibrinolytic activity (to break down clots) decreases during pregnancy. The platelet count may decrease slightly but generally remains within the normal range. These changes offer some protection from hemorrhage during childbirth but also increase the risk of thrombus formation. The risk is a particular concern if the woman must stand or sit for prolonged periods with stasis of blood in the veins of the legs (see Appendix A).

✔ **CHECK YOUR READING**

6. Why is expanded blood volume important during pregnancy?
7. How does physiologic anemia or pseudoanemia differ from iron deficiency anemia?
8. Why is it important for all caregivers to use the same techniques when measuring BP?
9. Why do some pregnant women feel faint when they are in a supine position?
10. Why is circulation to the kidneys and skin increased during pregnancy?

Respiratory System

The major respiratory changes in pregnancy are the result of three factors: increased oxygen consumption, hormonal factors, and physical effects of the enlarging uterus.

OXYGEN CONSUMPTION

Oxygen consumption increases by about 15% to 20% in pregnancy. Half the oxygen is used by the fetus and placenta, and the rest is consumed by the uterus, breast tissue, and increased maternal respiratory and cardiac demands. To compensate for the increased need for oxygen, progesterone causes the woman to hyperventilate slightly by breathing more deeply, although her respiratory rate remains unchanged. As a result the tidal volume (the volume of gas moved into or out of the respiratory tract with each breath) and respiratory minute volume (the volume of air inspired or expired in 1 minute) increase by about 40% (Whitty & Dombrowski, 2004). Although residual capacity decreases total vital capacity does not change in pregnancy.

As a consequence of the elevated minute volume, the partial pressure of carbon dioxide (PCO_2) is lowered. Excretion of bicarbonate from the kidneys partially compensates for the resulting respiratory alkalosis. Decreased partial pressure of PCO_2 also promotes the transfer of carbon dioxide from fetal to maternal circulation.

HORMONAL FACTORS

PROGESTERONE. Progesterone is considered a major factor in the respiratory changes of pregnancy. In addition to causing mild hyperventilation, progesterone, along with prostaglandins, helps decrease airway resistance by relaxing the smooth muscle in the respiratory tract (Blackburn, 2003). Progesterone is also believed to increase the sensitivity of the respiratory center (medulla oblongata) to carbon dioxide, therefore stimulating the increase in minute ventilation and lowering the PCO_2. These two factors are responsible for the heightened awareness of the need to breathe, or dyspnea, experienced by many women during pregnancy.

ESTROGEN. Estrogen causes increased vascularity of the mucous membranes of the upper respiratory tract. As the capillaries become engorged, edema and hyperemia develop within the nose, pharynx, larynx, and trachea. This congestion gives rise to several conditions commonly seen during pregnancy, such as nasal and sinus stuffiness, epistaxis (nose-

bleed), and changes in the voice. Increased vascularity also causes edema of the eardrum and eustachian tubes and may result in a sense of fullness in the ears or earaches.

PHYSICAL CHANGES

By the third trimester the enlarging uterus lifts the diaphragm by about 4 cm (1.6 in), preventing the lungs from expanding as fully as they normally do. The elevation of the diaphragm does not impede its movement, however, which is increased by about 1.5 cm (0.6 in) during respirations. The ribs flare, the substernal angle widens, and the circumference of the chest expands by about 6 cm (2.5 in) to compensate for the reduced space. These changes begin when the uterus is just beginning to enlarge. They result from the hormone relaxin, which causes relaxation of the ligaments around the ribs. Breathing becomes thoracic rather than abdominal, adding to the dyspnea experienced by many women.

Gastrointestinal System

The gastrointestinal system undergoes changes that are clinically significant because they may cause discomfort for the expectant mother.

APPETITE

Unless the woman is nauseated, her appetite is often increased during pregnancy. This helps her to take in the additional calories recommended during pregnancy.

MOUTH

Elevated levels of estrogen cause hyperemia of the tissues of the mouth and gums and may lead to gingivitis and bleeding gums. Some women develop severe vascular hypertrophy of the gums, which appear reddened and swollen and bleed easily. The condition regresses spontaneously after childbirth.

Some women experience ptyalism, or excessive salivation, that is unpleasant and embarrassing. The cause of ptyalism appears to be stimulation of the salivary glands by the ingestion of starch (Cunningham et al., 2005). Small, frequent meals and use of chewing gum and oral lozenges offer limited relief for some women.

Many women think that pregnancy adversely affects the teeth. However, the teeth do not lose minerals to the fetus and remain unaffected by pregnancy.

ESOPHAGUS

The lower esophageal sphincter tone decreases during pregnancy, primarily because of the relaxant activity of progesterone on the smooth muscles. The reduced tone and relaxation of the lower esophageal sphincter allows gastroesophageal reflux of acidic stomach contents into the esophagus and produces heartburn, or pyrosis.

STOMACH AND SMALL INTESTINE

Elevated levels of progesterone relax all smooth muscle, leading to decreased tone and motility of the gastrointestinal tract. The effect on emptying time of the stomach is unclear, with some studies showing a decrease and others showing no change during pregnancy.

LARGE AND SMALL INTESTINE

The small intestine takes longer to empty during pregnancy, which may allow additional time for nutrients to be absorbed. This slowed process benefits the growing fetus by allowing more time for digestion of nutrients, but it may cause bloating and abdominal distention. Calcium and iron are better absorbed during pregnancy, but absorption of some of the B vitamins is reduced. Decreased motility in the large intestine allows time for more water to be absorbed, which tends to make the stools hard and may lead to constipation. Constipation may cause or exacerbate hemorrhoids if the expectant mother must strain to have bowel movements.

LIVER AND GALLBLADDER

Although the size of the liver and gallbladder remains unchanged during pregnancy, functional changes occur, largely because of the effects of progesterone. The enlarging uterus pushes the liver upward and backward during the last trimester, and liver function is also altered. Serum alkaline phosphatase rises to two to four times that of nonpregnant women, whereas levels of serum albumin and total protein fall gradually (Gordon, 2002). These changes are primarily because of the effects of estrogen and hemodilution.

The gallbladder becomes hypotonic, and emptying time is prolonged. The bile becomes thicker and cholesterol crystals may be retained, predisposing to the development of gallstones. Reduced gallbladder tone also leads to a tendency to retain bile salts, which can cause itching (pruritus).

Urinary System

BLADDER

During the first and third trimesters, the woman experiences frequency and urgency of urination. Although uterine expansion within the pelvis is one cause of these urinary changes, frequency begins before the uterus is big enough to exert pressure on the bladder. Hormonal influences, the increased blood volume, and changes in glomerular filtration rate may play a significant role (Blackburn, 2003). The uterus extends into the abdominal cavity during the second trimester, which relieves pressure on the bladder and may decrease the frequent urge to void.

Bladder capacity doubles by term as the bladder, like all smooth muscle, relaxes in response to increasing levels of progesterone. Nocturia is common because sodium and water are retained when the woman is standing and excreted during the night when she is lying down. Many women experience stress incontinence that begins at any time during pregnancy and continues until after delivery (see Chapter 33).

Bladder mucosa becomes congested with blood, and the bladder walls become hypertrophied as a result of stimulation from estrogen. Decreased drainage of blood from the base of the bladder results in edema of its tissues and renders the area susceptible to trauma and infection during childbirth.

Late in the third trimester, lightening causes the fetus to settle into the pelvis and press against the bladder. Once again the woman experiences frequency, urgency, and nocturia. Although frequency and urgency are normal during pregnancy, they are also signs of infection and, if accompanied by burning sensations or pain, are cause for assessment for urinary tract infection.

KIDNEYS AND URETERS

CHANGES IN SIZE AND SHAPE OF THE KIDNEYS. During pregnancy the kidneys change in both size and shape because there is dilation of the renal pelves and calyces. The ureters also dilate above the pelvic brim. The dilation begins during the second month of pregnancy. It is caused by (1) the effect of progesterone, which causes the ureters to become elongated and relaxes the ureteral walls, making them more distensible and (2) compression of the ureters between the enlarging uterus and the bony pelvic brim.

The flow of urine through the ureters is partially obstructed, causing them to dilate and apply hydrostatic pressure against the renal pelvis, which also dilates. This occurs especially on the right side, because the uterus turns toward the right during pregnancy and the right ovarian vein crosses the ureter. The resulting stasis of urine is clinically significant because it allows time for bacteria to multiply. The risk of bacteriuria, which may be asymptomatic, is increased and urinary tract infection and pyelonephritis may result.

FUNCTIONAL CHANGES OF THE KIDNEYS. Renal plasma flow, or the total amount of plasma to flow through the kidneys, increases significantly. This change results from increases in plasma volume and cardiac output. The flow is highest when the woman is in a side-lying position. The glomerular filtration rate—the rate at which water and dissolved substances are filtered in the glomerulus—rises by as much as 50% by the end of the first trimester. This elevation results from the higher renal plasma flow and decreased colloid osmotic pressure caused by a reduction in the concentration of plasma proteins.

The increases in renal plasma flow and glomerular filtration rate are necessary for the excretion of additional metabolic waste from the mother and fetus, but they also affect the excretion of glucose. As the glomerular filtration rate rises, the filtered load of glucose exceeds the ability of the renal tubules to reabsorb it, and glucose spills into the urine. Therefore glycosuria is common during pregnancy, particularly after consumption of foods such as candy and cookies that are high in simple sugars. Furthermore, small quantities of amino acids and water-soluble vitamins are excreted. Bacteria thrive in urine that is rich in nutrients, and therefore glycosuria is another reason for the increased incidence of urinary tract infections during pregnancy.

Mild proteinuria is common and does not necessarily indicate abnormal kidney function or preeclampsia (Blackburn,

2003). Protein is monitored throughout pregnancy to identify increases that would indicate a problem. Tests of renal function may be misleading during pregnancy. As a result of increased glomerular filtration rate, plasma concentrations of both creatinine and urea normally decline.

✔ CHECK YOUR READING

11. Why do some women experience dyspnea during pregnancy?
12. How does the respiratory system compensate for upward pressure exerted on the diaphragm by the enlarging uterus?
13. How does pregnancy affect the gastrointestinal system?
14. Why are pregnant women at increased risk for urinary tract infection?

Integumentary System

SKIN

Circulation to the skin increases during pregnancy and encourages activity of the sweat and sebaceous glands. This helps dissipate excess heat produced by increased metabolism. Pregnant women feel warmer and perspire more, particularly during the last trimester. Accelerated activity by the sebaceous glands fosters the development of facial blemishes, which are usually reduced by careful cleansing of the face several times each day. Additional changes include hyperpigmentation and vascular changes in the skin.

HYPERPIGMENTATION. Increased pigmentation occurs in 90% of pregnant women (Blackburn, 2003). It may begin as early as the second month and may be the result of estrogen, progesterone, and elevated levels of melanocyte-stimulating hormone. Women with dark hair or skin exhibit more hyperpigmentation than women with very light skin.

Areas of pigmentation include brownish patches called *melasma, chloasma,* or the "mask of pregnancy," which involves the forehead, cheeks, and bridge of the nose. It may also occur in nonpregnant women taking oral contraceptives. Melasma increases with exposure to sunlight, but use of sunscreen may reduce the severity. Although melasma usually resolves after delivery when estrogen and progesterone decline, it continues for months or years in some women.

The linea alba—the line that marks the longitudinal division of the midline of the abdomen—darkens to become the linea nigra. This dark line of pigmentation may extend from the symphysis pubis to the top of the fundus. Preexisting moles (nevi), freckles, and the areolae become darker as pregnancy progresses. Hyperpigmentation usually disappears after childbirth when the levels of estrogen and progesterone decline.

CUTANEOUS VASCULAR CHANGES. Blood vessels dilate and proliferate during pregnancy. This change is thought to be largely because of the effect of estrogen. Changes in surface blood vessels are obvious during pregnancy, especially in women with fair skin. These include an-

giomas (vascular spiders, telangiectasia) that appear as tiny red elevations branching in all directions and appear most often on the face, neck, upper chest, and arms. Redness of the palms or soles of the feet, known as palmar erythema, also occurs in many white women and some African-American women. Vascular changes often occur simultaneously, and although they may be emotionally distressing for the expectant mother, they are clinically insignificant and usually disappear shortly after childbirth.

CONNECTIVE TISSUE

Linear tears may occur in the connective tissue, most often on the abdomen, breasts, and buttocks, appearing as slightly depressed, pink to purple streaks called *striae gravidarum* or "stretch marks" (Figure 7-5). Women are concerned about striae because they do not disappear after childbirth, although the marks usually fade to silvery lines. Laser therapy is sometimes used after childbirth to reduce or eliminate se-

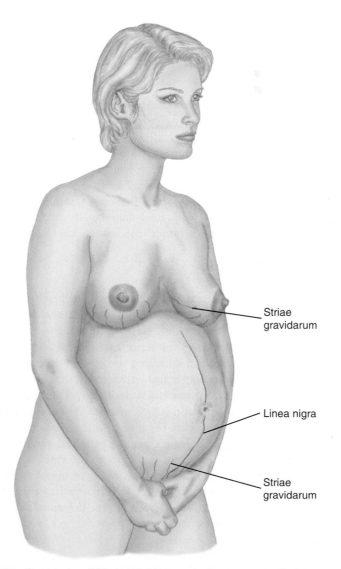

Striae gravidarum

Linea nigra

Striae gravidarum

Figure 7-5 ■ Striae gravidarum are linear tears that may occur in the connective tissue. Linea nigra, a dark pigmented line from above the umbilicus to the symphysis pubis, may also appear.

vere striae. Many women believe that striae can be prevented by massage with oil or vitamin E, but the effectiveness of this treatment has not been documented. Antipruritic creams may be effective in controlling the itching that accompanies severe striae.

HAIR AND NAILS

Because fewer follicles are in the resting phase, hair grows more rapidly and less hair falls out during pregnancy. After childbirth, hair follicles return to normal activity, and many women become concerned at the rate of hair loss that occurs 1 to 4 months postpartum. They need reassurance that more follicles have returned to the normal resting phase and excessive hair loss will not continue. Although as much as 35% of the scalp hair may be lost over that time, hair loss is not noticeable until 40% to 50% is lost (Rapini, 2004).

Nail growth increases during pregnancy. Many women notice thinning and softening of the nails as pregnancy progresses, although reasons for these changes are unclear.

Musculoskeletal System

CALCIUM STORAGE

During pregnancy, fetal demands for calcium increase, especially in the third trimester. Absorption of calcium from the intestine doubles during pregnancy, with the increase beginning in the first trimester. This allows maternal bone formation to increase during the first half of pregnancy.

Calcium is stored to meet the later needs of the fetus. During the third trimester, 25 to 30 g of calcium from maternal bone stores is transferred to the fetus, but this amount is small in comparison with total maternal stores and does not deplete the mother's bones (Blackburn, 2003; Gordon, 2002).

POSTURAL CHANGES

Musculoskeletal changes are progressive. They begin in the second trimester when relaxin and progesterone initiate gradual softening of the pelvic cartilage and connective tissue to facilitate passage of the fetus through the pelvis during birth. Loosening and widening of the symphysis pubis and the sacroiliac joints creates pelvic instability and may cause pain at the symphysis and inner thighs. The pregnant woman may assume a wide stance with the "waddling" gait of pregnancy, which occurs because of muscle fatigue and an effort to compensate for a changing center of gravity.

During the third trimester, as the uterus increases in size, the expectant mother must lean backward to maintain her balance. This creates a progressive lordosis, or curvature of the lower spine (Figure 7-6). The strain on the muscles and ligaments of the back often causes backache.

ABDOMINAL WALL

Pregnancy also affects the abdominal muscles, which may be stretched beyond their capacity during the third trimester, causing the rectus abdominis muscles to separate (diastasis recti). The extent of the separation varies from

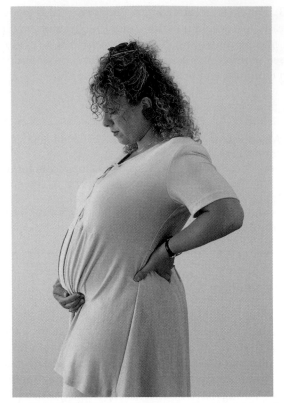

Figure 7-6 ■ Lordosis increases by the third trimester as the uterus grows larger, and the woman must lean backward to maintain her balance.

slight and not clinically significant to severe, when a large portion of the uterine wall is covered only by skin and fascia (see Chapter 17).

Endocrine System

Numerous changes in hormones occur in pregnancy (Table 7-1).

PITUITARY GLAND

Although the pituitary gland increases in size during pregnancy, most hormones from the pituitary gland are suppressed. The hormones FSH and LH, which stimulate ovulation in the nonpregnant woman, are unnecessary during pregnancy, and growth hormone from the anterior pituitary also decreases during pregnancy. However, prolactin increases to prepare the breasts to produce milk.

The posterior pituitary secretes oxytocin, also involved in lactation. Oxytocin stimulates the milk-ejection reflex after childbirth. Oxytocin also stimulates contractions of the uterus, but this action is inhibited during pregnancy by progesterone, which relaxes the smooth muscle fibers of the uterus. After childbirth, progesterone levels decline, and oxytocin plays an important role in keeping the uterus contracted and thereby preventing excessive bleeding.

THYROID GLAND

Early in the first trimester a rise in total thyroxine (T_4) occurs, along with a corresponding gain in thyroxine-binding globulin. Serum unbound or free T_4 increases early in preg-

TABLE 7-1 Hormones Related to Pregnancy

Hormone	Source	Major Effects
Aldosterone	Adrenals	Increased during pregnancy to conserve sodium and maintain fluid balance
Cortisol	Adrenals	Increased during pregnancy; active in metabolism of glucose, protein, and fats; antiinflammatory effect may be helpful in preventing rejection of pregnancy
Estrogen	Ovary, placenta	Stimulates uterine development to provide environment for fetus and stimulates breast to prepare for lactation
Follicle-stimulating hormone	Anterior pituitary	Initiates maturation of ovum; suppressed during pregnancy
Human chorionic gonadotropin	Trophoblasts (placenta)	Prevents involution of corpus luteum, thereby maintaining production of progesterone until placenta is formed
Human placental lactogen (human chorionic somatomammotropin)	Placenta	Stimulates metabolism of glucose and converts it to fat; antagonistic to insulin
Luteinizing hormone	Anterior pituitary	Stimulates ovulation of mature ovum in nonpregnant state
Melanocyte-stimulating hormone	Anterior pituitary	Increased during pregnancy; produces hyperpigmentation
Oxytocin	Posterior pituitary	Stimulates uterine contractions to initiate labor; stimulates milk-ejection reflex after birth
Prolactin	Anterior pituitary	Primary hormone of milk production
Progesterone	Ovary, placenta	Maintains uterine lining for implantation, relaxes smooth muscle, including uterus; develops acini cells and lobes to prepare breasts for lactation; increases resistance to insulin
Relaxin	Ovary, placenta	Softens muscles and joints of pelvis
Thyroxine	Thyroid	Increased during pregnancy to stimulate basal metabolic rate

nancy but returns to nonpregnant levels by the end of the first trimester. The gland itself enlarges because of hyperplasia and increased vascularity. Size may be greater if iodine intake is insufficient. The basal metabolic rate increases up to 25% primarily because of metabolic activity of the fetus (Cunningham et al., 2005).

PARATHYROID GLANDS

Parathyroid hormone, which is important in calcium homeostasis, is slightly decreased or at low normal levels during pregnancy. In spite of this, calcium is adequate for transfer to the fetus even though urinary excretion is increased. Although total calcium levels decrease because of the increased intravascular fluid and decreased albumin, ionized calcium—the physiologically active form—remains stable.

PANCREAS

Significant changes in the pancreas during pregnancy are the result of alterations in maternal blood glucose levels and consequent fluctuations in insulin production. Blood glucose levels during pregnancy are 10% to 20% lower than before pregnancy, and hypoglycemia may develop between meals and at night as the fetus continuously draws glucose from the mother (Blackburn, 2003).

During the second half of pregnancy, maternal tissue sensitivity to insulin begins to decline because of the effects of hormones such as human placental lactogen (hPL), prolactin, estrogen, progesterone, and cortisol. As a consequence of the tissue resistance to insulin, postprandial (after a meal) blood glucose levels are higher than before pregnancy. This rise in glucose makes more glucose available for fetal energy needs and stimulates the pancreas of a healthy woman to produce additional insulin. Insulin production more than doubles during meals, and 24-hour levels average 30% higher than usual by the third trimester to meet the insulin needs (Moore, 2004). Inadequate insulin production results in gestational diabetes (see Chapter 26).

ADRENAL GLANDS

Although the adrenal glands enlarge only slightly during pregnancy, significant changes occur in two adrenal hormones: cortisol and aldosterone. Levels of both total cortisol and free (unbound) cortisol, the metabolically active cortisol, are elevated because of elevated estrogen and a decrease in metabolic clearance rate. Cortisol regulates carbohydrate and protein metabolism. It stimulates gluconeogenesis (formation of glycogen from noncarbohydrate sources such as amino and fatty acids) whenever the supply of glucose is inadequate to meet the body's needs for energy.

Aldosterone regulates the absorption of sodium from the distal tubules of the kidneys. Production increases very early in pregnancy to maintain the necessary level of sodium in the greatly expanded blood volume and to meet the needs of the fetus. Aldosterone is closely related to water metabolism (see p. 120).

CHANGES CAUSED BY PLACENTAL HORMONES

HUMAN CHORIONIC GONADOTROPIN. In early pregnancy, human chorionic gonadotropin (hCG) is produced by the trophoblastic cells surrounding the developing embryo. The primary function of hCG in early pregnancy is to prevent deterioration of the corpus luteum so that it can continue producing progesterone until the placenta is sufficiently developed to assume this function. The presence of this hormone produces a positive pregnancy test result.

ESTROGEN. Estrogen is produced by the corpus luteum for the first few weeks of pregnancy, but primarily by the placenta after the sixth or seventh week of pregnancy. Functions of estrogen during pregnancy include the following:

- Stimulating uterine growth
- Increasing blood supply to uterine vessels
- Increasing uterine contractions near term
- Aiding in the development of the glands and ductal system in the breasts in preparation for lactation
- Causing hyperpigmentation, vascular changes in the skin, increased activity of the salivary glands, and hyperemia of the gums and nasal mucous membranes.

PROGESTERONE. Progesterone is produced first by the corpus luteum and then by the fully developed placenta. Progesterone is the most important hormone of pregnancy. Its major functions include the following:

- Maintaining the endometrial layer for implantation of the fertilized ovum
- Preventing spontaneous abortion by relaxing smooth muscles of the uterus
- Helping to prevent tissue rejection of the fetus
- Stimulating the development of the lobes and lobules in the breast in preparation for lactation
- Facilitating the deposit of maternal fat stores, which provide a reserve of energy for pregnancy and lactation

Progesterone relaxes not only the smooth muscle of the uterus but also other smooth muscle. Consequently, progesterone is associated with decreased motility of the bowel, dilation of the ureters, and increased bladder capacity. Progesterone raises the respiratory sensitivity to carbon dioxide and thereby stimulates increased ventilation.

HUMAN PLACENTAL LACTOGEN. Also called *human chorionic somatomammotropin*, hPL is present early in pregnancy and its level increases steadily throughout pregnancy. Its primary function is to increase the availability of glucose for the fetus. A potent insulin antagonist, hPL decreases the sensitivity of maternal cells to insulin and decreases maternal metabolism of glucose. This frees glucose for transport to the fetus, who needs a constant supply. In addition, hPL encourages the quick metabolism of free fatty acids to provide energy for the pregnant woman.

RELAXIN. Relaxin is produced by the corpus luteum and placenta and is present by the first missed menstrual period. Relaxin inhibits uterine activity, softens connective tissue in the cervix, and relaxes the cartilage and connective tissue of the pelvic joints.

CHANGES IN METABOLISM

WEIGHT GAIN. Because a correlation between infant mortality and low birth weight has been documented, women are encouraged to gain an average of 25 to 35 pounds during pregnancy (see Table 9-1). The fetus, placenta, and amniotic fluid make up less than half the recommended weight gain. The remainder is found in the increased size of the uterus and breasts, increased blood volume, increased interstitial fluid, and maternal stores of subcutaneous fat (see Figure 9-1).

WATER METABOLISM. The amount of water needed during pregnancy increases to meet the needs of the fetus, placenta, amniotic fluid, and increased blood volume. Fluid balance depends on adequate concentrations of sodium, and the kidneys must compensate for the many factors that favor excretion of sodium during pregnancy. Increased glomerular filtration rate, decreased concentration of plasma proteins, and increased progesterone levels all result in an increase in sodium excretion. However, increased concentrations of estrogen, cortisol, prolactin, and aldosterone all tend to promote the reabsorption of sodium. The net effect of the combined hormonal action is the maintenance of the sodium balance.

DEPENDENT EDEMA. Because of hemodilution, colloid osmotic pressure slightly decreases, which favors the development of edema during pregnancy. Edema further increases toward term when the weight of the uterus compresses the veins of the pelvis. This process delays venous return, causing the veins of the legs to become distended, and increases venous pressure, resulting in additional fluid shifts from the vascular compartment to interstitial spaces.

All women, including those without edema, accumulate water during pregnancy to allow for the added fluid needs of the fetus as well as those of the woman. Between 1.5 and 9 L of water are retained during pregnancy to meet the increased needs for expanded blood volume and the tissue needs of the mother and fetus (Blackburn, 2003; Monga, 2004). Water retention accounts for a large part of maternal weight gain.

When water in the interstitial spaces exceeds 1.5 L, edema is apparent. Edema of the feet and ankles is obvious at the end of the day (particularly if a pregnant woman stands for prolonged periods), and the force of gravity contributes to the pooling of blood in the veins of the legs. Dependent edema is clinically insignificant if no other abnormal signs are present.

CARPAL TUNNEL SYNDROME. Fluid retention is also associated with carpal tunnel syndrome, believed to result when edema compresses the median nerve at the point at which it passes through the carpal tunnel of the wrist. Symptoms include burning, numbness, or tingling of the hand and wrist. Splinting of the wrist at night may provide improvement. The condition usually resolves by 3 months postpartum.

CARBOHYDRATE METABOLISM. Carbohydrate metabolism changes markedly during pregnancy. More insulin is required as pregnancy progresses because the hormones hPL, prolactin, estrogen, progesterone, and cortisol cause maternal tissue resistance to insulin.

The decrease in the mother's ability to use insulin is a protective mechanism that allows an ample supply of glucose for transfer to the fetus. However, the mother's pancreas produces more insulin so that she can continue to metabolize enough glucose to meet her own energy needs and prevent hyperglycemia. Hyperglycemia occurs when blood glucose levels exceed available insulin, which is needed to transport glucose into cells.

For most women hyperglycemia is not a problem and insulin production is increased, particularly during the second and third trimesters. In some women, however, insulin production cannot be increased, and these women experience periodic hyperglycemia or gestational diabetes mellitus (see Chapter 26).

Sensory Organs

EYE

During pregnancy the cornea thickens because of edema, especially in the third trimester. Women who wear contact lenses may have some discomfort at this time. The problem resolves by 6 weeks postpartum, and women should not get new prescriptions for lenses until after that time. Intraocular pressure decreases, which may cause improvement and a need for less medication in women with glaucoma (Blackburn, 2003; Cunningham et al., 2005).

EAR

Changes in the mucous membranes of the eustachian tube brought about by estrogen may cause women to have blocked ears and a mild hearing loss that is temporary.

IMMUNE SYSTEM

Immune function is altered during pregnancy to allow the fetus, which is foreign tissue for the mother, to grow undisturbed without being rejected by the woman's body. Resistance to infection is decreased because of lessened WBC functioning. This may cause autoimmune conditions such as rheumatoid arthritis to improve during pregnancy (Gordon, 2002).

✔ CHECK YOUR READING

15. What causes the progressive changes in posture and gait during pregnancy?
16. Why don't women ovulate and have menstrual periods during pregnancy?
17. Why do maternal needs for insulin change during pregnancy?

CONFIRMATION OF PREGNANCY

When pregnancy occurs, women note changes that make them aware that they may be pregnant. Changes in the mother and fetus throughout pregnancy are summarized in Figure 7-7. Women usually wish to confirm a pregnancy as soon as possible. Confirmation of pregnancy is often made by ultrasonography, which makes it possible to view the fetal outline and observe the fetal heartbeat very early in pregnancy.

Traditionally, the diagnosis of pregnancy has been based on symptoms experienced by the woman and signs observed by the health care provider. These signs and symptoms are grouped into three classifications: presumptive, probable, and positive indications of pregnancy. A diagnosis of pregnancy cannot be made solely on the presumptive or probable signs because they may have other causes, listed in Table 7-2.

Presumptive Indications of Pregnancy

Presumptive indications are mainly subjective changes that are experienced and reported by the woman. Presumptive changes are the least reliable indicators of pregnancy because any can be caused by conditions other than pregnancy.

Gestational age 1 to 4 weeks

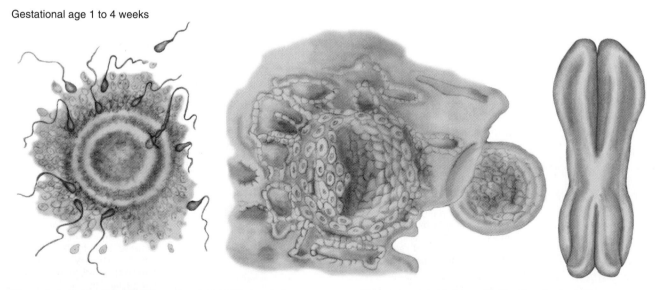

Woman's basal body temperature elevated; hCG elevated; pregnancy tests positive.

Crown-rump length 4 mm. Fertilization, implantation. Preembryonic stage.

Figure 7-7 ■ Fetal growth and development and maternal responses based on the date of the last menstrual period.

Continued

Gestational age 5 to 8 weeks

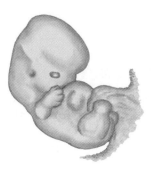

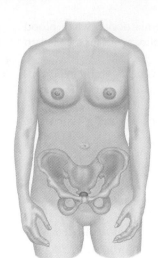

Crown-rump length 13 mm. Embryonic stage. Heart developed, beginning to pump. Arm and leg buds present. Head large, with facial features beginning to form.

Woman misses menstrual period. Nausea; fatigue. Tingling of breasts. Uterus is size of a lemon; positive Chadwick's, Goodell's and Hegar's signs. Urinary frequency; increased vaginal discharge.

Gestational age 9 to 12 weeks

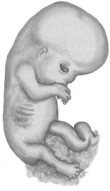

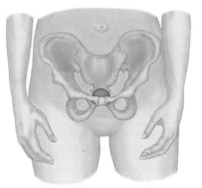

Crown-rump length 6 to 7 cm (2.4 to 2.8 in). Fetal stage begins at 10 weeks after last menstrual period. Extremities developed; fingers and toes differentiated; external genitalia show signs of male or female sex. Weight 14 g (0.5 oz). Heartbeat heard by Doppler at 10 weeks.

Nausea usually decreases after 12 weeks. Uterus is size of an orange; palpable above symphysis pubis. Vulvar varicosities may appear.

Gestational age 13 to 16 weeks

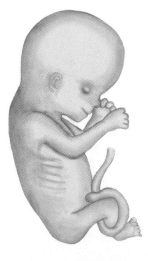

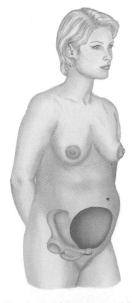

Crown-rump length 12 cm (4.7 in). Weight 110 g (4 oz). Fetus begins to move. Head and thorax can be identified by ultrasound; sexual organs formed. Urine formation begins.

Fetal movements may be felt at about 16 weeks. Uterus has risen into the abdomen; fundus midway between symphysis pubis and umbilicus. Urinary frequency decreases; blood volume increases; uterine souffle heard.

Figure 7-7, cont'd ■ For legend see page 121.

Gestational age 17 to 20 weeks

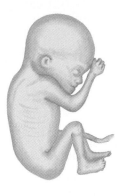

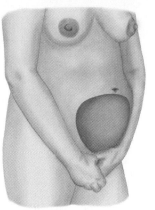

Crown-rump length 16 cm (6.3 in). Weight 320 g (11 oz). Heartbeat can be heard with fetoscope or electronic device. Meconium begins collecting in bowel. Period of very rapid growth.

Fetal movements felt. Skin pigmentation increases: areolae darken; chloasma and linea nigra may be obvious. Colostrum may be expressed. Braxton Hicks contractions palpable. Fundus at level of umbilicus at about 20 weeks.

Gestational age 21 to 24 weeks

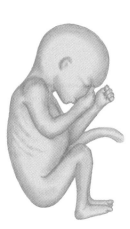

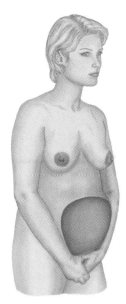

Crown-rump length 21 cm (8 in). Weight 630 g (1 lb 6 oz). Skin wrinkled and red; vernix present; head and body covered with lanugo.

Relaxation of smooth muscles of veins and bladder increases the chance of varicose veins and urinary tract infections. Woman is more aware of fetal movements.

Gestational age 25 to 28 weeks

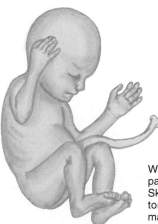

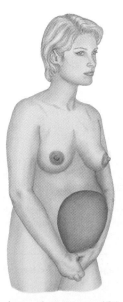

Crown-rump length 25 cm (9.8 in). Weight 1000 g (2 lb 3 oz). Eyes partially open; eyelashes present. Skin covered with vernix. Respiratory system immature, but fetus may survive if born.

Period of greatest weight gain and lowest hemoglobin level begins. Fundal height is 3 to 4 fingerbreadths above umbilicus. Lordosis may cause backache.

Figure 7-7, cont'd ■ For legend see page 121.

Continued

Gestational age 29 to 32 weeks

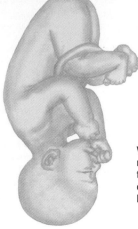

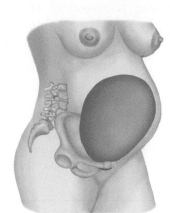

Crown-rump length 28 cm (11 in). Weight 1700 g (3 lb, 12 oz). Toenails present. Body filling out, testes descending. Iron, nitrogen, calcium stored. Vernix covers body. Chances of survival good.

Heartburn common as uterus presses on diaphragm and displaces stomach. Braxton Hicks contractions more noticeable. Lordosis increases; waddling gait develops due to increased mobility of pelvic joints.

Gestational age 33 to 36 weeks

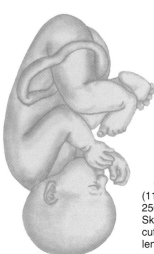

Crown-rump length 30 to 32 cm (11.8 to 12.6 in). Weight 2000 to 2500 g (4 lb, 6 oz to 5 lb, 8 oz). Skin thicker, less wrinkled as subcutaneous fat accumulates. Excellent chance for survival.

Shortness of breath caused by upward pressure on diaphragm; woman may have difficulty finding a comfortable position for sleep. Umbilicus protrudes. Varicosities more pronounced; pedal or ankle edema may be present. Urinary frequency noted following lightening when presenting part settles into pelvic cavity.

Gestational age 37 to 40 weeks

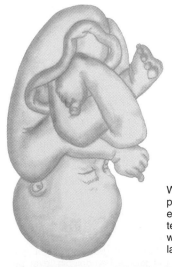

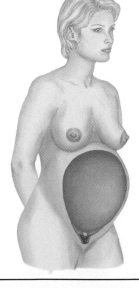

Crown-rump length 36 cm (14 in). Weight 3400 g (7 lb, 8 oz). Body plump; lanugo remains over shoulders; nails extend beyond nail beds; testes within scrotum; female labia well developed; labia majora cover labia minora.

Woman is uncomfortable; looking forward to birth of baby. Cervix softens, begins to efface; mucus plug is often lost.

Figure 7-7, cont'd ■ For legend see page 121.

AMENORRHEA

Absence of menstruation in a sexually active woman who regularly menstruates is one of the first changes noted and strongly suggests that conception has occurred. Menses cease after conception because progesterone and estrogen, secreted by the corpus luteum, maintain the endometrial lining in preparation for implantation of the fertilized ovum. A small amount of bleeding from implantation of the blastocyst may be interpreted as a period by the woman.

NAUSEA AND VOMITING

Many women experience nausea and vomiting that begins about 6 weeks after the last menstrual period began and usually disappears by about 14 weeks (Cunningham et al., 2005). Nausea and vomiting are believed to be caused by the increased levels of hormones (such as hCG and estrogen) and decreased gastric motility (an effect of progesterone).

FATIGUE

Many pregnant women experience extraordinary fatigue and drowsiness during the first trimester. The direct cause is unknown but it may be from changes in hormones such as progesterone.

URINARY FREQUENCY

Urinary frequency is first noticed by the expectant mother in the first few weeks of pregnancy and results from hormonal and fluid volume changes as well as pressure on the bladder by the expanding uterus. This effect abates during the second trimester when the uterus expands into the abdominal cavity. Late in the third trimester the fetus settles into the pelvic cavity, and the woman once again experiences frequency and urgency of urination as the uterus presses against the bladder.

BREAST AND SKIN CHANGES

Breast changes begin at about the sixth week of pregnancy. The expectant mother experiences breast tenderness, tingling, feelings of fullness, and increased size and pigmentation of the areolae. Breast changes result from the influence of estrogen and progesterone.

Many women observe increased pigmentation of the skin (such as chloasma, linea nigra, darkening of the areolae of the breasts) during pregnancy. These skin changes are the result of increased levels of melanocyte-stimulating hormone, which is an effect of estrogen.

VAGINAL AND CERVICAL COLOR CHANGES

The cervix, vagina, and labia change from pink to a dark bluish violet. This color change, called *Chadwick's sign*, results from increased vascularity of the pelvic organs. It is present by 8 weeks of pregnancy.

FETAL MOVEMENT

Unlike other presumptive indications of pregnancy, fetal movement (quickening) is not perceived until the second trimester. Although some women become aware of fetal movement sooner, most women notice subtle fetal movements, which gradually increase in intensity between 16 and 20 weeks of gestation.

Probable Indications of Pregnancy

Probable indications of pregnancy are objective findings that can be documented by an examiner. They are primarily related to physical changes in the reproductive organs. Al-

---

TABLE 7-2 Indications of Pregnancy and Other Possible Causes

Sign	Other Possible Causes
Presumptive Indications	
Amenorrhea	Emotional stress, strenuous physical exercise, endocrine problems, chronic disease, early menopause, anovulation, low body weight
Nausea and vomiting	Gastrointestinal virus, food poisoning, emotional stress
Fatigue	Illness, stress, sudden changes in lifestyle
Urinary frequency	Urinary tract infections
Breast and skin changes	Premenstrual changes, use of oral contraceptives
Cervical color changes	Infection or hormonal imbalance causing pelvic congestion
Quickening	Intestinal gas, peristalsis, or pseudocyesis (false pregnancy)
Probable Indications	
Abdominal enlargement	Abdominal or uterine tumors
Cervical softening	Hormonal contraceptives or imbalance
Changes in uterine consistency	Hormonal imbalance
Ballottement	Uterine or cervical polyps
Braxton Hicks contractions	Soft uterine fibroids (myomas)
Palpation of fetal outline	Large leiomyoma that feels like the fetal head, small soft leiomyoma that simulates fetal body parts
Positive result of pregnancy tests	Some medications, premature menopause, blood in urine, malignant tumors that produce human chorionic gonadotropin
Positive Indications	
Auscultation of fetal heart sounds	
Fetal movements felt by examiner	
Visualization of embryo or fetus	

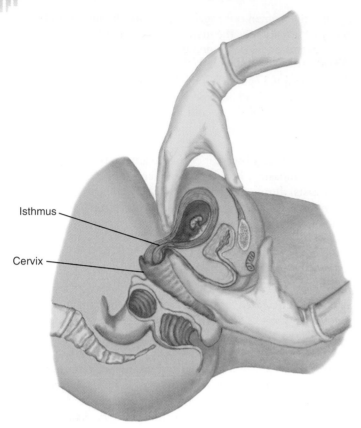

Isthmus

Cervix

Figure 7-8 ■ Hegar's sign demonstrates softening of the isthmus of the cervix.

though these signs are stronger indicators of pregnancy, a positive diagnosis cannot be made because they may have other causes.

ABDOMINAL ENLARGEMENT

Enlargement of the abdomen during the childbearing years is a fairly reliable indication of pregnancy, particularly if it corresponds with a slow, gradual increase in uterine growth. Pregnancy is even more likely when abdominal enlargement is accompanied by amenorrhea.

CERVICAL SOFTENING

In the early weeks of pregnancy the cervix softens as a result of pelvic vasocongestion (Goodell's sign). Cervical softening is noted during pelvic examination.

CHANGES IN UTERINE CONSISTENCY

About 6 to 8 weeks after the last menses the lower uterine segment is so soft that it can be compressed to the thinness of paper. This is called Hegar's sign (Figure 7-8). The body of the uterus can be easily flexed against the cervix.

BALLOTTEMENT

At about 20 weeks a sudden tap on the cervix during vaginal examination may cause the fetus to rise in the amniotic fluid and then rebound to its original position (Figure 7-9). This movement, called ballottement, is a strong indication of pregnancy, but it may also be caused by other factors.

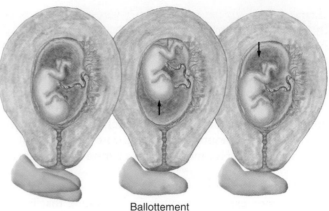

Ballottement

Figure 7-9 ■ When the cervix is tapped, the fetus floats upward in the amniotic fluid. A rebound is felt by the examiner when the fetus falls back.

BRAXTON HICKS CONTRACTIONS. Irregular, painless contractions occur throughout pregnancy, although many expectant mothers do not notice them until the third trimester. They increase in frequency as the woman nears term. It is important to differentiate Braxton Hicks contractions from the contractions of preterm labor. This is often difficult, and the woman should check with her health care provider if contractions continue, she has any other signs of early labor, or she is unsure if she might be in preterm labor.

PALPATION OF THE FETAL OUTLINE. Unless the woman is very obese, an experienced practitioner is able to palpate the outlines of the fetal body by the middle of pregnancy. Outlining the fetus becomes easier as the pregnancy progresses and the uterine walls thin to accommodate the growing fetus.

PREGNANCY TESTS

Pregnancy tests detect hCG or the beta subunit of hCG, which is secreted by the placenta and present in the blood and urine of the pregnant woman shortly after conception.

RADIOIMMUNOASSAY TESTS. Because radioimmunoassay tests use radioactively labeled markers to detect antibodies against beta-subunit hCG in blood or urine, they must be performed in a laboratory. This causes them to be more expensive than immunometric tests. They are accurate as early as 1 week after conception.

ENZYME-LINKED IMMUNOSORBENT ASSAY. The enzyme-linked immunosorbent assay (ELISA) uses antibodies to detect hCG in blood or urine. The test is quick and ideal for early diagnosis of pregnancy. It can detect hCG in serum at very low concentrations and is positive as early as 5 days before the woman misses a period (Buster & Carson, 2002).

HOME PREGNANCY TESTS. Pregnancy test kits, often based on ELISA, are available for purchase over the counter to be used in the home. They are uncomplicated and convenient. The woman places urine on a strip, wick, or other device and watches for an indicator such as a color change. Although the first morning void is most concentrated, samples from any time of day can be used for most kits.

Home-test kits are capable of greater than 97% accuracy, but their instructions must be followed precisely to obtain accurate results (Cunningham et al., 2005).

When pregnancy test results are reported as negative and the woman is in fact pregnant, the results are called *false negative*. False-negative results may occur when the instructions are not followed properly, it is too early in the pregnancy, the urine is too dilute, or the woman has an ectopic pregnancy or impending spontaneous abortion. Other sources of hCG may cause the test to give a false-positive result. Certain drugs may affect the accuracy of the test. The woman should check with the manufacturer's instructions or her health care provider if she is taking drugs.

Positive Indications of Pregnancy

Only three signs are accepted as positive confirmation of pregnancy: auscultation of fetal heart sounds, fetal movement felt by an examiner, and visualization of the fetus with sonography.

AUSCULTATION OF FETAL HEART SOUNDS

Fetal heart sounds can be heard with a fetoscope by 18 to 20 weeks of gestation. The electronic Doppler, which is used more often, detects heart motion and makes a sound that is audible by 10 weeks of gestation. (See Figure 14-1.)

The fetal heartbeat must be distinguished from the maternal pulse for a positive diagnosis of pregnancy to be made. The fetal heartbeat should be auscultated during palpation of the radial or apical pulse of the expectant mother to be sure that a difference in the rate exists. The fetal heart rate depends on gestational age. The normal range is between 110 and 160 bpm in the third trimester. The fetal heart rate is muffled by amniotic fluid, and the location changes because the fetus moves freely in the amniotic fluid.

FETAL MOVEMENTS FELT BY EXAMINER

Fetal movements vary from faint flutterings in early pregnancy to the characteristic kick or thrust of later pregnancy. These movements are considered a positive sign of pregnancy when felt by an experienced examiner who is not likely to be deceived by similar sensations produced by peristalsis in the large intestine.

VISUALIZATION OF THE FETUS

Confirmation of pregnancy has become much simpler since the development of ultrasonography, which makes it possible to view the fetal outline and observe the fetal heartbeat very early in pregnancy. Positive confirmation of pregnancy is possible by transvaginal ultrasonography as early as 4 weeks after the last menstrual period, when the gestational sac can be identified (Buster & Carson, 2002). Ultrasound testing is discussed further in Chapter 10.

CHECK YOUR READING

18. How do presumptive and probable indications of pregnancy differ?
19. Why is "fetal" movement felt by the pregnant woman not a positive sign of pregnancy?
20. What are the most common causes of false-negative pregnancy tests?

ANTEPARTUM ASSESSMENT AND CARE

The objective of antepartum care is to ensure that pregnancy ends in the birth of a healthy infant without impairing the health of the mother. Prenatal care involves early and continuing risk assessments, health education, counseling, and social support.

Antepartum care is considered adequate when it begins in the first trimester and continues on a regular basis thereafter. Inadequate antepartum care is associated with low birth weight and an increased incidence of prematurity in neonates, and these two complications lead to increased infant morbidity and mortality.

Approximately 84% of U.S. women begin antepartum care in the first trimester. The Healthy People 2010 goal is for at least 90% of U.S. women to begin antepartum care in the first trimester. The amount of prenatal care varies among groups. In 2002 prenatal care beginning in the first trimester was obtained most often by women who were Asian (87%) and white (89%) and least often by those of Hispanic (77%), African-American (75%), and American Indian or Alaska Native (70%) ethnicity (National Center for Health Statistics, 2004).

Clinical pathways provide guidelines and a time sequence for specific assessments and interventions. Pathways assist the multidisciplinary team—composed of nurses, nurse-midwives, nurse practitioners, physicians, social workers, nutritionists, and counselors—to coordinate care for each woman. Figure 7-10 provides an example of a clinical pathway for prenatal care. The most common family problems and risk factors are listed at the top of the pathway and alert the team that additional assessments or care may be required.

Preconception Visit

Ideally, the first visit takes place before conception. Preconception care is important for identification and mitigation of problems that might harm the mother or infant once pregnancy occurs. The early weeks of pregnancy are particularly important, because during that time the fetal organs are forming and are especially sensitive to harm. The first visit to the woman's health care provider to begin prenatal care may occur after this sensitive period, and damage may already have occurred. Because so many pregnancies are unintended, preconception counseling should be incorporated into visits for family planning or well-women checkups, times when there is a negative pregnancy test performed by a health care provider, or any visit to a health professional by a woman who might become pregnant.

YORK HEALTH SYSTEM
YORK, PENNSYLVANIA
PRENATAL CARE
CLINICAL PATHWAY

DEMOGRAPHIC LABEL

EDC _____

PRETERM LABOR RISK

1. ☐ Substance abuse   4. ☐ <90 lb prepregnancy weight   7. ☐ Multiple gestation
2. ☐ Prior preterm delivery 5. ☐ Placental anomaly   8. ☐ Persistent bleeding
3. ☐ >2 abortions   6. ☐ STD current pregnancy   9. ☐ Incompetent cervix

DOCUMENTATION CODES
Initialed box=Meets standard   ★=Exception on pathway identified   N=Not applicable

**CONSULTS/PROBLEM MANAGEMENT
FOR PATIENTS INCLUDE:**
- Social service prn
- Perinatologist prn
- Genetic counseling prn
- Nutritionist prn
- WIC prn
- Pastoral care prn
- Lactation consultant prn (3rd trimester)

**STANDARD OF CARE FOR
PRENATAL PATIENTS INCLUDES:**
- Activity ad lib
- Diet to meet needs of pregnancy.
- Prenatal vitamins
- $FeSO_4$, if needed

Clinical Path Visits	Expected Patient/ Family Outcomes	Multidisciplinary Assessment (Refer to STD-0011)	Tests	Education & DC Planning (Refer to STD-0011)
Nurse Interview Date _____ RN Name _____	☐ Referrals made as indicated following prenatal standard of care ☐ Verbalizes understanding of normal vs. abnormal signs and symptoms of pregnancy ☐ Verbalizes agreement to complete labs, obtain prenatal vitamins and keep scheduled appointments ☐ Verbalizes signs and symptoms of preterm labor ☐ No risk factors PTL identified ☐	• Refer to Standard 0011-Nurse interview • Weight, height • Physical, psych/social, behavioral, nutritional risk factors • Knowledge of normal vs. abnormal signs and symptoms of pregnancy • Premature labor risk assessment	• CCMS-UA, for nitr/leuk/ glucose C and S if applicable. • Prenatal group • HIV • Sickle cell if applicable • Dating ultrasound scheduled	☐ Childbirth ed., baby care and postpartum classes. Exercise during pregnancy. Effects of risk factors on pregnancy. Sexuality during pregnancy. Nutrition education. Normal effects of pregnancy on the body. Fetal growth/development. S and S of complications/preterm labor. Preadmission form. Contraceptives/STD Prevention/HIV counseling. Schedule return-to-clinic appointment. Orient to clinic hours/physical setup, emergency protocol.
1st OB Exam RN Name _____	☐ Prenatal group tests within normal limits. ☐ Demonstrates measures to relieve normal complaints of pregnancy. ☐ No change in preterm labor risk factors ☐	• Signs and symptoms of normal physical changes, complications • Behavioral risks • BP, weight • Urine dipstick for sugar/ ketone/protein • Fetal heart sounds • Fundal height • Pelvimetry	• Pap • GC • Chlamydia (if indicated) • Wet smear bacterial/ trich./vaginosis vaginal ph and Whiff Test	

Clinical Path Visits	Expected Patient/ Family Outcomes	Multidisciplinary Assessment (Refer to STD-0011)	Tests	Education & DC Planning (Refer to STD-0011)
(1-14 Weeks) Date _____ RN Name _____	☐ Demonstrates measures to relieve the normal complaints of pregnancy during 1st trimester ☐ Established exercise routine ☐ Exhibits minimum weight loss/gain ☐ 1st trimester test results within normal limits ☐ Avoids or demonstrates decrease in risk associated behavior (ie. smoking) ☐ No change in preterm labor risk factors ☐ Takes prenatal vitamins ☐ _____ ☐ _____	• Signs and symptoms of normal physical changes, complications • Behavioral risks • BP, weight • Urine dipstick for sugar, ketone, protein • Fetal heart sounds • Fundal height		☐ Reinforce (STD-0011) (Prenatal Standard of Care) Importance of compliance
(15-28 Weeks) RN Name _____	☐ Demonstrates measures to relieve the normal complaints of pregnancy during 2nd trimester. ☐ Exhibits normal weight gain. ☐ 2nd trimester test results within normal limits. ☐ Continues exercise routine. ☐ Avoids risk associated behavior. ☐ Demonstrates self-palpation technique and verbalizes signs and symptoms of preterm labor. ☐ No change in preterm labor risk factors. ☐ _____	• Signs and symptoms of normal physical changes, complications including: • Behavioral risks • BP, weight • Urine dipstick for sugar/ketone/ protein • Fetal heart sounds, fundal height • Fundal movement at 16-20 Weeks • Premature labor	• Triple Screen (16 to 19 weeks) • Ultrasound, as needed • Fibronectin (24 to 26 weeks) **ORDER AT 26 WEEKS:** • Trutol • Antibody screen (Rh Neg) • Repeat WCBC • RhoGAM at 28 weeks, if indicated	☐ Fetal growth/development for 2nd tri. Encourage childbirth, baby care and postpartum classes Reinforce (STD-0011) (Prenatal Standard of Care) Review S and S of preterm labor at 24 week appointment Importance of compliance Home visit
(29-42 Weeks) RN Name _____	☐ Demonstrates measures to relieve the normal complaints of pregnancy during 3rd trimester. ☐ Exhibits normal weight gain. ☐ Continues exercise routine. ☐ Normal physical changes of pregnancy w/o complications. ☐ Avoids risk associated behavior. ☐ Attends childbirth, baby care and postpartum classes ☐ Responds appropriately to signs and symptoms of preterm labor or other complications when indicated. ☐ Performing nipple preparation, if needed. ☐ No change in preterm labor risk factors. ☐ _____	• Signs and symptoms of normal physical changes, complications including: • Behavioral risks • BP, weight • Urine dipstick for sugar/ketone/protein • Fetal heart sounds, fundal height • Fetal movement • Planned method of infant feeding • Nipple exam, if planning to breast feed • Premature labor	• Ultrasound as needed **ORDER AT 36 WEEKS:** • Recto vaginal cultures for GBS Order at 41 Weeks: • NST and AFI Biweekly (amniotic fluid index)	☐ Fetal growth/development for 3rd trimester Review signs and symptoms and admission procedures for normal labor at 36 weeks. Reinforce (STD-11) (Prenatal Standard of Care) Review S and S of preterm labor Importance of compliance Update perinatal risk assessment Childbirth education, babycare and postpartum classes Tubal forms, if indicated by 34 weeks Treatment for inverted nipples if indicated Home visit

Figure 7-10 ■ The prenatal clinical pathway identifies outcomes, assessments, interventions, and consultations performed for pregnancy. (Courtesy Women and Children Services of the York Health System, York, Penn. Modified with permission.)

A complete history and physical examination are important to assess for health problems (such as diabetes, sexually transmissible infections), habits (such as use of alcohol or drugs), or social problems (such as domestic violence) that might unfavorably affect pregnancy. Previous reproductive problems and family history of possible genetic conditions are explored. When problems are discovered, treatment may be started before pregnancy to avoid complications of pregnancy or worsening of the woman's condition or situation because of pregnancy.

The woman is asked about her use of prescription and over-the-counter drugs, vitamins, and other supplements. It may be possible to change medications for chronic health problems if they are problematic during pregnancy. Use of complementary or alternative therapies is also addressed, because some that are safe at other times may be harmful during pregnancy. Avoidance of common teratogens or other harmful substances is discussed. Interventions for nutritional or weight problems are important. Referral to smoking cessation programs may be indicated.

Screening for rubella, varicella, and hepatitis B is performed, and the vaccines are given if indicated. The woman should be instructed to wait at least 1 month after receiving rubella and varicella vaccines before conceiving (Centers for Disease Control and Prevention [CDC], 2001; CDC, 2004). Many women are not aware of the need for folic acid before and during pregnancy. Women who might become pregnant are advised to consume 400 mcg (0.4 mg) of folic acid daily before conception and 600 mcg (0.6 mg) after conception to decrease the risk of neural tube defects.

Initial Prenatal Visit

If a preconception visit has occurred recently, many initial prenatal assessments will have been completed at that time. If not, a thorough history and physical examination must be completed. The primary objectives of the first antepartum examination are to:

- Verify or rule out pregnancy
- Evaluate the pregnant woman's physical health relevant to childbearing
- Assess the growth and health of the fetus
- Establish baseline data for comparison with future observations
- Establish trust and rapport with the childbearing family
- Evaluate the psychosocial needs of the woman and her family
- Assess the need for counseling or teaching
- Negotiate a plan of care to ensure both a healthy mother and a healthy baby

HISTORY

OBSTETRIC HISTORY. The obstetric history provides essential information about previous pregnancies that may alert the health care provider to possible problems in the present pregnancy. The usual components of this history include:

- Gravida, para, abortions, and living children
- Length of previous gestations
- Weight of infants at birth

- Labor experiences, type of deliveries, locations of births, and names of attending physicians or midwives
- Types of anesthesia and difficulties with anesthesia at any time in the past
- Maternal complications such as hypertension, diabetes, infection, and bleeding
- Infant complications
- Methods of infant feeding used in the past and currently planned (breastfeeding or formula)
- Special concerns

Gravida refers to a woman who is or has been pregnant, regardless of the length of the pregnancy. *Para* refers to the number of pregnancies that have ended at 20 or more weeks. The number of fetuses in a pregnancy does not change the para. Therefore a woman who gives birth to twins with her first pregnancy will be a gravida 1, para 1 if the birth occurred at 20 or more weeks of gestation. Para does not indicate whether the fetus was born alive or was stillborn.

Use of the GTPAL acronym is another way to describe pregnancy outcomes. GTPAL stands for pregnancies or gravida (G), term births [or pregnancies delivered] (T), preterm births (P), abortions (A), and living children (L). GTPAL may also be used to describe infants instead of pregnancies delivered. In this case (T) becomes term infants born and (P) becomes preterm infants born. Because the acronym is not used consistently, it can be confusing (Box 7-1).

Nurses must exercise caution when discussing gravida and para with the expectant mother in the presence of her family or significant other. Although the antepartum record indicates a previous pregnancy or childbirth, she may not have shared this information with her family, and her right to privacy could be jeopardized by probing questions. The pregnancy may have terminated in elective or spontaneous abortion or in the

BOX 7-1 Calculation of Gravida and Para

A method for calculating gravida and para is to separate pregnancies and their outcome using the acronym GTPAL: G = gravida, T = term, P = preterm, A = abortions, and L = living children.
The following examples illustrate the use of this method to obtain complete information.

- Sally Lam is pregnant for the fifth time. She had one spontaneous and one elective abortion in the first trimester. She has a son who was born at 40 weeks' gestation and a daughter who was born at 34 weeks'. She is gravida 5, para 2 and T = 1 (the son born at 40 weeks'); P = 1 (the daughter born at 34 weeks'), A = 2, L = 2. The two abortions are counted in the gravida but not included in the para because they occurred before 20 weeks'. Therefore Sally's GTPAL would be 5-1-1-2-2.
- Kathleen Eber gave birth to twins at 32 weeks' gestation and to a stillborn infant at 24 weeks' gestation. Approximately 2 years later, she experienced a spontaneous abortion at 12 weeks' gestation. If pregnant now, she is gravida 4, para 2 (the twins counting as 1 parous experience and the stillborn infant counting as 1 parous experience).
  If the GTPAL acronym is used to refer to pregnancies delivered, T = 0 (no pregnancies went to term), P = 2 (the twins and the stillborn infant counting as 2 pregnancies ending in preterm birth), A = 1, L = 2. The GTPAL would be 4-0-2-1-2.
  If the GTPAL acronym is used to refer to infants born, T = 0 (no pregnancies went to term), P = 3 (the twins and the stillborn infant born preterm), A = 1, L = 2. The GTPAL would be 4-0-3-1-2.

birth of an infant who was placed for adoption. The confidentiality of the pregnant woman must always be protected. The nurse should wait until the woman is alone if it is necessary to clarify information about her gravida or para.

MENSTRUAL HISTORY. A complete menstrual history is necessary to establish the EDD. Common practice is to determine the EDD on the basis of the first day of the last menstrual cycle, although ovulation and conception occur about 2 weeks after the beginning of menstruation in a regular 28-day cycle. The average duration of pregnancy from the first day of the last normal menstrual period (LNMP) is 40 weeks, or 280 days.

Nägele's rule is often used to establish the EDD. This method involves subtracting 3 months, adding 7 days to the first day of the LNMP, and correcting the year. For example:

- LNMP August 30, 2006
- Subtract 3 months: May 30, 2006
- Add 7 days and change the year: June 6, 2007

Many health care providers also use a gestational wheel or calculator to determine EDD quickly, although some wheels are prone to error (Cunningham et al., 2005). Calculations of EDD may be inaccurate in some situations. For example, Nägele's rule is less accurate when the woman's menstrual cycle is very irregular.

Many women have one or more ultrasounds during pregnancy. Ultrasound measurements taken early in pregnancy can more accurately determine the gestational age.

CONTRACEPTIVE HISTORY. Masculinization of female fetuses has been associated with inadvertent use of hormonal contraceptive during pregnancy (Briggs, Freeman, & Yaffe, 2002). Although the incidence is low, any woman who suspects she might be pregnant should stop taking hormonal contraceptives and use another contraceptive method until she has sought confirmation from a health care provider.

Although pregnancy with an intrauterine device (IUD) in place is unusual, it can cause complications such as spontaneous abortion and preterm delivery. The IUD is usually removed if the string is visible. In some cases the IUD may be left in place without apparent harm to the fetus (Speroff & Darney, 2001).

MEDICAL AND SURGICAL HISTORY. Chronic conditions such as diabetes mellitus, hypertension, and renal disease can affect the outcome of the pregnancy and

must be investigated. Infections, surgical procedures, and trauma that may complicate the pregnancy or childbirth should be documented. The history should include:

- Age, race, and ethnic background (relevant for groups at high risk for specific genetic problems such as sickle cell anemia, thalassemia, cystic fibrosis, and Tay-Sachs disease)
- Childhood diseases and immunizations
- Chronic illnesses such as asthma, heart disease, chronic hypertension, diabetes, lupus (onset and treatment)
- Previous illnesses, surgical procedures, and injuries (particularly of the pelvis and back)
- Previous infections such as hepatitis, sexually transmitted diseases, tuberculosis, and presence of group B streptococcus
- History of and treatment for anemia
- Bladder and bowel function (problems or changes)
- Amount of caffeine consumed each day (such as coffee, tea, chocolate, soft drinks)
- Alcohol intake (amount, type, frequency)
- Tobacco use (number of years and number of packs per day)
- Medications such as prescription or over-the-counter drugs and reasons for use
- Use of illicit drugs (name, amount, date, and time of last use)
- Complementary or alternative therapies used
- Overall health and energy
- Appetite, general nutrition, and history of eating disorders
- Contact with domestic pets, particularly cats (increases the risk for infections such as toxoplasmosis)
- Allergies and drug sensitivities
- Occupation and related risk factors

FAMILY HISTORY. A family history provides valuable information about the general health of the family, including chronic diseases such as diabetes and heart disease and infections such as tuberculosis and hepatitis. In addition, it may reveal information about patterns of genetic or congenital anomalies.

PARTNER'S HEALTH HISTORY. The partner's history helps determine whether the father of the expected child or his family has a history of significant health problems such as genetic abnormalities, chronic diseases, and infections. Use of drugs such as cocaine and alcohol may affect the ability of the family to cope with pregnancy and childbirth. Tobacco use by the father is of concern because both the mother and the infant are at risk for upper respiratory complications as a result of passive smoking.

In addition, the blood type and Rh factor of the father are important if the mother is Rh-negative and if blood incompatibility between the mother and fetus is possible.

PSYCHOSOCIAL HISTORY. The psychosocial history also should be elicited during the initial visit. It is discussed in Chapter 8.

PHYSICAL EXAMINATION

Because many women have never had a complete physical examination, a thorough evaluation of all body systems is necessary to detect previously undiagnosed physical prob-

CRITICAL THINKING EXERCISE 7-1

Wilma Turner gave birth to twin girls at 38 weeks of gestation 3 years ago. She had a spontaneous abortion last year at 12 weeks of gestation and thinks she may be pregnant now because she has missed a menstrual period and is experiencing nausea in the mornings. Wilma's LNMP began June 22.

Questions
1. If Wilma is pregnant now, what would be her gravida and para?
2. Explain to Wilma why amenorrhea and morning sickness are not positive indications of pregnancy.
3. Use Nägele's rule to compute the EDD.

lems that may affect the pregnancy outcome. It also allows the examiner to establish baseline levels that will guide the treatment of the expectant mother and fetus throughout pregnancy.

VITAL SIGNS

BLOOD PRESSURE. The method for obtaining BP should be the same for all caregivers within a practice setting because position affects BP in the pregnant woman. All staff members should use the same Korotkoff's phase to measure diastolic BP. The woman should be seated with her arm supported in a horizontal position at heart level. Documentation should include the position, arm used, and pressures obtained.

PULSE. The normal adult pulse rate is 60 to 90 bpm. Tachycardia is associated with anxiety, hyperthyroidism, and infection and should be investigated. Apical pulse should be assessed for at least 1 minute to determine the amplitude and regularity of the heartbeat and presence of murmurs. Pedal pulses are assessed to determine the presence of circulatory problems in the legs. Pedal pulses should be strong, equal, and regular.

RESPIRATORY EFFORT. Respiratory rate during pregnancy is in the range of 16 to 24 bpm. Tachypnea may indicate respiratory infection or cardiac disease. Breath sounds should be equal bilaterally, chest expansion should be symmetric, and lung fields should be free of abnormal breath sounds.

TEMPERATURE. Normal temperature during pregnancy is 36.6° C to 37.6° C (97.8° F to 99.6° F). Increased temperature suggests infection and may require medical management.

CARDIOVASCULAR SYSTEM

VENOUS CONGESTION. Additional assessment of the cardiovascular system includes observation for venous congestion, which can develop into varicosities. Venous congestion is most commonly noted in the legs, vulva, or rectum.

EDEMA. Edema of the legs may be a benign condition that reflects pooling of blood in the extremities, which results in a shift of intravascular fluid into interstitial spaces. When pressure exerted by a finger or thumb leaves a persistent depression, it is termed *pitting edema* (see Figure 17-9).

MUSCULOSKELETAL SYSTEM

POSTURE AND GAIT. Body mechanics and changes in posture and gait should be addressed. Body mechanics during pregnancy may place strain on the muscles of the lower back and legs.

HEIGHT AND WEIGHT. A determination of initial weight is needed to establish a baseline for evaluation of weight gain throughout pregnancy. Weight should be compared against the chart of ideal weight for height. Women who are underweight before pregnancy are at increased risk for having low-birth-weight infants and pregnancy loss. Those who are obese before pregnancy are at risk for in-

creased perinatal mortality, delivery complications, large-for-gestational-age infants, preeclampsia, and diabetes.

Recommendations for weight gain during pregnancy are often based on the woman's body mass index (see Chapter 9).

PELVIC MEASUREMENTS. The bony pelvis is evaluated early in the pregnancy to determine whether the diameters are adequate to permit vaginal delivery (see Chapter 12).

ABDOMEN. The contour, size, and muscle tone of the abdomen should be assessed. Fundal height should be measured if the fundus is palpable above the symphysis pubis. The bladder must be empty before the measurement is taken to ensure accuracy. The woman lies on her back with her knees slightly flexed. The top of the fundus is palpated, and a tape is stretched from the top of the symphysis pubis over the abdominal curve to the top of the fundus (Figure 7-11).

From 16 to 38 weeks the fundal height, measured in centimeters, is equal to the gestational age of the fetus in weeks, within 3 cm (Johnson & Niebyl, 2002). If fundal height is higher or lower than what is expected for the weeks of gestation, additional assessment is necessary to investigate the discrepancy. The cause may be an error in the EDD, a variation in the amount of amniotic fluid present, or an abnormality in fetal growth. Ultrasound may be performed to obtain further information.

If the pregnancy is advanced enough that the fetal heart rate is audible, the beats should be counted and the number documented.

NEUROLOGIC SYSTEM

A complete neurologic assessment is not necessary for young women who are free of signs or symptoms indicating a problem. However, deep tendon reflexes should be evaluated because hyperreflexia is associated with complications of pregnancy. (See Procedure 25-1 for assessment of deep tendon reflexes.)

INTEGUMENTARY SYSTEM

Skin color should be consistent with racial background. Pallor may indicate anemia. Jaundice may indicate hepatic disease. Lesions, bruising, rashes, areas of hyperpigmentation

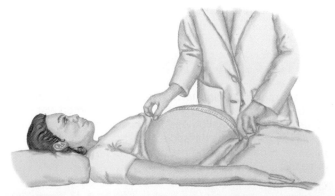

Figure 7-11 ■ Uterine measurements include the distance between the upper border of the symphysis pubis and the top of the fundus.

(such as melasma, linea nigra) related to pregnancy, and stretch marks (striae) should be noted. Nail beds should be pink with instant capillary return.

ENDOCRINE SYSTEM

The thyroid enlarges slightly during the second trimester. However, gross enlargement or tenderness may indicate hyperthyroidism and requires further medical evaluation.

GASTROINTESTINAL SYSTEM

MOUTH. Mucous membranes should be pink, smooth, glistening, and uniform. The lips should be free of ulcerations. The gums may be red, tender, and edematous from the effects of increased estrogen, which produces hyperplasia. The teeth should be in good repair. The woman should be referred for regular dental care because periodontal disease may result in infections that precipitate preterm labor. The second trimester may be the most comfortable time for dental care. However, if necessary, dental care can be performed during the third trimester if the woman is positioned to avoid supine hypotensive syndrome. Dental radiography should be avoided during pregnancy because it has been associated with low birth weight in infants (Mills & Moses, 2002).

INTESTINE. A warm stethoscope for assessing bowel sounds is most comfortable for the pregnant woman. Bowel sounds may be diminished because of the effects of progesterone on smooth muscle. Bowel sounds are often increased if a meal is overdue or diarrhea is present. Problems with constipation can be discussed during abdominal examination.

URINARY SYSTEM

Urine collected for testing should always be a clean-catch midstream sample. Urine is tested to detect signs of urinary tract infection and substances that may indicate a problem.

PROTEIN. Although a trace amount of protein may be present in the urine, the amount should not increase. Its presence may indicate contamination by vaginal secretions, kidney disease, or preeclampsia.

GLUCOSE. Small amounts of glucose may indicate physiologic "spilling" that occurs during normal pregnancy. Larger amounts require glucose screening of the blood.

KETONES. Ketones may be found in the urine after heavy exercise or as a result of inadequate intake of food and fluid.

BACTERIA. Increased bacteria in the urine is associated with urinary tract infection, which is common during pregnancy.

REPRODUCTIVE SYSTEM

BREASTS. Breast size and symmetry, condition of the nipples, and presence of colostrum should be noted. Any lumps, dimpling of the skin, or asymmetry of the nipples requires further evaluation.

EXTERNAL REPRODUCTIVE ORGANS. The skin and mucous membranes of the perineum, vulva, and anus are inspected for excoriations, growths, ulcerations, lesions, varicosities, warts, chancres, and perineal scars. Enlargement, tenderness, redness, or discharge from Bartholin's glands or Skene's glands may indicate gonorrheal or chlamydial infection. The examiner should obtain a specimen for culture of any discharge from lesions or inflamed glands to determine the causative organisms and to provide effective care.

INTERNAL REPRODUCTIVE ORGANS. A speculum inserted into the vagina permits the examiner to view the walls of the vagina and the cervix. The cervix should be pink in a nonpregnant woman and bluish in a pregnant woman (Chadwick's sign). The external cervical os is closed in primigravidas, but one fingertip may be admitted in multiparas. The cervix feels relatively firm except during pregnancy, when marked softening is noted (Goodell's sign). Routine cervical cultures for gonorrhea and chlamydial infection are standard practice during the initial pregnancy examination. The examiner also collects a specimen for a Papanicolaou (Pap) smear, to screen for cervical cancer.

A bimanual examination involves the use of both hands to palpate the internal genitalia. One hand is placed on the abdomen and the other is inserted into the vagina. The examiner palpates the uterus for size, contour, tenderness, and position. The uterus should be movable between the two examining hands and should feel smooth. The ovaries, if palpable, should be about the size and shape of almonds and nontender.

Pelvic measurements may be assessed at this time to determine if the shape and size of the bony pelvis are adequate for a normal birth (see Figure 12-4).

LABORATORY DATA

Table 7-3 lists laboratory examinations commonly performed during pregnancy and the purpose and significance of each test.

✓ CHECK YOUR READING

21. Why is a preconception visit important?
22. Why are a medical-surgical history and an obstetric history necessary?
23. How does fundal height relate to gestational age?

RISK ASSESSMENT

Risk assessment begins at the initial visit when the health care provider identifies factors that put the expectant mother or fetus at risk for complications and that require specialized care. Many women identified as high risk give birth to healthy full-term infants. Furthermore, risk factors change as pregnancy progresses, and risk assessment must be updated throughout pregnancy. Gestations categorized as low risk at the initial assessment may later become high risk. Table 7-4 lists major risk factors and their implications.

Subsequent Assessments

Ongoing antepartum care is important to the successful outcome of pregnancy. Although the recommended number of visits can be reduced for women without complica-

TABLE 7-3 Common Laboratory Tests

Test	Purpose	Significance
Blood grouping	To determine blood type and Rh	Identifies possible causes of incompatibility with the fetus that may cause jaundice
Hemoglobin (Hgb) or hematocrit (Hct)	To detect anemia; often checked several times during pregnancy	Hgb < 11 g/dl in the 1st and 3rd trimesters or < 10.5 g/dl in the 2nd trimester may indicate a need for additional iron supplementation.
Complete blood count (CBC)	To detect infection, anemia, or cell abnormalities	12,000/mm³ or more white blood cells or decreased platelets require follow-up
Rh factor and antibody screen	To check for possible maternal-fetal blood incompatibility	If mother is Rh-negative and father is Rh-positive or antibodies are present, additional testing and treatment are required; if Rh⁻ and unsensitized, RhoGAM will be given at 28 weeks
Venereal Disease Research Laboratory (VDRL) test or rapid plasma reagin (RPR)	To screen for syphilis	Treat if results are positive; retest at 36 weeks
Rubella titer	To determine immunity	If titer is 1:8 or less, mother is not immune; immunize postpartum if not immune
Skin test	To screen for tuberculosis	If results are positive, refer for additional testing or therapy
Hemoglobin electrophoresis	To screen for sickle cell trait if client is of African-American descent	If mother is positive, check partner; infant is at risk only if both parents are positive
Hepatitis B screen	To detect presence of antigens in maternal blood	If present, infants should be given hepatitis immune globulin and vaccine soon after birth
Human immunodeficiency virus (HIV) screen	Voluntary test encouraged at first visit to detect HIV antibodies	Positive results require retesting, counseling, and treatment to lower infant infection
Urinalysis	To detect renal disease or infection	Requires further assessment if positive for more than a trace protein (renal damage, preeclampsia, or normal), ketones (fasting or dehydration), or bacteria (infection)
Papanicolaou (Pap) test	To screen for cervical neoplasia	Treat and refer if abnormal cells are present
Cervical culture	To detect group B streptococci and sexually transmissible diseases	Treat and retest as necessary, treat group B streptococci during labor
Multiple marker screen: maternal serum alpha-fetoprotein, human chorionic gonadotropin (hCG), and estriol. May include other tests such as inhibin A.	To screen for fetal anomalies	Abnormal results may indicate Down syndrome or neural tube defects
Maternal blood glucose (glucose challenge test)	To screen for possible gestational diabetes	If elevated, a 3-hour glucose tolerance test is recommended

tions, the usual schedule for prenatal assessment in normal pregnancy is as follows:

- Conception to 28 weeks—every 4 weeks
- 29 to 36 weeks—every 2 to 3 weeks
- 37 weeks to birth—weekly

VITAL SIGNS

Deviations from the baseline value for vital signs indicate the need for further assessment. The BP should be measured in the same arm with the mother in the same position each time.

WEIGHT

Weight should be recorded to document that weight gain is progressing as expected (see Chapter 9). Inadequate weight gain may signify that the pregnancy is not as advanced as was thought or that the fetus is not growing as expected. Sudden, rapid weight gain may indicate excessive fluid retention.

URINALYSIS

Urine is tested at each visit for the presence of protein, glucose, ketones, and bacteria. A culture may be performed if the woman has a history or symptoms of uri-

nary tract infection or if a dipstick indicates the presence of bacteria.

FUNDAL HEIGHT

Measuring fundal height is an inexpensive and noninvasive method of evaluating fetal growth and confirming gestational age.

LEOPOLD'S MANEUVERS

Leopold's maneuvers provide a systematic method for palpating the fetus through the abdominal wall during the later part of pregnancy. These maneuvers provide valuable information about the location and presentation of the fetus (see Chapter 13).

FETAL HEART RATE

The fetal heart rate may be heard with a Doppler transducer in early pregnancy or with a fetoscope in later pregnancy (see Figure 14-1). The location of the fetal heart sounds provides information that helps determine the position in which the fetus is entering the pelvis. For instance, fetal heart sounds heard in an upper quadrant of the abdomen suggest that the fetus is in a breech presentation.

TABLE 7-4 Summary of High-Risk Factors in Pregnancy

Factors	Implications
Demographic Factors	
<16 years or >35 years of age	Increased risk for preterm labor, preeclampsia, congenital anomalies
Low socioeconomic status or dependence on public assistance	Increased risk for preterm labor, low-birth-weight infants
Nonwhite race	Incidence of infant and maternal death higher than that of whites
Multiparity: >4 pregnancies	Increasing parity increases risk of pregnancy loss, antepartum or postpartum hemorrhage, and cesarean birth
Social and Personal Factors	
Low prepregnancy weight	Associated with low-birth-weight infants
Obesity	Increased risk for preeclampsia, difficult labor and delivery, large-for-gestational-age infants, diabetes, and cesarean birth
Height <152 cm (5 feet)	Increased incidence of cesarean birth because of cephalopelvic disproportion
Smoking	Associated with increased infant mortality, low-birth-weight infants, intrauterine growth restriction, preterm birth, preterm labor, spontaneous abortion, and placental problems
Use of alcohol or unprescribed drugs	Increased risk of congenital anomalies, neonatal withdrawal syndrome, and fetal alcohol syndrome
Obstetric Factors	
Birth of previous infant >4000 g (8.8 pounds)	Increased need for cesarean birth; increased risk for infant birth injury, neonatal hypoglycemia, and maternal gestational diabetes
Previous fetal or neonatal death	Maternal psychological distress
Rh sensitization	Fetal anemia, erythroblastosis fetalis, kernicterus
Existing Medical Conditions	
Diabetes mellitus	Increased risk for preeclampsia, cesarean birth, infant either small or large for gestational age, neonatal hypoglycemia, fetal or neonatal death, congenital anomalies
Thyroid disorder	
Hypothyroidism	Increased incidence of spontaneous abortion, congenital anomalies, congenital hypothyroidism
Hyperthyroidism	Maternal risk for preeclampsia, thyroid storm, or postpartum hemorrhage; neonatal risk for thyrotoxicosis
Cardiac disease	Maternal risk for cardiac decompensation and increased death rate; increased risk for fetal and neonatal death
Renal disease	Maternal risk for renal failure and preterm delivery; fetal risk for intrauterine growth restriction
Concurrent infections	Severe fetal implications (heart disease, blindness, deafness, bone lesions) if maternal disease occurred in the first trimester, increased incidence of spontaneous abortion or congenital anomalies associated with some infections

FETAL ACTIVITY

Fetal movements (quickening) are usually first noticed by the expectant mother at 16 to 20 weeks of gestation and gradually increase in frequency and strength. In the last trimester the woman may be asked to count fetal movements, commonly called *kick counts*. In general, fetal activity indicates a physically healthy fetus. Therefore fetal activity is a reassuring sign.

SIGNS OF LABOR

The woman should be asked about signs of labor at each visit. A discussion of contractions, bleeding, and rupture of membranes will help the woman learn how to identify preterm labor. She should be cautioned to call the health care provider or hospital if she thinks any of the signs is occurring.

ULTRASOUND SCREEN

Although an ultrasound examination is not necessary for all women, the test is often performed at 12 to 20 weeks of gestation. Ultrasound helps determine gestational age and may show some fetal anomalies and determine the sex. (See Chapter 10.)

GLUCOSE SCREEN

The blood glucose level is screened between 24 and 28 weeks of gestation with a glucose challenge test using a 50-g glucose load followed by a 1-hour plasma glucose determination. If the result is 140 mg/dl or higher, the woman receives a 3-hour, 100-g glucose tolerance test to determine whether she has gestational diabetes (Cunningham et al., 2005). Some practitioners use a cutoff glucose value of 130 mg/dl to determine if a glucose tolerance test is necessary (American Diabetes Association, 2004).

Glucose screening may not be necessary in women who are less than 25 years of age and who are at low risk for developing gestational diabetes. Women at low risk are those with a body mass index less than 25, no history of abnormal glucose tolerance or adverse pregnancy outcomes that occur with gestational diabetes, and no close relative with diabetes (American Academy of Pediatrics [AAP] and American College of Obstetricians and Gynecologists [ACOG], 2002).

Those at high risk may be tested earlier in pregnancy and again at 24 to 28 weeks. See Chapter 26 for more information about diabetes and pregnancy.

ISOIMMUNIZATION

Antibody tests may be repeated in the third trimester in women who are Rh-negative if the father of the baby is Rh-positive. If unsensitized, the woman should receive anti-D immune globulin (RhoGAM) prophylactically at about 28 weeks of gestation (see Chapter 25).

PELVIC EXAMINATION

During the last month of pregnancy the physician or midwife may perform a pelvic examination to determine cervical changes. The descent of the fetus and the presenting part can also be assessed at this time.

Multifetal Pregnancy

A multifetal pregnancy is a pregnancy in which two or more embryos or fetuses are present simultaneously (see Chapter 6).

DIAGNOSIS

Multifetal pregnancies are more likely in women with a personal or family history, in older mothers, and especially in conceptions that result from infertility therapy.

Maternal symptoms of multifetal pregnancy include the woman's sensations of feeling larger than with previous pregnancies and of more fetal movement. A greater weight gain and more rapid uterine growth also increase the suspicion that more than one fetus is present. Fundal height is greater than expected on the basis of gestational age computed from the last menstrual period.

When more than one fetus is suspected, diagnosis should be confirmed by sonography. Separate gestational sacs may be seen as early as 6 weeks of gestation. Multiple fetal parts may be visible by the tenth week.

MATERNAL ADAPTATION TO MULTIFETAL PREGNANCY

The degree of maternal physiologic change is greater with multiple fetuses than with a single fetus. For instance, blood volume increases 500 ml more than the amount needed for a single fetus. This increase heightens the workload of the heart and may contribute to fatigue and activity intolerance. The additional size of the uterus intensifies the mechanical effects of pregnancy. The uterus may achieve a volume of 10 L or more and weigh more than 9 kg (20 lb) (Cunningham et al., 2005). Respiratory difficulty increases because the overdistended uterus causes greater elevation of the diaphragm.

The uterus may also cause more compression of the large vessels, resulting in more pronounced and earlier supine hypotension. Greater compression of the ureters can occur, and maternal edema and slight proteinuria are common. Compression of the bowel makes constipation a persistent problem.

ANTEPARTUM CARE IN MULTIFETAL PREGNANCY

Early diagnosis of multifetal pregnancy allows time for the family to be educated about the many ways in which the pregnancy will differ from those involving a single fetus. Special antepartum classes can explain the need for increased nutrition, rest, and fetal monitoring. Instruction about signs of preterm labor, a common complication, should begin early. Discussions of the possible need to reduce activity, frequent rest periods, and the potential family stress caused by a high-risk pregnancy should also be included.

Women with multifetal pregnancies have more frequent antepartum visits to allow early detection of common complications. These include anemia, gestational diabetes, preeclampsia, preterm labor, and congenital anomalies. Visits may be scheduled biweekly at 20 weeks of gestation and weekly at 24 weeks.

Diet also must be considered. The need for calories, iron, vitamins, and folic acid is higher than for single-fetus pregnancies. Iron is particularly important, as anemia is common. Education about foods high in iron and iron supplements is important. The Institute of Medicine has recommended that the target weight gain at term for women carrying twins should be 16 to 20.5 kg (35 to 45 lb).

The woman may have many concerns and may need more support than women with only one fetus. Discomforts of pregnancy, which are merely annoying to other women, are increased during multifetal pregnancies. In addition the financial burden of medical and hospital care during and after pregnancy is increased. The woman may need referral for assistance in this area.

✔ CHECK YOUR READING

24. What are major risk factors during pregnancy?
25. What is the recommended schedule for antepartum visits?
26. How does maternal adaptation differ in multifetal pregnancies?

Common Discomforts of Pregnancy

Many women experience discomforts of pregnancy that are not serious but detract from the woman's feeling of comfort and well-being. (Measures to help relieve these discomforts are discussed in "Women Want to Know: How to Overcome the Common Discomforts of Pregnancy.")

NAUSEA AND VOMITING

The nausea and vomiting of pregnancy are frequently called *morning sickness* because these symptoms are more acute on arising. However, they may occur at any time and may continue throughout the day. Morning sickness occurs in 70% to 85% of pregnant women (ACOG, 2004). Women need reassurance that although morning sickness is distressing, it is common and temporary and will not harm the fetus. Morning sickness must be distinguished from hyperemesis

How to Overcome the Common Discomforts of Pregnancy

NAUSEA AND VOMITING

- Eat crackers or dry toast before arising in the morning, and then get out of bed slowly.
- Eat small amounts of carbohydrates, such as crackers, every 2 hours to prevent an empty stomach, or eat five or six small meals per day rather than three full meals.
- Drink fluids frequently but separately from meals.
- Avoid odors that increase the nausea.
- Avoid fried, high-fat, greasy, or spicy foods and those with strong odors such as onion and cabbage.
- Experiment with different foods that may be helpful, such as ginger, peppermint, or tart and salty combinations.
- Eat a protein snack before bedtime.

HEARTBURN

- Eat several small meals daily and avoid fatty or spicy foods.
- Eliminate or curtail smoking and coffee, which stimulate acid formation in the stomach.
- Remain upright for at least an hour after eating to reduce reflux and relieve symptoms.
- Avoid eating or drinking at bedtime and sleep with an extra pillow under the head and shoulders.
- Try deep breathing and sipping water to help relieve the burning sensation.
- Use antacids, but avoid those that are high in sodium (such as Alka-Seltzer, baking soda) because excessive sodium may result in fluid retention. Antacids high in calcium (such as Tums, Alka-Mints) are a good choice. Liquid antacids may be more effective, as they coat the esophagus.

BACKACHE

- Maintain correct posture with the head up and the shoulders back.
- Avoid high-heeled shoes, to improve posture.
- When picking up objects, squat rather than bending from the waist.
- When sitting, use foot supports, arm rests, and pillows behind the back.
- Exercise: Tailor sitting, shoulder circling, and pelvic rocking strengthen the back and help prepare for labor.
- A maternity back binder for use in pregnancy may be helpful.

ROUND LIGAMENT PAIN

- Use good body mechanics and avoid very strenuous exercise.
- Avoid stretching and twisting at the same time. When getting out of bed, turn to the side first and then get up slowly.
- Bend toward the pain, squat, or bring the knees up to the chest to relieve pain by relaxing the ligament.
- Try a heating pad if discomfort persists.

URINARY FREQUENCY AND LOSS OF URINE

Performing Kegel's exercises helps maintain bladder control:

- Identify the muscles to be exercised when stopping the flow of urine midstream. Do not routinely perform the exercise while urinating, however, because it might cause urinary retention and increase the risk of urinary tract infection.
- Contract the muscles around the vagina and hold for 10 seconds. Relax for at least 10 seconds.
- Repeat the contraction-relaxation cycle 30 times each day.

VARICOSITIES

The key to prevention and treatment is to prevent pooling of blood in the large veins of the legs:

- Avoid constricting clothing or crossing the legs at the knees, which impede blood return from the legs.
- Take frequent rest periods with the legs elevated above the level of the hips.
- Apply support hose or elastic stockings that reach above the varicosities before getting out of bed each morning. Putting them on later makes them less effective because pooling begins on rising.
- If working in one position for prolonged periods, walk around for a few minutes at least every 2 hours to stimulate blood flow and relieve discomfort.

HEMORRHOIDS

- To prevent hemorrhoids, try to establish a regular pattern of bowel elimination that does not require straining. Drink plenty of water, eat foods rich in fiber, and exercise regularly.
- To relieve existing hemorrhoids, take frequent, tepid baths. Apply cool witch hazel compresses or anesthetic ointments. Use a side-lying position with the hips elevated on a pillow.
- Gently push any external hemorrhoids back into the rectum. To do so, put on a vinyl glove and lubricate the index finger. Maintain pressure for 1 to 2 minutes.
- If pain or bleeding persists, call your health care provider.

CONSTIPATION

Self-care measures generally are as effective as laxatives but do not interfere with absorption of nutrients or lead to laxative dependency:

- Drink at least eight glasses of water each day. These should not include coffee, tea, or carbonated drinks because of their diuretic effect. After drinking one of these beverages, drink a glass of water to counteract its diuretic effect.
- Additional fiber in the diet helps maintain bowel elimination. Foods high in fiber include unpeeled fresh fruits and vegetables, whole-grain cereals, bran muffins, oatmeal, baked potatoes with skins, and fruit juices. Four pieces of fruit and a large salad provide enough fiber requirements for 1 day (see Box 9-3).
- Restrict consumption of cheese, which causes constipation.
- Curtail the intake of sweets, which increases bacterial growth in the intestine and can lead to flatulence.
- Do not discontinue taking iron supplements if they have been prescribed. If constipation persists, consult the health care provider for advice about use of stool softeners.

Continued

- Exercise stimulates peristalsis and improves muscle tone. Walking briskly for at least 1 mile per day, swimming, or riding a stationary bicycle may be helpful.
- Establish a regular pattern by allowing a consistent time each day for elimination. One hour after meals is ideal to take advantage of the gastrocolic reflex (the peristaltic wave in the colon that is induced by taking food into the fasting stomach). Using a footrest during elimination provides comfort and decreases straining.

LEG CRAMPS

- To prevent cramps, elevate the legs frequently to improve circulation.
- To relieve cramps, extend the affected leg, keeping the knee straight. Bend the foot toward the body, or ask someone to assist. Stand and apply pressure on the affected leg. These measures lengthen the affected muscles and relieve cramping.
- Avoid excessive foods high in phosphorus, such as soft drinks.

- Supplemental calcium or magnesium may be helpful but should be taken only on the advice of the health care provider.

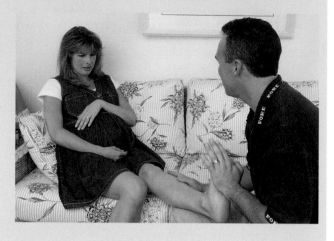

gravidarum, a condition with severe vomiting accompanied by weight loss, dehydration, electrolyte imbalance, and ketosis (see Chapter 25).

Although the cause of nausea and vomiting is unknown, it is believed to be related to increased levels of hCG and estrogen. Symptoms may be aggravated by odors (such as from cooking), fatigue, and emotional factors. Women under emotional stress are more likely to experience nausea.

Nausea usually ends by the second trimester, but some women experience it longer. Nausea and vomiting that significantly interfere with the woman's intake of nutrients may decrease nutrients available to the fetus. Taking a multivitamin at the time of conception may decrease the symptoms. Vitamin B_6 (pyridoxine) is safe during pregnancy (ACOG, 2004). Several antihistamines and phenothiazines may be prescribed safely for more severe nausea (Magee, Mazzota, & Korne, 2002). Various nonpharmacologic alternative therapies such as ginger may also be used for relief of nausea. The health care provider should be consulted about home remedies used.

HEARTBURN

Heartburn, an acute burning sensation in the epigastric and sternal regions, occurs in two thirds of pregnant women (Lu & Hobel, 2004). It may be associated with other gastrointestinal symptoms such as frequent belching, nausea, and epigastric pressure.

Heartburn occurs when reverse peristaltic waves cause regurgitation of acidic stomach contents into the esophagus. The underlying causes are diminished gastric motility and displacement of the stomach by the enlarging uterus. Improper diet and nervous tension may be precipitating factors.

◉ COMPLEMENTARY/ALTERNATIVE THERAPY

Nausea in Pregnancy

The following home treatments may be helpful for nausea and vomiting in pregnancy. The woman should check with her health care provider before using any complementary or alternative therapies.
- Combinations of salty and tart foods such as potato chips and lemonade or green apples
- Peppermint (tea or candy)
- Ginger (tea, cookies, soda)
- Acupressure over the Neiguan acupuncture point (approximately three fingerwidths above the wrist crease on the inner arm); devices that apply an electrical impulse over this point are available by prescription, and devices that apply pressure alone are available over the counter
- Acupuncture
- Hypnosis

BACKACHE

Backache is a common complaint during the third trimester. Prevention of backache with correct posture and body mechanics is a primary focus (Figure 7-12). Stooping or bending puts a great deal of strain on the muscles of the lower back. Instruction should include correct and incorrect methods for lifting (Figure 7-13) and exercises to relax the shoulders and thighs and help prevent backache (Figure 7-14).

ROUND LIGAMENT PAIN

Round ligament pain is a sharp pain in the side or inguinal area, usually on the right side, that results from softening and stretching of the ligament from hormones and uterine growth. The right round ligament is stretched more than the left because the uterus turns slightly to the right during pregnancy.

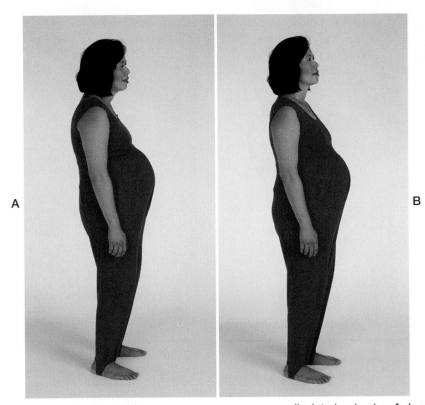

Figure 7-12 ■ Posture during pregnancy may cause or alleviate backache. **A,** Incorrect posture. The neck is jutting forward, the shoulders are slumping, and the back is sharply curved, creating back pain and discomfort. **B,** Correct posture. The neck and shoulders are straight, the back is flattened, and the pelvis is tucked under and slightly upward.

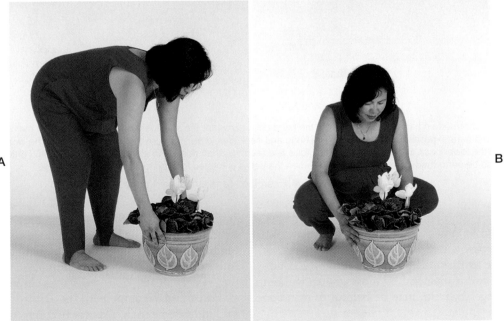

Figure 7-13 ■ Techniques for lifting. Squatting places less strain on the back. **A,** Incorrect technique. Stooping or bending places a great deal of strain on muscles of the lower back. **B,** Correct technique. Squatting and moving the object close permits the stronger muscles of the legs to do the lifting.

Shoulder circling

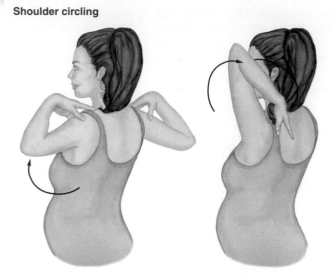

The fingertips are placed on the shoulders, then the elbows are brought forward and up during inhalation, back and down during exhalation. Repeat five times.

Tailor sitting

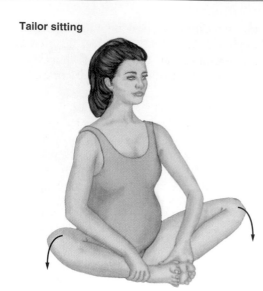

The woman uses her thigh muscles to press her knees to the floor. Keeping her back straight, she should remain in the position for 5 to 15 minutes.

Pelvic tilt or pelvic rocking

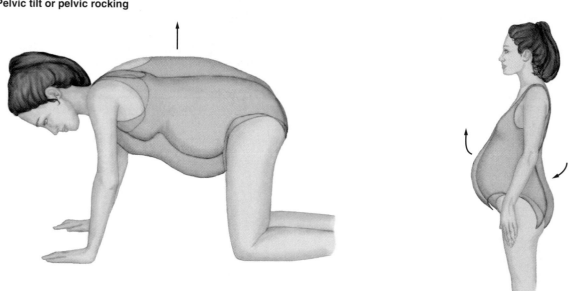

This exercise can be performed on hands and knees, with the hands directly under the shoulders and the knees under the hips. The back should be in a neutral position, not hollowed. The head and neck should be aligned with the straight back. The woman then presses up with the lower back and holds this position for a few seconds, then relaxes to a neutral position. Repeat 5 times. The exercise may also be performed in a standing position when the pelvis is rotated forward to flatten the lower back.

Figure 7-14 ■ Exercises to prevent backache.

URINARY FREQUENCY

Although urinary frequency is a common complaint of women during the first trimester and near term, the condition is temporary and is managed by most women without undue distress. Kegel exercises may be helpful to maintain bladder control.

VARICOSITIES

Varicosities occur in 40% of pregnancies and most often occur in women who are obese, are multiparas, or have a family history of varicose veins. During pregnancy the weight of the uterus partially compresses the veins returning blood from the legs, and estrogen causes elastic tissue to become more fragile (Blackburn, 2003). As blood pools the vessels dilate, and the valves in the veins become stretched and incompetent. The result is even more pooling, and in time the veins may become engorged, inflamed, and painful. Varicose veins are exacerbated by prolonged standing, during which the force of gravity makes blood return more difficult.

Varicosities are usually confined to the legs but may involve the veins of the vulva or rectum (hemorrhoids).

Signs and symptoms depend on the degree of engorgement and range from barely noticeable blemishes with minimal discomfort at the end of the day to large, tortuous veins that produce severe discomfort with any activity.

HEMORRHOIDS. Hemorrhoids are varicosities of the rectum and may be external (outside the anus) or internal (above the anal sphincter). Some common causes of hemorrhoids are vascular engorgement of the pelvis, constipation, straining at stool, and a prolonged sitting or standing position. The pushing that occurs during the second stage of labor aggravates the problem, which may continue into the postpartum period.

CONSTIPATION

Occasional constipation is not harmful, although it can cause feelings of abdominal fullness and flatulence and aggravate painful hemorrhoids. Intestinal motility is reduced during pregnancy as a result of progesterone and may result in hard, dry stools and decreased frequency of bowel movements. Iron supplementation often increases constipation.

LEG CRAMPS

Painful contractions of the muscles of the lower legs occur most often during sleep when the muscles are relaxed. Cramps are also likely to occur when the woman stretches and extends her feet with the toes pointed. Leg cramps may be caused by an imbalance of serum calcium and phosphorus, but this has not been proved. Low magnesium levels may also be a cause, and magnesium supplementation may be helpful (Shabert, 2004). A 1:1 ratio of calcium to phosphorus is desirable but difficult to achieve during pregnancy, when many women consume large amounts of dairy products that are high in calcium and phosphorus. Venous congestion in the legs during the third trimester also contributes to leg cramps.

Cultural Considerations

Although the physical changes of pregnancy are fairly universal, culture often determines the health beliefs, values, and expectations of the family when a woman becomes pregnant (see Chapter 8).

✓ CHECK YOUR READING

27. What causes morning sickness?
28. How can backache be alleviated during pregnancy?

Application of the Nursing Process
Family Responses to Physical Changes of Pregnancy

The nursing process focuses on identifying each family's unique responses to the physiologic changes of pregnancy, determining factors that might interfere with the ability to adapt to changes that occur, and finding solutions to problems that are identified.

Assessment

Assess the family's responses to the physiologic processes of pregnancy. During the third trimester explore the family's preparation for the birth. Use structured interviews and planned teaching sessions, as well as more informal discussions that occur spontaneously during the initial or subsequent assessments. Review the history and physical examination to obtain important data. Gather information from the expectant mother as well as from her partner and other significant family members, if appropriate.

Analysis

When analyzing data, nurses must use all their critical thinking skills before coming to a conclusion about the most significant nursing diagnoses (Box 7-2). One of the most common errors is an unexamined assumption. Nurses may assume that all families experience the same concerns during pregnancy. Such an assumption may lead to diagnoses that are irrelevant to the actual problems of a specific family.

In maternal-newborn nursing the nursing process must be adapted to a generally healthy population experiencing a life event that holds the possibility for growth as well as problems. Unlike medical-surgical nursing, much maternal-newborn nursing activity is devoted to assessing, diagnosing, and promoting family strengths and healthy functioning (see Nursing Care Plans 7-1 and 7-2).

Many problem-oriented nursing diagnoses do not address the healthy family preparing for the birth of a child. Most families express an intense desire to protect the health of the unborn child and well-being of the mother. Perhaps the most encompassing nursing diagnosis for the prenatal period is "Health-Seeking Behaviors: prenatal care and health practices that provide optimal benefit to the fetus and mother."

BOX 7-2 Common Nursing Diagnoses

Activity Intolerance
Constipation
Deficient Diversional Activity
Deficient Knowledge
Disturbed Sleep Pattern
Fatigue*
Deficient Fluid Volume*
Health-Seeking Behavior*
Ineffective Health Maintenance
Ineffective Sexuality Patterns
Nausea
Acute Pain (Backache)
Risk for Imbalanced Nutrition: Less than Body
   Requirements*
Risk for Imbalanced Nutrition: More than Body
   Requirements
Risk for Injury
Sleep Deprivation

*Nursing diagnoses that are explored in this chapter.

NURSING CARE PLAN 7-1   Discomfort during Early Pregnancy

ASSESSMENT: Maria Gomez, a thin, 21-year-old primigravida of 8 weeks' gestation, has dry, cracked lips and a pulse rate of 90 when she arrives at the prenatal clinic. She states that she is experiencing nausea with occasional vomiting throughout the day. She reports that the nausea is intensified by the odor of cooking food and she has little appetite. Although she is always thirsty, she restricts fluids because "they make me sicker." Her urine sample is concentrated, with a specific gravity of 1.030 and a small amount of ketones.

NURSING DIAGNOSIS: Risk for Imbalanced Nutrition: Less than Body Requirements related to nausea, vomiting, and anorexia

CRITICAL THINKING: Were all assessment data considered? Organize data and develop a second diagnosis. State outcomes for that diagnosis, and identify at least two interventions.

ANSWER: No. All data should be grouped and analyzed. Nausea throughout the day, occasional vomiting, and anorexia support the stated nursing diagnosis. Dry lips, tachycardia, thirst, and concentrated urine, however, suggest a second nursing diagnosis: Risk for Deficient Fluid Volume related to inadequate intake of fluids and fluid loss through vomiting.

GOALS/OUTCOME CRITERIA INCLUDE:
1. Increase intake of fluids to 2000 ml/day
2. Maintain urine specific gravity within normal range
3. Demonstrate no signs or symptoms of dehydration

INTERVENTIONS INCLUDE:
1. Suggest alternative sources of fluids, such as gelatin, frozen juice bars, ice cream, pudding, and watermelon.
2. Recommend frequent small amounts of ice chips or clear liquids.
3. Emphasize the importance of taking frequent small amounts of water instead of coffee or tea, which act as diuretics.
4. Ask Maria to return within 2 days if she is unable to retain recommended amounts of fluid. Waiting until the next scheduled prenatal visit is not prudent if she is dehydrated.

GOALS/EXPECTED OUTCOMES: Maria will:
1. Maintain adequate intake of calories and nutrients to meet her needs, as evidenced by sufficient energy to carry on the activities of daily living, and result in a weight gain of 4.5 kg (10 lb) by 20 weeks
2. Report less nausea and a decrease in the episodes of vomiting by the next clinic visit

INTERVENTION	RATIONALE
1. Recommend that Maria eat two dry crackers half an hour before arising in the morning and that she get out of bed slowly.	1. Food counteracts hypoglycemia resulting from overnight fasting and helps prevent an initial episode of nausea that may become difficult to control.
2. Suggest that she eat a high-protein bedtime snack, such as cottage cheese or half a turkey sandwich on whole wheat bread.	2. Proteins are metabolized at a slower rate and help prevent morning hypoglycemia.
3. Instruct Maria to eat small, dry meals five to six times a day rather than three large ones.	3. Frequent dry meals prevent the stomach from becoming empty and decrease the feeling of nausea.
4. Suggest that fluids be taken separately from solid foods and that she brush her teeth often, especially after vomiting.	4. Fluids overstretch the stomach and may precipitate vomiting. Brushing her teeth removes bad tastes and helps prevent damage to the enamel from stomach acids.
5. Recommend that she eat a dry cracker, unbuttered popcorn, or dry toast every 2 hours.	5. Nausea is more intense when the stomach is empty.
6. Advise her to avoid foods that are fried, greasy, highly seasoned, or high in fat and those with strong odors. Suggest that she try ginger teas or combinations of salty and tart flavors.	6. Odors and greasy textures are associated with nausea and increased episodes of vomiting. Some women find various foods or combinations helpful.
7. Suggest that Maria eat ice chips when she is most nauseated, followed by clear liquids such as water, clear juices, or popsicles. Recommend that she experiment with soups, shakes, smoothies, and vegetable drinks when she is feeling better.	7. Clear liquids are most easily tolerated during nausea. Foods that are usually tolerated well but are high in nutrients should be started in small amounts as soon as possible.
8. Reassure her that nausea and vomiting usually disappear by the second trimester and do not indicate a problem with the pregnancy.	8. Knowing that the condition is self-limiting and does not threaten the fetus reduces anxiety.
9. Teach Maria to keep a record of daily intake of food and fluids, episodes of vomiting, and measures that reduce nausea.	9. A record is essential to determine if adequate nutrients and fluids are being retained and to identify the most helpful measures to control nausea.

NURSING CARE PLAN 7-1 Discomfort during Early Pregnancy—cont'd

INTERVENTION	RATIONALE
10. Assess Maria's weight at each prenatal visit and compare weight gain with that expected for the weeks of gestation.	10. If weight gain is normal, the focus remains on relieving the discomfort of nausea and vomiting. If weight gain is too low or signs of dehydration are present, refer her for medical management.
11. Instruct her to call if her nausea and vomiting become worse.	11. Persistent vomiting may lead to dehydration, fluid and electrolyte imbalance, and inadequate nutrient intake.

EVALUATION: Maria's periodic nausea and vomiting continue throughout the first trimester but cease during the second trimester. At 20 weeks, she appears well hydrated and has gained 4.5 kg (approximately 10 lb).

ASSESSMENT: Maria says she is often very tired during the day even though she is sleeping 8 to 10 hours at night. Fatigue concerns her because she is normally very energetic. Her job is demanding and requires that she concentrate and balance many factors at the same time.

NURSING DIAGNOSIS: Fatigue related to inadequate rest periods to accommodate the physiologic demands of pregnancy.

> *CRITICAL THINKING: What assumption has the nurse made? What other factors should be considered before this diagnosis is made?*
>
> *ANSWER: Although extraordinary fatigue is common in early pregnancy, nurses must not assume that pregnancy is the only cause. Additional data, such as hemoglobin and hematocrit levels, should be obtained before this diagnosis is made. Information about increasing iron-rich foods or iron supplementation may be necessary.*

GOALS/EXPECTED OUTCOMES: Maria will:
1. Identify methods to cope with fatigue, such as negotiating a flexible work schedule or time for short rest periods while continuing employment during pregnancy.
2. Report increased energy by the second trimester.

INTERVENTION	RATIONALE
1. Acknowledge the fatigue and reassure Maria that this is self-limiting and a common experience during the first months because of the change in hormone levels.	1. Reassurance helps alleviate the concern that fatigue indicates a problem with her pregnancy.
2. Recommend that she lie down or sit comfortably with her feet elevated for a few minutes every 2 hours and consciously relax the muscles of the legs, abdomen, and shoulders.	2. This position renews energy even when sleep is not possible.
3. Suggest that she try deep breathing and visualizing a favorite location or pastime whenever possible. Progressive relaxation—conscious tensing and relaxing of groups of muscles beginning with those in the feet and working upward toward the head—may be helpful.	3. These exercises relieve physical tension that adds to fatigue and also provide mental distraction.
4. Recommend that she get as much sleep as she feels she needs when possible. Adequate rest may involve curtailing social activities and tasks that can be postponed.	4. Although recreation is important, the need for sleep is overwhelming for some women during the first weeks of pregnancy.
5. Suggest she explore a flexible schedule or routine with her employer. Advise a short nap after work before beginning other activities at home.	5. Often a very short nap in the morning or afternoon is all that is needed to continue to function effectively.
6. Recommend that she enlist the assistance of family, a significant other, and friends with home responsibilities.	6. Assistance can free her of all but the most essential tasks during this time.
7. Explain that during the second trimester Maria will probably have more energy, but that it is normal to be tired again near the end of pregnancy.	7. Knowing the normal course of fatigue during pregnancy helps a woman to plan ahead for ways to cope with it.

> *CRITICAL THINKING: What additional interventions are necessary if the hemoglobin level and hematocrit are low?*
>
> *ANSWER: If low levels of hemoglobin and hematocrit indicate that the client is anemic, the physician or nurse-midwife should be notified so that iron supplementation can be started. The nurse should provide education about iron-containing foods.*

EVALUATION: Maria was able to negotiate two short rest periods each day and, at 12 weeks of gestation, continues to use learned techniques to renew energy. Maria relates increased energy at the third prenatal visit (16 weeks).

NURSING CARE PLAN 7-2 Self-Care during Pregnancy

ASSESSMENT: Paula Orne, a primigravida at 28 weeks of gestation, has numerous questions about self-care. She is a courier and drives many hours each day. She is concerned about safety while driving. She also asks what sexual activity is allowed, and she is worried because her partner continues to smoke.

NURSING DIAGNOSIS: Health-Seeking Behaviors: Prenatal care related to travel, sexual activity, and effects of passive smoking

GOALS/EXPECTED OUTCOMES: Paula will:
1. Describe measures to decrease discomfort and promote safety while traveling by the next visit
2. Continue mutually satisfactory sexual activity during pregnancy
3. Modify the environment to eliminate exposure to passive smoking by (specific date)

INTERVENTION	RATIONALE
1. Recommend that Paula use lap and shoulder seat belts throughout pregnancy. Suggest that she keep the lap restraint under the abdomen.	1. Use of restraints prevents ejection from the car in case of an accident. The most serious injuries are sustained when a person is ejected at impact.
2. Suggest that she stop the car at least every 2 hours to walk for a few minutes and perform some gentle shoulder and upper body stretches. She should also empty her bladder at each stop.	2. Frequent stops improve circulation and relieve the muscles involved in prolonged sitting and driving. Frequent voiding promotes comfort and prevents bladder infection resulting from stasis of urine.
3. Instruct her to drink a glass of water at each stop but to avoid sweet drinks and caffeinated beverages.	3. Sweet drinks increase thirst, and caffeine drinks act as diuretics and increase thirst. Water refreshes and prevents dehydration.
4. Determine Paula's specific concerns about sexuality and respond to those in particular.	4. Concerns vary among couples. Some couples worry about harming the fetus or causing discomfort for the mother.
5. Reassure her that sexual activity poses no harm to either the mother or the fetus in a normal pregnancy. Explain the anatomy of the vagina, cervix, and uterus. Suggest she bring her partner to the next visit if he has concerns.	5. Knowledge of the separation between the vagina and fetus may relieve concern about the safety of vaginal intercourse during pregnancy.
6. Suggest that alternative positions, such as side-lying, woman-superior, and rear-entry, be used during the third trimester.	6. The male-superior position becomes uncomfortable for the woman when the uterus is large and heavy, and it increases the risk of supine hypotension.
7. Discuss the danger of passive smoking, and recommend that the partner curtail or eliminate smoking in the house, car, and other enclosed areas. This limitation is important during pregnancy and also after the infant is born.	7. Toxins in cigarette smoke affect those in the vicinity as well as the one who is smoking.

EVALUATION: Paula uses both shoulder and lap restraints and says she feels more comfortable while driving. She relates mutually satisfying sexual experiences. Her partner agrees to curtail smoking inside the house and whenever he is out with Paula.

CRITICAL TO REMEMBER

Danger Signs of Pregnancy

- Vaginal bleeding with or without discomfort
- Rupture of membranes (escape of fluid from the vagina)
- Swelling of the fingers (woman notices rings becoming tight) or puffiness of the face or around the eyes
- Continuous pounding headache
- Visual disturbances (such as blurred vision, dimness, flashing lights, spots before the eyes)
- Persistent or severe abdominal or epigastric pain
- Chills or fever
- Painful urination
- Persistent vomiting
- Change in frequency or strength of fetal movements
- Signs of preterm labor: uterine contractions, cramps, constant or irregular low backache, pelvic pressure

Planning

Goals for this nursing diagnosis are that the expectant mother, the family, or both will:

- Explain practices that promote the safety and well-being of the mother and fetus throughout pregnancy
- Describe measures that provide relief from the common discomforts of pregnancy
- Describe a realistic plan during the first trimester to modify behaviors or habits that could adversely affect the health of the mother and fetus

Interventions

After the initial assessment the woman is usually not seen by the health care provider for 4 weeks. Instruct her and her family about signs and symptoms that indicate a serious danger and should be reported immediately ("Critical to Remember: Danger Signs of Pregnancy").

■ Although making the expectant mother aware of the danger signs of pregnancy is crucial, the nurse must take care not to overly worry her. Avoid the term *danger signs* when talking to the woman and her family, because it may be frightening. It is less alarming to say "The signs I am about to explain to you are unusual, but if you notice them, notify the health care provider at once because they require immediate attention."

TEACHING HEALTH BEHAVIORS

All teaching should be focused on the mother's immediate questions and concerns. These will vary over the course of the pregnancy and should be addressed at each visit. Common concerns are discussed here.

BATHING. Daily bathing protects pregnant women from infections that may develop if bacteria normally present on the skin are allowed to remain and multiply. Bathing also promotes comfort by dissipating heat produced by increased metabolism. Advise the woman to use nonskid pads in the tub or shower especially during the last trimester, when her balance is altered by a changing center of gravity and she is prone to falls.

HOT TUBS AND SAUNAS. Although warm baths and showers help relax tense and tired muscles, pregnant women should avoid activities that may cause hyperthermia. Maternal hyperthermia, particularly during the first trimester, may be associated with fetal anomalies. Caution the woman not to be in a sauna for more than 15 minutes or a hot tub for more than 10 minutes and to keep her head and chest out of the water (AAP & ACOG, 2002).

DOUCHING. Despite increased vaginal discharge, douching is unnecessary before, during, or after pregnancy. Some women douche because they believe it increases cleanliness and prevents infection. However, douching is associated with infections, preterm labor, and low birth weight. Cultural differences exist with regard to douching. For example, African-American women are more likely to douche than white women (Cottrell, 2003). Discuss women's reasons for douching and explain the detrimental effects.

BREAST CARE. Instruct the expectant mother to avoid using soap on her nipples because it removes the natural lubricant that forms on the nipples. Advise her to wear a bra that fits well and supports her breasts to prevent loss of muscle tone that can occur as the breasts become heavier during pregnancy. Wide bra straps distribute the weight evenly across the shoulders and provide greater comfort.

Inform the couple that breast stimulation, which increases oxytocin secretion and therefore may cause uterine contractions, is unsafe if the woman has a history of preterm labor or existing signs of preterm labor, such as rhythmic pelvic pressure or uterine contractions that assume a regular pattern or increase in frequency or intensity.

CLOTHING. Recommend practical, comfortable, and nonconstricting clothing. Tight jeans or panty hose, which may impede venous circulation, should be avoided or worn only for short periods. Low heels are best because they do not interfere with balance. High heels increase the curvature of the lower spine (lordosis) that is prevalent during the last trimester.

EXERCISE. Exercise during pregnancy is generally beneficial and can strengthen muscles, reduce backache, reduce stress, and provide a feeling of well-being. The amount and type of exercise recommended depend on the physical condition of the woman and the stage of pregnancy. Women who have no medical or obstetric complications should exercise in moderation each day for 30 minutes or more during pregnancy (ACOG, 2002).

Walking is an ideal exercise because it stimulates muscular activity, gently increases respiratory and cardiovascular effort, and does not result in fatigue or strain. Swimming and water exercises are excellent forms of exercise during pregnancy because the buoyancy of the water helps prevent injuries.

Recreational sports generally can be continued if no risk of falling or abdominal trauma exists. Activities such as step aerobics, contact sports, gymnastics, horseback riding, downhill skiing, or scuba diving should be postponed until after delivery.

Women should not begin strenuous exercise programs or intensify training during pregnancy. Those who have been exercising strenuously before pregnancy should consult the health care provider but may be able to continue much of their usual routine. As pregnancy progresses, the exercise program may need modification because the change in the woman's center of gravity makes her more prone to falls. Therefore an activity that is safe in the first trimester may not be safe in the third trimester.

Exercise in the supine position is unsafe, particularly after the first trimester, because it may cause decreased cardiac output and hypotension. Warm-up and cool-down periods with stretching exercises should be included in each exercise session. Emphasize the importance of taking liquids before, during, and after exercise to prevent dehydration.

Exercise should be tailored to the way the woman feels to avoid overfatigue. The health care provider may suggest she take her pulse periodically and not exceed a certain heart rate range. She should stop exercising and seek medical advice if she has chest pain, dizziness, headache, decreased fetal movement, or signs of labor while exercising.

SLEEP AND REST. Finding a comfortable position for rest becomes a problem in the third trimester. Pillows can be used to support the abdomen and back and provide the best opportunity for sleep (Figure 7-15). Emphasize that frequent rest periods are beneficial, even if the woman does not fall asleep. Suggest relaxation exercises to use during the day and before bed.

SEXUAL ACTIVITY. Sexual intercourse is generally safe for the healthy pregnant woman (see Chapter 8).

NUTRITION. A discussion of nutrition should be part of each visit. Assess the woman's diet and use of prenatal vitamins. Answer any questions she may have (see Chapter 9).

EMPLOYMENT. Most women of childbearing age in the United States are employed outside the home, and most continue to work during pregnancy. Whether the expectant

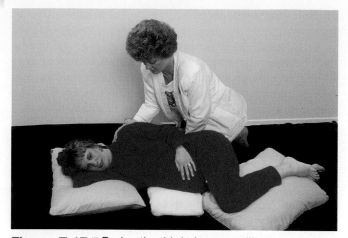

Figure 7-15 ■ During the third trimester, pillows supporting the abdomen and back provide a comfortable position for rest.

mother can or should work depends on the presence of environmental toxins and industrial hazards and the level of physical activity involved.

Maternal Safety. Work should not lead to undue fatigue. Frequent rest periods with the feet elevated are essential. Jobs that require constant standing or sitting are very tiring, and the pregnant woman should change positions often or walk briefly to stimulate circulation and reduce fatigue. Tasks that require balance may be hazardous because the center of gravity shifts as the uterus enlarges. Suggest curtailing these jobs during the last trimester. Heavy lifting should be avoided.

Working women often have many home responsibilities that, for some, do not decrease during pregnancy. The fatigue and stress of the home and employment workload may be difficult during pregnancy. Recommend that, if possible, the expectant mother adapt her home and employment workloads during pregnancy to reduce fatigue and stress.

Exposure to Teratogens. The problem of intrauterine exposure to toxic substances is of particular concern during the first trimester, which is the period of organogenesis. Advise clients to investigate their own occupational hazards. For example, hairdressers are exposed to toxic substances in hair dyes and aerosol sprays; painters may be exposed to benzene, lead, and toluene; nurses and hospital personnel may be exposed to radiation and anesthetic gases; and laundry and dry cleaning workers may be exposed to fetotoxic compounds. In addition, some women are exposed to smoke from other people's cigarettes (passive smoking) in the workplace. Passive smoking is known to be harmful to both mother and fetus.

TRAVEL. Although travel by car is generally safe, it may cause discomfort or fatigue. Frequent stops are necessary to allow the expectant mother to empty her bladder and walk. Instruct the woman to fasten the seat belt snugly with the lap belt below her abdomen and the shoulder belt in a diagonal position across her chest. This position is uncomfortable for some women, and it causes concern about internal injuries if a collision occurs. However, it is safer to wear the belt than to leave it off and risk ejection from the vehicle during an accident. In one large study, women who were in crashes were more likely to have a low-birth-weight infant, excessive maternal bleeding, or a fetal death if they did not wear a seat belt than if they were belted (Hyde, Cook, Olson, Weiss, & Dean 2003).

Travel by plane is generally safe, although some physicians discourage air travel after 36 weeks of gestation. If travel is necessary, advise the woman to walk frequently to maintain adequate peripheral circulation and avoid thromboembolism. Support stockings may also be helpful. The woman should not travel to remote locations where medical care is unavailable. Suggest she take a copy of her medical records if traveling a long distance.

IMMUNIZATIONS. In general, immunizations using live virus vaccines (such as measles, mumps, rubella, varicella, oral polio) are contraindicated during pregnancy because they may have teratogenic effects on the fetus. Inactivated vaccines are safe and can be used in women who have a risk of developing diseases such as tetanus, hepatitis A or B, and influenza (ACOG, 2003; Jones, 2002). The woman should be advised to divulge that she is pregnant before a vaccine is administered.

TEACHING ABOUT THE COMMON DISCOMFORTS OF PREGNANCY

Although pregnancy is a state of health, the numerous physiologic changes that occur during pregnancy often cause physical discomforts for which medical care does not exist. Relief depends on self-help measures that informed nurses are expected to teach. (See Figures 7-13 to 7-15 and "Women Want to Know: How to Overcome the Common Discomforts of Pregnancy.")

TEACHING NECESSARY LIFESTYLE CHANGES

Many expectant parents are willing to make changes in lifestyle to avoid adversely affecting the fetus. Discuss the use of substances that may be harmful during pregnancy.

PRESCRIPTION AND OVER-THE-COUNTER DRUGS. Advise pregnant women to consult with their health care providers before taking any drugs. This precaution is important for both over-the-counter and prescription drugs. Explain that information is inadequate with regard to safe use of some medications during pregnancy. When prescription drugs are necessary, the health care provider weighs the risks against the benefits to decide if a drug can safely be used or if changes are necessary. Advise the woman that over-the-counter drugs such as acetaminophen are considered safe, but she should not take more than 4 g per day (Weiner & Buhimschi, 2004). Acetaminophen is an ingredient in many other over-the-counter preparations, and women should read the labels carefully. Some nonsteroidal antiinflammatory drugs such as aspirin should be avoided because they may increase bleeding.

TOBACCO. An important aspect of prenatal care is assessment and intervention for smoking. In 2003 11% of women reported that they smoked during their pregnancies. Pregnant women who smoke have an increased risk for low-birth-weight infants, intrauterine growth restriction, increased infant mortality, preterm labor, spontaneous abortions, and placental dysfunction (Albrecht et al., 2004; Arias, Hamilton, Martin, & Sutton, 2004). These problems can be greatly reduced if the woman stops smoking, preferably before conception. However, even if smoking is stopped during pregnancy, it will help reduce complications.

Smoking tobacco affects fetal development for several reasons:

- Nicotine causes vasoconstriction of vessels in the placenta.
- Carbon monoxide, which is released in tobacco smoke, inactivates maternal and fetal hemoglobin, which are essential to transport oxygen to the fetus.
- Maternal appetite is decreased, causing a lower intake of calories.
- Plasma volume, needed to transport nutrients and oxygen to the fetus, is decreased.

The U.S. Public Health Service (Fiore et al., 2000) recommends the "5A" approach to smoking cessation; the five As are ask, advise, assess, assist, and arrange.

1. *Ask* the woman at each visit if she smokes, if there have been changes in the amount of smoking, and if she would like to quit. Pregnancy is a time when women are motivated to make changes that will benefit their health and that of the fetus.
2. *Advise* the woman about the importance of not smoking.
3. *Assess* the woman's willingness to try to stop smoking. Discuss motivational information if the woman is not willing to quit at this time. Refer the woman to a smoking cessation program if she is willing to try to stop smoking.
4. *Assist* the woman in making a plan to stop smoking, and provide practical counseling on how to solve the problems she may encounter—for example, avoidance of others who smoke and activities she associates with smoking may be helpful. Generally the use of drugs and nicotine replacement products is discouraged, because their effect during pregnancy is unknown.
5. *Arrange* follow-up contact in person or by telephone to discuss the woman's progress and any problems that may have occurred and to offer encouragement.

The 5A approach is also part of the evidence-based project of the Association for Women's Health, Obstetric and Neonatal Nurses to reduce smoking (Albrecht et al., 2004). See Chapters 9 and 24 for more information about smoking and pregnancy.

ALCOHOL. Alcohol is a known teratogen, and maternal alcohol use is a leading cause of mental retardation in the United States. Alcohol produces a characteristic cluster of developmental anomalies known as *fetal alcohol syndrome.* Children with fetal alcohol syndrome exhibit a typical pattern of prenatal and postnatal growth restriction with characteristic facial, cardiovascular, and limb defects (see Figure 24-3). Affected children also exhibit cognitive and fine-motor dysfunctions that are tragic and irreversible.

Conclusive data about fetal effects of social or moderate drinking are not available, but no amount of alcohol consumed is known to be safe. Therefore the best advice for women who are pregnant or who plan to become pregnant is to abstain from all alcohol (see Chapter 24).

ILLEGAL DRUGS. Use of so-called *street drugs* or *recreational drugs* such as cocaine, heroin, and methamphetamines is harmful to the fetus. Advise the pregnant woman to seek help to discontinue all illicit drug use (see Chapters 24 and 30).

COMPLEMENTARY AND ALTERNATIVE THERAPIES. Some complementary and alternative therapies are very safe and helpful during pregnancy. Some, however, can be harmful. For example, herbs such as black or blue cohash, juniper, rosemary, and raspberry tea may cause contractions if used in pregnancy (March of Dimes, 2004). Ask if the woman uses any of these and advise her to discuss them with her health care provider.

Evaluation

Interventions can be considered to effectively meet the established outcomes if the mother and her family (1) discuss and practice self-care measures taught them to promote safety and health of the mother and fetus, (2) explain methods to help relieve common discomforts of pregnancy, and (3) identify a plan early in pregnancy to modify habits that could adversely affect health, such as curtailing the use of alcohol or tobacco. If interventions are ineffective, the nurse collaborates with the family to define new plans and work out additional interventions.

ANTEPARTUM HOME CARE NURSING

Economic constraints in health care often limit or prevent antepartum nursing care for clients in the home setting. Home visits for women who have no complications are not common in the United States. Women with specific high-risk conditions who can be cared for in the home setting may receive home visits to help them manage intravenous fluids or other aspects of care.

SUMMARY CONCEPTS

- Pregnancy causes a predictable pattern of uterine growth. In general the uterus can be palpated halfway between the symphysis and the umbilicus at 16 weeks of gestation, at the level of the umbilicus at 20 weeks, and at the xiphoid process by 36 weeks.
- Thick mucus fills the softened connective tissue in the cervical canal and protects the fetus from infection caused by bacteria ascending from the vagina.
- Plasma volume expands faster and to a greater extent than red blood cells, resulting in a dilution of hematocrit concentration. This condition is referred to as *physiologic anemia (pseudoanemia)* because it does not reflect an inadequate number of red blood cells.
- Blood flow alters during pregnancy to include the uteroplacental unit. Increased renal plasma flow results in increased glomerular filtration rate, which effectively removes additional metabolic wastes produced by the mother and the fetus but often results in "spilling" of glucose and other nu-

trients in the urine. Increased blood flow to the skin attempts to reduce the additional heat generated by the fetus and the increased maternal metabolic rate.

- Although blood volume increases, blood pressure is not elevated during pregnancy.
- The gravid uterus partially occludes the vena cava and aorta when the mother is supine. The occlusion causes supine hypotensive syndrome, which can be prevented or corrected when she assumes a lateral position.
- During the last trimester the uterus pushes the diaphragm upward, decreasing lung capacity. To compensate, the ribs flare, the substernal angle widens, and the circumference of the chest increases.
- Estrogen and hCG are associated with nausea in early pregnancy. Morning sickness will not harm the fetus and usually ends by the second trimester.
- Increased progesterone is associated with relaxation of smooth muscles, including those of the ureters, bladder, and bowel. Resulting stasis of urine, rich in nutrients, increases the risk of urinary tract infections.
- Alterations in hormones are also responsible for cutaneous changes such as hyperpigmentation.
- The expanding uterus and the hormone relaxin result in progressive changes that can lead to muscle strain and backache during the last trimester.
- Progesterone maintains the uterine lining for implantation of the blastocyst, prevents uterine contractions during pregnancy, and helps prepare the breasts for lactation.
- Presumptive and probable signs of pregnancy may be caused by conditions other than pregnancy and therefore cannot be considered positive or diagnostic signs. Positive signs can have no other cause.
- A complete history and physical examination are necessary at the initial antepartum visit to determine the potential risks to the mother and fetus and obtain baseline data for a plan of care.
- Assessment for risk of problems is performed at each prenatal visit because pregnancies considered low risk in early pregnancy may later become high risk.
- Multifetal pregnancies impose greater physiologic changes than a single-fetus pregnancy and require extra vigilance to detect possible complications.
- Families need information related to self-care, health promotion, and coping with the common discomforts of pregnancy.
- Nurses must use the nursing process and critical thinking skills to assist the parents to make necessary changes in lifestyle.

ANSWERS TO CRITICAL THINKING EXERCISE 7-1, p. 131

1. If pregnant now, Wilma is gravida 3, para 1 (the twin birth counts as one parous experience). If the acronym GTPAL is used, more complete information about Wilma is: G = 3, T = 1, P = 0 (no preterm infants), A = 1 (one pregnancy ended before 20 weeks of gestation), L = 2 (living twins).
2. Amenorrhea and nausea and vomiting are only presumptive (subjective) indications of pregnancy because they can be caused by conditions other than pregnancy.
3. Count back 3 months to March 22, and add 7 days. This brings the date to March 29. Add 1 to the current year.

REFERENCES & READINGS

Albrecht, S.A. (2004). Achieving "success": Nursing care for pregnant women who smoke. *AWHONN Lifelines, 4*(1), 23-27.
Albrecht, S.A., Maloni, J.A., Thomas, K.K., Jones, R., Halleran, J., & Osborne, J. (2004). Smoking cessation counseling for pregnancy women who smoke: Scientific basis for practice for AWHONN's SUCCESS project. *Journal of Obstetric, Gynecologic & Neonatal Nursing, 33*(3), 298-305.
American Academy of Pediatrics (AAP) & American College of Obstetricians and Gynecologists (ACOG). (2002). *Guidelines for perinatal care* (5th ed.). Elk Grove Village, IL: Author.
American College of Obstetricians and Gynecologists (ACOG). (2002). ACOG committee opinion number 267: Exercise during pregnancy and the postnatal period. *Obstetrics & Gynecology, 99*(1), 171-173.
American College of Obstetricians and Gynecologists (ACOG). (2003). ACOG committee opinion number 282: Immunization during pregnancy. *Obstetrics & Gynecology, 101*, 207-212.
American College of Obstetricians and Gynecologists (ACOG). (2004). Nausea and vomiting of pregnancy, ACOG practice bulletin #52. ACOG: *Obstetrics & Gynecology, 103*, 803-815.
American Diabetes Association. (2004). Position statement: Gestational diabetes mellitus. *Diabetes Care, 27*(Suppl 1), S88-S90.
Arias, E., MacDorman, M.F., Strobino, D.M., & Guyer, B. (2003). Annual summary of vital statistics–2002. *Pediatrics, 112*(6), 1215-1230.
Association of Women's Health, Obstetric and Neonatal Nurses (AWHONN). (2003). *Standards and guidelines for professional nursing practice in the care of women and newborns* (5th ed.). Washington, DC: Author.
Barron, M.L. (2001). Antenatal care. In K.R. Simpson & P.A. Creehan, *AWHONN perinatal nursing* (2nd ed, pp. 125-160). Philadelphia: Lippincott.
Blackburn, S.T. (2003). *Maternal, fetal, and neonatal physiology* (2nd ed.). Philadelphia: Saunders.
Bond, L. (2004). Physiology of pregnancy. In Mattson, S., & Smith, J.E. (Eds.), *Core curriculum for maternal-newborn nursing* (3rd ed., pp. 96-123). Philadelphia: Saunders.
Briggs, G.G., Freeman, R.K., & Sumner, J.Y. (2002). *Drugs in pregnancy and lactation* (6th ed.). Baltimore: Williams & Wilkins.
Buster, J.E., & Carson, S.A. (2002). Endocrinology and diagnosis of pregnancy. In S.G. Gabbe, J.R. Niebyl, & J.L. Simpson (Eds.), *Obstetrics, normal and problem pregnancies* (4th ed., pp. 3-36). New York: Churchill Livingstone.
Carr, C.A. (2003). Use of a maternity support binder for relief in pregnancy-related back pain. *Journal of Obstetric, Gynecologic, & Neonatal Nursing, 32*(4),495-502.
Carsten, M.E., & Lu, M.C. Endocrinology of pregnancy and parturition. In N.F. Hacker, J.G. Moore, & J.C. Gambone, *Essentials of obstetrics and gynecology* (4th ed., pp. 57-64). Philadelphia: Saunders.
Centers for Disease Control and Prevention (CDC). (2001). Notice to readers: Revised ACIP recommendation for avoiding pregnancy after receiving a rubella-containing vaccine. *MMWR. Morbidity and Mortality Weekly Report, 50*(49), 1117.
Centers for Disease Control and Prevention. (2004). Varicella vaccine–Frequently asked questions related to pregnancy. Retrieved June 17, 2004, from http://www.cdc.gov/nip/vaccine/varicella/faqs-clinic-vac-preg.htm.
Cottrell, B.H. (2003). Vaginal douching. *Journal of Obstetric, Gynecologic, and Neonatal Nursing, 32*(1), 12-18.
Cunningham, F.G., Leveno, K.J., Bloom, S.L., Hauth, J.C., Gilstrap, L.C., & Wenstrom, K.D. (2005). *Williams obstetrics* (22nd ed.). New York: McGraw-Hill.
Fiore, M.C., Bailey, W.C., Cohen, S.J., & the Guideline Panel. (2000). *Treating tobacco use and dependence (Clinical Practice Guide-*

line). Rockville, MD: U.S. Department of Health and Human Services, Public Health Service.

Glover, D.D., Amonkar, M., Rybeck, B.F., & Tracy, T.S. (2003). Prescription, over-the-counter, and herbal medicine use in a rural, obstetric population. *American Journal of Obstetrics & Gynecology, 188,* 1039-1045.

Gordon, M.C. (2002). Maternal physiology in pregnancy. In S.G. Gabbe, J.R. Niebyl, & J.L. Simpson (Eds.), *Obstetrics, normal and problem pregnancies* (4th ed., pp. 63-91). New York: Churchill Livingstone.

Hamilton, B.E., Martin, J.A., & Sutton, P.D. (2004). Births: Preliminary data for 2003, National vital statistics reports 53(9). Hyattsville, MD: National Center for Health Statistics.

Hobbins, D. (2001). *Preconception care: Maximizing the health of women and their newborns.* Washington, DC: AWHONN.

Hujoel, P.P., Bollen, A., Noonan, C.J., & delAguila, M.A. (2004). Antepartum dental radiography and infant low birth weight. *Journal of the American Medical Association, 291*(16), 1987-1993.

Hyde, L.K., Cook, L.J., Olson, L.M., Weiss, H.B., & Dean, J.M. (2003). Effect of motor vehicle crashes on adverse fetal outcomes. *Obstetrics & Gynecology, 102*(2), 279-286.

Johnson, T.R.B., & Niebyl, J.R. (2002). Preconception and prenatal care: Part of the continuum. In S.G. Gabbe, J.R. Niebyl, & J.L. Simpson (Eds.), *Obstetrics, normal and problem pregnancies* (4th ed., pp. 139-159). New York: Churchill Livingstone.

Jones, T.B. (2002). Vaccines in pregnancy. In S.B. Ransom, M.P. Dombrowski, M.I. Evans, & K.A. Ginsburg (Eds.), *Contemporary therapy in obstetrics and gynecology* (pp. 57-64). Philadelphia: Saunders.

Katz, V.L. (2003). Prenatal care. In J.R. Scott, R.S. Gibbs, B.Y. Karlan, & A.F. Haney (Eds.), *Danforth's obstetrics and gynecology* (9th ed., pp. 1-33). Philadelphia: Lippincott Williams & Wilkins.

Koos, B.J., Nuwayhid, B.S., & Moore, J.G. (2004). Maternal physiologic and immunologic adaptation to pregnancy. In N.F. Hacker, J.G. Moore, & J.C. Gambone, *Essentials of obstetrics and gynecology* (4th ed., pp. 65-82). Philadelphia: Saunders.

Kronenberg, F., Murphy, P.A., & Wade, C. (2003). Select populations: Women. In J.W. Spencer & J.J. Jacobs, *Complementary and alternative medicine: An evidence-based approach* (2nd ed., pp. 458-481). St. Louis: Mosby.

Liu, J.H. (2004). Endocrinology of pregnancy. In R.K. Creasy & R. Resnik, *Maternal-fetal medicine: Principles and practice* (5th ed., pp. 121-134). Philadelphia: Saunders.

Lu, M.C., & Hobel, C.J. (2004). Antepartum care: Preconception and prenatal care, genetic evaluation and teratology, and antenatal fetal assessment. In N.F Hacker, J.G. Moore, & J.C. Gambone, *Essentials of obstetrics and gynecology* (4th ed., pp. 83-104). Philadelphia: Saunders.

Luppi, C.J. (2001). Physiologic changes of pregnancy. In K.R. Simpson & P.A. Creehan, *AWHONN perinatal nursing* (2nd ed, pp. 96-114). Philadelphia: Lippincott.

Magee, L.A., Mazzota, P., & Korne, G. (2002). Evidence-based view of safety and effectiveness of pharmacologic therapy for nausea and vomiting of pregnancy. *American Journal of Obstetrics & Gynecology, 186*(5), S256-S261.

Maloni, J.A., Albrecht, S.A., Thomas, K.K., Halleran, J., & Jones, R. (2003). Implementing evidence-based practice: Reducing risk for low birth weight through pregnancy smoking cessation. *Journal of Obstetric, Gynecologic, & Neonatal Nursing, 32*(5), 676-682.

March of Dimes. (2004). Herbal supplements: their safety, a concern for health care providers. Retrieved July 14, 2004, from www.marchofdimes.com/professionals/681_1815.asp.

Matteson, P.S. (2001). *Women's health during the childbearing years: A community-based approach.* St. Louis: Mosby.

Mills, L.W., & Moses, D.T. (2002). Oral health during pregnancy. *MCN: American Journal of Maternal/Child Nursing, 27*(5), 275-280.

Monga, M. (2004). Cardiovascular and renal adaptation to pregnancy. In R.K. Creasy & R. Resnik, *Maternal-fetal medicine: Principles and practice* (5th ed., pp. 111-120). Philadelphia: Saunders.

Moore, T.R. (2004). Diabetes in pregnancy. In R.K. Creasy & R. Resnik, *Maternal-fetal medicine: Principles and practice* (5th ed., pp. 1023-1061). Philadelphia: Saunders.

Moos, M. (2003). *Preconception health promotion: A focus for women's wellness.* White Plains, NY: March of Dimes Birth Defects Foundation.

National Center for Health Statistics. (2004). Healthy People 2010 Progress Reviews Retrieved November 6, 2004, from http://healthypeople.gov.

Parker, K.M., & Smith, S.A. (2003). Aquatic-aerobic exercise as a means of stress reduction during pregnancy. *Journal of Perinatal Education, 12*(1), 6-17.

Pivarnik, J.M., & Rivera, J.M. (2002). Exercise in pregnancy. In S.B. Ransom, M.P. Dombrowski, M.I. Evans, & K.A. Ginsburg (Eds.), *Contemporary therapy in obstetrics and gynecology* (pp. 85-89). Philadelphia: Saunders.

Rapini, R.P. (2004). The skin and pregnancy. In R.K. Creasy & R. Resnik, *Maternal-fetal medicine: Principles and practice* (5th ed., pp. 1201-1211). Philadelphia: Saunders.

Repke, J.T. (2002). Medication use during pregnancy. In S.B. Ransom, M.P. Dombrowski, M.I. Evans, & K.A. Ginsburg (Eds.), *Contemporary therapy in obstetrics and gynecology* (pp. 137-141). Philadelphia: Saunders.

Rosen, T., deVeciana, M., Miller, H.S., Stewart, L., Rebarber, A., & Stotnick, R.N. (2003). A randomized controlled trial of nerve stimulation for relief of nausea and vomiting in pregnancy. *Obstetrics & Gynecology, 102*(1), 129-135.

Shabert, J.K. (2004). Nutrition during pregnancy and lactation. In L.K. Mahan & S. Escott-Stump, *Krause's food, nutrition, and diet therapy* (11th ed., pp. 182-213). Philadelphia: Saunders.

Sherman, P.W., & Flaxman, S.M. (2002). Nausea and vomiting in an evolutionary perspective. *American Journal of Obstetrics & Gynecology, 186*(5), S190-S195.

Smith, C., Crowther, C., Wilson, K., Hotham, N., & McMillian, V. (2004). A randomized controlled trial of ginger to treat nausea and vomiting in pregnancy. *Obstetrics & Gynecology, 103*(4), 639-645.

Spellacy, C.E. (2001). Urinary incontinence in pregnancy and the puerperium. *Journal of Obstetric, Gynecologic, and Neonatal Nursing, 3*(6), 634-641.

Speroff, L., & Darnery, P.D. (2001). *A clinical guide for contraception* (3rd ed.). Philadelphia: Lippincott Williams & Wilkins.

Steele, N.M., French, J., Gatherer-Boyles, J., Newman, S., & Leclaire, S. (2001). Effect of acupressure by Sea-Bands on nausea and vomiting of pregnancy. *Journal of Obstetric, Gynecologic, and Neonatal Nursing, 30*(1), 61-70.

Tillett, J., Kostich, J.M., VandeVusse, L. (2003). Use of over-the-counter medications during pregnancy. *Journal of Perinatal and Neonatal Nursing, 17*(1), 3-18.

Tiran, D. (2002). Nausea and vomiting in pregnancy: safety and efficacy of self-administered complementary therapies. *Complementary Therapies in Nursing & Midwifery, 8,* 191-196.

U.S. Department of Health and Human Services. (2000). *Healthy people 2010* (Conference ed. in 2 volumes). Washington, DC: Author.

Watson-Blasioli, J. (2001). Doubletake–Defining the need for specialized prenatal care for women expecting twins: A Canadian perspective. *AWHONN Lifelines, 5*(2), 34-42.

Weiner, C.P. & Buhimschi, C. (2004). *Drugs for pregnant and lactating women.* Philadelphia: Churchill Livingstone.

Whitty, J.E., & Dombrowski, M.P. (2004). Respiratory diseases in pregnancy. In R.K. Creasy & R. Resnik, *Maternal-fetal medicine: Principles and practice* (5th ed., pp. 953-974). Philadelphia: Saunders.

Williams, S.R. (2003). Nutrition during pregnancy and lactation. In S.R. Williams and E.D. Schlenker, *Essentials of nutrition and diet therapy* (5th ed., pp. 269-292). St. Louis: Mosby.

Psychosocial Adaptations to Pregnancy

OBJECTIVES

After studying this chapter, you should be able to:

1. Describe the psychological responses of the expectant mother to pregnancy.
2. Identify the process of role transition.
3. Explain the maternal tasks of pregnancy.
4. Describe the developmental processes that a man completes to make the transition to the role of father.
5. Describe the responses of prospective grandparents and siblings to pregnancy.
6. Discuss factors that influence psychosocial adaptation to pregnancy, such as age, parity, absence of a partner, social support, abnormal situations, and socioeconomic status.
7. Describe the ways in which these factors affect nursing practice.
8. Describe cultural influences on pregnancy and cultural assessment and negotiation.

Go to your Student CD-ROM for Review Questions keyed to these Objectives.

DEFINITIONS

Ambivalence Simultaneous conflicting emotions, attitudes, ideas, or wishes.

Attachment Development of strong affectional ties as a result of interaction between an infant and a significant other (such as mother, father, sibling, caretaker).

Body Image Subjective image of one's own physical appearance and capabilities; derived from one's own observations and the evaluation of significant others.

Bonding Development of a strong emotional tie of a parent to a newborn; also called *claiming*, or *binding in*.

Couvade Pregnancy-related rituals or a cluster of symptoms experienced by some prospective fathers during pregnancy and childbirth.

Developmental Task A step in growth and maturation that one must complete before additional growth and maturation are possible.

Disturbance in Body Image Negative feelings about the characteristics, functions, or limitations of one's body.

Fantasy Mental images formed to prepare for the birth of a child.

Introversion Inward concentration on the self and body.

Mimicry Copying the behaviors of other pregnant women or mothers as a method of "trying on" the role of advanced pregnancy or motherhood.

Narcissism Undue preoccupation with oneself.

Role Transition Changing from one pattern of behavior and one image of self to another.

Becoming a parent who is capable of loving and caring for a totally dependent infant is more than a biologic event. The process begins before conception and involves major changes in the expectant mother, her partner, and the entire family. Although each couple adapts to pregnancy in a unique way, the psychological responses of prospective parents change as the pregnancy progresses. Although the initial reaction may be uncertainty, by the time the infant is born, the woman and her partner have completed developmental tasks that allow them to become parents in the true sense of the word. Both social and cultural factors influence their adjustment to pregnancy.

MATERNAL PSYCHOLOGICAL RESPONSES

A woman's psychological response to pregnancy changes with time. Initially she may be uncertain or ambivalent about the pregnancy, and her primary focus is on herself. Gradually her focus shifts, and she becomes increasingly concerned about protecting and providing for the fetus.

First Trimester

UNCERTAINTY

During the early weeks the woman is unsure if she is pregnant and tries to confirm it. She observes her body carefully for changes indicating pregnancy. She may confer with family and friends about the probability and may use an over-the-counter pregnancy test kit for validation.

Reaction to the uncertainty of pregnancy depends on the individual. A woman may be eager to find confirming signs, or she may dread the possibility and hope for signs indicating she is not pregnant. Usually she seeks confirmation from a physician, certified nurse-midwife, or nurse practitioner during the first trimester of pregnancy.

AMBIVALENCE

Because almost half of pregnancies are unintended, pregnancy is often unexpected. Once the pregnancy is confirmed, most women have conflicting feelings, or ambivalence, about being pregnant. Some feel that this is not the right time, even if the pregnancy is wanted and planned. Women who had planned to become pregnant often say they thought it would take longer for the pregnancy to become a reality and feel unprepared for it. Many pregnancies are desired but unplanned, and these women may wish they had completed some specific plan or goal before becoming pregnant.

Pregnancy causes permanent life changes for the woman, and she often begins to examine expected changes and how she will cope with them. If it is her first pregnancy, the woman may worry about the added responsibility and feel unsure of her ability to be a good parent. She may be apprehensive about how this pregnancy will affect her relationship with her other children and her partner. Ambivalence has usually changed to acceptance by the second trimester.

THE SELF AS PRIMARY FOCUS

Throughout the first trimester the woman's primary focus is on herself, not the fetus. Early physical responses to pregnancy, such as nausea and fatigue, confirm that something is happening to her, but the concept of the fetus seems vague and unreal. Because she has not gained weight to confirm a growing, developing fetus, she probably thinks more about being pregnant than about the coming baby.

Physical changes and increased hormone levels may cause emotional lability (unstable moods). Her mood can change quickly from contentment to irritation or from optimistic planning to an overwhelming sleepiness. This may be confusing to her partner and her family, who are accustomed to more stability.

Nurses should concentrate on the mother's physical and psychological needs during this period of maternal self-focus. Teaching should be aimed at the common early changes of pregnancy and their normality. Coping with morning sickness, sexuality, and mood swings are important subjects to explore with the couple. The nurse should assess how they are managing these changes and explain that these changes are normal and generally do not indicate problems.

Second Trimester

PHYSICAL EVIDENCE OF PREGNANCY

During the second trimester, physical changes occur in the expectant mother that make the fetus "real." The uterus grows rapidly and can be palpated in the abdomen, weight increases, and breast changes are obvious. Ultrasound examination allows her to see the fetus, and she may receive an ultrasound picture or video to share with her family. Quickening, the feeling of fetal movement, occurs during this time. This experience is important because it confirms the presence of the fetus with each movement. As a result, she no longer thinks of the fetus as simply a part of her body but now perceives it as separate although entirely dependent on her (Figure 8-1).

THE FETUS AS PRIMARY FOCUS

The fetus becomes the woman's major focus during the second trimester. The discomforts of the first trimester have usually decreased, and her size does not alter her activity. She is now concerned about producing a healthy infant. She is often interested in information about diet and fetal development. A feeling of creative energy and satisfaction is common.

NARCISSISM AND INTROVERSION

At this time, many women become increasingly concerned about their ability to protect and provide for the fetus. This concern is often manifested as narcissism and introversion. Selecting exactly the right foods to eat or the right clothes to wear may assume more importance than before. Some women lose interest in their jobs, which may seem alien compared with the events taking place inside them. Some

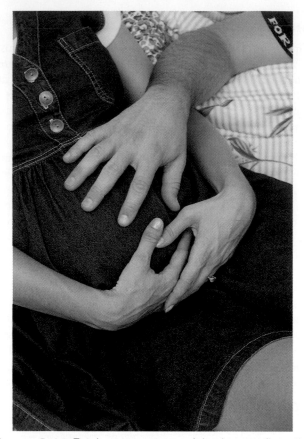

Figure 8-1 ■ Fetal movement, or quickening, confirms that a separate life is developing.

women may focus on the pregnancy and become less interested in current events, or they may become fearful that world events threaten them and therefore present a danger to the fetus.

If this is her first pregnancy, the woman wonders about the infant. She looks at baby pictures of herself and her partner and may want to hear stories about what they were like as infants. Although multiparas know more about infants in general, they are interested in this infant and concerned with this child's acceptance by siblings and grandparents. Expectant mothers may also examine their relationships with others and how they will change after the birth.

The woman often spends much time thinking about the fetus and daydreaming about what life will be like when it is born. She may call it by the name chosen for the baby and talk about the personality of the fetus. Some mothers enjoy reading about fetal development to see what changes are happening each week. This intense introspection may be confusing to her partner and family because it is so different from her usual behavior.

BODY IMAGE

Rapid and profound changes take place in the body during the second trimester. Changes in body size and contour are obvious with bulging of the abdomen, thickening of the waist, and enlargement of the breasts. The changes may be welcomed because they signify growth of the fetus and give the woman and her partner a feeling of pride. For some

women, however, the change in body size and shape, coupled with hyperpigmentation of the skin and striae gravidarum, may contribute to a negative body image. In addition, changes in body function such as altered balance, reduced physical endurance, and discomfort in the pelvis and lower back areas may also affect her image (Nursing Care Plan 8-1).

CHANGES IN SEXUALITY

The sexual interest and activity of pregnant women and their partners are unpredictable and may increase, decline, or remain unchanged. The woman's physical comfort and sense of well being are closely linked to her interest in sexual activity. The culture of the couple is also important. Intercourse during pregnancy is allowed and encouraged in some cultures but strictly forbidden in others. Unless complications exist, intercourse is safe throughout pregnancy.

During the first trimester, freedom from the worry of becoming pregnant or the need for contraception may provide a sense of freedom and enhance sexual interest for both partners. However, physical complaints such as nausea, fatigue, and breast tenderness may interfere with erotic feelings. Fear of miscarriage may cause couples to avoid intercourse, particularly if the woman has previously lost a pregnancy. Nurses can help reassure the couple that no evidence shows intercourse to be related to early pregnancy loss when no other complications are present.

In the second trimester, women experience increased sensitivity of the labia and clitoris and increased vaginal lubrication as a result of pelvic vasocongestion. Nausea is no longer a concern by this time for most women, and many have a general feeling of well-being and energy that may increase sexual responsiveness. Orgasm may occur more frequently and with greater intensity during pregnancy because of these changes. Although orgasm causes temporary uterine contractions, they are not harmful if the pregnancy has been normal.

During the third trimester the "missionary position" (male on top) may cause discomfort because of abdominal pressure. Heartburn, indigestion, and supine hypotensive syndrome also increase in this position. The pressure of the fetus low in the pelvis may add to discomfort. Moreover, fatigue, ligament pain, urinary frequency, and shortness of breath may be problems.

The nurse can suggest alternative positions such as female-superior, side-lying, or rear-entry for intercourse. The side-lying position may be the most comfortable and require the least amount of energy during the third trimester. Hugging, cuddling, kissing, and mutual massage or masturbation are other ways to express affection without vaginal intercourse.

As they become larger, some women believe their bodies are ugly and may worry about their partners' reactions to their increased size. Sexual response varies widely among men. Some men report heightened feelings of sexual interest, but others perceive the woman's body in late pregnancy as unattractive, and erotic feelings decrease. In addition, fear of harming the fetus or causing discomfort during pregnancy may interfere with sexual activity.

NURSING CARE PLAN 8-1 Body Image During Pregnancy

ASSESSMENT: Dolores White is a 34-year-old primigravida in the twenty-sixth week of pregnancy. Both she and her husband have been runners for several years. With her physician's permission Dolores continued running until 6 weeks ago and reports that she no longer runs because she finds it uncomfortable. She says she now walks "like other old ladies." Dolores verbalizes concern about the brown discoloration on her face and her increasing size and says she feels "fat, awkward, and ugly." She states, "I hate the way I look! I can't wait to get back into shape."

NURSING DIAGNOSIS: Disturbed Body Image related to changes in body size, contour, and function secondary to pregnancy

GOALS/EXPECTED OUTCOMES: By the end of her next prenatal visit Dolores will:
1. Make statements that indicate acceptance of expected body changes during her pregnancy.
2. Express her feelings about body changes to her husband and the health care team.
3. Set realistic goals for weight loss and the resumption of a running program after childbirth.

INTERVENTION	RATIONALE
1. Acknowledge Dolores' feelings. "I can see you're disappointed at not being able to run and concerned about how your body has changed as a result of pregnancy."	1. Feelings must be acknowledged, reflected, and dealt with before the underlying cause can be addressed.
2. Clarify her concerns. "You've always been an athlete. Women often wonder if changes in pregnancy will affect them permanently."	2. An underlying unvoiced concern may be that pregnancy will change the woman from an athlete to a mother who won't be able to continue athletics. This altered perception of herself causes fear, grief, or both.
3. Suggest that she share her feelings with her husband and seek his support. Model this interaction if necessary: "I feel awkward and left out of a big part of our lives. I need some reassurance from you now."	3. Although the woman may assume the partner observes and understands when negative feelings exist, this may not be true.
4. Discuss types of low-impact, moderate exercise, such as walking or swimming, that would be beneficial for Dolores.	4. Moderate daily exercise is permissible and encouraged during uncomplicated pregnancy.
5. Explain the expected pattern of weight gain from 26 weeks to full term and correlate this with the growth and development of the fetus.	5. Understanding that weight gain indicates the fetus is growing and knowledge of the expected weight gain may allay unexpressed fears of excessive weight gain.

6. Help Dolores make realistic plans to lose weight and recover her strength and endurance after childbirth.
  a. Discuss the expected pattern of weight loss after childbirth: an initial weight loss of 4.5 to 5.5 kg (10 to 12 lb). An additional 2.3 to 3.6 kg (5 to 8 lb) may be lost in the first few postpartum days. Many women return to near their prepregnancy weight within 6 to 12 months.
  b. Demonstrate graduated exercises that increase muscle tone and strength.
  c. Explain the purpose of adipose tissue gained during pregnancy and discuss a diet that meets her needs for breastfeeding.
	6. Adipose tissue provides a needed source of energy during birth and lactation. Many women are relieved to know that the adipose tissue has a purpose and that the added weight will be lost gradually. Breastfeeding requires additional calories.

7. Explain that the discoloration on her face is normal and should go away after pregnancy. Suggest she stay out of the sun and use sunscreen.	7. Melasma is normal in pregnancy. Avoiding exposure to the sun and using sunscreen may help decrease the severity.

EVALUATION: Dolores begins to speak with pride about how big the baby is growing and makes other statements showing more acceptance of body changes. She reports that her husband shows increased concern about her feelings and has been very supportive since she shared her feelings with him. Dolores has explored other types of exercises and has found several she will use during the rest of her pregnancy. She begins to plan a realistic schedule of diet and exercise for after the birth.

Despite the need for information, many women are reluctant to initiate a discussion about sexual activity. Unfortunately, most health professionals do not introduce the topic. They may fear offending the client or may be uncomfortable with their own sexuality and embarrassed to begin a discussion. They often lack time for any but the most pressing assessments. The result may be that an important aspect of care is ignored.

■ A broad opening statement may help initiate discussion about sexual activity—for example, "Sometimes couples are concerned about having sex during pregnancy." Such statements introduce the subject in a way that lets the woman feel comfortable pursuing it or letting it drop.

The couple should be made aware of the normal changes in sexual desire that occur during pregnancy and the importance of communicating their feelings openly with each other to find solutions to problems. The nurse can reassure the couple that their feelings are normal.

Many health care providers advise couples to avoid all sexual activity if the woman has a high risk for preterm labor. Although it is not proved, some believe that uterine contractions leading to labor might be initiated by nipple stimulation, orgasm, or semen. Bleeding, an incompetent cervix, and the rupture of membranes are other contraindications for intercourse. In addition, blowing into the vagina should be avoided at any time because it can cause an air embolus (Coverston, 2004).

Third Trimester

VULNERABILITY

The sense of well-being and contentment that dominates the second trimester gives way to increasing feelings of vulnerability that peak during the seventh month. Pregnant women often feel that the precious baby may be lost or harmed if not protected at all times (Figure 8-2). Many expectant mothers have fantasies or nightmares about having a deformed baby or harm coming to the infant and become very cautious as a result. They may avoid crowds because they feel unable to protect the infant from infectious diseases or potential physical dangers. They need reassurance

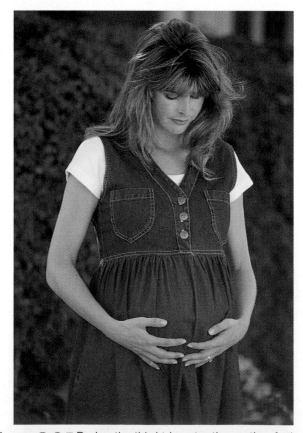

Figure 8-2 ■ During the third trimester the mother feels increasingly vulnerable. She cradles her fetus to signify her protectiveness.

that such dreams and fears are not unusual in pregnancy (Ramer & Frank, 2001).

INCREASING DEPENDENCE

The expectant mother often becomes increasingly dependent on her partner in the last weeks of pregnancy. She may insist that he be easy to reach at all times and may call him several times during the day just to be sure that he is available. Women often have fears about the safety of the partner and that something will happen to him. Her need for love and attention from her partner is even more pronounced in late pregnancy. She needs to be certain of his support and availability. When she is assured of his concern and willingness to provide assistance, she feels more secure and able to cope. She may rely on her partner and others more at this time and seek their help in making decisions. This may be frustrating if it is a marked change for her.

Although the woman may not be able to explain the increasing dependence, she expects her partner to understand the feeling and may become angry if he is not sympathetic. Irritability may increase because of her fatigue at this time, as well. The nurse can encourage couples to discuss fears and feelings openly so that misunderstandings can be avoided.

Some pregnant women have difficulty with tasks that require direct, sustained attention, particularly in the third trimester. Women may feel they have trouble concentrating or focusing on learning new material or skills at this time (Stark, 2000). Teaching should be clear and concise to help women learn most easily.

PREPARATION FOR BIRTH

Gradually the feelings of vulnerability decrease as the woman comes to terms with her situation. The fetus continues to grow, and fetal movements are no longer gentle. Pokes, jabs, and kicks are intrusive expressions of the baby's crowded condition and increasing activity. The woman's relationship with the fetus changes as she acknowledges that although she and the fetus are interrelated, the baby is a pervasive presence and not a part of herself. Although she may not consciously acknowledge the increasing feelings of separateness, she longs to see the baby and become acquainted with her child.

Most pregnant women are concerned with their ability to determine when they are in labor. They review the signs of labor and question friends and family members who are parents. Many couples are anxious about getting to the hospital or clinic in time for the birth, and they may be worried about coping with labor.

During the last few weeks the woman becomes increasingly concerned with her due date and the experience of labor and delivery. Some women fear labor and dread the due date, whereas others are so uncomfortable that they look forward to that day, expecting it to be the exact day the birth will occur. They often say they are tired of being pregnant and want the pregnancy to be over.

Women pregnant for the first time are more likely to fear childbirth than multiparas. Many women fear the pain of

TABLE 8-1 Progressive Changes in Maternal Responses to Pregnancy

First Trimester	Second Trimester	Third Trimester
Emotional Response		
Uncertainty, ambivalence, focus on self	Wonder, increased narcissism, introversion, concern about changes in her body and sexuality	Vulnerability, increased dependence, acceptance that fetus is separate but totally dependent
Physical Validation		
No obvious signs of fetal growth	Quickening, enlarging abdomen	Obvious fetal growth, discomfort, decreased maternal activity
Role		
May begin to seek safe passage for self and fetus	Seeks acceptance of fetus and her role as mother	Prepares for birth
"Self-Statement"		
"I am pregnant."	"I am going to have a baby."	"I am going to be a mother."

childbirth or that something will go wrong during labor (Melender, 2002a). If a previous pregnancy or birth experience was difficult, worry during the current pregnancy will be increased. Women may seek help for their fears by talking to members of their support system or by seeking information from health professionals, books, or television or on the Internet.

During the third trimester an expectant mother prepares for the infant, if that is appropriate in her culture. "Nesting" behavior includes obtaining and arranging a place for the infant to sleep. Negotiation of changes in how she and her partner will share household tasks are among the plans made at this time. In addition, many couples complete childbirth education classes at this time (see Chapter 11). Table 8-1 summarizes changes in maternal responses in pregnancy.

CHECK YOUR READING

1. Why might an expectant mother say "I am pregnant" during the first trimester and "I am going to be a mother" late in pregnancy?
2. How might pregnancy affect sexual responses of the mother and father?

MATERNAL ROLE TRANSITION

Becoming a mother involves more than giving birth and providing physical care for the newborn. Mothering also involves intense feelings of love, tenderness, and devotion that endure over a lifetime. How does a woman learn to be a mother?

The transition into mothering begins during pregnancy and increases with gestational age. Some aspects of this transition must be accomplished before the woman moves on to the next part of the process. She must accept the pregnancy and the changes that will result. She must develop a relationship with the unborn child, first as part of herself and then as a separate individual. Near the end of preg-

nancy she must prepare herself for the birth and for parenting the new baby (Ramer & Frank, 2001).

Transitions Experienced throughout Pregnancy

The woman undergoes transitions in relationships that continue throughout the pregnancy. She becomes more aware of herself and the changes occurring in her life. Alterations occur in her relationship with the father as they both prepare for parenthood. Her relationship with her own mother is examined and may change as the expectant mother develops a view of herself as a mother and what that role entails. In addition, she must develop a relationship with this particular child (Ramer & Frank, 2001).

Steps in Maternal Role Taking

Rubin (1984) observed specific steps that provide a framework for understanding the process of maternal role taking: mimicry, role play, fantasy, the search for a role fit, and grief work.

MIMICRY

Mimicry involves observing and copying the behavior of other women who are pregnant or mothers in an attempt to discover the characteristics of the role. Mimicry often begins in the first trimester, when the woman may wear maternity clothes before they are needed to understand the feelings of women in more advanced pregnancy and see how others react to her. She may also mimic the waddling gait or posture of a woman who is close to delivery long before these changes are necessary for her.

ROLE PLAY

Role play consists of acting out some aspect of what mothers actually do. The pregnant woman searches for opportunities to hold or give care to infants in the presence of another person. She does this to evaluate not only her comfort in the situation but also the response of the observer. Role playing gives her an opportunity to "practice" the expected role and receive validation from an observer that she has functioned well. She is particularly sensitive to the responses of her partner and her own mother.

FANTASY

Fantasies allow the woman to consider a variety of possibilities and daydream or "try on" a variety of behaviors. Fantasies often revolve around how the infant looks and what characteristics the infant will have. The woman may daydream about taking her child to the park or holding, reading to, or playing music for the child. She may also have vivid dreams at night.

At times, fantasies are fearful. What happens if something is wrong with the infant? What if the baby cries and will not stop? Fearful fantasies often provoke a pregnant woman to respond to the fears by seeking information or reassurance. For instance, she may ask her partner if he will love the baby even if it is not perfect, or she may strive to learn all she can about caring for a baby that is difficult to console.

Fantasies may change during each trimester and may be different for primigravidas and multigravidas. Women have the most frequent fantasies during the third trimester. Listening to women's fantasies helps the nurse show the woman acceptance and understanding. In addition, it provides a means of identifying potential concerns that may need further discussion.

THE SEARCH FOR A ROLE FIT

The search for a role fit is a process that occurs once the woman has built up a set of role expectations for herself and internalized a view of the behavior of a "good" mother. She then observes the behaviors of mothers and compares them with her own expectations of herself. She imagines herself acting in the same way and either rejects or accepts the behaviors, depending on how well they fit her idea of what is right. This process implies that the woman has explored the role of mother long enough to have developed a sense of herself in the role and to be able to select behaviors that reaffirm her idea of how she will fulfill the role.

GRIEF WORK

Although grief work seems incongruous with maternal role taking, women often experience a sense of sadness when they realize that they must give up certain aspects of their previous selves and can never go back. A mother will never again be a carefree woman who has not had a child. She must relinquish some of her old patterns of behavior to be able to move into the new identity as mother of an infant. Even simple things such as going shopping or to the movies will require planning to include the infant or find alternative care. Changes may be particularly difficult for the adolescent mother, who is unused to planning ahead and may have to give up or change school plans as well.

Maternal Tasks of Pregnancy

To become mothers, pregnant women spend a great deal of time and energy learning new behaviors. As the woman works to establish a relationship with the infant, she must also reorder her relationship with her partner and family.

This psychological work of pregnancy has been grouped into four maternal tasks of pregnancy: (1) seeking safe passage for herself and baby through pregnancy, labor, and childbirth; (2) securing acceptance of the baby and herself from her partner and family; (3) learning to give of herself; and (4) developing attachment and interconnection with the unknown child (Rubin, 1984).

SEEKING SAFE PASSAGE

Seeking safe passage for herself and her baby is the woman's priority task. If she cannot be assured of that safety, she cannot move on to the other tasks. Behaviors that ensure safe passage include seeking the care of a health care provider and following recommendations about diet, vitamins, rest, and subsequent visits to the office or clinic.

In addition to following the advice of health care professionals, the pregnant woman must adhere to cultural practices that ensure the safety of herself and the infant. For instance, a Hmong woman may avoid raising her arms above her head because she believes it may cause preterm labor; she does not cut her hair during pregnancy, as it might harm the fetus (Lee, 2003).

SECURING ACCEPTANCE

Securing acceptance is a process that begins in the first trimester and continues throughout pregnancy. The process involves reworking relationships so that the important persons in the family accept the woman in the role of mother and welcome the baby into the family constellation.

If this is a first pregnancy, the woman and the father of the baby must give up an exclusive relationship and make a place in their lives for a child. The woman feels valued and comforted when her partner expresses pride and joy in each pregnancy. This feeling is so important that many women retain a memory of the partner's reaction to the announcement of pregnancy for many years. Women with supportive partners are more likely to report the pregnancy is wanted (Kroelinger & Oths, 2000).

Support and acceptance from her own mother is especially important. The pregnant woman gains energy and contentment when her mother freely offers acceptance and support. Many expectant mothers gain a sense of increased closeness with their mothers during pregnancy (Figure 8-3). Previous conflicts may be resolved at this time (Matteson, 2001).

Problems may occur if the family strongly desires a child with particular characteristics and the woman believes that the family may reject an infant who does not meet the criteria. For example, if family members wish for a boy, will they accept a girl? Unconditional acceptance of the infant by the woman and her family is an important accomplishment by the third trimester (Coverston, 2004).

LEARNING TO GIVE OF HERSELF

Giving is one of the most idealized components of motherhood, but one that is essential. Learning to give to the coming infant begins in pregnancy when the woman allows her

special, exclusive relationship develops between the woman and fetus that simulates a secret, romantic love.

Mothers report feedback from their unborn infants during the third trimester and describe unique characteristics of the fetus with regard to sleep-wake cycles, temperament, and communication. Love of the infant becomes possessive and leads to feelings of vulnerability. The woman integrates the role of mother into her image of herself. She becomes comfortable with the idea of herself as mother and finds pleasure in contemplating the new role (Mercer & Ferketich, 1994).

✔ CHECK YOUR READING

3. What does "looking for a fit" mean in role transition?
4. Why is grief work part of maternal role transition?
5. How does the pregnant woman seek safe passage for herself and the baby?

PATERNAL ADAPTATION

Expectant fathers do not experience the biologic processes of pregnancy, but they also must make major psychosocial changes to adapt to a new role. These changes may be more difficult because the male partner is often neglected by both the health care team and his peer group when attention is focused on the woman. His concern and anxieties may remain unknown because of the lack of focus on him.

Variations in Paternal Adaptation

Wide variations exist in paternal responses to pregnancy. Some men are emotionally invested and comfortable as full partners and wish to explore every aspect of pregnancy, childbirth, and parenting. Others are more task oriented and view themselves as managers. They may direct the woman's diet and rest periods and act as coaches during childbirth but remain detached from the emotional aspects of the experience. Other men are more comfortable as observers and prefer not to participate. In some cultures men are conditioned to see pregnancy and childbirth as "women's work" and may not be able to express their true feelings about pregnancy and fatherhood.

Readiness for fatherhood is more likely in the presence of a stable relationship between the partners, financial security, and a desire for parenthood. Additional factors include the man's relationship with his own father, his previous experience with children, and his confidence in his ability to care for the infant.

Unplanned pregnancy is more likely to cause distress for fathers-to-be, as might be expected. Distress is also more likely in younger fathers and those whose relationship with the mother has lasted less than 2 years (Buist, Morse, & Durkin, 2003). In addition, coping with the expectant mother's emotional lability can be confusing and difficult.

Fathers have many concerns during a pregnancy. These include anxiety about the health of the mother and the

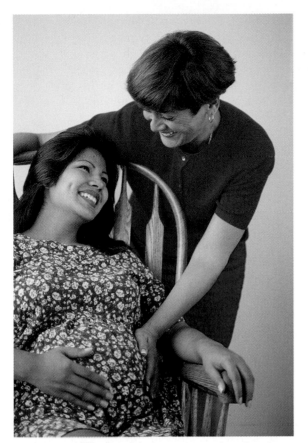

Figure 8-3 ■ The bond between a pregnant woman and her own mother is particularly important to the young mother.

body to give space and nurturing to the fetus. This involves considering the benefits and costs of motherhood in terms of the effect on her lifestyle. She also observes giving in others and then tests her own ability to derive pleasure from giving. This test often takes the form of providing food or care for her family, but also includes acts of thoughtfulness. The acceptance and enjoyment of the "gift" by the receivers enhance her pleasure and strengthen the role. She may explore further by giving small gifts to friends, especially those who are pregnant, and she feels pride and delight when the gift is appreciated.

Pregnant women also learn to give by receiving. Gifts received at "baby showers" are more than needed items. They also confirm continued interest and commitment from friends and family and enhance the ability of the woman to give. Intangible gifts from others, such as companionship, attention, and support, help increase her energy and affirm the importance of giving.

COMMITTING HERSELF TO THE UNKNOWN CHILD

The process of attachment begins in early pregnancy when the woman accepts or "binds in" to the idea that she is pregnant, even though the baby is not yet real to her. During the second trimester the baby becomes real when quickening occurs, and feelings of love and attachment surge. A baby, financial concerns, and worry about his role during the birth and about the changes that will result from the birth of the baby. Financial concerns may be especially acute in a two-income family if the mother develops complications that prevent her from working as long as expected. A reduction in income coupled with an increase in expenses can result in added stress for both parents. Fathers with only part-time employment are likely to have the added distress of worry about the costs of the pregnancy. Men with full-time employment may seek a second job or work overtime to prepare for the increased financial needs.

Other concerns common to expectant fathers include the responsibility parenthood will bring and whether he and his partner will be good parents. They also worry about how the mother will cope with staying at home after the baby is born and whether the mother will be lonely or bored, a concern shared by expectant mothers (Matthey et al., 2002).

Developmental Processes

The responses of the expectant father are dynamic, progressing through phases that are subject to individual variation. Jordan (1990) describes three developmental processes that an expectant father must address:

- Grappling with the reality of pregnancy and the new child
- Struggling for recognition as a parent from his family and social network
- Making an effort to be seen as relevant to childbearing

THE REALITY OF PREGNANCY AND THE CHILD

The pregnancy and the child must become real before a man can take on the identity of father. The process requires time and is often incomplete until the birth. Initially, the pregnancy is a diagnosis only, and changes in the expectant woman's behavior, such as nausea and fatigue, are perceived as symptoms of illness that have little to do with having a baby.

A man's initial reaction to the announcement of pregnancy may be pride and joy, but he often experiences the same ambivalence as his partner, particularly if he is unprepared for the added responsibility or commitment. Various experiences act as catalysts or "reality boosters" that make the child more real (Figure 8-4). The most frequently mentioned experiences are hearing the baby's heartbeat, feeling the infant move, and seeing the fetus on a sonogram.

Preparing the nursery or a space in the home and accumulating supplies for the new addition also reinforce the reality of the forthcoming child. These tasks often represent the first time that the expectant father has the opportunity to do something directly for the child. The birth itself is the most powerful reality booster, and the infant becomes real to the father when he has an opportunity to see and hold the infant.

THE STRUGGLE FOR RECOGNITION AS A PARENT

Men are often viewed by others as helpmates but not parents in their own right. During pregnancy and childbirth, their primary responsibility is to support their partners.

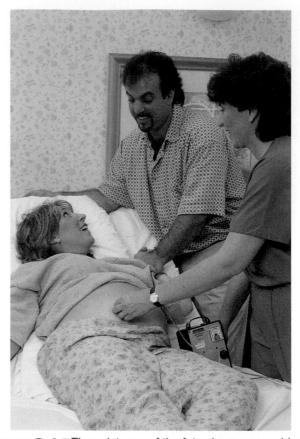

Figure 8-4 ■ The existence of the fetus becomes real (a reality booster) for the father when he hears the fetal heartbeat through the transducer.

Some men may be upset that their feelings are seldom validated and that they may not be recognized as parents as well as helpers. Many men accept that the focus should be on their partners, but others are frustrated by the lack of understanding of their own experiences.

Support groups or classes for expectant fathers are sometimes available. These groups allow a father-to-be to talk with other men about changes resulting from the pregnancy and how these changes have affected them. Knowing his experiences and feelings are shared by other men in the same situation is very helpful.

Expectant mothers play an important role in helping their partners gain recognition as parents. Women who openly share their physical sensations and emotions help expectant fathers feel that they are part of the process. These women often refer to it as "our" pregnancy and "our" baby rather than as "my" pregnancy or "my" baby. They also insist on including their partners in all discussions and decisions.

Nurses must learn to view the mother, father, and child as the client and not focus exclusively on the mother and fetus. Men may be concerned about the physical symptoms experienced by expectant mothers. The nurse should encourage men to ask questions about their partners' pregnancies. These men are entitled to as much advice and reassurance as expectant women (Figure 8-5).

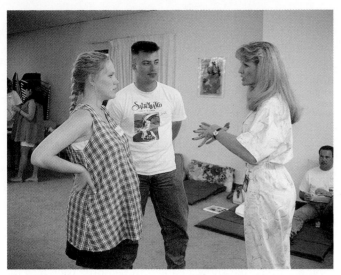

Figure 8-5 ■ The nurse who views the mother, father, and child as one client provides parents with the greatest opportunity to learn infant care and parenting skills.

The nurse can also guide the couple in discussion of the role the father will play during and after the birth. How actively will he participate during labor? Will he be involved in infant care from the start, or will he wait until the baby is older? Will he change diapers and help with nighttime care, or does he see those tasks as belonging to the mother? The expectant parents may be surprised to learn each other's views and will need to negotiate, taking the beliefs of each partner into consideration to determine the roles each will play.

THE ROLE OF THE INVOLVED FATHER

Men use various means to create a parenting role that is comfortable for them. They may seek closer ties with their own fathers to reminisce about their own childhoods. They may fantasize about their relationships with their children as they grow up. Some men change their self-images and even their appearances to fit their new images (Coverston, 2004).

Expectant fathers also observe men who are already fathers and "try on" fathering behaviors to determine whether they are comfortable and fit their own concepts of the father role. In addition, many men assertively seek information about infant care and growth and development so that they will be prepared for their new responsibilities.

PARENTING INFORMATION. Expectant fathers may not receive enough information on parenting for them to be ready to care for their infants after birth. Although adequate information may have been given to them, fathers may not be ready to learn the information at the time it is provided. As a result, they may be unprepared to care for their infants and have unrealistic expectations of the newborn. Nurses must review information about infant care and growth and development after the infant is born when the knowledge is immediately relevant.

COUVADE. The term *couvade* refers to pregnancy-related symptoms and behavior in expectant fathers. In primitive cultures, couvade took the form of rituals involving special dress, confinement, limitations of physical work, avoidance of certain foods, sexual restraint, and in some instances, performance of "mock labor."

In modern practice, expectant fathers sometimes experience physical symptoms similar to those experienced by pregnant women, such as loss of appetite, nausea and vomiting, headache, fatigue, and weight gain. Symptoms are more likely to occur in early pregnancy and lessen as the pregnancy progresses. They may be caused by stress, anxiety, or empathy for the pregnant partner. They are usually harmless but may persist and result in nervousness, insomnia, restlessness, and irritability. Although the symptoms are almost always unobserved by the health care team, anticipatory guidance is beneficial for both partners.

✔ CHECK YOUR READING

6. What are reality boosters? Why are they important for the expectant father's adjustment?
7. How can nurses help men in their struggle for recognition as parents?
8. Why should information relating to newborn care presented in prenatal classes be repeated after the infant is born?

ADAPTATION OF GRANDPARENTS

The initial reaction of grandparents depends on several factors such as their ages, the number and spacing of other grandchildren, and their perceptions of the role of grandparents.

Age

Age is a major determining factor in the emotional responses of prospective grandparents. By the time they become grandparents, many people have already dealt with their feelings about aging and react with joy when they find they are to become grandparents. They look forward to being able to love grandchildren, who signify the continuity of life and family.

Younger grandparents may not be happy with the stereotype of grandparents as old persons. They may experience conflict when they must resolve their self-image with the stereotype. They often have career responsibilities and may not be accessible because of the continuing demands of their own lives.

Number and Spacing of Other Grandchildren

The number and spacing of other grandchildren also determine grandparents' reactions. A first grandchild may be an exciting event that creates great joy. If the grandparents have other grandchildren, another may be welcomed, but the excitement is often less than for the first grandchild. The subdued reaction may be disappointing to the couple, who may desire the same excited reaction as that expressed for the first grandchild.

Perceptions of the Role of Grandparents

Grandparents' beliefs about their importance to grandchildren vary widely. Many grandparents see their relationships with grandchildren as second in importance only to the parent-child relationship. They want to be involved in the pregnancy, and grandmothers often engage in rituals such as shopping and gift-giving showers that confirm their role as important participants. Many grandparents are intimately involved in child care and offer unconditional love to the child. They offer to care for older children while the mother gives birth, and they assist during the first weeks after childbirth.

In the past, grandparents were often looked to for advice about childbearing and child rearing. Health care personnel have now become the "experts," and many grandparents have difficulty adjusting to this change. If the issue is not recognized, distance may develop as the grandparents withdraw, sensing that their participation is no longer valued. Other grandparents worry about their lack of familiarity with modern ways of childbearing and parenting. Special classes are often available to teach them about current childbearing practices.

On the other hand, some contemporary grandparents plan little participation in pregnancy or child care. A frequently heard comment is "I've raised my children, and I don't plan to do it again." This attitude often results in conflict with the parents, who are hurt and wish for the grandparents' help during the third trimester and after the birth.

Nurses can assist families to verbalize their feelings about the grandparents' responses to the pregnancy. Statements such as "It may seem that the grandparents aren't interested in the baby, but perhaps they are uneasy about what their role should be." Parents and grandparents may need to negotiate ways in which the grandparents can be involved without feeling that they must assume more care of the child than they desire. For instance, the couple may need suggestions to help the grandparents participate in family gatherings that do not involve baby-sitting or child care (see Chapter 18). Letting grandparents know that the parents want them to share in the joy the child brings without other expectations may ease the situation.

ADAPTATION OF SIBLINGS

Sibling adaptation to the birth of an infant depends largely on age and developmental level.

Toddlers

Very young children (2 years or younger) are unaware of the maternal changes occurring during pregnancy and are unable to understand that a new brother or sister is going to be born. Because toddlers have little perception of time, many parents delay telling them that a baby is expected until shortly before the birth.

Although preparing very young children for the birth of a baby is difficult, the nurse can make suggestions that may prove helpful. Any changes in sleeping arrangements should be made several weeks before the birth so that the child does not feel displaced by the new baby. Parents can prepare family and friends for the toddler's feelings of jealousy and resentment when the young child must share time and attention with a baby.

Until children feel secure in the affection of their parents, expecting 2-year-olds to welcome a new "stranger" is not realistic. Frequent reassurances of parental love and affection are of primary importance. The parents can be taught to accept strong feelings that the toddler may express, such as anger, jealousy, and frustration, without judgment and to continue to reinforce the child's feelings of being loved (see Chapter 18).

Older Children

Children from 3 to 12 are more aware of changes in the mother's body that show a baby is to be born. They may be interested in observing the mother's abdomen, feeling the fetus move, and listening to the heartbeat. They may have questions about how the fetus develops, the way it started, and how it will get out of the abdomen. Although they look forward to the baby's arrival, younger children may expect the infant to be a full-fledged playmate and may be shocked and disappointed when the infant is small and helpless. They need preparation for the fact that the mother will go away for several days when the baby is born.

School-age children are often told about the pregnancy during the second trimester and benefit from being included in preparations for the new baby. They enjoy following the development of the fetus, preparing space for the infant to sleep, and helping to accumulate supplies the infant will need. The children should be encouraged to feel the fetus move, and many come close to the mother's abdomen and talk to the fetus. School-age children may wonder how the birth will affect their role in the family. Parents should address these concerns and reassure the children on their continued importance. Providing time alone with the parents may help them gain a sense of security (Figure 8-6). Reading books about other children's experiences after the birth of a sibling may be helpful.

Children as young as 3 years can benefit from sibling classes. They are encouraged to bring a doll to simulate caring for the infant. The classes also provide an opportunity for them to discuss what newborns are like and what changes the new baby will bring to the family (see Chapter 11).

In some settings siblings are permitted to be with the mother during childbirth. If young children are to be present, they should attend a class that prepares them for the event. During the birth a familiar person who has no other role but to support and care for siblings should be available to explain what is taking place and to comfort or remove them if events become overwhelming.

Adolescents

The response of adolescents also depends on their developmental level. Some are embarrassed because the pregnancy confirms the continued sexuality of their parents. They may

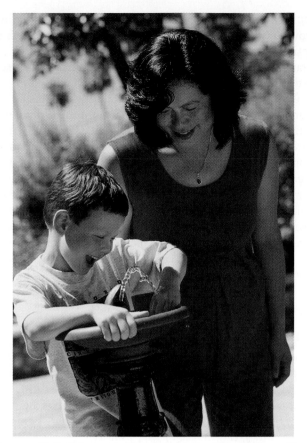

Figure 8-6 ■ A pregnant woman who spends time with an older child can provide affection and a sense of security.

be repelled by the obvious physical changes. Many adolescents are immersed in their own developmental tasks involving loosening ties to their parents and coming to terms with their own sexuality. They may be indifferent to the pregnancy unless it directly affects them or their activities. Other adolescents become very involved and want to help with preparations for the baby.

✔ **CHECK YOUR READING**

9. What determines the response of grandparents to the pregnancy?
10. How does the response to pregnancy differ for a toddler, a preschool child, and an adolescent?
11. How can parents prepare siblings for the addition of a newborn to the family?

FACTORS INFLUENCING PSYCHOSOCIAL ADAPTATIONS

Age

Pregnancy presents a challenge for teenagers who, as expectant parents, must cope with the conflicting developmental tasks of pregnancy and adolescence at the same time. The major developmental task of adolescence is to form and become comfortable with a sense of self. On the other hand,

one of the major tasks of pregnancy involves learning to "give of self," a process that includes sacrificing personal desires for the benefit of the fetus.

Nurses who work with pregnant teenagers should help them adjust to their changing bodies and the increasing presence of the developing fetus. Adolescents also need prompting to follow a lifestyle that promotes the best outcomes for them and their infants. Concerns relating to the pregnant adolescent and the woman over age 35 years are discussed further in Chapter 24.

Multiparity

The assumption that a multipara needs less help than a first-time mother is inaccurate. Pregnancy tasks are often more complex for the multipara than for the primigravida. When dealing with the task of negotiating safe passage for herself and the infant, the multipara does not have time to take special care of herself as she did during the first pregnancy. She is more likely to experience fatigue and may have serious worries about her other children accepting the infant and about finding time and energy for additional responsibilities. When seeking acceptance of the new baby, the multipara may find the family less excited than they were for the first child. The couple's celebration is also more subdued.

The woman spends a great deal of time working out a new relationship with the first child, who often becomes demanding. This behavior may foster feelings of guilt as she tries to expand her love to include the second child. Developing attachment for the coming baby is hampered by feelings of loss between herself and the first child. She senses that the child is growing up and away from her, and she may grieve for the loss of their special relationship.

Nurses must remember that some multiparas may need more help and understanding than primigravidas. The nurse cannot assume that the process is "old hat" and that information about labor, breastfeeding, and infant care is not needed. Special assistance may be necessary to help a multipara integrate an additional infant into the family structure.

CRITICAL THINKING ⚲**EXERCISE 8-1**

Emma Hastings, a 24-year-old gravida 2, para 1 of 32 weeks' gestation, appears apathetic and tired when she arrives at the prenatal clinic. She states that she is concerned about whether her 2-year-old son will accept the new baby and sometimes feels guilty that she is having this baby so soon.

Sara Nguyen, age 28, also has a prenatal visit. She is in her twenty-eighth week of pregnancy and has children who are 2, 4, and 6 years old.

Questions
1. How will the concerns of these multiparas likely differ from those of a primigravida?
2. How might the tasks of pregnancy differ between the two women?
3. What measures can each mother take to prepare other children before the new baby arrives?

Absence of a Partner

Single pregnant women may have special concerns. Although some unmarried women have the financial and emotional support of a partner, many do not. These women may experience more stress about telling their family and friends about the pregnancy. They may have to enlist more social support to substitute for that of a partner. Legal issues such as whom to list as the father on birth records and what arrangements must be made to allow paternal contact with the infant may be added concerns.

Single women without partners often live below the poverty level. They are more likely to delay prenatal care until the second or third trimester and are at increased risk for pregnancy complications and delivery of a low-birth-weight infant.

Nurses must recognize the single mother's needs for accessible and affordable prenatal care. In addition, nurses must be prepared to offer specialized supportive care for single mothers. Necessary social services may include Medicaid; the Special Supplemental Nutrition Program for Women, Infants, and Children (WIC) for food vouchers; and transportation to the prenatal clinic.

Some women are single by choice. They may have been inseminated to achieve pregnancy or may choose not to continue the relationship with the father. If the pregnancy was planned, these women may have fewer financial concerns.

Social Support

The presence of support persons in their lives is an important determinant in the woman's adaptation to pregnancy (Coverston, 2004). Social support includes that from the woman's partner, family, friends, and co-workers. Generally, support from the woman's partner and her mother are par-

ticularly important. Benefits of social support include improved coping, compliance with health care regimens, satisfaction with intimate relationships, and attachment to the infant. Reduced physical symptoms and increased breastfeeding are other effects (Logsdon, 2000).

Women who have little support during pregnancy are more likely to begin prenatal care late and to be depressed during and after pregnancy (Webster et al., 2000). When social support is inadequate the nurse can help the woman explore potential sources such as support groups, childbearing education classes, church, work, or school. In some situations nurses can provide social support during the pregnancy by telephone. This takes little time but can be very valuable to women who need extra support during pregnancy (Bullock, Browning, & Geden, 2002). Some community programs employ paraprofessionals to visit expectant mothers to provide teaching and social support when they do not have other means of social support (Logsdon & Davis, 2004).

Abnormal Situations

Other factors that influence psychosocial adaptation during pregnancy include abnormal situations such as abuse (discussed in Chapter 24) and depression (discussed in Chapter 28). All women should be screened for both of these risk factors during pregnancy so that appropriate referrals for help can be given.

Socioeconomic Status

One of the greatest influences on childbearing practices is the socioeconomic status of the family (Table 8-2). The term *socioeconomic status* refers to the resources of the family to meet the needs for food, shelter, and health care. Socioeconomic status can be divided into the categories of affluent, middle class, working poor, and new poor.

TABLE 8-2 Impact of Socioeconomic Factors on the Family's Response to Pregnancy

Affluent	Middle Class	Working Poor and Unemployed	New Poor
Resources			
Is confident of ability, has financial reserves to protect from economic fluctuations, owns or rents home in a safe neighborhood, has health insurance or can pay for health care, is able to provide enriched environment	Has relative security but fewer reserves and more debt, owns or rents home in relatively safe neighborhood, depends on employment for health insurance	Lacks skills and bargaining power, is most vulnerable to economic fluctuations, struggles to meet basic needs	Was previously self-sufficient but has lost prior resources; may have recently lost job and insurance; unused to public assistance
Value Placed on Health Care			
Values preventive care	Values health care but must rely on health insurance related to employment	May value health care but often does not see a way to improve situation	Values health care but may no longer have finances to access it
Time Orientation			
Is future-oriented and seeks prenatal care early; expects best possible care and education for children	Is future oriented and seeks early prenatal care; makes plans to provide best possible care and education for children	Priority is to meet needs of present; often seeks prenatal care late; uncertain future	Has middle-class time orientation but must meet present needs; may begin prenatal care late

THE AFFLUENT

Affluent families have resources to provide for their needs and purchase health care. They have a good income, secure shelter in a safe neighborhood, and the education and reserves to protect themselves from economic fluctuations. They are able to provide an enriched environment for children, and they can pay for health care through either private means or insurance.

The affluent family's attitudes toward health care reflect their ability to pay. They believe they deserve the best in health care and respect from health care providers, and they expect to be active participants in their care. They are future oriented and therefore value preventive care. In general, they seek early, regular antepartum care and comply with recommendations of the health care providers.

THE MIDDLE CLASS

The middle class constitutes the largest group of families in the United States. In fact, most health care workers fit into this class. Although these families do not have the reserves of the affluent, they usually are able to rent or own homes in relatively safe neighborhoods. They have adequate food and either education or skills that assist them to obtain and keep jobs for long periods. They often share child care with family and neighbors and develop a network of people who rely on one another for support and assistance.

Middle-class families rely on group insurance, obtained as part of their salaries, to shield themselves from exorbitant health care costs. A major concern is loss of a job that results in loss of health insurance.

These families are future oriented and seek health care early in pregnancy. They prepare for the birth and make plans to provide for their children's security and education.

THE WORKING POOR AND UNEMPLOYED

The working poor and unemployed include unskilled or unemployed workers who live with a great deal of uncertainty. They work for low wages and are often the last hired and the first fired. They frequently live below the poverty level and have barely enough to survive. Some have difficulty meeting the basic needs for food and shelter, and some become homeless families. They have few financial resources, and their limited skills give them little bargaining power.

Attitudes related to health care differ from those of the more affluent (Nursing Care Plan 8-2). Because of economic uncertainty, they place more emphasis on meeting present needs than on attaining future goals. As a result, they place less value on preventive (future-oriented) care. This often causes them to postpone prenatal care until the second or even the third trimester.

THE NEW POOR

The new poor constitute an expanding group of individuals and families who were previously self-sufficient but are now without resources because of such circumstances as loss of a job or health care insurance. These people must find their way into a health care system that is unfamiliar and frightening.

The values of the new poor are those of the middle class: self-sufficiency, hard work, and pride in the ability to succeed. Seeking public assistance is very difficult for this group. These families are devastated when they encounter the lack of respect and the rudeness that may occur when some health care workers interact with families unable to pay for health care.

BARRIERS TO PRENATAL CARE

Women's access to prenatal care is limited by financial, systemic, and attitudinal barriers. Financial barriers are among the most important factors limiting prenatal care. Many women have either no insurance or insufficient insurance to cover maternity care. Although Medicaid finances prenatal care for indigent women, the enrollment process is burdensome and lengthy. Some women do not register because they do not know how to access this resource.

Systemic barriers include negative institutional practices that interfere with consistent care. For instance, women must often wait weeks for their first visit. Prenatal visits are usually scheduled during daytime hours that conflict with working women's schedules. In addition, child care is rarely available, and women who must find child care are torn between being a mother and keeping clinic appointments.

An important barrier to health care results from the unsympathetic attitude of some health care workers toward those who are unable to pay for prenatal care. These clinics are often understaffed and overworked. Poor families may experience long delays, hurried examinations, rudeness, and arrogance from some members of the health care team. Many women report waiting hours for an examination that lasts only a few minutes. Many never see the same health care provider more than once. These women may not keep clinic appointments because they do not see the importance of the hurried examinations.

Nurses must understand the importance of treating each family with respect and consideration. They must insist that the care of poor families who are unable to pay adheres to the same standard as that of families who can pay. Nurses can work to determine which barriers apply to the clients with whom they work and find ways to meet the needs of the specific population being served. Scheduling prenatal visits in the evening or on weekends, setting aside times for walk-in prenatal visits, and offering other services such as applications for Medicaid and WIC might increase use of prenatal services (Beckmann, Buford, & Witt, 2000).

Some women may not obtain early prenatal care because they do not want the pregnancy confirmed, do not want anyone to know about the pregnancy, or are considering an abortion. One study found that only 17.5% of women who did not want to be pregnant began prenatal care during the first trimester. Poor housing and use of substances such as drugs or alcohol also decreased early prenatal care (Pagnini & Reichman, 2000).

NURSING CARE PLAN 8-2 Socioeconomic Problems during Pregnancy

ASSESSMENT: Theresa Matheny, a 19-year-old primigravida, is seen for initial prenatal care at 24 weeks of gestation. She took the day off from work in a factory and rode the bus to the clinic. She is currently living with her sister and brother-in-law, who receive Temporary Assistance for Needy Families. During the interview Theresa states that she will not be able to keep clinic appointments because she cannot afford to take more time off until the baby comes. She is unmarried and says the father of the baby is "gone." Physical assessment shows Theresa and her fetus are healthy. She declares she does not need further prenatal care and only needs to find someone to deliver the baby.

NURSING DIAGNOSIS: Risk for Ineffective Health Maintenance related to lack of a plan to obtain regular prenatal care and lack of understanding of the importance of care

GOALS/EXPECTED OUTCOMES: During the first prenatal visit, Theresa will:
1. Describe the benefits of prenatal care.
2. Verbalize a plan for obtaining regular prenatal care.

INTERVENTION	RATIONALE
1. Use active listening to show concern and empathy with the difficulties Theresa has in obtaining prenatal care.	1. Expressing interest in the client's situation may make her more likely to listen to health teaching.
2. Emphasize why regular prenatal care is essential: a. To monitor the growth and development of the baby b. To evaluate Theresa's health, which directly affects the health of the fetus c. To detect problems and intervene before they become severe.	2. Preventive care is often not a priority when the client has conflicting needs for food and shelter. Many women are unaware that complications such as preeclampsia or gestational diabetes, which may be identified and treated with routine care, are serious hazards if they remain undetected.
3. Assist Theresa in devising a plan to obtain regular prenatal care. a. Provide her with a list of prenatal clinics near her home or place of work and the hours they are open. b. Discuss transportation services and determine whether family or friends can help her keep prenatal appointments. c. Explore dates, times, and alternatives until she finds a schedule that works for her. d. Obtain a list of phone numbers (e.g., friends, family, employer) where she can be reached for follow-up.	3. Some clinics are open on weekends and evenings to accommodate working women. Unreliable transportation is a major reason for failure to keep scheduled appointments, and clinic schedules that allow some flexibility are helpful. Interest in a client's individual situation is highly motivating for her to find a way to continue prenatal care.

EVALUATION: Theresa is attentive as the nurse talks about the importance of health care. She shows interest in finding a way to have regular prenatal care and makes an appointment for the next visit. If she misses scheduled appointments, follow-up phone calls to arrange alternative appointments may be necessary.

CRITICAL THINKING: Although this diagnosis addresses Theresa's problem with managing prenatal care, what additional assessments should be made to determine how she is managing the psychosocial concerns of pregnancy? What additional nursing diagnosis might be relevant?

ANSWER: The nurse should assess Theresa's progress with the tasks of pregnancy. She has made the first step in seeking safe passage, but other tasks need attention, such as securing the acceptance of her family and learning to give of herself. It is important to assess for depression, which may begin in pregnancy and continue after birth (see Chapter 28). In addition, signs that she is developing attachment for the fetus are particularly important. An additional nursing diagnosis might be Risk for Impaired Parent-Infant Attachment related to lack of support from significant others or the presence of financial stress. Interventions might include helping her explore sources of emotional support such as women's groups, church members, or Internet web sites related to pregnancy.

Many women rely on advice from family and friends during pregnancy, and some believe prenatal care is unimportant, especially when they have no obvious problems with the pregnancy. Other reasons may include lack of child care, inability to take time off from work for financial reasons and because of lack of job security, and lack of transportation.

✔ CHECK YOUR READING

12. Why do many low-income women delay seeking health care until the second or third trimester?
13. How do the attitudes of health care workers affect the care of poor families?

CULTURAL INFLUENCES ON CHILDBEARING

More distinct cultural groups live in the United States than anywhere else in the world. Each culture has its own health and healing belief system for major life events such as pregnancy and childbirth. The success of health care depends on its ability to fit in with the beliefs of those being served. Therefore ignorance of culturally divergent beliefs may lead to failure in health care delivery.

Differences within Cultures

Wide variations of beliefs and practices exist within each culture, and nurses must recognize that people sharing a culture may not have identical beliefs. Families who have lived in Western societies for years or generations often do not exhibit behaviors prescribed by their culture. Nurses must be careful not to stereotype people or expect a certain set of behaviors from every person in a particular cultural group. Individual differences are as important as cultural variations.

A woman who does not normally follow certain beliefs of her culture may adhere to them during pregnancy. She may do this to avoid offending or to show respect for family members to whom these beliefs are especially important during pregnancy, or she may fear that some part of the belief may be true after all and that she will harm her baby if she does not follow it.

Cultural Differences Causing Conflict

Cultural differences that cause conflict between health care workers and families during pregnancy are observed most often in the areas of health care beliefs, communication, and time orientation. It is important to understand these beliefs to give culturally specific nursing care. When health professionals violate cultural norms, women are less likely to follow health instructions and education given (Ramer & Frank, 2001).

HEALTH BELIEFS

For many cultures, health is the balance of mind, body, and spirit. Health-promoting behaviors are the actions used in each of these dimensions to maintain health, prevent illness, and restore health (Spector, 2000).

HEALTH MAINTENANCE. The predominant U.S. culture treats pregnancy like an illness, with frequents visits to a physician, many laboratory tests, and hospitalization for delivery with numerous medical interventions. Many other cultures, however, view pregnancy as a natural condition with little or no need for medical care. Visits to a health care provider often occur later in pregnancy than for U.S. women.

Different cultures have various requirements for maintaining health during pregnancy. Practices that maintain health include wearing proper clothing, which is believed by some Hispanic women to ensure a safe birth. Puerto Rican women are often indulged by their families during pregnancy, and exercise is considered inappropriate at this time (Torres, 2004). American Indians may believe that eating berries while pregnant will cause the infant to have a birthmark. They may avoid tying knots during pregnancy to prevent complications of the umbilical cord (Cesario, 2001).

Avoidance of unclean things and strong emotions like anger is believed necessary by some groups to prevent harm to the fetus or a difficult childbirth. Concentration, silence, prayer, and meditation to maintain mental and spiritual health are practiced by some. In many cultures, women must avoid contact with illness and death and may not attend funerals during pregnancy. They also must surround themselves with beautiful things and positive people (Shilling, 2000).

BELIEF IN FATE. Some cultures (such as Southeast Asian, Middle Eastern) promote a strong belief in fate. Women often believe that the only way in which they can affect the outcome of pregnancy is by eating correctly and observing the taboos of their culture. Because of this belief, it may be difficult to convince women to seek early and regular prenatal care.

Advance preparation for the baby is also avoided in some cultures. Arabic Muslim women believe that preparing for the baby defies the will of Allah. Navajo families do not choose a name for the baby until after birth because they fear it will harm the infant (Callister, 2001). Some Jewish families select items needed for the new baby, but do not bring them home until after the birth (Lewis, 2003).

PREVENTING ILLNESS. Practices that prevent illness include the use of protective religious objects or charms, such as an amulet or talisman. Some women also believe that certain foods can prevent illness. For instance, people in many cultures eat raw garlic or onion or adhere to numerous food taboos and prescribed combinations of foods. Strict adherence to religious codes, morals, and practices is also believed to prevent illness.

MODESTY. Fear, modesty, and a desire to avoid examination by men may keep some women from seeking health care during pregnancy. In many cultures (such as Muslim, Hindu, Hispanic), exposure of the genitals to men is considered demeaning. In these cultures the reputations of women depend on their demonstrated modesty. If necessary, female health care providers can perform examinations. If this is not possible, the woman should be carefully draped with her legs completely covered. A female nurse needs to remain with the woman at all times. Obtaining permission from the husband may be necessary before any examination or treatment can be performed.

FEMALE GENITAL MUTILATION. Female genital mutilation is also called *female circumcision*. Common forms involve clitoridectomy (removal of the clitoris and part of the labia minora) or infibulation (removal of the clitoris, labia minora, and all or part of the labia majora) and is usually performed at some time during childhood. The procedure is widely practiced in parts of Africa and some areas of Asia and the Middle East. The practice has been associated with premarital chastity and is a prerequisite for marriage in some African cultures. Female genital mutilation is illegal in some countries, including the United States.

Women who have undergone the procedure and now live in North America need nurses and physicians who are knowledgeable about the custom and prepared for the woman to have abnormal-looking genitals. Pelvic examination is very painful because the introitus is so small and inelastic scar tissue makes the area especially sensitive. Women are more prone to pelvic and urinary tract infections, incontinence, infertility, and menstrual abnormalities after the procedure (Doyle & Faucher, 2002).

Nurses can assist the woman in finding a health care provider with whom she is comfortable. Pelvic examinations should be made as comfortable as possible by maintaining utmost privacy and using drapes to provide maximum coverage. The woman may not give any verbal or nonverbal sign of pain, but this lack of response does not indicate an absence of pain.

RESTORING HEALTH. Traditional ways to restore health include natural folk medicine such as herbs and plants. Women may often use charms, holy words, prescribed acts, and traditional healers before seeking other medical advice. Hispanics may consult with *curanderas* (faith healers), who work with women to maintain balance and harmony, which have been lost during illness (Spector, 2000). Some Africans and Haitians may rely on folk medicine that includes witchcraft, voodoo, and magic.

■ To be certain that all essential information about folk medicine is obtained, nurses should inquire whether the client is taking folk remedies with questions such as "What do pregnant women take to protect themselves and the baby? How often and how much of this do you take? What special foods and drinks are important?"

COMMUNICATION

LANGUAGE. Language is a major barrier to health care. Numerous dialects within many languages can make it difficult to find competent interpreters. The ideal is to have trained interpreters that are preferably women. Other persons may be used if necessary, but considerations of confidentiality, the use of medical jargon, and the possible need to discuss sensitive issues indicate the need for professional interpreters.

Adults who came to the United States as children may speak English well and can interpret for their parents and grandparents. Other family members or friends, as well as co-workers in the clinic or hospital, may be helpful but not fluent. They may misunderstand instructions, particularly if medical jargon is used (Nursing Care Plan 8-3). It is important not to use the woman's children to interpret if the topics are not usually discussed with children or are likely to embarrass the parent or child.

Telephone interpreter services are provided in many agencies. This is more awkward than having an interpreter at the bedside but ensures that both the nurse and the client receive accurate information.

COMMUNICATION STYLE. Styles in communication differ among cultures. For example, among Asians, nodding and smiling may mean "Yes, I hear you" but may not indicate agreement or even understanding. When presenting information, the nurse should validate the person's understanding by requesting that the listener repeat the information: "Tell me what you understood" or "Show me what you learned."

Hispanics are traditionally diplomatic and tactful. They frequently engage in "small talk" before bringing up questions they may have about their care. Nurses must remember that small talk is a valuable use of time. It establishes rapport and often helps to accomplish the goals of care. For example, women from Mexico try to avoid conflict. Although they may seem to agree with what is said, they may not follow instructions (Quinzanos, 2003).

Native Americans often converse in a low tone that may be difficult to hear in a noisy setting. They may consider note-taking taboo and expect the caregiver to remember what is said (Spector, 2000). Cherokee women generally do not volunteer information and may not disclose symptoms unless asked specifically because they do not think the symptoms are important and do not want to bother the caregiver. They may not ask for information because they consider asking questions rude because it calls attention to themselves (Moore & Moos, 2003).

EYE CONTACT. People in the United States and those from African-American families often consider eye contact important to communication and believe it denotes honesty. However, this belief is not held by some other groups. Some American Indian groups avoid direct eye contact, which is like looking into the soul and endangers both people (Moore & Moos, 2003). Southeast Asians often believe eye contact shows disrespect. Eye contact between unmarried men and women is considered seductive by those from the Middle East.

Eye-contact avoidance sometimes frustrates health care personnel who believe that eye contact denotes honesty. Eye-contact behavior is also important when nurses deal with Latino infants and children. *Mal ojo* (evil eye) is a sudden unexplained illness that may occur when an individual with special powers admires a child too openly. Eye contact between a woman and man may be considered seductive by those from Middle Eastern cultures.

TOUCH. Touch is also an important component of communication. In some cultures (such as Hindu, Muslim), touch by a woman other than the wife is offensive. In contrast, women from Haiti find touch supportive and reassuring, and gentle touch is particularly important during labor and birth. Hispanic women are from a "high touch" culture and generally appreciate touch (Mattson, 2003). Nurses must remain sensitive to the response of the person being touched and should refrain from touching if the person indicates it is not welcomed.

TIME ORIENTATION

Time orientation can create conflict between health care professionals, who parcel out care in discrete units of time measured in minutes, and groups that keep time by the

NURSING CARE PLAN 8-3 Language Barrier during Pregnancy

ASSESSMENT: Diep Tran, a young Vietnamese primigravida of 16 weeks' gestation, speaks very little English. She listens quietly to the nurse's health care instructions, and although she appears confused, she asks no questions. Her husband, Bao Nguyen, nods and smiles frequently and speaks more English than his wife but has difficulty responding to questions about her health.

CRITICAL THINKING: Why must additional assessments be made before a nursing diagnosis can be formulated?

ANSWER: Nodding and smiling do not always mean that persons from another culture understand health teaching. Instead, such actions may simply indicate that the information has been heard, or perhaps Mr. Nguyen is being polite and does not want the nurse to feel inadequate as an instructor. Before assuming that Mr. Nguyen can translate health care teaching for his wife, the nurse must validate his learning by asking him to explain it himself.

NURSING DIAGNOSIS: Impaired Verbal Communication related to foreign language barriers

GOALS/EXPECTED OUTCOMES: Throughout the pregnancy the family will:
1. Keep scheduled appointments.
2. Follow health care instructions.
3. Verbalize basic needs and concerns at each prenatal visit.

INTERVENTION	RATIONALE
1. Assess the couple's ability to speak, read, and write in English and determine if they are fluent in other languages.	1. Clients who are not fluent in speaking a language may be more adept at reading it.
2. Obtain the assistance of a fluent interpreter, preferably a woman.	2. A fluent interpreter is essential because Asians do not always reveal that they do not understand instructions. This hinders follow-up questions. Printed instructions reinforce information that was given verbally and may answer unasked questions. Written materials and communication cards in the client's language convey interest in communicating and provide a means of eliciting basic information.
a. Establish a list of bilingual staff members throughout the facility who are willing to interpret and be educated about the importance of confidentiality and exactness.	
b. Enlist the aid of adult family members or friends who can interpret for the couple, if a professional interpreter is not available.	
c. Use a translator to develop written material in languages most commonly encountered in the facility. Develop communication aids about common teaching topics in various languages. Use communication cards with questions and answers printed in Vietnamese with Diep and her husband.	
3. Face the client and direct conversation to the client rather than to the interpreter, using quiet tones. Use the same interpreter whenever possible.	3. Talking directly to the client while facing her shows respect and concern. Soft speech protects the client's privacy and modesty. A natural response when people do not understand is to raise the voice. This may convey impatience or anger. A consistent interpreter enhances communication.
4. Ask the interpreter to explain exactly what the nurse says as much as possible instead of paraphrasing.	4. If the interpreter paraphrases the nurse's words, important information may be lost.
5. Consider nonverbal factors when communicating.	5. Even subtle body language can indicate interest and empathy or impatience, annoyance, or hurry. Touch and eye contact are sensitive cultural variables, and nurses must be aware that they are not always welcomed.
a. Speak slowly and smile when appropriate.	
b. Keep an open posture. Avoid crossing the arms over the chest or turning away from the family.	
c. Attend carefully to what the family says by nodding, leaning forward, or encouraging continued talk with frequent "uh-huhs."	
d. Avoid fidgeting or watching a clock.	
e. Determine Diep's response to a light touch on the arm, and use or avoid touch depending on her response.	
f. Do not expect prolonged eye contact.	
6. Locate prenatal classes in Vietnamese. Explain what is included in such classes and encourage the couple to attend.	6. Information is more easily learned in one's own language. Appropriate cultural concerns are likely to be discussed in classes taught in Vietnamese.

EVALUATION: Diep keeps each prenatal appointment. She brings her husband or an English-speaking friend or family member with her to translate. She follows all recommendations and asks many appropriate questions at each visit.

progress of the sun or seasons. American Indians, Middle Eastern, Hispanic, and African-American women tend to emphasize the moment rather than the future. This attitude causes conflicts in a health care setting in which tests or appointments are scheduled at particular times. If a woman does not place the same importance on keeping appointments, she may encounter anger and frustration in the health care setting that leaves her bewildered and ashamed.

Culturally Competent Nursing Care

Culturally competent nursing care requires an awareness of, sensitivity to, and respect for the diversity of the clients served. It involves assessment of the family's culture and cultural negotiation when necessary.

CULTURAL ASSESSMENT

Although nurses cannot know all the precise details of every culture, they must be aware of the important aspects of the dominant cultures seen in their practice area and become adept at performing cultural assessment. Some specific questions such as the following may elicit information that helps the nurse understand the family's beliefs about appropriate care during pregnancy:

- How will you and your family prepare for the baby?
- What concerns do you have about the pregnancy?
- What would provide the greatest assistance?
- Where do you obtain most health care information?
- What foods are encouraged or discouraged?
- Who will be with you during labor and birth of the baby?
- Who will help you at home during the pregnancy and after birth?

CULTURAL NEGOTIATION

Cultural negotiation involves providing information while acknowledging that the family may hold views that are different from those of the nurse. If the family indicates that the information would be helpful, it can be incorporated into the teaching plan.

If the family indicates that the information is not helpful or is harmful in their opinion, the conflict must be acknowledged openly and clarified. "I sense that you are unsure about this. Tell me about your reluctance to try it." After allowing the family to express their beliefs, the nurse explains why the recommendation is valid and works with the family to find a compromise.

Cultural negotiation also involves sensitivity to specific concerns. For example, nurses must be aware of Islamic laws governing modesty when caring for Muslim women. A Muslim woman must cover her hair, body, arms to the wrist, and legs to the ankles at all times when in the presence of a man. She is not to be alone in the presence of a man other than her husband or a male relative.

Muslim women prefer a female health care provider and should be informed of the availability of female caregivers. Adequate drapes and covers should be available to allow

covering all areas of the body except those that must be exposed for examination. In addition, the woman's husband, a female friend, or a male relative should be allowed to be present during examinations.

When talking to the woman's significant others the nurse must be sure to call them by the correct name. For example, a Vietnamese woman keeps her maiden name when she marries. Therefore the husband and wife will have different last names.

✓ CHECK YOUR READING

14. What are some cultural differences that may cause conflict between health care workers and clients?
15. What is meant by the term *cultural negotiation*?

Application of the Nursing Process
Psychosocial Concerns
Assessment

The purpose of a psychosocial assessment is to monitor the adaptation of the family to pregnancy, which some consider a maturational "crisis" that requires a major transition in role function and relationships. Although not all agree that pregnancy is a crisis, it does initiate change and stress. The family's ability to cope is a primary concern. For some families, pregnancy offers the potential for growth. For others an alteration in family processes requires guidance and information. Specific needs can be discovered during a thorough psychosocial assessment. Some data, such as age, gravida, para, and general health status, are obtained during the physical assessment. Table 8-3 identifies areas for assessment, provides sample questions, and indicates nursing implications.

Analysis

Critical thinking is extremely important when analyzing psychosocial data that may be open to several interpretations. Nurses must be careful to examine their own assumptions and biases about proper responses to pregnancy. They must resist the urge to form an opinion before obtaining adequate information. In addition, they must validate data, particularly when assessing clients of different cultural backgrounds.

Nursing diagnoses are based on data obtained during individual assessments and can vary among families (Box 8-1). Most families strive to maintain the health of the expectant mother and fetus and complete developmental tasks that allow the couple to become parents. Perhaps the most encompassing nursing diagnosis is "Readiness for Enhanced Family Coping," which relates to the readiness and desire to meet added family needs and assume parenting roles.

Planning

Goals related to family coping include:
- The family will verbalize emotional responses that are appropriate to each trimester.

TABLE **8-3** Psychosocial Assessment

Findings (Normal and Unusual)*	SAMPLE QUESTIONS	NURSING IMPLICATIONS
Psychological Response First trimester: uncertainty, ambivalence, mood changes, self as primary focus Second trimester: wonder, joy, focus on fetus Third trimester: vulnerability, preparing for birth (fear, anger, apathy, ambivalence, lack of preparation)	"How do you and your partner feel about being pregnant?" "How will your lives change as a result of being pregnant?" "How do you feel about the changes in your body?" "What preparations have you made for the baby?"	Use active listening and reflection to establish a sense of trust. Reevaluate negative responses (fear, apathy, anger) in subsequent assessments.
Availability of Resources Financial concerns (lack of funds or insurance) Availability of grandparents, friends, family (family geographically or emotionally unavailable)	"What are your plans for prenatal care and birth?" "How do your parents feel about being grandparents?" "Who else can you depend on besides the family?" "Who provides strength when there is a problem?"	Determine adequacy of financial means. Refer to resources such as a public clinic for care, WIC for food. Help the couple discover alternative resources if the family is unavailable. Identify family conflicts early to allow time for resolution.
Changes in Sexual Practices Mutual satisfaction with changes (excessive concern with comfort or safety, excessive conflict)	"How have sexual patterns or satisfaction changed?" "How do you cope with the changes?" "What concerns you most?"	Offer reassurance that intercourse is safe if pregnancy is normal. Suggest alternative positions and open communication.
Educational Needs Many questions about pregnancy, childbirth, and infant care (no questions, absence of interest in educational programs)	"How do you feel about caring for an infant?" "What are your major concerns?" "Whom do you count on for information?"	Respond according to priority to needs that are expressed. Refer couple to appropriate child and parenting classes, reliable Internet sources of information.
Cultural Influences Ability of either the woman or her family to speak English or availability of fluent interpreters; cultural influences support a healthy pregnancy and infant (harmful cultural beliefs or health practices)	"What foods are recommended during pregnancy?" "What practices are recommended?" "What is forbidden?" "What is most important to you in your care?" "How do your religious beliefs affect pregnancy?"	Locate fluent interpreters if needed. Avoid labeling beliefs as "superstition." Reinforce beliefs that promote a good pregnancy outcome. Elicit help from accepted sources of information to overcome harmful practices.

*Findings that require additional assessment or intervention are shown in parentheses.

BOX **8-1** Common Nursing Diagnoses Used in Pregnancy

Anxiety
Deficient Knowledge
Disturbed Body Image*
Disturbed Personal Identity
Health-Seeking Behaviors
Risk for Ineffective Health Maintenance*
Ineffective Home Maintenance
Ineffective Role Performance
Ineffective Sexuality Patterns
Risk for Impaired Parent-Infant Attachment
Impaired Verbal Communication*
Interrupted Family Processes
Readiness for Enhanced Family Coping*
Situational Low Self-Esteem

*Nursing diagnoses explored in this chapter.

- The family will describe methods to help the expectant parents complete the developmental processes of pregnancy.
- The family will identify cultural factors that may produce conflicts and collaborate to reduce those conflicts.

Interventions

PROVIDING INFORMATION

Provide the prospective parents with information and anticipatory guidance to prepare them for the progressive changes that occur during pregnancy and reassure them that their feelings and behaviors are normal. Guidance also gives them an opportunity to ask questions and explore their feelings. Common subjects include the following:

- The emotional changes that occur during pregnancy (such as ambivalence, introversion, feelings of vulnerability)
- The developmental tasks of the mother (such as seeking safe passage, securing acceptance, forming an attachment with the unknown baby)
- Role transition (such as mimicry, role playing, fantasy, grief work)
- The developmental processes of the prospective father (such as grappling with the reality, struggling for recognition as a parent, creating the role of involved father)

ADAPTING NURSING CARE TO PREGNANCY PROGRESS

Adapt nursing care to the changes that occur in each trimester of pregnancy. During the first trimester, focus on the woman's acceptance of the pregnancy. Tailor teaching to her feelings (physical and psychological), as this is a period of self-focus. The second trimester is a time to concentrate more on the fetus and how the woman and her family will adapt to the changes the birth will bring. Ask about her fantasies about the baby and her relationships with significant others. The focus is on the woman's discomforts and readiness to give birth during the third trimester. Observe for signs that the mother is having difficulty with any of the tasks or steps throughout pregnancy.

DISCUSSING RESOURCES

Initiate a discussion of the adequacy of the financial situation and support systems and help couples without financial resources or insurance coverage find a convenient location to obtain prenatal care. This is particularly important for the new poor, who have little knowledge about how to obtain government-sponsored care. Emotional resources include those that help the new family adjust to the demands of pregnancy and parenting.

Discuss the responses and participation of the grandparents. Although emotional responses vary, the family unit is strengthened and the attachment of the grandparents to the child is enhanced when grandparents actively participate in the pregnancy.

If family members who traditionally offer support in times of stress are unavailable, refer the prospective parents to community resources such as support groups and childbirth education, sibling, breastfeeding, and new parenting classes.

HELPING THE FAMILY PREPARE FOR BIRTH

During the last trimester, discuss lifestyle changes that will occur when the infant is born. Unanticipated changes that accompany this dramatic life event may add stress and disrupt family processes. Help the prospective parents make practical plans for the infant, such as obtaining clothing and needed equipment and choosing the method of feeding.

Assist the parents in planning sibling preparation. Older siblings should be prepared several weeks or even months before the birth. Younger children have a poor concept of time and can be prepared for the arrival of a new baby shortly before the birth. The response of children depends on their ages and developmental levels. Children often benefit from participating in prenatal care and planning for the baby.

Suggest that the expectant parents determine how they will work out the division of household and parenting tasks and what they will do about child care if the mother must return to work after childbirth. If these issues are not resolved, the couple can experience frustration and anger when one parent, usually the mother, assumes total care of the infant and attempts to complete all household tasks. Ex-

haustion and frustration can overwhelm the joys of parenting when one parent must provide all care.

MODELING COMMUNICATION TECHNIQUE

When disagreements are evident, discuss and model therapeutic communication techniques that include all significant family members. Techniques to clarify, summarize, and reflect feelings can defuse negative feelings that might result in family disruption (see Chapter 2).

IDENTIFYING CONFLICTING CULTURAL FACTORS

Explore possible areas of conflict related to cultural beliefs and health practices that affect pregnancy.

> ■ Expectant mothers are reassured when nurses support beneficial health beliefs before confronting them with concerns about health care practices. For example, "The foods you are choosing are very good for you and the baby. I am worried, though, because you missed your last appointment."

If a conflict occurs because of differences in time orientation, acknowledge the problem, convey understanding of the differences, and emphasize the importance of calling when appointments cannot be kept. Many families do not realize that when they miss an appointment, another family misses the opportunity for health care.

Evaluation

When the family verbalizes concerns and emotions throughout pregnancy, the initial goal is met. Continued interest and involvement of the partner and significant family members are evidence that the family has completed the developmental tasks of pregnancy. Participation of the family with health care workers to find a compromise when differing cultural beliefs cause conflict confirms that the family will identify and initiate measures to reduce conflicts.

SUMMARY CONCEPTS

- Maternal psychological responses progress during pregnancy from uncertainty and ambivalence to feelings of vulnerability and preparation for the birth of the infant.
- As the fetus becomes real, usually in the second trimester, maternal focus shifts from the self to the fetus and the woman turns inward to concentrate on the processes taking place in her body.
- Changes in the maternal body during pregnancy may result in a negative body image that affects sexual responses. This change may be especially troubling if the couple does not discuss emotions and concerns related to the changes in sexuality.
- Making the transition to the role of mother involves mimicking the behavior of other mothers, fantasizing about the baby, grieving for the loss of previous roles, and developing a sense of self as mother.
- To complete the maternal tasks of pregnancy the woman must take steps to seek safe passage for herself and the

infant, gain acceptance of significant persons, and learn to be giving while forming an interconnection with and attachment to the unknown child.

- Paternal responses change throughout pregnancy and depend on the ability to perceive the fetus as real, gain recognition for the role of parent, and create a role as involved father.
- The most powerful reality boosters for the expectant father during pregnancy are hearing the fetal heartbeat, feeling the fetus move, and viewing the fetus on a sonogram.
- In primitive cultures *couvade* refers to pregnancy-related rituals performed by the man. Today, it refers to a cluster of pregnancy-related symptoms experienced by the man.
- The response of grandparents to pregnancy depends on their ages, the number and ages of other grandchildren, and their beliefs about the role of grandparents.
- The response of siblings to pregnancy depends on their ages and developmental levels.
- Completing the developmental tasks of pregnancy is more difficult for multiparas because they have less time, experience more fatigue, and must negotiate a new relationship with the older child or children.
- Socioeconomic status is a major factor in determining health practices during pregnancy. Poor families have competing priorities for food and shelter and seek prenatal care late in pregnancy.
- Cultural differences can create major conflicts between expectant families and health care workers. Language, time orientation, and health beliefs are the areas in which conflicts are most likely to occur.

ANSWERS TO CRITICAL THINKING EXERCISE 8-1, p. 161

1. These women will have more concerns about lack of time and increased fatigue. In addition, they will have concerns about the effect of another baby on their other children and the time and energy required to meet the needs of all children.
2. Although both have 2-year-olds, Ms. Hastings will be concerned about her son's response to sharing her time and attention. Ms. Nguyen has experienced this before and may be more worried about the effect of another baby on her economic situation, and her ability to manage yet another child.
3. Suggest that any changes in sleeping arrangements be made early so that other children will not feel displaced by the infant. Recommend that they plan ways to have time alone with the older child(ren) when the baby arrives, and review measures to reduce sibling rivalry. Ask Ms. Nguyen about measures that were helpful when her last two children were born, and suggest that she involve the older children in preparing for the new baby.

REFERENCES & READINGS

Association of Women's Health, Obstetric and Neonatal Nurses (AWHONN). (2000). Nurse providers of perinatal education: Competencies and program guide. Washington, DC: Author.

Beckmann, C.A., Buford, T.A., & Witt, J.B. (2000). Perceived barriers to prenatal care services. *MCN: American Journal of Maternal/Child Nursing, 25*(1), 43-46.

Braveman, P., Marchi, K., Egerter, S., Pearl, M., & Neuhaus, J. (2000). Barriers to timely prenatal care among women with insurance: The importance of prepregnancy factors. *Obstetrics & Gynecology, 95*(1), 874-880.

Buist, A., Morse, C.A., & Durkin, S. (2003). Men's adjustment to fatherhood: Implications for obstetrical health care. *Journal of Obstetric, Gynecologic, and Neonatal Nursing, 32*(2), 172-180.

Bullock, L.F.C., Browning, C., & Geden, E. (2002). Telephone social support for low-income pregnant women. *Journal of Obstetric, Gynecologic, and Neonatal Nursing, 31*(6), 658-664.

Callister, L.C. (2001). Integrating cultural beliefs and practices into the care of childbearing women. In K.R. Simpson & P.A. Creehan (Eds.). *AWHONN perinatal nursing* (2nd ed., pp. 68-94). Philadelphia: Lippincott.

Cesario, S.K. (2001). Care of the Native American woman: Strategies for practice, education, and research. *Journal of Obstetric, Gynecologic, and Neonatal Nursing, 30*(1), 13-19.

Coverston, C.R. (2004). Psychology of pregnancy. In S. Mattson & J.E. Smith (Eds.), *Core curriculum for maternal-newborn nursing* (3rd ed., pp. 124-143). Philadelphia: Saunders.

Doyle, E.I., & Faucher, M.A. (2002). Pharmaceutical therapy in midwifery practice: A culturally competent approach. *Journal of Midwifery & Women's Health, 47*(3), 122-129.

Driscoll, J.W. (2001). Psychosocial adaptation to pregnancy and postpartum. In K.R. Simpson & P.A. Creehan (Eds.), *AWHONN perinatal nursing* (2nd ed., pp. 115-124). Philadelphia: Lippincott.

Gichia, J.E.U. (2000). African-American women's preparation for motherhood. *MCN: American Journal of Maternal/Child Nursing, 25*(2), 86-91.

Jordan, P.L. (1990). Laboring for relevance: Expectant and new fatherhood. *Nursing Research, 39*(1), 11-16.

Kridli, S.A. (2002). Health beliefs and practices among Arab women. *MCN: American Journal of Maternal/Child Nursing, 27*(1), 178-182.

Kroelinger, C.D., & Oths, K.S. (2000). Partner support and pregnancy wantedness. *Birth, 27*(2), 112-119.

Lee, I. (2003). An Hmong perspective. In M.L. Moore & M. Moos (Eds.). *Cultural competence in the care of childbearing families* (pp. 73-74). White Plains, NY: March of Dimes Birth Defects Foundation.

Lewis, J.A. (2003). Jewish perspectives on pregnancy and childbearing. *MCN: American Journal of Maternal/Child Nursing, 28*(5), 306-312.

Logsdon, M.C. (2000). *Social support for pregnant and postpartum women.* Washington, DC: AWHONN.

Logsdon, M.C., & Davis, D.W. (2004). Paraprofessional support for pregnant and parenting women. *MCN: American Journal of Maternal/Child Nursing, 29*(2), 92-97.

Matteson, P.S. (2001). *Women's health during the childbearing years: A community-based approach.* St. Louis: Mosby.

Matthey, S., Morgan, M., Healey, L., Barnett, B., Kavanaugh, D.J., & Howie, P. (2002). Postpartum issues for expectant mothers and fathers. *Journal of Obstetric, Gynecologic, and Neonatal Nursing, 31*(4), 428-425.

Mattson, S. (2000). Providing culturally competent care: Strategies and approaches for perinatal clients. *AWHONN Lifelines, 4*(5), 39-41.

Mattson, S. (2003). Caring for Latino women. *AWHONN Lifelines, 7*(3), 258-260.

Mattson, S. (2004). Ethnocultural considerations in the childbearing period. In S. Mattson & J.E. Smith (Eds.), *Core curriculum for maternal-newborn nursing* (3rd ed., pp. 75-96). Philadelphia: Saunders.

Melender, H. (2002a). Experiences of fears associated with pregnancy and childbirth: a study of 329 pregnant women. *Birth, 29*(2), 101-111.

Melender, H. (2002b). Fears and coping strategies associated with pregnancy and childbirth in Finland. *Journal of Midwifery & Women's Health, 47*(4), 256-263.

Mercer, R.T. (1990). *Parents at risk*. New York: Springer.

Mercer, R.T. (1995). *Becoming a mother: Research on maternal identity from Rubin to the present*. New York: Springer.

Mercer, R.T., & Ferketich, S.L. (1994). Predictors of maternal role competence by risk status. *Nursing Research, 43*(1), 38-43.

Midmer, D. (2000). Psychosocial support for childbearing families. In H. Nichols & S.S. Humenick (Eds.). *Childbirth education: Practice, research, and theory* (2nd ed., pp. 476-500). Philadelphia: Saunders.

Moore, M.L., & Moos, M. (2003). *Cultural competence in the care of childbearing families*. White Plains, NY: March of Dimes Birth Defects Foundation.

Pagnini, D.L., & Reichman, N.E. (2000). Psychosocial factors and the timing of prenatal care among women in New Jersey's HealthStart program. *Family Planning Perspectives, 32*(2), 56-64.

Quinzanos, G.O. (2003). A Mexican perspective. In M.L. Moore & M. Moos. *Cultural competence in the care of childbearing families* (pp. 82-84). White Plains, NY: March of Dimes Birth Defects Foundation.

Ramer, L., & Frank, B. (2001). *Pregnancy: Psychosocial Perspectives*. White Plains, NY: March of Dimes Birth Defects Foundation.

Rubin, R. (1975). Maternal tasks in pregnancy. *MCN: The American Journal of Materna/Child Nursing, 4*(3), 143-153.

Rubin, R. (1984). *Maternal identity and the maternal experience*. New York: Springer.

Schneider, Z. (2001). An Australian study of women's experiences of their first pregnancy. *Midwifery, 18*, 238-249.

Shilling, T. (2000). Cultural perspectives on childbearing. In F.H. Nichols & S.S. Humenick (Eds.). *Childbirth education: Practice, research, and theory* (2nd ed., pp. 138-154). Philadelphia: Saunders.

Sleutel, M.R. (2003). Intrapartum nursing: Integrating Rubin's framework with social support theory. *Journal of Obstetric, Gynecologic, and Neonatal Nursing, 32*(1), 76-82.

Spector, R.E. (2000). *Cultural diversity in health and illness* (5th ed.). Norwalk, CT: Appleton & Lange.

Stark, M.A. (2000). Is it difficult to concentrate during the 3rd trimester and postpartum? *Journal of Obstetric, Gynecologic, and Neonatal Nursing, 29*(4), 378-389.

Torres, S. (2004). Puerto Rican Americans. In J.N. Giger & R.E. Davidhizar (Eds.). *Transcultural nursing: Assessment and intervention* (4th ed., pp. 617-631). St. Louis: Mosby.

Webster, J., Linnane, J.W.J., Dibley, L.M., Hinson, J.K., Starrenburg, S.E., Roberts, J.A. (2000). Measuring social support in pregnancy: Can it be simple and meaningful? *Birth, 27*(2), 97-101.

Wilkerson, N.N., & Shrock, P. (2000). Sexuality in the perinatal period. In F.H. Nichols & S.S. Humenick (Eds.). *Childbirth education: Practice, research, and theory* (2nd ed., pp. 48-65.) Philadelphia: Saunders.

Zwelling, E. (2000). The pregnancy experience. In F.H. Nichols & S.S. Humenick (Eds.). *Childbirth education: Practice, research, and theory* (2nd ed., pp. 35-47). Philadelphia: Saunders.

Nutrition for Childbearing

OBJECTIVES

After studying this chapter, you should be able to:

1. Explain the importance of adequate nutrition and weight gain during pregnancy.
2. Compare the nutrient needs of pregnant and nonpregnant women.
3. Describe common factors that influence a woman's nutritional status and choices.
4. Describe the effects of common nutritional risk factors on nutritional requirements during pregnancy.
5. Compare the nutritional needs of the postpartum woman who is breastfeeding with those of the woman who is not breastfeeding.
6. Apply the nursing process to nutrition during pregnancy, the postpartum period, and lactation.

Go to your Student CD-ROM for Review Questions keyed to these Objectives.

DEFINITIONS

Anorexia Nervosa Refusal to eat because of a distorted body image and feeling of obesity.

Bulimia Eating disorder characterized by ingestion of large amounts of food followed by purging behavior such as induced vomiting or laxative abuse.

Dietary Reference Intakes A label for several terms that estimate nutrient needs; includes recommended dietary allowance, adequate intake, tolerable upper intake level, and estimated average requirement.

Essential Amino Acids Amino acids that cannot be synthesized by the body and must be obtained from foods.

Gynecologic Age The number of years since menarche (first menstrual period).

Heme Iron Iron obtained from meat, poultry, or fish sources; the form most usable by the body.

Incomplete Protein Food Food that does not contain all the essential amino acids.

Kilocalorie A unit of heat; used to show the energy value in foods (commonly called calorie).

Lacto-Ovovegetarian A vegetarian whose diet includes milk products and eggs.

Lactose Intolerance Inability to digest most dairy products because of a deficiency of the enzyme lactase.

Lactovegetarian A vegetarian whose diet includes milk products.

Nonheme Iron Iron obtained from plant and fortified foods.

Nutrient Density The quality and quantity of protein, vitamins, and minerals per 100 calories in foods.

Ovovegetarian A vegetarian whose diet includes eggs.

Pica Ingestion of a nonnutritive substance such as laundry starch, dirt, or ice.

Recommended Dietary Allowances Levels of nutrient intake considered to meet the needs of healthy individuals.

Vegan A complete vegetarian who does not eat any animal products.

Vegetarian An individual whose diet consists wholly or mostly of plant foods and who avoids animal food sources.

At no other point in a woman's life is nutrition as important as during pregnancy and lactation. At this time she must nourish not only her own body but also that of her baby. Nutrition may affect the size of the fetus and determine whether it has adequate stores of some nutrients after birth. If the woman fails to consume sufficient nutrients during pregnancy, her own stores of some nutrients may be depleted so that she can meet the needs of the fetus, who also may be deprived of essential nutrients.

Nurses can provide ongoing education about nutritional needs throughout the childbearing period. This is especially important because studies show that many women do not adequately understand the nutritional needs of pregnancy (Fowles, 2002; Hilton, 2002). Nurses are often able to offer nutrition counseling before conception to women who are considering becoming pregnant. Such counseling increases the chances that a woman will be nutritionally healthy at the time of conception and will continue to practice good nutrition throughout pregnancy. It may also increase the level of nutrition the woman provides for her entire family. Therefore nutritional education is an essential part of nursing care.

WEIGHT GAIN DURING PREGNANCY

Weight gain during pregnancy, especially after the first trimester, is an important determinant of fetal growth, yet women often do not gain weight at the recommended levels. In one study only 38% of women had a weight gain within the recommended range (Olson & Strawderman, 2003). Other sources report that weight gain in the recommended range occurs in only 30% to 40% of pregnant women (Abrams, Minassian, & Pickett, 2004).

Low birth weight (less than 2.5 kg or 5.5 lb), preterm labor, and increased risk of fetal and newborn mortality and morbidity have been associated with insufficient weight gain during pregnancy. Poor maternal weight gain indicates lower caloric intake as well as decreased intake of other important nutrients.

Excessive weight gain also is a problem. It is associated with greater risk for higher birth weight (macrosomia), prolonged labor, birth trauma, and cesarean birth. An infant birth weight of 3 to 4 kg (6.5 to 8.8 lb) is associated with the lowest rates of infant mortality (Mitchell 2003; Strychar et al., 2000).

The nutrient intake that results in the weight gain is even more important than the weight gain itself. Weight gain from a diet lacking in essential nutrients is not as beneficial as weight gain from a balanced diet.

Recommendations for Total Weight Gain

Recommendations for weight gain during pregnancy have changed considerably over the years. In the late nineteenth century, rickets, a disease of the bones resulting from deficiencies of calcium and vitamin D, caused some women to have small, distorted pelves. Restricted weight gain kept the fetus small and facilitated delivery. Later, weight gain was limited because of the inaccurate belief that large gains caused preeclampsia.

Recommendations for weight gain in pregnancy are based on the woman's prepregnancy weight for her height or body mass index (BMI). BMI is calculated by dividing the weight in kilograms by the height in meters squared. Another method is to divide the weight in pounds by the height in inches squared and multiply the result by 704.5. For example, if a woman weighs 56 kg (124 lb) before pregnancy and is 1.63 meters (64 in) tall, her BMI is 21, which shows normal weight for height.

The recommended weight gain during pregnancy is 11.5 to 16 kg (25 to 35 lb) for women who begin pregnancy at normal weight for their height or have a BMI between 19.8 and 26. This weight gain is believed to reduce intrauterine growth restriction caused by inadequate maternal intake. The range allows for individual differences because no precise weight gain is appropriate for every woman. It provides a target while allowing for variations in individual needs.

Suggested gains vary according to the woman's BMI before pregnancy (Table 9-1). Low prepregnancy weight is associated with preterm labor and low-birth-weight infants. Women who have low BMIs (less than 19.8) should gain more during pregnancy to meet the needs of pregnancy as well as their own need to gain weight.

In the past, obese women (BMI above 29) were told to gain little or even to lose weight during pregnancy. Obesity in pregnant women is associated with increased incidence of gestational diabetes, preeclampsia, cesarean birth, and large-for-gestational-age infants (Cunningham et al., 2001). The current recommended gain for overweight women (BMI above 26 to 29) is 7 to 11.5 kg (15 to 25 lb), to provide sufficient nutrients for the fetus. The weight gain for obese women (BMI above 29) is at least 7 kg (15 lb), which is equivalent to the weight of the products of conception (fetus, placenta, amniotic fluid).

TABLE 9-1 Recommended Weight Gain During Pregnancy

Weight before Pregnancy	Total Gain	Total Gain (First Trimester)	Weekly Gain (Second and Third Trimesters)
Normal weight (BMI 19.8-26)	11.5-16 kg (25-35 lb)	1.6 kg (3.5 lb)	0.4 kg (0.88 lb)
Underweight (BMI <19.8)	12.5-18 kg (28-40 lb)	2.3 kg (5 lb)	0.49 kg (1.07 lb)
Overweight (BMI >26-29)	7-11.5 kg (15-25 lb)	0.9 kg (2 lb)	0.3 kg (0.67 lb)
Obese (BMI >29)	At least 7 kg (15 lb)	Individually determined	Individually determined
Twin pregnancies	16-20.5 kg (35-45 lb)	1.6 kg (3.5 lb)	0.75 kg (1.5 lb)

Based on data from National Academy of Sciences. (1990). *Nutrition during pregnancy, part I: Weight gain.* Washington, DC: National Academy Press.
BMI, Body mass index.

Women who are shorter than 157 cm (62 in) may not need to gain as much as taller women and should gain only to the lower limits of the recommended range. Young adolescents need to gain to the upper end of the range to provide for their own growth during pregnancy as well as that of the fetus.

Another variation is the woman who is pregnant with more than one fetus. Infants of a multifetal pregnancy are often born before term and tend to weigh less than those born of single pregnancies. A greater weight gain in the mother may help prevent low birth weight.

Pattern of Weight Gain

The pattern of weight gain is as important as the total increase in weight. Early and adequate prenatal care allows assessment of weight gain on a regular basis throughout pregnancy. The general recommendation is an increment of about 1.6 kg (3.5 lb) during the first trimester, when the mother may be nauseated and the fetus needs few nutrients for growth. During the rest of the pregnancy the expected weight gain is 0.44 kg (nearly 1 lb) per week.

Maternal and Fetal Distribution

Women often wonder why they should gain so much weight when the fetus weighs only 3.2 to 3.6 kg (7 to 8 lb). The nurse should explain the distribution of weight to help them understand this need (Figure 9-1).

FACTORS THAT INFLUENCE WEIGHT GAIN

The nurse can positively influence the expectant mother's weight gain by teaching her the importance of her diet for fetal growth. A discussion of the effects of maternal intake on fetal growth and storage of nutrients often motivates women to improve their nutrition. Knowing about factors that may negatively influence nutrient intake and weight gain helps the nurse devise plans for improving nutrition.

Women at risk for inadequate weight gain include those who are young, are unmarried, have a low income, are poorly educated, have poor general health, or are receiving insufficient prenatal care. African-American, Southeast Asian, and Hispanic women are at greater risk for low weight gain during pregnancy than white women. Adequate weight gain may be more important for African-Americans and teenagers, who tend to have smaller infants even when they gain the same amount of weight as white women and older mothers. The reasons for this difference are not fully understood. Multiparas are at higher risk for low weight gain than primiparas. Smoking and substance abuse may interfere with food intake and weight gain.

✓ CHECK YOUR READING

1. How does weight gain in the mother relate to the birth weight of the infant?
2. How much weight should the average woman gain during pregnancy? What factors might change this?
3. What pattern of weight gain is recommended for the average woman?

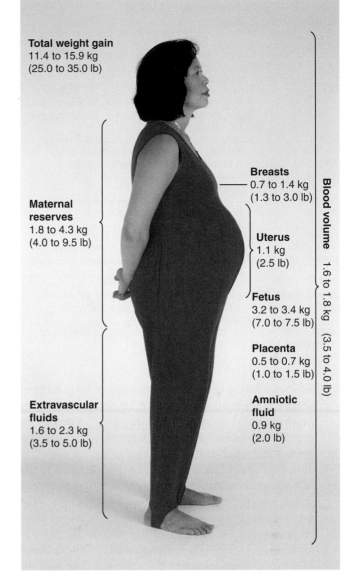

Figure 9-1 ■ Distribution of weight gain in pregnancy. The numbers represent a general distribution because variation among women is great. The component with the greatest fluctuation is the weight increase attributed to extravascular fluids (edema) and maternal reserves of fat.

Total weight gain
11.4 to 15.9 kg
(25.0 to 35.0 lb)

Maternal reserves
1.8 to 4.3 kg
(4.0 to 9.5 lb)

Extravascular fluids
1.6 to 2.3 kg
(3.5 to 5.0 lb)

Breasts
0.7 to 1.4 kg
(1.3 to 3.0 lb)

Uterus
1.1 kg
(2.5 lb)

Fetus
3.2 to 3.4 kg
(7.0 to 7.5 lb)

Placenta
0.5 to 0.7 kg
(1.0 to 1.5 lb)

Amniotic fluid
0.9 kg
(2.0 lb)

Blood volume 1.6 to 1.8 kg (3.5 to 4.0 lb)

NUTRITIONAL REQUIREMENTS

During pregnancy, nutrient needs increase to meet the demands of the mother and fetus. The amount of increase for each nutrient varies. In most cases the increases are not large and it is relatively easy to obtain the required nutrients through the diet (Table 9-2).

Dietary Reference Intakes

In the United States, Dietary Reference Intakes (DRIs) are used to estimate nutrient needs. DRIs include the following four categories:

- Recommended Dietary Allowance (RDA)–The amount of a nutrient that is sufficient to meet the needs of almost all (97% to 98%) healthy people in an age group

TABLE 9-2 Extra Foods Needed to Meet Pregnancy Requirements*

Energy (kcal)	1 carrot, 1 slice whole wheat bread, ½ banana, and 1 glass low-fat milk in the second trimester; add ½ banana in the third trimester.
Protein	1-2 oz meat, fish, or poultry *or* 3 c milk *or* 3 oz cheddar cheese *or* 1 c cottage cheese *or* 1 block (4 oz) tofu *or* 1 c brown rice and 1½ c beans
Iron	1 oz red meat *and* 1 c lima beans *and* ½ c cooked spinach *and* 1 c broccoli
Thiamine	½ c bran flakes *or* ¾ c peanuts *or* 1½ oz pecans *or* 1 oz ham *or* 1½ c rice *or* 1 c macaroni
Riboflavin	¾ c milk or cottage cheese *or* 2 oz oatmeal *or* 1½ oz beef *or* 1 c broccoli *or* 1 c spinach
Niacin	1 T peanut butter *or* 4 slices bread *or* 1 oz meat; also made by body from tryptophan
Vitamin C	2 t orange juice *or* ½ c peaches *or* ½ c apple *or* 1½ T tomato juice

Data from Grodner, M., Long, S., & DeYoung, S. (2004). *Foundations and clinical applications of nutrition: A nursing approach* (3rd ed.). St. Louis: Mosby.
c, Cup; *T*, tablespoon; *t*, teaspoon.
*Examples of foods that would meet the additional requirements for pregnancy for women between ages 19 and 50.

- Adequate Intake (AI)—The nutrient intake assumed to be adequate when an RDA cannot be determined; based on an observed average or experimentally set intake that appears to sustain nutritional status; AIs have been set for nutrients such as fluoride, fiber, and vitamin K
- Tolerable Upper Intake Level (UL)—The highest amount of a nutrient that can be taken without probable adverse health effects by most people—for example, the RDA for vitamin C during pregnancy for women aged 19 to 50 years is 85 mg/day, and the UL is 2000 mg/day
- Estimated Average Requirement (EAR)—The amount of a nutrient estimated to meet the needs of half the healthy people in an age group

Tables of recommendations are based on a reference individual, a hypothetical person of medium size. These tables are used to calculate nutrient needs based on age, gender, and size. For example, the reference woman for ages 19 to 30 years is 163 cm (64 in) tall and weighs 61 kg (133 lb). Actual needs of individuals, particularly for calories and protein, may vary according to body size, previous nutritional status, and usual activity level.

Energy

The energy provided by foods for body processes is calculated in kilocalories. Kilocalories (commonly called *calories*) are obtained from carbohydrates and proteins, which provide 4 calories in each gram, and fats, which provide 9 calories in each gram.

CARBOHYDRATES

Carbohydrates may be simple or complex. The most common simple carbohydrate is sucrose (table sugar), which is a source of energy but does not provide other nutrients. Fruits and vegetables contain simple sugars along with other nu-

trients. Complex carbohydrates are present in starches such as cereals and supply vitamins, minerals, and fiber. They should be the major source of carbohydrates in the diet because of their value in providing other nutrients.

Another type of carbohydrate is fiber, the nondigestible product of plant foods and an important source of bulk in the diet. Fiber absorbs water and stimulates peristalsis, causing food to pass more quickly through the intestines. Fiber helps prevent constipation and also slows gastric emptying, causing a sensation of fullness.

FATS

Fats provide energy and fat-soluble vitamins. When decreasing calories is necessary, a reduction, but not elimination, of carbohydrates and fats is important. If carbohydrate and fat intake does not provide sufficient calories, the body uses protein to meet energy needs. This use decreases the amount of protein available for building and repairing tissue.

Women often restrict fat to prevent weight gain. However, essential fatty acids such as docohexaenoic acid (DHA), an n-3 or omega-3 fatty acid, help in formation of the placenta, fetal brain development, and fetal visual function. DHA is transferred to the infant after birth during breastfeeding. Women should be encouraged to include fish and red meat that contain these fatty acids in their diets several times per week (Brooks, Mitchell, & Steffenson, 2000).

CALORIES

Approximately 68,000 to 80,000 additional calories are needed during pregnancy (Grodner, Long, & DeYoung, 2004). These extra calories furnish energy for production and maintenance of the fetus, placenta, added maternal tissues, and increased basal metabolic rate. The Estimated Energy Requirement (EER) for women of childbearing age is approximately 2400 calories per day. The *2005 Dietary Guidelines for Americans* recommends a caloric intake of 1800-2400 calories per day for women aged 19-50 years old. The number of calories for each woman depends on her activity level (U.S. Department of Health and Human Services and U.S. Department of Agriculture, 2005).

During the first trimester of pregnancy, no added calories are needed. However, the caloric intake for adolescent and adult pregnant women should increase by 340 calories during the second trimester and 452 calories during the third trimester (Institute of Medicine, 2002a). This is a change from previous recommendations of an increase of only 300 calories during the second and third trimesters. This increase can be achieved relatively easily with a variety of foods and only a small increase in food.

Nutrient density—the quantity and quality of the various nutrients in each 100 calories of food—must be considered when calories are added. Foods of high nutrient density have large amounts of quality nutrients per serving. During pregnancy the increased need for most nutrients may not be met unless calories are selected carefully. The term *empty calories* refers to foods that are high in calories but low in other nutrients. Many snack foods contain excessive calories and low nutrient density and are high in fat and sodium. In-

TABLE 9-3 Recommendations for Daily Energy and Protein Intakes for Women Age 15 to 50 Years

Nonpregnant Adult Female	Pregnancy	Lactation
Energy		
1800 to 2400 kcal (varies greatly according to body size, age, and physical activity level)	First trimester: No change from non-pregnant needs Second trimester: 340 kcal above non-pregnant needs Third trimester: 452 kcal above non-pregnant needs	First 6 months: 330 kcal above nonpregnant needs Second 6 months: 400 kcal above non-pregnant needs
Carbohydrate		
130 g	175 g	210 g
Protein		
46 g	71 g	71 g

Data from Institute of Medicine, Food and Nutrition Board. (2002). *Dietary reference intakes for energy, carbohydrates, fiber, protein and amino acids (macronutrients).* Washington, DC: National Academy Press; Kaiser, L.L., & Allen, L. (2002). Position of the American Dietetic Association: Nutrition and lifestyle for a healthy pregnancy outcome. *Journal of the American Dietetic Association, 102*(10), 1479-1490.

creased calories should be "spent" on foods that provide the nutrients needed in increased amounts during pregnancy.

Women often use sugar substitutes to reduce their caloric intake. Saccharin (Sweet 'n' Low), sucralose (Splenda), and aspartame (Equal or NutraSweet) are considered safe for normal women during pregnancy. Use of aspartame at any time by women with phenylketonuria can result in brain damage because they lack the enzyme to metabolize it (Shabert, 2004) (Table 9-3).

Protein

Protein is necessary for metabolism, tissue synthesis, and tissue repair. The RDA for adults is 0.8 g of protein per kilogram of body weight. This requirement averages to a daily need of 46 g for females depending on their age and size. During pregnancy a daily protein intake of 1.1 g/kg or approximately 71 g each day is recommended because of expansion of blood volume and growth of maternal and fetal tissues. This is an increase of 25 g of protein daily (Shabert, 2004).

Protein is generally abundant in diets in most industrialized nations, and many women obtain more than the required amount of this nutrient. Diets low in caloric intake may also be low in protein, however. If calories are low and protein is used to provide energy, fetal growth may be impaired.

The nurse should teach women at risk for eating diets poor in protein how to determine protein intake and increase food sources of protein. When a woman needs to increase her protein intake, she should eat more protein-rich foods rather than use high-protein powders or drinks. Protein substitutes increase protein but do not have the other nutrients provided by foods.

Vitamins

Although most people do not eat as much of every vitamin each day as they should, true deficiency states are uncommon in North America. During pregnancy, women usually get vitamins but they may not eat enough foods high in vitamins B$_6$, D, or E and folic acid to attain the recommended levels (Table 9-4).

FAT-SOLUBLE VITAMINS

Because the fat-soluble vitamins (A, D, E, and K) are stored in the liver, deficiency states are not as likely to occur as with the water-soluble vitamins. However, excessive intake of fat-soluble vitamins can be toxic. For example, too much vitamin A can cause fetal defects. The nurse should inquire about vitamins and medications taken by pregnant women and counsel them about the dangers of excess vitamins.

WATER-SOLUBLE VITAMINS

Water-soluble vitamins (vitamins B$_6$, B$_{12}$, and C, folic acid, thiamine, riboflavin, and niacin) are not stored in the body as easily as fat-soluble vitamins and therefore should be included in the daily diet. Because excess amounts are excreted in the urine, the chance of toxicity from ingestion of too much of these vitamins is less.

Water-soluble vitamins are easily transferred from food to water during cooking. Foods should be steamed, microwaved, or prepared in only small amounts of water. The remaining water can be used in other dishes such as soups. Vitamin C is supplemented in many juices, and riboflavin, vitamin B$_{12}$, and niacin are supplemented in many breads and cereals. Diets are less likely to be low in these nutrients.

FOLIC ACID

Folic acid (also called *folate*) can decrease the occurrence of neural tube defects in newborns. Adequate intake of folic acid is especially important just before conception and during the first trimester after conception. Because many pregnancies are unplanned, all women of childbearing age should consume at least 400 mcg (0.4 mg) of folic acid every day. Once pregnancy occurs, an intake of 600 mcg (0.6 mg) of folic acid is recommended. For women who have had a child with a neural tube defect previously, the recommended dose is 4 mg (4000 mcg) each day before conception (see Chapter 5).

However, women often do not realize the importance of folic acid in the diet before pregnancy begins and need instruction in this area. Healthy People 2010 goals are to increase the number of childbearing women with adequate

TABLE 9-4 Recommendations for Vitamins and Minerals

Nonpregnant Adult Females	Pregnancy and Lactation	Sources	Purpose	Importance in Pregnancy
Fat-Soluble Vitamins				

Vitamin A
Age 14-50:
  700 mcg (RDA)
	Pregnancy: Age 14-18:
	  750 mcg
	Age 19-50: 770 mcg
	Lactation: Age 14-18:
	  1200 mcg
	Age 19-50: 1300 mcg
		Dark green, yellow, or orange vegetables, whole or fortified low-fat or nonfat milk, egg yolk, butter and fortified margarine	Important for vision and cell reproduction, growth, and functioning of skin and mucous membranes	Fetal growth and cell differentiation; excessive intake causes spontaneous abortions or serious fetal defects; isotretinoin (Accutane), a vitamin A derivative for acne, should not be taken during pregnancy because it causes fetal defects

Vitamin D
Age 14-50:
  5 mcg (AI)
	Pregnancy and lactation:
	  Age 14-50: 5 mcg
		Fortified milk, margarine, and soy products, butter, egg yolks; synthesized in skin exposed to sunlight; vegans who are not exposed to sunlight and who do not eat fortified foods need supplements	Necessary for metabolism of calcium and prevention of rickets	Inadequate amounts may cause neonatal hypocalcemia, hypoplasia of tooth enamel, and maternal osteomalacia (softening of the bones); excessive intake causes hypercalcemia and possible fetal deformities; supplements should be taken cautiously

Vitamin E
Age 14-50:
  15 mg (RDA)
	Pregnancy: Age 14-50:
	  15 mg
	Lactation: Age 14-50:
	  19 mg
		Vegetable oils, whole grains, nuts, and green leafy vegetables	Antioxidant, important for tissue growth and integrity of cells, particularly red blood cell membranes	Rarely deficient in pregnant women, but can cause anemia in mother and fetus

Vitamin K
Age 14-18:
  75 mcg
Age 19-50:
  90 mcg (AI)
	Pregnancy and lactation: Age 14-18:
	  75 mcg
	Age 19-50: 90 mcg
		Dark green leafy vegetables; also produced by normal bacterial flora in small intestine	Necessary for blood clotting	Newborns are temporarily deficient and receive one dose by injection at birth to prevent hemorrhage

Water-Soluble Vitamins				

Vitamin B$_6$ (Pyridoxine)
Age 14-18:
  1.2 mg
Age 19-50:
  1.3 mg (RDA)
	Pregnancy: Age 14-50:
	  1.9 mg
	Lactation: Age 14-50:
	  2 mg
		Chicken, fish, pork, eggs, peanuts, whole grains, cereals	Important in amino acid metabolism and blood, nervous system, and immune function	Increased metabolism of amino acids during pregnancy

Vitamin B$_{12}$
Age 14-50:
  2.4 mcg (RDA)
	Pregnancy: Age 14-50:
	  2.6 mcg
	Lactation: Age 14-50:
	  2.8 mcg
		Meat, fish, poultry, eggs, milk, fortified soy, and cereal products	Amino acid and fatty acid metabolism, formation of hemoglobin; prevents megaloblastic (pernicious) anemia	Increased formation of red blood cells and protein synthesis

Folic Acid
Age 14-50:
  400 mcg
  (0.4 mg) (RDA)
	Pregnancy: Age 14-50:
	  600 mcg (0.6 mg)
	Lactation: Age 14-50:
	  500 mcg (0.5 mg)
		Green leafy vegetables, legumes, beans, peanuts, orange juice, asparagus, spinach, and fortified cereal and pasta; may be lost in cooking	Coenzyme in metabolism; important for cell replication, amino acid synthesis, and hemoglobin synthesis and for prevention of megaloblastic anemia	Expanded blood volume and tissue growth; deficiency in first weeks of pregnancy may cause spontaneous abortion and neural tube defects

Thiamine
Age 14-18: 1 mg
Age 19-50:
  1.1 mg (RDA)
	Pregnancy and lactation: Age 14-50:
	  1.4 mg
		Lean pork, whole or enriched grain products, legumes, seeds, nuts	Forms coenzymes necessary to release energy, aids in nerve and muscle functioning	Increased because of intake of calories

Data from Institute of Medicine (IOM), Food and Nutrition Board (FNB). (1998). *Dietary reference intakes for thiamin, riboflavin, niacin, vitamin B$_6$, folate, vitamin B$_{12}$, pantothenic acid, biotin, and choline.* Washington, DC: National Academy Press; IOM, FNB. (1997). *Dietary reference intakes for calcium, phosphorus, magnesium, vitamin D, and fluoride.* Washington, DC: National Academy Press; IOM, FNB. (2000). *Dietary reference intakes for vitamin C, vitamin E, selenium, and carotenoids.* Washington, DC: National Academy Press; IOM, FNB. (2002). *Dietary reference intakes for vitamin A, vitamin K, arsenic, boron, chromium, copper, iodine, iron, manganese, molybdenum, nickel, silicon, vanadium, and zinc.* Washington, DC: National Academy Press.

AI, Adequate Intake; *RDA,* Recommended Daily Allowances.

TABLE 9-4 Recommendations for Vitamins and Minerals—cont'd

Nonpregnant Adult Females	Pregnancy and Lactation	Sources	Purpose	Importance in Pregnancy
Water-Soluble Vitamins—cont'd				
Riboflavin Age 14-18: 1 mg Age 19-50: 1.1 mg (RDA)	Pregnancy: Age 14-50: 1.4 mg Lactation: Age 14-50: 1.6 mg	Milk, meat, fish, poultry, eggs, enriched grain products, deep green vegetables	Forms coenzymes necessary to release energy	Increased because of greater intake of calories
Niacin Age 14-50: 14 mg (RDA)	Pregnancy: Age 14-50: 18 mg Lactation: Age 14-50: 17 mg	Meats, fish, poultry, legumes, enriched grains, milk	Forms coenzymes necessary to release energy	Increased because of greater intake of calories
Vitamin C Age 14-18: 65 mg Age 19-50: 75 mg (RDA)	Pregnancy: Age 14-18: 80 mg Age 19-50: 85 mg Lactation: Age 14-18: 115 mg Age 19-50: 120 mg	Citrus fruit, peppers, strawberries, cantaloupe, green leafy vegetables, tomatoes, potatoes; destroyed by heat and oxidation	Important in collagen formation, tissue integrity, healing, immune response, and metabolism; severe deficiency causes scurvy	Necessary for formation of fetal tissue; need increased with smoking, drug or alcohol abuse, and aspirin use
Minerals				
Iron Age 14-18: 15 mg Age 19-50: 18 mg (RDA)	Pregnancy: Age 14-50: 27 mg Lactation: Age 14-18: 10 mg Age 19-50: 9 mg	Meats, green leafy vegetables, eggs, grain products, enriched bread and cereal, dried fruits, tofu, legumes, nuts, blackstrap molasses	Formation of hemoglobin and enzymes for metabolism	Expanded maternal blood volume, formation of fetal red blood cells, and storage in the fetal liver for use after birth
Calcium Age 14-18: 1300 mg Age 19-50: 1000 mg (AI)	Pregnancy and lactation: Age 14-18: 1300 mg Age 19-50: 1000 mg	Dairy products, salmon or sardines with bones, legumes, fortified juice and tofu, broccoli, kale, tofu	Needed in bone formation, cell membrane permeability, coagulation, and neuromuscular function	Mineralization of fetal bones and teeth
Phosphorus Age 14-18: 1250 mg Age 19-50: 700 mg (RDA)	Pregnancy and lactation: Age 14-18: 1250 mg Age 19-50: 700 mg	Dairy products, lean meat, fish, poultry, cereals; high in processed foods, snacks, carbonated drinks	Needed with calcium for bone formation and cell metabolism	Mineralization of fetal bones and teeth; excessive intake causes binding of calcium in intestines and prevents calcium absorption
Zinc Age 14-18: 9 mg Age 19-50: 8 mg (RDA)	Pregnancy: Age 14-18: 13 mg Age 19-50: 11 mg Lactation: Age 14-18: 14 mg Age 19-50: 12 mg	Meat, poultry, seafood, eggs, nuts, seeds, legumes, wheat germ, whole grains, yogurt	Used in cell differentiation and reproduction, DNA and RNA synthesis, metabolism, acid-base balance	Fetal and maternal tissue growth.
Magnesium Age 14-18: 360 mg Age 19-30: 310 mg Age 31-50: 320 mg (RDA)	Pregnancy: Age 14-18: 400 mg Age 19-30: 350 mg Age 31-50: 360 mg Lactation: Age 14-18: 360 mg Age 19-30: 310 mg Age 31-50: 320 mg	Whole grains, nuts, legumes, dark green vegetables, small amounts in many foods	Important in cell growth and neuromuscular function; activates enzymes for metabolism of protein and energy	Same as for nonpregnant; women; excessive intake may interfere with absorption of iron
Iodine Age 14-50: 150 mcg (RDA)	Pregnancy: Age 14-50: 220 mcg Lactation: Age 14-50: 290 mcg	Seafood, iodized salt	Important in thyroid function	Deficiency may cause abortion, stillbirth, congenital hypothyroidism, neurologic conditions

TABLE 9-5 Foods High in Folic Acid

Food	Amount of Folic Acid per 1-Cup Serving (in mcg)
Black beans	256
Kidney beans	126
Pinto beans	144
Peanuts	114
Orange	55
Orange juice	109
Avocado	93
Asparagus	171
Peas (cooked from frozen)	148
Broccoli	140
Spinach (raw)	58
Spinach (cooked)	262

Data from Grodner, M., Long, S., & DeYoung, S. (2004). *Foundations and clinical applications of nutrition, a nursing approach* (3rd ed.). St. Louis: Mosby.

intake of folic acid to 80% and to cut the incidence of neural tube defects in half by the year 2010 (U.S. Department of Health and Human Services, 2000).

A woman who has given birth to an infant with a neural tube defect should take higher doses of folic acid (Table 9-5). This practice can decrease the risk of recurrence of neural tube defects by 70% (American Academy of Pediatrics [AAP]/ American College of Obstetrics and Gynecology [ACOG], 2002).

✔ CHECK YOUR READING

4. How many more calories should a woman consume each day during pregnancy?
5. How much protein is recommended during pregnancy?
6. Which vitamins are most likely to be low in the diets of pregnant women?
7. Which vitamins are in the fat-soluble and water-soluble groups? What is the difference in the way the body stores them?
8. Why should all women of childbearing age consume 400 mcg of folic acid daily?

Minerals

Although most minerals are supplied in adequate amounts in normal diets, the intake of iron, calcium, zinc, and magnesium may drop below recommended levels for pregnancy (Giddens et al., 2000; Swensen, Harnack, & Ross, 2001).

IRON

Iron is important in the formation of hemoglobin to carry oxygen throughout the body, and it helps form some enzymes necessary for metabolism. During pregnancy approximately 1000 mg of iron are needed. Of this, 500 mg are used for the 25% to 33% increase in maternal red blood cells, 200 mg for normal daily losses, and 300 mg for transfer to the fetus for production of red blood cells and iron storage (Blackburn, 2003; Mitchell, 2003; Monga, 2004). Iron will be transferred to the fetus even if maternal iron intake is inadequate, but this causes depletion of the mother's iron stores. The fetus stores iron for the first 4 to 6 months after birth when the infant's intake of iron is low.

TABLE 9-6 Foods High in Iron Content*

Food and Amount	Average Amounts of Iron Supplied (mg)
Meats and Poultry (1 oz)	
Red meats (avg)	2
Chicken	0.9
Turkey	2
Legumes	
Kidney beans (½ c)	1.6
Lentils (½ c)	3.3
Peanuts (1 oz)	1.1
Sunflower seeds (1 oz)	1.1
Chickpeas (garbanzo beans) (½ c)	1.6
Lima beans (½ c) (frozen)	3
Peas (½ c)	2.5
Eggs	
Eggs (each)	0.4
Grains (1 c)	
Rice	
Brown	0.8
White	1.9
Bran flakes	8
with raisins	8.9
Bread, wheat (slice)	0.9
Fruits	
Raisins (⅓ c)	1.1
Prunes (¼ c)	1.5
Apricots, dried (½ c)	3
Vegetables (1 c)	
Asparagus (frozen)	1.2
Broccoli	2.4
Collards	0.9
Spinach	
Raw	0.8
Cooked (frozen)	3.3
Other	
Tofu, firm (1 oz)	1.2

Data from Grodner, M., Long, S., & DeYoung, S. (2004). *Foundations and clinical applications of nutrition, a nursing approach* (3rd ed.). St. Louis: Mosby.
*The Recommended Daily Allowance for iron during pregnancy is 30 mg. Although many women take supplements because they do not eat enough iron-containing foods in their daily diet to meet this need, iron in foods is often better absorbed. Therefore the nurse should suggest ways a woman can increase her dietary iron.

Iron is probably the only nutrient that cannot be supplied completely and easily by the diet during pregnancy. Iron is present in many foods, but in small amounts (Table 9-6). The average woman's daily diet contains only about 9 mg of iron, and she frequently enters pregnancy with low iron stores. In addition, some women restrict their intake of meats and grains in an effort to cut down on fat, carbohydrates, and calories. Therefore many adult women do not meet their daily nonpregnancy requirements for iron and are already anemic or have low iron stores when they begin pregnancy.

Absorption of iron is affected by intake of other substances. Calcium and phosphorus in milk and tannin in tea decrease iron absorption from plant sources and fortified foods (called *nonheme iron*) if they are consumed during the same meal. Coffee binds iron, preventing it from being fully absorbed. Foods cooked in cast-iron pans contain more iron. Foods containing ascorbic acid and meat, fish, or poultry eaten with nonheme iron–containing foods may increase absorption. Iron from animal sources (called *heme iron*) is more readily absorbed than iron from nonheme iron and is less affected by other foods.

Because of the difficulty in obtaining enough iron in the diet, health care providers often prescribe iron supplements of 30 mg daily during the second and third trimesters. Women who are anemic may need 60 to 120 mg daily (see Chapter 26). Women who take high doses of iron also need zinc and copper supplements because iron interferes with the absorption and uses of these minerals. Supplementation should begin during the second trimester when the need increases. The expectant mother can also tolerate the iron better because morning sickness usually ends by this time.

Iron taken between meals is absorbed more completely, but many women find it difficult to tolerate iron without some food. Iron taken at bedtime may be easier to tolerate. Milk, tea, coffee, and antacids taken with iron decrease absorption. For best results, it should be taken with water or orange juice. Side effects occur more often with higher doses and include nausea, vomiting, heartburn, epigastric pain, constipation, diarrhea, and black stools.

Women should be reminded to keep iron and all other medicines out of the reach of children. Accidental iron overdose is a leading cause of childhood poisoning.

CALCIUM

Calcium is necessary for bone formation, maintenance of cell membrane permeability, coagulation, and neuromuscular function. It is transferred to the fetus, especially in the last trimester, and is important for mineralization of fetal bones and teeth. The changes in progesterone, estrogen, and parathyroid hormone during pregnancy result in increased calcium absorption and retention. This provides enough calcium to meet the needs of pregnancy. The recommendations for calcium intake (1300 mg for women under age 18 and 1000 mg for those 18 and older) are the same as those for nonpregnant women.

Calcium is removed from the bones in women who do not have an adequate calcium intake. Because the total amount of calcium required is only a small part of that stored in the bones, mineralization of the woman's bones is not usually affected, and changes are reversed after pregnancy. A common myth is that calcium is removed from the teeth during pregnancy, leading to excessive decay. In reality, calcium in the teeth is stable and not affected by pregnancy.

Dairy products are the best source of calcium. Whole, low-fat, and skim milk all contain the same amount of calcium and may be used interchangeably to increase or reduce calorie intake. However, women with lactose intolerance (lactase deficiency resulting in gastrointestinal problems when dairy products are consumed) need other sources of calcium (Box 9-1).

Calcium is also present in legumes, nuts, dried fruits, dark green leafy vegetables, and broccoli. Although spinach contains calcium, it also contains oxalates that decrease calcium availability and make spinach a poor source. Blackstrap molasses and tofu processed with calcium sulfate are

BOX **9-1** Calcium Sources Approximately Equivalent to 1 Cup of Milk*

1 c yogurt
1¼ oz hard cheese
2 c low-fat cottage cheese
16 oz peanuts
¾ c almonds
3 c pinto beans
3 c tofu (soybean curd)
2¼ c broccoli
1 c cooked collard greens
1 c fortified orange juice
⅓ can salmon with bones
½ c sardines with bones
6 corn tortillas

Data from Grodner, M., Long, S., & DeYoung, S. (2004). *Foundations and clinical applications of nutrition, a nursing approach* (3rd ed.). St. Louis: Mosby.
*This list can be used to counsel women who are vegans or lactose intolerant. Lactose-intolerant women can often manage small amounts of yogurt and cheese without distress. Although the amounts of some foods listed are more than would be likely to be eaten within 1 day, they serve for comparison.

sources for vegans. Caffeine increases the excretion of calcium and decreases intestinal absorption.

Women who do not eat dairy products for cultural reasons, because of lactose intolerance, because they avoid eating animal products, or for other reasons should take supplements unless they can meet their needs with other calcium-rich foods. More calcium is needed by women younger than 18 years because their bone density is incomplete. Calcium should be taken with vitamin D, which increases its absorption. It is better absorbed when taken with meals, separately from iron supplements. Caffeine increases the excretion of calcium.

Sodium

Sodium needs are increased during pregnancy to provide for an expanded blood volume and the needs of the fetus. Although sodium is not restricted during pregnancy, excessive amounts should be avoided. Women are advised that a moderate intake of salt or the salting of foods to taste is acceptable, but that intake of high-sodium foods (Box 9-2) should be limited.

BOX **9-2** High-Sodium Foods*

- Products that contain the words *salt, soda,* and *sodium,* such as table salt, onion salt, monosodium glutamate, and bicarbonate of soda (baking soda)
- Foods that taste salty, including sauerkraut and snack foods like popcorn, potato chips, pretzels, and crackers
- Condiments and relishes such as catsup, chili sauce, horseradish, mustard, soy sauce, bouillon, pickles, and green and black olives
- Smoked, dried, and processed foods such as ham, bacon, lunch meats, and corned beef
- Canned soups, meats, and vegetables unless the label states that the contents are low in sodium
- Canned tomato and vegetable juices
- Packaged mixes for sauces, gravies, cakes, and other baked foods

*During pregnancy, foods high in sodium should be consumed in moderation. Expectant mothers should be taught to read labels and avoid products in which sodium is listed among the first ingredients.

- Take only vitamin and mineral supplements prescribed by your health care provider. Over-the-counter supplements may not be formulated to meet your individual needs and could be harmful to you and your baby.
- Take iron on an empty stomach if possible. If you have nausea, heartburn, constipation, or diarrhea, try taking your iron at different times of the day such as at bedtime

or 1 to 2 hours after meals. To increase absorption, take iron with orange juice or another source of vitamin C. Do not take iron with calcium supplements, milk, tea, or coffee because these substances decrease absorption.
- Keep all vitamin and mineral supplements away from children because they may cause accidental poisoning.

Nutritional Supplementation

PURPOSE

Food is the best source of nutrients. Health care providers usually prescribe prenatal vitamin-mineral supplements, and they are often seen as an important part of pregnancy by many women. However, women with adequate diets may not need supplements except for iron and folic acid, which are often not obtained in adequate amounts through normal food intake. Expectant mothers who are vegetarians, are lactose intolerant, or have special problems in obtaining nutrients through diet alone may need vitamin-mineral supplements. Assessment of each woman's individualized needs determines whether supplementation is appropriate.

DISADVANTAGES AND DANGERS

Because they believe supplements are a harmless way to improve their diets, some women take large amounts without consulting a health care provider. No standardization or regulation of the amounts of ingredients contained in supplements is available at this time. Some supplements may not have the amount of an ingredient that is listed on the label and may not fulfill the health claims made for it.

The use of supplements in addition to food may increase the intake of some nutrients to doses much higher than the recommended amounts. Excessive amounts of some vitamins and minerals may be toxic to the fetus. Vitamin A can cause fetal anomalies of the bones, urinary tract, and central nervous system when more than 10,000 international units are taken per day. This is double the amount in most prenatal vitamins. No more than 5000 international units per day should be taken during pregnancy (AAP/ACOG, 2002). High levels of vitamin A are taken by women using the drug isotretinoin (Accutane) for acne. Other nutrients that may cause harm in excessive amounts include vitamins B_6, C, and D and the minerals iron, selenium, and zinc (Cunningham, 2001).

High doses of some vitamins or minerals may interfere with the ability to use others. For example, a high calcium intake decreases absorption of iron and zinc. Excessive intake of vitamin C inhibits absorption and metabolism of vitamin B_{12}. If women understand this, they are more likely not to exceed recommended doses.

Some women believe their nutrient needs can be met in supplement form and are less concerned about their food

intake. Supplements do not contain protein and calories and may lack many necessary nutrients. Nurses must emphasize that supplements are not food substitutes and do not contain all the nutrients needed during pregnancy. In fact, some nutrients that are important to pregnancy and provided by foods may be unknown at this time.

Water

Water is important during pregnancy for the expanded blood volume and as part of the increased maternal and fetal tissues. Women should drink at least eight 8-oz glasses of fluids each day, with water constituting most fluid intake. Fluids low in nutrients (such as carbonated beverages, coffee, tea, or juice drinks that contain high amounts of sugar and little real juice) should be limited because they are filling and they replace other, more nutritional foods and drinks.

Food Guide Pyramid

The U.S. Department of Agriculture (USDA) food pyramid provides a guide for healthy eating for adults and children. The pyramid is shown in Figure 9-2. Table 9-7 lists portion sizes equivalent to one serving. Pregnancy needs are discussed below.

WHOLE GRAINS

Breads, cereals, rice, and pastas provide complex carbohydrates, fiber, vitamins, and minerals. Whole grains provide more nutrients than processed grain products. At least half of the servings of grains should be whole grains. Although foods can be enriched to replace some nutrients lost during processing, not all nutrients are restored by enrichment. The USDA recommends 6 to 11 servings of this group for healthy adults over age 25. Pregnant women should have at least seven servings.

VEGETABLES AND FRUITS

Vegetables and fruits are important sources of vitamins, minerals, and fiber. New dietary guidelines are for nonpregnant women to eat 2 c (4 servings) of fruits and 2.5 c (5 servings) of vegetables each day. Weekly fruit and vegetable recommendations include:

- 3 c dark green vegetables (broccoli, spinach, romaine)
- 2 c orange (or dark yellow) vegetables (carrots, sweet potatoes, winter squash)

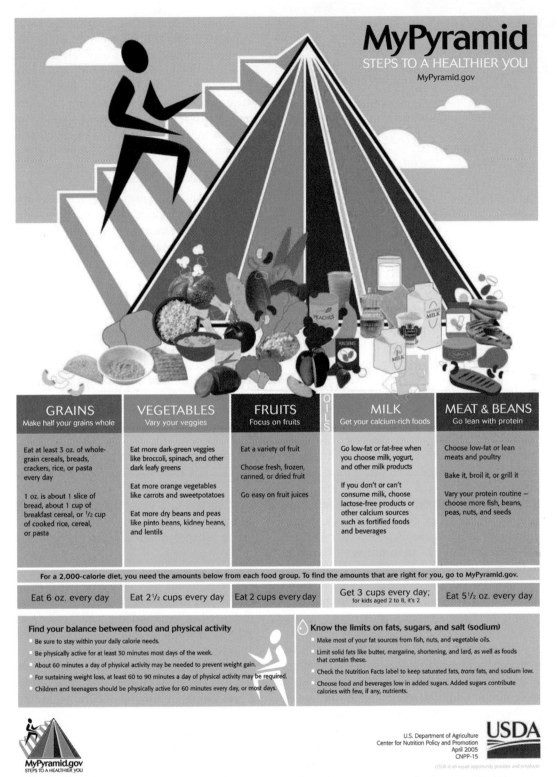

Figure 9-2 ■ Nutrient needs for the healthy adult. (Modified from U.S. Department of Health and Human Services and U.S. Department of Agriculture. *Dietary Guidelines for Americans, 2005,* 6th ed. Washington, DC: U.S. Government Printing Office and U.S. Department of Agriculture Center for Nutrition Policy and Promotion, April 2005, CNPP-16).

■ 3 c legumes (pinto or kidney beans, lentils, tofu). Legumes are included in both the protein and vegetable groups. A serving should be counted in only one group, however.

■ 3 c starchy vegetables (white potatoes, corn, green peas)

■ 6.5 c other vegetables (tomatoes, lettuce, green beans, onions)

The pregnant or lactating woman needs at least the same number of servings of vegetables and fruits as the nonpregnant woman.

TABLE **9-7** Food Group Examples and Portion Sizes

Food Group Examples	Portion Sizes
Dairy products	1 c milk or yogurt 1½ oz natural cheese (e.g., cheddar) 2 c cottage cheese
Protein sources (to make 1-oz serving)	1 oz or ¼ c cooked meat, poultry, fish ¼ c dried beans 1 egg ¼ c tofu 1 T peanut butter ½ oz nuts or seeds
Vegetables and fruits	1 medium piece or ½ c cooked or chopped raw ½ c juice 1 c raw, leafy vegetable ¼ c dried fruit
Whole grains	1 slice bread 1 c dry cereal ½ c cooked rice or pasta
Oils	1 t

C, Cup *T,* tablespoon; *t,* teaspoon.

DAIRY FOODS

Dairy foods include foods such as milk, yogurt, and cheese. They contain approximately the same nutrient values whether they are whole (4% fat), low fat (2% fat), or nonfat (skim), but calories and fat are less in the latter two. Dairy products are especially good sources of calcium. Adults older than age 25 need three servings from this group. Women who are pregnant or lactating need at least three servings.

In the past, calcium supplements and decreased milk intake were recommended to prevent leg cramps from an imbalance of calcium and phosphorous in the diet. However, the effectiveness of this treatment has not been proven. Magnesium supplementation may be helpful for leg cramps (Shabert, 2004). Because milk provides a large number of nutrients, women generally should not limit intake during pregnancy.

PROTEIN

Many adults think of meat, poultry, fish, and eggs as the only sources of protein. However, legumes (beans, peas, and lentils), nuts, and soybean products such as tofu are also good sources. Adults should consume 5.5 oz or the equivalent each day. Pregnant and lactating women need at least 7 oz of protein foods. A typical portion of meat, fish, and poultry varies in size and may contain several ounces. A 3-oz portion is about the size of a deck of playing cards.

Although fish are an excellent source of protein, certain precautions should be taken. Shark, swordfish, king mackerel, and tilefish often have high levels of mercury, which can damage the fetal central nervous system. Tuna and other types of fish may have smaller amounts of mercury. Other contaminants may be present in salmon and lake trout. Women should restrict their intake of fish during pregnancy to 6 to 12 ounces per week (Evans, 2002) and should check with their health care providers for changes in foods that should be avoided in pregnancy. Raw fish should also be avoided (James, Mahomed, Stone, van Wijngaarden, & Hill, 2003).

Some foods may be contaminated with *Listeria* monocytogenes, which may cause listeriosis. If contracted during pregnancy, listeriosis may result in abortion, stillbirth, or severe illness of the newborn. Foods that are more likely to be contaminated include cold cuts, hot dogs, deli meats, some cheeses (brie, feta, blue cheese, and Camembert), refrigerated pâté or meat spreads, and raw or undercooked meats and poultry (U.S. Food and Drug Administration, 2002).

OTHER ELEMENTS

Oils, fats and concentrated sugars should be taken sparingly. They provide calories for energy but few other nutrients. An adequate allowance for this group is 6 teaspoons (2 tablespoons) of unsaturated fats. Foods containing saturated fats and *trans* fatty acids should be avoided.

✔ **CHECK YOUR READING**

9. Which minerals are often below the recommended amounts in the diets of pregnant women?
10. Why is excessive use of vitamin-mineral supplements unnecessary and possibly dangerous?
11. How much fluid should a woman drink each day during pregnancy?
12. How many servings from each food group are recommended during pregnancy?

FACTORS THAT INFLUENCE NUTRITION

Age, knowledge about nutrition, exercise habits, and cultural background influence the food choices women make and their nutritional status. The nurse must consider these factors when counseling women about their diets.

Age

Extremes of age may influence the nutritional needs associated with pregnancy. The adolescent who is not fully mature needs nutritional support for her own growth. Older women who are in good health have the same nutritional requirements as younger pregnant women. They may have more knowledge about nutrition through life experiences or need as much teaching as younger women. They are more likely to be financially secure than very young women.

Nutritional Knowledge

Even women who have not been attentive to their diets before pregnancy often try to learn about the relationship between what they eat and the effect on the fetus once pregnancy is confirmed. Although women know they should "eat well" during pregnancy, they may have little idea of the meaning. Some women lack basic understanding of nutrition and have misconceptions based on common food myths that interfere with good nutritional choices. These expectant mothers may seek information about nutrition from books, magazine articles, or on the Internet. They benefit from help from nurses in learning about nutrition.

Exercise

Moderate exercise during pregnancy is encouraged. Women who are athletes or exercise more strenuously may need modifications of their diet to meet additional nutritional needs. Extra calories may be needed to make up for the energy used during exercise. A serving of fruit, yogurt, or pasta before and after exercise may be sufficient. Additional fluids should be taken during and after exercise as well. Depending on the amount of exercise and the trimester of pregnancy, more nutrients may also be needed. The woman should consult her health care provider for an evaluation of nutrition during exercise (Gunderson, 2003).

Culture

Food is important in all cultures and often has special meaning during pregnancy and childbirth when certain foods may be favored or discouraged. Nurses need to be aware of the habits of a variety of cultures so that they can provide culturally appropriate nutritional counseling. Before making assumptions about the influence of a woman's culture on her diet, the nurse must assess each woman individually. Not all women follow food practices considered typical for their cultures.

The nurse should assess the woman's age, how long she has lived in North America, and whether she has adopted any eating habits that are prevalent. Greater exposure to North American diet may cause younger members of a group to make more dietary changes than older relatives. Some women who usually follow an American diet may return to aspects of their traditional cultural diet during pregnancy to "make sure" they do not harm the fetus.

Nurses often give women pamphlets in the appropriate language during nutritional teaching.

■ Before giving a woman written materials, the nurse should determine if the woman can read English or her native language. People who cannot read may not readily admit it to others. In addition, the reading level may be too complicated for a woman with little education to understand. Having an interpreter discuss the material with the woman helps in the determination of how well she can read and aids in other teaching.

People of many cultures believe that certain foods, conditions, and medicines are "hot" or "cold" and must be balanced to preserve health (Table 9-8). Foods considered hot in one culture may not fit in that category in another culture, and the designation does not necessarily match the temperature of the food. In some Asian cultures, this belief is expressed with terms such as *yin* (Chinese) or *eum* (Korean) for cold and *yang* (Chinese or Korean) for hot and may influence what the mother eats during pregnancy and the postpartum period.

Food taboos may determine what some women eat during the childbearing period. For example, Korean women may avoid chicken, pork, and blemished fruits during pregnancy. These foods are believed to have a harmful effect on the infant's physical appearance. Special foods may be customary during pregnancy or after birth. A Korean family may bring the woman *miyuk-kuk*, a hot seaweed soup served after birth to new mothers (Kim-Godwin, 2003).

TABLE 9-8 Common "Hot" and "Cold" Foods in Southeast Asian and Hispanic Diets*

"Hot" Foods	"Cold" Foods
Southeast Asian	
Yang Foods	*Yin Foods*
Peppers, onions	Most fruits and juices
Pork and poultry	Flour
Fish and fish sauce	Cold fluids
Broth	Sour foods
Eggs	Noodles
Spices, salty foods	Beef
Rice	Green vegetables
Hispanic	
Potatoes, peas, onions, chili peppers, garlic	Most fruits and vegetables
Cheese, evaporated milk	Milk
Chicken, lamb	Fish
Flour tortillas	Corn tortillas
Chickpeas and kidney beans	Green and red beans

*Although variations exist within cultural groups, foods considered hot are used for conditions thought to be cold, and vice versa. This influences what women are willing to eat during pregnancy or illness, and such customs must be respected during nursing care.

Cultural preferences for foods are extremely varied. For instance, some African-Americans follow a diet similar to that of people living in the southeastern United States. This diet includes foods such as okra, collard greens, mustard greens, ham hocks, black-eyed peas, and hominy or grits. The diet of other African-Americans, however, varies according to the geographic area in which they live.

Iron-deficiency anemia occurs in 15% of African-American women of childbearing age, compared with 10% of white women (U.S. Department of Health and Human Services, 2000). Lactose intolerance is common and results in a lack of calcium if other sources are not present in the diet. Intake of high-sodium and fried foods may present health problems.

Some Jewish women follow a strictly kosher diet. They avoid meat from animals that do not have cloven hooves, which excludes pork and pork products. The meat must be processed to remove all blood and cannot be eaten in the same meal as milk. Muslim women also do not eat pork and may fast on certain days. Although the religion exempts pregnant and nursing women from obligatory fasting, the woman may choose to fast during this time so they do not have to make up the fasting days at another time (Earl, 2004).

The diet of Native American women may contain corn, beans, and squash but be low in fresh fruits and vegetables. Lactose intolerance is common, and milk and cheese are avoided. Fried dough ("fry bread") is frequently served (Earl, 2004). Fat, carbohydrate, sodium, and sugar intake is often high. Low-income Native Americans living on reservations may receive foods such as white flour, cornmeal, white rice, and processed meats from federal programs. Eating berries during pregnancy is thought to cause a birthmark, and eating liver is believed to darken the skin (Cesario, 2001).

Food preferences for two cultures, Southeast Asian and Hispanic, are explored further here to show the influence of culture on diet. Immigrants from Southeast Asia and their families are the third largest ethnic group in the United States. African-Americans are the largest group, and Hispanics are the next largest group (Earl, 2004). Nurses throughout the United States need information about food preferences prevalent in these groups.

SOUTHEAST ASIAN DIETARY PRACTICES

Southeast Asians come from Cambodia, Laos, and Vietnam. Traditional cooking methods in these countries include searing fresh vegetables quickly with small portions of meat, poultry, or fish in a little oil over high heat. Meals cooked in this manner are low in fat and retain vitamins. Most meals are accompanied by rice, which increases the intake of complex carbohydrates, and soup. A salty fish sauce called *nuoc mam* and fresh vegetables are also part of most meals. Tofu and fresh fruits are frequent additions.

Many Southeast Asians eat larger amounts of U.S. foods, such as eggs, beef, pork, and bread, which add nutrients but also fat to the diet. Candy, soft drinks, coffee, butter or margarine, and fast foods have been less favorable influences because they are low in nutrients but high in sugar or fat. The intake of fish, a low-fat source of protein has decreased (Williams, 2003a).

EFFECT OF CULTURE ON DIET DURING CHILDBEARING. In Southeast Asian cultures, pregnancy (especially the third trimester) is considered "hot," and the woman is encouraged to eat "cold" foods to maintain a balance. She eats more sour foods, fruits, noodles, spinach, and mung beans and avoids fish, excessively salty or spicy foods, alcohol, and rice. She avoids unfamiliar foods for fear that they may harm her or her fetus.

The postpartum period is considered "cold," partly because of the loss of blood, which is "hot." Mothers avoid losing more heat, which would negatively affect their health. They stay warm physically and choose "hot" foods to eat, including rice with fish sauce, broth, salty meats, fish, chicken, and eggs. They may avoid sour or greasy foods, beef, and fruits and green vegetables after birth (Davis, 2001; Mattson, 2004). Cold drinks may be refused, but women may welcome hot fluids, requesting tea or plain hot water. Families frequently bring food to the mother while she is in the hospital because hospital food may not meet her preferences.

The diet of Southeast Asians, especially those with low incomes, may be high in sodium but below recommended levels for energy, calcium, iron, zinc, magnesium, and vitamins B_6 and D. These deficiencies may be of special concern during pregnancy. The woman can often increase her intake of needed nutrients without deviating greatly from her usual diet.

INCREASING NUTRIENTS WITH TRADITIONAL FOODS. Milk products are not part of the traditional Southeast Asian diet, and lactose intolerance is common. Increasing the intake of commonly used dark green leafy vegetables such as mustard greens, bok choy, and broccoli, however, increases levels of calcium, iron, magnesium, and folic acid. Tofu is a good source of calcium and iron. A broth made from pork or chicken bones soaked in vinegar, which removes calcium from the bones, is frequently served. If the mother avoids fortified milk, she may need vitamin D supplementation. Increasing the intake of meats and poultry elevates levels of protein, iron, vitamin B_6, and zinc.

HISPANIC DIETARY PRACTICES

Spanish-speaking people such as Mexican-Americans, Puerto Ricans, and Cuban-Americans are often referred to as *Hispanics* or *Latinos*. Like many Asians, many Hispanics follow the theories of "hot" and "cold" foods and conditions. They also consider pregnancy to be "hot" and the postpartum period to be "cold" and adjust the diet accordingly. During pregnancy, Hispanic women may be encouraged to satisfy food cravings (Mattson, 2003).

Dried beans (especially pinto beans) are a staple of the Mexican-American diet and are part of most meals, served alone, in the form of refried beans, or mixed with other foods such as rice. The major grain is corn, which is ground and made into a dough called *masa* to make corn tortillas. The corn is treated with lime and is a good source of calcium. Corn and flour tortillas are eaten with most meals. Rice is also an important grain. Although milk is not commonly used except for infants, cheese is used in many dishes. Chili peppers and tomatoes are the most common vegetables in Hispanic diets. Green leafy and yellow vegetables are seldom included.

Hispanic foods are often hot, spicy, and fried. The diet is high in fiber and complex carbohydrates. However, it tends to be high in calories and fat, leading many Mexican-Americans to become overweight. The diet may be low in iron, calcium, and vitamins A and D, which should be increased through foods or supplements during pregnancy.

Puerto Rican and Cuban diets are similar to that of Mexican-Americans, with the addition of tropical fruits and vegetables from the homeland when available. Viandas, which are starchy fruits, and vegetables such as plantains, green bananas, sweet potatoes, yams, and breadfruit are common. They may be cooked with codfish and onion. Guava, papaya, mango, and eggplant also are used when available.

✔ CHECK YOUR READING

13. When the nurse assesses cultural influences on nutrition during pregnancy, what factors must be considered?
14. Compare the diet of Southeast Asian women with that of Hispanic women.

NUTRITIONAL RISK FACTORS

Many factors may interfere with a woman's ability to meet the nutritional needs of pregnancy. Some of these are discussed in the following sections.

Socioeconomic Status

POVERTY

Low-income women may have deficient diets because of lack of financial resources and nutritional education. Carbohydrate foods are often less expensive than meats, dairy products, fresh fruits, and vegetables. Therefore the diet may be high in calories but low in vitamins and minerals. A referral to Temporary Assistance to Needy Families (TANF) or the Special Supplemental Nutrition Program for Women, Infants, and Children (WIC) may be helpful if a woman's food intake is inadequate because of lack of money. Vitamin-mineral supplementation may be important for her, especially if her diet is likely to be inconsistent.

FOOD SUPPLEMENT PROGRAMS

The WIC program is administered by the USDA to provide nutritional assessment, counseling, and education to low-income women and children up to age 5 years who are at nutritional risk. The program also provides vouchers for foods such as milk, cheese, eggs, iron-fortified cereal, fruit juice, dried beans, peanut butter, and formula to qualified women and their children. Eligibility is based on an income at or below 185% of the federal poverty level. Women are eligible throughout pregnancy and for 6 months after birth if formula feeding or 1 year if breastfeeding.

Adolescence

Adolescent pregnancies are associated with higher risk for complications for both the expectant mother and the fetus (see Chapter 24). Adolescents at greatest risk for problem pregnancies are those who are the youngest in terms of gynecologic age (number of years since menarche) and those who are still growing. Maternal growth may interfere with placental blood flow and transfer of nutrients to the fetus. As a result the adolescent mother may add weight and fat to her own body rather than use it for support of the fetus. This leads to a tendency to have smaller infants even with good weight gains in the mother (Spear, 2004). Weight gain for the young pregnant adolescent should be in the upper part of the range suggested for her BMI.

NUTRIENT NEEDS

The DRIs for nutrients needed by pregnant adolescents are the same as those for older women for most nutrients. Adolescents need more calcium, phosphorus, magnesium, and zinc to meet their own growth needs. Individualized assessment of gynecologic age, nutritional status, and daily diet may indicate the need for increases in some other areas. Increased amounts of energy, protein, and iron may be necessary for some younger adolescents who are still growing.

COMMON PROBLEMS

The diets of teenagers before and during pregnancy are often low in vitamins C and A, folic acid, calcium, iron, and zinc (Schlenker, 2003). Supplements may be prescribed, but the adolescent may not take them regularly. This combination of poor intake and unreliable supplementation may further deplete nutrient stores and worsen general nutritional status.

Peer pressure is an important influence on nutritional status. Adolescents are often concerned about body image. If weight is a major focus for a teenager and her peers, she is more likely to restrict calories to prevent weight gain during pregnancy. Teenagers tend to skip meals, especially breakfast. The fetus requires a steady supply of nutrients, and the expectant mother's stores may be used if intake is not sufficient to meet energy needs.

Teenagers are often in a hurry and want foods that are fast and convenient. Meals may be irregular and are often eaten away from home. A significant part of the adolescent diet consists of fast foods from restaurants or snack machines. These foods are often high in calories and sodium, and many derive more than 50% of their calories from fats. Fast foods tend to be low in calcium, iron, riboflavin, folic acid, and vitamins A and C (Spear, 2004). Choosing fast foods that do not make her appear different from her peers yet meet her added nutrient needs are important for the pregnant adolescent. (See Nursing Care Plan 9-1.)

NURSING CARE PLAN **9-1** Nutrition for the Pregnant Adolescent

ASSESSMENT: Vicki, age 15, is 20 weeks pregnant and has gained 3.6 kg (8 lb). She attends school and lives at home but usually cooks for herself because "I don't like the stuff Mom cooks." She skips breakfast and eats from snack machines during breaks at school. She goes to fast food restaurants for lunch and after-school snacks. Vicki says she is disgusted with how heavy she is and wants to go on a diet to lose some weight. Her hemoglobin level is 10.4 g/dl. She listens with interest when the nurse discusses nutrition, especially when weight is mentioned. Her statements show concern about her baby's needs. Vicki was at a normal weight before her pregnancy, and a weight gain of approximately 16 kg (35 lb) is appropriate for her. Her gynecologic age is 2.5 years.

NURSING DIAGNOSIS: Imbalanced Nutrition: Less Than Body Requirements related to concern about weight gain and dietary choices inadequate to meet nutrient requirements of adolescent pregnancy

CRITICAL THINKING: What other information does the nurse need to complete the assessment? Is Vicki's weight gain what is expected for this point in pregnancy?

ANSWER: A 24-hour diet history is necessary for a better understanding of Vicki's diet. The nurse should also ask about her likes and dislikes to make a meaningful diet plan for Vicki. At 20 weeks of pregnancy, Vicki would be expected to have gained about 1.6 kg (3.5 lb) during the first trimester and another 0.4 kg (approximately 1 lb) a week for the other 7 weeks, for a total of approximately 4.8 kg (10.5 lb) by the time of this assessment. Therefore her weekly weight gain for the rest of pregnancy should be at least 0.4 kg (approximately 1 lb) or slightly greater.

The diet history reveals Vicki eats few dairy foods, although she says she does not dislike them. She dislikes cooked vegetables but will eat salads and some raw vegetables.

Continued

NURSING CARE PLAN 9-1 Nutrition for the Pregnant Adolescent—cont'd

GOALS/EXPECTED OUTCOMES: Vicki will:

1. Explain the weight gain pattern and number of servings from each food group optimal for adolescent pregnancy.
2. List foods she can choose at fast food restaurants that meet her nutrient needs and allow her to feel part of her peer group.
3. Gain approximately 0.4 to 0.57 kg (0.88 to 1.25 lb) per week for the rest of her pregnancy.
4. Attain and maintain a hemoglobin level of at least 11 g/dl during the third trimester of pregnancy.

INTERVENTION	RATIONALE
1. Praise Vicki for her interest in nutrition and her concern about gaining too much weight.	1. Praise helps foster rapport and may focus attention on learning.
2. Discuss the reasons for appropriate weight gain during pregnancy and its effect on the fetus. Explain the needs of the adolescent who is not finished growing and the importance of preventing the problems associated with low birth weight in the infant.	2. Adolescents may not understand how diet affects the fetus and expectant mother during pregnancy. Explanation of the potential effects of her actions should increase the expectant mother's interest in nutrition.
3. Assist Vicki in comparing her food intake with the recommended servings from each food group. Point out areas of strength, and praise her for them.	3. Active involvement of the learner and positive reinforcement help increase motivation.
4. Ask Vicki what problems she sees in her diet. Point out areas she may have missed. Explain the effect that lack of specific nutrients may have on the fetus.	4. Adolescents learn best when they see how the material applies to them.
5. Discuss the high caloric intake of fast foods in relation to her present diet, and explain the concept of nutrient density in terms of "spending calories" to "buy" nutrients needed during pregnancy.	5. Relating information to concepts already understood increases understanding.
6. Determine, from Vicki's food preferences, low-calorie foods that meet her nutrient needs and are acceptable to her. Point out fruits and vegetables high in vitamins A and C, yet low in calories.	6. Individualizing the recommended diet to meet the woman's likes and dislikes increases compliance.
7. Suggest nutritional foods that Vicki could choose at fast food restaurants, and ask which ones she would eat.	7. The adolescent needs to feel that she is part of her peer group. Including her input on what she likes to eat may increase her compliance.
8. Discuss the importance of breakfast during pregnancy. Explain that the fetus needs a steady supply of nutrients especially in the morning after the long fast during the night.	8. Prolonged periods without maternal food intake can lead to a state of ketosis that is hostile to the fetus.
9. Discuss breakfast foods that Vicki likes. Point out the nutrients found in whole grain breads and cereals (protein, iron, B vitamins) and their importance.	9. Whole grains are often a part of a well-balanced breakfast.
10. Suggest that Vicki eat foods not usually considered breakfast foods if she prefers. For example, cold pizza or a cheeseburger will provide calcium and protein.	10. Nontraditional methods of meeting the adolescent's nutritional needs may be very effective.
11. Suggest foods high in nutrient density that are available from snack dispensers. Ask which of these are agreeable to Vicki.	11. Adolescents are unlikely to give up foods that help them feel part of their peer group. Snacks can be important sources of nutrients.
12. After explaining the importance of dairy products to her and her baby, ask Vicki if she is willing to eat more of them. Help her choose those she will eat to meet her needs.	12. Compliance is increased when clients maintain a feeling of control.
13. Ask Vicki if she is taking her vitamin-mineral supplements and how she is tolerating them. Offer suggestions on how to deal with any problems she is having in this area. Reinforce the importance of consistent intake.	13. Adolescents generally need supplements but may take them inconsistently, especially if side effects are experienced.
14. Ask Vicki to bring in another 24-hour diet history on her next visit.	14. Reassessment of dietary intake identifies new or continuing problems.
15. Suggest that Vicki share with you any ways she has found to meet her dietary needs that you could tell other teenagers. Ask for feedback on the methods discussed.	15. It is important for the adolescent to feel that her thoughts and ideas are valued by the nurse.

EVALUATION: Vicki's 24-hour diet histories show that she is meeting the recommendations for each food group. She gains 1.8 to 2.7 kg (4 to 6 lb) per month throughout the rest of her pregnancy for a total weight gain of 15 kg (33 lb). She brings back ideas about ways to eat fast foods healthfully and seems to like educating the nurse about teenage diet preferences. Her hemoglobin level rises to 11 g/dl. A healthy 3.4-kg (7.5-lb) baby girl is born at term.

TEACHING THE ADOLESCENT

Teaching the adolescent about nutrition can be a challenge for nurses. It is essential to establish an accepting, relaxed atmosphere and show willingness to listen to the teenager's concerns. Her lifestyle, pattern of eating, and food likes and dislikes should be explored to determine if changes are necessary in the diet.

The adolescent's home life may affect her nutritional status. She may live at home with a mother who does the cooking, and the whole family may eat together. Or she may eat with the family only occasionally because she is often away at mealtimes. Some pregnant adolescents are homeless or in unstable situations. The number of other people in the home and the sufficiency of the food available also affect the dietary intake.

Suggestions should be kept to a minimum, and the nurse should focus on only those changes that are necessary. If an adolescent believes she must eliminate all her favorite foods, she is likely to rebel. Asking for the adolescent's input increases the likelihood that she will follow suggestions. When changes are necessary the nurse should explain why they are important for both the fetus and the expectant mother. Teenagers, like other pregnant women, often make changes for the sakes of their unborn children that they would not consider for themselves alone.

The need to be like her peers is of major importance to the adolescent, especially when she is going through the changes of pregnancy. With education about appropriate choices, she can eat fast foods with her friends and still maintain a nourishing diet. Giving her plenty of examples of alternatives from which she can choose should be very helpful (Table 9-9 and "Pregnant Adolescents Want to Know").

Vegetarianism

Although the knowledgeable vegetarian may eat a highly nutritious diet, she is at higher risk during pregnancy when her nutrient intake must nourish the fetus and herself. If she is new to vegetarian food practices, uninformed about pregnancy needs, or careless with her diet, she could fail to meet her nutrient needs. Guidelines for vegetarian foods during pregnancy (Table 9-10) are similar to those for nonvegetarians.

TABLE 9-9 Nutritious Choices from Snack Machines*

Food	Nutrients Provided
Yogurt, white or chocolate milk	Protein, calcium
Fruit juices or fresh fruits (usually apples or oranges)	Vitamins, fiber
Popcorn (best without butter or salt)	Fiber
Peanuts	Protein, vitamins, calcium, iron
Granola or granola bars	Fiber, protein
Crackers and cheese	Protein, calcium
Crackers and peanut butter	Protein

*Snack machines generally dispense foods high in calories, fats, and sodium and low in nutrients. The foods listed here, although somewhat high in calories, provide other worthwhile nutrients.

TABLE 9-10 Food Plan for Pregnant or Lactating Vegetarians*

Food	Number of Servings for Pregnancy	Number of Servings for Lactation
Whole and enriched grains	6	6
Protein-rich foods: legumes, nuts, soy, meat substitutes, eggs, dairy	7	8
Vegetables†	4	4
Fruits†	2	2
Fats	2	2
Calcium-rich foods (included in the above food group servings)	8	8
B_{12}-rich foods (may be included in above groups) or a B_{12} supplement	4	4

Data from Messina, V. Melina, V., & Mangels, A.R. (2003). A new food guide for North American vegetarians. *Journal of the American Dietetic Association, 103*(6), 771-775.
*A serving of a calcium-rich food is also counted as a serving of one of the other food groups. Adolescents need six servings of protein-rich foods and 10 servings of calcium-rich foods. Vegans need B_{12} supplementation. Vitamin and mineral supplements may be necessary according to individual needs.
†At least 1 additional serving of vegetables and 2 additional servings of fruits are needed to meet the 2005 Dietary Guidelines for Americans.

PREGNANT ADOLESCENTS WANT TO KNOW How Can I Eat Fast Foods and Still Maintain a Good Diet?

- Add cheese to hamburgers to increase calcium and protein. Include lettuce and tomato for vitamins A and C.
- Avoid dressings on hamburgers because they tend to be high in calories and fat.
- To reduce fat and calories, choose broiled, roasted, and barbecued foods (such as chicken breast, roast beef). Avoid fried foods (such as French fries, fried zucchini, onion rings) because they are high in fat and the high heat may destroy some vitamins. Breaded foods like chicken nuggets and breaded clams are high in calories and absorb more oil if they are fried.
- Baked potatoes with broccoli, cheese, and meat fillings provide better nutrition than French fries or even baked potatoes with sour cream and butter.

- Pizza is high in calories, but the cheese provides protein and calcium. Ask for vegetable toppings or add a salad to increase vitamins.
- Salad bars are often available at fast food restaurants and provide vitamins and minerals without adding too many calories. Use only a small amount of salad dressing, which is high in fat.
- Milk, milkshakes, and orange juice provide more nutrients than carbonated beverages, which are high in sodium and calories. Too much sodium may increase swelling of the ankles.
- Avoid pickles, olives, and other salty foods. Add only small amounts of salt to foods to prevent or decrease swelling.

Vegetarianism occurs in a variety of forms. Vegans avoid all animal products and may have the most difficulty meeting their nutrient needs. Their diet may be lacking in adequate calcium, iron, zinc, and vitamins D and B$_{12}$ (Grodner et al, 2000; Earl, 2004). Vegans must pay particular attention to obtaining these nutrients in food or supplement form. It is easier for lactovegetarians, ovovegetarians, and lacto-ovovegetarians to meet their nutrient needs.

Although not true vegetarianism, a diet that includes the elimination of red meats to decrease intake of saturated fats and cholesterol is a growing trend. Women who follow this type of diet usually eat small amounts of chicken, fish, and dairy products. The needs of women who follow any form of vegetarianism are different during pregnancy.

MEETING THE NUTRITIONAL REQUIREMENTS OF PREGNANCY

ENERGY. Vegetarian diets are low in calories and fat and may not meet the energy needs of pregnancy. The diets are high in fiber and may cause a feeling of fullness before enough calories are eaten. A pregnant woman can increase caloric intake by eating snacks and foods with higher caloric content. If carbohydrate and fat intake are too low, her body may use protein for energy, making it unavailable for other purposes.

PROTEIN. Although most vegetarians get enough protein, this area needs consideration, especially in vegan diets. "Complete" proteins contain all the essential amino acids the body cannot synthesize from other sources. Animal proteins are complete, but plant proteins lack one or more of the essential amino acids. Combining incomplete plant proteins with other plant foods that have complementary amino acids allows intake of all essential amino acids. Dishes that contain grains (wheat, rice, corn) and legumes (garbanzo, navy, kidney, pinto, or soy beans, peas, peanuts) provide complete proteins. Complementary proteins do not have to be eaten at the same meal if they are consumed in a single day.

Incomplete proteins can also be combined with small amounts of complete protein foods such as cheese to provide all amino acids. Therefore women who include even small amounts of animal products meet their protein needs more easily.

Many vegetarians use tofu, made from soybeans, which provides protein as well as calcium and iron. Meat analogs that have a taste and texture similar to meat but are made from textured vegetable protein are available. Some look and taste similar to hamburgers, bacon, lunch meats, chicken patties, and other commonly eaten foods. Meat analogs may be fortified with nutrients whose levels are often low in vegan diets.

CALCIUM. Vegetarians who include milk products in the diet may meet their pregnancy needs for calcium. Vegans obtain calcium from vegetables, but their high-fiber diet may interfere with calcium absorption. Calcium-fortified juices or soy products such as soy milk or tofu may meet the requirements. Calcium supplements may be necessary. Vitamin D supplementation is especially important if the woman drinks no milk and has little exposure to sunlight. Soy milks may be enriched with vitamin D.

IRON. Iron in the vegetarian diet is poorly absorbed because of the lack of heme iron from meats, which improves absorption. Absorption is enhanced by eating a source of vitamin C in the same meal as nonheme iron or cooking in cast-iron pans. Iron supplementation is particularly important for vegetarian women during pregnancy.

ZINC. Because the best sources of zinc are meat and fish, vegans may be deficient in this mineral. They may need zinc supplements to meet their needs.

VITAMIN B$_{12}$. Vitamin B$_{12}$ is obtained only from animal products. Because vegetarian diets contain large amounts of folic acid, the development of anemia from inadequate intake of vitamin B$_{12}$ may not be apparent at first. Vegans may eat fortified foods such as cereal and soy products or may take supplements.

VITAMIN A. Vitamin A is generally abundant in vegetarian diets. If a pregnant woman takes multiple vitamin-mineral supplements, her intake of vitamin A may be excessive, causing toxicity with anorexia, irritability, hair loss, and dry skin and damage to the fetus. Supplementation should be individualized for each woman based on her diet and needs.

Lactose Intolerance

Intolerance to lactose is caused by a deficiency of the small intestine enzyme lactase, which is necessary for absorption of lactose, a milk sugar. Some degree of lactose intolerance is normal for most of the world's population after early childhood. This includes many African-American, Hispanic, Asian, Native American, and Middle-Eastern women. Although women with lactose intolerance may tolerate cultured and fermented milk products such as aged cheese, buttermilk, and some brands of yogurt, symptoms may occur after drinking as little as a cup of milk. Symptoms include nausea, bloating, flatulence, diarrhea, and intestinal cramping.

Although the ability to tolerate lactose may increase during pregnancy, women who avoid dairy foods are at risk for not getting the recommended amounts of calcium. Most women can tolerate small amounts (½ cup) of milk, and they should increase their intake of other foods that provide calcium. Soy milk, low-lactose milk, and milk treated with lactase are available. The enzyme can be purchased to be added to milk or taken as a tablet. Calcium supplements may be necessary for some lactose-intolerant women.

Nausea and Vomiting of Pregnancy

Morning sickness usually disappears soon after the first trimester, although some women experience nausea at other times of the day and for longer than 12 weeks. Most women can consume enough food to maintain nutrition sufficiently. They are often able to manage frequent, small meals better than three large meals. Protein and complex carbohydrates are often tolerated best, but fatty foods increase nausea. Drinking liquids between meals instead of with meals often helps. Eating a bedtime protein snack such as cheese helps maintain glucose levels through the night. Eating a carbohydrate food such as dry toast or crackers before getting out of bed in the morning helps prevent nausea. (See Nursing Care Plan 7-1 on p. 142.)

Anemia

Anemia is a common concern during pregnancy. A Healthy People 2010 goal is to reduce iron deficiency anemia in females of childbearing age from the baseline of 11% to 7% and to reduce anemia in low-income pregnant women in the third trimester from the baseline of 29% to 20% (U.S. Department of Health and Human Services, 2000).

Hemoglobin values decrease during the second trimester of pregnancy as a result of the dilution of the blood caused by plasma increases. This physiologic anemia is normal (see Chapter 7). During the third trimester, hemoglobin levels generally rise to prepregnant levels because of increased absorption of iron from the gastrointestinal tract, even though iron is transferred to the fetus primarily during this time.

If fetal iron stores during the third trimester are sufficient, anemia will not develop in the newborn for the first 4 to 6 months after birth. However, if the woman's intake of iron is insufficient, her hemoglobin levels may not rise during the third trimester, nutritional anemia may develop, and transfer of iron to the fetus may be decreased.

Iron stores may be measured by determining the serum ferritin level in the blood. A ferritin level less than 12 micrograms per liter (mcg/L) indicates that the anemia is caused by iron deficiency (Kilpatrick & Laros, 2004). A woman may begin pregnancy with anemia or develop it during pregnancy. She is considered anemic if her hemoglobin is less than 11 g/dl during the first and third trimesters or less than 10.5 g/dl during the second trimester (Cunningham et al, 2001).

Anemic women need help choosing foods high in iron. They should take iron supplements because diet alone is unlikely to provide adequate amounts of iron. Iron supplements are better absorbed if taken at bedtime or between meals with a dietary source of vitamin C to increase absorption. Because high intakes of iron inhibit use of zinc and copper, anemic women may need to take these minerals also.

Abnormal Prepregnancy Weight

In addition to teaching about dietary changes, the nurse should be alert for problems associated with abnormal prepregnancy weight. The woman who is below normal weight may not have enough money for food or may have an eating disorder. In addition, obese woman may have other health problems such as hypertension that may affect the nurse's nutritional counseling plan.

Eating Disorders

Eating disorders include anorexia nervosa (refusal to eat because of a distorted body image and feelings of obesity) and bulimia (overeating sometimes followed by induced vomiting). These conditions can be a threat to pregnancy and fetal development and require close supervision during pregnancy (James, 2001). Some women with these disorders eat normally during pregnancy for the sake of the fetus. For others, old fears about obesity may be reactivated by the normal weight gain of pregnancy. They may return to their previous eating patterns during pregnancy or in the early postpartum period when they do not lose weight immediately. These women need a great deal of individual counseling to ensure that they meet the increased nutrient needs of pregnancy and understand normal postpartum weight loss.

Food Cravings and Aversions

Women may have a strong preference or a strong dislike for certain foods that is present only in pregnancy. Cravings for pickles, ice cream (not necessarily together), pizza, chocolate, cake, candy, spicy foods, and dairy products are common. Food aversions are most often to coffee, alcoholic beverages, highly seasoned or fried foods, and meats. The cause of cravings and aversions is not known, but they may be a result of changes in sense of taste and smell. They are generally not harmful, and some, like aversion to alcohol, may be beneficial (Kleinman, 2004; Mitchell, 2003).

PICA

Some women have cravings for nonnutritive substances. The practice of eating substances not normally considered food is called *pica*. Ice, clay or dirt, and laundry starch or cornstarch are the most common materials, but other items such as freezer frost, chalk, baking soda, burnt matches, or ashes may be included. Pica is more common in inner cities and in the rural areas of the southeastern United States, in African-Americans, in women who live in poverty and have poor nutrition, and in those with a childhood or family history of the practice. However, pica is not limited to any socioeconomic group or geographic area.

The cause of pica is unknown, although cultural values may make pica a common practice. Pica may be related to beliefs regarding a material's effects on labor or the baby. For example, some women believe that starch gives the skin a lighter tone or helps the baby to be born more easily. Pica is frequently associated with poor nutrition and may be a sign of iron deficiency anemia (Kilpatrick & Laros, 2004).

The major concern with pica is that it may decrease the intake of foods and essential nutrients. Clay and dirt may decrease absorption of other nutrients such as iron, may be contaminated with organisms, and may cause intestinal blockage. They may also be contaminated with toxins such as lead. Some women fear that their eating habits are harmful but are unable to ignore the cravings. They may hide their eating practices from caregivers who might disapprove.

CRITICAL THINKING ⚲EXERCISE 9-1

Joan very hesitantly confides in the nurse that the reason she is not gaining much weight is that she eats large amounts of ice. She buys bags of crushed ice each day. "I know I should be gaining more weight, but I'm just not hungry for anything besides ice," she says.

Questions
1. What might happen if Joan believes the nurse disapproves of her actions?
2. How should the nurse handle this situation?

Multiparity and Multifetal Pregnancy

The number and spacing of pregnancies and the presence of more than one fetus influence the nutritional requirements. The woman who has had five or more pregnancies may begin a pregnancy with a nutritional deficit. In addition, she may be too busy meeting the needs of her family to be attentive to her own nutritional needs.

Closely spaced pregnancies may not allow a woman to make up any nutritional deficits originating from a previous pregnancy. Therefore she begins a new pregnancy with inadequate nutrient stores to maintain both her own needs and fetal requirements. She is unable to draw from those stores as usual during pregnancy and must meet nutritional needs from her daily diet and supplementation alone. The development of morning sickness from a new pregnancy soon after delivery may further interfere with an expectant mother's ability to eat an adequate diet.

The woman with a multifetal pregnancy must provide enough nutrients to meet the needs of each fetus without depleting her own stores. She needs more calories to meet her weight gain and energy needs. An additional gain of 4.5 to 9 kg (10 to 20 lb) above that of single pregnancies is suggested for women who are pregnant with twins. Women pregnant with twins should gain 1.5 kg (3.3 lb) each week in the second and third trimesters. Women carrying triplets should gain 1.5 kg (3.3 lb) weekly throughout pregnancy (Abrams, Minassian, & Pickett, 2004). Supplementation with calcium, iron, and folic acid also may be necessary.

Substance Abuse

The damaging effects of smoking, alcohol, and drug use on the fetus are discussed in Chapter 24. Substance abuse often accompanies a lifestyle that is unlikely to promote healthy eating habits. The expense of supporting a substance abuse habit may decrease money available to purchase food. Therefore nutrition in pregnant women who abuse substances should be explored fully. Usually more than one substance is involved, and the effects on nutrition of various combinations of substances are not fully understood.

SMOKING

Cigarette smoking increases maternal metabolic rate and decreases appetite, which may result in a lower weight gain. Infant birth weight decreases despite an adequate diet as the amount of smoking increases. Prematurity, spontaneous abortion, and other complications may also result. Smoking causes vasoconstriction that interferes with blood flow through the placenta. The many chemicals found in cigarette smoke may also retard fetal growth. Smoking decreases the absorption of some vitamins and minerals, which makes vitamin-mineral supplements important during pregnancy. Counseling to help the woman stop smoking or at least de-

crease the number of cigarettes smoked during pregnancy is essential (see Chapter 7).

CAFFEINE

The effect of caffeine on nutrition during pregnancy is controversial. Most studies show no association between caffeine and preterm labor or congenital defects, but more research is needed. Mothers who consume more than 300 mg per day have an increased risk of having infants who are small for gestational age (Andres, 2004). Caffeine changes calcium, zinc, thiamin, and iron absorption or excretion. Until more is known about the effects of caffeine on nutrition and the fetus, daily caffeine intake should be limited during pregnancy to 300 mg per day (equal to two or three cups of coffee, six cups of tea, or five carbonated beverages with caffeine). The nurse should discuss other sources of caffeine, including chocolate and some over-the-counter medications.

ALCOHOL

Because of the association between drinking and fetal alcohol syndrome, women should avoid alcohol completely during pregnancy (see Chapter 24). Alcohol interferes with absorption and use of protein, thiamine, folic acid, and zinc; impairs metabolism; and often takes the place of food in the diet. Vitamin-mineral supplementation may be necessary for women who had large intakes of alcohol before pregnancy, even if they stop drinking after conception, because their nutrient stores may be depleted.

DRUGS

The use of drugs other than those prescribed during pregnancy increases danger to the fetus and may interfere with nutrition. Abusers often use a combination of various drugs, and they may not be pure. The interaction of various drugs with nutrients is not fully understood.

Marijuana increases appetite, but women may not satisfy their hunger with foods of good nutrient quality. Heroin interferes with insulin response to glucose and metabolism and may cause a woman to become malnourished. Cocaine acts as an appetite suppressant, interfering with nutrient intake. Vasoconstriction from cocaine use decreases nutrient flow to the fetus. Cocaine users also tend to drink more caffeine and alcoholic beverages. Amphetamines depress appetite. Women who use amphetamines for dieting should be warned that these drugs should be discontinued during pregnancy.

Other Risk Factors

Women who follow food fads may not meet the nutrient requirements for pregnancy. Women who have followed a severely restricted diet for a long time may have depleted nutrient stores. Nurses can help them understand the necessary diet changes to help ensure successful pregnancies.

Women with complications of pregnancy such as diabetes, heart disease, and preeclampsia may need dietary alterations. Those with other medical conditions such as extreme obesity, cystic fibrosis, and celiac disease may need nutritional counseling from a dietitian.

✔ CHECK YOUR READING

15. For what nutritional problems should the nurse assess when caring for low-income women?
16. What nutritional problems may the adolescent have during pregnancy?
17. What suggestions can the nurse give the vegan about diet during pregnancy?
18. How can lactose-intolerant women increase their intake of calcium?
19. What other conditions present nutritional risk factors during pregnancy?

NUTRITION AFTER BIRTH

Nutritional requirements after birth depend on whether the mother breastfeeds her infant or gives formula. The nurse should review the woman's nutritional knowledge as she returns to her prepregnancy diet and teach the breastfeeding mother ways to adapt her diet to meet the needs of lactation.

Nutrition for the Lactating Mother

The lactating mother must nourish both herself and her baby as she did during pregnancy. Therefore she continues to need a highly nutritious diet. The DRIs for lactation are higher for almost every nutrient compared with the needs of nonpregnant adult women. These recommendations are based on the assumption that the mother produces approximately 750 to 800 ml of breast milk daily. However, the amount of milk produced varies according to the infant's age and whether the infant is taking formula or solid foods with breast milk.

Lactating women with poor diets may have reduced milk levels of fatty acids, selenium, iodine, and some B vitamins (Shabert, 2004). Milk volume is usually adequate even when a mother's diet is less than optimal.

ENERGY

During the first 6 months of lactation, 500 calories are needed each day above prepregnancy requirements. Of that 500 calories, it is estimated that 170 calories per day are drawn from the woman's fat stores, aiding in weight loss. Therefore, the EER during the first 6 months of lactation is 330 calories each day in addition to normal needs for women according to age, weight, and height.

The EER for the second 6 months of lactation is 400 calories more than prepregnancy needs. Although the infant takes solids after 6 months and decreases the milk intake, it is assumed that maternal energy stores have been used and the calories should come from the woman's daily intake (Institute of Medicine, 2002a). Women who were underweight before pregnancy or those who had inadequate weight gain

during pregnancy need more calories. Those who are overweight may need fewer calories than the EER.

PROTEIN

The RDA for protein during lactation is 71 g each day, which is the same as that needed during pregnancy. Although no change in protein is needed, it is important for the woman to keep up her protein intake throughout the breastfeeding period.

VITAMINS AND MINERALS

The DRIs for lactating women are increased above pregnancy needs for vitamins A, B_6, B_{12}, C, and E and zinc, riboflavin, iodine, and selenium. Lactating women who take in at least 1800 calories (well below the energy intake recommended) probably consume adequate amounts of other essential nutrients to meet the infant's and their own needs. Although the quality of the milk is not affected by the mother's intake of most minerals, the vitamin content may be decreased if her diet is consistently low in vitamins. Vitamin D levels in the milk may be low if the mother has a low intake, is not exposed to the sun, or has dark skin (Shabert, 2004). Milk levels of some nutrients, such as calcium and folic acid, remain constant because some nutrients are drawn from the mother's stores if her intake is poor. Routine supplements are not necessary unless the diet is considered lacking in vitamins and minerals.

SPECIFIC CONCERNS

Some women have difficulty consuming all required nutrients and need special counseling. This group includes women who are dieting, adolescents, vegans, women who avoid dairy products, and those whose diet is inadequate for other reasons.

DIETING. Women who are concerned about losing weight after pregnancy need special consideration. After the initial losses in the first month, weight gradually decreases as maternal fat is used to meet a portion of the energy needs of lactation. Breastfeeding mothers tend to lose body fat even without dieting (Grodner et al., 2000). However, breastfeeding does not necessarily result in weight loss, and 20% of women maintain or even gain weight during lactation (Matteson, 2001). This is more likely when weight gain during pregnancy was excessive.

Dieting should be postponed for at least 3 weeks after birth to allow the woman to recover fully from childbirth and establish her milk supply if she is breastfeeding. Gradual weight loss is preferable and should be accomplished by a combination of moderate exercise and a diet high in nutrients with at least 1800 calories per day. Weight loss of approximately 0.45 kg (1 lb) a week is generally considered safe (Shabert, 2004).

Although moderate dieting does not affect the quantity of the milk, the mother should evaluate the infant's apparent satisfaction with feedings. She should not use liquid diet drinks or diets that severely restrict any nutrient because she will not meet her needs. Nursing mothers should avoid appetite suppressants, which may pass into the milk and harm the infant.

ADOLESCENCE. The problems of the adolescent diet continue to be of concern during lactation. The adolescent may be deficient in the same nutrients as other mothers during lactation and also lacking in iron. If she dislikes or cannot afford fruits and vegetables, she may have an inadequate vitamin A intake.

VEGAN DIET. The milk of the vegan mother may contain inadequate vitamin B_{12}, and she and her infant need supplementation. Vitamin D may also be low. Vegans can meet their need for other nutrients during lactation by diet alone with careful planning. Those who are not knowledgeable about nutrition should take supplements.

AVOIDANCE OF DAIRY PRODUCTS. The recommendation for calcium remains the same for pregnancy and lactation, and the calcium content of breast milk is not affected by maternal intake. Less calcium is excreted in the urine during lactation. Although calcium is removed from the mother's bones during lactation it is replaced when she is no longer breastfeeding (Witt & Mihok, 2003). Women who do not eat dairy products should obtain calcium from other sources or take a calcium supplement. Unless they consume foods fortified with vitamin D or are exposed to sunlight, they may also require vitamin D supplementation, which is necessary for calcium absorption.

INADEQUATE DIET. Women with cultural or other food prohibitions may need help choosing a diet adequate for lactation. Those with inadequate income may need referral to agencies such as WIC. If the mother must take medications that interfere with absorption of certain nutrients, her diet should be high in foods containing those nutrients.

ALCOHOL. Alcohol intake during lactation is another concern. Although the relaxing effect of alcohol was once considered helpful to the nursing mother, the damaging effects of alcohol are too important to consider this suggestion appropriate today. An occasional single glass of an alcoholic beverage may not be harmful, but larger amounts may interfere with the milk-ejection reflex and may be harmful to the infant. Alcohol in the milk peaks at 30 to 60 minutes after being ingested by the mother (Witt & Mihok, 2003).

CAFFEINE. Foods high in caffeine should also be limited. The mother should restrict her caffeine intake to two to three cups of coffee or the equivalent each day. Caffeine in excessive amounts can make some infants irritable.

FLUIDS. Nursing mothers should drink fluids sufficient to relieve thirst, which often increases in the early breastfeeding period. Eight to ten glasses of fluids that do not contain caffeine are adequate. Drinking large quantities of fluids, as was once recommended, is not necessary.

FOODS TO AVOID

Lactating mothers are often concerned about whether they should avoid certain foods that might adversely affect the infant. Except for foods to which the mother is allergic, no specific foods must be restricted in every case. Most mothers find that few foods affect the infant and fussiness is related to other factors. If the family history places the infant at risk for developing allergies, the woman should avoid highly allergenic foods including cow's milk, eggs, fish, and nuts (AAP, 2000).

Some infants react to a food in the mother's diet with excessive irritability, crying as if in pain, passing gas, diarrhea, or a rash. These signs may be caused when the mother has ingested cow's milk, cabbage, broccoli, onions, garlic, nuts, chocolate, large amounts of fresh fruits, and foods that are highly allergenic, spicy, or acidic (orange juice) during the previous 8 to 12 hours. Eliminating the suspected food from the mother's diet for a few days and then trying it again can often pinpoint whether it was the cause of the problem.

Nutrition for the Nonlactating Mother

The postpartum woman who is not breastfeeding can return to her prepregnancy diet, provided it meets the RDA for the adult woman. She should plan her diet so that it contains enough protein- and vitamin C–containing foods to promote healing. Many health care providers suggest that the woman continue to take her prenatal vitamin-mineral supplements until her supply is finished. This ensures adequate intake during the time involution occurs and helps renew nutrient stores.

The nurse should assess the mother's understanding of the number of servings she needs from each food group. A review of important nutrient sources for calcium and iron may be

---

BREASTFEEDING MOTHERS
WANT TO KNOW How Can I Tell Which Foods Are Affecting My Baby?

- Keep a list of any foods you eat that are new or different from your usual diet.
- Look for signs that the baby may be reacting to something you ate. Signs include excessive irritability, crying as if in pain, passing gas, diarrhea, and rash. These signs happen for other reasons than a reaction to your diet, so consider other causes as well.
- When your baby has a fussy period, note whether you ate anything new during the previous 8 to 12 hours.
- Watch the baby's reaction after you have eaten any food that sometimes causes problems for infants. These include foods in the cabbage family, onions, foods that are

highly allergenic (such as wheat, eggs, cow's milk) or acidic (such as orange juice), spicy foods, garlic, nuts, chocolate, and large amounts of fresh fruits.
- If you think there may be a connection between something you ate and distress in your baby, avoid that food for several days to 1 week. Then try a small amount of the food again. If the baby seems to be affected, eliminate that food from your diet.
- Eat all foods in moderation. Babies often tolerate small amounts of any food in their mother's diet but react to large amounts.

relevant. If the woman was anemic during pregnancy, she should continue to take an iron supplement until her hemoglobin level returns to normal. When her baby is born, a woman can expect to lose about 4.5 to 5.5 kg (10 to 12 lb) immediately. She loses approximately another 2.3 to 3.6 kg (5 to 8 lb) during involution (Scoggin, 2004). If her weight gain during pregnancy has not been excessive, she will probably lose all but about 1 kg (2.2 lb) within a year if she follows a well-balanced diet. She should decrease her caloric intake to her normal nonpregnant levels to avoid retaining weight.

Some women are impatient with slow weight loss and disappointed that they do not lose all their pregnancy weight gain soon after the baby is born. Because they need energy to meet the demands of infant care, new mothers should wait at least 3 weeks to start dieting to lose weight. Suggestions for sensible calorie reduction combined with exercise are appropriate. Women who gain a large amount of weight beyond that recommended during pregnancy may have difficulty losing it after birth and should be referred to a dietitian for help in planning a weight loss program.

Mothers are sometimes so involved with the needs of the infant during the early days that they fail to eat properly. They may snack instead of planning meals for themselves, especially if they are home alone with the baby during the day. The nurse should remind them that snacking often involves high caloric intake without meeting nutritional needs. During postpartum the mother needs to ensure her own good health so that she is able to care for her baby. Therefore meals and snacks should be high in nutrient content.

✔ CHECK YOUR READING

20. How do the nutritional needs of the lactating mother compare with those of the woman who is not lactating?
21. What foods should the breastfeeding woman avoid in her diet?
22. What changes should the woman who is not breastfeeding make after the birth of her baby?

Application of the Nursing Process
Nutrition for Childbearing

The nursing process focuses on determining the factors that might interfere with the woman's ability to meet the nutrient needs of pregnancy, the postpartum period, and lactation and finding solutions to any problems identified. This process primarily involves education of the woman.

Assessment

INTERVIEW

The interview provides an opportunity to develop rapport and identify any specific problems affecting dietary intake.

APPETITE. Begin the interview by discussing the woman's appetite. Has it changed during the pregnancy? How does it compare with her appetite before pregnancy? Morning sickness may decrease her food intake during the

first trimester. Determine the severity and duration of nausea and vomiting. For some women the discomfort is mild and occurs only during the morning or when they are fatigued. For others, severe nausea continues throughout the day and beyond the first trimester. Hyperemesis gravidarum is the most serious form of this problem and may require intravenous correction of fluid and electrolyte imbalance and parenteral nutrition (see Chapter 25).

EATING HABITS. Assess the usual pattern of meals to discover poor food habits such as skipping breakfast, eating only snack foods for lunch, or eating fast foods for most meals. Determine who cooks for the family. If a pregnant teenager's mother prepares meals for her, discuss nutritional needs during pregnancy with the mother. If the woman does the cooking herself, the likes and dislikes of other family members may influence what she serves, especially if she has little understanding of her own needs during pregnancy.

FOOD PREFERENCES. Ask the woman about her food preferences and dislikes. If she dislikes all fruits and vegetables, she needs another source of vitamins. Some women experience aversions to certain foods, such as meats, only during pregnancy. Careful counseling helps work around dislikes and aversions to find ways of obtaining the nutrients needed.

Discussing likes and dislikes provides an opening to ask about food cravings and pica. Cravings may be for nutritional foods or foods low in nutrient density or eaten in amounts that interfere with intake of other foods. Ask about pica in a matter-of-fact way to avoid giving an impression of disapproval. Food items such as ice are included in pica and should be asked about as well. Also ask whether the mother eats large amounts of a particular food or group of foods.

> ▪ When assessing for pica the nurse might say, "Have you had any cravings for special things to eat during your pregnancy?" This can be followed with, "Women sometimes eat things like ice, clay, and starch during pregnancy. What about you?" Some women are willing to make substitutions such as nonfat dry milk powder for laundry starch.

PSYCHOSOCIAL INFLUENCES. Ascertain whether cultural or religious considerations affect the diet. Do these apply only during pregnancy or at all times? Assess whether the woman follows all or only certain restrictions, and determine the effect on her nutrient intake.

Identify other factors that interfere with adequate nutrition. Women with low incomes may not know about sources of assistance. Inquire how long the vegetarian has followed her diet and determine her awareness of changes necessary during pregnancy. A woman's smoking habits, alcohol intake, and other substance abuse may become obvious during the interview. Determine if she takes medications that interfere with nutrient absorption. Other questions include the amount of time she has for food preparation and the frequency of fast food intake.

Ask the woman if she has any special concerns about her diet. This question may bring out fears about excessive weight gain and concerns that specific foods could hurt the fetus. It also allows her to discuss issues that have not yet been addressed.

DIET HISTORY

Diet histories provide information about a woman's usual intake of nutrients. Food intake records, food frequency questionnaires, and 24-hour diet histories can form a basis for counseling about any changes required to meet pregnancy needs. They also help the woman become more aware of her eating habits.

A 24-HOUR DIET HISTORY. Ask the woman to recall what she ate at each meal and snack during the previous 24 hours. Use specific questions about the size of portions, ingredients, and food preparation for each meal. Inquire about beverages and snacks between meals and at bedtime. Determine whether this sample is typical of her usual daily food intake. If it is not, ask what foods are more representative of her usual intake. Analyze her diet to determine whether the woman has met the recommendations for specific food groups, calories, and protein. Detailed analysis for individual nutrients is unnecessary because it is time consuming and daily variation in intake occurs.

The food history may be inaccurate if the woman cannot remember what she ate or is mistaken about amounts of food. Models of food items and measuring utensils may be helpful to determine portion sizes. The expectant mother may alter her reported intake to make it appear that she is eating better. She may be embarrassed about her inability to follow the diet prescribed because of lack of money or cooking facilities. The atmosphere created by the nurse is important in helping mothers feel free to be honest.

FOOD INTAKE RECORDS. Food intake records are used to report foods eaten during 1 or more days. Instruct the woman to list everything she eats throughout the day. The list is more accurate if she writes down each food immediately after eating. Some women eat more nutritious foods during the recording period when they are concentrating on good diet, then go back to a less-wholesome diet later.

FOOD FREQUENCY QUESTIONNAIRES. Food frequency questionnaires, which contain lists of common foods, may provide information about diet over a longer time. Review the questionnaire with the woman and ask her how often she eats each food. Foods consumed daily and weekly are her most common source of nutrients. Analyze the list to determine whether foods from each food group are eaten in adequate amounts to meet pregnancy needs and determine whether any major groups are omitted.

PHYSICAL ASSESSMENT

Information about nutritional status can be obtained during the physical assessment. This assessment includes measurement of weight and examination for signs of nutritional deficiency.

WEIGHT AT INITIAL VISIT. The woman's weight at the first prenatal visit provides a baseline value for future comparison if it is early in pregnancy. Ask her if this is her usual weight or if she has gained or lost weight. If her first visit is later in pregnancy, ask what her usual prepregnancy weight is. Measure her height without shoes because she may not have had a recent accurate measurement. Compare her prepregnancy weight for height to tables of normal values to help draw conclusions about her nutritional condition. If her weight is low for height, nutritional reserves are marginal. If it is high, she may be overweight or obese.

WEIGHT AT SUBSEQUENT VISITS. Assessment of weight gain at each prenatal visit provides an easy method of estimating whether nutrition is adequate and serves as a basis for counseling about nutrition. Weigh the woman at each visit on the same scale with approximately the same amount of clothing. She should remove her shoes and coat for an accurate measurement to be obtained.

Record the weight on a weight grid at each visit throughout the pregnancy (Figure 9-3). This grid allows examination of the pattern and total gain to date. It also helps keep track of the amount of gain between individual visits.

> Be careful not to overemphasize weight gain. In some instances a woman may be afraid that caregivers will be disapproving if she gains weight and consequently may diet or fast for 1 or 2 days before her prenatal visit.

SIGNS OF NUTRIENT DEFICIENCY. Other indications of nutritional status include any signs of deficiency. For example, bleeding gums may indicate inadequate intake of vitamin C. Actual deficiency states, however, are not likely to occur in women in most industrialized countries. Even though intake may not be enough to allow for optimal health and storage of nutrients, most women obtain enough nutrients to avoid signs of deficiency. The most important exception is iron-deficiency anemia, which is common in a mild form. Signs and symptoms include pallor, low hemoglobin level, fatigue, and increased susceptibility to infection.

LABORATORY TESTS

Laboratory tests for in-depth analysis of nutrient intake are generally impractical. Analysis of specific nutrients is expensive, and normal laboratory values during pregnancy have not been determined for all laboratory tests. Hemoglobin, hematocrit, and in some cases serum ferritin tests are most often used to determine anemia, particularly iron-deficiency anemia.

REASSESSING NUTRITIONAL STATUS AT EACH VISIT

At each prenatal visit the nurse should (1) reassess the woman's dietary status, (2) ask if she has any questions about her diet or has had any difficulty, (3) check her weight gain to see whether she is within the expected pattern, (4) evaluate her hemoglobin and hematocrit levels to detect anemia, and (5) explain what assessments are being made and why.

Analysis

Although some women consume more calories than necessary during pregnancy and risk obesity as a result, more women are likely to eat fewer nutrients than recommended.

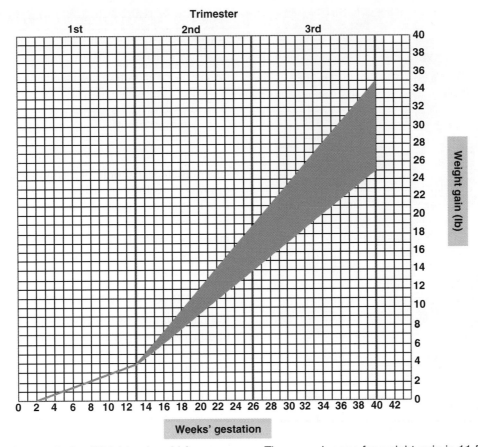

Figure 9-3 ▪ Weight gain grid for pregnancy. The normal range for weight gain is 11.5 to 16 kg (25 to 35 lb). Adolescents often need to gain in the higher end of the range. Women who are shorter than 157 cm (62 in) should gain in the lower portion.

The problem may be related to many factors, the most common of which is general lack of knowledge. Therefore the most important nursing diagnosis concerning nutrition is "Imbalanced Nutrition: Less than Body Requirements" related to lack of understanding about the nutrient needs of pregnancy.

Planning

Goals and expected outcomes for this nursing diagnosis include the following:

- The woman will consume a diet that includes the recommended number of servings from each food group throughout her pregnancy.
- The woman with a normal BMI before pregnancy will gain approximately 1.6 kg (3.5 lb) during the first trimester and 0.4 kg (0.88 lb) per week during the second and third trimesters for a total gain of 11.5 to 16 kg (25 to 35 lb).

Interventions

IDENTIFYING PROBLEMS

After analyzing food likes and dislikes and taking a 24-hour diet history, identify any obvious areas of potential deficiency and determine the woman's knowledge about the nutrient needs of pregnancy.

EXPLAINING NUTRIENT NEEDS

Use the woman's diet history as a basis to introduce information about nutrition during pregnancy. Explain the recommended servings from each food group, help the woman analyze her own diet so that she understands the process, and determine whether she meets the number of servings recommended for each food group. Explain which important nutrients are provided in each food group and why they are necessary for her and the fetus.

Make a rough estimate of calories, protein, iron, folic acid, and calcium in the diet for a general idea of intake of these nutrients. The usual sources of these major nutrients compared with her diet history and favorite foods can help determine whether the woman eats enough of these foods regularly. Suggest ways to increase nutrients she is lacking by increasing foods that are good sources. Advise the woman that adequate nutrition, especially intake of iron and folic acid, may help reduce fatigue during pregnancy and after birth.

PROVIDING REINFORCEMENT

Give frequent positive reinforcement when the woman is eating appropriately. Assist her in evaluating necessary changes in her diet, and plan ways to overcome weaknesses in her present diet (Figure 9-4). Ask her what problems she foresees in obtaining the nutrients she needs. Explore a va-

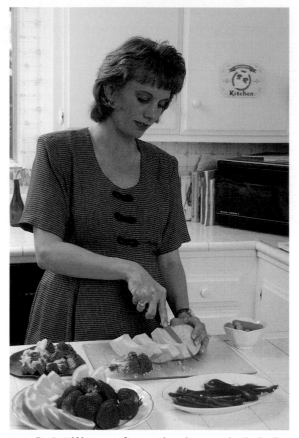

Figure 9-4 ■ Women often make changes in their diets for the sakes of their unborn children that they would not consider for themselves alone.

riety of options to overcome expected problems, and ask about how these changes will affect the rest of her family. Perhaps the changes she needs to make for her own needs would be beneficial to the entire family.

If the woman can read, give her written materials on nutrition during pregnancy and review them with her. If she can take the information home, she can review it to ensure that she is eating properly. A small pamphlet with pictures might be placed on the refrigerator to help her remember what foods she needs each day.

EVALUATING WEIGHT GAIN

Compare the woman's weight with a weight-gain grid to ascertain whether she has gained the appropriate amount of weight for this point in her pregnancy. Discuss the importance and expected pattern of weight gain and explain the importance of eating foods high in nutrient density when she is increasing calories. If she is greatly outside of normal ranges, discuss necessary diet modifications with her primary health care provider. For example, an obese woman is expected to gain some weight but the amount must be individualized according to her particular needs.

Although slight variations from the recommended weight gain have little significance, possible reasons for

---

> **BOX 9-3** **Common Sources of Dietary Fiber**
>
> Fruits and vegetables (with skins when possible): apples, strawberries, pears, carrots, corn, potatoes with skins, cabbage, and broccoli
> Whole grains and whole grain products: whole wheat bread, bran muffins, bran cereals, oatmeal, brown rice, and whole wheat pasta
> Legumes: peas, lentils, kidney beans, lima beans, baked beans, and peanuts

larger differences should be examined carefully. For women of normal weight a monthly gain of less than 1 kg (2.2 lb) should lead to a discussion of diet and possible problems in food intake. A gain of more than 2.9 kg (6.5 lb) per month may signify edema. However, errors in calculation of gestation may also reflect a pattern of weight gain different from that expected.

ENCOURAGING SUPPLEMENT INTAKE

If vitamin-mineral supplements have been prescribed, determine whether she is taking them regularly and, if not, explore reasons and possible solutions. Iron supplements often cause constipation, but dietary changes such as increased intake of fluids and fiber can help prevent this problem (Box 9-3). If the problem is forgetfulness, suggest that she take vitamin-mineral supplements with meals or iron supplements with orange juice at bedtime just before brushing her teeth. If she avoids iron supplements because of side effects such as nausea, she can take them with meals or snacks. Even though taking iron supplements with food decreases the absorption of the iron, it is preferred to not using the supplements at all. Let her know that black stools are a harmless side effect of iron supplements.

MAKING REFERRALS

The nurse can provide nutritional counseling that is more than adequate for most women, but some situations warrant referral to other sources. Women with health problems that affect nutrition (such as diabetes, celiac disease, extreme weight problems) may need an initial consultation with a dietitian and a follow-up consultation with the nurse. Women with inadequate financial resources to buy food can be referred to public assistance programs such as WIC. At the next visit, determine whether the woman obtained the help needed and if other assistance is necessary.

Evaluation

Ongoing evaluation of diet and pattern of weight gain throughout the pregnancy determines whether the goals have been met. The woman should meet the RDA for pregnancy by eating the recommended number of servings of foods from each food group. She should gain 1.6 kg (3.5 lb) during the first trimester and 0.4 kg (0.88 lb) per week during the second and third trimesters. Total weight gain should be 11.5 to 16 kg (25 to 35 lb).

SUMMARY CONCEPTS

- Nutritional education during the childbearing period may have long-term positive effects on the mother, infant, and entire family.
- Weight gain during pregnancy is an important determinant of fetal growth. Poor weight gain in pregnant women is associated with low birth weight in infants. Excessive weight gain may lead to macrosomia and labor complications.
- The recommended weight gain for women of normal weight during pregnancy is 11.5 to 16 kg (25 to 35 lb). The amount is greater for women who are underweight or who carry more than one fetus, and it is less for obese women.
- The pattern of weight gain is as important as the total increase in weight. The average should be 1.6 kg (3.5 lb) during the first trimester and 0.4 kg (0.88 lb) per week thereafter.
- The recommended increase in energy intake during pregnancy is 340 calories per day in the second trimester and 452 calories per day in the third trimester. Calorie increases should be attained by choosing foods high in nutrient density to meet other needs of pregnancy.
- Protein should be increased to 71 g daily during pregnancy, which is 25 g more than nonpregnancy needs.
- Women may not eat enough foods high in vitamins B_6, D, and E and folic acid to meet recommendations.
- Fat-soluble vitamins (A, D, E, K) are stored in the liver. Excess consumption may result in toxic effects.
- Daily intake of water-soluble vitamins (B, C) and folic acid is necessary because excesses are not stored but excreted.
- Minerals that may not be consumed at recommended amounts during pregnancy are iron, calcium, zinc, and magnesium. Iron is often added as a supplement, whereas calcium is added for women with low intake.
- Vitamin-mineral supplements must be used carefully to prevent excessive intake and toxicity. Increased intake of some nutrients interferes with use of others and may result in deficiencies.
- Pregnant women should drink at least eight 8-oz glasses of fluids each day. They should eat at least seven servings of whole grains, four servings of fruits and five servings of vegetables, three servings of dairy products, and seven ounces of protein foods daily.
- Culture can influence diet during pregnancy. The nurse should learn whether a woman follows traditional dietary practices and whether her food practices are consistent with good nutrition.
- Both Southeast Asian and Hispanic dietary practices include the importance of yin and yang (cold and hot) foods. The nurse must know which foods are acceptable at what times.
- Low-income women may not have enough money or knowledge to meet the nutrient needs of pregnancy. Nurses should refer them for financial assistance and nutritional counseling.
- Adolescents may skip meals and eat snacks and fast foods of low nutrient density. They are subject to peer pressure that may decrease their nutritional intake.
- Pregnant vegetarians may need help choosing an adequate diet that includes nonanimal sources of energy, protein, iron, calcium, vitamin B_{12}, and other nutrients. They may need vitamin-mineral supplements during pregnancy.
- Lactose-intolerant women should increase calcium intake from foods other than milk, such as calcium-rich vegetables.
- Abnormal prepregnancy weight, anemia, eating disorders, pica, multiparity, substance abuse, closely spaced pregnancies, and multifetal pregnancies are all nutritional risk factors that warrant adaptations of diet during pregnancy.
- Lactating women need more of almost every nutrient than women who are not lactating. Approximately 500 calories per day are needed for milk production during the first 6 months. This can be met by an added intake of 330 calories during the first six months, with the remaining 170 calories drawn from maternal stores. During the second six months of breastfeeding, an added intake of 400 calories is needed.
- Lactating women should avoid alcohol, caffeine, and foods that seem to cause distress in the infant.
- The postpartum woman who does not breastfeed should resume her prepregnant caloric intake and should eat a well-balanced diet to enhance recovery from childbirth. Weight loss should be accomplished slowly and sensibly.

ANSWERS   TO CRITICAL THINKING EXERCISE 9-1, p. 191

1. If Joan feels the nurse is disapproving of her actions, she is unlikely to trust the nurse with further confidences. Because she will probably not end her pica, especially without help, a disapproving nurse will cause her to withdraw and continue to practice it in secret.
2. Being accepting and nonjudgmental is important when responding to Joan. The nurse should use therapeutic communication to explore Joan's feelings about her cravings. A discussion of feelings can lead to teaching about nutrition. The nurse should determine the amount of ice Joan eats each day, whether she has other cravings, and how these affect her intake of important nutrients. A 24-hour diet history will help identify areas of deficiencies. Joan and the nurse can work together to find acceptable ways to modify the diet to include more of the food groups that are lacking. Joan should be referred to a dietitian for further counseling but the nurse should also continue to discuss the diet at each prenatal visit.

REFERENCES & READINGS

Abrams, B., Minassian, D., & Pickett, K.E. (2004). Maternal nutrition. In R.K. Creasy & R. Resnik, *Maternal-fetal medicine: Principles and practice* (5th ed., pp. 155-164). Philadelphia: Saunders.

American Academy of Pediatrics (AAP) Committee on Nutrition. (2000). Hypoallergenic infant formulas. *Pediatrics, 106*(2), 346-349.

American Academy of Pediatrics & American College of Obstetricians and Gynecologists. (2002). *Guidelines for perinatal care* (5th ed.). Elk Grove Village, IL: Author.

American Dietetic Association and Dietitians of Canada. (2003). Position of the American Dietetic Association and Dietitians of Canada: Vegetarian diets. *Journal of the American Dietetic Association, 103*(6), 748-765.

Andres, R.L. (2004). Effects of therapeutic, diagnostic, and environmental agents and exposure to social and illicit drugs. In R.K. Creasy & R. Resnik (Eds.), *Maternal-fetal medicine: Principles and practice* (5th ed., pp. 281-314). Philadelphia: Saunders.

Bond, L. (2004). Physiology of pregnancy. In S. Mattson & J.E. Smith (Eds.), *Core curriculum for maternal-newborn nursing* (3rd ed., pp. 96-123). Philadelphia: Saunders.

Blackburn, S.T. (2003). *Maternal, fetal, and neonatal physiology* (2nd ed.). Philadelphia: Saunders.

Brodeur, M.A. (2002). Understanding dietary supplement regulation. *AWHONN Lifelines, 6*(2), 106-109.

Bronner, Y.L., & Auerbach, K.G. (2005). Maternal nutrition during lactation. In J. Riordan, *Breastfeeding and human lactation* (3rd ed., pp 437-457). Boston: Jones & Bartlett.

Brooks, S.L., Mitchell, A., & Steffenson, N. (2000). Mothers, infants, and DHA: Implications for nursing practice. *MCN: American Journal of Maternal/Child Nursing, 25*(2), 71-75.

Cesario, S.K. (2001). Care of the Native American woman: Strategies for practice, education, and research. *Journal of Obstetric, Gynecologic, and Neonatal Nursing, 30*(1), 13-19.

Cesario, S.K. (2003). Obesity in pregnancy: What every nurse needs to know. *AWHONN Lifelines, 7*(2), 118-125.

Corbett, R.W., Ryan, C., & Weinrich, S.P. (2003). Pica in pregnancy: Does it affect pregnancy outcomes? *Journal of Obstetric, Gynecologic, and Neonatal Nursing, 28*(3), 183-189.

Cunningham, F.G., Gant, N.F., Leveno, K.J., Gilstrap, L.C., Hauth, J.C., & Wenstrom, K.D. (2001). *Williams obstetrics* (21st ed.). Norwalk, CT: Appleton & Lange.

Davis, R.E. (2001). The postpartum experience for Southeast Asian women in the United States. *MCN: American Journal of Maternal/Child Nursing, 26*(4), 208-213.

Earl, R. (2004). Guidelines for dietary planning. In L.K. Mahan & S. Escott-Stump (Eds.), *Krause's food, nutrition, and diet therapy* (10th ed., pp. 363-389). Philadelphia: Saunders.

Evans, E.C. (2002). The FDA recommendations on fish intake during pregnancy. *Journal of Obstetric, Gynecologic, and Neonatal Nursing, 31*(6), 715-720.

Fowles, E.R. (2002). Comparing pregnant women's nutritional knowledge to their actual dietary intake. *MCN: American Journal of Maternal/Child Nursing, 27*(3), 171-177.

Fowles, E.R. (2004). Prenatal nutrition and birth outcomes. *Obstetric, Gynecologic, and Neonatal Nursing, 33*(6), 809-822.

Giddens, J.B., Krug, S.K., Tsang, R., Guo, S., Miodovnik, M., & Prada, J.A. (2000). Pregnant adolescent and adult women have similarly low intakes of selected nutrients. *Journal of the American Dietetic Association, 100*(11), 1334-1340.

Grodner, M., Long, S., & DeYoung, S. (2004). *Foundations and clinical applications of nutrition, a nursing approach* (3rd ed.). St. Louis: Mosby.

Gunderson, E.P. (2003). Nutrition during pregnancy for the physically active woman. *Clinical Obstetrics and Gynecology, 46*(2), 390-402.

Hassenau, S.M., & Covington, C. (2002). Neural tube defects: prevention and folic acid. *MCN: American Journal of Maternal/Child Nursing, 27*(1), 87-91.

Hilton, J.J. (2002). Folic aid intake of young women. *Journal of Obstetric, Gynecologic, and Neonatal Nursing, 31*(2), 172-177.

Institute of Medicine, Food and Nutrition Board. (1997). *Dietary reference intakes for calcium, phosphorus, magnesium, vitamin D, and fluoride.* Washington, DC: National Academy Press.

Institute of Medicine, Food and Nutrition Board. (1998). *Dietary reference intakes for thiamin, riboflavin, niacin, vitamin B_6, folate, vitamin B_{12}, pantothenic acid, biotin, and choline.* Washington, DC: National Academy Press.

Institute of Medicine, Food and Nutrition Board. (2000). *Dietary reference intakes for vitamin C, vitamin E, selenium, and carotenoids.* Washington, DC: National Academy Press.

Institute of Medicine, Food and Nutrition Board (2002a) *Dietary reference intakes for energy, carbohydrates, fiber, protein and amino acids (macronutrients).* Washington, DC: National Academy Press.

Institute of Medicine, Food and Nutrition Board. (2002b). *Dietary reference intakes for vitamin A, vitamin K, arsenic, boron, chromium, copper, iodine, iron, manganese, molybdenum, nickel, silicon, vanadium, and zinc.* Washington, DC: National Academy Press.

Institute of Medicine, National Academy of Sciences, Food and Nutrition Board. (1990). *Nutrition during pregnancy. Part I: Weight gain. Part II: Nutrient supplements.* Washington, DC: National Academy Press.

Institute of Medicine, National Academy of Sciences, Food and Nutrition Board. (1991). *Nutrition during lactation.* Washington, DC: National Academy Press.

Institute of Medicine, National Academy of Sciences, Subcommittee for a Clinical Application Guide. (1992). *Nutrition during pregnancy and lactation, an implementation guide.* Washington, DC: National Academy Press.

James, D.C. (2001). Eating disorders, fertility, and pregnancy: Relationships and complications. *Journal of Perinatal and Neonatal Nursing, 15*(2), 36-48.

James, D.K., Mahomed, K., Stone, S., van Wijngaarden, W., & Hill, L.M. (2003). *Evidence-based obstetrics.* Philadelphia: Saunders.

Kaiser, L.L., & Allen, L. (2002). Position of the American Dietetic Association: Nutrition and lifestyle for a healthy pregnancy outcome. *Journal of the American Dietetic Association, 102*(10), 1479-1490.

Kilpatrick, S.J., & Laros, R.K. (2004). Maternal hematologic disorders. In R.K. Creasy & R. Resnik (Eds.), *Maternal-fetal medicine: Principles and practice* (5th ed., pp. 975-1004). Philadelphia: Saunders.

Kim-Godwin, Y.S. (2003). Postpartum beliefs and practices among non-western cultures. *MCN: American Journal of Maternal/Child Nursing, 28*(2), 74-78.

Kleinman, R.E. (Ed.). (2004). *Pediatric nutrition handbook* (5th ed.). Elk Grove Village, IL: American Academy of Pediatrics.

Matteson, P.S. (2001). *Women's health during the childbearing years: A community-based approach.* St. Louis: Mosby.

Mattson, S. (2003). Caring for Hispanic women. *AWHONN Lifelines, 7*(3), 258-260.

Mattson, S. (2004). Ethnocultural considerations in the childbearing period. In S. Mattson & J. E. Smith (Eds.), *Core curriculum for maternal-newborn nursing,* (3rd. ed., pp. 75-95). Philadelphia: Saunders.

Messina, V., Melina, V., & Mangels, A.R. (2003). A new food guide for North American vegetarians. *Journal of the American Dietetic Association, 103*(6), 771-775.

Mitchell, M.K. (2003). *Nutrition across the life span* (9th ed.). Philadelphia: Saunders.

Mohrbacher, N., & Stock, J. (2003). *The breastfeeding answer book* (3rd ed.). Schaumburg, IL: La Leche League International.

Monga, M. (2004). Maternal cardiovascular and renal adaptation to pregnancy. In R.K. Creasy & R. Resnik (Eds.), *Maternal-fetal medicine: Principles and practice* (5th ed., pp. 111-120). Philadelphia: Saunders.

Moore, M.L., & Moos, M. (2003). *Cultural competence in the care of childbearing families.* White Plains, NY: March of Dimes.

Mullaly, L.M. (2003). The 12-month pregnancy: Preconception care and information. In S.M. Levasseur & D.A. Raines (Eds.). *Perinatal nursing secrets* (pp. 35-48). Philadelphia: Hanley & Belfus.

National Research Council. (1989). *Recommended dietary allowances* (10th ed.). Washington, DC: National Academy Press.

Olson, C.M., & Strawderman, M.S. (2003). Modifiable behavioral factors in a biopsychosocial model predict inadequate and excessive gestational weight gain. *Journal of the American Dietetic Association, 103*(1), 48-54.

Peckenpaugh, N.J. (2003). *Nutrition essentials and diet therapy* (9th ed.). Philadelphia: Saunders.

Ramer, L., & Frank, B. (2001). *Pregnancy: Psychosocial perspectives.* White Plains, NY: March of Dimes Birth Defects Foundation.

Reifsnider, E., & Gill, S.L. (2000). Nutrition for the childbearing years. *Journal of Obstetric, Gynecologic, and Neonatal Nursing, 29*(1), 43-55.

Schlenker, E.D. (2003). Nutrition for growth and development. In S.R. Williams & E.D. Schlenker (Eds.), *Essentials of nutrition and diet therapy* (8th ed., pp. 293-319). St. Louis: Mosby.

Scoggin, J. (2004). Physical and psychological changes. In S. Mattson & J.E. Smith (Eds.), *Core curriculum for maternal-newborn nursing* (3rd ed., pp. 371-386). Philadelphia: Saunders.

Shabert, J.K. (2004). Nutrition during pregnancy and lactation. In L.K. Mahan & S. Escott-Stump (Eds.), *Krause's food, nutrition, and diet therapy* (11th ed., pp. 182-213). Philadelphia: Saunders.

Spear, B.A. (2004). Nutrition in adolescence. In L.K. Mahan & S. Escott-Stump (Eds.), *Krause's food, nutrition, and diet therapy* (11th ed., pp. 284-302). Philadelphia: Saunders.

Strychar, I.M., Chabot, C., Champagne, F., Ghadirian, P., Leduc, L., Lemonnier, M., & Raynauld, P. (2000). Psychosocial and lifestyle factors associated with insufficient and excessive maternal weight gain during pregnancy. *Journal of the American Dietetic Association, 100*(3), 353-356.

Swensen, A.R., Harnack, L.J., & Ross, J.A. (2001). Nutritional assessment of pregnant women enrolled in the Special Supplemental Program for Women, Infants, and Children (WIC). *Journal of the American Dietetic Association, 101*(8), 903-908.

U.S. Department of Health and Human Services. (2000). *Healthy People 2010* (Conference ed., 2 volumes). Washington, DC: Author.

U.S. Department of Health and Human Services and U.S. Department of Agriculture. (2005). *Dietary Guidelines for Americans* (6th ed.). Washington, D.C., U.S. Government Printing Office.

U.S. Food and Drug Administration. (2002). *Listeriosis and pregnancy: What is your risk?* Washington, DC: Author.

Wilkerson, N.N. (2000). Nutrition. In F.H. Nichols & S.S. Humenick (Eds.), *Childbirth education: Practice, research, & theory,* Philadelphia: Saunders.

Williams, S.R. (2003a). The food environment and food habits. In S.R. Williams & E.D. Schlenker (Eds.), *Essentials of nutrition and diet therapy* (8th ed., pp. 219-245). St. Louis: Mosby.

Williams, S.R. (2003b). Nutrition during pregnancy and lactation. In S.R. Williams & E.D. Schlenker (Eds.), *Essentials of nutrition and diet therapy* (8th ed., pp. 269-292). St. Louis: Mosby.

Witt, K.A., & Mihok, M.A. (2003). Lactation and breastfeeding. In M.K. Mitchell. *Nutrition across the life span* (9th ed., pp. 177-206). Philadelphia: Saunders.

Antepartal Fetal Assessment

After studying this chapter, you should be able to:

1. Identify indications for fetal diagnostic procedures.
2. Discuss the purpose, procedure, advantages, and risks of each diagnostic procedure discussed in this chapter.
3. Provide information for common questions that clients may have about antepartal fetal assessment procedures.
4. Apply the nursing process to care of clients undergoing antepartal fetal assessment procedures.

Go to your Student CD-ROM for Review Questions keyed to these Objectives.

Alpha-fetoprotein Plasma protein produced by the fetus.

Amniocentesis Transabdominal puncture of the amniotic sac to obtain a sample of amniotic fluid that contains fetal cells and biochemical substances for laboratory examination.

Amniotic Fluid Index (AFI) An ultrasound examination in which the vertical depth of the largest fluid pocket in each of the four quadrants of the uterus is measured and totaled.

Baseline Risk The risk, usually in reference to birth defects or spontaneous abortion, of the general population of pregnant women who have no identified high-risk factors or invasive procedures.

Biophysical Profile Method for evaluating fetal status during the antepartum period based on five variables originating with the fetus: fetal heart rate, breathing movements, gross body movements, muscle tone, and amniotic fluid volume.

Chorionic Villus Sampling Transcervical or transabdominal procedure to obtain a sample of chorionic villi (projections of the outer fetal membrane) for analysis of fetal cells.

Contraction Stress Test Method for evaluating fetal status during the antepartum period by observing response of the fetal heart to the stress of uterine con-

tractions that may induce recurrent episodes of fetal hypoxia.

Δ OD$_{450}$ A test used to measure the change (delta, or Δ) in optical density of the amniotic fluid caused by staining with bilirubin.

Karyotype A display of a cell's chromosomes, arranged from largest to smallest pairs.

Late Deceleration The slowing of the fetal heart rate after the onset of a uterine contraction and persisting after the contraction ends.

Lecithin/Sphingomyelin Ratio (L/S Ratio) Ratio of two phospholipids in amniotic fluid that is used to determine fetal lung maturity; ratio of 2:1 or greater usually indicates fetal lung maturity.

Multiple-Marker Screening Analysis of maternal serum for abnormal levels of alpha-fetoprotein, human chorionic gonadotropin, and estriols that may predict chromosomal abnormalities of the fetus; often called *triple-screen*. Addition of tests such as inhibin A have improved accuracy of the results, leading to alternate names for the package of tests.

Neural Tube Defect A congenital defect in closure of the bony encasement of the spinal cord or skull. Includes defects such as anencephaly, spina bifida, meningocele, myelomeningocele, and others.

D E F I N I T I O N S—cont'd

Nonstress Test A method for evaluating fetal status during the antepartum period by observing the response of the fetal heart rate to fetal movement.

Percutaneous Umbilical Blood Sampling (PUBS) Procedure for obtaining fetal blood through ultrasound-guided puncture of an umbilical cord vessel to detect fetal problems such as inherited blood disorders, acidosis, or infection; also called *cordocentesis*.

Phosphatidylglycerol (PG) A major phospholipid of surfactant whose presence in amniotic fluid indicates fetal lung maturity.

Phosphatidylinositol (PI) A phospholipid of surfactant that is produced and secreted in increasing amounts as the fetal lungs mature.

Placenta Previa Abnormal implantation of the placenta in the lower uterus located at or very near the cervical os.

Surfactant Combination of lipoproteins produced by the lungs of the mature fetus to reduce surface tension in the alveoli, thus promoting lung expansion after birth.

Ultrasonography Technique for visualizing deep structures of the body by recording the reflections (echoes) of high-frequency sound waves directed into the tissue.

Uteroplacental Insufficiency Inability of the placenta to exchange oxygen, carbon dioxide, nutrients, and waste products properly between the maternal and fetal circulations.

Vibroacoustic Stimulation Use of sound stimulation to elicit fetal movement and acceleration (speeding up) of the fetal heart rate.

Until relatively recently, only nonspecific methods were available to assess the condition and physical development rate of the fetus. Fundal height was measured to estimate fetal growth, the fetal heart rate (FHR) was auscultated, and the mother's perception of fetal movements was noted. The development of additional methods has allowed the detection of physical abnormalities in the fetus and greater accuracy in the monitoring of the fetal condition, including growth rate.

Antepartal fetal assessments offer reassurance for most expectant parents. If no fetal anomalies are found and the fetus appears to be in good condition, relief and reduced anxiety are usually immediate. If fetal health is uncertain, the woman often faces decisions about further testing. She may experience anxiety throughout the pregnancy if tests continue to raise questions about the well-being of the fetus. If tests identify fetal anomalies, the woman may face the choice of whether to continue the pregnancy. This decision can create emotional conflict as well as ethical dilemmas that are stressful for the family.

INDICATIONS FOR FETAL DIAGNOSTIC TESTS

Most fetal diagnostic procedures are reserved for pregnancies in which there is a reason to believe the fetus may experience developmental or physical problems. However, many physicians believe that some screening tests such as ultrasonography and maternal serum screening should be offered to all women.

Two broad reasons exist for antepartal fetal assessment testing: (1) to detect congenital anomalies and (2) to evaluate the condition of the fetus. Some procedures such as amniocentesis and ultrasonography may be used for both purposes.

Many factors increase the risk for the fetus during pregnancy. These include maternal medical conditions such as diabetes and hypertension, demographic factors such as age and poverty, and obstetric factors such as previous birth of an infant who was preterm, was stillborn, or had congenital anomalies (Box 10-1).

No antepartal testing or antepartal surveillance procedure can guarantee the birth of a perfect infant. The woman

---

BOX 10-1 Indications For Fetal Diagnostic Procedures

Medical Conditions
Preexisting diabetes mellitus or gestational diabetes
Hypertension (chronic or pregnancy-induced)
Acute or nonacute infections (e.g., pyelonephritis)
Sexually transmissible diseases
Severe anemia
Parents carry or express a genetic disorder (e.g., sickle cell anemia, cystic fibrosis)

Demographic Factors
Maternal age <16 or >35 years
Poverty
Nonwhite (greater risk for prematurity or neonatal or infant death)
Inadequate prenatal care (initial visit after 20 weeks' gestation or fewer than five prenatal visits to physician or nurse-midwife)

Obstetric Factors
History of low-birth-weight (<2500 g) or preterm (<37 completed weeks of pregnancy) infant
Multifetal pregnancy
Malpresentation (breech, shoulder)
Previous fetal loss or birth of infant with congenital anomaly
Previous infant >4000 g at birth
Hydramnios (>2000 ml at term; amniotic fluid index >18-20)
Oligohydramnios (<500 ml at term; amniotic fluid index <5)
Decrease in or absence of fetal movements
Uncertainty about gestational age
Suspected intrauterine growth restriction
Discordant (unequal) fetal growth of twins
Postmaturity (>42 weeks)
Preterm labor (>20 weeks and <38 weeks of gestation)
Grand multiparity (>5 pregnancies)

Concurrent Maternal Factors
Prepregnancy weight less than 45 kg (100 lb) or body mass index (BMI) less than 19.8
Prepregnancy weight more than 90 kg (200 lb) or more than 20% above ideal weight for height at conception
Inadequate weight gain or poor pattern of weight gain
Excessive weight gain
Use of drugs, alcohol, tobacco

and her support person must be counseled that prenatal diagnostic tests cannot detect all congenital defects. A baseline risk remains for congenital defects in every pregnancy.

The nurse should remember the woman's right to refuse antepartal testing even though she may have an increased risk for a baby with a birth defect that can be diagnosed with one of these tests. If a screening test suggests an abnormality that requires further testing to determine whether the abnormality is actually present, the woman has the right to accept or refuse further testing. Nurses must respect the woman's personal decisions.

ULTRASONOGRAPHY

When high-frequency sound waves of an ultrasonic beam are aimed at body tissues, they are deflected by tissues in their path and returned as echoes. The amount of energy returned as an echo depends on the properties of the tissues in the path of the ultrasonic beam and the angle and strength of the beam. In obstetrics the ultrasonic beam sent by a transducer is directed through tissues of the abdomen or vagina to provide two-dimensional images showing structures of different densities (Figure 10-1).

Technologic and software advances have refined ultrasound data, producing a three-dimensional image with greater clarity and visual depth than the two-dimensional image. Three-dimensional ultrasound images have greater detail to confirm normal features and identify congenital abnormalities, particularly those of surface features such as facial clefts. They provide more accurate identification of the extent and size of abnormalities. Ultrasound images in three dimensions are often easier to interpret because they are more realistic than two-dimensional flat images (Figure 10-2). A four-dimensional image is being studied because it allows study of both fetal anatomy and function of the organs (Manning, 2004). Methods that may be used to evaluate and store images include optical and magnetic media as well as thermal photographs.

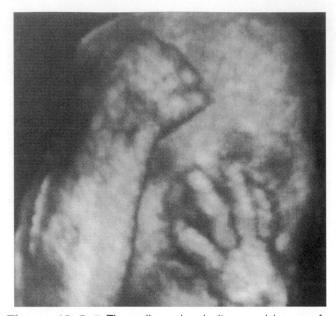

Figure 10-2 ■ Three-dimensional ultrasound image of a 30-week fetus holding normal hands in front of the face. (From Pretorius, D.H., Nelson, T.R., & Lev-Toaff, A.S. [2000]. Three dimensional ultrasound in obstetrics and gynecology. In P.W. Callen [Ed.], *Ultrasonography in obstetrics and gynecology* [4th ed.]. Philadelphia: Saunders.)

A simple written interpretation of the ultrasound image is done for each examination.

Today's procedures use real-time scanning, showing movement as it happens. Real-time ultrasound allows the observer to see fetal heart motion, fetal breathing activity, and fetal body movement. Real-time scanning also allows the observer to distinguish between moving tissues of the fetus and relatively fixed maternal tissues. Ultrasonography may be used during any trimester, but the procedure and the reasons for its use vary. Ultrasonography is also used in gynecology and infertility care.

Emotional Responses

In some countries a basic ultrasound scan is routine in all pregnancies, but ultrasonography is not considered a routine part of care in the United States, primarily because a major trial (RADIUS) failed to show a significant improvement in perinatal outcome when routine ultrasonography was used for screening during pregnancy. However, other studies have shown greater value of routine screening for detecting fetal anomalies early. In actual practice, almost 80% of women in the United States who have live births had at least one ultrasound examination (Manning, 2004; Martin et al., 2003). The procedure is so common that many women expect to have an ultrasound scan at some time during pregnancy.

Parents' responses to ultrasonography vary widely. Some expectant parents are excited and report feelings of love and protectiveness when they view the fetus. Others report more anxiety about the fetus and fear that something will be found wrong. Undoubtedly, parents breathe sighs of relief

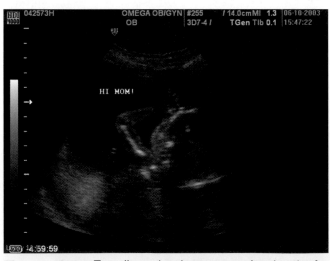

Figure 10-1 ■ Two-dimensional sonogram showing the fetal body profile and the details of the fetal arm, hand, and fingers. (Courtesy of Paul and Kerri Hamilton.)

when scans show normal results. Sometimes the presence of one or more "markers," findings that might indicate a problem, fails to give parents the expected reassurance and puts them on a path to other difficult choices they must make about their baby.

Both parents are usually fascinated by the quality of today's ultrasound images, which allows them to see their unborn baby with clarity. Many couples want to know the gender of the fetus. Others do not want to know the gender, even if it is obvious, and prefer to wait and "be surprised." The sonographer often provides parents with still images and sometimes a short videotape of their fetus. Images made for parents are keepsakes and are not used for medical diagnostics. Other views are archived for medical documentation purposes.

Levels of Obstetric Ultrasound

Three levels of obstetric ultrasound examination are as follows (Menihan, 2000; Stringer et al, 2003):

- Basic—The basic scan includes a general survey of the fetus, placenta, and amniotic fluid quantity and should be performed by a sonographer.
- Comprehensive—The comprehensive, or extended, scan is ordered if abnormalities are found during the basic scan. A maternal-fetal medicine physician often consults with the woman's primary provider when the comprehensive scan is required. The comprehensive scan targets the questionable finding to obtain greater detail and information than that found with the basic scan.
- Limited—Because nurses in labor units and emergency departments may need to quickly determine information during pregnancy, the American College of Obstetricians and Gynecologists (ACOG) has recognized limited ultrasound. The Association of Women's Health, Obstetric, and Neonatal Nurses provides specific guidelines for didactic and clinical training. The limited ultrasound scan is less detailed than a basic scan but is appropriate for gathering information such as fetal well being, number, presentation, and placenta location (Box 10-2).

First-Trimester Ultrasonography

During the first trimester, transvaginal ultrasonography allows clear visualization of the uterus, gestational sac, embryo, and pelvic structures such as the ovaries and fallopian tubes.

BOX **10-2** Indications for a Limited Ultrasound Scan

Determine placental location
Detect presence or absence of fetal cardiac activity
Assess volume of amniotic fluid
Determine fetal presenting part
Guide delivery of the second twin in a vaginal birth
Assist with amniocentesis and external cephalic version
Assess fetal well-being (such as a biophysical profile)
Identify problems if mother uses drugs, alcohol, or tobacco

PURPOSES

During the first trimester, ultrasonography is most frequently used to do the following:

- Confirm pregnancy
- Verify the location of the pregnancy (such as uterine, ectopic)
- Detect multifetal gestations
- Determine gestational age with measures such as crown-rump length, head measurements
- Confirm number and viability of fetuses
- Identify markers such as nuchal translucence that suggest chromosome or other abnormalities
- Determine the locations of the uterus, cervix, and placenta for procedures such as chorionic villus sampling (CVS)

During the first trimester, gestational age is based on the appearance of the gestational sac, which can be seen as early as 25 days after the last menstrual period. At this time the crown-rump length of the embryo is the most reliable indicator of gestational age. Fetal viability is confirmed by observation of fetal heartbeat, which is visible as early as 38 days after the last normal menstrual period (Manning, 2004). Maternal structures and abnormalities such as uterine fibroids, ovarian cysts, and bicornuate uteri can be seen.

PROCEDURE

The woman is placed in a lithotomy position for transvaginal ultrasonography. A transvaginal probe, which is encased in a disposable cover and coated with a gel that provides lubrication and promotes conductivity, is inserted into the vagina. The woman may feel more comfortable if she inserts the probe herself. The procedure takes about 10 to 15 minutes.

Second- and Third-Trimester Ultrasonography

Transabdominal ultrasonography is most often used during the second and third trimesters because the uterus extends out of the pelvis, allowing clear views of the fetus and placenta, which are no longer obstructed by pelvic bones.

PURPOSES

Ultrasonography is used throughout the second and third trimesters to do the following:

- Confirm fetal viability
- Evaluate fetal anatomy, including the umbilical cord, its vessels, and the insertion site
- Determine gestational age
- Assess serial fetal growth over several scans
- Compare growth of fetuses in multifetal gestations, and evaluate quantity of fluid in each amniotic sac
- Evaluate amniotic fluid volume (see also "Biophysical Profile," p. 217)
- Locate the placenta when placenta previa is suspected
- Determine fetal presentation
- Guide needle placement for amniocentesis or percutaneous umbilical blood sampling (PUBS)

Gestational age determination by ultrasonography is increasingly less accurate after the first trimester because the combination of individual growth potential and intrauterine environment causes greater variations among fetuses. Two methods improve accuracy of gestational age determination in later pregnancy:

- Multiple measurements are done, such as fetal head biparietal diameter, head circumference, abdominal circumference, and length of bones in extremities.
- If the woman is between 24 and 32 weeks' gestation, two or three ultrasound measurements may be taken 2 weeks apart to compare against standard fetal growth curves

Initial estimation of fetal age by ultrasonography after 32 weeks' gestation is subject to major error. The fetus is evaluated for other signs of well-being or compromise at this time (Manning, 2004).

Accurate gestational age is needed when testing the maternal serum alpha-fetoprotein (MSAFP) because the level of alpha-fetoprotein (AFP) is altered by fetal age and number of fetuses (see p. 207). Accurate gestational age is also important if intrauterine growth restriction is suspected or the expected date of delivery is questioned.

A comprehensive ultrasound in the second trimester is used to evaluate the fetus when risk factors are present or the basic examination shows abnormal findings. Examples include prior birth of an infant with anomalies or abnormal clinical findings such as hydramnios (excessive amniotic fluid), oligohydramnios (insufficient amniotic fluid), or abnormal levels of MSAFP or other tests in multiple-marker testing. Fetal anatomy is carefully and systematically examined to identify major system and organ anomalies. Anomalies that can be detected with comprehensive ultrasonography include most neural tube defects such as myelomeningocele and anencephaly, abdominal wall defects such as gastroschisis and omphalocele, malformed kidneys, hydrocephalus, obstruction in fetal bowel and urinary systems, cleft lip and palate, and limb abnormalities.

PROCEDURE

For a transabdominal ultrasound, the woman is positioned on her back with the head and knees supported. If she desires, a display panel can be positioned so that she (and her support person) can see the images on the screen. Her head should be elevated, and she should be turned slightly to one side to prevent supine hypotension, which may be caused by compression of the vena cava and aorta by the gravid uterus. A wedge or rolled blanket is placed under one hip to help her maintain this position comfortably. Warm mineral oil or transmission gel is spread over her abdomen, and the sonographer slowly moves a transducer over the abdomen to obtain a picture (Figure 10-3). The procedure takes 10 to 30 minutes.

During the second trimester a full bladder may be needed to displace the gas-filled intestines and elevate the uterus for better image quality. If a full bladder is necessary, the woman should be instructed to drink several glasses of clear fluid 1 hour before the examination and not void until after the examination. She may experience some discomfort as the transducer is moved over her distended bladder.

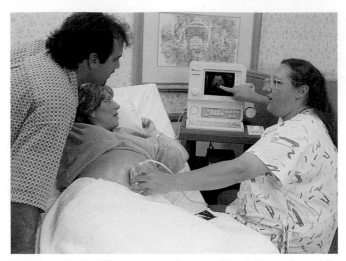

Figure 10-3 ■ The sonographer provides information while moving an ultrasound transducer over the mother's abdomen to obtain an image.

Advantages

Ultrasonography allows clear visibility of the fetus and surrounding structures and is safe. No clinically significant adverse effects have been reported (Manning, 2004). Ultrasonography is noninvasive and relatively comfortable. In addition, results are obtained immediately. It is widely available and portable.

Disadvantages

Depending on their health care coverage, women may have a problem with the cost of ultrasonography. Women who do not have prenatal care in the first trimester of pregnancy, including those with uncertain gestation, will not obtain all potential benefits from ultrasonography. Ultrasound cannot identify all defects of fetal structures and/or fetal function. Abnormal fetal function may affect the structure but ultrasound does not always find it.

The high quality of ultrasound images enables clinicians to identify several structural markers in the fetal anatomy that may predict a serious problem. For example, nuchal translucency, an area at the back of the fetal neck that does not return ultrasound echoes, has helped identify chromosome abnormalities and some heart defects early. Normal results are reassuring to parents, but suspicious or clearly abnormal images raise their anxiety levels. The physician must discuss with the expectant mother all ultrasound findings and further testing that may be indicated by these results.

DOPPLER ULTRASOUND BLOOD FLOW ASSESSMENT

When an ultrasound wave is directed at an acute angle to a moving target, as with blood flowing through a vessel, the frequency of echoes changes as the cardiac cycle goes through systole and diastole. This change, referred to as the *Doppler shift*, indicates forward movement of blood within a vessel.

Purpose

Pregnancies complicated by hypertension or fetal growth restriction may have Doppler ultrasound assessment of blood flow through the umbilical artery to identify abnormalities in the diastolic flow. In severe cases, diastolic flow may be absent or even reversed. Such findings are not diagnostic in themselves but provide additional information in tests for fetal well-being (Harman, 2004).

Color Doppler

The direction and velocity of the Doppler shift can be imaged in color depending on the direction of the flow to or from the transducer (Figure 10-4).

✓ CHECK YOUR READING

1. What are the major indications for ultrasonography during the first trimester? During the second and third trimesters?
2. How does the procedure for first-trimester ultrasonography differ from that performed during the second trimester?
3. What are the major advantages and disadvantages of ultrasonography?

ALPHA-FETOPROTEIN SCREENING

AFP is the predominant protein in fetal plasma and is synthesized by the embryonic yolk sac, developing fetal liver, and gastrointestinal tract. AFP diffuses from fetal plasma into fetal urine and is excreted into the amniotic fluid. Although a portion of the AFP in amniotic fluid is swallowed and digested by the fetus, the remainder crosses placental membranes into the maternal circulation. Therefore AFP can be measured in MSAFP and amniotic fluid (AFAFP). Abnormal concentrations of AFP are associated with serious fetal anomalies (Box 10-3). Knowing an accurate fetal gesta-

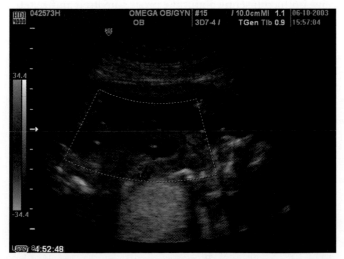

Figure 10-4 ■ Color Doppler imaging of the umbilical vein and two arteries. Blood flow toward the transducer is typically shown as red, and the flow away is shown as blue. (Courtesy of Paul and Kerri Hamilton.)

BOX 10-3 Conditions Associated with Abnormal Maternal Serum Alpha-Fetoprotein Levels

Elevated Levels of AFP
Open neural tube defects (anencephaly, spina bifida)
Esophageal obstruction
Abdominal wall defects (omphalocele, gastroschisis)
Increased amount leaked by fetal kidney (hydronephrosis)
Threatened abortion
Fetal demise
Normal fetus in conjunction with one or more of the following:
   Amniotic fluid contaminated with fetal blood (e.g., during amniocentesis, percutaneous umbilical blood sampling)
   Underestimation of fetal age
   Maternal insulin-dependent diabetes (such as type 1)
   Incorrect maternal weight (lower than the true weight)
   Multifetal gestation

Low Levels of AFP
Chromosomal trisomies (e.g., Down syndrome, or trisomy 21)
Gestational trophoblastic disease
Normal fetus in conjunction with:
   Overestimation of gestational age
   Increased maternal weight (higher than true weight)

AFP, Alpha-fetoprotein.

---

tional age and the correct number of fetuses is also essential for accuracy.

Purpose

Low levels of MSAFP suggest chromosomal abnormalities such as trisomy 21. Elevated MSAFP levels are associated with open neural tube defects and body wall defects. These anomalies leave internal tissues exposed to amniotic fluid, allowing large quantities of AFP to seep into amniotic fluid and enter maternal serum.

The most common open neural tube defects are:
- Anencephaly, in which the cranial vault is absent and most of the brain is undeveloped.
- Spina bifida, including meningocele and myelomeningocele. In meningocele the meninges protrude from the spinal canal. In myelomeningocele, the spinal cord and meninges protrude through the defect, and extensive nerve damage may be expected.

Spina bifida occulta is not an open neural tube defect and usually causes no problems. Open neural tube defects are fairly common; anencephaly occurred in 9.9 and spina bifida in 20 per 100,000 live births, respectively, in 2002. The rates for neural tube defects have declined since 1996, the year that folic acid supplementation and addition to food products was instituted (Martin et al., 2003).

Procedure

Initial screening is offered to all women between 16 and 18 weeks' gestation, when blood may be drawn to evaluate the concentration of MSAFP. Additional tests done at this time constitute a multiple-marker screening for defects (American Academy of Pediatrics [AAP] & ACOG, 2002). Gestational age, maternal weight, multifetal pregnancy, race, and maternal diabetes can affect MSAFP and must be considered when evaluating the levels. The mother is informed that MSAFP is a screening test rather than a diagnostic test and that further tests may be offered to explain abnormal concentrations. If

MSAFP levels are elevated, ultrasonography is offered to determine whether the abnormal concentration results from inaccurate gestational age, multifetal gestation, or fetal demise.

Advantages

Maternal serum AFP evaluation has several advantages:

- It is a simple procedure that requires only a sample of maternal blood.
- It is a noninvasive procedure to screen for open neural tube defects and other open defects in the fetal body wall.
- Addition of other tests (see "Multiple-Marker Screening"); AFP is part of a screening test for chromosome defects, as well.
- Screening at about 16 weeks' gestation allows time for more comprehensive testing if results for MSAFP are abnormal. Parents may examine their options or prepare for the birth of an infant who will need special care.

Limitations

Some major limitations of MSAFP are the following:

- Maternal serum AFP evaluation is a screening test only and must be viewed as the first step in a series of potential decisions about diagnostic procedures if abnormal concentrations are found.
- Because conditions such as inaccurate estimation of gestational age can result in apparently abnormal levels in a healthy fetus, the parents may experience a great deal of anxiety and expense if they choose to pursue follow-up testing.
- Timing also imposes some limits. Maternal serum AFP evaluation is performed between 16 and 18 weeks. Women may not seek care until late in pregnancy, missing the opportunity for MSAFP and related screening.
- Because closed neural tube and other closed defects do not produce elevated levels of AFP, normal levels of AFP do not guarantee a perfect baby.

MULTIPLE-MARKER SCREENING

Although MSAFP is a prominent noninvasive test for an open body wall defect such as a neural tube defect, low levels of the protein are linked to chromosome defects. Trisomy 21, or Down syndrome, is a common birth defect that occurred in 46.7 per 100,000 births in 2002 (Martin et al., 2003). The risk for having an infant with a chromosome defect increases with maternal age, rising sharply after age 35. The birth rate among women older than 35 is rising, but remains lower than the birth rate among younger women. Therefore, tests to identify chromosome abnormalities noninvasively are useful for both younger and older pregnant women.

Human chorionic gonadotropin (hCG) levels tend to be higher and unconjugated estriol levels lower in maternal serum when the fetus has trisomy 21. Adding these two tests—especially measurement of hCG, which is present at about twice normal levels in the fetus with trisomy 21— yields a higher detection rate and a lower false-positive rate than MSAFP screening alone. The three markers have also

been found to increase the detection of other trisomies such as trisomy 18. Including a fourth test for inhibin A, a product produced first by the corpus luteum and then the placenta, may further add to the detection rate for trisomy 21 (Jenkins & Wapner, 2004). Therefore what was once called a "triple screen" may now be called a "quad screen" or "tetra screen" or may be called "multiple-marker screening," as other screening tests are being evaluated and may be included. One disadvantage of using multiple screening tests is added costs, often incurred by women who are at a low risk for having an affected fetus.

✓ **CHECK YOUR READING**

4. Why is MSAFP considered a screening test?
5. What are possible causes for elevated levels of AFP?
6. What are possible causes for low levels of AFP?
7. What is multiple-marker screening? Why is it performed?

CHORIONIC VILLUS SAMPLING

Purpose

Chorionic villi are microscopic projections from the outer membrane (chorion) that develop and burrow into endometrial tissue as the placenta is formed. The villi are fetal tissues and reflect the chromosomal and genetic makeup of the fetus.

Indications

CVS is usually performed between 10 and 12 weeks of gestation to diagnose fetal chromosomal, metabolic, or DNA abnormalities. CVS is not used to detect open body wall defects such as spina bifida because an amniotic fluid sample is required (AAP & ACOG, 2002; Jenkins & Wapner, 2004).

Procedure

As with all diagnostic procedures, the woman should receive both counseling about the procedure itself and genetic counseling about the specific defect for which CVS is being performed. The risks and benefits of the procedure should be carefully explained, and a signed informed consent should be obtained.

CVS can often be performed by either the transcervical or the transabdominal approach. The transcervical approach is usually more comfortable for the woman, but it often results in minor postprocedure bleeding. The approach providing the easiest, most direct access to the villi is usually chosen (Jenkins & Wapner, 2004).

For transcervical aspiration the woman is placed in the lithotomy position. The vagina and cervix are washed with an antiseptic germicidal agent before the procedure, and strict aseptic technique is observed to decrease the chance of infection. Cultures for infections such as gonorrhea, chlamydia, and group B streptococcus may be required before CVS. Under ultrasound guidance a flexible catheter is inserted through the cervix, and a sample of chorionic villi

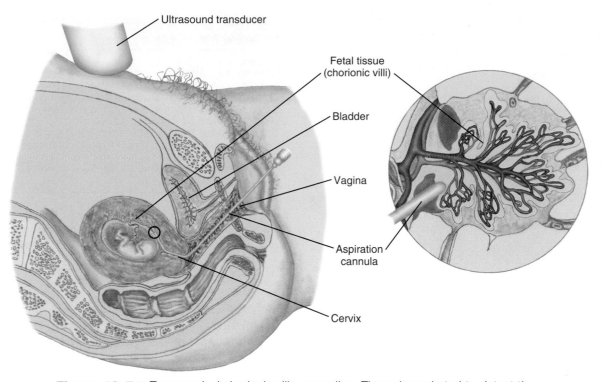

Figure 10-5 ■ Transcervical chorionic villus sampling. Tissue is aspirated to detect the presence of genetic defects in the fetus. Transabdominal aspiration is an alternative method.

is aspirated through the catheter into a syringe containing culture medium (Figure 10-5).

Transabdominal CVS is performed with the woman in a supine position. Ultrasound examination first determines the best entry position and angle of passage of the sampling needle. An area on the abdomen is cleansed with antiseptic solution. With ultrasound guidance the physician inserts a needle through the abdominal wall and myometrium, and the tip is advanced to the placenta. A sample of chorionic villi is withdrawn into the syringe containing culture medium.

After CVS, fetal heart activity is often documented to confirm viability. Maternal vital signs are assessed, and the woman is allowed to void. Rh$_o$(D) immune globulin (RhoGAM) is given to women who are Rh-negative because CVS increases the risk of Rh sensitization. A small amount of vaginal spotting may occur, but heavy bleeding or the passage of amniotic fluid, clots, and tissue should be reported. The woman needs to rest at home for several hours after the procedure. Sexual intercourse may be limited for a few days.

Advantages

CVS is performed between 10 and 12 weeks of gestation, so results are known earlier than early amniocentesis. As a result, CVS offers prenatal diagnosis to women who find later procedures unacceptable. Furthermore, if results are abnormal and the woman chooses abortion, she may consider the earlier abortion less physically and emotionally traumatic than a later procedure.

Risks

The rate of pregnancy loss after CVS is similar to that of amniocentesis. Fetal loss appears to be less frequent in centers that perform many CVS procedures. More than two attempts and bleeding during the week before the procedure increases the risk for fetal loss. Reports of limb reduction defects (LRD) associated with CVS performed before 10 weeks of gestation appeared in the early 1990s. Present data appear to confirm the safety of CVS at the gestational age of 10 to 12 weeks, but the risk for LRD must be shared with the parents (Jenkins & Wapner, 2004).

Preliminary results from CVS are available within 2 to 3 hours because the villi cells rapidly divide. For added quality villi cells are incubated for 2 to 4 days, with added cells placed in tissue culture for analysis within 7 days (Jenkins & Wapner, 2004). Tests other than karyotyping, such as those for metabolic disorders, may be available very quickly or may require a longer time for analysis. Clarifying questionable CVS results may require further testing with cells obtained by amniocentesis, adding expense, invasiveness, and anxiety to the prenatal diagnosis process.

✓ **CHECK YOUR READING**

8. What is the major advantage of CVS compared with amniocentesis?
9. What major risks are associated with CVS?

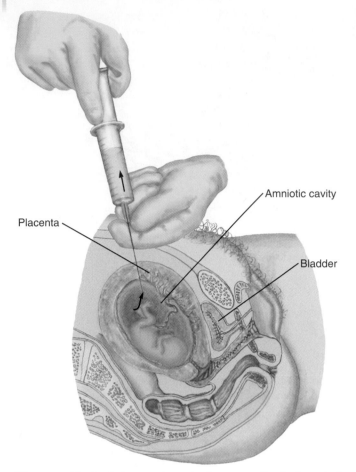

Placenta

Amniotic cavity

Bladder

Figure 10-6 ■ In amniocentesis a needle is inserted through the expectant mother's abdomen to aspirate fluid from the amniotic sac. The fluid can then be tested to determine fetal maturity, chromosomal abnormalities, and other possible problems.

AMNIOCENTESIS

Amniocentesis is the aspiration of amniotic fluid from the amniotic sac for examination (Figure 10-6). The procedure has been traditionally performed at 15 to 20 weeks of gestation. Current techniques allow early amniocentesis at 11 to 14 weeks' gestation. Fetal foot deformations are more likely to occur with removal of amniotic fluid at earlier gestation than 13 weeks.

Purposes

MIDTRIMESTER

The most common purpose for midtrimester amniocentesis is to examine fetal cells present in amniotic fluid to identify chromosome abnormalities. Other methods of genetic analysis, such as those for metabolic defects in the fetus, may be performed on the cells as well.

In addition to detecting chromosomal abnormalities, amniocentesis is used to evaluate the fetal condition when the woman is sensitized to Rh-positive blood, diagnose intrauterine infections, and investigate amniotic fluid AFP

BOX 10-4 Common Indications for Second-Trimester Amniocentesis

Maternal age ≥ 35 years
Chromosomal abnormality in close family member
Sex determination for maternal carrier of X-linked disorder (such as hemophilia, Duchenne's muscular dystrophy)
Birth of previous infant with chromosomal abnormalities or an open neural tube or body wall defect
Pregnancy after three or more spontaneous abortions
Elevated levels of maternal serum alpha-fetoprotein that remain unexplained
Rh sensitization of maternal Rh-negative blood to Rh-positive blood

---

and acetylcholinesterase (AChE), when the multiple-marker test done on maternal serum is not normal (Box 10-4).

THIRD TRIMESTER

The most common indications for amniocentesis during the third trimester are to determine fetal lung maturity and evaluate the fetal condition when the woman has Rh isoimmunization. Although several types of maternal-fetal blood incompatibilities exist, Rh incompatibility is most severe (see Chapter 25).

TESTS TO DETERMINE FETAL LUNG MATURITY. A test for fetal lung maturity is recommended when delivery is considered before 38 weeks of gestation or if the actual gestation is uncertain. Surfactant, a surface-active substance composed primarily of phospholipids, reduces the surface tension on the inner walls of the alveoli, allowing them to stay open slightly when the infant exhales. Without adequate surfactant, the walls adhere to one another, making it difficult to inflate the alveoli with the next breath. Each breath requires greater effort to reopen collapsed alveoli, and the infant soon tires.

The lecithin/sphingomyelin (L/S) ratio is a test for estimating fetal lung maturity. Lecithin is a phospholipid component of fetal lung fluid and surfactant, and sphingomyelin is a general amniotic membrane lipid. Lecithin and sphingomyelin are present in approximately equal amounts until about 30 weeks of gestation. At this time the level of sphingomyelin plateaus, while lecithin continues to rise. An L/S ratio of at least 2:1 generally indicates adequate surfactant and mature fetal lungs. However, an L/S ratio of 2:1 may not indicate lung maturity in some conditions such as maternal diabetes. Therefore amniotic fluid is usually tested for the presence of phosphatidylglycerol (PG) and phosphatidylinositol (PI), two other components of surfactant, in addition to the L/S ratio. Presence of PG and PI phospholipids supports the likelihood that the fetal lungs are mature. The accuracy of the three tests may be affected by presence of blood and meconium in the amniotic fluid (Glantz & Woods, 2004).

PG is also useful in evaluating the maturity of the fetal lungs from a sample of amniotic fluid taken from a vaginal pool when the membranes have ruptured prematurely. This test is noninvasive, but the fluid sample will also be contaminated by substances such as mucus, blood, and bacteria that may interfere with accuracy of lung maturity tests (Mercer, 2004).

TEST FOR FETAL HEMOLYTIC DISEASE. Amniocentesis is used to determine fetal bilirubin concentration with a Δ OD_{450} if the mother is Rh-negative and was sensitized after being exposed to Rh-positive blood. Antibodies of the sensitized woman can destroy Rh-positive blood of the fetus, leaving the fetus vulnerable to erythroblastosis fetalis and hydrops fetalis (see Chapter 25).

Erythroblastosis is marked by excessive destruction of mature erythrocytes capable of carrying oxygen and the proliferation of immature erythroblasts incapable of carrying oxygen. Bilirubin, which is released from erythrocyte breakdown, increases. The fetus becomes anemic, jaundiced, and edematous (hydrops fetalis) as the heart fails.

Procedure

Before the examination the woman is placed in a supine position and draped with her abdomen exposed. A rolled towel is placed under one buttock to shift the weight of the uterus to the side and off the vena cava and aorta. Maternal blood pressure and FHR are assessed for baseline levels.

Ultrasonography is used to locate the fetus and placenta and identify the largest pockets of amniotic fluid that can safely be sampled. The skin is prepared with antiseptic solution. A small amount of local anesthetic may be injected into the skin. The woman may feel pressure as the needle is inserted and mild cramping as the needle enters the myometrium.

A 3- to 4-inch, 20- or 21-gauge spinal needle is inserted into the pocket of fluid. After discarding 1 to 2 ml of fluid, approximately 20 ml of fluid are removed for analysis. A smaller volume of fluid (about 1 ml per week of gestation) is available for early amniocentesis at 11 to 14 weeks. The woman rests quietly for observation and ultrasound reassurance of the FHR and that fluid remains. She may then resume normal activities after 24 hours. Strenuous exercise such as jogging and other aerobic exercises should be deferred for 1 or 2 days. She should report persistent uterine contractions, vaginal bleeding, leakage of amniotic fluid, and fever (Cunningham et al., 2001).

As with CVS, $Rh_o(D)$ immune globulin is administered to prevent sensitization in nonsensitized Rh-negative women after amniocentesis.

Advantages

Amniocentesis has several advantages:
- It is a simple and reasonably safe procedure for diagnosis of many fetal abnormalities, maternal Rh-sensitization and its impact on the Rh-positive fetus, and fetal lung maturity.
- It is a relatively painless procedure that takes a short time.
- It has been performed for many years with few reported complications and is familiar to most obstetricians.

Disadvantages

Timing is a disadvantage of amniocentesis for genetic studies. Until recently the procedure was performed at approximately 15 to 16 weeks of gestation when the uterus is readily accessible and the volume of amniotic fluid permits removal of at least 20 ml. Analysis of the fluid, requiring active division of cells for an adequate number to karyotype, adds 3 to 7 days to the date of the amniocentesis, depending on the test. Techniques that may be possible for more rapid results include DNA probes to identify specific genes in a chromosome, such as fluorescence in situ hybridization (FISH). Spectral karyotyping (SKY) can be used to "paint" each of the 23 pairs of chromosomes with a specific color to identify extra or missing chromosomes. (See also Chapter 5.)

Abnormal results from amniocentesis usually are known in time to give the woman the choice of pregnancy termination before 20 weeks of gestation. However, this time frame is unacceptable to many women because of the increasing reality of pregnancy. Added tests such as high-quality ultrasound screening, biochemical screening through maternal serum, CVS, early amniocentesis, techniques for more rapid fetal chromosome analysis, and DNA analysis not requiring cell culture have helped identify birth defects that were not known to be at higher risk for the woman. However, the added techniques may seem simple at first, yet require many added decisions to reach a final decision about whether a birth defect exists.

Risks

The risks of amniocentesis include a pregnancy loss rate of less than 1%. A higher pregnancy loss rate of 2% to 5% has been noted after early amniocentesis between 11 and 13 weeks (AAP & ACOG, 2002). Ultrasound guidance of needle insertion reduces the incidence that the placenta or cord is pierced. Transfer of fetal blood to maternal circulation may occur, resulting in sensitization of the Rh-negative woman carrying an Rh-positive fetus. $Rh_o(D)$ immune globulin is administered to prevent sensitization in nonsensitized Rh-negative women after amniocentesis.

✔ **CHECK YOUR READING**

10. What factors make a pregnant woman a candidate for amniocentesis?
11. How is fetal lung maturity confirmed?
12. Why is bilirubin in amniotic fluid evaluated?
13. Why is early amniocentesis sometimes chosen over standard amniocentesis for prenatal diagnosis of genetic disorders?

PERCUTANEOUS UMBILICAL BLOOD SAMPLING (PUBS)

PUBS, also called *cordocentesis,* involves the aspiration of fetal blood from the umbilical cord for prenatal diagnosis or therapy (Figure 10-7). Major indications for PUBS include

THERAPEUTIC COMMUNICATIONS

Responding to Anxiety Related to Fetal Testing

Margaret Kitchner is a 35-year-old primigravida. She has postponed pregnancy to complete her education and establish a law practice. She has been referred for possible amniocentesis at 14 weeks because the risk for chromosome abnormalities increases beginning at age 35. Counseling has already been provided by a specialist in genetics, and the risks and benefits of the amniocentesis have been discussed. The genetic counselor has also discussed the option of multiple-marker screening and ultrasound rather than amniocentesis with Margaret and her husband. Together with ultrasound examination to look for signs associated with chromosome or other birth defects and the factor of Margaret's age, multiple-marker screening helps identify other possible birth defects, such as spina bifida.

Margaret: I'm here, but I'm not thrilled to be here.

Nurse: You wish you were somewhere else?

(Clarifying without attempting to lead.)

Margaret: The place isn't the problem really, but what about this test?

Nurse: You have some questions you'd like to ask about the amniocentesis?

(Seeking information, staying with the woman's comments by paraphrasing.)

Margaret: Well, my mother believes that if one thinks bad thoughts, bad things will come to pass.

Nurse: Bad thoughts?

(Knowing that the intergenerational belief system is powerful, the nurse focuses and seeks clarification.)

Margaret: Yes, you know, if we think something could be wrong with the baby, it's more likely to be true.

Nurse: I'd like to hear more.

("I" statement conveys interest and invites more discussion.)

Margaret: Well, my mother is not familiar with the tests, and she's just afraid that the test could hurt the baby.

Nurse: She must be very anxious about this test. How do you feel?

(The nurse notes that Margaret identifies her mother as the person who is concerned and avoids her own feelings. Acknowledging mother's feeling; focusing on woman's feeling by open-ended question.)

Margaret: She's anxious, and to tell you the truth, I'm anxious too.

Nurse: You would rather not be having the test.

(This makes an assumption; she said only that she was anxious. Saying "Tell me more about that" might be more therapeutic.)

Margaret: No, I want the test. I'm glad there is an option to having an amniocentesis for those who want to go that way. But having more decisions from several kinds of prenatal tests also makes me worry even more about whether I'm making the right choices. I want this baby so much and I've waited a long time.

Nurse: So the anxiety is really about whether the decision you made is the right one.

(The nurse "hears" the anxiety that Margaret didn't put into words; summarizes concerns and helps the woman identify and focus on what seems unclear to her.)

Margaret: That's for sure. It will be so hard to wait for the results, and I don't know what I would do if the news is bad or if I must decide about even more testing. I would also feel guilty if something happens to the baby because of the test.

Nurse: Waiting is difficult, but chances are that the news will be good.

(Acknowledging the difficulty is therapeutic, but offering reassurance blocks the interaction instead of focusing on the uncertainty expressed. The nurse might have said instead: "And it's very hard to imagine something is wrong with the baby." This response would have kept the interaction going and focused on the patient's feelings. Instead the blocking comment ended the interaction without allowing a full expression of feelings.)

Margaret: You think so? I hope so.

---

management of Rh disease, diagnosis of abnormal blood clotting factors, and acid-base status of the fetus. Fetal blood may be used to clarify questionable results of genetic testing by methods previously discussed. The PUBS technique can be used to treat blood diseases and deliver therapeutic drugs that cannot be delivered to the fetus in another way.

Procedure

High-resolution ultrasound is used to locate the fetus, placenta, and umbilical cord and guide needle insertion. The needle is inserted into the umbilical cord near the site at which the cord meets the placenta, which affords more cord stability. The umbilical vein is used more commonly than the umbilical arteries because it is larger and less likely to constrict during the procedure. Knowing which vessel (umbilical vein or artery) was sampled is important when testing fetal acid-base parameters. Blood returning to the fetus through the umbilical vein contains freshly-oxygenated blood and lower carbon dioxide content than blood leaving the fetus and going to the placenta through the umbilical arteries.

After needle withdrawal, the duration of bleeding from the umbilical cord is usually short and can be monitored by ultrasound examination. The fetal heart is monitored electronically for 30 to 60 minutes (Harman, 2004). The Rh-negative woman is given RhoGAM to prevent sensitization by any Rh-positive fetal blood that may have entered her circulation.

Risks

PUBS can occasionally result in a variety of life-threatening complications for the fetus. Therefore the perinatal team must be prepared for emergencies with a plan based on the indication for the sampling and fetal gestational age. This plan must be determined ahead of time and shared with the expectant woman and her support person.

Fetal bradycardia is the most common complication and is usually brief and has no long-term consequence. More severe bradycardia is associated with puncture of the umbilical artery. Less common complications include prolonged bleeding from the cord, cord laceration, cord hematoma,

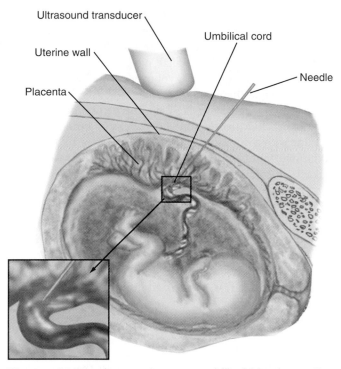

Figure 10-7 ■ In percutaneous umbilical blood sampling (PUBS, or cordocentesis) a needle is inserted through the expectant mother's abdomen and into an umbilical vessel (vein or artery) to withdraw a sample of fetal blood.

thrombosis, thromboembolism, preterm labor, and preterm rupture of membranes. Maternal blood sensitization, usually to the Rh factor, may occur if a fetal-to-maternal bleed exceeds 10 ml and inadequate RhoGAM is given for prevention. Sensitization to other blood factors may also occur (Harman, 2004).

ANTEPARTUM FETAL SURVEILLANCE

Antepartum fetal surveillance has three goals: (1) to determine fetal health or compromise as accurately as possible, (2) to reduce perinatal morbidity and mortality, and (3) to guide intervention by the obstetric team. The three most common methods of fetal surveillance are the nonstress test (NST), contraction stress test, and biophysical profile (BPP). A fourth method, maternal assessment of fetal movement, provides a way for the expectant mother to alert her health care provider to possible problems in her fetus. These methods are not expected to predict compromise caused by acute events such as abruptio placentae (premature separation of the placenta).

Nonstress Test

PURPOSE

The NST identifies whether an increase in the FHR occurs when the fetus moves, indicating adequate oxygenation, a healthy neural pathway from the fetal central nervous system to the fetal heart, and the ability of the fetal heart to respond to stimuli. FHR accelerations without fetal move-

ment are also considered a reassuring sign of adequate fetal oxygenation. If the fetal heart does not accelerate with movement, however, fetal hypoxemia and acidosis are concerns. In those cases an additional test such as the contraction stress test or BPP is necessary to evaluate the metabolic condition of the fetus. The test may help identify intraamniotic infection when the membranes have ruptured prematurely (Garite, 2004). The NST is often included as part of the BPP.

PROCEDURE

The NST takes about 40 minutes, allowing for most fetal sleep-wake cycles, although the fetus may show a reassuring pattern more quickly. A nurse with special preparation conducts the test in a hospital or an obstetrician's office. Before the test, the nurse discusses the test with the woman and explains why it is recommended. The test is termed *nonstress* because it consists of monitoring only. The fetus is not challenged or stressed by uterine contractions stimulated to obtain the necessary data.

For greatest accuracy the woman should not have smoked recently. Baseline vital signs should be done before the NST. To avoid supine hypotension the woman's head should be elevated at least 45 degrees or she should lie with uterine displacement from a lateral tilt. One study of 108 women found that NST results were more likely to be reactive if women were in sitting positions rather than lying on their left sides (Nathan, Haberman, Burgess, & Minkoff, 2000). If hypotension occurs, she should change her position to maintain the baseline pressure.

The nurse applies external electronic monitoring equipment. An ultrasound transducer to record fetal heart activity is secured on the woman's abdomen, where the fetal heart is heard most clearly. Next, a tocotransducer ("toco"), which detects uterine activity and fetal movement, is secured to the maternal abdomen (Figure 10-8). The woman may be given an event marker to press each time she senses movement, or the nurse may palpate the uterus to identify movements. Fetal heart activity and movements are

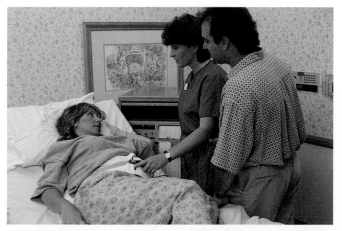

Figure 10-8 ■ A nonstress test is a noninvasive test that measures the response of the fetal heart to fetal movements. Here the nurse reassures the parents by pointing to fetal heart accelerations.

recorded on a moving strip of paper or an electronic strip in computerized systems (see Chapter 14). Contractions may be identified during an NST. These are often irregular, reflecting normal functions of the uterus as pregnancy progresses. However, frequent contractions in the preterm pregnancy may indicate increased uterine irritability that should be reported.

INTERPRETATION

Physicians must review and interpret NST results, although the nurse performs most NSTs. Results are classified as reactive (reassuring) or nonreactive (nonreassuring) (AAP & ACOG, 2002).

- Reactive (reassuring)—At least two fetal heart accelerations, with or without fetal movement detected by the woman, occur within a 20-minute period, peak at least 15 beats per minute (bpm) above the baseline, and last 15 seconds from baseline to baseline (Figure 10-9). Acoustic stimulation that elicits similar rate accelerations is also reassuring. Extending the testing time for an additional 40 minutes may be needed to allow for common fetal sleep-wake cycles.
- Nonreactive (nonreassuring)—Tracing does not demonstrate the required characteristics of a reactive tracing within a 40-minute period.

Fetal heart reactivity develops with maturation of the fetal autonomic nervous system. More than 15% of NSTs performed before 32 weeks of gestation are likely to be nonreactive even with normal fetal oxygenation. Criteria for reassuring status on the fetus younger than 32 weeks may be used, although these are not well established. Suggested criteria for a reassuring NST in the fetus younger than 32 weeks include accelerations that peak 10 bpm above the baseline with a duration of 10 seconds ("10 by 10") within a 30-minute time window (AAP & ACOG, 2002; Atterbury, Mikkelsen, & Santa-Donato, 2003).

ADVANTAGES

The NST is noninvasive and painless and believed to be without risk to mother or fetus. Consequently, it is the primary means of fetal surveillance in pregnancies at increased risk for uteroplacental insufficiency and consequent fetal hypoxia. The NST is easy to administer and often is repeated weekly and even daily if necessary. In addition, results are available immediately.

DISADVANTAGES

A disadvantage is a false-positive test result that occurs in a well-oxygenated term fetus that does not have accelerations reaching a peak of 15 bpm or that last less than 15 seconds

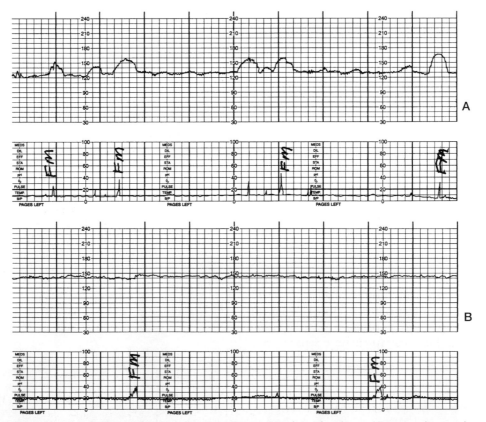

Figure 10-9 ■ **A,** Several accelerations have a duration of at least 15 seconds, reaching a peak of 25 to 30 beats per minute in this example of a reactive nonstress test. Comparable accelerations without fetal movement are also reassuring. **B,** In this recording of a nonreactive nonstress test, accelerations are absent after fetal movement *(FM).* (Courtesy Graphic Controls, Buffalo, New York.)

from baseline to baseline. Because of the high false-positive rate, women may undergo additional testing even though the fetus is actually healthy. Additional testing related to a nonreactive NST is usually a BPP or contraction stress test (CST).

Sleep is the usual reason for lack of fetal movement. Fetal sleep cycles average 20 to 40 minutes but other sleep cycles are longer. Acoustic stimulation reduces many false-positive results. Various methods have been used to stimulate the fetus and elicit accelerations in the FHR. These include having the mother drink orange juice to raise her glucose level, manipulating her abdomen, and using sound stimulation such as speakers placed on the abdomen. Of these, only acoustic stimulation has been shown by research to be both safe and effective in reducing false-positive results.

Vibroacoustic (Acoustic) Stimulation

PURPOSE AND PROCEDURE

Vibroacoustic stimulation (VAS), also called *acoustic stimulation,* can be used to confirm nonreactive NST findings and shorten the time required to obtain high-quality NST data during the last third of pregnancy. Reactive test results obtained with a vibroacoustic stimulator, similar to an electronic larynx, appear to predict fetal well-being without interfering with detection of the compromised fetus. Vibroacoustic stimulation can be used in intrapartum monitoring to verify questionable findings (see Chapter 14).

A vibroacoustic stimulator is applied to the maternal abdomen over the area of the fetal head, and stimulation with vibration and sound is given for up to 3 seconds. Vibroacoustic stimulation can be repeated at 1-minute intervals up to three times.

FETAL RESPONSES

Brain responses to auditory stimulation appear between 26 and 28 weeks of gestation. The sound of vibroacoustic stimulation does not appear to damage hearing in the fetus. Temporary changes in fetal body movements, breathing movements, and heart rate have been described. Fetuses near term show an increase in the number of gross (large and easily visible or felt) body movements to vibroacoustic stimulation, whereas fetuses between 26 and 32 weeks of gestation show no response. This suggests maturational change in response to vibroacoustic stimulation. Likewise, near-term fetuses appear to have fewer and more irregular breathing movements after vibroacoustic stimulation (Richardson & Gagnon, 2004).

RISKS

Vibroacoustic stimulation appears to be safe for the fetus in terms of hearing. The amniotic fluid and maternal tissues surrounding the fetus softens the sound of the stimulator.

✔ CHECK YOUR READING

14. What is a nonstress test, and why is it so named?
15. What is vibroacoustic stimulation and what is its expected result during the last third of pregnancy?

Contraction Stress Test

PURPOSE

A CST may be done if NST findings are nonreactive, or the test is sometimes the initial test of fetal well-being. Because a BPP often supplements both reassuring and nonreassuring NSTs, the CST is less often performed.

Uterine contractions compress the arteries that supply the placenta with oxygenated maternal blood, causing a recurrent decrease in fetal oxygen levels. The CST records the response of the FHR to stress induced by uterine contractions, identifying the fetus whose oxygen reserves are insufficient to tolerate the recurrent mild hypoxia of uterine contractions. Variability and accelerations of the FHR are expected as in the NST.

The fetus with adequate oxygen reserves tolerates the temporary hypoxia induced by uterine contractions, resulting in a reassuring FHR. However, if the fetus has inadequate reserves and substantial hypoxia has led to anaerobic metabolism, fetal acidosis results. This is likely to be manifested in nonreassuring fetal monitoring patterns.

Because contractions are induced, the CST is contraindicated in some situations (AAP & ACOG, 2002):

- Preterm labor or women who have a high risk for preterm labor
- Preterm membrane rupture
- History of extensive uterine surgery or classical uterine incision for cesarean birth (see Chapter 16)
- Placenta previa (see Chapter 25)

PROCEDURE

The nurse positions the woman in a supine position with her head comfortably elevated. Side-lying or uterine displacement reduces uterine pressure on her aorta and inferior vena cava. External electronic fetal monitoring devices are applied to record uterine activity and FHR. An initial recording is taken to determine if the woman is having at least three spontaneous contractions within a 10-minute time period, each with a duration of 40 seconds or longer. If spontaneous uterine contractions are adequate to interpret the test, uterine stimulation is not needed. If adequate uterine contractions are not present, either of two methods is used to achieve adequate contractions within a 10-minute period for interpretation of the test.

The breast self-stimulation test is based on the knowledge that stimulation of the nipples causes release of oxytocin from the posterior pituitary, which can cause uterine contractions. The woman brushes her palm across one nipple through her clothing for 2 minutes, stopping if a contraction begins. The nipple stimulation continues after a 5-minute rest period until an adequate contraction pattern is attained.

If the breast self-stimulation test does not effectively stimulate contractions or if the health care provider prefers this method the oxytocin challenge test may be performed. The oxytocin challenge test uses an intravenous infusion of dilute oxytocin to stimulate uterine contractions. The nurse inserts a primary intravenous line carrying plain fluid such as lactated Ringers and a long secondary (piggyback) line for administration of dilute oxytocin solution. The initial rate is low (0.5 to 1 milliunits/min) and increased every 15 to 20 minutes until the desired contraction frequency is attained (AAP & ACOG, 2002).

INTERPRETATION

CST results may be interpreted as negative (normal, or reassuring of fetal well-being), positive (abnormal, or nonreassuring that the fetus is healthy), equivocal, or unsatisfactory (AAP & ACOG, 2002) (Figure 10-10).

- Negative (reassuring)—No late decelerations (decreases in the FHR persisting after the contraction ends) although the fetus was stressed by three contractions of at least 40 seconds' duration in a 10-minute period
- Positive (abnormal)—Late decelerations accompanying at least 50% of contractions even when fewer than three contractions occur in 10 minutes

- Equivocal (suspicious)—Intermittent late decelerations and significant variable decelerations (sudden decreases in the FHR that quickly return to the baseline)
- Equivocal (hyperstimulation)—FHR decelerations occurring in the presence of contractions that are closer than every 2 minutes or last longer than 90 seconds
- Unsatisfactory—Fewer than three contractions in 10 minutes or a tracing that cannot be interpreted

ADVANTAGES

Contraction stress testing has several advantages:
- The test provides a minimally invasive follow-up of a nonreactive NST result or BPP.
- If findings are negative, CST offers more than 99% reassurance that the uteroplacental unit is likely to support life for at least 1 more week (ACOG, 1999).

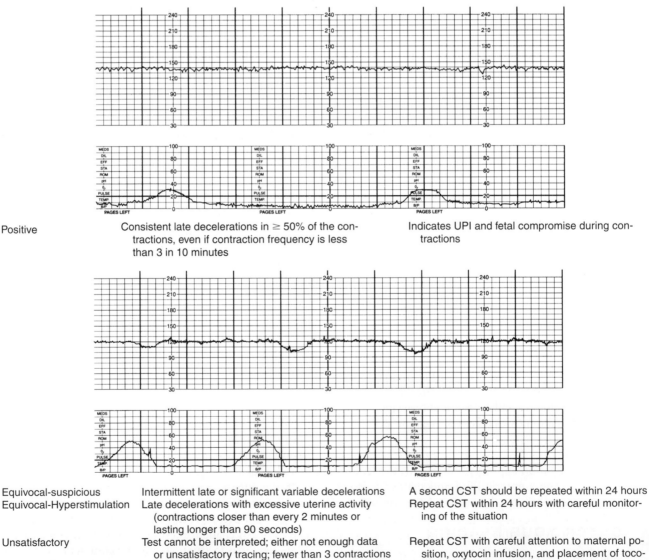

Negative — No late decelerations — Reassuring that the fetus can tolerate labor

Positive — Consistent late decelerations in ≥ 50% of the contractions, even if contraction frequency is less than 3 in 10 minutes — Indicates UPI and fetal compromise during contractions

Equivocal-suspicious — Intermittent late or significant variable decelerations — A second CST should be repeated within 24 hours

Equivocal-Hyperstimulation — Late decelerations with excessive uterine activity (contractions closer than every 2 minutes or lasting longer than 90 seconds) — Repeat CST within 24 hours with careful monitoring of the situation

Unsatisfactory — Test cannot be interpreted; either not enough data or unsatisfactory tracing; fewer than 3 contractions in 10 minutes — Repeat CST with careful attention to maternal position, oxytocin infusion, and placement of toco-transducer

Figure 10-10 ■ Interpretation of contraction stress test *(CST)*. *UPI,* Uteroplacental insufficiency. (Courtesy Graphic Controls; Buffalo, New York.)

- A positive CST result allows the physician to analyze available options for further testing and make plans for the birth of an infant who may be compromised because of decreased placental functioning during labor.

DISADVANTAGES

The CST has three major disadvantages:
- The test is more time consuming than the NST.
- The CST requires precision, needing either the participation of the woman in breast self-stimulation or careful infusion of oxytocin by the nurse to obtain an adequate contraction pattern without causing hyperstimulation of the uterus.
- The cost is higher than the NST, particularly if the oxytocin challenge test is used. It is usually performed in a hospital setting with a per-hour charge. Equipment and supplies such as intravenous lines, oxytocin, and infusion pumps add to the cost.

✓ CHECK YOUR READING

16. Why is initiating contractions necessary in a CST?
17. In a CST, what do late decelerations of FHR indicate?

Biophysical Profile

The condition of the fetus can be most accurately predicted if several parameters are evaluated. Unlike the NST and CST, which assess only fetal heart activity, the BPP assesses five parameters of fetal status: FHR, fetal breathing movements, gross fetal movements, fetal muscle tone, and amniotic fluid volume.

PURPOSE

The individual components of the examination are a combination of acute and chronic markers of fetal well-being. The acute or short-term markers are the FHR reactivity, fetal breathing movements, gross fetal movements, and fetal tone. The major chronic or long-term marker is the amount of amniotic fluid.

The acute markers are controlled by different central nervous system control centers that develop at different stages in gestation. Fetal tone is the earliest to develop, then fetal movements, then regular breathing movements. FHR reactivity develops last at the end of the second trimester or beginning of the third trimester.

The fetal central nervous system centers that control each individual parameter of the BPP react differently to hypoxemia. The control centers that develop later require higher oxygen levels than those developing earlier. Therefore FHR reactivity disappears first. Fetal breathing movements are affected next, and fetal movement and fetal tone are the last areas affected. Because of this, absence of fetal tone indicates advanced asphyxia and acidosis. This progression has been termed the *gradual hypoxia concept* (Figure 10-11).

The amount of amniotic fluid provides information about chronic hypoxia if loss of fluid is not the result of pre-

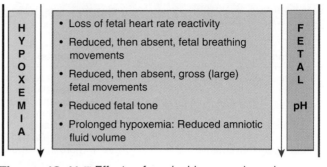

Figure 10-11 ■ Effects of gradual hypoxemia and worsening of fetal acidosis.

mature membrane rupture. During periods of hypoxemia the fetus shunts blood from areas not critical to fetal life, such as the kidneys and lungs, to vital organs such as the heart, brain, and placenta. If hypoxemia is prolonged, blood flow to the fetal kidneys and lungs, which produce much of the amniotic fluid, may virtually cease. Therefore oligohydramnios indicates prolonged fetal hypoxia and is a strong indication of fetal compromise. The amount of amniotic fluid is established by calculating the depth of the single maximum-sized pocket. A method that adds the depths of amniotic fluid in four uterine quadrants is the amniotic fluid index (AFI). Established normal values for the AFI do not exist, but volume sums greater than 10 cm are considered reassuring, and less than 5 cm volume is considered oligohydramnios. An AFI higher than 18 to 20 cm suggests excess amniotic fluid volume, or hydramnios (Harman, 2004; Hobel, 2004).

PROCEDURE AND INTERPRETATION

FHR reactivity is interpreted from an NST. The other four parameters are measured by real-time ultrasonography. A scoring technique is used to interpret the data, with each parameter contributing either 0 or 2 points. A score of 10 is perfect; a score of 0 is the worst score. A total score of 8 to 10 is considered normal unless oligohydramnios is present (Table 10-1). Oligohydramnios may indicate chronic fetal hypoxia and requires further evaluation (ACOG, 1999; Harman, 2004).

Modified Biophysical Profile

Some physicians now assess the fetus only by ultrasonography and omit the NST if other parameters are normal (ACOG, 1999). This shortens testing time without significantly compromising accuracy. In other medical centers the test is modified to include only two parameters, an AFI and an NST.

ADVANTAGES

The modified BPP is noninvasive and less costly than some tests because it can be performed on an outpatient basis. Results are immediately available and may decrease the number of false-positive NST findings. The BPP allows conservative treatment of high-risk patients because delivery can be delayed if fetal well-being is indicated. The BPP helps iden-

TABLE 10-1 Scoring the Biophysical Profile for a Term Fetus

	Points	
Criterion	Present (2 points)	Absent (0 points)
Nonstress test (NST) (if used)	Reactive NST (at least two fetal heart rate [FHR] accelerations peaking at least 15 beats per minute [bpm] above baseline for 15 sec within a 20-min period)	Nonreactive NST (absence of required characteristics for reactive test after 40 min of testing)
Fetal breathing movements (FBM)	One or more episodes of rhythmic FBM of 30 sec or more within 30 min	Absent FBM or none that meet criterion for "present"
Gross body movements	Three or more trunk movements in 30 min; limb and trunk movement is considered one movement	Two or fewer trunk movements in 30 min
Fetal tone	One or more episodes of fetal extremity extension with return to flexion; opening or closing of hand	Extension with return to partial flexion; absence of flexion
Amniotic fluid volume	At least one pocket of fluid that measures at least 2 cm in two planes perpendicular to each other	Amniotic fluid volume that does not meet this criterion

From American Academy of Pediatrics (AAP) & American College of Obstetricians and Gynecologists (ACOG). (2002). *Guidelines for perinatal care* (5th ed.). Elk Grove Village, IL, and Washington, DC: Author.
Interpretation: Normal (reassuring) = 8 to 10 points; equivocal = 6 points; abnormal = ≤4 points and delivery may be considered. If oligohydramnios is present, more frequent testing is warranted and delivery may be considered. If the NST is omitted from the BPP, the maximum score of the four remaining ultrasound criteria is 8.

tify the presence and severity of hypoxia and acidemia because it measures multiple variables.

The BPP may be used when membranes rupture prematurely and the risk for fetal infection increases. BPP evaluation may accompany other fetal assessment methods to determine whether intrauterine infection has developed after the amniotic sac ruptures at an early gestation (Garite, 2004).

DISADVANTAGES

Additional research is needed to refine interpretation of the test. For example, each variable is given equal weight, although some variables may be more important than others. The predictive accuracy of the BPP is best at the extremes, meaning that scores of 0 and 10 are highly predictive of the presence or absence of fetal acidosis, respectively. Scores toward the middle have less predictive accuracy.

Because perinatal asphyxia is a possible cause of cerebral palsy, antepartal surveillance techniques may allow fetal hypoxia to be identified and treated before it reaches critical levels. The BPP may be the main testing to identify problems before they result in permanent fetal injury, but other methods must often enter the diagnostic picture to best clarify fetal condition (Harman, 2004).

✔ CHECK YOUR READING

18. What is the relationship between loss of fetal tone and hypoxia?
19. Why is amniotic fluid volume an important parameter in the BPP?

MATERNAL ASSESSMENT OF FETAL MOVEMENT

Fetal movements detected by the mother are often called *kick counts*. The well-oxygenated fetus moves frequently. The fetus with a compromised oxygen supply conserves energy with fewer movements. Daily evaluation of these movements provides additional data from the fetus in the context of other assessment techniques such as nonstress or BPP testing. The nurse must teach the woman to promptly report any sudden change in usual fetal movements to her health care provider.

Procedure

Numerous protocols exist for assessing kick counts. The woman lies on her side, places her hands on the largest part of her abdomen, and concentrates on fetal movements. She uses a clock or timer and records the number of movements felt during that time. Examples of kick count protocols include the following:

- Count fetal movements for 30 minutes three times per day (Figure 10-12). Further evaluation is recommended if fewer than four movements occur in 30 minutes.
- Count fetal movements daily for 1 hour. If fewer than 10 movements are felt, continue counting for another hour. Fewer than 10 movements in a 2-hour period should be reported to the health care provider.
- The Cardiff count-to-10 method entails counting the first 10 movements and noting the time of day when the tenth movement is felt. The health care provider should be notified if the tenth movement occurs progressively later or if fewer than 10 movements occur in 12 hours.
- Count fetal movements for 30 minutes in the morning and evening to establish a baseline. If a 50% decrease or no fetal movement occurs, extend the counting period for 30 minutes.

Advantages

Counting fetal movement has obvious advantages:
- It is inexpensive.
- It is noninvasive.
- It may identify fetal problems early in the client who has no known pregnancy risk factors.
- It is convenient for the client and encourages her participation in her care.

Time of day	Sunday	Monday	Tuesday	Wednesday	Thursday	Friday	Saturday
Dates: 11/14/01 to 11/20/01							
Morning 8-9 AM	⊞⊞ ⊞⊞	⊞ //	⊞ ///				
Afternoon 1-2 PM	⊞ /	⊞ ///	⊞				
Evening 9-10 PM	⊞ // ⊞	⊞ ////					
Total	28	24					

Figure 10-12 ■ Daily fetal movement record in use. The mother counts the number of fetal movements (kicks) within a specified period several times per day and indicates each movement on a chart. She reports any abnormality to her health care provider.

Disadvantages

Many variables make interpretation of fetal movement counts difficult:

- Fetal resting state decreases movements.
- Maternal perception of movement may vary. The ability of women to perceive fetal movement varies considerably, even in the same woman at different times.
- The time of day may affect fetal movement (lower in the morning, higher in the evening).
- Drugs taken by the mother (such as methadone, heroin, cocaine, alcohol, tobacco) may affect fetal activity.
- The mother may evaluate fetal movements erratically, making her counts less informative.

Application of the Nursing Process
Diagnostic Testing

Perinatal nurses perform NSTs and CSTs. With additional education, nurses may perform limited ultrasound examinations. Basic ultrasound examinations, which usually occur in an office or a clinical setting, require education beyond that for limited ultrasound. Nurses explain testing procedures and the information that can be determined from the tests. Nurses also reduce anxiety by providing emotional support when decisions about repeated testing or a series of procedures becomes necessary.

Assessment

Collect as much information as possible about the woman and her reasons for having the tests. The information may be helpful when conducting the tests and interpreting the results. Necessary information includes the following:

- Gravida, para, living children, gestation (in weeks).
- Maternal health problems (such as hypertension, diabetes, heart disease).
- Current obstetric problems (such as vaginal bleeding, decreased fetal movement, multifetal gestation, intrauterine growth restriction, malpresentation, hydramnios, oligohydramnios).

- Prior obstetric problems (such as birth of a stillborn infant or an infant with congenital anomalies, birth of a low-birth-weight infant or a large-for-gestational age infant).
- History of substance abuse, including alcohol and tobacco.
- Knowledge of reasons for the test and the procedure to be performed: "What questions can I answer before we start the test?"
- Knowledge of surveillance regimen if additional testing is necessary: "Will you tell me what you understand about the need to repeat the test every week?" "What kinds of changes in your baby's movement are important to report?" "How soon should you report the changes?"
- Emotional response to the tests: "What are your major concerns?" "What can we do to make the tests easier for you?"
- The woman's or couple's expectations of the diagnostic tests. The risks and limitations of testing should be discussed, as well as the indications. It may also be necessary to remind the couple that results from one test may indicate that others are appropriate. They must decide at each step whether to continue.

Analysis

Women at increased risk for problems during pregnancy require fetal diagnostic procedures. Clients' responses vary depending on their levels of knowledge and their usual responses to stressful situations. Many women are concerned with both the test and the condition of the fetus. The relevant nursing diagnosis is "Anxiety related to lack of knowledge of diagnostic procedures and the uncertain condition of the fetus."

Planning

Goals and expected outcomes for this nursing diagnosis are that the woman (and her support person) will do the following:

- Describe how, when, and why she is to be tested before testing procedures are initiated
- Verbalize concerns about the condition of the fetus and seek information from her health care team at each appointment

Interventions

PROVIDING INFORMATION

The nurse may be the primary provider of information, such as for an NST, or the nurse may reinforce physician explanations. Provide simple, clear explanations of what the test measures and its purpose and frequency. Explain safety and the amount of discomfort the woman will experience. Describe the procedure, including its usual length of time, to minimize anxiety caused by lack of knowledge. The woman is less likely to forget important information if she is given verbal and written instructions about follow-up care and events that should be reported to the physician.

Parents often become concerned when screening test results are abnormal, such as an MSAFP or multiple-marker test. The nurse may need to remind them that other factors may cause abnormal results and that added tests help clarify the results. In addition, nurses often need to interpret technical information that parents receive from physicians because it may be confusing and cause the parents undue anxiety. Awaiting results from follow-up testing, even if very brief, often adds to parent's anxiety.

PROVIDING SUPPORT

Identify and respond to feelings expressed by expectant parents when antepartum testing procedures are recommended or fetal problems are confirmed. The woman often experiences frustration with the discomfort, limitations, and time-consuming demands of pregnancy and the regimen of fetal testing. Skill in therapeutic communication is never more important than during counseling about fetal diagnostic tests.

- Active listening conveys interest and concern.
- Paraphrasing allows for interpretation because it expresses in different words what concerns the family.
- Reflecting what the family conveys about feelings helps them "hear" their feelings.
- Clarifying helps the woman "see" the issues and available options.
- Comforting measures such as touch, if culturally acceptable to the woman, convey empathic concern and are especially important during difficult procedures.

Although nurses offer caring concern and careful reflection of feelings, they do not offer advice. The woman, along with her primary support person and other chosen persons, must make decisions about antepartal assessment. Nurses frequently help the family contact persons (such as a clergy member or close relative) to whom they turn in troubled times, such as when abnormal test results are verified.

HELPING CLIENTS SET REALISTIC GOALS

Women benefit from understanding how an antepartal surveillance regimen benefits the fetus. Although the repeated tests may seem tedious, they often offer the best chance for the fetus to be delivered at the best possible time. Explain to the woman that testing helps the perinatal team decide whether intervention is needed and choose the best possible intervention under the circumstances. The fetus has an im-proved chance of surviving and reaching maturity if test results remain reassuring.

If the woman is having testing to identify fetal abnormalities, help her understand that a baseline risk for abnormalities remains when tests show the fetus is normal. Even if performing all diagnostic tests for birth defects on a woman were possible, the background risk would remain.

SUPPORTING THE WOMAN'S DECISION

Prenatal genetic diagnosis sometimes leads a woman to choose pregnancy termination, often during the second trimester. The woman also has the right to indicated prenatal genetic diagnostic procedures even if she would not terminate her pregnancy for an abnormal fetus. Nurses must examine their own ethical beliefs before becoming involved in fetal diagnostic testing. They must be prepared to support whatever decision a family makes, even if it is not one they would make. A woman who decides to continue or terminate a pregnancy is entitled to compassionate care regardless of the nurse's personal views about her decision.

Evaluation

The goals and expected outcomes are successful if the woman verbalizes knowledge of why tests are recommended and how and when they will be performed. The second goal and expected outcome is met if the woman and family verbalize any concerns about the fetus and seek additional information from the perinatal team as needed.

SUMMARY CONCEPTS

- Ultrasonography is widely used during pregnancy to determine a variety of fetal and placental conditions and aid in the performance of other tests such as amniocentesis. It is also used in gynecology and infertility care. Doppler ultrasound is a variation that allows estimation of blood flow and vascular resistance in fetal structures.
- Alpha-fetoprotein assessment is performed on maternal serum or amniotic fluid with the primary goal of detecting open body wall defects such as neural tube defects. Additional tests are required if alpha-fetoprotein levels are abnormal. Other markers, human chorionic gonadotropin and estriol, are usually assessed with maternal serum alpha-fetoprotein in a triple-screen for chromosomal anomalies such as trisomy 21. Additional markers such as inhibin A are becoming more common, changing the triple-screen testing to multiple-marker testing.
- Chorionic villus sampling is performed at 10 to 12 weeks of gestation to provide parents with information about chromosomal and other congenital defects in the first trimester of pregnancy. Chorionic villus sampling does not provide a sample of amniotic fluid for alpha-fetoprotein testing.
- Amniocentesis is usually performed in the second trimester to identify fetal genetic defects or open defects such as neural tube defects. It may be used during the third trimester to evaluate fetal maturity or Rh incompatibility problems. Standard amniocentesis is performed at

15 to 20 weeks of gestation. Early amniocentesis (11 to 14 weeks) allows earlier diagnosis of genetic problems.

- Percutaneous umbilical blood sampling involves aspiration of blood from umbilical vessels to detect blood disorders, acid-base balance, or fetal disease. Therapeutic medications and blood products can also be injected by the same route. Fetal bradycardia is the most common complication.

- The nonstress test determines whether the fetal heart rate accelerates when the fetus moves. Accelerations of the heart rate, regardless of fetal movement, are a reassuring sign because they are associated with adequate fetal oxygenation and an intact neural pathway from the fetal brain to the heart. The healthy fetus younger than 32 weeks of gestation may not have accelerations that meet the criteria for a reactive nonstress test.

- Contraction stress tests evaluate response of the fetal heart to recurrent short interruptions in placental blood flow and oxygen supply that occur with uterine contractions.

- Maternal assessment of fetal movement ("kick counts") is an inexpensive and noninvasive method of evaluating the fetus. The poorly oxygenated fetus usually moves less than the well-oxygenated fetus. The woman may be advised to follow any of several protocols because no standard protocol exists.

- All perinatal nurses must be prepared to offer clear explanations of diagnostic procedures and any problems the woman should report. Support for the family requiring fetal diagnostic tests can reduce their anxiety.

REFERENCES & READINGS

American Academy of Pediatrics (AAP), & American College of Obstetricians and Gynecologists (ACOG). (2002). *Guidelines for perinatal care* (5th ed.). Elk Grove Village, IL: Author.

ACOG. (1999). *Antepartum fetal surveillance*, Practice Bulletin No. 9. Washington, DC: Author.

ACOG. (2004). *ACOG issues position on first-trimester screening methods*. Retrieved September 27, 2004, from www.acog.org/from_home/publications/press_releases/nr06-30-04.cfm.

Armour, K. (2004). Antepartum maternal-fetal assessment. *AWHONN Lifelines*, 8(3), 232-240.

Atterbury, J.L., Mikkelsen, G.M., & Santa-Donato, A. (2003). Antenatal fetal assessment and testing. *Fetal heart monitoring: Principles and practices* (3rd ed., pp. 261-288). Dubuque, IA: Kendall/Hunt.

Benn, P.A., Egan, J.F.X., Fang, M., & Smith-Bindman, R. (2004). Changes in the utilization of prenatal diagnosis. *Obstetrics & Gynecology, 103*(6), 1255-1260.

Cunningham, F.G., MacDonald, P.C., Gant, N.F., Leveno, K.J., Gilstrap, L.C., Hankins, G.D.V., et al. (2001). *Williams obstetrics* (21st ed.). New York: McGraw-Hill.

Filly, R.A. (2000). Obstetrical sonography: The best way to terrify a pregnant woman. *Journal of Ultrasound in Medicine, 19*(1), 1-5.

Garite, T.J. (2004). Premature rupture of the membranes. In R.K. Creasy, R. Resnik, & J.D. Iams (Eds.), *Maternal-fetal medicine: Principles and practice* (5th ed., pp. 723-739). Philadelphia: Saunders.

Gilbert, E.S., & Harmon, J.S. (2003). *Manual of high-risk pregnancy and delivery* (3rd ed.). St. Louis: Mosby.

Glantz, C., & Woods, J.R. (2004). Significance of amniotic fluid meconium. In R.K. Creasy, R. Resnik, & J.D. Iams (Eds.), *Maternal-fetal medicine: Principles and practice* (5th ed., pp. 441-450). Philadelphia: Saunders.

Goldberg, J.D., & Norton, M.E. (2001). Prenatal diagnostic techniques. In M.R. Harrison, M.I. Evans, N.S. Adzick, & W. Holzgreve (Eds.), *The unborn patient: The art and science of fetal therapy* (3rd ed., pp. 125-148). Philadelphia: Saunders.

Harman, C.R. (2004). Assessment of fetal health In R.K. Creasy, R. Resnik, & J.D. Iams (Eds.), *Maternal-fetal medicine: Principles and practice* (5th ed., pp. 357-401). Philadelphia: Saunders.

Hing, E., & Middleton, K. (2004). Ambulatory medical care survey: 2002 outpatient department summary. *Advance Data from Vital and Health Statistics*, No. 345. Hyattsville, MD: National Center for Health Statistics. Retrieved September 23, 2004, from www.cdc.gov/nchs/data/ad/ad345.pdf.

Hobel, C.J. (2004). Obstetric complications: Preterm labor, PROM, IUGR, postterm pregnancy, and IUFD. In N.F. Hacker, J.G. Moore, & J.C. Gambone, *Essentials of obstetrics and gynecology* (4th ed., pp. 167-182). Philadelphia: Saunders.

Jasper, M.L. (2004). Antepartum fetal assessment. In S. Mattson & J.E. Smith (Eds.), *Core curriculum for maternal-newborn nursing* (3rd ed., pp. 161-200). Philadelphia: Saunders.

Jenkins, T.M., & Wapner, R.J. (2004). Prenatal diagnosis of congenital disorders. In R.K. Creasy, R. Resnik, & J.D. Iams (Eds.), *Maternal-fetal medicine: Principles and practice* (5th ed., pp. 235-280). Philadelphia: Saunders.

Jobe, A.H. (2004). Fetal lung development. In R.K. Creasy, R. Resnik, & J.D. Iams (Eds.), *Maternal-fetal medicine: Principles and practice* (5th ed., pp. 209-222). Philadelphia: Saunders.

Jorde, L.B., Carey, J.C., Bamshad, M.J., & White, R.L. (2003). *Medical genetics* (3rd ed.). St. Louis: Mosby.

Manning, F.A. (2004). General principles and applications of ultrasonography. In R.K. Creasy, R. Resnik, & J.D. Iams (Eds.), *Maternal-fetal medicine: Principles and practice* (5th ed., pp. 315-355). Philadelphia: Saunders.

Martin, J.A., Hamilton, B.E., Sutton, P.D., Ventura, S.J., Menacker, F., & Munson, M.L. (2003). Births: Final data for 2002. *National Vital Statistics Reports, 52*(10). Hyattsville, MD: National Center for Health Statistics. Retrieved September 21, 2004, from www.cdc.gov/nchs/data/nvsr/nvsr52/nvsr52_10.pdf.

Menihan, C.A. (2000). Limited obstetric ultrasound in nursing practice. *Journal of Obstetric, Gynecologic, and Neonatal Nursing, 29*(3), 325-330.

Mercer, B.M. (2004). Assessment and induction of fetal pulmonary maturity. In R.K. Creasy, R. Resnik, & J.D. Iams (Eds.), *Maternal-fetal medicine: Principles and practice* (5th ed., pp. 451-463). Philadelphia: Saunders.

Moise, K.J. (2004). Hemolytic disease of the fetus and newborn. In R.K. Creasy, R. Resnik, & J.D. Iams (Eds.), *Maternal-fetal medicine: Principles and practice* (5th ed., pp. 537-561). Philadelphia: Saunders.

Nathan, E.B., Haberman, S., Burgess, T., & Minkoff, H. (2000). The relationship of maternal position to the results of brief nonstress tests: A randomized clinical trial. *American Journal of Obstetrics & Gynecology, 182*(5), 1070-1072.

National Center for Health Statistics. (2004). *Health, United States, 2004 with Chartbook on Trends in the Health of Americans*. Hyattsville, MD: Author.

Nelson, K.H., & Nelson, L.H. (2003). Ultrasound in obstetrics. In J.R. Scott, R.S. Gibbs, B.Y. Karlan, & A.F. Haney (Eds.), *Danforth's obstetrics and gynecology* (9th ed., pp. 143-158). Philadelphia: Lippincott Williams & Wilkins.

Parer, J.T., & Nageotte, M.P. (2004). Intrapartum fetal surveillance. In R.K. Creasy, R. Resnik, & J.D. Iams (Eds.), *Maternal-fetal medicine: Principles and practice* (5th ed., pp. 403-427). Philadelphia: Saunders.

Pretorius, D.H., Nelson, T.R., & Lev-Toaff, A.S. (2000). Three dimensional ultrasound in obstetrics and gynecology. In P.W. Callen (Ed.), *Ultrasonography in obstetrics and gynecology* (4th ed., pp. 747-762). Philadelphia: Saunders.

Richardson, B.S., & Gagnon, R. (2004). Fetal breathing and body movements. In R.K. Creasy, R. Resnik, & J.D. Iams (Eds.), *Maternal-fetal medicine: Principles and practice* (5th ed., pp. 181-197). Philadelphia: Saunders.

Simpson, J.L., & Elias, S. (2003). *Genetics in obstetrics and gynecology* (3rd ed.). Philadelphia: Saunders.

Spong, C.Y. (2003). Fetal monitoring. In J.R. Scott, R.S. Gibbs, B.Y. Karlan, & A.F. Haney. (Eds.), *Danforth's obstetrics and gynecology* (9th ed., pp. 159-171). Philadelphia: Lippincott Williams & Wilkins.

Stringer, M., Miesnik, S.R., Brown, L.P., Menei, L., & Macones, G.A. (2003). Limited obstetric ultrasound examinations: Competency and cost. *Journal of Obstetric, Gynecologic, and Neonatal Nursing, 32*(3), 307-312.

Tekay, A., & Campbell, S. (2000). Doppler ultrasonography in obstetrics. In P.W. Callen (Ed.), *Ultrasonography in obstetrics and gynecology* (4th ed., pp, 677-723). Philadelphia: Saunders.

Ward, K. (2003). Genetics and prenatal diagnosis. In J.R. Scott, R.S. Gibbs, B.Y. Karlan, & A.F. Haney (Eds.), *Danforth's obstetrics and gynecology* (9th ed., pp. 105-128). Philadelphia: Lippincott Williams & Wilkins.

Perinatal Education

OBJECTIVES

After studying this chapter, you should be able to:

1. List the goals of perinatal education.
2. Explain choices in childbearing and the effects of education on these choices.
3. Describe the various types of education for childbearing families.
4. Describe techniques for pain relief taught in Lamaze childbirth classes.
5. Describe the support person's role in helping women during labor and birth.
6. Explain the components frequently included in a birth plan.

Go to your Student CD-ROM for Review Questions keyed to these Objectives.

DEFINITIONS

Birth Plan A plan describing a couple's preferences for their birth experience (also called a *family preference plan*).

Doula A trained labor support person who provides labor or postpartum support.

Effleurage Massage of the abdomen or another body part performed during labor contractions.

Habituation Decreased response to a repeated stimulus.

Psychoprophylaxis Method of prepared childbirth that emphasizes mental concentration and relaxation to increase pain tolerance.

Perinatal education is important to help couples learn about pregnancy, birth, and parenting. Many classes not only focus on preparation for childbirth but also include information formerly received during the birth facility stay. Prenatal classes are often included in perinatal clinical pathways (see Figure 7-10, pp. 128-129).

GOALS OF PERINATAL EDUCATION

The goals of perinatal education are to help parents become knowledgeable consumers, take an active role in maintaining health during pregnancy and birth, and learn coping techniques to deal with pregnancy, childbirth, and parenting. Meeting these goals reduces fear of the unknown and increases parents' abilities to make decisions regarding childbirth and parenting with confidence and satisfaction.

Perinatal education classes are strongly recommended by the American Academy of Pediatrics and the American College of Obstetricians and Gynecologists (2002). A Healthy People 2010 goal is to increase the proportion of women who attend a series of prepared childbirth classes (U.S. Department of Health and Human Services, 2000).

PROVIDERS OF EDUCATION

Although most perinatal education classes are taught by registered nurses, physical therapists or others who have taken special courses also may become perinatal educators. Many instructors are certified by organizations such as the American Society for Psychoprophylaxis in Obstetrics (ASPO) or the International Childbirth Education Association (ICEA). Certification ensures that the instructors have received special preparation to provide sound education adhering to the certifying organization's general philosophy. The Association of Women's Health, Obstetric and Neonatal Nurses (AWHONN) has published guidelines for educator competencies and class curricula (AWHONN, 2000).

Teachers must be versed in adult education theory and techniques and skillful in handling groups of people of diverse ages and from diverse backgrounds. They must be familiar with the policies and daily routines of the agencies their students will use so the information they present will be current and accurate.

Education may be presented formally in classrooms. Nurses in offices, clinics, and birth sites also educate women informally. Teaching may occur in waiting rooms of clinics before women are called for their appointments or as part of routine care. Teaching methods involve discussion, demonstration and return demonstration, written material, role play, and use of visual aids such as videos, models, posters, and equipment. Material used should be evaluated frequently to ensure it is up to date and correct.

Classes may be sponsored by schools, health departments, civic organizations, medical groups, or hospitals. Teachers may be employed by a sponsoring agency or self-employed. Classes may also occur in less traditional sites. For example, some companies offer prenatal classes at the work site. Teaching women ways to reduce risk factors for complications is a way for employers to reduce costs associated with prematurity and low birth weight.

CLASS PARTICIPANTS

Participants in classes about childbearing have traditionally been middle-income couples who are older and better educated than those who do not take classes. Low-income women may not have money to pay for classes or transportation to get there. Although inexpensive or free classes are available in some areas, women with little or no prenatal care may not know about them. Classes in languages other than English are often available in areas where they are needed.

People take classes for a variety of reasons. Many have a strong desire to participate actively in all aspects of childbearing. For these people, making decisions about what happens to them is important, and they want the education to help them decide wisely. Others are looking for coping strategies to deal with their fears of childbirth and pain.

Some women develop a greater sense of control during labor and delivery when they have taken prepared childbirth classes. When women feel that they are informed and have some control over what happens to them, they are more likely to expect birth to be satisfying and fulfilling and to experience it as such.

CHOICES FOR CHILDBEARING

One purpose of perinatal education is to help parents learn what options are available so that they can make appropriate choices. Parents learn that many ways of birthing are possible and no one "right" method exists. Knowledgeable parents can communicate assertively with their health care providers about their needs and desires.

Health Care Professional

Women contemplating pregnancy and birth may choose a certified nurse-midwife (CNM), nurse practitioner (NP), obstetrician, or family practice physician to be their health care providers. They need to know what to expect from each of these practitioners.

A CNM cares for women at low risk for complications and refers them to a back-up physician if problems develop. CNMs, NPs, and physicians treat women during pregnancy and the postpartum period, but NPs do not usually perform deliveries. NPs usually work in a physician's office and see women for routine prenatal care, but the delivery is performed by the physician. A CNM, NP, or family practice physician may also care for the newborn. A physician generally arrives for the birth near the end of labor, whereas the CNM is often present through most of labor and birth.

Some couples visit several different care providers before choosing the one they feel is best for them. They may ask about the provider's usual practices and the provider's beliefs about areas that are important to them, such as medication, use of episiotomies, or separation from the infant.

Setting

The woman and her partner must choose a birth setting and select a care provider who practices in that setting. Hospitals are the most frequent setting for birth in North America. They often have birthing suites that provide a homelike atmosphere. There may also be traditional labor and delivery rooms. A freestanding birth center provides an atmosphere that is less institutional than the hospital. Home birth allows the woman to give birth in her own surroundings with delivery managed by a midwife (see "Current Settings for Childbirth" in Chapter 1). Couples may visit the birth setting before making a choice. Their insurance may limit their selection of a setting.

Support Person

During labor the woman needs to have someone with her to help her through the experience. The support person is most often the father of her baby, but a relative or friend may also take this role (Figure 11-1). Some women wish to share the birth experience with several relatives and close friends. If the birth setting is traditional, only one person is permitted to be present. In less traditional settings, more support people are usually allowed. Some women hire a support person such as a doula to provide support during labor.

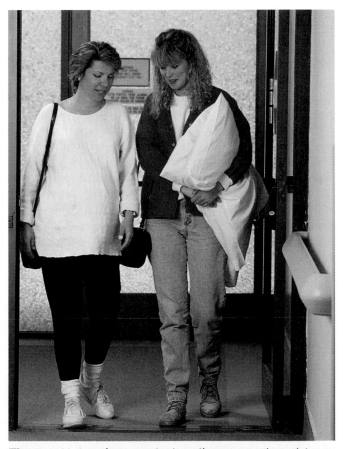

Figure 11-1 ■ An expectant mother may ask a sister or close female friend to be her labor partner and attend classes with her.

A doula is a trained labor support person who is employed by the mother to provide labor support. She gives physical support such as massage and helping with relaxation and provides emotional support and advocacy throughout labor. Some doulas also help during the postpartum period.

Siblings

The presence of children at birth is controversial. Some believe that children become closer to their new siblings when they are present at birth. Others believe that the sights of the birth process, blood, and their mothers in pain may be too frightening for children. Some debate centers on the age of the child attending the birth.

Children who participate in the birth of a sibling may attend all or part of the labor and birth or may join the parents just after the birth to participate in the immediate celebration. An adult support person is necessary to stay with the child throughout the experience. The support person should have no role other than attending to the child. This role includes gauging the child's response, providing explanations and reassurance, and taking the child out of the room as needed.

Education

Expectant mothers must also decide on prenatal education classes. Their decisions are based on the classes available in the area, costs, and types of information they need. A wide variety of classes is available to women in most areas.

Small classes of a few women and their partners are ideal but may be too expensive or unavailable. If the class includes more than 10 couples, the teacher should have an assistant to help with individual instruction. The teacher is usually a registered nurse who has experience in maternity nursing and is certified by a nationally known organization such as ASPO or ICEA.

✔ CHECK YOUR READING

1. What are the goals of perinatal education?
2. What major decisions must couples make in preparation for childbirth?

TYPES OF CLASSES AVAILABLE

Although most people think of perinatal education primarily as preparation for the birth experience, classes are available in all areas of pregnancy, childbirth, and parenting. An added benefit of prenatal classes is the opportunity for women to meet others with similar concerns.

Preconception Classes

Classes for couples who are thinking about having a baby are designed to help such couples have a healthy pregnancy from the beginning. Information about nutrition before conception, signs of pregnancy, healthy lifestyle, and choosing a caregiver are presented. The effects of pregnancy and childbirth on a woman's relationships and career are discussed. Preconception classes emphasize early and regular prenatal care and ways to reduce risk factors for poor pregnancy outcome.

Early Pregnancy Classes

Early pregnancy classes focus on the first two trimesters (Box 11-1). First-trimester classes are sometimes called *early bird* or *right start classes.* They cover information on adapting to pregnancy, dealing with early discomforts such as morning sickness and fatigue, and understanding what to expect in the months ahead. Emphasis is placed on how to have a healthy pregnancy by obtaining prenatal care and avoiding hazards to the fetus.

Second-trimester classes focus on changes that occur during middle pregnancy, fetal development, and alterations in roles. Information on body mechanics, work during pregnancy, and what to expect during the third trimester are included. Teachers discuss childbirth choices and information to help students become more knowledgeable consumers.

Parents may begin to learn about the needs of the mother and infant after birth in these classes or may attend other classes to meet this need. This information is especially important because of the short birth facility stay after birth.

Exercise Classes

Exercise classes help women keep fit and healthy during pregnancy. Some classes also continue into the postpartum period. Written consent from the primary caregiver may be required to ensure that the woman can participate safely. The instructor should understand the special needs of pregnancy and teach low-impact exercises preceded by warm-up routines. Women should avoid excessive heart rate elevation to prevent diversion of blood away from the uterus.

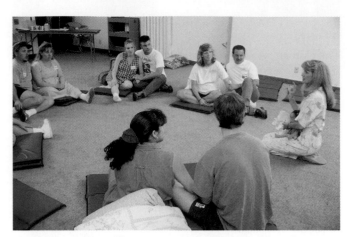

Figure 11-2 ■ The nurse teaching this class discusses movement of the fetus through the pelvis.

Childbirth Preparation Classes

Women and their support persons learn self-help measures and what to expect for labor and birth in childbirth preparation classes during the third trimester (Figure 11-2). Although once referred to as "natural childbirth classes," they are now called *prepared childbirth classes* to denote the woman's preparation for all aspects of childbirth, including complications. Couples learn coping methods to help them approach childbirth in a positive manner. Teachers do not promise prevention of all pain in labor. However, the increased confidence and the techniques learned in prepared childbirth classes may help decrease perception and increase tolerance of pain during labor.

Prepared childbirth classes based in birth facilities include detailed information on what to expect in that particular setting but may not cover options that are unavailable at that agency. Hospital classes have sometimes been criticized for teaching clients to be "good" or compliant patients. A woman may wish to talk to the instructor before taking a class to ask about class size and the teacher's philosophy, background, and teaching methods.

The amount of material and specific topics included in prepared childbirth classes varies by the number and length of the classes and the needs of the clients. Classes generally include information about labor and pharmacologic and nonpharmacologic methods of pain relief. Common complications are also discussed. If the class is held in a birth setting, a tour of the maternity areas is offered. Supervised practice of relaxation, breathing techniques, and coping strategies in "labor rehearsals" is part of every class (Figure 11-3). Videos assist women to develop a realistic picture of the birth process (Box 11-2).

The teacher describes advantages and disadvantages of various options in birthing. For example, couples may learn that epidural anesthesia, which is almost routine in many areas, usually removes most pain but may increase the length of labor, cause less effective pushing, and make catheterization and administration of oxytocin more likely. On the other hand, use of relaxation techniques avoids the disad-

---

BOX 11-1 Topics Covered in Early Pregnancy Classes

The amount of material and specific topics included will vary by the length of the class and the needs of the clients.
Pregnancy changes
  Anatomy and physiology
  Physiologic and psychological changes
  Fetal development
  Hazards to the mother and fetus (such as drugs, alcohol, smoking, environmental hazards)
  Medical care (such as importance, what to expect at each visit)
  Communication with the provider
  Prenatal screening tests
Self-care
  Hygiene
  Nutrition
  Exercise and body mechanics
  Discomforts of pregnancy
  Danger signs and what to do
  Sexuality
  Work and pregnancy
Infant care
  Selection of a pediatrician
  Infant development
  Infant feeding
Birth
  Birth options (such as birth plan, costs)
  Preterm labor

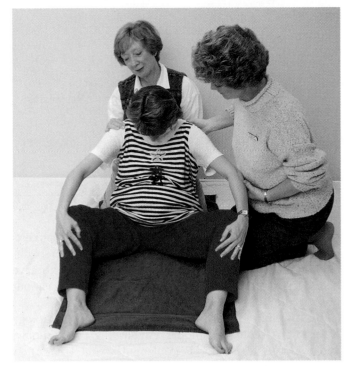

Figure 11-3 ■ The teacher helps each couple, individually and together, with pushing during a labor rehearsal.

vantages of analgesic drugs and anesthesia but does not remove all pain. When women have balanced views of their options, they are able to discuss them intelligently with caregivers and make better decisions. It is important to emphasize that the decision to use medications or not to use them is an individual choice and there is no right or wrong decision.

In recent years many women have chosen to have epidural anesthesia during childbirth. However, even women who plan to have an epidural as soon as possible should learn and practice methods of pain relief. The woman may not be able to receive an epidural as soon as she wants it if the anesthesiologist is unavailable at that time or labor is moving too fast. The anesthesia may not be complete for some women who may still have some pain. Knowing how to use nonpharmacologic pain relief measures is very helpful in these situations.

Information about the postpartum period, breastfeeding, and infant care may be included in this class or taught in separate classes. Class series range from a 1-day class to four to nine meetings depending on the content included. Some classes also include discussion of the postpartum period, breastfeeding, and infant care.

Refresher Courses

Women whose last prepared childbirth was more than 2 or 3 years ago often take a refresher class for an update of current practices and a review of techniques. Classes consist of one to three sessions in which supervised practice is the major focus. Courses also include discussion of role changes in the family and sibling adjustment.

BOX 11-2 Topics Included in Prepared Childbirth Classes

Physical and psychological changes of the last trimester
    Common discomforts and concerns
    Nutrition
    Exercise and body mechanics
    Sexuality
    Danger signs and what to do
Antepartum testing
    Common third trimester tests
Labor and birth
    Anatomy and physiology of labor
    Plans for the birth (such as consumerism, options, birth plan)
    Signs of labor and when to go to the hospital
    Hospital admission and procedures
    Physical and emotional aspects of labor
    Labor variations (such as back labor)
    Medical procedures (such as inductions, amniotomies, episiotomies, vacuum extraction)
    Birthing process
    Recovery
    Tour of maternity unit
    Role of the labor partner
    Techniques for support
Coping techniques for labor
    Relaxation and breathing techniques
    Comfort measures
    Labor rehearsals
    Pain relief (both pharmacologic and nonpharmacologic)
Complications
    High-risk pregnancy
    Cesarean birth
Postpartum
    Birth agency stay
    Postpartum physiologic and psychological changes
    Role adaptation, postpartum blues and depression
    Family planning
Normal newborn
    Characteristics
    General care and safety
    Feeding (breast and formula)

CRITICAL THINKING ⌇ EXERCISE 11-1

Liz, gravida 2, para 1, tells you that she does not plan to attend prepared childbirth classes because she took classes before her son, Danny, was born 5 years ago. What should you discuss with her?

Cesarean Birth Preparation Classes

Education about cesarean birth should be included in general childbirth classes. Some classes are conducted separately for those expecting a cesarean birth (Box 11-3).

GENERAL CESAREAN CLASSES

In 2003, 27.6% of births in the United States were by cesarean delivery (Hamilton, Martin, & Sutton, 2004). Therefore, women need preparation for this possibility. Cesarean birth is usually discussed briefly during general prepared childbirth classes. Topics include indications, options, surgical procedure, and postoperative course.

Reasons for cesarean births should be discussed in detail. A woman might view the terms *failed induction* and *failure to progress* as casting blame on her. She may believe that if she had used relaxation techniques better or been more tolerant of pain, she might have avoided the need for surgery. Teach-

---

BOX 11-3 Topics Included in Cesarean Birth Classes

Indications
Prenatal tests
Preparation (such as nothing by mouth [NPO], shave, Foley catheter)
Anesthesia
Surgical procedure
Role of support person during surgery
Options
Postsurgical care and pain relief
Relaxation techniques
Postpartum course
Future birth options

BOX 11-4 Topics Included in Breastfeeding Classes

Anatomy and physiology
Preparation for breastfeeding
First feedings
Positioning and latch-on
Establishment of milk supply
Problems and prevention: engorgement, sore nipples, nipple confusion, insufficient milk supply, and mastitis
Nutrition
Use of bottles and storage of breast milk
Breast pumps
Role of support person(s)
Work and breastfeeding
Weaning

---

ers often point out that the causes of cesarean births are conditions over which the woman has no control.

> ■ Couples are sometimes inattentive during discussions about cesarean birth because they think "it can't happen to me." Teachers can gain their attention by pointing out the number of couples in the class who may have cesarean births based on the 2003 rate of 26.7% for all women and 19.1% for women who had not had a cesarean birth previously (Hamilton, Martin, & Sutton, 2004). Written materials may be helpful for later review if the need for surgery develops.

PLANNED CESAREAN BIRTH CLASSES

Women who know they will have a cesarean birth may attend planned cesarean birth classes. The class offers those who have had a previous cesarean birth an opportunity to share experiences and feelings and clarify misconceptions. These women may remember little about the preparation for the procedure because they were frightened and exhausted. Couples anticipating their first cesarean birth may appreciate hearing from others who have had the experience.

Class content includes indications for cesarean births, surgical procedure, postoperative course, and possible options. A woman who wishes to go into labor to ensure maturity of the fetus and experience labor should discuss this decision with her caregiver. Class discussion helps couples feel that they have some control over events and provides a basis for discussion with caregivers.

Vaginal Birth after Cesarean Birth

The number of vaginal births after a previous cesarean birth, as well as classes to prepare for this type of birth, has decreased in recent years. Women who wish to have a vaginal birth after cesarean (VBAC) or a trial of labor after cesarean (TOLAC) may take a special class. Content includes explanations of the precautions taken, rationale, and coping techniques. Situations that might necessitate another cesarean birth and the emotional aspects of a "failed VBAC" are also discussed.

Breastfeeding Classes

Prenatal breastfeeding education is important because of the short time available to help breastfeeding mothers in the birth facility after birth. Classes help increase a

woman's confidence in her ability to breastfeed successfully and provide her with resources if she encounters difficulties. Teachers are often lactation consultants who have had special education and have advanced knowledge about breastfeeding.

Breastfeeding classes include information on physiology of lactation, feeding techniques, establishing a milk supply, and solutions to common problems (Box 11-4). Partners who attend learn methods of providing support during breastfeeding. Some teachers hold additional sessions after the birth to provide ongoing counseling at a time when mothers may experience unexpected problems. These sessions allow discussion of problems as they occur.

Parenting Classes

Instruction on parenting and newborn care may be included in prepared childbirth classes or provided separately. Content typically includes infant safety, general care, and common concerns such as infant crying and advantages and disadvantages of circumcision (Box 11-5). Baby equipment such as infant car seats is often displayed. Practice with dolls may also be included. Classes may continue after the birth of the infant.

CLASSES FOR FATHERS

Classes for fathers often focus on the male perspective of pregnancy, birth, and parenting. They provide an opportunity for men to meet other expectant fathers and ask questions they might not ask in classes that include expectant mothers. Some classes are called "Boot Camp for Dads" and

---

BOX 11-5 Topics Included in Parenting Classes

Normal newborn characteristics: marks, rashes, normal behavior
General care: diapering, cord care, circumcision care, bathing
Feeding methods and problems, schedules, colic
Other concerns: crying, sleeping through the night
Safety: car seats, "baby proofing" the home
Baby equipment
Early growth and development: expectations, infant stimulation, immunization
Illness: signs of common conditions, taking a temperature, calling the physician
Infant cardiopulmonary resuscitation (CPR)
Family and relationship changes

---

involve practicing infant care techniques such as diapering and bathing with dolls.

Postpartum Classes

Although the postpartum period is discussed in prepared childbirth classes, the mother can also attend classes after birth. Content includes the physiologic and psychological changes of the postpartum period, role transition, sexuality, and nutrition. Signs of postpartum depression are often discussed, with emphasis on when the woman should seek help. Some classes are informal support groups led by a knowledgeable professional. Other classes focus primarily on exercise for the postpartum period. Because many women return to work soon after childbirth, sessions are often held at night and on weekends and include the concerns of working mothers. Breastfeeding infants are usually welcome.

Classes for Other Family Members

SIBLINGS

Sibling classes are usually for children aged 3 to 12 years. The classes help them learn about newborn characteristics and help decrease anxiety about the approaching birth (Figure 11-4).

Many young children have never seen a newborn and are expecting a child near their age who can be a playmate. A tour of the nursery or visit with a newborn infant allows them to see newborns at close range and learn to be safe helpers. Videos and stories promote discussion about normal feelings of jealousy and anger. Emphasis is placed on the important role of big brothers and sisters and the fact that a baby could not replace them in their parents' affection.

A separate parent discussion provides suggestions for further preparation and ways to cope with the transition after birth. Concerns about sibling rivalry and meeting the needs of more than one child are common topics (see Chapter 18). Sibling visitation during hospitalization to help decrease the child's anxiety is also discussed.

Special sibling classes may be held for children who will be present at the birth. These help prepare the child for the

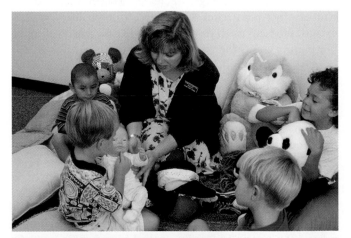

Figure 11-4 ■ During sibling classes, children learn about the new babies coming into their lives.

sights and sounds of birth. The child's support person also attends the class.

GRANDPARENTS

Classes for grandparents provide updates about recent developments in childbirth and parenting practices. Grandparents compare parenting in the past and present in a supportive environment with others in similar situations. Topics generally focus on family-centered childbirth and infant care. Changes in infant care practices such as positioning the newborn on the back for sleep are emphasized. Discussions also review current views of feeding, early growth and development, and accident prevention. The art of grandparenting and the importance of grandparents are particularly emphasized.

✔ **CHECK YOUR READING**

3. How are early pregnancy classes different from later pregnancy classes?
4. Why should all women learn about cesarean childbirth?
5. Why are sibling and grandparent classes important?

EDUCATION FOR CHILDBIRTH

Many studies have attempted to determine whether education for childbirth affects the outcome with regard to client satisfaction, pain relief, length of labor, and frequency of complications. The results of these studies vary. Many show less need for pharmacologic pain relief measures, reduced tension, and a feeling of less pain. Others report no difference between prepared and unprepared women. Most studies agree that couples receiving prenatal preparation for childbirth are more satisfied with their birth experiences and have greater feelings of control, even when unexpected complications occur.

Methods of Pain Management

EDUCATION

One of the most important aspects of any childbirth preparation class is education to increase the woman's confidence in her ability to cope with birth. Confidence may be increased with classes that provide detailed information about childbirth, vicarious experiences such as videos and reports of others' births, and techniques to increase coping ability during labor.

By learning what to expect during labor and birth, women and their support persons are able to rehearse the experience in their minds in preparation for the actual event. They practice coping techniques during simulated contractions. Realistic, valid class information and discussion of possible variations are essential so that couples are adequately prepared.

RELAXATION

Tension and anxiety during labor cause tightening of abdominal muscles, impeding contractions and increasing pain by stimulation of nerve endings that heighten awareness of pain. Prolonged muscle tension causes fatigue and increased pain perception. When anxiety and tension are high, uterine contractions are less effective and the length of labor increases. A woman who is able to remain relaxed is likely to have more efficient and less painful labor and have increased ability to use other techniques to help herself. A number of different techniques are taught to enhance relaxation during labor. Many of these techniques can be used at other stressful times, as well.

CONDITIONING

Many techniques for prepared childbirth are based partially on theories of conditioned response, in which certain responses to stimuli become automatic through frequent association. Women learn to associate uterine contractions with relaxation by practicing relaxation techniques with mental images of contractions. Because effective conditioning requires a great deal of practice, women are encouraged to practice their techniques daily. For some women, the intensity of real uterine contractions is surprisingly different from their experiences during practice sessions. They may have difficulty with relaxation as a result and may need to use other methods along with conditioning.

METHODS OF CHILDBIRTH EDUCATION

Although all methods of prepared childbirth education use some combination of pain management techniques, each method has its unique aspects. Some differences exist in types of classes and class content, depending on geographic area. Many classes have a holistic approach, providing a variety of techniques from many sources from which couples can choose those that work best for them.

Dick-Read Childbirth Education

Grantly Dick-Read was an English physician who was one of the first to use education and relaxation techniques to help women through childbirth. His theory was that fear of childbirth results in tension and pain. To prevent the fear-tension-pain cycle, he developed a method of slow abdominal breathing in early labor and rapid chest breathing in advanced labor. His methods were the first to be called *natural childbirth*.

Bradley Childbirth Education

The Bradley method was the first to include the father as a support person for "husband-coached childbirth." Abdominal breathing to increase relaxation and breath control is taught in these classes, which usually last for 12 weeks. The Bradley method also emphasizes avoidance of all medication and other interventions.

LeBoyer Method of Childbirth

The LeBoyer childbirth method sometimes called *birth without violence,* views birth as a traumatic experience for the newborn. To decrease the trauma at birth, lights are dimmed and noise is decreased to help the newborn adapt to ex-

trauterine life more easily. The infant receives a warm bath immediately after birth to help relaxation.

Lamaze Childbirth Education

The Lamaze method is often called *psychoprophylaxis* because it uses the mind to prevent pain. It involves concentration and conditioning to help the woman respond to contractions with relaxation and various techniques to decrease pain. The Lamaze method is the most popular method used today. A variety of techniques are taught, and women should feel free to choose those that they feel work best for them. Women should not be taught that there is only one right way of responding to labor.

CLASS CONTENT

The content of specific Lamaze classes may differ, but most follow a similar pattern. Although the focus is on the childbirth experience, other topics such as the postpartum period and infant care are often included. Techniques for coping with labor include education to prevent fear of the unknown and activities that promote relaxation during labor.

Lamaze teachers acknowledge that labor is painful and do not promise these techniques will produce a pain-free birth. Instead, the techniques are used to increase the woman's ability to cope with pain by relieving some of the accompanying distress.

EXERCISES

Women learn toning and conditioning exercises to prepare for childbirth and help prevent discomfort in late pregnancy. Because the classes are taken during the third trimester of pregnancy, the instructor must consider the changes in center of gravity and joint stability that occur at that time when selecting exercises (see Chapter 7 for exercises for pregnancy).

RELAXATION TECHNIQUES

The ability to relax during labor is one of the most important components of coping effectively with childbirth. Relaxation conserves energy, decreases oxygen use, and enhances other pain relief techniques. Women learn various exercises to help them recognize and release tension. The labor partner assists the woman by providing feedback during exercise sessions and labor. The partner is alert to ways in which the woman shows tension. For example, she may tighten her shoulders, frown, or jiggle her foot when stressed. Her partner helps her focus on areas she finds difficult to relax. Positive feedback from the partner and teacher encourages women to increase relaxation.

Relaxation exercises must be practiced frequently to be useful during labor. Couples begin practice sessions in a quiet, comfortable setting. Later, they practice in other places that simulate the noise and unfamiliar setting of the hospital. Relaxation exercises may also be combined with other techniques such as imagery and massage (Figure 11-5).

PROGRESSIVE RELAXATION. Progressive relaxation involves contracting and then consciously releasing

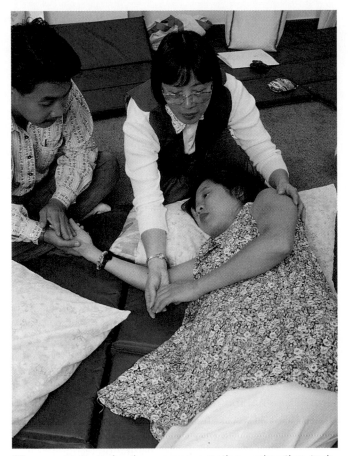

Figure 11-5 ■ As the woman practices relaxation techniques for labor, the partner massages her hand and the nurse checks for muscle tension.

different muscle groups. The exercise is repeated throughout the body until all voluntary muscles are relaxed. The woman learns to differentiate between the feelings of tense and relaxed muscles. With this knowledge, she can systematically assess and then release muscle tension throughout her body.

NEUROMUSCULAR DISASSOCIATION. Neuromuscular disassociation (also called *differential relaxation*) helps the woman learn to relax her body even when one group of muscles is strongly contracted. This process helps prepare her to relax during the powerful uterine contractions of labor. The woman contracts an area such as an arm or a leg and then concentrates on releasing tension from the rest of her body. After a short time of contracting one area, she relaxes it and moves on to another. Her partner checks for unrecognized tension by gently moving areas to see that they are limp.

TOUCH RELAXATION. The purpose of touch relaxation is to help the woman learn to loosen taut muscles when they are touched by her partner. The woman tenses an area and then relaxes it as her partner strokes and massages it. With frequent practice of this exercise, the woman becomes conditioned to respond to touch with relaxation. During labor, her partner's touch is a signal for release of tension.

RELAXATION AGAINST PAIN. Because first-time mothers have difficulty imagining the pain and strength of labor contractions, they may occasionally practice use of relaxation against pain. The pain is caused by her partner, who

exerts pressure against a tendon or large muscle of the arm or leg. The pressure is applied gradually to simulate the gradual increase, peak, and decrease of a uterine contraction. Sometimes ice is applied as another type of discomfort to simulate contractions.

OTHER TECHNIQUES

Other techniques to aid the woman in relaxation include cutaneous and mental stimulation. Touch stimulates large-diameter sensory nerve fibers and interferes with transmission of pain impulses to the brain through small-diameter sensory nerve fibers. Mental focusing and distraction also interfere with pain messages reaching the brain.

CUTANEOUS STIMULATION TECHNIQUES

EFFLEURAGE. Effleurage is the slow massage of the abdomen during contractions (Figure 11-6). Women learn to perform effleurage using both hands in a circular motion. If fetal monitor belts are in place during labor, the woman can massage her abdomen between the belts. When she lies on her side, she uses only one hand to massage her abdomen. In the side-lying position, she may be more comfortable

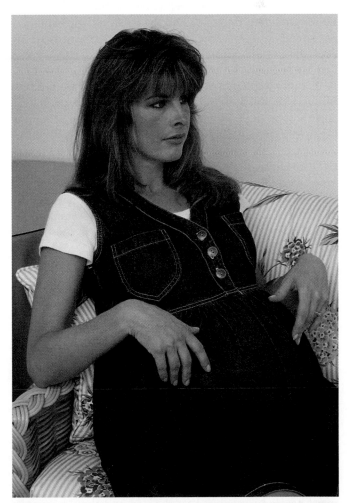

Figure 11-6 ■ The woman begins effleurage with the hands at the symphysis and then slowly moves around the sides and down the center toward the symphysis again. As an alternative she can go up the center of the abdomen and around the sides.

making smaller movements on her abdomen or massaging her thigh so that her arm and shoulder remain relaxed.

Massage and pressure on the palms and fingertips stimulate large-diameter nerve fibers. Relief is temporary because stimulation of these fibers results in habituation, a decreased response to stimuli. When habituation occurs, pain is more readily perceived. Periodically changing the type and area of stimulation increases effectiveness.

The woman and her partner may alternate effleurage to provide more variety in sensory input and decrease habituation. The woman can massage her thigh instead of her abdomen and use her fingertips to trace circles and figure-eight patterns on the bed. The use of specific patterns of effleurage provides sources of concentration and increased input to the brain. This exercise may also interfere with transmission of pain impulses.

SACRAL PRESSURE. Firm pressure against the sacral area may help relieve strain on the sacroiliac joint from a fetal occiput posterior position (often called "back labor"). It is also effective in women who do not have back labor. The partner begins to increase pressure on the sacrum as soon as the contraction begins. If a fetal monitor is in place, the partner can watch the line depicting the contraction to determine when to begin and end the pressure. The hand may be moved slowly over the area or remain positioned directly over the sacrum, but pressure should be continuous and firm throughout the contraction.

The partner should place the other hand over the woman's hip and steady her during sacral pressure. Care should be taken not to jiggle the woman, which may be irritating. Between contractions the woman gives her partner feedback about hand placement. Often, moving the hands a fraction of an inch increases effectiveness. This technique can be combined with thermal stimulation to increase effectiveness. Tennis balls may also be used to apply pressure to the back.

OTHER MASSAGE. Massage of the temples and shoulders by the labor partner may help relax these areas. The palms and soles of the feet are particularly sensitive to touch, and firm massage of these areas may be helpful. Types of stimuli should be changed whenever they no longer seem effective, generally every 15 to 30 minutes.

THERMAL STIMULATION. Application of heat and cold stimulates thermoreceptors and may decrease pain sensation. Cool cloths used to wipe the woman's face, ice chips offered to the woman for eating, and ice in a glove applied to the woman's lower back may be effective. Alternating cold with heat over the back prevents habituation. In early labor a whirlpool bath or shower with warm water directed against the back may be soothing. A warm bath blanket, moist towel, or glove filled with warm water can be held against the sacrum for pressure and warmth. Cloth bags or socks filled with rice and heated may also be used. Any device for providing heat or cold should be covered with a washcloth or towel before being placed on the skin and should never be applied to any anesthetized area because injury could result.

POSITIONING. Position changes during labor also provide cutaneous stimulation. Women are taught to practice their techniques using a variety of positions and to change positions frequently during labor. Ambulation and an upright position make contractions more efficient and less painful. Position changes approximately every 30 to 60 minutes increase comfort and decrease muscle fatigue.

MENTAL STIMULATION TECHNIQUES

Various methods decrease pain by increasing mental concentration. They may modify pain perception as a result of interference with pain impulses in the spinal cord or in the brain itself.

FOCAL POINT. A focal point is an object on which the woman centers her attention during contractions (Figure 11-7). It helps her direct her thoughts away from the contractions. During the contraction, she looks at the focal point and thinks about its shape, size, and gradations of colors. Women often use pictures of infants and restful scenic landscapes as focal points. If a video player is available during labor, a video tape of scenery, perhaps combined with music, may increase interest in the focal point.

Women who do not bring focal points to the birth setting may use anything in their lines of vision, such as a pattern on the wallpaper or the support person's face. Because the fetal monitor is directly next to the bed, many women focus on it. Watching the contraction pattern on the monitor usually is not soothing and tends to increase attention to the strength of the contraction. Focusing on a button or knob on the monitor may be more helpful.

Women who are familiar with meditation techniques may prefer closing their eyes and using an internal focal point during contractions. This allows them to shut out light and movement around them and focus on a mental picture.

IMAGERY. Another technique to enhance relaxation is imagery. During imagery exercises, childbirth educators often talk about a pleasant scene or experience while the woman imagines herself in that setting. A walk through a garden is portrayed by describing the flowers, the warmth of the sun, the sound of birds, and a feeling of peacefulness. Couples are encouraged to practice imagery with scenes of their own choosing. While practicing relaxation techniques, the woman can picture oxygen entering her body to nourish her baby every time she inhales and tension leaving each time she exhales.

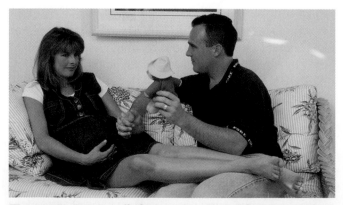

Figure 11-7 ■ A stuffed toy or any other object can serve as a focal point on which the expectant mother can fix her attention during labor.

Other imagery suggestions are given for use during labor. The woman might picture a flower bud opening into full bloom to simulate the opening of the cervix. She can imagine the cervix pulling over the infant's head and the infant moving lower in the pelvis with each contraction. Teachers usually advise women to save images of cervical dilation and childbirth until labor actually begins.

MUSIC. Some women find that music and other sounds, like rainfall and waves at the seashore, help them relax. They may use tapes and CDs during practice and bring them with headphones when they are in labor and come to the birth setting. Headphones have the added benefit of obscuring surrounding noise. The rhythm of the music may assist the woman in pacing her breathing. Music is often used with other techniques such as imagery to increase relaxation.

SPECIAL TECHNIQUES

Special techniques may be discussed briefly in classes. Some techniques require further preparation elsewhere. Acupressure or reflexology applies pressure over specific points on the body to raise endorphin levels to reduce pain. Biofeedback may lower pain by reducing tension of abdominal muscles. Some women find transcutaneous electrical nerve stimulation helpful. This process provides pain relief through the use of electrodes on the lower back to deliver low-intensity, high-frequency electrical stimulation of the nerves. Aromatherapy, the use of special fragrances, is sometimes used to cover hospital odors and promote relaxation. Some women find yoga helpful. Yoga may help women learn to relax, which is important during labor and birth (White, 2001).

In hydrotherapy the woman is immersed in a tub of water or a Jacuzzi. The water helps the woman relax, decreases muscle tension and pressure on the abdomen, and reduces the perception of pain.

BREATHING TECHNIQUES

Although they were once the major focus of many classes, focused or controlled breathing techniques are now considered just one of many coping strategies used to enhance the woman's ability to work with her labor during birth (see the discussion on breathing techniques in Chapter 15, pp. 342-343).

Classes may teach very specific breathing techniques or may teach the woman to breathe in a pattern that is comfortable to her during labor (Matteson, 2001). If they plan to use specific breathing patterns, the woman and her partner should practice the techniques frequently to gain comfort with them. If the woman has not practiced, they may not be helpful during labor.

Focused breathing techniques should not be used in labor until they are actually needed, which is usually when the woman can no longer walk and talk during a contraction. If breathing techniques are used too early, the woman tends to move through the different techniques too quickly, and she may stop using them. In addition, use of the more complex breathing patterns in latent labor may increase fatigue. Women should be encouraged to adapt the techniques to their own comfort and needs.

✔ **CHECK YOUR READING**

6. How can education, relaxation, and conditioning decrease pain?
7. How do cutaneous stimulation and imagery help reduce pain?
8. What is the purpose of breathing techniques in labor?

THE LABOR PARTNER

Almost all methods of childbirth preparation encourage the participation of someone who remains with the woman throughout labor. This person may be called a *labor partner, support person,* or *labor companion.* The presence of a labor partner may help the woman cope more effectively, decrease her distress during labor, and result in greater satisfaction with the childbirth experience. The support person shares the experience and helps the woman remain focused and calm during labor.

The person who takes on this role may be the baby's father, a friend, or a relative. The labor partner generally attends classes with the mother to learn about labor, birth, and techniques to assist during labor. By practicing together, the woman and her partner learn to work smoothly as a team during labor. Classes may increase confidence for support persons, who learn specific techniques to use during labor. When the labor partner is the father, communication and a sense of closeness between the expectant parents may be enhanced.

The woman may wish to have a doula in addition to her support person. A doula has education and experience to provide assistance during childbirth. Some have national certification by specialty organizations like ICEA to perform the role. The doula is most often employed by the expectant parents to provide continuous labor support. Doulas help the woman with physical support such as relaxation and massage and provide emotional support and advocacy throughout labor. Some doulas also help in the home during the postpartum period.

Role of the Labor Partner

Not all labor partners play identical roles during labor. Some take a major part in assisting the mother, but others provide support in less active ways. They may confine their support to giving verbal encouragement and some physical care such as back rubs when requested. Others feel more comfortable with passive support by being present but not actively participating. Even with education, the support person may feel somewhat helpless and look to others to provide help to the laboring woman. Expectant fathers often have concerns about the health of the baby and safety of the mother during labor and may feel more comfortable when others provide support.

Some men and women believe that active involvement in labor is not an acceptable role for men because of cultural values. For example, Hispanic couples may expect the partner to offer support by being present and encouraging the woman during labor rather than taking a more active role. Middle Eastern men also may not participate because of cultural reasons.

Encourage couples to think about the support person's labor role before labor begins and then encourage the partner in whatever role is chosen (Nursing Care Plan 11-1). Labor partners should not feel responsible for more than is included in the role. Teachers should discuss the duties of the labor nurse and encourage labor partners to seek assistance when they are uncertain. The labor nurse may have helpful suggestions and adaptations of techniques.

NURSING CARE PLAN 11-1 Planning For Childbirth

ASSESSMENT: Carmen Sanchez, age 19, is 4 months pregnant with her first baby. She and her husband, Ramon, "want to be the best parents possible." Carmen works as a teacher's aide in a primary school. Ramon, age 26, manages a small restaurant. Both Carmen and Ramon are the youngest in their families and have little actual experience with infants. Carmen plans to have her baby at the local hospital in a birthing suite.

Carmen tells the nurse that Ramon tends to favor the "old ways" and is unsure whether he should be involved during childbirth. She is most anxious for him to participate during her labor. Ramon seems embarrassed and says, "Having a baby is for women." He seems very loving toward Carmen and later says, "I want to help Carmen, but I don't know anything about these things. I'd just be in the way."

NURSING DIAGNOSIS: Decisional Conflict related to father's ambivalence toward his anticipated role in childbirth

CRITICAL THINKING: Is this an appropriate use of a nursing diagnosis? If Carmen is the client, should the nurse make a nursing diagnosis that focuses on her husband?

ANSWER: Although Carmen is the primary client, family-centered nursing involves care of all family members, especially when their needs affect those of the primary client. If the nurse can help Carmen and Ramon resolve this problem, Carmen will be able to focus more positively on preparing for the birth of their baby.

GOALS/EXPECTED OUTCOMES: Ramon will:
1. Explore various options regarding his role during Carmen's labor and the birth of his baby.
2. Make a decision about his role during childbirth by 1 month before the baby is expected.

INTERVENTION	RATIONALE
1. Explore Ramon's concerns before beginning discussion of educational opportunities with Carmen.	1. In some cultures the man is the head of the family and makes many of the decisions. Showing respect for his authority is important if health teaching is to be accepted.
2. Use therapeutic communication techniques (such as reflection, paraphrasing) to help Ramon discuss his feelings about participating in childbirth.	2. Use of therapeutic communication shows that the nurse is willing to listen and thinks that the client's feelings are important.
3. Ask Ramon how he views childbirth and the role of the support person during labor and birth.	3. Asking the partner about his perception of his role during birth helps the nurse adapt teaching to his needs.
4. Explain various labor support roles. Include the options of actively participating by providing encouragement and comfort measures or merely being present for the labor, birth, both, or neither.	4. The nurse must encourage and accept whatever role the support person chooses.
5. Ask Ramon to consider the advantages and disadvantages of each role. Clarify misinformation and discuss additional advantages and disadvantages if necessary.	5. Participation increases learning.
6. Present all information in a nonjudgmental atmosphere.	6. If the nurse remains nonjudgmental, the client does not feel pressured to make a particular decision.
7. Encourage Ramon to discuss this new information with Carmen, his friends, and family. If possible, refer him to other men who have played various roles during labor and birth.	7. Discussion with family and friends is important when making decisions and provides sources for other viewpoints.
8. Suggest that Ramon think about his options and make a decision at a later date. Provide written information for Ramon and Carmen to review at home.	8. Processing new information and making decisions takes time. Written information provides a readily available source for review.
9. Include Carmen in the discussion and ask for her input as well.	9. A couple may be unaware of each other's concerns and feelings. Hearing the partner talk about them helps each understand the other's point of view.

EVALUATION: Ramon reports 2 months later that he has decided to go with Carmen to classes to learn more about childbirth. He is unsure about his degree of participation during labor and birth and says that he will decide when the time arrives. Carmen says that she feels comfortable with Ramon's decision and is glad he will go to prepared childbirth classes with her.

Class discussion of complications should include the role of the support person. For example, partners should understand circumstances that would allow and preclude their presence during a cesarean birth.

Support Techniques

Knowledge of specific, practical measures to assist the woman in labor often helps labor partners feel more comfortable in the birth setting. They learn ways to time contractions at home and to work with the fetal monitor in the birth setting. Telling the woman when the monitor shows the peak of the contraction is over can be particularly helpful. If the woman is sleeping between contractions, the monitor may show a contraction beginning before she feels it. The labor partner can alert her to begin her focused breathing before the contraction becomes strong.

The partner suggests ways to make the environment less stressful, such as listening to tapes and CDs with headphones to obscure surrounding noise and turning down the lights to promote rest between contractions.

Providing comfort measures is an important role of the support person. These measures include offering ice chips, wiping the woman's face with a cold cloth, using cold and warm packs, and helping her change positions. The partner applies sacral pressure and gives back rubs and other types of massage. Partners learn ways to provide feedback about breathing and relaxation and make suggestions during practice sessions and labor. They learn the importance of encouraging the woman and giving directions in a positive manner.

The woman and her support person may pack a bag of items that may help comfort the expectant mother during labor (Box 11-6). As labor progresses, the couples use each article as it seems appropriate.

✔ CHECK YOUR READING

9. How does having someone with her help the woman in labor?
10. What are the various roles that the support person might take?
11. What specific techniques do labor partners learn to help the woman in labor?

Application of the Nursing Process
Education for Childbirth

The nursing process focuses on assisting the woman and her partner to obtain the knowledge necessary to plan for a birth experience that is realistic and meets their individual needs. Preparation helps each family progress through the childbearing experience as knowledgeable consumers and full participants in their own health care.

Assessment

Assess the educational needs of the woman and her partner. Some couples are quite knowledgeable about available prenatal classes and childbirth options, but others need direc-

---

BOX 11-6 What to Take to the Hospital

Items to be Included in the Labor Bag
Focal point
Lotion, oil, or powder to make massage more comfortable
Warm socks for cold feet
Colored washcloths for washing the face (white ones might be lost)
Hand-held fan
Rubber bands and clips for hair
Tennis balls in a sock for sacral pressure
Sugarless sour lollipop for dry mouth
Mouthwash
Lip balm, unflavored
Instruction sheets or reminder checklists
Paper and pencil
Playing cards or simple games for early labor
Camera
Snack for labor partner
Tape or CD player with headphones
Cell phone, change or telephone card and telephone numbers for calls after birth
Pillows (use colored pillowcases to prevent loss)
Rice bags in a sock (to warm in a microwave)

Items for after Birth
Robe and nightgown or pajamas that open in the front
Nursing bras
Slippers
Toiletries
Loose fitting clothes to wear home
Clothes for the baby to wear home
Baby blanket

---

tion in choosing classes that are right for them. The couple may come to the nurse with a birth plan already made or may need help in thinking through their expectations and desires.

Determine whether special factors require adaptation of the usual educational approaches. Examples are the pregnant adolescent and the woman with a physical disability. Cultural factors may be very influential in determining individual educational needs. Assessing cultural expectation during pregnancy and birth can help determine the focus of teaching sessions.

Next, assess the needs of support persons and the degree of participation they wish to have in the birth. They may have concerns about their role, especially during labor and birth. These must be addressed to decrease their anxiety and help them be more effective in supporting their partner.

Analysis

The nursing diagnosis pertaining to the couple who is not unusually anxious about childbirth but desires more information is "Health-Seeking Behaviors related to desire for education about pregnancy, childbirth, and/or parenting."

Planning

The goals and expected outcomes for this nursing diagnosis are that the woman and her partner will:
- Write a birth plan that is realistically based on available options and meets their needs
- Verbalize a plan for obtaining education for pregnancy, childbirth, and parenting

■ Report feelings of increased confidence in their ability to cope with pregnancy, childbirth, and parenting after educational preparation is completed

Interventions

MAKING A BIRTH PLAN

Help couples write a plan for their birth experience if they so wish. The birth plan, sometimes called a *family preference plan,* helps women and their partners examine their options and take an active part in planning their birth experience. The plan may be very simple, such as the desire to keep the infant with the mother at all times, or it may be a list of very specific items to be included in the childbirth experience. Cultural preferences can be incorporated into the birth plan.

The birth plan is a tool for expanding communication with health professionals. It ensures that the couple's wishes are known before labor begins. The plan may help the couple choose a provider, a setting, and classes that are most conducive to meeting specific needs. The couple should discuss their wishes and concerns with the health care provider

during pregnancy and with the nurse in the labor and delivery unit when they are admitted.

Help the couple learn about locally available choices and explain any restrictions. For example, insurance coverage may dictate which facility a woman must use. Those without insurance are concerned about the cost of various options. In addition, the health care provider or birth agency may have set policies on certain issues. Complications during labor and birth may necessitate changes in the plan.

Suggest that couples interview several physicians or nurse-midwives to learn about the provider's usual practices and possible exceptions. With discussion, the couple and provider can create a plan that is satisfactory to all.

CHOOSING CLASSES

Help the woman and her partner find classes suited to their educational needs. Give them a list and description of classes in the community and suggest that they talk with others who have taken various classes. They may wish to interview teachers to learn about their preparation and philosophies. Some couples want classes that consider

---

PARENTS WANT TO KNOW   What Options Should We Consider for Our Birth Plan?

Whether the following options are available may depend on the policies of the birth facility and health care provider. Discuss them with your provider to learn more about the choices available to you.

Monitoring—Do you have strong feelings about using electronic fetal monitoring? Some women find it reassuring because it provides continuous information about the fetus. Others believe that it interferes with their ability to remain active during labor. Intermittent use of monitoring and auscultation may be possible if no complications occur.

Intravenous (IV) fluids—Some health care professionals consider IV fluids necessary to replace fluids lost during labor and to give pain medications and emergency drugs. Some women find them painful and intrusive, whereas others do not mind them. Alternatives include waiting until active labor to begin IV fluids, avoiding them unless complications occur, and using a saline lock so that you can move about more freely.

Food and oral fluids—Other than ice chips, food and fluids often are not allowed during active labor because of decreased gastric motility, vomiting, and the possibility of aspiration if general anesthesia is suddenly needed. Clear fluids or hard candy may be an option.

Enemas—A very-small-volume enema may or may not be routine. An enema may stimulate contractions, but many women dislike them and have loose stools in early labor.

Activity—You may prefer to walk, shower or bathe, sit in a rocking chair, and remain active rather than staying in bed throughout labor. Some women wish to squat, kneel, or lie on their sides for birth. A birthing ball may be comfortable during labor. A birthing bed or chair may allow a comfortable and effective delivery position.

Episiotomy—Although an episiotomy is frequently performed, you may wish to avoid it unless absolutely necessary. Discuss the use of episiotomy with your birth attendant.

Pain relief—You may plan to avoid medication for pain relief completely, use it only if absolutely necessary, or take it as

soon as possible to avoid pain. You may expect to use relaxation techniques throughout labor or only until you can receive anesthesia. Specific ideas about available types of pain relief should also be considered.

Support person—You may wish only the infant's father, a relative, a close friend, or a doula to be with you during labor and birth, or you may prefer to have a number of people present for some or all of the experience.

Medical interventions—Some women prefer to have labor induced or augmented and use other medical interventions, if possible. Others prefer to avoid oxytocin stimulation of labor, amniotomy, and other interventions unless they are necessary.

Breastfeeding—Many women want to begin breastfeeding immediately after birth or within the first hour. You may prefer that no water or formula be given to your baby unless a problem develops. Some mothers ask that the nursery staff feed the baby during the night.

Siblings—You may want your other children to be present at the birth, to arrive immediately after the birth, or to visit you during your hospital stay.

Care of the newborn—Having your baby stay with you at all times to promote bonding may be possible if there are no complications. To get more rest, you may prefer to care for the baby only during the day and evening hours. The infant may spend the night in the nursery or be returned to you for night feedings.

Discharge—Your insurance coverage may influence your discharge time. Mothers usually go home within 48 hours after a vaginal birth or 96 hours after a cesarean birth. You may decide to stay the full time allowed so you can rest before assuming full care of the newborn along with other responsibilities, or you may prefer earlier discharge with follow-up visits from a home visit nurse, in a clinic, or in your provider's office.

avoidance of medication a primary goal of childbirth. Many prefer those that consider a variety of tools, including medication, for coping with pain.

SUGGESTING CLASSES FOR SPECIAL NEEDS

Refer women with special needs to specific courses. If none are available, suggest ways to adapt the information presented in regular classes to their own situations.

ADOLESCENTS. Although adolescents may attend regular prenatal classes, those designed especially to meet their needs are most effective. High schools with programs for school-aged mothers, hospitals, clinics, and community agencies may offer courses. Teens may find that separate classes for their age group are more comfortable because they learn with peers with similar problems and concerns. Fathers and other support persons may also attend.

Education for pregnant adolescents is similar to that for adults, but it focuses on the teenager's perceptions of childbearing. Clarification of misconceptions in a nonjudgmental manner makes classes more meaningful. Young women need information about the importance of prenatal care, nutrition, weight gain, body image, labor, birth, and contraception. The effects of substance abuse and sexually transmissible diseases on pregnancy and the fetus are other important topics for discussion.

Although the decision about whether to keep the infant is usually made before classes begin, options may be discussed. Because of their lack of experience and unrealistic expectations of infants, adolescents, particularly younger adolescents, have a greater need for information about parenting and infant care than do older mothers. Provide an opportunity for discussion of ways in which the infant will affect the adolescent's life, future goals, and schooling.

Teenagers with academic problems may have difficulty reading material and understanding abstract concepts. Use of concrete terms and simple language helps to increase understanding. Models, videos, demonstrations, and presentations by those who have previously taken classes make the course more relevant. Presentations should include interactive activities such as games and demonstrations because teenagers often become bored easily.

OLDER WOMEN. Women older than age 35 may feel "different" from the younger women in their prenatal class and isolated from their friends who have completed childbearing. Because delayed parenthood is quite common today, classes for older mothers provide opportunities for these women to make friends with others with similar backgrounds. Older couples may want more sophisticated information than that usually included in regular prenatal classes, and they have many questions about the chances of complications related to age. Offer realistic reassurance and direct them to books and articles that meet their need for in-depth information.

WOMEN WITH HIGH-RISK PREGNANCIES. The woman with a high-risk pregnancy has activity restrictions and may be unable to attend regular perinatal classes. If possible, help her arrange for individual instruction. Audio and video tapes, written materials, and phone contact with an instructor are ways for her to learn and practice techniques without attending classes.

WOMEN WHO MUST MAKE CULTURAL ADAPTATIONS. Women from other cultures, especially those who do not speak English, are at a disadvantage when they enter birth settings in the United States. Classes in other languages are often available in communities in which large groups with this need exist. They contain the same basic information as the English versions, but the content and process are adapted to meet the cultural needs of the students. The teacher usually has the same cultural background as the students. This cultural match ensures fluency in their language and understanding of their needs, increasing the likelihood that the instructor and the information presented are accepted.

The instructor discusses childbirth in the United States and compares it with that in the couples' countries of origin. Students learn the importance of prenatal care, which may not have been emphasized in their own cultures. They discuss expectations of health care providers and the birthing experience. Misconceptions about needs and care throughout the childbearing period are clarified. Many cultures focus on certain foods or actions that will help protect the mother and baby. Nurses can point out how various practices help protect the woman and the infant to increase the woman's understanding and compliance with suggestions.

WOMEN WITH OTHER NEEDS. If necessary, refer the woman and her support person to classes that address other needs. Classes for adoptive couples and women with multifetal pregnancies and disabilities may be available. Women who are concerned about continuing their careers after birth may enroll in courses for working mothers to help them choose child care and learn to balance the needs of family and work. Classes for fathers may provide a comfortable environment for discussions of fathering, sexuality, and roles during labor and birth, breastfeeding, and the postpartum period in the company of other men with similar concerns.

Evaluation

If goals have been achieved, the woman and her partner will do the following:

- Write a realistic birth plan
- Attend classes that are appropriate for their needs
- Verbalize increased confidence in coping with pregnancy, childbirth, and parenting

SUMMARY CONCEPTS

- Education for childbearing helps couples become knowledgeable consumers and active participants in pregnancy and childbirth.
- Women must make many decisions about childbirth, including choosing a birth attendant, a birth setting, a support person for labor, and the type of educational classes to attend.
- Many classes are available for pregnant women and their support persons. Early pregnancy classes emphasize ways to have a healthy pregnancy. Classes conducted in later pregnancy focus on preparation for childbirth, breastfeeding, and early parenting.
- Because more than 27% of all births are cesarean, women in all prepared childbirth classes should be made aware of this possibility and learn about the procedure.

- Classes for siblings and grandparents help all family members prepare for the birth.
- Education, relaxation, and conditioning are used to increase coping ability for childbirth. Other techniques act to decrease transmission of pain impulses from the spinal cord to the brain.
- Exercises in relaxation help women recognize and learn to reduce tension during labor.
- Cutaneous and mental stimulation techniques help to reduce pain perception. Techniques need to be varied to prevent habituation.
- Women learn a variety of focused breathing techniques for labor with the purpose of increasing relaxation.
- Having a support person increases a woman's satisfaction with childbirth. The educated support person may find labor less stressful and feel increased confidence.
- The support person may participate in labor actively, minimally, or only by being present. The nurse should accept all roles taken by support persons.
- Specific support techniques include assisting with relaxation and breathing, encouraging the woman, and using sacral pressure, massage, and comfort measures.

ANSWERS TO CRITICAL THINKING EXERCISE 11-1, p. 227

Women and their support people should attend classes before each birth, especially if more than 2 to 3 years have passed since the previous childbirth class, because they may have forgotten some information. Birthing care and options may have changed since the last birth. Couples often have concerns and questions about their last experience, and the nurse can discuss these issues and help them feel more positive about the pending birth. The needs of other children can also be addressed, including practical suggestions about easing the transition.

REFERENCES & READINGS

American Academy of Pediatrics & American College of Obstetricians and Gynecologists. (2002). *Guidelines for perinatal care* (5th ed.). Elk Grove Village, IL: Author.

Arias, E., MacDorman, M.F., Strobino, D.M., & Guyer, B. (2003). Annual summary of vital statistics–2002. *Pediatrics, 112*(6), 1215-1230.

Association of Women's Health, Obstetric and Neonatal Nurses (AWHONN). (2000). *Nurse providers of perinatal education: Competencies and program guide.* Washington, DC: Author.

AWHONN. (2003). *Standards and guidelines for professional nursing practice in the care of women and newborns* (6th ed.). Washington, DC: Author.

Barron, M.L. (2001). Antenatal care. In K.R. Simpson & P.A. Creehan (Eds.), *AWHONN perinatal nursing* (2nd ed., pp. 125-160). Philadelphia: Lippincott Williams & Wilkins.

Brown, C. (2001). Pregnancy and labor support for the high-risk woman. *International Journal of Childbirth Education, 16*(2), 24-27.

Coverston, C.R. (2004). Psychology of pregnancy. In S. Mattson & J.E. Smith (Eds.), *Core curriculum for maternal-newborn nursing* (3rd ed., pp. 124-143). Philadelphia: Saunders.

Creehan, P.A. (2001). Pain relief and comfort measures during labor. In K.R. Simpson & P.A. Creehan (Eds.), *AWHONN perinatal nursing* (2nd ed., pp. 417-444.) Philadelphia: Lippincott Williams & Wilkins.

Englestad, C.D. (2003). Perinatal consumer education. In S.M. Levasseur & D.A. Raines (Eds.), *Perinatal nursing secrets* (pp. 11-20). Philadelphia: Hanley & Belfus.

Freedman, L.H. (2000). Honoring childbirth: Birth as a healing experience. *Lifelines, 4*(32), 70-72.

Goodfriend, C. (2001). Aromatherapy for pregnancy and birth. *International Journal of Childbirth Education, 16*(3), 18-27.

Hamilton, B.E., Martin, J.A., & Sutton, P.D. (2004). Births: Preliminary data for 2003. *National vital statistics reports, 53*(9). Hyattsville, MD: National Center for Health Statistics.

Humenick, S.S., Shrock, P., & Libresco, M.M. (2000). Relaxation. In F.H. Nichols & S.S. Humenick (Eds.), *Childbirth education: Practice, research, and theory* (2nd ed., pp. 179-199). Philadelphia: Saunders.

International Childbirth Education Association (ICEA). (1999). *ICEA position paper: The role of the childbirth educator and the scope of childbirth education.* Minneapolis, MN: Author.

ICEA. (1999). *ICEA position paper: The role and scope of the doula.* Minneapolis, MN: Author.

Jimenez, S.L. (2000). Comfort and pain management. In F.H. Nichols & S.S. Humenick (Eds.), *Childbirth education: Practice, research, and theory* (2nd ed., pp. 157-177). Philadelphia: Saunders.

Johnson, T.R.B., & Niebyl, J.R. (2002). Preconception and prenatal care: Part of the continuum. In S.G. Gabbe, J.R. Niebyl, & J.L. Simpson (Eds.), *Obstetrics, normal and problem pregnancies* (4th ed., pp. 139-159). New York: Churchill Livingstone.

Keenan, P. (2000). Benefits of massage therapy and use of a doula during labor and childbirth. *Alternative Therapies, 6*(1), 66-74.

Keppler, A.B., & Simpson, K.R. (2001). Discharge planning. In K.R. Simpson & P.A. Creehan (Eds.), *AWHONN perinatal nursing* (2nd ed., pp. 610-632). Philadelphia: Lippincott Williams & Wilkins.

Lamaze International. (2001). *Position paper: Lamaze for the twenty-first century.* Washington, DC: Author.

Lamaze International. (2003). *Position paper: Promoting, protecting, and supporting normal birth.* Washington, DC: Author.

Matteson, P.S. (2001). *Women's health during the childbearing years: A community-based approach.* St. Louis: Mosby.

Ottani, P.A. (2002). When childbirth preparation isn't a cultural norm. *International Journal of Childbirth Education, 17*(2), 12+.

Redman, B.K. (2001). *The practice of patient education* (9th ed.). St. Louis: Mosby.

Riordan, J., & Bocar, D.L. (2005). Breastfeeding education. In J. Riordan (Ed.), *Breastfeeding and human lactation* (3rd ed., pp. 689-712). Boston: Jones and Bartlett.

Ryser, F.G., & King, E. (2002). Nursing students providing prenatal education to pregnant teens: An innovative approach to adolescent childbirth education. *International Journal of Childbirth Education, 17*(4), 18-19.

Schneider, Z. (2001). An Australian study of women's experiences of their first pregnancy. *Midwifery, 18*, 238-249.

Schwartz, J. (2002). Enhancing the birth experience: The doula as part of the hospital maternity program. *International Journal of Childbirth Education, 17*(1), 18-19.

Shilling, T. (2000). Cultural perspectives on childbearing. In F.H. Nichols & S.S. Humenick (Eds.), *Childbirth education: Practice, research, and theory* (2nd ed., pp. 138-154). Philadelphia: Saunders.

Spiby, H., Slade, P., Escott, D., Henderson, B., & Fraser, R.B. (2003). Selected coping strategies in labor: An investigation of women's experiences. *Birth, 30*(3), 189-194.

Steffes, S.A. (2000). Relaxation: Imagery. In F.H. Nichols & S.S. Humenick (Eds.), *Childbirth education: Practice, research, and theory* (2nd ed., pp. 227-252). Philadelphia: Saunders.

U.S. Department of Health and Human Services. (2000). *Healthy People 2010* (Conference ed., 2 volumes). Washington, DC: Author.

Wallace, K.E. (2000). The Bradley method. *International Journal of Childbirth Education, 15*(1), 9-10.

White, M. (2001). Yoga for pregnancy. *International Journal of Childbirth Education, 16*(4), 5-9.

Worzer, L. (2004). Stress and sleep deprivation in pregnancy. *International Journal of Childbirth Education, 19*(1), 16-18.

Processes of Birth

OBJECTIVES

After studying this chapter, you should be able to:

1. Describe the woman's physiologic and psychological responses to labor.
2. Describe fetal responses to labor.
3. Explain the ways each component of the birth process affects the course of labor and birth and the interrelation of these components.
4. Relate the mechanisms of labor to the process of vaginal birth.
5. Explain premonitory signs of labor.
6. Compare true labor with false labor.
7. Describe common differences in the labors of nulliparous and parous women.
8. Compare each stage of labor and the phases within the first stage.

Go to your Student CD-ROM for Review Questions keyed to these Objectives.

DEFINITIONS

Acme Peak, or period of greatest strength, of a uterine contraction.

Attitude Relationship of fetal body parts to one another.

Bloody Show Mixture of cervical mucus and blood from ruptured capillaries in the cervix; often precedes labor and increases with cervical dilation.

Braxton Hicks Contractions Irregular, mild uterine contractions that occur throughout pregnancy and become stronger in the last trimester.

Decrement Period of decreasing strength of a uterine contraction.

Duration Period from the beginning of a uterine contraction to the end of the same contraction.

Engagement Descent of the widest diameter of the fetal presenting part to at least a zero station (the level of the ischial spines in the maternal pelvis).

Fontanel Space at the intersection of sutures connecting fetal or infant skull bones.

Frequency Period from the beginning of one uterine contraction to the beginning of the next.

Increment Period of increasing strength of a uterine contraction.

Intensity Strength of a uterine contraction.

Interval Period between the end of one uterine contraction and the beginning of the next.

Lie Relationship of the long axis of the fetus to the long axis of the mother.

Lightening Descent of the fetus toward the pelvic inlet before labor.

Lochia Vaginal drainage after birth.

Molding Shaping of the fetal head during movement through the birth canal.

Nullipara A woman who has not completed a pregnancy to at least 20 weeks' gestation.

Para A woman who has given birth after a pregnancy of at least 20 weeks' gestation; also designates the number of pregnancies that end after at least 20 weeks' gestation (multifetal gestation such as that of twins is considered as one birth when calculating parity).

Position Relation of a fixed reference point on the fetus to the quadrants of the maternal pelvis.

Presentation Fetal part that enters the pelvic inlet, or the presenting part.

Ripening Softening of the cervix as labor nears as the result of an increase in water content and the effects of relaxin on its connective tissue.

Station Measurement of fetal descent in relation to the ischial spines of the maternal pelvis (see also *engagement*).

Sutures Narrow areas of flexible tissue that connect fetal skull bones, permitting slight movement during labor.

VBAC Acronym for *vaginal birth after cesarean.*

Family roles and relationships are forever altered by birth, making nursing care related to this event rewarding. Understanding the physiologic and psychological components of the birth process helps the nurse provide safe, effective care for the childbearing family through evidence-based practice. Awareness of expected changes allows the nurse to support the laboring woman when these changes occur and provides a basis for identifying abnormal occurrences. This chapter focuses on the changes that occur during normal birth.

PHYSIOLOGIC EFFECTS OF THE BIRTH PROCESS

The birth process affects the physiologic systems of the mother and fetus. The maternal reproductive system and systems related to fetal and neonatal oxygenation are most obviously affected.

Maternal Response

The most obvious changes of pregnancy and birth occur in the woman's reproductive system, but her other systems also respond in various ways. Significant changes occur during labor in her cardiovascular, respiratory, gastrointestinal, urinary, and hematopoietic systems.

REPRODUCTIVE SYSTEM

CHARACTERISTICS OF CONTRACTIONS. Normal labor contractions are coordinated, involuntary, and intermittent.

Coordinated. The uterus can contract and relax in a coordinated way, like the heart and other smooth muscles. Contractions during pregnancy are of low intensity and uncoordinated. As the woman approaches full term, contractions become organized and gradually assume a regular pattern of increasing frequency, duration, and intensity during labor. Coordinated labor contractions begin in the uterine fundus and spread downward toward the cervix to propel the fetus through the pelvis.

Involuntary. Uterine contractions are involuntary in that they are not under conscious control, unlike movement of skeletal muscles. The mother cannot cause labor to start and stop by conscious effort. However, walking and other activities may stimulate existing labor contractions. Anxiety and excessive stress can diminish them, whereas relaxation can facilitate natural processes.

Intermittent. Labor contractions are intermittent rather than sustained, allowing relaxation of the uterine muscle and resumption of blood flow to and from the placenta to permit gas, nutrient, and waste exchange for the fetus.

CONTRACTION CYCLE. Each contraction consists of three phases (Figure 12-1). The increment occurs as the contraction begins in the fundus and spreads throughout the uterus. The peak, or acme, is the period during which the contraction is most intense. The decrement is the period of decreasing intensity as the uterus relaxes.

The contraction cycle and pattern of contractions are also described in terms of frequency, duration, and intensity. Frequency is the period from the beginning of one uterine contraction to the beginning of the next. It is expressed in minutes and fractions of minutes (such as "contractions are $3\frac{1}{2}$ to 4 minutes apart").

Duration is the length of each contraction from beginning to end. It is usually expressed in seconds. For example, the nurse might say, "Her contractions last 55 to 65 seconds."

Intensity is the strength of the contractions. The terms *mild, moderate,* and *strong* describe contraction intensity as palpated by the nurse. Different descriptions of intensity apply when an internal fetal monitor is used to record contractions (see Chapter 14).

The interval is the period between the end of one contraction and the beginning of the next. Most fetal exchange of oxygen, nutrients, and waste products occurs in the placenta at this time.

UTERINE BODY. Uterine activity during labor is characterized by opposing features. The upper two thirds of the uterus contracts actively to push the fetus down. The lower third of the uterus remains less active, promoting downward passage of the fetus. The cervix is similar to the lower uterine segment in that it is also passive. The net effect of labor contractions is enhanced because the downward push from the upper uterus is accompanied by reduced resistance to fetal descent in the lower uterus.

Myometrial (pertaining to the uterine muscle) cells in the upper uterus remain shorter at the end of each contraction

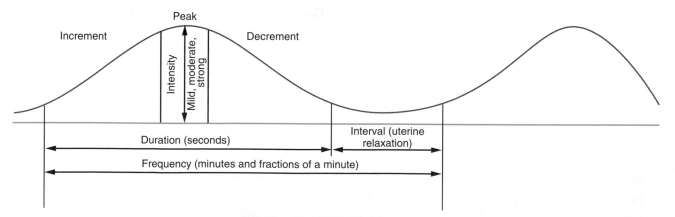

Figure 12-1 ■ Contraction cycle.

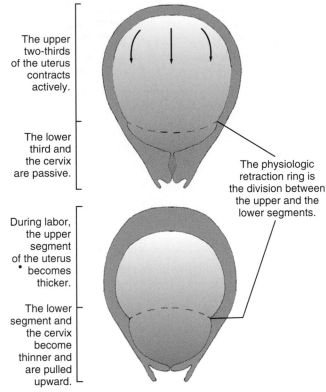

The upper two-thirds of the uterus contracts actively.

The lower third and the cervix are passive.

During labor, the upper segment of the uterus becomes thicker.

The lower segment and the cervix become thinner and are pulled upward.

The physiologic retraction ring is the division between the upper and the lower segments.

Figure 12-2 ■ Opposing characteristics of uterine contraction in the upper and lower segments of the uterus.

rather than returning to their original length. In contrast, myometrial cells in the lower uterus become longer with each contraction. These two characteristics enable the upper uterus to maintain tension between contractions to preserve the cervical changes and downward fetal progress made with each contraction.

The opposing characteristics of myometrial contraction in the upper and lower uterine segments cause changes in the thickness of the uterine wall during labor. The upper uterus becomes thicker while the lower uterus becomes thinner and is pulled upward during labor. The physiologic retraction ring marks the division between the upper and lower segments of the uterus (Figure 12-2).

Opposing characteristics of contractions in the upper and lower uterine segments change the shape of the uterine cavity, which becomes more elongated and narrow as labor progresses. This change in uterine shape straightens the fetal body and efficiently directs it downward in the pelvis.

CERVICAL CHANGES. Effacement (thinning and shortening) and dilation (opening) are the major cervical changes during labor. Effacement and dilation occur concurrently during labor but at different rates. The nullipara completes most cervical effacement early in the process of cervical dilation. In contrast, the cervix of a parous woman is usually thicker than that of a nullipara at any point during labor.

Effacement. Before labor the cervix is a cylindric structure about 2 cm long at the lower end of the uterus. Labor contractions push the fetus downward against the cervix

while pulling the cervix upward. If the membranes are intact, hydrostatic (fluid) pressure of the amniotic sac adds to the force of the presenting part on the cervix. The cervix becomes shorter and thinner as it is drawn over the fetus and amniotic sac (Figure 12-3). The cervix merges with the thinning lower uterus rather than remaining a distinct cylindric structure. Effacement is estimated as a percentage of the original cervical length. A fully thinned cervix is 100% effaced. Effacement also may be documented as the cervical length estimated during vaginal examination.

Dilation. As the cervix is pulled upward and the fetus is pushed downward, the cervix dilates. Dilation is expressed in centimeters. Full dilation is approximately 10 cm, sufficient to allow passage of the average-sized full-term fetus. The action during effacement and dilation can be likened to pushing a ball out through the cuff of a sock.

CARDIOVASCULAR SYSTEM

During each uterine contraction, blood flow to the placenta gradually decreases, causing a relative increase in the woman's blood volume. This temporary change increases her blood pressure slightly and slows her pulse. Therefore the woman's vital signs are best assessed during the interval between contractions because slight alterations in her blood pressure and pulse may occur during a contraction. Supine hypotension (see p. 113) may occur during labor if the woman lies on her back. The woman should be encouraged to rest in positions other than the supine to promote blood return to her heart and therefore enhance blood flow to the placenta and promote fetal oxygenation.

RESPIRATORY SYSTEM

The depth and rate of respirations increase, especially if the woman is anxious or in pain. A woman who breathes rapidly and deeply may experience symptoms of hyperventilation if respiratory alkalosis occurs as she exhales too much carbon dioxide. She may feel tingling of her hands and feet, numbness, and dizziness. The nurse should help her slow her breathing and breathe into a paper bag or her cupped hands to restore normal blood levels of carbon dioxide and relieve these symptoms.

GASTROINTESTINAL SYSTEM

Gastric motility is reduced during labor to varying degrees, which can result in nausea and vomiting. Most women are not hungry but are thirsty and have dry mouths. Ice chips are commonly provided, and small amounts of other clear liquids and juices, popsicles, and hard candy on a stick may be permitted. Solid food is usually withheld to prevent vomiting and aspiration of undigested food in the event that general anesthesia is required (see Chapter 15).

URINARY SYSTEM

The most common change in the urinary system during labor is a reduced sensation of a full bladder. Because of intense contractions and the effects of regional anesthesia, the woman may be unaware that her bladder is full, yet it may

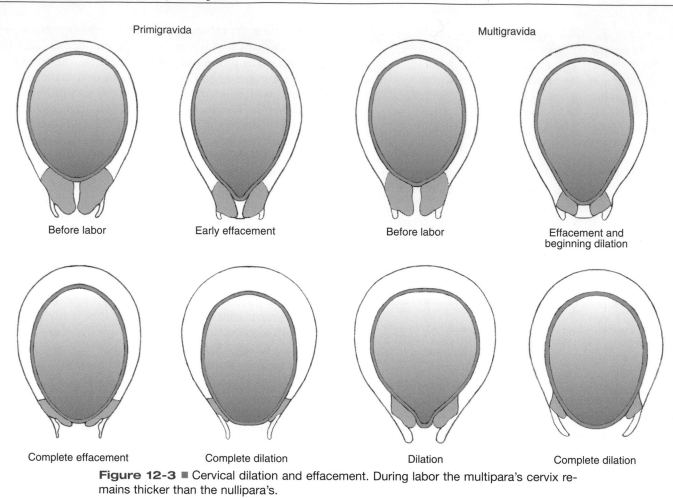

Primigravida

Before labor   Early effacement

Complete effacement   Complete dilation

Multigravida

Before labor   Effacement and beginning dilation

Dilation   Complete dilation

Figure 12-3 ■ Cervical dilation and effacement. During labor the multipara's cervix remains thicker than the nullipara's.

contribute to discomfort, especially that which persists after regional anesthesia. A full bladder can inhibit fetal descent because it occupies space in the pelvis.

The normal hypervolemia of pregnancy is reversed during the first 5 days postpartum, and large quantities of urine are excreted. The bladder may fill rapidly during the first few days after birth, even if the woman has not had an intravenous infusion during labor.

HEMATOPOIETIC SYSTEM

Most authorities recognize 500 ml as the maximum normal blood loss during vaginal birth. Women usually tolerate this loss well because the blood volume increases during pregnancy by 1 to 2 L (Guyton & Hall, 2000). A woman who is anemic at the beginning of labor has less reserve for normal blood loss and a poor tolerance for excess bleeding. A hemoglobin level of 10.5 g/dl and a hematocrit of 33% or higher give most women an adequate margin of safety for blood loss associated with normal birth. The leukocyte count averages 14,000 to 16,000/mm^3 but may be as high as 25,000 mm^3 or more during active labor with no other evidence of infection (Blackburn, 2003; Cunningham et al., 2001; Duffy, 2004).

Levels of several clotting factors, especially fibrinogen, are elevated during pregnancy and continue to be higher during labor and after delivery. The greater number of clotting factors provides protection from hemorrhage but also increases the mother's risk for a venous thrombosis during pregnancy and after birth.

Fetal Response

Responses to labor are most notable in the placental circulation, cardiovascular system, and pulmonary system.

PLACENTAL CIRCULATION

The exchange of oxygen, nutrients, and waste products between the mother and fetus occurs in the intervillous spaces without the mixing of maternal and fetal blood (see Chapter 6). During strong labor contractions, the maternal blood supply to the placenta decreases and eventually stops temporarily as the spiral arteries supplying the intervillous spaces are compressed by the uterine muscle. Therefore most placental exchange occurs during the interval between contractions. The placental circulation usually has enough reserve compared with fetal basal needs to tolerate the periodic interruption of blood flow.

Fetal protective mechanisms include the following:
- Fetal hemoglobin (hemoglobin F), which more readily takes on oxygen and releases carbon dioxide
- High hemoglobin and hematocrit levels that can carry 20% to 50% more oxygen than adult hemoglobin. The

fetal hemoglobin level averages 14.5 to 22.5 g/dl, and the hematocrit is approximately 48% to 69%.
- A high cardiac output of 250 ml/kg/min

The fetus may not tolerate labor contractions well in conditions associated with reduced placental function, such as maternal diabetes and hypertension, and conditions associated with reduced fetal oxygen-carrying capacity, such as fetal anemia.

CARDIOVASCULAR SYSTEM

The fetal cardiovascular system reacts quickly to events during labor. Alterations in the rate and rhythm of the fetal heart may result from normal labor effects or suggest fetal intolerance to the stress of labor. The fetal heart rate is rapid and ranges from 110 to 160 beats per minute (bpm) at term (Cyber, Adelsperger, & Torgersen, 2003; Feinstein, Sprague, & Trépanier, 2000; King & Simpson, 2001). The preterm fetus usually has a rate in the higher end of this range.

PULMONARY SYSTEM

The fetal lungs produce fluid to allow normal development of the airways. Lung fluid must be cleared to allow normal air breathing after birth. As term nears, production of fetal lung fluid decreases to about 65% of its maximum production and its absorption into the interstitium of the lungs increases. Labor speeds the absorption of lung fluid, so about 35% of the maximum amount remains in the airways at birth. Some fluid is expelled from the upper airways as the fetal head and thorax are compressed during passage through the birth canal. Most remaining lung fluid is absorbed into the interstitial spaces of the newborn's lungs and then into the circulatory system. A small amount is cleared by the lymphatic circulation (Cunningham et al., 2001; Jobe, 2004).

Catecholamines (primarily epinephrine and norepinephrine) produced by the fetal adrenal glands in response to the stress of labor appear to contribute to the infant's adaptation to extrauterine life. They stimulate cardiac contraction and breathing; quicken the clearance of remaining lung fluid, and aid in temperature regulation. Infants born by cesarean birth not preceded by labor are more likely to have transient breathing difficulty (see pp. 800-801).

✔ CHECK YOUR READING

1. How do labor contractions cause the cervix to efface and dilate? How do they cause fetal descent?
2. What differences in effacement are expected in the parous woman compared with the woman who has not previously given birth?
3. What changes occur in the maternal cardiovascular, respiratory, gastrointestinal, renal, and hematopoietic systems during labor?
4. Why are intermittent rather than sustained uterine contractions important?
5. How does the normal process of vaginal birth benefit the newborn after birth?

COMPONENTS OF THE BIRTH PROCESS

Four major factors interact during normal childbirth. These factors are often called the *four Ps:* powers, passage, passenger, and psyche.

Powers

UTERINE CONTRACTIONS

During the first stage of labor (onset to full cervical dilation), uterine contractions are the primary force that moves the fetus through the maternal pelvis.

MATERNAL PUSHING EFFORTS

During the second stage of labor (full cervical dilation to birth of the baby), uterine contractions continue to propel the fetus through the pelvis. In addition, the woman feels an urge to push and bear down as the fetus distends her vagina and puts pressure on her rectum. She adds her voluntary pushing efforts to the force of uterine contractions in second-stage labor.

Passage

The birth passage consists of the maternal pelvis and soft tissues. The bony pelvis is usually more important to the outcome of labor than the soft tissue because the bones and joints do not readily yield to the forces of labor. However, softening of the cartilage linking the pelvic bones occurs at term because of increased levels of the hormone relaxin.

The linea terminalis (pelvic brim) divides the bony pelvis into the false pelvis (top) and true pelvis (bottom) (see Chapter 4). The true pelvis is most important in childbirth. The true pelvis has three subdivisions: (1) the inlet, or upper pelvic opening; (2) the midpelvis, or pelvic cavity; and (3) the outlet, or lower pelvic opening. During birth, the true pelvis functions like a curved cylinder with different dimensions at different levels (Figure 12-4).

Passenger

The passenger is the fetus, membranes, and placenta. Several fetal anatomic and positional variables influence the course of labor.

FETAL HEAD

The fetus enters the birth canal in the cephalic presentation 96% of the time. The fetal shoulders are also important because of their width, but they usually can be moved to adapt to the pelvis.

BONES, SUTURES, AND FONTANELS. The bones of the fetal head involved in the birth process are the two frontal bones on the forehead, two parietal bones at the crown of the head, and occipital bone at the back of the head (Figure 12-5). The five major bones are not fused but are connected by sutures composed of strong but flexible fibrous tissue. The fontanels are wider spaces at the intersections of the sutures.

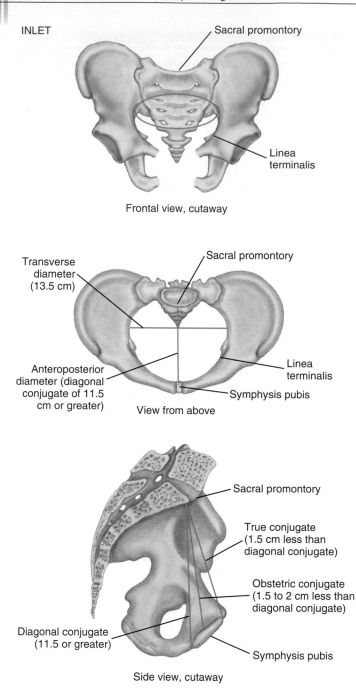

INLET

Sacral promontory

Linea terminalis

Frontal view, cutaway

Transverse diameter (13.5 cm)

Sacral promontory

Anteroposterior diameter (diagonal conjugate of 11.5 cm or greater)

Linea terminalis

Symphysis pubis

View from above

Sacral promontory

True conjugate (1.5 cm less than diagonal conjugate)

Obstetric conjugate (1.5 to 2 cm less than diagonal conjugate)

Diagonal conjugate (11.5 or greater)

Symphysis pubis

Side view, cutaway

If the inlet is small, the fetal head may not be able to enter it. Because it is almost entirely surrounded by bone, except for cartilage at the sacroiliac joint and symphysis pubis, the inlet cannot enlarge much to accommodate the fetus. The bony measurements are essentially fixed.

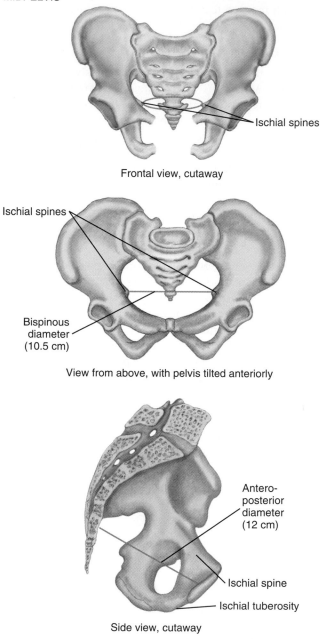

MIDPELVIS

Ischial spines

Frontal view, cutaway

Ischial spines

Bispinous diameter (10.5 cm)

View from above, with pelvis tilted anteriorly

Antero-posterior diameter (12 cm)

Ischial spine

Ischial tuberosity

Side view, cutaway

The boundaries of the inlet are the symphysis pubis anteriorly, the sacral promontory posteriorly, and the linea terminalis on the sides. The inlet is slightly wider in its transverse diameter (13.5 cm) than in its anteroposterior (diagonal conjugate) diameter (11.5 cm or greater).

The diagonal conjugate is slightly larger than both the obstetric and true conjugates. The obstetric conjugate is the narrowest of the three conjugate diameters but cannot be measured directly. The obstetric conjugate is estimated by first measuring the diagonal conjugate and then subtracting 1.5 to 2 cm.

The midpelvis, or pelvic cavity, is the narrowest part of the pelvis through which the fetus must pass during birth. Midpelvic diameters are measured at the level of the ischial spines. The anteroposterior diameter averages 12 cm.

The transverse diameter (bispinous or interspinous) averages 10.5 cm. Prominent ischial spines that project into the midpelvis can reduce the bispinous diameter.

Figure 12-4 ■ Pelvic divisions and measurements.

OUTLET

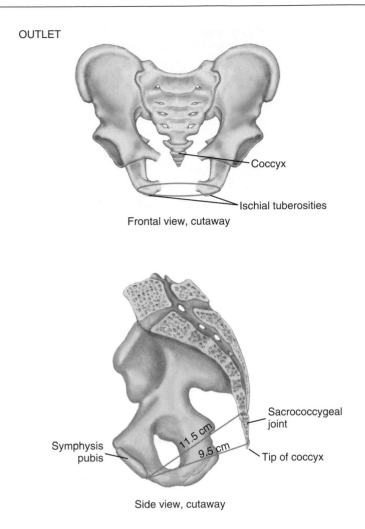

Frontal view, cutaway

Side view, cutaway

Three important diameters of the pelvic outlet are (1) the anteroposterior, (2) the transverse (bi-ischial or intertuberous), and (3) the posterior sagittal. The angle of the pubic arch is also an important pelvic outlet measure.

The anteroposterior diameter ranges from 9.5 to 11.5 cm, varying with the curve between the sacrococcygeal joint and the tip of the coccyx. The anteroposterior diameter can increase if the coccyx is easily movable.

The transverse diameter is the bi-ischial, or intertuberous, diameter. This is the distance between the ischial tuberosities ("sit bones"). It averages 11 cm.

The posterior sagittal diameter is normally at least 7.5 cm. It is a measure of the posterior pelvis. The posterior sagittal diameter measures the distance from the sacrococcygeal joint to the middle of the transverse (bi-ischial) diameter.

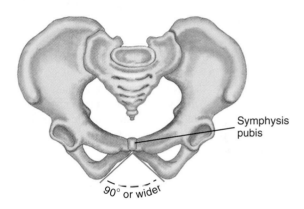

Frontal view, with pelvis tilted anteriorly

The angle of the pubic arch is important because it must be wide enough for the fetus to pass under it. The angle of the pubic arch should be at least 90 degrees. A narrow pubic arch displaces the fetus posteriorly toward the coccyx as it tries to pass under the arch.

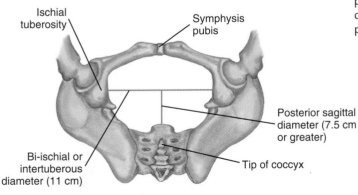

View from below (woman is in lithotomy position)

Figure 12-4, cont'd ■ Pelvic divisions and measurements.

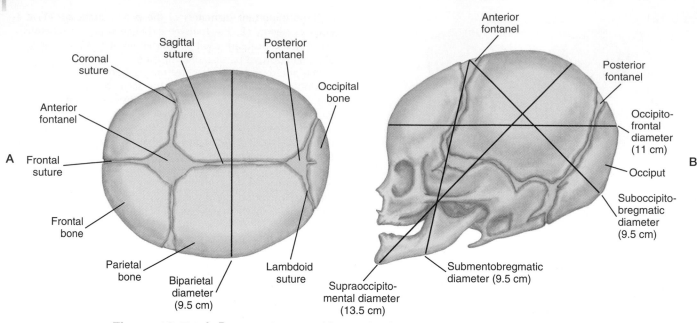

Figure 12-5 ■ A, Bones, sutures, and fontanels of the fetal head. Note that the anterior fontanel has a diamond shape, whereas the posterior fontanel is triangular. B, Lateral view of the fetal head demonstrating that anteroposterior diameters vary with the amount of flexion or extension.

The anterior fontanel has a diamond shape formed by the intersection of four sutures: the two coronal, frontal, and sagittal, which connect the two frontal and two parietal bones. The posterior fontanel has a triangular shape formed by the intersection of three sutures, one sagittal and two lambdoid, which connect the two parietal bones and occipital bone. The posterior fontanel is very small and often looks more like a slight indentation in the skull. The sutures and fontanels allow the bones to move slightly, changing the shape of the fetal head so that it can adapt to the size and shape of the pelvis by molding. The sutures and different shapes of the fontanels provide important landmarks to determine fetal position and head flexion during vaginal examination.

FETAL HEAD DIAMETERS. Most fetuses enter the pelvis in the cephalic presentation, but several variations are possible. The major transverse diameter of the fetal head is the biparietal, measured between the two parietal bones. The biparietal diameter averages 9.5 cm in a term fetus.

The anteroposterior diameter of the head varies with the degree of flexion. In the most favorable situation, the head becomes fully flexed during labor and the anteroposterior diameter is suboccipitobregmatic, averaging 9.5 cm (see Figure 12-5, *B*).

VARIATIONS IN THE PASSENGER

FETAL LIE. The orientation of the long axis of the fetus to the long axis of the woman is called the *fetal lie* (Figure 12-6). In more than 99% of pregnancies, the lie is longitudinal and parallel to the long axis of the woman. In the longitudinal lie, either the head or the buttocks of the fetus enters the pelvis first. A transverse lie exists when the

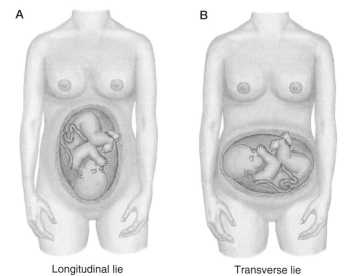

Longitudinal lie   Transverse lie

Figure 12-6 ■ Fetal lie. A, In a longitudinal lie the long axis of the fetus is parallel to the long axis of the woman. B, In a transverse lie the long axis of the fetus is at right angles to the long axis of the mother. The woman's abdomen has a wide, short appearance.

long axis of the fetus is at a right angle to the woman's long axis. This occurs in fewer than 1% of pregnancies. An oblique lie is at some angle between the longitudinal lie and the transverse lie.

ATTITUDE. The relation of fetal body parts to one another is the attitude of the fetus (Figure 12-7). The normal fetal attitude is one of flexion, with the head flexed toward the chest and the arms and legs flexed over the thorax. The

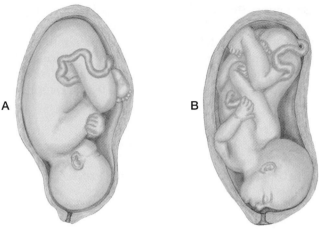

A   Flexion

B   Extension

Figure 12-7 ■ Attitude. **A,** The fetus is in the normal attitude of flexion, with the head, arms, and legs flexed tightly against the trunk. **B,** The fetus is in an abnormal attitude of extension. The head is extended, and the right arm is extended. A face presentation is illustrated.

back is curved in a convex **C** shape. Flexion remains a characteristic feature of the term newborn.

PRESENTATION. The fetal part that first enters the pelvis is termed the *presenting part.* Presentation falls into three categories: (1) cephalic, (2) breech, and (3) shoulder. The cephalic presentation with the fetal head flexed is the most common (Figure 12-8). Other presentations are associated with prolonged labor and other problems and are more likely to require cesarean birth.

Cephalic Presentation. The cephalic presentation is more favorable than others for several reasons:

- The fetal head is the largest single fetal part, although the breech (buttocks), with the legs and feet flexed on the abdomen, is collectively larger than the head. After the head is born, the smaller parts follow easily as the extremities unfold.
- During labor, the fetal head can gradually change shape, molding to adapt to the size and shape of the maternal pelvis.
- The fetal head is smooth, round, and hard, making it a more effective part to dilate the cervix, which is also round.

Cephalic presentation has four variations (Figure 12-8):

- Vertex—This is the most common type of cephalic presentation, in which the fetal head is fully flexed. It is called a *vertex* or an *occiput presentation* in everyday usage. This presentation is the most favorable for normal progress of labor because the smallest suboccipitobregmatic diameter is presenting.
- Military—The head is in a neutral position, neither flexed nor extended. The longer occipitofrontal diameter is presenting.
- Brow—The fetal head is partly extended. The brow presentation is unstable, usually converting to a vertex presentation if the head flexes or a face presentation if it extends. The longest supraoccipitomental diameter is presenting.
- Face—The head is extended, and the fetal occiput is near the fetal spine. The submentobregmatic diameter is presenting.

Vertex presentation   Military presentation   Brow presentation   Face presentation

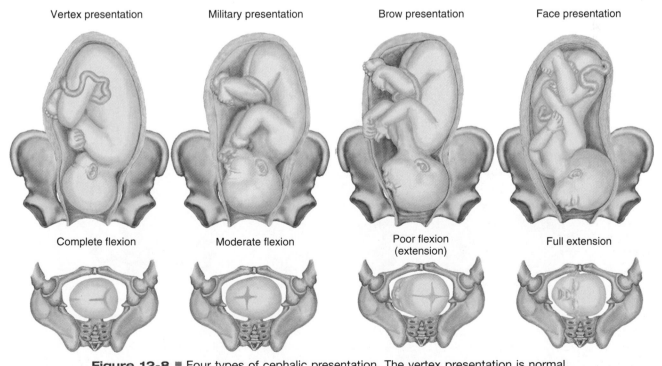

Complete flexion   Moderate flexion   Poor flexion (extension)   Full extension

Figure 12-8 ■ Four types of cephalic presentation. The vertex presentation is normal. Note positional changes of the anterior and posterior fontanels in relation to the maternal pelvis.

Breech Presentation. A breech presentation occurs when the fetal buttocks enter the pelvis first, which happens in about 3% of births. Breech presentation is more common in preterm births and when a fetal abnormality such as hydrocephalus (enlargement of the head with fluid) prevents the head from entering the pelvis. Breech presentation is also more likely to occur with abnormalities of the maternal uterus and pelvis and with placenta previa (placenta in the lower uterus).

Breech presentations are associated with several disadvantages:

- The buttocks are not smooth and firm like the head and are less effective at dilating the cervix.
- The fetal head is the last part to be born. By the time the fetal head is deep in the pelvis, the umbilical cord is outside the mother's body and is subject to compression between the head and maternal pelvis.
- Because the umbilical cord can be compressed after the fetal chest is born, the head must be delivered quickly to allow the infant to breathe. This does not permit gradual molding of the fetal head as it passes through the pelvis.

The breech presentation has three variations, depending on the relationship of the legs to the body (Figure 12-9):

- Frank breech—This is the most common variation, occurring when the fetal legs are extended across the abdomen toward the shoulders.
- Full (complete) breech—This is a reversal of the usual cephalic presentation. The head, knees, and hips are flexed, but the buttocks are presenting.
- Footling breech—This occurs when one or both feet are presenting.

Shoulder Presentation. The shoulder presentation is a transverse lie and accounts for only 0.2% of births (Cunningham et al., 2001). It occurs more often with preterm birth, high parity, prematurely ruptured membranes, hydramnios, and placenta previa. A cesarean birth is necessary in a viable fetus (one of a gestational age that might survive).

✓ CHECK YOUR READING

6. What are the two powers of labor?
7. What are the three divisions of the true pelvis?
8. Why is the vertex presentation best during birth?

POSITION

Fetal position describes the location of a fixed reference point on the presenting part in relation to the four quadrants of the maternal pelvis (Figure 12-10). The four quadrants are the right and left anterior and right and left posterior. The fetal position is not fixed but changes during labor as the fetus moves downward and adapts to the pelvic contours. Abbreviations indicate the relationship between the fetal presenting part and maternal pelvis.

RIGHT (R) OR LEFT (L). The first letter of the abbreviation describes whether the fetal reference point is to the right or left of the mother's pelvis. If the fetal reference point is neither to the right nor to the left of the pelvis, this letter is omitted.

OCCIPUT (O), MENTUM (M), OR SACRUM (S). The second letter of the abbreviation refers to the fixed fetal reference point, which varies with the presentation. The occiput is used in a vertex presentation. The chin, or men-

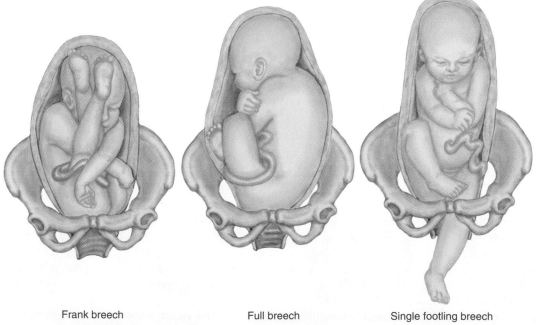

Frank breech   Full breech   Single footling breech

Figure 12-9 ■ Three variations of a breech presentation. Frank breech is the most common variation. Footling breeches may be single or double.

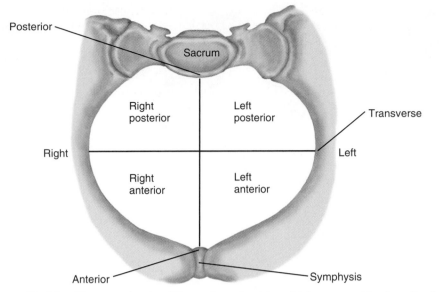

Figure 12-10 ■ Four quadrants of the maternal pelvis, which are used to describe fetal position.

tum, is the reference point in a face presentation. The sacrum is used for breech presentations. Letters may also designate the less common brow (F for fronto) and shoulder (Sc for scapula) presentations.

ANTERIOR (A), POSTERIOR (P), OR TRANSVERSE (T). These letters describe whether the fetal reference point is in the anterior or posterior quadrant of the mother's pelvis. If the fetal reference point is in neither an anterior nor a posterior quadrant, it is described as transverse. If the fetal occiput is located in the left anterior quadrant of the mother's pelvis, the position is described as left occiput anterior (LOA). If the occiput is in the mother's anterior pelvis, neither to the right nor to the left, it is described as occiput anterior (OA). If the fetal sacrum is located in the mother's right posterior pelvis, the abbreviation is R (right) S (sacrum) P (posterior) (Figure 12-11).

✓ **CHECK YOUR READING**

9. For each fetal position listed, describe the fetal landmark. Where is this landmark located in relation to the mother's pelvis: ROP? OA? RSA? LMA?
10. If the fetus is in a face presentation, why is using the occiput to determine position within the pelvis not possible?

Psyche

The psyche is a crucial part of childbirth. Marked anxiety and fear decrease a woman's ability to cope with pain in labor. Maternal catecholamines secreted in response to anxiety and fear can inhibit uterine contractility and placental blood flow. In contrast, relaxation augments the natural process of labor. Preparation for childbirth can enhance a woman's ability to work with her body's efforts rather than resist the natural forces. Much of the nurse's care during labor involves promoting relaxation and reducing anxiety and fear. Information and a positive sense of control and mastery over the birth increases the woman's sense of satisfaction with her birth experience (Nichols & Gennaro, 2000).

INDIVIDUAL AND CULTURAL VALUES

A woman in childbirth is more than a physical being. She is a blend of her experiences, present status, and future expectations. She is an individual, a member of a family and cultural group, and a part of her larger society.

A woman's culture affects her views of birth and the practices surrounding it. Culture shapes the values that people hold, their expectations of birth experiences, and their responses to birth. A woman's culture influences her reaction to labor and her expectations of interaction with her newborn. If the woman, her family, and her caregivers have similar viewpoints, little conflict in their values and expectations is likely. However, if these individuals hold markedly different viewpoints, confusion may result because each expects something different of the other. Cultural differences are most obvious when newly immigrated women give birth. After time and exposure to other cultural groups, the distinctive cultural practices and values often become blurred.

Within a culture a childbearing woman is an individual. The nurse's familiarity with a group's cultural values and practices related to birth provides a foundation for culturally competent care. Cultural knowledge provides a framework to assess and care for the woman and her family as individuals. However, the nurse must assess the personal expectations and values of each woman and her support person related to birth within this general framework. Cultural assessment questions for the intrapartum period might include the following:

■ How long have the woman and her family been in the area? Are they recent immigrants, or have their relatives and friends lived in the area for generations?

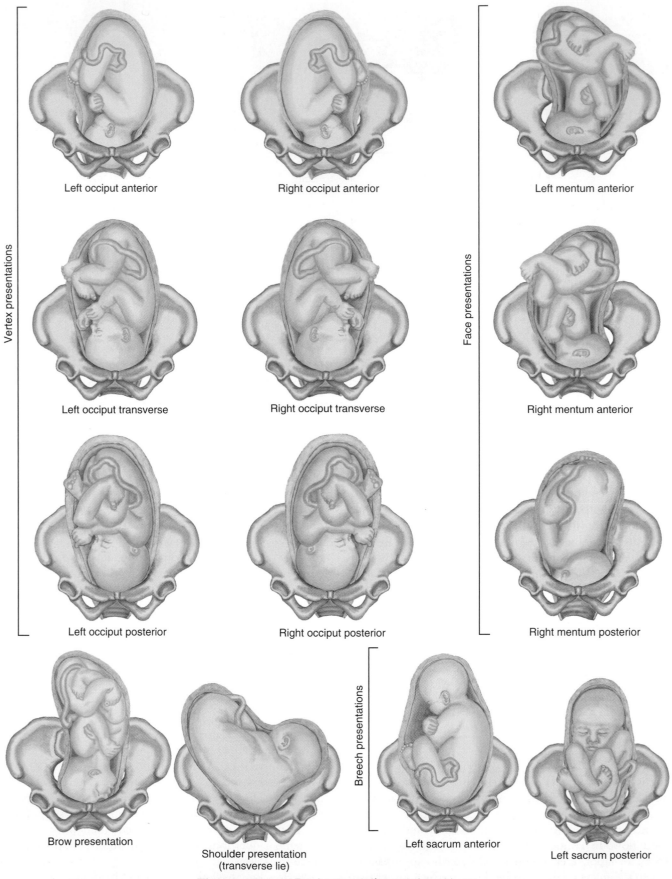

Left occiput anterior

Right occiput anterior

Left mentum anterior

Left occiput transverse

Right occiput transverse

Right mentum anterior

Left occiput posterior

Right occiput posterior

Right mentum posterior

Vertex presentations

Face presentations

Breech presentations

Brow presentation

Shoulder presentation
(transverse lie)

Left sacrum anterior

Left sacrum posterior

Figure 12-11 ■ Fetal presentations and positions.

- What is the primary language used? Do the woman and her support person speak the same language or does only one of them speak the dominant language? Are they relatively comfortable communicating in the nurse's language if that is not their usual language? If an interpreter is needed, what people would the woman or her family consider to be unacceptable interpreters (e.g., men or members of certain religious groups)?
- Who is the woman's primary support person for labor? What is that person's role? Will that person actively support the laboring woman (e.g., by coaching her breathing), or will he take a less active role? Who will be present at the birth?
- Who is the decision maker in the family, or who must be consulted about important decisions?
- Will another relative (such as a grandmother) assume primary care for the infant?
- Is a professional caregiver (such as a nurse or physician) of the same gender and cultural group essential?
- What are the woman's feelings about touch? Is she comfortable telling the nurse when she does not welcome touch?
- Are specific symbols, practices, and ceremonies used during the birth period? Who will conduct any ceremonies?

Other cultural assessments are needed as labor progresses and birth occurs (see Chapters 15 and 18).

BIRTH AS AN EXPERIENCE

Childbirth is a physical and an emotional experience. It is an irrevocable event that forever changes a woman and a family. Families describe the births of their children as they describe other pivotal events in life, such as marriages, anniversaries, religious events, and even deaths. They do not talk about childbirth as they might discuss an illness or surgery. With the prevalence of smaller families, parents have greater expectations about the experience of childbirth than in the past. A woman who has more realistic expectations about the birth is more likely to have a positive experience. Nursing measures that increase the woman's sense of control and mastery during birth help her perceive the birth as a positive event. The nurse must attend to the psychological and emotional needs of the woman during birth to promote a positive birth experience for the woman.

A number of variables influence the meaning of the birth experience for the woman (Nichols & Gennaro, 2000):

- Relatively constant variables such as the woman's cultural and ethnic beliefs and values, spiritual beliefs, personal history (including whether this is her first baby), and age, education, and socioeconomic class
- Variables that the health care team can influence, such as anxiety and fear, pharmacologic pain management, the birthing environment, labor support, and promotion of the woman's confidence, sense of mastery and control, and self-esteem

- Variables that the health care team may influence in some situations, including obstetric risk factors and the type of birth

IMPACT OF TECHNOLOGY

The goal of maternity care is to protect the health of the mother, fetus, and newborn and to support and enrich the woman's birth experience. Technology helps caregivers identify problems and intervene quickly to protect the health of the mother and fetus. However, extensive use of sophisticated technology may make maternity care seem impersonal. Women may feel that their feelings are less important than data from the monitors and infusion pumps attached to them for normal childbirth. Technology may make some nurses feel less necessary to the well-being of the woman. The nurse must guard against "nursing the machines" or internal feelings of being unnecessary to the woman's birth experience. Most nurses become intrapartum nurses because they enjoy helping women give birth. If the nurse can keep the focus on the woman as the childbearer and the machine as a tool, frustration for all concerned is less likely.

Uncomplicated birth is a natural process that does not demand routine use of complex technology. Indeed, interventions during birth can lead to other interventions that may inhibit the natural process. For example, epidural analgesia is now almost routine in births. Although epidural analgesia can provide dramatic pain relief, it also requires infusion of large amounts of intravenous fluids and usually confines the woman to bed. Because the bladder fills quickly, urinary catheterization is usually another part of the process. Many upright positions such as walking and standing are not possible during epidural pain relief.

Although normal labor and birth do not require routine use of sophisticated technology, many women subordinate their preferences for low-intervention birth experiences to their desires for what they believe offers maximal safety for their babies. Other women simply have not thought of a low-technology birth, possibly because many friends and relatives have had a high-technology birth. The intrapartum nurse can be the bridge between the technology and humanity of the birth experience. The nurse must continue to provide support and reassurance even if the woman has minimal pain because of an epidural block. The nature of nursing support is simply different in this case than if the woman were not using medication. The nurse must maintain the nursing focus on the woman, fetus, and support person rather than the technology.

Interrelationships of Components

The four Ps have been described separately but are actually an interrelated whole. For instance, a woman with a small pelvis (passage) and a large fetus (passenger) can have a normal labor and birth if the fetus is ideally positioned and the uterine contractions and maternal bearing-down efforts (powers) are vigorous. The nurse's supportive attitude strengthens positive psychological elements (psyche) and enhances the processes of birth. The nurse can act as an advocate for the laboring woman and her support person to increase their sense of control and mastery of labor, which often reduces anxiety and fear and helps them achieve their desired birth experience.

NORMAL LABOR

Theories of Onset

Despite continuing research, the exact mechanisms that initiate labor remain unknown. Labor normally starts when the fetus is mature enough to adjust easily to extrauterine life but before it grows so large that vaginal birth is impossible. This stage (term gestation) occurs between 38 and 42 weeks after the first day of the woman's last menstrual period. One or more sonograms during pregnancy may have influenced the "due date," especially for the woman who often has irregular periods.

Labor begins when forces favoring continuation of pregnancy are offset by forces favoring its end. Research is ongoing in this area because this knowledge is essential to developing effective measures to treat preterm labor. Factors that appear to have a role in starting labor include the following:

- Changes in the relative effects of estrogen and progesterone encourage onset of labor. Progesterone, a hormone that relaxes the uterus, remains stable in the blood while the estrogen levels rise until the onset of labor. With labor's onset, a functional or actual fall in the progesterone level allows the now stronger estrogen effects to increase sensitivity to substances that stimulate contractions. As estrogen effects increase and progesterone effects decrease, uterine stimulants such as progesterone from the fetal membranes and oxytocin from the maternal posterior pituitary increase. Estrogens increase the number of gap junctions, connections that allow the individual muscle cells of the uterus to contract as a coordinated unit (Challis & Lye, 2004; Cunningham et al., 2001; Guyton & Hall, 2000).
- An increase in prostaglandins produced by the decidua and the membranes may have a role in preparing the uterus for stimulation by oxytocin at term. Prostaglandins are secreted from the lower area of the fetal membranes (forebag) during labor and may reflect inflammation caused by contact with microorganisms from the woman's vagina.
- Increased secretion of oxytocin appears to maintain labor once it has begun. Oxytocin alone does not appear to start labor but may play a part in labor's initiation in conjunction with other substances. Evidence of fetal oxytocin secretion also exists (Challis & Lye, 2004; Cunningham et al., 2004).
- Oxytocin receptors increase markedly as labor begins; the increase continues during labor and peaks at delivery. Oxytocin has little effect on the uterine muscle if the receptors have not developed.
- A fetal role in the initiation of labor appears likely. The fetal membranes release prostaglandin in high concentrations during labor. In addition to fetal oxytocin secretion, large quantities of cortisol are secreted by the fetal adrenal, possibly acting as a uterine stimulant (Guyton & Hall, 2000).
- Stretching, pressure, and irritation of the uterus and cervix increase as the fetus reaches term size. During the rest of pregnancy the uterus has not reacted to stretching by contracting as smooth muscle normally does. A feedback loop is probably responsible for labor contractions at term; the fetal head stretches the cervix, causing the fundus of the uterus to contract, pushing the fetal head against the cervix, and causing more fundal contractions. Cervical stretching also causes secretion of oxytocin (Guyton & Hall, 2000).

Premonitory Signs

BRAXTON HICKS CONTRACTIONS

Contractions occurring throughout pregnancy are irregular and mild. As term approaches, contractions become more noticeable and even painful. Parous women often describe more uterine activity preceding labor than do nulliparous women.

Increased perception of Braxton Hicks contractions often makes sleep difficult at the end of pregnancy. The contractions may become regular at times, only to decrease spontaneously. Because contractions are often uncomfortable but sometimes regular, the woman may be confused about whether labor has really begun.

LIGHTENING

As the fetus descends toward the pelvic inlet ("dropping"), the woman notices that she breathes more easily because upward pressure on her diaphragm is reduced. However, increased pressure on her bladder causes her to urinate more frequently. Pressure of the fetal head in the pelvis also may cause leg cramps and edema. Lightening is most noticeable in nulliparas and occurs about 2 to 3 weeks before the onset of labor.

INCREASED VAGINAL MUCOUS SECRETIONS

An increase in clear and nonirritating vaginal secretions occurs as fetal pressure causes congestion of the vaginal mucosa. The woman may need to wear a perineal pad because of the quantity of mucus.

CERVICAL RIPENING AND BLOODY SHOW

As full term nears, the cervix softens because of the effects of the hormone relaxin and increased water content. These changes (ripening) allow the cervix to yield more easily to the forces of labor contractions. As the fetal head descends with lightening, it puts pressure on the cervix, starting the process of effacement and dilation. Effacement and dilation cause expulsion of the mucus plug that sealed the cervix during pregnancy, rupturing small cervical capillaries in the process. Bloody show is a mixture of thick mucus and pink or dark brown blood. It may begin several days to a few weeks before the onset of labor, especially in the nulliparous woman, or it may not begin until labor starts.

A recent vaginal examination or sexual intercourse also may result in small amounts of bloody show because it disrupts these small vessels. Bloody show increases during labor as the cervix completes dilation and effacement. Women who have previously had a vaginal birth often have less bloody show than nulliparas.

ENERGY SPURT

Some women have a sudden increase in energy, which is called "nesting." They should be cautioned to conserve their energy so that they are not exhausted when labor actually begins.

WEIGHT LOSS

A small weight loss of 2.2 to 6.6 kg (1 to 3 lb) may occur because the altered estrogen and progesterone ratio causes excretion of some of the extra fluid that accumulates during pregnancy.

CRITICAL THINKING EXERCISE 12-1

Alan Lindsey phones you when you are working in the birth unit of your hospital one night. He says, "My wife's baby is due. Heather has been having some contractions off and on all day, and they're keeping her awake now. Should we come to the hospital?"

Questions
1. Do you need any other information? If so, what information do you need? (Assume that your hospital has a protocol for telephone triage that allows nurses to answer and document similar phone inquiries.)
2. What should you tell Heather about her symptoms? What advice can you give her?

True Labor and False Labor

False labor, also called *prodromal labor*, is common because the exact time of labor's onset is rarely known and usually is gradual. False labor often causes women to go to the birth center, thinking that labor has started, only to be disappointed when it has not. The term *false labor* is discouraging to women because they do not realize that these "false" contractions are preparation for true labor.

Several characteristics distinguish true labor from false labor: contractions, discomfort, and cervical change. The best distinction between true and false labor is that contractions of true labor cause progressive change in the cervix. An increase in effacement and dilation occurs with true labor contractions.

Some women experience membrane rupture as the first sign of labor's onset. If this occurs, the woman should go to the birth center for evaluation. Infection and compression of the fetal umbilical cord are possible complications.

Mechanisms of Labor

The mechanisms (cardinal movements) of labor occur as the fetus is moved through the pelvis during birth. The fetus undergoes several positional changes to adapt to the size and shape of the mother's pelvis at different levels (Figure 12-12). Although the mechanisms of labor are described separately in Figure 12-12, some occur concurrently. In a vertex presentation the mechanisms include the following:
- Descent of the fetal presenting part through the true pelvis
- Engagement of the fetal presenting part as its widest diameter reaches the level of the ischial spines of the mother's pelvis
- Flexion of the fetal head, allowing the smallest head diameters to align with the smaller diameters of the midpelvis as it descends

WOMEN WANT TO KNOW — How to Know Whether Labor Is "Real"

True labor differs from false labor in three categories.

False Labor	True Labor
CONTRACTIONS	
Are inconsistent in frequency, duration, and intensity	Usually have a consistent pattern of increasing frequency, duration, and intensity
Do not change or may decrease with activity (such as walking)	Tend to increase with walking
	Begins in lower back and gradually sweeps around to lower abdomen
DISCOMFORT	
Is felt in the abdomen and groin	May persist as back pain in some women; often resembles menstrual cramps during early labor
May be more annoying than truly painful	
CERVIX	
Does not significantly change in effacement or dilation	Includes progressive effacement and dilation (most important characteristic)

DESCENT, ENGAGEMENT, AND FLEXION

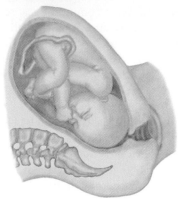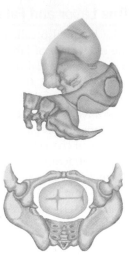

Descent of the fetus is a mechanism of labor that accompanies all the others. Without descent, none of the mechanisms will occur.

STATION

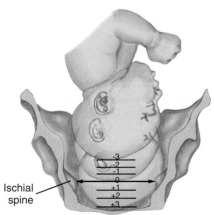

Ischial spine

Station describes the descent of the fetal presenting part in relation to the level of the ischial spines. The level of the ischial spines is a zero station. Other stations are described with numbers representing the approximate number of centimeters above (negative numbers) or below (positive numbers) the ischial spines. As the fetus descends through the pelvis, the station changes from higher negative numbers (–3, –2, –1) to zero to higher positive numbers (+1, +2, +3, etc.) Sometimes the terms *floating* or *ballottable* may describe a fetal presenting part that is so high that it is easily displaced upward during abdominal or vaginal examination, similar to tossing a ball upward.

Engagement

Engagement occurs when the largest diameter of the fetal presenting part (normally the head) has passed the pelvic inlet and entered the pelvic cavity. Engagement is presumed to have occurred when the station of the presenting part is zero or lower. Engagement often takes place before onset of labor in nulliparous women. In many parous women and in some nulliparas, it does not occur until after labor begins.

Flexion

As the fetus descends, the fetal head is flexed further as it meets resistance from the soft tissues of the pelvis. Head flexion presents the smallest anteroposterior diameter (suboccipito-bregmatic) to the pelvis.

INTERNAL ROTATION

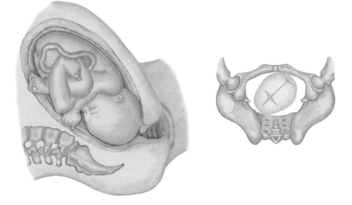

The fetus enters the pelvic inlet with the sagittal suture in a transverse or oblique orientation to the maternal pelvis because that is the widest inlet diameter. Internal rotation allows the longest fetal head diameter (the anteroposterior) to conform to the longest diameter of the maternal pelvis as the fetus descends.

The longest pelvic outlet diameter is the anteroposterior. As the head descends to the level of the ischial spines, it gradually turns so that the fetal occiput is in the anterior of the pelvis (OA position, directly under the maternal symphysis pubis). When internal rotation is complete, the sagittal suture is oriented in the anteroposterior pelvic diameter (OA). Less commonly, the head may turn posteriorly so that the occiput is directed toward the mother's sacrum (OP).

Figure 12-12 ■ Mechanisms (cardinal movements) of labor.

EXTENSION

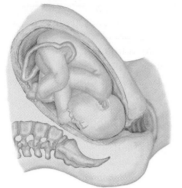
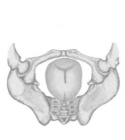

Extension beginning (internal rotation complete)

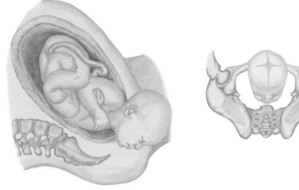

Extension complete

Because the true pelvis is shaped like a curved cylinder, the fetal head is directed posteriorly toward the rectum as it begins its descent. To negotiate the curve of the pelvis, the fetal head must change from an attitude of flexion to one of extension.

While still in flexion, the fetal head meets resistance from the tissues of the pelvic floor. At the same time, the fetal neck stops under the symphysis, which acts as a pivot. The combination of resistance from the pelvic floor and the pivoting action of the symphysis causes the fetal head to swing anteriorly, or extend, with each maternal pushing effort. The head is born in extension, with the occiput sliding under the symphysis and the face directed toward the rectum. The fetal brow, nose, and chin slide over the perineum as the head is born.

EXTERNAL ROTATION

When the head is born with the occiput directed anteriorly, the shoulders must rotate internally so that they align with the anteroposterior diameter of the pelvis.

After the head is born, it spontaneously turns to the same side as it was in utero as it realigns with the shoulders and back (through a process called *restitution*). The head then turns further to that side in external rotation as the shoulders internally rotate and are positioned with their transverse diameter in the anteroposterior diameter of the pelvic outlet. External rotation of the head accompanies internal rotation of the shoulders.

EXPULSION

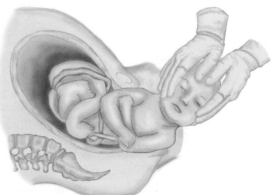

Expulsion occurs first as the anterior, then the posterior, shoulder passes under the symphysis. After the shoulders are born, the rest of the body follows.

Figure 12-12, cont'd ■ Mechanisms (cardinal movements) of labor.

- Internal rotation to allow the largest fetal head diameters to align with the largest maternal pelvic diameters
- Extension of the fetal head as the neck pivots on the inner margin of the symphysis pubis, allowing the head to align with the curves of the pelvic outlet
- External rotation of the fetal head, aligning the head with the shoulders during expulsion
- Expulsion of the fetal shoulders and fetal body

The mechanisms of labor are different in presentations other than the vertex, but the reason is the same: to effectively use the available space in the maternal pelvis.

✔ **CHECK YOUR READING**

11. What are some signs and symptoms that a woman might experience before labor begins?
12. What are the differences between true and false labor? Which difference is the most significant?
13. Why does the fetus enter the pelvis with the sagittal suture aligned with the transverse diameter of the woman's pelvic inlet?
14. Why does the fetal head turn during labor until the sagittal suture aligns with the anteroposterior diameter of the mother's pelvic outlet?

TABLE 12-1 Characteristics of Normal Labor

	First Stage	Second Stage	Third Stage	Fourth Stage
Work accomplished	Effacement and dilation of cervix	Expulsion of fetus	Separation of placenta	Physical recovery and bonding with newborn
Forces	Uterine contractions	Uterine contractions and voluntary bearing-down efforts	Uterine contractions	Uterine contraction to control bleeding from placental site
Average duration				
Nullipara	8-10 hr (range 6-18 hr) after reaching active phase; dilation averages 1 cm/hr	Average 50 min (range, 30 min-3 hr)	5-10 min; up to 30 min is normal for unassisted placental separation	1-4 hr after birth
Multipara	6-7 hr (range, 2-10 hr) after reaching active phase; dilation averages 1.2 cm/hr	Average 20 min (range, 5-30 min)	Same as for nullipara	Same as for nullipara
Cervical dilation	*Latent phase:* 0-3 cm *Active phase:* 4-7 cm *Transition phase:* 8-10 cm	10 cm (complete dilation)	Not applicable	Not applicable
Uterine contractions	*Latent phase:* Initially mild and infrequent; progress to moderate strength, every 5 min with a regular pattern; duration increases to 30-40 sec by end of latent phase *Active phase:* Increase in frequency, duration, and intensity until every 2-5 min, 40-60 sec, and moderate to strong intensity *Transition phase:* Strong, every 1½-2 min, 60 sec	Strong, every 2-3 min, lasting 40-60 sec; may be slightly less intense than during transition phase of first stage; may pause briefly as second stage begins	Firmly contracted	Firmly contracted
Discomfort*	Often begins with a low backache and sensations similar to those of menstrual cramps; back discomfort gradually sweeps to the lower abdomen in a girdlelike fashion, discomfort intensifies as labor progresses	Urge to push or bear down with contractions, which becomes stronger as fetus descends; distention of vagina and vulva may cause a stretching or splitting sensation	Little discomfort; sometimes slight cramp is felt as placenta is passed	Discomfort varies; some women have afterpains, more common in multigravidas or those who have had a large baby; as anesthesia wears off, perineal discomfort may become noticeable
Maternal behaviors*	Sociable, excited, and somewhat anxious during early labor; becomes more inwardly focused as labor intensifies; may lose control during transition	Intense concentration on pushing with contractions; often oblivious to surroundings and appears to doze between contractions	Excited and relieved after baby's birth; usually very tired; often cries	Tired, but may find it difficult to rest because of excitement; eager to become acquainted with her newborn

*Maternal discomfort and behaviors often vary with pain-relief method chosen.

STAGES AND PHASES OF LABOR

Labor is divided into four stages. Each stage has its unique qualities (Table 12-1). This chapter describes typical physiologic characteristics and maternal behaviors in the average woman. Individual women vary in their labor patterns and responses to labor. The woman who chooses an epidural block is likely to behave differently because of this method of pain management.

FIRST STAGE

Cervical effacement and dilation occur in the first stage, or stage of dilation. It begins with the onset of true labor contractions and ends with complete dilation (10 cm) and effacement (100%) of the cervix.

The first stage of labor is the longest for both nulliparous and parous women (Hobel & Chang, 2004; Kendrick & Simpson, 2001; Kilpatrick & Laros, 1989). The duration of first-stage labor averages 8 to 10 hours (range of 6 to 18 hours) for the nullipara and 6 to 7 hours (range of 2 to 10 hours) for the parous woman. The rate of labor progress is also important. When the active phase begins, the cervix of the nullipara usually dilates about 1 cm per hour and that of the multipara dilates about 1.2 cm per hour. Labor progress is often plotted on a labor progress graph called a *Friedman curve* (Figure 12-13).

First-stage labor differs from the other stages because it has three phases: latent (early), active, and transition. Each phase is characterized by changing maternal behaviors. These behaviors vary with the woman's preparation, use of coping skills, and use of medication.

LATENT PHASE. The latent phase is the first 3 cm of cervical dilation. Its length varies among women but averages 8.6 hours for the nullipara and 5.3 hours for the multipara (Kendrick & Simpson, 2001). Latent labor may be quite long, and much of it may pass unnoticed by the pregnant woman. Cervical effacement and fetal positional change occur during latent phase, preparing for the more rapid changes of active labor.

Contractions gradually increase in frequency, duration, and intensity. The interval between contractions shortens until contractions are about 5 minutes apart as the woman progresses to the active phase. Duration increases to 30 to 40 seconds by the end of the latent phase. With regard to intensity, labor begins with mild contractions, during which the contracting uterus can be easily indented with the fingertips, and progresses to moderate contractions, during which the uterine muscle is indented with more difficulty. The contractions gradually build to their peak intensity and remain at the peak briefly before diminishing.

During latent labor the woman may notice discomfort in her back with each contraction. As labor progresses, back discomfort encircles the lower abdomen with each contraction. Many women describe the discomfort as similar to menstrual cramps, especially during early labor.

The woman is usually sociable, excited, and cooperative. She is anxious as she realizes that these contractions are not Braxton Hicks contractions but the "real thing," yet she is usually relieved that her pregnancy is finally about to end.

ACTIVE PHASE. The active phase of labor is so named because the pace of labor increases. The cervix dilates from 4 to 7 cm and at a more rapid rate than in the latent phase. The duration averages 4.6 hours for the nullipara and 2.4 hours for the multipara (Kendrick & Simpson, 2001). Effacement of the cervix is completed. The fetus descends in the pelvis, and internal rotation begins.

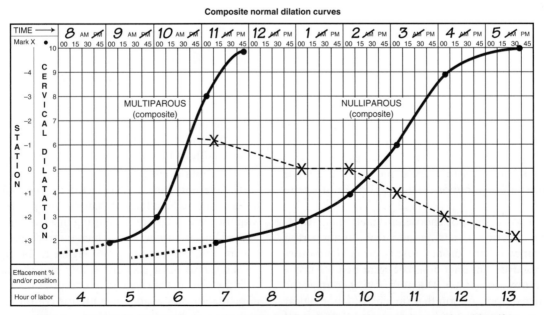

Figure 12-13 ■ A labor curve, often called a *Friedman curve,* may be used to identify whether a woman's cervical dilation is progressing at the expected rate. The symbol for station *(X)* may be added to the labor curve. Typical labor curves for a multiparous woman and a nulliparous woman are illustrated for comparison of patterns.

Contractions average 2 to 5 minutes apart, with a duration of about 40 to 60 seconds and an intensity that ranges from moderate to strong. Active labor contractions reach their peak intensity quickly and stay at the peak longer than during the latent phase.

As contractions intensify, discomfort also increases if the woman has not had analgesia such as epidural block. The site of discomfort during the active phase is similar to that during the latent phase.

The woman's behavior changes. She becomes more anxious and may feel helpless as the contractions intensify. The sociability that characterized early labor is gone and is replaced with a serious, inward focus. She is unlikely to initiate interactions unless she has specific requests. Her behaviors are typical of a person concentrating intently on a demanding task. Women who choose to take pain medication and regional analgesia usually do so during this phase. The nurse helps the woman maintain her concentration, supports her coping techniques, and helps her find alternatives for methods that do not work for her.

TRANSITION PHASE. The cervix dilates from 8 to 10 cm, and the fetus descends further into the pelvis. Bloody show often increases with the completion of cervical dilation. Transition is a short but intense phase, averaging 3.6 hours in the nullipara and having a variable length in the multipara (Kendrick & Simpson, 2001).

Contractions are very strong. They may be as frequent as 1.5 to 2 minutes apart, and their duration is 60 to 90 seconds. Strong contractions combined with fetal descent may cause the woman to have an urge to push and bear down during contractions. If she pushes before cervical dilation is complete, the cervix may swell and labor may be prolonged. Leg tremors, nausea, and vomiting are common.

The woman who does not choose epidural analgesia often finds the transition phase to be the most difficult part of her labor. She may be irritable and lose control. Her partner may be confused because actions that were helpful just a short time ago now bother her. The nurse can encourage the woman and her support person that the end of labor is near and help them use coping techniques most effectively. If premature bearing down is a problem, the nurse can help the woman blow outward with each breath until the urge passes.

SECOND STAGE

The second stage (expulsion) begins with complete (10 cm) dilation and full (100%) effacement of the cervix and ends with the birth of the baby. The duration averages 30 minutes to 3 hours in nulliparas and 5 to 30 minutes in parous women.

Contractions may diminish slightly or even pause briefly as the second stage begins. They are still strong, about 2 to 3 minutes apart, with a duration of 40 to 60 seconds.

As the fetus descends, pressure of the presenting part on the rectum and the pelvic floor causes an involuntary pushing response in the mother. She may say that she needs to have a bowel movement or say "the baby's coming" or "I have to push." Her voluntary pushing efforts augment involuntary uterine contractions. As the fetus descends low in the pelvis and the vulva distends with the crowning of the fetal head, she may feel a sensation of stretching or splitting even if no trauma occurs.

The woman often regains a feeling of control during the second stage of labor. Contractions are strong, but she may feel more in control and know that she is doing something to complete the process by pushing with them. The word *labor* aptly describes the second stage. The woman exerts intense physical effort to push her baby out. Between contractions, she may be oblivious to her surroundings and appear asleep. She feels tremendous relief and excitement as the second stage ends with the birth of the baby.

THIRD STAGE

The third (placental) stage begins with the birth of the baby and ends with the expulsion of the placenta (Figure 12-14). This stage is the shortest, lasting up to 30 minutes, with an average length of 5 to 10 minutes. No difference in duration exists between nulliparas and parous women.

When the infant is born, the uterine cavity becomes much smaller. The reduced size decreases the size of the placenta site, causing it to separate from the uterine wall. Four signs suggest placenta separation:

- The uterus has a spherical shape.
- The uterus rises upward in the abdomen as the placenta descends into the vagina and pushes the fundus upward.
- The cord descends further from the vagina.
- A gush of blood appears as blood trapped behind the placenta is released.

The placenta may be expelled in one of two ways. In the more common Schultze mechanism, the placenta is expelled with the shiny fetal side presenting first (see Figure 12-14, *A*). In the Duncan mechanism, which is less common, the rough maternal side is presenting (see Figure 12-14, *B*).

The uterus must contract firmly and remain contracted after the placenta is expelled to compress open vessels at the implantation site. Inadequate uterine contraction after birth may result in hemorrhage.

Pain during the third stage of labor results from uterine contractions and brief stretching of the cervix as the placenta passes through it.

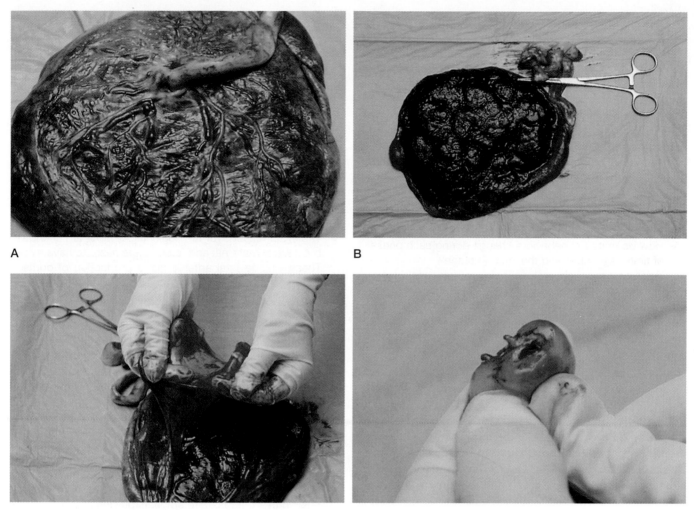

Figure 12-14 ■ **A,** Fetal side of the placenta. **B,** Maternal side of the placenta. **C,** Separating membranes. **D,** Umbilical cord vessels, two arteries, and one vein.

FOURTH STAGE

The fourth stage of labor is the stage of physical recovery for the mother and infant. It lasts from the delivery of the placenta through the first 1 to 4 hours after birth.

Immediately after birth, the firmly contracted uterus can be palpated through the abdominal wall as a firm, rounded mass about 10 to 15 cm (4 to 6 inches) in diameter at or below the level of the umbilicus. Uterine size varies with the size of the infant and parity of the mother and is larger when the infant is large or the mother is a multipara. A full bladder or blood clot in the uterus interferes with uterine contraction, increasing blood loss. A soft (boggy) uterus and increasing uterine size are associated with postpartum hemorrhage because large blood vessels at the placenta site are not compressed (see Chapter 28).

The vaginal drainage after childbirth is called *lochia*. The three stages are lochia rubra, lochia serosa, and lochia alba (see p. 395). Lochia rubra, consisting mostly of blood, is present in the fourth stage of labor.

Many women are chilled after birth. The cause of this reaction is unknown but probably relates to the sudden decrease in effort, loss of the heat produced by the fetus, decrease in intraabdominal pressure, and fetal blood cells entering the maternal circulation. The chill lasts for about 20 minutes and subsides spontaneously. A warm blanket, a hot drink, or soup may help shorten the chill and make the woman more comfortable.

Discomfort during the fourth stage usually results from birth trauma and afterpains. Localized discomfort from birth trauma such as lacerations, an episiotomy, edema, or a hematoma is evident as the effects of local and regional anesthetics diminish. Ice packs on the perineum limit this edema and hematoma formation.

Afterpains are intermittent uterine contractions occurring after birth as the uterus begins to return to the prepregnancy state. The discomfort is similar to menstrual cramps. Afterpains are more common in multiparas, women who breastfeed, women who have large babies or other uterine overdistention during pregnancy, and cases involving interference with uterine contraction because of a full bladder or blood clot that remains in the uterus.

The mother is simultaneously excited and tired after birth. She may be exhausted but too excited to rest. The fourth stage of labor is an ideal time for bonding of the new family because the interest of both the parents and the newborn is high. It is the best time to initiate breastfeeding if no maternal and infant problems are present. The baby is alert and seeks eye contact with the new parents, giving powerful reinforcement for the parents' attachment to their newborn.

✔ CHECK YOUR READING

15. How do maternal behaviors change during each phase of first-stage labor and the second stage?
16. What are typical characteristics of contractions during each phase of first-stage and second-stage labor?
17. What four signs may indicate that the placenta has separated?
18. What complications may occur if the uterus does not contract firmly and remain contracted after the placenta is expelled?

Duration of Labor

The total duration of labor is significantly different for women who have never given birth and those who have previously given birth vaginally. The parous woman usually delivers more quickly than the nulliparous woman. However, women are individuals. Some nulliparas progress through labor quickly, whereas labor for some parous women resembles that of women who have never given birth. A woman who experienced a long labor with her first child may not have a long labor with every baby. If she has a history of rapid labor, however, later births are often rapid as well.

Although fewer women have a vaginal birth after cesarean (VBAC) than a few years ago, a parous woman may have had no vaginal births. In this situation, the woman is likely to have a labor more like that of the nullipara, particularly if she did not labor before her previous cesarean birth.

SUMMARY CONCEPTS

- Labor contractions are intermittent, which allows oxygen, nutrients, and waste products to be exchanged between maternal and fetal circulations during the interval between contractions.
- The upper uterus contracts actively during labor, maintaining tension to pull the more passive lower uterus and cervix over the fetal presenting part. These actions bring about cervical effacement and dilation.
- Maternal vital signs are best assessed between contractions because slight alterations in the woman's blood pressure and pulse may occur during a contraction.
- Hyperventilation may occur if the woman breathes deeply and rapidly. Its manifestations include tingling of the hands and feet, numbness, and dizziness.
- The fetal heart rate and rhythm respond rapidly to events occurring during labor.

- Several occurrences during late pregnancy and labor aid the newborn in making adaptations to extrauterine life: reduced production of fetal lung fluid and increased absorption of lung fluid into the interstitium of the fetal lungs; expulsion of fluid from upper airways during the compression forces of labor; and increased catecholamine secretion by the fetal adrenals to stimulate cardiac contraction and breathing, speed clearance of remaining lung fluid, and aid in temperature regulation.
- Four interrelated components affecting the process of birth are the powers, passage, passenger, and psyche. Presentation and position further describe the relation of the fetus (passenger) to the maternal pelvis (passage).
- The mechanisms of labor favor the most efficient passage of the fetus through the mother's pelvis.
- The exact reasons for the beginning of labor are unknown, but several maternal and fetal factors seem to have a role. These include fetal adrenal gland production of cortisol; changes in the ratio of estrogen to progesterone effects so that estrogen's effect is higher than progesterone's effect; increased uterine oxytocin receptors and gap junctions; and stretching of the uterus and cervix.
- As labor approaches, the woman may notice one or more premonitory signs preceding its onset: increase in frequency and intensity of Braxton Hicks contractions, lightening, increased vaginal secretions, bloody show, a spurt of energy, and weight loss.
- The conclusive difference between true labor and false labor is that progressive effacement and dilation of the cervix occur with true labor.
- The four stages and phases of labor are characterized by different physiologic events and maternal behaviors: first stage, cervical dilation and effacement; second stage, expulsion of the fetus; third stage, expulsion of the placenta; and fourth stage, maternal physiologic stabilization and parent-infant bonding.
- Normal labor is characterized by consistent progression of uterine contractions, cervical dilation and effacement, and fetal descent.

ANSWERS TO CRITICAL THINKING EXERCISES 12-1, p. 253

1. You need to speak directly to Heather rather than Alan because she is the one who is pregnant and having the symptoms. You need to know which baby this is for her (gravida and para), her due date, whether her membranes have ruptured, and the characteristics of her contractions (for example, frequency, duration, intensity, and effect of activity). After you gather assessment data, you learn that Heather's first baby is due the following week, she has had no leaking of fluid from her vagina, and her baby has been normally active. She says, "My contractions are coming every 2 to 10 minutes, and most of them last about 30 seconds. They didn't bother me much until I tried to go to sleep, but now they are keeping me awake. I'm so tired of all this!"

2. Heather's symptoms sound like those of false labor: irregular contractions that are mild, fairly short, and more annoying than truly painful. Although not harmful, these frequent contractions in late pregnancy interrupt the woman's rest. You should tell Heather that these contractions do not sound like true labor, then review with her the

typical signs and symptoms of true labor. Advise her to come to the hospital if her contractions intensify and become more consistent, her "water breaks," the baby seems to move less, or she has vaginal bleeding other than bloody show. Remind her that labor cannot be diagnosed over the phone, and tell her to come to the hospital if she has any continuing concerns.

ANSWERS TO CRITICAL THINKING EXERCISES 12-2, p. 258

Mrs. Saenz's cervix is about 2 to 3 cm dilated and has effaced to about one fourth of its original length (now about 0.5 cm long, or 75% effaced). The widest part of the fetal head (the biparietal diameter) is at the level of the ischial spines (0 station) and has passed the pelvic inlet.

The vertex presentation means that the fetal head is well flexed, which is most favorable because it presents the smallest anteroposterior diameter to the maternal pelvis. ROP means that the fetal occiput is in Mrs. Saenz's right posterior pelvic quadrant.

During the early part of first-stage labor (latent phase), you would expect Mrs. Saenz to be relatively comfortable. She may be visiting with her husband and other family members and friends. Although rapid progress is unlikely with the first baby, be alert to behaviors such as sudden grunting and bearing down (usually accompanied by a marked increase in bloody show), crying out "the baby's coming" or "I've got to push," and inability to maintain control with techniques that have previously been helpful. Summon an experienced nurse or her nurse-midwife by using the call signal at once if any of these behaviors occur. Do not leave her unattended in case the baby arrives unexpectedly.

REFERENCES & READINGS

American Academy of Pediatrics (AAP) & American College of Obstetricians and Gynecologists (ACOG). (2002). *Guidelines for perinatal care* (5th ed.). Elk Grove Village, IL: Author.

Association of Women's Health, Obstetric, and Neonatal Nurses (AWHONN). (2003). *Fetal heart monitoring: Principles & practices* (3rd ed.). Dubuque, IA: Kendall/Hunt Publishing.

Bashore, R.A., & Hayashi, R.H. (2004). Uterine contractility and dystocia. In N.F. Hacker, J.G. Moore, & J.C. Gamboni (Eds.), *Essentials of obstetrics and gynecology* (4th ed., pp. 159-166). Philadelphia: Saunders.

Bernstein, D. (2004). The fetal to neonatal circulatory transition. In R.E. Behrman, R.M. Kliegman, & H.B. Jenson (Eds.), *Nelson textbook of pediatrics* (17th ed., pp. 1479-1481). Philadelphia: Saunders.

Blackburn, S.T. (2003). *Maternal, fetal, and neonatal physiology: A clinical perspective* (2nd ed.). Philadelphia: Saunders.

Bowes, W.A., & Thorp, J.M. (2004). Clinical aspects of normal and abnormal labor. In R.K. Creasy, R. Resnik, & J.D. Iams (Eds.), *Maternal-fetal medicine: Principles and practice* (5th ed., p. 671-705). Philadelphia: Saunders.

Challis, J.R.G., & Lye, S.J. (2004). Characteristics of parturition. In R.K. Creasy, R. Resnik, & J.D. Iams (Eds.), *Maternal-fetal medicine: Principles and practice* (5th ed., 79-89). Philadelphia: Saunders.

Creehan, P.A. (2001). Pain relief and comfort measures during labor. In K.R. Simpson & P.A. Creehan, *AWHONN perinatal nursing* (2nd ed., pp. 417-444). Philadelphia: Lippincott Williams & Wilkins.

Cunningham, F.G., Gant, N.F., Leveno, K.J., Gilstrap, III. L.C., Hauth, J.C., & Wenstrom, K.D. (2001). *Williams obstetrics* (21st ed.). New York: McGraw-Hill.

Cyber, R.L., Adelsperger, D., & Torgersen, K.L. (2003). Interpretation of fetal heart rate patterns. In N. Feinstein, K.L. Torgersen, & J. Atterbury (Eds.), *AWHONN fetal heart monitoring principles and practices* (3rd ed., pp. 113-158). Dubuque, IA: Kendall Hunt Publishing.

Duffy, T.P. (2004). Hematologic aspects of pregnancy. In G.N. Burrow, T.P. Duffy, & J.P. Copel (Eds.), *Medical complications during pregnancy* (6th ed., pp. 69-86). Philadelphia: Saunders.

Feinstein, N.F., Sprague, A., & Trépanier, M.J. (2000). *Fetal heart rate auscultation.* Washington, DC: Association of Women's Health, Obstetric, and Neonatal Nurses.

Guyton, A.C., & Hall, J.C. (2000). *Textbook of medical physiology* (10th ed.). Philadelphia: Saunders.

Haddad, G.G., & Pérez Fontán, J.J. (2004). Development of the respiratory system. In R.E. Behrman, R.M. Kliegman, & H.B. Jenson (Eds.), *Nelson textbook of pediatrics* (17th ed., pp. 1357-1359). Philadelphia: Saunders.

Hobel, C.J., & Chang, A.B. (2004). Normal labor, delivery, and postpartum care. In N.F. Hacker, J.G. Moore, & J.C. Gambone (Eds.), *Essentials of obstetrics and gynecology* (4th ed., pp. 104-135). Philadelphia: Saunders.

Jobe, A.H. (2004). Fetal lung development, tests for maturation, induction of maturation, and treatment. In R.K. Creasy, R. Resnik, & J.D. Iams (Eds.), *Maternal-fetal medicine: Principles and practice* (5th ed., pp. 209-222). Philadelphia: Saunders.

Kendrick, J.M., & Simpson, K.R. (2001). Labor and birth. In K.R. Simpson & P.A. Creehan (Eds.), *AWHONN perinatal nursing* (2nd ed., pp. 298-377). Philadelphia: Lippincott Williams & Wilkins.

Kilpatrick, S.J., & Laros, R.K. (1989). Characteristics of normal labor. *Obstetrics & Gynecology, 74*(1), 85-87.

King, T.L., & Simpson, K.R. (2001). Fetal assessment during labor. In K.R. Simpson & P.A. Creehan (Eds.), *AWHONN'S perinatal nursing* (2nd ed., pp. 378-416). Philadelphia: Lippincott Williams & Wilkins.

Mayberry, L.J., Wood, S.H., Strange, L.B., Lee, L., Heisler, D.R., & Nielsen-Smith, K. (2000). *AWHONN symposium. Second stage labor management: Promotion of evidence-based practice and a collaborative approach to patient care.* Washington, DC: AWHONN.

Monga, M., & Sanborn, B.M. (2004). Biology and physiology of the reproductive tract and control of myometrial contraction. In R.K. Creasy, R. Resnik, & J.D. Iams (Eds.), *Maternal-fetal medicine: Principles and practice* (5th ed., pp. 69-78). Philadelphia: Saunders.

Nichols, F.H., & Gennaro, S. (2000). The childbirth experience. In F.H. Nichols & S.S. Humenick (Eds.), *Childbirth education: Practice, research and theory* (2nd ed., pp. 66-83). Philadelphia: Saunders.

Noah, Z., & Budek, C. (2004). Fetal-to-neonatal circulatory transition. In R.E. Behrman, R.M. Kliegman, & H.B. Jenson (Eds.), *Nelson textbook of pediatrics* (17th ed., pp. 1479-1481). Philadelphia: Saunders.

Parer, J.T., & Nageotte, M.P. (2004). Intrapartum fetal surveillance. In R.K. Creasy, R. Resnik, & J.D. Iams (Eds.), *Maternal-fetal medicine: Principles and practice* (5th ed., pp. 403-427). Philadelphia: Saunders.

Rouse, D.J., & St. John, E. (2003). Normal labor, delivery, newborn care, and puerperium. In J.R. Scott, R.S. Gibbs, B.Y. Karlan, & A.F. Haney (Eds.), *Danforth's obstetrics and gynecology* (9th ed., pp. 35-56). Philadelphia: Lippincott Williams & Wilkins.

Stoll, B.J., & Kliegman, R.M. (2004). The newborn infant. In R.E. Behrman, R.M. Kliegman, & H.B. Jenson (Eds.), *Nelson textbook of pediatrics* (17th ed., pp. 523-531). Philadelphia: Saunders.

Winslow, E.H., & Crenshaw, J. (2000). Managing labor: Does walking help or hurt? *American Journal of Nursing, 100*(3), 50-51.

The Childbirth Story

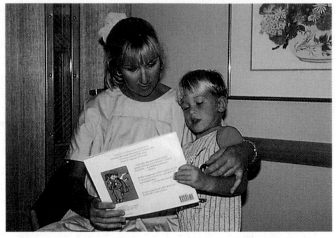

1 ■ Shari, in early labor with her second child, spends time with her 5-year-old son, Adam, in the labor-delivery-recovery room.

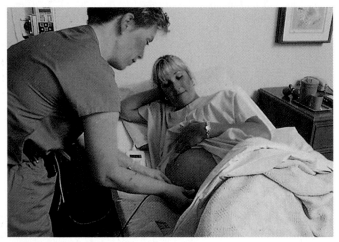

2 ■ The nurse frequently assesses the condition of both the mother and the fetus. Here she listens to the fetal heart rate.

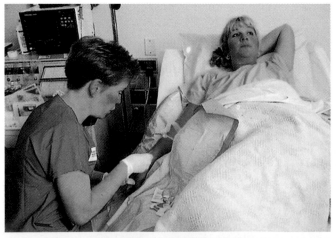

3 ■ Although intravenous fluids are not always necessary, most physicians order them to prevent dehydration and for access to a vein in case an emergency develops.

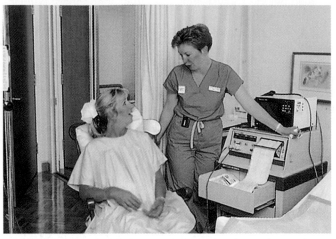

4 ■ The nurse establishes a relationship of trust by assisting Shari into a comfortable position and explaining information obtained by electronic fetal monitoring.

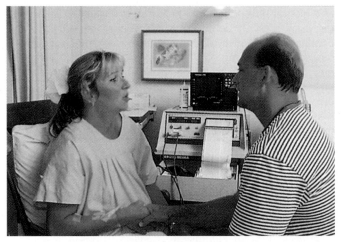

5 ■ Shari plans a childbirth without anesthesia. Darren, the father, uses skills learned in childbirth education classes to help her cope with discomfort.

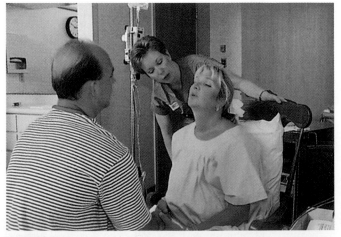

6 ■ Maintaining control is more difficult for Shari as the contractions become stronger. The nurse praises the couple's efforts and reviews measures to reduce discomfort.

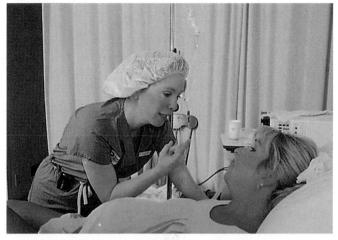

7 ▪ During transition, often the most difficult phase of labor, the nurse remains in close contact with Shari and assists her through each contraction.

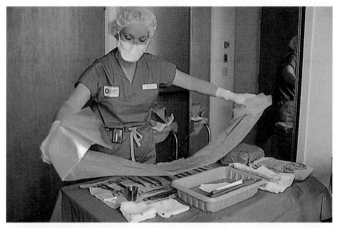

8 ▪ The nurse prepares the sterile instruments that will be used during the birth. A mask is not always needed when preparing the table for vaginal birth but should be used as needed for the birth.

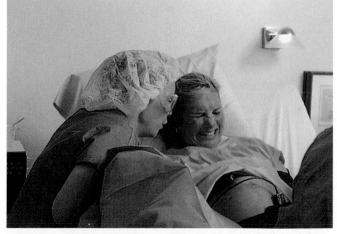

9 ▪ As birth approaches, the nurse positions Shari and assists her to push with each contraction. Note that the nurse now wears protective glasses.

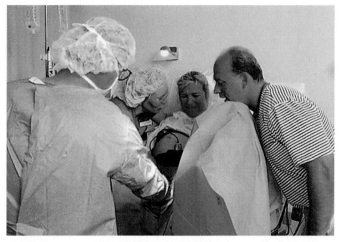

10 ▪ The nurse also encourages Darren to remain in close contact with the mother and continue to participate in the birth.

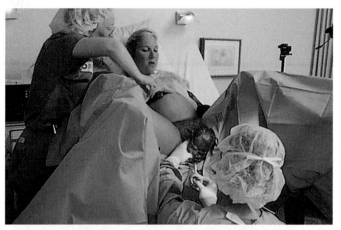

11 ▪ The physician suctions secretions from the nose and mouth of the infant when the head is delivered.

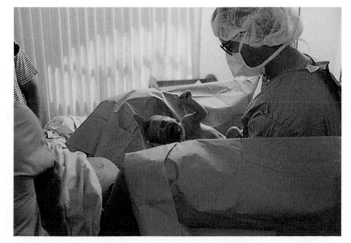

12 ▪ The physician holds the infant so that the parents can get their first look at their newborn son.

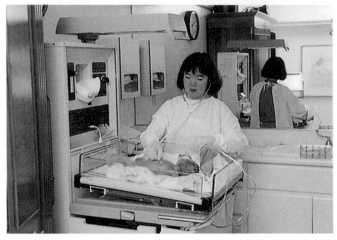

13 ■ A nurse counts the apical pulse and observes the newborn's pink color, which makes the administration of oxygen unnecessary.

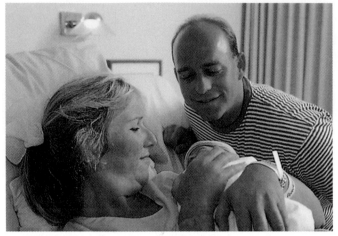

16 ■ Nurses are aware of the importance of early contact, and as soon as possible after birth the mother, father, and newborn are brought together.

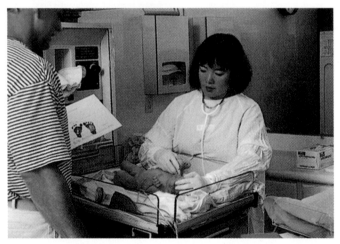

14 ■ The father observes as the nurse suctions secretions from the newborn's nose and mouth and completes identification procedures such as footprinting.

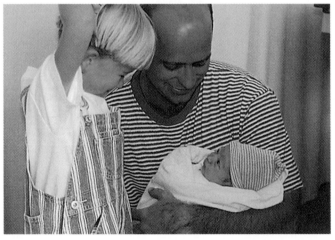

17 ■ Although Adam was not present at the birth, within a short time he meets the wide-eyed baby, who gazes intently at his older brother.

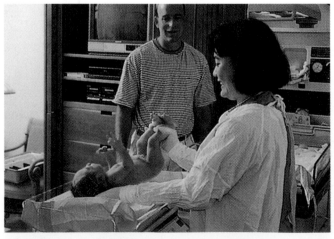

15 ■ Darren is an interested observer as the nurse weighs and measures the newborn.

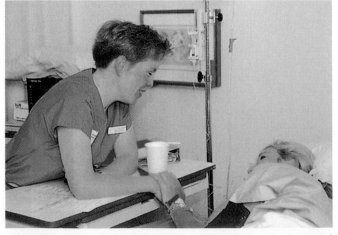

18 ■ Shari and the nurse demonstrate the mutual regard that developed as they shared the intense experience of labor and birth.

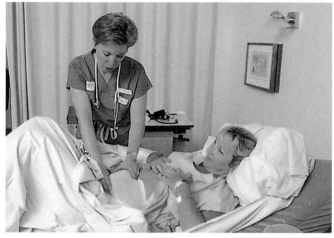

19 ■ The nurse palpates the fundus frequently during the first hour after childbirth to confirm that the uterus is firmly contracted and thus prevent excessive bleeding.

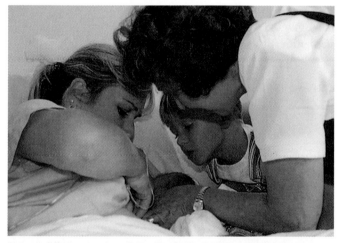

20 ■ Adam watches intently as his mother and grandmother put the baby to breast for the first time.

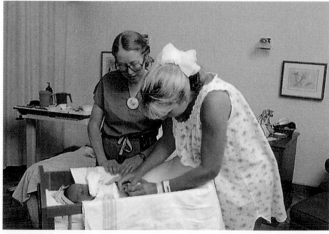

21 ■ Nurses must teach mothers how to care for themselves and their infants within a very short time. Here the nurse instructs Shari in cord care.

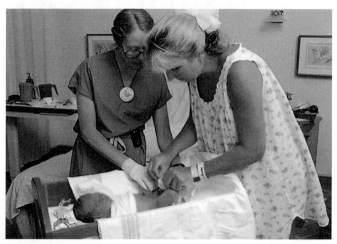

22 ■ Shari gains confidence in circumcision care when the nurse allows a return demonstration.

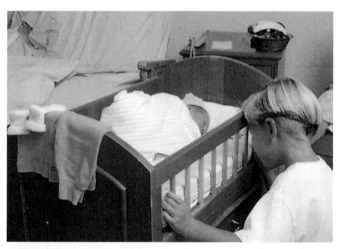

23 ■ Adam peeks at his baby brother while the family receives additional instructions.

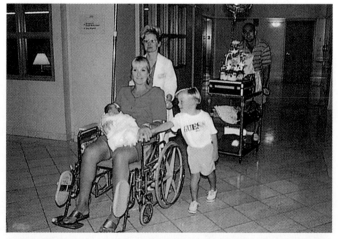

24 ■ Twenty-four hours after her admission, Shari and the infant are discharged from the postpartum unit.

13 Nursing Care during Labor and Birth

OBJECTIVES

After studying this chapter, you should be able to:

1. Analyze issues that may face the new nurse who cares for women during the intrapartum period.
2. Explain teaching guidelines for going to the hospital or birth center.
3. Describe admission and continuing intrapartum nursing assessments.
4. Describe common nursing procedures used when caring for women during the intrapartum period.
5. Identify nursing priorities when assisting the woman to give birth under emergency circumstances.
6. Relate therapeutic communication skills to care of the intrapartum woman and her significant others.
7. Apply the nursing process to care of the woman experiencing false or early labor.
8. Apply the nursing process to care of the woman and her significant others during the intrapartum period.

Go to your Student CD-ROM for Review Questions keyed to these Objectives.

DEFINITIONS

Abortion A pregnancy that ends before 20 weeks' gestation, either spontaneously (miscarriage) or electively. *Miscarriage* is a lay term for spontaneous abortion that is being more frequently used by health professionals.

Amniotomy Artificial rupture of the membranes (amniotic sac).

Caput Succedaneum Area of edema over the presenting part of the fetus or newborn that results from pressure against the cervix (usually called *caput*).

Crowning Appearance of the fetal scalp or presenting part at the vaginal opening.

EDD Abbreviation for *estimated date of delivery;* also may be abbreviated *EDB* (estimated date of birth).

Episiotomy Incision of the perineum to enlarge the vaginal opening.

Ferning Microscopic appearance of amniotic fluid resembling fern leaves when the fluid is allowed to dry on a microscope slide; also called *fern test*.

Gravida A pregnant woman; also refers to a woman's total number of pregnancies, including the one in progress, if applicable.

Multipara A woman who has given birth after two or more pregnancies of at least 20 weeks' gestation; also informally used to describe a pregnant woman before the birth of her second child.

Nitrazine Paper Paper used to test pH; helps determine whether the amniotic sac has ruptured.

Nuchal Cord Umbilical cord around the fetal neck.

Nullipara A woman who has not completed a pregnancy to at least 20 weeks' gestation.

Para A woman who has given birth after a pregnancy of at least 20 weeks' gestation; also designates the number of a woman's pregnancies that have ended after at least 20 weeks' gestation. (A multifetal gestation, such as twins, is considered one birth when calculating parity.)

Primipara A woman who has given birth after a pregnancy of at least 20 weeks' gestation; also used informally to describe a pregnant woman before the birth of her first child.

Care of the woman and her family during labor and birth is a rewarding yet demanding specialty within nursing. The birth of a baby is more than a physical event. Birth has deep personal and social significance for the family, whose roles and relationships are forever altered by this event.

The nurse must support natural physical processes, promote a meaningful experience for the family, and be alert for complications. Additionally, the nurse cares for two clients, one of whom—the fetus—cannot be observed directly.

The intrapartum area is typically a happy place, and good outcomes for mothers and infants are usual. Most women have accepted their pregnancies and look forward to meeting their infants. Yet some women have had stressful pregnancies because of physical and substance abuse, economic hardship, unsupportive personal relationships, and other problems (see Chapter 24).

ISSUES FOR NEW NURSES

New nurses and nursing students often approach care of laboring women with apprehension. They may face several common issues when caring for families during birth.

Pain Associated with Birth

Working with people in pain is difficult, and most nurses feel compelled to relieve pain promptly. Yet pain is expected in labor and cannot always be eliminated. Some women choose to have unmedicated births. Helping the woman manage the pain of birth is a critical part of nursing care, and many nurses find this to be the most creative aspect of their roles.

Inexperience and Negative Experiences

The nurse who has never given birth may feel inadequate to care for laboring women, even though the same nurse rarely thinks that experiencing a fracture is necessary to care for someone with that problem. Nursing skills needed by the intrapartum nurse are basic: observation, critical thinking, problem solving, therapeutic communication, comfort promotion, empathy, and common sense.

Nurses also may be anxious because of their own difficult experiences during birth. They must be careful not to convey negative attitudes to the laboring woman and her significant other.

Unpredictability

Birth follows its own timetable, even with efforts to "manage" it. Some nurses find the uncertain nature of an intrapartum area troubling, whereas others find it exciting. Some occurrences cannot be predicted or explained. In addition, the number of women needing care and the levels of care they require can change quickly.

Intimacy

The intimate nature of intrapartum care and its sexual overtones make some nurses uncomfortable. They may feel that they are intruding on a private time.

The male nurse often is anxious about this aspect of intrapartum care. Although he may have cared for other female clients, his care rarely has been so focused on the reproductive system. He often wonders whether a woman's male partner will accept him as a care provider.

Both male nurses and female nurses should maintain professional conduct and take cues from the couple. If the couple wants privacy, the nurse should intervene only as needed to assess the woman and fetus. In more advanced labor, both partners often welcome the presence of a competent, caring nurse of either gender.

ADMISSION TO THE BIRTH CENTER

The Decision to Go to the Hospital or Birth Center

During the last trimester, the woman needs to know when she should go to the hospital or birth center. Factors to consider include:

- Number and duration of any previous labors
- Distance from the hospital
- Available transportation
- Child care needs

Nurses instruct women to distinguish between false and true labor. Nurses teach guidelines for going to the birth center and reinforce those given by the physician or nurse-midwife ("Women Want to Know: When to Go to the Hospital or Birth Center"). Not everyone has a typical labor, so a woman should be encouraged to go to the birth center if she is uncertain or has other concerns.

WOMEN WANT TO KNOW

When to Go to the Hospital or Birth Center

These are guidelines for providing individualized instruction to women about when to enter the hospital or birth center.

Contractions—A pattern of increasing regularity, frequency, duration, and intensity.
- Nullipara—Regular contractions, 5 minutes apart, for 1 hour
- Multipara—Regular contractions, 10 minutes apart, for 1 hour

Ruptured membranes—A gush or trickle of fluid from the vagina should be evaluated, regardless of whether contractions are occurring.

Bleeding—Bright-red bleeding should be evaluated promptly. Normal bloody show is thicker, pink or dark red, and mixed with mucus.

Decreased fetal movement—If you notice a substantial decrease in the baby's movement, notify your physician or nurse-midwife or come to the labor unit.

Other concerns—These guidelines cannot cover all situations and do not replace specific instructions given to you by your birth attendant. Therefore please go to the hospital for evaluation of any concerns and feelings that something may be wrong.

THERAPEUTIC COMMUNICATIONS

Establishing a Therapeutic Relationship

Sandra Hall is a nursing student assigned to the intrapartum unit. A woman walks toward Sandra. The woman is leaning on a man and breathing rapidly. She says to Sandra, "I think I'm in labor, and my water broke on the way to the hospital."

Sandra: It sounds like today's the day! Let's find you a room.

Sandra asks the woman's name (Amy James) and that of her birth attendant (Donna Moore, CNM, a nurse-midwife) as they walk to a room.

Sandra: I'm Sandra Hall, a nursing student. What names do you want us to call each of you? *(Questioning for information. Shows respect by not assuming how the couple wants to be addressed.)*

Amy: I'm Amy, and my husband is Jeff.

Sandra: Is this your first baby, Amy, or have you had others? *(Questioning in a way that avoids "yes" or "no" answers.)*

Amy: It's my second, and the first took forever! I've been having contractions off and on since midnight, but they didn't get regular till about 6:00 this morning. They are coming every 3 minutes now and starting to hurt a lot.

Sandra helps Amy put a gown on and applies the external fetal monitor while they wait for the RN. She does not follow up on Amy's implied concern about having a long labor, however.

Amy: Oh no . . . the monitor . . . .

Sandra: You have a problem about the monitor? *(Clarifying the nonspecific remark that Amy made about the monitor.)*

Amy: I hated having that thing on with my last baby. I had to lie the same way all the time or they couldn't hear the baby. I know it's best for the baby, though.

Sandra: You seem to have mixed feelings about the monitor. *(Reflecting what Amy seems to be feeling.)*

Amy: Yes, I didn't like it, but I do feel better knowing the baby's okay.

Sandra: We can usually find ways so it doesn't bother you so much. We don't want you to feel tied down because that will make you more uncomfortable. *(Giving information without promising that Amy will be totally comfortable with the external fetal monitor.)*

Sandra observes that Amy's contractions are every 3 minutes and strong. She finds an experienced nurse to help evaluate Amy. Sandra uses critical thinking and wisely seeks help from an experienced nurse because Amy seems to be in active labor and this is her second baby. The fact that Amy's first labor "took forever" does not necessarily mean that this labor will be long.

Nursing Responsibilities during Admission

The two nursing priorities when the woman arrives at the birth center are to (1) establish a therapeutic relationship and (2) assess the condition of the mother and fetus.

ESTABLISHING A THERAPEUTIC RELATIONSHIP

The nurse must quickly establish a therapeutic relationship with the woman and her significant other. The woman's first impression influences her perception of the quality of her entire birth experience.

MAKING THE FAMILY FEEL WELCOME. A warm greeting makes the woman and her significant other feel valued. Even if the unit is busy, the nurse should communicate interest, friendliness, caring, and competence. People understand if the nurse is busy, but they do not understand rudeness and insensitivity to their needs.

Nurses often encounter women who speak a language other than English. Arranging for a culturally acceptable interpreter who is fluent in the woman's language makes the woman and her family feel welcome and promotes safety because it enhances understanding among the woman, her family, and the nurse.

- When caring for a woman who has not had prenatal care or childbirth classes, which are behaviors that most nurses value, the nurse must not be judgmental in either words or actions. The woman's priorities and values may be different from those of the nurse, but she deserves the same respect, support, and care as the woman who made every preparation for her baby's birth.

DETERMINING FAMILY EXPECTATIONS ABOUT BIRTH. Regardless of their number of children, women and their partners have expectations about the birth experience. The partners may have studied their options extensively and planned a birth that best fits their ideals. Those who have not made specific plans also have expectations shaped by contact with relatives and friends and previous birth experiences. A couple may want to repeat a previous satisfying experience or avoid repeating a poor experience. Sometimes one part of a past birth has negatively influenced the couple's impression of the entire experience.

CONVEYING CONFIDENCE. From the first encounter, the nurse should convey confidence and optimism in the woman's ability to give birth and the ability of her significant other to support her. Women having their first baby may be overwhelmed by the power of normal labor contractions. The nurse can reassure these women that intense contractions are normal in active labor while helping them manage contractions and watching for true problems.

- Think about the different perspectives implied by the phrases *give birth* and *be delivered*. The woman who gives birth is an active and able participant; she is the principal action figure. However, the language of *be delivered* implies that the woman is passive. The nurse might ask "Who will attend you as you give birth?" rather than "Who will deliver your baby?"

ASSIGNING A PRIMARY NURSE. Having one nurse give care during all of labor is ideal but often unrealistic. However, changes in caregivers should be as limited as possible. The woman should know the name of and what to expect from each caregiver. For example, the primary nurse might explain the role of a nursing student in the woman's care. Common roles of nursing students in the intrapartum area include promoting comfort, giving emotional support, and helping the primary nurse observe for maternal and fetal problems.

USING TOUCH FOR COMFORT. Touch can communicate acceptance and reassurance and provide physical and emotional comfort to many laboring women. Women who usually do not welcome touch may appreciate it during labor. Cultural norms and personal history influence a woman's comfort with touch from an unrelated person. The nurse should not assume that the woman desires touch but instead ask her if she welcomes or benefits from touch. As labor progresses, the woman's desire for touch may change, and touch may become irritating rather than comforting.

RESPECTING CULTURAL VALUES. Cultural beliefs and practices give structure, meaning, and richness to the birth experience. They influence the behavior of both the childbearing family and the professional staff. Most cultural groups have specific practices related to childbearing. The nurse should incorporate a family's beneficial and neutral cultural practices into care as much as possible.

■ People naturally believe that their own cultural values are best. The nurse should avoid using an attitude that is superior or diminishes the validity of another person's cultural beliefs. Trust in technology is a common value of many caregivers in the United States, but such reliance on technology is considered unnecessary, odd, and even harmful by many other cultures.

✔ CHECK YOUR READING

1. What communication skills can the nurse use to establish a therapeutic relationship when the woman and her family enter the hospital or birth center?
2. How can the nurse incorporate a couple's cultural practices into intrapartum care?

MAKING ASSESSMENTS AT THE TIME OF ADMISSION

A paper or computerized record of prenatal care is sent to the center where the woman plans to give birth and added to her chart when she is admitted. Admission information can be obtained from the prenatal record and verified or updated as needed. Women who have not had prenatal care or who had care with a provider other than one who practices at the facility she enters need more extensive assessment by the nurse and physician (Table 13-1).

FOCUSED ASSESSMENT

A focused assessment is performed before the broader database assessment in the intrapartum unit, opposite of the usual order. Assessment priorities are to determine the condition of the mother and fetus and whether birth is imminent.

FETAL HEART RATE. For assessment of a term fetus using intermittent auscultation, the following fetal heart rate (FHR) guidelines are considered reassuring (Feinstein, Sprague, & Trépanier, 2000):

■ A lower limit of 110 beats per minute (bpm) and an upper limit of 160 bpm
■ Regular rhythm
■ Presence of accelerations in the FHR
■ Absence of decelerations from the baseline

These findings also would be reassuring in an electronically monitored fetus (see Chapter 14).

MATERNAL VITAL SIGNS. Maternal vital signs are assessed to identify signs of hypertension and infection. Hypertension during pregnancy is defined as a sustained blood pressure increase to 140 mm Hg systolic or 90 mm Hg diastolic. The hypertension may be a disorder that is specific to pregnancy or it may be chronic (American Academy of Pediatrics [AAP] & American College of Obstetricians and Gynecologists [ACOG], 2002; ACOG, 2001; ACOG, 2002) (see Chapter 25 for more information). A temperature of 38° C (100.4° F) or higher suggests infection.

IMPENDING BIRTH. Grunting sounds, bearing down, sitting on one buttock, and saying urgently, "The baby's coming" suggest imminent birth. The nurse abbreviates the initial assessment and collects other information after birth. While the nurse cares for the mother, the following minimal information can be quickly gathered if birth is imminent:

■ Names of mother and support person(s)
■ Name of her physician or nurse-midwife if she had prenatal care
■ Number of pregnancies and prior births, including whether the birth was vaginal or cesarean
■ Status of membranes
■ Expected date of delivery
■ Any problems during this or other pregnancies
■ Allergies to medications, foods, or other substances
■ Time and type of last oral intake
■ Maternal vital signs and FHR
■ Pain: location, intensity, factors that intensify or relieve, duration, whether constant or intermittent, whether the pain is acceptable to the woman

If focused assessments of mother and fetus are normal and birth is not imminent, a more complete admission assessment is taken. If the initial assessments show that birth is near or another urgent condition is identified, the physician or nurse-midwife is notified promptly with essential assessment information.

✔ CHECK YOUR READING

3. What are the two assessment priorities when a woman comes to the intrapartum unit?
4. What FHR characteristics (when auscultated) are reassuring?
5. What observations suggest that a woman is going to give birth very soon? What should the nurse do in that case?

Text continued on p. 275.

TABLE 13-1 Intrapartum Assessment Guide

Women who have had prenatal care have much of this information available on their prenatal record. The nurse need only verify it or update it as needed.

Assessment, Method (Selected Rationales)	Common Findings	Significant Findings, Nursing Action
Interview		
Purpose: To obtain information about the woman's pregnancy, labor, and conditions that may affect her care. The interview is curtailed if she seems to be in late labor.		
Introduction: Introduce yourself, and ask the woman how she wants to be addressed. Ask her if she wants her partner and/or family to remain during the interview and assessment. (Shows respect for the woman and gives her control over those she wants to remain with her.)	Many women prefer to be addressed by their first names during labor.	The surname (family name) precedes the given name in some cultures. Clarify which name is used to properly address the woman and to properly identify both mother and newborn.
Culture and language: If she is from another culture, ask what her preferred language is and what language(s) she speaks, reads, or verbally understands. (Identifies the need for an interpreter and enables the most accurate data collection.)	Common non-English languages of women in the United States are Spanish and some Asian dialects. The most common non-English language varies with location.	Try to secure an interpreter fluent in the woman's primary language. Ask her if there are people who are not acceptable to her as interpreters (e.g., males or members of a group in conflict with her culture). Family members may not be the best interpreters because they may interpret selectively, adding or subtracting information as they see fit. Telephone interpreters are available in many facilities. Hearing-impaired women may read lips well, or they may need sign-language interpreters or other assistance.
Communication: Ask the woman to tell you when she has a contraction, and pause during the interview and physical assessment. (Shows sensitivity to her comfort and allows her to concentrate more fully on the information the nurse requests.)	Women in active labor have difficulty answering questions or cooperating with a physical examination while they are having a contraction.	If contractions are very frequent, assess the woman's labor status promptly rather than continuing the interview. Ask only the most critical questions.
Nonverbal cues: Observe the woman's behaviors and interactions with her family and the nurse. (Permits estimation of her level of anxiety. Identifies behaviors indicating that she should have a vaginal examination to determine whether birth is imminent.)	*Latent phase:* Sociable and mildly anxious. *Active phase:* Concentrating intently with contractions; often uses prepared childbirth techniques.	The unprepared or extremely anxious woman may breathe deeply and rapidly, displaying a tense facial and body posture during and between contractions. These behaviors suggest that birth is imminent: 1. Her statement that the baby is coming 2. Grunting sounds (low-pitched, guttural sounds) 3. Bearing down with abdominal muscles 4. Sitting on one buttock Euphoria, combativeness, or sedation suggests recent illicit drug ingestion.
Reason for admission: "What brings you to the hospital/birth center today?" (Open-ended question promotes more complete answer.)	Labor contractions at term, induction of labor, or observation for false labor are common reasons for admission.	Bleeding, preterm labor, pain other than labor contractions. Report these findings to the physician or nurse-midwife promptly.
Prenatal care: "Did you see a doctor or nurse-midwife during your pregnancy?" "Who is your doctor or nurse-midwife?" "How far along were you in your pregnancy when you saw the physician or nurse-midwife?" "Have you ever been admitted here before during this pregnancy?" (Enables location of prenatal record and prior visit records.)	Early and regular prenatal care promotes maternal and fetal health.	No prenatal care or care that was irregular or begun in late pregnancy means that complications may not have been identified.

TABLE 13-1 Intrapartum Assessment Guide—cont'd

Assessment, Method (Selected Rationales)	Common Findings	Significant Findings, Nursing Action
Interview—cont'd		
Estimated date of delivery (EDD): "When is your baby due?" (Determines if gestation is term.) "When did your last menstrual period begin?" (For estimation of EDD if woman did not have prenatal care.)	*Term gestation:* 38-42 wk. The woman's gestation may have been confirmed or adjusted during pregnancy with an ultrasound or other clinical examination.	Gestations earlier than the beginning of the 38th week (preterm) or later than the end of the 42nd week (postterm) are associated with more fetal or neonatal problems. The physician may try to stop labor that occurs earlier than 36 weeks.
Gravidity, parity, abortions: "How many times have you been pregnant?" "How many babies have you had? Were they full term or premature?" "How many children are now living?" "Have you had any miscarriages or abortions?" "Were there any problems with your babies after they were born?" (Helps estimate probable speed of labor and anticipate neonatal problems.)	Labor may be faster for the woman who has given birth before than for the nullipara. *Miscarriage* is used to describe a spontaneous abortion because many lay people associate the term *abortion* with only induced abortions.	Parity of 5 or more (grand multiparity) is associated with placenta previa (see Chapter 25) and postpartum hemorrhage (see Chapter 28). Women who have had several spontaneous abortions or who have given birth to infants with abnormalities may face a higher risk for an infant with a birth defect.
Pregnancy history (Identifies problems that may affect this birth.)		
Present pregnancy: "Have you had any problems during this pregnancy, such as high blood pressure, diabetes, infections, or bleeding?"	Complications are not expected.	Women who have diabetes or hypertension may have poor placental blood flow, possibly resulting in fetal compromise. Some complications of past pregnancies, such as gestational diabetes, may recur in another pregnancy. The woman who plans a VBAC may need more support and reassurance to give birth vaginally.
Past pregnancies: "Were there any problems with your other pregnancy(ies)?" "Were your other babies born vaginally or by cesarean birth?"	Women who had previous cesarean birth(s) may have a trial of labor and vaginal birth (VBAC). A woman who previously had a difficult labor or a cesarean birth may be more anxious than one who had an uncomplicated labor and birth.	Although the VBAC is less common, it may be chosen for a variety of reasons. The nurse should be aware of the need for support and for complications that may be more likely in the current pregnancy.
Other: "Is there anything else you think we should know so that we can better care for you?"	This open-ended question gives the woman a chance to share information that may not be elicited by other questions.	
Labor status: "When did your contractions become regular?" "What time did you begin to think you might really be in labor?" (Facilitates a more accurate estimation of the time labor began.)	Varies among women. Many women go to the birth facility when contractions first begin. Others wait until they are reasonably sure that they are really in labor.	Women who say they have been "in labor" for an unusual length of time (e.g., "for 2 days") have probably had false labor. These women may be very tired from the annoying, nonproductive contractions.
Contractions: "How often are your contractions coming?" "How long do they last?" "Are they getting stronger?" "Tell me if you have a contraction while we are talking." (Obtains the woman's subjective evaluation of her contractions. Alerts the nurse to palpate contractions that occur during the interview.)	Varies according to her stage and phase of labor. Labor contractions are usually regular and show a pattern of increasing frequency, duration, and intensity.	Irregular contractions or those that do not increase in frequency, duration, or intensity are more likely to represent false labor. Contractions that are too frequent or too long can reduce placental blood flow. Incomplete uterine relaxation between contractions also can reduce placental blood flow (see Chapter 14).
Membrane status: "Has your water broken?" "What time did it break?" "What did the fluid look like?" "About how much fluid did you lose—was it a big gush or a trickle?" (Alerts the nurse of the need to verify whether the membranes have ruptured if it is not obvious. Identifies possible prolonged rupture of membranes or preterm rupture.)	Most women go to the birth facility for evaluation soon after their membranes rupture. If a woman is not already in labor, contractions usually begin within a few hours after the membranes rupture at term.	If the woman's membranes have ruptured and she is not in labor or if she is not at term, a vaginal examination is often deferred. Labor may be induced if she is at term with ruptured membranes.

VBAC, Vaginal birth after cesarean.

Continued

TABLE **13-1**   Intrapartum Assessment Guide—cont'd

Assessment, Method (Selected Rationales)	Common Findings	Significant Findings, Nursing Action
Interview—cont'd		
Allergies: "Are you allergic to any foods, medicines, or other substances?" "Do you have an allergy to latex?" "What kind of reaction do you have?" "Have you ever had a problem with anesthesia when you have had dental work?" (Determines possible sensitivity to drugs that may be used.)	Record any known allergies to food, medication, or other substances. As needed, describe how they affected the woman.	Allergy to seafood, iodized salt, or x-ray contrast media may indicate iodine allergy. Because iodine is used in many "prep" solutions, alternative ones should be used. Allergy to latex is becoming more common. Allergy to dental anesthetics may indicate possible allergy to the drugs used for local or regional anesthetics. These drugs usually end in the suffix *-caine*.
Food intake: "When was the last time you had something to eat or drink?" "What did you have?" (Provides information needed to most safely administer general anesthesia if required. Identifies possible fluid or energy deficit.)	Record the time of the woman's last food intake and what she ate. Include both liquids and solids.	If the woman says she has not had any intake for an unusual length of time, question her more closely: "Is there any food you may have forgotten, such as a snack or a drink of water or other liquid?"
Recent illness: "Have you been ill recently?" "What was the problem?" "What did you do for it?" "Have you been around anyone with a contagious illness recently?"	Most pregnant women are healthy. An occasional woman may have had a minor illness such as an upper respiratory tract infection.	Urinary tract infections are associated with preterm labor. The woman who has had contact with someone having a communicable disease may become ill and possibly infect others in the facility.
Medications: "What drugs do you take that your doctor or nurse-midwife has prescribed?" "Are there any over-the-counter drugs that you use?" "I know this may be uncomfortable to discuss, but we need to know about any illegal substances that you use, to more safely care for you and your baby." (Permits evaluation of the woman's drug intake and encourages her to disclose nonprescribed use.)	Prenatal vitamins and iron are commonly prescribed. Record all drugs the woman takes, including time and amount of last ingestion. Women who use illegal substances often conceal or diminish the extent of their use because they fear reprisals.	Drugs may interact with other medications given during labor, especially analgesics and anesthetics. Substance abuse is associated with complications for the mother and infant (see Chapter 24). If the woman discloses that she uses illegal drugs, ask her what kind and the last time she ingested them (often referred to as "taking a hit"). A nonjudgmental approach is more likely to result in honest information.
Tobacco or alcohol: "Do you smoke or use tobacco in any other form? About how many cigarettes a day?" "Do you use alcohol? About how many drinks do you have each day (or week)?" (Evaluates use of these legal substances.)	As in substance abuse, women may underreport the extent of their use of tobacco or alcohol.	Infants of heavy smokers are often smaller and may have reduced placental blood flow during labor. Infants of women who use alcohol may show fetal alcohol effects (see Chapter 30).
Birth plans (shows respect for the woman and her family as individuals and promotes achievement of their expectations; enables more culturally appropriate care):		
Coach or primary support person: "Who is the main person you want to be with you during labor?" Ask that person how he or she wants to be addressed, such as "Mr. Ramos," or "Carlos."	This is usually the woman's husband or the baby's father, but it may be her mother, her sister, or a friend, especially if she is single.	The woman who has little or no support from significant others probably needs more intense nursing support during labor and after the birth. These clients are more likely to have problems with parent-infant attachment.
Other support: "Is there anyone else you would like to be present during labor?"	Women often want another support person present.	
Preparation for childbirth: "Did you attend prepared childbirth classes?" "Did someone go with you?"	Ideally, the woman and a partner have had some preparation in classes or self-study. Women who attended classes during previous pregnancies do not always repeat the classes during subsequent pregnancies.	The unprepared woman may need more support with simple relaxation and breathing techniques during labor. Her partner may need to learn techniques to assist her.
Preferences: "Are there any special plans you have for this birth?" "Is there anything you want to avoid?" "Did you plan to record the birth with pictures or video?"	Some women or couples have strong feelings regarding certain interventions. Common ones are (1) analgesia or anesthesia; (2) intravenous lines; (3) fetal monitoring; (4) use of episiotomy or forceps.	Conflict may arise if the woman has not previously discussed her preferences with her physician or nurse-midwife or if she is unaware of what services are available where she gives birth.
Cultural needs: "Are there any special cultural practices that you plan when you have your baby?" "How can we best help you to fulfill these practices?"	Women from Asian and Hispanic cultures may subscribe to the "hot-and-cold" theory of illness and want specific foods after birth, such as soft-boiled eggs. They may not want their water or other fluids iced.	Try to incorporate all positive or neutral cultural practices. If a practice is harmful, explain why and try to find a way to work around it if the family does not want to give it up.

TABLE 13-1 Intrapartum Assessment Guide—cont'd

Assessment, Method (Selected Rationales)	Common Findings	Significant Findings, Nursing Action
Fetal Evaluation *Purpose:* To determine if the fetus seems to be healthy and tolerating labor well. *Fetal heart rate* (FHR): Assess by intermittent auscultation, or apply an external fetal monitor if that is the facility's policy (most common in the United States). Document FHR according to the risk status and stage of labor (see Chapter 14). *Guidelines include:* Low risk: q 1 h (latent phase), q 30 min (active phase), q 15 min (2nd stage). High risk: q 30 min (latent phase), q 15 min (active phase), q 5 min (2nd stage).	Average rate at term is 110-160 bpm. Rate usually increases when the fetus moves and is reassuring.	These signs may indicate fetal stress and should be reported to the physician or nurse-midwife: 1. Rate outside the normal limits 2. Slowing of the rate that persists after the contraction ends 3. No increase in rate when the fetus moves 4. Irregular rhythm More frequent assessments should be made of the FHR and contractions if any finding is questionable.
Labor Status *Purpose:* To identify whether the woman is in labor and if birth is imminent. If she displays signs of imminent birth, this assessment is done as soon as she is admitted. *Contractions* (yields objective information about labor status): In addition to asking the woman about her contraction pattern, assess the contractions by palpation with the fingertips of one hand. Contractions should be assessed each time the FHR is assessed.	See interview section earlier in table.	See interview section earlier in table. Women who have intense contractions or who are making rapid progress should be assessed more frequently.
Vaginal examination (Determines cervical dilation and effacement; fetal presentation, position, and station; bloody show; and status of the membranes.)	Varies according to the stage and phase of labor. It may not be possible to determine the fetal position by vaginal examination when membranes are intact and bulging over the presenting part.	A vaginal examination is not performed if the woman reports or has evidence of active bleeding (not bloody show) and may not be done if her gestation is 36 weeks or less and she does not seem to be in active labor. Report reasons for omitting a vaginal examination to the physician or nurse-midwife.
Status of membranes: During a vaginal examination a flow of fluid suggests ruptured membranes. A nitrazine test and/or fern test may be done, often using a sterile speculum exam. (Test is not needed if it is obvious that the membranes have ruptured.)	Amniotic fluid should be clear, possibly containing flecks of white vernix. Its odor is distinctive but not offensive. The nitrazine test with a color change of blue-green to dark blue (pH >6.5) suggests true rupture of the membranes but is not conclusive. The fern test is more diagnostic of true rupture of membranes because it is less likely to be affected by vaginal infections, recent intercourse, or other factors.	A greenish color indicates meconium staining, which may be associated with fetal compromise or postterm gestation. Thick meconium with heavy particulate matter ("pea soup") is most significant (see Chapter 30). Thick green-black meconium may be passed by the fetus in a breech presentation and is not necessarily associated with fetal compromise. Cloudy, yellowish, strong-, or foul-smelling fluid suggests infection. Bloody fluid may indicate partial placental separation (see Chapter 25).
Leopold's maneuvers: Often done before assessing the FHR to locate the best place for assessment. (Identifies fetal presentation and position. Most accurate when combined with information from vaginal examination.)	A cephalic presentation with the head well flexed (vertex) is normal. The fetal head is often easily displaced upward ("floating") if the woman is not in labor. When the head is engaged, it cannot be displaced upward with Leopold's maneuvers.	A hard, round, freely movable object in the fundus suggests a fetal head, meaning the fetus is in a breech presentation. Less commonly, the fetus may be crosswise in the uterus: a transverse lie.
Pain: Note discomfort during and between contractions. Note tenderness when palpating contractions. (Distinguishes between normal labor pain and abnormal pain that may be associated with a complication.)	There may be verbal or nonverbal evidence of pain with contractions, but the woman should be relatively comfortable between contractions. The skin around the umbilicus is often sensitive.	Constant pain or a tender, rigid uterus suggests a complication, such as abruptio placentae (separated placenta) (see Chapter 25) or, less commonly, uterine rupture (see Chapter 27).
Physical Examination *Purpose:* To evaluate the woman's general health and identify conditions that may affect her intrapartum and postpartum care.		

bpm, Beats per minute.

Continued

TABLE 13-1 Intrapartum Assessment Guide—cont'd

Assessment, Method (Selected Rationales)	Common Findings	Significant Findings, Nursing Action
Physical Examination—cont'd		
General appearance: Observe skin color and texture, nutritional state, and appearance of rest or fatigue. Examine the woman's face, fingers, and lower extremities for edema. Ask her if she can take her rings off and put them on.	Women are often fatigued if their sleep has been interrupted by Braxton Hicks contractions, fetal activity, or frequent urination. Mild edema of the lower extremities is common in late pregnancy.	Pallor suggests anemia. Substantial edema of the face and fingers or extreme (pitting) edema of the lower extremities is associated with preeclampsia although it may occur in the absence of this hypertensive disorder (see Chapter 25).
Vital signs: Take the woman's temperature, pulse, respirations, and blood pressure. Reassess the temperature every 4 hr (every 2 hr after membranes rupture or if elevated); reassess blood pressure, pulse, and respirations every hour.	*Temperature:* 35.8°-37.3° C (96.4°-99.1° F). *Pulse:* 60-100/min. *Respirations:* 12-20/min, even and unlabored. Blood pressure near baseline levels established during pregnancy. Transient elevations of blood pressure are common when the woman is first admitted, but they return to baseline levels within about ½ hr.	Report abnormalities to physician or nurse-midwife. Temperature of 38° C (100.4° F) or higher suggests infection. Pulse and respirations may also be elevated. Pulse and blood pressure may be elevated if the woman is extremely anxious or in pain. A blood pressure ≥140 mm Hg or ≥90 mm Hg diastolic or higher is considered hypertensive. For women who did not have prenatal care, there is no baseline for comparison.
Heart and lung sounds: Auscultate all areas with a stethoscope.	Heart sounds should be clear with a distinct S_1 and S_2. A physiologic murmur is common because of the increased blood volume and cardiac output. Breath sounds should be clear, with respirations even and unlabored.	The woman who is breathing rapidly and deeply may have symptoms of hyperventilation: tingling and spasm of the fingers, numbness around the lips.
Breasts: Palpate for a dominant mass.	Breasts are full and nodular. Areola is darker, especially in dark-skinned women. Breasts may leak colostrum (clear, sticky, straw-colored fluid) during labor.	Report a dominant mass to the physician or nurse-midwife.
Abdomen: Observe for scars at the same time Leopold's maneuvers and the FHR are assessed. It is usually sufficient to assess the fundal height by observing its relation to the xiphoid process.	Striae (stretch marks) are common. If scars are noted, ask the woman what surgery she had and when. The fundus at term is usually slightly below the xiphoid process but varies with maternal height and fetal size and number.	Report a previous cesarean birth to the physician or nurse-midwife. Transverse uterine scars are least likely to rupture if the woman is in labor (see Chapter 27). Measure the fundal height (see p. 132) if the fetus seems small or if the gestation is questionable.
Deep tendon reflexes: Assess patellar reflex (see Chapter 25). Upper extremity deep tendon reflexes should be used if epidural block analgesia is planned because they are normally not as strong as the patellar reflex.	A brisk jerk without spasm or sustained muscle contraction is normal. Some women normally have hypoactive reflexes, but at least a slight twitch is expected. Obese women may appear to have diminished reflexes because of the fat tissue over the tendon.	Report absent (uncommon unless the woman is receiving magnesium sulfate) or hyperactive reflexes. Hyperactive reflexes and clonus (repeated tapping when the foot is dorsiflexed) are associated with pregnancy-induced hypertension and often precede a seizure (see Chapter 25).
Midstream urine specimen: Assess protein and glucose levels with a dipstick. Follow instructions on the package for waiting times. Check for ketones if the woman has not eaten for a prolonged period or has been vomiting. Send for urinalysis if ordered.	Negative or trace of protein; negative glucose and ketones.	Proteinuria is associated with pregnancy-induced hypertension but may also be associated with urinary tract infections or a specimen that is contaminated with vaginal secretions. Glucosuria is associated with diabetes. Ketonuria is common in poorly controlled diabetes or if the woman does not eat adequate carbohydrates to meet her energy needs.
Laboratory tests: Women who have had prenatal care may not need as many admission tests. Common tests include: 1. Complete blood cell count (or hematocrit done on unit).	1. Hemoglobin at least 11 g/dl; hematocrit at least 33%.	1. Values lower than these reduce maternal reserve for normal blood loss at birth.
2. Blood type and Rh factor.	2. The woman who is Rh-negative receives Rh immune globulin at 28 weeks' gestation to prevent formation of anti-Rh antibodies if she has regular prenatal care.	2. Rh-negative mothers need Rh immune globulin after birth if the infant is Rh-positive.
3. Serologic tests for syphilis.	3. Negative.	3. A positive test indicates that the baby could be infected and needs treatment after birth. The mother should be treated if she has not been treated already.

CRITICAL THINKING ⁇EXERCISE 13-1

During a labor admission assessment, a woman quickly denies her use of drugs and herbal preparations other than her prescribed prenatal vitamins. She becomes quiet, answering the nurse's questions in a terse manner.

Questions
What might explain the woman's change in behavior? Should the nurse alter the assessment interview?

DATABASE ASSESSMENT. In addition to performing the focused assessment, the nurse should assess the mother, fetus, and available maternal support persons.

Basic Information. Intrapartum admission forms guide the nurse to obtain required information. Typical information includes the following:

- The woman's reason for coming to the hospital or birth center (such as contractions, rupture of membranes)
- Prenatal care: when it began, her most recent visit, and her physician or nurse-midwife's name
- Estimated date of delivery (EDD)
- Number of pregnancies, births, spontaneous pregnancy losses, and abortions
- Allergies: medications, food, other substances such as latex
- Food intake: what food and when it was eaten
- Medical, surgical, and pregnancy history
- Recent illness, including treatment
- Medications, including prescription and over-the-counter drugs, tobacco, alcohol and other substances of abuse
- Complementary or alternative therapy; use of herbal and botanical preparations and their purpose
- Use of tobacco, alcohol, and illicit substances
- Her subjective evaluation of her labor
- Birth plans, including planned pain management methods
- Support persons: who they are and the role of each
- Potential domestic violence (ask only when the woman is alone)

Women often bring several people with them to the birthing room and want them to stay during admission. However, be careful about asking for sensitive information, such as prior pregnancies and births and potential abuse, when others are present. A woman may have had an abortion or relinquished a baby for adoption, and her family may not know about it. Even if her partner knows about previous pregnancies, her family or friends may not. Asking about domestic violence when the abuser is present will result in a quick denial and can be dangerous for the woman. Delay asking sensitive information until the woman is alone for confidentiality, safety, and accuracy.

Fetal Assessments. The fetal presentation and position are assessed using a combination of vaginal examination and Leopold's maneuvers (Figure 13-1 and Procedure 13-1). The FHR is assessed by intermittent auscultation and electronic monitoring (see Chapter 14). The nurse documents the color and odor of the amniotic fluid and the time of rupture if the membranes ruptured before admission.

Labor Status. The woman's labor status is determined by assessing her contraction pattern, performing vaginal examination if there are no contractions, and determining whether her membranes have ruptured. Contractions are assessed by palpation (Procedure 13-2), the fetal monitor, or both. Cervical dilation and effacement and the fetal station, presentation, and position are evaluated by vaginal examination. The vaginal examination may also reveal whether the membranes have ruptured if fluid is not obviously leaking from the vagina. Vaginal examination is not performed if the woman has active bleeding (other than bloody show) because the procedure can increase bleeding.

Physical Examination. A brief physical examination evaluates the woman's overall health. Other important observations relating to birth include the presence and location of edema, abdominal scars, and height of the fundus.

✔ CHECK YOUR READING

6. Which tests may be done if the nurse is not certain whether the woman's membranes have ruptured? (See Table 13-1.)
7. Which characteristics of contractions may reduce blood flow to the placenta? (See Procedure 13-2.)

USING ADMISSION PROCEDURES

NOTIFYING THE BIRTH ATTENDANT. After assessment the nurse notifies the woman's birth attendant to report the woman's status and obtain orders. The nurse includes the following data in the report:

- Gravidity, parity, abortions, and term and preterm births
- EDB and fundal height if it conflicts with the EDB
- Contraction pattern
- Results of vaginal examination
  - Cervical dilation and effacement
  - Fetal presentation and position
  - Station of the presenting part
- Fetal heart rate and pattern
- Maternal vital signs
- Any identified abnormalities and concerns about the maternal or fetal condition
- Pain, anxiety, or other reactions to labor

If the birth attendant admits the woman, any of several procedures may be performed.

CONSENT FORMS. The woman signs consent for care during labor, such as anesthesia, vaginal birth and/or cesarean birth, blood transfusion, testing for human immunodeficiency virus (HIV). A separate consent for tubal ligation must be signed by the woman if she desires permanent sterilization at the time of birth. Consent for newborn care and circumcision of male infants is often completed at this time.

Text continued on page 280.

CARE PATH FOR STAGES OF LABOR 1 & 2

NANDA Problem Number	LOCATION	PREADMIT	ADMISSION	LATENT PHASE (0-4 cm)
IV 5, 8, 9, 16 I 5, 6 III I I	Assessments	High risk screening with referrals prn: – MFM – Homecare – Genetic Counsel – Social Services	T, P, R, BP Deep tendon reflexes / clonus Labor status: – admit for labor per protocol: CRITERIA FOR LABOR: 1. complete effacement; or 2 cm in nullipara 2. cervical change 3. rupture of membranes s̄ labor 4. contractions at least 5 min apart – cervix: sterile vaginal exam unless contraindicated – uterine activity (toco / palpation) – membrane status, color, amount, odor of fluid Fetus: – presentation (ultrasound prn) – FHR: 20 min or electronic fetal monitoring strip (continue electronic fetal monitoring if non-reassuring pattern) Urine – dip for protein & ketones Level of childbirth preparation Family interaction Beta-strep risk factors – preterm labor – rupture of membranes < 37 wk – previous baby c̄ Beta-strep	P, R, BP q̄ 1 hr T q̄ 2 hr if rupture of membranes, q̄ 4 hr if bag of waters intact BP, P q̄ 15 min if epidural anesthetic Bladder status q̄ 2 hr Urine protein/ketones dip-stick prn Deep tendon reflexes/clonus prn Fetal monitoring: electronic fetal monitor or electronic fetal monitoring while in bed or intermittent auscultation Labor status: – frequency, duration, strength, resting tone of contractions q̄ 1 hr by toco/palpation or intrauterine pressure catheter – membrane status; color, amount and odor of fluid – sterile vaginal exam prn & prior to meds as indicated Fetus: – low risk: FHR q̄ 30 min – high risk: FHR q̄ 15 min In and out catheterization **Progress to active phase c̄ in 6° of admission** verified _____
IV 5, 6	Procedures/ Tests		CBC, VDRL, ABO-Rh stat on admission HBSAG if not on prenatal record	**If intrauterine pressure catheter labor pattern shows > 250 Montevideo unit** verified _____
	Treatments		Initiate Labor Curve Initiate "Active Management of Labor Protocol" if criteria are met. Notify Special Care Nursery of potential problems.	Consider amniotomy for prolonged latent phase. Consider use of intrauterine pressure catheter if inadequate cervical change.
VI 3 XI 5	Medication			PAIN CONTROL: Parenteral analgesia as ordered. (Consider Stadol or Nubain). If inadequate pain control, anesthesia consult, re-evaluate for epidural _____ Narcotic epidural _____ Anesthetic epidural
	Signatures	____/____ ____/____	____/____ ____/____	____/____ ____/____

MED REC NO. _____

PATIENT _____

PHYSICIAN _____

BAYLOR UNIVERSITY MEDICAL CENTER

DALLAS, TEXAS

CARE PATH FOR STAGES OF LABOR 1 & 2

PAGE 1 OF 4

Figure 13-1 ■ Care path for stages 1 and 2 of labor.

CARE PATH FOR STAGES OF LABOR 1 & 2

NANDA Problem Number	LOCATION	PREADMIT	ADMISSION	LATENT PHASE (0-4 cm)
III 11	Elimination			Encourage voiding q̄ 2-3 hr In and out catheterization if unable to void & bladder is distended Bladder remains nondistended
II 7	Nutrition Hydration		Clear liquids/ice chips, hard candy if desired	Clear liquids/ice chips, hard candy if desired IV fluids prn and as ordered for T > 101 on 2 consecutive readings (notify attending MD) IV (18G) or heplock if VBAC Hydration status will be maintained
IV 11	Activity			Bag of waters intact or rupture of membranes with presenting part engaged: encourage up ad lib; chair prn Ambulates frequently

VI 2, 5, 6	PT/Family Education	At 1st OB appt, give info on:
		  – Labor warnings
		  – Kick counts
		  – Prepared childbirth classes
		  – Optional classes:
		    VBAC
		    Baby care
		    Breastfeeding
		Advise in selection of a pediatrician
		Goal: By 28 wks, pt identifies when to call the doctor & describes when & how to do kick counts
			Ambulation & position changes
			Electronic Fetal Monitor
			Breathing & Relaxation (B & R) techniques
			Analgesia & Anesthesia (A & A) options
			Labor progress & expectations
			
			Verbalizes understanding
			verified _____
				Appropriate B & R maintained
				verified _____

VIII 7, 8	Psycho Social Emotional		**Support person identified** verified _____	Support person identified
	Signatures	Initials for these signatures will be found throughout the care path.	____ / _____ ____ / _____	____ / _____ ____ / _____

MED REC NO. _____

PATIENT _____

PHYSICIAN _____

BAYLOR UNIVERSITY MEDICAL CENTER

DALLAS, TEXAS

CARE PATH FOR STAGES OF LABOR 1 & 2

PAGE 2 OF 4

Figure 13-1, cont'd ■ For legend see opposite page.

Continued

CARE PATH FOR STAGES OF LABOR 1 & 2

NANDA Problem Number	LOCATION	ACTIVE PHASE (4-10 cm)	SECOND STAGE (10 cm – Delivery)
IV 5, 8, 9, 16 I 5, 6 III I I	Assessments	T, q̄ 4° if bag of waters intact; q̄ 2° if rupture of membranes BP, P, R, q̄ 1 hr BP, P q̄ 15 min if epidural anesthetic Bladder status q̄ 2 hr Urine protein/ketones dipstick prn Deep tendon reflexes/clonus prn Fetal monitoring: electronic fetal monitoring while in bed, or intermittent auscultation Labor status: – frequency, duration, strength, resting tone of contraction q̄ 1 hr by toco/palpation or intrauterine pressure catheter – membrane status; color, amount and odor of fluid – sterile vaginal exam prn & prior to meds Fetus: – low risk: FHR q̄ 30 min – high risk: FHR q̄ 15 min In and out catheterization **If intrauterine pressure catheter, labor pattern shows > 250 Montevideo units** verified _____ **Cervix changes at a rate of > 1.2 cm/hr for nullips; > 1.5 cm/hr for multips** verified _____	T, q̄ 4° if bag of waters intact; q 2° if rupture of membranes BP, P, R, q̄ 1 hr BP, P q̄ 15 min if epidural anesthetic Bladder status q̄ 2 hr Urine protein/ketones dipstick prn Deep tendon reflexes/clonus prn Fetal monitoring: electronic fetal monitoring while in bed, or intermittent auscultation Labor status: – frequency, duration, strength, resting tone of contraction q̄ 1 hr by toco/palpation or intrauterine pressure catheter – membrane status; color, amount and odor of fluid – sterile vaginal exam prn & prior to meds Fetus: – low risk: FHR q̄ 15 min – high risk: FHR q̄ 5 min – VBAC continous electronic fetal monitor or electronic fetal monitoring Effectiveness of expulsive efforts – descent of presenting part – position; document if abnormal presentation – caput
IV 5, 6	Procedures / Tests		
	Treatments	Plot cervical dilation q̄ 2 hours or per exam Consider use of intrauterine pressure catheter if inadequate cervical change	
VI 3 XI 5	Medications	PAIN CONTROL: Parenteral analgesics as ordered. (Consider Stadol or Nubain). Anesthesia consult; epidural prn Oxytocin augmentation, if indicated per protocol If rupture of membranes > 24 hr antibiotics as ordered **Maintains control; utilizes B & R techniques prn** verified _____	**Maintains control; utilizes B & R techniques prn** verified _____
	Signatures	____/____ ____/____	____/____ ____/____ ____/____ ____/____

MED REC NO. _____

PATIENT _____

PHYSICIAN _____

BAYLOR UNIVERSITY MEDICAL CENTER
DALLAS, TEXAS

CARE PATH FOR STAGES OF LABOR 1 & 2
PAGE 3 OF 4

Figure 13-1, cont'd ■ Care paths for stages 1 and 2 of labor.

CARE PATH FOR STAGES OF LABOR 1 & 2

NANDA Problem Number	LOCATION	ACTIVE PHASE (4-10 cm)	SECOND STAGE
IIII I I	Elimination	Encourage voiding q̄ 2-3 hr In and out catheterization if unable to void & bladder is distended Bladder remains nondistended	Encourage voiding q̄ 2-3 hr In and out catheterization if unable to void & bladder is distended Bladder remains nondistended
II 7	Nutrition Hydration	Clear liquids/ice chips IV fluids prn and as ordered for T > 101 on 2 consecutive readings (notify attending MD) IV (18G) or heplock if VBAC Hydration status will be maintained	Clear liquids/ice chips IV fluids prn: and as ordered for T > 101 on 2 consecutive readings (notify attending MD) IV (18G) or heplock if VBAC Hydration status will be maintained
IV 11	Activity	Bag of waters intact or rupture of membranes with presenting part engaged: encourage up ad lib; chair prn Facilitate frequent position changes (q̄ 1-2 hr) while in bed	Facilitate frequent position changes (q̄ 1-2 hr) while in bed
VI 2, 5, 6	PT/Family Education		
		Appropriate B & R maintained verified _____	**Appropriate B & R maintained** verified _____
	Psycho Social Emotional	Support person identified	Support person identified
	Signatures	_____/_____ _____/_____	_____/_____ _____/_____ _____/_____ _____/_____

MED REC NO. _____

PATIENT _____

PHYSICIAN _____

BILLING NO. _____

BAYLOR UNIVERSITY MEDICAL CENTER

DALLAS, TEXAS

CARE PATH FOR STAGES OF LABOR 1 & 2

PAGE 4 OF 4

Figure 13-1, cont'd ■ For legend see opposite page.

13-1 Leopold's Maneuvers

PURPOSE: **To determine presentation and position of the fetus and aid in location of fetal heart sounds**

1. Explain the procedure to the woman and the rationale for each step as it is performed. Tell her what is found at each step. *Gives information, teaches the woman, and reassures her when the assessment findings are normal.*
2. Ask the woman to empty her bladder if she has not done so recently. Have her lie on her back with her knees flexed slightly. Place a small pillow or folded towel under one hip. *Decreases discomfort of a full bladder during palpation and improves ability to feel fetal parts in the suprapubic area. Knee flexion helps the woman relax her abdominal muscles to enhance palpation. Uterine displacement prevents aortocaval compression, which could reduce blood flow to the placenta.*
3. Wash your hands with warm water. Wear gloves if contact with secretions is likely. *Prevents transmission of microorganisms. Warm hands are more comfortable during palpation and prevent tensing of abdominal muscles.*
4. Stand beside the woman, facing her head, with your dominant hand nearest her. *The first three maneuvers are most easily performed in this position.*

FIRST MANEUVER

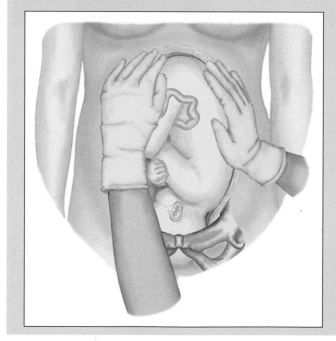

5. Palpate the uterine fundus. The breech (buttocks) is softer and more irregular in shape than the head. Moving the breech also moves the fetal trunk. The head is harder and has a round, uniform shape. The head can be moved without moving the entire fetal trunk. *Distinguishes between a cephalic and breech presentation. If the fetus is in a cephalic presentation, the breech is felt in the fundus. If the presentation is breech, the head is felt in the fundus.*

SECOND MANEUVER

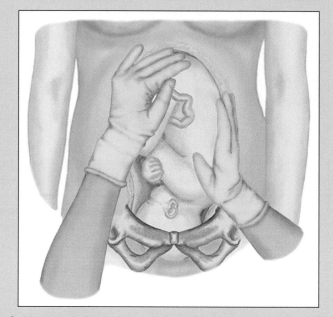

6. Hold the left hand steady on one side of the uterus while palpating the opposite side of the uterus with the right hand. Then hold the right hand steady while palpating the opposite side of the uterus with the left hand. The fetal back is a smooth, convex surface. The fetal arms and legs feel nodular, and the fetus often moves them during palpation. *Determines on which side of the uterus is the back and on which side are the fetal arms and legs ("small parts").*

LABORATORY TESTS. Women who had regular prenatal care need laboratory tests only for specific indications, whereas those who did not have prenatal care need more extensive laboratory tests. Simple tests that are often performed on the unit include the following:

■ Hematocrit obtained by finger stick
■ Midstream urine specimen to assess protein and glucose levels—usually obtained before notifying the birth attendant

INTRAVENOUS ACCESS. If used, intravenous (IV) access is started with at least an 18-gauge catheter. A saline lock may be used, or the woman may receive continuous infusion of fluids. The lock eases walking during early labor but provides quick access if fluids or drugs are needed. Continuous fluid infusion prevents and relieves dehydration and is necessary if epidural block analgesia is used. IV solutions containing electrolytes, such as lactated Ringer's solution, are most common.

13-1 Leopold's Maneuvers—cont'd

PURPOSE: To determine presentation and position of the fetus and aid in location of fetal heart sounds

THIRD MANEUVER

7. Palpate the suprapubic area. If a breech was palpated in the fundus, expect a hard, rounded head in this area. Attempt to grasp the presenting part gently between the thumb and fingers. If the presenting part is not engaged, the grasping movement of the fingers moves it upward in the uterus. *Confirms the presentation determined in the first maneuver. Determines whether the presenting part is engaged (widest diameter at or below a zero station) in the maternal pelvis.*

8. Omit the fourth maneuver if the fetus is in a breech presentation. *Is performed only in cephalic presentations to determine whether the fetal head is flexed.*

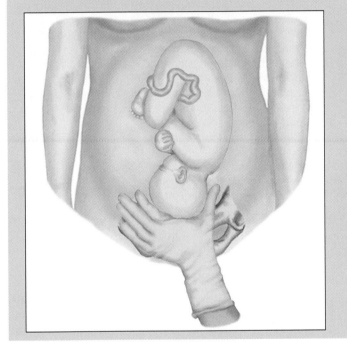

FOURTH MANEUVER

9. Turn so that you face the woman's feet. *Is most easily performed in this position.*

10. Place your hands on each side of the uterus with fingers pointed toward the pelvic inlet. Slide hands downward on each side of the uterus. On one side, your fingers easily slide to the upper edge of the symphysis. On the other side, your fingers meet an obstruction, the cephalic prominence. *Determines whether the head is flexed (vertex) or extended (face). The vertex presentation is normal. If the head is flexed, the cephalic prominence (the forehead in this case) is felt on the opposite side from the fetal back. If the head is extended, the cephalic prominence (the occiput in this case) is felt on the same side as the fetal back.*

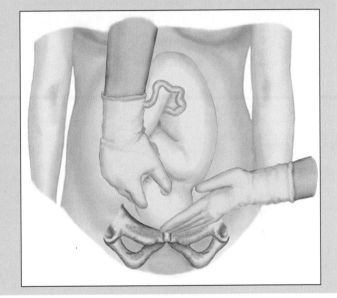

Other procedures are no longer common but are occasionally indicated:

- Perineal preparation—Hair in the immediate area of an episiotomy may be removed by shaving or clipping the hair near the skin with a shaver or disposable scissors. This judgment may not be made until near vaginal delivery.
- Enema—A small-volume enema (such as Fleet enema) may be given if stool in the rectum causes the woman discomfort or would interfere with fetal descent. Extra lubricant on the enema tip reduces discomfort from hemorrhoids.

MAKING ASSESSMENTS AFTER ADMISSION

The woman is usually observed if whether she is in true labor is unclear after the initial assessment. After 1 or 2 hours, progressive cervical change (effacement, dilation, or both) strongly suggests true labor. The woman and fetus are assessed during the observation period as if in early labor.

After the admission assessment the woman and fetus need regular assessments based on their risk status and whether they have interventions such as oxytocin stimulation or epidural analgesia. General guidelines for continuing assessments are listed here.

FETAL ASSESSMENTS. Fetal assessments are performed to identify signs of well-being and those that suggest compromise. The principal fetal assessments include the FHR and patterns and character of the amniotic fluid. Abnormalities revealed in these assessments may be associated with impaired fetal gas exchange and infection.

Fetal Heart Rate. The FHR is assessed using either intermittent auscultation or electronic fetal monitoring. Frequency of assessment and documentation depends on the risk status of the mother and fetus.

Amniotic Fluid. A spontaneous rupture of membranes (SROM) may occur, or the birth attendant may perform an amniotomy. The FHR is assessed for at least 1 minute when the membranes rupture. The umbilical cord could be dis-

13-2 Palpating Contractions

PURPOSE: **To determine whether a contraction pattern is typical of true labor; to identify abnormal contractions that may jeopardize the health of the mother or fetus**

1. Assess at least three contractions in a row at the time the fetal heart rate (FHR) is checked. Guidelines for minimal frequency of assessments are therefore:
   a. Hourly during latent phase
   b. Every 30 minutes during active phase and transition
   c. Every 15 minutes during second stage
   Assess more frequently if abnormalities are identified. Assessment of at least three sequential contractions permits better evaluation of the pattern. Palpate contractions periodically when an external fetal monitor is used because it is less accurate for intensity as a result of thickness of the abdominal fat pad, maternal position, and fetal position.
2. Place fingertips of one hand on the uterine fundus, using light pressure. Keep fingertips relatively still rather than moving them over the uterus. The fingertips are more sensitive to the first tightening of the uterus. Contractions usually begin in the fundus, although the mother usually feels them in her lower abdomen and back. Constant moving of the hand over the uterus may stimulate contractions and give an inaccurate assessment of their true pattern.
3. Note the time when each contraction begins and ends.
   a. Determine frequency by noting the average time that elapses from the beginning of one contraction to the beginning of the next one.
   b. Determine duration by noting the average time in seconds from the beginning to the end of each contraction.
   c. Determine interval by noting the average time between the end of one contraction and the beginning of

the next one. *Contractions are expected to increase in frequency, duration, and intensity as labor progresses. False labor is usually characterized by contractions that are irregular and do not increase in frequency, duration, and intensity.*

4. Estimate the average intensity of contractions by noting how easily the uterus can be indented during the peak of the contraction:
   a. With mild contractions the uterus can be easily indented with the fingertips. They feel similar to the tip of the nose.
   b. With moderate contractions the uterus can be indented with more difficulty. They feel similar to the chin.
   c. With firm contractions the uterus feels "woody" and cannot be readily indented. The contractions feel similar to the forehead. Contractions during labor are expected to intensify progressively. If they do not the woman may not be in true labor or she may be experiencing dysfunctional labor (see Chapter 27).
5. Report hypertonic contractions:
   a. Occurring less than 2 minutes apart and no more than 5 contractions in 10 minutes
   b. Durations longer than 90 to 120 seconds
   c. Intervals shorter than 30 seconds
   d. Incomplete relaxation of the uterus between contractions
   Hypertonic contractions reduce placental blood flow by prolonged compression of the vessels that supply the intervillous spaces.

---

placed in a large fluid gush, resulting in compression and interruption of blood flow through it (prolapsed cord; see p. 724). Charting related to membrane rupture includes the time, FHR, and character of the fluid.

Amniotic fluid should be clear and may include bits of vernix, the creamy white fetal skin lubricant. Cloudy, yellow, and foul-smelling amniotic fluid suggests infection. Green fluid indicates that the fetus passed meconium before birth. Meconium passage may have been in response to transient hypoxia, although the cause is often unknown. The newborn often will need extra respiratory suctioning at birth if the fluid is heavily stained with meconium.

CRITICAL THINKING ⌇ EXERCISE 13-2

Chloe Green is in labor with her second baby. The baby is in a left occiput anterior (LOA) position, and Chloe's cervix is 5 cm dilated and completely effaced. Her membranes rupture at the end of a strong contraction. You note that the fluid is green and watery.

Question
What nursing actions are most important at this time? Why?

Quantity should be described in approximate terms; for example, at term, a "large" amount is more than 1000 ml, a "moderate" amount is about 500 to 1000 ml, and "scant" amniotic fluid is a trickle, barely enough to detect. If the fetus is well down into the pelvis when the membranes rupture, a small amount of fluid in front of the fetal head may be discharged (forewaters), with the rest lost at birth.

MATERNAL ASSESSMENTS. Several maternal assessments also relate to the health of the fetus, such as vital signs and contractions.

Vital Signs. Abnormalities should be reported and the assessment frequency increased (see Table 13-1).

Contractions. Contractions can be assessed by palpation or with the electronic fetal monitor.

Progress of Labor. A vaginal examination is done periodically to determine cervical dilation and effacement and fetal descent (Figure 13-2). The frequency of vaginal examinations depends on the woman's parity, status of her membranes, and overall speed of her labor. Vaginal examinations are limited to avoid the introduction of microorganisms from the perineal area into the uterus.

PURPOSES

To determine whether membranes have ruptured.
To determine cervical effacement and dilation.
To determine fetal presentation, position, and station.

METHOD

Vaginal examination is not performed by the inexperienced nurse except when training for graduate nursing practice in the intrapartum area.

EQUIPMENT

Sterile gloves, sterile lubricant. If nitrazine paper is being used to test for ruptured membranes, lubricant is not used to avoid altering the test paper.

HAND POSITION

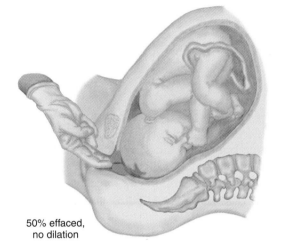

50% effaced,
no dilation

The nurse usually uses the index and middle fingers of the dominant hand for vaginal examination. The thumb and other fingers are kept out of the way to avoid carrying microorganisms into the vagina.

DETERMINING WHETHER MEMBRANES HAVE RUPTURED

Intact membranes feel like a slippery membrane over the fetal presenting part. No leakage of amniotic fluid can be detected.
Bulging membranes feel like a slippery, fluid-filled balloon over the presenting part. It may be difficult to feel the presenting part clearly if the membranes are bulging tensely.
Ruptured membranes show drainage of fluid from the vagina as the nurse manipulates the cervix and presenting part.

DETERMINING CERVICAL EFFACEMENT AND DILATION

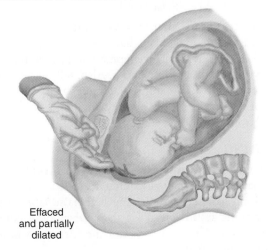

Effaced
and partially
dilated

The nurse determines *effacement* by estimating the thickness of the cervix. The uneffaced cervix is about 2 cm long. If it is 50% effaced, it is about 1 cm long. Effacement is expressed as a percentage (0% to 100%), or it may be described as the length in centimeters.
Dilation is determined by sweeping the fingertips across the cervical opening. The average woman's index finger is about 1.5 cm in diameter.

DETERMINING THE PRESENTING PART

The fetal skull feels smooth, hard, and rounded in a cephalic presentation. The fetal buttocks are softer and more irregular in a breech presentation. If the membranes are ruptured, the fetus in a breech presentation may expel thick, green-black meconium. (Presence of meconium in a breech presentation is *not* necessarily a sign of fetal compromise. The nurse must evaluate other signs of fetal condition.)

DETERMINING THE FETAL POSITION

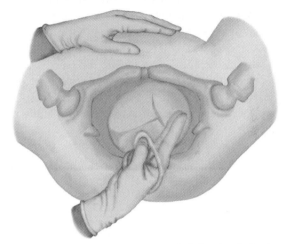

In a cephalic presentation, the nurse feels for the distinctive features of the fetal skull. The posterior fontanel is usually felt in a vertex presentation and is triangular with three suture lines (two lambdoid and one sagittal) leading into it. The anterior fontanel is not felt unless the head is poorly flexed or is in the mechanism of extension in late labor. It feels like a diamond-shaped depression with four suture lines (one frontal, two coronal, and one sagittal) leading into it.

DETERMINING THE STATION

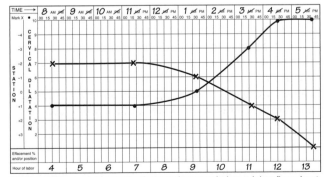

Findings of the vaginal examination may be recorded on a labor flow sheet, narrative, or a graph. The graph may be termed a *Friedman curve*, a *partogram*, or a *labor curve*.

Figure 13-2 ■ Vaginal examination during labor.

Intake and Output. Oral and IV intake and each voiding are recorded. Labor may reduce a woman's urge to void, so her suprapubic area should be checked every 2 hours or more frequently to identify bladder distention if she has received large quantities of IV fluids.

Pressure of the fetal head on the rectum in late labor makes many women feel the need to defecate. The nurse should look at the perineum for crowning of the fetal head if the woman suddenly expresses a strong need to defecate during a contraction.

Response to Labor. The woman's behavioral responses change as labor intensifies, especially if she has not had epidural analgesia. She withdraws from interactions but needs more nursing presence and reassurance. She may become more anxious because of pain and fear of bodily injury, unknown outcome, loss of control, unresolved psychological issues that influence her readiness to give birth (such as sexual abuse, previous birth experiences), and unexpected occurrences during labor.

Women vary in their ability to handle the pain of labor. The nurse constantly must assess whether additional pain control measures are needed. Behaviors that suggest the woman may want help with pain management include the following:

- Specific requests for medication and other pain control measures such as epidural analgesia (see Chapter 15)
- Statements that nonpharmacologic measures are ineffective
- Tension of her muscles and arching of her back during contractions
- Persistence of muscle tension between contractions
- A tense facial expression, rolling in the bed
- Expressions such as "I can't take it anymore"

THE SUPPORT PERSON'S RESPONSE. Labor is stressful for the woman's support person, who often is the baby's father. He may become anxious, fearful, or tired. He feels a responsibility to protect and support the woman but may have limited resources for doing so. Watching the woman he loves in pain is difficult, even if the pain is normal. He may respond to stress in many ways, including being quiet, suffering silently, or reacting with pacing and anger. Some fathers respond by leaving the room frequently or for long periods, whereas others resist even short breaks.

Nurses encourage and value the father's presence during labor and birth. However, this may conflict with a couple's cultural norms dictating that birth is a strictly female activity. The father may be pulled in two directions, wanting to be included but hesitating because men in his culture are not customarily involved with birth. The nurse should respect the values of each couple and their wishes about father involvement.

The support person also may be a parent or another relative, a friend of either gender, or a homosexual partner. The nurse must remember that anyone who assists the woman during labor may have feelings of anxiety and helplessness at times. Reassurance and care for the labor partner strengthen the person's ability to support the woman and enhance the likelihood that both will view the birth experience as positive.

✔ **CHECK YOUR READING**

8. What is the routine frequency for FHR assessment in uncomplicated labor? Why should the FHR be assessed after the membranes rupture?
9. What is the significance of greenish amniotic fluid? Of cloudy, yellowish, or foul-smelling amniotic fluid?
10. Why are frequent vaginal examinations undesirable during labor?
11. What observations suggest that the woman may need additional help with pain management during labor?

Application of the Nursing Process
False or Early Labor

Assessment

After observation, the nurse may realize that the woman is not in true labor. If findings are normal and the woman's membranes are intact, she is usually discharged. The woman who is in very early labor may be discharged to await active labor, especially if she is a nullipara and lives nearby.

Analysis

A woman may be frustrated because she cannot tell whether labor is real. She may resist returning to the birth center, possibly causing needless delay of care. She often is tired of being pregnant and just wants it to be over. A nursing diagnosis applicable to many women with false labor contractions is "Deficient Knowledge: Characteristics of True Labor."

Planning

An expected outcome for this nursing diagnosis is that before discharge, the woman and her support person will describe reasons for returning to the birth center for evaluation.

Interventions
PROVIDING REASSURANCE

A woman sent home after observation may feel foolish and frustrated. She may want to have labor induced to "get it over." Reassure her that even professionals cannot always identify true labor and false labor. Also, tell her that important preparation occurs during late pregnancy, such as softening of the cervix, even if obvious progress like cervical dilation has not yet occurred.

TEACHING

Review guidelines for returning to the birth center and explain that these are only guidelines and she should return if she has any concerns. Returning with false labor is better than entering in advanced labor or developing complications at home. The woman is not the first and will not be the last in this situation.

Evaluation

The woman and her support person should describe guidelines for returning to the birth center. These include regular contractions, leaking of amniotic fluid, bleeding other than bloody show, and decreased fetal movement.

Application of the Nursing Process
True Labor

The admission assessment may confirm that the woman is in true labor, or true labor may be evident after observation. Nursing diagnoses and collaborative problems change during labor because the intrapartum period is an active process. Problems covered in this chapter relate to fetal oxygenation, maternal discomfort, and maternal injury.

Nursing diagnoses often interact during labor. For example, high anxiety reduces effectiveness of pain-relief measures by interfering with relaxation. A maternal fluid volume deficit can alter fetal oxygenation because less blood is available to circulate to the placenta.

FETAL OXYGENATION

Assessment

The main assessments related to fetal well-being are the following (see Table 13-1 and Box 13-1):

- Fetal heart rate evaluation
- Amount and character of amniotic fluid and time of rupture
- Maternal vital signs
- Contractions: frequency, duration, intensity, and resting interval

Analysis

Several factors can reduce fetal oxygen, nutrient, and waste exchange, such as maternal hypotension and hypertension, maternal fever, excessively strong and long contractions (tetanic), and compression of the umbilical cord. The healthy fetus usually tolerates labor well, and the nurse simply needs to be alert for problems. Therefore a valid collaborative problem is "Potential Complication: Fetal Compromise" (see box). See Chapter 14 for other FHR characteristics associated with fetal compromise.

Planning

Client-centered goals are not made for collaborative problems as they are for nursing diagnoses. Planning includes nursing responsibilities to (1) promote normal placental function and (2) observe for and report problems to the physician or nurse-midwife.

Interventions

PROMOTING PLACENTAL FUNCTION

Maternal positioning is the primary measure to promote placental function during normal labor. The supine position should be avoided because it can cause the woman's

---

BOX 13-1 Assisting with an Emergency Birth

The inexperienced nurse rarely must deliver a baby in the hospital or birth center but occasionally helps the more experienced nurse do so. Unplanned out-of-hospital births are not common, but they do occasionally occur.

Nursing Priorities for an Emergency Birth in Any Setting
Prevent or reduce injury to the mother and infant.
Maintain the infant's airway and temperature after birth.

Preparing for an Emergency Birth
Study the delivery sequence in Figures 13-7 and 13-8.
Locate the emergency delivery tray ("precip" tray) on the unit.

During the Birth
Remain with the woman to assist her in giving birth. Use the call bell, or ask her partner to call for help. Stay calm to reduce the couple's anxiety.
Put on gloves, preferably sterile, to prevent contact with blood and other secretions. Sterile gloves reduce transmission of environmental organisms to the mother and infant. However, the nurse will be "catching" the infant in this situation. No invasive procedure is performed.

After the Birth
Observe the infant's color and respirations for distress. Suction excess secretions with a bulb syringe.
Dry the infant, and place skin-to-skin with the mother or cover with warmed blankets to maintain warmth.
Put the infant to the mother's breast, and encourage suckling to promote uterine contraction, facilitating expulsion of the placenta and controlling bleeding.

CRITICAL TO REMEMBER

Conditions Associated with Fetal Compromise

- Fetal heart rate outside the normal range for a term fetus: 110-160 bpm for a term fetus
- Meconium-stained (greenish) amniotic fluid
- Cloudy, yellowish, or foul-smelling amniotic fluid (suggests infection)
- Excessive frequency or duration of contractions (reduces placental blood flow)
- Incomplete uterine relaxation and intervals shorter than 30 seconds between contractions (reduces placental blood flow)
- Maternal hypotension (may divert blood flow away from the placenta to ensure adequate perfusion of the maternal brain and heart)
- Maternal hypertension (may be associated with vasospasm in spiral arteries, which supply the intervillous spaces of the placenta)
- Maternal fever (38° C [100.4° F] or higher)

---

uterus to compress her aorta and inferior vena cava (aortocaval compression), reducing blood flow to the placenta. If she must be in the supine position for a procedure such as catheterization, a small pillow or folded blanket under one hip shifts her uterus to maintain good placental blood flow.

OBSERVING FOR CONDITIONS ASSOCIATED WITH FETAL COMPROMISE

If conditions associated with fetal compromise are identified, assess the fetus more frequently and notify the birth attendant.

Evaluation

Evaluation of client goals and expected outcomes does not apply to a collaborative problem. Throughout labor, compare actual data with the norms for the mother and fetus.

DISCOMFORT

Assessment

See Table 13-1 for continuing assessments of the laboring woman.

Analysis

Women vary in their responses to labor's pain and the choices of pain management methods. The woman with choices for pain management and support for her choices has an increased sense of control over her birth experience. The woman who successfully masters the pain and other physical demands of labor is more likely to view her experience as positive. Her support person also is likely to feel more satisfaction with the experience.

Pain and anxiety are related nursing diagnoses. Excess anxiety reduces pain tolerance, and pain worsens anxiety. The nurse clusters assessment data to determine which is the primary problem. For example, several cues suggest that anxiety is primary, such as a previous poor experience during birth and expressions of worry and concern. However, if contractions are intense and labor is progressing quickly, the primary nursing diagnosis would be pain. Of these two options, the nursing diagnosis selected for this discussion is "Pain related to effects of uterine contractions."

Planning

The elimination of labor's pain is not realistic. Although highly effective pharmacologic methods exist, they cannot be implemented until the woman is in established labor. Therefore appropriate goals and expected outcomes related to pain include the following:
1. During labor the woman will state that her chosen method or methods of pain management are satisfactory and will tell the nurse if others are needed.
2. By discharge from the birth facility the woman's support person will express satisfaction with having provided labor support.
3. By discharge from the birth facility the woman will describe her birth experience as positive.

Interventions

Labor pain management includes measures to promote comfort and specific methods to relieve pain, such as breathing techniques and medication (see Chapters 11 and 15).

PROVIDING COMFORT MEASURES

Ordinary measures reduce irritating surroundings that impair a woman's ability to relax and use coping skills.

LIGHTING. Soft, indirect lighting is soothing, whereas a bright overhead light is irritating. Bright lights imply a hospital ("sick") atmosphere rather than a normal event like birth. A bright, overhead light should be used only when needed. A small flashlight is handy if the woman wants her room dark.

TEMPERATURE. Labor is work, and women in labor are often hot and perspiring. Cool, damp washcloths on the woman's face and neck promote comfort (Figure 13-3). Keep an ample supply of damp washcloths available and change them often to keep them cool. The woman should wear socks if her feet are cold. An electric fan circulates air in the labor room and directs a breeze on the woman. Be sure that the fan does not blow on the infant after birth, which might cause hypothermia.

CLEANLINESS. Bloody show and amniotic fluid leak from the woman's vagina during labor. The nurse should change the sheets and gown as needed to keep her dry and comfortable. Her preferences should be the guide because she may not want to be disturbed during late labor. Change the disposable underpad regularly to reduce microorganisms that may ascend into the vagina. A folded towel or bath blanket absorbs larger quantities of amniotic fluid than the pad alone.

MOUTH CARE. Ice chips (Figure 13-4), frozen juice bars, and hard candy on a stick reduce the discomfort of a dry mouth. If oral intake is contraindicated, brushing the teeth (without swallowing water) and simply rinsing the mouth is helpful to the woman. Many women appreciate a moist washcloth applied to their lips.

BLADDER. A full bladder intensifies pain during labor and can delay fetal descent. It may cause pain that remains

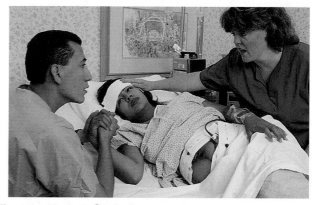

Figure 13-3 ■ Cool, damp washcloths placed where the woman finds them most comforting help her relax during each contraction. Several washcloths should be kept near the area to maintain their cool dampness.

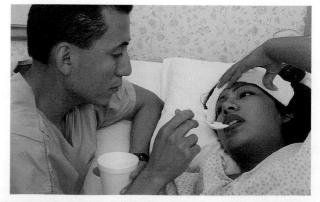

Figure 13-4 ■ Most laboring women welcome ice chips to ease their dry mouths.

after an epidural is instituted. Remind the woman to empty her bladder at least every 2 hours, and check her suprapubic area that often or more frequently if she has had large amounts of fluids.

POSITIONING. Occasionally, a specific maternal position is helpful to reduce discomfort and assist the labor process. Encourage the woman to assume any position she finds comfortable (other than the supine) and change positions frequently (Figure 13-5). Frequent changes reduce discomfort from constant pressure, help the fetus adapt to the pelvic contours, and promote fetal descent.

Upright positions benefit labor by adding the force of gravity to uterine contractions. Women who labor upright often need less analgesia and have more effective contractions. Studies also have shown improved blood gases and pH levels in the newborns of women who labored upright (Mayberry et al., 2000b).

POSITIONS FOR FIRST STAGE

Standing

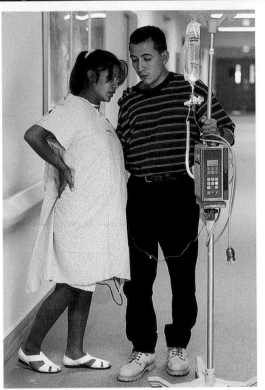

Sitting Upright

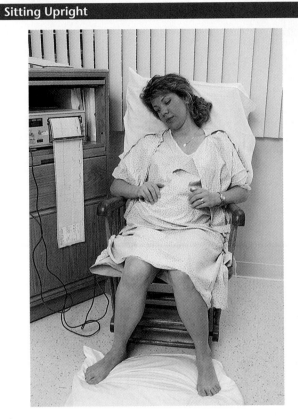

ADVANTAGES
Adds gravity to force of contractions to promote fetal descent.
Contractions are less uncomfortable and more efficient.
Variation: Standing, leaning forward with support reduces back pain because fetus falls forward, away from the sacral promontory.

DISADVANTAGES
Tiring over long periods.
Continuous electronic fetal monitoring is not possible without telemetry.

NURSING IMPLICATIONS
If the woman has intravenous fluid infusing, give her a rolling pole. Encourage her to alternate walking with other positions whenever she tires or desires to do so.
Remind the woman and her partner when she should return to the labor area for evaluation of the fetal heart rate and her labor status.

ADVANTAGES
Uses gravity to aid fetal descent.
Can be done when sitting on side of bed, in a chair, or on the toilet.
Can be used with continuous electronic fetal monitoring.
Avoids supine hypotension.

DISADVANTAGES
May increase suprapubic discomfort.
Contractions are the most efficient when the woman alternates sitting with other positions.

NURSING IMPLICATIONS
A rocking chair is soothing.
Place a pillow on a chair with a disposable underpad over the pillow to absorb secretions.
Use pillows or a footstool to keep the short woman's legs from dangling.
Encourage the woman to alternate positions periodically; for example, she can alternate walking with sitting or sitting with side lying.

Figure 13-5 ■ Common maternal positions for labor. Many maternal labor positions can be adapted for the first stage and second stage of labor. A. Positions for first stage. B. Positions for pushing in second stage.

Continued

Sitting, Leaning Forward with Support

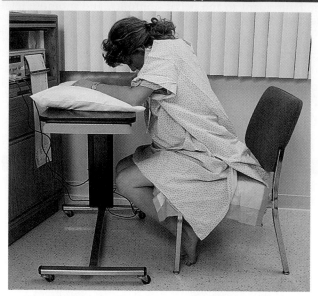

ADVANTAGES

Same as for sitting.
Reduces back pain because fetus falls forward, away from sacral promontory.
Partner or nurse can rub back or give sacral pressure to relieve back pain.

DISADVANTAGES

Same as for sitting.

NURSING IMPLICATIONS

Same as for sitting.

Semi-Sitting

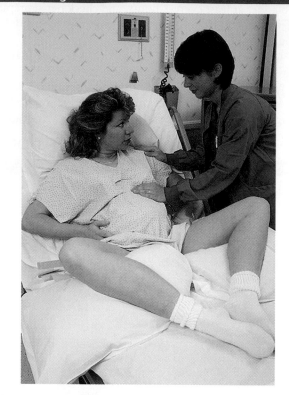

ADVANTAGES

Same as for sitting.
Aligns long axis of uterus with pelvic inlet, which applies contraction force in the most efficient direction through pelvis.

DISADVANTAGES

Same as for sitting.
Does not reduce pain as well as the forward-leaning positions.

NURSING IMPLICATIONS

Same as for sitting.
Raise bed to about a 30- to 45-degree angle.
Encourage the woman to use sitting (leaning forward) or side lying if she has back pain so that the caregiver can rub her back or apply sacral pressure.

Figure 13-5, cont'd ■ For legend see page 287.

Side-Lying

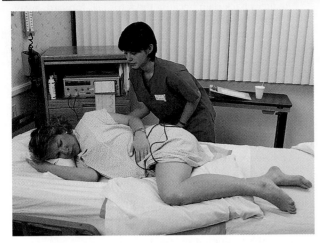

ADVANTAGES

Is a restful position.
Prevents supine hypotension and promotes placental blood
    flow.
Promotes efficient contractions, although they may be less
    frequent than with other positions.
Can be used with continuous fetal monitoring.

DISADVANTAGES

Does not use gravity to aid fetal descent.

NURSING IMPLICATIONS

Teach the woman and her partner that although the con-
    tractions are less frequent, they are more effective.
This position offers a break from more tiring positions.
Use pillows for support and to prevent pressure: at her back,
    under her superior arm, and between her knees.
Use disposable underpads to protect the pillow between the
    woman's knees from secretions.
Some women like to put their superior leg on the bed rail; if
    the woman wants this variation, pad the bed rail with a
    blanket to prevent pressure.
If she wants to remain recumbent, she should use this posi-
    tion to promote placental blood flow.

Kneeling, Leaning Forward with Support

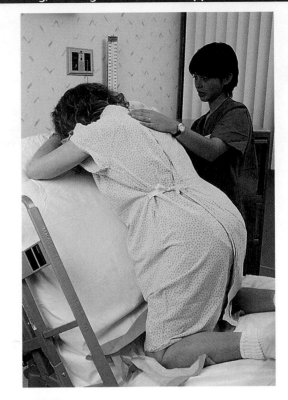

ADVANTAGES

Reduces back pain because fetus falls forward, away from
    sacral promontory.
Adds gravity to force of contractions to promote fetal de-
    scent.
Can be used with continuous fetal monitoring.
Caregivers can rub her back or apply sacral pressure.
Promotes normal mechanisms of birth.

DISADVANTAGES

Knees may become tired or uncomfortable.
Tiring if used for long periods.

NURSING IMPLICATIONS

Raise the head of the bed, and have the woman face the
    head of the bed while she is on her knees.
Another method is for the partner to sit in a chair, with the
    woman kneeling in front, facing her partner, and leaning
    forward on him or her for support.
Use pillow under the knees and in front of the woman's
    chest, as needed, for comfort.
Encourage her to change positions if she becomes tired.

Figure 13-5, cont'd ■ For legend see page 287.

Continued

Hands and Knees

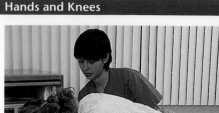
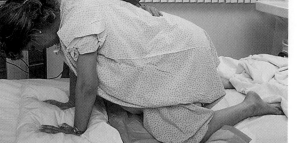

ADVANTAGES

Reduces back pain because the fetus falls forward, away from the sacral promontory.

Promotes normal mechanisms of birth.

The woman can use pelvic rocking to decrease back pain.

Caregivers can rub the woman's back or apply sacral pressure easily.

DISADVANTAGES

The woman's hands (especially wrists) and knees can become uncomfortable.

Tiring when used for a long time.

Some women are embarrassed to use this position.

NURSING IMPLICATIONS

Encourage the woman to change to less tiring positions occasionally.

Ensure privacy when encouraging the reluctant woman to try this position if she has back pain.

A second hospital gown with the opening in front covers her back and hips but may be too warm.

The birthing ball can provide support when in a kneeling position.

POSITIONS FOR PUSHING IN SECOND STAGE

Adaptations of First Stage Positions for Pushing

STANDING

This position may be tiring, and access to the woman's perineum is difficult. Because the infant could fall to the ground if birth occurs rapidly, provide padding under the mother's feet. Gravity aids fetal descent.

HANDS AND KNEES

Advantages and disadvantages are similar to those during first-stage labor. In addition, caregivers must reorient themselves because the landmarks are upside down from their usual perspective.

A variation is for the mother to kneel and lean forward against a beanbag or the side of the bed. This variation reduces some of the strain on her wrists and hands.

Semi-Sitting

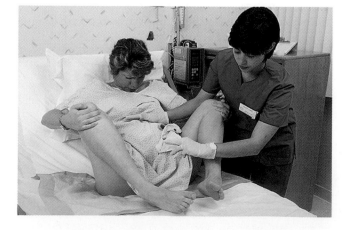

Side-Lying

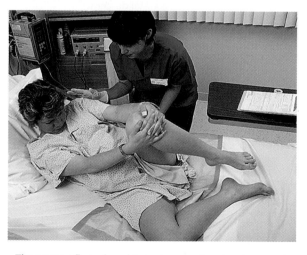

The woman flexes her chin on her chest and curls around her uterus as she pushes. She pulls on her flexed knees or the knee of the superior leg as she pushes.

Many women prefer this because they have the security of a back rest; it is also familiar to caregivers and allows easy observation of the perineum. Elevate the woman's back at least 30 to 45 degrees so that gravity aids fetal descent. The woman pulls on her flexed knees (behind or in front of them) as she pushes. She should keep her head flexed and her sacrum flat on the bed to straighten the pelvic curve.

Squatting

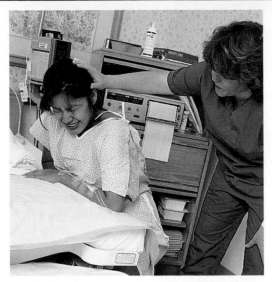

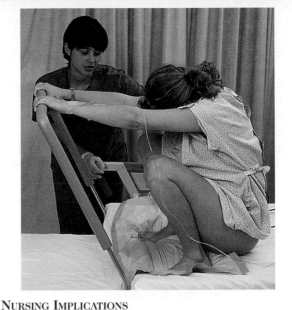

ADVANTAGES

Adds gravity to force of contractions to promote fetal descent.

Straightens the pelvic curve slightly for more direct fetal descent.

Increases dimensions of pelvis slightly.

Promotes effective pushing efforts in the second stage.

Caregivers can rub back or provide sacral pressure.

DISADVANTAGES

Knees and hips may become uncomfortable because of prolonged flexion.

Tiring over a long time.

NURSING IMPLICATIONS

Provide support with a squat bar attached to the bed or by two people standing on each side of the woman.

If she becomes tired, or between contractions, she can lean back into the sitting position.

Variation: Have the woman squat beside the bed as she pushes.

Figure 13-5, cont'd ■ For legend see page 287.

"Back labor" commonly occurs, in which the back of the fetal head puts pressure on the woman's sacral promontory (occiput posterior position). The discomfort of back labor is difficult to relieve with medication alone. Positions that encourage the fetus to move away from the sacral promontory, such as those in which the mother uses the hands-and-knees position or leans forward over a birthing ball (a sturdy ball similar to a beach ball), reduce back pain and enhance the internal rotation mechanism of labor. Smaller versions of the birthing ball are available for use when the mother is sitting and leaning forward.

WATER. Water in the form of a shower, tub, or whirlpool is relaxing for many women (see Chapter 15). However, a bath may slow labor if used in latent labor. It should be used in active labor or if persistent, nonproductive contractions during early labor have caused the woman to become very fatigued (Simkin, 2002).

TEACHING

Teaching the woman in labor is a continuously changing task.

FIRST STAGE. Many women become discouraged because several hours are needed to reach 4 or 5 cm of cervical dilation. They believe that the last 5 cm will take as long as the first 5 cm. From a time standpoint, 5 cm is more like two thirds of the way through first-stage labor rather than

half of the way because the rate of dilation increases during the active phase.

A woman's urge to push usually occurs when her cervix is fully dilated and effaced and the fetus descends to about a +1 station and internally rotates. However, as she nears the second stage, the fetus may descend enough to give her an urge to push before full cervical dilation. If her cervix, which is usually 8 or 9 cm dilated at this time, yields easily to downward pressure, pushing in response to her spontaneous urge rarely causes problems, especially if this is a second or later vaginal birth.

Either of two problems may occur if she pushes against a cervix that does not easily yield to pressure from the fetal presenting part:

■ The cervix may become edematous, which can block progress.

■ The cervix may be lacerated.

Teach the woman to exhale in short breaths if pushing is likely to injure her cervix or cause cervical edema.

SECOND STAGE. The woman may need help to trust the sensations from her body and push most effectively during second-stage labor. Nursing research is growing in labor nursing support and has resulted in inclusion of care based on more solid evidence. Examples of evidence-based practice for second stage labor include actions that do not try to arbitrarily shorten this stage and actions that consider each woman's sensations of actions she should take.

Two hours was once accepted as the upper limit for the duration of the second stage, with little evidence of the benefits of restricting the second stage or the accuracy of this time limit. A second stage longer than 2 hours is now recognized as safe as long as the mother and fetus show no signs of compromise.

Women push most effectively when they feel the reflexive urge to do so. Women having epidural analgesia with modern techniques usually detect an urge to push, although the urge may not be as strong as in women who did not have regional analgesia. Many women do not immediately feel the urge to push when the cervix is fully dilated, even if no regional analgesia such as an epidural is administered. A brief slowing of contractions often occurs at the beginning of the second stage. Pushing vigorously sooner than the onset of the reflexive urge may contribute to birth canal injury because her vaginal tissues are stretched more forcefully and rapidly than if she pushed spontaneously and in response to her body's signals. The mother may be frustrated and uncomfortable because she is asked to do something that does not feel right to her.

The technique of delaying pushing until the reflex urge to push occurs may be called any of several names, including *delayed pushing, laboring down, rest and descend,* and *passive pushing.* Delayed pushing has been shown to have a lower incidence of variable FHR decelerations, less maternal fatigue, and Apgar scores equal to those of women who pushed immediately on full cervical dilation (Mayberry et al., 2000a; Minato, 2000/2001; Roberts, 2003).

Positions. Squatting is an ideal position for pushing because it enlarges the pelvic outlet slightly and adds the force of gravity to the mother's efforts, which is an advantage if she has a small pelvis or the fetus is large. Some women push effectively while sitting on the toilet because that is where they are accustomed to giving in to the sensation of rectal pressure. Pushing while sitting on a birthing ball and pulling against a squatting bar on the bed or playing "tug of war" with another person provides a similar gravitational advantage. Women may find that pulling on something from above is efficient. Her upper torso should be in front of her pelvis to allow her coccyx to move backward as the fetus descends deeply into her pelvis (Simkin, 2003). Squatting is not possible for all women having epidurals because the block may cause leg weakness, although women can gain some of the position's advantages using sitting and semi-sitting positions.

If the mother pushes in a sitting or semi-sitting position, teach her to curve her body around her uterus in a C shape rather than arching her back. For greatest effectiveness the woman should pull on her knees, handholds, or a squatting bar while pushing. She should maintain a similar C shape to her upper body if she pushes on her side.

Method and Breathing Pattern. Support the woman's spontaneous pushing techniques if they are effective. The woman should push with her abdominal muscles while relaxing her perineum. If she needs coaching, teach her to begin by taking a breath and exhaling and then to take another breath and exhale while pushing for 4 to 6 seconds at a time. Sustained pushing while holding a breath (Valsalva maneuver or "purple pushing") or pushing more than four times per contraction reduces blood flow to the placenta and is fatiguing. Another deep breath that is more like a sigh helps her relax after the contraction.

■ A woman who is modest or fears losing control may inhibit her best pushing efforts if she is instructed to push as if she were having a bowel movement, particularly if she is in a bed or chair. An anatomically correct image is to teach the woman to push down and out under her symphysis (pubic bone), following the pelvic curve. Seeing a diagram of the pelvis helps her to visualize the curve.

PROVIDING ENCOURAGEMENT

Success breeds success. Tell the woman when her labor is progressing. If she can see that her efforts are effective, she has more courage to continue. Help her touch or see the baby's head with a mirror as crowning occurs.

Praise the woman and her support person when they use breathing and other coping techniques effectively. This reinforces their actions, gives them a sense of control, and conveys the respect and support of the nurse. If one technique is not helpful after a reasonable trial (three to five contractions), encourage them to try other techniques.

GIVING OF SELF

The importance of the nurse's caring presence cannot be overlooked as a component of labor support. Even independent women may become dependent during labor and need human contact. Many times the woman simply needs reassurance that all is going well and the nurse is there for her. The nurse's presence helps to allay her fears of abandonment and conveys safety, acceptance, support, and comfort.

Although the woman and her support person may have prepared for childbirth, they often welcome suggestions and affirmation from the nurse. They are more likely to use the techniques they learned if the nurse helps them use them. The nurse's presence, gentle coaching, and encouragement help the woman have confidence in her own body and fitness to give birth.

■ Labor nursing is a contact sport. Laboring women need the human support of a skilled, empathic, and intuitive nurse at the bedside—coaching them, reassuring them, and most of all, being there for them. This degree of support cannot be matched by the nurse who spends more time observing a fetal monitor at a central nurses' station than in the company of the laboring mother.

OFFERING PHARMACOLOGIC MEASURES

Birth is usually a normal process, and the prepared woman and labor partner can deliver their infant without medication if they choose to do so. However, many do choose pharmacologic pain management. The nurse must be informative but neutral when explaining about available pain medication.

Some women may have a firm goal of avoiding pain medication during labor. A woman who planned an unmedicated birth may interpret the nurse's information about available medication as pressure for her to take medication. If the woman takes the medication offered, she may later feel that she "gave in" at a "weak moment," thus reducing her sense of mastery over her birth. She may feel disappointed and guilty because she took medication despite her planned unmedicated birth.

Other women may plan to use a specific method such as epidural analgesia. If something prevents use of a chosen method, the woman may be upset about this unexpected development in her birth experience. Although the event may not be what she wanted, encouraging the woman to express her feelings helps her put it into perspective.

CARING FOR THE BIRTH PARTNER

The woman's support person is an integral part of her labor care. Her labor partner can provide care and comfort, which support the woman's ability to give birth. However, do not expect too much of the support person or make assumptions about the type and amount of involvement desired.

Some partners are coaches in the true sense of the word, actively assisting the woman through labor. Others want the woman and nurse to lead them and tell them how to help. They are eager to do what they can but expect instructions about methods and timing. Many couples see the partner's role as encouraging, offering moral support, and simply being there for the woman.

Imposing unrealistic expectations of leadership, care, and comfort on the partner makes the birth experience unnecessarily stressful. To ensure a positive experience for both, accept whatever pattern of support the partner is able and willing to provide and is comfortable to the couple. Without taking over or diminishing this role, provide any support that the partner cannot.

Encourage the partner to conserve physical strength, eat, and drink liquids. The partner may have missed sleep during the hours of early labor and may need a break. Encouraging the partner to eat a meal or snack may be necessary. Some partners think that they should not eat because the laboring woman is not doing so. However, hypoglycemia has caused more than one support person to faint at the time of birth and miss the main event.

Evaluation

Achievement of the three goals or expected outcomes occurs if the following conditions are met:

1. The woman indicates satisfaction with her method of pain management or requests nursing assistance to find other, more satisfactory methods.
2. The woman's support person expresses satisfaction with having provided labor support by the time of discharge.
3. The woman describes her birth experience as positive by the time of discharge.

The first nursing diagnosis regarding pain management is continually reevaluated throughout labor. The ability of the woman's support person is also continually evaluated. The last nursing diagnosis is evaluated after the woman and her significant other have had time to begin putting the birth experience into perspective.

PREVENTION OF INJURY

Assessment

Nursing assessments of the mother and fetus continue as the woman nears birth. During the second stage, observe the woman's perineum to determine when to make final birth preparations.

The exact time for final birth preparations varies according to the woman's parity, overall speed of labor, and fetal station. Preparations are usually completed when crowning in the nullipara reaches a diameter of about 3 to 4 cm. The multipara is prepared sooner, usually when her cervix is fully dilated and the fetal head is well down in the pelvis but before much crowning has occurred.

Analysis

The woman is vulnerable to injury immediately before and after birth for several reasons: (1) altered physical sensations such as intense pressure and effects of medication, (2) positional changes for birth, and (3) unexpectedly rapid progress. The nursing diagnosis selected for the laboring woman near the time of birth is "Risk for Injury (maternal) related to altered sensations and positional or physical changes."

Planning

The nurse's primary objective is to prevent and minimize injuries that can occur during final birth preparations and because of a sudden birth. The goal or expected outcome for this nursing diagnosis is that the woman does not have a preventable injury such as muscle strains, thrombosis, and lacerations during birth.

Interventions

Transferring the woman to the delivery site and positioning her in the birthing bed is the first step in the sequence of events that culminates in the birth of the baby (Figures 13-6 to 13-8). During the period around birth, the nurse reduces factors that contribute to maternal injuries.

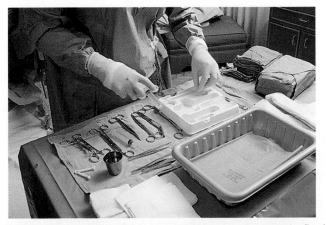

Figure 13-6 ■ The physician arranges instruments in final preparation for birth. Although the vagina is not sterile, a sterile table is prepared to limit introduction of outside organisms into the birth canal. Included on the sterile table are infant care materials (e.g., cord clamp, cord blood tube), instruments for repair of maternal injury or episiotomy, and anesthesia materials (if needed).

Transfer and Positioning for Birth

Action: When the woman is almost ready to give birth, transfer her to the delivery room or position the birthing bed. The exact time varies with several factors (such as overall speed of labor and rate of fetal descent). *Rationale:* Rushed, last-moment preparations are anxiety-producing for the woman, her partner, and the nurse. Remaining in the birth position for a long time can be tiring.

Action: Continue observing her perineum while making final preparations for birth. *Rationale:* Birth may occur unexpectedly, and the nurse should be prepared to "catch" the infant if the attendant (physician or nurse-midwife) is not in the room.

Action: Continue observing the fetal heart rate (FHR) with continuous monitoring or intermittent auscultation. *Rationale:* Detects changes in fetal condition that may require interventions by the attendant to speed birth.

Action: Elevate the woman's back, shoulders, and head with a wedge (on a delivery table) or by raising the head of the birthing bed. *Rationale:* Allows more effective maternal pushing and uses gravity to aid fetal descent.

Action: Stirrups or foot rests to support the woman's legs and feet may be used on a birthing bed. Pad the surface. *Rationale:* Padding reduces pressure, preventing venous stasis and possible thrombus formation.

Action: When placing the woman's legs in stirrups, elevate them and remove them simultaneously. Do not separate her legs widely. *Rationale:* Reduces strain on muscles and ligaments.

Prepping and Draping

Action: After the woman is in position, cleanse the perineal area with a sterile iodophor and water preparation unless she is allergic. Use warm water to dilute the iodophor scrub. *Rationale:* Removes secretions and feces from perineal area.

Action: After hand washing, apply sterile gloves for the prep procedure. Take a fresh sponge to begin each new area, and do not return to a clean area with a used sponge. Six sponges are needed. The proper order and motions are as follows:

1. Use a zig-zag motion from clitoris to lower abdomen just above the pubic hairline.

2, 3. Use a zig-zag motion on the inner thigh from the labia majora to about halfway between the hip and knee. Repeat for the other inner thigh.

4, 5. Apply a single stroke on one side from clitoris over labia, perineum, and anus. Repeat for the other side.

6. Use a single stroke in the middle from the clitoris over the vulva and perineum.

Rationale: Prevents cross-contamination or recontamination of an area that is already clean.

Action: The attendant may apply sterile drapes if desired. *Rationale:* A vaginal birth is a clean procedure rather than a sterile one because the vagina is not sterile. Sterile drapes are unnecessary, but some attendants may prefer to use them.

Birth of the Head

Action: If an episiotomy is needed, the attendant will perform it when the head is well crowned (see Chapter 20). *Rationale:* Minimizes blood loss from the episiotomy.

Action: As the vaginal orifice encircles the fetal head, the attendant applies gentle pressure to the woman's perineum with one hand while applying counterpressure to the fetal head with the other hand (Ritgen's maneuver). The attendant may ask the mother to blow so that she avoids pushing, or to push gently. *Rationale:* Controls the exit of the fetal head so that it is born gradually rather than popping out; this minimizes trauma to the maternal tissues.

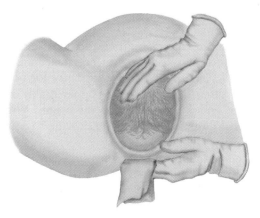

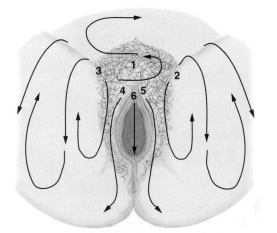

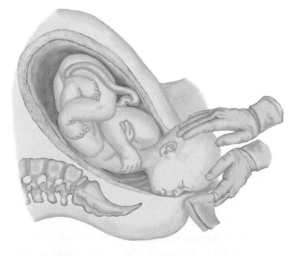

Figure 13-7 ■ Sequence for delivery.

Action: The attendant wipes secretions from the infant's face and suctions the nose and mouth with a bulb syringe. *Rationale:* Removes blood and secretions, preventing the infant from aspirating them with the first breaths.

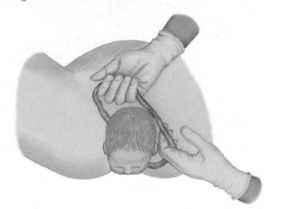

Action: The attendant feels for a cord around the fetal neck (nuchal cord). If it is loose, it is slipped over the head. If tight, it is clamped and cut between two clamps before the rest of the baby is born. *Rationale:* Allows the rest of the birth to occur and prevents stretching or tearing the cord.

Birth of the Shoulders

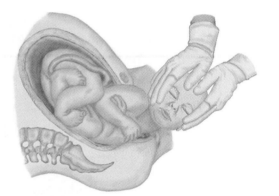

Action: After external rotation, the attendant applies gentle traction on the fetal head in the direction of the mother's perineum. *Rationale:* External rotation allows the shoulders to rotate internally and aligns their transverse diameter with the anteroposterior diameter of the mother's pelvic outlet. Traction on the head in the direction of her perineum allows the anterior fetal shoulder to slip under the symphysis pubis.

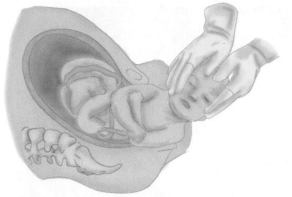

Action: The attendant then lifts the head toward the mother's symphysis pubis. *Rationale:* Permits the posterior fetal shoulder to be eased over the perineum, minimizing trauma to the maternal tissues.

Clearing the Infant's Airway and Cutting the Cord

Action: The rest of the infant's body is born quickly after the shoulders are born. The attendant maintains the infant in a slightly head-dependent position while suctioning excess secretions with a bulb syringe. The infant is often placed on the mother's abdomen. *Rationale:* Gravity aids spontaneous drainage of secretions and prevents aspiration of oral mucus and secretions.

Action: The attendant clamps the cord. Either the father or the attendant cuts the cord above the clamp. *Rationale:* Allows parents to interact more freely with their infant. Prevents flow of blood between placenta and infant, which might result in anemia (if infant is higher than placenta) or polycythemia (if infant is below the placenta).

Delivery of the Placenta

Action: After the placenta separates, it can usually be delivered if the mother bears down. The attendant may pull gently on the cord. *Rationale:* Excess traction on the cord may cause it to break, making the placenta harder to deliver.

Action: The attendant inspects both sides of the placenta. *Rationale:* Ensures that no fragments remain inside the uterus that might cause hemorrhage and infection.

After the infant and placenta are born, the attendant inspects the birth canal for injuries. If needed, any injuries and the episiotomy (if one was done) are repaired.

Figure 13-7, cont'd ■ For legend see opposite page.

TRANSFERRING TO A DELIVERY ROOM

Most births occur in a combination labor, delivery, and recovery room. Occasionally the woman must be transferred to a separate room for vaginal birth. If so, she should be transferred early to avoid rushed, last-minute preparations that cause anxiety for everyone.

POSITIONING FOR BIRTH

Upright positions promote effective pushing and take advantage of gravity. Squatting is a good position for uncomplicated birth but limits accessibility to the woman's perineum and may not be an option for women having epidural analgesia. Squatting, during which the upper body leans forward, promotes expulsive efforts, directs the fetus

efficiently toward the pelvic outlet, and increases the diameters of the pelvic outlet.

Other upright positions for the birth include standing and kneeling upright positions. The semirecumbent position limits movement of the coccyx as the fetus descends during birth but maintains some advantages of gravity. Sitting on a birthing bed with a cutout for the perineal area maintains many advantages of squatting and may be less tiring. The hands-and-knees position may be helpful if the fetus is in the occiput posterior position and to rotate wide fetal shoulders.

Many women and birth attendants are more comfortable using stirrups and foot rests to support the woman's legs and feet and make her perineum more accessible. If she cannot move her legs because of motor block from anesthesia,

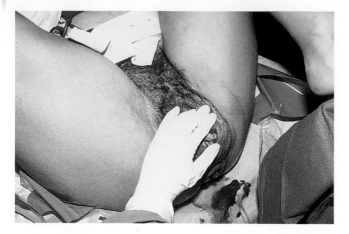

A. Crowning. The fetal head distends the labial and perineal tissues. The anus is stretched wide, and it is not unusual to see the woman's anterior rectal wall at this time. Any feces expelled are wiped posteriorly to avoid contaminating the vulva. The attendant (physician or nurse-midwife) is not holding the fetal head back but rather controlling its exit by using gentle pressure on the fetal occiput.

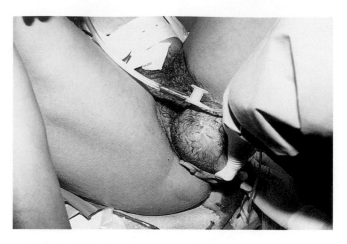

C. Birth of the head. As the head emerges, the attendant prepares to suction the nose and mouth to avoid aspiration of secretions when the infant takes the first breath.

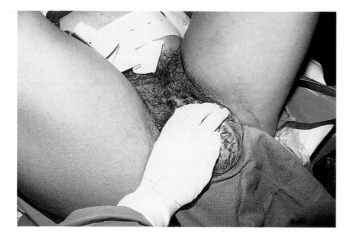

B. Ritgen maneuver. Pressure is applied to the fetal chin through the perineum at the same time pressure is applied to the occiput of the fetal head. This action aids the mechanism of extension as the fetal head comes under the symphysis.

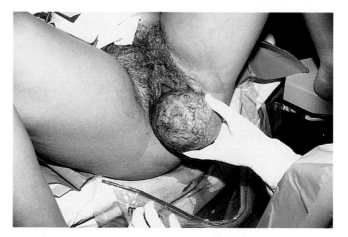

D. Restitution and external rotation. After the head emerges, it realigns with the shoulders (restitution). External rotation occurs as the fetal shoulders internally rotate, aligning their transverse diameter with the anteroposterior diameter of the pelvic outlet.

Figure 13-8 ■ Vaginal birth.

raise and lower her legs together and do not separate them too widely. Surfaces that contact the popliteal space behind the knee should be padded because of veins near the surface, on which pressure could lead to thrombus formation. The woman's upper body should be in a semi-reclining or sitting rather than a flat position.

OBSERVING THE PERINEUM

The exact time at which a woman is ready to give birth is an educated guess. A woman who has been having a slow labor may suddenly make rapid progress. Birth is near when the fetal head swings anteriorly in the mechanism of extension as the occiput slips under the symphysis pubis. Observe the woman's perineum, especially during late second-stage labor.

A classic sign of imminent birth is the mother's urgent cry, "The baby's coming!" Look at her perineum, and if the baby will be born before the physician or nurse-midwife arrives, remain calm and support the infant's head and body with gloved hands as it emerges (Table 13-2). The support person should push the call button to summon help.

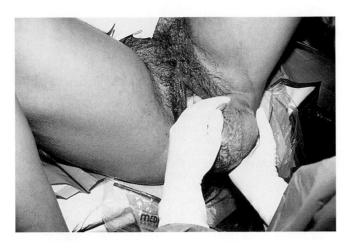

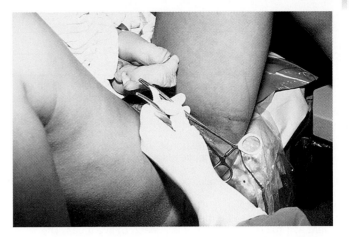

E. Birth of the anterior shoulder. The attendant gently pushes the fetal head toward the woman's perineum to allow the anterior shoulder to slip under her symphysis. The bluish skin color of the fetus is normal at this point; it becomes pink as the infant begins air breathing.

H. Cord clamping. While the infant is in skin-to-skin contact on the mother's abdomen, the attendant doubly clamps the umbilical cord. The cord is then cut between the two clamps. Samples of cord blood are collected after it is cut.

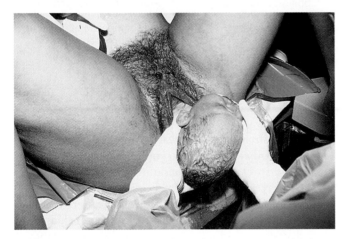

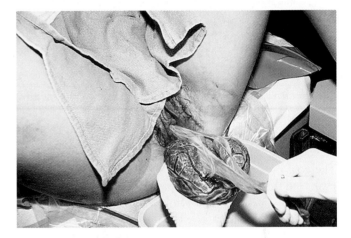

F. Birth of the posterior shoulder. The attendant now guides the fetal head upward toward the woman's symphysis to allow the posterior shoulder to slip over her perineum.

I. Birth of the placenta. The attendant applies gentle traction on the cord to aid expulsion of the placenta. This placenta is expelled in the more common Schultze mechanism, with the shiny fetal surface and membranes emerging. Note the fetal membranes that surrounded the fetus and amniotic fluid during pregnancy. The chorionic vessels that branch from the umbilical cord are readily visible on the fetal surface of the placenta.

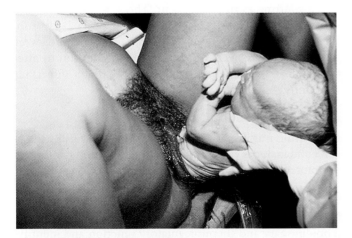

G. Completion of the birth. The attendant supports the fetus during expulsion. Note that the fetus has excellent muscle tone, as evidenced by facial grimacing and flexion of the arms and hands.

Figure 13-8 ■ Vaginal birth.

TABLE 13-2 Apgar Score*

Assessment	Points		
	0	1	2
Heart rate	Absent	Below 100/min	100/min or higher
Respiratory effort	No spontaneous respirations	Slow respirations or weak cry	Spontaneous respirations with a strong, lusty cry
Muscle tone	Limp	Minimal flexion of extremities; sluggish movement	Flexed body posture; spontaneous and vigorous movement
Reflex response	No response to suction or gentle slap on soles	Minimal response (grimace) to suction or gentle slap on soles	Responds promptly to suction or a gentle slap to the sole with cry or active movement
Color	Pallor or cyanosis	Bluish hands and feet only	Pink (light skinned) or absence of cyanosis (dark skinned); pink mucous membranes

*The Apgar score is a method for rapid evaluation of the infant's cardiorespiratory adaptation after birth. The nurse scores the infant at 1 minute and 5 minutes in each of five areas. The assessments are arranged from most important (heart rate) to least important (color). The infant is assigned a score of 0 to 2 in each of the five areas, and the scores are totaled. Resuscitation should not be delayed until the 1-minute score is obtained. However, general guidelines for the infant's care are based on three ranges of 1-minute scores:

0	1	2	3	4	5	6	7	8	9	10

Infant needs resuscitation.

Gently stimulate by rubbing the infant's back while administering oxygen. Determine whether mother received narcotics, which may have depressed infant's respirations. Have naloxone (Narcan) available for administration.

Provide no action other than support of the infant's spontaneous efforts and continued observation.

Note: Neonatal resuscitation measures, if needed, do not await 1-minute Apgar scoring but are instituted at once.

Evaluation

The goal or expected outcome for this nursing diagnosis is evaluated throughout the postpartum period because injuries such as muscle strains or thrombus formation are not evident until later (see Chapter 17). The birth attendant notes lacerations after the baby's birth and makes necessary repairs.

✔ CHECK YOUR READING

12. How might maternal hypotension or hypertension affect the fetus?
13. What position should the woman avoid during labor? Why? What if the woman must be in this position temporarily?
14. What general measures can make the woman more comfortable during labor? How can the nurse support the woman's labor partner?
15. Why is watching the perineum as a woman pushes important?

NURSING CARE DURING THE LATE INTRAPARTUM PERIOD

Responsibilities during Birth

The nurse's responsibilities during birth may include the following:

- Preparation of a delivery table with sterile gowns, gloves, drapes, solutions, and instruments (see Figure 13-6)
- Perineal cleansing preparation
- Initial care and assessment of the newborn

- Administration of medications (usually oxytocin) to contract the uterus and to control blood loss (see Drug Guide 16-1). The anesthesiologist or nurse-anesthetist also may give maternal medications.

A nurse or resuscitation team from the nursery is usually present if the newborn is at risk for problems such as respiratory depression and if problems occurred during labor. A person certified to provide neonatal resuscitation must be present at all births.

Personal protective equipment, including eye shields, should be worn as protection from fluid splashing and blood spurting as the cord is cut. The newborn is covered with blood, amniotic fluid, vernix, and other body substances. Persons involved in infant care should wear gloves and other needed protective equipment until after the first bath to avoid contact with potentially infectious secretions.

Responsibilities after Birth

Intrapartum nursing care extends through the fourth stage of labor and includes care of the infant, mother, and family unit (for more information, see also Chapters 17 through 23).

CARE OF THE INFANT

Nursing care of the newborn includes supporting cardiopulmonary and thermoregulatory function and identifying the infant. In addition, assess the infant for approximate gestational age (see p. 495) and examine for obvious anomalies and birth injuries. A full neonatal assessment may be delayed for about 1 hour to give the family a chance to meet their new member and initiate breastfeeding.

MAINTAINING CARDIOPULMONARY FUNCTION. Assess the infant's Apgar score (see Table 13-2) at 1 and 5 minutes (and at 10 minutes if response is poor) after birth for rapid evaluation of early cardiopulmonary adaptation. If the Apgar score is 8 or higher, no intervention is needed other than promoting normal respiratory efforts. If the infant is obviously in distress (no or low heart rate and respirations, limp muscle tone, lack of response to stimulation, blue or pale color), interventions to correct the problem are instituted immediately rather than waiting for the 1-minute Apgar score.

Place the infant on a prewarmed warmer, suctioning secretions from the mouth and nose with a bulb syringe as needed. Avoid keeping the infant in a head-dependent position without a specific indication; the position limits diaphragmatic movement because of upward pressure from the intestines. When a vigorous cry and minimal secretions are established, place the baby in a flat position or turned to one side with the head flat or slightly elevated. Suction secretions from the infant's mouth and nose with a bulb syringe as needed. Suction with a catheter may be necessary for more copious secretions.

SUPPORTING THERMOREGULATION. Hypothermia raises the infant's metabolic rate and oxygen consumption, worsening any respiratory problems. Place the infant on a prewarmed warmer and quickly dry with warm towels to reduce evaporative heat loss. The head should be dried well because substantial heat loss can occur from the head, which is about one fourth of the neonate's body surface area. The stimulus of drying the skin promotes vigorous crying and lung expansion in most healthy infants.

Skin-to-skin contact with a parent also maintains the infant's temperature and promotes bonding between the infant and parent. Avoid coming between the infant and the radiant heat source in the warmer. The infant should be wrapped in dry warm blankets when not in the warmer or making skin-to-skin contact. Remove wet linens, replacing them with warm and dry ones. A stockinette cap further reduces heat loss if it is placed on the baby's *dry* head. A cap is not worn while the infant is in the radiant warmer because the cap slows transfer of heat to the baby.

IDENTIFYING THE INFANT. Bands with matching imprinted numbers and identifying information are the primary means to ensure that the right baby goes to the right mother after any separation (Figure 13-9). Check that imprinted band number and mother's name are identical on each set of bands and have the parent(s) verify this information at the time of banding. Apply two bands on the infant, one on an arm and another on an ankle, or one on each ankle to prevent facial scratching. Infant bands are applied more snugly than those worn by an adult, with about one adult fingerwidth of slack in the bands. Trim the excess band ends and apply the longer band to the mother's wrist. The mother's primary support person usually wears a fourth band. The infant will not be released to any adult who is not wearing a band with a matching name and number. A set of bands is needed for each baby in a multiple birth. Some facilities take an early photo of the infant, when the infant is

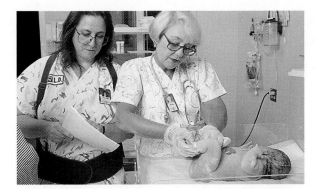

Figure 13-9 ■ When the birthing room nurse turns over care of the infant to the nurse who will provide ongoing newborn care, both nurses check the identification bands and record the same information.

often alert, which serves two purposes: as a keepsake for the parents and identification in the event of abduction.

CARE OF THE MOTHER

Nursing care of the mother during the fourth stage of labor focuses on observing for hemorrhage and relieving discomfort (Table 13-3).

OBSERVING FOR HEMORRHAGE. Important assessments related to hemorrhage are the woman's vital signs, uterine fundus, bladder, lochia, and perineal and labial areas (see Chapter 17).

Vital Signs. Assess the woman's temperature when fourth-stage care begins. Blood pressure, pulse, and respirations should be assessed every 15 minutes during the first hour. A rising pulse is an early sign of excessive blood loss because the heart pumps faster to compensate for reduced blood volume. The blood pressure falls as the blood volume diminishes, but this is a late sign of hypovolemia. A rising pulse may also reflect medications administered.

Fundus. The most common reason for excessive postpartum bleeding is that the uterus does not firmly contract and compress open vessels at the placental site. Assess the firmness, height, and positioning of the uterine fundus with each vital sign assessment. The fundus should be firm, in the midline, and below the umbilicus (about the size of a large grapefruit). If the fundus is firm, no massage is needed; if it is soft (boggy), it should be massaged until it is firm. Nipple stimulation from the infant's sucking releases oxytocin from the mother's posterior pituitary gland to maintain firm uterine contraction. Oxytocin in IV solution or administered intramuscularly has the same effect.

Bladder. A full bladder interferes with contraction of the uterus and may lead to hemorrhage. A full bladder is suspected if the fundus is above the umbilicus or displaced to one side, usually the right. The first two voidings are often measured until it is evident that she voids without difficulty and empties her bladder completely. Each voiding is usually at least 300 to 400 ml if she is emptying her bladder. If no contraindication such as altered sensation is present, the mother can walk to the bathroom (with assistance the first few times). She should sit on the side of the bed to make sure she is not lightheaded, move her legs back and

TABLE 13-3 Maternal Problems during the Fourth Stage of Labor

Sign	Potential Problem	Immediate Nursing Action
Rising maternal pulse rate and/or falling blood pressure; possibly accompanied by low or no urine output	An early sign of hypovolemia caused by excessive blood loss (visible or concealed)	Identify the probable cause of the blood loss, usually a poorly contracted uterus. Take steps to correct it (see below). Indwelling catheter may be inserted to observe urine output.
Soft (boggy) uterus	A poorly contracted uterus does not adequately compress large open vessels at the placental site, resulting in hemorrhage.	With one hand securing the uterus just above the symphysis and the other on the fundus, massage the uterus until firm. Push downward on the firm uterus to expel any clots. Empty the woman's bladder (by voiding or catheterization) if that is contributing to the uterine atony.
High uterine fundus, often displaced to one side	Suggests a full bladder, which can interfere with uterine contraction and result in hemorrhage.	Massage the uterus if it is not firm. Help the woman urinate in the bathroom or on the bedpan. If she cannot void, catheterize her (usually a routine postpartum order).
Lochia exceeding one saturated perineal pad per hour during the fourth stage	Suggests hemorrhage; however, perineal pads vary in their absorbency, and this must be considered.	Identify cause of hemorrhage, usually uterine atony, which is manifested by a soft uterus. Correct the cause. If lacerations are the suspected cause (excess bleeding with a firm fundus), notify the birth attendant. Keep the woman NPO until the birth attendant evaluates her.
Intense perineal or vaginal pain, poorly relieved with analgesics	Hematoma, usually of vaginal wall or perineum; signs of hypovolemia may occur with substantial blood loss into tissues.	If the hematoma is visible, apply cold packs to the area to slow bleeding into tissues. Notify the birth attendant, and anticipate possible surgical drainage. Keep the woman NPO.

NPO, Nothing by mouth.

forth, and raise her knees to be sure she has adequate strength and movement before ambulation.

Lochia. Assess for lochia with each vital sign and fundal assessment. The amount of lochia seems large to the inexperienced nurse and new mother. Perineal pads vary in their absorbency, but saturation of one standard pad (one that does not contain a cold pack) within the first hour is a guideline for the maximal normal lochia flow. Turn her to check for lochia pooling under the mother's buttocks and back. Small clots may be present, but the presence of large clots is not normal and the physician or nurse-midwife should be notified.

Perineal and Labial Areas. Observe these areas for hematoma formation. Small hematomas usually are easily limited by ice packs that are also applied for comfort. Large and rapidly expanding hematomas may cause significant enlargement of the tissues involved, a bluish color, and pain.

PROMOTING COMFORT

Uterine contractions (afterpains) and perineal trauma are common causes of pain after birth. A postpartum chill often adds to discomfort. Pain usually is mild and readily relieved by simple measures. Notify the birth attendant if pain is intense or does not respond to common relief measures.

ICE PACKS. Apply an ice pack to the perineum promptly after vaginal birth to reduce edema and limit hematoma formation. Some perineal pads include chemical cold packs. These pads absorb less lochia than ordinary pads, so this should be considered when estimating pad saturation. Ice packed into a glove is cheaper and colder than a chemical cold pack, although it melts quickly.

ANALGESICS. Afterpains and perineal pain respond well to mild oral analgesics. Regular urination reduces the

severity of afterpains because the uterus contracts most effectively. The nurse should encourage the woman to take analgesics on a regular schedule to stay ahead of both perineal and afterpain discomfort.

WARMTH. A warm blanket shortens the chill common after birth. A portable radiant warmer provides warmth to both the mother and infant. The mother may enjoy warm drinks initially.

PROMOTING EARLY FAMILY ATTACHMENT

The first hour after birth is ideal for parent-infant attachment because the healthy neonate is alert and responsive. Provide privacy while unobtrusively observing the parents and infant. The infant can remain in the parent's arms while the nurse takes vital signs and suctions small amounts of secretions. Many newborn admission assessments can be performed while the parent holds the baby. (See Box 13-2 for possible nursing diagnoses for the intrapartum family.)

BOX 13-2 Common Nursing Diagnoses for Intrapartum Families

Anxiety*
Fear
Deficient Fluid Volume
Impaired Verbal Communication
Coping (individual or family; ineffective, compromised, disabled, or readiness for enhanced)
Deficient knowledge*
Pain (acute or chronic)*
Risk for Injury*
Powerlessness (actual or risk)

*Nursing diagnoses explored in this chapter.

NURSING CARE PLAN 13-1 Normal Labor and Birth

ASSESSMENT: Cathy Taggart, 17 years old, is a gravida 1, para 0, who is admitted in early labor. Her cervix is 3 cm dilated and completely effaced, and the fetus is at a 0 station. Her membranes are intact. Cathy's husband, Tim, is with her. They did not attend childbirth classes. Cathy is holding Tim's hand tightly and breathing rapidly with each contraction. She says in a shaky voice, "I'm so scared. I've never been in a hospital before. I just don't know if I can do this."

NURSING DIAGNOSIS: Anxiety related to unfamiliar environment and lack of birth preparation

GOALS/EXPECTED OUTCOMES: Cathy will:
1. Express being less anxious after admission procedures are completed.
2. Have a relaxed facial expression and body posture between contractions.

INTERVENTION	RATIONALE
1. Maintain a calm and confident manner when caring for Cathy. Express confidence in her ability to give birth.	1. Calm provides reassurance that labor is normal and that she has the resources within her to manage it.
2. Use therapeutic communication when talking with Cathy. Adapt communication to the situation, simplifying explanations and directions as labor intensifies.	2. Clarity identifies dominant concerns so that they can be properly addressed. Intense physical sensations reduce the ability to comprehend complex information.
3. Determine the couple's plans for birth, and work within them as much as possible.	3. Determining their plan enhances their sense of control and helps them have a satisfying birth experience.
4. Stay with Cathy as much as possible during labor.	4. A nurse can provide reassurance through human contact and can reduce fears of abandonment.
5. Orient Cathy to the labor room, and explain procedures and equipment she will encounter.	5. Information reduces fear of the unknown.

EVALUATION: Cathy relaxes a bit after talking with the nurse and slows her breathing. Cathy says, "I feel a little better now. I hope I can have my baby before you go home."

ASSESSMENT: Cathy's admission vital signs are all normal: temperature, 37.1° C (98.8° F); pulse, 88; respirations, 20; and blood pressure, 112/70 mm Hg. The fetal heart rate averages 140 to 150 beats per minute (bpm). Her contractions occur every 4 minutes, last 50 seconds, and are of moderate intensity.

POTENTIAL COMPLICATION: Fetal compromise

GOALS/EXPECTED OUTCOMES: Goals are not formulated for a potential complication because the nurse cannot independently manage fetal compromise. The nurse will:
1. Take actions to promote normal placental function.
2. Observe for and report signs associated with fetal compromise.

INTERVENTION	RATIONALE
1. Encourage Cathy to use any position she desires except the supine. If she lies flat, a wedge should be placed under one hip to displace her uterus to one side.	1. The supine position can cause aortocaval compression, reducing blood flow to the placenta.
2. Assess and document the fetal heart rate using the guidelines in Table 13-1. Report rates or patterns that are not reassuring. Assess the fetal heart rate more frequently if deviations from normal are identified. (Refer to Chapter 14 for detailed information.)	2. Observation allows prompt identification of changes in the rate or of abnormal rates. Fetal heart rate assessments that are outside expected limits need corrective action and should be reported for possible medical intervention.
3. When the membranes rupture, observe the color, odor, and approximate amount of fluid, and note the time of rupture. Note the fetal heart rate after rupture.	3. Meconium-stained fluid may be associated with fetal compromise and should be reported. Cloudy, yellow, or foul-smelling fluid suggests infection. Prolonged rupture of membranes increases the risk of infection. A low fetal heart rate suggests significant cord compression.
4. Assess contractions when the fetal heart rate is assessed. Report incomplete uterine relaxation between contractions or excessively strong or long contractions (longer than 90-120 sec or having <30 sec of full relaxation). Keep in mind that the fetus with risk factors may not tolerate even less-than-normal labor contractions.	4. Most placental exchange occurs during the interval between contractions. Contractions that are too long or have an inadequate interval between them decrease the time available for the intervillous spaces of the placenta to eliminate wastes and refill with oxygenated blood and nutrients.

Continued

NURSING CARE PLAN 13-1 Normal Labor and Birth—cont'd

INTERVENTION	RATIONALE
5. Assess Cathy's blood pressure, pulse, and respirations every hour. Assess her temperature every 4 hr until her membranes rupture, then every 2 hr. If elevated, assess temperature every 2 hr or more frequently.	5. Maternal hypotension or hypertension can decrease blood flow to the placenta. Maternal fever increases the fetal temperature and metabolic rate, possibly raising fetal demand for oxygen beyond the mother's ability to supply it. A rising maternal pulse or fetal heart rate may precede the temperature elevation.
6. See the nursing care plan in Chapter 14, pp. 330–332, for additional interventions if signs of fetal compromise occur.	6. This nursing care plan addresses basic actions to promote fetal oxygenation and identify possible problems.

EVALUATION: Because no client goal is established for a potential complication, evaluation is not done as in the nursing diagnosis. The fetal heart rate remains approximately the same, and there are no signs of fetal compromise. Cathy finds that sitting in a rocking chair is most comfortable.

ASSESSMENT: In 1½ hours Cathy's cervical dilation progresses to 5 cm and the fetus descends to a +1 station. Her contractions occur every 3 minutes, last 60 seconds, and are of strong intensity. The fetal heart rate remains near its admission level. Cathy is having difficulty relaxing between contractions and is complaining of back pain. She is relieved that her labor is progressing normally.

NURSING DIAGNOSIS: Pain related to effects of uterine contractions

GOALS/EXPECTED OUTCOMES: Cathy will express assurance that she can manage labor pain satisfactorily.

INTERVENTION	RATIONALE
1. Encourage Cathy to try positions such as standing or sitting and leaning forward, side-lying, leaning over the back of the bed, or on her hands and knees. Remind her to change positions about every half hour or when she feels the need for a change.	1. These positions shift the weight of the fetus away from the sacral promontory, reducing back pain. Alternating positions relieves strain and constant pressure and also helps the fetus adapt to the pelvis.
2. Teach Tim to rub or apply firm pressure to Cathy's back. Ask her where the best place is and how hard to press. Apply powder to the area rubbed.	2. Back rubs or firm pressure counteract some of the back pain. Powder decreases friction and promotes skin comfort.
3. Offer thermal pain management options: a. A warm blanket or warm pack applied to her back. b. Cold packs applied to her back. c. Alternating warm and cold packs, or use of them for 20 minutes on and 20 minutes off. d. Warm water in a shower or whirlpool.	3. Thermal stimulation interferes with transmission of pain impulses. Changing the thermal stimulation prevents habituation. Nipple stimulation in a shower or whirlpool causes release of oxytocin from the posterior pituitary and enhances contractions.
4. Teach Cathy simple breathing and relaxation techniques (see Chapters 11 and 15).	4. Breathing techniques provide distraction from pain and give her a sense of control. Relaxation enhances a woman's ability to manage pain and enhances normal labor processes.
5. Observe Cathy's suprapubic area and palpate for a full bladder at least every 2 hours. Remind her to void if she has not done so recently.	5. A full bladder contributes to discomfort and can prolong labor by obstructing fetal descent.
6. Tell Cathy about her progress in labor. Explain that she will probably begin to dilate faster now that she has entered active labor.	6. Encouragement and the knowledge that her efforts are having the desired results increase a woman's willingness to continue.
7. Tell Cathy what pharmacologic pain relief measures are available to her.	7. Knowing available options gives the woman a sense of control because she can choose whether she wants these measures. (This action may be done during early labor to give a woman more time to consider her options.)

EVALUATION: Cathy continues to have back pain that is 6 on a 0-to-10 scale but says that she is more comfortable sitting on the side of the bed with her head on a pillow on the overbed table. Tim rubs her back during contractions. She says she is able to manage the pain because it is less between contractions and does not want medication yet.

NURSING CARE PLAN 13-1 Normal Labor and Birth—cont'd

ASSESSMENT: After another 2 hours Cathy is quite uncomfortable and requests pain medication. She is occasionally feeling an urge to push. Cathy cries and says she is "losing it" and "can't take it anymore." Tim asks anxiously, "What's wrong? Is Cathy OK? Why is she acting this way?" The fetal heart rate remains near the admission range and shows no signs suggesting fetal compromise. Contractions occur every 2 minutes, last 70 seconds, and are strong.

Cathy's cervix is now 8 cm dilated and the station is +1. She asks for pain relief but does not want an epidural. Butorphanol (Stadol), 1 mg slow IV push, helps her regain control and work with her contractions. She avoids pushing by blowing out at the peak of each contraction.

Cathy is fully dilated in 45 minutes, and the fetal station is +2. She pushes spontaneously several times with each contraction but tends to stiffen her back and push on the bed with her arms with each push. She pushes for about 10 to 15 seconds at a time, holding her breath each time. She prefers a semi-sitting position.

NURSING DIAGNOSIS: Deficient knowledge: Effective pushing techniques

GOALS/EXPECTED OUTCOMES: After instruction in more effective pushing techniques, Cathy will use the techniques until the birth occurs.

INTERVENTION	RATIONALE
1. Observe Cathy's perineum for fetal crowning with each push.	1. A woman having her first baby can still give birth rapidly. Observation permits the nurse to maintain her safety and that of the baby should rapid birth occur.
2. Encourage Cathy to exhale as she pushes strongly for about 4-6 sec at a time.	2. Prolonged pushing against a closed glottis reduces blood return to the heart and maternal oxygen saturation and decreases placental blood flow, especially if it is done with every contraction.
3. Teach Cathy techniques to make each push more effective: a. Instruct her to flex her head with each push.	a. Flexing her head directs each push downward into the pelvic cavity.
b. Instruct her to pull against her flexed knees (or handholds on the bed) as she pushes, curving her body around her uterus. Encourage upright positions, including squatting.	b. Pulling provides leverage to gain a more effective push from the abdominal muscles. Upright positions take advantage of gravity, and squatting enlarges the pelvic outlet slightly.
c. Have her push toward the vaginal outlet.	c. The vagina is the anatomically correct direction.
d. Help her relax her perineum as she pushes down.	d. Relaxation reduces soft-tissue resistance to fetal descent.
e. Keep her sacrum flattened against the bed when she pushes in a semi-sitting position.	e. A flat sacrum straightens the pelvic curve somewhat (and is similar to squatting).
4. Do not talk to Cathy unnecessarily between contractions.	4. Silence allows her to conserve her energy for pushing efforts.

EVALUATION: Cathy pushes more effectively with the nurse coaching her during each contraction. In another hour she gives birth to a 3346-g (7-lb, 6-oz) boy. The baby's Apgar scores are 9 at both 1 and 5 minutes. Cathy has a small first-degree laceration that is sutured with a local anesthetic. The new family gets acquainted during the recovery period.

Assist the mother to nurse during the recovery period if she plans to breastfeed. The infant is usually attentive and nurses briefly. Early nipple stimulation helps initiate milk production and contract the uterus.

When the parents are ready, siblings, other family members, and friends should be allowed to visit. Help siblings see and touch their new brother or sister by putting a stool at the bedside or letting them sit on the bed.

Toddlers are often upset by the separation from their mother and may not be interested in the new baby. With supervision, children of preschool age or older may sit in a chair and hold the baby. School-age children are often fascinated by the new baby and surroundings and ask many questions. Adolescents react in various ways. They may be excited and eager to be a substitute parent, or they may be embarrassed about their parents' obvious sexuality "at their age."

Observe for signs of early parent-infant attachment. Parent behaviors are tentative at first, progressing from fingertip touch to palm touch to enfolding of the infant. Parents usually make eye contact with the infant and talk to the baby in higher-pitched, affectionate tones.

Cultural variations should be considered when assessing early attachment (see Chapters 18 and 21). The nurse should be knowledgeable about the typical practices of the populations commonly served. In some cultures great attention to the newborn is considered unlucky ("evil eye"). (See p. 531.)

- Some women do not have symptoms typical of true labor. They should enter the birth center for evaluation if they are uncertain and have concerns other than those listed in the guidelines.
- The childbearing family's first impression on admission to the intrapartum unit is important to promote a therapeutic relationship with caregivers and a positive birth experience.
- Initial intrapartum assessments quickly evaluate maternal and fetal health and labor status.
- The fetus is the more vulnerable of the maternal-fetal pair because of complete dependence on the mother's physiologic systems.
- The normal fetal heart rate at term averages 110 beats per minute (bpm) at the lower limit and 160 bpm at the upper limit. Other reassuring signs include regular rhythm, presence of accelerations, and absence of decelerations.
- Persistent contraction frequencies closer than every 2 minutes or more than 5 contractions in 10 minutes, durations of longer than 90 to 120 seconds, and intervals shorter than 30 to 60 seconds may reduce placental blood flow and fetal oxygen, nutrient, and waste product exchange.
- A maternal supine position can reduce placental blood flow because the uterus compresses the aorta and inferior vena cava.
- General comfort measures promote the woman's ability to relax and cope with labor.
- Regular changes in position during labor promote maternal comfort and help the fetus adapt to the pelvis.
- The nurse must be alert for signs of impending birth: The woman may state, "The baby's coming," make grunting sounds, and bear down.
- The priority nursing care of the newborn immediately after birth is to promote normal respirations, maintain normal body temperature, and promote attachment.
- The priority nursing care of the mother after birth is to assess for hemorrhage and promote firm uterine contraction, promote comfort, and promote parent-infant attachment.

ANSWERS TO CRITICAL THINKING EXERCISE 13-1, p. 275

The woman's behavior may have changed for several reasons, so the nurse must not make assumptions. For example, she may have felt insulted that the nurse found it necessary to ask her questions about illicit drug use. Or she may use other drugs and herbal preparations (legal or illicit) but prefer not to admit it. However, she may simply have been surprised at the question about drug use. The nurse should delay asking any sensitive questions until alone with the woman. Women often want their family to remain with them during the admission assessment but may not admit substance use and physical abuse in their presence. Nonverbal cues, such as a quick denial, avoidance of eye contact, and vague responses, are clues that the woman may not be answering these questions truthfully. The nurse should follow up on maternal behaviors privately to clarify underlying facts. A nurse may also be surprised that a woman does not hesitate to answer questions about her illegal drug use, regardless of who is present.

ANSWERS TO CRITICAL THINKING EXERCISE 13-2, p. 282

Assess the fetal heart rate for at least 1 minute to identify any abnormal rate or pattern. Note the time of rupture and the appearance, odor, and approximate amount of amniotic fluid. Report the findings to the physician or nurse-midwife because green, meconium-stained amniotic fluid may be associated with fetal compromise. A foul or strong odor is associated with infection. The fetal heart rate should be assessed more often, and an electronic fetal monitor is usually applied if not already in place. Notify the resuscitation team for possible endotracheal suctioning immediately after birth.

REFERENCES & READINGS

American Academy of Pediatrics (AAP) & American College of Obstetricians and Gynecologists (ACOG). (2002). *Guidelines for perinatal care* (5th ed.). Elk Grove Village, IL, & Washington, DC: Author.

ACOG. (2001). *Chronic hypertension in pregnancy,* Practice Bulletin No. 29. Washington, DC: Author.

ACOG. (2002). *Diagnosis and management of preeclampsia and eclampsia,* Practice Bulletin No. 33. Washington, DC: Author.

Adachi, K., Mieko, S., & Usui, A. (2003). The relationship between the parturient's positions and perceptions of labor pain intensity. *Nursing Research, 52*(1), 47-51.

Arnold, E., & Boggs, K.U. (2003). *Interpersonal relationships: Professional communication skills for nurses.* Philadelphia: Saunders.

Association of Women's Health, Obstetric and Neonatal Nurses (AWHONN). (2003). *Fetal heart monitoring: Principles & practices* (3rd ed.). Dubuque, IA: Kendall/Hunt Publishing.

Bashore, R.A., & Hayashi, R.H. (2004). Uterine contractility and dystocia. In N.F. Hacker, J.G. Moore, & J.C. Gamboni (Eds.), *Essentials of obstetrics and gynecology* (4th ed., pp. 159-166). Philadelphia: Saunders.

Bernstein, D. (2004). The fetal to neonatal circulatory transition. In R.E. Behrman, R.M. Kliegman, & H.B. Jenson (Eds.), *Nelson textbook of pediatrics* (17th ed., pp. 1479-1481). Philadelphia: Saunders.

Blackburn, S.T. (2003). *Maternal, fetal, and neonatal physiology: A clinical perspective* (2nd ed.). Philadelphia: Saunders.

Bowes, W.A., & Thorp, J.M. (2004). Clinical aspects of normal and abnormal labor. In R.K. Creasy, R. Resnik, & J.D. Iams (Eds.), *Maternal-fetal medicine: Principles and practice* (5th ed., p. 671). Philadelphia: Saunders.

Challis, J.R.G., & Lye, S.J. (2004). Characteristics of parturition. In R.K. Creasy, R. Resnik, & J.D. Iams (Eds.), *Maternal-fetal medicine: Principles and practice* (5th ed., pp. 79-89). Philadelphia: Saunders.

Creehan, P.A. (2001). Pain relief and comfort measures during labor. In K.R. Simpson & P.A. Creehan (Eds.), *AWHONN perinatal nursing* (2nd ed., pp. 417-444). Philadelphia: Lippincott Williams & Wilkins.

Cude, G. (2004). Do men have a role in maternal-newborn nursing? The male student nurse experience. *AWHONN Lifelines, 8*(4), 342-347.

Cunningham, F.G., Gant, N.F., Leveno, K.J., Gilstrap, L.G., Hauth, J.C., & Wenstrom, K.D. (2001). *Williams obstetrics* (21st ed.). New York: McGraw-Hill.

D'Avanzo, C.E., & Geissler, E.M. (2003). *Mosby's pocket guide: Cultural assessment* (3rd ed.). St. Louis: Mosby.

Feinstein, N.F., Sprague, A., & Trépanier, M.J. (2000). *AWHONN Symposium: Fetal heart rate auscultation.* Washington, DC: Author.

Hobel, C.J., & Chang, A.B. (2004). Normal labor, delivery, and postpartum care. In N.F. Hacker, J.G. Moore, & J.C. Gambone (Eds.), *Essentials of obstetrics and gynecology* (4th ed., pp. 104-135). Philadelphia: Saunders.

Hunter, L.P. (2002). Being with woman: A guiding concept for the care of laboring women. *Journal of Obstetric, Gynecologic, and Neonatal Nursing, 31*(6), 650-657.

Kendrick, J.M., & Simpson, K.R. (2001). Labor and birth. In K.R. Simpson & P.A. Creehan (Eds.), *AWHONN perinatal nursing* (2nd ed., pp. 298-377). Philadelphia: Lippincott Williams & Wilkins.

King, T.L., & Simpson, K.R. (2001). Fetal assessment during labor. In K.R. Simpson & P.A. Creehan (Eds.), *AWHONN's perinatal nursing* (2nd ed., pp. 378-416). Philadelphia: Lippincott Williams & Wilkins.

Mattson, S. (2000). Striving for cultural competence. *AWHONN Lifelines, 4*(3), 48-52.

Mayberry, L.J., Wood, S.H., Strange, L.B., Lee, L., Heisler, D.R., & Nielsen-Smith, K. (2000a). *AWHONN Symposium: Second stage labor management: Promotion of evidence-based practice and a collaborative approach to patient care.* Washington, DC: AWHONN.

Mayberry, L.J., Wood, S.H., Strange, L.B., Lee, L., Heisler, D.R., & Nielsen-Smith, K. (2000b). Managing second stage labor: Exploring the variables during the second stage. *AWHONN Lifelines, 3*(6), 28-34.

Minato, J.F. (2000/2001). Is it time to push? Examining rest in second stage labor. *AWHONN Lifelines, 4*(6), 20-23.

Roberts, J.E. (2003). A new understanding of the second stage of labor: Implications for nursing care. *Journal of Obstetric, Gynecologic, and Neonatal Nursing, 31*(6), 721-732.

Simkin, P. (2002). Supportive care during labor: A guide for busy nurses. *Journal of Obstetric, Gynecologic, and Neonatal Nursing, 32*(6), 794-801.

Simkin, P. (2003). Maternal positions and pelves revisited. *Birth, 30*(2), 1063-1067.

Simpson, K.R. (2004). Monitoring the preterm fetus during labor. *MCN: Maternal-Child Nursing, 29*(6), 380-388.

Smith, K.V. (2004). Normal childbirth. In S. Mattson & J.E. Smith (Eds.), *Core curriculum for maternal-newborn nursing* (3rd ed., pp. 271-302). St. Louis: Elsevier.

Torgersen, K.L. (2004). Intrapartum fetal assessment. In S. Mattson & J.E. Smith (Eds.), *Core curriculum for maternal-newborn nursing* (3rd ed., pp. 303-368). St. Louis: Elsevier.

Woolley, D., & Nelsson-Ryan, S. (2000). Second stage labor. In F.H. Nichols & S.S. Humenick (Eds.), *Childbirth education: Practice, research, & theory* (pp. 342-375). Philadelphia: Saunders.

Intrapartum Fetal Surveillance

OBJECTIVES

After studying this chapter, you should be able to:

1. Identify the purposes of intrapartum fetal surveillance.
2. Explain the normal and pathologic mechanisms that influence fetal heart rate.
3. Identify the advantages and limitations of each method of intrapartum fetal surveillance: auscultation and electronic monitoring.
4. Explain the types of equipment used for auscultation and electronic fetal monitoring during labor and the advantages and limitations of each.
5. Describe the interpretation of intrapartum fetal assessment data.
6. Explain the methods that may be used in addition to electronic fetal monitoring to judge fetal well-being.
7. Describe appropriate responses to nonreassuring fetal heart rate patterns.
8. Use the nursing process to plan care for a woman undergoing intrapartum fetal assessment.

Go to your Student CD-ROM for Review Questions keyed to these Objectives.

DEFINITIONS

Acidosis Condition resulting from accumulation of acid (hydrogen ions) or depletion of base (bicarbonate); acid-base balance measured by pH.

Amnioinfusion Infusion of a sterile isotonic solution into the uterine cavity during labor to reduce umbilical cord compression; also done to dilute meconium in amniotic fluid, reducing the risk that the infant will aspirate thick meconium at birth.

Asphyxia Insufficient oxygen and excess carbon dioxide in the blood and tissues.

Baroreceptors Cells that are sensitive to blood pressure changes.

Chemoreceptors Cells that are sensitive to chemical changes in the blood, specifically changes in oxygen and carbon dioxide levels, and changes in acid-base balance.

Hypercapnia Excess carbon dioxide in the blood, evidenced by an elevated PCO_2.

Hypertonic Contractions Uterine contractions that are too long or too frequent, have too short a resting interval, or have an inadequate relaxation period to allow optimal uteroplacental exchange.

Hypoxemia Reduced oxygenation of the blood, evidenced by a low PO_2.

Hypoxia Reduced availability of oxygen to the body tissues.

Intermittent Monitoring Variation of electronic fetal monitoring in which an initial strip is obtained on admission. If patterns are reassuring the woman is remonitored for 15 minutes at regular intervals (such as every 30 to 60 minutes).

Montevideo Unit Method to quantify intensity of labor contractions with uterine activity monitoring. The baseline intrauterine pressure for each contraction in a 10-minute period is subtracted from the peak pressure. The resulting net pressures (peak minus baseline) are added to calculate Montevideo units, or MVUs.

Nadir Lowest point, such as the lowest pulse rate in a series.

Nuchal Cord Umbilical cord around the fetal neck.

Telemetry Wireless transmission of electronic fetal monitoring data to the bedside or central monitor unit.

Tocolytic Drug that inhibits uterine contractions.

Transducer Device that translates one physical quantity to another, such as fetal heart motion into an electrical signal for rate calculation, generation of sound, or a written record.

Uterine Resting Tone Degree of uterine muscle tension when the woman is not in labor or during the interval between labor contractions.

Intrapartum fetal assessment is the process of fetal surveillance to identify signs associated with well-being and with compromise. Accurate identification of these signs permits appropriate and timely care to reduce hazards to the fetus. At a minimum, intrapartum fetal assessment includes evaluation of the fetal heart rate (FHR) and the mother's uterine activity. More comprehensive monitoring includes assessment of fetal activity, fetal response to stimulation, and fetal pulse oximetry.

The purposes of intrapartum fetal assessment are to evaluate how the fetus tolerates labor and to identify hypoxic insult to the fetus during labor. However, no method of fetal assessment can identify every compromised fetus.

Fetal assessment data plays a major role in malpractice claims. These lawsuits may be brought many years, often decades, after the birth of a neurologically handicapped child. The nurse's documentation must prove that the standard of care was met at the time of birth. The nurse should detect signs associated with fetal hypoxia and inform the physician or nurse midwife in a timely manner. The nurse should contact administrators in the facility's chain of command if the birth attendant does not respond promptly to the nurse's report of fetal problems. The perinatal nurse must obtain initial competency in fetal assessment that meets standards of care and facility policy and must maintain currency in fetal assessment. Documentation of data must be complete and clear to provide proper communication among professionals and to facilitate the best defense in any future lawsuit.

Two basic approaches to intrapartum fetal monitoring are taken: low technology and high technology. Each has advantages and limitations. The nurse may use either or both of these approaches to assess a fetus during labor, depending on the woman's wishes, risk status, and facility policy.

The low-technology approach uses intermittent auscultation (IA) of the FHR and palpation of uterine activity. In the United States this type of fetal observation is more often used in home births and birth centers. It also may be used during hospital births.

Electronic fetal monitoring (EFM) is the high-technology approach to intrapartum fetal surveillance. In 2002 over 85% of live births in the United States were electronically monitored (Martin et al., 2003). Despite the almost routine use of electronic monitoring, its benefits to the fetus over IA have not been established.

FETAL OXYGENATION

Adequate fetal oxygenation needs five related factors:
- Normal maternal blood flow and volume to the placenta
- Normal oxygen saturation in maternal blood
- Adequate exchange of oxygen and carbon dioxide in the placenta
- An open circulatory path between the placenta and the fetus through vessels in the umbilical cord
- Normal fetal circulatory and oxygen-carrying functions

An understanding of the dynamics of uteroplacental exchange and fetal circulation is critical to the understanding of fetal responses to labor (see Chapter 6).

Uteroplacental Exchange

Oxygen-rich and nutrient-rich blood from the mother enters the intervillous spaces of the placenta via the spiral arteries (see Figure 6-7). Oxygen and nutrients in the maternal blood pass into the fetal blood that circulates within capillaries inside the chorionic villi in the intervillous spaces. Carbon dioxide and other waste products pass from the fetal blood into the maternal blood at the same time. Maternal blood carrying fetal waste products drains from the intervillous spaces through endometrial veins and returns to the mother's circulation for elimination by her body. Substances pass back and forth between mother and fetus without mixing of maternal and fetal blood.

During labor, contractions gradually compress the spiral arteries, temporarily stopping maternal blood flow into the intervillous spaces at the peak of strong contractions. The fetus depends on the oxygen supply already present in body cells, fetal erythrocytes, and the intervillous spaces during contractions. The oxygen supply in these areas is enough for about 1 to 2 minutes. As each contraction relaxes, fresh oxygenated maternal blood reenters the intervillous spaces and blood containing carbon dioxide and other fetal waste products drains out.

Fetal Circulation

The fetal heart circulates oxygenated blood from the placenta throughout the body and returns deoxygenated blood to the placenta. The umbilical vein carries oxygenated blood to the fetus, and the two umbilical arteries carry deoxygenated blood from the fetus to the placenta (see Figure 6-7).

Regulation of Fetal Heart Rate

Mechanisms that regulate the heart rate are balanced to maintain cardiac output at a level that keeps the fetal heart and brain oxygenated. Fetal cardiac output increase is primarily accomplished by an increase in the heart rate. Conversely, a marked decrease in FHR decreases fetal cardiac output.

Five fetal factors interact to regulate the FHR:
1. Autonomic nervous system
2. Baroreceptors
3. Chemoreceptors
4. Central nervous system
5. Adrenal glands

The balance among forces that increase and those that slow the heart rate result in the characteristic fluctuations in FHR during the last third of pregnancy.

AUTONOMIC NERVOUS SYSTEM

The sympathetic and parasympathetic branches of the autonomic nervous system are balanced forces that regulate the FHR. Sympathetic stimulation increases the heart rate and strengthens myocardial contractions through release of epinephrine and norepinephrine. The net result of sympathetic stimulation is an increase in cardiac output.

The parasympathetic nervous system, through stimulation of the vagus nerve, reduces the FHR and maintains variability (see p. 317). The parasympathetic branch gradually exerts greater influence as the fetus matures, beginning between 28 and 32 weeks of gestation. Therefore the average FHR in the term fetus is lower than in the preterm fetus.

BARORECEPTORS

Cells in the carotid arch and major arteries respond to stretching when the fetal blood pressure increases. The baroreceptors stimulate the vagus nerve to slow the FHR and decrease the blood pressure, thus lowering cardiac output.

CHEMORECEPTORS

Cells that respond to changes in oxygen, carbon dioxide, and acid-base levels, or pH, are found in the medulla oblongata and in the aortic and carotid bodies. Decreased oxygen, increased carbon dioxide content, or a lower pH in the blood or cerebrospinal fluid triggers an increase in the heart rate. However, prolonged hypoxia, hypercapnia, and acidosis depress the FHR.

ADRENAL GLANDS

The adrenal medulla secretes epinephrine and norepinephrine in response to stress, causing a sympathetic response that accelerates the FHR. The adrenal cortex responds to a fall in the fetal blood pressure with release of aldosterone and retention of sodium and water, resulting in an increase in the circulating fetal blood volume.

CENTRAL NERVOUS SYSTEM

The fetal cerebral cortex causes the heart rate to increase during fetal movement and decrease when the fetus is quiet. As the fetus becomes mature enough to have distinct wake and sleep states, the FHR responds with variations in rate. For example, the rate is slower, with little variability during deep fetal sleep, but faster and with greater variability and accelerations when the fetus is awake.

The hypothalamus coordinates the two branches of the autonomic nervous system, the sympathetic and parasympathetic. The medulla oblongata maintains the balance between stimuli that speed and slow the heart rate.

Pathologic Influences on Fetal Oxygenation

Compromise of fetal oxygenation may occur because of alterations in any of the placental or fetal factors or those of the pregnant woman.

MATERNAL CARDIOPULMONARY ALTERATIONS

Actual or relative reductions in the mother's circulating blood volume impair perfusion of the intervillous spaces with oxygenated maternal blood. Hemorrhage causes an actual decrease in her blood volume. Relative reductions in maternal circulating volume involve altered distribution of the blood volume without blood loss. For example, epidural

block analgesia may cause vasodilation, which increases the capacity of the maternal vascular bed. However, the amount of blood available to fill her vessels is unchanged. Hypotension results, with reduction of placental blood flow.

Aortocaval compression can occur when a pregnant woman lies in the supine position and the weight of the uterus compresses the aorta and inferior vena cava. Aortocaval compression reduces blood return to her heart, lowers her cardiac output (supine hypotension), and can reduce placental perfusion.

Maternal hypertension may reduce blood flow to the placenta because of vasospasm and narrowing of the spiral arteries. Hypertension may be pregnancy induced or chronic or may result from ingestion of drugs such as cocaine.

A lowered oxygen level in the mother's blood reduces the amount available to the fetus. Maternal acid-base alterations that accompany respiratory problems also can compromise exchange in the placenta. A lower maternal oxygen tension may result from respiratory disorders, such as asthma, or from smoking.

Uterine Activity

Hypertonic uterine activity reduces the time available for exchange of oxygen and waste products in the placenta. Contractions may be too long or too frequent or have too short an interval. The uterus may not fully relax between contractions, applying continuous compression to the spiral arteries and reducing maternal-fetal exchange in the intervillous spaces. Hypertonic uterine activity may occur spontaneously or with uterine stimulants such as oxytocin (Pitocin), prostaglandins, or misoprostol (Cytotec).

PLACENTAL DISRUPTIONS

Conditions such as abruptio placentae (partial separation before birth) and infarcts reduce the placental surface area available for exchange. The amount and location of placental disruption relate to the degree of impairment in uteroplacental exchange. Large infarcts or separations cause greater impairment than smaller ones. Central infarcts or separations usually cause greater impairment than those on edges of the placenta.

INTERRUPTIONS IN UMBILICAL FLOW

The usual cause of interrupted blood flow through the umbilical cord is compression. Blood flow through the umbilical cord may be reduced by compression between the fetal presenting part and the pelvis, a nuchal cord or one that is wrapped around the fetal body, or a knot in the cord. It may occur with oligohydramnios, because the amount of amniotic fluid is inadequate to cushion the cord. The umbilical cord also may become entangled between fetal body parts or it may have inadequate Wharton's jelly for cushioning.

The thin-walled umbilical vein is compressed initially, resulting in a reduced inflow of more highly oxygenated blood to the fetus. This results in initial hypoxia with hypotension. Baroreceptors and chemoreceptors respond by accelerating the FHR. Flow through the firmer-walled umbilical arteries that carry blood from the fetus to the placenta is reduced as cord compression continues, resulting in hypertension. Baroreceptors respond to hypertension by stimulating the vagus nerve, thus reducing blood pressure and slowing the fetal heart. The FHR again accelerates as pressure is relieved on the arteries and then on the vein.

FETAL ALTERATIONS

Fetal cells may be hypoxic despite adequate oxygen supply from the woman and adequate exchange within the placenta. A low circulating fetal blood volume, fetal hypotension, or fetal anemia may result in cellular hypoxia. Central nervous system or cardiac abnormalities may cause an abnormal rate or rhythm. For example, a fetus with complete heart block may not respond to stimuli that would normally cause a rate increase.

A prolonged rate lower than 50 beats per minute (bpm) may reduce fetal cardiac output enough to impair brain and heart perfusion. However, a persistent heart rate faster than 200 bpm also decreases cardiac output, because the ventricles do not have time to refill with oxygenated blood during diastole.

Risk Factors

When conditions associated with reduced fetal oxygenation exist (Box 14-1), assessments by either IA and palpation or EFM are done more often. No absolute indications, including the presence of risk factors, require the use of EFM during labor. Properly performed IA is equivalent to continuous electronic monitoring in assessing fetal condition (American Academy of Pediatrics [AAP] & American College of Obstetricians and Gynecologists [ACOG], 2002).

✔ CHECK YOUR READING

1. What five factors influence fetal oxygenation?
2. What changes in the FHR occur when the umbilical cord is compressed?
3. How is the FHR related to fetal cardiac output?
4. What risk factors indicate that fetal monitoring should be done more frequently? (See Box 14-1.)

AUSCULTATION AND PALPATION

IA of the FHR can be done using either the nonelectronic fetoscope or Doppler ultrasound fetoscope (Figure 14-1). The nurse's expert fingertips palpate uterine activity (see Procedure 13-2).

Advantages

Mobility is a major advantage of auscultation and palpation for intrapartum fetal assessment. The woman is free to change position and walk around. Nothing restricts her freedom to move and she is likely to change positions more often, which promotes normal labor. The nurse must have regular, close, and frequent personal contact with the woman when performing IA and palpation. Water-based methods

---

BOX 14-1 Potential Maternal, Fetal, or Neonatal Risk Factors

Antepartum Period
Maternal History
   Prior stillbirth (unexplained or potentially recurrent cause)
   Prior cesarean birth
   Poor nutrition, low prepregnancy weight, poor weight gain
   Chronic diseases, such as cardiac disease, anemia, hypertension, diabetes, asthma, and autoimmune diseases
   Acute infections, such as urinary tract, pneumonia, gastrointestinal
   Hematologic problems, such as anemia, deep vein thrombosis
   Drug use (includes prescription agents, over-the-counter drugs, herbal preparations, and illegal drugs)
   Psychosocial stress, domestic violence
Problems Identified during Pregnancy
   Intrauterine growth restriction
   Gestation >42 weeks
   Marked decrease in fetal movement
   Multifetal gestation
   Preeclampsia, eclampsia
   Gestational diabetes
   Placental abnormalities (placenta previa, abruptio placentae)
   Severe maternal anemia
   Maternal infection
   Maternal trauma

Intrapartum Period
Maternal Problems
   Hypotension or hypertension
   Hypertonic uterine contractions
   Abnormal labor: preterm or dysfunctional
   Prolonged rupture of membranes
   Chorioamnionitis
   Fever
Fetal or Placental Problems
   Fetal anemia
   Abnormal fetal heart rate or pattern
   Meconium-stained amniotic fluid
   Abnormal presentation or position
   Prolapsed cord
   Abruptio placentae

---

of pain management, such as whirlpool baths or showers, can be used more freely. The atmosphere is more natural than technologic and less invasive, which is important to some women during their birth experience. Some trials that compared auscultation and palpation with EFM noted a lower cesarean birth rate in the women having auscultation and palpation during labor (Feinstein, Sprague, & Trépanier, 2000b; Moffatt & Feinstein, 2003). The equipment is less costly than EFM equipment, but staffing to achieve the needed 1:1 nurse-client ratio may offset this cost advantage.

Limitations

A disadvantage of auscultation and palpation as the primary method of fetal assessment is that FHR and uterine activity are assessed for a small percentage of the total labor. The fetus is most stressed during contractions because of normal reduction of blood flow to the placenta at that time. The FHR is assessed during some contractions but is not recorded during every contraction. No continuous printed or computer-archived record exists to show the fetal response throughout labor or to identify subtle trends in the response.

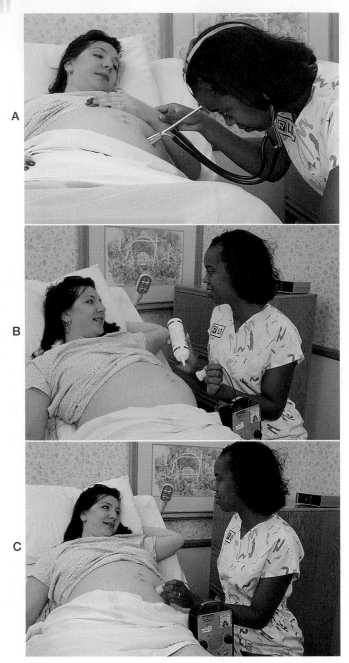

Figure 14-1 ▪ Low-intervention methods for evaluating the fetal heart rate during labor. **A,** Fetoscope, showing the head attachment to enhance conduction of faint fetal heart sounds. **B,** Transmission gel improves the clarity of the fetal heart movement sensed by the Doppler ultrasound transducer. **C,** The nurse moves the transducer until the sounds representing fetal heart motion are heard clearly. This location is usually over the fetal back, which is most likely to be located in the woman's right or left lower abdomen.

Some women find that interruptions for auscultation are distracting. The pressure of the instrument on the abdomen is uncomfortable for some, and it may require several moves to locate the best place for auscultation. Maternal obesity or large amniotic fluid volume may make it difficult to hear the fetal heart sounds.

IA is more staff-intensive than electronic monitoring, with a 1:1 nurse-client ratio recommended in clinical trials. When this nurse-client ratio cannot be achieved, auscultation may not be a realistic option as the primary method of intrapartum fetal surveillance.

Auscultation Equipment

Two basic types of auscultation equipment are used: a fetoscope and a Doppler ultrasound transducer. When listening with a fetoscope, the listener hears actual fetal heart sounds. The Doppler device senses motion and translates that motion into a sound that represents the cardiac events. An external fetal monitor, which is the same technology as the Doppler transducer, can be used, but the recording must be turned off, including computer archiving, for this to be valid as IA. If the FHR is recorded on a paper or computer monitor strip, the nurse must interpret that added data (Feinstein, Sprague, & Trépanier, 2000b).

Evaluation of Auscultated Fetal Heart Rate Data

Both the fetoscope and Doppler transducer can be used to identify the FHR baseline, rhythm, and changes from the baseline. Because the fetoscope is detecting actual fetal heart sounds, it can also detect dysrhythmias. The Doppler transducer (and external fetal monitor if it is being used for IA) also can be used to detect baseline, rhythm, and changes in the baseline. However, the Doppler transducer or external fetal monitor cannot be used to reliably detect dysrhythmias. (Procedure 14-1 explains auscultation of the FHR with the fetoscope and the Doppler transducer.)

ELECTRONIC FETAL MONITORING

EFM may be continuous, starting shortly after the woman is admitted; intermittent, with a short strip taken at regular intervals during labor; or intermittent during early labor and continuous during late labor.

Advantages

The electronic monitor supplies more data about the fetus than auscultation and archives a permanent record on paper, computer media, or both (Figure 14-2). Continuous EFM shows how the fetus responds before, during, and after each contraction rather than occasional contractions.

Many women in the United States expect electronic monitoring and find the constant sound of the fetal heartbeat comforting. Their support person can use the tracing of contractions on the monitor strip to help the woman anticipate the beginning and end of each contraction.

Electronic monitoring allows one nurse to observe two laboring women, primarily during uncomplicated early labor, while maintaining patient privacy. A 1:1 nurse-client ratio is needed during the second stage, regardless of the monitoring method used. Pregnancy complications may require a 1:1 nurse-client ratio even if the woman is not in labor. Electronic monitoring can give the nurse more time for teaching and supporting the laboring woman with breathing

PROCEDURE

14-1 Auscultating the Fetal Heart Rate

PURPOSE: **To evaluate the fetal condition and tolerance of labor**

1. Explain the procedure to give information to the woman and her partner. Wash your hands with warm water to reduce the transmission of microorganisms and to make your hands more comfortable when touching the woman's abdomen.
2. Use Leopold's maneuvers to identify the fetal back (Procedure 13-1) because it usually is closest to the surface of the maternal abdomen, where fetal heart sounds are clearest. Illustrations show approximate locations of the fetal heart rate in different presentations and positions.
3. Assess the fetal heart rate with a fetoscope or Doppler transducer. The external fetal monitor may be used but is more often used for intermittent electronic fetal monitoring (short periods of electronic monitoring interspersed with periods with no fetal surveillance, such as maternal ambulation).
4. Fetoscope (see Figure 14-1, *A*): Place the bell of the fetoscope over the fetal back with the head plate pressed against your forehead to add bone conduction to the sound coming through the earpieces. Move the fetoscope until you locate where the sound is loudest. Use your forehead to maintain pressure during auscultation to enhance the faint fetal heart sounds.
5. Doppler transducer (see Figure 14-1, *B*): Review the manufacturer's instructions for operating the Doppler device. Place water-soluble conducting gel over the transducer to make an interface for clear signal transmission, and turn it on. Place the transducer over the fetal back and move it until you hear clear sounds that represent the fetal heart motion.
6. With one hand, palpate the mother's radial pulse to verify that the fetal heart rate is what is actually heard. If her pulse is synchronized with the sounds from the fetoscope or Doppler transducer, try another location for the fetal heart. Other sounds that may be represented by the Doppler are the funic souffle (blood flowing through the umbilical cord) or uterine souffle (blood flowing through the uterine vessels). The funic souffle is synchronized with the fetal heart and has the same rate; the uterine souffle is synchronized with the mother's pulse.

AUSCULTATING THE FETAL HEART RATE

7. Count the baseline fetal heart rate for 30 to 60 seconds between contractions. Assessment during a contraction may clarify findings, but auscultation is difficult during contractions. Note accelerations or slowing of the rate.
8. Note reassuring signs that suggest the fetus is tolerating labor well:
   a. An average rate of 110 to 160 beats per minute
   b. Regular rhythm
   c. Accelerations from the baseline rate
   d. No decrease in rate from the baseline rate

9. Note nonreassuring signs, and make more frequent assessments. Notify the physician or nurse-midwife for further evaluation.
   a. Heart rate outside normal limits; unexplained tachycardia or bradycardia for 10 minutes or longer
   b. Irregular rhythm
   c. Gradual or abrupt decrease in rate

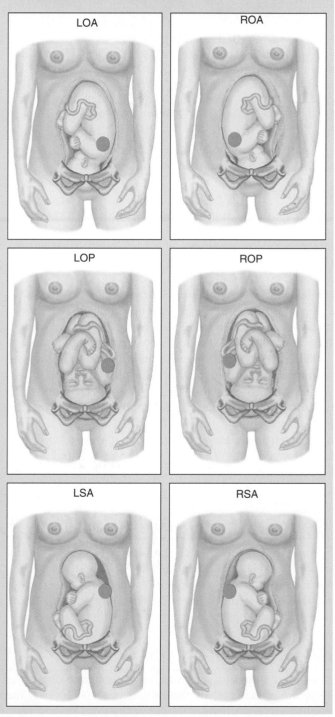

LOA ROA

LOP ROP

LSA RSA

Modified from Feinstein, N.F., Torgersen, K.L., & Atterbury, J. (Eds.). (2003). *AWHONN's fetal heart monitoring: Principles and practices* (3rd ed.). Dubuque, IA: Kendall/Hunt.

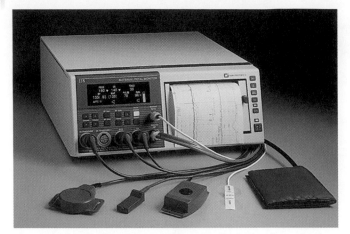

Figure 14-2 ■ Bedside unit for electronic fetal monitoring. In addition to fetal heart rate and uterine activity, the unit can help the nurse evaluate the woman's pulse, blood pressure, and saturation of oxygen in her blood. Both fetuses in a twin gestation can be assessed. (Courtesy Corometrics Medical Systems, Inc., Wallingford, Connecticut.)

and relaxation techniques if the nurse maintains the primary focus on the woman and not on the machine.

Limitations

Reduced mobility is a limitation of EFM. Telemetry or intermittent monitoring gives the woman more freedom of movement than continuous electronic monitoring without telemetry. Otherwise the woman is limited to her bed or a nearby chair if EFM is continuous.

Frequent maternal position changes or an active fetus often requires constant adjustment of equipment. The belts or stockinette band, used to keep sensors positioned properly for external monitoring, are uncomfortable for some women.

The high-tech atmosphere created by the electronic fetal monitor may be objectionable to a woman and her partner.

EFM, though used in more than 80% of U.S. births, has not proved to be consistently reliable at identifying the fetus who is truly in trouble. EFM best identifies the well-oxygenated fetus, but it does not as reliably identify the compromised fetus. Therefore EFM must be considered to be a screening rather than a diagnostic tool.

ELECTRONIC FETAL MONITORING EQUIPMENT

EFM equipment consists of the bedside monitor unit and sensors for FHR and uterine activity (see Figure 14-2). Sensors for each function may be either internal or external. Additional equipment may include data entry devices, remote screens, and computer interfaces to store information confidentially.

Bedside Monitor Unit

The bedside monitor unit receives information about the FHR and uterine activity from the sensors. It processes the information and provides output in the form of a numeric display and a printed strip (Figure 14-3). Current units can

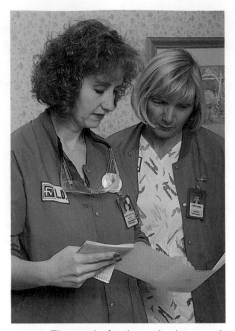

Figure 14-3 ■ Electronic fetal monitoring can be continuous and provides nurses with monitor strips, either paper or computer based, on which uterine activity and fetal heart rate are permanently recorded.

record rates for both fetuses in a twin pregnancy and have inputs for maternal blood pressure, pulse, and blood oxygen saturation. (The maternal blood pressure may be signified on the strip by the acronym NIBP, which means noninvasive blood pressure.)

Paper Strip

Data about the FHR and uterine activity are printed on a paper strip having a horizontal grid for the FHR and another for the uterine activity (Figure 14-4). Segments of paper between perforations are numbered for identification and reassembly of a multipart strip. The FHR is recorded on the upper strip. The range of rates is from 30 to 240 bpm. Other countries may use a strip with a slightly different configuration and paper speed.

Uterine activity is recorded on the lower grid as bell-shaped curves. Contraction intensity and uterine resting tone from 0 to 100 mm Hg are recorded on the lower grid.

Vertical lines on both upper and lower grids are time divisions. At a paper speed of 3 cm/min, dark vertical lines are 1 minute apart. Lighter lines subdivide the 1-minute divisions into six 10-second segments. The vertical lines are used to time contraction frequency and duration and to identify the fetal response in relation to the contractions.

Sometimes the "paper" is a computer's monitor screen with the same appearance as the paper strip. The strip may not be routinely printed on paper at all. The nurse moves backward or forward through the strip on the screen using keyboard arrows or a pointing device such as a mouse or light pen or by setting a time and date to go to a specific location. Maintenance or malfunction in the computer system often requires printing of the records until function is restored.

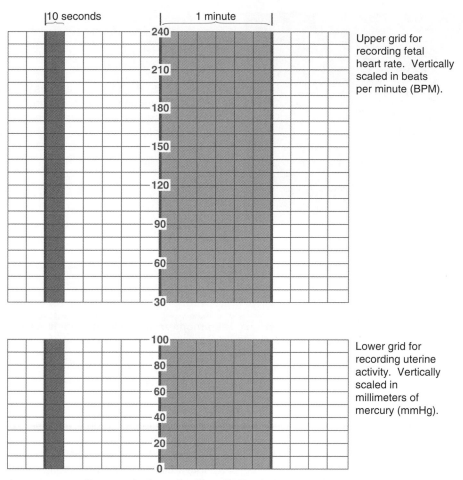

Figure 14-4 ■ Paper strip for recording electronic fetal monitoring data. Each dark vertical line represents 1 minute, and each lighter vertical line represents 10 seconds. Paperless computer displays that depict the fetal heart rate and uterine activity patterns have a similar appearance.

Data Entry Devices and Computer Software

Monitors print some notations automatically, such as the date, time, paper speed, and type of device being used to detect the FHR and uterine activity. Most also have data entry devices, allowing entry of data to be printed on the strip. Computer software is commonly used to archive fetal monitoring information plus other information relating to the care of mother and fetus. The software may extend beyond the intrapartum stay and be used for documentation in the postpartum and newborn periods.

Computer-assisted analysis of EFM data uses software to interpret patterns the nurse sees on the electronic fetal monitor. Automated analysis is likely to become a common adjunct in the review of EFM data and in suggesting possible interventions for problems. The professional person–nurse, nurse-midwife, or physician–chooses whether to accept the software analysis.

Remote Surveillance

Many facilities have display units at the nursing station or other locations to allow surveillance when the nurse is not at the bedside. These units display the tracing on a screen and have settings for alerts, such as upper and lower limits for the heart rate, decelerations, and end of the paper.

Devices for External Fetal Monitoring

Both the FHR and uterine activity can be monitored by external sensors, or transducers. External devices are secured on the mother's abdomen by elastic straps, a tube of wide stockinette, or an adhesive ring (Figure 14-5). External devices are slightly less accurate than internal ones but are noninvasive. They do not require ruptured membranes or cervical dilation, making them useful for women who should not have devices placed in the vagina or uterus, such as the woman with preterm membrane rupture. (Procedure 14-2 contains instructions for using the external electronic fetal monitor.)

FETAL HEART RATE MONITORING WITH AN ULTRASOUND TRANSDUCER

The Doppler ultrasound device detects movements other than fetal heart motion, such as fetal or maternal activity or blood flow through the umbilical cord and the woman's aorta. Today's monitors filter these extraneous sounds to provide a clean tracing.

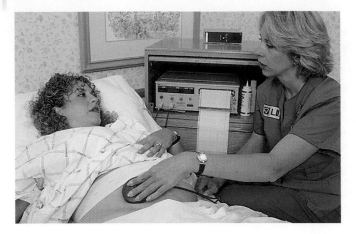

Figure 14-5 ■ The nurse applies the uterine activity transducer on the woman's upper abdomen, in the fundal area. The Doppler transducer for sensing the fetal heart rate is usually placed on her lower abdomen when the fetus is in the cephalic presentation.

PROCEDURE

14-2 External Fetal Monitor

PURPOSE: **To properly apply the external electronic fetal monitor; to perform a basic evaluation of the fetal heart rate and uterine activity patterns**

1. Read instruction manual for equipment. *Become familiar with proper operation of the equipment and identify all parts.*
2. Perform a function test following manufacturer's instructions. Press "TEST" button and observe for result. Common correct test results are the following:
   a. Fetal heart rate (FHR): The monitor prints a line at 120, 150, or 200 beats per minute (bpm), depending on the model.
   b. Uterine activity: The monitor adds 50 to uterine activity display.
   A correct function test ensures that the bedside monitor unit is calibrated properly so that caregivers are assured of accurate data to interpret. Each manufacturer sets standards for indicators of proper function.
3. Explain the basic procedure of electronic fetal monitoring to the woman and her partner or family. Vary instructions according to equipment being used and hospital protocols. A sample is:
   a. Using the electronic fetal monitor is the way we normally assess the baby's response to labor contractions.
   b. Two belts go around your abdomen, one for the FHR sensor and one for contractions.
   c. Feel free to move with the monitor on. If the tracing is poor, we can adjust the sensors.
   Knowledge decreases the woman's fear of the unknown. Teaching her that she can move with the monitor in place enhances her comfort and promotes normal labor.
4. Apply belts or stockinette if an adhesive ring is not used:
   a. Slide both belts under the woman's back without the sensors attached. Be sure to keep the belts smooth under her back.
   b. Cut a length of stockinette tubing about 15 to 18 inches long for the average-sized woman. Cut a longer length of wide stockinette for a heavier woman. Slide the stockinette up from her feet to her abdomen.
   Smooth application of straps or stockinette enhances a woman's comfort and improves contact of external sensors with her abdomen. Good contact improves the quality of the tracing and may reduce the number of adjustments needed.

5. Use Leopold's maneuvers (see Procedure 13-1) to locate the fetal back as in intermittent auscultation, Procedure 14-1.
6. Apply ultrasound gel to the Doppler ultrasound transducer and place it on the woman's abdomen at the approximate location of the fetus' back. Move the transducer until a clear signal is heard. Most bedside units have a green light or flashing heart shape to indicate a good signal. *Gel improves transmission and reception of the ultrasound waves to provide more accurate data.*
7. Place the uterine activity sensor in the fundal area or the area where contractions feel the strongest when palpated. This is often near the umbilicus. When the woman has a contraction, observe the tracing for the bell shape. The line for uterine activity is jagged because it also senses the rise and fall of the abdomen with breathing. Fetal or maternal movement, coughing, or sneezing causes a spike in the line. Observe through several contractions. *The external uterine activity monitor senses the change in the abdominal contour as the uterus rotates forward with each contraction. Contractions are usually strongest in the fundus of the uterus. Observation of the uterine activity line (on the lower grid) through several contractions verifies correct placement and identifies needed changes in placement of the sensor.*
8. Observe the strip for baseline FHR, presence of variability, periodic changes, and uterine activity (contraction duration and frequency). Palpate contractions for intensity and relaxation between contractions. Notify the physician or nurse-midwife of nonreassuring patterns. Identifies reassuring and nonreassuring FHR patterns (see Table 14-1). *Contractions having a frequency greater than every 2 minutes, a duration longer than 90 to 120 seconds, a resting interval shorter than 30 seconds, or incomplete uterine relaxation between contractions may reduce maternal blood flow into the intervillous spaces and impair exchange of oxygen and waste products. The external uterine activity sensor is useful only for contraction frequency and duration. It is not accurate for actual intensity or uterine resting tone.*

The Doppler transducer produces a two-part muffled sound that resembles the galloping of horses. The two closely linked sounds represent closure of the heart valves during systole (mitral and tricuspid valves) and diastole (aortic and pulmonic valves). Fetal or maternal activity produces a rough, erratic sound rather than the crisp, rhythmic sound characteristic of the fetal heart. Fetal hiccups have a distinct and rhythmic thumping sound.

UTERINE ACTIVITY MONITORING WITH A TOCOTRANSDUCER

A tocotransducer (also called a *tocodynamometer* or simply a "toco") with a pressure-sensitive area detects changes in abdominal contour to measure uterine activity. The uterus pushes outward against the mother's anterior abdominal wall with each contraction. The monitor calculates changes in this signal and prints them as bell shapes on the lower grid of the strip.

Movement other than uterine activity also registers on the monitor. For example, maternal respirations cause the uterine activity line to have a zigzag appearance. Other fetal or maternal movements, such as fetal hiccups, appear as spikes on the uterine activity tracing.

Uterine activity is sensed through the woman's abdomen and is therefore useful for observing the frequency and duration of contractions. It does not reliably measure actual contraction intensity and uterine resting tone. Several factors affect apparent intensity as printed on the strip.

- Fetal size—The uterus will not push firmly against the abdominal wall with each contraction when the fetus is small, making contractions appear less intense.
- Abdominal fat thickness—A thick layer of abdominal fat absorbs energy from uterine contractions, reducing their apparent intensity on the printed strip. The uterine activity recording of a thin woman whose uterus rotates sharply forward with each contraction may appear to be more intense than it actually is.
- Maternal position—Different maternal positions may increase or decrease the pressure against the transducer, changing the apparent intensity of contractions on the tracing.
- Location of the transducer—Uterine activity is best detected where it is strongest and where the fetus lies close to the uterine wall. This is usually over the fundus. Changes during contractions may not be detectable if the transducer is located elsewhere.

Devices for Internal Fetal Monitoring

Accuracy is the main advantage of using internal devices for EFM. However, their use requires ruptured membranes and about 2 cm of cervical dilation. The devices are invasive, and the risk of infection is slightly increased.

FETAL HEART RATE MONITORING WITH A SCALP ELECTRODE

The fetal scalp electrode (or spiral electrode) detects electric signals from the fetal heart (Figure 14-6). Fetal or maternal movement does not interfere with accuracy because the rate is calculated from electrical events in the fetal heart. The monitor unit generates a beeping sound with each fetal

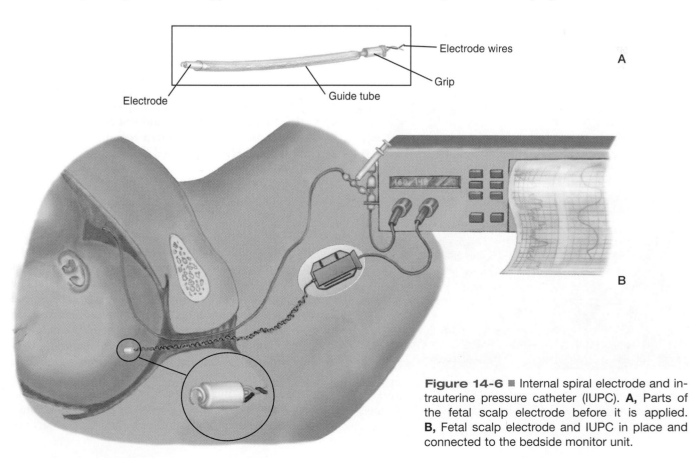

Figure 14-6 ■ Internal spiral electrode and intrauterine pressure catheter (IUPC). **A,** Parts of the fetal scalp electrode before it is applied. **B,** Fetal scalp electrode and IUPC in place and connected to the bedside monitor unit.

heartbeat, but this sound can be silenced, as can sounds from the Doppler transducer.

Although called a *fetal scalp electrode*, the device may be applied to the buttocks in a breech presentation. Areas to avoid for electrode application are the fetal face, fontanels, and genitals. The electrode wire protrudes from the mother's vagina and is attached to a leg plate on the woman's thigh. A cord from the leg plate connects to the bedside unit.

Because it barely penetrates the fetal skin (about 1 mm), the electrode is easily displaced. The tracing then becomes erratic or stops if the electrode is fully detached. Secure attachment of the electrode is often difficult if the fetus has thick hair. The electrode is removed by turning it counterclockwise about one and one half turns until it detaches.

UTERINE ACTIVITY MONITORING WITH AN INTRAUTERINE PRESSURE CATHETER

Two kinds of intrauterine pressure catheters (IUPC) can be used to measure uterine activity, including contraction intensity and resting tone:

- A solid catheter with a pressure transducer in its tip (Figure 14-7), which may have an additional lumen for amnioinfusion
- A hollow, fluid-filled catheter that connects to a pressure transducer on the bedside monitor unit

Both types sense intrauterine pressure and increases in intraabdominal pressure, such as with coughing or vomiting.

The solid catheter is not affected by height because its transducer is in the catheter. However, the sensor in its tip measures hydrostatic pressure from the amniotic fluid above the fetal presenting part as well as the pressure from uterine activity. Therefore recorded intrauterine pressures from the solid catheter are higher than those from the fluid-

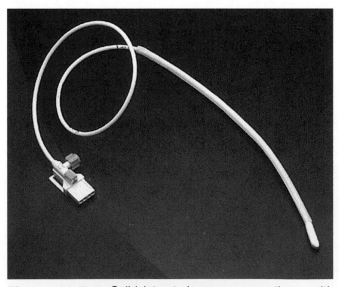

Figure 14-7 ■ Solid intrauterine pressure catheter with transducer in its tip. This model also has a lumen for amnioinfusion and is shown with its introducer over the catheter. (Courtesy Utah Medical Products, Midvale, Utah.)

filled catheter, and the nurse must consider this fact when assessing whether uterine activity is normal or hypertonic. Because it is simpler to use, the solid catheter is more commonly used.

The tip of the fluid-filled catheter in the uterus should be at the level of the transducer on the outside for best accuracy. If the tip is lower than the transducer, the recorded pressure is lower than the actual intrauterine pressure. If the tip is higher, the recorded pressure may be artificially high. Changes in the mother's position may alter the height of the catheter tip, requiring adjustment of the transducer's height.

✓ CHECK YOUR READING

5. What are the advantages and limitations of each fetal monitoring method?
6. Which grid on the paper or computer monitor strip of the electronic fetal monitor is used to record the FHR? Uterine activity? What other information may be recorded on the monitor strip?
7. Which EFM sensor uses heart motion to measure FHR?
8. What are some variables that can affect the accuracy of the external uterine activity sensor?
9. What are the two types of internal uterine activity catheters? Which one tends to record higher intrauterine pressures? Which one is affected by its height in relation to the mother's position?

EVALUATING INTERMITTENT AUSCULTATION AND PALPATION DATA

Data about FHR and uterine activity obtained by IA of the FHR and palpation of uterine activity should be evaluated in an orderly way to identify reassuring and nonreassuring signs. Some characteristics of FHR data obtained by IA are also evaluated when the data are obtained by EFM. However, characteristics unique to EFM strips, such as variability or deceleration patterns, should not be evaluated when IA is used (Feinstein, 2000; Moffatt & Feinstein, 2003).

The baseline FHR is evaluated for the following:
- Rate
- Regularity of rhythm
- Absence of decrease from the baseline

A reassuring rate is between 110 and 160 bpm and regular. If the rate is within normal limits but has changed significantly from the previous assessment, a longer listening period or more frequent assessments may clarify whether the rate is a change in the baseline. Accelerations in the rate may be heard and are a reassuring sign. An abrupt decrease in rate from the baseline rate is not reassuring and should be followed with other measures to clarify the fetal condition.

Contractions are palpated for frequency, duration, intensity, and rest interval and rest tone. If the fetus begins labor well oxygenated, then contractions that are no more frequent than every 2 minutes, are 90 to 120 seconds or less in duration, and have a resting interval of at least 30 seconds will allow adequate reoxygenation for the next contraction.

Also, the uterus must fully relax for the intervillous spaces to refill with maternal oxygenated blood.

EVALUATION OF ELECTRONIC FETAL MONITORING STRIPS

The nurse evaluates the FHR tracing for baseline rate, variability, and presence of periodic changes. Uterine activity is evaluated by determining the frequency, duration, and intensity of contractions and by assessing uterine resting, or baseline, tone. FHR and uterine activity patterns must be evaluated together.

Between 1995 and 1996 a series of workshops was held to clarify and standardize definitions for EFM data (National Institute of Child Health and Human Development [NICHD] Research Planning Workshop, 1997). A major purpose was to have standard definitions to make research data that was more comparable among studies. Many health care facilities have adopted these definitions in their policies. A simplified version is used here.

Other data are relevant to strip interpretation, such as maternal vital signs, pulse oximeter data, maternal position and position changes, drug or oxygen administration, character of the amniotic fluid, labor status, and procedures performed. These are customarily recorded on the EFM strip.

Fetal Heart Rate Baseline

The FHR baseline is the average heart rate, rounded to 5 bpm, measured over at least 2 minutes within a 10-minute window. During this 2 or more minutes the uterus must be at rest (Figure 14-8). During this 2 or more minutes the uterus must be at rest and episodes of significant increases or decreases in rate must not occur (see Figure 14-6). The baseline also excludes periodic and nonperiodic changes (see p. 319) or segments of the baseline that differ by more than 25 bpm. The baseline rate is classified as follows (Cypher, Adelsperger, & Torgersen, 2003; NICHD Research Planning Workshop, 1997):

- Normal—A rate that averages from 110 to 160 bpm. The preterm fetus at 26 to 28 weeks often averages a rate at the upper end of this range because the parasympathetic nervous system, which slows the rate, is immature. Some healthy full-term fetuses have a rate that averages 100 to 110 bpm.
- Bradycardia—Less than 110 bpm, persisting for at least 10 minutes.
- Tachycardia—More than 160 bpm, persisting for at least 10 minutes.

Some healthy term fetuses have bradycardia between 100 and 110 bpm with no other signs of compromise. A normal preterm fetus may have a baseline rate at the higher end of this range because the parasympathetic nervous system is immature.

Baseline Fetal Heart Rate Variability

Variability denotes the fluctuations in the baseline FHR that cause the printed line to have an irregular rather than a smooth appearance (Figure 14-9). Two types of variability, short-term and long-term, are often described, but the NICHD consensus does not distinguish between the two types because they occur together. Facilities that distinguish between the two types look for the following characteristics in each type:

- Short-term variability (STV)—changes in the FHR from one beat to the next (beat-to-beat variability). This variability is most accurately assessed with an internal spiral electrode because it detects cardiac electrical activity rather than heart motion. Presence of STV gives the line for the FHR a rough appearance, whereas the line is smooth if STV is absent.

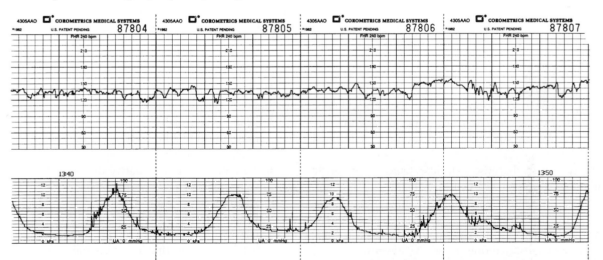

Figure 14-8 ■ Electronic fetal monitor strip showing a reassuring pattern of fetal heart rate (FHR) and uterine activity. The FHR baseline is 130 to 140 beats per minute (bpm), variability is about 10 bpm. There are no periodic changes in this strip. Contraction frequency is every 2 to 3 minutes, duration is about 50 to 60 seconds, intensity is 75 to 90 mm Hg with the internal spiral electrode, and uterine resting tone is approximately 10 mm Hg. (Courtesy Corometrics Medical Systems, Inc., Wallingford, Connecticut. Redrawn with permission.)

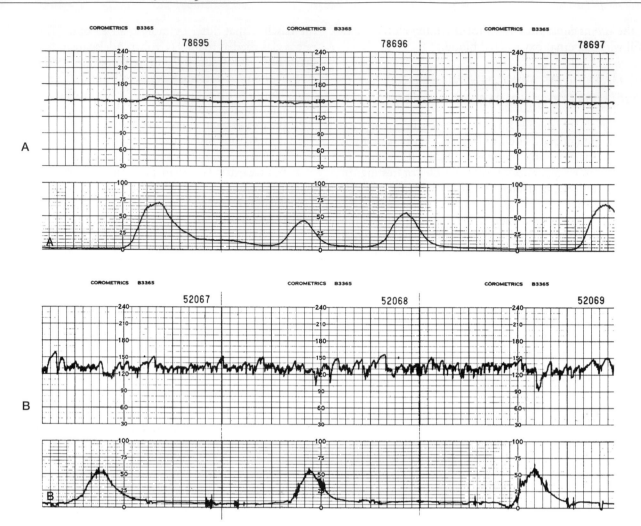

Figure 14-9 ■ Contrasts in fetal heart rate (FHR) variability. A fetal scalp electrode is being used. **A,** Minimal variability (less than 3 beats per minute [bpm]). Note the smooth, flat line in the upper graph for the FHR. **B,** Moderate variability (average 20 bpm). Note the marked zigzag appearance of the FHR line compared with the flat appearance in A. (Courtesy Corometrics Medical Systems, Inc., Wallingford, Connecticut. Redrawn with permission.)

■ Long-term variability (LTV)—broader fluctuations that are apparent over 1-minute intervals. About three to six of these broad rate changes occur each minute. LTV may be assessed with either external or internal placement.

Variability occurs because multiple factors constantly speed and slow the fetal heart in a push-and-pull manner. Evaluation of variability helps to clarify how a fetus is tolerating the stress of labor, including factors that cause hypoxia. Variability is a significant component of the FHR tracing on the electronic monitor for two reasons:

■ Adequate oxygenation promotes normal function of the autonomic nervous system and helps the fetus adapt to the stress of labor.
■ Variability evaluates the function of the fetal autonomic nervous system, especially the parasympathetic branch.

Variability may be decreased by both nonpathologic and pathologic factors, such as the following:

■ Fetal sleep (usually lasting 40 min or less at term, but may last up to 2 hours [Blackburn, 2003; Cunningham et al., 2001; Harman, 2004])
■ Narcotics or other sedative drugs, such as magnesium sulfate, given to the woman
■ Alcohol, illicit drugs
■ Fetal tachycardia
■ Gestation less than 28 weeks
■ Fetal anomalies that affect central nervous system regulation of the heart rate, such as anencephaly
■ Hypoxia that is severe enough to affect the central nervous system
■ Abnormalities of the central nervous system, heart, or both
■ Maternal acidemia or hypoxemia

The following descriptions classify variability in beats per minute:

- Absent–Undetectable
- Minimal–Undetectable to ≤5 bpm
- Moderate–6 to 25 bpm
- Marked–>25 bpm

Periodic Patterns in the Fetal Heart Rate

Periodic patterns are transient and recurrent changes from the baseline rate associated with uterine contractions. They include accelerations and decelerations. Periodic patterns are evaluated with baseline characteristics (rate and variability).

ACCELERATIONS

An acceleration is an abrupt, temporary increase in the FHR that peaks at least 15 bpm above the baseline and lasts at least 15 seconds (Figure 14-10). Accelerations often occur with fetal movement. They may be nonperiodic (having no relation to contractions) as well as periodic. They may occur with vaginal examinations, uterine contractions, and mild cord compression and when the fetus is in a breech presentation. Accelerations are usually a reassuring sign, reflecting a responsive, nonacidotic fetus.

The healthy preterm fetus may have accelerations that are less striking. Before 32 weeks of gestation, temporary increase in the FHR that peaks at least 10 bpm above the baseline and lasts at least 10 seconds is considered an acceleration. However, the younger preterm fetus often has the 15-bpm-for-15-seconds acceleration pattern that is expected at 32 weeks (NCHID, 1997; Simpson, 2004).

Accelerations lasting longer than 2 minutes but less than 10 minutes are prolonged accelerations. Accelerations that last longer than 10 minutes are a change in the baseline rate or may reflect a merging of several accelerations that later return to the previous baseline.

DECELERATIONS

Periodic decelerations are classified into three types based on their shape and relationship to uterine contractions.

EARLY DECELERATIONS. Fetal head compression briefly increases intracranial pressure, causing the vagus nerve to slow the heart rate. Early decelerations are not associated with fetal compromise and require no intervention. They occur during contractions as the fetal head is pressed against the woman's pelvis or soft tissues, such as the cervix.

Early decelerations have a gradual, rather than abrupt, decrease from the baseline. They have a consistent appearance in that one early deceleration looks similar to others. The early decelerations mirror the contraction, beginning near its onset and returning to the baseline by the end of the contraction, with the low point (nadir) of the deceleration occurring near the contraction's peak (Figure 14-11). The rate at the lowest point of the deceleration is usually no lower than 30 to 40 bpm from the baseline.

LATE DECELERATIONS. Deficient exchange of oxygen and waste products in the placenta (uteroplacental insufficiency) may result in a pattern of late (delayed) decelerations. This nonreassuring pattern suggests that the fetus has reduced reserve to tolerate the recurrent reductions in oxygen supply that occur with contractions. The cause of uteroplacental insufficiency may be acute, such as maternal hypotension. It may also occur with chronic conditions that impair placental exchange, such as maternal hypertension or diabetes.

Late decelerations are similar to early decelerations in the degree of FHR slowing and lowest rate (30 to 40 bpm) but are shifted to the right in relation to the contraction. They often begin after the peak of the contraction. The FHR returns to the baseline *after* the contraction ends

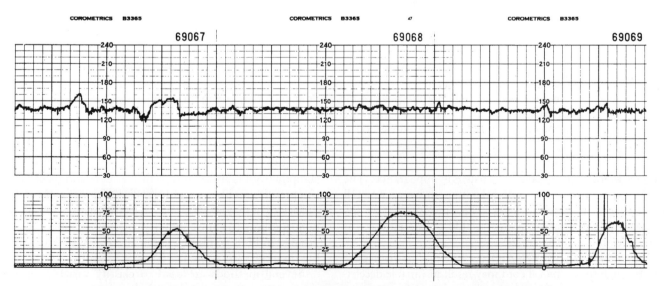

Figure 14-10 ■ Acceleration of the fetal heart rate. (Courtesy Corometrics Medical Systems, Inc., Wallingford, Connecticut. Redrawn with permission.)

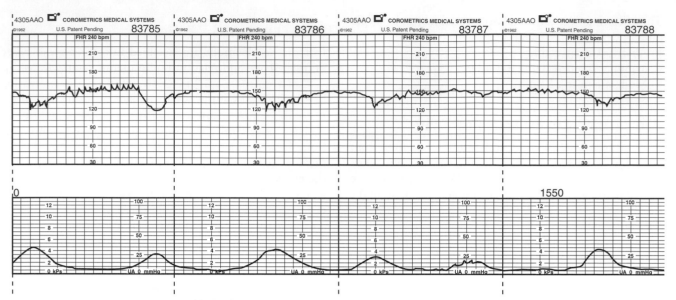

Figure 14-11 ■ Early decelerations. Note that the slowing of the fetal heart rate mirrors the contraction. It begins near the beginning of the contraction and returns to the baseline by the end of the contraction. Cause: fetal head compression. (Courtesy Corometrics Medical Systems, Inc., Wallingford, Connecticut.)

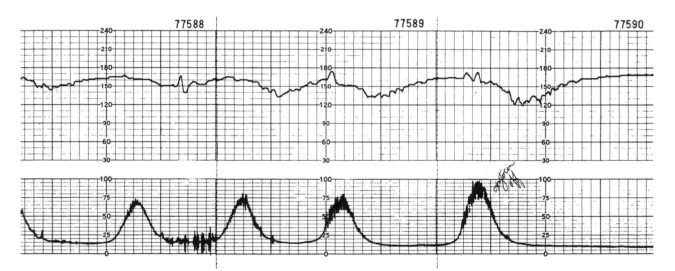

Figure 14-12 ■ Late decelerations. Note that the decelerations look similar to early decelerations but are offset to the right. They begin at about the peak of the contraction, and the nadir occurs well after the peak of the contraction, often during the interval. Cause: Uteroplacental insufficiency. (Courtesy Corometrics Medical Systems, Inc., Wallingford, Connecticut. Redrawn with permission.)

(Figure 14-12). They have a consistent appearance. The FHR may remain in the normal range and may not fall much below its baseline level. The amount of rate decrease from the baseline is not related to the amount of uteroplacental insufficiency.

VARIABLE DECELERATIONS. Conditions that reduce flow through the umbilical cord may result in variable decelerations. These decelerations do not have the uniform appearance of early and late decelerations. Their shape, duration, and degree of fall below baseline rate vary. They fall and rise abruptly (within 30 seconds) with the onset and relief of cord compression, unlike the gradual fall and rise of early and late decelerations (Figure 14-13). Variable decelerations also may be nonperiodic, occurring at times unrelated to contractions. The decrease in FHR is at least 15 bpm and lasts at least 15 seconds but no more than 2 minutes (Parer & Nageotte, 2004).

Several methods are used to classify variable decelerations according to depth and duration, but no uniform agreement exists. Baseline rate and variability are also considered in the evaluation of variable decelerations.

CRITICAL TO REMEMBER

Differences between Early and Late Decelerations

Both Early and Late Decelerations

Decrease from the baseline fetal heart rate and return to baseline are gradual (onset to nadir of at least 30 seconds).
Occur with contractions.
Rate decrease is rarely more than 30 to 40 beats per minute below the baseline.

Early Decelerations

Are mirror images of the contraction (lowest point in the fetal heart rate occurs with the peak of the contraction).
Return to the baseline fetal heart rate by the end of the contraction.
Maternal position changes usually have no effect on pattern.
Associated with fetal head compression.
Are not associated with fetal compromise and require no added interventions.

Late Decelerations

Look similar to early decelerations but begin after the contraction begins (often near the peak).
Nadir occurs after the peak of the contraction.
Reflect possible impaired placental exchange (uteroplacental insufficiency).
Occasional late decelerations accompanied by moderate variability, and accelerations are not ominous.
Persistent late decelerations, especially with no accelerations and absent or minimal variability, should be addressed by nursing interventions to improve placental blood flow and fetal oxygen supply.
The degree of fall in rate from baseline is unrelated to the amount of uteroplacental insufficiency.
Should be addressed by nursing interventions to improve placental blood flow and fetal oxygen supply.

Uterine Activity

Assessment of uterine activity involves four components: frequency, duration, and intensity of the contractions and uterine resting tone. Contraction frequency may be measured with the electronic monitor as with palpation (beginning of one contraction to beginning of the next) or from peak to peak. Duration is calculated from the beginning to end of each contraction.

Palpation is used to estimate contraction intensity and uterine resting tone when an external uterine activity monitor is used (see Procedure 13-2). Contraction intensity is described as mild, moderate, or strong.

With either type of IUPC the scale on the paper is used to describe intensity and resting tone. Intensity increases as labor progresses. Uterine contraction intensity with the IUPC is about 50 to 75 mm Hg during labor, although it may reach 110 mm Hg with pushing during the second stage. Average resting tone is 5 to 15 mm Hg.

Montevideo units (MVUs) may be used to describe contraction intensity in mm Hg when an IUPC is used. The MVU is calculated by noting the contraction intensity in mm Hg above the resting tone and multiplying by the number of contractions in 10 minutes. For example, if a woman has three contractions in 10 minutes, each of which has an intensity of 110 mm Hg and a resting tone of 15 mm Hg, the result in MVUs is 285. Excess uterine activity during labor would be 400 MVU (Cypher, Adelsperger, & Torgersen, 2003).

✔ CHECK YOUR READING

10. What is the significance of FHR accelerations?
11. What are the differences between early and late decelerations? Which pattern is nonreassuring?
12. What do variable decelerations look like? What is their cause?

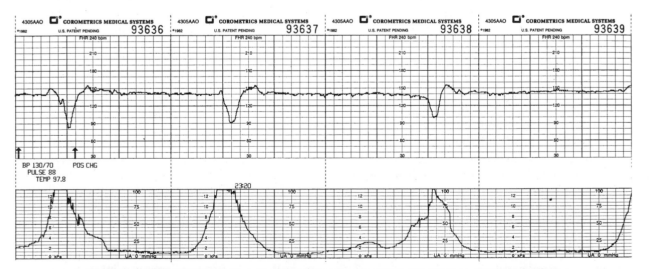

Figure 14-13 ■ Variable decelerations. The decelerations are sharp in onset and offset. Note slight rate accelerations (shoulders) after each variable deceleration. Cause: Umbilical cord compression. (Courtesy Corometrics Medical Systems, Inc., Wallingford, Connecticut. Redrawn with permission.)

CRITICAL THINKING ✑ EXERCISE 14-1

Nancy Joe is having her labor induced with oxytocin and is having internal electronic fetal monitoring. Her contractions are, on average, 2 to 2.5 minutes apart, are 90 to 100 seconds in duration, and reach 75 mm Hg on the scale for the intrauterine pressure catheter. Uterine resting tone between contractions is about 20 mm Hg. The baseline fetal heart rate is 135 to 145 bpm with about 7 bpm variability.

Her nurse, Jackie Brown, notes a pattern of uniform decelerations that begin at the peak of each contraction. The rate falls to 125 bpm before returning to the previous baseline about 30 seconds after the contraction ends.

Questions
1. What pattern does this describe?
2. What is the most appropriate nursing response?

SIGNIFICANCE OF FETAL HEART RATE PATTERNS

As with IA, FHR patterns on the electronic monitor are classified as either "reassuring" or "nonreassuring." Between these two classifications are patterns that are "equivocal," neither clearly reassuring nor clearly nonreassuring. For equivocal (ambiguous) patterns or for questionable IA data, several methods may be used to further evaluate the fetal condition. Table 14-1 summarizes reassuring and nonreassuring patterns.

Reassuring Patterns

Reassuring patterns, such as accelerations with fetal movement, are associated with fetal well-being. No intervention is required because the pattern suggests that the fetus has adequate reserves to tolerate intrapartum stressors.

Nonreassuring Patterns

Nonreassuring patterns occur if favorable signs are absent or if signs that are associated with fetal hypoxia or acidosis are present. Nonreassuring patterns do not necessarily indicate that fetal hypoxia or acidosis has occurred. They indicate that steps should be taken to identify possible causes for the nonreassuring patterns and correct those causes.

Nonreassuring patterns are more significant if they occur together and are persistent. For example, bradycardia with variability of less than 3 bpm and late decelerations suggests greater fetal stress than bradycardia alone. The healthy fetus may demonstrate occasional late decelerations, but a persistent pattern of late decelerations is more likely to represent compromise in a fetus, especially if it is combined with other nonreassuring patterns. Nonreassuring patterns include but are not limited to the following:

- Tachycardia
- Bradycardia
- Absent or minimal variability
- Late decelerations
- Variable decelerations that persistently fall to less than 60 bpm for longer than 60 seconds

- Prolonged decelerations
- Hypertonic uterine activity, whether spontaneous or stimulated by drugs

Nonreassuring patterns do not always indicate that labor should end immediately. Several interventions may be used to clarify the fetal condition and to determine the best course of action. Other interventions can increase fetal oxygenation.

CLARIFICATION OF DATA

Four methods may clarify data about the fetal condition. Two methods are used during the intrapartum period: vibroacoustic stimulation (VAS) and fetal scalp stimulation. Fetal scalp blood sampling is less common. A fourth method, analysis of umbilical cord blood gases and pH, is used immediately after birth.

In addition to these methods, fetal oxygen saturation monitoring, similar to pulse oximetry used in adult and pediatric care, is a new method that is being added to the fetal monitoring units of many intrapartum facilities.

VIBROACOUSTIC STIMULATION. Vibroacoustic, or simply acoustic (or sound), stimulation may be used by the nurse, physician, or nurse-midwife as the initial method to stimulate the fetus or to supplement fetal scalp stimulation, or it may be used if scalp stimulation is contraindicated.

An artificial larynx or vibroacoustic stimulator is applied to the mother's lower abdomen, and it is turned on for up to 3 seconds. A reassuring response is an acceleration that peaks at 15 bpm for 15 seconds or more. An absent response, however, does not necessarily mean that the fetus is suffering from hypoxia or acidosis.

FETAL SCALP STIMULATION. Scalp stimulation is used to evaluate the fetus' response to tactile stimulation (Figure 14-14). The nurse, physician, or nurse-midwife may perform this procedure. The examiner applies pressure to the scalp (or other presenting part) with a gloved finger or fingers and sweeps the fingers in a circular motion. An FHR acceleration, as in VAS, is a reassuring response that suggests the fetus is in normal oxygen and acid-base balance. The acceleration may be delayed rather than immediate.

Fetal scalp stimulation is not done in some cases:
- Preterm fetus (may cause contractions)
- Prolonged rupture of membranes (higher risk of infection)
- Chorioamnionitis (intrauterine infection)
- Placenta previa (placenta overlies the cervix, and hemorrhage is likely)
- Maternal fever of unknown origin (possibility of introducing microorganisms into the uterus)

FETAL SCALP BLOOD SAMPLE. Occasionally the physician may obtain a sample of fetal scalp blood to evaluate the pH. Normal scalp pH is 7.25 to 7.35. Scalp sampling is less common because it is invasive and the results are not available immediately.

FETAL OXYGEN SATURATION MONITOR. This type of fetal surveillance, also called *fetal pulse oximetry*, is

TABLE 14-1 Reassuring and Nonreassuring Fetal Surveillance Assessments

Reassuring Assessments

Baseline FHR: Stable, rate 110-160

Moderate variability (6-25 bpm)

Accelerations: Peaking at least 15 bpm above the baseline with a duration of 15 sec or more (10 bpm and 10 sec if gestation is 32 weeks or less)

Variable decelerations of less than 60 sec with rapid return to baseline, accompanied by normal baseline rate and moderate variability

Uterine Activity

Contraction frequency: No more frequent than every 2 min

Contraction duration: No longer than 90-120 sec

Interval between contractions: At least 30 sec

Uterine resting tone: Uterus relaxed between contractions (by palpation when intermittent auscultation or external fetal monitoring is used); uterine resting tone <20 mm Hg (with intrauterine pressure catheter)

Montevideo units <400

Nonreassuring Assessments

Pattern and Description	Possible Cause or Causes
Tachycardia Baseline FHR >160 bpm for at least 10 min	Maternal fever (fetal tachycardia may precede fever or other signs of infection) Maternal dehydration Maternal or fetal hypoxia Fetal acidosis Maternal or fetal hypovolemia Fetal cardiac arrhythmias Severe maternal anemia Maternal hyperthyroidism Drugs administered to mother (such as terbutaline, bronchodilators, decongestants, stimulant drugs)
Bradycardia Baseline FHR <110 bpm for at least 10 min; baseline rates between 100 and 110 bpm are usually not associated with fetal compromise if there are no nonreassuring patterns in the term fetus	Fetal head compression Fetal hypoxia Fetal acidosis Fetal heart block Umbilical cord compression Late second-stage labor with maternal pushing

Decreased or Absent Variability
FHR baseline has a smooth, flat appearance
	Fetal sleep episodes (usually 40 min or less; occasionally as long as 2 hr)
	Fetal hypoxia with acidosis
	Drug effects:
	  CNS depressants
	  Local anesthetic agents

Late Decelerations
Gradual decelerations having a uniform appearance and a consistent relation to the contraction
Onset to nadir of 30 sec or longer
Nadir occurs after the peak of the contraction
	Uteroplacental insufficiency, which may be secondary to:
	  Maternal hypotension or hypertension
	  Excess uterine activity, spontaneous or stimulated
	  Placental interruption, such as abruptio placentae or placenta previa
	  Maternal diabetes
	  Severe maternal anemia
	  Maternal cardiac disease

Variable Decelerations
Sharp in onset and offset
May occur as a periodic or nonperiodic (random) pattern
Nonreassuring if:
  Fall to <60 bpm for >60 sec
  Return to baseline prolonged
  Overshoots (exceeding baseline after deceleration) are present
  Accompanied by tachycardia and/or loss of variability
	Umbilical cord compression, which may be secondary to:
	  Prolapsed cord
	  Nuchal cord (around fetal neck)
	  Cord around fetal body parts
	  Oligohydramnios (abnormally small amount of amniotic fluid)
	  Cord between fetus and mother's uterus or pelvis, without obvious prolapse
	  Knot in cord

bpm, Beats per minute; *CNS,* central nervous system; *FHR,* fetal heart rate.

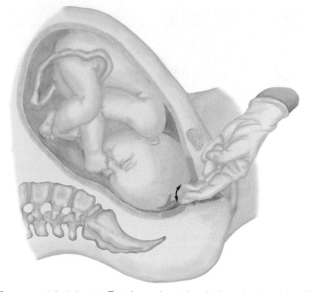

Figure 14-14 ■ Fetal scalp stimulation helps identify whether the fetus responds to gentle massage. An acceleration in the FHR peaking 15 beats per minute above the baseline suggests that the fetus is in normal oxygen and acid-base balance. Accelerations often occur with vaginal examination unrelated to a nonreassuring FHR pattern.

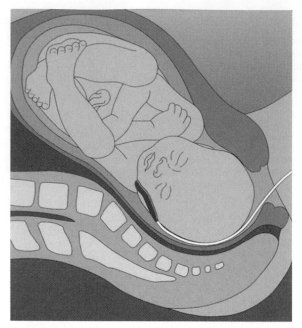

Figure 14-15 ■ The sensor for the fetal pulse oximeter is inserted vaginally so that it lies against the fetal cheek or temple. The sensor is held in place by the wall of the uterus. (Courtesy Nellcor Puritan Bennett.)

relatively new in the United States. Ideally, fetal pulse oximetry would help caregivers make better judgments about whether a nonreassuring FHR pattern is one that requires immediate operative intervention (cesarean or forceps birth) or if labor can safely continue. Further clinical research after its introduction to practice has indicated that fetal oxygen saturation monitoring should be considered as only one type of data to evaluate how the fetus is tolerating labor. Fetal oxygen saturation monitoring should be considered in conjunction with rate, variability, and presence of reassuring or nonreassuring patterns in the FHR, not as a single diagnostic measure for fetal well-being (Cypher & Adelsperger, 2003; Simpson, 2003b; Simpson, 2004; Simpson & Porter, 2001; Williams & Galerneau, 2003).

The technique is similar to that used for the mother's pulse oximetry. A special sensor is placed alongside the fetal cheek or temple area to pick up the fetal pulse for calculation of oxygen saturation (Figure 14-15). An oxygen saturation of 30% to 70% is considered normal for fetuses because of their high hemoglobin and hematocrit (compared with a normal value of 95% to 100% oxygen saturation for an adult). Technical difficulties have included the normally faint pulses of a fetus, interference of vernix and other debris between fetal skin and the sensor, and displacement of the sensor.

CORD BLOOD GASES AND pH. Umbilical cord blood analysis is used to assess the infant's oxygenation and acid-base balance immediately after birth. The samples are analyzed for pH, Pco_2, Po_2, and bicarbonate and for base deficit. This information helps identify whether acidosis exists and whether it is respiratory (short-term), metabolic (prolonged), or mixed. Normal cord blood gases and pH

can confirm that the fetus was adjusting normally to the stresses of labor even though the fetal monitoring pattern may have been nonreassuring. Arterial cord blood best reflects fetal oxygenation because this blood is leaving the fetus on its way to the placenta.

The cord is promptly double-clamped (within 20 to 30 seconds of birth) and cut to isolate a 10- to 30-cm (4- to 12-inch) segment. Blood samples from an umbilical artery provide the most accurate information about the newborn's acid-base status. The sample can also be obtained from a fetal artery on the surface of the placenta. Blood is drawn into heparinized syringes to prevent coagulation, and the syringes are capped to avoid altering values by exposure to room air (Figure 14-16). Samples kept at room temperature are reliable for up to 60 minutes.

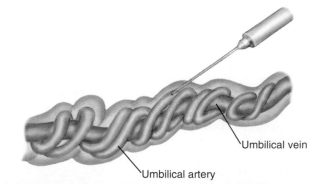

Umbilical vein

Umbilical artery

Figure 14-16 ■ Obtaining a blood sample for umbilical cord blood gases and pH after birth. Samples are drawn from the umbilical artery, vein, or both. The samples in capped syringes may be kept for up to 60 minutes at room temperature and 3 hours on ice.

CRITICAL TO REMEMBER

Nursing Responses to Nonreassuring Fetal Heart Rate Patterns

1. Identify the cause of the nonreassuring pattern to plan the best interventions:
   a. Evaluate the pattern to determine its probable cause (late or variable decelerations, bradycardia or tachycardia, absent variability).
   b. Evaluate maternal vital signs to identify hypotension, hypertension, or fever.
   c. Perform vaginal examination to identify a prolapsed umbilical cord.
2. Stop oxytocin infusion if the drug is being administered.
3. Reposition the woman, avoiding the supine position, for patterns associated with cord compression; repositioning may improve other nonreassuring patterns as well.
4. Increase the rate of a nonadditive intravenous fluid to expand the mother's blood volume and improve placental perfusion.
5. Administer oxygen by face mask at 8 to 10 L/min to increase her blood oxygen saturation, making more oxygen available to the fetus.
6. Initiate electronic fetal monitoring if intermittent auscultation data are questionable.
7. Initiate continuous electronic fetal monitoring with internal devices if no contraindication exists.
8. Notify physician or nurse-midwife as soon as possible. Report and document the following:
   a. The pattern that was identified
   b. Nursing interventions taken in response to the pattern
   c. The fetal response after nursing interventions
   d. The response of the physician or nurse-midwife (orders, other response)
9. If the nonreassuring pattern is severe, other staff members should begin preparing for immediate delivery (usually cesarean birth unless vaginal birth is imminent). Preparation for birth should include staff members for neonatal resuscitation.

INTERVENTIONS FOR NONREASSURING PATTERNS

Any of several nursing or medical interventions or both may be indicated if a nonreassuring FHR pattern is present. All are directed toward identifying the cause of the nonreassuring pattern and improving fetal oxygenation.

IDENTIFYING THE CAUSE OF A NONREASSURING PATTERN. Careful examination of the strip may suggest a cause for the nonreassuring FHR pattern and direct the most appropriate interventions. For example, a pattern of late decelerations suggests uteroplacental insufficiency. However, uteroplacental insufficiency may be secondary to a variety of causes, such as maternal hypotension or excessive uterine activity. Different causes require different corrective interventions. Checking the mother's vital signs identifies hypotension, hypertension, and fever. Maternal sedative medications may alter variability in a well-oxygenated fetus.

A vaginal examination may identify a prolapsed cord, which may cause variable decelerations, bradycardia, or both, as it is compressed. A vaginal examination also evaluates the woman's labor status, which helps the birth attendant decide if labor should continue. For example, labor may be allowed to continue or it may be ended with forceps or a vacuum extractor if a nonreassuring pattern occurs during late labor. If the same nonreassuring pattern persisted during early labor despite interventions to correct it, a cesarean birth would be more likely.

Internal monitoring is often chosen for greater accuracy if a nonreassuring pattern develops when external devices are used. The fetal scalp electrode gives a clear picture of variability, and the IUPC allows the most precise determination of actual contraction intensity and resting tone.

INCREASING PLACENTAL PERFUSION. The woman is placed in a nonsupine position to eliminate aortocaval compression, which can reduce placental blood flow and increase maternal discomfort. Increasing infusion of nonadditive intravenous fluids such as lactated Ringer's solution increases the maternal blood volume to better perfuse the placenta if maternal hypotension is the problem.

Uterine activity reduces blood flow into the intervillous spaces, and a fetus with little reserve for stress may be unable to tolerate even normal contractions. Persistent hypertonic uterine activity may compromise a fetus with normal reserves. If a woman is receiving oxytocin, it is discontinued, or its rate may be slowed so that uterine activity is not stimulated. A tocolytic drug, such as terbutaline (0.125 to 0.25 mg intravenously or 0.25 mg subcutaneously), may be given to reduce uterine activity.

INCREASING MATERNAL BLOOD OXYGEN SATURATION. Administration of 100% oxygen through a snug face mask makes more oxygen available for transfer to the fetus. A commonly suggested rate is 8 to 10 L/min.

REDUCING CORD COMPRESSION. If cord compression is suspected, the woman is repositioned. She may be turned from side to side, or her hips may be elevated to shift the fetal presenting part toward her diaphragm. A hands-and-knees position may reduce compression on the cord that is entrapped behind the fetus. Several position changes may be required before the pattern improves or resolves.

Amnioinfusion increases the fluid around the fetus and cushions the cord. Lactated Ringer's solution or normal saline is infused into the uterus through an IUPC. The underpads must be changed regularly because fluid leaks out constantly. Possible complications include overdistention of the uterus and increased uterine resting tone. These complications are relieved by releasing some of the fluid. Amnioinfusion also may be used to wash out and dilute fluid that contains thick meconium so that the infant does not aspirate it at birth.

✔ CHECK YOUR READING

13. What is the rationale for performing fetal scalp stimulation or VAS? What is the expected fetal response to these actions?
14. What is the purpose of blood gas and pH determinations on cord blood samples?
15. What nursing actions are appropriate for a nonreassuring FHR pattern? Why are they performed?
16. How can a tocolytic drug increase oxygen supply to the fetus?
17. What are the two purposes of amnioinfusion?

CRITICAL THINKING ✍ EXERCISE 14-2

LaShonda Blair is in active labor and is having external electronic fetal monitoring. LaShonda has not had medication, and her labor has been normal so far. Her membranes ruptured about 1 hour ago, and the amniotic fluid was clear. Contractions occur every 3 minutes, are 60 seconds in duration, and are of moderate intensity. Her uterus fully relaxes between each contraction.

The nursing student who is helping to care for LaShonda notes abrupt slowing of the fetal heart rate to about 90 bpm during the next 2 contractions, each episode lasting about 30 seconds.

Questions
1. How should the nursing student manage this development?
2. Are any nursing actions needed?
3. If nursing actions are needed, what are they and in what order should they be done?

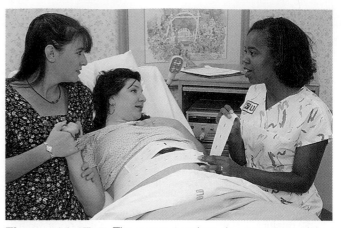

Figure 14-17 ■ The nurse teaches the woman and her partner about electronic fetal monitoring to limit her anxiety and promote her comfort during labor. The nurse should help the woman understand that the electronic fetal monitor is only one method used to evaluate the fetal well-being during labor.

Application of the Nursing Process
Intermittent Auscultation and Electronic Fetal Monitoring

Assessment of the fetus using either IA or EFM requires additional education after entering the intrapartum nursing specialty. The novice nurse or student usually provides care in the form of applying the external monitor, recording maternal vital signs, and assisting in position changes and ambulation. The experienced nurse should be notified promptly if questionable or nonreassuring findings such as bradycardia occur, because they cannot always be anticipated.

The nurse may identify any of several nursing problems related to intrapartal fetal assessment. The woman or couple preferring a nontechnical environment for birth may encounter a decisional conflict if EFM is routine in the birth facility. The woman may become anxious if she does not understand the data, if a change from IA is needed, or if complications develop. Pain may be increased and labor could be impeded by the reduced mobility that can occur with continuous EFM, even if the reduced mobility is self-imposed by the woman.

Two nursing care needs related to intrapartum fetal assessment by either technique are the woman's (and support person's) learning needs and an expansion of nursing care related to fetal oxygenation. Care related to fetal monitoring by either auscultation or electronic means should be combined with that for normal or complicated intrapartum nursing as needed.

LEARNING NEEDS

Assessment

Identify what the woman and her support person already know about auscultation and the electronic fetal monitor (Figure 14-17). Women who have attended prepared child-birth classes or have given birth before may have a basic understanding of the purpose and limitations of the fetal monitor. Identifying what clients already know allows you to build on their knowledge and correct any inaccurate information.

If the woman is not familiar with either technique of intrapartum fetal assessment, assess her perception of each. For example, does she believe that use of the electronic fetal monitor indicates the development of a complication, or does she expect its use? Is the woman comfortable with IA for fetal assessment or does she worry that something important will be missed?

Lack of knowledge contributes to anxiety. Note the anxiety level of the woman when the monitor is used. For example, is the woman afraid to move because the fetal heart sounds and tracing skip at that time? Does she place the monitor's data above her own comfort? Note questions about the monitor and its data and then reassess after teaching to identify information that is still unclear or is causing anxiety.

Analysis

Many women expect to have continuous EFM during labor. They have often been introduced to it during prepared childbirth classes or have friends and family members who have had it. Most women have additional questions, however, and some women know little about this mode of fetal surveillance. Others may be quite surprised to learn that IA during birth is a valid choice.

Because of the prevalence of EFM for labor, the nursing diagnosis chosen for this discussion is "Deficient Knowledge: Fetal monitoring." A comparable nursing diagnosis could be made for the woman who has IA and palpation.

Planning

A goal or expected outcome for this nursing diagnosis is that, after being taught about intrapartum fetal surveillance, the woman and her partner will express understanding of the equipment, procedures, limitations, and expected data.

Interventions

EXPLAINING FETAL HEART RATE AUSCULTATION WITH UTERINE PALPATION

Many women are surprised to know that auscultation and palpation are accepted modes of fetal surveillance during labor because they do not know of anyone who had this "low-tech" approach. Explain that the frequency of assessment by either method varies with risk status and stage of labor. Also explain that the physician or midwife may recommend EFM for several reasons and that this does not necessarily indicate a complication.

EXPLAINING THE ELECTRONIC FETAL MONITOR

Education continues as circumstances change. Explain the purposes of the monitor and the equipment to be used. A simple explanation is to tell the parents that the monitor is a tool to assess how the fetus reacts to labor, especially during contractions. If true, assure the woman that its use does not mean something is wrong with her baby. Explain why changes in the fetal assessment mode (IA to EFM; external to internal EFM) are done. Also helpful may be an explanation that the fetal monitor strip is only one of many factors evaluated during labor.

ADDRESSING PARENTS' SAFETY CONCERNS

Explain how the equipment functions. Some women are afraid of being attached to an electrical device, especially because cords and electrodes are wet with amniotic fluid and vaginal secretions. Reassure the woman that the connections to her and those to the wall current are isolated from each other.

The woman may be concerned about attachment of the scalp electrode to the fetal presenting part. Show her that the electrode is a fine wire that penetrates the outer layer of skin only (about 1 mm, or the thickness of a dime). The IUPC lies beside the fetus, next to the inner wall of the uterus.

COPING WITH MISLEADING DATA

Teach the woman that the monitor sometimes gives data that suggest a problem when no problem exists. For example, the FHR may suddenly fall to zero and the audible tone may stop if the sensor (external or scalp electrode) is displaced. The patient should call the nurse for adjustment or replacement of the sensor.

The woman may be discouraged because the curves representing contractions do not look as strong on the strip as they feel to her. This situation is common with use of an external transducer. Explain the factors that cause the contraction curves to appear stronger or weaker than they really are, such as her position, the fetal position, or the amount of abdominal fat. Tell her the strip is used mainly to assess the timing of

---

PARENTS WANT TO KNOW
About Electronic Fetal Monitoring

When women have electronic fetal monitoring during labor, they often have questions that the nurse may answer. Here are some frequently asked questions and suggested answers.

Can I move around with the monitor?

You can move freely with the monitor. If you notice that you can't hear the fetal heart sounds or see the contractions as well, call me and I'll readjust it. Make yourself comfortable; then we'll adjust the machine if necessary.

What if I need to go to the bathroom?

If you need to go to the bathroom, we'll unplug the cords from the machine or we can roll the monitor to the door of the bathroom and you can walk in there.

Will the monitor shock me? I don't know if I want to be hooked to an electrical outlet, especially because my water has broken and I have bloody show.

The part of the monitor that is attached to you and your baby transmits information only into the machine for processing. The sensors on your body are separated from electrical parts in the monitor.

Why is the baby's heart beating so fast?

A baby's heart normally beats faster than an adult's, both before and after birth. The normal rate is about 110 to 160 beats per minute. A rate outside these boundaries does not always mean that the baby has a problem, but we do look at the monitor strip closely to see if we need to check for other problems.

Why do those numbers for the baby's heart rate change so much?

The heart rate of a healthy baby near full term who is awake changes constantly. When the baby moves, the heart speeds up, just as yours does.

What do those numbers for contractions (external monitor) mean? They change all the time.

The numbers reflect a change in the pressure that the monitor senses. The monitor senses many changes in pressure other than those from contractions, such as changes from breathing, coughing, or movement of you or the baby.

My contractions don't look very strong, but they sure feel strong to me! (External uterine activity monitor is being used.)

The external monitor senses contractions indirectly, rather than sensing the actual pressure within the uterus. Their appearance on the tracing varies because of many factors, such as your position, the position of the sensor on your abdomen, and the thickness of your abdominal wall. You may notice spikes on the line and the sound of a "bump" at regular intervals when the baby has hiccups, which is very common.

Will the internal monitor hurt my baby?

The spiral electrode attaches only to the outer layer of skin on the baby's head. We are careful to avoid sensitive areas on the head, such as the fontanels (soft spots) or the face. The uterine catheter slides up beside the baby.

contractions and the fetus's reaction to contractions when an external tocotransducer is used. Explain that an IUPC may be recommended if knowledge of true intrauterine pressure is crucial and her membranes are ruptured.

Reassure the woman that her perception of her contractions and discomfort is important. Data from the woman are as important as the machine-generated data. Palpate contractions at intervals and evaluate their appearance on the monitor strip.

Your attention is naturally drawn to the electronic fetal monitor when entering a woman's room. However, focus on the woman and her family rather than devoting excessive attention to the monitoring equipment. The woman is having the baby, not the monitor.

INCLUDING THE LABOR PARTNER

Tell the partner how to identify the onset and peak of contractions from the strip. During active labor, some women discover that contractions become intense before they can prepare for them. If this is the case, instruct the support person to tell the woman when each contraction begins, to prepare her. This person can also encourage her by telling her when the peak has passed.

ENHANCING COMFORT

Nursing care involves finding ways to make the mother comfortable and the monitor as nonintrusive as possible. Teach the woman ways to improve comfort while still allowing an adequate tracing to be obtained.

Explain that staying in one position not only is uncomfortable but also does not promote normal labor. The woman may assume any position except supine in most cases. She can sit in a chair, stand beside the bed, and assume most positions in the labor bed. She should find her most comfortable position, then the nurse can adjust the external devices to best detect contractions and the fetal heartbeat. Internal devices may be an option if external devices cannot be adjusted to provide useful data.

If the woman finds the sound produced by the electronic fetal monitor distracting or inconsistent with the atmosphere she wants, lower the sound or turn it off. The auditory cues for rate accelerations and decelerations are absent if the sound is muted, so the pattern on the strip must be noted.

If no other contraindications to walking exist, the woman may go to the bathroom to urinate or defecate. Unplug the sensors at the machine, let her walk to the bathroom, and reconnect and adjust the sensors when she returns. Alternatively, roll the machine to the door of the bathroom to keep the cords connected. Document ambulation and any interruption in monitoring on the strip. If the fetus has a nonreassuring pattern, it is preferable not to interrupt the recording. Computerized storage for EFM strips may result in alarms when the monitor is disconnected, even for a short time.

Evaluation

The evaluation of knowledge is continuous because most women think of questions after initial explanations and as conditions change. Achievement of the goal or expected outcome is evident if the partners indicate their understanding after each explanation. Their understanding also may be accompanied by a decrease in signs of anxiety.

FETAL OXYGENATION

Assessment

Evaluate the fetal monitoring strip systematically for the elements noted previously. Assessment and documentation intervals recommended are similar for IA and EFM:

- Low-risk women—Every 30 minutes during the active phase and every 15 minutes during the second stage
- High-risk women—Every 15 minutes during the active phase and every 5 minutes during the second stage

See Table 14-2 for other times when the FHR should be evaluated and documented.

Take the woman's temperature every 4 hours (every 2 hours after membranes rupture). Maternal fever increases the fetal temperature and fetal oxygen requirements. The nurse should assess the woman's pulse, respirations, and blood pressure hourly. Hypotension or hypertension may reduce maternal blood flow to the intervillous spaces.

Assessment of mother and fetus is continuous during the dynamic process of labor. Compare data about FHR patterns, uterine activity, and maternal vital signs with baseline data and normal ranges. Observe for subtle trends in the data, and distinguish between patterns that have similar appearances, such as early and late decelerations.

Vaginal examination may be performed to evaluate specific FHR patterns, for example, to check for a prolapsed cord if a pattern of variable decelerations occurs (see p. 320).

Analysis

The collaborative problem "Potential Complication: Fetal Compromise" is selected for nursing care related to fetal oxygenation when EFM is used.

TABLE 14-2 Guidelines for Assessment and Documentation of Fetal Heart Rate Using Auscultation

Women Without Risk Factors	Women With Risk Factors Present on Admission or That Develop During Labor
Active First-Stage Labor	
At least every 30 min, just after a contraction	At least every 15 min, just after a contraction
Second-Stage Labor	
At least every 15 min	At least every 5 min

Other Times to Document Fetal Heart Rate
- Before artificial rupture of the membranes; after rupture of the membranes, either artificially or spontaneously
- Before and after ambulation
- If contractions become too frequent or last too long or if there is an inadequate interval between them
- Before administration of oxytocin and when evaluating the dose for increase, maintenance, or decrease
- Before administration of sedative medications or central nervous system depressants and at time of peak action
- Before epidural analgesia is started and every 15 min for 1 hr after it is started

Planning

Because the nurse does not manage fetal compromise independently, client (fetal) goals are not made. The nurse's responsibility includes planning to do the following:

- Promote adequate fetal oxygenation.
- Take corrective actions to increase fetal oxygenation if nonreassuring patterns are identified.
- Report nonreassuring patterns to the physician or nurse-midwife.
- Support the woman and her partner if a complication develops.
- Document assessments and care.

Interventions

Measures to promote fetal oxygenation are also discussed with the care of the woman in normal labor (see Chapter 13) and the woman having an epidural or subarachnoid block (see Chapter 15).

TAKING CORRECTIVE ACTIONS

The priority of nursing care is to improve fetal oxygenation. If a nonreassuring pattern is noted, identify its cause and improve fetal oxygenation (see p. 307). Birth facilities have protocols to give nurses a framework for steps to take if nonreassuring patterns develop. Nursing interventions may include both independent nursing actions and delegated medical actions.

REASSURING PARENTS

Parents understandably become anxious when a nonreassuring pattern occurs. Remain calm at the bedside to avoid increasing their anxiety. The call signal can be used to summon other nurses to help with corrective actions and to notify the physician or nurse-midwife if it is impossible to leave.

Explain any problems and the reason for corrective actions in simple, concise language. Severe anxiety reduces the parents' ability to understand information. Inform them if the FHR returns to a reassuring pattern. Some corrective actions, such as oxygen administration and positioning, may continue after a reassuring pattern returns. Tell the woman she may talk while wearing the oxygen mask. Document parental response to teaching about care for nonreassuring patterns.

NONREASSURING PATTERNS

Notify the birth attendant of nonreassuring patterns as soon as possible after taking corrective actions. In addition, document the time and content of all consultations with the physician or nurse-midwife about the mother or fetus and the birth attendant's response.

DOCUMENTING ASSESSMENTS AND CARE

Record data related to fetal well-being according to facility policy. Box 14-2 shows guidelines for documentation on the monitor and labor records. Documentation and charting may be done on computer media rather than paper. Record-

---

BOX 14-2 Documenting Electronic Fetal Monitoring

Documentation When Monitoring Initiated
Monitor Strip
Woman's name
Physician's or nurse-midwife's name
Date and time of admission
Date and time electronic monitoring is begun (verify date and time if this information is automatically printed by monitor)
Gravidity, parity, abortions, living children
Gestation in weeks
Presence of identified risk factors
Character of amniotic fluid (if membranes are ruptured)
Function test of monitor accuracy
Initial mode of monitoring (external or internal devices)
Labor Record
Same information as on monitor strip
First panel number when a paper strip is begun

Continuing Documentation
Monitor Strip
Maternal vital signs
Vaginal examinations, including cervical dilation and effacement and fetal station
Rupture of membranes (spontaneously or artificially)
Color, quantity, and character (such as foul odor or cloudiness) of amniotic fluid
Maternal position changes
Maternal or fetal movement
Maternal vomiting, coughing, or other movement that affects tracing
Adjustment of equipment
Medication and anesthesia, including related interventions
Changes of equipment mode (such as external to internal device)
Interventions for nonreassuring patterns
Temporary interruptions in strip, such as woman walking
Labor Record
Same information as on monitor strip
Periodic summary of the baseline rate, variability, periodic changes, and uterine activity (frequency, duration, and intensity of contractions and uterine resting tone)
Communications with physician or nurse-midwife, including his or her response to reports of problems
Actions taken in chain of command if the physician or nurse-midwife fails to respond appropriately to the nurse's report of a problem

---

ing data carefully can demonstrate good nursing care and show that the standard of care has been met.

Record the woman's name, the date, and the time on the paper or electronic strip when electronic fetal monitoring begins. If a break in the paper strip occurs, such as to change paper, label the new strip with the woman's name, the date, and the time. Record the last panel number of the previous strip on the new strip so that the entire record can be reassembled sequentially.

Continue documenting the heart rate and maternal observations until vaginal birth occurs. If a cesarean birth is needed, continue monitoring by auscultation or electronic means as long as practical while preparing the woman for surgery. Remove internal devices before securing her legs to the operating table with a strap. Document the time at which monitoring is stopped and the time of abdominal incision. (See Nursing Care Plan 14-1.)

NURSING CARE PLAN 14-1 Intrapartum Fetal Compromise

ASSESSMENT: Glenda Brown is a 30-year-old African-American woman. She is a gravida 2, para 1 and has a 7-year-old son. Glenda had early and regular prenatal care. She had a biophysical profile during her pregnancy because of a slight blood pressure elevation. Glenda's labor is being induced with oxytocin (Pitocin) at 37 weeks' gestation because of preeclampsia, a type of hypertension during pregnancy. Her admission blood pressure was 148/94, and repeat assessments have been about the same level. Glenda's fetus will be monitored with electronic fetal monitoring. Glenda is accompanied by her husband, Paul. Glenda said they did not take classes because they felt that they remembered enough from their first birth. Chris Lowe is Glenda's intrapartum nurse.

CRITICAL THINKING: What nursing diagnosis is appropriate at this time? Should the nurse include Paul when considering the initial nursing diagnosis?

ANSWER: Although the Browns have had one successful pregnancy, the nurse should not assume that they know about current use of fetal monitoring in labor, because their son was born 7 years ago. The fact that they did not attend classes also increases the likelihood that they need teaching about newer versions of electronic fetal monitors.

NURSING DIAGNOSIS: Knowledge Deficit: Electronic fetal monitoring

GOALS/EXPECTED OUTCOMES: Glenda and Paul will state that they understand the reason for electronic monitoring, related equipment and procedures, and the data that are expected.

INTERVENTION	RATIONALE
1. Assess the parents' present knowledge about electronic fetal monitoring.	1. This builds on existing accurate knowledge and allows correction of misunderstandings.
2. Explain information about the monitor to Glenda and Paul.	2. Explain that the use of the electronic fetal monitor does not mean something is wrong with Glenda or the baby.
a. Purpose: To record the fetal response to labor and guide interventions if nonreassuring patterns are identified.	a. This provides a realistic explanation of how the monitor is used.
b. Safety: The monitoring sensors are electrically isolated from the wall current. The fetal scalp electrode (if used) penetrates the outer layer of skin, about a dime's thickness. The intrauterine pressure catheter lies between the baby and the wall of the uterus.	b. This addresses possible safety concerns of parents. One millimeter, or a dime's thickness, is less than the thickness of the outer layer of skin on the fetal scalp.
c. Encourage Glenda to call for assistance if she is concerned about anything related to the monitor, such as being unable to hear the fetal heartbeat. Tell her that a nurse will adjust her monitor as needed.	c. Sensors, especially external devices, are easily displaced. Preparing Glenda and Paul for this possibility reduces their fears if they should stop hearing the fetal heartbeat.
d. Encourage Glenda to move about freely. Explain that she should urinate at least every 2 hours and that the nurse can help her roll the monitor to the bathroom door or temporarily disconnect the sensors.	d. Maternal movement and regular urination enhance normal labor processes. A woman is likely to become anxious and uncomfortable if she concentrates more on maintaining data from the monitor than on coping with labor.

EVALUATION: Glenda and Paul say they expected electronic fetal monitoring during labor and are familiar with the external monitor because it was used for the biophysical profile. Glenda agrees to have internal monitoring if needed, saying that she understands that greater accuracy is important because of her higher risk status.

ASSESSMENT: Chris applies the external fetal monitor, which shows irregular spontaneous contractions. The fetal heart rate (FHR) baseline averages 125 to 135 beats per minute (bpm) with accelerations. The nurse begins an oxytocin infusion to induce labor. Glenda's blood pressure is 160/96, pulse is 76, and respirations are 18.

CRITICAL THINKING: Does the nurse need other data at this point?

ANSWER: Added information would help clarify whether the elevation in Glenda's blood pressure is in response to anxiety or pain or is a part of her preeclampsia. The nurse should assess Glenda for hyperactive reflexes and edema, particularly of her face and fingers (see Chapters 13 and 25).

POTENTIAL COMPLICATION: Fetal compromise.

GOALS/EXPECTED OUTCOMES: Client goals for the fetus are inappropriate because nurses cannot independently manage fetal compromise. Chris's planning for Glenda should reflect the need to do the following:
1. Compare FHR and uterine activity data with baseline levels before oxytocin induction.
2. Promote normal fetal oxygenation.
3. Take corrective actions for nonreassuring patterns.
4. Notify Glenda's physician if nonreassuring patterns develop.

NURSING CARE PLAN 14-1 Intrapartum Fetal Compromise—cont'd

INTERVENTION	RATIONALE
1. Identify relevant risk factors for fetal compromise.	**1.** The development of preeclampsia is a risk factor that means Glenda should have increased frequency of fetal assessments.
2. Encourage Glenda to assume any comfortable position other than the supine position. Encourage her to change positions regularly, about every half hour.	**2.** The supine position can reduce blood return to the heart by compressing the inferior vena cava. Compression of the aorta and reduced cardiac output reduce placental perfusion. Regular changes of position promote normal labor progress and comfort.
3. Evaluate the tracing at the following times, signing or initialing the paper strip or using computer documentation each time. Document a summary of the evaluation on the labor record.	**3.** Documents that assessment was done. Documenting on both strip and labor record allows each to stand alone (if that is facility policy).
a. Every 15 minutes during the first stage and every 5 minutes during the second stage	**a.** This situation involves a high-risk pregnancy, and the fetus should be evaluated by those guidelines.
b. Before and after procedures such as amniotomy, medications, epidural anesthesia	**b.** Rupture of membranes (spontaneously or by amniotomy) may result in cord compression. Medications may alter the rate or variability of the fetal heartbeat. Epidural anesthesia may cause hypotension, which can decrease uteroplacental perfusion.
c. With changes of activity, such as urination and repositioning	**c.** Changes in activity or position could alter the uterine or umbilical cord blood flow. Sensors may slip and need adjustment with activity.
4. Use a four-step approach to evaluate the strip:	**4.** Systematic framework allows evaluation of the fetal response to labor.
a. Baseline FHR.	**a.** Tachycardia may be an early response to hypoxia. Bradycardia may occur in response to vagal stimulation or prolonged hypoxia.
b. Variability.	**b.** Normal variability suggests that the fetus is well oxygenated and not in acidosis.
c. Periodic changes: Accelerations, decelerations. (Note relationship of periodic changes to fetal movement, contractions, and the woman's status and activity. Note nonperiodic [random] accelerations or variable decelerations.)	**c.** Accelerations are a reassuring sign of fetal well-being. Early decelerations are a response to head compression. Late (uteroplacental insufficiency) and variable (umbilical cord compression) decelerations are nonreassuring. The nurse should attempt to identify their cause, correct it if possible, and take steps to improve fetal oxygenation.
d. Uterine activity. (Evaluate frequency and duration using either external or internal devices. When external uterine activity monitoring is done, palpate three or more contractions. Note whether the uterus relaxes between contractions for at least 60 seconds. If an intrauterine pressure catheter is used, read contraction intensity and uterine resting tone from scale on strip. Calculate Montevideo units [MVUs] if that is the policy in the facility.)	**d.** The presence of contractions that are too long (more than 90 to 120 seconds in duration) or too frequent (closer than every 2 minutes), a resting interval of less than 30 seconds, or a baseline (resting) intrauterine pressure of more than 20 mm Hg reduces the time available for normal uteroplacental exchange. Because of diabetes and pregnancy-induced hypertension, uteroplacental exchange may be reduced before labor begins. Oxytocin stimulates uterine activity and adds to risk.
5. For a fetal pulse oximeter, evaluate for a reassuring reading of 30% to 70%.	**5.** Pulse oximeter readings between 30% and 70% are currently considered normal for the fetus because of their high hemoglobin and hematocrit.
6. If nonreassuring patterns develop, take appropriate corrective actions such as discontinuing the oxytocin, increasing the rate of the nonadditive intravenous solution, repositioning Glenda, and administering oxygen. Notify physician of nonreassuring patterns, corrective actions taken, and the fetal response. Document physician response and any orders.	**6.** The first priority is to identify the cause of the nonreassuring pattern and improve fetal oxygenation. The physician should be notified of the maternal-fetal status for needed medical orders or interventions as soon as possible.

EVALUATION: Goals are not established for collaborative problems. Chris compared data from the fetal monitor and other nursing evaluations with the baseline data before Glenda started receiving oxytocin to start contractions. For the first 4 hours of the oxytocin induction, the FHR continued near its baseline of 125 to 135 bpm, with variability averaging 10 bpm. FHR accelerations continue. No nonreassuring patterns were noted.

Continued

NURSING CARE PLAN 14-1 Intrapartum Fetal Compromise—cont'd

ASSESSMENT: The physician ruptures Glenda's membranes and inserts internal devices for the FHR and uterine activity. Glenda's blood pressure is 145/90, and her oxytocin infusion continues. She is having contractions every 4 minutes; they are of 50 seconds' duration and 50 mm Hg intensity, and she has a uterine resting tone of 10 mm Hg. One hour after Glenda's membranes are ruptured, Chris notes that the baseline FHR has risen to approximately 145 to 150 bpm with variability averaging 3 bpm. A pattern of repeated late decelerations develops. Chris stops the oxytocin infusion and increases the rate of lactated Ringer's intravenous fluid, positions Glenda on her left side, and administers 100% oxygen at 10 L/min with a snug face mask. The physician is notified. Baseline variability improves to 5 bpm, but repeated late decelerations continue. Glenda is holding Paul's hand tightly and breathing rapidly. Her vital signs are blood pressure, 158/96; pulse, 90; respirations, 32. Uterine activity is unchanged.

CRITICAL THINKING: *What new nursing diagnosis or collaborative problem seems apparent based on the latest assessment data? Why?*

ANSWER: *Glenda displays several behaviors typical of anxiety: rapid pulse and respiratory rates and gripping her husband's hand. The rise in her blood pressure could be due to anxiety or to the disease process. Because of added complications and the minimal improvement in fetal status superimposed on her higher-risk status, anxiety seems appropriate. Helping her control her anxiety can promote a more normal labor as well as make her more comfortable.*

NURSING DIAGNOSIS: Anxiety related to unexpected development of complications

GOALS/EXPECTED OUTCOMES:
1. Glenda will have a reduced respiratory rate (12-20/min) after interventions.
2. Glenda will have a more relaxed face and body posture after interventions.

INTERVENTION	RATIONALE
1. Maintain calm behavior while performing corrective actions and notifying the physician.	1. Calm behavior nonverbally communicates competence to parents. Anxious behavior on the part of caregivers tends to increase the parents' anxiety.
2. Use simple, concise language for all explanations.	2. High anxiety or intense physical sensations impair a person's ability to comprehend explanations.
3. Explain the following to Glenda and Paul: a. The problem that was identified b. The usual cause of the problem c. Reasons for corrective actions d. Expected results e. That Glenda can talk with oxygen mask on	3. If Glenda and Paul understand what is happening and why the corrective actions are taken, they are more likely to comply with the care. Knowledge decreases fear of the unknown. Assuring Glenda that she can talk with the oxygen mask on allows her to ask questions and express feelings to reduce anxiety and fear.
4. Inform Glenda and Paul if the pattern improves or is resolved. For example, tell them when baseline variability improves and that the fetal pulse oximetry readings remain normal.	4. This decreases anxiety about the fetus's condition.
5. Allow Glenda and Paul to express their feelings about the labor and birth during the postpartum period. Explain any gaps in their understanding about what happened.	5. This helps the couple accept and put unexpected occurrences in perspective. It decreases the possibility that one or both parents feel like "a failure" if emergency intervention (cesarean birth) became necessary.

EVALUATION: Over the next hour the FHR pattern gradually improves. The baseline rate slows (130 to 140 bpm), and late decelerations are sporadic. Baseline short-term variability improves to about 8 bpm and fetal pulse oximetry readings remain in the normal range. Glenda gradually relaxes her grip on Paul's hand and her body relaxes. Her respiratory rate slows to 20 breaths per minute. Glenda requires a cesarean birth because her cervix does not dilate to greater than 7 cm, despite adequate contractions.

Evaluation

Client-centered goals are not formulated for a collaborative problem. Compare data with established standards to determine whether they are within normal limits. If nonreassuring patterns are identified, the nurse should:

- Take measures to increase fetal oxygenation
- Notify the physician or nurse-midwife of nonreassuring patterns
- Document all relevant data

SUMMARY CONCEPTS

- The purpose of intrapartum fetal assessment is to identify fetal well-being and to identify the fetus who may be having hypoxic stress beyond the ability to compensate for it.
- The two approaches to intrapartum fetal assessment are intermittent auscultation with palpation of uterine activity and electronic fetal monitoring. Each type has advantages and limitations. Electronic fetal monitoring has not been shown to be superior to auscultation with palpation, but

staffing needed to achieve safe intermittent auscultation with palpation may be higher.

- Fetal oxygenation depends on a normal flow of oxygenated maternal blood into the placenta, normal exchange within the placenta, patent umbilical cord vessels, and normal fetal circulatory and oxygen-carrying function.

- Stimulation of the sympathetic nervous system increases the FHR and strengthens the heart contraction. Stimulation of the parasympathetic nervous system slows the heart rate and maintains short-term variability. The parasympathetic nervous system matures later than the sympathetic, beginning at about 28 to 32 weeks of gestation.

- An advantage of the fetoscope over Doppler ultrasound devices is that the fetoscope assesses actual fetal heart sounds and therefore can identify fetal cardiac dysrhythmias. Doppler devices sense cardiac motion and convert the motion into sound that represents the cardiac activity.

- External electronic fetal monitoring is less accurate for fetal heart rate and uterine activity patterns than internal monitoring, but it is noninvasive.

- Greater accuracy is the main advantage of internal electronic fetal monitoring devices.

- Nursing responsibilities related to intrapartum fetal monitoring include promoting fetal oxygenation, identifying and reporting nonreassuring findings, supporting parents, communicating with the physician or nurse-midwife, and documenting all care.

ANSWERS TO CRITICAL THINKING EXERCISES 14-1, p. 322

The pattern described is one of late decelerations, probably caused by excess uterine activity secondary to the use of oxytocin. Jackie's initial action should be to stop the oxytocin infusion and increase the rate of nonadditive IV fluid, which is Ringer's lactate in Nancy's case. Oxygen should be given through a snug face mask at 8 to 10 L/min. Nancy should be placed on her side, if she is not already in this position, to increase placental blood flow. After the immediate corrective actions are completed, Jackie should contact Nancy's physician or nurse-midwife, documenting her interventions and the content of the call.

ANSWERS TO CRITICAL THINKING EXERCISES 14-2, p. 326

The nursing student should call the RN to the room to evaluate the patient. A change of position may relieve cord compression. These changes include turning from side to side or assuming a hands-and-knees position to release the cord from its entrapped position. Positioning LaShonda with her hips higher than her head may also relieve pressure on the cord. The monitoring strip should be evaluated by an experienced RN or the physician to clarify whether a variable deceleration pattern truly exists or if the pattern was an isolated dip in the rate. Evaluation should continue to determine if the decreases in FHR are repetitive or isolated.

LaShonda's oxygenation and hydration should be considered as well. Oxygen at 8 to 10 L/min by face mask and increasing the plain intravenous fluid can correct inadequacies in these areas.

REFERENCES & READINGS

Adelsperger, D., & Waymire, V.J. (2003). Physiological interventions for fetal heart rate patterns. In N. Feinstein, K.L. Torgersen, & J. Atterbury (Eds.), *AWHONN's fetal heart monitoring: Principles and practices* (3rd ed., pp. 159-175). Dubuque, IA: Kendall/Hunt Publishing.

American Academy of Pediatrics (AAP) & American College of Obstetricians and Gynecologists (ACOG). (2002). *Guidelines for perinatal care* (5th ed.). Elk Grove Village, IL, and Washington, DC: Author.

Blackburn, S.T. (2003). *Maternal, fetal, and neonatal physiology: A clinical perspective* (2nd ed.). Philadelphia: Saunders.

Challis, J.R.G., & Lye, S.J. (2004) Characteristics of parturition. In R. Creasy, R. Resnik, & J.D. Iams (Eds.), *Maternal-fetal medicine: Principles and practice* (5th ed., pp. 79-87). Philadelphia: Saunders.

Cunningham, F.G., MacDonald, P.C., Gant, N.F., Leveno, K.J., Gilstrap, L.C., Hankins, G.D.V., et al. (2001). *Williams obstetrics* (21st ed.). New York: McGraw-Hill.

Cypher, R.L., & Adelsperger, D. (2003). Assessment of fetal oxygenation and acid-base status. In N. Feinstein, K.L. Torgersen, & J. Atterbury (Eds.), *AWHONN's fetal heart monitoring: Principles and practices* (3rd ed., pp. 177-198). Dubuque, IA: Kendall/Hunt.

Cypher, R.L., Adelsperger, D., & Torgersen, K.L. (2003). Interpretation of fetal heart rate patterns. In N. Feinstein, K.L. Torgersen, & J. Atterbury (Eds.), *AWHONN'S fetal heart monitoring: Principles and practices* (3rd ed., pp. 113-158). Dubuque, IA: Kendall/Hunt Publishing.

Feinstein, N.F. (2000). Fetal heart rate auscultation: Current and future practice. *Journal of Obstetric, Gynecologic, and Neonatal Nursing, 29*(3), 306-315.

Feinstein, N.F., Sprague, A., & Trépanier, M.J. (2000a). *AWHONN Symposium: Fetal heart rate auscultation.* Washington, DC: Author.

Feinstein, N.F., Sprague, A., & Trépanier, M.J. (2000b). Fetal heart rate auscultation. *AWHONN Lifelines, 4*(3), 35-44.

Garite, T.J., Dildy, G.A., McNamara, H., Nageotte, M.P., Boehm, F.H., Dellinger, E.H., et al. (2000). A multicenter controlled trial of fetal pulse oximetry in the intrapartum management of nonreassuring fetal heart rate patterns. *American Journal of Obstetrics & Gynecology, 183*(5), 1049-1058.

Gilstrap, L.C. (2004). Fetal acid-base balance. In R. Creasy, R. Resnik, & J.D. Iams (Eds.), *Maternal-fetal medicine: Principles and practice* (5th ed., pp. 429-439). Philadelphia: Saunders.

Glantz, J.C., & Woods, J.R. (2004). Significance of amniotic fluid meconium. In R. Creasy & R. Resnik (Eds.), *Maternal-fetal medicine: Principles and practice* (5th ed., pp. 441-450). Philadelphia: Saunders.

Gorenberg, D.M. (2003). Fetal pulse oximetry: Correlation between oxygen desaturation, duration, and frequency and neonatal outcomes. *American Journal of Obstetrics & Gynecology, 189*(1), 136-138.

Guyton, A.C., & Hall, J.E. (2000). *Textbook of medical physiology* (10th ed.). Philadelphia: Saunders.

Harman, C.R. (2004). Assessment of fetal health. In R.K. Creasy, R. Resnik, & J.D. Iams (Eds.), *Maternal-fetal medicine: Principles and practice* (5th ed., pp. 357-401). Philadelphia: Saunders.

King, T.L., & Simpson, K.R. (2001). Fetal assessment during labor. In K.R. Simpson & P.A. Creehan (Eds.), *AWHONN perinatal nursing* (2nd ed., pp. 378-416). Philadelphia: Lippincott Williams & Wilkins.

Mahoney, K., Torgersen, K.L., & Feinstein, N. (2003). Maternal-fetal assessment. In N. Feinstein, K.L. Torgersen, & J. Atterbury (Eds.), *AWHONN's fetal heart monitoring: Principles and practices* (3rd ed., pp. 61-76). Dubuque, IA: Kendall/Hunt.

334 **PART III** The Family during Birth

Martin, J.A., Hamilton, B.E., Sutton, P.D., Ventura, S.J., Menacker, F., & Munson, M.L. (2003). Births: Final data for 2002. *National Vital Statistics Reports, 50*(5). Hyattsville, MD: National Center for Health Statistics.

Moffatt, F.W., & Feinstein, N. (2003). Techniques for fetal heart assessment. In N. Feinstein, K.L. Torgersen, & J. Atterbury (Eds.), *AWHONN'S fetal heart monitoring: Principles and practices* (3rd ed., pp. 77-110). Dubuque, IA: Kendall/Hunt Publishing.

Murray, M.L. (2004). Maternal or fetal heart rate? Avoiding intrapartum misidentification. *Journal of Obstetrics, Gynecology, & Neonatal Nursing, 33*(1), 93-104.

National Institute of Child Health and Human Development Research Planning Workshop. (1997). Electronic fetal monitoring: Research guidelines for interpretation. *Journal of Obstetric, Gynecologic, and Neonatal Nursing, 26*(6), 635-640.

Parer, J., & Nageotte, M.P. (2004). Intrapartum fetal surveillance. In R. Creasy, R. Resnik, & J.D. Iams (Eds.), *Maternal-fetal medicine: Principles and practice* (5th ed., pp. 403-427). Philadelphia: Saunders.

Priddy, K.D. (2004). Is there logic behind fetal monitoring? *Journal of Obstetric, Gynecologic, and Neonatal Nursing, 33*(5), 550-553.

Simpson, K.R. (2003a). Fetal pulse oximetry update. *AWHONN Lifelines, 7*(5), 411-412.

Simpson, K.R. (2003b). Second opinion: Is fetal pulse oximetry ready for clinical practice? *MCN: American Journal of Maternal/Child Nursing, 28*(2), 64-65.

Simpson, K.R. (2004). Monitoring the preterm fetus during labor. *MCN: American Journal of Maternal/Child Nursing, 29*(6), 380-388.

Simpson, K.R., & Porter, M.L. (2001). Fetal oxygen saturation monitoring: Using this new technology for fetal assessment in labor. *AWHONN Lifelines, 5*(2), 27-33.

Stiller, R., von Mering, R., König, V., Huch, A., & Huch, R. (2002). How well does reflectance pulse oximetry reflect intrapartum fetal acidosis? *American Journal of Obstetrics & Gynecology, 186*(6), 1351-1357.

Williams, K.P., & Galerneau, F. (2003). Intrapartum fetal heart rate patterns in the prediction of neonatal acidemia. *American Journal of Obstetrics & Gynecology, 188*(3), 820-823.

Wood, S.H. (2003). Should women be given a choice about fetal assessment in labor? *MCN: American Journal of Maternal/Child Nursing, 28*(5), 292-298.

Pain Management during Childbirth

OBJECTIVES

After studying this chapter, you should be able to:

1. Compare childbirth pain with other types of pain.
2. Describe the way excessive pain can affect the laboring woman and her fetus.
3. Examine how physical and psychological forces interact in the laboring woman's pain experience.
4. Describe use of nonpharmacologic pain management techniques in labor.
5. Describe the way medications may affect a pregnant woman and the fetus or neonate.
6. Identify benefits and risks of specific pharmacologic pain control methods.
7. Explain nursing care related to different types of intrapartum pain management, both nonpharmacologic and pharmacologic.

Go to your Student CD-ROM for Review Questions keyed to these Objectives.

DEFINITIONS

Agonist Substance that causes a physiologic effect.

Analgesic Systemic agent that relieves pain without causing loss of consciousness.

Anesthesia Loss of sensation, especially to pain, with or without loss of consciousness.

Anesthesiologist Physician who specializes in administration of anesthesia.

Antagonist Drug that blocks the action of another drug or of body secretions.

Aspiration Pneumonitis Chemical injury to the lungs that may occur with regurgitation and aspiration of acidic gastric secretions.

Endorphin Substance similar to opioids that occurs naturally in the central nervous system and modifies pain sensations; related to enkephalins.

Enkephalin Substance similar to opioids that occurs naturally in the central nervous system and modifies pain sensations; related to endorphins.

Epidural Space Area outside the dura, between the dura mater and the vertebral canal.

Gate Control Theory A theory about pain based on the premise that a gating mechanism in the dorsal horn of the spinal cord can open or close a "gate" for transmission of pain impulses to the brain.

General Anesthesia Systemic loss of sensation with loss of consciousness.

Motor Block Loss of voluntary movement caused by regional anesthesia.

Nurse Anesthetist A registered nurse who has advanced education and certification in administration of anesthetics; also, certified registered nurse anesthetist (CRNA).

Pain Threshold (or Pain Perception) The lowest level of stimulus one perceives as painful; relatively constant under different conditions.

Pain Tolerance Maximum pain one is willing to endure. Pain tolerance may increase or decrease under different conditions.

Regional Anesthesia Anesthesia that blocks pain impulses in a localized area without loss of consciousness.

Sensory Block Loss of sensation caused by regional anesthesia.

Subarachnoid Space Space between the arachnoid mater and the pia mater containing cerebrospinal fluid.

Each woman has unique expectations about birth, including expectations about pain and her ability to manage it. The woman who successfully deals with the pain of labor is more likely to view her experience as a positive life event. A woman's experience with labor pain varies with several physical and psychological elements, and each woman responds differently. Nonpharmacologic and pharmacologic methods offer a selection of pain management techniques from which the laboring woman may choose.

UNIQUE NATURE OF PAIN DURING BIRTH

Pain is a universal experience but is difficult to define. It is an unpleasant sensation of distress resulting from stimulation of sensory nerves. Pain involves two components:

- A physiologic component including reception by sensory nerves and transmission to the central nervous system
- A psychological component, which involves recognizing the sensation, interpreting it as painful, and reacting to the interpretation

Pain is subjective and personal. No one can feel another's pain. Evidence of pain is a person's reaction to it. Childbirth pain, however, differs from other types of pain in several important respects:

- It is part of a normal process. Childbirth pain is part of a normal process, whereas other types of pain are connected with injury or illness. Pain may lead a woman to assume different positions in labor, favoring descent of the fetus through her pelvis.
- Preparation time exists. The pregnant woman has several months to prepare for labor, including acquiring skills to help manage pain. Realistic preparation and knowledge about the birth process help her develop skills to cope with labor pain.
- It is self-limiting. Labor pain has a foreseeable end. Although it is intense, a woman can expect her labor to end in hours, rather than days, weeks, or months. Other kinds of pain may also be brief, but the baby's birth brings a rapid decrease in pain.
- Labor pain is not constant but intermittent. A woman may describe little discomfort with contractions during early labor. Even during late labor, a woman may be relatively comfortable between contractions.
- Labor ends with the birth of a baby. The emotional significance of the child's birth cannot be ignored when trying to understand a woman's response to pain. Care about her fetus often motivates a woman to tolerate more pain during labor than she otherwise might be willing to endure.

ADVERSE EFFECTS OF EXCESSIVE PAIN

Although expected during labor, pain that exceeds a woman's tolerance can have harmful effects on her and the fetus.

Physiologic Effects

Excessive pain can heighten a woman's fear and anxiety, which stimulates sympathetic nervous system activity and results in increased secretion of catecholamines (epinephrine and norepinephrine). Catecholamines stimulate alpha and beta receptors, causing effects on the blood vessels and uterine muscles. Epinephrine stimulates both alpha and beta receptors, whereas norepinephrine stimulates primarily alpha receptors.

Stimulation of the alpha receptors causes uterine and generalized vasoconstriction and an increase in the uterine muscle tone. These effects reduce uterine blood flow as they raise the maternal blood pressure.

Stimulation of the beta receptors relaxes the uterine muscle and causes vasodilation. However, uterine vessels are already dilated in pregnancy, so dilation of other maternal vessels allows her blood to pool in them. The pooling of blood reduces the amount of blood available to perfuse the placenta.

The combined effects of excessive catecholamine secretion are therefore the following:

- Reduced blood flow to and from the placenta, restricting fetal oxygen supply and waste removal
- Reduced effectiveness of uterine contractions, slowing labor progress

Labor increases a woman's metabolic rate and her demand for oxygen. Pain and anxiety increase her already high metabolic rate. She breathes fast to obtain more oxygen, exhaling too much carbon dioxide in the process. Significant changes, more than those expected during labor, can occur in the woman's PaO_2 and $PaCO_2$ and in her arterial pH. These maternal respiratory and metabolic changes alter placental exchange. The fetus may have less oxygen available for uptake and have less ability to unload carbon dioxide to the mother. The net result is that the fetus shifts to anaerobic metabolism, with buildup of hydrogen ions (acidosis). This type of acidosis is metabolic and does not resolve as quickly after birth as respiratory acidosis, which results from shorter periods of hypoxia.

Psychological Effects

Poorly relieved pain lessens the pleasure of this extraordinary life event for both partners. The mother may find it difficult to interact with her infant because she is depleted from a painful labor. Unpleasant memories of the birth may affect her response to sexual activity or another labor. Her support person may feel inadequate during birth. The woman's partner may feel helpless and frustrated when her pain is unrelieved.

✔ CHECK YOUR READING

1. How does the pain of childbirth differ from other kinds of pain?
2. How can excessive pain adversely affect a laboring woman and her fetus?

VARIABLES IN CHILDBIRTH PAIN

A variety of physical and psychosocial factors contribute to a woman's pain response during labor. These factors provide possibilities for nursing interventions for pain relief.

Physical Factors

Childbirth pain is of two types—visceral and somatic. Visceral pain is a slow, deep, poorly localized pain that is often described as dull or aching. Visceral pain dominates during first-stage labor as the uterus contracts and the cervix dilates.

Somatic pain is a quick, sharp pain that can be precisely localized. Somatic pain is most prominent during late first-stage labor and during second-stage labor as the descending fetus puts direct pressure on maternal tissues.

SOURCES OF PAIN

Four sources of labor pain exist in most labors. Other physical factors may modify labor pain, increasing or decreasing it.

TISSUE ISCHEMIA. The blood supply to the uterus decreases during contractions, leading to tissue hypoxia and anaerobic metabolism. Ischemic uterine pain has been likened to ischemic heart pain.

CERVICAL DILATION. Dilation and stretching of the cervix and lower uterus are a major source of pain. Pain stimuli from cervical dilation travel through the hypogastric plexus, entering the spinal cord at the T10, T11, T12, and L1 levels (Figure 15-1).

PRESSURE AND PULLING ON PELVIC STRUC-TURES. Some pain results from pressure and pulling on pelvic structures, such as ligaments, fallopian tubes, ovaries, bladder, and peritoneum. The pain is a visceral pain; a woman may feel it as referred pain in her back and legs.

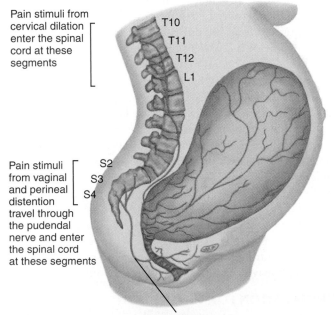

Pain stimuli from cervical dilation enter the spinal cord at these segments

T10
T11
T12
L1

Pain stimuli from vaginal and perineal distention travel through the pudendal nerve and enter the spinal cord at these segments

S2
S3
S4

Pudendal nerve

Figure 15-1 ■ Pathways of pain transmission during labor.

DISTENTION OF THE VAGINA AND PERINEUM. Marked distention of the vagina and perineum occurs with fetal descent, especially during the second stage. The woman may describe a sensation of burning, tearing, or splitting (somatic pain). Pain from vaginal and perineal distention and pressure and pulling on adjacent structures enters the spinal cord at the S2, S3, and S4 levels (see Figure 15-1).

FACTORS INFLUENCING PERCEPTION OR TOLERANCE OF PAIN

Although physiologic processes cause labor pain, a woman's tolerance of pain is affected by other physical influences.

INTENSITY OF LABOR. The woman who has a short, intense labor may complain of severe pain because each contraction does so much work (effacement, dilation, and fetal descent). A rapid labor may limit her options for pharmacologic pain relief as well.

CERVICAL READINESS. If prelabor cervical changes (softening, with some dilation and effacement) are incomplete, the cervix does not open as easily as it does when it is soft and dilation and effacement have begun. More contractions are needed to achieve dilation and effacement, resulting in a longer labor and greater fatigue in the laboring woman.

FETAL POSITION. Labor is likely to be longer and more uncomfortable when the fetus is in an unfavorable position. An occiput posterior position is a common variant seen in otherwise normal labors. In this position, each contraction pushes the fetal occiput against the woman's sacrum. She experiences intense back discomfort (back labor) that persists between contractions. A woman may not be able to deliver her baby until it rotates to the occiput anterior position. The fetal head must therefore rotate a wider arc before the mechanisms of extension and expulsion occur, so labor is often longer (see Figure 12-12). Back pain may decrease dramatically when a fetus rotates into the more favorable position. The rate of labor progress usually increases as well.

CHARACTERISTICS OF THE PELVIS. The size and shape of a woman's pelvis influence the course and length of her labor. Abnormalities may cause a difficult and longer labor and may contribute to fetal malpresentation or malposition.

FATIGUE AND HUNGER. Fatigue reduces a woman's ability to tolerate pain and to use coping skills she has learned. She may be unable to focus on techniques that would otherwise help her tolerate labor. An extremely fatigued woman may have an exaggerated response to contractions, or she may be unable to respond to sensations of labor such as the urge to push. Because oral intake is limited, her energy reserves are also likely to be depleted in a long labor.

Many women find that sleep is difficult during the last weeks of pregnancy. A woman's shortness of breath when lying down, frequent urination, and fetal activity interrupt sleep so that she often begins labor with a sleep deficit. If labor begins late in the evening, she may have been awake more than

24 hours by the time she gives birth. Even if a woman begins labor well rested, slow progress may exhaust her.

INTERVENTION OF CAREGIVERS. Although they may be appropriate for the well-being of a woman and fetus, some interventions add discomfort to the natural pain of labor.

Intravenous (IV) lines cause pain when inserted and remain noticeable to many women during labor. Fetal monitoring equipment is uncomfortable to some women. Both may hamper a woman's mobility, which she might use to assume a more comfortable position.

A woman whose labor is induced or augmented often reports more pain and increased difficulty coping with it because contractions reach peak intensity quickly. Vaginal examinations, amniotomy, and insertion of internal fetal monitoring devices also increase a woman's discomfort briefly because of vaginal and cervical stretching. Vaginal manipulation often stimulates a contraction because of a reflex known as *Ferguson's reflex.*

Psychosocial Factors

Several psychosocial variables influence a woman's experience of pain.

CULTURE

A woman's sociocultural roots influence how she perceives, interprets, and responds to pain during childbirth. Some cultures encourage loud and vigorous expression of pain, whereas others value self-control. However, women are individuals within their cultural groups. The experience of pain is personal, and caregivers should not make assumptions about how a woman will behave during labor.

Women should be encouraged to express themselves in any way they find comforting, and the diversity of their expressions must be respected. Accepting a woman's individual response to labor and pain promotes a therapeutic relationship.

The nurse should avoid praising some behaviors (such as stoicism) while belittling others (such as noisy expression). This restraint is difficult because noisy women are challenging to work with and may disturb others.

CRITICAL THINKING ✍ EXERCISE 15-1

Truc Pham is a Vietnamese-American in labor with her first baby. Her cervix is dilated 6 cm, effacement is 100%, and the fetus is at a +1 station. Truc's contractions occur every 3 minutes, last 50 to 60 seconds, and are of strong intensity. She smiles at the nurse each time the nurse talks to her but does not talk much herself. Truc stiffens her body during contractions and interacts little with her husband or the nurse at those times.

Questions
1. How should the nurse interpret Truc's assessment and behavior?
2. Does the nurse need additional data?
3. What nursing actions are appropriate?

The unique nature of childbirth pain and women's diverse responses to it make nursing management complex. The nurse can miss important cues if the woman is either stoic or outspoken about her pain. With either extreme the nurse may not readily identify critical information such as impending birth or symptoms of a complication.

ANXIETY AND FEAR

Mild or moderate anxiety can enhance attention and learning. However, high anxiety and fear magnify sensitivity to pain and impair a woman's ability to tolerate it. They consume energy she needs to cope with the birth process, including its painful aspects.

Anxiety and fear increase muscle tension, diverting oxygenated blood to the brain and skeletal muscles. Tension in pelvic muscles counters the expulsive forces of uterine contractions and the laboring woman's pushing. Prolonged tension results in general fatigue, increased pain perception, and reduced ability to use skills to cope with pain.

If a previous pregnancy had a poor outcome, such as a stillborn infant or one with abnormalities, a woman is probably more anxious during labor and for a time after birth. She is likely to examine and reexamine her infant to assure herself that this baby is normal.

PREVIOUS EXPERIENCES WITH PAIN

Early in life a child learns that pain means bodily injury. Consequently, fear and withdrawal are a woman's natural reactions to pain during labor. Learning about the normal sensations of labor, including pain, helps a woman suppress her natural reactions of fear and withdrawal, allowing her body to do the work of birth.

A woman who has given birth previously has a different perspective. If she has had a vaginal delivery, she is probably aware of normal labor sensations and is less likely to associate them with injury or abnormality. Also, time has a way of blunting the memory of painful experiences. A woman who had a previous long and difficult labor may be anxious about the outcome of the present one. She may be surprised that her second labor moves more quickly than her first.

Fewer women today have the option of choosing vaginal birth after cesarean (VBAC). However, a woman who plans a VBAC but has never experienced labor may be particularly anxious. The experience of cesarean birth is known to her, even if she does not want to repeat it, whereas labor is unknown. A repeat cesarean birth may seem to be the quicker and less painful option at times, yet she strongly prefers to have a "normal" vaginal birth if possible. She may have difficulty yielding to the normal forces of birth.

Previous experiences may positively affect a woman's ability to deal with pain. She may have learned ways to cope with pain during other episodes of pain or during other births and may use these skills adaptively during labor.

PREPARATION FOR CHILDBIRTH

Preparation for childbirth does not ensure a pain-free labor. A woman should be prepared for pain realistically, including reasonable expectations about analgesia and anesthesia.

She may feel that unexpected events during labor may invalidate her childbirth preparation.

Preparation reduces anxiety and fear of the unknown. It allows a woman to rehearse for labor and learn a variety of skills to master pain as labor progresses. She and her partner learn about expected behavioral changes during labor, and their knowledge decreases their anxiety when those changes occur.

SUPPORT SYSTEM

An anxious partner is less able to provide the support and reassurance that the woman needs during labor. In addition, anxiety in others can be contagious, increasing her anxiety. She may assume that if others are worried, something is wrong.

The birth experiences of a woman's family and friends cannot be ignored. Those individuals can be an important source of support if they express realistic information about labor pain and its control. If they describe labor as intolerable, however, she may have needless distress. Hearing that labor is painless is equally detrimental. No two labors are alike, even in the same woman.

✔ CHECK YOUR READING

3. How may physical and psychological factors interact in a woman's labor pain experience?
4. What four sources of pain are present in most labors?
5. How can each of these physical factors influence the pain a woman experiences during childbirth: (a) Labor intensity? (b) Cervical readiness? (c) Fetal position? (d) Maternal pelvis? (e) Fatigue?
6. How do psychosocial factors influence a woman's experience with labor pain?

STANDARDS FOR PAIN MANAGEMENT

The Joint Commission on Accreditation of Healthcare Organizations (JCAHO) has recognized that pain management is an essential part of the care of all clients in health care settings. The organization has added a number of explicit pain management standards related to the following:

- The rights of all patients to pain management
- Staff competency in pain assessment and management
- Establishment of policies and procedures that support prescription of appropriate pain medications
- Education of patients and families about effective pain management
- Discharge planning related to pain management

NONPHARMACOLOGIC PAIN MANAGEMENT

The nurse who cares for women in labor and birth can offer many nonpharmacologic and pharmacologic pain management methods. Education about nonpharmacologic pain management is the foundation of prepared childbirth classes. Most women use these methods to complement pharmacologic methods, although some use them as their only pain management techniques.

To be most helpful to women and their labor partners, the intrapartum nurse should know methods that are taught in local childbirth classes. Teaching techniques during labor that conflict with what a woman learned and practiced may confuse her. Other techniques can be reserved for use if a woman finds learned techniques ineffective.

Advantages

Nonpharmacologic methods have several advantages over pharmacologic methods if pain control is adequate. They do not slow labor and have no side effects or risk of allergy.

The woman who chooses analgesia needs alternate pain management until she receives it, usually after labor is established. Also, some pharmacologic methods may not eliminate labor pain, and a woman needs these techniques to control the pain that remains, even if it is greatly reduced.

Nonpharmacologic methods may be the only realistic option for a woman who enters the hospital in advanced, rapid labor. Drugs might not have enough time to take effect, or there may not be time needed to administer an effective epidural block before birth. The time of peak drug action in terms of newborn respiratory effort must be considered if an analgesic drug is given.

Limitations

Nonpharmacologic methods also have limitations, especially as the sole method of pain control. Women do not always achieve their desired level of pain control using these methods alone. Because of the many variables in labor, even a well-prepared and highly motivated woman may have a difficult labor and need analgesia or anesthesia.

Gate Control Theory

A discussion of nonpharmacologic pain management techniques would not be complete without discussion of the gate control theory of pain. According to this theory, transmission of nerve impulses is controlled by a neural mechanism in the dorsal horn of the spinal cord that acts like a gate to control impulses transmitted to the brain. Transmission is affected by stimulation of large- or small-diameter sensory nerve fibers and descending impulses from the brain. This mechanism opens or closes the "gate" to pain sensation by allowing or preventing some impulses from reaching the brain, where they are recognized as pain.

Pain is transmitted through small-diameter sensory nerve fibers. Stimulation of large-diameter fibers in the skin blocks conduction of pain through small-diameter fibers, thereby "closing the gate" and decreasing the amount of pain felt. Examples of this stimulation include tactile stimulation such as massage, thermal stimulation, or hydrotherapy.

Impulses from the brain have a similar ability to impede transmission through the dorsal horn using visual and auditory stimulation techniques. Examples of visual or auditory stimulation include use of a focal point or breathing techniques.

Memory and cognitive processes affect the perception of stimuli as painful. Education and support during labor are used to increase the woman's relaxation, confidence, and feeling of control. Although these methods may not completely prevent pain, they may decrease the severity of perceived pain (Creehan, 2001).

Preparation for Pain Management

The ideal time to prepare for nonpharmacologic pain control is before labor. During the last few weeks of pregnancy, the woman learns about labor, including its painful aspects, in childbirth classes. She can prepare to confront the pain, learning a variety of skills to use during labor. Her support person learns specific methods to encourage and support her. After admission, the nurse can review and reinforce what the partners learned in class.

The nurse can teach the unprepared woman and her support person nonpharmacologic techniques. The latent phase of labor is the best time for intrapartum teaching because the woman is usually anxious enough to be attentive and interested, yet comfortable enough to understand. The nurse must usually teach one contraction at a time during late labor because the woman's focus is very narrow.

No one method or combination of methods helps every woman. Most methods may become less effective (habituation) after prolonged use, and changing techniques counters this problem. Knowing a variety of methods gives the nurse a selection.

Application of Nonpharmacologic Techniques

Techniques that can be applied during labor include relaxation, cutaneous stimulation, hydrotherapy, mental stimulation, and breathing techniques.

RELAXATION

Promoting relaxation is a basis for all other methods, both nonpharmacologic and pharmacologic, because it does the following:

- Promotes uterine blood flow, improving fetal oxygenation
- Promotes efficient uterine contractions
- Reduces tension that increases pain perception and decreases pain tolerance
- Reduces tension that can inhibit fetal descent

ENVIRONMENTAL COMFORT. Comfortable surroundings support relaxation. The nurse can reduce irritants such as bright lights and uncomfortable temperature and can change soiled underpads.

Music masks outside noise and provides a background for use of imagery and breathing techniques. This distraction shifts the woman's attention from pain perception. Television has a similar effect for some women.

GENERAL COMFORT. Promoting the woman's personal comfort helps her focus on using pain management techniques during labor (Figure 15-2). This includes actions to increase comfort and reduce the effects of irritants.

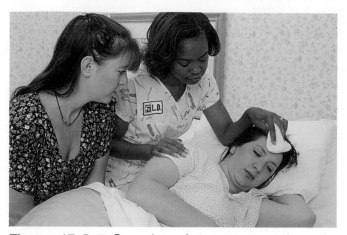

Figure 15-2 ■ General comfort measures such as the nurse's reassuring presence or a cool cloth to the face supplement other methods of nonpharmacologic and pharmacologic pain control.

REDUCING ANXIETY AND FEAR. The nurse may reduce a woman's anxiety and increase her self-control by providing accurate information and focusing on birth as a normal process. Simple nursing actions keep the focus on the normality of childbirth. For example, calling the woman by her name rather than calling her a "patient" (implying "sick") helps her to see birth as a normal process. Empowering the woman by giving her choices whenever possible helps her to see herself as competent and capable of giving birth.

IMPLEMENTING SPECIFIC RELAXATION TECHNIQUES. Many techniques discussed in Chapters 11 and 13 are most successful if practiced before labor. However, during labor, caregivers can watch a woman for signs of tension and help her focus on relaxing tense muscles. Her partner often recognizes subtle signs of tension and can be guided to massage the area or call attention to the tension, thereby helping the laboring woman to release it. Pillows that provide support for extremities are positioned for minimal tension.

CUTANEOUS STIMULATION

Cutaneous stimulation has several variations that are often combined with each other or with other techniques.

SELF-MASSAGE. The woman may rub her abdomen, legs, or back during labor (effleurage) to counteract discomfort. Some women find abdominal touch irritating, especially near the umbilicus. Women in labor may find firm stroking more helpful than light stroking (see Figure 11-6).

Some women benefit from firm palm or sole stimulation during labor. They may like someone to rub their palms vigorously; independently to rub their hands or feet together; or to bang their palms on or grip a cool surface. They may hold another's hand tightly during a contraction. The nurse should determine if these actions indicate excess pain or if they are a woman's way of countering pain and therefore useful.

MASSAGE BY OTHERS. Massage increases circulation and reduces muscle tension. The support person or nurse can rub the woman's back, shoulders, legs, or any area where she finds massage helpful. Body powder on the skin

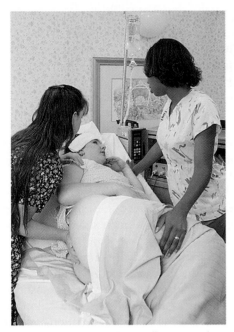

Figure 15-3 ■ The coach applies sacral pressure to counter back pain, common during labor.

BOX **15-1** Benefits and Cautions Related to Hydrotherapy during Labor

Benefits
Promotes relaxation; reduces muscle spasms and cramps
Reduces stress resulting in catecholamine secretion
Promotes a sense of well-being
Reduces pain by increasing pain threshold
Reduces pressure of abdominal muscles on uterus, reducing pain
Upright position favors fetal descent
Buoyancy allows greater freedom of movement
Nipple stimulation promotes oxytocin stimulation from the posterior pituitary
Reduces blood pressure by causing diuresis

Cautions
Hydrotherapy may slow labor if used during the latent phase but is useful if the woman needs rest and relaxation. During active labor, nipple stimulation from whirlpool bubbles or shower spray causes natural oxytocin secretion that can stimulate contractions. If contractions become hypertonic, remove nipples from the stimulating water.
Water temperature should be maintained between 35° and 37.8° C (95° and 100° F) to avoid maternal hyperthermia or hypothermia, each of which could increase her metabolic rate, reducing fetal oxygen supply and increasing glucose demand.
The woman should have generous hydration to prevent dehydration from the diuresis that occurs with water immersion.
A nurse or support person should remain with the woman while she is in the tub. Underwater birth may not be planned in the facility, but labor could proceed rapidly with relaxation and pain relief. If birth occurs, bring the infant immediately, but gently, to the surface. Cut the cord outside the water.
Have a shower chair available to the woman if she uses a shower.
Clean tubs with hospital-approved germicide between uses, ensuring that it circulates through whirlpool jets and filters. Culture equipment periodically.

From Kabler, J. (2000). Water immersion during labor and birth. In *Childbirth education: Practice, research, and theory* (2nd ed., pp. 284-294). Philadelphia: Saunders; and Teschendorf, M.E., & Evans, C.P. (2000). Hydrotherapy during labor: An example of developing a practice policy. *MCN: American Journal of Maternal/Child Nursing, 25*(4), 198-203.

reduces friction during massage. Powder should be kept away from the nose and mouth of the newborn.

COUNTERPRESSURE. Sacral pressure may help when the woman has back pain, usually most intense when her fetus is in an occiput posterior position. Sacral pressure may be applied using the palm of the hand, the fist or fists, or a firm object such as two tennis balls in a sock (Figure 15-3). A variation of sacral pressure is a double hip squeeze, in which the palms are placed on the woman's hips and pressed down and inward toward the symphysis (Simkin & Frederick, 2000). When pressure is used, the woman should guide the support person as to the exact location and amount of pressure.

TOUCH. Nonclinical touch by the nurse is a powerful tool if the woman does not object to it. Holding her hand, stroking her hair, or similar actions convey caring, comfort, affirmation, and reassurance at this vulnerable time.

THERMAL STIMULATION. Many women appreciate warmth applied to the back, abdomen, or perineum during labor. Warmth increases local blood flow, relaxes muscles, and raises the pain threshold. Massage is often more comfortable to a tense woman after her skin is warmed (Simkin & Frederick, 2000). A sock filled with dry rice and microwaved provides gentle warmth and can be used to apply warm pressure to the sacral area.

Cool, damp washcloths provide comforting coolness if the woman feels hot. She may put them on her head, throat, abdomen, or any place she wants. She also may want to put them in her mouth to relieve dryness. Ice chips cool the mouth and provide hydration.

HYDROTHERAPY

A shower, tub bath, or whirlpool bath is relaxing and provides thermal stimulation. Several studies have shown benefits of water therapy during labor, including immersion in a tub or whirlpool (jet hydrotherapy, or Jacuzzi). The major concern about immersion therapy has been newborn and postpartum maternal infections caused by microorganisms in the water. The organisms may be from ascending vaginal organisms or organisms from previous births if the tub has not been cleaned properly between births. However, several studies have not found a significant association between newborn or postpartum maternal infections and use of immersion hydrotherapy with proper cleaning (Kabler, 2000; Teschendorf & Evans, 2000). More research is needed to clarify both the benefits and the concerns about hydrotherapy (Box 15-1). Facility policies should be written to outline specific guidelines based on most recent evidence for use of hydrotherapy.

MENTAL STIMULATION

Mental techniques occupy the woman's mind and compete with pain stimuli. They also aid relaxation by providing a tranquil imaginary atmosphere.

IMAGERY. If the woman has not practiced a specific imagery technique, the nurse can help her create a relaxing mental scene. Most women find images of warmth, softness, security, and total relaxation most comforting.

Imagery can help the woman dissociate herself from the painful aspects of labor. For example, the nurse can help her visualize the work of labor: the cervix opening with each contraction or the fetus moving down toward the outlet each time she pushes. This technique is like visualizing success or movement toward a goal with each contraction. The nurse can help the woman visualize being in a pleasant and relaxing place.

FOCAL POINT. When using nonpharmacologic techniques, a woman may prefer to close her eyes or may want to concentrate on an external focal point. Classes may emphasize that keeping the eyes open on a focal point helps her concentrate on something outside her body and thus away from the pain of contractions. She may bring a picture of a relaxing scene or an object to use as a focal point and to aid in the use of imagery. She can use any point in her room as a focal point.

✔ CHECK YOUR READING

7. How does the gate control theory of pain relate to non-pharmacologic methods of pain control?
8. What are some nursing actions to encourage relaxation during labor?
9. How can the nurse reduce a laboring woman's anxiety or fear?
10. How might each of these cutaneous stimulation techniques be used to aid relaxation during labor: Self-massage? Massage by others? Counterpressure? Warmth or cold?
11. When hydrotherapy is used during labor, why are cautions related to the following required: Adequate maternal hydration? Control of water temperature?

BREATHING TECHNIQUES

Breathing techniques give a woman a different focus during contractions, interfering with pain sensory transmission (Figure 15-4). They begin with simple patterns and progress to more complex ones as greater distraction is needed. No universal right time exists to change patterns during labor. However, complex patterns are fatiguing if used for a long time.

For best results, the woman and her partner must practice the techniques frequently. If patterns are too complicated or if the woman has not practiced, they may not be helpful during labor. Breathing techniques should be used only when needed, usually when the woman can no longer walk or talk during a contraction. The woman should not change from a simpler technique to the next, more complex, technique until necessary so that use of the most complex techniques is limited to the shortest time possible.

FIRST-STAGE BREATHING. Breathing in the first stage of labor consists of a cleansing breath and progressively more complex techniques of paced breathing.

Taking a Cleansing Breath. Each contraction begins and ends with a deep inspiration and expiration known as the *cleansing breath*. Like a sigh, a cleansing breath helps the woman release tension. It provides oxygen to help reduce myometrial hypoxia, one cause of pain in labor. The cleansing breath also helps the woman clear her mind to focus on relaxing and signals her labor partner that the contraction is beginning or ending. The woman may inhale through the nose and exhale through the mouth or take her cleansing breath in any way comfortable for her. When electronic monitors are used, a partner may help ease the discomfort of rapid contractions by watching for the rise in the lower part of the strip that signals the beginning of the contraction and telling the woman to take a cleansing breath.

Slow-Paced Breathing. The first breathing is slow-paced breathing, a slow, deep breathing that increases relaxation (Figure 15-5). The woman should concentrate on relaxing her body rather than on regulating the rate of her breathing. Relaxation naturally brings about slower breathing, similar to that during sleep. She can use nose, mouth, or a combination, depending on which is most comfortable.

Slow-paced breathing should be used as long as possible during labor because it promotes relaxation and oxygenation. Labor nurses often teach the technique to women who enter labor unprepared. It is easy to learn between contractions and, with the support of the nurse, helps even a frightened woman become calm and able to work with her contractions.

As with all techniques, variety prevents habituation. Adding other pain-relief approaches such as effleurage may help prolong the effectiveness of slow-paced breathing. Using another type of breathing for a short time may allow the woman to return to slower breathing again later.

Modified-Paced Breathing. When slow-paced breathing is no longer effective, the woman begins modified-paced breathing (Figure 15-6). This chest breathing at a faster rate matches the natural tendency to use more rapid breathing during stress or physical work, such as labor. Although modified-paced breathing is more shallow than slow-paced breathing, the faster rate allows oxygen intake to remain about the same. As with slow-paced breathing, the focus is on release of tension rather than on the actual number of breaths taken.

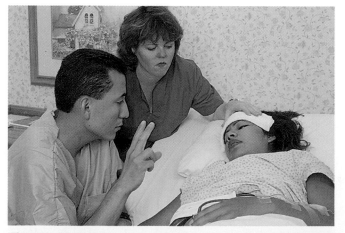

Figure 15-4 ■ A woman and her partner who are prepared for labor have learned a variety of skills to master pain as labor progresses. The coach uses hand signals to tell the woman how to change her pattern of paced breathing.

Women sometimes learn to combine slow and modified-paced breathing during a contraction (Figure 15-7). They begin slowly and use shallow, faster breathing over the peak of the contraction. During labor, women often do this naturally. The most important concern is that the breathing not interfere with relaxation but enhance it.

Patterned-Paced Breathing. Patterned-paced breathing (sometimes called *pant-blow breathing*) involves focusing on the pattern of breathing (Figure 15-8). It is similar to modified-paced breathing. After a certain number of breaths, however,

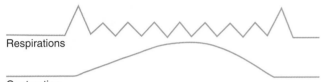

Figure 15-5 ■ Slow-paced breathing. Although a specific rate may or may not be used, slow-paced breathing should be *no slower than half* the woman's usual respiratory rate to ensure adequate oxygenation. This pace is generally about six to nine breaths per minute.

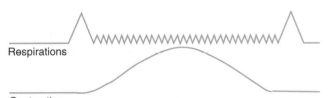

Figure 15-6 ■ Modified-paced breathing. The pattern for modified-paced breathing should be comfortable to the woman and *no faster than twice* her normal respiratory rate to prevent hyperventilation or interference with relaxation.

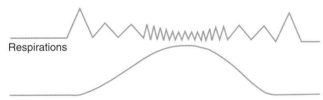

Figure 15-7 ■ Combining techniques. Slow and modified-paced breathing can be combined by using the slower breathing at the beginning and end of the contraction and the more rapid breathing over the peak of the contraction.

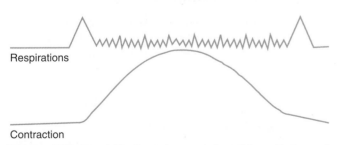

Figure 15-8 ■ Patterned-paced breathing. Patterned-paced breathing adds a slight emphasis or "blow" on the exhalation in a pattern. The diagram shows the emphasis after every third inhalation.

the woman exhales with a slight emphasis or blow and then begins the modified-paced breathing again. This addition causes her to focus more on her breathing and reduces habituation. The mouth should remain relaxed, and the woman should not try to make specific sounds that would tighten her vocal cords. Relaxation of her entire body is the goal.

The number of breaths before the blow may remain constant (usually between two and six) or may change in a pattern. Variations include a set pattern such as "3-1, 5-1, 3-1" or a decreasing, "stair-step," pattern such as "6-1, 5-1, 4-1, 3-1." Some couples use a random pattern determined by the coach, who uses hand signals to show the number of breaths the woman should take before each blow. The coach holds up fingers to show the total breaths to be taken or a single finger for each breath. Use of the random pattern, however, may be ineffective without sufficient practice to enable the two to work together well.

Breathing to Prevent Pushing. If a woman pushes strenuously before the cervix is completely dilated, she risks injury to her cervix and the fetal head. Blowing prevents closure of the glottis and breath holding, helping to overcome the urge to push strenuously. The woman blows repeatedly using short puffs when the urge to push is strong. The support person may learn to blow along with her to help the woman concentrate. Some women vary the blowing by using one short breath and one blow.

Overcoming Common Problems. Hyperventilation and mouth dryness are common when breathing techniques are used. Hyperventilation results from rapid deep breathing that causes excessive loss of carbon dioxide and therefore respiratory alkalosis. The woman may feel dizzy or lightheaded and may have impaired thinking. Vasoconstriction leads to tingling and numbness in fingers and lips. If hyperventilation continues, tetany resulting from decreased calcium in tissues and blood may result in stiffness of the face and lips and carpopedal spasm.

Women are taught to blow into a paper bag or their own cupped hands if they begin to feel dizzy. This kind of blowing increases the carbon dioxide levels by having the woman rebreathe her exhaled air. The woman should slow her rate of breathing to reduce the loss of carbon dioxide.

The woman's mouth becomes dry with prolonged mouth breathing. To avoid dryness, she can place her tongue gently against the roof of her mouth to moisturize entering air. The support person can offer ice, mouthwash, sugarless suckers, or liquids if they are allowed.

SECOND-STAGE BREATHING Care in the second stage of labor encourages a physiologic completion of labor, assisting the mother to respond to her urge to push rather than directing her to push as soon as her cervix is completely dilated even if she does not feel the urge. Lengthy pushing in second stage has been shown to result in greater maternal fatigue, more operative births, and nonreassuring fetal heart rate (FHR) patterns and does not significantly shorten the second stage (Mayberry et al., 2000).

With newer techniques of epidural block, women who choose this method of labor pain control often feel the urge to push, although not as strongly as unmedicated women.

Using their natural urge to push, even if reduced, helps them push with contractions most effectively. Delaying pushing for up to 1 to 2 hours after complete dilation has shown benefits similar to those in women who do not have epidural analgesia.

Prolonged breath-holding while pushing (more than 6 to 8 seconds) with a closed glottis involves use of the Valsalva maneuver. Closed-glottis pushing causes recurrent increases in intrathoracic pressure with a resulting fall in cardiac output and blood pressure. The woman's lower blood pressure then causes less blood to be delivered to the placenta, resulting in fetal hypoxia that is reflected in nonreassuring fetal heart patterns. Repeating this pushing technique more than 4 times per contraction further increases the adverse effects.

Promoting a physiologic second stage involves several variations of breathing rather than a specific technique. The woman may grunt, groan, sigh, or moan as she pushes, and the nurse should validate that these sounds are normal. Either open-glottis pushing or limiting breath-holding to under 6 to 8 seconds promotes best fetal oxygenation.

✔ CHECK YOUR READING

12. Why is it important to avoid advancing to more complex breathing techniques sooner than needed?
13. What is the purpose of a cleansing breath?

PHARMACOLOGIC PAIN MANAGEMENT

Most laboring women want pharmacologic pain relief, even if they use nonpharmacologic methods. Pharmacologic methods for pain management include systemic drugs, regional pain management techniques, and general anesthesia.

Special Considerations for Medicating a Pregnant Woman

Medicating a woman when she is pregnant is not as simple as before pregnancy, for the following reasons:
- Any drug taken by the woman is likely to affect her fetus.
- Drugs may have effects in pregnancy that they do not have in the nonpregnant person.
- Drugs can affect the course and length of labor.
- Pregnancy complications may limit the choice of pharmacologic pain management methods.
- Women who require other therapeutic drugs, use herbal or botanical preparations, or practice substance abuse may have fewer safe choices for pain relief.

EFFECTS ON THE FETUS

Effects on the fetus of drugs given to the mother may be direct, resulting from passage of the drug or its metabolites across the placenta to the fetus. An example of a direct effect on the fetus is decreased FHR variability after administration of an analgesic to the woman.

Effects on the fetus may be indirect, or secondary to drug effects in the mother. For example, if a drug causes maternal hypotension, blood flow to the placenta is reduced. Fetal hypoxia and acidosis may result.

MATERNAL PHYSIOLOGIC ALTERATIONS

Normal pregnancy changes in four body systems have the greatest implications for pharmacologic pain management methods.

CARDIOVASCULAR CHANGES. Compression of the aorta and inferior vena cava by the uterus can occur when a woman lies in the supine position (aortocaval compression). If the woman must be in the supine position temporarily, the uterus is displaced to one side with the hands or with a small wedge or towel roll under one hip. Displacement is often to the left (left uterine displacement, or LUD). Operating room tables are often tilted slightly to one side for a cesarean birth to provide the uterine displacement.

RESPIRATORY CHANGES. A pregnant woman's full uterus reduces her respiratory capacity. To compensate she breathes more rapidly and deeply. As a result she is more vulnerable to reduced arterial oxygenation during induction of general anesthesia and is more sensitive to inhalational anesthetic agents. The normal edema of pregnancy is also present in her upper airways and may present difficulty if she must be intubated for general anesthesia.

GASTROINTESTINAL CHANGES. A pregnant woman's stomach is displaced upward by her large uterus and has a higher internal pressure. Progesterone slows peristalsis and reduces the tone of the sphincter at the junction of the stomach and esophagus. These changes make a pregnant woman vulnerable to regurgitation and aspiration of gastric contents during general anesthesia.

NERVOUS SYSTEM CHANGES. During pregnancy and labor, circulating levels of endorphins and enkephalins, natural substances with analgesic properties, are high. These substances modify pain perception and reduce requirements for analgesia and anesthesia.

The epidural and subarachnoid spaces are smaller during pregnancy, enhancing the spread of anesthetic agents used for epidural blocks or subarachnoid blocks (SABs). Cerebrospinal fluid (CSF) pressure is higher during a contraction and when the woman is pushing. Nerve fibers are more sensitive to local anesthetic agents. High intraabdominal pressure causes engorgement of the epidural veins, increasing the risk for intravascular injection of anesthetic agents. The net result of these changes is that a reduced volume of local anesthetic is needed to achieve satisfactory epidural block or SAB.

EFFECTS ON THE COURSE OF LABOR

Ideally, analgesics are given when labor is well established to avoid slowing progress. However, caregivers must consider the adverse effects of excessive pain on labor progress, regardless of the cervical dilation. Regional analgesia, primarily the epidural block, can slow progress during the second stage by impairing the laboring woman's natural urge to push.

EFFECTS OF COMPLICATIONS

Complications during pregnancy may limit the choices of analgesia or anesthesia. For example, large volumes of IV fluids are infused to prevent hypotension with regional analgesia and anesthesia. If a pregnant woman has heart disease, this fluid load could be detrimental. Yet without it, she is vulnerable to hypotension.

INTERACTIONS WITH OTHER SUBSTANCES

A woman who ingests drugs (therapeutic, over-the-counter, or illicit), herbal or botanical preparations, or other substances may have fewer options because of interactions between these substances and analgesics or anesthetics. For example, recent alcohol use increases the depressant effects of opioid analgesics, making both the mother and newborn susceptible to respiratory depression.

✔ CHECK YOUR READING

14. How can drugs taken by the expectant mother affect the fetus?
15. How do changes in the following maternal body systems affect pharmacologic pain management: Cardiovascular system? Respiratory system? Gastrointestinal system? Nervous system?
16. Why is it important to know about a woman's intake of drugs, botanical medicines, legal substances (such as alcohol), and illegal drugs?

Regional Pain Management Techniques

Regional pain control methods may be used for intrapartum analgesia, surgical anesthesia, or both. These methods provide pain relief without loss of consciousness. Depending on the specific technique, it may be used for only labor, for only birth, or for both labor and birth.

Epidural block provides pain control during much of labor and for the birth itself. Intrathecal opioids are used for pain control during labor; additional measures are needed during late labor and for the birth. Another regional block, the SAB, is used only at birth. A newer technique, combined spinal-epidural (CSE) analgesia, allows subarachnoid injection of opioids via a spinal needle followed by ongoing pain relief from anesthetics injected through the epidural catheter.

The major advantage of regional pain management methods is that the woman can participate in birth yet have good pain control. The woman usually feels some pressure and discomfort, although these sensations are greatly reduced. She does not lose her protective airway reflexes, as can happen with general anesthesia. Disadvantages depend on the specific technique. The effects on the fetus depend primarily on how the woman responds rather than on direct drug effects.

EPIDURAL BLOCK

The lumbar epidural block is a popular regional block that provides analgesia and anesthesia for labor and birth without sedation of the woman and fetus. It is used for both vaginal and cesarean births. Epidural blocks are started and maintained by an anesthesiologist or nurse-anesthetist. The obstetrician may do this, but this is becoming less common.

The epidural space is outside the dura mater, between the dura and the spinal canal. It is loosely filled with fat, connective tissue, and epidural veins that are dilated during pregnancy (Figure 15-9).

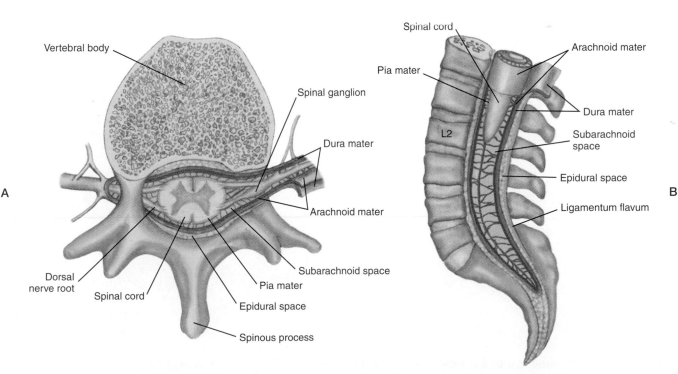

Figure 15-9 ■ **A,** Cross-section of spinal cord, meninges, and protective vertebra. The dura and arachnoid lie close together. The pia mater is the innermost of the meninges and covers the brain and spinal cord. The subarachnoid space is between the arachnoid and pia mater. **B,** Sagittal section of spinal cord, meninges, and vertebrae. The epidural and subarachnoid spaces are illustrated. Note that the spinal cord ends at the L2 vertebra.

An epidural block is performed by injecting local anesthetic agent, usually combined with an opioid, into the tiny epidural space. It provides substantial relief of pain from contractions and birth canal distention. The level of the epidural block can be extended upward to provide anesthesia for a cesarean birth or tubal ligation after birth. Analgesia, rather than full anesthesia that results in complete loss of movement and sensation, is preferred for labor. Lower concentrations of the anesthetic agent and an epidural opioid provide adequate pain relief without complete motor block for most women. Higher concentrations of the anesthetic agent used for abdominal surgery result in greater loss of both motor and sensory functions.

TECHNIQUE. The exact time to begin an epidural block is individualized. It is started just before a scheduled cesarean birth. For labor the best time to start the block is when the woman is in active labor, to avoid slowing progress. A number of ways are available to customize the epidural block for different pain management needs, however. If she is in early labor and needs pain relief, the woman may be given parenteral opioids until her labor is more active. Or she may be given a preservative-free epidural opioid via the epidural catheter, supplemented with a stronger epidural anesthetic agent when labor becomes more active. In this way she obtains pain relief and relaxation in early labor with less likelihood that labor progress will be slowed.

The epidural space is entered at about the L3-L4 interspace (below the end of the spinal cord), and a catheter is passed through the needle into the epidural space (Figure 15-10). The catheter allows continuous infusion or intermittent injection of medication to maintain pain relief during labor and vaginal or cesarean birth. The infusion of epidural medication may also be regulated by a patient-controlled epidural analgesia (PCEA) pump (Brown & Gottumukkala, 2004; Polley & Glosten, 2004).

Epidural block requires a larger volume of anesthetic agent than the SAB because it is outside the meninges. Before the full epidural dose is given, a small (3-ml) test dose of anesthetic is injected by the anesthesia provider to determine if the epidural catheter has inadvertently punctured a blood vessel or the dura. If a large dose of anesthetic reaches the subarachnoid space instead of the epidural space, the woman experiences rapid, intense motor and sensory block. Numbness of the tongue and lips, light-headedness, dizziness, and tinnitus may occur with intravascular injection. Epinephrine in the test dose produces tachycardia if injected intravascularly, although the tachycardia can have other causes, such as pain.

Epidural opioids used during labor include fentanyl (Sublimaze), sufentanil (Sufenta), and morphine (Duramorph, Astramorph). *All drugs injected into the epidural or subarachnoid spaces must be preservative free.*

A single dose of a long-acting epidural analgesic such as morphine is often given after cesarean birth before removal of the epidural catheter to provide long-acting pain relief with a low dose of opiate. The mother may require no added analgesics for almost 24 hours, or oral ones may be sufficient. The mother's respiratory status must be monitored for an extended time after the long-acting epidural analgesic, up to 24 hours based the duration of action for the long-acting drug.

DURAL PUNCTURE. Because the tough dura and the fragile weblike arachnoid membranes lie close together, dural puncture also punctures the arachnoid. If the dura is

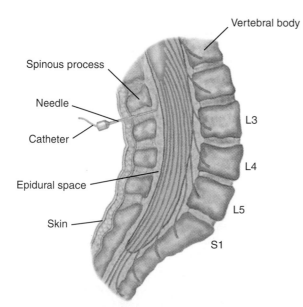

The epidural space is entered with a needle below where the spinal cord ends. A fine catheter is threaded through the needle.

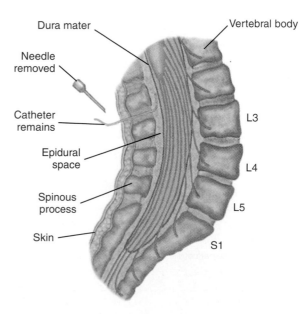

After the catheter is threaded into the epidural space, the needle is removed. Medication can then be injected into the epidural space intermittently or by continuous infusion for pain relief during labor and birth.

Figure 15-10 ■ Technique for epidural block.

unintentionally punctured with the needle used to introduce the epidural catheter, leakage of CSF can occur, which may result in a postdural puncture ("spinal") headache (see p. 350). Dural puncture and headache also can occur without obvious CSF leakage.

CONTRAINDICATIONS AND PRECAUTIONS. Epidural block is not suitable for all laboring women, and some refuse the block. Contraindications include coagulation defects, uncorrected hypovolemia, an infection in the area of insertion or a severe systemic infection, allergy, or a fetal condition that demands immediate birth.

ADVERSE EFFECTS OF EPIDURAL BLOCK. Epidural block can have several adverse effects.

Maternal Hypotension. Sympathetic nerves are blocked along with pain nerves, which may result in vasodilation and hypotension. Before the epidural, expanding the woman's blood volume by infusing 500 to 1000 ml of warmed IV solution such as lactated Ringer's solution offsets vasodilation by filling her vascular system. If hypotension occurs, additional fluids are infused. IV ephedrine in 5- to 10-mg increments may be required to cause vasoconstriction and raise her blood pressure.

Bladder Distention. A woman's bladder fills quickly because of the large quantity of IV solution, yet her sensation to void is reduced. Bladder distention may cause pain that remains after initiation of the block.

Prolonged Second Stage. The urge to push may be less intense than if a woman does not have an epidural block, particularly if she has an intense motor block. The pelvic muscles may be relaxed, which can interfere with the mechanism of internal rotation (see Figure 12-12). These factors increase the chance of forceps- and vacuum extractor–assisted births.

Catheter Migration. After accurate placement, the epidural catheter may move. A woman may then have symptoms of intravascular injection, an intense block or one that is too high, absence of anesthesia, or a unilateral block. The anesthesia professional should be notified of any question about catheter placement.

Cesarean Births. Results of research on whether epidural analgesia is associated with an increase in cesarean births have been mixed. Reasons for cesarean birth are often complex and interrelated. For example, abnormal labor may result in a cesarean birth but also may cause more severe labor pain that requires epidural block.

Maternal Fever. For reasons that are not totally clear, fever after epidural analgesia during labor is common. The fever associated with epidural analgesia is usually not caused by infection but may result from the reduced hyperventilation and decreased heat dissipation, such as reduced sweating, that occur when the woman's pain is relieved. Also, women who are having prolonged labors may be more likely to have epidural block analgesia. However, maternal fever increases the fetal temperature and the fetal demand for oxygen, which can lead to fetal hypoxia and acidosis.

Fever is also a marker for infection. To avoid needless administration of antibiotics and sepsis evaluations in the newborn, other indicators for infection should be sought as well, such as amniotic fluid with a cloudy or yellow color and a foul or strong odor and fetal tachycardia. One study found that a maternal temperature of more than 101° F (38.3° C) was associated with the need for infant resuscitation at birth and 1-minute Apgar scores less than 7. Medical and nursing personnel should try to lower the mother's temperature to a normal level and to identify and treat a suspected infection (Lieberman et al., 2000; Segal, Carp, & Chestnut, 2004).

ADVERSE EFFECTS OF EPIDURAL OPIOIDS. Adverse effects associated with epidural opioids may include nausea and vomiting, pruritus, and delayed maternal respiratory depression.

Nausea and Vomiting. Adjunctive drugs such as promethazine (Phenergan) reduce nausea and vomiting that can occur with epidural opioids.

Pruritus. Itching of the face and neck is an annoying side effect that may occur with epidural opioids. Although she may not specifically complain of itching, a woman may rub or scratch her face and neck. Diphenhydramine (Benadryl), naloxone (Narcan), or naltrexone (Trexan) may relieve pruritus (Table 15-1, p. 348) (Ayoub & Sinatra, 2004).

Delayed Respiratory Depression. The possibility of late respiratory depression exists for up to 24 hours after the administration of an epidural opioid, depending on the duration of action of the drug used.

NURSING CARE. The nurse should record baseline maternal vital signs and FHR and patterns for comparison with prenatal levels and those after the block. Intravenous access is ensured, and the prescribed preload of fluid is given. The nurse supports the woman in the correct position and tells the anesthesia provider when the woman is having a contraction. The woman may feel a brief "electric shock" sensation as the catheter is passed. The nurse should assist her in remaining still while the block is completed. After the medication is injected, the nurse observes for signs of subarachnoid puncture or intravascular injection.

Newest evidence-based practice guidelines from the Association of Obstetric, Gynecologic, and Neonatal Nurses (AWHONN) suggests assessing the maternal blood pressure and fetal heart rate every 5 minutes during the first 15 minutes after initiation of the epidural or any additional bolus doses of epidural medication. Individual facilities may use these guidelines or develop their own guidelines (AWHONN, 2001). As in any labor, maternal and fetal assessments are done more frequently if needed in the situation, such as maternal bleeding or a nonreassuring FHR pattern.

The woman's bladder must be assessed frequently because of the large IV fluid load and her reduced sensation to void. Intermittent or indwelling catheterization is usual.

The nurse should observe for signs associated with catheter migration from the epidural space and for adverse effects from epidural opioids, such as nausea and vomiting and pruritus. Reassurance about the harmless and temporary nature of pruritus is often sufficient.

TABLE **15-1** Drugs Commonly Used For Intrapartum Pain Management

Drug and Dose	Comments
Opioid Analgesics	
Meperidine (Demerol)	Respiratory depression (primarily in the neonate) is the main side effect.
12.5-50 mg every 2-4 hr IV; may be given by PCA	
Fentanyl (Sublimaze)	Onset is quick (5 min for administration IV), but duration of action is short.
50-100 mcg; may be repeated every hour; may be given by PCA	Less nausea, vomiting, and respiratory depression occurs than with meperidine.
Adjunct to epidural analgesia during labor (dose individualized)	Epidural use may cause pruritus.
Butorphanol (Stadol)	Has some narcotic antagonist effects; should not be given to the opiate-dependent woman (may precipitate withdrawal) or after other narcotics such as meperidine (may reverse their analgesic effects); also a respiratory depressant.
1 mg every 3-4 hr; range 0.5-2 mg IV; may be given by PCA	
Nalbuphine (Nubain)	Same as butorphanol.
10 mg every 3-6 hr IV; may be given by PCA	5-10 mg may be given to relieve pruritus associated with epidural narcotics.
Adjunctive Drugs	
Promethazine (Phenergan)	Given for nausea and vomiting in labor.
12.5-25 mg every 4-6 hr IV	Duration of action is longer than most narcotics; may enhance respiratory depressant effects of narcotics.
Diphenhydramine (Benadryl)	Given to relieve pruritus caused by epidural narcotics.
10-50 mg every 4-6 hr IV	
Hydroxyzine (Atarax, Vistaril)	See promethazine.
25-100 mg IM Z-track only	
Narcotic Antagonists	
Naloxone (Narcan)	Action shorter than most narcotics it reverses; must observe for recurrent respiratory depression and be prepared to give additional doses.
Adult:	
To reduce respiratory depression induced by opioids: 0.4-2 mg IV	
To reverse pruritus from epidural opioids: 0.04-0.2 mg IV or IV infusion 5-10 mcg/kg/hr	Small doses (0.04-0.08 mg) may be given to reduce pruritus from epidural opioids.
Neonatal resuscitation:	Neonatal resuscitation dose (see Chapter 30).
0.1 mg/kg IV (umbilical vein) or intratracheal	
Naltrexone (Trexan)	Long-acting drug to relieve pruritus from epidural narcotics.
3-6 mg PO × 1 dose	May reduce some analgesic effect when given for pruritus.

IM, Intramuscularly; *IV*, intravenously; *PCA*, patient-controlled analgesia; *PO*, orally.

INTRATHECAL OPIOID ANALGESICS

Intrathecal injection of an opioid analgesic provides another option for pain management without sedation. The drug is injected into the subarachnoid space, where it binds to opiate receptors, allowing much smaller doses than would be adequate if given systemically. The woman can feel her contractions but not the pain they would otherwise cause.

Advantages of intrathecal analgesics include the following:

- Rapid onset of pain relief without sedation
- No motor block, enabling the woman to ambulate during labor
- No sympathetic block, with its hypotensive effects

Disadvantages may include the following:

- Limited duration of action, possibly requiring another procedure for continued pain relief
- Inadequate pain relief for late labor and the birth, requiring added measures to manage pain at that time

Use of intrathecal opioids may also be combined with epidural block in a CSE, in which the woman receives the intrathecal opioid for rapid pain control at the time an epidural catheter is placed. Epidural drugs are then given to provide a long-acting block for labor.

TECHNIQUE. The subarachnoid space is entered with a spinal needle, as in the SAB. A preservative-free opioid analgesic is then injected. The drug chosen depends on the expected duration of labor at the time it is given. Drugs that may be used by this route include fentanyl, sufentanyl, and morphine.

One technique for performing the CSE is to insert the epidural needle into the epidural space. The much thinner spinal needle is then inserted through the larger epidural needle to reach the subarachnoid space for injection of the intrathecal opioid. The smaller needle is then withdrawn and an epidural catheter placed for injection of epidural medication.

ADVERSE EFFECTS OF INTRATHECAL OPIOIDS. As with epidural opioids, nausea, vomiting, and pruritus may occur. Delayed maternal respiratory depression may occur, depending on the drug used.

NURSING CARE. Vital signs and FHR are taken at the usual intervals for the woman's stage of labor. Side effects, such as nausea and vomiting or pruritus, are reported and managed similarly to those occurring with the epidural block. Reduced effectiveness suggests that the drug's duration of action is ending or that the woman is in late labor. Other pain management methods may be needed for the remainder of labor and for birth.

Care for the woman undergoing a CSE block is the same as that for a noncombined block.

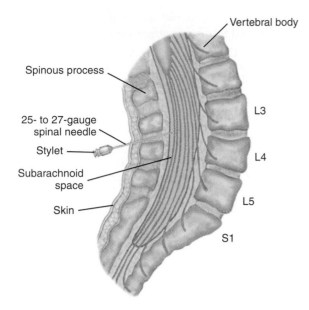

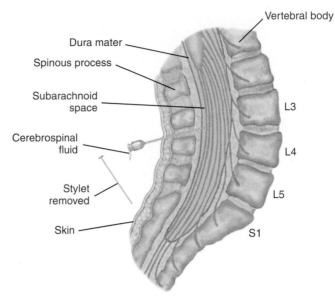

A 25- to 27-gauge spinal needle with a stylet occluding its lumen is passed into the subarachnoid space below where the spinal cord ends.

The stylet is removed, and one or more drops of clear cerebrospinal fluid at needle hub confirm correct needle placement. Medication is then injected, and the needle is removed.

Figure 15-11 ■ Technique for subarachnoid block.

SUBARACHNOID (SPINAL) BLOCK

An SAB is a simpler procedure than the epidural block and may be performed when a quick cesarean birth is necessary and an epidural catheter is not in place. It is similar to local infiltration and pudendal block. SAB is performed just before birth, providing no pain relief during most of labor.

The physician or nurse-anesthetist injects local anesthetic into the subarachnoid space in a single dose. The woman loses both sensory and motor function below the level of the SAB, with relief of pain from contractions.

TECHNIQUE. A 25- to 27-gauge spinal needle is placed in the subarachnoid space. Appearance of CSF at the needle hub assures correct placement, and the local anesthetic is injected (Figure 15-11).

The level of anesthesia for both epidural blocks and SABs is determined by the volume, concentration, and density of the drug (Figure 15-12).

CONTRAINDICATIONS AND PRECAUTIONS. Contraindications and precautions are similar to those for epidural block: the woman's refusal, coagulation defects, uncorrected hypovolemia, infection in the area of insertion, systemic infection, and allergy. SAB can be performed more quickly than an epidural block if prompt birth is necessary.

ADVERSE EFFECTS. Three adverse effects of an SAB are maternal hypotension, bladder distention, and postdural puncture headache. Hypotension is more likely with the SAB than with the epidural block and is treated in the same manner.

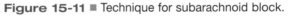

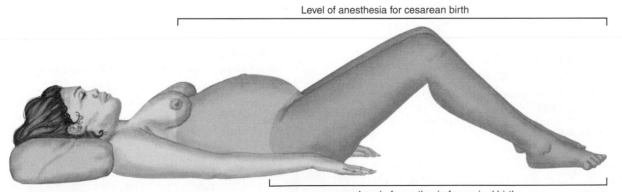

Figure 15-12 ■ Levels of anesthesia for epidural and subarachnoid blocks. A level of T10 through S5 is adequate for vaginal birth. A higher level to T4 to T6 is needed for cesarean birth.

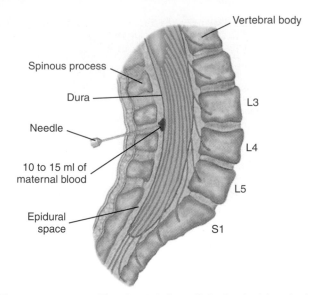

Figure 15-13 ■ Blood patch for relief of spinal headache. To seal a dural puncture, 10 to 15 ml of the woman's blood is injected into the epidural space. Other fluids such as normal saline or dextran may be injected using a similar technique.

Postdural Puncture Headache. Postdural puncture headache may occur after SAB in some women because of CSF leakage at the site of dural puncture. A spinal headache is postural. It is worse when a woman is upright and may disappear when she is lying flat. Headache is less likely if a small-gauge needle is used.

Bed rest with oral or IV hydration helps relieve the postdural puncture headache. Caffeine is another oral therapy. A blood patch may provide definitive relief. The blood patch involves injection of 10 to 15 ml of the woman's blood (obtained with sterile technique) into the epidural space. The blood forms a gelatinous seal over the hole in the dura, stopping spinal fluid leakage (Figure 15-13). The blood patch can be repeated if needed. Epidural injection of dextran, sterile saline, or fibrin glue created from pooled human plasma also has resulted in some success (Weeks, 2004).

Systemic Drugs for Labor

Systemic drugs have effects on multiple systems because they are distributed throughout the body. These intrapartum drugs include opioid analgesics and adjunctive drugs. Although general anesthesia is also systemic, it is discussed separately because it is used only at birth and causes loss of consciousness.

PARENTERAL ANALGESIA

Opioid analgesics are the most common parenteral medications given to reduce perception of pain without loss of consciousness. Analgesics that may be used for labor are meperidine (Demerol), fentanyl (Sublimaze), butorphanol (Stadol) (see Drug Guide), and nalbuphine (Nubain) (see Table 15-1).

Although the drug may be prescribed for labor analgesia, meperidine often produces a dysphoric rather than an analgesic effect in the woman. She may be restless or irritable and have twitching, jerking, shaking, tremors, or even delirium. Of more concern is that meperidine produces a longlasting active metabolite, normeperidine, which has a half-life of 3 to 6 hours in the woman but 15 to 23 hours in the newborn (Bricker & Lavender, 2002; Britt & Pasero, 1999).

Meperidine and fentanyl are pure opioid agonists, but butorphanol and nalbuphine have mixed opioid agonist and antagonist effects. A woman who is dependent on opiates (such as heroin) should avoid agonist-antagonist drugs,

---

DRUG GUIDE

BUTORPHANOL (STADOL)

Classification: Opioid analgesic.

Action: Opioid analgesic with some agonist-antagonist effects; exact mechanism of action unknown; produces respiratory depression that does not increase markedly with larger doses.

Indications: Systemic pain relief during labor.

Dosage and Route: Intravenous: 1 mg every 3-4 hr; range 0.5-2 mg; may be given undiluted.

Absorption: Onset of analgesia almost immediate with intravenous administration, peaks after about 30 min, and lasts about 3 hr; faster onset and shorter duration of action than meperidine or morphine.

Excretion: Excreted in urine; crosses placental barrier; secreted in breast milk.

Contraindications and Precautions: Contraindicated in persons who are hypersensitive; not used in opiate-dependent persons because antagonist activity of the drug may cause withdrawal symptoms in the woman or newborn; cautiously used during birth of preterm infant; drug actions potentiated (enhanced) by barbiturates, phenothiazines, cimetidine, and other tranquilizers.

Adverse Reactions: Respiratory depression or apnea (woman or newborn), anaphylaxis; dizziness, light-headedness, sedation, lethargy, headache, euphoria, mental clouding, fainting, restlessness, excitement, tremors, delirium, insomnia; nausea, vomiting, constipation, increased biliary pressure, dry mouth, anorexia; flushing, altered heart rate and blood pressure, circulatory collapse; urinary retention; sensitivity to cold.

Nursing Considerations: Assess for allergies and opiate dependence. Observe vital signs and respiratory function in woman (12 per minute or more) and newborn (30 per minute or more). Have naloxone and resuscitation equipment available for treatment of respiratory depression in woman and neonate. Report nausea or vomiting to the birth attendant for a possible order for an antiemetic. Antiemetics or other central nervous system depressants may enhance the respiratory depressant effects of butorphanol.

because they may cause withdrawal effects in her and the newborn. They should not be given if the woman has already received a pure opioid, because some analgesic effect of the first drug will be reversed. Agonist-antagonist drugs have a "ceiling effect" on the amount of analgesia they provide and are unsuitable for the increasing pain of the entire labor for many women (Britt & Pasero, 1999).

The primary side effect of opioids is respiratory depression, which is more likely to affect the newborn. Timing of administration is important to reduce neonatal respiratory depression. An infant who is born at the peak of the drug's action is more likely to have respiratory depression than if born earlier or later. Meperidine's metabolite, normeperidine, is active for a long time in the newborn and can cause delayed respiratory depression.

Opioid analgesics are given in small, frequent doses by the IV route during labor to provide a rapid onset of analgesia and a predictable duration of action. A woman benefits from rapid pain control, with less likelihood of neonatal respiratory depression. Starting the injection at the beginning of the contraction, when blood flow to the placenta is normally reduced, limits transfer to the fetus. When placental blood flow resumes, much of the drug is in maternal tissues. The drugs also may be delivered by patient-controlled analgesia (PCA) pump.

OPIOID ANTAGONISTS

Naloxone (Narcan) reverses opioid-induced respiratory depression, although it is seldom needed in obstetrics. Naloxone does not reverse respiratory depression from other causes, such as barbiturates, anesthetics, nonopioid drugs, or pathologic conditions. Naloxone has a shorter duration of action than most of the opioids it reverses, and respiratory depression may recur. In an opiate-dependent woman or newborn, naloxone can induce withdrawal symptoms. Naloxone is used with other measures as needed to support cardiopulmonary function (see Chapter 30).

Naloxone is most often given to the neonate. The neonatal resuscitation dose is 0.1 mg/kg by the recommended IV or intratracheal route for most reliable absorption. Airway management (i.e., bag-and-mask ventilation) takes precedence over use of naloxone, and the drug is not given unless there is reason to believe that maternal opioids are the reason for the newborn's respiratory depression (American Academy of Pediatrics [AAP] & American Heart Association, 2000; AAP & American College of Obstetricians and Gynecologists, 2002). The adult dose is 0.4 to 2 mg.

Small doses of naloxone may be given to the woman to relieve the pruritus that occurs with intrathecal or epidural narcotics. Naltrexone (Trexan), another opioid antagonist, and diphenhydramine (Benadryl), an antihistamine, may also be given for relief of pruritus.

ADJUNCTIVE DRUGS

Adjunctive drugs during the intrapartum period include those with antiemetic and tranquilizing effects and sedatives. These drugs are given to reduce nausea and anxiety and to promote rest (see Table 15-1).

Promethazine (Phenergan) relieves nausea and vomiting, which may occur when opioid drugs are given. Parenteral promethazine administration may be either the intramuscular or IV route. Promethazine does not potentiate the opioid's analgesic effects but can add to the opioid's respiratory depressant effects.

Hydroxyzine (Atarax, Vistaril) is also an antihistamine with antiemetic effects. Parenteral hydroxyzine can be given only into a large muscle with a deep Z-track technique. *Hydroxyzine is not given by the IV route.*

SEDATIVES

Sedatives such as barbiturates are not routinely given because they have prolonged depressant effects on the neonate. However, a small dose of a short-acting barbiturate may be given to promote rest if a woman is fatigued from false labor or a prolonged latent phase.

✔ CHECK YOUR READING

17. What is the primary adverse effect of opioid administration? How can this effect be reduced?
18. What should the nurse watch for after birth in the infant who received naloxone?

Vaginal Birth Anesthesia

LOCAL INFILTRATION ANESTHESIA

Infiltration of the perineum with a local anesthetic is done by the physician or nurse-midwife just before he or she performs an episiotomy or sutures a laceration (Figure 15-14). Local infiltration does not alter pain from uterine contractions or distention of the vagina. The local agent provides anesthesia in the immediate area of the episiotomy or laceration. A short delay occurs between anesthetic injection and onset of numbness, and the drug burns before its anesthetic action begins. Local infiltration rarely has adverse effects on either mother or infant.

PUDENDAL BLOCK

A pudendal block anesthetizes the lower vagina and part of the perineum to provide anesthesia for an episiotomy and vaginal birth, using low forceps if needed. A pudendal block does not block pain from uterine contractions, and the mother feels pressure. The pudendal block is a highly localized type of regional block, similar to a dental anesthetic that provides numbness for dental procedures.

The physician or nurse-midwife injects the pudendal nerves near each ischial spine with a local anesthetic (Figure 15-15). The perineum is infiltrated with local anesthetic because the pudendal block does not fully anesthetize this area. As in local infiltration, a delay occurs between injection and onset of numbness. Possible maternal complications include a toxic reaction to the anesthetic, rectal puncture, hematoma, and sciatic nerve block. If maternal toxicity is avoided, the fetus is usually not affected.

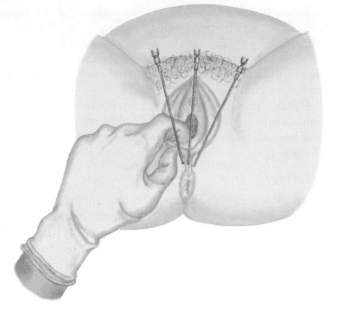

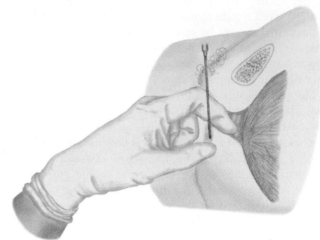

Figure 15-14 ■ Local infiltration anesthesia numbs the perineum just before birth for an episiotomy or after birth for suturing of a laceration. The birth attendant protects the fetal head by placing a finger inside the vagina while injecting the perineum in a fanlike pattern or as needed.

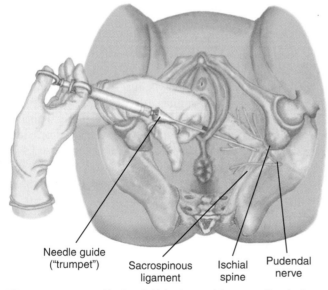

Needle guide ("trumpet")   Sacrospinous ligament   Ischial spine   Pudendal nerve

Figure 15-15 ■ Pudendal block provides anesthesia for an episiotomy and use of low forceps. A needle guide ("trumpet") protects the maternal and fetal tissues from the long needle needed to reach the pudendal nerve. Only about 1.25 cm (½ in) of the long needle protrudes from the guide.

GENERAL ANESTHESIA

General anesthesia is systemic pain control that involves loss of consciousness. It is rarely used for vaginal births, but it still has a place in cesarean birth. Some women either refuse or are not good candidates for epidural block or SAB for cesarean birth. Occasionally a planned epidural block or SAB proves to be inadequate for surgical anesthesia. General anesthesia may be needed unexpectedly and quickly for emergency procedures at any stage of pregnancy, such as to repair injury that results from an accident or domestic violence or to perform an appendectomy.

TECHNIQUE. Before induction of anesthesia, a woman breathes oxygen for 3 to 5 minutes, or at least four deep breaths, to increase her oxygen stores and those of her fetus for the short period of apnea during rapid anesthesia induction. The woman has a wedge under her right side (or the operating table is tilted toward her left side) to reduce aortocaval compression and increase placental blood flow.

ADVERSE EFFECTS. Major adverse effects are possible with the use of general anesthesia.

Maternal Aspiration of Gastric Contents. Regurgitation with aspiration of acidic gastric contents is a potentially fatal complication of general anesthesia. Aspiration of food particles may result in airway obstruction. Aspiration of acidic secretions results in a chemical injury to the airways—aspiration pneumonitis. Infection often occurs after the initial lung injury.

Respiratory Depression. Respiratory depression may occur in either the mother or the infant but is more likely in the baby. This is more likely to occur if the interval between induction of anesthesia and cord clamping is long.

Uterine Relaxation. Some inhalational anesthetics may cause uterine relaxation. This characteristic is desirable for some complications, such as replacing an inverted uterus (see p. 727). However, postpartum hemorrhage may occur if the uterus relaxes after birth.

METHODS TO MINIMIZE ADVERSE EFFECTS. Measures to reduce the risk of maternal aspiration or to limit lung injury if aspiration occurs include the following:

■ Restricting intake to clear fluids or maintaining nothing-by-mouth (NPO) status if surgery is expected, such as with a scheduled cesarean

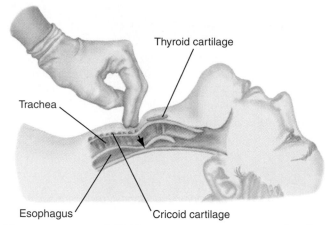

Figure 15-16 ■ Sellick's maneuver to prevent vomitus from entering the woman's trachea while she is being intubated for general anesthesia. An assistant applies pressure to the cricoid cartilage to obstruct the esophagus. Once the woman is successfully intubated with a cuffed endotracheal tube, gastric secretions cannot enter the trachea.

(Labels on figure: Thyroid cartilage, Trachea, Esophagus, Cricoid cartilage)

- Administering drugs to raise the gastric pH and make secretions less acidic, such as sodium citrate and citric acid (Bicitra), ranitidine (Zantac), cimetidine (Tagamet), or famotidine (Pepcid)
- Administering drugs to reduce secretions, such as glycopyrrolate (Robinul)
- Administering drugs to speed gastric emptying, such as metoclopramide (Reglan)
- Using cricoid pressure (Sellick maneuver) to block the esophagus by pressing the rigid trachea against it (Figure 15-16)

Neonatal respiratory depression may be prevented by doing the following:
- Reducing the time from induction of anesthesia to clamping of the umbilical cord
- Keeping use of sedating drugs and anesthetics to a minimum until the cord is clamped

To reduce the time from induction of anesthesia to cord clamping, the woman is prepared and draped and the physicians are ready before anesthesia is begun. The anesthesia is kept light until the infant is born and the woman may move slightly on the table, although she usually has no memory of the experience. The anesthesia level is deepened as soon as the cord is clamped.

✓ CHECK YOUR READING

19. What are two major advantages of using regional pain management techniques during childbirth?
20. What is the major adverse effect of the epidural block or SAB? How can the fetus be affected? How may this effect be reduced?
21. What are common side effects of epidural or intrathecal opioid analgesics, and how are these managed?
22. What are the major adverse effects of general anesthesia? What measures reduce the risks?

Application of the Nursing Process
Pain Management

Nursing care related to pain management should be combined with support for normal labor and any complications that arise. Care of the fetus remains important (see Chapter 14). Two problems that affect many women are pain and care related to epidural analgesia (Nursing Care Plan 15-1).

PAIN

Assessment

Pain assessment begins at admission and continues throughout labor (see Table 13-1). Pain-related assessments include the following:
- Preferences for pain management
- Previous surgeries, type of anesthesia, and any anesthesia-associated problems
- Maternal vital signs
- FHR and electronic fetal monitor patterns
- Allergies, focusing especially on allergy to opioid analgesics, dental anesthetics, and iodine (used in some preparation solutions)
- Oral intake—Time and type of last intake
- Evidence of pain—Verbal statement, requests for pain relief measures, crying, moaning; and nonverbal evidence such as tense, guarded posture or facial expression

LABOR STATUS

In addition to these routine assessments, ask the woman if she needs help with pain management. A stoic woman may give little evidence of pain yet may say she wants medication or other pain control if asked.

When assessing pain, clarify the words a woman uses. When asked if she has "pain," the woman may deny it. Yet changing the word used to "discomfort," "cramping," "aching," "pressure," or other words that may describe labor pain may bring a different response. Do not assume that everyone uses the same words to describe their pain. Pain is an individual experience, and so is the expression of pain.

Asking a woman to rate her pain on a scale of 0 to 10 (or your facility's standard scale) helps clarify her pain's intensity. A 0 represents no pain, whereas 10 is the worst possible pain. Ask the woman to rate her pain on this scale before and after pain relief measures to evaluate their effectiveness. Multilingual and picture scales are available for those who do not speak the dominant language. A surprising number of women have difficulty using a pain scale because they have little experience with pain. They may want to allow for an increase in the number later in labor, possibly underrating current pain. Or, they may say that they have no idea what the "worst pain imaginable" is and therefore cannot guess what pain rated as 10 feels like. A scale does, however, provide one measure of how pain feels before and after relief measures.

NURSING CARE PLAN 15-1 Intrapartum Pain Management

ASSESSMENT: Beth Anderson is a 28-year-old gravida 1, para 0 who was admitted 1 hour ago. Beth's cervix is 3 cm dilated and 100% effaced, the station is −2, and her membranes are intact. Contractions occur every 3 minutes, last 40 to 50 seconds, and are of moderate intensity. The fetal heart rate averages 135 to 145 beats per minute (bpm) and has no nonreassuring patterns. Beth says that back pain is most troubling. Beth and her husband Sam attended prepared childbirth classes and are using breathing techniques they learned.

NURSING DIAGNOSIS: Pain related to effects of uterine contractions and pressure on pelvic structures

GOALS/EXPECTED OUTCOMES: During labor, Beth will:
1. Continue to use techniques she learned in prepared childbirth classes.
2. Have a relaxed facial and body posture between contractions.

CRITICAL THINKING: At this time, what methods for pain management are most appropriate to suggest, nonpharmacologic or pharmacologic?

ANSWER: If no one has already done so, the nurse should explore Beth's preferences for pain relief with her before labor becomes more intense. Nonpharmacologic methods are ideal in early labor if they provide adequate pain management. Walking or other upright positions often ease back discomfort and aid fetal descent. However, Beth's ability to use these would be reduced if she were to receive some pharmacologic methods of pain control, such as systemic analgesics. Her labor pattern is normal, membranes are intact, and the fetal heart rate is stable and within normal limits, so walking is not contraindicated.

INTERVENTION	RATIONALE

1. Adjust the environment for comfort:
  a. Adjust room thermostat.
  b. Add warm blankets and socks for warmth.
  c. Offer small electric fan or hand-held fan if Beth is hot.
	1. A comfortable environment is conducive to relaxation. Relaxation underlies all other interventions because it increases a woman's ability to use her coping skills to tolerate discomfort.

2. Reduce distractions:
  a. Close door to reduce outside noise.
  b. Play music of Beth's choice to mask external noise.
  c. Do not stand in front of her focal point.
  d. Try to delay assessments or questions until after a contraction is over.
	2. Distractions interfere with use of the skills for pain management taught in prepared childbirth classes.

3. Reduce irritating stimulants:
  a. Keep sheets and underpads dry.
  b. Dim the lights as Beth desires. Use bright lights only when necessary.
  c. Perform all procedures and nursing interventions as gently as possible.
  d. Avoid bumping the bed.
  e. Limit visitors as the couple wishes.
	3. Irritating stimulants are distractions that decrease the woman's ability to use learned childbirth skills and add to her discomfort.

4. Encourage Beth to assume the most comfortable positions and to change positions regularly (about every 30 to 60 minutes). If there is no contraindication, she may walk around or sit in a chair or on a birth ball at the bedside. A rolled pillow or blanket provides a wedge in a side-tilt position.	4. Frequent position changes favor fetal descent by encouraging the fetal head to adapt to the pelvic diameters most efficiently. Position changes also reduce muscle tension and unrelieved pressure:
	  a. Upright positions enhance descent with gravity.
	  b. If lying down, a side-lying or side-tilt position is more comfortable and reduces aortocaval compression with decreased placental perfusion.

5. Check for bladder distention hourly or more often if she has had large quantities of intravenous (IV) or oral fluid. Encourage voiding at least every 2 hours. With an order, catheterize her if her bladder is full and she cannot void.	5. The sensation to void may be decreased during labor. A full bladder contributes to overall discomfort and may impede fetal descent and prolong labor.
6. Give Beth small amounts of clear fluids such as ice chips. If oral intake is prohibited or she does not want fluids, moisten her mouth with a damp washcloth or have her rinse her mouth with water.	6. Women often use rapid mouth breathing during labor, resulting in a dry mouth. These methods may relieve some of the discomfort associated with a dry mouth. Clear liquids limit the risk of aspiration if general anesthesia is needed.
7. Offer a back rub or firm, constant sacral pressure. Ask Beth where and how firm pressure should be applied. Use baby powder when rubbing her back. Have her tell caregivers if this technique becomes uncomfortable or if the location on her back needs to be changed. If Sam is rubbing her back, offer to relieve him occasionally and encourage him to take a break.	7. Back rubs may somewhat reduce discomfort associated with back labor by stimulating large-diameter fibers and interfering with transmission of the pain impulse to the brain. As labor continues, back rubs may become less effective or even uncomfortable. Powder reduces friction, which could be another source of discomfort. The partner needs a break to conserve energy and better help the woman in later labor.

NURSING CARE PLAN 15-1 Intrapartum Pain Management—cont'd

INTERVENTION	RATIONALE
8. Keep Beth and Sam informed about the progress of labor and their baby's condition.	8. Information reduces anxiety and fear of the unknown. Anxiety and fear increase pain perception and reduce pain tolerance.

EVALUATION: Beth concentrates on her breathing techniques with each contraction but has a relaxed body posture between them. She continues to use learned skills effectively for about 2 hours, when she begins to have more difficulty coping with her contractions.

ASSESSMENT: Three hours after admission, Beth's cervix is 4 cm dilated and 100% effaced and the fetal station is −1. Membranes have ruptured, and the amniotic fluid is clear. Contractions occur every 2 to 3 minutes, last 50 seconds, and are firm. Fetal heart rate and monitor patterns are reassuring. Back discomfort persists, and she is having difficulty relaxing between contractions and is discouraged that labor is not progressing as quickly as she expected. She is no longer able to use prepared childbirth techniques effectively and rates her labor pain as 8 on a 0-to-10 scale. Beth reluctantly requests an epidural block, which will be given by continuous infusion.

CRITICAL THINKING: At this time, what are some advantages and disadvantages of having an epidural? Are added measures needed to safeguard the fetus because of an epidural block?

ANSWER: An epidural may slow labor if performed earlier than this, but labor progress may benefit from the relief of pain and tension if done at this point or later. A disadvantage of the epidural block is that Beth's activity is limited, reducing her options for positions that might improve fetal descent and rotation through the pelvis.

To safeguard the fetus, the nurse gives Beth an IV preload of at least 500 ml of lactated Ringer's before the block is started, offsetting the hypotensive effects of the epidural. Fetal monitoring, usually by continuous electronic means, helps identify nonreassuring patterns that may occur. Beth may assume several positions but she should avoid a supine position that can cause aortocaval compression.

NURSING DIAGNOSIS: Risk for Injury related to altered sensation in her lower extremities

GOALS/EXPECTED OUTCOMES: Beth will not fall or suffer other injury while experiencing the effects of epidural block. The fetus will not be born in an uncontrolled manner.

INTERVENTION	RATIONALE
1. Assist Beth to change positions regularly. Ambulation after birth should be delayed until movement and strength return, and assistance should be available until her legs have normal strength.	1. Changing positions reduces constant pressure on one area and helps prevent muscle strain. The epidural block causes a varying degree of motor block and weakness. An assistant helps prevent falls when the woman first ambulates.

2. Observe for signs of labor progress:
  a. Contractions increasing in frequency, duration, and intensity
  b. Fetal heart rate changes such as early or variable decelerations that reflect head or cord compression
  c. Increase in bloody show
  d. Statement reflecting urge to push (not always present)
	2. Rectal pressure associated with fetal descent may be reduced. To prevent the fetus from being born unattended, the nurse must observe for other signs that birth is near.

3. Support Beth's pushing efforts. Teach her to avoid holding her breath while pushing longer than 6 to 8 seconds at a time. Explain to Beth and Sam that she may make grunting, moaning, or other sounds when pushing to avoid excessive breath-holding.	3. The urge to push may not be as strong but it is usually felt when the fetus descends low in the pelvis. Prolonged breath-holding or multiple long pushing efforts (see also Chapter 13) can cause fetal hypoxia and nonreassuring fetal heart rate patterns. Women may make a variety of sounds when they push.

EVALUATION: Beth is satisfied with her pain relief after the epidural block, rating her pain as "0 out of 10." She has little motor block. Her blood pressure and the fetal heart rate remain within expected limits. Cervical dilation progresses to 10 cm (complete) without injury to Beth or her fetus. However, despite her vigorous pushing efforts, the fetal station remains at 0. Beth has a cesarean birth, delivering a 3912-g (8-lb, 10-oz) girl.

ADDITIONAL NURSING DIAGNOSES AND COLLABORATIVE PROBLEMS TO CONSIDER:
Anxiety
Risk for Aspiration
Powerlessness
Situational Low Self-Esteem
Urinary Retention
Potential Complication: Fetal Compromise

Body language gives a clue to comfort level. Moaning, crying, thrashing, and an inability to use nonpharmacologic techniques are obvious indicators that a woman needs help with pain control, including pharmacologic pain relief. However, more subtle clues such as remaining tense between contractions also suggest difficulty coping with pain.

Evaluate the woman's labor status to help her choose the most appropriate method of pain control. Inform her if she has reached a decision point in labor to use or not use a specific pharmacologic method. No standard time or amount of cervical dilation serves as a guideline for this critical point. This is estimated based on projected time of birth, amount of time needed to establish a specific method, and the pharmacology of the drug or drugs.

Avoid making assumptions about a woman's pain based on her rate of labor progress, cervical dilation, or apparent intensity of contractions. Do not assume that a woman whose cervix is 2 cm dilated has little pain and that a woman whose cervix is dilated 8 cm has intense pain. An obese woman's contractions may be strong, but they may seem mild if they are assessed by palpation or an external monitor because of her thick abdominal fat pad. *Labor progress or contraction intensity cannot be equated with a woman's pain perception or tolerance.*

A woman's need for pain relief should not be based only on her outward expression. A quiet woman may need medication but may be reluctant to ask, whereas the expressive woman may be satisfied with only nonpharmacologic measures. Because women who do not speak the prevailing language may not know what is available, seek an interpreter to communicate effectively.

Observe for and report pain that is not typical of normal labor. Although labor pain is often intense, it should come and go with each contraction. The uterus should not be tender or boardlike between contractions and should not cause constant intense pain.

Analysis

Pain is expected in normal childbirth, and most laboring women have nursing needs that relate to its management. The nursing diagnosis is: Pain related to effects of uterine contractions and fetal descent.

Planning

Because pain is a subjective experience and expected in labor, two goals or expected outcomes are realistic. The woman will do the following:

1. Describe pain relief measures, both nonpharmacologic and pharmacologic, as satisfactory during labor
2. Effectively use breathing and relaxation techniques learned in childbirth class or from nurse during labor

Interventions

Nursing care related to intrapartum pain management focuses on reducing factors that hinder the woman's pain control and enhancing those that benefit it (see Chapter 13).

PROMOTING RELAXATION

Simple attention to details promotes relaxation. Make the environment more comfortable. If noise is a problem, suggest music or television to mask it. A warm blanket, a cool cloth, or a hot pack provides tangible comfort and conveys the nurse's caring attitude. Change the linens or underpads as needed to keep the woman reasonably clean and dry.

Offer the woman a warm shower or bath, especially if she is tense and if no contraindications exist (see Box 15-1). In general, walking is good during early labor, and water therapy is better during active labor. The mild nipple stimulation that occurs in a whirlpool or shower may intensify contractions in a woman whose labor has slowed, causing her posterior pituitary gland to secrete oxytocin.

Reduce intrusions as much as possible. For example, wait until a contraction is over before asking questions or performing a procedure. Longer assessments and procedures may span several contractions, but try to stop during each contraction if possible.

REDUCING OUTSIDE SOURCES OF DISCOMFORT

Anesthetize the IV site with lidocaine (Xylocaine) before inserting the line if the woman is not allergic and if policy permits. Normal saline infiltration of the site has a similar effect. Remind her to change position regularly to reduce tension and discomfort from constant pressure. Support her with pillows.

Observe the woman's bladder for distention hourly, and encourage her to void every 2 hours or more often if she has received a large quantity of IV fluids. Most intrapartum orders include one for catheterization if she cannot void and her bladder is full. An indwelling catheter may be inserted for women who have an epidural to reduce repeated catheterizations.

REDUCING ANXIETY AND FEAR

Accurate information reduces the negative psychological impact of the unknown. Tell the woman about her labor and its progress. You cannot predict when she will give birth, but tell her if labor progress is or is not on course. Sometimes she needs only the reassurance from an experienced nurse that her intense contractions are indeed normal. The woman may be willing to endure more discomfort than she otherwise would if she is making progress.

Be honest if problems do occur. A woman usually knows if a problem exists and is more anxious if she does not know what it is. Explain all measures taken to correct the problem, and inform her of the results.

HELPING THE WOMAN USE NONPHARMACOLOGIC TECHNIQUES

If the nonpharmacologic method is safe for the woman and fetus and if it is effective, do not interfere with its use. Try not to distract the woman from whatever technique she is using.

MASSAGE. Fetal monitor belts hinder abdominal effleurage. Encourage the woman to do effleurage on uncovered areas of her abdomen or to stroke her thighs. Consider using intermittent auscultation or intermittent electronic fetal monitoring (see Chapter 14).

Use powder to avoid friction and seek feedback from the woman about the best location and amount of pressure to use for sacral pressure or other massage. Because this information may change during labor or massage may become uncomfortable rather than helpful, seek the woman's feedback regularly.

MENTAL STIMULATION. Use a low, soothing voice when helping a woman use imagery. Speaking close to her ear is often helpful when trying to create a tranquil imaginary scene or to calm her. Use of a low, soothing voice during an emergency has a calming effect as well. Music can enhance mental stimulation techniques.

BREATHING. Women often modify the techniques they learn in class or invent some of their own during labor. Encourage the woman to change techniques when she needs to, but save the complex ones for later labor. If she has trouble maintaining her concentration, the nurse or her support person may try to make eye contact (if culturally appropriate) and breathe the pattern with her.

Symptoms of hyperventilation (dizziness, tingling and numbness of the fingers and lips, carpopedal spasm) are likely if a woman breathes fast and deep. If she hyperventilates, she should breathe into her cupped hands, a paper bag, or a washcloth placed over her nose and mouth. Talk to her gently to slow her breathing.

Teach breathing techniques to the unprepared woman when she is admitted. Review them when she seems to need a different method. If she makes up a breathing technique that works, leave it alone.

When teaching pain management techniques to the unprepared woman who is in advanced labor, follow these guidelines:

- Teach one method at a time.
- Demonstrate the method between contractions.
- Use breathing techniques with the woman while maintaining eye contact.

- Give her control over her labor: who is present, what technique she will use, and so on.
- Speak in a soft, calm tone of voice.

INCORPORATING PHARMACOLOGIC METHODS

All pharmacologic methods require collaboration with medical personnel for orders. Tell the woman soon after admission what medication is available if she needs it. This is intended not to undermine her self-confidence but to allow her to make an informed choice about medication when necessary. Analgesia is most effective if it is given before pain is severe.

Tell her that her preferences about pain relief methods will be honored if possible, but predicting the course of her labor is impossible. Her preferred method of pain management may be inappropriate if labor has unexpected developments. Assure her that no pharmacologic method will be used without her understanding and consent ("Parents Want to Know: How Will This Medicine Affect Our Baby?").

If a woman finds nonpharmacologic methods inadequate, help her try other ones or offer her available medication. When contacting the birth attendant for medication orders, report the fetal and maternal status and vital signs, labor status, and her request for medication. If she has a continuous epidural block, contact the person who inserted it if problems occur. Observe special nursing considerations associated with the method used (Table 15-2).

Evaluation

Labor is not expected to be painless, even with the most effective pharmacologic methods. The first goal or expected outcome is achieved if the woman is satisfied with her ability to manage her pain. Many women have occasional difficulty using breathing or other techniques, even if they have practiced faithfully. How did her pain scale rating change before and after the pain relief method, whether nonpharmacologic or pharmacologic, was used? Is she satisfied with her level of pain relief?

PARENTS WANT TO KNOW

How Will This Medicine Affect Our Baby?

Women and their partners often ask whether pain medication or anesthesia will harm their baby. The nurse can help parents choose wisely from available options by providing honest information:

- Pain that you cannot tolerate is not good for you or your baby, and it reduces the joy of this special event.
- Some risk is associated with every type of pain medication or anesthesia, but careful selection and the use of preventive measures minimize this risk. If complications occur, corrective measures can reduce the risk to you and your baby.
- Some pain relievers can cause your baby to be slow to breathe at birth, but carefully controlling the timing and

dose of the medication reduces the likelihood that this will occur. We can use another medication to reverse this effect if needed.

- Epidural or spinal anesthesia can cause your blood pressure to fall, which can reduce the blood flow to your baby. However, we give you lots of intravenous fluids to reduce this effect. We have other medications to increase your blood pressure if the fluids are not enough.
- General anesthesia can cause your baby to be slow to breathe at birth. To reduce this risk, the anesthesia will not be started until everything is ready for the surgery and the doctors will clamp the baby's umbilical cord as quickly as possible.

TABLE 15-2 Pharmacologic Methods of Intrapartum Pain Management

Method and Uses	Nursing Considerations
Opioid Analgesics Systemic analgesia during labor and for postoperative pain after cesarean birth. May be combined with an adjunctive drug such as promethazine to reduce the nausea and vomiting that sometimes occur with narcotic use and after surgery. May be given by epidural injection just before the epidural catheter is removed at the end of surgery. Often delivered by PCA pump in postoperative period.	1. Assess the woman for drug use at admission. Women who are opiate dependent should not receive analgesics that have mixed agonist and antagonist actions (butorphanol and nalbuphine). 2. Observe neonate for respiratory depression, especially if the mother had opioid narcotics within 4 hr of birth or at time of the drug's peak action or if the mother received multiple opioid doses during labor: • Delay in initiating or sustaining normal depth and rate of respirations • Respiratory rate <30/min • Poor muscle tone: limp, floppy 3. The use of adjunctive drugs for nausea, such as promethazine, enhances respiratory depressant effects. 4. Have naloxone available for infants exposed to opioids during labor. Respiratory and cardiac support precedes drug administration in neonatal resuscitation. Observe for recurrent respiratory depression after administration of naloxone.
Epidural Opioids *Labor:* Mixed with a local anesthetic agent to give better pain relief with less motor block. *Postoperatively:* Gives long-acting analgesia without sedation, allowing the mother and infant to interact more easily.	1. Observe same nursing implications as with epidural block. 2. Do not give additional opioids or other CNS depressants except as ordered by the anesthesia provider. Nonsteroidal antiinflammatory drugs or oral analgesics are often prescribed in routine orders. 3. Maternal respiratory depression may be delayed for up to 24 hr and varies with drug given. Observe respiratory rate, depth, oxygen saturation, and arousability hourly for 24 hr or according to hospital standards for the drug administered. Notify anesthesia provider for rate <12/min, persistent oxygen saturation <95% on pulse oximetry, reduced respiratory effort, difficulty arousing, or as ordered by the provider. Cyanosis is a late sign of respiratory depression. 4. Have naloxone, 0.4 mg, an oral airway, and an Ambu bag and mask immediately available, such as on a "crash cart." 5. Observe for pruritus or rubbing of the face and neck. Routine postoperative orders to relieve pruritus are usually provided. Notify anesthesia provider if these are insufficient. 6. Urinary retention may occur after indwelling catheter removal. Observe for adequacy of voiding, as in all postpartum women. 7. Notify anesthesia provider for relief of nausea or vomiting. 8. Assess sensation and mobility before allowing ambulation.
Intrathecal Opioid Analgesics Provides analgesia for most of first-stage labor without maternal sedation. A very small dose of the drug is needed because it is injected very near the spinal cord where sensory fibers enter. Usually not adequate for late labor or the birth itself. Often combined with epidural block for the CSE technique for labor.	1. Observe for the common side effects of nausea, vomiting, and pruritus. Notify the anesthesia provider if these effects occur, and have an antagonist such as naloxone or naltrexone available. 2. Observe for delayed respiratory depression, depending on the drug given. Use a pulse oximeter as indicated. 3. Observe for nonreassuring fetal heart rate patterns that may be associated with reduced maternal oxygenation.
Local Infiltration Anesthesia Numbs perineum for episiotomy or repair of laceration at vaginal birth. No relief of labor pain. Not adequate for forceps-assisted birth.	1. Assess for drug allergies, especially to dental anesthetics because they are related to those used in maternity care. 2. Apply ice to perineum after birth to reduce edema and hematoma formation and to increase comfort.
Pudendal Block Numbs the lower vagina and perineum for vaginal birth. No relief of labor pain because it is done just before birth. Provides adequate anesthesia for many forceps-assisted births.	1. Use the same interventions as for local infiltration. A woman or her partner may be alarmed if she notices the long needle (about 15 cm [6 in]). Teach her that it must be long to reach the pudendal nerve through the vagina and that it will be inserted only about 1.25 cm (½ in) near the location of the nerve. Tell her that a guide ("trumpet") will be used to avoid injuring her vaginal tissue or the baby.

CNS, Central nervous system; *CSE,* combined spinal-epidural; *PCA,* patient-controlled analgesia.

TABLE **15-2** Pharmacologic Methods of Intrapartum Pain Management—cont'd

Method and Uses	Nursing Considerations
Epidural Block *Labor:* Insertion of catheter provides pain relief for labor and vaginal birth (T10-S5 levels). *Cesarean birth:* If epidural was used during labor, block can be extended upward (T4-T6 level). Also used for planned cesarean birth and post-birth tubal ligation.	1. Prehydrate the woman with warmed nonglucose crystalloid solution such as Ringer's lactate solution. Common minimum amounts: 500-1000 ml for labor and vaginal birth; 1500-2000 ml for planned cesarean birth. 2. Displace uterus to left manually or with a wedge placed under the woman's right side to enhance placental perfusion. 3. Assess for hypotension at least every 5 min for 15 min after block is begun and with each new dose until vital signs are stable. Report to anesthesia provider: systolic BP <110 mm Hg or a fall of 20% or more from baseline levels, pallor, or diaphoresis. Facility procedures give further guidance. 4. Assess fetal heart rate for signs of impaired placental perfusion, and report to anesthesia provider and nurse-midwife: tachycardia (>160/min for 10 min) or bradycardia (<110/min for 10 min), late decelerations (see Table 14-1, p. 323.). 5. If hypotension or signs of impaired placental perfusion occur, increase the rate of infusion of nonadditive IV fluid, reposition the woman on her side, and administer oxygen by face mask (8-10 L/min). Have ephedrine available (usually included in epidural tray). 6. Observe for a full bladder, and catheterize as ordered. 7. Leg movement and strength vary after an epidural block. Transfer with help to avoid muscle strains to nurse or woman. 8. Ambulate only after sensation and movement have returned. Use another person's assistance with the first ambulation.

Subarachnoid Block
Cesarean birth: Can be established slightly faster than epidural block.
May rarely be used for complicated vaginal birth.
Does not provide pain relief for labor because it is done just before birth.
May be combined with an epidural block in a CSE. See "Intrathecal Opioid Analgesics" for more information.
	1. See "Epidural Block" for these interventions:
	  • IV prehydration
	  • Uterine displacement
	  • Observation of BP and fetal heart rate
	  • Care for hypotension or signs of impaired placental perfusion
	  • Observation and intervention for bladder distention
	  • Transfer and ambulation precautions
	2. Observe for postspinal headache: a headache that is worse when the woman is upright and that may disappear when she is lying flat. Notify anesthesia provider if it occurs (a blood patch may be done).
	3. Nursing interventions for postspinal headache: Encourage bed rest, increase oral fluids if not contraindicated, give oral caffeine, and give analgesics as ordered.

General Anesthesia Cesarean birth if epidural or spinal block is not possible or if the woman refuses regional anesthesia. May be required for emergency procedures such as replacement of inverted uterus.	1. Determine type and time of last food intake on admission. 2. Restrict oral intake to clear liquids or as ordered. Consult with physician or nurse-midwife if surgical intervention is likely. 3. Report to anesthesia provider: oral intake before and during labor, vomiting. 4. Displace uterus (see "Epidural Block"). 5. Give ordered drugs such as sodium citrate and citric acid (Bicitra). 6. Maintain cricoid pressure (Sellick maneuver) during intubation. 7. The woman will remain intubated until protective (gag) reflexes have returned. Have oral airway and suction immediately available. Oxygen by face tent or face mask should be given after extubation. 8. Interventions for postoperative respiratory depression: give positive-pressure oxygen by face mask; observe oxygen saturation with pulse oximetry until woman is awake and alert; have woman take several deep breaths if oxygen saturation falls below 95%. Notify anesthesia provider.

BP, Blood pressure; *IV,* intravenous.

EPIDURAL ANALGESIA

Many women choose epidural analgesia for pain relief during labor because of its effectiveness without sedation. Epidural block analgesia requires a number of specific nursing assessments and interventions.

Assessment

The admission assessment focuses on possible allergies to local anesthetics or opioid drugs that might be used in the block. Determine baseline maternal vital signs and the FHR and pattern. Assess for any skin infection in the area of the back where the epidural will be inserted.

Analysis

The primary risks associated with epidural analgesia are maternal hypotension and injury. These result in a collaborative problem and a nursing diagnosis:

- Potential complication–maternal hypotension with secondary fetal hypoxia
- Risk for Injury related to reduced sensation and movement secondary to anesthetic effects

Planning

Goals or expected outcomes are not appropriate for collaborative problems such as the potential complication of hypotension. The nurse's responsibility is to observe for hypotension and report its occurrence to the professional who is in charge of the anesthetic for definitive treatment. However, a goal or expected outcome is appropriate for the risk for injury nursing diagnosis: The woman has achieved the goal if she does not have a treatment-related injury while her sensation and mobility are reduced.

Interventions

MATERNAL HYPOTENSION

Maternal hypotension reduces blood supply to the placenta, decreasing fetal oxygen and nutrient supply and waste removal. Birth facilities will have policies that provide specific guidelines for care when women receive epidural block. Infuse the prescribed IV solution, at least 500 to 1000 ml before the block's initiation. If the woman has not received the full amount when the block is begun, notify the anesthesia professional.

The epidural may be placed with the woman in a sitting or side-lying position based on the decision of the anesthesia provider. If she is in a sitting position, hugging a pillow or a small birth ball helps her hold the correct position. Tell the anesthesia clinician when the woman is having a contraction. She may feel a brief "electric shock" sensation as the catheter is passed. After the epidural is initiated, maintain her position so that aortocaval compression is avoided, such as by placing a pillow under her right hip.

Take the woman's blood pressure and pulse (often an automatic cuff is used) every 2 to 3 minutes, or according to the facility's protocol, for 15 to 20 minutes after the initial injection of medication, comparing it with her baseline pressure. Maintain continuous electronic fetal monitoring. A significant blood pressure decrease is a 20% fall from her baseline or a fall to 100 mm Hg systolic. Hypotension of any degree accompanied by FHR decelerations is significant. If hypotension occurs, increase the rate of her IV fluid, keeping her positioned to avoid aortocaval compression. Ephedrine, 5 to 10 mg, is ordered if hypotension is significant and a fluid increase does not quickly improve it. When the blood pressure is stable, assess it every 15 minutes. Pulse oximetry identifies a fall in maternal oxygenation status to below 95%. Most electronic fetal monitors have the options of automatic blood pressure and pulse oximetry.

Continue observing the FHR. Signs of reduced placental perfusion may be evident before the woman shows signs of hypotension. These include fetal tachycardia (more than 160 bpm) or bradycardia (less than 110 bpm) and late decelerations (see Chapter 14). Take the mother's temperature to identify elevations that may also contribute to fetal tachycardia.

AVOIDANCE OF INJURY

Epidural block reduces lower extremity sensation and movement to varying degrees. Some women have such a light motor block that theirs is called a "walking epidural." However, to prevent falls, these women should not walk alone. Most women must remain in bed or sometimes a nearby chair after their epidural is begun because of reduced sensation.

Assess the degree of motor block and sensation hourly. If a distinct increase or change is noted, report it to the anesthesia clinician because this may indicate catheter migration or another complication.

A woman who has reduced mobility and sensation should be moved so that she maintains an anatomic position. Avoid prolonged pressure on one area. Remember that changing position often improves labor progress, even if the woman does not need to change positions for comfort. If surgery is needed, pad bony prominences to reduce pressure on those areas.

Before any ambulation, such as urination after birth, test the woman's ability to raise and move her legs. Have her push her legs against your hands to determine her leg strength. When she ambulates, accompany her, observing for her ability to move and her strength the entire time until the epidural's effects have worn off.

Evaluation

The collaborative problem is not evaluated, but the nurse compares the woman's baseline blood pressure and FHR to those after the block is begun to identify any significant changes. The goal or expected outcome related to injury is achieved if the woman does not have an injury related to her altered sensation and mobility while the epidural block is exerting its effects.

RESPIRATORY COMPROMISE

Assessment

General anesthesia may be needed any time during birth, most often for cesarean birth. Document the type (solids or liquids) and time of the woman's last food intake. Question her closely if she reports an unusually long interval since her last oral intake. Anesthesia providers can anticipate and prevent problems better if they know the actual oral intake.

Analysis

Nursing care of pregnant women who may require general anesthesia includes monitoring for the short-term risk for aspiration. It is impossible to predict every laboring woman who will require general anesthesia. In addition, surgery that requires general anesthesia may be required at any point during pregnancy.

Planning

The nursing diagnosis appropriate to minimize respiratory compromise that may affect both the woman and her fetus is Risk for Aspiration related to impaired protective laryngeal reflexes.

The expected outcome is that the woman will not aspirate gastric contents during the perioperative period.

Interventions

Nursing interventions relate to identifying factors that increase a woman's risk for aspiration and collaborative and nursing measures to reduce the risk of aspiration or lung injury.

IDENTIFYING RISK FACTORS

Report oral intake both before and after admission to the anesthesia provider. Oral intake during labor is often restricted to medications, clear liquids, ice chips, Popsicles, or hard candies.

Vomiting is a common occurrence during normal labor, regardless of the mother's oral intake. If vomiting occurs, chart the time, quantity, and character (amount, color, presence of undigested food).

REDUCING RISK FOR ASPIRATION OR LUNG INJURY

Nursing and medical personnel collaborate to reduce a woman's risk for pulmonary complications.

PERIOPERATIVE CARE

Restrict oral intake as ordered if surgery is expected. Give ordered medications such as sodium citrate and citric acid (Bicitra). Either the nurse or anesthesia provider may give parenteral drugs, such as glycopyrrolate (Robinul), depending on when they are administered.

An experienced nurse or a trained anesthesia assistant provides cricoid pressure (Sellick maneuver) to block the esophagus until the woman is intubated and the cuff of the endotracheal tube is inflated. Successful intubation with the cuffed endotracheal tube blocks passage of any gastric contents into the trachea.

POSTOPERATIVE CARE

Birth facility protocols guide postoperative care, including preextubation and postextubation care for the woman who has had general anesthesia. The woman is extubated when her protective laryngeal reflexes have returned. Suction equipment and an Ambu bag with appropriate-size mask should be immediately available. Administer oxygen by mask or face tent for 2 to 5 minutes until the woman is awake and alert, because the agents used for general anesthesia are respiratory depressants. Monitor oxygen saturation with a pulse oximeter. If her oxygen saturation falls below 95%, have her take several deep breaths. Deep breathing also helps her eliminate inhalational anesthetics and reduces stasis of pulmonary secretions.

Assess the woman's pulse, respiration, and blood pressure every 15 minutes for 1 hour or until stable; then continue according to policy. Observe her color for pallor or cyanosis, which suggests shock or hypoventilation.

Evaluation

Interventions for this nursing diagnosis are preventive and short-term because it is a temporary high-risk situation. The goal is met if the woman does not aspirate gastric contents during the perioperative period.

SUMMARY CONCEPTS

- Childbirth pain is unique because it is normal and self-limiting, can be prepared for, and ends with a baby's birth.
- Excess or poorly relieved pain may be harmful to the mother and fetus.
- Pain is a complex physical and psychological experience. It is subjective and personal.
- Four sources of pain are present in most labors, but other physical and psychological factors may increase or decrease the pain felt from these sources. These sources are cervical dilation, uterine ischemia, pressure and pulling on pelvic structures, and distention of the vagina and perineum.
- Relaxation enhances all other pain management techniques.
- Several nonpharmacologic pain management techniques supplement relaxation—cutaneous stimulation, hydrotherapy, mental stimulation, and breathing techniques.
- Physiologic alterations of pregnancy may affect a woman's response to medications.
- Any drug that the expectant mother takes, whether therapeutic or abused, including herbal or botanical preparations, also may affect the fetus. Fetal effects may be direct or indirect.
- The nurse should observe for respiratory depression, primarily in the newborn, when the mother has received opioid analgesics during labor.
- The major advantages of regional pain management methods are that the woman can participate in the birth and that she retains her protective airway reflexes.

- The nurse should observe for and take actions to prevent maternal hypotension with the epidural or subarachnoid block.
- The nurse should observe for fetal heart rate changes associated with impaired placental perfusion if the woman receives a regional technique that carries the risk for maternal hypotension.
- The main nursing observations for the woman who receives epidural or intrathecal opioids are for nausea and vomiting, pruritus, and delayed respiratory depression.
- Regurgitation with aspiration of acidic gastric contents is the greatest risk for a woman who receives general anesthesia.

ANSWERS TO CRITICAL THINKING EXERCISE 15-1, p. 338

1. Truc's labor progress and pattern of contractions and her tension suggest that she needs assistance with pain management. However, the nurse should not assume that she needs or wants medication, either. Truc may prefer non-pharmacologic measures, and these may also complement medication.

   The nurse cannot make assumptions about Truc's needs for pain relief based on her behavior. Asian women often value stoicism and are concerned with harmonious relationships. Truc may be smiling to please the nurse rather than because she is comfortable.

2. The nurse needs additional data about Truc's real needs and preferences for pain management.

3. The nurse can share observations about Truc's body posture during contractions. If Truc does not speak English well, an interpreter or picture-type pain scale may improve assessment of her need for pain relief. The nurse might demonstrate simple breathing and relaxation techniques, offer hydrotherapy in the form of a shower, tub, or whirlpool, and suggest position changes or ambulation.

REFERENCES & READINGS

Adachi, K., Shimada, M., & Usui, A. (2003). The relationship between the parturient's position and perceptions of labor pain intensity. *Nursing Research, 52*(1), pp. 47-51.

American Academy of Pediatrics (AAP) & American College of Obstetricians and Gynecologists (ACOG). (2002). *Guidelines for perinatal care* (5th ed.). Elk Grove Village, IL, and Washington, DC: Authors.

American Academy of Pediatrics & American Heart Association. (2000). *Neonatal resuscitation textbook* (4th ed.). Dallas, TX, and Elk Grove Village, IL: Authors.

American College of Obstetricians and Gynecologists. (2002). *Obstetric analgesia and anesthesia*. Practice Bulletin No. 36. Washington, DC: Author.

Association of Women's Health, Obstetric and Neonatal Nurses (AWHONN). (2001). *Evidence-based clinical practice guideline: Nursing care of the woman receiving regional analgesia/anesthesia in labor*. Washington, DC: Author.

AWHONN. (2000). *Symposium: Second stage labor management: Promotion of evidence-based practice and a collaborative approach to patient care*. Washington, DC: Author.

Ayoub, C.M., & Sinatra, R.S. (2004). Postoperative analgesia: Epidural and spinal techniques. In D.H. Chestnut (Ed.), *Obstetric anesthesia: Principles and practice* (3rd ed., pp. 472-506). St. Louis: Mosby.

Bricker, L., & Lavender, T. (2002). Parenteral opioids for labor pain relief: A systematic review. *American Journal of Obstetrics & Gynecology, 186*(5), S94-S109.

Britt, R., & Pasero, C. (1999). Pregnancy, childbirth, postpartum, and breastfeeding: Use of analgesics. In M. McCaffery & C. Pasero, *Pain: Clinical manual* (2nd ed., pp. 608-625). St. Louis: Mosby.

Brown, D.L., & Gottumukkala, V. (2004). Spinal, epidural, and caudal anesthesia: Anatomy, physiology, and technique. In D.H. Chestnut (Ed.), *Obstetric anesthesia: Principles and practice* (3rd ed., pp. 171-189). St. Louis: Mosby.

Chapman, L.L. (2000). Expectant fathers and labor epidurals. *MCN: American Journal of Maternal/Child Nursing, 25*(3), 133-138.

Chestnut, D.H. (2004a). Alternative regional anesthetic techniques: Paracervical block, lumbar sympathetic block, pudendal block, and perineal infiltration. In D.H. Chestnut (Ed.), *Obstetric anesthesia: Principles and practice* (3rd ed., pp. 387-396). St. Louis: Mosby.

Chestnut, D.H. (2004b). Epidural and spinal analgesia/anesthesia: Section III: Effect on the progress of labor and method of delivery. In D.H. Chestnut (Ed.), *Obstetric anesthesia: Principles and practice* (3rd ed., pp. 408-426). St. Louis: Mosby.

Creehan, P.A. (2001). Pain relief and comfort measures during labor. In K.R. Simpson & P.A. Creehan (Eds.), *AWHONN perinatal nursing* (2nd ed., pp. 417-444). Philadelphia: Lippincott Williams & Wilkins.

Cunningham, F.G., MacDonald, P.C., Gant, N.F., Leveno, K.J., Gilstrap, L.C., Hauth, J.C., & Wenstrom, K.D. (2001). *Williams obstetrics* (21st ed.). New York: McGraw-Hill.

Eckert, K., Turnbull, D., & MacLennan, A. (2001). Immersion in water in the first stage of labor: A randomized controlled trial. *Birth, 28*(2), 84-93.

Faucher, M.A., & Brucker, M.C. (2000). Intrapartum pain: Pharmacologic management. *Journal of Obstetric, Gynecologic, and Neonatal Nursing, 29*(2), 169-180.

Grabowska, C. (2000). Alternative therapies for pain relief. In M. Yerby (Ed.), *Pain in childbearing*, pp. 93-109. Edinburgh: Baillière Tindall.

Hobel, C.J., & Chang, A.B. (2004). Normal labor, delivery, and postpartum care: Anatomic considerations, obstetric analgesia and anesthesia, and resuscitation of the newborn. In N.F. Hacker, J.G. Moore, & J.C. Gambone (Eds.), *Essentials of obstetrics and gynecology* (4th ed., pp. 104-135). Philadelphia: Saunders.

Joint Commission on Accreditation of Healthcare Organizations. (2003). *Improving the quality of pain management through measurement and action*. Retrieved December 5, 2004, from www.jcaho.org.

Kabler, J. (2000). Water immersion during labor and birth. In F.H. Nichols & S.S. Humenick (Eds.), *Childbirth education: Practice, research, and theory* (2nd ed., pp. 284-294). Philadelphia: Saunders.

Lieberman, E., Lang, J., Richardson, D.K., Frigoletto, F.D., Heffner, L.J., & Cohen, A. (1999). Epidurals and cesareans: The jury is still out. *Birth, 26*(3), 196-198.

Lieberman, E., Lang, J., Richardson, D.K., Frigoletto, F.D., Heffner, L.J., & Cohen, A. (2000). Intrapartum maternal fever and neonatal outcome. *Pediatrics, 105*(1), pp. 8-13.

Mayberry, L.J., Clemmens, D., & De, A. (2002). Epidural analgesia side effects, co-interventions, and care of women during childbirth: A systematic review. *American Journal of Obstetrics and Gynecology, 186*(5), S81-S93.

Mayberry, L.J., Strange, L.B., Suplee, P.D., & Gennaro, S. (2003). Use of upright positioning with epidural analgesia: Findings from an observational study. *MCN: The American Journal of Maternal/Child Nursing, 28*(3), 152-159.

Mayberry, L.J., Wood, S.H., Strange, L.B., Lee, L., Heisler, D.R., & Nielsen-Smith, K. (2000). *Second-stage labor management: Promotion of evidence-based practice and a collaborative approach to patient care.* Washington, DC: Association of Women's Health, Obstetric, and Neonatal Nurses.

Naughton, N.N., & Cohen, S.E. (2004). Nonobstetric surgery during pregnancy. In D.H. Chestnut (Ed.), *Obstetric anesthesia: Principles and practice* (3rd ed., pp. 255-272). St. Louis: Mosby.

Pasero, C., Portenoy, R.K., & McCaffery, M. (1999). Opioid analgesics. In M. McCaffery & C. Pasero (Eds.), *Pain: Clinical manual* (2nd ed., pp. 161-299). St. Louis: Mosby.

Paull, J. (2000). Epidural analgesia for labor. In D.J. Birnbach, S.P. Gatt, & S. Datta (Eds.), *Textbook of obstetric anesthesia* (pp. 145-156). New York: Churchill Livingstone.

Polley, L.S., & Glosten, B. (2004). Epidural and spinal analgesia/anesthesia: Section I: Local anesthetic techniques. In D.H. Chestnut (Ed.), *Obstetric anesthesia: Principles and practice* (3rd ed., pp. 324-348). St. Louis: Mosby.

Poole, J.H. (2003). Analgesia and anesthesia during labor and birth: Implications for mother and fetus. *Journal of Obstetric, Gynecologic, and Neonatal Nursing, 32*(6), 780-793.

Riley, E.T., & Ross, B.K. (2004). Epidural and spinal analgesia/anesthesia: Section II: Opioid techniques. In D.H. Chestnut (Ed.), *Obstetric anesthesia: Principles and practice* (3rd ed., 349-368). St. Louis: Mosby.

Robinson, J.N., Norwitz, E.R., Cohen, A.P., McElrath, T.F., & Lieberman, E.S. (2000). Epidural analgesia and third- or fourth-degree lacerations in nulliparas. *Obstetrics and Gynecology, 94,* 259-262.

Segal, S., Carp, H., & Chestnut, D.H. (2004). Fever and infection. In D.H. Chestnut (Ed.), *Obstetric anesthesia: Principles and practice* (3rd ed., 647-661). St. Louis: Mosby.

Simkin, P., & Frederick, E. (2000). Labor support. In F.H. Nichols & S.S. Humenick (Eds.), *Childbirth education: Practice, research, and theory* (2nd ed., pp. 307-341). Philadelphia: Saunders.

Simkin, P.P., & O'Hara, M. (2002). Nonpharmacologic relief of pain during labor: Systematic reviews of five methods. *American Journal of Obstetrics & Gynecology, 186*(5), S131-S159.

Teschendorf, M.E., & Evans, C.P. (2000). Hydrotherapy during labor: An example of developing a practice policy. *MCN: American Journal of Maternal/Child Nursing, 25*(4), 198-203.

Wakefield, M.L. (2004). Systemic analgesia: Parenteral and inhalational agents. In D.H. Chestnut (Ed.), *Obstetric anesthesia: Principles and practice* (3rd ed., pp. 311-323). St. Louis: Mosby.

Weeks, S.K. (2004). Postpartum headache. In D.H. Chestnut (Ed.), *Obstetric anesthesia: Principles and practice* (3rd ed., pp. 562-578). St. Louis: Mosby.

Woolley, D., & Nelsson-Ryan, S. (2000). Second-stage labor. Labor support. In F.H. Nichols & S.S. Humenick (Eds.), *Childbirth education: Practice, research, and theory* (2nd ed., pp. 342-375). Philadelphia: Saunders.

Nursing Care during Obstetric Procedures

After studying this chapter, you should be able to:

1. Identify clinical situations in which specific obstetric procedures are appropriate.
2. Explain risks, precautions, and contraindications for each procedure.
3. Identify nursing considerations for each procedure.
4. Identify methods to provide effective emotional support to the woman undergoing an obstetric procedure.
5. Apply the nursing process to care for the woman having a cesarean birth.

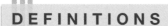

Go to your Student CD-ROM for Review Questions keyed to these Objectives.

DEFINITIONS

Abruptio Placentae Premature separation of a normally implanted placenta.

Amniotomy Artificial rupture of the amniotic sac (fetal membranes).

Augmentation of Labor Artificial stimulation of uterine contractions that have become ineffective.

Cephalopelvic Disproportion Fetal head size that is too large to fit through the maternal pelvis at birth (also called *fetopelvic disproportion*).

Cesarean Birth Surgical birth of the fetus through an incision in the abdominal wall and uterus.

Chignon Newborn scalp edema created by a vacuum extractor.

Chorioamnionitis Inflammation of the amniotic sac (fetal membranes); usually caused by bacterial and viral infections (also called *amnionitis*).

Dystocia Difficult or prolonged labor; often associated with abnormal uterine activity and cephalopelvic disproportion.

Episiotomy Surgical incision of the perineum to enlarge the vaginal opening.

Hydramnios Excessive volume of amniotic fluid, more than about 2000 ml at term (also called *polyhydramnios*).

Iatrogenic Term used to describe an adverse condition resulting from treatment.

Induction of Labor Artificial initiation of labor.

Montevideo Unit A unit of measure expressing the intensity of uterine contractions in mm Hg as measured with an intrauterine pressure catheter; the contraction intensity minus the resting tone multiplied by the number of contractions in 10 minutes.

Nuchal Cord Umbilical cord around the fetal neck.

Oligohydramnios Abnormally small quantity of amniotic fluid, less than about 500 ml at term.

Placenta Previa Abnormal implantation of the placenta in the lower uterus.

Premature Rupture of the Membranes Spontaneous rupture of the membranes before the onset of labor (term, preterm, or postterm gestation).

Version Turning the fetus from one presentation to another before birth, usually from breech to cephalic.

Although labor is a normal process, some women require special procedures to help them and their fetuses. A physician or nurse-midwife performs these procedures. Nursing considerations for each procedure are addressed in this chapter.

AMNIOTOMY

Indications

Amniotomy is usually performed in conjunction with induction and augmentation of labor and to allow internal electronic fetal monitoring (see Chapter 14). Amniotomy is not often used as the sole means to induce and augment labor, and more data are needed to determine its effectiveness when used in this way (Simpson & Poole, 1998). Amniotomy also is associated with risks that must be considered by the birth attendant before performing the procedure.

Risks

Amniotomy is performed by the physician or nurse-midwife. The nurse must observe for three risks associated with amniotomy and must assist in emergency procedures.

PROLAPSE OF THE UMBILICAL CORD

The primary risk is that the umbilical cord will slip down in the gush of fluid. The cord can be compressed between the fetal presenting part and the woman's pelvis, obstructing blood flow to and from the placenta and reducing fetal gas exchange.

INFECTION

With interruption of the membrane barrier, vaginal organisms have free access to the uterine cavity and may cause chorioamnionitis. The risk is low at first but increases as the interval between membrane rupture and birth increases. Birth within 24 hours of membrane rupture is desirable, although infection does not occur at any absolute time.

ABRUPTIO PLACENTAE

Abruptio placentae can occur if the uterus is distended with excessive amniotic fluid when the membranes rupture. As the uterus collapses with discharge of the amniotic fluid, the area of placental attachment shrinks. The placenta then no longer fits its implantation site and partially separates. A large area of placental disruption can significantly reduce fetal oxygenation, nutrition, and waste disposal.

Technique

A disposable plastic hook (such as AmniHook) is commonly used to perforate the amniotic sac (Figure 16-1). The birth attendant performs a vaginal examination to determine cervical dilation and effacement, fetal station, and fetal presenting part. Amniotomy is often deferred if the fetal presenting part is high or the presentation is not cephalic. The risk of a prolapsed cord is higher in these situations because more room is available for the cord to slip down. The fetus in a noncephalic presentation is more likely to be born by cesarean birth and an amniotomy is done at the time of surgery through the abdominal and uterine incisions.

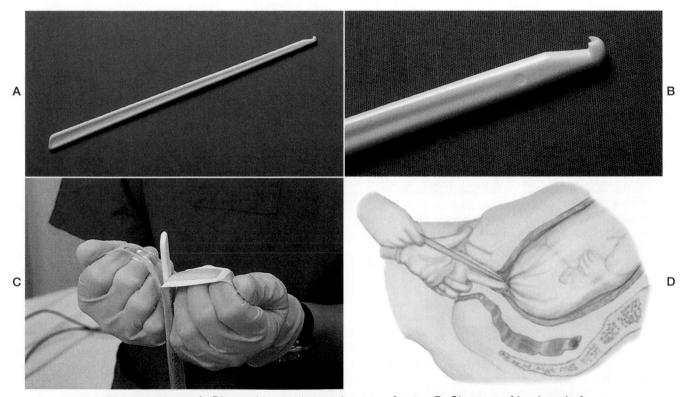

Figure 16-1 ■ **A,** Disposable plastic membrane perforator. **B,** Close-up of hook end of plastic membrane perforator. **C,** Correct method to open the package. **D,** Technique for artificial rupture of membranes.

The hook is passed through the cervical opening, snagging the membranes. The opening in the membranes is enlarged with the finger, allowing fluid to drain.

Nursing Considerations

OBTAINING BASELINE INFORMATION

The fetal heart rate (FHR) is assessed with electronic monitoring or auscultation to verify a reassuring rate and pattern before amniotomy is performed. The initial fetal assessment provides a baseline to compare with later assessments. A minimum of 20 to 30 minutes is needed for adequate baseline fetal evaluation.

ASSISTING WITH AMNIOTOMY

Before amniotomy, two or three underpads should be placed under the woman's buttocks to absorb the fluid and overlapped to extend from her waist to her knees. A folded bath towel under the buttocks absorbs more amniotic fluid.

Other supplies needed are a disposable plastic hook, sterile glove for the birth attendant, and a packet of sterile lubricant. The nurse should partly open the package containing the plastic hook at the handle end and hold back the package until the birth attendant takes the hook with a sterile, gloved hand.

PROVIDING CARE AFTER AMNIOTOMY

Nursing care after amniotomy is the same as that after spontaneous membrane rupture.

IDENTIFYING COMPLICATIONS. The FHR is assessed for at least 1 full minute after amniotomy. Nonreassuring monitor patterns or significant changes from previous assessments are reported promptly to the birth attendant. Cord compression is usually accompanied by a rate less than 100 beats per minute (bpm), which further falls during contractions.

The quantity, color, and odor of the amniotic fluid are charted. The fluid should be clear (often with bits of vernix) and have a mild odor. A large amount of vernix in the fluid

suggests that the fetus may be preterm. Greenish, meconium-stained fluid may be seen in postterm gestation or placental insufficiency. Fluid with a foul or strong odor, cloudy appearance, or yellow color suggests chorioamnionitis. Hydramnios is associated with some fetal abnormalities. Oligohydramnios may be associated with placental insufficiency or fetal urinary tract abnormalities.

Adequate amniotic fluid is necessary for lung development. The fetus with prolonged oligohydramnios may have respiratory problems after birth because the lungs cannot expand normally.

The woman's temperature should be assessed at least every 2 to 4 hours after the membranes rupture. Elevations above 38° C (100.4° F) should be reported. A rising FHR and fetal tachycardia (above 160 bpm) may precede maternal fever.

PROMOTING COMFORT. Amniotic fluid continues to leak from the woman's vagina. Regularly changed underpads keep her drier and reduce the moist environment that favors bacterial growth.

✓ **CHECK YOUR READING**

1. What are three risks associated with amniotomy?
2. Why is the FHR assessed before and after the membranes rupture?
3. What is the significance of green amniotic fluid?
4. What maternal and fetal signs are associated with chorioamnionitis?

INDUCTION AND AUGMENTATION OF LABOR

Induction and augmentation of labor use artificial methods to stimulate uterine contractions. Techniques and nursing care are similar for both induction and augmentation.

Induction of labor is an increasingly common procedure in intrapartum units and has more than doubled in just over a decade. In 1989 9% of live births were induced, compared with 19.9% in 2002. Augmentation rates have increased from 10.9% in 1989 to 20.6% in 2002 (Martin et al., 2003).

Indications

Induction of labor is performed when a continued pregnancy may jeopardize the health of the woman or fetus and labor and vaginal birth are considered safe. Labor induction is not done if the fetus must be delivered more quickly than the process permits, in which case a cesarean birth is performed. Induction is indicated in these conditions (American College of Obstetricians and Gynecologists [ACOG], 1999a):

- Conditions in which the intrauterine environment is hostile to fetal well-being (e.g., intrauterine fetal growth restriction, maternal-fetal blood incompatibility)
- Spontaneous rupture of the membranes at or near term without onset of labor, also called *premature rupture of the membranes* (PROM)
- Postterm pregnancy
- Chorioamnionitis (inflammation of the amniotic sac)

CRITICAL THINKING ⁇ EXERCISE 16-1

A physician performs an amniotomy on a laboring woman whose cervix is dilated to 5 cm. The amniotic fluid is pale yellow and moderate in amount, and it has a strong odor. The baseline fetal heart rate ranges from 155 to 165, accelerating when the fetus moves. Maternal vital signs are as follows: temperature, 99.7° F (37.6° C); pulse, 92; respirations, 22; blood pressure, 116/80. Contractions are of moderate to firm intensity, every 3 to 4 minutes, with a duration of 50 to 60 seconds and complete uterine relaxation between contractions.

Questions

1. Which of these observations should the nurse regard as normal? Which factors are abnormal?
2. Should the nurse modify routine labor care based on the postamniotomy assessments?

- Hypertension associated with pregnancy or chronic hypertension, both of which are associated with reduced placental blood flow
- Abruptio placentae (large abruptions require immediate delivery; see Chapter 25)
- Maternal medical conditions that worsen with continuation of the pregnancy (such as diabetes, renal disease, pulmonary disease, heart disease)
- Fetal death

Induction solely for convenience is not recommended. However, factors such as having a history of rapid labors and living a long distance from the hospital are valid reasons to induce labor because of the real possibility that the baby would be born in uncontrolled circumstances. Considerations such as maternity leave also may be valid.

Prenatal testing sometimes identifies a fetal anomaly that will require specialized neonatal care at a distant facility. The mother may be transported to that facility for labor induction or cesarean with needed equipment and specialists to care for the newborn.

Augmentation of labor with oxytocin is considered when labor has begun spontaneously but progress has slowed or stopped, even if contractions seem to be adequate.

Contraindications

Any contraindication to labor and vaginal birth is a contraindication to induction or augmentation of labor. Possible contraindications and cautions associated with induction may include:

- Placenta previa, which would result in hemorrhage during labor
- Vasa previa, in which fetal umbilical cord vessels branch over the amniotic sac rather than inserting into the placenta; fetal hemorrhage is a possibility if the membranes rupture
- Umbilical cord prolapse, because immediate cesarean is indicated to stop cord compression
- Abnormal fetal presentation for which vaginal birth is often more hazardous
- Fetal presenting part above the pelvic inlet, which may be associated with cephalopelvic disproportion or a preterm fetus
- Previous surgery in the upper uterus, such as a previous classical cesarean incision (see pp. 380-381) or extensive surgery for uterine fibroids

Other maternal or fetal conditions are not contraindications to induction but require individual evaluation:

- One or more previous low-transverse cesarean deliveries (see pp. 380-381)
- Breech presentation (vaginal birth may be more hazardous; also, the fetus may turn to a normal position by the time spontaneous labor occurs)
- Conditions in which the uterus is overdistended, such as a multifetal pregnancy and hydramnios, because the risk of uterine rupture is higher
- Severe maternal conditions such as heart disease and severe hypertension

- Fetal presenting part above the pelvic inlet, which may be associated with cephalopelvic disproportion or a preterm fetus
- Nonreassuring FHR patterns, because the added stress of stimulated contractions will reduce placental perfusion

Risks

Induction and augmentation of labor, like spontaneous labor, are associated with risks:

- Hypertonic uterine activity (excessive frequency, duration, or intensity of contractions) that can reduce placental perfusion and fetal oxygenation. Uterine hyperstimulation may or may not be accompanied by a nonreassuring FHR pattern.
- Uterine rupture, more likely with overdistension of the uterus.
- Maternal water intoxication, which is more likely if a hypotonic intravenous (IV) solution is used to dilute the oxytocin and with rates greater than 20 milliunits/min (ACOG, 1999a; Cunningham, et al., 2001; Simpson & Atterbury, 2003)
- Greater risk for cesarean birth

Evidence is accumulating that links labor induction to increased risk for cesarean birth. Studies have demonstrated that women who have their labor induced are two to three times more likely to have a surgical birth. Women having a Bishop score of less than 5 at the time of induction, indicating a cervix that is not favorable, had a greater risk for cesarean than women who had a score of 5 or more. Approximately 25% of inductions had no clearly documented medical or obstetric indication but were elective. The risk for cesarean after failed induction was similar whether women had medical or elective inductions (Johnson, Davis, & Brown, 2003; Martin et al., 2003; Seyb, Berka, Socol, & Dooley, 1999; Yeast, Jones, & Poskin, 1999).

Technique

Surgical and medical methods may be used for labor induction and augmentation. Amniotomy is the method of surgical induction and augmentation because rupturing membranes stimulates uterine contractions and occasionally may be adequate in itself if the cervix is very favorable. Medical methods for induction and augmentation use drugs such as prostaglandins, IV oxytocin (Pitocin), or both to stimulate contractions.

DETERMINING WHETHER INDUCTION IS INDICATED

The birth attendant evaluates whether the benefits of ending the pregnancy outweigh those of continuing it for the woman and fetus. Labor is not induced if the fetus is younger than 39 weeks unless a compelling reason exists. Also, induction is more likely to be successful at term because prelabor cervical changes favor dilation.

Cervical assessment estimates whether the cervix is favorable for induction. The Bishop scoring system (Table 16-1) is

TABLE **16-1** Bishop Scoring System to Evaluate the Cervix*

	Score			
Factor	0	1	2	3
Dilation	0 cm	1-2 cm	3-4 cm	5-6 cm
Effacement	0%-30%	40%-50%	60%-70%	≥80%
Fetal station	−3	−2	−1 or 0	+1 or +2
Cervical consistency	Firm	Medium	Soft	
Cervical position	Posterior	Middle	Anterior	

Modified from Bishop, E.H. (1964). Pelvic scoring for elective induction. *Obstetrics & Gynecology, 24*(2), 266-268.

*This system is used to estimate how easily a woman's labor can be induced. Higher scores are associated with a greater likelihood of successful induction because her cervix has undergone prelabor changes, often called *ripening*. A woman who has given birth before usually has a successful induction when her Bishop score is 5 or higher. Delivery in a woman who is having her first baby is most successfully induced if her score is 7 or higher.

used to estimate cervical readiness for labor with five factors: cervical dilation, effacement, consistency, position, and fetal station. Vaginal birth is more likely to result if a Bishop score is higher than 8 (ACOG 1999a).

The Bishop score is subjective and depends on the experience of the examiner. One objective method to evaluate a woman's readiness for induction of labor is assessment of fetal fibronectin (fFN) in the cervical and vaginal secretions. fFN is a protein concentrated at the junction of the decidua and chorion. It is found in the vaginal secretions in decreasing amounts until about 20 weeks' gestation but then reappears in these secretions about 2 weeks before the onset of term labor (Guinn & Gibbs, 2003). fFN appears promising in the determination of which women will have the most successful induction, particularly if induction is not urgent.

CERVICAL RIPENING

Procedures to ripen (soften) the cervix and make it more likely to dilate with the forces of labor are a common adjunct to induction. Most are done the day before the scheduled induction.

MEDICAL METHODS. Prostaglandin is a drug that may be used to cause cervical ripening. Prostaglandin E_2 (PGE$_2$) preparations may be given as an intravaginal gel, an intracervical gel, and a timed-release vaginal insert (Table 16-2).

TABLE **16-2** Prostaglandin Preparations for Cervical Ripening at Term

Prostaglandin Gel (dinoprostone [Prepidil])	Vaginal Insert (dinoprostone [Cervidil])	Misoprostol (Cytotec)
Dosage*		
0.5 mg applied to cervix; may be repeated 6-12 hr later. 2.5 mg vaginally.	10 mg in a time-release vaginal insert.	One quarter of 100-mcg tablet vaginally (approximately 25 mcg; see cautions below). Also used for labor induction by repeating 25-mcg dose every 3-6 hr. A 50-mcg dose is associated with hypertonic contractions.
Actions for Hypertonic Contractions, with or without Nonreassuring Fetal Heart Rate Pattern		
Place woman in side-lying position. Provide oxygen by face mask at 8-10 L/min. Administer tocolytic drug such as terbutaline or magnesium sulfate. Typically begins 1 hr after gel application. Higher incidence with vaginal application.	Same as for dinoprostone gel. Remove insert. Hypertonic uterine activity may occur up to 9½ hr after insert placement. Greater incidence than with lower-dose intracervical dinoprostone gel.	Same as for dinoprostone gel. Higher dose or more frequent administration is more likely to cause excessive contractions, which may or may not be accompanied by a nonreassuring fetal heart rate pattern.
When Oxytocin Induction May Begin		
Safe interval has not been established. Delaying oxytocin administration for 6-12 hr after total intracervical dose of 1.5-mg or 2.5-mg vaginal dose recommended.	30-60 min after removal of insert.	At least 4 hr after last dose.
Precautions and Comments		
Limit dinoprostone gel to maximum of 1.5 mg in 24 hr. Woman should remain recumbent with lateral uterine displacement for 15-30 min after application. Has increased effect if combined with other oxytocics such as oxytocin (Pitocin). Increases hypertensive effect of the herb ephedra. Use caution in women with asthma, hypertension, glaucoma, severe renal or hepatic dysfunction, or ischemic heart disease.	Remove after 12 hr or when active labor begins. Adverse effects can be reduced within 15 min of removal. Most expensive of the prostaglandin options.	Misoprostol is currently FDA-approved only for treatment of peptic ulcers but is widely used for cervical ripening and induction of labor. Manufacturer does not intend to seek approval, but American College of Obstetricians and Gynecologists supports its use for these purposes. 100-mcg tablet is not scored. Hospital pharmacy should prepare the 25-mcg dose for greater accuracy. Cost is about 1%-2% that of other prostaglandin preparations. Contraindicated in the woman with a previous cesarean or other uterine surgery.

From American College of Obstetricians and Gynecologists (ACOG). (1999). *Induction of labor.* Practice Bulletin No. 10. Washington, DC: Author.
FDA, Food and Drug Administration.
*Doses may be higher in cases of fetal death.

Misoprostol (Cytotec) is a prostaglandin E_1 (PGE_1) analog usually given for gastric ulcers. Misoprostol can be used for both cervical ripening and induction of labor. Misoprostol for cervical ripening is currently an unlabeled use, and its manufacturer does not plan to seek U.S. Food and Drug Administration approval for these purposes. In addition to its effectiveness, misoprostol is attractive for its lower cost and stability at room temperature (ACOG, 1999a; ACOG, 1999b). However, it should not be given to a woman who has had a previous cesarean birth.

Misoprostol is available in 100- and 200-mcg tablets. The usual dose is 25 mcg, one quarter of the already tiny, unscored 100-mcg tablet. The quarter-tablet is placed high in the vagina.

The major adverse reaction to prostaglandins is hyperstimulation of uterine contractions. Prostaglandins are administered in a setting in which fetal monitoring and emergency care, including cesarean birth, are immediately available. Prostaglandin should be given cautiously to women who have asthma, glaucoma, or pulmonary, hepatic, or renal disease. To reduce leakage the woman should lie flat for 15 to 20 minutes after the gel form of prostaglandin is inserted. The FHR should be monitored for at least 30 minutes for changes, and the uterus should be assessed for excessive contractions.

MECHANICAL METHODS. The most common mechanical method for cervical ripening involves placing hydrophilic (moisture-attracting) inserts into the cervical canal, where they absorb water and swell, gradually dilating the cervix. Examples of these dilators are the following:

- Dilapan—a synthetic material
- Lamicel—a synthetic sponge containing 450 mg of magnesium sulfate
- Laminaria tents—sterile, cone-shaped preparations of dried seaweed

OXYTOCIN ADMINISTRATION

Oxytocin is the most common drug given for induction and augmentation of labor (Drug Guide). Oxytocin is a powerful drug, and predicting a woman's response to it is impossible. Several precautions reduce the chance of adverse reactions in the mother and fetus.

- Oxytocin is diluted in an isotonic solution and given as a secondary (piggyback) infusion so that it can be stopped quickly if complications develop (Figure 16-2).
- The oxytocin line is inserted into the primary (nonadditive or maintenance) IV line as close as possible to the venipuncture site (the proximal port) to limit the amount of drug infused after changing to the nonadditive fluid.
- Oxytocin is started slowly, increased gradually, and regulated with a pump.
- Uterine activity, FHR, and fetal heart patterns are monitored when oxytocin is given.

The woman's uterus becomes more sensitive to oxytocin as labor progresses. Therefore the rate of oxytocin infusion may be gradually reduced when she is in the active phase of labor (about 5 to 6 cm of cervical dilation). It may be stopped or reduced after her membranes rupture. When labor is augmented with oxytocin, a lower total dose usually is needed to achieve adequate contractions.

SERIAL INDUCTION OF LABOR

Serial induction of labor is a variation that the nurse may occasionally encounter. Serial induction may be performed when the woman's cervix is not favorable and she has an indication for induction but same-day birth is not imperative. Risk of induction versus cesarean birth may also be considered. For example, serial induction may be performed for postdate pregnancy (gestation past the expected delivery date).

Oxytocin solution is given over a 2- to 3-day period for about 8 to 10 hours each day. If the woman's labor has not made progress during the day, the oxytocin is stopped, she is given a light meal, and the infusion is resumed the next morning. At the end of the third day, the woman is reevaluated if she is not yet in labor.

ACTIVE MANAGEMENT OF LABOR

Active management of labor is a protocol for labor augmentation created in Ireland. It applies only to nulliparous women in spontaneous labor at term and is aimed at reducing the cesarean birth rate in this group. Active labor management is not induction of labor. The goal of active labor management is to achieve birth within 12 hours of admission. Strict criteria for diagnosing labor and defining abnormal labor progress exist. Although cesarean rates have been found to be lower in many studies of active labor management, the process has not achieved success in the United States.

If the membranes remain intact, amniotomy is performed within 1 hour of admission. Oxytocin augmentation is begun if the rate of progress is less than 1 cm per hour after amniotomy. Oxytocin dosages given by the Irish protocol are higher than those typical in the United States. Cesarean delivery may be performed 12 hours after admission if birth is not imminent (Dudley, 2003).

Nursing Considerations

When providing care during cervical ripening and labor induction or augmentation, the nurse observes the woman and fetus for complications and takes corrective actions if abnormalities are noted. The nurse has a great responsibility when administering uterine stimulants to a pregnant woman. The nurse must decide when to start, change, and stop an oxytocin infusion using the facility's protocols and medical orders. This responsibility requires additional education and refinement of the nurse's critical thinking skills.

OBSERVING THE FETAL RESPONSE

Oxytocin stimulates uterine contractions, and they may become too strong or hypertonic (hyperstimulation). Uterine hyperstimulation can reduce placental blood flow (uteroplacental insufficiency), which decreases exchange of fetal oxygen and waste products. Before induction and augmentation of labor, the nurse determines whether the FHR and fetal

DRUG GUIDE

OXYTOCIN (PITOCIN)

Classification: Oxytocic.

Action: Synthetic compound identical to the natural hormone from the posterior pituitary. Stimulates uterine smooth muscle, resulting in increased strength, duration, and frequency of uterine contractions. Uterine sensitivity to oxytocin increases gradually during gestation. Oxytocin has vasoactive and antidiuretic properties.

Indications: Induction or augmentation of labor at or near term. Maintenance of firm uterine contraction after birth to control postpartum bleeding. Management of inevitable or incomplete abortion.

Dosage and Route

Induction or Augmentation of Labor

1. *Intravenous infusion* via a secondary (piggyback) line. Oxytocin infusion is controlled with a pump. Various dilutions of oxytocin and balanced electrolyte solution may be used. Mixtures having 60 milliunits/ml are convenient because the ml/hr setting on the infusion pump is the same number as the milliunits/min infused, reducing the chance for errors. Common mixtures that provide 60 milliunits/ml of oxytocin include (1) 15 units of oxytocin (1.5 ml) plus 250 ml of solution; (2) 30 units (3 ml) of oxytocin plus 500 ml of solution; and (3) 60 units (6 ml) of oxytocin plus 1000 ml of solution. Lower concentrations, such as 10-20 units of oxytocin plus 1000 ml of solution, may also be used. The drug may be given in 10-minute pulsed infusions rather than continuously.
2. Guidelines for oxytocin administration from the American College of Obstetricians and Gynecologists* provide examples of low- and high-dose oxytocin labor induction protocols. Depending on the protocol followed, the following

recommendations are provided: (1) starting doses of 0.5 to 6 milliunits/min, and (2) increasing the dose in 1- to 2-milliunits/min increments every 15 to 40 minutes. High-dose protocols may increase the dose in increments of up to 6 milliunits/min. The actual oxytocin dose is based on uterine response and absence of adverse effects. Higher starting doses, higher dose increases, and shorter intervals between dose increases are most likely to result in uterine hyperstimulation. A lower starting dose and lower rate increase increments are usually required to augment labor.

3. After an adequate contraction pattern is established and the cervix is dilated 5 to 6 cm, the oxytocin may be reduced by similar increments.

Control of Postpartum Bleeding

Intravenous infusion: Dilute 10 to 40 units in 1000 ml of intravenous solution. The rate of infusion must control uterine atony. Begin at a rate of 20 to 40 milliunits/min, increasing or decreasing the rate according to uterine response and the rate of postpartum bleeding. Any identifiable cause of the hemorrhage should also be corrected.

Intramuscular injection: Inject 10 units after delivery of the placenta.

Inevitable or Incomplete Abortion

Dilute 10 units in 500 ml of intravenous solution and infuse at a rate of 10 to 20 milliunits/min. Other dilutions are acceptable.

Absorption: Intravenous, immediate; intramuscular, 3 to 5 minutes.

Excretion: Liver and urine.

Contraindications and Precautions: Include, but are not limited to, placenta previa, vasa previa, nonreassuring

*American College of Obstetricians and Gynecologists. (1999). *Induction of labor.* Practice Bulletin No. 10. Washington, DC: Author.

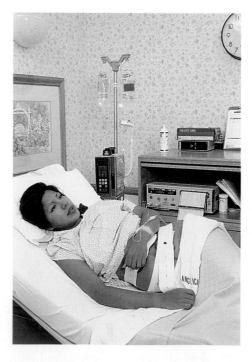

Figure 16-2 ■ Intravenous oxytocin setup for induction or augmentation of labor. The primary line (nonadditive, or maintenance line) on the left side of the pole contains no medication. The secondary line with the orange "medication added" label contains oxytocin. The secondary oxytocin line is regulated by the infusion pump and is inserted into the lowest port in the primary fluid line. An external fetal monitor is used to assess the fetal response to oxytocin-stimulated contractions. The woman lies on her side to promote uterine blood flow.

DRUG GUIDE

OXYTOCIN (PITOCIN)—cont'd

fetal heart rate patterns, abnormal fetal presentation, prolapsed umbilical cord, presenting part above the pelvic inlet, previous classic or other fundal uterine incision, active genital herpes infection, pelvic structural deformities, invasive cervical carcinoma.

Adverse Reactions: Most result from hypersensitivity to drug or excessive dosage. Adverse reactions include hypertonic uterine activity, impaired uterine blood flow, uterine rupture, and abruptio placentae. Uterine hypertonicity may result in fetal bradycardia, tachycardia, reduced fetal heart rate variability, and late decelerations. Fetal asphyxia may occur with diminished uterine blood flow. Fetal or maternal trauma, or both, may occur from rapid birth. Prolonged administration may cause maternal fluid retention, leading to water intoxication. Hypotension (seen with rapid intravenous injection), tachycardia, cardiac dysrhythmias, and subarachnoid hemorrhage are rare adverse reactions.

Drug interactions include vasopressors and the herb ephedra, causing hypertension.

Nursing Considerations

Intrapartum: Assess the fetal heart rate for at least 20 minutes before induction to identify reassuring or nonreassuring patterns. Perform Leopold's maneuvers, a vaginal examination, or both, to verify a cephalic fetal presentation. If nonreassuring fetal heart rate patterns are identified or if fetal presentation is other than cephalic, notify the physician and do not begin induction until an ultrasound is done to ascertain fetal presentation.

Observe uterine activity for establishment of effective labor pattern: contraction frequency every 2 to 3 minutes, duration of 40 to 90 seconds, intensity of 50 to 80 mm Hg (if

measured with an intrauterine pressure catheter). Observe for hypertonic uterine activity: contractions less than 2 minutes apart, rest interval shorter than 30 seconds, duration longer than 90 to 120 seconds, or an elevated resting tone greater than 20 mm Hg (if measured with an intrauterine pressure catheter).

Observe fetal heart rate for nonreassuring patterns such as tachycardia, bradycardia, decreased variability, and late decelerations.

If uterine hypertonicity or a nonreassuring fetal heart rate pattern occurs, intervene to reduce uterine activity and increase fetal oxygenation: stop the oxytocin infusion; increase the rate of nonadditive solution; position the woman in a side-lying position; and administer oxygen by snug facemask at 8 to 10 L/min. Notify the physician of adverse reactions, nursing interventions, and response to interventions. Record the maternal blood pressure, pulse, and respirations every 30 to 60 minutes or with each dose increase. Record intake and output.

Postpartum: Observe uterus for firmness, height, and deviation. Massage until firm if uterus is soft ("boggy"). Observe lochia for color, quantity, and presence of clots. Notify birth attendant if uterus fails to remain contracted or if lochia is bright red or contains large clots. Assess for cramping. Assess vital signs every 15 minutes or according to protocol for the recovery period. Monitor intake and output and breath sounds to identify fluid retention or bladder distention.

Inevitable or Incomplete Abortion: Observe for cramping, vaginal bleeding, clots, and passage of products of conception. Observe maternal vital signs, intake, and output as noted under postpartum nursing implications.

---

heart patterns are reassuring. The FHR is charted in the labor record at least every 15 minutes during first-stage labor and every 5 minutes during second-stage labor (King & Simpson, 2001; Simpson & Atterbury, 2003; Simpson & Poole, 1998).

The nurse remains alert for fetal heart patterns that suggest reduced placental exchange secondary to hypertonic contractions. Examples are fetal bradycardia (rate

<110 bpm at term), tachycardia (persistent rate >160 bpm at term), late decelerations (slowing after the peak of the contraction), and decreased FHR variability (reduced rate fluctuations). Reduced placental exchange also may have causes other than excess uterine activity, such as maternal hypotension or fetal sleep. The nurse must assess the woman and fetus carefully to identify the most likely cause of the problem and institute corrective actions.

If nonreassuring patterns occur or contractions are hypertonic, the nurse takes steps to reduce uterine activity and increase fetal oxygenation.

1. Reduce or stop the oxytocin infusion and increase the rate of the primary nonadditive infusion.
2. Keep the woman in a nonsupine position (usually side-lying) to prevent aortocaval compression and increase placental blood flow.
3. Give 100% oxygen by face mask at 8 to 10 L/min to increase the woman's oxygen saturation, making more available for the fetus.

The physician may order a drug to reduce uterine activity, such as terbutaline (Brethine) and magnesium sulfate. Terbutaline, 0.25 mg subcutaneously, can be given quickly to reduce uterine hyperstimulation.

CRITICAL THINKING ⟨⟩ EXERCISE 16-2

A woman is having labor induced with oxytocin. Her cervix is 4 cm dilated and fully effaced, and the fetal head is at station 0. The nurse notes that the fetal heart rate (internal monitor) is near its baseline of 120 to 130 beats per minute (bpm), with a variability of 10 bpm. Contractions are firm, occur every 1½ to 2 minutes, and typically last 80 to 100 seconds. The baseline uterine activity reference (external monitor) is 30 to 40 mm Hg between contractions.

Questions
1. What is the correct interpretation of these assessments?
2. What are appropriate nursing actions in this situation, and why are they done?

OBSERVING THE MOTHER'S RESPONSE

Uterine activity must be assessed for hypertonus that may reduce fetal oxygenation and contribute to uterine rupture. Contractions are assessed for frequency, duration, and intensity, and uterine resting tone is assessed for relaxation of at least 30 seconds between contractions. Uterine activity observations are charted at the same intervals as the FHR. Corrective actions for hypertonic uterine activity are the same as those listed in the discussion of the fetal response.

If the oxytocin must be discontinued, the decision about resuming it is individualized. The oxytocin infusion may be restarted at the same or a lower dose if the contractions are no longer hypertonic and the FHR is reassuring. If the oxytocin has been discontinued for as long as 40 minutes, the drug that was in the woman's system has been metabolized. Therefore it should be restarted at the beginning dose ordered and advanced more slowly to prevent a recurrence of uterine hyperstimulation and nonreassuring FHR patterns.

The woman's blood pressure and pulse are taken every 30 minutes or with each oxytocin dose change increase to identify changes from her baseline. Her temperature is checked every 2 to 4 hours to identify infection.

The woman may need to use pharmacologic and non-pharmacologic pain management techniques sooner. Although the goal of induced and augmented labor is to mimic natural labor, stimulated contractions often increase in intensity more quickly.

Recording intake and output identifies fluid retention, which may precede water intoxication. Signs and symptoms of water intoxication include headache, blurred vision, behavioral changes, increased blood pressure and respirations, decreased pulse, rales, wheezing, and coughing.

After birth the mother is observed for postpartum hemorrhage caused by uterine relaxation, as is the mother who had spontaneous labor. Postpartum uterine atony is more likely if she has received oxytocin for a long time because the uterine muscle becomes fatigued and does not contract effectively to compress vessels at the placental site. It is manifested by a soft uterine fundus and excess amounts of lochia, usually with large clots. Hypovolemic shock may occur with hemorrhage.

✓ CHECK YOUR READING

5. What precautions are taken to enhance the safety of oxytocin administration for the woman and fetus?
6. How may oxytocin administration differ if labor is being augmented rather than induced?
7. What signs may indicate an abnormal fetal response to oxytocin stimulation?
8. What are the signs of hypertonic uterine activity?
9. How can induction of labor with oxytocin contribute to postpartum hemorrhage?

CRITICAL TO REMEMBER

Signs of Hypertonic Uterine Activity

- Contraction duration longer than 90 to 120 seconds
- Contractions occurring less than 2 minutes apart or relaxation of less than 30 seconds between contractions
- Uterine resting tone higher than 20 mm Hg (with intrauterine pressure catheter)
- Peak pressure higher than 90 mm Hg during first-stage labor (with intrauterine pressure catheter)
- Montevideo units exceeding 400
- A fetal heart rate pattern of late decelerations accompanying hypertonic uterine activity

Nursing Actions for Hypertonic Uterine Activity

- Reduce or stop the oxytocin infusion
- Increase the rate of the primary nonadditive infusion
- Keep the laboring woman in a lateral position
- Give oxygen by face mask, 8 to 10 L/min
- Notify the physician or nurse-midwife

VERSION

Either of two methods may be used to change fetal presentation: external cephalic version (ECV) and internal version. Each has different indications and technique. ECV is the more common.

Indications

EXTERNAL CEPHALIC VERSION

The goal of ECV is to change the fetal position from a breech, shoulder (transverse lie), or oblique presentation. Successful version may allow the woman to avoid a cesarean birth by increasing her chance for vaginal birth (American Academy of Pediatrics [AAP] & ACOG, 2002; ACOG, 2000a; Cruikshank, 2003). However, another study concluded that the rate of cesarean for dystocia was increased after a woman had a successful ECV that changed the fetal position to cephalic (Vézina, Bujold, Varin, Marquette, & Boucher, 2004).

INTERNAL VERSION

Malpresentation in twin gestations is usually managed by cesarean birth, but internal version is sometimes used for the vaginal birth of the second twin.

Contraindications

ECV is not done if a woman is unlikely to deliver vaginally, which is the goal of the procedure. Contraindications are similar for internal and external procedures. Maternal conditions that may contraindicate ECV or reduce its success include:

- Uterine malformations that limit the room available to perform the version and may be the reason for the abnormal fetal presentation
- Previous cesarean birth with a vertical uterine incision. Manipulation of the fetus within the uterus may strain and rupture the old incision. A vertical uterine incision is most likely to rupture.
- Disproportion between fetal size and maternal pelvic size

Fetal conditions that may contraindicate the use of version include:

- Placenta previa. Manipulation of the fetus within the uterus may cause hemorrhage, endangering both mother and fetus. Placenta previa other than marginal is an indication for cesarean birth, even if no excessive bleeding has occurred (see Chapter 25).
- Multifetal gestation, which reduces the room available in which to turn the fetus or fetuses. ECV may be attempted after the first twin is born vaginally in a cephalic presentation.
- Oligohydramnios, ruptured membranes, and a cord around the fetal body or neck (nuchal cord). These conditions limit the room to turn the fetus and may lead to cord compression and fetal hypoxia.
- Uteroplacental insufficiency. Uterine contractions occurring during the version and labor may worsen the insufficiency and cause fetal compromise.
- Engagement of the fetal head into the pelvis

Risks

Few risks to the woman are present, and few serious fetal risks exist. Changes to FHR pattern are common, but the pattern usually returns to normal after the version. A serious risk is that the fetus may become entangled in the umbilical cord, compressing its vessels and resulting in hypoxia. Abruptio placentae may occur if fetal manipulation disrupts the placental site. Fetal and maternal blood could become mixed within placental vessels, possibly resulting in maternal sensitization to the fetal blood type. Cesarean birth may be needed for fetal compromise at the time of the external version or later if the fetus returns to an abnormal presentation.

Technique

EXTERNAL CEPHALIC VERSION

ECV is performed at a location and time to allow emergency cesarean delivery if necessary. A nonstress test or biophysical profile (see Chapter 10) is done before the procedure to evaluate fetal health and placental function. If nonreassuring fetal signs are present, the version is not performed. ECV would add stress to the fetus, who already is functioning with reduced physiologic reserve. An ultrasound examination confirms fetal gestational age and presentation and identifies adequacy of amniotic fluid.

ECV usually is attempted after 37 weeks' gestation but before the woman is in labor, for the following reasons:

- As term nears, the fetus may spontaneously turn to a cephalic presentation.
- The fetus is more likely to return to an abnormal presentation if version is attempted before 37 weeks' gestation.
- If fetal compromise and onset of labor occur, a fetus born after 37 weeks' gestation is not likely to have major problems associated with preterm birth, such as respiratory distress syndrome.

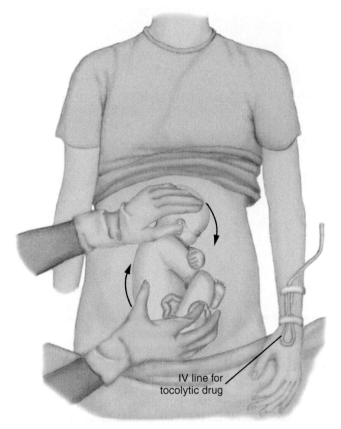

IV line for tocolytic drug

Figure 16-3 ■ External cephalic version.

The woman often is given a tocolytic drug such as terbutaline to relax the uterus while the version is performed. Epidural block analgesia or other analgesia may be given to reduce discomfort during the procedure.

Ultrasonography guides fetal manipulations during ECV and monitors the FHR about every 2 minutes. The physician gently pushes the breech out of the pelvis in a forward or backward roll (Figure 16-3).

If indicated, Rh immunoglobulin (RhoGAM) is given to the Rh-negative woman after external version to prevent Rh sensitization.

Labor induction may be done immediately after successful ECV, or the woman may await spontaneous labor or a later induction.

INTERNAL VERSION

Internal version is an unexpected, urgent procedure. The physician reaches into the uterus with one hand and, with the other hand on the maternal abdomen, moves the fetus into a longitudinal lie (cephalic or breech) to allow delivery (Figure 16-4).

Nursing Considerations

When caring for the woman having external version, the nurse provides information, assesses the woman and fetus, and helps reduce her anxiety.

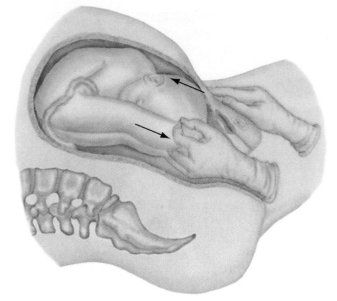

Figure 16-4 ■ Internal version for vaginal birth of a second twin.

PROVIDING INFORMATION

The birth attendant explains the indications and risks for ECV to the woman before she signs an informed consent. The purposes and side effects of any planned tocolytic drug are reviewed. Tachycardia and tremors are common but brief side effects of tocolytics such as terbutaline and stop shortly after the end of the procedure. If epidural or other analgesia is planned, its purposes and side effects are explained by the person who will administer the treatment, and the woman signs additional consents. The nurse verifies the woman's understanding of the purposes, risks, and limitations of the procedure and related treatments. Because cesarean birth may suddenly be required, the woman usually signs permits to allow the surgery and initial care of her newborn.

PROMOTING MATERNAL AND FETAL HEALTH

Admission information is collected as if the woman were in labor or having a cesarean birth because the need for operative intervention may arise suddenly. The woman should have nothing by mouth 4 hours before and during this short procedure in case a cesarean is needed quickly. An IV line is placed for possible drug administration or resuscitation.

Maternal vital signs are assessed, and fetal monitoring is begun to obtain baseline values and evaluate the initial nonstress test or biophysical profile. Nonreassuring FHR patterns should be reported promptly. Fetal bradycardia may occur during the procedure, but the FHR usually returns to normal when manipulation ends. The nurse administers the tocolytic drug. Terbutaline's onset of action is 6 to 15 minutes after subcutaneous injection. The blood pressure and pulse are checked every 5 minutes.

Ultrasonography is used to guide the ECV and check the FHR periodically.

The mother and fetus are observed for at least 1 hour after the procedure for a return of their vital signs to baseline values. Reassuring fetal signs are a heart rate within about the same range as on admission, resolution of any bradycardia, and the presence of FHR accelerations. Maternal vital signs are taken every 15 minutes until they return to her baseline level. The presence of regular contractions suggests onset of labor. Spontaneous rupture of membranes sometimes occurs, with leakage of fluid from the mother's vagina. Rh immune globulin is given if indicated. The IV line is discontinued after the maternal and fetal conditions return to normal unless labor will be induced the same day.

Discomfort should diminish quickly after the version. Persistent and continuous pain suggests a complication such as abruptio placentae.

Because the woman having ECV is near term, the nurse should review the signs of true labor with her and explain guidelines for returning to the hospital if she will be discharged (see Chapter 13).

REDUCING ANXIETY

The woman may be anxious before version because its success is not certain and complications may require emergency cesarean delivery. Afterwards, she still may be anxious because the fetus can return to its previous position and vaginal birth is not certain, as it is not certain with the woman who did not have ECV. The nurse should keep her informed about what is occurring during the version to reduce her fear of the unknown.

The expectant mother and her partner are probably concerned about the fetal condition. The nurse can point out reassuring fetal monitor patterns such as a normal rate and rate accelerations to help reduce anxiety about the baby. If a problem develops, such as bradycardia, the nurse should explain what has happened, what steps are being done to relieve it, and the result of these interventions.

✔ CHECK YOUR READING

10. Why is observing the FHR important during and after ECV?
11. Why should the uterine activity be monitored after ECV?

OPERATIVE VAGINAL BIRTH

Operative vaginal birth, also called *forceps* or *vacuum extraction,* may be used by the physician to apply traction to the fetal head during birth, aiding the woman's expulsive efforts. Both techniques assist descent only or both descent and rotation of the fetal head from an occiput posterior or occiput transverse position to the occiput anterior position. The use of forceps has fallen, whereas use of vacuum extractors has risen. The rate of births assisted by vacuum extraction is now double the rate of forceps-assisted births (Kozak & Weeks, 2002). However, as the rate of cesarean births has risen, vaginal births assisted by either vacuum extractor or forceps have decreased since 1996 (Martin et al., 2003).

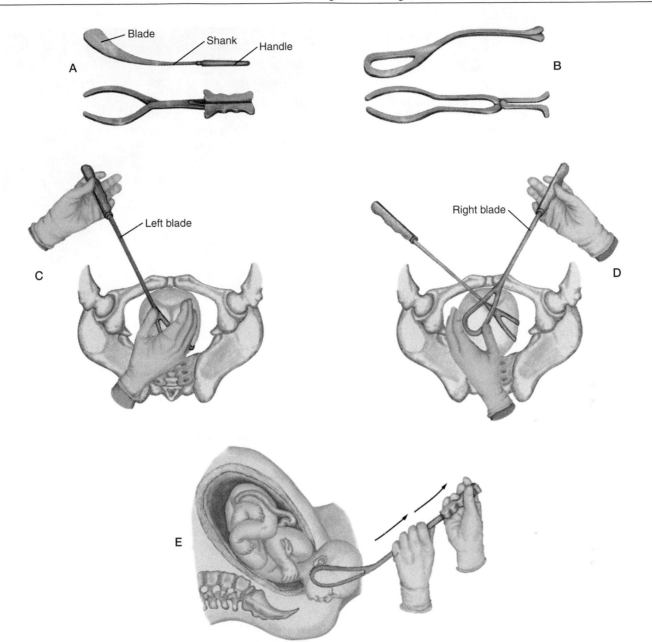

Figure 16-5 ■ Obstetric forceps and their application. **A,** Solid blade Tucker-McLean forceps. **B,** Piper forceps, used to deliver the head when the fetus is in a breech presentation. **C and D,** Application of forceps with an open (fenestrated) blade, first to the left side of the maternal pelvis **(C)** and then to the right side of the maternal pelvis **(D). E,** Direction of traction in a forceps-assisted birth.

Forceps are curved, metal instruments with two curved blades that can be locked in the center. Many styles are available for different needs. The blades may be closed or open and are shaped to grasp the fetal head (Figure 16-5). Foam pads are available to cushion the fetal head from the blades. Piper forceps are a special type used to assist birth of the head as it is born last in a vaginal breech birth. Forceps and a vacuum extractor also may be used during cesarean birth.

A vacuum extractor uses suction to grasp the fetal head while traction is applied (Figures 16-6 and 16-7). It is not used to deliver the fetus in a nonvertex presentation such as breech or face; otherwise, its use is similar to that of forceps. It also is not used for the very preterm fetus because the suc-

tion is more likely to injure the head, scalp, and intracranial vessels (Chmait & Moore, 2004).

Indications

Forceps or vacuum extraction is considered if the second stage should be shortened for the well-being of the woman, fetus, or both and if vaginal birth can be accomplished quickly without undue trauma. Maternal indications may include exhaustion, inability to push effectively, and cardiac and pulmonary disease. Fetal indications may include nonreassuring FHR patterns, failure of the fetal presenting part to fully rotate and descend in the pelvis, or partial separation of the placenta or nonreassuring FHR patterns near the time of birth.

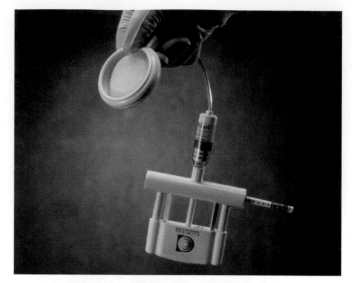

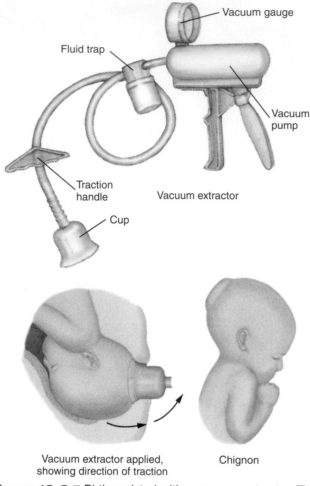

Vacuum extractor applied,
showing direction of traction

Chignon

Figure 16-6 ■ Birth assisted with a vacuum extractor. The chignon is scalp edema that often forms under the suction cup when the vacuum extractor is used.

Contraindications

Cesarean birth is preferable if the maternal and fetal conditions mandate a more rapid birth than can be accomplished with forceps or vacuum extraction and if the procedure would be too traumatic. Examples of these conditions are severe fetal compromise, acute maternal conditions such as congestive heart failure and pulmonary edema, a high fetal station, and disproportion between the size of the fetus and maternal pelvis.

Risks

The main risk of forceps and vacuum extraction is trauma to maternal and fetal tissues. Because of the relative safety of cesarean birth, the attempt at an instrumental birth usually is abandoned if the fetal head does not descend easily.

Maternal risks include laceration and hematoma of the vagina. The infant may have ecchymoses, facial and scalp lacerations and abrasions, facial nerve injury, cephalhematoma, subgaleal hemorrhage, and intracranial hemorrhage. A vacuum extractor may create scalp edema called a *chignon* at the application area (see Figure 16-6).

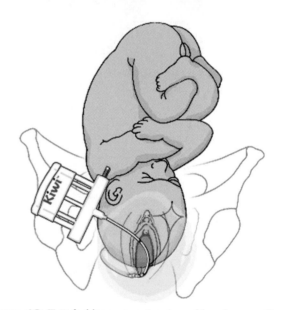

B

Figure 16-7 ■ **A,** Vacuum extractor with a low-profile cup that can be used for occiput posterior fetal positions. Note the green band that denotes adequate suction and the red band that warns of excess suction. **B,** Application of the low-profile cup to the fetal head in an occiput posterior position. (Courtesy of A. Vacca, Choices with Childbirth CD and Courtesy of Clinical Innovations, Inc.)

Technique

Preparation for forceps or vacuum extraction is similar to that for any vaginal birth. The presentation, position, and station of the fetal presenting part are verified. Membranes must be ruptured and the cervix completely dilated for forceps or vacuum extraction birth. The woman needs adequate anesthesia, usually a regional block such as an epidural.

Forceps and vacuum extractor–assisted births are classified according to the extent of descent of the fetal head into the pelvis during the procedure and necessary degree of rotation for the fetal head to be born (AAP & ACOG, 2002).

- Outlet operative vaginal delivery—The fetal head is on the perineum, with the scalp visible at the vaginal opening without separating the labia. The position is occiput anterior or either right or left occiput anterior (ROA, LOA) or posterior (ROP, LOP).
- Low operative vaginal delivery—The leading edge of the fetal skull is at station +2 (about 4 cm below the level of the mother's ischial spines) or lower. Low operative vaginal birth is subdivided according to the amount of rotation of the fetal head needed. Births requiring 45 degrees or less of fetal head rotation are simpler.
- Midpelvis operative vaginal delivery—The leading edge of the fetal skull is between a 0 (at the level of the ischial spines) and a +2 station.

The physician determines the presentation, position, and station of the fetal head and amount of cervical dilation. When the blades are correctly applied, the long axis of the blades lies over the fetal cheeks and parietal bones. After checking for proper application, the physician locks the two blades in the center and pulls gently as the woman pushes, following the curve of the pelvis. An episiotomy may be performed as the fetal head distends the perineum. The physician may keep the forceps on until the head is born or may remove the blades just before expulsion. The rest of the fetus is born in the usual way.

A hand pump is used to create suction to hold the vacuum cup on the fetal head in the midline of the occiput. The physician applies traction intermittently, as in a forceps-assisted birth. A vacuum release allows removal of the cup. Hospital policies often limit to three the number of times the vacuum cup can be applied.

Nursing Considerations

When a forceps or vacuum extraction birth is anticipated, a catheter is added to the instrument table for the birth unless the woman has an indwelling catheter. The physician specifies the type of forceps and vacuum cup. If the nurse must apply the suction to the cup, suction should not go outside the green zone on the suction indicator. FHR should be assessed and any rate lower than 100 bpm reported.

After birth the mother and infant are observed for trauma. The mother may have vaginal wall lacerations or hematoma. Vaginal wall lacerations bleed brighter red than normal lochia and somewhat continuously. The fundus usually is firm unless uterine atony also is present. Women with vaginal wall hematomas complain of severe and unrelenting pain and may have edema and discoloration of the labia and perineum. Cold applications for the first 12 hours reduce pain by numbing the area and limit bruising and edema of the tissues. Heat applications after 12 hours aid resolution of the edema and bruising.

The infant often has reddening and mild bruising of the skin where the forceps were applied. These areas do not need treatment. Cold treatment is not done for an infant because of hypothermia. Skin breaks that allow entry of microorganisms should be noted and kept clean. Facial asymmetry, which is most obvious when the infant cries, suggests facial nerve injury.

■ After a forceps birth a parent may ask why the baby's cheeks are reddened or bruised. A good response is to explain that the pressure of the forceps on the baby's delicate skin may cause minor bruising that usually resolves without treatment. Point out improvement in the area during the postpartum stay.

EPISIOTOMY

Episiotomy was performed on almost 800,000 women who gave birth in 2002 (Hing & Middleton, 2004). Routine performance of an episiotomy remains controversial. However, the decision about whether to do an episiotomy must be made just before birth, and indications are not always clear.

Indications

Fetal indications for episiotomy are similar to those for forceps and vacuum extraction. Episiotomy may be performed to reduce pressure on the head when a small, preterm infant is born.

Maternal benefits are less clear. Episiotomy was once thought to limit perineal trauma and reduce relaxation of pelvic floor muscles. Pelvic floor relaxation is associated with uterine prolapse and stress incontinence. Better-controlled studies have questioned these benefits, however. Although an episiotomy provides some control over the direction and extent of any opening in the perineum, a midline episiotomy, the most common kind, is associated with a higher incidence of the more severe third- and fourth-degree lacerations extending from the episiotomy. Other studies also showed that episiotomies did not exert a protective effect in preventing stress incontinence (Nager & Helliwell, 2001; Webb & Culhane, 2002). However, the episiotomy has clean edges rather than irregular edges like a laceration, making for simpler repair.

Risks

Infection is the main risk of episiotomy. Perineal pain occurs with both episiotomy and spontaneous tears. However, perineal pain may last longer with episiotomy, mainly because of its tendency to extend into deeper lacerations. Prolonged perineal pain impairs resumption of sexual intercourse and makes it uncomfortable for the woman.

Technique

An episiotomy is done when the fetal presenting part has crowned to a diameter of about 3 to 4 cm. The two types of episiotomies have different advantages and disadvantages: median (midline) and mediolateral (Figure 16-8).

Nursing Considerations

An episiotomy sometimes can be avoided or limited in length with nursing measures. An upright position while pushing promotes gradual stretching of the woman's perineum. Daily perineal massage and stretching by the woman

Median or Midline

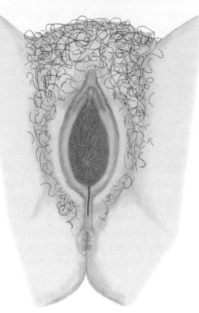

Mediolateral

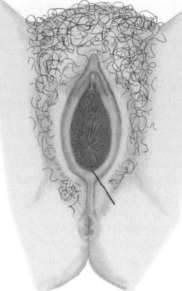

Advantages
Minimal blood loss
Neat healing with little scarring
Less postpartum pain than the
    mediolateral episiotomy

Disadvantages
An added laceration may ex-
    tend the median episiotomy
    into the anal sphincter
Limited enlargement of the va-
    ginal opening because peri-
    neal length is limited by the
    anal sphincter

Advantages
More enlargement of the vagi-
    nal opening
Little risk that the episiotomy
    will extend into the anus

Disadvantages
More blood loss
Increased postpartum pain
More scarring and irregularity
    in the healed scar
Prolonged dyspareunia (pain-
    ful intercourse)

Figure 16-8 ■ Types of episiotomies.

from about 34 weeks' gestation until birth has been shown to reduce the risk for perineal trauma during birth (Eason, Labrecque, Wells, & Feldman, 2000). The birth attendant must promote this action on the woman's part.

Nursing interventions during the recovery and postpartum periods are similar for episiotomy and perineal laceration. The perineum should be observed for hematoma and edema. As with use of forceps, perineal cold applications are done for at least the first 12 hours and followed by perineal heat.

✓ CHECK YOUR READING

12. What are the similarities in the uses of forceps and vacuum extractors? What are the differences?
13. Why should the nurse add a urinary catheter to the instrument table if a forceps-assisted birth is expected?
14. A woman has a forceps birth with a median episiotomy. What nursing interventions can make her more comfortable?
15. What injury is suggested by an asymmetric facial appearance when the infant cries?

CESAREAN BIRTH

In 1965 the cesarean birth rate in the United States was 4.5% of all births, rising to 24% in the late 1980s. Preliminary data for 2003 show that the rate of cesarean deliveries

was 27.6% of all births, a 6% increase from 2002. Of these cesareans 19.1% were primary or first cesarean births (Hamilton, Martin, & Sutton, 2004).

Many factors contributed to the rise in the national cesarean birth rate, some of which include:

■ Women having their first baby are more likely to deliver by cesarean than women who have had one or more previous births vaginally.

■ The high primary cesarean rate adds to the overall rate because more women will have repeat cesareans rather than attempting vaginal birth for their next children.

■ Women are having children later, and cesareans are more common in the older pregnant woman.

■ Electronic fetal monitoring often prompts concerns about fetal oxygen and acid-base status or progress of labor.

■ Cesarean birth may be chosen if the baby remains in a breech presentation.

■ A high threat of litigation if birth outcomes are not good causes physicians to opt for surgery quickly if the maternal or fetal condition or both seem to be at risk.

Evidence that links labor induction to increased risk for cesarean birth is accumulating. Studies have demonstrated that women who have their labor induced are two to three times more likely to have a surgical birth. Women having a Bishop score of less than 5 at the time of induction, indicating a cervix that is not favorable, had a greater risk for cesarean than women who had a score of 5 or more. Approximately 25% of inductions had no clearly documented medical or obstetric indication but were elective. The risk for cesarean after failed induction was similar whether women had medical or elective inductions (Johnson et al., 2003; Martin et al., 2003; Yeast et al., 1999).

A national goal for the *Healthy People 2010* initiative is to reduce the rate of first-time cesarean births in low-risk women to no more than 15% and reduce the percentage of repeat cesarean births from the 1997 rate of 71% to 63% (U.S. Department of Health and Human Services, 2000). Promotion of vaginal birth after cesarean (VBAC) in women for whom it is appropriate is a major way to accomplish the goal. Other possibilities include more careful evaluation of dystocia of labor as a reason for cesarean and careful selection of women who are appropriate candidates for vaginal breech birth. ECV (p. 373) is an option to attempt to change the presentation of a near-term fetus in the breech presentation to a cephalic presentation.

Experience with electronic fetal monitoring has improved knowledge of normal fetal responses to labor, promoting interventions for fetal benefit that may avoid cesarean delivery. Labor professionals increasingly recognize that simple interventions such as walking and squatting during the second stage may promote normal labor progress. However, epidural analgesia, the most popular choice, limits use of these measures.

Controversy exists about the wisdom of setting a numeric goal for cesarean births, and the issue is complex (ACOG, 1999c; Lowe, 2002; Sachs, Kobelin, Castro, & Frigoletto, 1999; Young, 1999). One part of the plan to achieve the Healthy People 2010 cesarean birth target is to promote VBAC when appropriate. Recent evidence has shown that maternal and newborn complications are more frequent if VBAC is not successful. Also, some women do not want to attempt VBAC but prefer an elective repeat cesarean birth. For these reasons some physicians argue against any target percentage set by the government and managed care. See p. 386 for additional information about VBAC.

Indications

Cesarean birth is performed when awaiting vaginal birth would compromise the mother, fetus, or both. Possible indications for cesarean birth include but are not limited to the following:

- Dystocia
- Cephalopelvic (fetopelvic) disproportion
- Hypertension if prompt delivery is necessary
- Maternal diseases such as diabetes, heart disease, or cervical cancer if labor is not advisable
- Active genital herpes
- Some previous uterine surgical procedures such as a classic cesarean incision
- Persistent nonreassuring FHR patterns
- Prolapsed umbilical cord
- Fetal malpresentations such as breech or transverse lie
- Hemorrhagic conditions such as abruptio placentae or placenta previa

A prior cesarean birth alone is not an indication for another cesarean birth for most women. Many women will choose repeat cesarean rather than a trial of labor even if they are appropriate candidates for VBAC, because of the small, but real, added risk for uterine rupture. In other cases they choose elective (scheduled) repeat cesarean to avoid another unsuccessful experience or the pain of labor. For other women, trying to deliver their next baby vaginally—whether successful or not—is important to them.

Contraindications

Few absolute contraindications exist, but cesarean birth in some conditions is not desirable because the risks to the woman are too great compared with the potential benefits to the woman and fetus. These conditions include fetal death, a fetus that is too immature to survive, and maternal coagulation defects.

Risks

Cesarean birth is one of the safest major surgical procedures. However, it poses greater risk for the mother than vaginal birth. Maternal risks include the following:

- Infection
- Hemorrhage
- Urinary tract trauma or infection
- Thrombophlebitis, thromboembolism
- Paralytic ileus
- Atelectasis
- Anesthesia complications

Cesarean delivery poses added risks to the infant, which may include the following:

- Inadvertent preterm birth
- Transient tachypnea of the newborn caused by delayed absorption of lung fluid (see Chapter 30)
- Persistent pulmonary hypertension of the newborn (see Chapter 30)
- Injury such as laceration, bruising, and other trauma

Lung immaturity is the greatest risk if the fetus is delivered preterm. Therefore tests for fetal lung maturity (see Chapter 10) are done if elective cesarean birth is planned. Other criteria for assuring fetal lung maturity at the time of cesarean birth include (AAP & ACOG, 2002):

- Documentation of fetal heart tones for 20 weeks by nonelectronic fetoscope or for 30 weeks by Doppler
- Passage of 36 weeks since positive results from a pregnancy test performed by a laboratory
- Ultrasound measurement of the crown-rump length at 6 to 11 weeks that supports a gestation of 39 weeks or more
- Clinical examinations between 12 and 20 weeks that support a gestation of 39 weeks or more

Technique

PREPARATION

Regional anesthesia such as an epidural block is commonly used for cesarean birth. However, general anesthesia, with its risk for vomiting and aspiration of gastric contents, may be needed unexpectedly. Placement of the regional block may not be possible, and an inadequate block may necessitate supplemental general anesthesia. Therefore the woman receives nothing by mouth. A drug such as famotidine (Pepcid) or sodium citrate (Bicitra) is given to reduce gastric acidity before surgery. The woman does not have routine premedication other than drugs to control gastric and respiratory secretions.

The fetus is monitored for at least 20 to 30 minutes after admission if the woman is having a scheduled cesarean birth. If electronic fetal monitoring is being used when a cesarean birth becomes necessary, it continues as long as possible before the surgery. A fetal scalp electrode should be removed before birth so that it is not pulled from the vagina through the uterus as the infant is delivered. A wedge under one hip and a tilted operating table avoid aortocaval compression and promote placental blood flow.

Routine laboratory studies vary with the mother's condition and type of anesthesia but often include complete blood count, clotting studies such as prothrombin and activated partial thromboplastin times, and blood typing and screening. The physician may order one or more units of blood typed and cross-matched to be available for transfusion if the woman's hemoglobin and hematocrit values are low or if she is at greater risk for hemorrhage, such as with grand multiparity (five or more births).

A single IV dose of a prophylactic antibiotic such as ampicillin or a cephalosporin is often ordered. Additional antibiotic doses are given to a woman who has an increased risk for infection, such as one who has had prolonged rupture of membranes.

If a Pfannenstiel (transverse or bikini) skin incision is planned, the woman's abdomen is shaved from about 7.5 cm (3 in) above the pubic hairline to the mons pubis, about where her legs come together. For a vertical skin incision, the upper border of the shave is just above the umbilicus. Some units shave the larger abdominal area for all skin incisions. Cordless electric clippers with disposable heads reduce skin nicks that provide an entry point for microorganisms.

An indwelling catheter inserted before the surgery keeps the bladder away from the operative area, reducing the risk for injury. The catheter allows accurate observation of urine output during and after surgery, which helps evaluate maternal circulatory status. To reduce discomfort, insertion may be delayed until an epidural block has taken effect.

An abdominal scrub is done just before sterile draping. As in other surgical skin preparations, the direction is circular from the center of the operative area outward and from the pubic area downward to each upper thigh. It may be necessary to use wide tape to hold excess abdominal fat (the pannus, or "apron") upward, pulling it away from the skin incision area.

Preoperative preparations are completed before a general anesthetic is begun to reduce neonatal exposure to anesthesia. The team scrubs, puts on gowns and gloves, and drapes the woman before general anesthesia is induced.

INCISIONS

Two incisions are made, one in the abdominal wall (skin incision) and the other in the uterine wall. Either of two skin incisions are used: a midline vertical incision between the umbilicus and the symphysis or a Pfannenstiel incision just above the symphysis (Figure 16-9).

Three types of uterine incisions are possible, each with different indications and limitations: (1) low transverse, (2) low vertical, and (3) classic, a vertical incision into the upper uterus (Figure 16-10). The low transverse uterine incision is preferred. The uterine incision does not always

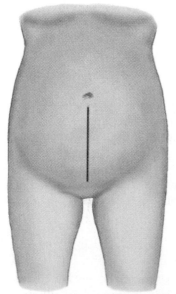

Vertical

Advantages
Quicker to perform
Better visualization of the uterus
Can quickly extend upward for greater visualization if needed
Often more appropriate for obese women

Disadvantages
Easily visible when healed
Greater chance of dehiscence and hernia formation

Pfannenstiel

Advantages
Less visibility when healed and the pubic hair grows back
Less chance of dehiscence or formation of a hernia

Disadvantages
Less visualization of the uterus
Cannot be done as quickly, which may be important in an emergency cesarean birth
Cannot easily be extended to give greater operative exposure
Re-entry at a subsequent cesarean birth may require more time

Figure 16-9 ■ Skin (abdominal wall) incisions for cesarean birth.

Low Transverse

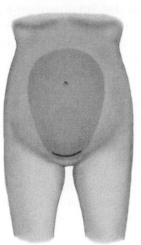

Low Vertical

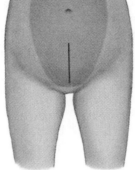

Classic

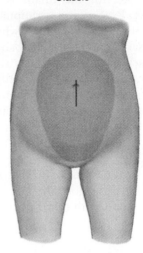

Advantages
Unlikely to rupture during a subsequent
    birth
Makes VBAC possible for subsequent
    pregnancy
Less blood loss
Easier to repair
Less adhesion formation

Disadvantage
Limited ability to extend laterally to en-
    large the incision

Advantage
Can be extended upward to make a larger
    incision if needed

Disadvantages
Slightly more likely to rupture during a
    subsequent birth
A tear may extend the incision downward
    into the cervix

Advantages
May be the only choice in these
    situations:
- Implantation of a placenta previa on
    the lower anterior uterine wall
- Presence of dense adhesions from
    previous surgery
- Transverse lie of a large fetus with the
    shoulder impacted in the mother's
    pelvis

Disadvantages
Most likely of the uterine incisions to
    rupture during a subsequent birth
Eliminates VBAC as an option for birth
    of a subsequent infant

Figure 16-10 ■ Uterine incisions for cesarean birth. The abdominal and uterine incisions
do not always match. *VBAC,* Vaginal birth after cesarean.

match the skin incision. For example, a woman may have a vertical skin incision and a low transverse uterine incision, particularly if she is obese.

The low transverse uterine incision may not be suitable if the fetus is very large. The length of this incision is limited because the uterine artery and vein enter the uterus at its lower right and left sides. The low transverse incision may not be large enough to deliver a large fetus without tearing these large vessels. Sometimes a vertical uterine incision must be added to a transverse one (making an inverted T) to deliver a very large baby.

A classic uterine incision occasionally must be used when the other two incisions are not possible, such as when a placenta previa is located in the lower anterior uterus. The vertical uterine incision, especially the classic one, is more likely to rupture during later pregnancies.

SEQUENCE OF EVENTS IN A CESAREAN BIRTH

The sequence of events in cesarean birth is similar to that in a vaginal birth. When the woman is anesthetized and draped, the physician makes the skin incision. If general anesthesia is required, the level is very light until the fetus is delivered and is deepened after the umbilical cord is clamped.

The bladder is separated from the uterine wall and held downward with a wide bladder retractor. The uterus is incised, usually in a low transverse incision. If the membranes are intact, they are ruptured with a sharp instrument and amniotic fluid is suctioned from the operative field. As in vaginal births, the color, odor, and quantity of the amniotic fluid are noted and the time of rupture is recorded.

The physician lifts the fetal presenting part through the uterine incision. An assistant may push on the uterine fundus to help deliver the fetus through the abdominal incision. A vacuum extractor or forceps may be needed to facilitate birth of the fetal head.

The infant's face is wiped, and the mouth and nose are suctioned to remove secretions that would impair breathing. The cord is quickly clamped and cut. The physician collects cord blood for analysis.

After the infant's birth, the physician removes the placenta. Oxytocin is given IV to contract the uterus firmly. The physician then closes the uterine and abdominal incisions, approximating each layer separately. Some physicians flush the operative area with saline or antibiotic solution before abdominal closure.

Nursing care for the infant is similar to that after vaginal birth. Resuscitation equipment should be readied for use. Professional personnel who care for the infant born by cesarean vary with the baby's anticipated condition and facility policy. A pediatrician, neonatal nurse-practitioner, or neonatal team usually attends the infant at the time of cesarean birth. Newborn care personnel must be prepared for unexpected resuscitation measures as in any birth.

Nursing Considerations

Nursing care for a woman who has a cesarean birth varies according to the situation. She may be planning a cesarean birth, or a surgical birth may be unexpected. Even in these

---

BOX 16-1 Nursing Care for a Woman Having Cesarean Birth

Before the Cesarean Birth
1. Assess the time of last oral intake and what was eaten.
2. Assess for allergies. Include drug, food, and substance (e.g., latex) allergies.
3. Determine medications taken and last dose. Include herbal preparations.
4. Have the woman sign informed consents for surgery, anesthesia, and usually blood transfusion.
5. Obtain ordered laboratory work.
6. Do preoperative teaching: what the woman can expect in the operating and recovery rooms, infant care, and who will be present.
7. Start ordered intravenous infusion and begin bolus dose for regional anesthetic at appropriate time (see discussion of epidural block in Chapter 15).
8. Perform abdominal shave (or use electric clipper).
9. Administer ordered medication to control gastric secretions if not done by anesthesiologist.
10. Insert an indwelling urinary catheter (or insert in operating room after regional block).
11. Assist woman to operating table, positioning her with a wedge under her hip to displace the uterus if the table is flat.
12. Apply grounding pad for electrocautery.
13. Perform sterile preparation of abdomen.
14. Call infant care team if it is routine in the facility or if newborn complications are anticipated.

During the Recovery Period
1. Begin anesthesia-related interventions: pulse oximeter, oxygen administration, cardiac monitor.
   a. Assess for return of sensation and movement if regional anesthesia was used.
   b. Assess level of consciousness if general anesthesia was used.
2. Do routine assessments every 15 minutes for the first hour, every 30 minutes during the second hour, and hourly thereafter until the woman is transferred to the postpartum unit. Assess:
   a. Vital signs; oxygen saturation
   b. Electrocardiogram (ECG) pattern
   c. Uterine fundus for firmness, height, and deviation (massage if poorly contracted)
   d. Lochia for color, quantity, and presence of large clots
   e. Urine output for color, quantity, and patency of the catheter and tubing
   f. Abdominal dressing for drainage
3. Assess need for analgesia, and administer as ordered.
4. Change position hourly if no contraindication exists. Have her breathe deeply and cough at each routine assessment time. Provide a small pillow to support her incision when coughing or turning if sensation is present.

---

two situations, women differ. For example, is the planned cesarean her first, or has she had a cesarean birth before? Was her previous cesarean planned? An unplanned cesarean birth may occur after hours of unsuccessful labor or may be needed quickly in an emergency.

Nursing care is similar for women having cesarean childbirth, but the approach in each situation is different (Box 16-1). For example, although preoperative teaching is important, it must be abbreviated or even omitted in a true emergency.

PROVIDING EMOTIONAL SUPPORT

Emotional support may begin before and extend after the birth. A mother who has had a previous cesarean birth may harbor unresolved feelings of grief, guilt, or inadequacy because she perceives that she somehow failed in her expected birth experience. Therapeutic communication techniques help identify stressors and misunderstandings to promote a positive childbirth experience (Box 16-2).

■ The nurse in the prenatal setting can open the subject of a woman's previous cesarean birth with a broad lead such as, "Tell me about your experience with the birth of your other baby."

Anxiety is an expected and normal reaction to surgery and is useful within limits. For example, mild to moderate anxiety may prompt the woman who expects a cesarean birth to learn more about her upcoming experience. However, high anxiety inhibits concentration. The woman who has an emergency cesarean birth is more likely to have high levels of anxiety, but the woman who expects the surgery also is vulnerable.

The staff's behavior can either reduce or increase the woman's anxiety. A calm and confident manner helps her feel that she is being cared for by competent professionals. A quiet, low voice is calming.

The nurse and the woman's significant others are important sources of emotional support. The nurse should remain with her and let her express her fears. Therapeutic communication helps clarify her concerns, so explanations to reduce her fear of the unknown can be most effective.

The father or other support person should be encouraged to remain with her during surgery if she has regional anesthesia. In some hospitals the support person may come into the operating room after the woman is intubated for general anesthesia to foster attachment with the infant and help the mother integrate her birth experience afterward.

BOX 16-2 Nursing Diagnoses for the Woman Undergoing an Operative Obstetric Procedure

Anxiety*
Fear
Pain
Risk for Impaired Spontaneous Ventilation (mother or newborn)
Risk for Aspiration (general anesthesia)
Risk for Injury*
Hypothermia (mother or newborn)
Readiness for Enhanced Family Coping

*Nursing diagnoses explored in this chapter.

Nurses also support a woman's partner and significant others during the cesarean birth. The partner may be as anxious as the woman but afraid to express it because she needs so much support. The partner may be physically exhausted after hours of labor coaching. The staff should not expect more support from partners than can be reasonably provided.

■ Although cesarean births are routine in the intrapartum unit they are not routine to women who undergo them and to their families. Avoid belittling their fears by telling women and their families not to worry and that everything will be all right, especially if an emergency occurs.

After birth, visiting the mother and her family allows the nurse to answer questions about the surgery and fill in any gaps in their understanding. This helps them understand the experience and promotes a positive perception of the birth (Nursing Care Plan 16-1).

TEACHING

Knowledge may reduce fear of the unknown and increase a woman's sense of control over her infant's birth. The nurse cannot assume that a woman who had a previous cesarean birth already knows what will happen and why. If her previous surgery was done after a long labor or in an emergency, she may recall only parts and not understand those parts she does remember. Teaching should be given in simple language and include her support person.

The nurse explains preoperative procedures and their purposes, such as the abdominal shave, indwelling catheter, IV lines, and dressings. The catheter and IV lines usually remain in place no longer than 24 hours after birth. The nurse may need to reinforce information provided by others, such as an anesthesiologist.

Women who have regional anesthesia, such as an epidural or a subarachnoid block, often fear that they will feel pain during surgery. They do feel pressure and pulling, but these sensations do not mean that the anesthesia is wearing off. The nurse reassures her that her pain management is regularly assessed by the anesthesiologist.

If a woman is having general anesthesia, the nurse explains why operative preparations are completed before she is anesthetized. She should be reassured that her surgery will not begin until she is asleep and she will not wake up during the procedure.

The nurse describes the operating room and everyone who will be present to make it less intimidating to her. The operating room is very cool, and the surgery table is narrow. Her labor nurse often is the circulating nurse during surgery and reassures her with a familiar face and voice.

The support person should be told when to expect to come into the operating room. If it is not already in place, an epidural block often is established after the woman goes to the operating room. The partner may not be brought in until the regional block and other preparations such as the indwelling catheter are complete. These preparations may take 30 to 45 minutes if no rush exists. Support persons should be told that they will not be forgotten and that apparent delays do not indicate problems.

The recovery room and any equipment that will be used, such as a pulse oximeter, electrocardiogram monitor, and automatic blood pressure cuff are explained to the couple. The nurse reviews routine assessments and interventions such as fundus and lochia checks, coughing, and deep breathing. The woman is taught simple exercises to promote normal circulation. The nurse reassures her that every effort will be made to promote her comfort with medication, positioning, and other interventions.

PROMOTING SAFETY

The woman's food intake is assessed for type and time on admission because general anesthesia occasionally is necessary. Oral intake and emesis during labor are recorded and reported to the anesthesia clinician. Oral intake other than ordered medications and possibly ice chips is discontinued if a cesarean birth becomes likely. Drugs to control gastric and respiratory secretions are administered as ordered.

The woman is transferred and positioned carefully to prevent injury, especially if she has received regional anesthesia that reduces motor control and sensation. An extra-large operating table is used if indicated by her size and weight. Bony prominences are cushioned. A safety strap placed across her thighs secures her on the narrow operating table. A wedge under one hip or a tilted operating table avoids aortocaval compression and reduced placental blood flow. During positioning the drain tube of the indwelling catheter should be routed under her leg to promote drainage and keep the tubing away from the operative area. The catheter bag is placed near the head of the table so that the anesthesia clinician can monitor urine output, an important measure of fluid balance.

The nurse verifies proper function of equipment such as suction devices, monitors, and electrocautery. Leads for the cardiac monitor, temperature, and pulse oximeter are placed to observe vital functions. A grounding pad permits safe use of an electrocautery.

After the surgery, the incision area is cleansed with sterile water and a sterile dressing is applied. Blood and amniotic fluid are cleaned from the woman's abdomen, buttocks, and back before she is transferred to a bed. Smooth transfers reduce pain and hypotension.

PROVIDING POSTOPERATIVE CARE

Postoperative care for the mother who has had a cesarean birth is similar to that for one who has had a vaginal birth, with added interventions related to the incision. Her temperature is assessed on admission and according to protocol thereafter. If her condition is stable, other assessments are done every 15 minutes during the first 1 to 2 hours and progress to every 30 minutes to 1 hour until she is transferred to her postpartum room. In addition to temperature, routine postoperative assessments include the following:

- Vital signs, respiratory character, and oxygen saturation
- Return of motion and sensation if a regional block was given
- Level of consciousness, particularly if general anesthesia and sedating drugs were given

NURSING CARE PLAN 16-1 Cesarean Birth

ASSESSMENT: Christina Cole is 22 years old and expecting her first baby. Her due date is 2 weeks from today and a cesarean was scheduled for 1 week from today because her baby remains in a complete (full) breech presentation. Because her membranes ruptured this afternoon and she is in early labor, she will have her cesarean today. Epidural anesthesia is planned for her surgery. Although her physician has discussed cesarean birth with her, Christina is anxious and has many questions about what will happen to her and her baby. She says she is very nervous about the upcoming surgery. She has never been a patient in a hospital. Christina's mother and husband Bruce are with her.

NURSING DIAGNOSIS: Anxiety related to unfamiliarity with the setting and procedures for cesarean birth

GOALS/EXPECTED OUTCOMES: After interventions Christina will:
1. State that she feels less apprehensive.
2. Verbalize understanding of preoperative and postoperative care.
3. Demonstrate postoperative techniques for coughing and deep breathing.

INTERVENTION	RATIONALE
1. Assess Christina's level of anxiety. Mild to moderate levels of anxiety are expected.	1. Assessment enables the nurse to approach preoperative care of the woman in the most appropriate manner. Mild to moderate anxiety may facilitate learning, but higher levels impair learning.
2. Remain with Christina as much as possible. Allow her to express her fears. Encourage her mother and Bruce to remain with her.	2. When the woman expresses her fears, it enables the nurse to answer the woman's concerns specifically. Support comes from significant others and a caring nurse.
3. Elicit Christina's feelings about surgery by using broad leads such as, "What were your thoughts when you found out you might have your baby by cesarean?"	3. This identifies expectations of the birth experience so that actions can be taken to make it a positive one. If a woman's expected and actual experience closely match, she is likely to be more satisfied with it. Identifies misunderstandings and possible feelings of inadequacy and anger.

4. Explain preoperative preparations using simple language, verifying Christina's understanding, and giving her the opportunity to ask questions.
  a. The anesthesiology professional visits her to explain anesthesia. The epidural anesthetic will be given in the operating room.
  b. Shave preparation (a Pfannenstiel incision is planned): from about 3 inches above the pubic hair to the level where the thighs meet.
  c. Indwelling urinary catheter, which is usually inserted after epidural anesthesia is begun.
  d. Operating room: appearance, narrow table, wedge under one hip (or tilted table), cool temperature, equipment.
  e. People who will be in the operating room: circulating nurse, scrub nurse, surgeon's assistant, neonatal nurse, pediatrician, any others.
	4. Knowledge decreases anxiety and fear of the unknown. Simple language facilitates understanding when a woman's attention is narrowed from anxiety. These interventions show respect and give the woman a greater sense of control.

5. Explain what to expect postoperatively, demonstrating as needed.
  a. Oxygen mask will be used briefly.
  b. Pulse oximeter on finger. Automatic blood pressure cuff.
  c. Frequent checks of her vital signs, fundus, lochia, and anesthesia-related assessments. Emphasize that nurses will be as gentle as possible when palpating her fundus.
  d. Catheter usually remains in place up to 24 hours.
  e. She will be kept as comfortable as possible with analgesics. For greatest effectiveness she should tell the nurse if she needs pain medication before pain is too bad.
  f. She will be asked to move and change position several times.
  g. Demonstrate effective coughing (splinting the abdomen with a pillow) and deep breathing techniques. Ask Christina to demonstrate each.
	5. Explanations reduce anxiety and fear of the unknown and promote understanding and acceptance that care will be painful while providing reassurance of pain control. Return demonstration verifies learning and identifies the need for additional teaching. Analgesics are most effective if given before pain is severe.

NURSING CARE PLAN 16-1   Cesarean Birth—cont'd

INTERVENTION	RATIONALE

6. Reduce unnecessary stimulation:
  a. Keep lights low and noise to a minimum.
  b. Limit unnecessary visitors and staff.
  c. Plan operative preparations so that they are done efficiently.
  d. Maintain calm and friendly behavior.
	6. These measures avoid adding to her anxiety and emphasize that a cesarean delivery is a birth, not just a surgical procedure.

EVALUATION: Christina says she believes that a cesarean birth is best for her baby, although she would have preferred to have her baby "naturally." She asks a few other questions and then states that she understands preoperative and postoperative care. She demonstrates effective coughing and deep breathing techniques.

ASSESSMENT: Christina had soup and a sandwich about 2 hours before admission. She will have epidural anesthesia for the birth. Her vital signs are as follows: temperature, 37.2° C (99° F); pulse, 88 beats per minute (bpm); respirations, 20 breaths per minute; blood pressure, 122/70. The fetal heart rate (FHR) is 130 to 140 bpm and accelerates with fetal movement.

CRITICAL THINKING: Does this assessment suggest another nursing diagnosis? What interventions should the nurse institute for the nursing diagnosis?

ANSWER: Risk for Aspiration would apply during the intraoperative period because general anesthesia might be needed unexpectedly and Christina has food in her stomach that might be vomited and aspirated. The woman is given nothing by mouth if general anesthesia is a possibility. The nurse should expect orders for a drug to reduce gastric acidity.

ASSESSMENT: Christina is transferred to the operating room, and epidural anesthesia is begun. She gives birth to a 3856-g (8-lb, 8-oz) baby. Christina is transferred to the recovery room for postoperative care.

NURSING DIAGNOSIS: Risk for Injury related to altered sensation from epidural anesthesia and use of electrical equipment during surgery

GOALS/EXPECTED OUTCOMES: Christina will not have injury such as pressure areas, muscle strains, and electrical injury during the perioperative period.

INTERVENTION	RATIONALE
1. Pad the operating table carefully, particularly under bony prominences. Avoid obstructing her popliteal area.	1. Padding reduces potential for tissue damage caused by pressure and venous stasis with possible thrombus formation.
2. Transfer Christina to and from the operating table carefully, using enough staff members to keep her body in alignment. Brace the bed and operating table to keep them from separating.	2. These measures reduce the risk of fall and muscle strains for both Christina and the staff.
3. After anesthesia is begun, position Christina on the operating table and secure her legs with a safety strap. She should have a wedge under one hip, or the table should be tilted.	3. Securing her legs prevents falls or displacement of legs that have lost sensation. A hip wedge or tilting the table reduces aortocaval compression, which might reduce placental blood flow.
4. Apply grounding pad if electrocautery is to be used.	4. A grounding pad avoids electrical shock or burn.

EVALUATION: During surgery Christina's body was secured in proper alignment with proper padding of all her bony prominences. The grounding pad ensured electrical safety for electrocautery. Christina was transferred to the recovery room without incident. During the recovery period she showed no signs of pressure, electrical, or musculoskeletal injury.

- Abdominal dressing
- Uterine firmness and position (midline or deviated to one side)
- Lochia (color, quantity, presence and size of any clots)
- Urine output (quantity, color, other characteristics)
- IV infusion (fluid, rate, condition of IV site)
- Pain relief needs

The nurse observes for return of motion and sensation if the woman had epidural or subarachnoid block anesthesia. The level of consciousness and respiratory status (skin and mucous membrane color, rate and quality of respirations, pulse oximeter readings) are important observations if she had general anesthesia. Respiratory observations also are important if the woman received epidural opioid narcotics, which can cause delayed respiratory depression. Naloxone (Narcan) should be available to reverse opioid-induced respiratory depression (see Chapter 15).

The pulse, respirations, blood pressure, and oxygen saturation provide important clues to the woman's circulatory and respiratory status. If oxygen saturation falls below 95%, it usually can be raised with several deep breaths. A persistent respiratory rate of less than 12 breaths per minute suggests respiratory depression. Deep breathing and coughing move secretions out of the lungs. A small pillow to support her incision reduces pain when she coughs. Position changes every 2 hours improve ventilation; reduce pooling of lung secretions, and decrease discomfort from constant pressure.

As with vaginal birth, the fundus is assessed for height, firmness, and position. This examination is painful after regional anesthesia wears off, but the postcesarean mother also can have uterine atony. To relax her abdominal muscles and thus reduce pain from fundus checks, she should flex her knees and take slow, deep breaths. The nurse can gently "walk" the fingers toward the fundus to determine uterine firmness. The woman who has a Pfannenstiel skin incision usually has less pain with fundus checks than the woman with a vertical skin incision. A firm fundus does not need massage. The dressing is checked for drainage with each fundus check.

The nurse assesses the lochia and urine output with other assessments. Lochia may pool under the mother's buttocks and lower back. Urine may be bloody temporarily if the cesarean delivery was done after a long labor or an attempted forceps delivery. The urine drain tubing should be observed for gradual clearing of the blood. Urine should drain freely to prevent bladder distention, which worsens pain and increases the risk for postpartum hemorrhage. The nurse must remember that falling urine output is an early sign of hypovolemia.

The woman's needs for pain relief should be regularly assessed. The woman who received an epidural opioid may not need other analgesia during the early postpartum period. If she needs added pain relief while the epidural opioid is still in effect, the dose ordered often is lower than if she had not had that form of analgesia. If she did not receive an epidural opioid, analgesia usually is given by patient-controlled analgesia pump. Oral analgesics usually replace parenteral ones the day after surgery.

VAGINAL BIRTH AFTER CESAREAN

The decision about whether to have a VBAC has never been more difficult than at present. At one time the dictum "once a cesarean, always a cesarean" was accepted without question. For many years, the only women who had VBACs were those who entered the hospital in such advanced labor that no time was available to perform a repeat cesarean.

As low transverse uterine incisions became the norm for almost all women having cesarean births, the safety of a trial of labor became established. Gradually, VBAC became accepted as a way to lower the overall cesarean birth rate (ACOG, 2004).

Recent studies have found that VBAC is associated with a small but significant risk of uterine rupture resulting in a poor outcome for the mother and infant. An unsuccessful trial of labor resulting in a cesarean birth also is associated with more maternal and infant complications (ACOG, 2004). For these reasons many physicians are now more conservative when recommending VBAC.

Women may be anxious about attempting vaginal birth in a later pregnancy. A woman may know that she is a good candidate for VBAC but find it impossible to disregard even small risks. Scheduling a repeat cesarean may seem safer, simpler, and something on which she can count. The prospect of laboring and perhaps still needing a cesarean birth is worrisome as well.

The physician discusses VBAC during prenatal care, and the nurse reinforces these explanations and identifies misunderstandings. If the woman chooses VBAC, the nurse should reinforce the appropriateness of attempting VBAC and advantages of a vaginal birth, such as fewer overall complications. VBAC should be presented in a positive way if it is a real option, yet the possibility of cesarean delivery should be acknowledged because the surgery can be needed unexpectedly in any birth. (See Box 16-3.)

✓ CHECK YOUR READING

16. Why is the low transverse uterine incision preferred for cesarean birth?
17. What should a woman who expects a cesarean birth be taught about the operating room? The recovery room?
18. How should the nurse modify recovery room care of the mother who had a cesarean birth from that of the mother who had a vaginal delivery?

BOX 16-3 Vaginal Birth after Cesarean Birth

Approximately 60% to 80% of women with one low transverse uterine incision from a previous cesarean birth have successful vaginal births.
Women who had their previous cesarean for a nonrecurring reason, such as breech presentation, are more likely to have a successful vaginal birth after cesarean birth (VBAC) than women who had their previous cesarean because of dystocia.
Women who have had a vaginal birth, before or since the prior cesarean birth, are more likely to have successful VBAC.

Candidates and Requirements for VBAC
A woman who has one or two previous low transverse uterine incisions
Absence of other uterine scars (e.g., removal of fibroid tumors) or a previous uterine rupture
A pelvis that is clinically adequate for the estimated fetal size
Immediate availability of a physician during active labor if an emergency cesarean is needed
Availability of anesthesia and personnel to perform an emergency cesarean

Management of Women Who Plan VBAC
External cephalic version may be as successful for women having a previous cesarean as for women with an unscarred uterus.
Epidural analgesia and anesthesia may be used.
Induction and augmentation of labor with oxytocin may be done. Use of prostaglandin gel appears to be safe. Misoprostol (Cytotec) is currently contraindicated.
Most authorities recommend electronic fetal monitoring.

Data from American College of Obstetricians and Gynecologists. (2004). *Vaginal delivery after previous cesarean birth*. Practice Bulletin No. 54. Washington, DC: Author.
American Academy of Pediatrics & American College of Obstetricians and Gynecologists. (2002). *Guidelines for perinatal care* (5th ed.). Elk Grove, IL: Authors.

SUMMARY CONCEPTS

- Prolapse and compression of the umbilical cord are the primary risks of amniotomy. As the fluid gushes out, the cord can become compressed between the fetal presenting part and the expectant woman's pelvis.
- Infection is more likely to occur when membranes have been ruptured for a long time (such as 24 hours).
- Induction of labor may be done if continuing the pregnancy is more hazardous to the maternal and fetal health than the induction. It is not done if a maternal or fetal contraindication to labor and vaginal birth exists.
- Oxytocin-stimulated uterine contractions may be hypertonic, decreasing placental perfusion.
- External cephalic version is done to promote vaginal birth by changing the fetal presentation from a breech or transverse lie to a cephalic presentation. Internal version sometimes is used to change presentation of a second twin after the birth of the first twin.
- Trauma to maternal and fetal tissue is the primary risk associated with use of forceps and vacuum extraction. Possible trauma to the mother includes vaginal wall laceration and hematoma. Trauma to the infant may include ecchymoses, lacerations, abrasions, facial nerve injury, and intracranial hemorrhage.
- The median episiotomy is less painful but more likely to extend into the rectum than the mediolateral episiotomy.
- The preferred uterine incision for cesarean birth is the low transverse incision because it is least likely to rupture in a subsequent pregnancy. The skin incision does not always match the uterine incision and is unrelated to the risk of later uterine rupture.
- Some women have feelings of guilt and inadequacy if they have a cesarean birth. Therapeutic communication and sensitive, family-centered care are essential to help them achieve a positive perception of their birth experience.

ANSWERS TO CRITICAL THINKING EXERCISE 16-1, p. 366

1. The amount of amniotic fluid is normal, but the pale yellow color and strong odor suggest chorioamnionitis, or infection of the amniotic sac. The risk for chorioamnionitis increases as the duration of ruptured membranes increases, but it can be apparent at any time, including at initial rupture. The FHR is slightly elevated from the normal upper rate at term of 160 bpm. Accelerations with fetal movement are a reassuring sign. The maternal temperature, pulse, and respirations are slightly elevated. Accurately interpreting these values is difficult because the baseline values at the time of admission are not stated. The contractions are typical for a woman entering the active phase of first-stage labor.
2. The nurse should continue to assess the fetus for tachycardia, which often precedes maternal fever. Assess the woman's temperature at least every 2 hours for temperature of 100.4° F (38° C) or higher. Report abnormalities to the physician. Also observe for fetal tachycardia and signs of fetal compromise that may occur with maternal infection.

ANSWERS TO CRITICAL THINKING EXERCISE 16-2, p. 371

1. The nurse must consider that the FHR and fetal heart pattern are internally monitored, whereas the uterine activity is monitored externally. Evidence of hypertonic uterine activity is that the duration of contractions is 90 to 120 seconds and the rest interval is no longer than 40 seconds. External monitoring of uterine activity may vary with maternal position and placement of the tocotransducer ("toco"; see Chapter 14), but another possibility is that too little uterine relaxation may be present. Oxytocin stimulation is the probable cause of the excessive frequency and duration of contractions as well as possible incomplete relaxation between contractions. The normal FHR suggests that the fetus is now tolerating the excessive contractions.
2. Fetal oxygenation may be compromised if the excessive contractions continue. Reduce or stop the oxytocin infusion to decrease uterine stimulation. Increase the primary (nonadditive) IV infusion as needed to maintain adequate circulating volume and ensure maximum uterine blood flow. Keep the woman in a lateral position to reduce aortocaval compression and increase placental blood flow. Oxygen at 8 to 10 L/min with a snug facemask increases her blood oxygen saturation, making more available to the fetus.

REFERENCES & READINGS

Alexander, J.M., McIntire, D.D., & Leveno, K. (2001). Prolonged pregnancy: Induction of labor and cesarean births. *Obstetrics & Gynecology, 97*(6), 911-915.

American College of Obstetricians and Gynecologists (ACOG). (1999a). *Induction of labor.* Practice Bulletin No. 10. Washington, DC: Author.

American College of Obstetricians and Gynecologists. (1999b). *Induction of labor with misoprostol.* Committee Opinion No. 228. Washington, DC: Author.

American College of Obstetricians and Gynecologists. (2000a). *External cephalic version.* Practice Bulletin No. 13. Washington, DC: Author.

American College of Obstetricians and Gynecologists. (2000c). *Operative vaginal delivery.* Practice Bulletin No. 17. Washington, DC: Author.

American College of Obstetricians and Gynecologists. (2003). *Dystocia and augmentation of labor.* Practice Bulletin No. 49. Washington, DC: Author.

American College of Obstetricians and Gynecologists. (2004). *Vaginal birth after previous cesarean delivery.* Practice Bulletin No. 54. Washington, DC: Author.

American Academy of Pediatrics (AAP) & American College of Obstetricians and Gynecologists (ACOG). (2002). *Guidelines for perinatal care* (5th ed.). Elk Grove Village, IL: Authors.

Bachman, J., & Kendrick, J.M. (2001). Labor and birth. In K.R. Simpson & P.A. Creehan (Eds.), *AWHONN perinatal nursing* (2nd ed., pp. 298-377). Philadelphia: Lippincott Williams & Wilkins.

Belfort, M.A. (2003). Operative vaginal delivery. In J.R. Scott, R.S. Gibbs, B.Y. Karlan, & A.F. Haney (Eds.), *Danforth's obstetrics and gynecology* (9th ed., pp. 419-447). Philadelphia: Lippincott Williams & Wilkins.

Bishop, E.H. (1964). Pelvic scoring for elective abortion. *Obstetrics & Gynecology, 24*(2), 266-268.

Boucher, M., Bujold, E., Marquetter, G.P., & Vézina, Y. (2003). The relationship between amniotic fluid index and successful external cephalic version: A 14-year experience. *American Journal of Obstetrics & Gynecology, 189*(3), 751-754.

Bowes, W.A., & Thorpe, J.M. (2004). Clinical aspects of normal and abnormal labor. In R. Creasy, R. Resnik, & J.D. Iams (Eds.), *Maternal-fetal medicine: Principles and practice* (5th ed., pp. 671-705). Philadelphia: Saunders.

Chmait, R.H., & Moore, T.R. (2004). Obstetric procedures. In N.F. Hacker, J.G. Moore, & J.C. Gambone (Eds.), *Essentials of obstetrics and gynecology* (4th ed., pp. 247-255). Philadelphia: Saunders.

Cruikshank, D.P. (2003). Breech, other malpresentations, and umbilical cord complications. In J.R. Scott, R.S. Gibbs, B.Y. Karlan, & A.F. Haney (Eds.), *Danforth's obstetrics and gynecology* (9th ed., pp. 381-395). Philadelphia: Lippincott Williams & Wilkins.

Cunningham, F.G., Gant, N.F., Leveno, K.J., Gilstrap, L.C., Hauth, J.C., & Wenstrom, K.D. (2001). *Williams obstetrics* (21st ed.). New York: McGraw-Hill.

Dauphinee, J.D. (2004). VBAC: Safety for the patient and the nurse. *Journal of Obstetric, Gynecologic, and Neonatal Nursing, 33*(1), 105-115.

Dudley, D.J. (2003). Complications of labor. In J.R. Scott, R.S. Gibbs, B.Y. Karlan, & A.F. Haney (Eds.), *Danforth's obstetrics and gynecology* (9th ed., pp. 397-417). Philadelphia: Lippincott Williams & Wilkins.

Eason, E., & Feldman, P. (2000). Clinical commentary: Much ado about a little cut: Is episiotomy worthwhile? *Obstetrics & Gynecology, 95*(4), 616-618.

Eason, E., Labrecque, M., Wells, G., & Feldman, P. (2000). Preventing perineal trauma during childbirth: A systematic review. *Obstetrics & Gynecology, 95*(3), 464-471.

Flamm, B.L., Berwick, D.M., & Kabcenell, A. (1998). Reducing cesarean section rates safely: Lessons from a "breakthrough series" collaborative. *Birth, 25*(2), 117-124.

Fleming, N., Newton, E.R., & Roberts, J. (2003). Changes in postpartum perineal function in women with and without episiotomies. *Journal of Midwifery & Women's Health, 48*(1), 53-59.

Goer, H. (2003). "Spin doctoring" the research. *Birth, 30*(2), 124-129.

Guinn, D.A., & Gibbs, R.S. (2003). Preterm labor and delivery. In J.R. Scott, R.S. Gibbs, B.Y. Karlan, & A.F. Haney (Eds.), *Danforth's obstetrics and gynecology* (9th ed., pp. 173-190). Philadelphia: Lippincott Williams & Wilkins.

Hamilton, B.E., Martin, J.A., & Sutton, P.D. (2004). Births: Preliminary data for 2003. *National Vital Statistics Reports, 53*(9). Retrieved December 26, 2004, from www.cdc.gov/nchs/pressroom/04facts/birthrates.htm.

Hing, E., & Middleton, K. (2004). National Hospital Ambulatory Medical Care Survey: 2002 Outpatient Department Summary. *Advance Data from Vital and Health Statistics:* No. 345. Hyattsville, MD: National Center for Health Statistics.

Hobel, C.J., & Chang, A.B. (2004). Normal labor, delivery, and postpartum care: Anatomic considerations, obstetric analgesia and anesthesia, and resuscitation of the newborn. In N.F. Hacker, J.G. Moore, & J.C. Gambone (Eds.), *Essentials of obstetrics & gynecology* (4th ed., pp. 104-135). Philadelphia: Saunders.

Johnson, D.P., Davis, N.R., & Brown, A.J. (2003). Risk of cesarean delivery after induction at term in nulliparous women with an unfavorable cervix. *American Journal of Obstetrics & Gynecology, 188*(6), 1565-1672.

King, T.L., & Simpson, K.R. (2001). Fetal assessment during labor. In K.R. Simpson & P.A. Creehan (Eds.), *AWHONN perinatal nursing* (2nd ed., pp. 378-416). Philadelphia: Lippincott Williams & Wilkins.

Kozak, L.J., & Weeks, J.D. (2002). U.S. trends in obstetric procedures, 1990-2000. *Birth, 29*(3), 157-161.

Lowe, N. (2002). The institutional factor in cesarean section rates [editorial]. *Journal of Obstetric, Gynecologic, and Neonatal Nursing, 31*(3), 245.

Lowe, N. (2003). Amazed or appalled, apathy or action? [editorial]. *Journal of Obstetric, Gynecologic, and Neonatal Nursing, 32*(3), 281-282.

Martin, J.A., Hamilton, B.E., Sutton, P.D., Ventura, S.J., Menacker, F., & Munson, M.L. (2003). Births: Final data for 2002. *National Vital Statistics Reports, 52*(10). Retrieved December 19, 2004, from www.cdc.gov/nchs/data/nvsr52/nvsr52_10.pdf.

Nager, C.W., & Helliwell, J.P. (2001). Episiotomy increases perineal laceration length in primiparous women. *American Journal of Obstetrics & Gynecology, 185*(2), 444-450.

Porter, T.F., & Scott, J.R. (2003). Cesarean delivery. In J.R. Scott, R.S. Gibbs, B.Y. Karlan, & A.F. Haney (Eds.), *Danforth's obstetrics and gynecology* (9th ed., pp. 449-460). Philadelphia: Lippincott Williams & Wilkins.

Rayburn, W.F., & Zhang, J. (2002). Rising rates of labor induction: Present concerns and future strategies. *Obstetrics & Gynecology, 100*(1), 164-167.

Ridley, R.T., Davis, P.A., Bright, J.H., & Sinclair, D. (2002). What influences a woman to choose vaginal birth after cesarean? *Journal of Obstetric, Gynecologic, and Neonatal Nursing, 31*(6), 665-672.

Sachs, B.P., Kobelin, C., Castro, M.A., & Frigoletto, F. (1999). The risks of lowering the cesarean delivery rate. *New England Journal of Medicine, 340*(1), 54-57.

Sanchez-Ramos, L., Oliver, F., Delke, I., & Kaunitz, A.M. (2003). Labor induction versus expectant management for postterm pregnancies: A systematic review with meta-analysis. *Obstetrics & Gynecology, 101*(6), 1312-1316.

Seyb, S.T., Berka, R.J., Socol, M.L., & Dooley, S.L. (1999). Risk of cesarean delivery with elective induction of labor at term in nulliparous women. *Obstetrics & Gynecology, 94*(4), 600-607.

Simpson, K.R., & Atterbury, J. (2003). Trends and issues in labor induction in the United States: Implications for clinical practice. *Journal of Obstetric, Gynecologic, and Neonatal Nursing, 32*(6), 767-779.

Simpson, K.R., & Poole, J.H. (1998). *Practice resource: Cervical ripening and induction and augmentation of labor.* Washington, DC: Association of Women's Health, Obstetric and Neonatal Nurses.

U.S. Department of Health and Human Services. (2000). Healthy People 2010: *Reduce cesarean births among low-risk (full term, singleton, vertex presentation) women.* Retrieved December 26, 2004, from www.healthypeople.gov/document/html/objectives/16-09.htm.

Vézina, Y., Bujold, E., Varin, J., Marquette, G.P., & Boucher, M. (2004). Cesarean delivery after successful external cephalic version of breech presentation at term: A comparative study. *American Journal of Obstetrics & Gynecology, 190*(3), 763-768.

Webb, D.A., & Culhane, J. (2002). Hospital variation in episiotomy use and the risk of perineal trauma during childbirth. *Birth, 29*(2), 132-136.

Williams, D.R., & Shah, M.A. (2003). Soaring cesarean section rates: A cause for alarm [editorial]. *Journal of Obstetric, Gynecologic, and Neonatal Nursing, 32*(3), 283.

Yeast, J.D., Jones, A., & Poskin, M. (1999). Induction of labor and the relationship to cesarean delivery. *American Journal of Obstetrics & Gynecology, 180*(3 Pt. 1), 626-633.

Young, D. (1999). Whither cesareans in the new millennium? *Birth, 26*(2), 67-70.

The Cesarean Birth Story

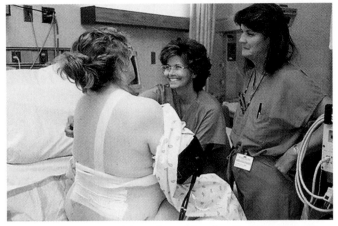

1 ■ Vicky is in active labor. An epidural catheter allows injection of medications to provide analgesia during labor. Additional epidural medications can be used to provide anesthesia if surgery becomes necessary. An intravenous infusion precedes placement of the epidural block to offset the tendency of the block to cause hypotension.

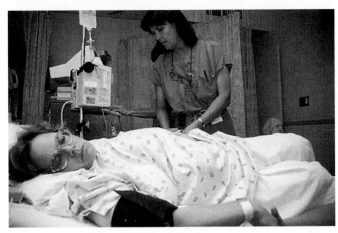

2 ■ Support under her left hip displaces Vicky's uterus, thus avoiding pressure on her inferior vena cava and aorta and enhancing placental circulation. An automatic blood pressure cuff helps keep up with the frequent blood pressure assessments that are necessary when an epidural block is first begun.

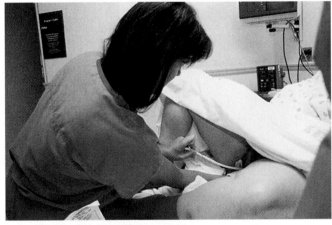

3 ■ After rupturing the membranes, the nurse-midwife applies a spiral electrode to the fetal scalp to improve the accuracy of the fetal heart tracing on the monitor.

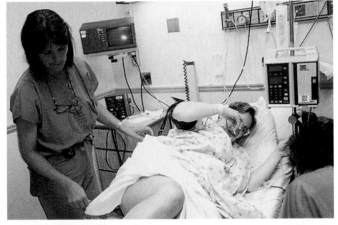

4 ■ Because the fetal monitor shows patterns suggesting fetal compromise, Vicky will need a cesarean birth. Monitors for her blood pressure, pulse, and cardiac rhythm help identify maternal factors contributing to the fetal heart rate patterns. She receives oxygen by facemask to provide the maximal amount to her fetus.

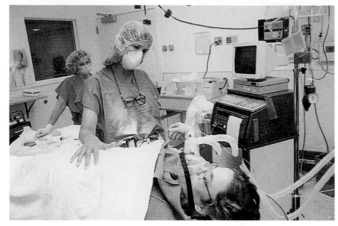

5 ■ While Vicky is prepared for surgery, fetal monitoring and maternal oxygen administration continue. If possible, the same nurses accompany the woman to the operating room so that she has a continuing relationship during the cesarean birth, as she would have for vaginal birth in most circumstances.

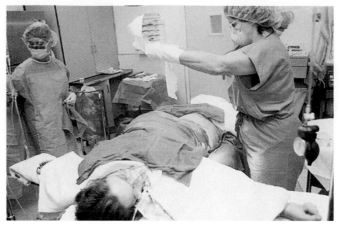

6 ■ Vicky's abdomen is shaved to prepare for the surgery and then is cleansed with an antimicrobial prep solution. Shaving extends from just above the umbilicus to the point where the legs come together if a vertical incision is expected. If a Pfannenstiel (transverse) incision is expected, the top border can be about 3 inches above the upper pubic hairline.

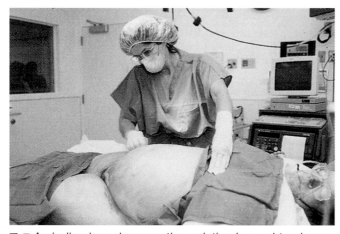

7 ■ An iodine-based preparation solution is used to cleanse the abdomen using a circular motion beginning at the incisional area and extending outward. The cleansing sponge should not be returned toward the center. During preparations for surgery, Vicky's trunk is tilted slightly toward her left side by a wedge under her right hip to promote circulation to the placenta. The internal fetal scalp electrode is removed before the incision is made so that it is not brought from the unsterile vagina through the incision as the baby is born.

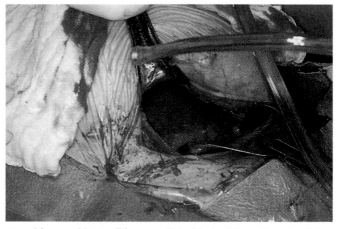

8 ■ After making a Pfannenstiel skin incision, the physician separates the layers until the uterus is reached. The uterus is then opened in a low transverse incision. Wide retractors hold the mother's tissues back to expose an area large enough to allow the fetus to emerge. A suction device is available to suction blood and amniotic fluid from the uterus when it is incised.

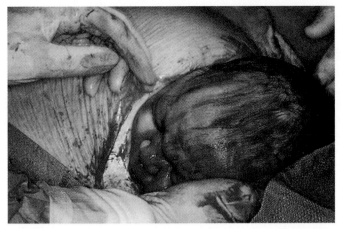

9 ■ The fetal head is first brought through the incision. The bluish skin color is normal at this point.

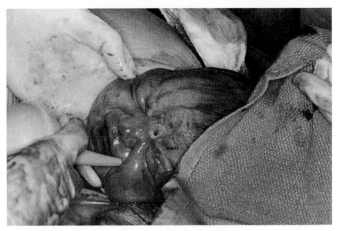

10 ■ After birth of the head has occurred, the mouth and nose are suctioned to remove blood and other secretions before the infant takes his first breath. This baby is grimacing with the suction, which usually is associated with adequate oxygenation.

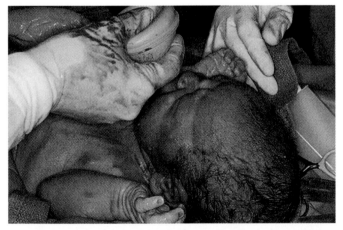

11 ■ Further infant suctioning is done after the baby emerges.

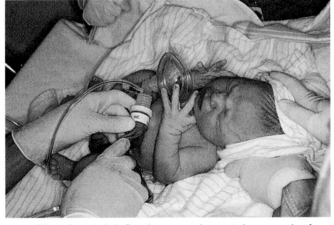

12 ■ The infant is briefly given supplemental oxygen by face mask. His color is becoming pinker than it was immediately after birth because he has a larger proportion of oxygenated hemoglobin. At the same time, another nurse dries the baby to prevent cold stress, which could increase his oxygen needs. Note that nurses handling the baby wear gloves to protect them from blood and other secretions.

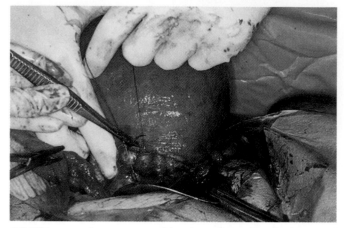

13 ■ Heavy sutures are used to close the muscular layers of the transverse uterine incision.

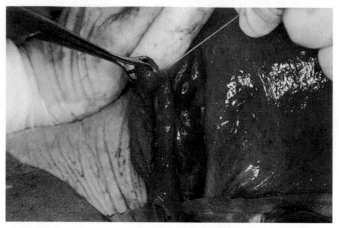

14 ■ Vicky is having a bilateral tubal ligation for sterilization. One fallopian tube is identified by its connection to the uterus to distinguish it from her ureter. It then is doubly tied, and a segment of the tube is cut away and sent to the pathology laboratory for analysis.

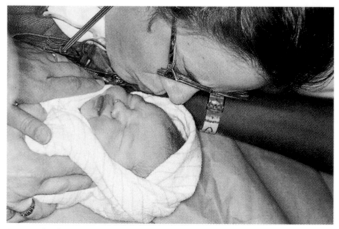

15 ■ As her surgery continues and the infant's condition is stable, Vicky sees her baby up close for the first time.

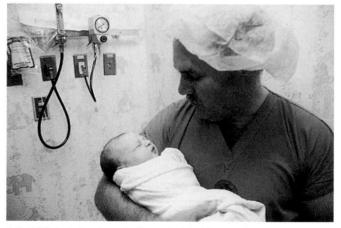

16 ■ Vicky's husband, Greg, holds his newborn son shortly after birth.

CHAPTER 17

Postpartum Physiologic Adaptations

OBJECTIVES

After studying this chapter, you should be able to:

1. Explain the physiologic changes that occur during the postpartum period.
2. Identify the purpose of clinical pathways in postpartum care.
3. Describe nursing assessments and nursing care during the postpartum period.
4. Recount expected outcomes and interventions for the most common nursing diagnoses.
5. Discuss the role of the nurse in health education, and identify important areas of teaching.
6. Describe postpartum home and community care in terms of criteria for discharge, common problems, and available health care services.
7. Compare nursing assessments and care for women who have undergone cesarean birth and vaginal birth.
8. Use critical thinking exercises to improve selected nursing care plans.

Go to your Student CD-ROM for Review Questions keyed to these Objectives.

DEFINITIONS

Afterpains Cramping pain after childbirth caused by alternate relaxation and contraction of uterine muscles.

Atony Absence or lack of usual muscle tone.

Catabolism Destructive process that converts living cells into simpler compounds; process involved in involution of the uterus after childbirth.

Decidua Name applied to the endometrium during pregnancy. All except the deepest layer is shed after childbirth.

Diastasis Recti Separation of the longitudinal muscles of the abdomen (rectus abdominis) during pregnancy.

Dyspareunia Difficult or painful coitus in women.

Engorgement Swelling of the breasts resulting from increased blood flow, edema, and presence of milk.

Episiotomy Surgical incision of the perineum to enlarge the vaginal opening.

Fundus Part of the uterus that is farthest from the cervix, above the openings of the fallopian tubes.

Involution Retrogressive changes that return the reproductive organs, particularly the uterus, to their nonpregnant size and condition.

Kegel Exercises Alternate contracting and relaxing of the pelvic muscles. These movements strengthen the pubococcygeal muscle, which surrounds the urinary meatus and vagina.

Lactation Secretion of milk from the breasts; also describes the period of breastfeeding.

Lochia Alba White or cream-colored vaginal discharge that follows lochia serosa. Occurs when the amount of blood is decreased and the number of leukocytes is increased.

Lochia Rubra Reddish vaginal discharge that occurs immediately after childbirth; composed mostly of blood.

Lochia Serosa Pink or brown-tinged vaginal discharge that follows lochia rubra and precedes lochia alba; composed largely of serous exudate, blood, and leukocytes.

Milk-Ejection Reflex Release of milk from the alveoli into the ducts; also known as the *letdown reflex.*

Oxytocin Posterior pituitary gland hormone that stimulates uterine contractions and the milk-ejection reflex. Also prepared synthetically.

Prolactin Anterior pituitary hormone that promotes growth of breast tissue and stimulates production of milk.

Puerperium Period from the end of childbirth until involution of the reproductive organs is complete; approximately 6 weeks.

REEDA Acronym for redness, ecchymosis, edema, discharge, and approximation; useful for assessing wound healing or the presence of inflammation or infection.

Subinvolution Delayed return of the uterus to its non-pregnant size and consistency.

The first 6 weeks after the birth of an infant are known as the *postpartum period,* or puerperium. During this time, mothers experience numerous physiologic and psychosocial changes. Physiologic and psychosocial changes and their implications are presented in separate chapters, although in actual practice they occur at the same time. (See Appendix C, "Keys to Clinical Practice," for a summary of postpartum assessment and care.)

Many of the physiologic changes are retrogressive in nature: changes that occurred in body systems during pregnancy are reversed as the body returns to the nonpregnant state. Progressive changes also occur, most obviously in the initiation of lactation.

REPRODUCTIVE SYSTEM

Involution of the Uterus

Involution refers to the changes the reproductive organs, particularly the uterus, undergo after childbirth to return to their nonpregnant size and condition. Uterine involution depends on three processes: (1) contraction of muscle fibers, (2) catabolism, and (3) regeneration of uterine epithelium. Involution begins immediately after delivery of the placenta, when uterine muscle fibers contract firmly around maternal blood vessels at the area where the placenta was attached. This contraction controls bleeding from the area left denuded when the placenta separated. The uterus decreases in size as muscle fibers, which have been stretched for many months, contract and gradually regain their former contour and size.

Although the total number of cells remains unchanged, the enlarged muscle cells of the uterus undergo catabolic changes in protein cytoplasm that cause a reduction in individual cell size. The products of the catabolic process are absorbed by the bloodstream and excreted in the urine as nitrogenous waste.

Regeneration of the uterine epithelial lining begins soon after childbirth. The outer portion of the endometrial layer is expelled with the placenta. Within 2 to 3 days, the remaining decidua separates into two layers. The first layer is superficial and is shed in the lochia. The basal layer con-

taining the residual endometrial glands remains intact to provide the source of new endometrium. Regeneration of the endometrium, except at the site of placental attachment, occurs by 2 to 3 weeks.

The placental site, which is about 7 cm (2.7 in) in diameter, heals by a process of *exfoliation* (scaling off of dead tissue). New endometrium is generated at the site from glands and tissue that remain in the lower layer of the decidua after separation of the placenta (Cunningham et al., 2005). This process leaves the endometrial layer smooth and spongy, as it was before pregnancy, and leaves the uterine lining free of scar tissue, which would interfere with implantation of future pregnancies. Healing at the placental site occurs more slowly and requires approximately 6 to 7 weeks.

DESCENT OF THE UTERINE FUNDUS

The location of the uterine fundus helps determine whether involution is progressing normally. Immediately after delivery, the uterus is about the size of a large grapefruit or softball and weighs approximately 1000 g (2.2 lb). The fundus can be palpated midway between the symphysis pubis and umbilicus (James, 2001). Within 12 hours the fundus rises to the level of the umbilicus, or slightly above or below the umbilicus (Blackburn, 2003).

By the second day, the fundus descends by approximately 1 cm, or one fingerbreadth, per day. Usually the fundus has descended into the pelvic cavity by the tenth day and cannot be palpated abdominally (Figure 17-1). This process is normally slower when the uterus was distended during pregnancy with more than one fetus, a large fetus, or hydramnios (excessive amniotic fluid). When the process of involution does not occur properly, subinvolution occurs.

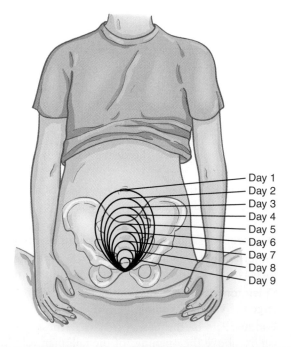

Day 1
Day 2
Day 3
Day 4
Day 5
Day 6
Day 7
Day 8
Day 9

Figure 17-1 ■ Involution of the uterus. Height of the uterine fundus decreases by approximately 1 cm per day.

Subinvolution can cause postpartum hemorrhage (see Chapter 28).

Descent is documented in relation to the umbilicus. For instance, *U-1* or ↓ 1 indicates that the fundus is palpable about 1 cm below the umbilicus. Within a week, the weight of the uterus decreases to about 500 g (1 lb); at 6 weeks, the uterus weighs 60 g (2 oz), which is roughly the prepregnancy weight.

AFTERPAINS

Intermittent uterine contractions, known as *afterpains,* are a source of discomfort for many women. The discomfort is more acute for multiparas because repeated stretching of muscle fibers leads to loss of muscle tone that results in repeated contraction and relaxation of the uterus. The uterus of a primipara tends to remain contracted, but she may also experience severe afterpains if her uterus has been overdistended during pregnancy or if retained blood clots are present.

SEVERITY. Afterpains are particularly severe during breastfeeding. Oxytocin, released from the posterior pituitary to stimulate the milk-ejection reflex, stimulates strong contractions of uterine muscles.

NURSING CONSIDERATIONS. Analgesics are frequently used to lessen the discomfort of afterpains. Medication that a breastfeeding mother takes just before nursing the infant may not reach the milk for 30 minutes or more. Many breastfeeding mothers are reluctant to take medication for fear that the infant will be harmed by the medication in breast milk. However, health care experts generally agree that analgesics may be used for short-term pain relief without harm to the infant. The benefits of pain relief, such as comfort and relaxation, facilitate the milk-ejection reflex and usually outweigh the small effect of the medication on the infant.

Some mothers find that lying in a prone position with a small pillow or folded blanket under the abdomen helps keep the uterus contracted and provides relief. The nurse can reassure the mother that afterpains are self-limiting and decrease rapidly after 48 hours.

LOCHIA

Changes in the color and amount of lochia also provide information about whether involution is progressing normally.

CHANGES IN COLOR. For the first 3 days after childbirth, lochia consists almost entirely of blood, with small particles of decidua and mucus. It is called *lochia rubra* because of its red color. The amount of blood decreases by about the fourth day, when leukocytes begin to invade the area, as they do any healing surface. The color of lochia then changes from red to pink or brown-tinged (lochia serosa). Lochia serosa is composed of serous exudate, erythrocytes, leukocytes, and cervical mucus. By about the eleventh day, the erythrocyte component decreases. The discharge becomes white, cream, or light yellow in color (lochia alba). Lochia alba contains leukocytes, decidual cells, epithelial cells, fat, cervical mucus, and bacteria. It is present in most women until the third week after childbirth but may persist for 6 weeks.

AMOUNT. Because estimating the amount of lochia on a peripad (perineal pad) is difficult, nurses frequently document lochia in terms that are difficult to quantify, such as *scant, moderate,* and *heavy.* Agreement on the meanings of terms in an agency is important to make charting accurate. One method for recording the amount of lochia in 1 hour uses the following labels:

- Scant—Less than a 2.5-cm (1-in) stain on the peripad
- Light—2.5- to 10-cm (1- to 4-in) stain
- Moderate—10- to 15-cm (4- to 6-in) stain
- Heavy—Saturated peripad in 1 hour
- Excessive—Saturated peripad in 15 minutes (Scoggin, 2004)

Determining the time a peripad has been in place is important when assessing lochia. What appears to be a moderate amount of lochia may be only a light flow if the peripad has been in use for more than an hour (Figure 17-2). The amount of lochia absorbed by a peripad varies according to the brand used.

The time between delivery and assessment of lochia also is important. Lochia flow will be greater immediately after delivery but will gradually decrease. It is less after cesarean birth because some of the endometrial lining is removed during surgery. The lochia of the cesarean mother will go through the same phases as that of the woman who had a vaginal birth, even though the amount may be reduced.

Lochia flow often is heavier when the new mother first gets out of bed after birth or after sleeping because gravity allows blood that pooled in the vagina during the hours of rest to flow freely when she stands.

Table 17-1 summarizes the characteristics of normal and abnormal lochial discharge.

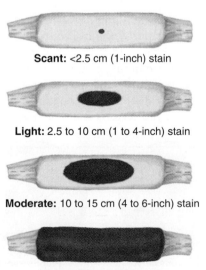

Scant: <2.5 cm (1-inch) stain

Light: 2.5 to 10 cm (1 to 4-inch) stain

Moderate: 10 to 15 cm (4 to 6-inch) stain

Heavy: Saturated in 1 hour

Figure 17-2 ■ Guidelines for assessing the amount of lochia on the perineal pad.

TABLE 17-1 Characteristics of Lochia

Time and Type	Normal Discharge	Abnormal Discharge
Days 1-3: lochia rubra	Bloody; small clots; fleshy, earthy odor	Large clots; saturated perineal pads; foul odor
Days 4-10: lochia serosa	Decreased amount; serosanguineous; pink or brown	Excessive amount; foul smell; continued or recurrent reddish color
Days 11-21: lochia alba	Cream, white, or light yellow color; decreasing amounts	Persistent lochia serosa; return to lochia rubra, foul odor; discharge continuing

Cervix

Immediately after childbirth the cervix is formless, flabby, and open wide enough to admit the entire hand. This allows manual extraction of the placenta, if necessary, and manual examination of the uterus. Small tears or lacerations may be present, and the cervix is often edematous. Rapid healing takes place, and by the end of the first week the cervix feels firm and the external os is the width of a pencil. The internal os closes as before pregnancy, but the shape of the external os is permanently changed. It remains slightly open and appears slit-like rather than round, as in the nulliparous woman (Figure 17-3).

Vagina

The vagina and vaginal introitus are greatly stretched during birth to allow passage of the fetus. Soon after childbirth, the vaginal walls appear edematous, and multiple small lacerations may be present. Very few vaginal rugae (folds) are present. The hymen is permanently torn and heals with small, irregular tags of tissue visible at the vaginal introitus.

Although the vaginal mucosa heals and rugae are regained by 3 weeks, the entire postpartum period (6 weeks) is needed for the vagina to complete involution and to gain approximately the same size and contour it had before pregnancy. The vagina does not entirely regain the nulliparous size, however.

During the postpartum period, vaginal mucosa becomes atrophic and vaginal walls do not regain their thickness until estrogen production by the ovaries is reestablished. Because ovarian function, and therefore estrogen production, is not well established during lactation, breastfeeding mothers are likely to experience vaginal dryness and may experience dyspareunia or discomfort during intercourse.

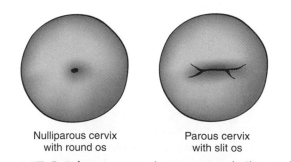

Nulliparous cervix
with round os

Parous cervix
with slit os

Figure 17-3 ■ A permanent change occurs in the cervical os after childbirth.

Perineum

The muscles of the pelvic floor stretch and thin greatly during the second stage of labor, when the fetal head applies pressure as it descends, rotates, and then extends to be delivered. After childbirth, the perineum may be edematous and bruised. In the United States many women who give birth also have a surgical incision (episiotomy) of the perineal area. The episiotomy site may take 4 to 6 months to heal completely (Blackburn, 2003).

Generally, the episiotomy is median or midline, extending straight back from the lower edge of the introitus toward the anus. A mediolateral incision, begun at the introitus and directed laterally and downward away from the rectum to either the right or the left side, may be performed to provide additional room for birth of the infant. This type of episiotomy results in more blood loss and pain but less likelihood of extension of the incision (Cunningham et al, 2005).

Lacerations of the perineum may also occur during delivery. Lacerations and episiotomies are classified according to tissue involved (Box 17-1). (See Chapter 16 for further discussion of episiotomy and lacerations.)

BOX 17-1 Lacerations of the Birth Canal

Perineum
Perineal lacerations are classified in degrees to describe the amount of tissue involved. Some physicians or nurse-midwives also use degrees to describe the extent of midline episiotomies.
- *First-degree:* Involves the superficial vaginal mucosa or perineal skin
- *Second-degree:* Involves the vaginal mucosa, perineal skin, and deeper tissues, which may include muscles of the perineum
- *Third-degree:* Same as second-degree lacerations but involves the anal sphincter
- *Fourth-degree:* Extends through the anal sphincter into the rectal mucosa

Periurethral Area
A laceration in the area of the urethra may cause a woman to have difficulty urinating after birth. An indwelling catheter may be necessary for a day or two.

Vaginal Wall
A laceration involving the mucosa of the vaginal wall.

Cervix
Tears in the cervix may be a source of significant bleeding after birth.

DISCOMFORT

Although the episiotomy is relatively small, the muscles of the perineum are involved in many activities (for example, walking, sitting, stooping, squatting, bending, urinating, and defecating). An incision in this area can cause a great deal of discomfort. In addition, many pregnant women are affected by hemorrhoids (distended rectal veins), which are pushed out of the rectum during the second stage of labor.

NURSING CONSIDERATIONS

Hemorrhoids, as well as perineal trauma, episiotomy, or lacerations, can make physical activity or bowel elimination difficult during the postpartum period. Relief of perineal discomfort is a nursing priority that may include teaching self-care measures such as sitz baths, perineal care, use of topical anesthetics, cooling astringent pads, and ordered analgesics.

✔ **CHECK YOUR READING**

1. Which three processes are involved in involution of the uterus?
2. How is the fundus expected to descend after childbirth?
3. Which mothers are most likely to experience afterpains? How are they treated?
4. What are the differences among lochia rubra, lochia serosa, and lochia alba in appearance and expected duration?

CARDIOVASCULAR SYSTEM

Hypervolemia, which produces a 40% to 50% increase in blood volume at term, allows the woman to tolerate a substantial blood loss during childbirth without ill effect. On average, up to 500 ml of blood is lost in vaginal deliveries and up to 1000 ml is lost in cesarean births (Blackburn, 2003).

Cardiac Output

Despite the blood loss, a transient increase in maternal cardiac output occurs after childbirth. This increase is caused by (1) an increased flow of blood back to the heart when blood from the uteroplacental unit returns to the central circulation, (2) decreased pressure from the pregnant uterus on the vessels, and (3) the mobilization of excess extracellular fluid into the vascular compartment.

The rise in cardiac output, which persists for about 48 hours after childbirth, is caused by an increase in stroke volume (Resnik, 2004). As a result, bradycardia (a pulse rate of 50 to 60 beats per minute [bpm]) is often noted during the early postpartum period. Gradually, cardiac output decreases and returns to normal nonpregnant levels by 6 to 12 weeks after childbirth (Blackburn, 2003).

Plasma Volume

The body rids itself of excess plasma volume that was necessary during pregnancy by two methods: diuresis and diaphoresis.

- Diuresis (increased excretion of urine) is facilitated by a decline in the adrenal hormone aldosterone, which is increased during pregnancy to counteract the salt-wasting effect of progesterone. As aldosterone production decreases, sodium retention declines and fluid excretion accelerates. A decrease in oxytocin, which promotes reabsorption of fluid, also contributes to diuresis. A urinary output of 3000 ml per day is common, especially on days 2 through 5 postpartum (Blackburn, 2003).
- Diaphoresis (profuse perspiration) also rids the body of excess fluid. Although not clinically significant, diaphoresis can be uncomfortable and unsettling for the mother who is not prepared for it. Explanations of the cause and provision of comfort measures, such as showers and dry clothing, are generally sufficient.

Coagulation

Significant changes that occur during pregnancy also affect the body's ability to coagulate blood and form clots. During pregnancy, plasma fibrinogen and other factors necessary for coagulation increase as a protection against postpartum hemorrhage. As a result the mother's body has a greater ability to form clots and thus prevent excessive bleeding. Fibrinolytic activity (to break down clots) is decreased during pregnancy. Although fibrinolysis increases shortly after delivery, elevations in clotting factors continue for several days or longer, causing a continued risk of thrombus formation. It takes 3 to 4 weeks before the hemostasis returns to normal prepregnant levels (Blackburn, 2003).

Although the incidence of thrombophlebitis has declined greatly as a result of early postpartum ambulation, new mothers are still at increased risk for thrombus formation. Women who have varicose veins or a history of thrombophlebitis or who have experienced a cesarean birth are at further risk, and the lower extremities should be monitored closely. Antiembolism hosiery or sequential compression devices are often applied before a cesarean birth or if the mother is at particular risk because of a history of previous phlebitis or the presence of varicosities (see Chapter 28).

Blood Values

Besides clotting factors, other components of the blood change during the postpartum period. Marked leukocytosis occurs, with the white blood cell (WBC) count increasing to as high as 30,000/mm^3 (Cunningham et al., 2005). The average increase is to 14,000 to 16,000/mm^3 (Scoggin, 2004). The white blood count falls to normal values by 4 to 7 days after birth (Blackburn, 2003). Neutrophils, which increase in response to inflammation, pain, and stress to protect against invading organisms, account for the major increase in WBCs.

Maternal hemoglobin and hematocrit values are difficult to interpret during the first few days after birth because of the remobilization and rapid excretion of excess body fluid. The hematocrit is low when plasma increases and dilutes the concentration of blood cells and other substances carried by the plasma. As excess fluid is excreted, the dilution gradually is reduced. Hematocrit should return to normal limits within 4 to 8 weeks unless excessive blood loss has occurred (Blackburn, 2003).

GASTROINTESTINAL SYSTEM

Soon after childbirth, digestion begins to be active. The new mother usually is hungry because of the energy expended in labor. She is thirsty because of the decreased oral intake during labor, the fluid loss from exertion, mouth breathing, and early diaphoresis. Nurses anticipate the mother's needs and provide food and fluids soon after childbirth.

Constipation is a common problem during the postpartum period for a variety of reasons. Bowel tone, which was diminished during pregnancy as a result of progesterone, remains sluggish for several days. Restricted food and fluid intake during labor often results in small, hard stools. Perineal trauma, episiotomy, and hemorrhoids cause discomfort and interfere with effective bowel elimination. In addition, many women anticipate pain when they attempt to defecate and are unwilling to exert pressure on the perineum. Women who are taking iron have an added cause of constipation.

Temporary constipation is not harmful, although it can cause a feeling of abdominal fullness and flatulence. Many women become extremely concerned about constipation, and stool softeners and laxatives frequently are prescribed to prevent or treat constipation (Table 17-2). The first stool usually occurs within 2 to 3 days postpartum. Normal patterns of bowel elimination usually resume by 8 to 14 days after birth (Blackburn, 2003).

URINARY SYSTEM

Physical Changes

The kidneys return to normal function by 4 to 6 weeks after delivery (Resnik, 2004; Scoggin, 2004). The dilation of the renal pelvis, calyces, and the ureters may continue for 3 or more months (Resnik, 2004). Both protein and acetone may be present in the urine in the first few postpartum days. Acetone suggests dehydration that often occurs during the exertion of labor. Mild proteinuria usually is the result of the catabolic processes involved in uterine involution. Sugar in the form of lactose also is sometimes present.

Changes during pregnancy cause the bladder of the postpartum woman to have increased capacity and decreased muscle tone. During childbirth, the urethra, bladder, and tissue around the urinary meatus may become edematous and traumatized as the fetal head passes beneath the bladder. This often results in diminished sensitivity to fluid pressure, and many new mothers have little or no sensation of needing to void even when the bladder is distended.

The bladder fills rapidly because of the diuresis that follows childbirth. As a consequence the mother is at risk for overdistention of the bladder, incomplete emptying of the bladder, and retention of residual urine. Women who have received regional anesthesia are at particular risk for bladder distention and difficulty in voiding until sensation returns.

Urinary retention and overdistention of the bladder may cause two complications: urinary tract infection and postpartum hemorrhage. Urinary tract infection occurs when urinary stasis allows time for bacteria to multiply. Risk of postpartum hemorrhage increases because uterine ligaments, which were stretched during pregnancy, allow the uterus to be displaced upward and laterally by the full bladder (Figure 17-4). The displacement results in an inability of the uterine muscles to contract (uterine atony), a primary cause of excessive bleeding.

Stress incontinence occurring during pregnancy usually improves within 3 months after birth (James, 2001). For some women the problem resolves with exercises (for exam-

---

TABLE 17-2 Commonly Recommended Laxatives for the Postpartum Period

Types	Examples	Comments
Fecal wetting agents	Docusate calcium (Surfak), Docusate sodium (Colace)	Detergent-like action, permit easier mixing of fats and fluids with fecal mass; produce softer, more easily passed stools.
Saline laxatives	Milk of magnesia	Work by osmotic action, drawing water through the intestinal wall to soften stool. May decrease absorption of some medications.
Stimulant laxatives	Bisacodyl (Dulcolax), casanthranol (Peri-Colace), senna (Senokot)	Increases fluid and electrolyte accumulation in the colon to promote peristalsis. Should not be taken within 1 hour of taking other medications (may decrease effectiveness), antacids, or milk products. Do not chew or crush.
Suppositories	Glycerine, bisacodyl	Chill and moisten with water or water-soluble lubricant before insertion.
All laxatives		Teach client to increase fluid intake and that prolonged use may result in dependence.

Data from Hodgson, B.B., & Kizior, R.J. (2005). *Saunders nursing drug handbook 2005.* Philadelphia: Saunders.

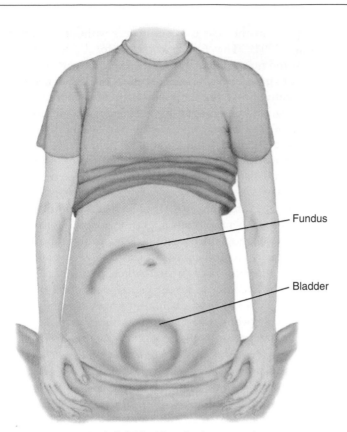

Figure 17-4 ■ A full bladder displaces and prevents contraction of the uterus.

ple, Kegel) and time for healing. Others have continued problems (see Chapter 33).

MUSCULOSKELETAL SYSTEM

Muscles and Joints

In the first 1 to 2 days after childbirth, many women experience muscle fatigue and aches, particularly of the shoulders, neck, and arms, because of exertion during labor. Warmth and gentle massage increase circulation to the area and provide comfort and relaxation.

During the first few days, levels of the hormone relaxin gradually subside, and ligaments and cartilage of the pelvis begin to return to their prepregnancy positions. These changes can cause hip and joint pain that interferes with ambulation and exercise. The mother should be told that the discomfort is temporary and does not indicate a medical problem. Good body mechanics and correct posture are extremely important during this time to help prevent low back pain and injury to the joints (see Figures 7-12 and 7-13 on p. 139).

Abdominal Wall

During pregnancy the abdominal walls stretch to accommodate the growing fetus, and muscle tone is diminished. Many women, expecting that the abdominal muscles will return to the prepregnancy condition immediately after

childbirth, are dismayed to find the abdominal muscles weak, soft, and flabby.

In addition, the longitudinal muscles of the abdomen may separate (diastasis recti) during pregnancy (Figure 17-5). The separation may be minimal or severe. The mother can determine the amount of separation by placing the fingertips at the umbilicus and raising the head and shoulders while in a supine position. She may benefit from gentle exercises to strengthen the abdominal wall, which usually returns to normal position by 6 weeks after birth (Scoggin, 2004; Figure 17-6).

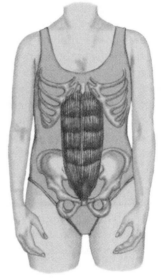 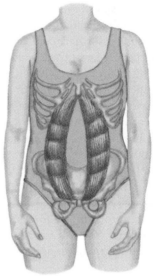

Normal location of rectus muscles of the abdomen

Diastasis recti: separation of the rectus muscles

Figure 17-5 ■ Diastasis recti occurs when the longitudinal muscles of the abdomen separate during pregnancy.

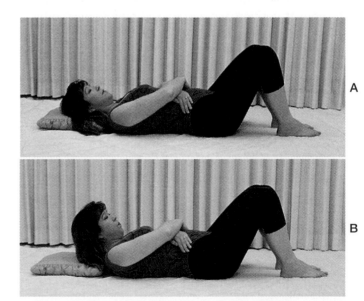

Figure 17-6 ■ Abdominal exercises for diastasis recti. **A,** The woman inhales and supports the abdominal wall firmly with her hands. **B,** Exhaling, the woman raises her head as she pulls the abdominal muscles together.

INTEGUMENTARY SYSTEM

Many skin changes that occur during pregnancy are caused by an increase in hormones. When the hormone levels decline after childbirth, the skin gradually reverts to the prepregnancy state. For example, levels of estrogen, progesterone, and melanocyte-stimulating hormone, which caused hyperpigmentation during pregnancy, decrease rapidly after childbirth, and pigmentation begins to recede. This change is particularly noticeable when the "mask of pregnancy" (melasma or chloasma) and linea nigra fade and disappear for most women. In addition, spider nevi and palmar erythema, which may develop during pregnancy as a result of increased estrogen levels, gradually disappear.

Striae gravidarum (stretch marks), which develop during pregnancy when connective tissues in the abdomen and breasts are stretched, gradually fade to silvery lines but do not disappear. Increased loss of hair may especially concern the woman. This is a normal response to the hormonal changes that caused decreased hair loss during pregnancy. Hair loss peaks at 3 to 4 months after birth but regrowth generally occurs by 9 months after birth (Rapini & Jordan, 2004).

NEUROLOGIC SYSTEM

Anesthesia or analgesia may produce temporary neurologic changes such as lack of feeling in the legs and dizziness. During this time, prevention of injury from falling is a priority.

Complaints of headache require careful assessment. Frontal headaches are not unusual in the first week postpartum (Blackburn, 2003). Severe headaches are not common, but may be postpuncture headaches resulting from regional anesthesia. They may be most severe when the woman is in an upright position and are relieved by a supine position. They should be reported to the appropriate health care provider, usually an anesthesiologist. Headache, along with blurred vision, photophobia, proteinuria, and abdominal pain, also may indicate development or worsening of preeclampsia (see Chapter 25).

ENDOCRINE SYSTEM

After expulsion of the placenta, a fairly rapid decline occurs in placental hormones such as estrogen, progesterone, human placental lactogen, and human chorionic gonadotropin. Adrenal hormones such as aldosterone return to prepregnancy levels. If the mother is not breastfeeding, the pituitary hormone prolactin, which stimulates milk secretion, returns to nonpregnant levels in about 2 weeks.

Resumption of Ovulation and Menstruation

The average time for nonnursing mothers to resume menstruation is within 7 to 9 weeks after childbirth, although this varies widely (Blackburn, 2003). Menstruation that takes place in the first 6 weeks occurs without ovulation (Resnik, 2004). The first few cycles for both lactating women and nonlactating women are often anovulatory, but ovulation may occur before the first menses. Therefore contraceptive measures are important considerations when sexual relations are resumed for both lactating and nonlactating women.

Breastfeeding delays the return of both ovulation and menstruation. Menses while lactating may resume as early as 12 weeks or as late as 18 months (Scoggin, 2004). The length of the delay depends on several factors including the frequency of breastfeeding, use of supplements, and duration of lactation. Generally, women who breastfeed more often and use fewer supplements are likely to ovulate and menstruate later than women who breastfeed less often, use more supplements, and wean earlier (Kennedy, 2005). Women who breastfeed for less than 28 days ovulate at approximately the same time as nonnursing mothers (Resnik, 2004). For the woman who is breastfeeding frequently and without supplements, contraception should be used by the time the infant is 6 months old or earlier because ovulation and menses are increasingly likely by that time.

Lactation

During pregnancy, estrogen and progesterone prepare the breasts for lactation. Although prolactin also rises during pregnancy, lactation is inhibited at this time by the high levels of estrogen and progesterone. After expulsion of the placenta, estrogen and progesterone decline rapidly, and prolactin initiates milk production within 2 to 3 days after childbirth. Once milk production is established, it continues because of frequent removal of milk from the breast. That is, the more the infant nurses, the more milk the mother produces.

Oxytocin is necessary for milk ejection or "let-down." This hormone, which is secreted by the posterior pituitary gland, causes milk to be expressed from the alveoli into the lactiferous ducts during suckling (see Chapter 22).

Weight Loss

Approximately 4.5 to 5.5 kg (10 to 12 lb) are lost during childbirth. This includes the weight of the fetus, placenta, and amniotic fluid and blood lost during the birth. An additional 2.3 to 3.6 kg (5 to 8 lb) are lost as a result of diuresis in the early postpartum days and as the reproductive organs undergo the process of involution (Scoggin, 2004).

Adipose (fatty) tissue that was gained during pregnancy to meet the energy requirements of labor and breastfeeding is not lost initially, and the usual rate of loss is slow. Most women approach their prepregnancy weight about 6 months after childbirth, but it may be a year before almost all weight is lost. Many mothers are frustrated during this time because they desire an immediate return to prepregnancy weight. Nurses can provide information about diet and exercise that will produce an acceptable weight loss without depleting the mother's energy or impairing her health.

CHECK YOUR READING

5. Why is the mother at risk for urinary retention? Which two complications may result?
6. Why does hyperpigmentation decrease after childbirth?
7. How does breastfeeding affect the resumption of ovulation and menstruation?
8. Should the nurse be concerned if a woman who delivered a baby yesterday has a WBC count of 16,000? Why or why not?
9. When should a woman who is formula feeding her infant expect her menses to resume? The woman who is breastfeeding?
10. How much weight will the woman lose during childbirth? How much can she expect to lose by 6 weeks after childbirth?

POSTPARTUM ASSESSMENTS

Providing essential, cost-effective postpartum care to new families is a challenge for maternity nurses. Legislation allows women and their health care providers to determine the length of stay and provides for insurance payments for covered care. This allows most women to stay in the birth facility for 48 hours after an uncomplicated vaginal birth and 96 hours after a cesarean birth. Some women, however, choose to go home at an earlier time.

Although the length of stay is short, the family's need for care and information remains the same. This need causes nurses a great deal of concern for families who are discharged without adequate preparation or support. Nurses are actively involved in developing ways to provide continuing care in the home. They use measures such as clinical pathways to structure assessments, care, and teaching during the birth facility stay.

Clinical Pathways

Many institutions use clinical pathways (also called *critical pathways, care maps, care paths,* or *multidisciplinary action plans*) to guide necessary care while reducing the length of stay. Clinical pathways identify expected outcomes and establish time frames for specific assessments and interventions that prepare the mother and infant for discharge. The clinical pathway is a guideline and documentation tool (Figure 17-7).

Initial Assessments

Caring for postpartum clients exposes the nurse to the risk of coming into contact with body fluids such as colostrum, breast milk, amniotic fluid, and lochia from the mother as well as urine, stool, and blood from the infant. Therefore the recommendations of the Centers for Disease Control and Prevention (CDC) for standard blood and body fluid precautions must be maintained diligently.

Postpartum assessments begin during the fourth stage of labor (the first 1 to 2 hours after childbirth). The mother is examined to determine whether she is physically stable. Initial assessments include the following:

- Vital signs
- Skin color
- Location and firmness of the fundus
- Amount and color of lochia
- Perineum (edema, episiotomy, lacerations, hematoma)
- Presence and location of pain
- Intravenous (IV) infusions: type of fluid, rate, added medications (type and amount), patency of the IV line, and redness, pain, or edema of the site
- Urinary output: time and amount of last void or catheterization, presence of a catheter, color and character of urine
- Status of abdominal incision and dressing, if present
- Level of feeling and ability to move if regional anesthesia was administered

Chart Review

When the initial assessments confirm that the mother's physical condition is stable, nurses should review the chart to obtain pertinent information and determine if there are factors that increase the risk of complications during the postpartum period. Relevant information includes the following:

- Gravida, parity
- Time and type of delivery (use of vacuum extractor, forceps)
- Presence and degree of episiotomy or lacerations
- Anesthesia or medications administered during labor
- Significant medical and surgical history, such as diabetes, hypertension, heart disease
- Medications given during labor or delivery or routinely taken and the reasons for their use
- Food and drug allergies
- Chosen method of infant feeding
- Condition of the baby

Laboratory data also are examined. Of particular interest are the prenatal hemoglobin and hematocrit values, blood type and Rh factor, hepatitis B surface antigen, rubella immune status, syphilis screen, and group B streptococcus status (see Chapter 26).

NEED FOR RH$_o$(D) IMMUNE GLOBULIN

Prenatal and neonatal records are checked to determine whether Rh$_o$(D) immune globulin (RhoGAM) should be administered. Rh$_o$(D) immune globulin may be necessary if the mother is Rh-negative, the newborn is Rh-positive, and the mother is not already sensitized. Rh$_o$(D) immune globulin should be administered within 72 hours after childbirth to prevent the development of maternal antibodies that would affect subsequent pregnancies (see Chapter 25 for Rh incompatibility and Rh$_o$[D] immune globulin drug guide).

NEED FOR RUBELLA VACCINE

A prenatal rubella antibody screen is performed on each pregnant woman to determine whether she is immune to rubella. If she is not immune, rubella vaccine is recommended after

Text continued on p. 406

Date:

CARE PATH FOR POSTPARTUM VAGINAL DELIVERY

Problem Number	LOCATION	2 TO 8 HR p̄ DELIVERY	8 TO 16 HR p̄ DELIVERY	16 TO 24 HR p̄ DELIVERY

I 5
II 7,8
IV 16
	Assessments	q̄ 4 hr:
		  TPR, BP
		  PP check (fundus–location & tone; lochia–amount, color, odor, clots)
		  Bladder status
		q̄ shift
		Perineum–epis, ± hematoma, ± edema
		Homan's sign, redness, swelling, tenderness of calf
		Lungs, breasts
		Bowel sounds, abd distention
		If tubal, incision site
		Bladder checks × 3:
		
		time _____, _____
		
		amount of void _____, _____
		
		fundus @ _____, _____
		
		bladder _____, _____
		(NP–nonpalpable; P–palpable)
			q̄ 4 hr:
			  TPR, BP
			  PP check
			  Bladder status
			
			q̄ shift
			Perineum–epis, ± hematoma, ± edema
			Homan's sign, redness, swelling, tenderness of calf
			Lungs, breasts
			Bowel sounds, abd distention
			If tubal, incision site
			
			time _____, _____
			
			amount of void _____, _____
			
			fundus @ _____, _____
			
			bladder _____, _____
			(NP–nonpalpable; P–palpable)
				q̄ 4 hr:
				  TPR, BP
				  PP check
				  Bladder status
				
				q̄ shift
				Perineum–epis, ± hematoma, ± edema
				Homan's sign, redness, swelling, tenderness of calf
				Lungs, breasts
				Bowel sounds, abd distention
				± BM
				If tubal, incision site

		Fundus firm @ U or lower **Lochia min to mod s̄ clots, odor** **Bladder nonpalpable p̄ void × 3** **Perineum intact s̄ hematoma** verified _____	**Fundus firm @ U or lower** **Bladder nonpalpable p̄ void** **Perineum intact s̄ hematoma** verified _____	**Fundus firm @ U or lower** **Bladder nonpalpable p̄ void** **Perineum intact s̄ hematoma** verified _____
	Procedures/ Tests	HCT the AM p̄ delivery	HCT the AM p̄ delivery result _____	
I 5,7,21	Treatments	Ice to perineum Fundal massage prn to maintain uterine tone Pericare q̄ void Performs self peri care Assist c̄ breastfeeding	Ice to perineum Fundal massage prn to maintain uterine tone Pericare q̄ void Assist c̄ breastfeeding	Sitz bath prn Fundal massage prn to maintain uterine tone Pericare q̄ void Assist c̄ breastfeeding
VI 3 XI 5	Activity	**Up c̄ assistance × 1 then ad lib** verified _____	**Ad lib** verified _____	**Ad lib** verified _____
	Signatures	_____/_____ _____/_____ _____/_____ _____/_____ _____/_____	_____/_____ _____/_____ _____/_____ _____/_____ _____/_____	_____/_____ _____/_____ _____/_____ _____/_____ _____/_____

MED REC NO. _____

PATIENT _____

PHYSICIAN _____

BILLING NO. _____

BAYLOR UNIVERSITY MEDICAL CENTER

DALLAS, TEXAS

CARE PATH FOR POSTPARTUM VAGINAL DELIVERY

PAGE 1 OF 4

Figure 17-7 ■ Clinical pathway for uncomplicated vaginal birth. (Copyright © and courtesy of Baylor University Medical Center, Dallas, Texas.)

Date: _____

CARE PATH FOR POSTPARTUM VAGINAL DELIVERY

Problem Number	LOCATION	2 TO 8 HR p̄ DELIVERY	8 TO 16 HR p̄ DELIVERY	16 TO 24 HR p̄ DELIVERY

VI 3
III 1
	Meds/IV's	Analgesics: For _____ pain
		  Pain level ____ on pain scale
		  ____ Lortab 1-2
		  q̄ 3-4 hr prn Time ____
		                 Time ____
		  ____ Darvocet N 100
		  1-2 po q̄ 4-6 hr prn
		  Time ____ Time ____
		  ____ Tylenol __ Tabs Time ____
		Local anesthetics
		  ____ Epifoam tid prn
		  ____ Proctofoam tid prn
		Stool softener
		  ____ Doxidan 1 hs prn
		  ____ Senokot 1 hs prn
		  ____ Dulcolax supp. 1 pr prn
			Analgesics: For _____ pain
			  Pain level ____ on pain scale
			  ____ Lortab 1-2
			  q̄ 3-4 hr prn Time ____
			                 Time ____
			  ____ Darvocet N 100
			  1-2 po q̄ 4-6 hr prn
			  Time ____ Time ____
			  ____ Tylenol __ Tabs Time ____
			Local anesthetics
			  ____ Epifoam tid prn
			  ____ Proctofoam tid prn
			Stool softener
			  ____ Doxidan 1 hs prn
			  ____ Senokot 1 hs prn
			  ____ Dulcolax supp. 1 pr prn
				Analgesics: For _____ pain
				  Pain level ____ on pain scale
				  ____ Lortab 1-2
				  q̄ 3-4 hr prn Time ____
				                 Time ____
				  ____ Darvocet N 100
				  1-2 po q̄ 4-6 hr prn
				  Time ____ Time ____
				  ____ Tylenol __ Tabs Time ____
				Local anesthetics
				  ____ Epifoam tid prn
				  ____ Proctofoam tid prn
				Stool softener
				  ____ Doxidan 1 hs prn
				  ____ Senokot 1 hs prn
				  ____ Dulcolax supp. 1 pr prn
				Rhogam ____ given ____
				na verified ____

		Comfort maintained @ ≤ 2 on pain scale verified _____	**Comfort maintained @ ≤ 2 on pain scale** verified _____	**Comfort maintained @ ≤ 2 on pain scale** verified _____
	Nutrition	General diet	General diet	General diet
		Tolerates verified _____	**Tolerates** verified _____	**Tolerates** verified _____

VI 2
I 4
	PT/Family Education	Assess current knowledge; teach/reinforce:
		  Postpartum routine
		  Safety (assistance c̄ 1st time out
		    of bed, infant security)
		  Bladder checks
		  Postpartum checks
		  Fundal massage
		  Breast feeding
		  Pain control/comfort measures
		  Pericare
			Assess current knowledge; teach/reinforce:
			All previous teaching +:
			  Breasts/nipple care
			  Nutrition
			  Elimination
			  Uterine regression
			  Lochia changes
				Assess current knowledge; teach/reinforce:
				All previous teaching +:
				  Kegel exercises
				  S&S of illness/complications
				  Activity/exercise
				  Contraception
				  Nothing in vagina
				  FU MD visit
				  Take home meds

		Demonstrates/verbalizes understanding verified _____	**Demonstrates/verbalizes understanding** verified _____	**Demonstrates/verbalizes understanding** verified _____
	Discharge Planning	**Baseline educational needs identified by pt & nurse** verified _____	Discuss homecare needs	Provide c̄ written discharge instructions
		Initiate SW consult if inidicated _____	Pastoral care visit	
VIII 2,7	Psycho-Social Emotional Spiritual	**Parents will demonstrate + interactions c̄ infant (hold, establish eye contact)** verified _____ **Identifies support person/system** verified _____	**Parents will demonstrate + interactions c̄ infant (hold, establish eye contact)** verified _____	**Parents will demonstrate + interactions c̄ infant (hold, establish eye contact)** verified _____
	Signatures	_____ / _____ _____ / _____	_____ / _____ _____ / _____	_____ / _____ _____ / _____

MED REC NO. _____

PATIENT _____

PHYSICIAN _____

BILLING NO. _____

BAYLOR UNIVERSITY MEDICAL CENTER

DALLAS, TEXAS

CARE PATH FOR POSTPARTUM VAGINAL DELIVERY

PAGE 2 OF 4

Figure 17-7, cont'd ■ For legend see opposite page.

Date: _____

CARE PATH FOR POSTPARTUM VAGINAL DELIVERY

Problem Number	LOCATION	24 TO 32 HR p̄ DELIVERY	32 TO 40 HR p̄ DELIVERY	40 TO 48 HR p̄ DELIVERY	DC CRITERIA
I 5 II 7,8 IV 16	Assessments	q̄ 8 hr: TPR, BP PP check Bladder status q̄ shift Perineum–epis, ± hematoma, ± edema Homan's sign, redness, swelling, tenderness of calf Lungs Breasts Bowel sounds, abd distention ± BM If tubal, incision site	q̄ 8 hr: TPR, BP PP check Bbladder status q̄ shift Perineum–epis, ± hematoma, ± edema Homan's sign, redness, swelling, tenderness of calf Lungs Breasts Bowel sounds, abd distention ± BM If tubal, incision site	q̄ 8 hr: TPR, BP PP check Bladder status q̄ shift Perineum–epis, ± hematoma, ± edema Homan's sign, redness, swelling, tenderness of calf Lungs Breasts Bowel sounds, abd distention ± BM If tubal, incision site	VSS, Temp ≤ 100.4 **Verified** _____ Fundus firm, at U or lower **Verified** _____ Lochia minimal to moderate s̄ clots **Verified** _____ Emptying bladder s̄ difficulty + Bowel sounds + Flatus **Verified** _____
		Fundus firm @ U or lower Bladder nondistend p̄ void Perineum intact s̄ hematoma verified _____	**Fundus firm @ U or lower Bladder nondistend p̄ void Perineum intact s̄ hematoma** verified _____	**Fundus firm @ U or lower Bladder nondistend p̄ void Perineum intact s̄ hematoma** verified _____	
	Procedures/ Tests				
I 5,7,21	Treatments	Sitz bath prn Fundal massage prn to maintain uterine tone Pericare q̄ void Assist c̄ breastfeeding	Sitz bath prn Fundal massage prn to maintain uterine tone Pericare q̄ void Assist c̄ breastfeeding	Sitz bath prn Fundal massage prn to maintain uterine tone Pericare q̄ void Assist c̄ breastfeeding	
IV 2	Activity	**Ad lib** verified _____	**Ad lib** verified _____	**Ad lib** verified _____	**Able to perform self & infant care** verified _____
	Signatures	_____/_____ _____/_____ _____/_____ _____/_____	_____/_____ _____/_____ _____/_____ _____/_____	_____/_____ _____/_____ _____/_____ _____/_____	_____/_____ _____/_____ _____/_____ _____/_____

MED REC NO. _____

PATIENT _____

PHYSICIAN _____

BILLING NO. _____

BAYLOR UNIVERSITY MEDICAL CENTER

DALLAS, TEXAS

CARE PATH FOR POSTPARTUM VAGINAL DELIVERY

PAGE 3 OF 4

Figure 17-7, cont'd ■ Clinical pathway for uncomplicated vaginal birth.

Date: _____

CARE PATH FOR POSTPARTUM VAGINAL DELIVERY

Problem Number	LOCATION	24 TO 32 HR p̄ DELIVERY	32 TO 40 HR p̄ DELIVERY	40 TO 48 HR p̄ DELIVERY	DC CRITERIA
VI 3 III 1	Meds/IV's	Analgesics: For _____ pain Pain level ___ on pain scale _____ Lortab 1-2 q̄ 3-4 hr prn Time ____ Time ____ _____ Darvocet N 100 1-2 po q̄ 4-6 hr prn Time ____ Time ____ __ Tylenol __ Tabs Time __ Local anesthetics _____ Epifoam tid prn _____ Proctofoam tid prn Stool softener _____ Doxidan 1 hs prn _____ Senokot 1 hs prn _____ Dulcolax supp. 1 pr prn	Analgesics: For _____ pain Pain level ___ on pain scale _____ Lortab 1-2 q̄ 3-4 hr prn Time ____ Time ____ _____ Darvocet N 100 1-2 po q̄ 4-6 hr prn Time ____ Time ____ __ Tylenol __ Tabs Time __ Local anesthetics _____ Epifoam tid prn _____ Proctofoam tid prn Stool softener _____ Doxidan 1 hs prn _____ Senokot 1 hs prn _____ Dulcolax supp. 1 pr prn	Analgesics: For _____ pain Pain level ___ on pain scale _____ Lortab 1-2 q̄ 3-4 hr prn Time ____ Time ____ _____ Darvocet N 100 1-2 po q̄ 4-6 hr prn Time ____ Time ____ __ Tylenol __ Tabs Time __ Local anesthetics _____ Epifoam tid prn _____ Proctofoam tid prn Stool softener _____ Doxidan 1 hs prn _____ Senokot 1 hs prn _____ Dulcolax supp. 1 pr prn Rubella____given ____na **verified** _____	
		Comfort maintained @ ≤2 on pain scale verified _____	**Comfort maintained @ ≤2 on pain scale** verified _____	**Comfort maintained @ ≤2 on pain scale** verified _____	
	Nutrition	General diet	General diet	General diet	Tolerates general diet
		Tolerates verified _____	**Tolerates** verified _____	**Tolerates** verified _____	

VI 2
I 4
	PT/Family Education	Assess current knowledge; teach/reinforce:
		All previous teaching +:
		  Kegel exercises
		  S&S of illness/
		    complications
		  Activity/exercise
		  Contraception
		  Nothing in vagina
		  FU MD visit
		  Take home meds
			Assess current knowledge; teach/reinforce:
			All previous teaching +:
			  Kegel exercises
			  S&S of illness/
			    complications
			  Activity/exercise
			  Contraception
			  Nothing in vagina
			  FU MD visit
			  Take home meds
				Assess current knowledge; teach/reinforce:
				All previous teaching +:
				  Kegel exercises
				  S&S of illness/
				    complications
				  Activity/exercise
				  Contraception
				  Nothing in vagina
				  FU MD visit
				  Take home meds
					Verbalizes/demonstrates knowledge of self care:
					  Breast/nipple care
					  Breastfeeding
					  Activity/exercise
					  Elimination
					  Diet
					  S&S of comps

		Demonstrates/verbalizes understanding verified _____	**Demonstrates/verbalizes understanding** verified _____	**Demonstrates/verbalizes understanding** verified _____	**Verbalizes/demonstrates knowledge of Infant care—see infant discharge teaching.** verified _____
	Discharge Planning	Provide c̄ written discharge instructions	Provide c̄ written discharge instructions	Provide c̄ written discharge instructions	Expresses confidence in ability to care for self & infant. Identifies FU appt date. **verified** _____
VIII 2,7	Psycho-Social Emotional Spiritual	**Parents will demonstrate + interactions c̄ infant (hold, establish eye contact)** verified _____	**Parents will demonstrate + interactions c̄ infant (hold, establish eye contact)** verified _____	**Parents will demonstrate + interactions c̄ infant (hold, establish eye contact)** verified _____	**Identifies at least 1 person or service to assist with self and infant care at home** verified _____
	Signatures	_____ / _____ _____ / _____	_____ / _____ _____ / _____	_____ / _____ _____ / _____	_____ / _____ _____ / _____

MED REC NO. _____

PATIENT _____

PHYSICIAN _____

BILLING NO. _____

BAYLOR UNIVERSITY MEDICAL CENTER

DALLAS, TEXAS

CARE PATH FOR POSTPARTUM VAGINAL DELIVERY

PAGE 4 OF 4

Figure 17-7, cont'd ■ For legend see opposite page.

DRUG GUIDE

RUBELLA VACCINE

Classification: Attenuated live virus vaccine.

Action: Vaccination produces a modified rubella (German measles) infection that is not communicable, causing the formation of antibodies against rubella virus.

Indications: The vaccine is administered after childbirth or abortion to women whose antibody screen shows they are not immune to rubella. This prevents rubella infection and possible severe congenital defects in the fetus during a subsequent pregnancy.

Dosage and Route: The entire reconstituted volume of a single-dose vial or 0.5 ml from a multiple dose vial. Inject subcutaneously in the upper outer aspect of the upper arm.

Absorption: Well absorbed.

Contraindications and Precautions: The vaccine is contraindicated in women who have a respiratory or febrile infection, active untreated tuberculosis, or conditions that affect the bone marrow or lymphatic systems or are immunosuppressed, pregnant, or sensitive to neomycin or

eggs. The attenuated virus may appear in breast milk and some infants develop a rash, but this is not a contraindication to vaccination of lactating women. It should be deferred for 3 months in clients receiving immune globulin or blood transfusions. Although it can be given after $Rh_o(D)$ immune globulin, women receiving the vaccine should be tested for immune status at 6-8 wk to be sure they are immune (Centers for Disease Control and Prevention, 2003).

Adverse Reactions: Transient stinging at site, fever, lymphadenopathy, arthralgia, and transient arthritis are the most common adverse reactions.

Nursing Implications: Previously, the woman and her partner were warned to avoid pregnancy for at least 3 months after vaccination because of the possibility that a fetus might be affected by the live virus in the vaccine. The CDC has changed this time period to 4 weeks. Signed informed consent is usually required.

Vials should be refrigerated. Reconstitute only with diluent supplied with the vial. Use immediately after reconstitution and discard if not used within 8 hours. Protect from light. Do not give at the same time as immune globulin.

---

childbirth to prevent her from acquiring rubella during subsequent pregnancies, when it can cause serious fetal anomalies. Although defects in infants born to mothers who received rubella vaccine during pregnancy have not been reported, the vaccine is a live virus and there is a theoretic risk of fetal defects if the mother becomes pregnant soon after it is administered.

In the past the mother and her partner were warned to avoid pregnancy for at least 3 months after vaccination because of the possibility that a fetus might be affected by the live virus in the vaccine. This time period was shortened to 28 days by the CDC (2003).

Before administration, some agencies require that the mother give written permission to receive the vaccine. Some agencies require that she sign a statement indicating she understands the risks of becoming pregnant again too soon after the injection. If a written statement from the mother is not required, the nurse should document in the chart that the risk has been explained and that the parents have verbalized their understanding (see Drug Guide).

RISK FACTORS FOR HEMORRHAGE AND INFECTION

Nurses must be aware of conditions that increase the risk of hemorrhage and infection, the two most common complications of the puerperium.

Focused Assessments after Vaginal Birth

Nurses perform postpartum assessments according to facility protocol. One example is as follows:
- First hour: every 15 minutes
- Second hour: every 30 minutes
- First 24 hours: every 4 hours
- After 24 hours: every 8 hours (Scoggin, 2004)

Although assessments vary depending on the particular problems presented by the mother, a focused assessment for a vaginal delivery generally includes the vital signs, fundus, lochia, perineum, bladder elimination, breasts, and lower extremities. The assessment for women whose infants were born vaginally differs from that performed for postcesarean mothers (see p. 415).

CRITICAL TO REMEMBER

Postpartum Risk Factors

Hemorrhage
Grand multiparity (five or more)
Overdistention of the uterus (large baby, twins, hydramnios)
Precipitous labor (less than 3 hours)
Prolonged labor
Retained placenta
Placenta previa or abruptio placentae
Induction or augmentation of labor
Administration of tocolytics to stop uterine contractions
Operative procedures (vacuum extraction, forceps, cesarean birth)

Infection
Operative procedures (cesarean birth, vacuum extraction, forceps)
Multiple cervical examinations
Prolonged labor (more than 24 hours)
Prolonged rupture of membranes
Manual extraction of placenta
Diabetes
Catheterization
Anemia (hemoglobin less than 10.5 mg/dl)

VITAL SIGNS

BLOOD PRESSURE. Blood pressure varies with position, and to obtain accurate results it should be measured with the mother in the same position each time. Therefore nurses must document both the mother's position when blood pressure is taken and the pressure obtained. Postpartum blood pressure should be compared with that of the predelivery period so that deviations from what is normal for the mother can be quickly identified. An increase from the baseline suggests preeclampsia. A decrease may indicate dehydration or hypovolemia resulting from excessive bleeding.

ORTHOSTATIC HYPOTENSION. After birth a rapid decrease in intraabdominal pressure results in dilation of blood vessels supplying the viscera. The resulting engorgement of abdominal blood vessels contributes to a rapid fall in blood pressure of 15 to 20 mm Hg when the woman moves from a recumbent to a sitting position. As a result of the sudden drop in blood pressure, mothers feel dizzy or light-headed and may faint when they stand. The nursing diagnosis "Risk for Injury" applies to women with orthostatic hypotension (Nursing Care Plan 17-1).

Hypotension may also indicate hypovolemia. Careful assessments for hemorrhage (location and firmness of the

---

NURSING CARE PLAN 17-1 Postpartum Hypotension, Fatigue, and Pain

ASSESSMENT: Lani Tilden, gravida II, para II, gave birth to a baby girl weighing 3400 g (7.5 lb) 4 hours ago. She became weak and dizzy and said, "Everything is going black" when she attempted to ambulate the first time. Her gait was unsteady, and the nurse had to lower her back to bed to prevent her from fainting. Her color was pale, and her pulse was rapid.

NURSING DIAGNOSIS: Risk for Injury related to physiologic effects of orthostatic hypotension

CRITICAL THINKING: Does the nurse have enough data to make this diagnosis? If not, what other data are necessary? Why?

ANSWER: Although dizziness and feeling faint may indicate orthostatic hypotension, they may also indicate hypovolemia. The nurse must also assess Lani for signs of excessive blood loss, such as evidenced by the location and firmness of the uterine fundus, the amount of lochia, the pulse rate at rest, and hemoglobin and hematocrit levels. If these data are within expected levels, a diagnosis of "Risk for Injury related to the effects of orthostatic hypotension" is appropriate.

GOALS/EXPECTED OUTCOME: Lani will remain free of injury caused by fainting and falling during the postpartum period.

INTERVENTION	RATIONALE
1. Obtain the assistance of another staff person each time ambulation is attempted until Lani is able to ambulate without dizziness or feeling faint.	1. A second person is necessary to help prevent injury to the client and the staff if Lani should start to fall.
2. Check Lani's blood pressure using the same arm while she is in a supine position and in a sitting position before getting her out of bed again. Use the same arm each time the blood pressure is taken.	2. A decrease of 20 mm Hg in systolic pressure in the upright position indicates orthostatic hypotension. Measuring from the same arm provides more accurate information because the reading may differ slightly in each arm.
3. Elevate the head of the bed for a few minutes before Lani attempts to stand. Help her to sit on the edge of the bed for several minutes before standing, and help her to stand slowly.	3. Sitting and standing slowly allows time for the blood pressure to stabilize before she is fully upright, thus maintaining circulation to the brain.
4. Instruct Lani to move her feet constantly when she first stands.	4. Moving the feet increases venous return from the lower extremities to maintain cardiac output and increase cerebral circulation.
5. Suggest that she take brief, tepid (not hot) showers and that she bend her knees and "march" during the shower. Provide a chair for her to use while in the shower.	5. Hot water dilates peripheral blood vessels, allowing additional blood to remain in the vessels of the legs. Moving the feet and legs increases blood return from the legs and increases blood to the brain. Sitting takes less energy if she is feeling weak.
6. Initiate measures to prevent injuries that could be sustained if she fainted: a. Stay with Lani when she ambulates, and be prepared to assist her in sitting down and lowering her head or to lower her gently to the floor if she becomes faint. b. Call for additional assistance, if needed, before attempting to return her to bed. c. Remind her to call for assistance before trying to ambulate. Check to see that the call light is conveniently located.	6. Gravity increases blood flow to the brain when the head is lowered and thus prevents fainting. Adequate assistance prevents falling and possible injury during a fainting episode.

EVALUATION: Lani has participated in self-care and has sustained no injury during her hospital stay.

Continued

NURSING CARE PLAN 17-1 Postpartum Hypotension, Fatigue, and Pain—cont'd

ASSESSMENT: On the second day after delivery Lani demonstrates skill in breastfeeding but wonders how she will be able to care for her baby girl and her 18-month-old boy when she gets home. She states that he "is busy every minute." She has a third-degree episiotomy and asks what can be done to prevent the pain she experienced during intercourse for several months after the last child was born.

NURSING DIAGNOSIS: Anxiety related to anticipated fatigue and discomfort

> **CRITICAL THINKING:** *What assumption is the nurse making? How might the nurse validate the assumption? Can you identify another diagnosis that is more specific?*
>
> **ANSWER:** *The nurse assumes the client is anxious. Neither signs nor symptoms of anxiety are part of the assessment data. The nurse can validate the assumption by asking Lani if she is anxious. "Anxiety" is a very broad diagnostic category. Based on data available, a more specific and therefore more helpful nursing diagnosis might be "Risk for Ineffective Sexuality Patterns related to fatigue and pain."*

GOALS/EXPECTED OUTCOMES: The couple will:
1. Verbalize measures to promote comfort during sexual activity by discharge.
2. Verbalize a plan to reduce fatigue, which interferes with interest in and energy for sexual activity, by discharge.

INTERVENTION	RATIONALE
1. Recommend that the parents postpone vaginal intercourse until the perineum is well healed, usually about 3 weeks. Suggest that the mother continue perineal care, sitz baths, and the use of topical agents until the perineum is healed.	1. These measures promote rapid healing and reduce pain or fear of pain when sexual activity is resumed.
2. Suggest that Lani breastfeed the infant shortly before the parents initiate sexual activity.	2. Breastfeeding reduces the chance of leaking milk, which interferes with sexual pleasure for some couples. Feeding the infant may also allow uninterrupted time while the infant sleeps.
3. Suggest the use of a water-soluble vaginal lubricant (K-Y Jelly, Lubrin, Replens) if the mother is planning to breastfeed for longer than 6 weeks.	3. Breastfeeding delays the resumption of ovarian hormones, including estrogen, which may result in vaginal dryness that is most noticeable after 6 weeks of breastfeeding.
4. Prior to vaginal intercourse, as part of foreplay, suggest that one finger be inserted into the vaginal introitus to determine areas of tenderness or pain.	4. Locating areas of discomfort and stretching the perineal scar gently help increase comfort.
5. Suggest that the woman assume the superior position during intercourse.	5. In the superior position, the woman controls the depth and location of penetration and can reduce her discomfort.
6. Explain that sexual arousal may be slower because of decreased hormones and fatigue. More stimulation may be required before the mother is sexually aroused.	6. Knowledge of the physiologic changes reduces the anxiety and tension that occur if the parents are unprepared for them.
7. Remind the mother to perform Kegel exercises until she can comfortably do 30 contraction-relaxation cycles each day.	7. Kegel exercises strengthen the muscles around the vagina and promote increased sexual satisfaction.

8. Suggest measures that may lessen fatigue:
  a. Recommend a 30-minute nap for each partner during the day or evening.
  b. Suggest that sexual activity be resumed in the morning or afternoon rather than at the end of a tiring day.
  c. Suggest that parents rest when the infant sleeps and that they postpone major home projects that will increase fatigue until the infant is sleeping through the night.
	8. Fatigue is a major cause of decreased interest in sexual activity after childbirth for both mothers and fathers.

9. Discuss the need for frank communication between partners about measures that reduce discomfort as well as specific concerns and needs.	9. Communication facilitates understanding and fosters a feeling of closeness that can enhance sexual interest.

EVALUATION: The parents express interest in trying various measures to reduce fatigue and discomfort. They verbalize a plan to use the instructions provided.

fundus, amount of lochia, pulse rate for tachycardia) should be made if the postpartum blood pressure is significantly less than the prenatal baseline blood pressure.

PULSE. Bradycardia, defined as a pulse rate of 50 to 60 bpm, may occur; the average range is 60 to 90 bpm. The lower pulse rate reflects the large amount of blood that returns to the central circulation after delivery of the placenta. The increase in central circulation results in increased stroke volume and allows a slower heart rate to provide adequate maternal circulation.

Tachycardia may indicate excitement, pain, fatigue, dehydration, hypovolemia, anemia, pain, or infection. If tachycardia is noted, additional assessments should include blood pressure, location and firmness of the uterus, amount of lochia, estimated blood loss at delivery, hemoglobin, and hematocrit values. The objective of the additional assessments is to rule out excessive bleeding and intervene at once if hemorrhage is suspected. Tachycardia is also one sign of infection.

RESPIRATIONS. A normal respiratory rate of 12 to 20 breaths per minute should be maintained. Assessing breath sounds is not necessary if the mother has had a normal vaginal delivery, is ambulatory, and is without signs of respiratory distress. Breath sounds always should be auscultated if the birth has been cesarean or if the mother is receiving magnesium sulfate (see Chapter 25), is a smoker, has a history of frequent or recent upper respiratory infections, or has a history of asthma.

TEMPERATURE. A temperature of up to 38° C (100.4° F) is common during the first 24 hours after childbirth and may be caused by dehydration or normal postpartum leukocytosis. If the elevated temperature persists for longer than 24 hours or if it exceeds 38° C (100.4° F), the nurse should suspect infection and report the fever to the physician or nurse-midwife.

PAIN. Pain, the fifth vital sign, should be assessed along with other vital signs to determine the type, location, and severity on a pain scale. Some new mothers are too excited by the birth of their child to complain of discomfort. Others don't want to "bother the nurse" or may come from cultures in which complaining is not acceptable. Nurses must remain alert to signs of afterpains, perineal discomfort, and breast tenderness. Signs of discomfort include an inability to relax or sleep, a change in vital signs, restlessness, irritability, and facial grimaces. Women should be encouraged to take prescribed medications for afterpains and perineal discomfort. The nurse should also assess the effectiveness of pain relief measures.

FUNDUS

The fundus should be assessed for consistency and location (Procedure 17-1). It should be firmly contracted and at or near the level of the umbilicus. If the uterus is above the expected level or shifted from the middle of the abdomen or midline position (usually to the right), the bladder may be distended. The location of the fundus should be rechecked after the woman has emptied her bladder.

If the fundus is difficult to locate or is soft or "boggy," the nurse stimulates the uterine muscle to contract by gently massaging the uterus. The nondominant hand must support and anchor the lower uterine segment if the massaging of an uncontracted uterus is necessary. Uterine massage is not necessary if the uterus is firmly contracted.

The uterus can contract only if it is free of intrauterine clots. To expel clots, the nurse must support the lower uterine segment to prevent inversion of the uterus (turning inside out) when the nurse applies firm pressure downward toward the vagina. This expresses clots that have collected in the uterus. Nurses should observe the perineum for the number and size of clots expelled. (Table 17-3 describes normal and abnormal findings of the uterine fundus and includes follow-up nursing actions for abnormal findings.)

Drugs sometimes are needed to maintain contraction of the uterus and thus prevent postpartum hemorrhage. The most commonly used drugs are methylergonovine (Methergine) and oxytocin (Pitocin) (Table 17-4). In addition, a drug guide for methylergonovine is presented on p. 736 and for oxytocin on p. 371.

LOCHIA

Important assessments include the amount, color, and odor of lochia. Nurses observe the amount and color of lochia on peripads and while checking the perineum. They also watch vaginal discharge while palpating or massaging the fundus to determine the amount of lochia and the number and size of any clots expressed during these procedures. Important guidelines include:

- A constant trickle or dribble of lochia indicates excessive bleeding and requires immediate attention.
- Excessive lochia in the presence of a contracted uterus suggests lacerations of the birth canal. The health care provider must be notified so that lacerations can be located and repaired.

The odor of lochia is usually described as fleshy, earthy, and musty. A foul odor suggests endometrial infection, and assessments should be made for additional signs of infection. These signs include maternal fever, tachycardia, and uterine tenderness and pain.

Absence of lochia, like the presence of a foul odor, may also indicate infection. If the birth was cesarean, lochia may be scant because the uterine cavity was wiped by sponges, removing some of the endometrial lining. Lochia should not be entirely absent, however.

PERINEUM

The acronym *REEDA* is used as a reminder that the site of an episiotomy or a perineal laceration should be assessed for five signs: redness (R), edema (E), ecchymosis (E) (bruising), discharge (D), and approximation (A) (the edges of the wound should be close, as though stuck or glued together).

Redness of the wound may indicate the usual inflammatory response to injury. If accompanied by excessive pain or tenderness, however, it may indicate the beginning of localized infection. Ecchymosis or edema indicates soft-tissue

PROCEDURE

17-1   Assessing the Uterine Fundus

PURPOSE: To determine the location and firmness of the uterus

1. Explain the procedure and rationale for each step before beginning the procedure. *Explanations reduce anxiety and elicit cooperation.*
2. Ask the mother to empty her bladder if she has not voided recently. *A distended bladder lifts and displaces the uterus.*
3. Place the mother in a supine position with her knees slightly flexed. *This relaxes the abdominal muscles and permits accurate location of the fundus.*
4. Put on clean gloves and lower the perineal pads to observe lochia as the fundus is palpated. *Gloves are recommended whenever the possibility exists of coming into contact with body fluids.*
5. Place your nondominant hand above the woman's symphysis pubis. *This supports and anchors the lower uterine segment during palpation or massage of the fundus.*

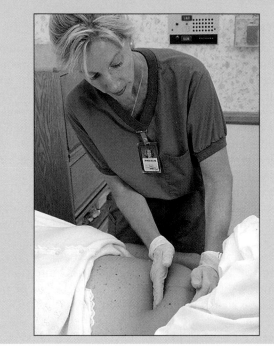

6. Use the flat part of your fingers (not the fingertips) for palpation. *The larger surface provides more comfort. Palpation may be painful, particularly for the mother who had a cesarean birth.*
7. Begin palpation at the umbilicus, and palpate gently until the fundus is located. The hand "cups" the uterus to determine firmness and location of the fundus. *The fundus should be firm, in the midline, and approximately at the level of the umbilicus. Locating the fundus is more difficult if the woman is obese or if the abdomen is distended.*
8. If the fundus is difficult to locate or is soft or "boggy," keep the nondominant hand above the woman's symphysis pubis and massage the fundus with the dominant hand until the fundus is firm. *The nondominant hand anchors the lower segment of the uterus and prevents trauma while the uterus is massaged. The uterus contracts in response to tactile stimulation, and this helps control excessive bleeding.*
9. After the boggy fundus is massaged until it is firm, press firmly to expel clots. Keep one hand pressed firmly just above the symphysis (over the lower uterine segment) during the entire time. *Removing clots allows the uterus to contract properly. Providing pressure over the lower uterine segment prevents uterine inversion.*
10. If the fundus is above or below the umbilicus, use your fingers to determine the number of fingerbreadths between the fundus and the umbilicus. *Using the fingers to measure allows an approximation of the number of centimeters.*
11. Document the consistency and location of the fundus. Consistency is recorded as "fundus firm," "firm with massage," or "boggy." Fundal height is recorded in fingerbreadths or centimeters above or below the umbilicus. For example, "fundus firm, midline, ↓ 1" (one fingerbreadth or 1 cm below the umbilicus). As another example, "fundus firm with light massage, U + 2 (two fingerbreadths or 2 cm above the umbilicus), displaced to right." *This promotes accurate communication and identifies deviations from expected so that potential problems can be identified early.*

TABLE 17-3 Observations of the Uterine Fundus Requiring Nursing Actions

Normal Findings	Abnormal Findings	Nursing Actions
Fundus firmly contracted	Fundus is soft, "boggy," uncontracted, or difficult to locate	Support the lower uterine segment. Massage until firm.
Fundus remains contracted when massage is discontinued	Fundus becomes soft and uncontracted when massage is stopped	Continue to support the lower uterine segment. Massage until firm and apply pressure to the fundus to express clots that may be accumulating in the uterus. Notify the health care provider and begin oxytocin administration, as prescribed, to maintain a firm fundus.
Fundus is located at the level of the umbilicus and midline	Fundus is above the umbilicus and/or displaced from the midline	Assess bladder elimination. Assist the mother in urinating or catheterize, if necessary, to empty the bladder. Recheck the position and consistency of the fundus after the bladder is empty.

TABLE **17–4** Commonly Used Drugs during the Postpartum Period

Indications	Usual Dosage	Nursing Considerations
Methylergonovine Maleate (Methergine)		
Prevention and treatment of hemorrhage caused by uterine atony	0.2 mg IM q2-4h for no more than five doses or 0.2 mg PO q6-8h	Monitor and record BP, P, and uterine response. Do not give if BP elevated. Report any sudden change in vital signs, continued uterine relaxation, or excessive lochia.
Oxytocin (Pitocin, Syntocinon)		
Reduction of bleeding after expulsion of the placenta	10-40 units in 1000 ml of normal saline, lactated Ringer's, or 5% dextrose water IV at a rate to control bleeding (usually 20 to 40 milliunits/minute) or 10 units IM	Administer by infusion (diluted in solution), not by bolus (a concentrated mass). Monitor and record uterine contraction, heart rate, and BP every 15 minutes. Assess and record the amount of lochia.
Simethicone (Mylicon)		
Flatulence, abdominal distention	40- to 80-mg in chewable tablet form and at bedtime	Assess for bowel activity, relief of distention.
Ibuprofen (Motrin, Advil)		
Mild to moderate pain	200-400 mg PO q4-6h	Assess for nausea, vomiting, diarrhea. Increases effects of anticoagulants.
Ketorolac (Toradol)		
Mild to moderate pain	30 mg IV or IM q6h 10 mg PO q4-6h	Assess for nausea, cramping, diarrhea. Increases effects of anticoagulants. Watch for bleeding.
Acetaminophen (Tylenol, Panadol)		
Mild to moderate pain	325-650 mg PO q4-6h	Side effects rare; assess for allergic reaction, such as skin rash.
Darvocet-N (325 or 650 mg acetaminophen and 50 or 100 mg propoxyphene)		
Mild to moderate pain	1 tablet q4h	Determine sensitivity to acetaminophen or oxycodone. Observe for signs of respiratory depression. Watch for nausea, vomiting, vertigo. Do not administer with sedatives.
Tylenol with Codeine # 3 (325 mg acetaminophen with 30 mg codeine)		
Moderate pain	Tylenol # 3, one or two tablets q3-4h	Determine sensitivity to acetaminophen or codeine. Do not administer with sedatives.
Percocet (325 mg acetaminophen and 5 mg oxycodone) **Tylox (500 mg acetaminophen and 5 mg oxycodone)**		
Moderate pain	One or two tablets PO q4h	Determine sensitivity to acetaminophen or oxycodone. Observe for signs of respiratory depression. Watch for nausea, vomiting, vertigo. Do not administer with sedatives.
Lortab (2.5, 5, or 7.5 mg hydrocodone and 500 mg acetaminophen) **Vicodin (5 mg hydrocodone and 500 mg acetaminophen)** **Vicodin ES (7.5 mg hydrocodone and 750 mg acetaminophen)**		
Moderate to moderately severe pain	One or two tablets PO q4-6h	Determine sensitivity to acetaminophen or hydrocodone. Observe for signs of respiratory depression. Watch for nausea, vomiting, vertigo. Do not administer with sedatives.
Rh$_o$(D) Immune Globulin (RhoGAM, Rhophylac, BayRho-D)		
Prevention of sensitization to Rh factor in Rh-negative mothers who gave birth to Rh-positive infants	One vial (one standard dose) IM within 72 hr after childbirth	Confirm that administration is necessary. Check with second licensed personnel that medication is cross-matched for the specific woman. Record lot number and manufacturer. Do not give with live virus vaccines.
Rubella Virus Vaccine, Live (Meruvax II)		
See drug guide, p. 406		

Data from Hodgson, B.B., & Kizior, R.J. (2005). *Saunders nursing drug handbook 2005*. Philadelphia: Saunders.
BP, Blood pressure; *IM*, intramuscularly; *IV*, intravenously; *P*, pulse; *PO*, by mouth.

Jenny Wilson, a 27-year-old gravida 4, para 4, was admitted from the labor, delivery, and recovery unit 2 hours after the birth of an 8-lb (3600-g) baby boy. An hour later her fundus is boggy, located three fingerbreadths above the umbilicus, and displaced to the right. Her perineal pads, which were changed just before transfer, are saturated.

Questions
1. What do these data suggest? Why?
2. What nursing action should be taken first? What follow-up assessments are necessary?
3. Why is it necessary to remind and assist Jenny to void?

CRITICAL TO REMEMBER

Signs of a Distended Bladder

Location of fundus above the baseline level (determined when the bladder is empty)
Fundus displaced to the side from midline
Excessive lochia
Bladder discomfort
Bulge of bladder above symphysis
Frequent voidings of less than 150 ml of urine, which may indicate urinary retention with overflow

damage that can delay healing. No discharge should come from the wound. Rapid healing necessitates that the edges of the wound be closely approximated. (Procedure 17-2 describes the perineal examination.)

BLADDER ELIMINATION

Because the mother may not experience the urge to void even if the bladder is full, nurses must rely on physical assessment to determine whether the bladder is distended. Bladder distention often produces an obvious or palpable bulge that feels like a soft, movable mass above the symphysis pubis. Other signs include an upward and lateral displacement of the uterine fundus and increased lochia. Frequent voidings of less than 150 ml suggest urinary retention with overflow. Signs of an empty bladder include a firm fundus in the midline and a nonpalpable bladder.

Two to three voidings after birth or the removal of a catheter should be measured to determine whether normal bladder function has returned. When the mother can void at least 300 to 400 ml, the bladder usually is empty. Regardless of the amount voided, however, the fundus must be assessed after the woman voids to confirm that the bladder is empty after the first few voidings. Subjective symptoms of urgency, frequency, or dysuria suggest urinary tract infection and should be reported to the health care provider.

BREASTS

For the first day or two after delivery, the breasts should be soft and nontender. After that, breast changes depend largely on whether the mother is breastfeeding or taking measures to prevent lactation. The breasts should be examined even if she chooses formula feeding because engorgement may occur despite preventive measures. The size, symmetry, and shape of the breasts should be observed. Some

PROCEDURE

17-2   Assessing the Perineum

PURPOSE: **To observe perineal trauma and the state of healing**

1. Provide privacy, and explain the purpose of the procedure. This elicits cooperation and reduces anxiety about the procedure.
2. Put on clean gloves. Implement standard precautions to provide protection from possible contact with body fluids.
3. Ask the mother to assume a Sims (side-lying) position and flex her upper leg. Lower the perineal pads and lift her superior buttock. If necessary, use a flashlight to inspect the perineal area. Position provides an unobstructed view of the perineum; light allows better visualization.
4. Note the extent and location of edema or bruising. Extensive bruising or asymmetric edema may indicate formation of a hematoma (see Chapter 28).
5. Examine the episiotomy or laceration for redness, ecchymosis, edema, discharge, and approximation ("REEDA"). Redness, edema, or discharge may indicate infection of the wound; extensive bruising may delay healing; wound edges must be in direct contact for uncomplicated healing to occur.

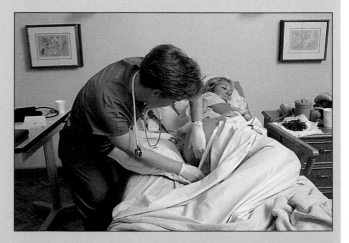

6. Note the number and size of hemorrhoids. Swollen, painful hemorrhoids interfere with activity and bowel elimination.

mothers need reassurance that breast size has no relationship to successful breastfeeding. The skin should be inspected for dimpling or thickening, which, although rare, can indicate breast tumor.

The areola and nipple should be carefully examined for potential problems such as flat or retracted nipples, which may make breastfeeding more difficult. Signs of nipple trauma (redness, blisters, or fissures) may be noted during the first days of breastfeeding, especially if the mother needs assistance in positioning the infant correctly (see Chapter 22).

The breasts should be palpated for firmness and tenderness, which indicate increased vascular and lymphatic circulation that may precede milk production. The breasts may feel "lumpy" as various lobes begin to produce milk.

The breast assessment is an excellent opportunity to provide information or reassurance about breast care and breastfeeding techniques.

LOWER EXTREMITIES

The legs are examined for varicosities and signs and symptoms of thrombophlebitis. Indications of thrombophlebitis include localized areas of redness, heat, edema, and tenderness. Pedal pulses may be obstructed by thrombophlebitis and should be palpated with each assessment (see Chapter 28).

HOMANS' SIGN

Discomfort in the calf with sharp dorsiflexion of the foot is a positive Homans' sign (Figure 17-8) and may indicate deep vein thrombosis. Absence of discomfort indicates a negative Homans' sign. A positive Homans' sign (presence of discomfort) should be reported to the health care provider. Confusion arises because a deep venous thrombosis may not produce calf pain with dorsiflexion. In addition, women may report pain that is caused by strained muscles from positioning and pushing during delivery.

EDEMA AND DEEP TENDON REFLEXES

Pedal or pretibial edema may be present for the first day or two, until excess interstitial fluid is remobilized and excreted. (Figure 17-9 shows how to assess for pitting edema.) Diuresis is highest between the second and fifth days after birth and should be complete by 21 days (Blackburn, 2003).

Deep tendon reflexes should be 1+ to 2+. Report brisker-than-average and hyperactive reflexes (3+ to 4+), which suggest preeclampsia (see p. 640 for a description of assessing deep tendon reflexes).

✔ CHECK YOUR READING

11. What additional assessments are necessary when tachycardia is noted? Why?
12. What causes orthostatic hypotension? What are the typical onset and signs and symptoms of orthostatic hypotension?
13. When is uterine massage necessary? How is the uterus supported during massage?
14. What does excessive bleeding suggest when the uterus is firmly contracted?

CARE IN THE IMMEDIATE POSTPARTUM PERIOD

The postpartum period often is divided into three periods. The first 24 hours is the immediate postpartum period, the first week is the early postpartum period, and the second to the sixth week is the late period. Care of the mother during the immediate postpartum period focuses on maintaining physiologic safety of the mother through frequent assessments (discussed previously), providing comfort measures, establishing bladder elimination, and providing health education.

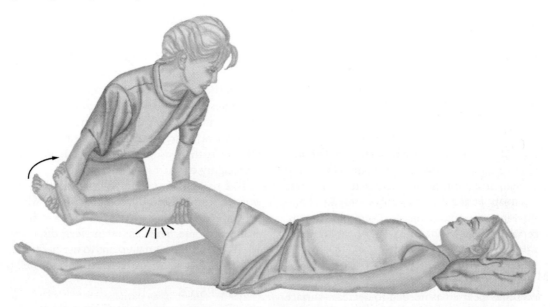

Figure 17-8 ■ Homans' sign is positive when the mother experiences discomfort in the calf on sharp dorsiflexion of the foot.

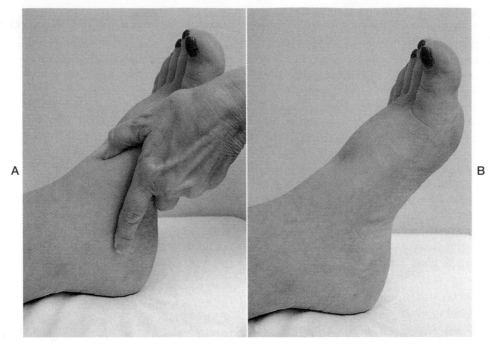

Figure 17-9 ■ Pedal edema. **A,** Apply pressure to foot. **B,** "Pit" appears when fluid moves into adjacent tissue and away from point of pressure.

Providing Comfort Measures

ICE PACKS

Both cold and warmth are used to alleviate perineal pain after childbirth. Ice causes vasoconstriction and is most effective if applied soon after the birth to prevent edema and to numb the area. Chemical ice packs and plastic bags or clean gloves filled with ice may be used during the first 12 hours after a vaginal birth. The ice pack is wrapped in paper before it is applied to the perineum. It should be left in place until the ice melts. It is removed for 10 minutes before a fresh pack is applied. Some peripads have cold packs incorporated in them. Condensation from ice may dilute lochia and make it appear heavier that it actually is.

Some women have varicosities of the vulva and wish to use ice packs at home. An inexpensive way for women to apply cold to the perineum is to freeze a wet washcloth placed in a plastic bag and wrap it in a paper towel before applying it to the perineum.

PERINEAL CARE

Perineal care consists of squirting warm water over the perineum after each voiding or bowel movement. This is important for all postpartum mothers whether the birth was vaginal or by cesarean. Perineal care cleanses, provides comfort, and prevents infection of an area that often has an episiotomy or lacerations. The perineum is gently patted rather than wiped to dry.

TOPICAL MEDICATIONS

Anesthetic sprays may be used as needed to decrease surface discomfort and allow more comfortable ambulation. The mother is instructed to hold the nozzle of a benzocaine spray such as Americaine or Dermoplast 6 to 12 inches from her body and direct it toward the perineum. An anesthetic and steroid combination such as Epifoam may also be used. The medication should be used after perineal care and before clean pads are applied.

SITTING MEASURES

The mother should be advised to squeeze her buttocks together before sitting and lower her weight slowly onto her buttocks. This measure prevents stretching of the perineal tissue and avoids sharp impact on the traumatized area.

SITZ BATHS

Sitz baths, which provide continuous circulation of water, cleanse and comfort the traumatized perineum. They also increase circulation to the area to help healing. Cool water reduces pain caused by edema and may be most effective within the first 24 hours. Warm water increases circulation, promotes healing, and may be most effective after 24 hours. Nurses must be sure that the emergency bell is within easy reach in case the mother feels faint during the sitz bath. If the sitz bath is used by more than one client, it must be thoroughly cleaned after each use.

Sitz baths may be offered two to three times a day for women with episiotomies, painful hemorrhoids, or perineal edema. Women are instructed about ways to continue the procedure at home. They are often given disposable sitz baths to take home. If the woman plans to use her tub at home for sitz baths, she should be instructed to clean it well before using it.

ANALGESICS

Mothers should be encouraged to take prescribed medications for afterpains and perineal discomfort. Analgesics such as acetaminophen (Tylenol, Panadol) and nonsteroidal antiinflammatory drugs (NSAIDs) such as ibuprofen (Motrin, Advil) frequently are prescribed to provide relief for mild to moderate discomfort. Acetaminophen with codeine (Tylenol No. 3), acetaminophen and oxycodone (Percocet, Tylox) and hydrocodone and acetaminophen (Lortab, Vicodin) often are prescribed for more severe discomfort (see Table 17-4). NSAIDs such as ketorolac (Toradol) may be given intravenously for several doses to help relieve cesarean incisional pain. Because a side effect of ketorolac is prolonged bleeding, the nurse should monitor lochia carefully.

In some agencies, women receive self-medication kits for use during their postpartum stays. The kit may include routine stool softeners, gas-relieving drugs, and nonnarcotic analgesics or a limited supply of certain narcotic pain medications. Women are instructed on how to take their medications and given a log to record each dose. This allows them to receive pain medication quickly when they need it because they don't have to wait for a nurse to bring it to them and helps them develop an understanding of the medications available for them (Werrbach & Wroblewski, 2003).

Promoting Bladder Elimination

Many new mothers have difficulty voiding because of edema and trauma of the perineum and diminished sensitivity to fluid pressure in the bladder. As soon as they are able to ambulate safely, mothers should be assisted to the bathroom. Providing privacy and allowing adequate time for the first voiding is important. Common measures to promote relaxation of the perineal muscles and stimulate the sensation of needing to void include:

- Medicating the woman for pain to help her relax
- Running water in the sink or shower, placing the mother's hands in water, and pouring water over the vulva
- Encouraging urination in the shower or sitz bath
- Providing hot tea or fluids of choice
- Asking the mother to blow bubbles through a straw

A nonpalpable bladder and firm fundus at or below the level of the umbilicus and in the midline confirm that the bladder is empty and rule out urinary retention with overflow.

A distended bladder lifts and displaces the uterus, making it difficult for it to remain contracted. Thus, urinary retention is a major cause of uterine atony (loss of tone), which permits excessive bleeding. In addition, stasis of urine in the bladder predisposes the woman to urinary tract infection. Therefore the mother must be catheterized in these circumstances:

- She is unable to void.
- The amount voided is less than 150 ml, and the bladder can be palpated.
- The fundus is elevated or displaced from the midline.

Repeated catheterizations increase the chance of urinary tract infection because bacteria may be pushed into the bladder despite scrupulous aseptic technique. To decrease the risk of infection, an indwelling catheter often is inserted for 24 hours if catheterization is necessary more than once.

CRITICAL THINKING *EXERCISE* **17-2**

Elizabeth Brown has made good progress since she delivered her first baby yesterday by cesarean. Her Foley catheter was removed 3 hours ago, and she was medicated with two Percocet (325 mg acetaminophen and 5 mg oxycodone) tablets for pain 1 hour ago. Now she is wincing and moaning with pain and asking for more pain medication. She says she got up to the bathroom with her husband's help a short time after her catheter was removed and urinated but did not measure it. Her fundus is slightly above the umbilicus and slightly to the right. A thick pressure dressing covers the lower abdomen making it difficult to palpate the bladder. Elizabeth says she doesn't have to urinate.

Questions
1. What other assessments should the nurse make?
2. What should the nurse do?
3. What are possible causes of Elizabeth's pain?

Providing Fluid and Food

Adequate fluids help restore the balance altered by fluid loss during labor and the birth process. Women should be encouraged to drink approximately 2500 ml of fluids each day. Offering warm fluids may be more culturally appropriate for some women. They may prefer hot or room-temperature water to ice water.

If a woman is unable to tolerate oral fluids, IV administration may be necessary. Women usually are able to have ice chips soon after cesarean birth, and, although protocols vary, most are able to progress to a regular diet in a short time.

New mothers generally have a hearty appetite, and nurses should encourage healthy food choices with respect for ethnic background. Meals and snacks should be available at all times.

Preventing Thrombophlebitis

The mother should be assisted to ambulate early after childbirth to prevent the development of thrombi. Frequent trips to the bathroom will help accomplish this.

NURSING CARE AFTER CESAREAN BIRTH

Many facilities have developed clinical pathways or care maps for cesarean births that are similar to those used for uncomplicated vaginal births. The clinical pathway identifies outcomes and establishes a time frame for assessments and interventions for postcesarean mothers and their infants (Figure 17-10). Clinical pathways or care maps are guidelines only. If a problem, sometimes called a *variance*, arises, additional assessments and interventions are necessary. The usual length of stay for mothers after a cesarean birth is 72 to 96 hours after surgery.

Assessment

In addition to the usual postpartum assessments, the postcesarean mother must be assessed like any other postoperative patient.

Clinical Path Day		Interdisciplinary Assessment	Nutrition	Activities/ Interventions	Tests
Phase	**Date**				
Day of Surgery		T, P, R, B/P q 4h × 6 Fundus, lochia, incision, breath sounds q 4h × 3 Bowel sounds, I & O's QS Level of comfort	Sips & chips to clears	Deep breathe q 2h Leg exercises q 2h Dangle then assist OOB × 1 I & O's, foley care Assist with hygiene	
	Date				
Post-op Day 1		T, P, R, B/P q 4h × 6 then BID Breasts, breath & bowel sounds, incision, fundus, lochia BID I & O's QS Level of comfort Knowledge of mother and newborn care	Advance diet as tolerated	D/C foley D/C IV Dressing removed Assist OOB to ambulate Assist with bath/shower	WCBC
	Date				
Post-op Day 2		T, P, R, B/P BID Breasts, bowel sounds, fundus, Incision, bladder, lochia BID Level of comfort Pt/SO/Family Knowledge of mother and newborn care	Regular	OOB ad lib Shower	
	Date				
Post-op Day 3		T, P, R, B/P BID Breasts, bowel sounds, fundus, Incision, bladder, lochia BID Level of comfort Pt/SO/Family knowledge of mother and newborn care	Regular	OOB ad lib Shower	
	Date				
Post-op Day 4		T, P, R, B/P BID Breasts, bowel sounds, fundus, Incision, bladder, lochia BID Level of comfort Knowledge of self & baby care	Regular	OOB ad lib Shower	

KEY: Patient/family potential problems related to expected outcomes:

1. Pain   2. Anxiety   3. Knowledge deficit   4. Altered maternal/fetal homeostasis

5. Ineffective parenting skills   6. _____

Figure 17-10 ■ Clinical pathway for cesarean birth. Figure shows only the postpartum aspects of care, although the pathway begins during the prenatal period. (Courtesy York Health System, York, Pennsylvania, with adaptations.)

Clinical Path Day		Medications	Consults	Education & Discharge Planning	Expected Outcomes
Phase	**Date**				
Day of Surgery		IV with Pitocin Analgesia prn		Continue post-op teaching Initiate/continue maternal-newborn education record	_____ Achieves desired level of pain relief (1) _____ >30cc/hr urine output (4) _____ Incision site clean, dry and intact (4) _____ Postpartum parameters stable (4)
	Date				
Post-op Day 1		Analgesia prn Rhogam, if ordered, give within 72 hours of delivery		Continue maternal-newborn education record Home support system	_____ Achieves desired level of pain relief (1) _____ >30cc/hr urine output (4) _____ Incision site clean, dry and intact (4) _____ Postpartum parameters stable (4) _____ Anmbulate TID w/assist (4) _____ Pt verbalizes available home support (5)
	Date				
Post-op Day 2		Analgesia prn		Continue and reinforce maternal-newborn education record	_____ Achieves desired level of pain relief (1) _____ Voiding QS (4) _____ Postpartum parameters stable (4) _____ Cares for self & infant(3) _____ Incision clean & dry (4) _____ Verbalizes D/C plan (3)
	Date				
Post-op Day 3		Analgesia prn		Continue and reinforce maternal-newborn education record Review and complete all discharge instructions with patient, SO & family	_____ Achieves desired level of pain relief (1) _____ Voiding QS (4) _____ Postpartum parameters stable (4) _____ Cares for self & infant(3) _____ Incision clean & dry (4) _____ Verbalizes D/C plan (3)
	Date				

Post-op Day 4		Analgesia prn
		
		Rubella, if ordered
		
		Depo Provera, if ordered
				Completion of maternal-newborn education record
				
				Discharge instructions given
				Support services initiated prn
					_____ Achieves desired level of pain relief (1)
					_____ Postpartum physiologic parameters meet discharge guidelines (4)
					_____ Incision site clean, dry, intact (4)
					_____ PT/SO Fam verbalizes understanding of discharge instructions (3)
					_____ Discharge within 4 days after delivery
					_____ Support services initiated
					   ___ Follow-up phone call
					   ___ Lactation Consult follow-up
					   ___ Perinatal Coaching
					   ___ City/State Health Department
					   ___ WIC
					   ___ Other _____

York Hospital

York, PA

Cesarean Delivery - Clinical Pathing

Figure 17-10, cont'd ■ For legend see opposite page.

PAIN RELIEF

Assessment of the level and effectiveness of pain relief is important to nursing care of postcesarean clients, who differ from typical postoperative clients in three important ways. First, they often are eager to be alert so that they can interact with their newborn infants. Second, they are concerned that the analgesics they receive may pass into their breast milk and potentially harm their infants. Third, compared with other postoperative patients, postcesarean clients want to have more input and control of their care.

Pain relief is provided in various ways. Patient-controlled analgesia (PCA) is administered by continuous intravenous infusion of a low-concentration narcotic solution using a pump specifically designed for that purpose. If analgesia is insufficient, the woman can self-administer intermittent small doses of narcotic from the infusion pump. The machine is programmed to administer only a certain amount of the narcotic within a specified time interval to prevent an overdose. This allows the woman to have pain relief immediately when she needs it without waiting for a nurse to administer it. Side effects include respiratory depression, itching (pruritus), nausea and vomiting, and urinary retention.

A single dose of opioid (such as preservative-free morphine or fentanyl) injected into the epidural or subarachnoid space immediately after surgery provides about 24 hours of postcesarean analgesia. Itching is a major side effect, with an incidence as high as 84%. Other side effects are the same as for PCA use (Zuspan, 2000). Oral analgesics usually are effective if women need additional pain relief measures.

Pain relief can also be provided by local anesthetic delivered into the incision site through a catheter attached to a pump. This allows the woman to move about more freely than with a PCA and avoids the side effects of narcotics. Oral analgesics may also be required. Occasionally, intramuscular analgesics are given for one or two doses with epidural medications or local anesthetics.

RESPIRATIONS

When mothers receive epidural narcotics for postoperative pain relief, respirations must be assessed frequently because narcotics depress the respiratory center. In some facilities a pulse oximeter is used for 18 to 24 hours to detect decreased oxygen saturation from a decreased respiratory rate or depth. An apnea monitor also may be used. Both will emit an alarm if respirations decrease. If a pulse oximeter or apnea monitor is not used, the respiratory rate and depth should be checked every 15 minutes for the first hour, every 30 minutes for 3 to 6 hours, and every 30 to 60 minutes for the remainder of the first 24 hours. Oxygen saturation or respiratory rate is documented according to facility policy.

In addition to observation of respiratory rate and depth, the mother's breath sounds should be auscultated because depressed respirations and a longer period of immobility allow secretions to pool in the bronchioles.

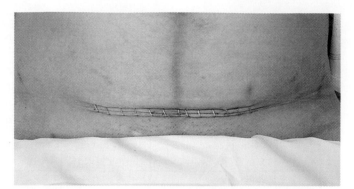

Figure 17-11 ■ This cesarean incision is closed with staples. Note the absence of all signs of infection, such as redness, edema, bruising (ecchymosis), discharge, and loss of approximation.

ABDOMEN

Nurses assess gastrointestinal function by auscultating for bowel sounds until normal peristalsis is noted in all abdominal quadrants. Although paralytic ileus (lack of movement in the bowel) is rare after cesarean birth, nurses must be aware of the signs, which include abdominal distention, absent or decreased bowel sounds, and failure to pass flatus or stool.

If a surgical dressing is present, it should be observed for intactness and discharge. When the dressing is removed, nurses observe the incision, which should be approximated, and use the acronym REEDA to assess for signs of infection such as redness and edema (Figure 17-11).

It is just as important to assess the fundus after cesarean birth as it is with vaginal birth. However, palpation must be gentle because of increased discomfort caused by the uterine incision.

INTAKE AND OUTPUT

The IV infusion should be monitored for the rate of flow and the condition of the IV site. Any signs of infiltration such as edema and coolness at the site and signs of infection such as edema, redness, warmth, and pain should be reported. Ice chips and clear fluids are allowed soon after birth. The amount, color, and clarity of urine should be monitored.

Interventions

THE FIRST 24 HOURS

Nursing care for the mother who gave birth by cesarean is similar to that for other postoperative clients.

PROVIDING PAIN RELIEF. The nurse should offer pain medication on a regular basis if the woman is not using a PCA. If a woman has a PCA, the nurse should check how often she is using it. The effectiveness of the analgesics should be determined. Relief of pain increases the woman's ability to increase her activity, helps prevent thrombophlebitis, and promotes healing. For women with epidural or spinal opioids, the nurse should continue to assess the respiratory status. If the respiratory rate begins to decline or is less than 12 per minute, the nurse should:

- Notify the anesthesiologist immediately.
- Elevate the head of the bed to facilitate lung expansion, and have the woman breathe deeply.
- Administer oxygen, and apply a pulse oximeter (if not already in place) to measure oxygen saturation.
- Follow facility protocol to administer narcotic antagonists, such as naloxone hydrochloride (Narcan).
- Observe for recurrence of respiratory depression because the duration of naloxone is only approximately 30 minutes.
- Recognize that naloxone reduces the level of pain relief.

OVERCOMING EFFECTS OF IMMOBILITY. The new mother is on bed rest for the first 8 to 12 hours. To prevent pooling of secretions in the airway, she must be assisted to turn, cough, and to expand the lungs by breathing deeply at least every 2 hours while she is awake. Splinting the abdomen with a small pillow reduces incisional discomfort when the woman coughs. Incentive spirometers help expand the lungs and thus prevent hypostatic pneumonia that can result from immobility and shallow, slow respirations.

Antiembolism stockings or sequential compression devices may be used to prevent the pooling of blood in the lower extremities while the woman is on bed rest. Activity will be gradually increased. The woman needs assistance to sit and dangle her feet for the first few times before she gets out of bed. She should be helped to get out of bed and walk a short distance within 24 hours to decrease risk for thrombophlebitis. She will need support ambulating when the IV and catheter are still in place.

PROVIDING COMFORT. Placing a pillow behind her back and one between her knees prevents strain and discomfort when the woman is lying on her side. Excellent physical care (such as oral hygiene, perineal care, a sponge bath, clean linen) comforts and refreshes her.

AFTER 24 HOURS

RESUMING NORMAL ACTIVITIES. After 24 hours several normal functions return as postcesarean women are able to participate more actively in their own care:

- Both the indwelling catheter and IV infusion are usually discontinued.
- The dressing, if present, is removed on the first or second day, and often any staples present are removed before discharge. Steri-Strips, a small nonstick dressing, or a peripad may be placed over the incision to protect it from friction from clothing or adipose tissue, or the incision may be left open to air.
- The mother is helped to ambulate by the first postpartum day and is comfortable sitting in a chair for brief periods of time.
- Clear liquids may be changed to a soft diet when bowel sounds are audible. In some agencies solids are provided earlier. If abdominal distention is minimal, the diet then progresses to a regular regimen.

Nurses must encourage the mother to increase her activity and ambulation each postpartum day. By the second day she usually is allowed to shower, if she wishes. Some health care providers request that the incision be covered with plastic; others permit showering without covering the incision.

ASSISTING THE MOTHER WITH INFANT FEEDING. Helping the mother find a comfortable position for holding and feeding her infant is important. Some mothers prefer sitting with a pillow on the lap to protect the incisional area. A side-lying position and football hold may be more comfortable because the infant is not putting pressure against the incision and causing discomfort. In addition, the side-lying position allows the mother to rest while feeding (see Chapter 22).

PREVENTING ABDOMINAL DISTENTION. Abdominal distention is a major source of discomfort. Measures to prevent and minimize it include:

- Early, frequent ambulation.
- Pelvic lifts—Lying supine with her knees bent, the woman lifts her pelvis from the bed and repeats the exercise up to 10 times, several times each day.
- Tightening and relaxing of the abdominal muscles.
- Avoidance of carbonated beverages and the use of straws, which increase the accumulation of intestinal gas.
- Simethicone to help disperse upper gastrointestinal flatulence.
- Rectal suppositories to help stimulate peristalsis and passage of flatus.

✔ CHECK YOUR READING

15. What additional assessments are necessary for the postcesarean mother?
16. How can hypostatic pneumonia be prevented?
17. Which measures are used to prevent or minimize abdominal distention?

Application of the Nursing Process
Knowledge of Self-Care

Assessment

Nurses are responsible for providing health education about a long list of subjects before the family is discharged from the birth facility. This task causes concern because so much must be taught during this short time, which is not ideal for teaching mothers who are not fully recovered from the birth process. Some women feel they have difficulty concentrating during the first week postpartum, although studies show they function better than they did during the last trimester of pregnancy (Stark, 2000).

Before beginning teaching, determine the learning needs and the major concerns of each family. Multiparas remember some aspects of self-care but often benefit from a review. Primiparas may be anxious about self-care measures and all aspects of infant care. They may require more thorough teaching and more time for practice. Identify the most common barriers to learning: age and developmental level, cultural factors, and difficulty understanding the language.

Analysis

In general, mothers adapt to the physiologic changes after childbirth, and most nursing care is wellness oriented. Some new mothers, however, lack knowledge of self-care and therefore are at risk for a disruption in health. Because of the need for health education, a nursing diagnosis that applies to many women and forms the basis for nursing interventions is "Risk for Ineffective Health Maintenance related to insufficient knowledge of self-care, signs of complications, and preventive measures." (The diagnoses "Risk for Injury" and "Ineffective Sexuality Patterns" appear in Nursing Care Plan 17-1. Common nursing diagnoses are listed in Box 17-2.)

Planning

Goals and expected outcomes for the nursing diagnosis "Risk for Ineffective Health Maintenance" related to insufficient knowledge of self-care, signs of complications, and preventive measures are that the mother will:

- Verbalize or demonstrate understanding of self-care instructions by (date).
- Verbalize understanding of practices that promote maternal health by discharge.
- Describe plans for follow-up care and signs and symptoms that should be reported to the health care provider by discharge.

BOX 17-2 Common Nursing Diagnoses for Postpartum Women

Risk for Ineffective Health Maintenance*
Risk for Ineffective Sexuality Patterns*
Risk for Injury*
Imbalanced Nutrition More (or Less) Than Body Requirements
Impaired Urinary Elimination
Constipation
Health-Seeking Behaviors
Ineffective Breastfeeding
Parental Role Conflict
Sleep Deprivation

*Nursing diagnoses discussed in this chapter.

Interventions
DETERMINING TEACHING TOPICS

Make a teaching plan with the mother to include topics most important to her. The mother's perceptions of what is most important may differ from those of the nurse. Determining the mother's educational needs ensures her interest in the subjects selected and makes best use of the short time available. Topics of less interest may require just a brief review. The review may elicit questions from the mother and interest in more in-depth information.

TEACHING THE PROCESS OF INVOLUTION

Provide the woman with basic information about involution, including how to assess lochia and how to locate and palpate the fundus. This information allows her to recognize abnormal signs such as prolonged lochia, reappearance of bright-red lochia after lochia rubra has ended, and uterine tenderness, which should be reported to the health care provider. If the mother is a very young adolescent, another family member also may need the information.

TEACHING SELF-CARE

HANDWASHING. Emphasize the importance of thoroughly washing her hands before the woman touches her breasts, after diaper changes, after bladder and bowel elimination, and always before handling the infant. Observing nurses model this behavior reinforces this teaching for parents.

BREAST CARE FOR LACTATING MOTHERS. Instruct the breastfeeding mother to avoid using soap on her nipples because it will remove the natural lubrication secreted by Montgomery's glands. Keeping the nipples dry between feedings helps prevent tissue damage, and wearing a good bra provides necessary support as breast size increases (see Chapter 22).

MEASURES TO SUPPRESS LACTATION. If the mother chooses not to breastfeed, initiate measures to suppress lactation. Binding the breasts or having the mother wear a snug-fitting bra 24 hours per day until the breasts become soft can help reduce breast distention. A support bra is often more comfortable, allows less leaking, and is as effective in reducing engorgement as binding the breasts (Swift & Janke, 2003).

THERAPEUTIC COMMUNICATIONS
Teaching Self-Care Measures

Clare Beauchamp gave birth to a baby boy 48 hours ago. Terry Meyer is a nurse preparing to teach Clare self-care measures before discharge from the birth facility.

Clare: Look at me! I still look pregnant, and my husband calls me Tubby.

Terry: You were looking forward to your abdomen being flat after the baby was born.

This clarifies the woman's concern by reflecting content.

Clare: Well, I was always so flat. I'm really disappointed.

Terry: Remember, it took 9 months for those muscles to stretch. You can't expect them to snap back in a few days.

This blocks communication by ignoring the feeling expressed. A more helpful response would be to acknowledge the disappointment and to delay giving information until feelings have been expressed. For example: "It is upsetting! When you are ready, we can discuss some exercises that will help."

Manage breast discomfort by application of ice, which reduces vasocongestion, and administration of analgesics. Advise the woman to refrain from actions such as allowing warm water to fall on the breasts during showers and pumping or massaging the breasts, as these will stimulate milk production.

CARE OF THE CESAREAN INCISION. If the birth was by cesarean, the woman may have concerns about care of the incision. Staples, if used, have usually been removed before the woman is discharged. If adhesive strips have been applied, teach the woman that they will gradually detach and it is all right to shower with the strips in place.

A topical skin adhesive may be applied in surgery instead of staples or adhesive strips. No dressing is required over the site, and the woman can shower when the topical adhesive is in place. For each method, explain that the incision is closed and is unlikely to come apart. There should be little or no drainage from the incision. Instruct her to call her provider if the incision separates or drainage increases or has a foul smell.

PERINEAL CARE. Teach the woman how to cleanse her perineum. The most common method is to fill a squeeze bottle with warm water and spray the perineal area from the front toward the back. Warm water alone or with a small amount of cleansing solution added is used. Remind the new mother not to separate the labia during this procedure because that would allow water to enter the vagina. If a commercial product that includes a nozzle attached to the faucet is used, teach the mother that the nozzle should not touch the perineum during use.

Toilet paper or moist antiseptic towelettes are used in a patting motion to dry the perineum. Teach the mother to dry from front to back to prevent fecal contamination of the vaginal introitus from the anal area. She should perform perineal cleansing and change peripads after each voiding or defecation.

Some women do not use peripads for menstrual protection and must be taught to use them correctly. Mesh panties and adhering pads are used in most facilities. Careful handling of the pads is important to prevent perineal infection.

- Thorough handwashing is important before and after changing pads.
- Unused pads should be stored inside their packages.
- Pads should be applied without touching the side that contacts the perineum.
- The pads should be applied and removed in a front-to-back direction to prevent contamination of the vagina and perineum.
- Used pads must be disposed of properly.

KEGEL EXERCISES. All women should become familiar with Kegel exercises (see Chapter 33). These movements strengthen the pubococcygeal muscle, which surrounds the vagina and urinary meatus. This exercise helps prevent the loss of muscle tone that can occur after childbirth and that sometimes leads to urinary incontinence.

The exercise involves contracting muscles around the vagina (as though stopping the flow of urine), holding tightly for 10 seconds, and then relaxing for 10 seconds. Each contraction should be of moderate to near maximum intensity, and a full 10 seconds should be allowed for relaxation between each contraction. The woman should work up to 30 contraction-relaxation cycles each day.

PROMOTING REST AND SLEEP

Many women experience fatigue after childbirth that continues for weeks or months (Troy, 2003). The extreme fatigue new mothers feel has a variety of causes. Women are often tired when they begin the postpartum period because they slept poorly during the third trimester, and they are further exhausted by the exertion of labor. Feelings of excitement and euphoria after childbirth interfere with their ability to rest. Periods of rest are interrupted by numerous visitors and phone calls, hospital routines, noise, and an unfamiliar environment. Afterpains, discomfort from an episiotomy or incision, muscle aches, and breast engorgement also contribute to a woman's discomfort and inability to sleep.

Most mothers are discharged from the facility within 24 to 48 hours after vaginal birth or 72 to 96 hours after cesarean birth, and they go home with a tremendous deficit in sleep and energy. Yet new parents may be unprepared for the conflict between their need for sleep and the infant's need for care and attention. The joys of parenting can easily be overshadowed by the exhaustion and frustration that result.

REST AT THE BIRTH FACILITY. Hospital routines continue around the clock, making uninterrupted rest difficult and increasing the probability that the mother is fatigued when she is discharged. Make every attempt to allow the mother adequate time for uninterrupted rest periods. Group assessments and care, and try to correlate them with times when the mother would be awake, such as just before or after meals, infant feeding times, and visiting hours. If the room is shared, providing care for both women at the same time also reduces activities that interrupt sleep.

Try to persuade the mother to select a time when phone calls and visitors are restricted so that she can use this time for napping. Encourage the mother to use a side-lying position for breastfeeding to allow her to rest during feedings. A quiet, softly lit environment also promotes sleep.

REST AT HOME. Help the mother understand the impact that her physical discomfort and the demands of the newborn and other family members will have on her energy during the first few weeks. If she understands that fatigue is common and will continue for some time, she can plan ways to obtain extra help and conserve her energy. Suggest the following energy-saving measures:

- Maintain a relaxed, flexible routine that focuses on care of the mother and infant.
- Nap or rest when the infant sleeps, if possible.
- Plan simple meals and flexible meal times.
- Limit visitors when she is feeling too tired.
- Accept assistance with food shopping, meal preparation, laundry, and housework.

- Put off housework that isn't absolutely necessary.
- Postpone major household projects.
- Involve friends and family to provide care for other children.

Explain to the mother that she should delay her return to employment, if possible, until the infant sleeps through the night (usually by 4 months) or later. It takes time to recover from the birth, as well as to adjust to the changes that occur with a new baby. Advise all mothers to restrict intake of coffee, tea, colas, and chocolate, which contain the stimulant caffeine, or use caffeine-free versions for the first few weeks. Suggest total relaxation exercises (lying quietly, alternately tightening and relaxing the muscles of the neck, shoulders, arms, legs, and feet), which are helpful when a nap is not possible.

Emphasize to the mother the importance of asking for help when she begins to feel exhausted or overwhelmed. Encourage her to share these feelings with family, friends, and other new mothers.

INFANT SLEEP AND FEEDING SCHEDULES. Many families require information about infant sleep cycles, frequency of feeding, and probable crying episodes during the first weeks. Although newborns sleep much of the time, they may awaken every 2 to 3 hours for feeding (see Chapter 22 regarding infant feeding and Chapter 23 regarding parenting during the early weeks).

PROVIDING NOURISHMENT AND NUTRITION COUNSELING

FOOD SUPPLY. Determining the amount and type of food that is available to the mother and her family sometimes is appropriate. This is particularly true for families of low socioeconomic status, who might benefit from referral to government-sponsored programs, such as food stamps or the Special Supplemental Nutrition Program for Women, Infants, and Children (WIC). Determining the facilities available for cooking and storing food also may be necessary. The new family may need referral to a social worker to identify the best solutions for its unique problems.

DIET. Although many women are unsatisfied with slow weight loss, they should avoid severe restriction of caloric intake. Advise the mother to select foods that provide adequate calories to meet her energy needs, taking into account the time and energy required to care for a newborn.

Women often lose weight by decreasing consumption of carbohydrates. However, their fat intake may increase if they skip meals and eat high-fat snacks or fast foods because of time constraints (Gennaro & Fehder, 2000). A balanced, low-fat diet with adequate protein, complex carbohydrates, fruits, and vegetables provides the energy and nutrients needed (see Chapter 9).

PROMOTING REGULAR BOWEL ELIMINATION

Explain the role of progressive exercise, adequate fluid, and dietary fiber in preventing constipation. Walking is an excellent exercise, and the distance can be increased as strength and endurance build. Drinking at least eight glasses of water daily helps maintain normal bowel elimination.

Unpeeled fruits and vegetables are good sources of dietary fiber, and prunes are a natural laxative. Additional fiber is found in whole grain cereals, bread, and pasta.

A regular schedule of bowel elimination is important in overcoming constipation. For instance, bowel elimination after breakfast allows the mother to take advantage of the gastrocolic reflex (stimulation of peristalsis induced in the colon when food is consumed on an empty stomach). In addition, measures that reduce perineal and hemorrhoidal pain, such as sitz baths, prepackaged witch hazel astringent compresses, and hydrocortisone ointments facilitate bowel elimination.

PROMOTING GOOD BODY MECHANICS

EXERCISE. Exercise has beneficial physical and psychological effects during the postpartum period. Teach exercises in the early postpartum period to strengthen the abdominal muscles and firm the waist (Figure 17-12). These mild exercises can be started soon after childbirth. At first, each exercise should be repeated five times, twice each day. Gradually the number of exercises is increased as the mother gains strength.

Instruct postcesarean mothers to follow the instructions of their health care provider. They may need to avoid a vigorous exercise program for 4 to 6 weeks but can participate in less strenuous activities such as walking. The woman should not exercise if it causes her pain.

PREVENTION OF BACK STRAIN. Back strain often can be prevented if the mother and father find a location for infant care, such as a kitchen table or bathroom counter, that does not require bending and leaning forward. For lifting objects, teach mothers to hold the back straight as they squat and use their legs rather than bending at the waist (see Figure 7-13).

COUNSELING ABOUT SEXUAL ACTIVITY

The couple may have concerns about the resumption of sexual intercourse and contraceptive choices. Fatigue, perineal pain, fear of pregnancy, concerns about the baby, and a feeling of unattractiveness may interfere with a woman's sexual desire. In one study, women who had a second-degree or more extensive laceration or episiotomy were 80% to 270% more likely to report dyspareunia at 3 months postpartum. When the birth involved a vacuum extractor or forceps, pain during intercourse was still significant at 6 months postpartum (Signorello, Harlow, Chekos, & Repke, 2001).

Many new parents are reluctant to ask about when to resume sexual activity and potential changes in sexuality resulting from pregnancy and childbirth. Nurses must be sensitive to unasked questions and should try to provide anticipatory guidance.

- If couples do not indicate such concerns, introduce the topic in a general, nonspecific manner, such as "You have an episiotomy that may cause some discomfort with intercourse until it is completely healed" or "Sometimes couples are not aware that some vaginal dryness occurs as a result of breast-feeding." Such broad opening statements permit the couple to pursue the topic as they desire.

ABDOMINAL BREATHING

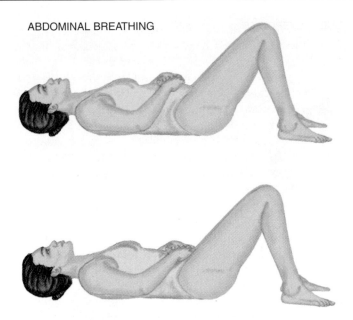

This is one of the simplest exercises and can be started on the first postpartum day. The woman assumes a supine position with knees bent. She inhales through the nose, keeps the rib cage as stationary as possible, and allows the abdomen to expand. She then contracts the abdominal muscles as she exhales slowly through the mouth.

HEAD LIFT

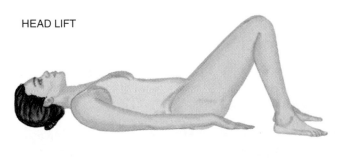

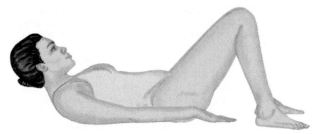

This exercise can be started within a few days after childbirth. The mother is supine with knees bent and arms outstretched at her side. She inhales deeply to begin, then exhales while lifting the head slowly; she holds the position for a few seconds and relaxes.

MODIFIED SIT-UPS

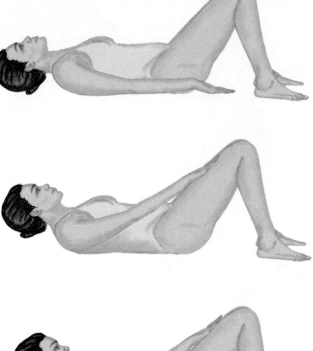

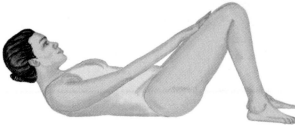

Head lifts may progress to modified sit-ups with the approval of the health care provider; the mother should follow the advice of the health care provider about the number of repetitions.

The exercise begins with the mother supine with arms outstretched and the knees bent. She raises her head and shoulders as her hands reach for her knees. She raises the shoulders only as far as the back will bend; her waist remains on the floor.

Figure 17-12 ■ Postpartum exercises. Exercises should be approved by the woman's physician, nurse-midwife, or nurse practitioner before she begins them.

Continued

KNEE AND LEG ROLLS

CHEST EXERCISES

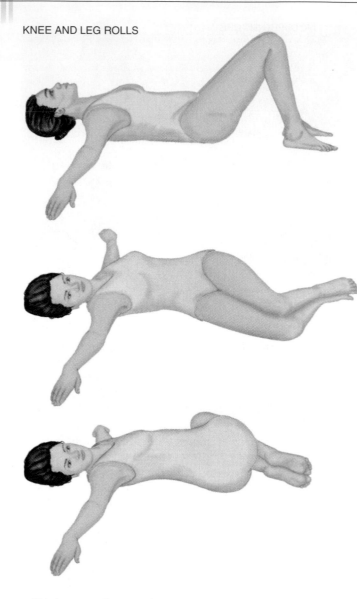

This is an excellent exercise to begin firming the waist. The mother lies flat on her back with knees bent and feet flat on the floor or bed; she keeps the shoulders and feet stationary and rolls the knees to touch first one side of the bed, then the other. She maintains a smooth motion as the exercise is repeated five times. Later, as flexibility increases, the exercise can be varied by the rolling of one knee only. The mother rolls her left knee to touch the right side of the bed, returns to center, and rolls the right knee to touch the left side of the bed.

This is an excellent exercise to strengthen the chest muscles. The mother lies flat with arms extended straight out to the side; she brings the hands together above the chest while keeping the arms straight; she holds for a few seconds and returns to the starting position. She repeats the exercise five times initially and follows the advice of the health care provider for increasing the number of repetitions.

Isometric exercises also increase strength and tone; the mother bends her elbows, clasps her hands together above her chest, and presses her hands together for a few seconds. This is repeated at least five times.

Figure 17-12, cont'd ■ Postpartum exercises. Exercises should be approved by the woman's physician, nurse-midwife, or nurse practitioner before she begins them.

Interventions for parental concerns about sexual activity are discussed in Nursing Care Plan 17-1 (p. 407).

Cultural or religious convictions may restrict the choice of contraceptive method for some couples, whereas availability of health care or inadequate finances may dictate the choice for others. Discuss previous experience with contraceptives and the satisfaction with that method. Some women choose to have a tubal ligation before discharge after birth (see Chapter 31).

INSTRUCTING ABOUT FOLLOW-UP APPOINTMENTS

Remind the new mother to make an appointment with her physician or nurse-midwife for a postpartum examination at the time suggested by her provider. This is often 2 to 6 weeks after childbirth. Emphasize that the postpartum examination allows early identification and treatment of problems that may be developing. Women who have had complications during the pregnancy or postpartum period may need to see their health care provider sooner or for more extensive follow-up than those without complications.

TEACHING ABOUT SIGNS AND SYMPTOMS THAT SHOULD BE REPORTED

Teach new mothers and at least one family member which physical signs and symptoms should be reported to the health care provider immediately. These signs and symptoms include:

- Fever
- Localized area of redness, swelling, or pain in either breast that is not relieved by support or analgesics
- Persistent abdominal tenderness
- Feelings of pelvic fullness or pelvic pressure
- Persistent perineal pain
- Frequency, urgency, or burning on urination
- Abnormal change in character of lochia (increased amount, resumption of bright red color, passage of clots, foul odor)
- Localized tenderness, redness, swelling, or warmth of the legs
- Swelling of, redness in, drainage from, or separation of an abdominal incision

ENSURING A THOROUGH EDUCATION

Before beginning teaching sessions, be sure the woman is comfortable. Give pain medication, if necessary, to prevent her being distracted by discomfort. Time teaching so that it does not interfere with meals, infant care, needs or visiting. Insert small teaching segments throughout the day rather than planning long teaching sessions.

Although there are many topics to discuss in parent teaching, avoid covering too much information at a time. Interspersing small segments of teaching into normal care throughout the day will keep the woman from being overwhelmed and help her remember information better.

Organize information so that it can be presented and absorbed in the time available. Group instruction and hospital classes, such as those that demonstrate infant care and provide breastfeeding instructions, make efficient use of the nurse's time.

Individual instruction is also necessary. In some agencies, women are given some information pertaining to postpartum self-care during the prenatal period. During the hospital stay the nurse reviews and rechecks the mothers' understanding of previous teaching.

DOCUMENTING TEACHING

Documentation is an important aspect of teaching, just as it is for other aspects of nursing care. Documentation that discharge teaching was performed and that the client has indicated comprehension of teaching is required by accrediting agencies. To prevent omissions, many hospitals use teaching checklists to record topics that must be taught (Box 17-3) (see Chapter 21 for teaching about infant care).

BOX 17-3 Postpartum Discharge Teaching Topics

Uterine massage
Lochia norms
Involution
Episiotomy care
Care of abdominal incisions
Breast care for lactating and nonlactating women
Bowel function
Urinary function
Nutrition
Rest
Exercise
Contraception
Sexual activity
Postpartum danger signs
Follow-up care
Medications
Emotional responses
Infant care and feeding
Family adjustment
Available resources

Evaluation

- The mother's demonstration of correct breast and perineal hygiene provides evidence of her ability to perform self-care measures.
- The mother's ability to discuss practices that promote health in the areas of diet, exercise, rest, and sleep confirm understanding of these measures.
- Her plan for future appointments with the health care provider for examinations or follow-up of complications increases the likelihood that she will experience an uncomplicated recovery.

Postpartum Home and Community-Based Care

CRITERIA FOR DISCHARGE

Most women leave the hospital when they are just beginning to recover from giving birth and starting to learn how to care for themselves and their infants. Criteria for discharge of mothers have been developed by The American Academy of Pediatrics and the American College of Obstetricians and Gynecologists (2002):

- The mother has no complications, and assessments (including vital signs, lochia, fundus, urinary output, incisions, ambulation, ability to eat and drink, and emotional status) are normal.
- Pertinent laboratory data including hemoglobin or hematocrit have been reviewed, and immune globulin has been administered, if necessary.
- The mother has received instructions on self-care, deviations from normal, and proper response to danger signs and symptoms.
- The mother demonstrates readiness to care for herself and her baby.
- The mother has received instructions on postpartum activity, exercises, and relief measures for common postpartum discomforts.
- Arrangements have been made for postpartum care.
- Family members or other support persons are available to the mother for the first few days after discharge.

HOME CARE SERVICES

New parents must be made aware of local home care services. Information lines, follow-up telephone calls, home visits, and nurse-managed postpartum outpatient clinics are often available. In addition, some facilities offer breastfeeding and parenting classes, "baby and me" walks, exercise sessions, and postpartum support groups (see Chapter 23 for information about community care).

INFORMATION LINES. Ideally, information lines should be open 24 hours a day, 7 days a week. They should be staffed by qualified nurses who use agency protocols to respond to the family's questions. In addition, the nurses must be prepared to "triage." That is, they must be skilled at soliciting information to identify problems and determining the priority of the problems identified. For instance, does the information obtained indicate that the family should come to the office or clinic for a more thorough assessment by their health care provider? Should they come now or can they wait? Can their problem be solved by information or advice?

Legal liability is a concern for all agencies and personnel who identify problems, set priorities, and provide information by telephone. The staff must be educated and evaluated for the task. Protocols must be devised, a documentation system must be developed, and adequate consultation or "back-up" support must be available.

A major disadvantage of information lines is that they rely on families to initiate a request for assistance. Not all families recognize when a problem begins to develop and, as a result, may delay seeking information.

TELEPHONE CALLS. Nurses at some facilities initiate telephone interviews to assess and provide information to families at home. The calls usually are made 1 to 3 days after discharge. As with information lines, a qualified nurse, following the facility protocol, conducts a systematic assessment of the mother and infant. The nurse solicits questions and reinforces important information. Telephone calls are relatively inexpensive. The major disadvantage is that the nurse cannot confirm data but must rely on observations made by the family.

HOME VISITS. Home visits allow physical examination of the mother and infant and assessment of family adaptation and the home environment. Maternal assessment should include the breasts, fundus, lochia, perineum, abdominal incision (if applicable), and psychosocial status (Figure 17-13). If possible, nurses should allow time to observe breastfeeding and provide encouragement and reassurance that is badly needed during the first days before lactation is well established.

The newborn's weight, color, elimination pattern, and feeding history are important parts of the home visit. Postpartum visits provide an added opportunity for teaching. Ample time should be allowed to reinforce previous learning, answer questions, and introduce new topics, such as home safety. Although home visits are expensive, they provide the most comprehensive nursing care.

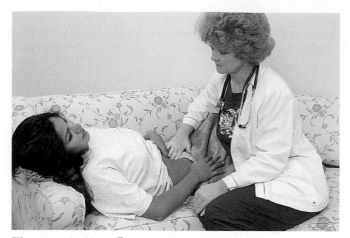

Figure 17-13 ■ Postpartum home visits include assessments and health education. Here the nurse evaluates involution while teaching the mother how to palpate her fundus.

OUTPATIENT CLINICS. Nurse-managed outpatient clinics offer another option for postpartum care. Although transportation is a problem for some families, clinic visits are less costly for the agency than home visits and more clients can be seen in a day than with home visits. Clinic visits may be used either to replace or to supplement home visits. Like home care, clinic visits include an examination of the mother and infant. Adequate time is provided to answer questions about maternal self-care, provide assistance with infant feeding, and deal with special concerns such as care of the umbilical cord or circumcision and postpartum blues.

✓ CHECK YOUR READING

18. How is lactation suppressed when the mother elects not to breastfeed?
19. What is the major challenge nurses have in preparing new mothers for discharge? How do clinical pathways affect nursing care?
20. What are the criteria for discharge of the mother?
21. What are the advantages and disadvantages of information lines, telephone calls, home visits, and nurse-managed outpatient clinics?

SUMMARY CONCEPTS

■ After childbirth the uterus returns to its nonpregnant size and condition by involution, which involves contraction of stretched muscle fibers, catabolic processes that reduce enlarged muscle cells, and regeneration of uterine epithelium.

■ The site of placental attachment heals by a process of exfoliation, which leaves the endometrium smooth and without scars.

■ Involution can be evaluated by measuring the descent of the fundus (about 1 cm/day). By about the tenth day after childbirth the fundus should be located in the pelvic cavity and should no longer be palpable abdominally.

- Afterpains, or intermittent uterine contractions, cause discomfort for many women, particularly multiparas who breastfeed.
- Vaginal discharge (lochia) progresses from lochia rubra (mostly blood) to lochia serosa (serous exudate, blood, and leukocytes) to lochia alba (increased amounts of leukocytes and decidual cells) in a predictable time frame. Lochia should be assessed for volume, type, and odor. Foul odor suggests endometrial infection.
- Although vaginal mucosa heals within 3 weeks, it takes 6 weeks for the vagina to regain its nonpregnant size and contour.
- Hemorrhoids and perineal trauma, including edema, bruising, episiotomy, and lacerations, can cause a great deal of discomfort and interfere with bladder and bowel elimination.
- Cardiac output increases when blood from the uterus and placenta returns to central circulation and extracellular fluid moves into the vascular compartment. Excess fluid is excreted by diuresis and diaphoresis.
- Increased clotting factors predispose the postpartum woman to thrombus formation. Early, frequent ambulation is the best method for preventing thrombophlebitis.
- Constipation may occur as a result of decreased fluid intake during labor, reduced activity, decreased muscle tone, diminished bowel tone, and fear of pain during defecation.
- Increased bladder capacity and decreased sensitivity to fluid pressure may result in urinary retention. Stasis of urine allows time for bacteria to grow and can lead to urinary tract infection.
- A distended bladder lifts and displaces the uterus and can interfere with uterine contraction and cause excessive bleeding.
- Exercises to strengthen the abdominal muscles and good posture and body mechanics may reduce musculoskeletal discomfort.
- As hormone levels decline, the skin gradually reverts to its prepregnancy state.
- Breastfeeding may delay the return of ovulation and menstruation but is not a reliable method of family planning. Both lactating and nonlactating mothers need information about family planning.
- Breastfeeding mothers are more likely to experience dyspareunia as a result of vaginal dryness that results from inadequate estrogen.
- Lactation may be suppressed by wearing a snug bra and avoiding stimulation of the breasts.
- The postpartum woman should be afebrile, but her temperature may be higher during the first 24 hours after delivery because of exertion, dehydration, and leukocytosis.
- Bradycardia is expected. Tachycardia may be caused by excitement, infection, dehydration, pain, and hypovolemia. Additional assessments (for example, lochia, fundus) are required to determine whether excessive bleeding is the cause.
- Orthostatic hypotension occurs when the mother goes from a supine to standing position quickly. It may result in injury if precautions to protect her are not initiated.
- The postcesarean woman requires postoperative and postpartum assessments and care. She is at increased risk for problems associated with immobility and discomfort.

- The common practice of early discharge challenges nurses to streamline information and develop a plan for teaching self-care and infant care in a short time.

ANSWERS TO CRITICAL THINKING EXERCISE 17-1, p. 412

1. The birth of a large infant and the fact that Jenny is a multipara increase the risk of postpartum hemorrhage. Saturation of pads in a short time suggests heavy bleeding. Location of the fundus above the umbilicus and displaced to the side indicates that the cause of bleeding might be a distended bladder.
2. Assisting the mother to void is the most appropriate nursing action. If, after voiding, the fundus is located at the level of the umbilicus and firmly contracted, the nurse can be relatively certain that the cause of the bleeding was a distended bladder, which made it difficult for the uterus to contract firmly. The location and consistency of the uterus, amount of lochia, blood pressure, and pulse should be assessed frequently so that further excessive bleeding can be promptly identified and controlled.
3. Jenny does not experience the urge to void because the bladder has not regained the muscle tone lost during pregnancy and the sensitivity to pressure is decreased.

ANSWERS TO CRITICAL THINKING EXERCISE 17-2, p. 415

1. Any time a client has more pain than would be expected, further assessment is necessary to determine the cause. Ask Elizabeth whether she urinated a large or small amount. Ask her to rate her pain. Exactly where is the pain located? What type of pain is it? Burning, pressure, dull ache? How much lochia does she have compared with previous assessments?
2. Regardless of the amount she thinks she voided previously and Elizabeth's lack of the sensation of needing to void, assist her to the bathroom to see if she can void. If she urinates, measure the amount to see if it is adequate (approximately 300 ml) and determine if she feels relief after voiding. If she is unable to void and an order exists, catheterize her. If no order exists, call the health care provider to obtain an order.
3. A distended bladder is the most likely cause of Elizabeth's pain. However, she may have a very low pain tolerance or need a different kind of analgesic. In this case, however, Elizabeth had surgery yesterday and has received pain medication since that time. A low pain tolerance or a drug that was ineffective for her would already have been noted. Some surgical complication may exist. If the pain continues, refer the problem to the provider.

REFERENCES & READINGS

American Academy of Pediatrics & American College of Obstetricians and Gynecologists. (2002). *Guidelines for perinatal care* (5th ed.). Elk Grove Village, IL: Author.

American College of Obstetricians and Gynecologists. (2002). Exercise during pregnancy and the postpartum period. *Obstetrics & Gynecology, 99*(1), 171-173.

Association of Women's Health, Obstetric and Neonatal Nurses (AWHONN). (2000a). *Evidence-based clinical practice guideline: Breastfeeding support: Prenatal care through the first year* (Monograph). Washington, DC: Author.

AWHONN. (2000b). *Evidence-based clinical practice guideline: Breastfeeding support: Prenatal care through the first year. Practice guidelines.* Washington, DC: Author.

AWHONN. (2003). *Standards & guidelines for professional nursing practice in the care of women and newborns* (6th ed.). Washington, DC: Author.

Blackburn, S.T. (2003). *Maternal, fetal, and neonatal physiology* (2nd ed.). Philadelphia: Saunders.

Bowes, W.A., & Katz, V.L. (2002). Postpartum care. In S.G. Gabbe, J.R. Niebyl, & J.L. Simpson (Eds.), *Obstetrics, normal and problem pregnancies* (4th ed., pp. 701-725). New York: Churchill Livingstone.

Buist, A., Morse, C.A., & Durkin, S. (2003). Men's adjustment to fatherhood: implications for obstetrical health care. *Journal of Obstetric, Gynecologic, and Neonatal Nursing, 32*(2), 172-180.

Callister, L.C. (2001). Integrating cultural beliefs and practices into the care of childbearing women. In K.R. Simpson & P.A. Creehan, *AWHONN Perinatal Nursing* (2nd ed, pp. 68-94). Philadelphia: Lippincott Williams & Wilkins.

Cartwright, Y. (2004). Battling excess postpartum weight retention. *Journal of the American Dietetic Association, 104*(7), 1108-1109.

Centers for Disease Control and Prevention. (2003). *Epidemiology & prevention of vaccine-preventable diseases* (8th ed.). Retrieved September 18, 2004 from www.cdc.gov/nip/publications/pink/def_pink_full.htm.

Cesario, S.K. (2001). Care of the Native American woman: Strategies for practice, education, and research. *Journal of Obstetric, Gynecologic, and Neonatal Nursing, 30*(1), 13-19.

Chagnon, L., & Wehmeyer, J. (2004). After the birth: Providing comprehensive services in a hospital outpatient setting. *AWHONN Lifelines, 8*(4), 334-138.

Cunningham, F.G., Leveno, K.J., Bloom, S.L., Hauth, J.C., Gilstrap, L.C., Wenstrom, K.D. (2005). *Williams obstetrics* (22nd ed.). New York: McGraw-Hill.

Dana, S.N., & Wambach, K.A. (2003). Patient satisfaction with an early discharge home visit program. *Journal of Obstetric, Gynecologic, and Neonatal Nursing, 32*(2), 190-198.

Gennaro, S., & Fehder, W. (2000). Health behaviors in postpartum women. *Family & Community Health, 22*(4), 16-26.

Hayashi, R.H., & Zettelmaier, M.A. (2000). Postpartum management. In S.B. Ransom, M.P. Dombrowski, S.G. McNeeley, K.S. Moghissi, & A.R. Munkarah (Eds.), *Practical strategies in obstetrics and gynecology* (pp. 321-325). Philadelphia: Saunders.

James, D.C. (2001). Postpartum care. In K.R. Simpson & P.A. Creehan, *AWHONN Perinatal Nursing* (2nd ed, pp. 446- 472). Philadelphia: Lippincott Williams & Wilkins.

Kennedy, K.I. (2005). Fertility, sexuality, & contraception during lactation. In J. Riordan (Ed.), *Breast-feeding and human lactation* (3rd ed., pp. 621-651). Boston: Jones and Bartlett.

Keppler, A.B., & Simpson, K.R. (2001). Discharge planning. In K.R. Simpson & P.A. Creehan (Eds.), *AWHONN perinatal nursing* (2nd ed, pp. 610-632). Philadelphia: Lippincott Williams & Wilkins.

Lieu, T.A., Braveman, P.A., Escobar, G.J., Fischer, A.F., Jensvold, N.G., & Capra, A.M. (2000). A randomized comparison of home and clinic follow-up visits after early postpartum hospital discharge. *Pediatrics, 105*(5), 1058-1065.

Martell, L.K. (2003). Postpartum women's perceptions of the hospital environment. *Journal of Obstetric, Gynecologic, and Neonatal Nursing, 32*(4), 478-485.

Matteson, P.S. (2001). *Women's health during the childbearing years: a community-based approach.* St. Louis: Mosby.

Nelson, A.M. (2003). Transition to motherhood. *Journal of Obstetric, Gynecologic, and Neonatal Nursing, 32*(4), 465-477.

Perla, L. (2002). Patient compliance and satisfaction with nursing care during delivery and recovery. *Journal of Nursing Care Quality, 16*(2), 60-66.

Pivarnik, J.M., & Rivera, J.M. (2002). Exercise in pregnancy. In S.B. Ransom, M.P. Dombrowski, M.I. Evans, & K.A. Ginsburg (Eds.), *Contemporary therapy in obstetrics and gynecology* (pp. 85-89). Philadelphia: Saunders.

Rapini, R.P., & Jordon, R.E. (2004). The skin and pregnancy. In R.K. Creasy & R. Resnik (Eds.), *Maternal-fetal medicine: Principles and practice* (5th ed., pp. 1201-1211). Philadelphia: Saunders.

Resnik, R. (2004). The puerperium. In R.K. Creasy & R. Resnik (Eds.), *Maternal-fetal medicine: principles and practice* (5th ed., pp. 165-168). Philadelphia: Saunders.

Ruchala, P.L. (2000). Teaching new mothers: Priorities of nurses and postpartum women. *Journal of Obstetric, Gynecologic, and Neonatal Nursing, 29*(3), 265-273.

Scoggin, J. (2004). Physical and psychological changes. In S. Mattson & J.E. Smith (Eds.), *Core curriculum for maternal-newborn nursing* (3rd ed., pp. 371-386). Philadelphia: Saunders.

Signorello, L.B., Harlow, B.L., Chekos, A.K., & Repke, J.T. (2001). Postpartum sexual functioning and its relationship to perineal trauma: A retrospective cohort study of primiparous women. *American Journal of Obstetrics & Gynecology, 184*(5), 881-890.

Simpson, K.R., & James, D.C. (2005). *Postpartum care.* White Plains, NY: March of Dimes.

Spellacy, C.E. (2001). Urinary incontinence in pregnancy and the puerperium. *Journal of Obstetric, Gynecologic, and Neonatal Nursing, 3*(6), 634-641.

Stark, M.A. (2000). Is it difficult to concentrate during the third trimester and postpartum? *Journal of Obstetric, Gynecologic, and Neonatal Nursing, 29*(4), 378-389.

Swenson, D.E. (2001). *Telephone triage for the obstetric patient.* Philadelphia: Saunders.

Swift, K., & Janke, J. (2003). Breast binding . . . is it all that it's wrapped up to be? *Journal of Obstetric, Gynecologic, and Neonatal Nursing, 32*(3), 332-339.

Troy, N.W. (2003). Is the significance of postpartum fatigue being overlooked in the lives of women? *MCN: American Journal of Maternal/Child Nursing, 28*(4), 252-257.

Werrbach, K., & Wroblewski, M. (2003). Self-administered pain medications: A practical approach in an OB/GYN setting. *AWHONN Lifelines, 7*(2), 132-138.

Wilkerson, N.N., & Shrock, P. (2000). Sexuality in the perinatal period. In F.H. Nichols & S.S. Humenick (Eds.), *Childbirth education: Practice, research, and theory* (2nd ed., pp. 48-65). Philadelphia: Saunders.

Zuspan, K. (2000). Control of postpartum pain. In F.P. Zuspan & E.J. Quilligan (Eds.), *Current therapy in obstetrics and gynecology* (5th ed., pp. 261-263). Philadelphia: Saunders.

Postpartum Psychosocial Adaptations

OBJECTIVES

After studying this chapter, you should be able to:

1. Explain the process of bonding and attachment, including maternal touch and verbal interactions.
2. Describe the progressive phases of maternal adaptation to childbirth and the stages of maternal role attainment.
3. Identify maternal concerns and the way they change over time.
4. Discuss the cause and manifestations of and the interventions related to postpartum blues.
5. Describe the processes of family adaptation to the birth of a baby.
6. Explain factors that affect family adaptation.
7. Discuss cultural influences on family adaptation.
8. Describe assessments and interventions related to postpartum psychosocial adaptations.
9. Discuss the need for additional care of the mother and infant after discharge from the birth facility.

Go to your Student CD-ROM for Review Questions keyed to these Objectives.

DEFINITIONS

Attachment Development of strong affectional ties as a result of interaction between an infant and a significant other.

Bonding Development of a strong emotional tie of a parent to a newborn; also called *claiming* or *binding-in*.

En Face Position that allows eye-to-eye contact between the newborn and a parent.

Engrossment Intense fascination and close face-to-face observation between the father and newborn.

Entrainment Newborn movement in rhythm with adult speech, particularly high-pitched tones, which are more easily heard.

Fingertipping First tactile (touch) experience between the mother and newborn in which the mother explores the infant's body, mainly with her fingertips.

Fourth Trimester First 12 weeks after birth; a time of transition for parents and siblings.

Letting-Go A phase of maternal adaptation that involves relinquishment of previous roles and assumption of a new role as a parent.

Postpartum Blues Temporary, self-limited period of tearfulness experienced by many new mothers beginning in the first week after childbirth.

Reciprocal Bonding Behaviors Repertoire of infant actions that promotes attachment between the parent and newborn.

Sibling Rivalry Feelings of jealousy and fear of replacement when a young child must share the attention of the parents with a newborn infant.

Taking-Hold Second phase of maternal adaptation during which the mother assumes control of her own care and initiates care of the infant.

Taking-In First phase of maternal adaptation during which the mother passively accepts care, comfort, and details about the newborn.

Perhaps no other event requires such rapid change in family structure and function as the birth of a baby. The mother progresses through restorative phases to replenish the energy lost during labor and childbirth and to gain confidence in her role as mother. Both the mother and the father begin the process of attachment with the newborn. Siblings must adapt to a new standing in the family structure and cope with feelings of jealousy and rivalry that may occur with the birth. Numerous factors such as previous experience, the availability of a strong support system, and culture influence the family's adaptation.

The role of maternity nurses includes not only the care of the mother-infant dyad but the well-being of the entire family, as well. Nurses are concerned with the family's adjustment to childbearing during the hospital stay and during the early weeks at home. The first 12 weeks, as the family makes the transition to parenthood and adapts to changes in the family structure after childbirth, are often called the *fourth trimester*.

THE PROCESS OF BECOMING ACQUAINTED

Nursing literature has described the way parents and newborns become acquainted and progress to develop feelings of love, concern, and deep devotion that last throughout life. The terms *bonding* and *attachment* are commonly used to describe the initial steps. Although the terms are sometimes used interchangeably, their meanings differ.

Bonding

The term *bonding* refers to the rapid initial attraction felt by parents soon after childbirth. It is unidirectional, from parent to child, and is enhanced when parents and infants are permitted to touch and interact during a so-called *sensitive period* extending through the first 30 to 60 minutes after birth. During this time the infant is in a quiet, alert state and seems to gaze directly at the parents (Figure 18-1).

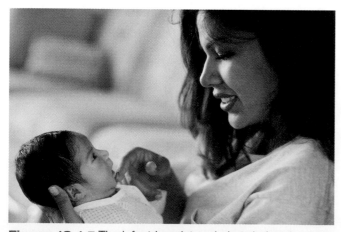

Figure 18-1 ■ The infant is quiet and alert during the initial sensitive period. The newborn gazes at the mother and responds to her voice and touch.

Nurses frequently delay procedures, such as instillation of prophylactic eye medication, administration of vitamin K injections, and measurements, that would interfere with this time, so that parents can focus on their newborn baby.

The concept of a sensitive period can be misinterpreted by parents and health care workers, who may believe it is the only time for the process of attachment to begin. Early and sustained contact between the parents and infant can enhance bonding and attachment. But if early contact between parent and infant is limited because of an obstetric emergency or neonatal illness, bonding and attachment can still occur at a later time.

Attachment

Attachment is the process by which an enduring bond between a parent and child is developed through pleasurable, satisfying interaction. The process begins in pregnancy and extends for many months after childbirth. The infant receives warmth, food, and security from the parent. The parent, usually the mother, accepts responsibility for the infant's care and places the child's needs above her own for years to come. In return, she receives enjoyment and establishes her identity as a mother. Both benefit from the formation of irreplaceable links that continue long after the child ceases to be dependent.

Attachment follows a progressive or developmental course that changes over time. It is rarely instantaneous. Attachment behaviors of inexperienced or first-time mothers do not differ significantly from those of experienced mothers (Mercer & Ferketich, 1994).

Attachment occurs through mutually satisfying experiences. Therefore if the newly delivered mother is in pain or physically exhausted, she needs pain relief and assistance so she is able to enjoy the early experiences with the baby.

Unlike bonding, attachment is reciprocal—it occurs in both directions between parent and infant. It is facilitated by positive feedback, either real or perceived, from the infant. Alert infants have a repertoire of responses called *reciprocal attachment behaviors*. An infant's grasp reflex around a parent's finger means "I love you" to the parent. These behaviors are the infant's part in the process of early attachment that progresses to lifelong, mutual devotion.

CRITICAL TO REMEMBER

Reciprocal Attachment Behaviors

Newborn infants have the ability to do the following:
- Make eye contact and engage in prolonged, intense, mutual gazing
- Move their eyes and attempt to "track" the parent's face
- Grasp and hold the parent's finger
- Move synchronously in response to rhythms and patterns of the parent's voice (called *entrainment*)
- Root, latch onto the breast, and suckle
- Be comforted by the parent's voice or touch

Maternal Touch

Maternal behavior, particularly maternal touch, changes rapidly as the mother progresses through a discovery phase with her infant. Initially the mother may not reach for the infant, but if the infant is placed in her arms, she holds the baby in an *en face* position with the infant's face in the same vertical plane as her own. When the infant is awake, the two engage in prolonged, mutual gazing (see Figure 18-1).

The mother needs time to get acquainted with the tiny stranger. She may gently explore the infant's face, fingers, and toes with her fingertips only. This exploration, called *fingertipping*, is common during the early minutes (Figure 18-2).

After fingertipping the infant, the mother begins to stroke the baby's chest and legs with the palm. Next, she uses her entire hand to enfold the infant and to bring her baby close to her body (Figure 18-3). She holds the newborn closer, strokes the baby's hair, presses her cheek against the infant's cheek, and finally feels comfortable enough to engage in a full range of consoling behaviors.

The mother next begins to identify specific features of the newborn: "Look at how bright his eyes are." Then she begins to relate features to family members: "He has his father's chin and nose" (Figure 18-4). This identification process has been termed *claiming* or *binding-in* (Rubin, 1977).

Verbal Behaviors

Verbal behaviors are important indicators of maternal attachment. Most mothers speak to the infant in a high-pitched voice. Although some mothers have called the baby by name since seeing it on an ultrasound scan during pregnancy, others begin by referring to the baby as "it," then use "he or she," and then progress to using the given name. "I can't believe it's here" rapidly becomes "Michele is such a good baby." Verbal behaviors may provide clues to a mother's early psychological relationship with her infant. Nurses observe interactions of mothers and their infants and, if necessary, teach and model interactions that foster early attachment between them.

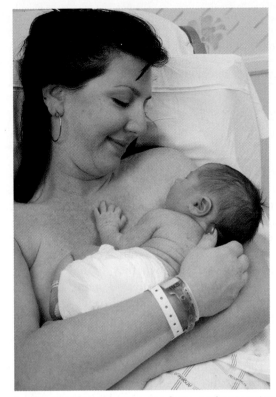

Figure 18-3 ■ Mothers progress from exploratory touching to enfolding the infant. Their pleasure is enhanced by skin-to-skin contact.

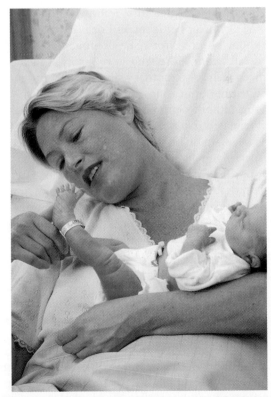

Figure 18-4 ■ During the binding-in or claiming process the mother identifies her baby's specific features and relates them to other family members. This mother states, "His long toes are exactly like mine."

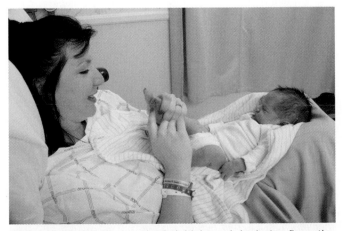

Figure 18-2 ■ The mother's initial touch includes fingertipping, whereby she becomes acquainted with her infant by touching only with her fingertips.

1. How do bonding and attachment differ?
2. How does maternal touch change over time?
3. How does verbal interaction change over time?

THE PROCESS OF MATERNAL ADAPTATION

Puerperal Phases

In the early 1960s Rubin identified restorative phases that the mother must go through to replenish the energy lost during labor and attain comfort in the role of mother. The puerperal phases are called *taking-in, taking-hold,* and *letting-go* and provide one method to observe progressive change in maternal behavior. Although they should not be used as strict guidelines for maternal assessment, the phases can help the nurse anticipate maternal needs and intervene to meet those needs.

TAKING-IN PHASE

During the taking-in phase the mother is focused primarily on her own need for fluid, food, and sleep. Inexperienced nurses may be puzzled by the mother's passive, dependent behavior as she receives, or takes in, attention and physical care. She also takes in every detail of the neonate but seems content to allow others to make decisions.

A major task for the mother during this time is to integrate her birth experience into reality. To do this she recounts the details of her labor and delivery many times on the telephone or for visitors. She attempts to piece together all the details from those who were involved in the birth. This process helps the mother realize that the pregnancy is over and the newborn is now a separate individual.

Although Rubin believed that the taking-in phase lasts for approximately 2 days, it probably lasts a day or less today. The taking-in phase may be prolonged when a cesarean birth, especially in an emergency, has been necessary. These women may have difficulty assimilating the unfamiliar and intrusive procedures that occurred in rapid succession and may have negative perceptions of the birth experience. Women who have had cesarean births need continued attention and sensitive care that takes into account their physical and psychological needs.

TAKING-HOLD PHASE

The mother becomes more independent during the taking-hold phase. She exhibits concern about managing her own body functions and assumes responsibility for her own care. When she feels more comfortable and in control of her body, she shifts her attention from her own needs to the performance of the infant. She compares her infant with other infants to validate wellness and wholeness. She welcomes information about the wide variety of behaviors exhibited by newborns.

During the taking-hold phase, the mother may verbalize much anxiety about her competence as a mother. She may compare her caretaking skills unfavorably with those of the nurse.

> ■ Nurses must be careful not to assume the mothering role, but instead should allow the mother to perform as much of the caretaking as possible and should praise each attempt, even if the mother's early care is awkwardly performed.

The taking-hold phase, which extends over several days, has been called the "teachable, reachable, referable moment." Nurses who provide home or clinic care can take advantage of this ideal time to review previously taught material and provide additional instructions and demonstrations.

LETTING-GO PHASE

The letting-go phase is a time of relinquishment for the mother and often for the father. If this child is their first, the couple must give up their previous role as a childless couple and acknowledge the loss of their lifestyle. Many mothers also must give up idealized expectations of the birth experience. For example, they may have planned to have a vaginal birth with minimal or no anesthesia, but instead they required a cesarean birth.

In addition, some mothers and fathers are disappointed in the size, gender, and characteristics of the infant who does not "match up" with the fantasy baby of pregnancy. They must relinquish the infant of their fantasies and accept the real infant.

🔊 **THERAPEUTIC** COMMUNICATIONS

Anxiety about Caretaking Skills

Liz Jackson is a nurse in the postpartum unit. When she enters a room she finds Claire Bradley, a new mother, in tears.

Claire (crying): I can't do anything right. The pediatrician just asked me a bunch of questions, and I couldn't answer any of them.

Liz: Actually, you've been doing a lot right, but it's upsetting when you feel you don't have all the answers. *(Offering reassurance and acknowledging feelings.)*

Claire: He just fired the questions at me and I couldn't think that fast!

Liz: You feel that you're not measuring up because you couldn't answer the questions. *(Paraphrasing and focusing on Claire's feelings.)*

Claire: Well, I want to be a good mother, but I'm so worried that I won't know what to do.

Liz: You have some concerns. *(Reflecting feelings without leading.)*

Claire: There's just so much to taking care of a baby. I don't know where to start.

Liz: It can be overwhelming at first. Which areas worry you most? *(Reflecting feelings and inviting the mother to describe specific concerns. By allowing Claire to express her feelings, Liz has helped dissipate the feelings and set the stage for effective teaching.)*

These losses often provoke subtle feelings of grief that may be unexamined or unacknowledged. Both parents may benefit, however, if given the opportunity to talk about unexpected feelings and realize that these feelings are common. If the mother is very young or the pregnancy was unplanned, the feelings of loss and grief may be acute.

Maternal Role Attainment

Role attainment is a process by which the mother achieves confidence in her ability to care for her infant and becomes comfortable with her identity as a mother. The process begins during pregnancy and continues for several months after childbirth.

The transition to the maternal or paternal role includes four stages (Mercer, 1995b):

1. The anticipatory stage begins during the pregnancy when pregnant women choose a physician or nurse-midwife and a location for the infant's birth. Women often attend childbirth classes to be prepared and have some control over the birth experience. They seek out role models to help them learn the role of a mother.

2. The formal stage begins with the birth of the infant and continues for approximately 4 to 6 weeks (Mercer, 1995a). During this stage, behaviors are largely guided by others such as health professionals, close friends, and parents. A major task during this stage is for parents to become acquainted with their infants so that they can mesh their caregiving with cues from their infants.

3. The informal stage may overlap the formal stage. It begins once the woman has learned appropriate responses to her infant's cues and signals. The mother begins to respond according to the unique needs of the infant and develops the maternal role that fits her rather than following the directives of textbooks or health professionals.

4. The personal stage is attained when the woman feels a sense of harmony in the role, enjoys the infant, sees the infant as a central person in her life, and has internalized the parental role. The mother or father accepts the role of parent and feels comfortable in this role. The range of time for achieving the parental role is highly variable, with some parents reaching that point in the first month and others taking much longer.

Heading toward a New Normal

Martell (2001) provides another view of early postpartum changes with "Heading toward a New Normal" as the theme. This view also has three phases as the woman reorganizes her life as a mother. Although the phases have distinctive characteristics, they are continuous rather than separate.

APPRECIATING THE BODY

This phase centers on the way the woman feels physically. She must cope with discomfort such as nipple and perineal pain. Her sleep is disrupted by excitement, hospital routines, and her physical discomfort, leaving her fatigued. Changes in her body function as she begins lactation and the differences in her appearance make her more aware of her physical self. The phase also involves dealing with emotional lability and changes in the way women think and retain information.

SETTLING-IN

Settling-in involves becoming competent, developing confidence, and accommodating and integrating the infant into the parents' lives. A mother's desire to settle into her own environment may lead her to leave the hospital as soon as possible. During this phase a mother becomes more secure with her infant. As she gradually gains competence, her reliance on past methods of solving problems relaxes into comfort with the tasks of newborn care.

A mother may have little confidence in her own parenting abilities just after the birth and is glad to have help available. When immediate help is no longer available because her partner returns to work or her mother leaves, the new mother is concerned about being able to care for her baby alone. Confidence builds as the infant gains weight and the mother is able to soothe and care for the infant without help from others.

A mother must accommodate her needs and activities to meet the needs of the infant. After a period of adjustment, some mothers find ways to integrate the infant into their usual activities with only minor changes.

BECOMING A NEW FAMILY

As women work toward becoming part of a new family, they modify relationships with their partners and other family members and develop new routines to include the infant. Although they are grateful for help from others, they are glad to be on their own and enjoy spending time alone with their newly developed family.

Redefined Roles

The mother is particularly concerned about redefining roles and focuses on maintaining a strong, adaptive relationship with her partner. She observes him carefully for any change in behavior and is acutely sensitive to his interaction with the infant. From the father's perspective, anxieties about succeeding in his new role put added pressure on the family. Conflicting demands between work and home, feelings of exclusion, and concerns about his relationship with his partner present additional challenges.

The new parents may need to agree on a division of tasks and responsibilities that was not necessary before the birth of the infant. This process is accomplished quickly and with very little discord in some families. Role assignment in other families is much less flexible, and any change can be a source of tension and frustration.

Although nurses are not actively involved in redefining family roles, they can use their communication skills to assist the family in expressing their feelings and concerns so that the changes can be accomplished with minimum stress.

NURSING CARE PLAN 18-1 Adaptation of the Working Mother

ASSESSMENT: Rebecca Sanders, a 30-year-old single mother, gave birth to a baby boy, Derrek, by cesarean delivery 5 days ago. Breastfeeding is going well. During her visit at a nurse-managed postpartum clinic, Rebecca discusses her need to return to work as a sales executive in 6 weeks. She states that she does not want to leave the baby with someone else while she works. "I've always wanted to stay home when I had a baby, but it's impossible. How can I be a mother and work full time?"

NURSING DIAGNOSIS: Anticipatory Grieving related to inability to perform role of mother as she wishes because of the need to return to full-time employment

---

CRITICAL THINKING: *Grieving is related to loss. What has Rebecca lost, or what must she give up?*

ANSWER: *Rebecca must give up her idealized picture of motherhood. She also must give up mothering tasks and time with the infant to another caregiver. She will have to modify her self-concept based on the perception of these losses.*

GOALS/EXPECTED OUTCOMES: Rebecca will:
1. Describe the concerns and feelings that result from her need to leave her infant with a secondary caregiver by (specific date).
2. Verbalize plans to achieve maximal satisfaction in her role as mother by the time she returns to work.

INTERVENTION	RATIONALE
1. Allow Rebecca to describe her perception of her role as a mother and express concerns about the way employment will interfere with her ability to fulfill this role.	1. Role conflict, stress, and grief can result when a mother who envisions her role as the primary caregiver must leave the infant with another caregiver and return to her job.
2. Suggest free expression of feelings of anxiety, guilt, and jealousy to significant others and the care provider who is selected.	2. Candid expression of feelings helps to resolve them and allows for a discussion of measures that will help in overcoming the intense feelings that cause conflict.
3. Acknowledge the feelings Rebecca expresses, and reassure her that the feelings are common.	3. Knowledge that the feelings are not trivial and are experienced by others reinforces their validity and importance.

4. Help Rebecca develop a schedule that allows her maximal time with the infant:
  a. Make a list of errands and supplies needed to avoid frequent stops that delay getting home from work.
  b. Double the recipe when cooking, and freeze half for future use.
  c. Pick up nutritious takeout meals to avoid cooking each evening.
  d. Purchase nutritious prepackaged frozen meals to have available when needed.
  e. Schedule appointments on the same day when possible.
  f. Include the baby in daily walks, exercise, and social visits.
	4. Feelings of frustration and stress can be alleviated if the mother has a plan that allows her long periods of uninterrupted time with the infant.

5. Recommend that Rebecca allow 30 to 45 minutes when she first gets home to hold the infant. Delay all other activities until this need is satisfied for both mother and infant.	5. Time is needed to make the transition between work and home. It helps to reestablish feelings of closeness, comfort, and attachment.
6. Suggest that Rebecca delay her return to employment, if possible, until the infant is at least 16 weeks old.	6. By 16 weeks most infants are able to sleep through the night, reducing the sleep deprivation that often adds to the stress of working and infant care.
7. Recommend that Rebecca investigate several daycare providers before choosing. She should check references, make unannounced visits, see required licenses and certification, discuss the number and ages of children cared for and the daily schedule, determine the provider's philosophy of infant care, determine if the care provider is trained in emergency measures, and know what emergency plans are in place.	7. A great deal of stress is eliminated if parents feel confident that a competent and nurturing daycare provider has been found.
8. Suggest that Rebecca leave the infant with the chosen daycare provider for 2 to 3 days before full-time employment is resumed.	8. Allowing both mother and infant to "practice separating" while their schedules are still somewhat flexible helps ease the transition.
9. Recommend that Rebecca pump her breasts and feed the infant by bottle at least once per day in the week or two before returning to work.	9. Becoming proficient at pumping the breasts and introducing the infant to bottle feeding prepares both the mother and infant for all-day separation.

EVALUATION: Rebecca freely expressed her feelings of guilt, anxiety, and concern about leaving her infant. She made a plan to investigate daycare in her area and discussed plans to reorganize her work and social schedule so that she can spend more time with her son.

Role Conflict

Role conflict occurs when a person's perception of role responsibilities differs significantly from reality. For example, if the mother perceives her responsibility as providing most of the care and comfort for the infant, but reality dictates that she must place the infant with another caregiver and return to full-time employment, role conflict may occur. In the United States 53.7% of women with children under 1 year of age are employed (U.S. Department of Labor, 2004).

Mothers often report that it took them 3 to 6 months to feel they really knew their infants (Nelson, 2003). If possible, women should put off employment until they are comfortable in the parenting role and know the infant's unique needs.

Primiparas often fail to realize how strong their attachment to the infant will be and do not recognize how difficult it will be for them to leave the infant to return to work (Nelson, 2003). Many mothers experience feelings of guilt for leaving their infant and experience intense "separation grief" when they first leave the infant with a caregiver. Some report feeling jealous of the caregiver, whom they fear will supplant them in the infant's affection.

One study of women who returned to work shortly after giving birth found that women experienced role overload. This involved difficulty with work and family strains and guilt about leaving the infant. In addition, there were stressors involving competing demands and concerns about childcare, finances, and emotional issues (Nichols & Roux, 2004).

The nurse may help by acknowledging these feelings and reassuring the mother that her emotions are normal. Anticipatory guidance from the nurse is important. The mother needs time to reestablish feelings of closeness when she comes home from work, and she needs to develop a schedule that allows maximum time with the infant when she is at home. She may have to negotiate with another family member to take over some of the household tasks until she feels more comfortable with the situation (Nursing Care Plan 18-1).

Major Maternal Concerns

Nurses plan follow-up care based on the knowledge that mothers' major concerns change over time after childbirth. As the woman gains confidence in her ability to care for the infant and her physical discomfort decreases, emotional concerns related to the self become more intense. Body image and the experience of postpartum blues are particularly important.

BODY IMAGE

Women are very concerned about regaining their normal figures. Some mothers have unrealistic expectations about weight loss and the time it takes for the body to regain its nonpregnant shape. Nurses must emphasize that weight loss should be gradual and that about 6 to 12 months is usually required to lose most weight gained during pregnancy. Rigid

THERAPEUTIC COMMUNICATIONS

Body Image

Mary Kay Beauchamp gave birth to a baby boy 48 hours ago. Yvonne Meyer is a nurse reviewing self-care measures before Mary Kay's discharge from the birth facility.

Mary Kay: Look at me! I still look pregnant, and my husband calls me Tubby.

Yvonne: You were looking forward to your abdomen being flat after the baby was born.

This clarifies the woman's concern by reflecting content.

Mary Kay: Well, I never had a big belly before. I thought it would all go away after I had the baby. I can't believe I look this fat.

Yvonne: Remember, it took 9 months for those muscles to stretch. You can't expect them to snap back in a few days.

This blocks communication by ignoring the feeling expressed. A more helpful response would be to acknowledge Mary Kay's distress and to delay giving information until feelings have been expressed. For example: "How disappointing for you! If you like, we can discuss some exercises that will help."

restriction of calories can lead to depleted energy and decreased immunity. A diet that meets the mother's needs should be discussed by the nurse (see Chapter 9).

In addition, nurses should teach the importance of safe activities such as walking and graduated exercises to regain muscle tone. Some birth facilities offer classes for postpartum mothers that include exercise and nutrition, as well as the opportunity to share concerns with other postpartum women. Mothers should seek the advice of a health care professional before initiating a rigorous exercise program (see Chapter 17).

POSTPARTUM BLUES

Mild depression, also known as *postpartum blues, baby blues,* or *maternity blues,* is a frequently expressed concern. This mild, transient condition affects more than 70% of U.S. women who have given birth (American Academy of Pediatrics & American College of Obstetricians and Gynecologists, 2002). The condition begins in the first week and usually lasts no longer than 2 weeks. It is characterized by insomnia, irritability, fatigue, tearfulness, mood instability, and anxiety. The symptoms are usually unrelated to events, and the condition does not seriously affect the ability of the mother to care for the infant.

Although the direct cause is unknown, postpartum blues may be a result of the emotional letdown that occurs after birth, postpartum discomforts, fatigue, anxiety about her ability to care for the infant, and concern about her attractiveness (Cunningham et al., 2005). Hormonal fluctuations are often considered to be the source of the problem, but they have not been proven to be a cause.

Although postpartum blues is self-limiting, mothers benefit greatly when empathy and support are freely given by the family and the health care team. Because the condition is so common in postpartum women, caregivers or family members may not be as empathetic as they would be for a condition deemed more serious. Yet, the mother needs adequate attention to move through this period. She should be encouraged to rest, take some time for herself, and discuss her feelings. In addition, reassurance should be given that such feelings are normal and generally last less than 2 weeks. Complementary or alternative therapy such as therapeutic touch helps some women feel more calm and relaxed during the early weeks after birth (Kieman, 2002).

Postpartum blues must be distinguished from postpartum depression and postpartum psychosis, which are disabling conditions and require therapeutic management for full recovery (Chapter 28). Nurses should teach family and the woman to call the health care provider if depression becomes severe or lasts longer than 2 weeks or if she is unable to cope with daily life.

✔ CHECK YOUR READING

4. How do maternal behaviors in the taking-in phase differ from those in the taking-hold phase?
5. What does the mother (and the father) relinquish in the letting-go phase?
6. How do the parents progress through the stages of role attainment?
7. What are the phases of "heading toward a new normal"?
8. What causes postpartum blues? How can nurses intervene for this common emotional response?

THE PROCESS OF FAMILY ADAPTATION

The birth of an infant requires the reorganization of roles and relationships within the family. The previously childless couple now must integrate a new member into the family unit. Fathers learn new skills and often adjust to new roles. Siblings must adapt to a new standing in the family structure. Expectations and involvement of grandparents vary widely.

Fathers

The father's developing bond with his newborn is facilitated by engrossment. Engrossment is characterized by intense interest in how the infant looks and responds, along with a desire to touch and hold the baby. Many fathers comment on the baby's distinctive features and view the baby as perfect. They experience strong attraction to the infant and express elation after the baby's birth. Attachment behaviors of the father increase when the infant is awake, makes eye contact, and responds to the father's voice (Figure 18-5).

Many fathers eagerly look forward to co-parenting with their mates. However, they may lack confidence in providing infant care and are sensitive to exclusion from instructions and demonstrations of infant care. They may feel that others see their role only as providing support to the mother. The nurse can assist the new father by involving him in child care activities soon after birth to help him feel more confident and competent (Matteson, 2001).

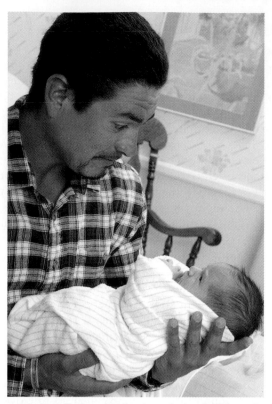

Figure 18-5 ■ Fathers' behaviors during initial contact with their infants often correspond to maternal behaviors. The intense fascination that fathers exhibit is called *engrossment*. Note eye-to-eye contact between the father and infant.

Some fathers have difficulty adapting to the changes in role the birth brings. Those with unsteady or part-time jobs and those whose relationship with the mother is of shorter length or is less satisfactory are more likely to experience distress than those with steady jobs and longer relationships both during and after pregnancy. Most fathers have resolved these issues by the time of the birth. However, fathers who experience more distress in the postpartum period may have underestimated the changes that would occur and must begin to cope with them after the birth (Buist, Morse, & Durkin, 2003).

Although fathers may attend prenatal classes about parenting, they often do not know what to expect from infants and need more information about normal growth and development during infancy. A review of information about child care presented in the prenatal period is helpful after the baby is born, when the information is more relevant and the father is ready to learn.

The additional work involved in care of a newborn may be a source of concern for both mothers and fathers. One study showed that fathers maintained the same level of functioning in child care and household tasks as they had before the birth, but did not increase their participation even though the need was greater (McVeigh, Baafi, & Williamson, 2002). Parents should be encouraged to negotiate the division of household chores during pregnancy or shortly after delivery.

Siblings

Siblings' response to the birth of a new brother or sister depends on their age and developmental level. Toddlers usually are not completely aware of the impending birth. They may view the infant as competition or may fear that they will be replaced in the parents' affection. Negative behaviors may indicate the degree of stress experienced by the youngster. These behaviors include sleep problems, an increase in attention-seeking efforts, and regression to more infantile behaviors such as renewed bed-wetting and thumbsucking. Some toddlers exhibit hostile behaviors toward the mother, particularly when she holds or feeds the newborn. These behaviors are manifestations of the jealousy and frustration that young children feel as they observe the mother's attention being given to another. Parents must find opportunities to affirm their continued love and affection for the very vulnerable sibling.

Preschool siblings may engage in more looking than touching. Most spend at least some time in proximity to the infant and talk to the mother about the infant (Figure 18-6). Older children may adapt more easily. All siblings need extra attention from the parents and reassurance that they are loved and important. Sibling classes, available in many agencies, may help ease the transition (see Chapter 11). Siblings often visit the mother and new baby in the birth agency.

At home a relaxed approach without time constraints may facilitate interactions between young children and infants. Special care must be taken by the parents, visitors, and nurses to pay as much attention to the sibling as to the new baby. Parents can emphasize the advantages of being an older sibling and can allow siblings to participate in age-appropriate aspects of infant care.

Grandparents

The involvement of grandparents with grandchildren depends on many factors. One of the most important is proximity. Grandparents who live near the child frequently develop strong attachment that evolves into unconditional love and a special relationship that brings joy to the grandparents and an added sense of security to the grandchildren.

When grandparents live many miles from grandchildren and have sporadic contact, forming a close attachment is more difficult. Grandparents must try to devise ways to foster a relationship with grandchildren they seldom see.

Expectations of the role of grandparents are also a factor in the adaptation of the grandparents to the birth of a grandchild. Many grandparents strive to be fully involved in the care and upbringing of the child, but others desire less involvement. The degree of grandparent involvement may cause some conflict with parents, or it may be a comfortable arrangement for both families.

Grandparents often are a major part of the support system that new parents need. Grandmothers in particular provide assistance with household tasks and infant care, which allows the mother to recover from childbirth and make the transition to parenthood. Grandfathers who were very busy providing for their own children may enjoy the opportunity to nurture their grandchildren (Figure 18-7).

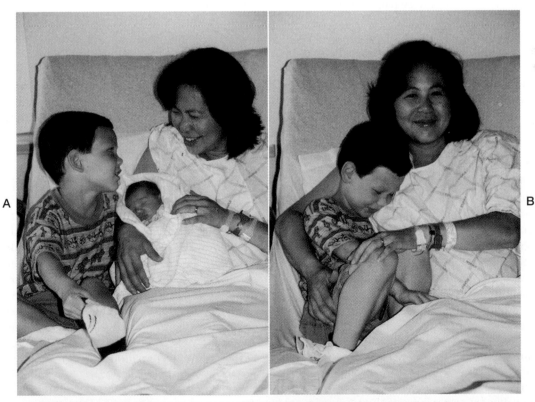

Figure 18-6 ■ **A,** Although they may hesitate to touch the infant, children often want to be close. **B,** This boy's relief and joy are obvious as he reclaims a favorite spot.

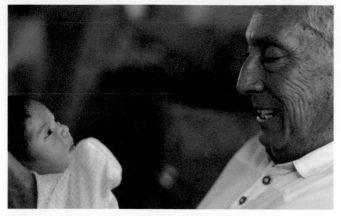

Figure 18-7 ■ Grandfathers may develop strong bonds with grandchildren.

FACTORS THAT AFFECT FAMILY ADAPTATION

Numerous factors influence the family's adjustment. Some, such as discomfort and chronic fatigue, can be anticipated because they are so common. Additional factors include knowledge of infant needs, expectations of the infant, previous experience, age of the parents, and temperaments of the mother and infant. Unanticipated events such as cesarean birth, birth of a preterm or ill infant, and birth of more than one infant also affect the ease and speed with which the family adjusts.

Discomfort and Fatigue

Normally, discomforts such as perineal pain and afterpains resolve within the first days after the birth. However, discomfort may make it difficult to focus on the needs of the newborn. Fatigue often remains a problem during the first few weeks and months, when the infant's schedule is erratic and the chance for uninterrupted sleep is minimal. When the infant begins to sleep through the night (at about 16 weeks), the parents usually can reestablish familiar patterns, and fatigue often becomes less of a factor.

Knowledge of Infant Needs

Parents experience powerful feelings of protectiveness when they discover that they can console their infant and the infant responds to their care. First-time parents, who are unsure of how to care for a newborn, become very anxious if they are unable to console a crying infant. In addition, many are concerned about feeding and specific procedures such as care of the umbilical cord and circumcision. Breastfeeding benefits both the mother and the infant but may add to the stress initially experienced by parents who lack sufficient knowledge and support (see Chapter 22 for information on breastfeeding and Chapter 23 for information on early parenting).

Some parents have concerns about spoiling the infant. They may believe that responding each time the infant cries causes the child to cry to get attention. It may be necessary to teach parents that infants cry to indicate hunger, cold, wetness, and a need for cuddling or gentle stimulation and that responding to crying does not spoil the child. Suggest-

ing a variety of methods to cope with crying may be helpful. Prompt, gentle response to crying helps the infant develop trust in the world as a safe, secure place. Trust is a basic developmental task of infancy and depends on the child's learning that caregivers respond consistently and gently.

Previous Experience

Previous experience with newborns also may affect family adjustment. Multiparas are more comfortable with infants and exhibit attachment behaviors earlier than primiparas, who may spend many more hours in the early discovery phase of attachment. Because they know what to expect, multiparas are more relaxed in caring for the new baby but have to establish new routines that fit the expanded family. The mother may find it more difficult to find time alone with her partner. She may need more help from family and friends than the primipara because of the lack of sleep and the time and energy involved in meeting the needs of all family members (O'Reilly, 2004). Women with one or more other children may need encouragement to take time for themselves and time alone with their partner. Support groups for multiparas may be helpful.

Mothers who have had a long interval between pregnancies may have forgotten much of the teaching received with the first birth and may need more instruction. Those who previously gave birth to infants with anomalies or infants that did not survive may need more time to feel comfortable with this infant.

Expectations for the Newborn

Unrealistic expectations of the infant also may influence adjustment. Parents who have little experience with newborns may be disappointed at the newborn's appearance. They are unprepared for the normal newborn characteristics such as cranial molding, blotchy skin, and newborn rash. Nurses must teach normal growth and development and assist parents in working through misconceptions about normal infant behavior. For instance, the capacity of an infant's stomach is small, and the infant must be fed frequently. Also, infants are neurologically unable to sleep through the night during the early weeks. Increasing the time the mother spends with the infant during the postpartum stay provides extra opportunities for her to gain comfort with the physical characteristics as well as learning infant care when a nurse is available to help her.

Some mothers may be very disappointed in the gender of their infants or sense that their partners are disappointed. These feelings must be acknowledged and resolved before attachment can take place. For example, a mother of four sons might be so disappointed that the fifth child is a boy that she cries and refuses to pick out a boy's name at first. Later, when she holds the baby and begins to observe differences between this infant and her other sons, she can begin her discovery period with this unique child.

Maternal Age

Adjustment to parenthood is a challenge for the teenager who has not achieved a strong sense of her own identity. In general, adolescents tend to talk less, respond less, appear more passive, and sometimes appear less affectionate with their children than older parents. They need special assistance to develop necessary parenting skills that promote optimal development of the infant (see Chapter 24).

Maternal Temperament

Maternal personality traits greatly influence attachment. Mothers who are calm, secure in their abilities to learn, and free from unnecessary anxiety adjust more easily to the demands of motherhood. Conversely, mothers who are excitable, insecure, and anxious have more difficulty.

Temperament of the Infant

The infant's temperament also affects the mother's adjustment. Infants who are calm, are easily consoled, and enjoy cuddling increase parental confidence and feelings of competence. Conversely, irritable infants who are difficult to console and do not respond to cuddling increase parental frustration and interfere with attachment.

Availability of a Strong Support System

A strong, consistent support system is a major factor in the adjustment of the new mother. Friends and relatives who are parents can provide role modeling that is particularly important to first-time mothers. They can also provide encouragement, praise, and reassurance that she is a good mother. That others see the baby as special and demonstrate love and affection is very important to the new mother. Support may be needed for an extended period of time after childbirth. In addition, the mother needs practical assistance with household tasks such as meal preparation, laundry, and shopping.

Postpartum support groups are often available and can help the mother with early concerns of this period. They provide an opportunity for women to share their experiences with others who are having similar experiences. Some groups are focused on breastfeeding or exercise, but others simply provide an opportunity for interacting with other new mothers. Fathers may be included at all meetings or occasionally.

Unanticipated Events

CESAREAN BIRTH

A cesarean birth, especially one that was not anticipated, can make parental adjustment more difficult. Consequences of birth by cesarean include a longer recovery time for the mother, additional discomfort, increased stress for the family, and possible financial strain. The mother's need for recovery and attachment with her newborn must be considered in planning nursing care.

PRETERM OR ILL INFANT

Birth of a preterm or ill infant results in additional concerns about the condition of the infant. Prolonged separation of parents and child may be necessary. Although attachment can occur in these situations, the separation may delay the process and create stress on the normally functioning family. (See Chapter 29.)

BIRTH OF MULTIPLE INFANTS

Even when parents know during pregnancy that more than one baby will be born, problems of attachment may occur. Parents attach to each infant separately as they get to know the infant's unique characteristics. Nurses must help the parents relate to each infant as an individual rather than part of a unit by pointing out the individual responses and characteristics of each infant. Arranging time for the parents to interact with each child alone, especially in the early, getting-acquainted period, is important.

Multiple birth often follows a high-risk pregnancy in which the mother was confined to restricted activity or bed rest. There may have been one or more hospitalizations for preterm labor, and the infants may have been born prematurely and have health problems. This often results in financial strain, because the mother had to stop work earlier than expected and because expenses associated with the birth and in the future are higher. In addition, birth of more than one infant makes family relationships more complex, especially if there are other children.

Early, frequent contacts or rooming-in helps the parents gain confidence in caretaking and facilitates the attachment process. Mothers may be overwhelmed at the prospect of breastfeeding more than one infant. They need reassurance that they will produce an ample supply of milk for each infant because supply increases with demand (see Nursing Care Plan 18-2 and Chapter 22 for information regarding breastfeeding after multiple birth).

✔ CHECK YOUR READING

9. What does a father mean when he says he feels "out of place"?
10. What feelings may siblings experience when a new baby is born into the family?
11. How does the birth of multiple infants affect parental attachment?

🔲 CRITICAL TO REMEMBER

Factors That Affect Adaptation

- Lingering discomfort or pain
- Chronic fatigue
- Knowledge of infant needs
- Available support system
- Expectations of the newborn
- Previous experience with infants
- Maternal temperament
- Infant characteristics
- Unanticipated events: cesarean birth, preterm or ill infant, or birth of more than one infant (such as twins or triplets)

NURSING CARE PLAN 18-2 Adaptation to the Birth of Twins

ASSESSMENT: Maureen Parry, a 32-year-old primipara, gave birth to twin girls 22 hours ago. Her labor began at 39 weeks, and she delivered vaginally.

Both she and her husband are inexperienced in caring for infants. They attended breastfeeding and parenting classes during her pregnancy. Both infants are in the room, and she moves anxiously from one to the other. She has examined both infants but has not had individual time with each infant. She touches the infants cautiously and asks, "How in the world will I be able to take care of two babies?"

NURSING DIAGNOSIS: Risk for Altered Parent-Infant Attachment related to inadequate time with individual infants and lack of confidence in ability to provide care for two infants

CRITICAL THINKING: What data (behaviors) led to this diagnosis? What other data would confirm the diagnosis?

ANSWER: Time to learn an infant's characteristics is necessary for attachment. Maureen has not had time with each child individually. Observing the way she touches and interacts verbally with each child and noting that names have not been selected might confirm the diagnosis.

GOALS/EXPECTED OUTCOMES: Maureen will:
1. Demonstrate progressive bonding behaviors with each infant before discharge.
2. Collaborate with nursing staff and her husband to devise a plan for caring for the infants during the early weeks at home.
3. Verbalize increased confidence in her ability to care for the infants before discharge.

INTERVENTION	RATIONALE
1. Promote bonding and attachment with individual infants by arranging separate time with each infant and pointing out the unique characteristics of each child.	1. Parents attach more easily to one infant at a time. They must go through the getting-acquainted phases separately.
2. Make sure that the parents have contact with the infant who is awake and responsive.	2. The infant must respond to the parent by some signal, such as eye contact or gazing, for attachment to occur.
3. Foster a relaxed atmosphere that permits unlimited contact between the parents and twins. Model behaviors such as holding, consoling, and talking to the infants.	3. A relaxed atmosphere and prolonged contact with the twins enhance interaction that promotes bonding. Modeling is a very effective teaching strategy for demonstrating appropriate interactions.
4. Encourage participation in infant care. Demonstrate infant care, and praise all maternal efforts to provide care.	4. Caring for the infant or successfully consoling a crying infant elicits feelings of nurturing and greatly increases feelings of confidence and competence.

5. Assist Maureen in making a plan for caring for the twins.
  a. Provide instruction on breastfeeding twins and refer parents to a lactation consultant for continuing support.
  b. Suggest that the parents keep a record of care for each baby for the first few days at home so that they do not become confused.
  c. Reassure parents that a daily bath for the infants is unnecessary. Suggest bathing every other day because the face, neck, and diaper area are bathed as necessary.
	5. During the time that breastfeeding is being established, the mother needs information and encouragement. Collaborating on a plan for providing and recording care increases the parents' confidence in their ability to care for the infants. This is particularly true when the parents receive reassurance that care does not have to be on a strict schedule.

6. Emphasize the importance of obtaining adequate rest. Suggest that the mother sleep when the infants sleep and the parents take turns caring for the infants. Recommend that they accept assistance with household tasks from family and friends so that they can concentrate on care of the twins.	6. Sleep deprivation and chronic fatigue can interfere with the joys of parenting unless the parents anticipate the problem and make plans to deal with it.

EVALUATION: Maureen went from fingertipping to enfolding her baby girls and selected names for them. By discharge on the second postpartum day she stated she was feeling more confident with breastfeeding and caring for the infants but would need continued help. Both parents participated in infant care and identified family members who would assist them during the early weeks at home.

CULTURAL INFLUENCES ON ADAPTATION

An important goal of nursing practice in the postpartum period is to provide nursing care that is culture specific; that is, it fits the health beliefs, values, and practices of each client. This is difficult because of the wide ethnic diversity in countries such as the United States and Canada. A major challenge for nurses is to be aware of cultural beliefs and acknowledge their importance in family adaptation. The postpartum period often is thought to be a time of vulnerability for the woman and infant (Mattson, 2004).

NURSING CARE PLAN 18-2   Adaptation to the Birth of Twins—cont'd

ASSESSMENT: During discharge teaching, Maureen states that she does not work outside the home and always has assumed total responsibility for household tasks. She reveals that a perfectly maintained home is important to her and especially to her husband. She wonders about his possible reaction to the disruption that the twins will create.

NURSING DIAGNOSIS: Risk for Altered Family Processes related to the impact of the twins on family functioning

GOALS/EXPECTED OUTCOMES: The couple will:
1. Share concerns with each other and identify family strengths by (specific date).
2. Identify measures that reduce stress and promote family adjustment to the birth of twins by discharge.
3. Renegotiate responsibilities as necessary during the first few weeks at home.

INTERVENTION	RATIONALE
1. Determine whether Maureen has shared her concerns with her husband. If she has not, suggest that she tell him she is worried about the effect of the twins on their normal life.	1. Open communication is the first step in identifying stressors and clarifying feelings.
2. Discuss what family members or others might do to help. Attempt to determine overlooked resources, such as community resources or the ability to afford hired help with the housework for a few weeks.	2. Many families develop a higher level of functioning during times of stress, and individual members participate actively. Families often overlook community resources such as neighbors and friends.
3. Assist the family in identifying measures to reduce stress that may occur when family patterns are disrupted: a. Recommend simple meals that are easy to prepare and use of disposable dishes for a few weeks. b. Emphasize the importance of good nutrition and daily exercise. c. Review measures to obtain rest, but point out that fatigue is likely to persist until the twins sleep through the night. d. Recommend that both parents continue to participate in activities that provide recreation and relaxation, both together and separately.	3. During times of stress many parents overlook the benefits of good nutrition, exercise, and recreation. Even short periods of recreation can refresh spirits and replenish energy.
4. Suggest that the couple negotiate sharing household tasks such as meal preparation during the first few weeks, even though this is not part of their usual roles.	4. Sharing tasks reduces fatigue and helps prevent frustration and arguments during this time of stress.
5. Recommend that the couple negotiate child care activities so that both parents are involved in the day-to-day care as much as possible.	5. When both parents are involved in child care, they co-parent more effectively. Continued shared responsibility for the twins provides each parent with individual time with the infants. It also reduces fatigue.
6. Refer Maureen to groups for parents of multiples. Provide her with local phone numbers and websites (such as the Mothers of Twins website: www.nomotc.org).	6. Interacting with other parents in their situation may provide information to help Maureen and her husband adjust to their family changes.

EVALUATION: Maureen discussed with her husband her concerns about the effect of the twins on the usual pattern of family life and was surprised to learn that he was very willing to assume many of the household tasks while the infants require so much care. Maureen's mother is available to babysit, so Maureen and her husband can have some time for exercise and recreation.

Many cultural factors relevant to the postpartum period can be grouped into communication, dietary practices, and health beliefs.

Communication

Verbal communication may be difficult because of the numerous dialects and languages spoken. An interpreter should be fluent in the language, of the same religion, and of the same country of origin, if possible. This compatibility is particularly important for Middle-Eastern families, whose religious orientation may vary widely and who come from countries with long histories of social and religious conflicts with some other groups.

Respect for privacy and modesty of all people is important, but modesty is especially important in Hispanic, Middle-Eastern, and Asian cultures. Laws of modesty require that Muslim women cover their hair, body, arms to the wrists, and legs to the ankles except when at home with family or in all-female company (Giger & Davidhizar, 2004).

Health care workers often place a premium on efficiency and come directly to the point, but direct communication can be distressing, particularly for some Hispanics and Native Americans. Clients from these cultures may approach a subject only after exchanging polite and gracious comments. In Native American families, decisions are often made by the women in the family. Therefore the matriarch of the family should be included in teaching (Cesario, 2001).

> When the nurse and family speak different primary languages, verifying the family's understanding is important. An affirmative nod may be a sign of courtesy rather than understanding or agreement. To be certain the message has been received, the nurse should ask family members to repeat in their own words what they have been told.

A woman may not indicate that she disagrees with what the nurse tells her to do because she does not want to show disrespect. She may simply not follow the nurse's instructions. She might also follow cultural requirements that differ with nursing expectations. This may occur even if she does not really believe the requirements are necessary, but she may do it to avoid offending close relatives.

Health Beliefs

Cultural beliefs and practices provide a sense of security for new mothers. Provision of care for the mother and baby by female relatives is a common thread among cultures. A woman from Japan may practice *satogaeri bunben*, in which she stays in her parents' home from near the end of pregnancy until 1 to 2 months after birth (Moore & Moos, 2003). Women from parts of India also return to the parent's home and stay there for 16 weeks postpartum while the new mother is cared for by her own mother (Bowes & Katz, 2002). Caregiving may be performed by the mother-in-law for Korean women. Much attention is given to the woman's need for rest, and she may have no other duties than to eat, sleep, and recover for the first month (Kim-Godwin, 2003).

For many Southeast Asians the postpartum period is important to ensure health in later years. New mothers are expected to rest for 1 to 3 months while the grandmother or other female relatives take over the mother's usual responsibilities of cooking or housework and care for the mother, her baby, and other children. Lack of an adequate period of rest or the proper diet during this period is believed to cause varicose veins, early aging, problems with eyesight and digestion, and head and back pain. In later life, early signs of aging may be viewed as a sign that the woman did not receive adequate care after childbirth (Davis, 2001).

Health beliefs relating to hygiene may cause conflict in the postpartum period. Some Southeast Asian, Hispanic, Chinese, and Haitian women believe that the mother should be kept warm to avoid upsetting the balance of hot and cold. Korean women may believe that a new mother must keep warm to protect her loose bones and to prevent bone pain in later years (Kim-Godwin, 2003). Use of ice for perineal edema or breast engorgement may not be acceptable to these women.

Some Asian women do not wish to take baths or showers or wash their hair during the postpartum period. This practice is upsetting for nurses who are concerned about hygiene. If a sitz bath is indicated and this is explained to the mother, she may agree, if she is kept warm throughout the process. A heat lamp may be more acceptable, or a hot pack, if necessary (Mattson, 2004). Although an opportunity to wash or shower should be offered, it is up to the woman to decide her preference.

On the other hand, some Haitian women bathe in herb water at specific times after childbirth (Cosgray, 2004). Some women from India take daily hot baths during the weeks after childbirth, but cold baths are taboo (Bowes & Katz, 2002). Tact and sensitivity are necessary to determine what care is appropriate for each woman and to find a compromise, if necessary.

Specific religious practices should be accepted and supported. For instance, Muslim mothers are exempted from their obligation to pray while they are bleeding. However, the father and other family members kneel, place their heads on the floor, and pray five times per day. If possible, a clean, quiet room should be provided so that this obligation can be fulfilled without having to leave the birthing center.

Dietary Practices

Some cultural dietary practices to consider center on the hot-cold theory of health and diet. This theory concerns intrinsic properties of certain foods, which may not correlate with the temperature or spiciness of foods. For example, some Southeast Asians (including Cambodians, Vietnamese, Hmong, Laotians) believe that after childbirth the woman should eat only "hot" foods such as chicken, pork, and rice.

Some Chinese women believe that a combination of yin and yang maintains balance. Yin foods include bean sprouts, broccoli, carrots, and cauliflower. Yang foods include broiled meat, chicken, soup, and eggs.

Although ice water is commonly given to hospital clients, it is not acceptable to many Asians. For example, Southeast Asian women may refuse cold water because they believe it may cause weakness, prolonged healing, and clotting (Davis, 2001). They may prefer hot water or other warm beverages to keep warm.

Food brought from home is a welcome sign of caring in many cultures. This is especially true if traditional foods are eaten after a woman gives birth. Nurses should encourage the bringing of foods from home and should discuss any dietary restrictions with the family.

HOME AND COMMUNITY-BASED CARE

Because many mothers and infants are discharged from the birth facility soon after childbirth, many assessments and interventions described in this chapter occur in the home or clinic setting. Mothers may leave the birth facility when they still have discomfort and are just beginning to recover from the childbirth experience. Consequently, most psychosocial concerns such as family adaptation and postpartum blues surface later, when support from health care professionals is not as available.

Many methods currently are used to provide care for mothers and infants who leave the birth facility within hours after childbirth. These methods include telephone calls, nurse-managed postpartum clinics, home visits, and "baby lines" staffed by nurses who provide information and guidance for callers (see Chapters 1, 17, and 23). Some programs use paraprofessionals to help extend the work of nurses in providing support to postpartum women. All methods have advantages and disadvantages.

The overlap between nursing care in the birth facility and home makes communication among nurses extremely important. Nurses in the birth facility, who perform the initial assessments, should make information such as nursing diagnoses available to nurses who give follow-up care.

Application of the Nursing Process
Maternal Adaptation

Assessment

Several factors such as the mother's progression through the puerperal phases, her mood, her interaction with the infant, and unanticipated events affect maternal adaptation to the birth (Table 18-1).

Analysis

Parenting involves the parents' ability to create an environment that nurtures the growth and development of the infant. Parenting may be altered when one or more caregivers experience difficulty creating or continuing a nurturing en-

vironment. This difficulty occurs most often when factors such as maternal discomfort, fatigue, and lack of knowledge or confidence in infant care come into play. Therefore a common nursing diagnosis is "Risk for Impaired Parenting related to multiple factors such as fatigue, discomfort, and lack of knowledge of infant care" (Box 18-1).

Planning

Expected outcomes for this nursing diagnosis are that the mother will do the following:

- Verbalize feelings of comfort and support as she progresses through the phases of recovery.
- Demonstrate progressive attachment behaviors by (specific date).
- Participate in care of the newborn by discharge.

BOX 18-1 Common Nursing Diagnoses for Postpartum Period

Anticipatory Grieving*
Anxiety
Deficient Diversional Activity
Health-Seeking Behaviors
Ineffective Role Performance
Impaired Parenting*
Interrupted Family Processes*
Parental Role Conflict
Risk for Impaired Parent-Infant Attachment

* Nursing diagnoses discussed in this chapter.

TABLE 18-1 Assessing Maternal Adaptation

Assessments	Nursing Considerations
Progression through Puerperal Phases Taking-in (passive, dependent) Taking-hold (autonomous, seeks information) Letting-go (relinquishes fantasy baby, begins to see self as mother)	Consider the mother's need to rest, her need to tell the details of her labor and childbirth, and her readiness to learn infant care and assume control of her own care.
Maternal Mood Mood and energy level, eye contact, posture, and comfort	Tense body posture, crying, or anxiety (may indicate fatigue, discomfort or the beginning of postpartum blues).
Factors That Affect Maternal Adaptation Age of mother Previous experience	May need additional support if under 18 years of age. Primaparas progress through puerperal phases more slowly and may need more assistance than multiparas, who have more experience and knowledge. Birth of an infant with anomalies or death of a previous infant may delay adaptation.
Maternal and infant temperaments	Mothers who are calm, secure, and free from anxiety need less assistance. More teaching is necessary for parents of infants who are difficult to console.
Unanticipated events	Cesarean birth causes increased discomfort and longer recovery. Attachment problems may occur with birth of a preterm or ill infant or more than one infant.
Interaction with Infant Maternal touch	Progression from fingertipping to enfolding and a variety of comforting behaviors.
Verbal interaction	Mother may call infant "it" initially but progresses quickly to using given name and identifying specific characteristics.
Response to infant cues or signals	Prompt, gentle, consistent response indicates progressive adaptation to parenting role.
Preparation for Parenting Classes in breastfeeding, parenting, and infant care	Many mothers feel more prepared after completing classes and participate in care sooner.

Interventions

ASSISTING THE MOTHER THROUGH RECOVERY PHASES

"MOTHER" THE MOTHER. The early, taking-in phase is a time to mother the mother to help her move on to more complex tasks of maternal adjustment. During the first few hours after childbirth, she has a great need for physical care and comfort. Provide ample fluids and favorite foods. Keep linens dry, tuck warm blankets around her until chilling has stopped, and use warm water for perineal care.

MONITOR AND PROTECT. The new mother is dependent on nurses to monitor and protect her. Remind her of the need to void and assist her to ambulate. Assess her level of comfort frequently and offer analgesia before discomfort is severe and analgesia is less effective. Instruct her not to delay requesting analgesia because it is more effective and the postpartum course is smoother if her pain stays well controlled. At the first signs of fatigue, encourage her to sleep.

LISTEN TO THE BIRTH EXPERIENCE. Be prepared to listen to details of the birth experience and offer sincere praise for her efforts during labor. Use open-ended questions to determine the woman's perception of the birth. The opportunity to discuss her feelings about the experience helps her to integrate it and to clarify concerns. Women who are able to talk with others about their experiences and get needed explanations gain an understanding of their own strengths and a feeling of mastery (Callister, 2004).

Many mothers spend so much time on the telephone that completing assessments and care is difficult. The mother's need to relate her experiences to family and friends is important, and nurses may be reluctant to interrupt. When assessments and care are needed to ensure the mother's physical safety, a compromise can be effective. Offering a choice is often helpful: "Excuse me for a moment. I will need to check you soon. I can do it now or come back in 10 minutes."

FOSTERING INDEPENDENCE

As the mother becomes more independent, allow her to schedule her care as much as possible. Collaborate with her to plan when procedures such as sitz baths will be performed. Help her to assume responsibility for her self-care, and emphasize that the nurse's role at this point is to assist and teach.

PROMOTING BONDING AND ATTACHMENT

Early, unlimited contact between parents and infants is of primary importance to facilitate the attachment process. In many hospitals and birth centers, infants remain in the room with the parents all or most of the time, unless complications intervene. This arrangement may be called *mother-baby care, couplet care,* or *dyad care.*

In mother-baby care, one nurse is responsible for both the mother and the baby and is able to provide teaching and help with bonding as part of ongoing nursing care (Fig-

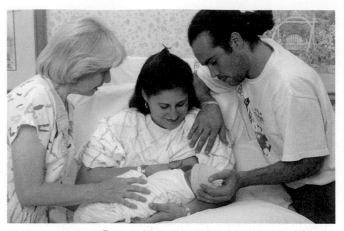

Figure 18-8 ■ By teaching about the newborn and family, the nurse helps parents develop confidence in their ability to provide care for the infant.

ure 18-8). The mother participates as she is able. If she does not feel well for a short period or is too tired to care for the infant, the nurse provides all care for the infant in the mother's room. Mother-baby care reduces fragmentation of care, provides extensive time for parent-infant interaction, and helps prepare the parents for discharge.

Prolonged contact between mothers and infants leads to more touching and caring for infants as the mothers learn their infants' characteristics and needs. Nursing measures to promote bonding and attachment include the following:

- Assist the parents in unwrapping the baby to inspect the toes, fingers, and body. Inspection fosters identification and allows the parents to become acquainted with the "real" baby, which must replace the fantasy baby that many parents imagined during the pregnancy.
- Position the infant in an *en face* position and discuss the infant's ability to see the parent's face. Face-to-face and eye-to-eye contact is a first step in establishing mutual interaction between the infant and parent.
- Point out the reciprocal bonding activities of the infant: "Look how she holds your finger." "He hasn't taken his eyes off you."
- Encourage the parents to take as much time as they wish with the infant. This allows them to progress at their own speed through the discovery or getting-acquainted phase.
- Assist the mother in putting the infant to the breast if she plans to breastfeed. If necessary, reassure her that many infants do not latch onto the breast right away. If she is using formula, assist her in positioning the infant securely and reassure her that holding and cuddling the infant provides comfort and security.
- Model behaviors by holding the infant close, making eye contact with the infant, and speaking in high-pitched, soothing tones.
- Point out the characteristics of the infant in a positive way: "She has perfectly shaped ears and such a lot of dark hair."

- Provide comfort and ample time for rest, because the mother must replenish her energy and be relatively free of discomfort before she can progress to initiating care of the infant. A mother who seems uninterested may just need a period of rest or pain intervention to be comfortable enough to focus on the infant.

INVOLVING PARENTS IN INFANT CARE

Providing care for the infant fosters feelings of responsibility and nurturing and is an important component of attachment. In addition, it allows parents to develop confidence in their ability to care for the infant before they go home. Begin with demonstrations, as necessary, and provide assistance while the parents gradually take over all infant care as their confidence in their abilities grows.

Although teaching begins during pregnancy, review information and repeat demonstrations if time allows. Demonstrate the simpler tasks such as care of the cord before progressing to more complicated procedures such as bathing. When the parents receive positive reinforcement for the simple tasks, they are more willing to try the more complicated ones (see Chapters 21 and 23).

Agreement among the entire staff about how to teach basic care is important. Mothers seek confirmation of information, and they become confused and lose faith in the credibility of the staff if information varies. Allow time for practice and repeated encouragement. Parents become easily discouraged if they feel unsuccessful with early attempts to care for their infants.

Suggestions for care must be tactfully phrased to avoid the implication that the parents are inept. "You burped that baby like a professional. There are a couple of little hints I can share about diapering."

Evaluation

- Independent self-care confirms the mother's progression through the phases of recovery.
- Progressive attachment behaviors include enfolding the infant, calling the infant by name, and responding gently when the infant cries.
- Participation in infant care includes diapering, feeding, and care of the umbilical cord and circumcision.

Application of the Nursing Process
Family Adaptation

Assessment
FATHERS

The father's emotional status and interaction with the infant are particularly important because he usually serves as the mother's primary support person. Is the father involved with the mother and infant? How does he interact with the infant? How much information does he have about infant characteristics and care? What are his expectations about his partner's recovery? Unrealistic expectations of the infant

(will sleep through the night, smile, be easily consoled) may lead to problems. In addition, if he expects the mother to recover her energy and libido rapidly, he may become resentful if her recovery takes longer than anticipated.

SIBLINGS

Note the ages of siblings and their reactions to the newborn. Are they interested and helpful? Are they hostile and aggressive? How do the parents react to sibling behaviors?

SUPPORT SYSTEM

Family members often provide a powerful support system, and their involvement is important to the adaptation of the family. Are grandparents available and involved? Do sisters and brothers live nearby? Are they available to help the new parents? If the family is unavailable, who provides support? What arrangements have been made for assistance?

NONVERBAL BEHAVIOR

Nonverbal behavior is equally important. Are the parents' words congruent with their actions? For example, does the mother verbalize satisfaction with her infant's characteristics but respond slowly to infant signals?

Validate impressions and conclusions arrived at during a psychosocial assessment. One of the best ways to do this is to ask questions such as, "How much experience have you had with newborns?" "You really thought you were having a girl, and a boy is a big surprise?" "How are newborns fed in Vietnam until the mother's milk comes in?" "What are your plans when you go home? How long can your mother stay?"

Ask questions over a period of time during normal caregiving. The mother should not be made to feel she is being interrogated because the nurse asks so many questions at once.

Analysis

Family assessment identifies family strengths and areas in which nursing interventions could promote family adaptation or prevent disruptions in family functioning (Table 18-2). Sometimes a family that usually functions effectively is unable to cope because of a specific event. An example is the birth of a baby and the need to integrate the newborn into the existing family structure. Therefore a common nursing diagnosis is "Interrupted Family Processes related to lack of knowledge of infant needs and behaviors, stress during the early weeks at home, and sibling rivalry."

Planning

Goals and expected outcomes for this nursing diagnosis may overlap with care after discharge because they often cannot be evaluated before the family leaves the birth facility.

By (specific date) the family will do the following:
- Verbalize understanding of infant needs and behaviors.
- Identify methods for reducing stress during the early weeks at home.

TABLE 18-2 Assessing Family Adaptation	
Assessment	**Nursing Considerations**
Characteristics of Infant That May Affect Family Adaptation	
Sex and size of infant	The sex of an infant may be very important for some families. Disappointment about the sex or concern about the small size may interfere with bonding.
Unexpected characteristics (cephalhematoma, jaundice, cranial molding, newborn rash)	Be prepared to explain unexpected appearance or behavior in language the parents can comprehend.
Infant behavior (irritable, easily consoled, cuddles)	An infant who is easy to manage increases bonding and attachment.
Paternal Adaptation	
Response to the mother and infant	The father often provides the most important support for the mother. His involvement with the infant indicates acceptance of the parenting role.
Knowledge of infant care	Such knowledge is useful in planning teaching that includes the father.
Response to infant cues or signals (crying, fussing)	Many fathers feel awkward handling the infant but want to become proficient in infant care so that they can co-parent.
Ages and Developmental Levels of Siblings	
Reaction of siblings	Young children often fear that the newborn will replace them in the affection of parents. The parents may need anticipatory guidance about sibling rivalry.
Support System	
Interest and availability of family or friends to assist during early weeks	Families may need assistance in identifying available support.
Plans for first few days at home	Suggest that parents plan for support and rest. Provide lists of resources such as telephone "hot lines," postpartum clinics, or support groups.
Follow-up plans	Appointments are generally scheduled at 2 to 6 weeks with the clinic or health care provider.
Cultural Factors	
Cultural beliefs and practices that may affect nursing care	Culture-specific care can be planned for hygiene, dietary preferences, usual care and feeding of infants, and role of mate and family in child care.
Expectations of the health care team	Expectations may vary in different cultures.

- Describe measures to reduce sibling rivalry.
- Identify external resources and support system.

Interventions

TEACHING THE FAMILY ABOUT THE NEWBORN

INFANT NEEDS. Some new parents have unrealistic expectations of the newborn. Provide them with information about the infant's capabilities as well as the infant's emotional and physical needs. For example, parents sometimes are surprised to hear that infants must be fed every 2 to 4 hours and will not sleep through the night for 12 to 16 weeks.

INFANT SIGNALS. Discuss the importance of responding promptly and gently to cues such as crying and fussing that indicate the infant needs attention. Reassure parents that responding to cues does not "spoil" their child but helps the child learn to trust that the world is a safe, secure place.

Help parents recognize signals that indicate when their infant has had enough and wants to avoid further stimulation. These *avoidance cues*, such as looking away, splaying the fingers, arching the back, and fussiness, indicate that the infant needs a quiet time.

HELPING THE FAMILY ADAPT

PROVIDING ANTICIPATORY GUIDANCE ABOUT STRESS REDUCTION. Help the family adjust to the demands of the first weeks at home by providing anticipatory guidance. This is a time when the need for rest is great but the opportunity for uninterrupted sleep is minimal. As a result, fatigue is a common problem for both parents. The nurse can assist as follows:

- Emphasize that the priority during the first 4 to 6 weeks should be caring for mother and baby.
- Recommend that mothers establish a relaxed home atmosphere and flexible meal schedule, because attempts to maintain a rigid schedule or meticulous environment increase tension within the family.
- Recommend that the mother sleep when the infant sleeps and conserve her energy for care of the baby.
- Encourage family members to let friends and relatives know sleep and nap times and request that they telephone and visit at other times. Adequate rest is necessary for mental and physical restoration and integration of new information into the memory.
- Advise parents to place a "Do Not Disturb" sign on the door and to set an answering machine to pick up immediately when the phone rings during rest times.
- Instruct the family about the need to limit coffee, tea, colas, and chocolate because they contain the stimulant caffeine and will interfere with rest.
- Teach breathing exercises and progressive relaxation to reduce stress and energize, especially when a nap is not possible.
- Encourage both parents to delay tiring projects until the infant is older. Remind them that although sched-

ules are chaotic for a while, the infant's behavior is generally more predictable by 12 to 16 weeks of age.

- Encourage open expression of feelings between parents as a first step in coping with stress.
- Remind parents of the need for healthy nutrition and recreation. Fatigue and tension easily can overwhelm the anticipated joys of parenting if no respite is available from constant care.
- Suggest that new parents enlist grandparents, other relatives, and friends to help with meal preparation and shopping.

HELPING THE FATHER CO-PARENT. Fathers often later remember the early interactions with their infants as being significant events in their lives (de Montigny & Lacharite, 2004). Help the father become involved with his

CRITICAL THINKING ⟨?⟩ EXERCISE 18-1

Carol, a 35-year-old primipara, had an infant daughter by cesarean birth after failure to progress in labor. Carol is very tired, although she is relatively comfortable. Her husband was present during the labor and birth and is excited about being a father. He has no experience with children, and his job requires almost constant travel. Carol has never taken care of a newborn.

On the day of delivery, Carol readily accepts assistance with hygiene. She passively follows the nurse's requests to turn, cough, and breathe deeply. She discusses the details of her labor and wonders why the physician did not perform a cesarean birth earlier. She examines her baby girl closely and touches the face and hands gently with her fingertips. She remarks that she plans to breastfeed and is surprised that the infant sleeps so much.

Questions
1. What are Carol's priority needs at this time?
2. What phase of recovery is she manifesting? Why does she "fingertip" the infant?

The first postoperative day, Carol's indwelling catheter is removed and intravenous (IV) fluids are discontinued. Carol ambulates with minimal assistance and is pleased to be able to urinate without difficulty. She asks about bowel function and requests the prescribed stool softener. She spends a great deal of time getting the baby to breastfeed. She is very frustrated that the infant does not breastfeed well and asks for assistance from the lactation educator.

Questions
3. What are Carol's priority needs now?
4. How have her behaviors changed?

Before discharge, Carol is breastfeeding well. The infant latches on and nurses for 10 to 15 minutes on each breast, and Carol's nipples are free of tenderness or signs of trauma. Carol has no relatives in the area, and her husband is home for the weekend only. She states that she will just have to get along by herself after that.

Questions
5. What anticipatory guidance should Carol receive before she goes home?
6. What further nursing interventions would be most helpful to her and the baby?

infant by including him in teaching and providing opportunities for him to participate in diapering, comforting activities, and feeding the infant or helping the mother breastfeed. Offer frequent encouragement and praise.

PROVIDING WAYS TO REDUCE SIBLING RIVALRY. Suggest that parents plan time alone with older children. Frequent praise and expressions of love and affection help reassure older children of their places in the family. Suggest that visitors and relatives avoid focusing exclusively on the infant and include older children in their gift giving and exclamations about the newborn.

Emphasize the importance of responding calmly and with understanding when a child regresses to more infantile behaviors or expresses hostility toward the infant. Acknowledging the child's feelings and offering prompt reassurance of continued love are the most valuable actions.

Some children, particularly those older than 3 years of age, enjoy being a big brother or sister and respond well when they are included in infant care. This participation may not be possible with younger children, and setting aside separate time to participate in a favorite activity may be more worthwhile for the parents.

IDENTIFYING RESOURCES. In many homes women assume the major responsibilities of day-to-day homemaking. With the birth of an infant, this task becomes more difficult. A division of labor must be negotiated to prevent undue stress and fatigue. This division of labor is particularly important when there are other children whose needs for time, attention, and comfort must also be met.

Although the mother's primary support often is the father of the baby, extended family members, particularly grandmothers and sisters, also provide valuable support. Community resources such as daycare centers, parenting classes, and breastfeeding support are available in many areas. In addition, close friends and neighbors often share solutions to specific problems. Remind the mother that resources are available when she begins to feel isolated and exhausted.

Evaluation

A prompt, gentle response to infant crying and fussing indicates a parent's understanding of the infant's need. Devising a plan for obtaining rest and lessening anxiety in siblings is a first step in reducing stress. Identifying resources in the family, neighborhood, and community may help the family function to meet its needs during the early weeks at home.

SUMMARY CONCEPTS

- Bonding and attachment are gradual processes that begin before childbirth and progress to feelings of love and deep devotion lasting all through life. Nurses foster bonding and attachment by providing early, unlimited contact between the parents and infant and modeling attachment behaviors.
- For bonding and attachment to occur, interaction between parents and the infant is required. Contact is particularly important when the infant is awake, alert, and able to in-

teract with the parents. Nurses often delay care that can be postponed so that the parents and infant can have this time together.

- Maternal touch changes over time as many mothers progress from exploratory "fingertipping" to enfolding and finally demonstrating a full range of comforting behaviors.
- Verbal behaviors are important indicators of maternal attachment. Nurses often model the way to speak to the infant and point out the infant's response to the verbal stimulation.
- Maternal adjustment to parenthood is a gradual process involving restorative phases of taking-in, taking-hold, and letting-go. Nurses play a valuable role in the process by first "mothering the mother" and fostering independence as the mother becomes ready.
- Mothers (and fathers) usually progress through four stages of role attainment—anticipatory, formal, informal, and personal—before they attain a sense of comfort and structure their parenting behaviors to mesh with the unique needs of their children.
- The mother develops a "new normal" as she goes through phases of appreciating her body, settling-in with the new baby, and becoming part of a new family.
- Many women experience role conflict when they must leave the infant with a caregiver and return to work. Nurses can offer anticipatory guidance that makes the conflict less difficult.
- Postpartum blues, a temporary, self-limiting period of tearfulness, often is ignored by the health care team. Explanations and support can assist the mother through this distressing episode.
- The birth of a baby necessitates reorganization of family structure and renegotiation of family responsibilities. Nurses can assist the father in co-parenting the infant and can help the new parents identify family resources.
- Siblings may be jealous and fearful that they will be replaced by the newborn in the affection of the parents. Nurses can reduce the negative feelings by providing information about ways to reduce sibling rivalry.
- Attention to cultural concerns of women after birth is important in helping them meet cultural, physical, and psychosocial needs.
- Nurses recognize that families leave the birth facility with unmet needs, and nursing care in the facility overlaps with follow-up care provided in the home.

ANSWERS TO CRITICAL THINKING EXERCISE 18-1, p. 447

1. Carol's priority needs are for physical care and comfort. She also needs to make the experience of childbirth part of her reality and does this by recounting the details of the birth and trying to fill in the missing pieces about the cesarean birth.
2. Carol is in the taking-in phase. She is getting acquainted with her "real" baby by exploring with her fingertips. This usually is the first maternal touch observed.
3. Carol's priorities are to assume control of her own body functions and manage her care so that she can "take hold" and assume care of the baby.
4. Carol has become more independent and now initiates breastfeeding. She demonstrates readiness to learn by requesting the assistance of the lactation educator.

5. Anticipatory guidance should focus on ways she can manage the care of the infant while still getting adequate rest and nutrition. Keeping a flexible schedule, resting while the infant rests, and preparing easy meals are some of the most important items to emphasize.
6. Assisting her in identifying friends and neighbors who could provide some support while her husband is away would be most helpful. If this is not possible, she should have telephone numbers for community resources such as the hospital "baby line." A follow-up home visit, visit to a postpartum clinic, or telephone call initiated by the nurse would be very helpful. The nurse could assess the mother and infant, reinforce teaching, and provide encouragement.

REFERENCES & READINGS

American Academy of Pediatrics and American College of Obstetricians and Gynecologists. (2002). *Guidelines for perinatal care* (5th ed.). Elk Grove Village, IL, and Washington, DC: Author.

Bowes, W.A., & Katz, V.L. (2002). Postpartum care. In S.G. Gabeb, J.R. Nimbly, & J.L. Simpson (Eds.), *Obstetrics, normal and problem Pregnancies* (4th ed., pp. 701-725). New York: Churchill Livingstone.

Buist, A., Morse, C.A., & Durkin, S. (2003). Men's adjustment to fatherhood: implications for obstetrical health care. *Journal of Obstetric, Gynecologic, and Neonatal Nursing, 32*(2), 172-180.

Callister, L.C. (2001). Integrating cultural beliefs and practices into the care of childbearing women. In K.R. Simpson & P.A. Creehand (Eds.), *AWHONN perinatal nursing* (2nd ed, pp. 68-94). Philadelphia: Lippincott Williams & Wilkins.

Callister, L.C. (2004). Making meaning: Women's birth narratives. *Journal of Obstetric, Gynecologic, and Neonatal Nursing, 33*(4), 508-518.

Cesario, S.K. (2001). Care of the Native American woman: Strategies for practice, education, and research. *Journal of Obstetric, Gynecologic, and Neonatal Nursing, 30*(1), 13-19.

Cosgray, R.E. (2004). Haitian Americans. In J.N. Giger & R.E. Davidhizar (Eds.)., *Transcultural nursing: Assessment and intervention* (4th ed., pp. 517-543). St. Louis: Mosby.

Cunningham, F.G., Leveno, K.J., Bloom, S.L., Hauth, J.C., Gilstrap, L.C., Wenstrom, K.D. (2005). *Williams obstetrics* (22nd ed.). New York: McGraw-Hill.

Damato, E.G. (2004). Predictors of prenatal attachment in mothers of twins. *Journal of Obstetric, Gynecologic, and Neonatal Nursing, 33*(4), 436-445.

Davis, R.E. (2001). The postpartum experience for Southeast Asian women in the United States. *MCN: American Journal of Maternal/Child Nursing, 26*(4), 208-213.

de Montigny, F., & Lacharite, C. (2004). Father's perceptions of the immediate postpartum period. *Journal of Obstetric, Gynecologic, and Neonatal Nursing, 33*(3), 328-339.

Driscoll, J.W. (2001). Psychosocial adaptation to pregnancy and postpartum. In K.R. Simpson & P.A. Creehan, *AWHONN perinatal nursing* (2nd ed, pp. 115-124). Philadelphia: Lippincott Williams & Wilkins.

Ewy-Edwards, D. (2000). Transition to parenthood. In F.H. Nichols & S.S. Humenick, *Childbirth education: Practice, research, and theory* (2nd ed., pp. 84-113). Philadelphia: Saunders.

Gennaro, S. & Fehder, W. (2000). Health behaviors in postpartum women. *Family & Community Health, 22*(4), 16-26.

Gichia, J.E.U. (2000). African-American women's preparation for motherhood. *MCN: American Journal of Maternal/Child Nursing, 25*(2), 86-91.

Giger, J.N., & Davidhizar, R. (Eds.). (2004). *Transcultural nursing assessment and intervention* (4th ed.). St. Louis: Mosby.

Hayashi, R.H., & Zettelmaier, M.A. (2000). Postpartum management. In S.B. Ransom, M.P. Dombrowski, S.G. McNeeley, K.S. Moghissi, & A.R. Munkarah. *Practical strategies in obstetrics-gynecology* (pp. 321-325). Philadelphia: Saunders.

James, D.C. (2001). Postpartum care. In K.R. Simpson & P.A. Creehan (Eds.), *AWHONN perinatal nursing* (2nd ed, pp. 446-472). Philadelphia: Lippincott Williams & Wilkins.

Kieman, J. (2002). The experience of therapeutic touch in the lives of five postpartum women. *MCN: American Journal of Maternal/Child Nursing, 27*(1), 47-53.

Killien, M.G., Habermann, B., & Jarrett, M. (2001). Influence of employment characteristics on postpartum mothers' health. *Women & Health, 33*(1/2).

Kim-Godwin, Y.S. (2003). Postpartum beliefs and practices among non-western cultures. *MCN: American Journal of Maternal/Child Nursing, 28*(2), 74-78.

Kridli, S.A. (2002). Health beliefs and practices among Arab women. *MCN: American Journal of Maternal/Child Nursing, 27*(3), 178-182.

Logsdon, M.C. (2000). *Social support for pregnant and postpartum women.* Washington, DC: Association of Women's Health, Obstetric and Neonatal Nurses (AWHONN).

Logsdon, M.C., & Davis, D.W. (2004). Paraprofessional support for pregnant and parenting women. *MCN: American Journal of Maternal/Child Nursing, 29*(2), 92-99.

Martell, L.K. (2001). Heading toward the new normal: a contemporary postpartum experience. *Journal of Obstetric, Gynecologic, and Neonatal Nursing, 30*(5), 496-506.

Martell, L.K. (2003). Postpartum women's perceptions of the hospital environment. *Journal of Obstetric, Gynecologic, and Neonatal Nursing, 32*(4), 478-485.

Matteson, P.S. (2001). *Women's health during the childbearing years: A community-based approach.* St. Louis: Mosby.

Mattson, S. (2003). Caring for Latino women. *AWHONN Lifelines, 7*(3), 258-260.

Mattson, S. (2004). Ethnocultural considerations in the childbearing period. In S. Mattson & J.E. Smith (Eds.), *Core curriculum for maternal-newborn nursing* (3rd ed., pp. 75-95). Philadelphia: Saunders.

McVeigh, C.A. (2000). Investigating the relationship between satisfaction with social support and functional status after childbirth. *MCN: American Journal of Maternal/Child Nursing, 25*(1), 25-30.

McVeigh, C.A., Baafi, M., & Williamson, M. (2002). Functional status after fatherhood: An Australian study. *Journal of Obstetric, Gynecologic, and Neonatal Nursing, 31*(2), 165-171.

Mercer, R.T. (1990). *Parents at risk.* New York: Springer.

Mercer, R.T. (1995a). *Becoming a mother: Research on maternal identity from Rubin to the present.* New York: Springer.

Mercer, R.T. (1995b). Predictors of maternal role attainment. *Nursing Research, 34*(4), 198-204.

Mercer, R.T., & Ferketich, S.L. (1990). Predictors of parental attachment during early parenthood. *Journal of Advanced Nursing, 15*, 268-280.

Mercer, R.T., & Ferketich, S.L. (1994). Maternal-infant attachment of experienced and inexperienced mothers during infancy. *Nursing Research, 43*(6), 344-351.

Metzger, M.E., & Shocker, B.A. (2003). Creating postpartum support groups. *International Journal of Childbirth Education, 19*(1), 12-15.

Moore, M.L., & Moos, M. (2003). *Cultural competence in the care of childbearing families.* White Plains, NY: March of Dimes Birth Defects Foundation.

Morin, K.H., Brogan, S., & Flavin, S.K. (2002). Attitudes and perceptions of body image in African American women. *MCN: American Journal of Maternal/Child Nursing, 23*(1), 20-25.

Nelson, A.M. (2003). Transition to motherhood. *Journal of Obstetric, Gynecologic, and Neonatal Nursing, 32*(4), 465-477.

Nichols, M.R., & Roux, G.M. (2004). Maternal perspectives on postpartum return to the workplace. *Journal of Obstetric, Gynecologic, and Neonatal Nursing, 33*(4), 463-471.

O'Reilly, M.M. (2004). Achieving a new balance: Women's transition to second-time parenthood. *Journal of Obstetric, Gynecologic, and Neonatal Nursing, 33*(4), 455-462.

Rubin, R. (1961). Puerperal change. *Nursing Outlook, 9*(12), 743-755.

Rubin, R. (1977). Binding-in in the postpartum period. *MCN: American Journal of Maternal/Child Nursing, 6*(1), 65-75.

Rubin, R. (1984). *Maternal identity and the maternal experience.* New York: Springer.

Scoggin, J. (2004). Physical and psychological changes. In S. Mattson & J.E. Smith (Eds.), *Core curriculum for maternal-newborn nursing* (3rd ed., pp. 371-386). Philadelphia: Saunders.

Simpson, K.R. & James, D.C. (2005). *Postpartum care.* White Plains, New York: March of Dimes.

Stark, M.A. (2000). Is it difficult to concentrate during the third trimester and postpartum? *Journal of Obstetric, Gynecologic, and Neonatal Nursing, 29*(4), 378-389.

Troy, N.W. (2003). Is the significance of postpartum fatigue being overlooked in the lives of women? *MCN: American Journal of Maternal/Child Nursing, 28*(4), 252-257.

U.S. Department of Labor, Bureau of Labor Statistics. (2004). Labor force participation of mothers with infants in 2003. *Monthly Labor Review.* Retrieved October 4, 2004, from http://stats.bls.gov/news.release/famee.t06.htm.

Normal Newborn: Processes of Adaptation

OBJECTIVES

After studying this chapter, you should be able to:

1. Explain the physiologic changes that occur in the respiratory and cardiovascular systems during the transition from fetal to neonatal life.
2. Describe thermoregulation in the newborn.
3. Compare gastrointestinal functioning in the newborn and adult.
4. Explain the causes and effects of hypoglycemia.
5. Describe the steps in normal bilirubin excretion and the development of physiologic, pathologic, and breast milk jaundice.
6. Describe kidney functioning in the newborn.
7. Explain the functioning of the newborn's immune system.
8. Describe the periods of reactivity and the six behavioral states of the newborn.

Go to your Student CD-ROM for Review Questions keyed to these Objectives.

DEFINITIONS

Asphyxia Insufficient oxygen and excess carbon dioxide in the blood and tissues.

Bilirubin Unusable component of hemolyzed erythrocytes.

Brown Fat (or Brown Adipose Tissue) Highly vascular specialized fat found in the newborn that provides more heat than other fat when metabolized.

Fetal Lung Fluid Fluid that fills the fetal lungs, expanding the alveoli and promoting lung development.

First Period of Reactivity Period beginning at birth in which newborns are active and alert. It ends when the infant first falls asleep.

Hyperbilirubinemia Excessive amount of bilirubin in the blood.

Jaundice Yellow discoloration of the skin and sclera caused by excessive bilirubin in the blood.

Neutral Thermal Environment Environment in which body temperature is maintained without an increase in metabolic rate or oxygen use.

Nonshivering Thermogenesis Process of heat production, without shivering, by oxidation of brown fat.

Polycythemia Abnormally high number of erythrocytes.

Second Period of Reactivity Period of 4 to 6 hours after the first sleep after birth when the newborn may have an elevated pulse and respiratory rate and excessive mucus.

Surfactant Combination of lipoproteins produced by the lungs of the mature fetus to reduce surface tension in the alveoli, thereby promoting lung expansion after birth.

Thermogenesis Heat production.

Thermoregulation Maintenance of body temperature.

At birth neonates must make profound physiologic changes to adapt to extrauterine life and meet their own respiratory, digestive, and regulatory needs. This chapter focuses on these changes and will assist nurses in identification of behaviors that signify problems or abnormalities. It provides a foundation for discussion of nursing assessment and care related to those changes, detailed in Chapters 20 and 21.

INITIATION OF RESPIRATIONS

The first vital task the newborn must accomplish is the initiation of respirations. Forces occurring throughout pregnancy and during birth bring about this change.

Development of the Lungs

During fetal life the alveoli produce fetal lung fluid that expands the alveoli and is essential for normal development of the lungs. Some of the fluid empties from the lungs into the amniotic fluid. The fluid is continuously produced at a rate of 4 to 6 ml/kg/hour, with a total amount of 20 to 30 ml/kg, which is approximately the amount of functional residual capacity after birth (Guttentag & Ballard, 2005). As the fetus nears term, production of fetal lung fluid decreases, so that by the time of birth only about 35% of the original amount remains (Blackburn, 2003).

During labor, the fluid begins to move into the interstitial spaces, where it is absorbed. Absorption of fetal lung fluid is accelerated by secretion of fetal epinephrine but may be delayed by cesarean birth without labor. The removal of the fluid helps reduce pulmonary resistance to blood flow that was present before birth and enhances the advent of air breathing.

At about 22 weeks' gestation the lungs begin to produce surfactant, a slippery, detergent-like lipoprotein (Hagedorn, Gardner, & Abman, 2002). Surfactant lines the inside of the alveoli and reduces surface tension within. This allows the alveoli to remain partially open when the infant begins to breathe at birth. Without surfactant the alveoli collapse as the infant exhales and must be reexpanded with each breath, greatly increasing the work of breathing and possibly resulting in atelectasis. At 34 to 36 weeks of gestation sufficient surfactant is usually produced for most infants born at that time to breathe without difficulty. Surfactant production increases during labor and immediately after birth to enhance the transition from fetal to neonatal life.

Steroids given to the mother in preterm labor help increase surfactant production and speed maturation of the lungs. The fetus who has intrauterine growth restriction or is stressed by conditions such as maternal hypertension or prolonged rupture of membranes may have accelerated lung maturation too. Infants of mothers with diabetes have slower lung maturation.

Causes of Respirations

At birth the infant's first breath must force fetal lung fluid into the interstitial spaces around the alveoli so that air can enter the respiratory tract. This requires a much larger nega-tive pressure (suction) than subsequent breathing. Breathing is initiated by chemical, mechanical, thermal, and sensory factors that stimulate the respiratory center in the medulla of the brain and trigger respirations (Figure 19-1).

CHEMICAL FACTORS

Chemoreceptors in the carotid arteries and the aorta respond to changes in blood chemistry brought about by the hypoxia that occurs with normal birth. A decrease in the blood oxygen level (PO_2) and pH and an increase in blood carbon dioxide level (PCO_2) cause impulses from these receptors to stimulate the respiratory center in the medulla. In addition, occlusion of the vessels in the cord ends the flow of a placental substance that may inhibit respirations (Hansen & Corbet, 2005.) A forceful contraction of the diaphragm results, causing air to enter the lungs. However, stimulation of the respiratory center and breathing do not occur if prolonged hypoxia causes central nervous system depression.

MECHANICAL FACTORS

During a vaginal birth the fetal chest is compressed by the narrow birth canal. A small amount of the fetal lung fluid is forced out of the lungs into the upper air passages during birth. The fluid passes out of the mouth or nose or is suctioned as the head emerges from the vagina. When the pressure against the chest is released, recoil of the chest draws air into the lungs and helps remove some of the viscous fluid in the airways.

THERMAL FACTORS

The temperature change that occurs with birth is an important stimulus to the initiation of respirations. At birth the infant moves from the warm, fluid-filled uterus into an environment where the temperature is more than 20° F cooler. Sensors in the skin respond to this sudden change in temperature by sending impulses to the brain that stimulate the respiratory center and breathing.

SENSORY FACTORS

Tactile stimuli that occur during birth stimulate skin sensors. Nurses hold, dry, and wrap infants in blankets, providing further stimulation to skin sensors. The stimulation of the sound, light, smell, and pain at delivery may also aid in initiating respirations.

Continuation of Respirations

Once the alveoli expand, surfactant acts to keep them partially open between respirations. About half of the air from the first breath remains in the lungs to become the functional residual capacity. Because the alveoli remain partially expanded with this residual air, subsequent breaths require much less effort than the first one.

With each cry of the newborn, pressure within the lungs increases, keeping alveoli open and causing remaining fetal lung fluid to move into the interstitial spaces, where it is absorbed by the pulmonary circulatory and lymphatic systems.

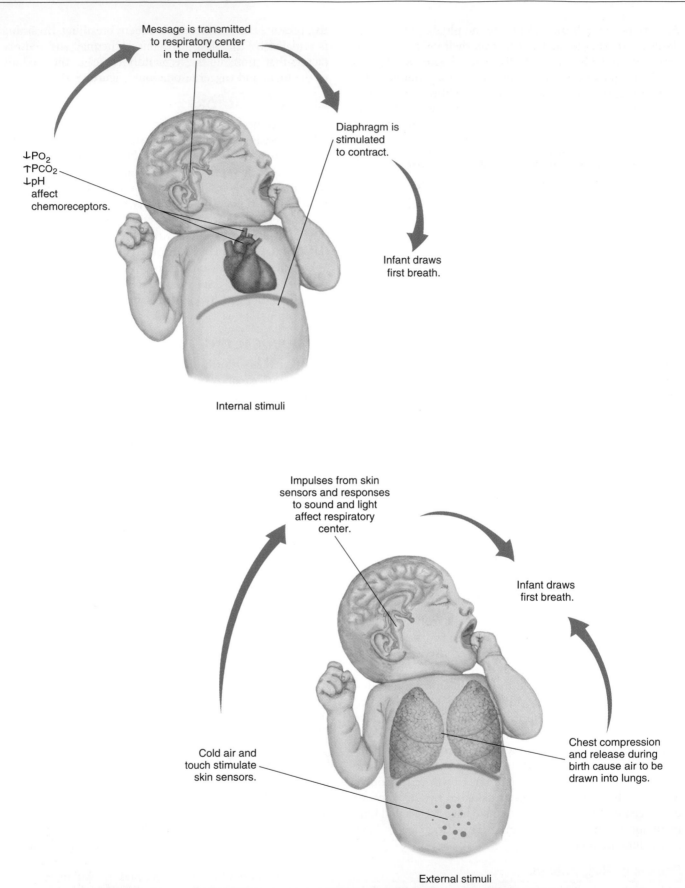

Figure 19-1 ■ Internal causes of the initiation of respirations are the chemical changes that take place at birth. External causes of respirations include thermal and mechanical factors.

Absorption is accelerated by the process of labor and may be delayed after cesarean birth. Although most fluid is absorbed within a few hours, complete absorption may take as long as 24 hours. This explains why the lungs may sound moist when first auscultated but become clear a short time later.

✔ CHECK YOUR READING

1. How do hypoxia during birth, a cool delivery room, and handling at birth stimulate the newborn to breathe?
2. Why is surfactant important to the newborn's ability to breathe easily?
3. How is fetal lung fluid removed before and after birth?

CARDIOVASCULAR ADAPTATION: TRANSITION FROM FETAL TO NEONATAL CIRCULATION

During fetal life three shunts—the ductus venosus, foramen ovale, and ductus arteriosus—carry blood away from the lungs and liver. At birth, changes in blood oxygen level, shifts in pressure within the heart and pulmonary and systemic circulations, and clamping of the umbilical cord allow the infant's blood to circulate to the lungs for oxygenation and to the liver for filtration (see Chapter 6, p. 106). The alterations necessary for transition from fetal to neonatal circulation occur simultaneously within the first few minutes after birth. They are discussed separately here (Table 19-1; see also Figure 6-9, pp. 104-105).

Ductus Venosus

Oxygenated blood from the placenta enters the fetal circulation through the umbilical vein. Because filtration of the blood by the liver is unnecessary during fetal life, the ductus venosus directs part of the blood flow from the umbilical vein away from the liver and directly to the inferior vena cava. The amount of blood shunted away from the liver varies during pregnancy. At 20 weeks about a third of blood passes through the ductus venosus, but in later pregnancy the liver needs more perfusion and up to 80% of the oxygenated blood goes to the liver instead of the ductus venosus (Blackburn, 2003).

Blood from the ductus venosus enters the inferior vena cava, where it joins blood from the lower part of the body, but travels to the heart in a separate stream within the inferior vena cava, so there is little mixing with blood from the lower body. As the more highly oxygenated blood flows into the right atrium, a flap of tissue directs most of it across the foramen ovale (Fineman, Clyman, & Heymann, 2004).

TABLE 19-1 Circulatory Changes at Birth

Structure	Purpose in Fetal Life	Change at Birth	Cause of Change at Birth	Results of Change at Birth	Time of Functional and Permanent Change
Ductus venosus	Shunts 50% of blood from umbilical vein to inferior vena cava and away from the immature liver.	Blood flow occluded with end of umbilical circulation.	Occlusion of cord stops flow of blood from placenta through umbilical vein to ductus venosus.	Blood travels through liver to be filtered as in adult circulation.	Functional: when cord is clamped. Permanent: 1-2 weeks. Becomes ligamentum venosum.
Foramen ovale	Provides opening between RA and LA so blood can bypass nonfunctioning lungs and go directly to LV and aorta; opens only in R-to-L direction because of high RA pressure and low LA pressure.	Closes when pressure in LA becomes higher than pressure in RA.	Cord occlusion elevates systemic resistance. Blood returns from PV to LA. Both increase L heart pressure. Decreased pulmonary resistance allows free flow of blood into lungs and decreased pressure in RA.	Blood entering RA can no longer pass through to LA; instead it goes to RV and through PA to the lungs.	Functional: within minutes. Permanent: 3 months. Becomes fossa ovale.
Pulmonary blood vessels	Narrowed vessels increase resistance in lungs to blood flow.	Dilation of all vessels in lungs.	Elevated blood oxygen level and removal of fetal lung fluid.	Decreased pulmonary resistance allows blood to enter freely to be oxygenated.	Beginning with first breath.
Ductus arteriosus	Is widely dilated to carry blood from PA to aorta and avoid nonfunctioning lungs.	Constriction preventing entrance of blood from PA.	Increase of oxygen level in blood.	Blood in PA is directed to lungs for oxygenation.	Functional: beginning within minutes after birth. Complete closure in 15 to 24 hr. Permanent: 3 to 4 weeks. Becomes ligamentum arteriosum.

L, Left; *LA,* left atrium; *LV,* left ventricle; *PA,* pulmonary artery; *PV,* pulmonary veins; *R,* right; *RA,* right atrium; *RV,* right ventricle.

When the umbilical cord is clamped at birth, little blood enters the ductus venosus. Fibrosis of the ductus venosus occurs by 1 to 2 weeks after birth, forming the *ligamentum venosum* (Lott, 2003).

Foramen Ovale

The foramen ovale is a flap in the septum between the right and the left atria of the fetal heart. As blood returns to the heart, most of the oxygenated blood from the inferior vena cava enters the right atrium and crosses the foramen ovale to the left side of the heart. The blood flows from the left atrium to the left ventricle and leaves through the aorta. The majority of the blood in the ascending aorta flows to the heart, brain, head, and upper body. Therefore most of the better-oxygenated blood bypasses the nonfunctioning lungs before birth.

The foramen ovale opens only from right to left. It remains open in the fetal heart because of the difference in pressures between the right and left atria. Blood flow from the right ventricle to the lungs is restricted by the narrow pulmonary artery and pulmonary blood vessels. The result is that pressure in the right side of the heart is higher than that in the left side of the heart. Pressure is low on the left side of the heart because there is little resistance as blood leaves the left ventricle to travel to the rest of the body and into the widely dilated placental vessels.

At birth, pressures are reversed between the right and the left sides of the heart. The sudden dilation of the vessels of the lungs allows blood to enter freely from the right ventricle and decreases pressure in the right side of the heart.

As blood enters the left atrium from the pulmonary vein, pressure in the left side of the heart builds. Systemic resistance increases when blood flow to the placenta ceases with cord clamping, further elevating the pressure in the left side of the heart. In addition, cooling of the skin causes vasoconstriction of the peripheral vessels, increasing the systemic vascular resistance even more. Because the foramen ovale opens only from right to left, it closes when the pressure in the left heart is higher than that in the right heart.

Closure of the foramen ovale forces the blood from the right atrium into the right ventricle and pulmonary artery. Because the ductus arteriosus is also closing, the blood continues into the lungs for oxygenation and returns to the left atrium through the pulmonary veins. It enters the left ventricle and leaves through the aorta to circulate to the rest of the body.

The foramen ovale is functionally closed soon after birth because the unequal pressures between the atria usually prevent it from opening. However, conditions such as asphyxia may reverse the pressures in the heart and cause the foramen ovale to reopen. It is permanently closed after several months in most infants but may stay open for 9 month or longer in some infants (Blackburn, 2003). Once it is permanently closed it is called the *fossa ovale*.

Pulmonary Blood Vessels

When the infant begins to breathe, the pulmonary blood vessels respond to the increased oxygenation by dilating. As fetal lung fluid shifts into the interstitial spaces and is re-

moved by the blood and lymph systems, more room is available for dilation of the pulmonary blood vessels. These changes decrease the pulmonary vascular resistance that prevented blood flow into the lungs during fetal life and allow the vessels within the lungs to accommodate the suddenly increased blood flow from the pulmonary artery.

Ductus Arteriosus

The ductus arteriosus connects the pulmonary artery and the descending aorta during fetal life. Prostaglandins from the placenta and low blood oxygen keep the ductus arteriosus widely dilated. All but about 10% to 12% of the blood that enters the pulmonary artery travels through the ductus arteriosus into the aorta and bypasses the nonfunctioning lungs (Blackburn, 2003).

As the infant takes the first breaths at birth the ductus arteriosus, which responds to a rise in oxygen by constricting, begins to close, preventing blood from the pulmonary artery from entering. At the same time, resistance within the pulmonary circulation decreases and resistance throughout the systemic circulation increases. These changes cause blood to flow from the pulmonary artery into the lungs for oxygenation.

The ductus arteriosus closes gradually as oxygenation improves and prostaglandins are metabolized in the lungs. Functional closure occurs within 15 to 24 hours (Lott, 2003). Until closure is complete, the blood that does flow through the vessel reverses, moving from the aorta to the pulmonary artery and increasing blood flow to the lungs. This occurs as pressure in the aorta becomes higher than that in the pulmonary artery. A murmur may be heard as a result of blood flow through the partially open vessel.

The ductus arteriosus closes permanently by 3 to 4 weeks (Lott, 2003). Once closed, it is called the *ligamentum arteriosum*. Until permanent closure occurs, low levels of oxygen in the blood may cause the ductus arteriosus to dilate and the pulmonary vessels to constrict. This may cause a return to fetal blood flow patterns and is a serious complication. A patent ductus arteriosus may occur in the infant who experiences asphyxia at birth, becomes hypoxic, or is preterm (see Chapter 30, p. 827).

CRITICAL THINKING ⚗ EXERCISE 19-1

Understanding the changes that occur during the transition from fetal to neonatal circulation helps in predicting the effect on blood flow of various defects in the heart.

Question
What would be the effect on neonatal blood flow of an opening in the septum of the atria of the heart?

✔ **CHECK YOUR READING**

4. What brings about the closure of the ductus arteriosus, foramen ovale, and ductus venosus at birth?
5. What causes the pulmonary blood vessels to dilate and the ductus arteriosus to constrict?

NEUROLOGIC ADAPTATION: THERMOREGULATION

At birth the infant must assume thermoregulation, the maintenance of body temperature. Although the fetus produces heat in utero, the consistently warm temperature of the amniotic fluid makes thermoregulation unnecessary. However, the temperature of the delivery room may be more than 20° F lower than that of the uterus, and the infant's temperature may drop rapidly. Neonates must produce and maintain enough heat to prevent cold stress, which can have serious and even fatal effects.

Newborn Characteristics That Lead to Heat Loss

Several newborn characteristics predispose them to lose heat. The skin is thin, and blood vessels are close to the surface. Little subcutaneous or white fat is present to serve as a barrier to heat loss. The percentage of subcutaneous fat in a neonate is only half that in an adult (Blackburn, 2003). Heat is readily transferred from the warmer internal areas of the body to the cooler skin surfaces and then to the surrounding air. Newborns have three times more surface area to body mass than adults do, which provides more area for heat loss. Newborns lose heat at a rate four times greater than that for adults (Stoll & Kliegman, 2004b).

The healthy full-term infant remains in a position of flexion, reducing the amount of skin surface exposed to the surrounding temperatures and decreasing heat loss. This is not the case for sick or preterm infants, who have decreased muscle tone and are unable to maintain a flexed position. Preterm infants also have thinner skin and even less white subcutaneous fat than full-term infants. Therefore they are at increased risk for cold stress (see Chapter 29).

Methods of Heat Loss

Heat is lost in four ways: evaporation, conduction, convection, and radiation (Figure 19-2). The nurse can prevent heat loss by each method and must be watchful for situations in which intervention is needed.

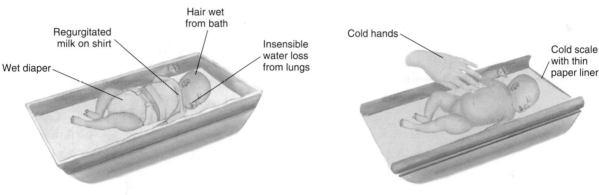

Evaporation can occur during birth or anytime the infant is wet, and from insensible water loss.

Conduction occurs when the infant comes in contact with cold objects or surfaces such as a scale.

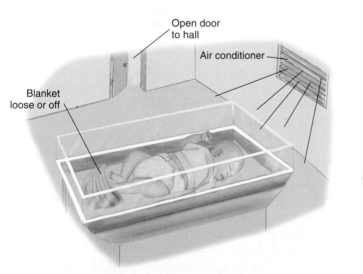

Convection occurs when drafts come from open doors, air conditioning, or even air currents created by people moving about.

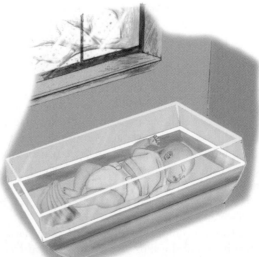

Heat is lost by radiation when the infant is near cold surfaces. Thus heat is lost from the infant's body to the sides of the crib or incubator and to the outside walls and windows.

Figure 19-2 ■ Methods of heat loss.

EVAPORATION

Evaporation occurs when wet surfaces are exposed to air. As the surfaces dry, heat is lost. At birth the infant loses heat when amniotic fluid on the skin evaporates. Evaporation also occurs during bathing. Drying the infant, especially the head, as quickly as possible at birth and after bathing helps prevent excessive heat loss. Insensible water loss from the skin and respiratory tract increases heat loss.

CONDUCTION

Movement of heat away from the body occurs when newborns come in direct contact with objects that are cooler than their skin. Placing infants on cold surfaces or touching them with cool objects causes this type of heat loss. The reverse is also true: contact with warm objects increases body heat by conduction. Warming the objects that will touch the infant or placing the unclothed infant against the mother's skin helps prevent conductive heat loss.

CONVECTION

Convection occurs when heat is transferred to air surrounding the infant. Air currents from air conditioning or people moving around increase the loss of heat. Keeping the newborn out of drafts, maintaining warm environmental temperatures, and warming oxygen before prolonged administration help prevent this type of heat loss. When infants are in incubators, the circulating warm air helps keep them warm by convection.

RADIATION

Radiation is the transfer of heat to cooler objects that are not in direct contact with the infant. For example, infants placed near cold windows lose heat by radiation. Infants in incubators transfer heat to the walls of the incubator. If the walls of the incubator are cold, the infant is cooled, even when the temperature of the air inside the incubator is warm. To combat this problem, incubators have double walls. Placing cribs and incubators away from windows and outside walls minimizes radiant heat loss. Newborns can gain heat by radiation, too. Using a radiant warmer transfers heat from the warmer to the cooler infant (Figure 19-3).

Nonshivering Thermogenesis

When adults are cold, they shiver, increasing muscle activity to produce heat. Newborns rarely shiver except at low temperatures, and shivering is not an effective method of heat production (Sahni & Schulze, 2004). Instead they cry and become restless. Their increased activity and flexion help generate some warmth and reduce the loss of heat from exposed surface areas of the body.

Exposure to cool temperatures also results in decreased flow of warm blood to the skin because of vasoconstriction. This helps prevent heat loss from the skin and causes the skin to feel cool to the touch. Acrocyanosis may occur. In addition, a drop in temperature increases the metabolic rate markedly, causing above-normal oxygen and glucose use (Blackburn, 2003).

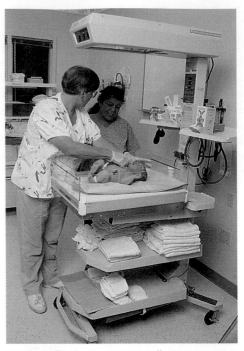

Figure 19-3 ■ Radiant warmers allow easy access to the infant without increasing heat loss resulting from exposure. The nurse should be careful not to come between the infant and the overhead source of heat when caring for the infant.

CRITICAL THINKING ⚲ EXERCISE 19-2

Look at a newborn's environment and the care given over a day. What are possible sources of heat loss for each method of heat loss?

The primary method of heat production in infants is nonshivering thermogenesis, the metabolism of brown fat to produce heat. Brown fat (also called *brown adipose tissue* or BAT) is a special kind of highly vascular fat found in newborns. It contains an abundant supply of blood vessels, which cause the brown color. Brown fat is located primarily around the back of the neck; in the axillae; around the kidneys, adrenals, and sternum; between the scapulae; and along the abdominal aorta (Figure 19-4). As brown fat is metabolized, it generates more heat than other fats. Blood passing through brown fat is warmed and carries heat to the rest of the body.

Nonshivering thermogenesis begins when thermal receptors in the skin detect a skin temperature of 35° to 36° C (95° to 96.8° F) (Blackburn, 2003). Thermal receptor stimulation is transmitted to the hypothalamus thermal center. As a result, norepinephrine is released in brown fat, initiating its metabolism.

Nonshivering thermogenesis goes into effect even before a change occurs in skin temperature or in core (interior) body temperature, as measured with a rectal thermometer. Activating thermogenesis before core temperature decreases allows the body to maintain internal heat at an even level. Therefore nonshivering thermogenesis may begin in an infant when skin temperature has been cooled, even though

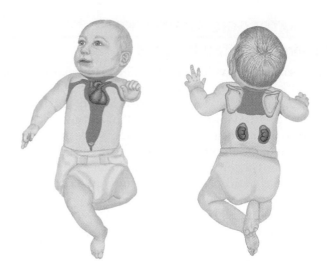

Figure 19-4 ■ Sites of brown fat in the neonate.

core and skin temperature measurements show normal readings. A decreased core temperature will not occur until nonshivering thermogenesis is no longer effective.

Some infants have inadequate brown fat stores. Preterm infants may be born before stores of brown fat have accumulated. Intrauterine growth restriction may deplete brown fat stores before birth. The fat may be consumed in newborns exposed to prolonged cold stress. These infants are not able to raise their body temperature if they are subjected to further episodes of cold stress and may have serious complications. Although it continues to develop until 3 to 5 weeks after birth, brown fat is generally used up during early infancy and is gradually replaced by white adipose tissue (Blackburn, 2003). Hypoxia, hypoglycemia, and acidosis may interfere with the infant's ability to use brown fat to generate heat.

Effects of Cold Stress

Cold stress causes many body changes. The increased metabolic rate and metabolism of brown fat that result from cold stress increase the need for oxygen (Figure 19-5). Just a 2° C (3.6° F) drop in the temperature of the environment can double the newborn's oxygen need (Blackburn, 2003). Cold stress also causes a diminished production of surfactant, impeding lung expansion. Prolonged cold stress can cause respiratory difficulty even in a healthy full-term infant. Mild respiratory distress can become severe hypoxia if oxygen must be used for heat production.

Glucose is also necessary in larger amounts when the metabolic rate rises to produce heat. When glycogen stores are converted to glucose, they may be quickly depleted, causing hypoglycemia. Infants who must use glucose for temperature maintenance have less available for growth.

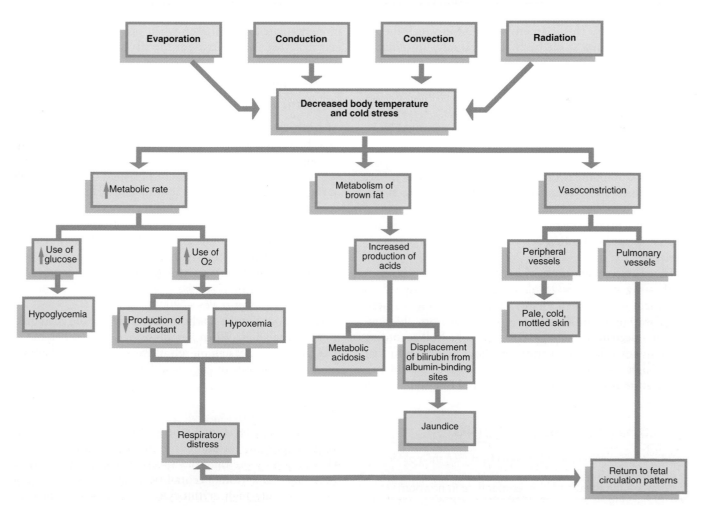

Figure 19-5 ■ Effects of cold stress.

Hazards of Cold Stress

Increased oxygen need
Decreased surfactant production
Respiratory distress
Hypoglycemia
Metabolic acidosis
Jaundice

Metabolism of brown fat and of glucose in the presence of insufficient oxygen causes increased production of acids. This release can cause metabolic acidosis, which can be a life-threatening condition. Elevated fatty acids in the bloodstream can interfere with transport of bilirubin to the liver, increasing the risk of jaundice.

As the infant's body attempts to conserve heat, vasoconstriction of the peripheral blood vessels occurs to reduce heat loss from the skin surface. Decreased oxygen in the blood, however, may also cause vasoconstriction of the pulmonary vessels. A result may be a return to fetal circulation patterns with shunting of blood from the left side of the heart to the right side, further increasing respiratory distress.

Neutral Thermal Environment

A neutral thermal environment helps prevent heat loss or gain in newborns. This is an environment in which the infant can maintain a stable body temperature with minimal oxygen need and without an increase in metabolic rate. The range of environmental temperature that allows this is called the *thermoneutral zone*. In healthy full-term newborns, an environmental temperature of 32° to 33.5° C (89.6° to 92.3° F) provides a thermoneutral zone (Blackburn, 2003).

Hyperthermia

Infants also respond poorly to hyperthermia. With an elevated temperature the metabolic rate rises, causing an increased need for oxygen and glucose. In addition, peripheral vasodilation leads to increased insensible fluid losses. Sweating may occur but is often delayed because sweat glands are immature.

The most frequent cause of hyperthermia in newborns is overheating by poorly regulated equipment designed to keep them warm. When infants are under radiant warmers, under warming lights, or in warmed incubators, the temperature mechanism must be set to vary the heat according to the infant's skin temperature and thus prevent heat that is too high or too low. Alarms to signal that the infant's temperature is too high or too low should be functioning properly.

CHECK YOUR READING

6. Why are neonates more prone to heat loss than older children or adults?
7. What are the effects of low temperature in newborns?

HEMATOLOGIC ADAPTATION

Factors That Affect the Blood

The average blood volume of the full-term newborn is 85 to 100 ml/kg. This may vary, however, depending on the time of clamping of the cord. The placenta contains approximately 75 to 100 ml of fetal blood (Sniderman & Taeusch, 2005). If the cord is not clamped for a few minutes, approximately 75 ml from the placenta may enter the infant's circulation (Guyton & Hall, 2000). Holding the infant below the level of the placenta before the cord is clamped also increases the blood volume.

Controversy exists about whether early or late cord clamping is best. Some think the extra blood volume may improve the transition to extrauterine life by opening the lungs, increasing pulmonary perfusion and removal of lung fluid, and providing additional iron stores (Blackburn, 2003; Mercer & Skovgaard, 2002). The added erythrocytes may, however, cause polycythemia and increase the risk of jaundice when they break down.

The various components found in the blood also depend on the time of cord clamping and the site from which the blood is drawn. The erythrocyte count and the hemoglobin level are higher after a delay in cord clamping. Blood samples drawn from the heel, where the circulation is sluggish, indicate higher levels of hemoglobin and hematocrit than samples taken from central areas. Venous blood samples are more accurate and are taken when precise measurement is essential. (See Appendix B for specific laboratory values.)

Blood Values

ERYTHROCYTES AND HEMOGLOBIN

At birth the infant has comparatively more erythrocytes (red blood cells [RBCs]) and higher hemoglobin and hematocrit levels than the adult. This difference is necessary because the partial pressure of oxygen of fetal blood in the umbilical vein is only about 30 mm Hg, much lower than the normal adult level. Adequate oxygenation of the cells is possible because fetal hemoglobin (hemoglobin F) carries 20% to 50% more oxygen than adult hemoglobin (Guyton & Hall, 2000). The large number of erythrocytes (4 to 6.6 million/mm^3) and higher hemoglobin level (14.5 to 22.5 g/dl) also enable the fetal cells to receive enough oxygen (Nicholson & Pesce, 2004).

Erythrocytes in the newborn have a shorter life span than those of the adult. When hemolysis occurs, hemoglobin is broken down, releasing bilirubin. Excess bilirubin resulting from the hemolysis of large numbers of RBCs may lead to jaundice.

HEMATOCRIT

The hematocrit level in the normal infant is 48% to 69% from peripheral sites during the first day and ranges from 44% to 72% by the third day (Nicholson & Pesce, 2004). A level above 65% from a central site indicates polycythemia (an abnormally high erythrocyte count). Polycythemia increases the risk of jaundice and damage to the brain and other organs as a result of blood stasis. Respiratory distress and hypoglycemia are more common in these infants (See Chapter 30, p. 816.)

Routine hematocrit testing is unnecessary in neonates. The hematocrit should be tested only if the infant has risk factors or signs of polycythemia or anemia (American Academy of Pediatrics [AAP] and American College of Obstetricians and Gynecologists [ACOG], 2002).

LEUKOCYTES

The leukocyte (white blood cell [WBC]) count at birth is 9000 to 30,000/mm³ (Nicholson & Pesce, 2004). The average WBC count is 18,000/mm³ in term infants. The leukocytes normally rise during the first 12 hours after birth and then decline slowly (Shaw, 2003). In newborns an elevated WBC count does not necessarily indicate infection. In fact, the WBC count may decrease in infections. Increased numbers of immature leukocytes are a sign of infection or sepsis in the neonate. Platelets may also decrease as a result of infections.

Risk of Clotting Deficiency

Newborns are at risk for clotting deficiency during the first few days of life because they lack vitamin K, which is necessary to activate several of the clotting factors (factors II [prothrombin], VII, IX, and X). Vitamin K is synthesized in the intestines, but food and normal intestinal flora are necessary for this process. At birth the intestines are sterile and therefore unable to produce vitamin K. To decrease the risk of hemorrhagic disease of the newborn, vitamin K is administered intramuscularly to most infants during initial care. Drugs such as phenytoin (Dilantin), phenobarbital, and aspirin taken by the mother during pregnancy interfere with clotting ability in the infant after birth.

Platelet (thrombocyte) levels range from 84,000/mm³ to 478,000/mm³ at birth. After the first week platelet levels are the same as in the adult—150,000/mm³ to 400,000/mm³ (Nicholson & Pesce, 2004). Although platelet counts in term newborns are near adult levels, platelet response to stimuli is decreased during the first few days of life.

GASTROINTESTINAL SYSTEM

Newborns must begin to take in, digest, and absorb food after birth because the placenta no longer performs these functions for them.

Stomach

The newborn's stomach capacity is about 6 ml/kg at birth (Blackburn, 2003) but expands to approximately 90 ml within the first week. Gastric emptying may be delayed at first. It is twice as rapid after ingestion of human milk as for formula but is slow if the infant has swallowed mucus. The gastrocolic reflex is stimulated when the stomach fills, causing increased intestinal peristalsis. Infants frequently pass a stool during or after a feeding. The cardiac sphincter between the esophagus and the stomach is relaxed, which explains the tendency to regurgitate feedings easily.

Intestines

The intestines of the newborn are long in proportion to the infant's size and compared with those of the adult. The added length allows more surface area for absorption. However, it makes infants more prone to water loss should diarrhea develop. Air enters the gastrointestinal tract soon after birth, and bowel sounds are present within the first hour.

The digestive tract is sterile at birth. Once the infant is exposed to the external environment and begins to take in fluids, bacteria enter the gastrointestinal tract. Normal intestinal flora is established within the first few days of life.

Digestive Enzymes

Maturation of the ability to digest and absorb occurs at different rates for various nutrients. Pancreatic amylase, needed to digest complex carbohydrates, is deficient for the first 4 to 6 months after birth (Blackburn, 2003). As a result, newborn digestion of complex carbohydrates such as those in cereals is decreased. Amylase is also produced by the salivary glands, but in low amounts until about the third month of life. Amylase is present in breast milk.

The newborn is also deficient in pancreatic lipase, limiting fat absorption significantly. Lipase present in the mouth and stomach helps with some digestion of fat. Lipase is also found in breast milk, which may make it more digestible for the newborn than formula. Protein and lactose, the major carbohydrate in the infant's milk diet, are both well digested.

Stools

Meconium is the first stool excreted by the newborn. It consists of particles from amniotic fluid such as vernix, skin cells, and hair, along with cells shed from the intestinal tract, bile, and other intestinal secretions. Meconium, which is greenish black with a thick, sticky, tarlike consistency, accumulates in the fetal intestines throughout gestation. The first meconium stool is usually passed within the first 12 hours of life, and 99% of neonates pass meconium within 48 hours (Stoll & Kliegman, 2004b). Failure to pass meconium within that time leads to suspicion of obstruction.

The second type of stool excreted by the newborn is called *transitional stool*. Transitional stools are a combination of meconium and milk stools. They are greenish brown and of a looser consistency than meconium. They are followed by milk stools characteristic of the type of feeding the infant eats.

The stools of infants fed with breast milk are seedy and the color and consistency of mustard, with a sweet-sour smell. The breastfed infant generally has more frequent stools than the infant who is formula fed. Breastfed newborns excrete as many as 10 small stools each day, although some older infants pass only one stool every 2 to 3 days. The normal breastfed newborn should have at least three stools daily.

The formula-fed infant excretes pale yellow to light brown stools. They are firmer in consistency than those of the breastfed infant. The infant may excrete several stools daily, or only one or two. The stools have the characteristic odor of feces.

✓ CHECK YOUR READING

8. Why do newborns have higher levels of erythrocytes, hemoglobin, and hematocrit than adults?
9. How do the stools change over the first few days after birth?

HEPATIC SYSTEM

The liver assumes many different functions after birth. Some of the most important include maintenance of blood glucose levels, conjugation of bilirubin, production of factors necessary for blood coagulation, storage of iron, and metabolism of drugs.

Blood Glucose Maintenance

Throughout gestation, glucose is supplied to the fetus by the placenta. During the last 4 to 8 weeks of pregnancy, glucose is stored as glycogen primarily in the fetal liver and skeletal muscles for use after birth. Glucose is used more rapidly in the newborn than in the fetus because energy is needed during the stress of delivery and for breathing, heat production, movement against gravity, and activation of all the functions that the neonate must take on at birth.

Until newborns begin regular feedings and their intake is adequate to meet energy requirements, the glucose present in the body is used. As the blood glucose level falls, stored glycogen is converted by the liver to glucose for use. Although the brain can use alternative fuels such as ketone bodies, lactic acids, fatty acids, and glycerol if necessary, glucose is the primary source of energy (Armentrout, 2004). Therefore the liver's ability to convert glycogen to glucose is essential. Glucose in the blood commonly falls to the lowest levels by 60 to 90 minutes after birth but rise within a few hours.

In the term infant, glucose levels should be 40 to 60 mg/dl on the first day and 50 to 90 mg/dl thereafter (Nicholson & Pesce, 2004). There is no general consensus about the level of blood glucose that defines hypoglycemia, but a level below 40 to 45 mg/dl in the term infant is often used (Blackburn, 2003; McGowan, Hagedorn, & Hay, 2002).

Many newborns are at increased risk for hypoglycemia. In the preterm and small-for-gestational-age infant, adequate stores of glycogen or even fat for metabolism may not have accumulated. Stores of glycogen may be used up before birth in the postterm infant because of poor intrauterine nourishment from a deteriorating placenta.

Large-for-gestational-age newborns may produce excessive insulin that consumes available glucose quickly. This is particularly true if the mother is diabetic. Infants of diabetic mothers receive large amounts of glucose from the mother throughout pregnancy and must produce enough insulin to use the glucose. Although the supply of glucose is cut off at birth, the infants may continue to produce more insulin than needed, which results in hypoglycemia soon after birth (see Chapter 30 for discussion of the infant of a diabetic mother).

When infants are exposed to such stressors as asphyxia or infection, the glycogen in the liver may be exhausted quickly, causing signs of hypoglycemia. Infants who become cold may deplete glycogen to increase metabolism and raise body temperature (see "Critical to Remember: Signs of Hypoglycemia," p. 488).

Conjugation of Bilirubin

A major function of the liver is the conjugation of bilirubin (Figure 19-6). The newborn's liver may not be mature enough to prevent jaundice during the first week of life. Jaundice occurs in 60% of term newborns and 80% of preterm infants (Stoll & Kliegman, 2004a).

SOURCE AND EFFECT OF BILIRUBIN

The principal source of bilirubin is the hemolysis of erythrocytes. This is a normal occurrence after birth, when fewer erythrocytes are needed than during fetal life. The breakdown of RBCs releases their components into the bloodstream to be reused by the body. Only bilirubin remains as an unusable residue in the blood. This substance is toxic to the body and must be excreted.

Bilirubin is released in an unconjugated form. Unconjugated bilirubin, also called *indirect bilirubin*, is soluble in fat but not in water. Before excretion can occur, the liver must change it to a water-soluble form by a process called *conjugation*. The bilirubin is then known as *conjugated* or *direct bilirubin*.

Because unconjugated bilirubin is fat soluble, it may be absorbed by the subcutaneous fat, causing the yellowish discoloration of the skin called jaundice. If enough unconjugated bilirubin accumulates in the blood, it may cause staining of the tissues in the brain resulting in kernicterus, or bilirubin encephalopathy, which may cause severe brain damage.

NORMAL CONJUGATION

When unconjugated bilirubin is released into the bloodstream, it attaches to binding sites on albumin in the plasma and is carried to the liver. There it binds to ligandin and other proteins and is changed to the conjugated form by the enzyme glucuronyl transferase in the smooth endoplasmic reticulum of the liver cells. Conjugated bilirubin is excreted into the bile and then into the duodenum. In the intestines the normal flora acts on bilirubin to reduce it to urobilinogen and stercobilin, which are excreted in the stools. Some urobilinogen is excreted by the kidneys.

A small percentage of conjugated bilirubin may be deconjugated, or converted back to the unconjugated state, by the intestinal enzyme β-glucuronidase. This enzyme is important in fetal life because bilirubin is transported to the placenta for conjugation by the mother's liver. The placenta can clear only unconjugated bilirubin. In the newborn, de-

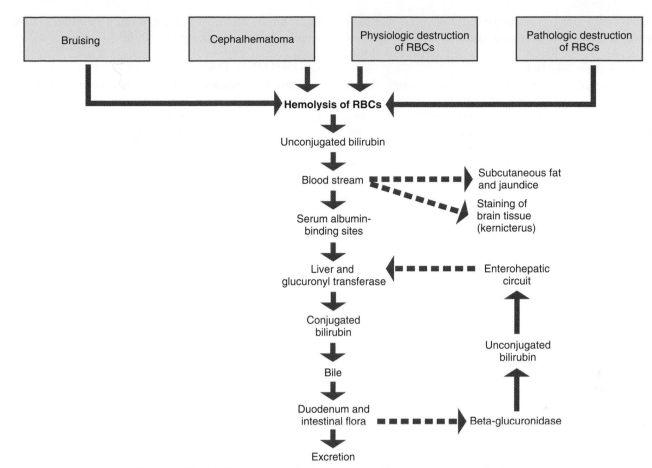

Figure 19-6 ▪ Sources of bilirubin and how it is removed from the body.

conjugated bilirubin in the intestines is reabsorbed into the portal circulation and carried directly back to the liver, where it again undergoes the conjugation process. This recirculation of bilirubin is called the *enterohepatic circuit*. It creates additional work for the liver.

Blood tests for bilirubin measure total bilirubin and direct (conjugated) bilirubin in the serum. Total bilirubin is a combination of indirect (unconjugated) and direct bilirubin.

FACTORS IN INCREASED BILIRUBIN

A number of factors lead to the production of excessive amounts of bilirubin or interfere with the normal process of conjugation, resulting in an increased incidence of jaundice during the first week of life.

EXCESS PRODUCTION. Approximately 6 to 8 mg/kg of bilirubin is produced in infants each day during the first 2 weeks of life, a rate 2.5 times that in adults (Maisels, 2001). Newborns have more RBCs per kilogram of weight than adults. This is because oxygen levels are low during fetal life and more erythrocytes are needed to carry enough oxygen to the cells.

RED BLOOD CELL LIFE. Fetal RBCs break down more quickly than adult erythrocytes. They last 80 to 100 days in term infants and 60 to 70 days in preterm infants, as compared with RBCs in adults, which last 120 days (Blackburn, 2003). In addition, erythrocytes are more fragile and suscepti-

ble to damage than those in the adult. For their size, neonates have more RBCs breaking down faster and producing greater amounts of bilirubin to excrete than adults.

LIVER IMMATURITY. The newborn's immature liver may not produce adequate amounts of glucuronyl transferase during the first few days of life. Insufficient availability of this enzyme limits the amount of bilirubin that can be conjugated.

INTESTINAL FACTORS. At birth the intestines of the newborn are sterile. Conjugated bilirubin cannot be reduced to urobilinogen or stercobilin for excretion without the action of intestinal flora. In addition, the newborn intestines have a large amount of the enzyme β-glucuronidase, which changes bilirubin back to the unconjugated state. These two factors may result in high levels of unconjugated bilirubin, which is reabsorbed into the blood circulation.

DELAYED FEEDING. Feeding the newborn helps establish the normal intestinal flora and promotes passage of meconium, which is high in bilirubin. When feeding is delayed or stools are not passed, exposure to β-glucuronidase is longer, increasing the chance that conjugated bilirubin will be converted to the unconjugated state and absorbed into the blood.

TRAUMA. Trauma during birth may result in increased hemolysis of RBCs. This is particularly true in cases of bruising, which may be caused by use of a vacuum extractor. The infant born in a breech position may also have bruising. A cephalhematoma contains a large number of erythrocytes. As the RBCs in the bruised areas break down, they add to the bilirubin load.

FATTY ACIDS. Free fatty acids have a greater affinity than bilirubin for the binding sites on albumin and bind to albumin in place of bilirubin. Fatty acids are released when brown fat is used to increase heat during cold stress. During asphyxia, anaerobic metabolism also produces free fatty acids. Therefore in infants who experience cold stress or asphyxia, unbound unconjugated bilirubin is increased and jaundice may develop.

OTHER FACTORS. Plasma albumin is lower in newborns and offers fewer binding sites than in adults. It increases rapidly during the first few days after birth. Bilirubin levels are more likely to be elevated in infants who are Asian, Native American, or preterm or whose mothers have diabetes (Madan, MacMahon, & Stevenson, 2005). Some drugs given to the mother during pregnancy or to the infant also increase jaundice. Swallowing blood during birth causes more breakdown of erythrocytes and increased bilirubin.

Hyperbilirubinemia

PHYSIOLOGIC JAUNDICE

Physiologic jaundice, also called *nonpathologic* or *developmental jaundice*, results from the transient hyperbilirubinemia. The jaundice is not present during the first 24 hours of life in term infants but appears on the second or third day after birth and is considered a normal phenomenon.

Jaundice becomes visible when it reaches 5 to 7 mg/dl (Blackburn, 2003). A rough guide to the total bilirubin level is that jaundice of the face occurs at 5 to 7 mg/dl, of the midabdomen at about 15 mg/dl, and of the soles of the feet at about 20 mg/dl (Stoll & Kliegman, 2004a).

The rate at which bilirubin in the blood rises and falls is important because it helps determine whether the rate for a particular infant is following the expected curve for age and birth weight. Cord blood has an average bilirubin level of less than 2 mg/dl.

In physiologic jaundice the indirect bilirubin rises rapidly, peaking at 5 to 6 mg/dl between the second and fourth days of life. The bilirubin then begins to fall, declining to adult indirect levels of 1 mg/dl by 10 to 14 days of age. For preterm infants jaundice begins at the same time or slightly later and lasts longer. Peak levels of 8 to 12 mg/dl

CRITICAL TO REMEMBER

Factors That Increase Hyperbilirubinemia

Hemolysis of excessive erythrocytes
Short red blood cell life
Liver immaturity
Lack of intestinal flora
Delayed feeding
Trauma resulting in bruising or cephalhematoma
Fatty acids from cold stress or asphyxia

occur on the fifth to seventh day and may last until 10 days after birth (Stoll & Kliegman, 2004a).

PATHOLOGIC JAUNDICE

Jaundice that appears during the first 24 hours after birth is generally from a pathologic process. Any of the following may indicate a nonphysiologic cause (Madan, MacMahon, & Stevenson, 2005):

- A direct bilirubin level above 1.5 to 2 mg/dl
- A total serum bilirubin concentration increasing by more than 0.2 mg/dl per hour or 5 mg/dl per day
- Total serum bilirubin concentration above the ninety-fifth percentile for the infant's age in hours
- Clinical jaundice that lasts more than 2 weeks in a full-term infant

Some authors also include a total serum bilirubin concentration higher than 12 mg/dl in a full-term infant or 10 to 14 mg/dl in a preterm infant (Stoll & Kliegman, 2004a).

Pathologic jaundice is most commonly a result of abnormalities causing excessive destruction of erythrocytes. These include incompatibilities between the mother's and infant's blood types (see p. 654), infection, and metabolic disorders (see discussion of pathologic jaundice, p. 805).

JAUNDICE ASSOCIATED WITH BREASTFEEDING

More than 50% of breastfed infants develop jaundice (Halamek & Stevenson, 2002). There are two types: breastfeeding jaundice and true breast milk jaundice.

BREASTFEEDING JAUNDICE. Bilirubin levels above 12 mg/dl develop in 13% of breastfed infants by 1 week of age (Stoll & Kliegman, 2004a). The most common cause of jaundice in breastfed infants is insufficient intake. Jaundice begins within the first week of life, and serum bilirubin may rise above 12 mg/dl and reach dangerous levels if intake is not increased.

Infants who are sleepy, who have a poor suck, or who nurse on an infrequent schedule may not receive enough colostrum—the substance that precedes true breast milk—to take advantage of its normal laxative effect. This delays the elimination of meconium, which is high in bilirubin. When meconium is not eliminated, the bilirubin may be deconjugated by β-glucuronidase in the intestine, absorbed, and recirculated to the liver for conjugation again.

Lack of adequate suckling depresses production of breast milk and increases the problem further. Helping the mother with breastfeeding to increase the infant's intake and stimulate milk production may be the most important treatment. If this is not possible, temporary formula supplementation is necessary. Dextrose water will not reduce bilirubin levels and should be avoided.

TRUE BREAST MILK JAUNDICE. True breast milk jaundice, also called *late-onset breast milk jaundice*, occurs after the first 3 to 5 days of life. The serum bilirubin usually peaks at 5 to 10 mg/dl at approximately 2 weeks, but some infants (less than 1%) reach levels over 20 mg/dl. Serum bilirubin falls gradually over several months (Halamek & Stevenson, 2002).

In true breast milk jaundice substances in the breast milk such as pregnanediol and fatty acids may interfere with conjugation. β-glucuronidase may be increased, causing deconjugation and absorption of bilirubin from the intestine. However, no proven cause is known. This may be a form of physiologic jaundice in breastfed infants.

Treatment of breast milk jaundice includes close monitoring of bilirubin levels in the blood and at least 8 to 10 feedings each 24 hours. If bilirubin levels become too high, phototherapy is begun. Breastfeeding may be continued with help to ensure the infant's intake is adequate, or formula may be used to supplement breast milk. If necessary, breastfeeding may be discontinued for 24 to 48 hours while the mother uses a breast pump to maintain lactation. Temporarily switching to formula causes a rapid drop in bilirubin. The level may rise again when breastfeeding is resumed but generally not high enough to interfere with further breastfeeding.

Blood Coagulation

Prothrombin and coagulation factors II, VII, IX, and X are produced by the liver and activated by vitamin K, which is deficient in the newborn. This is discussed on p. 459.

Iron Storage

Iron is stored in the liver during the last weeks of pregnancy. Full-term infants who are breastfeeding usually do not need added iron until 6 months of age. At that time, they should begin consuming iron-containing foods or iron supplements. All infants who are not breastfeeding should be given iron-fortified formula (AAP & ACOG, 2002).

Metabolism of Drugs

The liver metabolizes drugs inefficiently in the newborn. This must be considered when drugs are given to the neonate. In addition, a breastfeeding mother should alert her primary caregiver before taking medications, as harmful amounts may be transferred to the infant via the breast milk.

✔ **CHECK YOUR READING**

10. Why is hypoglycemia a problem for the newborn?
11. Why are infants more likely than adults to become jaundiced?
12. What are the differences among physiologic, pathologic, and breast milk jaundice?

URINARY SYSTEM

Kidney Development

The kidneys begin to produce urine at 9 to 10 weeks of gestation and become the major source of amniotic fluid by the second half of pregnancy (Blackburn, 2003). Fetal urine is not actually a waste product because the placenta elimi-

nates wastes for the fetus. Failure to produce adequate urine causes oligohydramnios, or lack of sufficient amniotic fluid.

Although the formation of nephrons is complete at 34 to 36 weeks' gestation, full kidney function does not occur until after birth when the kidneys take over the elimination of wastes. Blood flow to the kidneys increases after birth because of decreased resistance in the renal vessels. The improved perfusion results in a steady improvement in kidney function during the first few days of life.

Kidney Function

The newborn's kidney function at birth is immature compared with that of the adult. The ability of the glomeruli to filter and the renal tubules to reabsorb is considerably less than in adults. The glomerular filtration rate doubles during the first weeks of life but does not reach adult levels until 1 to 2 years of age (Swinford, Bonilla-Felix, Cerda, & Portman, 2002). Therefore infants have a decreased ability to remove waste products from the blood.

Small amounts of substances such as glucose and protein may escape into the urine of the neonate. They disappear within the first few days of life as kidney function improves. Urate crystals may give a pink or reddish color to the urine that is sometimes mistaken for blood.

The first voiding occurs within 12 hours of birth in most newborns and within 24 hours in 95% of newborns (Stoll & Kliegman, 2004b). Failure to void within that time may be a result of hypovolemia from inadequate intake of fluids. Absence of kidneys or anomalies that interfere with excretion of urine are usually discovered before birth because lack of urine excretion causes oligohydramnios, a deficiency of amniotic fluid volume. This generally prompts investigation into the cause during pregnancy. Only one to two voidings may occur during the first 2 days of life, although a higher number is common. The infant voids at least six times a day by the fourth day.

Fluid Balance

Newborns have a lower tolerance for changes in total volume of body fluid than do older infants. This is because of the location of water within the newborn's body and the inability of the kidneys to adapt to large changes in body fluids. In addition, the fluid turnover rate is greater than that in adults. To maintain fluid balance, full-term newborns need 40 to 60 ml/kg (18 to 27 ml/lb) daily during the first 2 days of life and then 100 to 150 ml/kg (45

⌐ CRITICAL TO REMEMBER

Intake and Output in the Newborn

First 2 Days of Life
Intake: 40 to 60 ml/kg (18 to 27 ml/lb) per day
Output: At least one or two voidings

After the First 2 Days
Intake: 100 to 150 ml/kg (45 to 68 ml/lb) per day
Output: At least six voidings by the fourth day

to 68 ml/lb) a day (Tsang, DeMarini, & Rath, 2003). For example, an infant who weighs 3.4 kg (7.5 lb) on the third day of life needs approximately 340 to 510 ml of fluid each day.

WATER DISTRIBUTION

Seventy-eight percent of the infant's body is composed of water. By 1 year of age, total body water decreases to the approximately 60% of weight seen in adults.

Body water is distributed differently in newborns than in adults (Table 19-2). Intracellular water constitutes 34% of body weight (Blackburn, 2003). Extracellular water (located in the interstitial or intravascular spaces) constitutes 44% of body weight. This is more than twice as much extracellular water as in adults, in whom it constitutes 20% of body weight. Although fluid within the cells is relatively stable, extracellular water is easily lost from the body. Because infants have more fluid for their size than adults, and because a larger proportion of it is located outside the cells, total body water is easily depleted. Conditions such as vomiting and diarrhea can quickly result in life-threatening dehydration.

INSENSIBLE WATER LOSS

Water lost from the skin and respiratory tract contributes to insensible water loss. Insensible water losses are increased in the newborn because of the large surface area of the body and the rapid respiratory rate. Fluid losses increase greatly when infants are placed under radiant heaters, which accelerate evaporation from the skin. An elevated respiratory rate or low humidity in the air surrounding the infant raises insensible water losses even further.

URINE DILUTION AND CONCENTRATION

The ability of a newborn's kidneys to dilute urine is similar to that in adults, to a specific gravity of 1.001 to 1.005 (Swinford et al, 2002). However, a newborn's kidneys cannot handle large increases in fluids, which result in fluid overload. This is most likely to happen if infants receive too much intravenous fluid. Normal urine output is 1 to 3 ml/kg/hr (Brodsky & Martin, 2003).

Because they have only half the adult's ability to excrete concentrated urine, newborns have more difficulty preventing loss of fluid in the urine than do adults (Blackburn, 2003; Guyton & Hall, 2000). Neonates can concentrate urine only to a specific gravity of 1.015 to 1.020 (Swinford et al., 2002), compared with the adult level of 1.040. When

abnormal conditions such as diarrhea cause excessive loss of fluid, the newborn's limited ability to conserve water may result in dehydration more quickly than in the older infant or child.

Acid-Base and Electrolyte Balance

The maintenance of acid-base and electrolyte balance is a primary function of the kidneys and may be precarious in neonates. Newborns tend to lose bicarbonate at lower levels than adults, increasing their risk for acidosis. The excretion of solutes is less efficient in newborns as well. Although newborns conserve needed sodium well, they are limited in excretion of sodium. This is particularly a problem if they receive excessive amounts (Blackburn, 2003).

IMMUNE SYSTEM

The neonate is less effective in fighting off infection than the older infant or child. WBCs respond slowly and inefficiently when the body is invaded by organisms. Leukocytes are delayed in moving to the site of invasion and are not efficient in destroying the invader. The infant's decreased ability to localize infection leads to a tendency toward generalized sepsis.

Fever and leukocytosis, which occur during infection of the older child, are often not present in the newborn with infection. This lack of response occurs because the hypothalamus and inflammatory responses are immature. Nonspecific signs such as changes in activity, tone, or feeding may be the only signs of sepsis.

Because of their immature immune system, infants are susceptible to pathogens that do not usually affect older children, such as group B streptococci and *Escherichia coli*. Full-term newborns received antibodies from the mother during the last trimester of pregnancy. The mother continues to give the infant antibodies in her milk, if she chooses to breastfeed. This transfers passive immunity to the infant. Immunoglobulins (serum globulins with antibody activity) help protect the newborn from infection. The major immunoglobulins are IgG, IgM, and IgA, each of which performs a different function. At birth the infant's total immunoglobulin levels range from 55% to 80% of the adult levels.

Immunoglobulin G

Immunoglobulin G (IgG), the only immunoglobulin that crosses the placenta, provides the fetus with passive temporary immunity to bacteria, bacterial toxins, and viruses to which the mother has developed immunity. IgG begins to cross the placenta during the first trimester. Preterm infants have less IgG because transfer is greatest during the third trimester. The full-term infant has IgG levels that are the same or above those of the mother.

Although the fetus begins to make its own IgG early in pregnancy, very little is produced until after 6 months of age (Blackburn, 2003). The infant gradually produces larger quantities of the immunoglobulin to replace IgG from the

TABLE **19-2** Distribution of Water in Newborns and Adults*		
	Newborn	**Adult**
Total body water	78%	50% females 60% males
Extracellular water	44%	20%
Intracellular water	34%	40%

*Comparison of distribution of body water in newborns and adults as a percent of body weight.

mother, which is being catabolized. The passive immunity gradually disappears at about 6 to 8 months of age (Buckley, 2004).

Immunoglobulin M

Immunoglobulin M (IgM) is the first immunoglobulin produced by the body when the newborn is challenged. This immunoglobulin helps protect against gram-negative bacteria. Small amounts of IgM are produced beginning at 20 weeks of gestation. Production increases rapidly beginning a few days after birth as a result of exposure to environmental antigens and rises to adult levels by 1 year of age (Buckley, 2004). IgM cannot cross the placenta because the molecules are too large. If IgM is found in larger-than-normal amounts, exposure to infection in utero is probable.

Immunoglobulin A

Immunoglobulin A (IgA) does not cross the placenta and must be produced by the infant. Because IgA is important in protection of the gastrointestinal and respiratory systems, newborns are particularly susceptible to infections of those systems. IgA may also help limit absorption of antigenic proteins in the diet. A form of IgA is present in colostrum and breast milk. Therefore breastfed infants may receive protection that formula-fed infants do not.

✔ CHECK YOUR READING

13. How does the distribution of fluid in the newborn compare with that in the adult?
14. Why are IgG, IgM, and IgA important to the newborn?

PSYCHOSOCIAL ADAPTATION

Periods of Reactivity

In the early hours after birth the infant goes through changes called the *periods of reactivity*. The two periods of reactivity are separated by a period of sleep.

FIRST PERIOD OF REACTIVITY

The first period of reactivity begins at birth. Infants are active at this time and appear wide awake, alert, and interested in their surroundings. Parents enjoy watching the infant gaze directly at them when held in the *en face* (face-to-face) position. Infants move their arms and legs energetically, root, and appear hungry. If allowed to nurse, many infants latch on to the nipple and suck well. The newborn may not demonstrate a period of quiet alert behavior this prolonged again for several days (Southgate & Pittard, 2001).

Respirations during the first period of reactivity may be as high as 80 breaths per minute. The heart rate may be elevated to 180 beats per minute. Crackles, retractions, nasal flaring, and increased mucous secretions may be present. The pulse and respirations gradually slow, and the infant becomes sleepy after about 30 minutes to 2 hours.

PERIOD OF SLEEP

After the first period of reactivity, infants become quiet and fall into a deep sleep, which lasts as long as 2 to 4 hours. During this time the pulse and respirations drop into the normal range, but the temperature may be low.

SECOND PERIOD OF REACTIVITY

When infants awaken from the period of sleep, they enter the second period of reactivity, which lasts only a short time or several hours. Infants are alert, and parents may enjoy the opportunity to get to know them at this time. Infants become interested in feeding and may pass meconium. The pulse and respiratory rates may increase, and some infants become cyanotic or have periods of apnea. Mucous secretions increase, and infants may gag or regurgitate.

Behavioral States

Six gradations in the behavioral state of the infant have been identified, ranging from deep sleep to crying. The amount of time infants spend in the different sleep-wake states varies and is a key to their individuality. Infants tend to move from one state to the next in the following sequence.

QUIET SLEEP STATE

During the quiet sleep state the infant is in a deep sleep with closed eyes and no eye movements. Respirations are quiet, regular, and slower than in the other states. Although startles occur at intervals, the infant's body is quiet. Little or no response to noise or stimuli occurs, and the infant returns to deep sleep quickly if not disturbed.

ACTIVE SLEEP STATE

The active sleep state is a lighter sleep in which infants move their extremities, stretch, change facial expressions, and make sucking movements and may fuss briefly. During this period, respirations tend to be more rapid and irregular and rapid eye movements (REM) occur. Infants are more likely to startle from noise or disturbances and may return to sleep or move to an awake state.

DROWSY STATE

The drowsy state is a transitional period between sleep and waking similar to that experienced by adults as they awaken. The eyes may remain closed or, if open, appear glazed and unfocused. Infants startle, move their extremities slowly, and whimper. They may go back to sleep or, with gentle stimulation, gradually awaken.

QUIET ALERT STATE

Parents should learn to identify the quiet alert state (also called *alert inactivity*), which is an excellent time for bonding. Infants focus on objects or people, respond to the parents with intense gazing, and seem bright and interested in their surroundings. Body movements are minimal as infants seem to concentrate on the environment.

ACTIVE ALERT STATE

In the active alert state infants are often fussy. They seem restless, have faster and more irregular respirations, and seem more aware of feelings of discomfort from hunger or cold. Although their eyes may be open, infants seem less focused on visual stimuli than during the quiet alert state.

CRYING STATE

The crying state may quickly follow the active alert state if no intervention occurs to comfort the infant. The cries are continuous and lusty, active body movement occurs, and the infant does not respond positively to stimulation. It may take a period of comforting to move the infant to a state in which feeding or other activities can be accomplished.

✔ CHECK YOUR READING

15. What are newborns like during the first and second periods of reactivity?
16. How do infant behavioral states vary?

SUMMARY CONCEPTS

- Chemical, thermal, and mechanical factors combine to stimulate the respiratory center in the brain and initiate respirations at birth.
- Surfactant lines the alveoli and reduces surface tension to keep the alveoli open. Fetal lung fluid moves into the interstitial spaces before, during, and after birth and is absorbed by the lymphatic and vascular systems.
- Increases in blood oxygen levels, shifts in pressure in the heart and lungs, and closing of the umbilical vessels cause closure of the ductus arteriosus, foramen ovale, and ductus venosus at birth.
- Infants are predisposed to heat loss because they have thin skin with little subcutaneous fat, blood vessels close to the surface, and a large skin surface area. They lose heat by evaporation, conduction, convection, and radiation.
- Heat is produced in newborns by an increased activity and flexion, vasoconstriction, and nonshivering thermogenesis. These factors increase oxygen and glucose consumption and may cause respiratory distress, hypoglycemia, acidosis, and jaundice.
- Laboratory values for erythrocytes, hemoglobin, and hematocrit are higher for newborns than for adults because oxygen available to them in fetal life was less than after birth.
- After birth, the stools progress from thick, greenish-black meconium to loose, greenish-brown transitional stools to milk stools. Stools of breastfed infants are frequent, soft, seedy, and mustard-colored, whereas those of formula-fed infants are pale yellow to light brown, firmer, and less frequent.
- The neonate uses glucose rapidly and is at risk for hypoglycemia.
- Physiologic jaundice occurs in normal newborns after the first 24 hours of life as a result of hemolysis of red blood cells and immaturity of the liver. Pathologic jaundice is abnormal, begins within the first 24 hours, and often requires treatment with phototherapy. Breast milk jaundice begins later than physiologic jaundice and may be attributable to substances in the milk.
- The newborn's kidneys filter, reabsorb, and monitor fluid and electrolyte balance less efficiently than the adult's kidneys. The newborn's body is composed of a greater percentage of water, with more located in the extracellular compartment, than in the adult.
- Newborns receive passive immunity when immunoglobin G crosses the placenta in utero. After birth, immunoglobin M and immunoglobin A are produced to protect against infection.
- During the first and second periods of reactivity, newborns are active and alert and may be interested in feeding. Their pulse and respiratory rates may be elevated, and they may show some transient signs of respiratory distress.
- Newborns progress through six behavioral states: quiet sleep, active sleep, drowsy, quiet alert, active alert, and crying.

ANSWERS TO CRITICAL THINKING EXERCISE 19-1, p. 454

If an opening was present between the right and left atria after birth, blood would flow from the left atrium, where pressures are high after birth, into the right atrium, where pressures are low after birth. This is the reverse of the blood flow through the foramen ovale during fetal life. The blood would then flow to the right ventricle, the pulmonary artery, and to the lungs. This would cause an increased workload on the lungs and could lead to serious complications.

ANSWERS TO CRITICAL THINKING EXERCISE 19-2, p. 456

Some sources of heat loss are:
- Evaporation—liquid on the body at birth or during bathing, contact with wet towels or blankets, regurgitation, leakage of urine, increased insensitive water loss while under a radiant warmer or under phototherapy lights
- Conduction—cool blankets, clothing, mattress, stethoscope, circumcision restraint board, cold hands of caregivers
- Convection—air conditioning or fans, drafts, open windows, cold oxygen
- Radiation—placement of crib or being held near an outside wall or window (open or closed), cool walls in poorly heated room

REFERENCES & READINGS

American Academy of Pediatrics (AAP) & American College of Obstetricians and Gynecologists (2002). *Guidelines for perinatal care* (5th ed.). Elk Grove, IL: AAP.

Armentrout, D. (2004). Glucose management. In M.T. Verklan & M. Walden (Eds.), *Core curriculum for neonatal intensive care nursing* (3rd ed., pp. 192-204). Philadelphia: Saunders.

Askin, D.F. (2002). Complications in the transition from fetal to neonatal life. *Journal of Obstetric, Gynecologic, & Neonatal Nursing, 31*(3), 318-327.

Blackburn, S.T. (2003). *Maternal, fetal, and neonatal physiology: A clinical perspective* (2nd ed.). Philadelphia: Saunders.

Blake, W.W., & Murray, J.A. (2002). Heat balance. In G.B. Merenstein & S.L. Gardner (Eds.), *Handbook of neonatal intensive care* (5th ed., pp. 100-115). St. Louis: Mosby.

Brodsky, D., & Martin, C. (2003). *Neonatology review*. Philadelphia: Hanley & Belfus.

Buckley, R.H. (2004). The T lymphocytes, B lymphocytes, and natural killer cells. In R.E. Behrman, R.M. Kliegman, & A.M. Arvin (Eds.), *Nelson textbook of pediatrics* (17th ed., pp. 683-689). Philadelphia: Saunders.

Buschbach, D., & Bordeaux, M.S. (2002). *Newborn physiological and developmental transitions: integrating key components of perinatal and neonatal assessment*. Washington DC: Association of Women's Health, Obstetric and Neonatal Nurses.

Cheffer, N.D. (2004). Adaptation to extrauterine life and immediate nursing care. In S. Mattson & J.E. Smith, (Eds.), *Core curriculum for maternal-newborn nursing* (3rd ed., pp. 421-436). Philadelphia: Saunders.

Fineman, J.R., Clyman, R., & Heymann, M.A. (2004). Fetal cardiovascular physiology. In R.K. Creasy & R. Resnik (Eds.), *Maternal-fetal medicine: Principles and practice* (5th ed., pp. 169-180). Philadelphia: Saunders.

Frank, C.G., Cooper, S.C., & Merenstein, G.B. (2002). Jaundice. In G.B. Merenstein & S.L. Gardner (Eds.), *Handbook of neonatal intensive care* (5th ed., pp. 443-461). St. Louis: Mosby.

Gardner, S.L., Johnson, J.L., & Lubchenco, L.O. (2002). Initial nursery care. In G.B. Merenstein & S.L. Gardner (Eds.), *Handbook of neonatal intensive care* (5th ed., pp. 70-99). St. Louis: Mosby.

Greenbaum, L.A. (2004). Pathophysiology of body fluids and fluid therapy. In R.E. Behrman, R.M. Kliegman, & A.M. Arvin (Eds.), *Nelson textbook of pediatrics* (17th ed., pp. 191-242). Philadelphia: Saunders.

Guttentag, S., & Ballard, P.L. (2005). Lung development: Embryology, growth, maturation, and developmental biology. In H.W. Taeusch, R.A. Ballard, & C.A. Gleason (Eds.), *Avery's diseases of the newborn* (8th ed., pp. 601-615). Philadelphia: Saunders.

Guyton, A.C., & Hall, J.E. (2000). *Textbook of medical physiology* (10th ed.). Philadelphia: Saunders.

Hackman, P.S. (2001). Recognizing and understanding the cold-stressed term infant. *Neonatal Network, 20*(8), 35-41.

Hagedorn, M.I., Gardner, S.L., & Abman, S.H. (2002). Respiratory diseases. In G.B. Merenstein & S.L. Gardner (Eds.), *Handbook of neonatal intensive care* (5th ed., pp. 485-575). St. Louis: Mosby.

Halamek, L.P., & Stevenson, D.K. (2002). Neonatal jaundice and liver disease. In A.A. Fanaroff & R.J. Martin (Eds.), *Neonatal-perinatal medicine* (Vol. 2, 7th ed., pp. 1309-1350). St. Louis: Mosby.

Hansen, T.N., & Corbet, A. (2005). Control of breathing. In H.W. Taeusch, R.A. Ballard, & C.A. Gleason (Eds.), *Avery's diseases of the newborn* (8th ed., pp. 616-633). Philadelphia: Saunders.

Hernandez, J.A., Fashaw, L., & Evans, R. (2005). Adaptation to extrauterine life and management during transition. In P.J. Thureen, J. Deacon, J. Hernandez, & D.M. Hall (Eds.), *Assessment and care of the well newborn* (2nd ed., pp. 83-109). Philadelphia: Saunders.

Jobe, A.H. (2002). Lung development and maturation. In A.A. Fanaroff & R.J. Martin (Eds.), (2002). *Neonatal-perinatal medicine* (Vol. 2, 7th ed.). St. Louis: Mosby.

Kenner, C. (2003). Resuscitation and stabilization of the newborn. In C. Kenner & J.W. Lott (Eds.), *Comprehensive neonatal nursing: A physiologic perspective* (3rd ed., pp. 210-227). Philadelphia: Saunders.

Lott, J.W. (2003). Assessment and management of the cardiovascular system. In C. Kenner & J.W. Lott (Eds.). *Comprehensive neonatal nursing: A physiologic perspective* (3rd ed., pp. 376-408). Philadelphia: Saunders.

Madan, A., MacMahon, J.R., & Stevenson, D.K. (2005). Neonatal hyperbilirubinemia. In H.W. Taeusch, R.A. Ballard, & C.A. Gleason (Eds.), *Avery's diseases of the newborn* (8th ed., pp. 1226-1256). Philadelphia: Saunders.

Maisels, M.J. (2001). Neonatal hyperbilirubinemia. In Klaus, M.H., & Fanaroff, A.A. (Eds.), *Care of the high-risk neonate* (5th ed., pp. 324-362). Philadelphia: Saunders.

McGowan, J.E., Hagedorn, M.I.E., & Hay, W.W. (2002). Glucose homeostasis. In G.B. Merenstein & S.L. Gardner (Eds.), *Handbook of neonatal intensive care* (5th ed., pp. 298-313). St. Louis: Mosby.

Mercer, J.S., & Skovgaard, R.L. (2002). Neonatal transitional physiology: a new paradigm. *Journal of Perinatal and Neonatal Nursing, 15*(4), 56-75.

Nicholson, J.F., & Pesce, M.A. (2004). Reference ranges for laboratory tests and procedures. In R.E. Behrman, R.M. Kliegman, & A.M. Arvin (Eds.), *Nelson textbook of pediatrics* (17th ed., pp. 2396-2421). Philadelphia: Saunders.

Noerr, B. (2004). Thermoregulation. In S. Mattson & J.E. Smith (Eds.), *Core curriculum for maternal-newborn nursing* (3rd ed., pp. 125-134). Philadelphia: Saunders.

Reiser, D.J. (2001). *Hyperbilirubinemia: Identification and management in healthy term and near term newborns*. White Plains, NY: March of Dimes Birth Defects Foundation.

Sahni, R., & Schulze, K. (2004). Temperature control in newborn infants. In R.A. Polin, W.W. Fox, & S.H. Abman (Eds.), *Fetal and neonatal physiology* (Vol I, 3rd ed., pp. 548-569). Philadelphia: Saunders.

Shaw, N.M. (2003). Assessment and management of the hematologic system. In C. Kenner & J.W. Lott (Eds.), *Comprehensive neonatal nursing: A physiologic perspective* (3rd ed., pp. 580-623). Philadelphia: Saunders.

Sniderman, S., & Taeusch, H.W. (2005). Initial evaluation: History and physical examination of the newborn In H.W. Taeusch, R.A. Ballard, & C.A. Gleason (Eds.), *Avery's diseases of the newborn* (8th ed., pp. 301-322). Philadelphia: Saunders.

Southgate, W.M., & Pittard, W.B. (2001). Classification and physical examination of the newborn infant. In M.H. Klaus & A.A. Fanaroff (Eds.), *Care of the high-risk neonate* (5th ed., pp. 100-129). Philadelphia: Saunders.

Stoll, B.J., & Kliegman, R.M. (2004a). Digestive system disorders. In R.E. Behrman, R.M. Kliegman, & H.B. Jenson (Eds.), *Nelson textbook of pediatrics* (17th ed., pp. 588-599). Philadelphia: Saunders.

Stoll, B.J., & Kliegman, R.M. (2004b). The newborn infant. In R.E. Behrman, R.M. Kliegman, & H.B. Jenson (Eds.), *Nelson textbook of pediatrics* (17th ed., pp. 523-531). Philadelphia: Saunders.

Swinford, R.D., Bonilla-Felix, M., Cerda, R.D., & Portman, R.J. (2002). Neonatal nephrology. In G.B. Merenstein & S.L. Gardner (Eds.), *Handbook of neonatal intensive care* (5th ed., pp. 609-643). St. Louis: Mosby.

Tsang, R.C., DeMarini, S., Rath, L.L. (2003). Fluids, electrolytes, vitamins, and trace minerals. In C. Kenner & J.W. Lott (Eds.), *Comprehensive neonatal nursing: A physiologic perspective* (3rd ed., pp. 409-424). Philadelphia: Saunders.

Verklan, M.T. (2004). Adaptation to extrauterine life. In M.T. Verklan & M. Walden (Eds.), *Core curriculum for neonatal intensive care nursing* (3rd ed., pp. 80-101). Philadelphia: Saunders.

Watson, R.L. (2004). Gastrointestinal disorders. In M.T. Verklan & M. Walden (Eds.), *Core curriculum for neonatal intensive care nursing* (3rd ed., pp. 643-702). Philadelphia: Saunders.

Assessment of the Normal Newborn

OBJECTIVES

After studying this chapter, you should be able to:

1. Describe the initial assessments of the newborn.
2. Explain the nurse's responsibilities in cardiorespiratory and thermoregulatory assessments.
3. Describe nursing assessments of body systems.
4. Explain the importance and components of gestational age assessment.

Go to your Student CD-ROM for Review Questions keyed to these Objectives.

DEFINITIONS

Acrocyanosis Bluish discoloration of the hands and feet because of reduced peripheral circulation.

Café-au-Lait Spots Light-brown birthmarks.

Caput Succedaneum Area of edema over the presenting part of the fetus or newborn resulting from pressure against the cervix; often called simply *caput.*

Cephalhematoma Bleeding between the periosteum and skull from pressure during birth; does not cross suture lines.

Choanal Atresia Abnormality of the nasal septum that obstructs one or both nasal passages.

Craniosynostosis Premature closure of the sutures of the infant's head.

Cryptorchidism Failure of one or both testes to descend into the scrotum.

Epispadias Abnormal placement of the urinary meatus on the dorsal side of the penis.

Erythema Toxicum Benign rash of unknown cause in newborns, with blotchy red areas that may have white or yellow papules or vesicles in the center.

Hypospadias Abnormal placement of the urinary meatus on the ventral side of the penis.

Lanugo Fine, soft hair that covers the fetus.

Milia White cysts, 1 to 2 mm in size, from distended sebaceous glands.

Molding Shaping of the fetal head during movement through the birth canal.

Mongolian Spots Bruiselike marks that occur mostly in newborns with dark skin tones.

Nevus Flammeus Permanent purple birthmark; also called *port-wine stain.*

Nevus Simplex Flat, pink area on the nape of the neck, midforehead, or over the eyelids resulting from dilation of the capillaries; also called *stork bites, salmon patches,* or *telangiectatic nevi.*

Nevus Vasculosus Rough, red collection of capillaries with a raised surface that disappears with time; also called *strawberry hemangioma.*

Periodic Breathing Cessation of breathing lasting 5 to 10 seconds without changes in color or heart rate.

Point of Maximum Impulse Area of the chest in which the heart sounds are loudest when auscultated.

Polydactyly More than 10 digits on the hands or feet.

Pseudomenstruation Vaginal bleeding in the newborn, resulting from withdrawal of placental hormones.

Strabismus A turning inward ("crossing") or outward of the eyes because of poor muscle tone in the muscles that control eye movement.

Syndactyly Webbing between fingers or toes.

Tachypnea Respiratory rate above 60 breaths per minute in the newborn after the first hour of life.

Vernix Caseosa Thick, white substance that protects the skin of the fetus.

A very important role of the nurse is assessing the newborn to identify abnormalities and problems in adapting to life outside the uterus. The first complete assessment of the newborn often is called an *admission assessment*. Subsequent assessments are less detailed (Table 20-1). "Keys to Clinical Practice" (Appendix C) describes the order of initial assessments and care.

EARLY FOCUSED ASSESSMENTS

Immediately after birth the nurse performs assessments that are most immediately crucial to determining the neonate's health status. These include the cardiorespiratory status, thermoregulation, and the presence of anomalies. The nurse determines whether resuscitation (p. 800) or other immediate interventions are necessary. When the infant is stable and oxygenating well, a more thorough assessment can be performed.

> When newborns have been dried at birth, it is easy to forget that their skin is contaminated with blood and amniotic fluids. The nurse should wear gloves when handling newborns until they are bathed and all blood is removed from the skin and hair. Wearing gloves helps protect the nurse from bloodborne infections.

Assessment of Cardiorespiratory Status

Assessments of respiratory and cardiovascular status are performed together because transitional changes take place in both systems at birth. Problems of adaptation in one system are likely to result in problems in the other system.

HISTORY

Information about the pregnancy, labor, and delivery is important in assessing the infant's cardiovascular and respiratory status and likelihood of problems at birth. For example, if the mother received narcotic analgesics late in labor, depression of the fetal central nervous system may interfere with initiation of respirations in the neonate. Preterm infants may not produce adequate amounts of surfactant, and atelectasis may occur because the alveoli do not remain open.

AIRWAY

During birth, some fetal lung fluid is forced into the upper airway. Excessive fluid and mucus in the infant's respiratory passages may cause respiratory difficulty for several hours after birth.

RESPIRATORY RATE. The nurse assesses respirations at least once every 30 minutes until the infant has been stable for 2 hours after birth (American Academy of Pediatrics [AAP] & American College of Obstetricians and Gynecologists [ACOG], 2002). If abnormalities are noted, respirations are assessed more often. The normal respiratory rate is 30 to 60 breaths per minute, with an average rate of 40 breaths per minute. The infant may breathe faster immediately after birth, during crying, and during the first and second periods of reactivity. Respirations should not be labored, and the chest movements should be symmetric. Because the pattern and depth of respirations are irregular, they must be counted for 1 full minute for accuracy (Procedure 20-1).

Counting the rapid, shallow, irregular respirations of a newborn can be a challenge at first. Differentiating between the respirations and other movements may be difficult while observing the infant's chest. Observation, auscultation, or palpation, alone or in combination, may be used to obtain an accurate respiratory rate.

The nurse observes for periodic breathing, which are pauses in breathing lasting 5 to 10 seconds without other changes. This occurs is some full-term infants during the first few days but most often in preterm infants. Apnea lasting longer than 20 seconds or accompanied by cyanosis, heart rate changes, or other signs of difficult breathing is abnormal.

BREATH SOUNDS. The anterior and posterior lung fields are auscultated for breath sounds, which should be present equally throughout. Breath sounds should be clear over most areas. However, hearing sounds of moisture in the lungs during the first hour or two after birth is not unusual because fetal lung fluid has not been completely absorbed. Infants born by cesarean may not experience the changes that occur in the lungs during labor and birth and are more likely to have coarse breath sounds. Wheezes, crackles, rhonchi, or stridor that persists should be reported.

Abnormal and diminished sounds always should be reported to the primary care provider if they continue. They may indicate a pneumothorax. Bowel sounds in the chest may be a sign of diaphragmatic hernia.

SIGNS OF RESPIRATORY DISTRESS. Throughout the assessment, the nurse must be alert for signs of respiratory distress, which may be present at birth or may develop later. They include tachypnea, retractions, flaring nares, central cyanosis, grunting, moaning, and seesaw respirations. Whenever one sign of labored breathing is present, the assessment must be carefully expanded to identify others.

Tachypnea. Tachypnea, a respiratory rate above 60 breaths per minute, is the most common sign of respiratory distress. It is not unusual during the first hour after birth and during the second period of reactivity, but continued tachypnea is abnormal.

Retractions. When the infant's weak chest wall muscles are used to help draw air into the lungs, retractions result. The soft tissue around the bones of the chest is drawn in with the effort of pulling air into the lungs. Xiphoid (substernal) retractions occur when the area under the sternum retracts each time the infant inhales. When the muscles between the ribs are pulled in so that each rib is outlined, intercostal retractions are present. The muscles above the sternum and around the clavicles also may be used to aid in respirations (supraclavicular retractions). Retractions may be mild or severe, depending on the degree of respiratory difficulty. Occasional mild retractions are common immediately after birth but should not continue after the first hour.

Text continued on p. 475.

TABLE 20-1 Summary of Newborn Assessment

Normal	Abnormal (Possible Causes)	Nursing Considerations
Initial Assessment Assess for obvious problems first. If infant is stable and has no problems that require immediate attention, continue with complete assessment.		
Vital Signs *Temperature* 36.5°-37.5° C (97.7°-99.5° F) axillary; 36.5°-37.6° C (97.7°-99.7° F) rectal. Axilla is preferred site.	Decreased (cold environment, hypoglycemia, infection, CNS problem). Increased (infection, environment too warm).	*Decreased:* Institute warming measures and check in 30 min. Check blood glucose. *Increased:* Remove excessive clothing. Check for dehydration. *Decreased or increased:* Look for signs of infection. Check radiant warmer temperature setting. Check thermometer for accuracy if skin is warm or cool to touch. Report abnormal values to physician.
Pulses Heart rate 120-160 bpm (100 sleeping, 180 crying). Rhythm regular. PMI at third to fourth intercostal space, slightly to left of midclavicular line. Brachial, femoral, and pedal pulses present and equal bilaterally.	Tachycardia (respiratory problems, anemia, infection, cardiac conditions). Bradycardia (asphyxia, increased intracranial pressure). PMI to right (dextrocardia, pneumothorax). Murmurs (functional or congenital heart defects). Arrhythmias. Absent or unequal pulses (coarctation of the aorta).	Note location of murmurs. Refer abnormal rates, rhythms and sounds, pulses.
Respirations Rate 30-60 (average 40) per min. Respirations irregular, shallow, unlabored. Chest movements symmetric. Breath sounds present and clear bilaterally.	Tachypnea, especially after the first hour. Slow respirations (maternal medications). Nasal flaring. Grunting (respiratory distress syndrome). Gasping (respiratory depression). Periods of apnea more than 20 sec or with change in heart rate or color (respiratory depression, sepsis, cold stress). Asymmetry or decreased chest expansion (pneumothorax). Intercostal, xiphoid, or supraclavicular retractions or seesaw respirations (respiratory distress). Moist, coarse breath sounds (crackles, rhonchi, fluid in lungs). Bowel sounds in chest (diaphragmatic hernia).	Mild variations require continued monitoring and usually clear in early hours after birth. If persistent or more than mild, suction, give oxygen, call physician, and initiate more intensive care.
Blood Pressure Average BP 65-95 mm Hg systolic, 30-60 mm Hg diastolic. Varies with activity and gestational age and size.	Hypotension (hypovolemia, shock, sepsis). Difference of 15 mm Hg between arms and legs (coarctation of the aorta).	Refer abnormal blood pressures. Prepare for intensive care if very low.
Measurements *Weight* 2500-4000 g (5 lb, 8 oz to 8 lb, 13 oz). Weight loss less than 10%.	High (LGA, maternal diabetes). Low (SGA, preterm, multifetal pregnancy, medical conditions in mother that affect fetal growth). Weight loss above 10% (dehydration, feeding problems).	Determine cause. Monitor for complications common to cause.
Length 48-53 cm (19-21 in).	Below normal (SGA, congenital dwarfism). Above normal (LGA, maternal diabetes).	Determine cause. Monitor for complications common to cause.
Head Circumference 33-35.5 cm (13-14 in). Head approximately one fourth of infant's length.	Small (SGA, microcephaly, anencephaly). Large (LGA, hydrocephalus, increased intracranial pressure).	Determine cause. Monitor for complications common to cause.
Chest Circumference 30.5-33 cm (12-13 in). Is 2-3 cm less than head circumference.	Large (LGA). Small (SGA).	Determine cause. Monitor for complications common to cause.

bpm, Beats per minute; *CNS,* central nervous system; *LGA,* large for gestational age; *PMI,* point of maximum impulse; *SGA,* small for gestational age.

TABLE 20-1 Summary of Newborn Assessment—cont'd

Normal	Abnormal (Possible Causes)	Nursing Considerations
Posture Flexed extremities resist extension, return quickly to flexed state. Hands usually clenched. Movements symmetric. Slight tremors on crying. Breech: extended, stiff legs. "Molds" body to caretaker's when held, responds by quieting when needs met.	Limp, flaccid, "floppy," or rigid extremities (preterm, hypoxia, medications, CNS trauma). Hypertonic (neonatal abstinence syndrome, CNS damage). Jitteriness or tremors (low glucose or calcium level). Opisthotonus, seizures, stiff when held (CNS damage).	Seek cause, refer abnormalities.
Cry Lusty, strong.	High-pitched (increased intracranial pressure). Weak, absent, irritable, catlike "mewing" (neurologic problems). Hoarse or crowing (laryngeal irritation).	Observe for changes, report abnormalities.
Skin Color pink or tan with acrocyanosis. Vernix caseosa in creases. Small amounts of lanugo over shoulders, sides of face, forehead, upper back. Skin turgor good with quick recoil. Some cracking and peeling of skin. Normal variations: Milia. Erythema toxicum ("flea bite" rash). Puncture on scalp (from electrode). Mongolian spots. Telangiectatic nevi (nevus simplex, salmon patch, or "stork bites").	*Color:* Cyanosis of mouth and central areas (hypoxia). Facial bruising (nuchal cord). Pallor (anemia, hypoxia). Gray (hypoxia, hypotension). Red, sticky, transparent skin (very preterm). Ruddy (polycythemia). Greenish-brown discoloration of skin, nails, cord (possible fetal compromise, postterm). Harlequin color (normal or cardiac problems, sepsis.) Mottling (normal or cold stress, hypovolemia, sepsis). Yellow vernix (blood incompatibilities). Jaundice (pathologic if first 24 hr). Thick vernix (preterm). *Delivery marks:* Bruises on body (pressure), scalp (vacuum extractor), or face (cord around neck). Petechiae (pressure, low platelets, infection). Forceps marks. *Birthmarks:* Mongolian spots. Telangiectatic nevi ("stork bites"). Nevus flammeus (port-wine stain). Nevus vasculosus (strawberry hemangioma). Café-au-lait spots (six or more or >0.5 cm in size, neurofibromatosis). *Other:* Excessive lanugo (preterm). Excessive peeling, cracking (postterm). Skin tags. Milia. Erythema toxicum. Pustules, or other rashes (infection). "Tenting" of skin (dehydration).	Differentiate facial bruising from cyanosis. Central cyanosis requires suction, oxygen, and further treatment. Refer jaundice in first 24 hr. Watch for respiratory problems in infants with meconium staining. Look for other signs and complications of preterm or postterm birth. Record location, size, shape, color, type of rashes and marks. Differentiate Mongolian spots from bruises. Check for facial movement with forceps marks. Watch for jaundice with bruising. Point out and explain normal skin variations to parents.
Head Sutures palpable with small separation between each. Anterior fontanel diamond shaped, 2-4 cm, soft and flat. May bulge slightly with crying. Posterior fontanel triangular, 0.5-1 cm. Hair silky and soft with individual hair strands. Normal variations: Overriding sutures (molding). Caput succedaneum or cephalhematoma (pressure during birth).	Head large (hydrocephalus, increased intracranial pressure) or small (microcephaly). Widely separated sutures (hydrocephalus) or hard, ridged area at sutures (craniosynostosis). Anterior fontanel depressed (dehydration, molding), full or bulging at rest (increased intracranial pressure). Woolly, bunchy hair (preterm). Unusual hair growth (genetic abnormalities).	Seek cause of variations. Observe for signs of dehydration with depressed fontanel, increased intracranial pressure with bulging of fontanel and wide separation of sutures. Refer for treatment. Differentiate caput succedaneum from cephalhematoma and reassure parents of normal outcome. Observe for jaundice with cephalhematoma.
Ears Ears well formed and complete. Area where upper ear meets head even with imaginary line drawn from inner to outer canthus of eye. Startle response to loud noises. Alerts to high-pitched voices.	Low-set ears (chromosomal disorders). Skin tags, preauricular sinuses, dimples (kidney or other anomalies). No response to sound (deafness).	Check voiding if ears abnormal. Look for signs of chromosomal abnormality if position abnormal. Refer for evaluation if no response to sound.

Continued

TABLE **20-1** Summary of Newborn Assessment—cont'd

Normal	Abnormal (Possible Causes)	Nursing Considerations
Face Symmetric in appearance and movement. Parts proportional and appropriately placed.	Asymmetry (pressure and position in utero). Drooping of mouth or one side of face, "one-sided cry" (facial nerve damage). Abnormal appearance (chromosomal abnormalities).	Seek cause of variations. Check delivery history for possible cause of damage to facial nerve.
Eyes Symmetric. Eyes clear. Transient strabismus. Scant or absent tears. Pupils equal, react to light. Alerts to interesting sights. Follows objects across midline. Doll's-eye sign, red reflex present. May have subconjunctival hemorrhage or edema of eyelids from pressure during birth.	Inflammation or drainage (chemical or infectious conjunctivitis). Constant tearing (plugged lacrimal duct). Unequal pupils. Failure to follow objects (blindness). White areas over pupils (cataracts). Setting-sun sign (hydrocephalus). Yellow sclera (jaundice). Blue sclera (osteogenesis imperfecta).	Clean and monitor any drainage; seek cause. Reassure parents that subconjunctival hemorrhage and edema will clear. Refer other abnormalities.
Nose Both nostrils open to air flow. May have slight flattening from pressure during birth.	Blockage of one or both nasal passages (choanal atresia). Malformations (congenital conditions). Flaring, mucus (respiratory distress).	Observe for respiratory distress. Report malformations.
Mouth Mouth, gums, tongue pink. Tongue normal in size and movement. Lips and palate intact. Sucking pads. Sucking, rooting, swallowing, gag reflexes present. Normal variations: Precocious teeth, Epstein's pearls.	Cyanosis (hypoxia). White patches on cheeks or tongue (candidiasis). Protruding tongue (Down syndrome). Diminished movement of tongue, drooping mouth (facial nerve paralysis). Cleft lip or palate, or both. Absent or weak reflexes (preterm, neurologic problem). Excessive drooling (tracheoesophageal fistula, esophageal atresia).	Oxygen for cyanosis. Expect loose teeth to be removed. Obtain order for nystatin medication for candidiasis. Check mother for vaginal or breast infection. Refer anomalies.
Feeding Good suck-swallow coordination. Retains feedings.	Poorly coordinated suck and swallow. Duskiness or cyanosis during feeding (cardiac defects). Choking, gagging, excessive drooling (tracheoesophageal fistula, esophageal atresia).	Feed slowly. Stop frequently if difficulty occurs. Suction and stimulate if necessary. Refer infants with continued difficulty.
Neck and Clavicles Short neck turns head easily side to side. Infant raises head when prone. Clavicles intact.	Weakness, contractures, or rigidity (muscle abnormalities). Webbing of neck, large fat pad at back of neck (chromosomal disorders). Crepitus, lump, or crying when clavicle palpated, diminished or absent arm movement (fractured clavicle).	Fracture of clavicle occurs especially in large infants with shoulder dystocia at birth. Immobilize arm. Look for other injuries. Refer abnormalities.
Chest Cylindric. Xiphoid process may be prominent. Symmetric. Nipples present and located properly. May have engorgement, white nipple discharge (maternal hormone withdrawal).	Asymmetry (diaphragmatic hernia, pneumothorax). Supernumerary nipples. Redness (infection).	Report abnormalities.
Abdomen Rounded, soft. Bowel sounds present soon after birth. Liver palpable 1-3 cm below costal margin. Skin intact. Three vessels in cord. Clamp tight and cord drying. Meconium passed within 12-48 hr. Urine passed within 12-24 hr. Normal variation: "Brick dust" staining of diaper (urate crystals).	Sunken abdomen (diaphragmatic hernia). Distended abdomen or loops of bowel visible (obstruction, infection, enlarged organs). Absent bowel sounds after first hour (paralytic ileus). Masses palpated (kidney tumors, distended bladder). Enlarged liver (infection, heart failure, hemolytic disease). Abdominal wall defects (umbilical or inguinal hernia, omphalocele, gastroschisis, extrophy of bladder). Two vessels in cord (other anomalies). Bleeding (loose clamp). Redness, drainage from cord (infection). No passage of meconium (imperforate anus, obstruction). Lack of urinary output (kidney anomalies) or inadequate amounts (dehydration).	Refer abnormalities. Look for other anomalies if only two vessels in cord. Tighten or replace loose cord clamp. If stool and urine output abnormal, check to see none was unrecorded, increase feedings, report.

TABLE 20-1 Summary of Newborn Assessment—cont'd

Normal	Abnormal (Possible Causes)	Nursing Considerations
Genitals		
Female		
Labia majora dark, cover clitoris and labia minora. Small amount of white mucous vaginal discharge. Urinary meatus and vagina present. Normal variations: Vaginal bleeding (pseudomenstruation). Hymenal tags.	Clitoris and labia minora larger than labia majora (preterm). Large clitoris (ambiguous genitalia). Edematous labia (breech birth).	Check gestational age for immature genitalia. Refer anomalies.
Male		
Testes within scrotal sac, rugae on scrotum, prepuce nonretractable. Meatus at tip of penis.	Testes in inguinal canal or abdomen (preterm, cryptorchidism). Lack of rugae on scrotum (preterm). Edema of scrotum (pressure in breech birth). Enlarged scrotal sac (hydrocele). Small penis, scrotum (preterm, ambiguous genitalia). Urinary meatus located on upper side of penis (epispadias), underside of penis (hypospadias), or perineum.	Check gestational age for immature genitalia. Refer anomalies. Explain to parents why no circumcision can be performed with abnormal placement of meatus.
Extremities		
Upper and Lower Extremities		
Equal and bilateral movement of extremities. Correct number and formation of fingers and toes. Nails to ends of digits or slightly beyond. Flexion, good muscle tone.	Crepitus, redness, lumps, swelling (fracture). Diminished or absent movement, especially during Moro reflex (fracture, nerve damage, paralysis). Polydactyly (extra digits). Syndactyly (webbing). Fused or absent digits. Poor muscle tone (preterm, neurologic damage, hypoglycemia, hypoxia).	Refer all anomalies, look for others.
Upper Extremities		
Two transverse palm creases.	Simian crease (Down syndrome). Diminished movement of arm with extension and forearm prone (Erb-Duchenne paralysis).	Refer all anomalies, look for others.
Lower Extremities		
Legs equal in length, abduct equally, gluteal and thigh creases and knee height equal, no hip "clunk." Normal position of feet.	Ortolani and Barlow tests abnormal, unequal leg length, unequal thigh or gluteal creases (developmental dysplasia of the hip). Malposition of feet (position in utero, talipes equinovarus).	Refer all anomalies, look for others. Check malpositioned feet to see if they can be manipulated back to normal position.
Back		
No openings observed or felt in vertebral column. Anus patent. Sphincter tightly closed.	Failure of vertebra to close (spina bifida), with or without sac with spinal fluid and meninges (meningocele) or cord (myelomeningocele) enclosed. Tuft of hair over spina bifida occulta. Pilonidal dimple or sinus. Imperforate anus.	Refer abnormalities. Observe for movement below level of defect. If sac, cover with sterile dressing wet with sterile saline. Protect from injury.
Reflexes		
Moro, palmar and plantar grasp, rooting, sucking, swallowing, tonic neck, Babinski, Gallant, and stepping reflexes present (see Table 20-2).	Absent, asymmetric, or weak reflexes.	Observe for signs of fractures, nerve damage, or injury to CNS.

PROCEDURE

20-1 Assessing Vital Signs in the Newborn

PURPOSE: To obtain an accurate measurement of newborn vital signs

RESPIRATIONS

1. Assess respirations when the infant is quiet or sleeping and before disturbing the infant for other assessments, if possible. *Allows the lung sounds to be heard more clearly.*

2. Observe, auscultate, and palpate the chest and abdomen. *The rapid, shallow, irregular respirations can be confused with other movements in an active infant. A combination of methods increases accuracy of the assessment.*

3. Lift the infant's blanket and shirt to see the chest and abdomen. Observe the pattern of respirations before beginning to count. *Respirations are often irregular, but a basic pattern is present. Observation of the pattern makes it easier to count the rate.*

4. If desired, place a hand lightly over the infant's chest or abdomen to feel the movement. Avoid covering the chest completely so that the chest excursions can be watched as well as palpated. *Palpation helps keep track of the rate.*

5. To auscultate respirations, move a stethoscope over the chest until the respirations are easily heard. This is often toward the right side of the infant's chest. After counting, move the stethoscope to listen to breath sounds in all areas. *Allows the sounds of the lungs to be heard with less interference from heart sounds.*

6. Count for a full minute. *Respirations are normally irregular in the newborn. Counting for a full minute increases accuracy.*

7. If the infant is crying, allow the infant to suck on a pacifier or gloved finger. If crying continues, count the respirations and note on the chart that the infant was crying. Recheck later when the infant is quiet. *Sucking may quiet the infant. Although respirations are most easily assessed on a quiet infant, they can be counted when the infant is crying. Respirations may be faster on a crying infant.*

8. Expect the respiratory rate to be 30 to 60 breaths/min when the infant is at rest. Observe and report signs of respiratory distress, including tachypnea, retractions, flaring, cyanosis, grunting, seesawing, apneic periods, and asymmetry of chest movements. Continue to watch infants whose respiratory rate is near the extremes of the normal range. *Allows early identification and follow-up of abnormalities. Rates near abnormal may become abnormal in a short time.*

PULSE

1. Listen to the apical pulse while the infant is quiet and before disturbing the infant for other assessments, if possible. *The heart sounds are heard more clearly in a quiet or sleeping infant.*

2. Use a pediatric head on the stethoscope to listen to the apical pulse. *Although a larger head may be used if necessary, the small head allows better contact between the stethoscope and the chest wall and eliminates some of the sounds from the lungs and intestines.*

3. If the infant is crying, insert a pacifier or a gloved finger into the infant's mouth. *Sucking often quiets infants.*

4. If the infant cannot be quieted, increase concentration and time spent listening. *Concentration helps to separate the sounds heard and to focus in on the heartbeat.*

5. Listen briefly before beginning to count. Tapping a finger in rhythm with the beat may be helpful. Count for a full minute. Expect the heart rate to be 120 to 160 bpm at rest. *Listening to the pattern allows time to get used to the rapid heartbeat before counting. Counting for a full minute increases chances of identifying abnormalities.*

6. Move the stethoscope over the entire heart area. Assess for arrhythmias, murmurs, or other abnormal sounds. Refer any abnormalities. *Listening over the entire area increases chances of hearing abnormal sounds. Reporting abnormalities to the pediatrician allows further investigation.*

TEMPERATURE

Axillary

1. Place the thermometer vertically along the chest wall with the tip of the thermometer against the skin in the center of the axillary space, with the infant's arm held firmly against the body over the probe. *If the thermometer is held horizontally, it may protrude behind the axilla and give an inaccurate reading. Holding the arm keeps the thermometer positioned correctly and prevents accidental injury if the infant moves unexpectedly.*

2. Read the thermometer at the proper time: electronic or digital, when indicator sounds; other types according to manufacturer's direction. Normal range: 36.5 to 37.5°C (97.7 to 99.5° F). *Ensures an accurate reading.*

Rectal

Note: Taking rectal temperatures is not recommended under most circumstances.

1. Take a rectal temperature only when necessary and according to birth facility policy. Use the axillary method whenever possible. *Rectal and axillary readings are very similar. Taking the temperature rectally involves the potential for perforation of the rectum, which can be life threatening.*

2. Place the infant in a supine position and hold the ankles firmly in one hand. Bend the infant's knees against the abdomen and raise the legs to expose the anus. Alternatively, place the infant prone or on the side and separate the buttocks. *Provides visualization and prevents excessive movement that might dislodge the thermometer, resulting in injury to delicate tissues.*

3. Lubricate the tip of the thermometer with water-soluble lubricant. *Allows the thermometer to be inserted without irritation to the sphincter. Water-soluble lubricant dissolves and washes away.*

4. Insert the thermometer carefully and gently into the rectum. *The rectum turns to the right 3 cm (1.2 in) from the sphincter. Inserting the thermometer farther may cause perforation.*

5. Do not force the thermometer if it does not insert easily. *An obstruction may be preventing insertion of the thermometer.*

6. Hold the thermometer securely throughout the time it remains in the rectum. *Maintains control to avoid inserting the thermometer too far and prevents injury if the infant moves.*

7. Read the thermometer at the proper time: electronic, when indicator sounds; other types according to manufacturer's directions. Normal range: 36.5 to 37.6° C (97.7 to 99.7° F). *Ensures accurate reading.*

Flaring of the Nares. A reflexive widening of the nostrils occurs when the infant is receiving insufficient oxygen. Nasal flaring helps decrease airway resistance and increase the amount of air entering the lungs. Intermittent flaring may occur in the first hour after birth. Continued flaring indicates a more serious respiratory problem.

Cyanosis. Cyanosis is a purplish blue discoloration indicating that the infant is not getting enough oxygen. It may be preceded by a dusky or gray hue to the skin. Central cyanosis involves the lips, tongue, mucous membranes, and trunk and shows true hypoxia. This sign indicates that not enough oxygen is reaching the vital organs and requires immediate attention. Bruising of the face may occur from a tight nuchal cord or pressure during birth and may look like central cyanosis. To differentiate cyanosis from bruising, apply pressure to the area. A cyanotic area will blanch, but a bruised area remains blue. Central cyanosis in infants with dark skin tones can be checked by looking at the color of the mucous membranes. A pulse oximeter may be used to determine oxygen saturation in infants with cyanosis.

Central cyanosis must be differentiated from peripheral cyanosis (acrocyanosis), which involves only the extremities. Acrocyanosis is normal during the first day after birth and if the infant becomes cold. It results from poor perfusion of blood to the periphery of the body (Figure 20-1).

Cyanosis may be present at birth or may become apparent later. It is not unusual to see a purplish blue discoloration at birth that quickly turns pink as the infant begins to breathe. Cyanosis occurs whenever the infant's breathing is impaired. It may occur during feedings because of difficulty in coordinating sucking, swallowing, and breathing. Infants who become cyanotic on exertion or crying may have a congenital heart defect.

Grunting. *Grunting* describes a noise made on expiration when air crosses partially closed vocal cords. This increases the pressure within the alveoli, which keeps the alveoli open and enhances the exchange of gases in the lungs. Grunting may be very mild and heard only with a stethoscope or loud enough to hear unaided in an infant having severe respiratory difficulty. Persistent grunting is a common sign of respiratory distress syndrome and necessitates expanded assessment and referral for treatment.

Seesaw Respirations. Normally the chest and abdomen rise and fall together during respiration. In the infant with severe respiratory difficulty, the chest falls when the abdomen rises and the chest rises when the abdomen falls, causing a seesaw effect. Seesaw respirations in infants without other signs of respiratory difficulty should not cause alarm (Southgate & Pittard, 2001).

Asymmetry. Chest expansion should be equal on both sides. Asymmetry or decreased movement on one side may indicate the collapse of a lung (pneumothorax).

CHOANAL ATRESIA. Assessment for choanal atresia is important because newborns are preferential nose breathers for approximately the first 3 weeks of life. This means that they breathe mostly through the nose except when crying. In choanal atresia, one or both nasal passages are blocked or narrowed by bone or membrane that protrudes into the area.

Bilateral choanal atresia causes severe respiratory distress and requires surgery. Blockage of one side puts the infant at risk for respiratory distress if the other side becomes occluded by mucus or edema.

The nurse can assess for choanal atresia by closing the infant's mouth and occluding one nostril at a time. The infant is observed for breathing, and breath sounds are auscultated while each nostril is occluded. Another method of assessment is to place a cold metal object under the nostrils and observe for fogging. Passing a catheter (No. 5 to 8 Fr) through each nostril to check for patency may be performed if there is a question with other methods. Infants with choanal atresia may become cyanotic when quiet but pink when crying because air is then drawn in through the mouth.

COLOR

In addition to cyanosis, the nurse assesses for pallor and ruddiness.

PALLOR. Some infants have a pale skin color. Pallor can indicate that the infant is slightly hypoxic or anemic. The physician may order a laboratory examination of hemoglobin and hematocrit or a complete blood count.

RUDDY COLOR. In contrast to pallor, a ruddy color (plethora) occurs in some infants. This reddish color of the skin may indicate polycythemia, an excessive number of red blood cells. A hematocrit above 65% confirms polycythemia. Infants with elevated hematocrits are at increased risk for jaundice from the normal destruction of excessive red blood cells that occurs after birth.

HEART SOUNDS

The heart is auscultated for rate, rhythm, and the presence of murmurs or abnormal sounds. The nurse should count the apical pulse for a full minute for accuracy and listen for abnormalities. The rate should range between 120 and 160 beats per minute (bpm) with normal activity. It may elevate to 180 bpm when infants are crying or drop as low as 100 bpm when they are in deep sleep.

If no problems are present at birth, the heart rate should be recorded at least once every 30 minutes until the infant has been stable for 2 hours after birth (AAP &

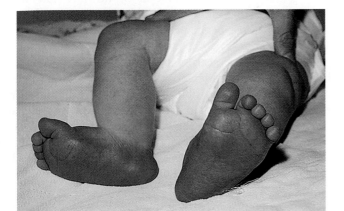

Figure 20-1 ■ Acrocyanosis. (From Eichenfeld, L.F., Frieden, I.J., & Esterly, N.B. [2001]. *Textbook of neonatal dermatology.* Philadelphia: Saunders.)

ACOG, 2002). Monitoring is more frequent if abnormalities are present. Once stable the heart rate is checked once every 8 hours or according to hospital policy unless a reason for more frequent assessment develops.

POSITION. An experienced examiner can determine the position of the heart in the chest by the location of heart sounds and the point of maximum impulse. The apex of the heart is located at the point of maximum impulse, where the pulse is most easily felt and the sound is loudest. This is at the third or fourth intercostal space, slightly left of the midclavicular line (a line drawn from the middle of the left clavicle). Conditions that affect the position of the heart include pneumothorax and dextrocardia (a right-to-left reversal from normal of the heart position).

RHYTHM AND MURMURS. The rhythm of the heart should be regular, and the first and second sounds (*lub* and *dub*) should be heard clearly. Abnormalities in rhythm and sounds such as murmurs should be noted. Murmurs are sounds of abnormal blood flow through the heart and may indicate openings in the septum of the heart or problems with blood flow through the valves. Most murmurs in the newborn are temporary and result from incomplete transition from fetal to neonatal circulation. A murmur is common until the ductus arteriosus is functionally closed. Although it may be a normal or functional murmur, any abnormal sounds of the heart are investigated because they may be signs of cardiac defects.

BRACHIAL AND FEMORAL PULSES

The brachial and femoral pulses should be present and equal bilaterally. The brachial pulse is located over the antecubital space, and the femoral pulse is located at the groin. Femoral pulses that are weaker than the brachial pulses may result from impaired blood flow in coarctation of the aorta, a congenital heart defect. In this condition, a narrowed area of the aorta impedes blood flow to the lower part of the body and causes weaker pulses in the lower extremities.

BLOOD PRESSURE

Measurement of blood pressure is not a necessary part of a routine assessment of the newborn, according to the AAP (AAP & ACOG, 2002). The blood pressure is taken on all extremities, however, if the infant has unequal pulses, murmurs, or other signs of cardiac complications. Doppler ultrasonography and other electronic measurement techniques are used to obtain an accurate blood pressure. For accurate measurement to be ensured, the infant should be quiet when the blood pressure is taken because crying elevates it. The width of the blood pressure cuff should cover the upper arm or leg without encroaching on the joints (Swinford, Bonilla-Felix, Cerda, & Portman, 2002). A cuff that is too narrow gives a false high reading, whereas a cuff that is too wide gives a false low reading.

The average blood pressure for full-term newborns is 65 to 95 mm Hg systolic and 30 to 60 mm Hg diastolic, al-

though variation exists according to the infant's weight (Hernandez, Fashaw, & Evans, 2005). It normally is lower in smaller babies. Hypotension may occur in the sick infant. The blood pressure of the lower extremities should be the same as or slightly higher than that of the upper extremities. A blood pressure in the upper extremities that is over 15 mm Hg higher than that in the lower extremities may indicate coarctation of the aorta (Gardner, Johnson, & Lubchenco, 2002).

CAPILLARY REFILL

Capillary refill is assessed to help determine if perfusion is adequate. It is checked by depressing the skin over the chest, the abdomen, or an extremity until the area blanches. The color should return in less than 3 seconds (Sansoucie & Cavaliere, 2003).

Assessment of Thermoregulation

The neonate's temperature is taken soon after birth while the infant is being held by the mother or is in a radiant warmer with a skin probe attached to the abdomen. The probe, which should not be attached over bony prominences, allows the warmer to measure and display the infant's temperature continuously. The temperature control is set to regulate the amount of heat produced according to the infant's skin temperature. The temperature should be assessed at least once every 30 minutes until the infant has been stable for 2 hours after birth (AAP & ACOG, 2002). It often is checked again at 4 hours and then once every 8 hours or according to facility policy as long as it remains stable (Procedure 20-2).

The most common method of taking the neonate's temperature is axillary measurement, which provides readings close to rectal measurements (Figure 20-2). The normal range for axillary temperature is 36.5 to 37.5° C (97.7 to 99.5° F). Taking axillary temperatures is safer than taking rectal temperatures because it avoids the possibility of irritation or damage to the rectum, which turns at a sharp right angle approximately 3 cm (1.2 in) from the anal sphincter (Blake & Murray, 2002).

If a rectal temperature is necessary, the nurse should use great care to avoid inserting the thermometer too far because potentially fatal perforation of the intestinal wall could result. A thermometer should never be forced into the rectum because of the possible presence of an imperforate (closed) anus.

Temperatures are usually measured with an electronic digital thermometer. Mercury thermometers are no longer used because of the possibility of injury or contamination with mercury if the thermometer breaks. Inexpensive digital thermometers used while the infant is in the hospital sometimes are given to the parents for home use. Disposable plastic strips that change color to indicate temperature readings are used less often than electronic models. Tympanic thermometers are used in some facilities but may be less accurate in newborns, especially those with fevers or in radiant warmers (Blackburn, 2003).

PROCEDURE

20-2 Weighing and Measuring the Newborn

PURPOSE: To obtain accurate measurements of the newborn

WEIGHT

1. Cover the scale with a blanket. Place a paper cover over the blanket if desired. *Prevents conductive heat loss from contact between the infant and a cold surface, helps prevent cross-contamination, and makes cleaning easier.*
2. Balance or adjust the scale to zero after the covering is placed. Electronic scale: Push the "on" button, and check to see that the digital readout is at zero. The electronic scale is usually self-adjusting. Balance scale: Adjust until the balance arm is horizontal. *Results in accurate weighing of the infant without including weight of the scale covering.*
3. Remove clothing and blankets from the infant, and place the infant in supine position on the scale. Keep one hand just above the infant and watch him or her carefully throughout the procedure. *Infants often are upset when first placed on the scale, and the startle or Moro reflex may occur. They may be in danger of sliding off the scale.*

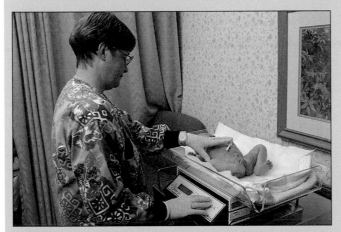

4. Wait until the infant is somewhat quiet. The electronic scale displays weight in pounds and ounces or in grams. Some electronic scales display an indicator when an accurate weight has been obtained. For a balance scale, move weights slowly until the arm is level. *Waiting until the infant is quiet increases accuracy.*
5. Write the numbers down immediately. If the scale is covered with paper, the weight can be written on the paper and taken with the infant to the warmer. Write it on the nurses' notes when the infant is safely settled. *Prevents forgetting the weight.*
6. Compare weight with the normal range for term infants: 2500 to 4000 g (5 lb, 8 oz to 8 lb, 13 oz). *Shows whether the infant is within expected range.*

LENGTH

Ruler Printed on Scale or Crib

1. Place the infant in supine position with his or her head at the upper edge of the ruler. *Places the infant in the proper position.*

2. While holding the infant with one hand so that the head does not move, use the other hand to fully extend the infant's leg along the ruler. Note the length at the bottom of the heel. *Holding the infant firmly ensures safety and allows an accurate measurement.*

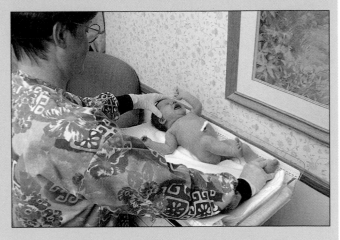

Tape Measure

1. Check that a paper tape has no partial tears in it. *A torn measuring tape would give an inaccurate measurement.*
2. Place tape beside the infant, with the upper end at the top of the head. Tuck it beneath the shoulder, and extend it down to the feet. *Helps prevent movement of the tape and ensures accurate measurements.*
3. Hold the tape straight alongside the infant's body while extending one of the infant's legs to its full length. Be sure that the tape has not moved from the top of the head. *Careful attention to tape placement ensures accurate measurement.*

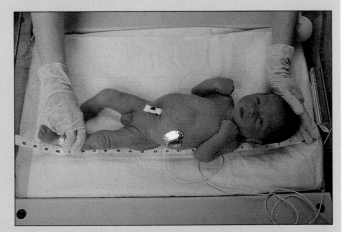

4. Another method is to mark the paper on which the infant is lying at the top of the head and the end of the extended leg. Then measure the distance between the two marks. *(Makes measuring more accurate when the infant is very active.)*

Continued

5. Compare with the normal range of 48 to 53 cm (19 to 21 in). *Helps determine abnormalities.*

HEAD AND CHEST CIRCUMFERENCE

1. Measure around the fullest part of the head, with the tape placed around the occiput and just above the eyebrows. *Allows measurement of the largest diameter of the head.*

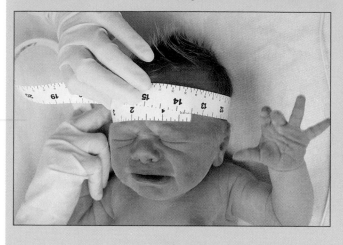

2. Move tape down to measure the chest at the level of the nipples. Be sure that the tape is even and taut. *Ensures accurate measurement.*

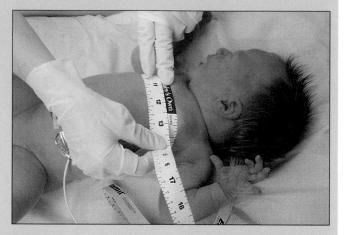

3. Remove tape by lifting or rolling the infant instead of pulling the tape. *Pulling tape can cut the infant's skin.*
4. Compare measurements with normal range. Head: 33 to 35.5 cm (13 to 14 in). Chest: 30.5 to 33 cm (12 to 13 in). *Determines whether the infant's measurements are normal.*

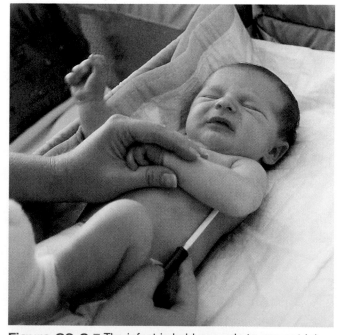

Figure 20-2 ■ The infant is held securely to prevent injury and obtain an accurate reading when taking the temperature.

CRITICAL TO REMEMBER

Normal Vital Signs in the Newborn

- Temperature: 36.5° to 37.5° C (97.7° to 99.5° F) axillary, 36.5° to 37.6° C (97.7° to 99.7° F) rectal
- Apical pulse: 120 to 160 bpm (100 sleeping, 180 crying)
- Respirations: 30 to 60 breaths/min

CHECK YOUR READING

1. What is the purpose of the early focused assessments of the infant after birth?
2. What is included in assessment of the newborn's cardiovascular status?
3. Why is taking a rectal temperature dangerous in an infant?

Assessment for Anomalies

If major abnormalities are present at birth, the nurse must maintain a calm, quiet demeanor to avoid frightening the parents. The physician should be alerted quietly and will explain the condition and possible plan of treatment to the parents.

HEAD AND NECK

The newborn's head makes up one fourth of the length of the body (Gardner et al., 2002). It is much larger in proportion to the rest of the body than that of the adult. The head is palpated to assess the shape and identify abnormalities. The newborn who was delivered by cesarean not preceded by labor usually has a round head, whereas the infant born vaginally usually has some molding. The head of infants who were in a breech position may be flattened on the top. The degree of molding, size of the fontanels, and presence of caput succedaneum or later development of a cephalhematoma are noted.

The hair should be fine with a consistent hair pattern. Abnormal hair growth patterns may indicate genetic abnormalities. The nurse separates the hair, if necessary, to display bruises, rashes, and other marks on the scalp. A small, red mark is apparent if a fetal monitor electrode was inserted into the skin of the scalp. Later, a small scab forms. Occasionally this area becomes infected and a topical antibiotic is applied.

MOLDING. The term *molding* refers to changes in the shape of the head that allow it to pass through the birth canal. It is caused by overriding of the cranial bones at the sutures and is common, especially after a long second stage of labor. The parietal bones often override the occipital and frontal bones, and a ridge can be felt at those areas. The condition generally resolves within a few days to 1 week after birth. Often, dramatic improvement is seen by the end of the first day of life. Parents may need reassurance that the infant's head is normal.

All suture lines should be palpated. Separation may be the temporary result of molding or, if it persists or widens, may indicate increased intracranial pressure. If no space is found between suture lines, it may be the result of molding and overriding of the bones. However, a hard, ridged area that is not the result of molding may indicate premature closure. This condition, called *craniosynostosis,* may impair brain growth and the shape of the head and necessitates surgery.

FONTANELS. The fontanels are the areas of the head where sutures between the bones meet. In the newborn the areas are not calcified but are covered by membrane. This allows space for the brain to grow.

The anterior fontanel is a diamond-shaped area where the frontal and parietal bones meet. It measures 2 to 4 cm, although this varies because of molding and individual differences. The fontanel closes between 12 and 18 months of age.

The nurse palpates the fontanels and notes the position in relation to the other bones of the skull (Figure 20-3). The anterior fontanel should be flat (level with the surrounding bones) or slightly sunken and should feel soft. When the anterior fontanel is palpated, the infant's head is elevated for accurate assessment. The infant may be placed in a semisitting position or held in an upright position. The fontanel should be palpated when the infant is quiet, because vigorous crying may cause it to protrude.

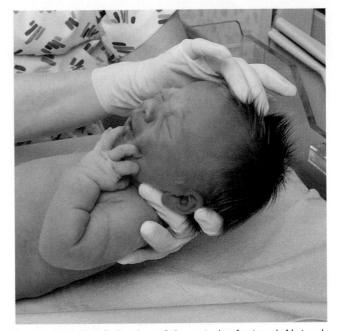

Figure 20-3 ■ Palpation of the anterior fontanel. Note elevation of the head.

Although the anterior fontanel may bulge slightly when the infant cries, bulging at rest may indicate increased intracranial pressure. A fontanel that is between flat and bulging is termed *full.* A larger-than-normal fontanel may be a sign of increased pressure within the skull. A depressed fontanel is unusual in a newborn unless it is the result of molding. After molding resolves, a depressed fontanel is a sign of dehydration. Abnormal signs are reported to the primary care provider.

The posterior fontanel is a triangular area where the occipital and parietal bones meet. It is much smaller than the anterior fontanel, measuring 0.5 to 1 cm. Molding may complicate the identification of the posterior fontanel because the overlapping bones impinge on that space. The posterior fontanel feels like a dimple at the juncture of the occipital and parietal bones. This fontanel closes by the time the infant is 2 to 3 months of age.

CAPUT SUCCEDANEUM. A caput succedaneum often appears over the vertex of the newborn's head as a result of pressure against the mother's cervix during labor (Figure 20-4). The pressure interferes with blood flow from the area, causing localized edema at birth. The edematous area crosses suture lines, is soft, and varies in size. It resolves quickly and disappears within 12 hours to several days after birth. Caput also may occur when a vacuum extractor is used to hasten second stage labor. When a vacuum is used, the caput corresponds to the area where the extractor was placed on the skull. The amount of edema and presence of bruising are assessed.

CEPHALHEMATOMA. A cephalhematoma, bleeding between the periosteum and the skull, occurs in 1% to 2% of newborns and is the result of pressure during birth (Southgate & Pittard, 2001). It occurs on one or both sides of the head over the parietal bones, although it occasionally

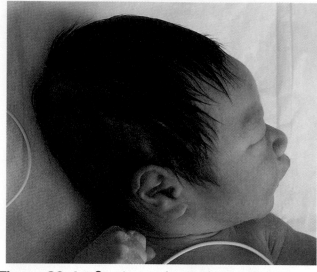

Figure 20-4 ■ Caput succedaneum is an edematous area on the head from pressure against the cervix. It may cross suture lines.

forms over the occipital bone (Figure 20-5). The swelling is not present at birth but develops within the first 24 to 48 hours.

The area is carefully palpated to determine whether the swelling crosses suture lines. A cephalhematoma has clear edges that end at the suture lines. It does not cross the suture lines, unlike a caput succedaneum, because the bleeding is held between the bone and its covering, the periosteum. A cephalhematoma reabsorbs slowly and may take a few weeks to months to completely resolve. Because of the breakdown of the red blood cells within the hematoma, affected infants are at greater risk for jaundice.

Both caput succedaneum and cephalhematoma may be frightening to parents. During the assessment, the nurse can reassure parents that the conditions are not harmful to the infant. Even if parents do not ask, they need information about the causes and length of time required for the areas to resolve.

FACE. The face is examined for symmetry, positioning of the facial features, movement, and expression. A transient asymmetry from intrauterine pressure may occur, lasting a few weeks or months. Irregularities of the facial features should be reported.

NECK AND CLAVICLES

The nurse assesses the infant's neck visually and notes the ease with which the head turns from side to side. The neck is very short. Webbing may indicate Turner's or Down syndrome (see Chapter 5). An unusually large fat pad between the occiput and the shoulders may indicate Down syndrome. When lying in a prone position, the newborn should be able to raise the head briefly and turn it to the other side.

Fractures of the clavicle are more likely to occur in large infants, especially when shoulder dystocia occurred. Sliding the fingers along each clavicle while moving the infant's arm helps identify a fractured clavicle. If a fracture is present, a lump or tenderness over the area of the fracture may be observed. Crepitus (grating of the bone) and movement of the bone may be felt during palpation. Swelling of the area and decreased movement of the arm on the affected side also may occur. A difference in the movement of the arms is especially noticeable when the Moro reflex is elicited. Damage to the brachial plexus may cause paralysis of the arm on the side of the fracture. Treatment of a fractured clavicle includes immobilization of the affected arm for a short time. The fracture heals quickly (Figure 20-6). In asymptomatic fractures, no treatment may be necessary.

CORD

The umbilical cord should contain three vessels. The two arteries are small and may stand up at the cut end. The single vein is larger than the arteries and resembles a slit because its walls are more easily compressed. If only one artery is

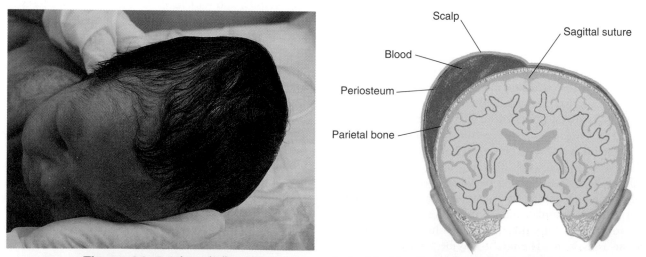

Figure 20-5 ■ A cephalhematoma is characterized by bleeding between the bone and its covering, the periosteum. It may occur on one or both sides and does not cross suture lines.

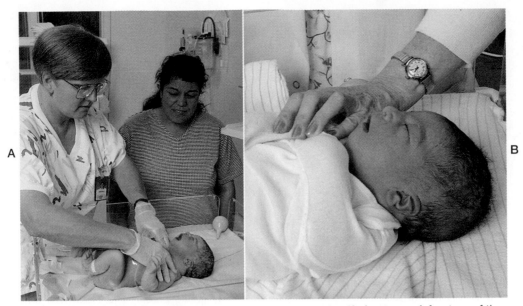

Figure 20-6 ■ A, The nurse palpates the clavicles to identify fractures. A fracture of the left clavicle is present. **B,** The arm on the side of the fractured clavicle is immobilized by pinning the sleeve to the shirt.

present, the infant is carefully assessed for other anomalies. A two-vessel cord is associated with chromosomal, renal, and gastrointestinal defects. The amount of Wharton's jelly in the cord is noted. If the cord appears thin, the infant may have been poorly nourished in utero. A yellow-brown or green tinge to the cord indicates that meconium was released at some time before birth, perhaps as a result of fetal compromise.

EXTREMITIES

The normal infant should actively move the extremities equally in a random manner. The extremities of a term infant should remain sharply flexed and resist extension during examination. Poor muscle tone results in a limp or "floppy" infant, which may be the result of inadequate oxygen during birth but should resolve within a few minutes as oxygen intake increases. Continued poor muscle tone may result from prematurity or neurologic damage. Infants with previously good muscle tone may show decreased flexion if they become hypoglycemic or experience respiratory difficulty.

All extremities are examined for signs of fractures such as crepitus, redness, lumps or swelling, and lack of use. Independent movement of each extremity should be determined to identify possible nerve injury that may occur with or without fractures.

Injury to the brachial nerve plexus may result in Erb's palsy (Erb-Duchenne paralysis), paralysis of the shoulder and arm muscles. Instead of the usual flexed position, the affected arm is extended at the infant's side with the forearm prone. Movement of this arm is diminished during the Moro reflex. The condition is treated by exercise, splinting, or both.

HANDS AND FEET. The fingers and toes are examined for extra digits (polydactyly) and webbing between dig-

its (syndactyly). Extra digits often are small and may not have bones. Tying the extra digits with sutures causes them to atrophy. Presence of a bone in the extra digit requires surgical removal. Webbed fingers or toes may be corrected by surgery. Nails in a term infant should extend to the end of the fingers or slightly beyond.

The creases in the hands also are examined. Normally, two long transverse creases extend most of the way across the palm. A single crease that crosses the palm without a break parallel with the base of the fingers is called a *simian crease* or *line*. It may be seen with incurving of the little finger in Down syndrome. The simian line alone is not diagnostic of Down syndrome, however, and may occur in normal infants, usually on one hand only.

The feet are assessed for talipes equinovarus, or clubfoot, a common malformation of the foot and lower leg. If a foot looks abnormal, it should be gently manipulated. If it moves to a normal position, the abnormality is probably temporary, resulting from the position of the infant in the uterus. In true clubfoot, the foot turns inward and down and cannot be moved to a midline position. Splints or casts are the usual treatment, but sometimes surgery is necessary.

HIPS. The hips are examined for signs of developmental dysplasia. In this condition, instability of the hip joint occurs and the head of the femur can be moved in and out of the acetabulum. Partial dislocation and inadequate development of the acetabulum may occur. The condition occurs more often in breech presentation and if prolonged oligohydramnios prevented normal movement. Identifying a hip problem early is important to prevent permanent damage to the joint.

Barlow and Ortolani tests are methods of assessing for hip instability in the newborn period (Figure 20-7). Both legs should abduct equally in normal infants. Abducting the

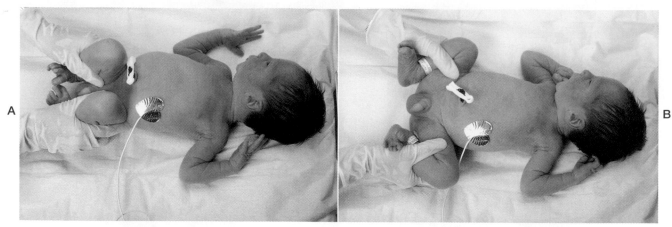

Figure 20-7 ■ Assessment of the hips. Place the fingers over the infant's greater trochanter and thumbs over the femur. Bend the knees and hips at a 90-degree angle. **A,** Barlow test. Adduct the hips, and apply gentle pressure down and back with the thumbs. In hip dysplasia the examiner can feel the femoral head move out of the acetabulum. **B,** Ortolani test. Abduct the thighs, and apply gentle pressure forward over the greater trochanter. A "clunking" sensation indicates a dislocated femoral head moving into the acetabulum. A hip click may be heard but is usually normal.

affected hip may be difficult. A hip click may be felt or heard but is usually normal and different from the "clunk" of hip dysplasia (Thompson, 2004).

The infant's knees should be bent with the feet flat on the bed to compare the height of the knees. If the hip is dislocated, the knee on the affected side is lower. The legs are extended while the infant is in a prone position to determine whether they are equal in length and thigh and gluteal creases are symmetric (Figure 20-8). If the hip is dislocated, the leg on the affected side is shorter and the

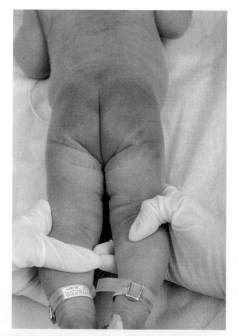

Figure 20-8 ■ Note the symmetry of gluteal and thigh creases.

creases are asymmetric. Because the hip may be unstable but not yet dislocated, these signs are not usually present at birth.

Treatment of developmental dysplasia of the hip involves immobilizing the leg in a flexed, abducted position, usually with a harness. Early identification and treatment is essential to provide the best results in correcting the problem. Treatment may involve surgery and casting if the condition is not discovered early.

VERTEBRAL COLUMN

The nurse palpates the entire length of the newborn's vertebral column to discover any defects in the vertebrae. An indentation is a sign of spina bifida occulta (failed closing of a vertebra). The defect is not obvious on visual inspection because it is covered with skin, but sometimes a tuft of hair grows over the area. Other, more obvious neural tube defects include meningoceles and myelomeningoceles, which are protrusions of nerves, the spinal cord, or both through the defect in the vertebrae. They appear as a sac on the back and may be covered by skin or only the meninges. The tissue should be covered with moist, sterile, saline dressings immediately after birth (p. 826). A pilonidal dimple may be present at the base of the spine. It should be examined for a sinus and the depth noted.

Measurements

Measurements provide information about the infant's growth in utero. The weight, length, and head and chest circumference are part of the initial assessment (see Procedure 20-1). The measurements are compared with the norms for the infant's gestational age. When a difference is noted between the expected and actual values, expanded assessments are necessary.

WEIGHT

The newborn's weight ranges between 2500 and 4000 g (5 lb, 8 oz and 8 lb, 13 oz) (Cheffer & Rannalli, 2004). The average weight of a full-term newborn is 3400 g (7.5 lb). If the infant's weight is outside the average range, possible causes are assessed. Factors affecting weight include gestational age, placental functioning, genetic factors such as race and parental size, and maternal diabetes, hypertension, or substance abuse.

Infants are weighed each day they are in the birth facility and at follow-up visits. They should lose less than 10% of their birth weight during the first 7 to 10 days of life (Berryman & Glass, 2005). The loss results from excretion of meconium from the bowel and normal loss of extracellular fluid. In addition, newborns often do not consume enough calories to maintain their weight during the first few days. However, many infants have regained their birth weight by the tenth day of life. Thereafter they gain about 25 g to 30 g per day during the early months (Walker & Creehan, 2001).

LENGTH

The infant's length is measured from the top of the head to the end of the outstretched leg. The average length of a full-term newborn is 48 to 53 cm (19 to 21 in) (Cheffer & Rannalli, 2004). Some agencies also record the crown-to-rump measurement, which is approximately equal to the head circumference.

HEAD AND CHEST CIRCUMFERENCE

The diameter of the head is measured around the occiput just above the eyebrows. The average head circumference of the term newborn is 33 to 35.5 cm (13 to 14 in) (Cheffer & Rannalli, 2004). The measurement may be affected by molding of the skull during the birth process. If a large amount of molding occurred, the head is remeasured when it regains its normal shape. An abnormally small head may indicate poor brain growth and microcephaly. A very large head may be a sign of hydrocephalus.

The chest is measured at the level of the nipples. It usually is 2 to 3 cm smaller than the head. The average circumference of the chest is 30.5 to 33 cm (12 to 13 in) (Cheffer & Rannalli, 2004). If molding of the head is present, the head and chest measurement may be equal at birth.

✔ CHECK YOUR READING

4. What are the differences among molding, caput succedaneum, and cephalhematoma?
5. Why are measurements of the neonate important?

ASSESSMENT OF BODY SYSTEMS

Neurologic System

REFLEXES

Assessment of the presence and strength of the reflexes is important to determine the health of the newborn's central nervous system. The nurse notes the strength of the reflexes

CRITICAL THINKING ❓ EXERCISE 20-1

What might be the effect on normal development if reflexes are retained beyond the age when they should disappear?

and whether both sides of the body respond symmetrically (Figure 20-9). A diminished overall response occurs in preterm and ill infants. Absence of reflexes may indicate a serious neurologic problem. Asymmetric responses may indicate that trauma during birth caused nerve damage, paralysis, or fracture. For example, trauma to the facial nerve from forceps or pressure during birth may cause unilateral drooping of the mouth. The infant may appear to have a one-sided cry and may have no rooting reflex on the affected side. Some newborn reflexes gradually weaken and disappear over a period of months (Table 20-2).

SENSORY ASSESSMENT

EARS. The ears are assessed for placement, overall appearance, and maturity. An imaginary line drawn from the outer canthus of the eye should be even with the area where the upper ear joins the head (Figure 20-10). Low-set ears may indicate chromosomal abnormalities.

The nurse examines the ears for skin tags and preauricular sinuses and dimples. Abnormalities of the ear may indicate chromosomal abnormalities, mental retardation, hearing problems, and kidney defects. The stiffness of the cartilage and degree of incurving of the pinna are checked as part of the gestational age assessment.

Infants can hear by the last trimester of pregnancy, and their hearing is very good after birth. Hearing is assessed by noting the infant's reaction to sudden loud noises, which should cause a startle response. Infants should respond to the sound of voices and prefer a high-pitched tone of voice and rhythmic sounds. They will turn toward the sound of the mother's voice or another interesting sound. A hearing screening is performed before discharge from most birth facilities (see Chapter 21).

EYES. The eyes should be symmetric and of the same size. The usual slate gray-blue color of the eyes of infants with light skin tones gradually changes to the true color by 3 to 12 months of age. Infants with dark skin may have brown eyes. The eyes are examined for abnormalities and signs of inflammation. Slanting of the epicanthal folds in a non-Asian infant may be a sign of Down syndrome. Edema of the eyelids and subconjunctival hemorrhages (reddened areas of the sclera) result from pressure on the head during birth, which causes capillary rupture in the sclera. The edema diminishes in a few days, and the hemorrhages resolve in 1 or 2 weeks.

The sclera should be white or bluish-white. A yellow color indicates jaundice. A blue color occurs in osteogenesis imperfecta, a congenital bone condition.

Conjunctivitis may result from infection and chemical reaction to medications. *Staphylococcus, Chlamydia,* and *Neisseria gonorrhoeae* are common organisms that cause infection.

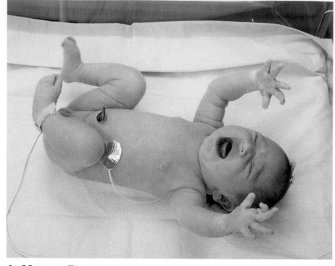

A, Moro reflex.

The Moro reflex is the most dramatic reflex. It occurs when the infant's head and trunk are allowed to drop back 30 degrees when the infant is in a slightly raised position. The infant's arms and legs extend and abduct, with the fingers fanning open and thumbs and forefingers forming a C position. The arms then return to their normally flexed state with an embracing motion. The legs may also extend and then flex.

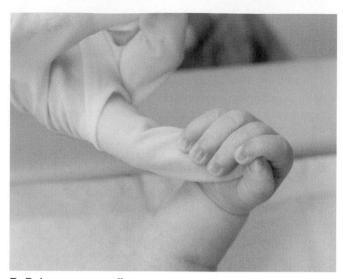

B, Palmar grasp reflex.

The palmar grasp reflex occurs when the infant's palm is touched near the base of the fingers. The hand closes into a tight fist. The grasp reflex may be weak or absent if the infant has damage to the nerves of the arms.

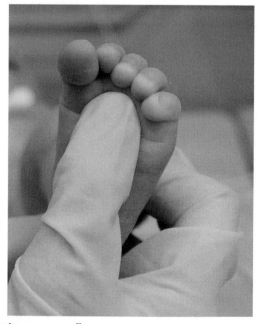

C, Plantar grasp reflex.

The plantar grasp reflex is similar to the palmar grasp reflex. When the area below the toes is touched, the infant's toes curl over the nurse's finger.

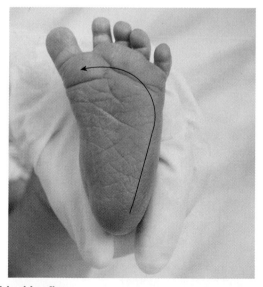

D, Babinski reflex.

The Babinski reflex is elicited by stroking the lateral sole of the infant's foot from the heel forward and across the ball of the foot. This causes the toes to flare outward and the big toe to dorsiflex.

Figure 20-9 ■ Reflexes.

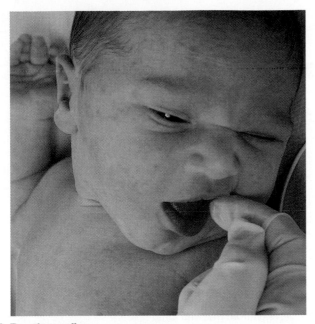

E, Rooting reflex.
The rooting reflex is important in feeding and is most often demonstrated when the infant is hungry. When the infant's cheek is touched near the mouth, the head turns toward the side that has been stroked. This helps the infant find the nipple for feeding. The reflex occurs when either side of the mouth is touched. Touching the cheeks on both sides at the same time confuses the infant.

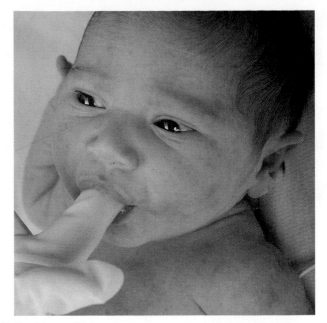

F, Sucking reflex.
The sucking reflex is essential to normal life. When the mouth or palate is touched by the nipple or a finger, the infant begins to suck. The sucking reflex is assessed for its presence and strength. Feeding difficulties may be related to problems in the infant's ability to suck and to coordinate sucking with swallowing.

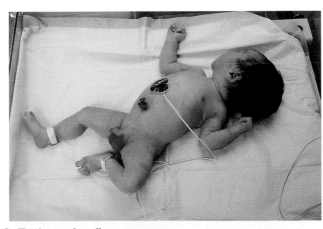

G, Tonic neck reflex.
The tonic neck reflex refers to the posture assumed by newborns when in a supine position. The infant extends the arm and leg on the side to which the head is turned and flexes the extremities on the other side. This is sometimes referred to as the "fencing reflex" because the infant's position is similar to that of a person engaged in a fencing match.

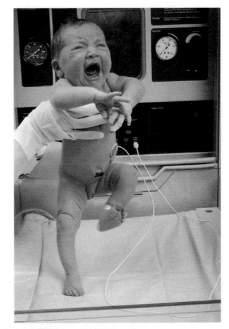

H, Stepping reflex.
The stepping reflex occurs when infants are held upright with their feet touching a solid surface. They lift one foot and then the other, giving the appearance that they are trying to walk.

Figure 20-9, cont'd ■ Reflexes.

TABLE **20-2** Summary of Neonatal Reflexes

Reflex	Method of Testing	Expected Response	Abnormal Response and Possible Cause	Time Reflex Disappears
Babinski	Stroke lateral sole of foot from heel to across base of toes.	Toes flare with dorsiflexion of the big toe.	No response. Bilateral: CNS deficit. Unilateral: local nerve damage.	12 mo.
Gallant (trunk incurvation)	Lightly stroke the back, lateral to the vertebral column.	Entire trunk flexes toward side stimulated.	No response: CNS deficit.	1 mo.
Grasp reflex (palmar and plantar)	Press finger against base of fingers or toes.	Fingers curl tightly; toes curl forward.	Weak or absent: neurologic deficit or muscle damage.	Palmar grasp lessens by 3 mo. Plantar grasp lessens by 8 mo.
Moro	Let infant's head drop back approximately 30 degrees.	Sharp extension and abduction of arms with thumbs and forefingers in C position. Followed by flexion and adduction to "embrace" position. Legs follow similar pattern.	Absent: CNS dysfunction. Asymmetry: brachial plexus injury, paralysis, or fractured bone of extremity. Exaggerated: maternal drug use.	6 mo.
Rooting	Touch or stroke from side of mouth toward cheek.	Infant turns to side touched. Difficult to elicit if infant sleeping or just fed.	Weak or absent: prematurity, neurologic deficit, depression from maternal drug use.	3-4 mo.
Startle	Make a loud noise.	Similar to Moro, but hands remain clenched.	Weak or absent: neurologic damage, deafness.	4 mo.
Stepping	Hold infant so feet touch solid surface.	Infant lifts alternate feet as if walking.	Asymmetry: fracture of extremity, neurologic deficit.	4-7 mo.
Sucking	Place nipple or finger in mouth, rub against palate.	Infant begins to suck. Weak if recently fed.	Weak or absent: prematurity, neurologic deficit, maternal drug use.	Disappears by 1 yr.
Swallowing	Place fluid on the back of the tongue.	Infant swallows fluid. Should be coordinated with sucking.	Coughing, gagging, choking, cyanosis: tracheoesophageal fistula, esophageal atresia, neurologic deficit.	Present throughout life.
Tonic neck reflex	Gently turn infant's head to one side while he or she is supine.	Extension of extremities on side to which head is turned, with flexion on opposite side.	Prolonged period in position: neurologic deficit.	May be weak at birth. Disappears by 4 mo.

CNS, Central nervous system.

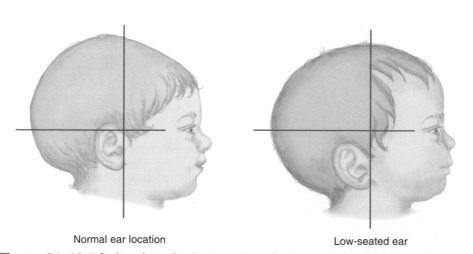

Normal ear location   Low-seated ear

Figure 20-10 ■ An imaginary line is drawn from the outer canthus of the eye to the ear. The line should intersect with the area where the upper ear joins the head.

Gonorrhea in the mother can cause infection of the infant during birth. The resulting ophthalmia neonatorum may result in blindness. To prevent this condition, all infants are treated prophylactically with antibiotics to the eyes. Any discharge from the eyes is reported for possible culture and treatment.

Transient strabismus (crossed eyes) is common for the first 3 to 4 months after birth because infants have poor control of their eye muscles. The doll's-eye sign is a normal finding in the newborn: When the head is turned quickly to one side, the eyes move toward the other side. The setting-sun sign (the iris appears low in the eye and part of the sclera can be seen above the iris) may be an indication of hydrocephalus.

The pupils should be equal in size and react equally to light. Cataracts (opacities of the lens) appear as white areas over the pupils. They may develop in infants of mothers who had rubella or other infections during the pregnancy. When a light is directed into the eyes, the normal red reflex may not be seen if large cataracts are present. Tears are scant or absent for the first 2 to 4 weeks of life. Excessive tearing may indicate a plugged lacrimal duct, which is treated with massage or surgery.

Although visual acuity is not well developed and the eyes cannot accommodate for distance, newborns should show a visual response to the environment. They should make eye contact when held in a cradle position during a period of alertness and focus best on objects that are 20 to 30 cm (8 to 12 in) away. Newborns can see objects up to 0.76 m (2.5 feet) away less well and follow interesting objects horizontally across midline and vertically. They should respond well to human faces and geometric patterns of black and white or medium bright colors but show little interest in pastel colors.

Newborns should blink or close their eyes in response to bright lights. Any infant who does not respond to visual stimuli should be reported to the physician or nurse practitioner for further investigation.

SENSE OF SMELL. Newborns have a good sense of smell, and discrimination develops quickly. They can identify the odor of the mother's breast milk within 5 days after birth (Cheffer & Rannalli, 2004). The ability of infants to distinguish taste is shown by their increased suck when given sweet liquids and rejection of sour liquids.

OTHER NEUROLOGIC SIGNS

The newborn is assessed for tremors or jitteriness. If tremors are present, the blood glucose level should be checked because hypoglycemia is the most common cause. If blood glucose is within normal range, the cause may be low calcium levels or prenatal exposure to drugs. Tremors increase each time the infant is touched or moved but stop briefly if the extremity is flexed and held firmly.

Seizures indicate central nervous system abnormality. To differentiate between tremors and seizures, the infant's extremities are held in a flexed position. This causes tremors to stop, whereas a seizure continues. Seizure activity also

CRITICAL TO REMEMBER

Differentiating Tremors and Seizures

Jitteriness or Tremors
- Stop when the extremities are held firmly in a flexed position
- Are commonly caused by low glucose or calcium levels

Seizures
- Continue even if extremities are held
- May include abnormal mouth or eye movements
- Indicate central nervous system abnormality

may include abnormal movements of the eyes and mouth and other subtle signs. Any infant thought to be having seizures is referred for further assessment and treatment.

The pitch of the cry is important. Cries that are shrill, high-pitched, hoarse, and catlike (mewing) are abnormal. These cries may indicate a neurologic disorder or other problem.

Normal infants are quiet and appear content when their needs are met. Infants should respond to soothing, gentle touch and holding. Rocking motions often are effective in quieting an irritable infant. Most infants nestle or mold their bodies to those of the people holding them, making them easy to hold and cuddle. Neonates who stiffen the body, seem to pull away from contact, and arch the back when held may be showing signs of central nervous system injury or may just have a different but normal way of responding.

Infants should react to painful stimuli with crying and an increase in vital signs. Excessive irritability and a high-pitched cry also may be signs of damage to the central nervous system. All such abnormal signs are reported for further neurologic assessment.

Hepatic System

The major early assessments of the hepatic system are related to blood glucose and bilirubin conjugation.

BLOOD GLUCOSE

The nurse must be alert for newborns at increased risk for hypoglycemia, which can cause brain damage. Factors that might have caused the infant to deplete available glucose are noted. A quick estimate to determine whether the newborn appears to be near term and of appropriate size for gestational age is performed at birth.

The AAP and the ACOG (2002) state that screening for the blood glucose level is necessary only for infants in risk categories and those showing early signs of hypoglycemia. Normal blood glucose during the first day of life is 40 to 60 mg/dl and 50 to 90 mg/dl thereafter (Nicholson & Pesce, 2004). Because capillary blood is used in screening tests, these tests are less accurate than laboratory tests using venous blood. Therefore a laboratory analysis (per agency policy) often is used to verify readings of 40 to 45 mg/dl or below.

CRITICAL TO REMEMBER

Risk Factors for Hypoglycemia

- Prematurity
- Postmaturity
- Intrauterine growth restriction
- Size large or small for gestational age
- Asphyxia
- Problems at birth
- Cold stress
- Maternal diabetes
- Maternal intake of terbutaline or ritodrine

CRITICAL TO REMEMBER

Signs of Neonatal Hypoglycemia

- Jitteriness
- Poor muscle tone
- Diaphoresis
- Poor suck
- Tachypnea
- Respiratory distress
- Tachycardia
- Dyspnea
- Cyanosis
- Apnea
- Low temperature
- High-pitched cry
- Irritability
- Lethargy
- Seizures, coma
- No signs (some infants may be asymptomatic)

Observing for signs of hypoglycemia is necessary throughout routine assessment and care. Early signs include jitteriness and other central nervous system signs and signs of respiratory difficulty, a decrease in temperature, and poor feeding. Some infants with hypoglycemia show no signs at all.

PROCEDURE

20-3   Obtaining Blood Samples from the Newborn by Heel Puncture

PURPOSE: To obtain a sample of an infant's blood by heel puncture for analysis of blood glucose, newborn screening tests, or other tests

1. Wash hands. *Helps prevent spread of infection.*
2. If the infant has not received a bath after birth, bathe the infant or wash the area to be used before puncturing the skin. *Avoids contamination of the puncture site with maternal blood on the infant's skin. This is especially important should the mother have a known or unknown infection such as hepatitis B or human immunodeficiency virus.*
3. Gather supplies needed. Supplies may vary with different glucose meters and for different types of tests. Common supplies include gloves, alcohol wipe, 2- × 2-in gauze, microlancet or commercial lancing device, adhesive bandage, cotton balls, pipettes, blood-collecting devices (glucose screening reagent strips, blotting paper for PKU tests, capillary tubes), cloth or commercial warming pack to warm heel. *Having all supplies ready allows efficient performance of the procedure.*
4. Calibrate or program the glucose meter and use quality control measures according to the manufacturer's guidelines. *Ensures proper functioning of the machine.*
5. Warm the infant's foot for a few minutes if it is cold or if blood is needed for several tests. Dampen a cloth with warm water and fasten it over the heel, or use a heel warming pack according to directions. Use caution to prevent burning the infant's skin. *Warming causes vasodilation and allows blood to flow more easily. This avoids having to make more than one puncture because of insufficient blood flow. Hot packs can cause burns to the infant's delicate skin.*
6. Provide comforting measures such as swaddling, providing a pacifier, allowing the mother to hold the infant, or giving oral sucrose (according to hospital policy). Rate the infant's pain level before the procedure using

an infant pain scale according to hospital policy. *Comfort measures help decrease the infant's pain. Rating the pain before the procedure helps determine the effectiveness of pain relief measures during and after the procedure.*
7. Apply gloves. *Prevents contamination of the hands with blood and is part of standard precautions.*

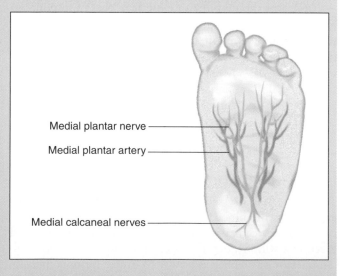

Medial plantar nerve
Medial plantar artery
Medial calcaneal nerves

8. Hold the heel in one hand. Palpate the bone of the heel and place the thumb or finger over the walking surface of the foot. Choose a puncture site that has not been used before. *Stabilizes the heel to prevent movement and inadvertent injury from the lancet.*

PKU, phenylketonuria

Avoiding injuries to the infant's foot is important when taking blood from the heel (Procedure 20-3). If the lancet goes into the calcaneus bone, osteomyelitis may result. The skin should be punctured to a depth of less than 2 mm to avoid piercing the bone for the full-term infant and less than 1.5 mm for the preterm infant (Meehan, 1998). Piercing in very small preterms should be according to their size. Commercial devices for heel puncture are designed to puncture the heel to the proper depth. The chosen site must avoid damage to major nerves and arteries in the area. Other complications include cellulitis, abscess, scarring, bruising, and pain.

Infants are usually fed if the reading is 40 to 45 mg/dl to prevent a further decrease in glucose, especially if the infant shows signs of hypoglycemia. The blood glucose is rechecked 30 minutes to an hour after the feeding and again before feedings until the level is above 50 mg/dl twice or according to hospital policy (Townsend, 2005).

BILIRUBIN

The nurse assesses for jaundice and watches for its development, particularly in infants at risk for hyperbilirubinemia. Jaundice is identified by pressing the infant's skin over a firm surface, such as the end of the nose or the sternum. The skin blanches as the blood is pressed out of the tissues, making it easier to see the yellow color that remains. Jaundice is more obvious when the nurse assesses in natural light. Because jaundice begins at the head and moves down the body, the severity of the problem can be roughly estimated by noting the areas of the body involved. Jaundice of the face occurs when the bilirubin level reaches 5 to 7 mg/dl, the midabdomen at about 15 mg/dl, and the soles of the feet at about 20 mg/dl (Stoll & Kliegman, 2004a).

In physiologic jaundice, the bilirubin level peaks at 5 to 6 mg/dl between the second and fourth days of life and then begins to drop. Jaundice appearing before the second day of life may indicate that the bilirubin is rising more

---

PROCEDURE

20-3 Obtaining Blood Samples from the Newborn by Heel Puncture—cont'd

Locating the bone helps avoid puncturing the calcaneus bone, which could result in osteomyelitis. Covering the walking surface avoids damage to nerves and arteries of this area. Avoiding a site that was punctured previously decreases the chance of infection and scarring.

9. Clean the lateral heel with alcohol. Allow to dry or wipe dry with sterile gauze. *Alcohol reduces contaminants. Drying prevents irritation to the tissues and dilution of the specimen with alcohol.*

10. Puncture side of heel with a lancet that punctures to a depth of less than 2 mm. Place lancet in a sharps container. *Insertion to the proper depth avoids injury to the infant and ensures blood flow so that further punctures are unnecessary. Proper disposal prevents injury to the infant and injury or unnecessary exposure of others to the infant's blood.*

11. If an automatic puncture device is used, place over appropriate site and activate according to manufacturer's directions. *Ensures proper use of device.*

12. Follow agency policy or manufacturer's directions for the type of test being performed about whether to wipe away the first drop of blood, how to collect sample, amount of blood to collect, proper handling, and reading of results. *Correct procedure promotes accuracy of test results.*

13. Avoid excessive squeezing of the foot. Apply gentle pressure at a point higher than the puncture site if necessary. *Excessive squeezing causes bruising and dilution of the sample with fluid from the tissues.*

14. Apply adhesive bandage. Check site frequently and remove the bandage when the bleeding stops. *A bandage helps prevent bleeding and infection of the site. Checking ensures no further bleeding has occurred.*

15. Document the procedure and results. Send specimens to the laboratory as appropriate. Report abnormal readings and follow up according to agency policy. *Helps ensure proper handling of specimens and proper care of the infant if results are abnormal.*

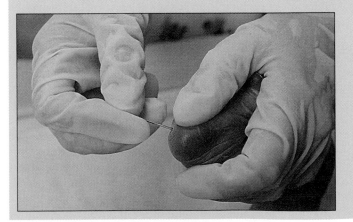

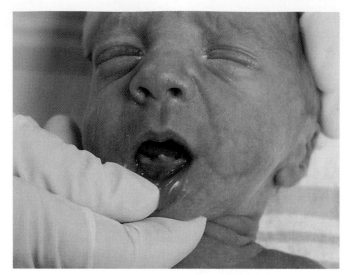

Figure 20-11 ■ A precocious tooth.

quickly and to higher levels than normal and may not be physiologic. The physician or nurse practitioner may order laboratory determinations of the bilirubin level based on the nurse's assessment. If serial bilirubin assays are ordered, the nurse notes changes from one reading to the next and correlates the results with the infant's age.

✔ CHECK YOUR READING

6. What are some signs of hypoglycemia?
7. Why is using the correct site for heel punctures to obtain blood samples important?

Gastrointestinal System

The initial assessment of the gastrointestinal tract occurs during the first hours after birth, when the nurse visualizes the parts that can be seen and the infant takes the initial feeding. Abnormalities and normal variations in structure and function are identified.

MOUTH

The mouth is inspected visually and by palpation. Some infants are born with precocious teeth, usually lower incisors (Figure 20-11). If the teeth are loose, the physician usually removes them to prevent aspiration. Epstein's pearls may be present on the hard palate and gums. These small, white, hard, inclusion cysts are accumulations of epithelial cells and disappear within a few weeks without treatment. They are similar to milia.

The nurse examines the tongue for size and movement. A large, protruding tongue is present in hypothyroidism and some chromosomal disorders such as Down syndrome. Paralysis of the facial nerve causes unilateral drooping of the mouth and affects the movement of the tongue. The tongue may appear to be tongue-tied because of the short frenulum, but this is normal and usually has no effect on the infant's ability to feed. In a true tongue-tie, there is limited tongue movement and the tip of the tongue has an inverted V shape. Clipping of the frenulum seldom is practiced because of the potential for infection.

Although candidiasis (thrush) is not apparent in the mouth immediately after birth, it may appear a day or two later. The lesions resemble milk curds on the tongue and cheeks that bleed if attempts are made to wipe them away. Newborns may become infected with *Candida albicans* during passage through the birth canal if the mother has a candidal vaginal infection. The infant is treated with nystatin suspension.

A cleft lip or palate results if the lip or palate fails to close. Cleft palate may involve the hard palate, soft palate, or both and may appear alone or with a cleft lip. The palate is inspected when the infant cries. A gloved finger is inserted into the mouth to palpate the hard and soft palates. A very small cleft of the soft palate may be missed if only a visual examination is done (see p. 824).

SUCK

The normal full-term infant should have a strong suck reflex, which is elicited when the lips or palate are stimulated. The reflex is weaker in the neonate who is preterm, is ill, or has just been fed. The newborn's cheeks have well-developed muscles and sucking pads that enhance the ability to suck. These fatty sucking pads last until late in infancy, when sucking is no longer essential. Blisters may be present on the newborn's hands or arms because of strong sucking before birth.

INITIAL FEEDING

The initial feeding is an opportunity to further assess the newborn. If the mother is breastfeeding, the nurse can observe the infant's response unobtrusively while assisting the mother to position the infant. A LATCH score should be given to all breastfeeding infants to identify problems with feeding (see Chapter 22, p. 545). To decrease regurgitation from overdistention of the stomach, an initial formula feeding should be no more than 1 oz.

The nurse evaluates the infant's ability to suck, swallow, and breathe in a coordinated manner. Although the fetus sucks and swallows in utero, these acts may not have been performed together. The addition of breathing to sucking and swallowing is a new experience. Choking, coughing, cyanosis, or excessive oral secretions may indicate a connection between the trachea and esophagus, such as tracheoesophageal fistula.

Some newborns choke or gag during the first feeding. Others may become dusky or cyanotic because they become apneic while they are feeding. In either case the nurse should stop the feeding immediately, suction if necessary, and stimulate the infant to cry by rubbing the back.

Most infants learn to coordinate sucking, swallowing, and breathing by the time the first feeding is finished. Neonates who continue to have difficulty may have a cardiac anomaly, tracheoesophageal fistula, or esophageal atresia (see pp. 823-825).

ABDOMEN

The abdomen should be soft and rounded and should protrude slightly but should not be distended. The stomach may be distended by mucus, blood, and amniotic fluid swallowed during birth. Fluid may be emptied through a feeding tube, if necessary. An abdomen so distended that the skin is stretched and shiny may indicate obstruction. Loops of bowel should not be visible through the abdominal wall. Visible bowel could indicate that air, meconium, or both are not passing through the intestines normally.

A sunken or scaphoid appearance of the abdomen occurs in diaphragmatic hernia, in which the intestines are located in the chest cavity instead of the abdomen. This condition interferes with development of the lungs, resulting in respiratory difficulty at birth. The nurse listens over the abdomen for bowel sounds, which usually appear within the first hour after birth. Bowel sounds heard in the chest may indicate diaphragmatic hernia.

An umbilical hernia occurs when the intestinal muscles fail to close around the umbilicus, allowing the intestines to protrude through the weak area. The condition is more common in African-American infants. By the time the infant is walking well, the muscles are usually strong enough that the hernia no longer is present. Some umbilical hernias require surgical repair.

Palpating the abdomen is easiest when the infant is relaxed and quiet. The abdomen should feel soft because the muscles are not yet well developed. Masses may indicate tumors of the kidneys. Palpation of the liver and kidneys is performed by the health care provider and generally is not part of routine nursing assessment of the abdomen. The liver normally is no more than 1 to 2 cm below the right costal margin. If the organ seems large, it should be reported to the physician or nurse practitioner because it may be a sign of congestive heart failure or congenital infection.

STOOLS

Stools should be assessed for color, type, and consistency. Meconium stools are dark greenish-black. They are soft but thick and tend to adhere to the skin. The infant may pass

CRITICAL THINKING ❓ **EXERCISE 20-2**

You are caring for an infant who was born 20 hours ago, and you hear on report that the infant has not passed meconium yet.

Question
What should you do?

meconium at delivery or after the initial feeding. Meconium stools are followed by transitional loose, greenish-brown stools on the second or third day.

Breastfed infants pass very soft, seedy, mustard-yellow stools after transitional stools. Formula-fed infants excrete stools that are more solid and pale yellow to light brown. A "water ring" should never occur around the solid part of any stool. A water ring is a wet, stained area on the diaper where watery stool has been absorbed into the diaper. There may be an area of more solid stool in addition, or all stool may have soaked into the diaper. A water ring may be caused by formula intolerance or infection.

The nurse should be aware of whether any stools have been passed since birth and, if so, when the infant's last stool occurred. Neonates usually pass the first meconium stool within 12 hours of birth, and 99% have the first stool within 48 hours (Stoll & Kliegman, 2004b). If there is a question about whether the infant has excreted a stool, the nurse must investigate further. Feeding may cause the infant to pass a stool. Although rectal temperatures are not recommended, a thermometer may be gently inserted into the rectum to determine patency and stimulate stool passage.

✓ CHECK YOUR READING

8. Why is assessment of newborn reflexes important?
9. Why is it important for the nurse to observe the first feeding carefully?
10. When do newborns pass the first stool? What can be done to stimulate stool passage?

Genitourinary System

KIDNEY PALPATION

Palpation of the kidneys is usually performed by the health care provider rather than being a part of the routine newborn nursing assessment. The kidneys may be felt 1 to 2 cm above the level of the umbilicus on each side of the abdomen during the first hours after birth. Abdominal masses may indicate enlargement or tumors of the kidneys.

The kidneys have more anomalies than any other organ (Swinford, et al., 2002). Kidney anomalies may accompany other defects because a problem early in fetal development may affect several organs vulnerable at that time. For example, infants with only one umbilical artery or defects involving the ears may have renal anomalies. The nurse should observe carefully for urinary output in these infants to determine whether the kidneys are functioning.

URINE

Most newborns void within 12 hours of birth, and 95% void by 24 hours (Stoll & Kliegman, 2004b). Because absence of urine output during this time may indicate anomalies, the first void is recorded on the chart. The newborn's bladder empties as little as once or twice during the first 2 days, although more frequent voiding is common. Because of the small amount, the first void may be missed. Sometimes it occurs in the delivery room but goes unnoticed because attention is focused on the infant's overall condition.

If there is a concern about whether the newborn has urinated, the delivery notes should be carefully read to see if the infant voided at birth. The nurse should ask the mother if she has changed a wet diaper. Increasing the infant's fluid intake often can initiate urination. If no void occurs in the expected time, the physician or nurse practitioner is alerted.

By the fourth day of life, at least six wet diapers can be expected daily. Each void is recorded in the infant's chart, including the number of diapers changed by the mother. The total number is correlated with that appropriate for the age of the infant. Mothers should be taught that at least six wet diapers after the first 3 days indicate the infant is taking adequate fluid.

If an infant is having feeding difficulties, noting the number of wet diapers is especially important. Disposable diapers are very absorbent, and determining whether the diaper is wet is sometimes difficult. The pale color of the newborn's urine may cause very little color change on the diaper. Wet diapers generally feel heavier than dry ones. If necessary, the nurse can put on gloves and take the diaper apart to examine it. The absorbent inner lining is damp if urine is present. Cotton balls and tissue placed in the diaper also may be used to increase visibility of small amounts of urine.

The newborn's urine may contain urate crystals that cause a reddish or pink stain on the diaper. This is known as "brick dust staining" and may be frightening to parents, who may think the infant is bleeding. It does not continue beyond the first few days as the kidneys mature.

GENITALIA

The nurse examines the newborn's genitalia for size, maturation, and presence of any abnormalities.

FEMALE. In the full-term female infant the labia majora should be large and should completely cover the clitoris and labia minora. The labia may be darker than the surrounding skin, a normal response to exposure to the mother's hormones before birth. Edema of the labia and white mucous vaginal discharge are normal. A small amount of vaginal bleeding, known as *pseudomenstruation,* may occur from the sudden withdrawal of the mother's hormones at birth. Hymenal (vaginal) tags are small pieces of tissue at the vaginal orifice. These are normal and disappear in a few weeks. The urinary meatus and vagina should be present.

MALE. The scrotum should be pendulous at term and may be dark brown from maternal hormones. Pressure during a breech delivery may cause it to be edematous. Rugae (creases in the scrotum) are deep and cover the entire scrotum in the full-term infant.

Enlargement of one or both sides of the scrotum may result from a hydrocele. This collection of fluid around the testes may make palpating the testes difficult. Placing a flashlight against the sac may outline the testes. Parents should be told that hydroceles are not painful and often reabsorb within 1 year. Some require later surgery.

The testes begin to descend through the inguinal canal at about 30 weeks of gestation and should be within the scrotal sac at 36 weeks. Palpation of the scrotum determines whether the testes have descended (Figure 20-12). Testes feel like small, round, movable objects that "slip" between the fingers. If the testes are not present in the scrotal sac, they may be felt in the inguinal canal. An empty scrotal sac appears smaller than one with testes. Undescended testes (cryptorchidism) occurs on one or both sides in approximately 3.4% of full-term and about 30% of preterm newborn boys. Most undescended testes will descend within 3 months. If the testes do not descend within 6 to 9 months, surgery is performed to preserve fertility (Elder, 2004).

The meatus should be at the tip of the glans penis. It may be abnormally located on the underside of the penis (hypospadias), on the upper side (epispadias), or on the perineum. The prepuce or foreskin of the penis covers the glans and is adherent to it. Attempts to retract it in the newborn are unnecessary and can cause damage. Abnormal placement of the meatus may not be visible because it is covered by the prepuce, but often the prepuce in these infants is incompletely formed. Hypospadias may be accompanied by chordee, a condition in which fibrotic tissue causes the penis to curve downward. These abnormalities are later corrected by surgery.

Parents are very concerned about any abnormalities of the genitalia. If the meatus is abnormally positioned, they need an explanation of the condition and why the infant should not be circumcised. The foreskin may be needed for later plastic surgery to repair the defect.

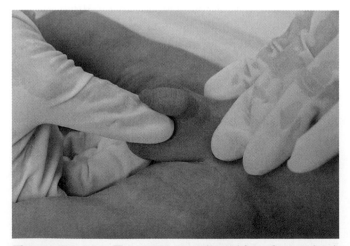

Figure 20-12 ■ The testes are palpated from front to back with the thumb and forefinger. Placing a finger over the inguinal canal holds the testes in place for palpation.

Integumentary System

SKIN

The newborn's skin is fragile and shows marks easily, especially in infants with fair coloring. Because the skin is so sensitive, reddened areas and rashes may develop during the early days of life. The nurse must examine every inch of skin surface carefully during the initial assessment and at the beginning of each shift. Marks should be documented and explained to parents who may be upset about the marks and need emotional support.

COLOR. The skin color should be pink or tan. Red, thin skin occurs in preterm infants. Redness in the full-term infant may indicate polycythemia. Acrocyanosis is common during the first day as a result of poor peripheral circulation. The infant's mouth and central body areas should not be cyanotic at any time. Blanching the skin over the nose or chest shows the presence of jaundice. Jaundice is abnormal during the first day of life but common during the first week.

A greenish-brown discoloration of the skin, nails, and cord results if meconium was passed before birth. The color may indicate that the infant was compromised at some time before birth, and it is more common in the postterm infant. These infants must be watched for other complications such as respiratory difficulty.

Harlequin coloration is a clear color division over the body from the head to the abdomen with one half deep pink or red and the other half pale or of normal color. The cause is unknown and it is usually transient and benign. It may indicate shunting of blood with cardiac problems or sepsis. Redness may occur on the lower side when the infant lies on the side.

Mottling (cutis marmorata) is a lacy, red pattern from dilated blood vessels under the skin. It is usually normal but may be a sign of cold stress, overstimulation, hypovolemia, or sepsis. If persistent, it may indicate a chromosomal abnormality.

VERNIX CASEOSA. Vernix, a thick, white substance that resembles cream cheese, provides a protective covering for the fetal skin in utero. The full-term infant has little vernix left on the body except small amounts in the creases. A thick covering of vernix may indicate a preterm infant, but a postterm infant may have none at all. Most vernix is removed when the infant is dried at birth or during the first bath. The remaining vernix is absorbed by the skin. Yellow-tinged vernix may indicate elevated bilirubin levels in utero, and green-tinged vernix is the result of meconium staining.

LANUGO. Lanugo is fine hair that covers the fetus during intrauterine life (Figure 20-13). As the fetus nears term, the lanugo becomes thinner. The term infant may have a small amount of lanugo on the shoulders, forehead, sides of the face, and upper back. Dark-skinned infants often have more lanugo than infants with lighter coloring, and their darker hair is more visible.

MILIA. Milia are white cysts, 1 to 2 mm in size, resulting from distention of sebaceous glands (oil glands) that are not yet functioning properly. They occur on the face over the forehead, nose, cheeks, and chin and disappear within 2 months without treatment (Figure 20-14).

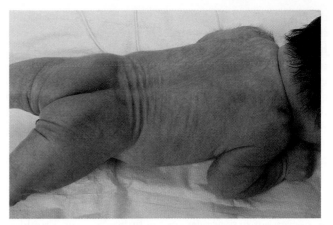

Figure 20-13 ■ Lanugo is abundant on this slightly preterm infant.

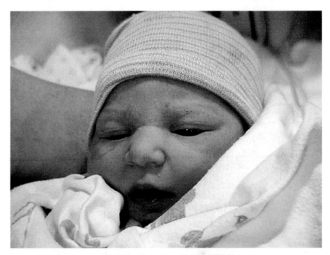

Figure 20-14 ■ Milia.

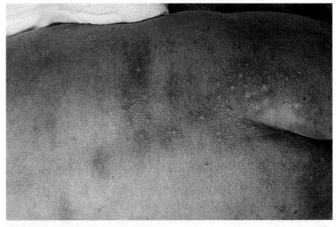

Figure 20-15 ■ Erythema toxicum. (From Hurwitz, S. [1993]. *Clinical pediatric dermatology* [2nd ed., p. 13]. Philadelphia: Saunders.)

ERYTHEMA TOXICUM. The nurse notes the presence of erythema toxicum, red, blotchy areas that may have white or yellow papules or vesicles in the center (Figure 20-15). It is commonly called *fleabite rash* or *newborn rash* and resembles small bites or acne. The rash appears during the first 24 to 48 hours after birth, although occasionally not until 1 to 2 weeks. It is most common over the face, back, shoulders, and chest. The condition does not result from infection but should be differentiated from a pustular rash caused by staphylococcal infection or vesicles from herpes simplex. The cause of erythema toxicum is unknown, but it occurs in 50% of full-term infants and disappears within hours or up to 10 days.

BIRTHMARKS. The size and location of all birthmarks should be carefully documented. Some more common birthmarks are listed here.

- Mongolian spots are bluish-black marks that resemble bruises (Figure 20-16). They usually occur in the sacral area but may appear on the buttocks, arms, shoulders, and other areas. Mongolian spots occur most frequently in newborns with dark skin and usually disappear after the first few years of life. Some continue into adulthood.
- A nevus simplex is also called *salmon patch, stork bite,* or *telangiectatic nevus* (Figure 20-17). It is a flat, pink or reddish discoloration from dilated capillaries that occur over the eyelids, just above the bridge of the nose, or at the nape of the neck. The color blanches when the area is pressed and is more prominent during cry-

ing. Stork bites disappear by 2 years of age, although those at the nape of the neck may persist.
- Nevus flammeus (port-wine stain) is a permanent, flat, dark, reddish-purple mark (Figure 20-18). It varies in size and location and blanches minimally or not at all with pressure. If it is large and in a visible area, it can be removed by laser surgery. Those located over the forehead and upper eyelid may be associated with Sturge-Weber syndrome, a serious neurologic condition that also may involve eye problems.
- Nevus vasculosus (strawberry hemangioma) consists of enlarged capillaries in the outer layers of skin. It is dark red and raised with a rough surface, giving a strawberry-like appearance. The hemangioma usually is located on the head. It may grow larger for 5 to 6 months but usually disappears by the early school years. No treatment is necessary.
- Café-au-lait spots are permanent, light-brown areas that may occur anywhere on the body. Although they are harmless, the number and size are important. Six or more spots or spots larger than 0.5 cm are associated with neurofibromatosis, a genetic condition of neural tissue.

MARKS FROM DELIVERY. The infant is inspected for marks that may have occurred from injury or pressure during labor or delivery.

- Petechiae, pinpoint bruises that resemble a rash, may appear over areas such as the back, face, and groin. They result from increased intravascular pressure during the birth process, such as occurs with a nuchal cord (cord around the neck) during delivery. Widespread or continued formation of petechiae may indicate infection or a low platelet count.
- Bruises may occur on any part of the body where pressure occurred during delivery. This is especially true when second-stage labor was difficult. Bruising or petechiae of the face may be present if the cord was wrapped tightly around the neck during birth.

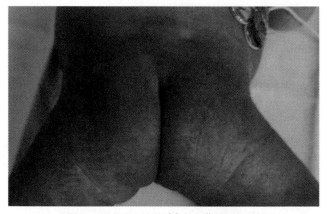
Figure 20-16 ■ Mongolian spots.

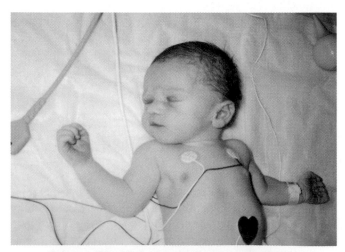
Figure 20-17 ■ Nevus simplex or stork bite.

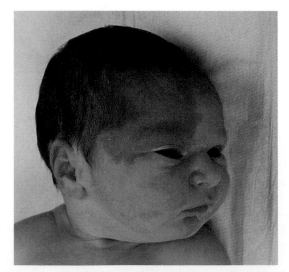
Figure 20-18 ■ Port-wine stain (nevus flammeus).

Bruising on the head may occur from use of a vacuum extractor.

- A small puncture mark is present on the newborn's head if a fetal monitor scalp electrode was attached. The area should scab and heal normally but should be observed for signs of infection.
- Forceps marks occur over the cheeks and ears where the instruments were applied. Their size, color, and location are carefully documented. Lack of movement or asymmetry of the face may indicate injury of the facial nerve.

OTHER ASPECTS. Other aspects of the skin that may indicate abnormalities should be recorded. Localized edema may be caused by trauma of delivery. Generalized edema indicates more serious conditions such as heart failure. Peeling of the skin is normal in full-term newborns. Excessive amounts of peeling may indicate a postterm infant.

BREASTS

The nurse notes the placement of the nipples and looks for extra (supernumerary) nipples, which may appear on the chest or in the axilla. Occasionally, the breasts become engorged 2 or 3 days after birth and secrete a small amount of white fluid (sometimes called "witch's milk") a few days later. This condition results from maternal hormones and resolves within a few weeks without treatment. The breasts should not be expressed or manipulated, as this could cause infection.

HAIR AND NAILS

The hair on the full-term infant should be silky and soft, whereas that on the preterm infant is woolly or fuzzy. The nails come to the end of the fingers or beyond. Very long nails may indicate a postterm infant.

DOCUMENTATION

All marks, bruises, rashes, and other abnormalities of the skin must be recorded in the nurses' notes. The location, size, color, elevation, and texture of each mark are described. Subsequent changes in appearance from previous descriptions also are noted on the chart.

The nurse may not always know the proper name for each type of mark on the infant's skin. Most agencies have books with pictures of the common skin variations.

- When in doubt about the name of a mark, a description is sufficient. For example, a stork bite (nevus simplex) might be described as a "flat, reddened area 1 × 2 cm in size over right eyelid that blanches with pressure."

ASSESSMENT OF GESTATIONAL AGE

The gestational age assessment is an examination of the newborn's physical and neurologic characteristics to determine the number of weeks from conception to birth. It is important because neonates born before or after term and those whose sizes are not appropriate for gestational age are at increased risk for complications. Although the gestational age often is calculated from the mother's last menstrual period and by ultrasonography during the pregnancy, the date of the last menstrual period is not always accurate, and ultrasonography is not always performed.

Because the times of development for various fetal characteristics are known, the presence or absence of these characteristics can help estimate gestational age. The estimated age then can be compared with the newborn's weight, length, and head circumference to determine whether the neonate is large, appropriate (average), or small in size for gestational age.

Assessment Tools

Several different tools are used to assess gestational age. The Dubowitz scoring system is an in-depth, detailed assessment tool that includes examination of physical, neurologic, and behavioral characteristics. The New Ballard Score (Figure 20-19) is a simplified adaptation of the Dubowitz tool that has been revised to include characteristics of very preterm infants. It can be performed quickly yet provides accurate information within 1 week when performed by an experienced examiner (Southgate & Pittard, 2001). The Ballard tool focuses on physical and neuromuscular characteristics, eliminating the behavioral characteristics. With each tool, a score is given to each assessment and the total score is used to determine the gestational age of the infant. The New Ballard Score is described in the following section.

Neuromuscular Characteristics
POSTURE

The posture and degree of flexion of the extremities are scored before the quiet infant is disturbed for the remainder of the examination (Figure 20-20). Preterm neonates have immature flexor muscles and little energy or muscle tone. Therefore they have extended, limp arms and legs that offer little resistance to movement by the examiner. Flexor tone improves as the gestational age increases, and it moves in a cephalocaudal manner down the infant's body. Full-term infants hold their arms close to the body with the elbows sharply flexed. The legs should be flexed at the hips, knees, and ankles. Posture is scored from zero for a limp, flaccid posture to 4 if the newborn demonstrates good flexion of all extremities. The legs of infants who were in a frank breech position are more likely to remain more extended than flexed even when they are full term.

SQUARE WINDOW

The square window sign is elicited by bending the hand at the wrist until the palm is as flat against the forearm as possible with gentle pressure (Figure 20-21). The angle between the palm and forearm is measured. If the palm bends only 90 degrees (which is the extent of flexion in the adult wrist and looks like a square window), the score is 0. The gestational age of the infant is probably 32 weeks or less. The more mature the neonate, the smaller the angle until the palm folds flat against the forearm at term, the result of maternal hormones at the end of pregnancy.

NEWBORN MATURITY RATING & CLASSIFICATION

ESTIMATION OF GESTATIONAL AGE BY MATURITY RATING
Symbols: X - 1st Exam   O - 2nd Exam

Gestation by Dates_____wks

Birth Date_____Hour_____ am/pm

APGAR_____1 min_____5 min

NEUROMUSCULAR MATURITY

	-1	0	1	2	3	4	5
Posture							
Square Window (wrist)	>90°	90°	60°	45°	30°	0°	
Arm Recoil		180°	140°-180°	110°-140°	90°-110°	<90°	
Popliteal Angle	180°	160°	140°	120°	100°	90°	<90°
Scarf Sign							
Heel to Ear							

PHYSICAL MATURITY

Skin	sticky friable transparent	gelatinous red, translucent	smooth pink, visible veins	superficial peeling &/or rash, few veins	cracking pale areas rare veins	parchment deep cracking no vessels	leathery cracked wrinkled
Lanugo	none	sparse	abundant	thinning	bald areas	mostly bald	
Plantar Surface	heel-toe 40-50mm:-1 <40mm:-2	>50mm no crease	faint red marks	anterior transverse crease only	creases ant. 2/3	creases over entire sole	
Breast	imperceptible	barely perceptible	flat areola no bud	stippled areola 1-2mm bud	raised areola 3-4mm bud	full areola 5-10mm bud	
Eye/Ear	lids fused loosely:-1 tightly:-2	lids open pinna flat stays folded	sl. curved pinna; soft; slow recoil	well-curved pinna; soft but ready recoil	formed &firm instant recoil	thick cartilage ear stiff	
Genitals male	scrotum flat, smooth	scrotum empty faint rugae	testes in upper canal rare rugae	testes descending few rugae	testes down good rugae	testes pendulous deep rugae	
Genitals female	clitoris prominent labia flat	prominent clitoris small labia minora	prominent clitoris enlarging minora	majora & minora equally prominent	majora large minora small	majora cover clitoris & minora	

MATURITY RATING

score	weeks
-10	20
-5	22
0	24
5	26
10	28
15	30
20	32
25	34
30	36
35	38
40	40
45	42
50	44

SCORING SECTION

	1st Exam=X	2nd Exam=O
Estimating Gest Age by Maturity Rating	_____Weeks	_____Weeks
Time of Exam	Date____ Hour____am/pm	Date____ Hour____am/pm
Age at Exam	_____Hours	_____Hours
Signature of Examiner	_____M.D.	_____M.D.

Figure 20-19 ■ New Ballard Score. (Courtesy Bristol-Myers Company, Evansville, Indiana. From Ballard, J.L., Khoury, J.C., Wedig, K., Wang, L., Eilers-Walsman, B.L., & Lipp, R. [1991]. New Ballard score, expanded to include extremely premature infants. *Journal of Pediatrics, 19*[3], 417-423.)

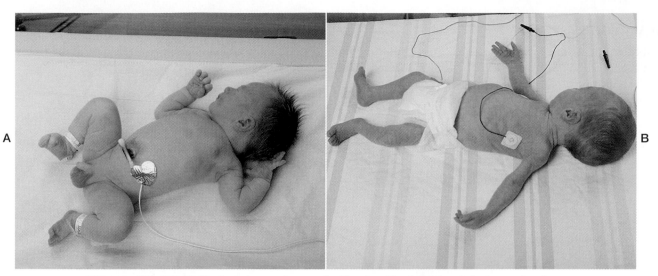

Figure 20-20 ■ Posture in newborns. **A,** The healthy full-term infant remains in a strongly flexed position. **B,** The preterm infant's extremities are extended.

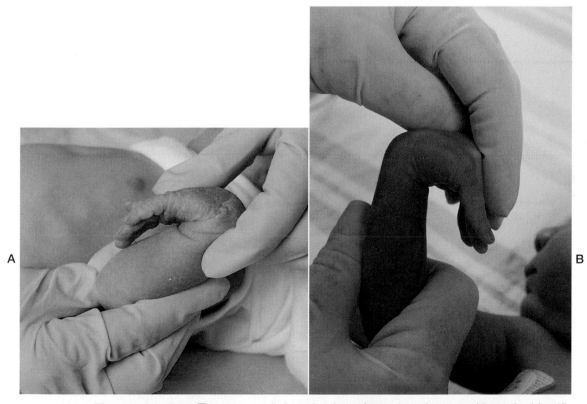

Figure 20-21 ■ The square window sign is performed on the arm without the identification bracelet. The nurse bends the wrist and measures the angle. **A,** Infant near full term. **B,** Preterm infant.

ARM RECOIL

Full-term infants resist extension of the arms. In testing for arm recoil, the nurse holds the neonate's arms fully flexed at the elbows for 5 seconds, then extends the arms by pulling the hands straight down to the sides (Figure 20-22). The hands are quickly released and the degree of flexion is measured as the arms return to their normally flexed position. Preterm infants may not move the arms at all and re- ceive a score of 0. Somewhat older infants have a sluggish recoil, with only partial return to flexion. If the arms move briskly to an angle of less than 90 degrees at the elbows, the score is 4.

POPLITEAL ANGLE

To measure the popliteal angle, the newborn's lower leg is folded against the thigh, with the thigh on the abdomen (Figure 20-23). The infant's hips must remain flat on the

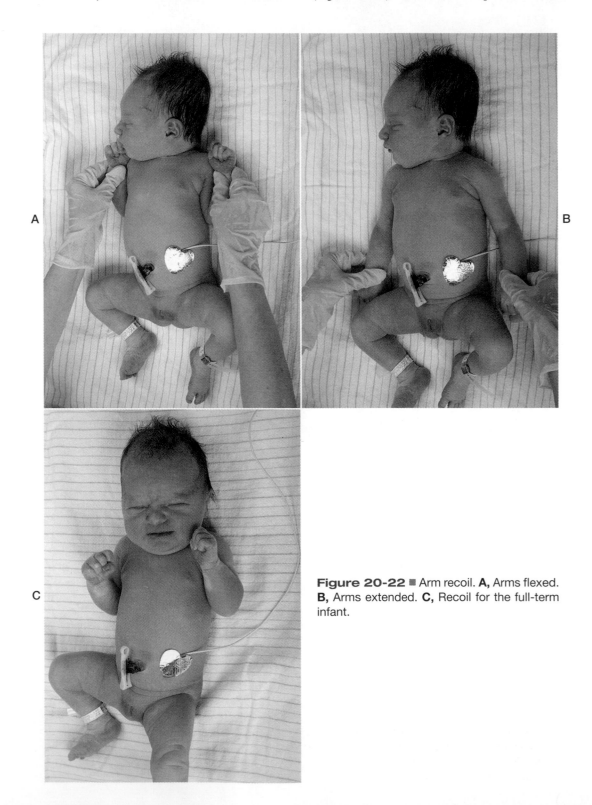

Figure 20-22 ■ Arm recoil. **A,** Arms flexed. **B,** Arms extended. **C,** Recoil for the full-term infant.

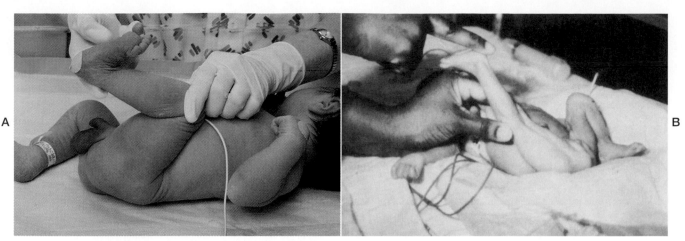

Figure 20-23 ■ The popliteal angle is measured by flexing the thigh against the abdomen and extending the lower leg to the point of resistance. **A,** Full-term infant. **B,** Preterm infant.

bed. With the thigh still flexed on the abdomen, the lower leg is straightened just until resistance is met. Continued pressure causes the infant to further extend the leg and results in an inaccurate score. The angle at the popliteal space when resistance is first felt is scored on a scale of 1 (if the leg can be fully extended) to 5 (if the angle at the popliteal space is less than 90 degrees). The leg may extend with little resistance if the infant was in a frank breech position at birth.

SCARF SIGN

For the scarf sign, the nurse grasps the infant's hand and brings the arm across the body to the opposite side, keeping the shoulder flat on the bed and the head in the middle of the body (Figure 20-24). The position of the elbow in relation to the midline of the infant's body is noted. The infant receives a score of 1 if muscle tone is so poor that the arm wraps across the body like a scarf with the elbow beyond the edge of the body. A full score (4) shows that the elbow fails to reach near to midline.

HEEL TO EAR

The heel-to-ear assessment is similar to the measurement of the popliteal angle. However, in this case, the nurse grasps the infant's foot and pulls it straight up alongside the body toward the ears while the hips remain flat on the surface of the bed (Figure 20-25). When resistance is felt, the position of the foot in relation to the head and the amount of flexion of the leg are compared with the diagrams. The more resistance and flexion, the more mature the infant.

Record the position when resistance is first felt because the neonate may relax the leg if pressure continues. This assessment also may be inaccurate in infants who were in a breech position at delivery.

Physical Characteristics

SKIN

The skin is assessed for color, visibility of veins, and peeling and cracking. The very preterm infant's skin is translucent because it is thin and has little subcutaneous fat beneath the

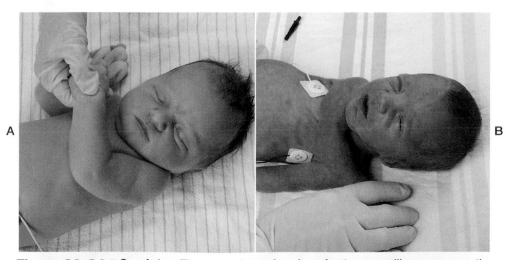

Figure 20-24 ■ Scarf sign. The nurse determines how far the arm will move across the chest and observes the position of the elbow when resistance is felt. **A,** Full-term infant. **B,** Preterm infant. (Note the many visible veins in the preterm infant and the absence of visible veins in the full-term infant.)

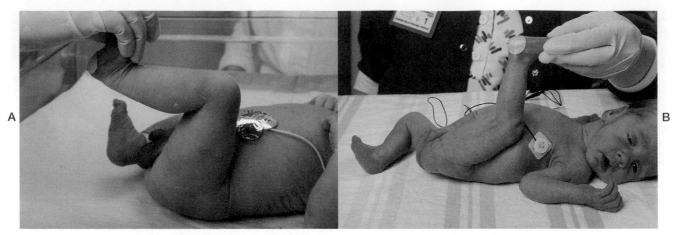

Figure 20-25 ■ Heel-to-ear assessment. The nurse grasps the foot and brings it up toward the ear, keeping the hips flat. The score is recorded when resistance is felt. **A,** Full-term infant. **B,** Preterm infant.

surface. The skin is red, sticky, and fragile, with easily visible veins. In the mature newborn the skin is thicker and the color is paler. Few veins are visible, usually over the chest and abdomen (see Figure 20-24). At term, vernix is present only in the creases.

The full-term infant exhibits some peeling and cracking of the skin, especially around areas with creases, such as the ankles and feet. The postmature infant has deeply cracked skin that appears as dry and thick as leather. Peeling becomes even more apparent during the hours after birth as the skin loses moisture.

LANUGO

Lanugo appears at 20 weeks of gestation and increases in amount until 28 weeks (see Figure 20-13). At that time it begins to disappear until little is left at term. A small amount

may remain over the upper back and shoulders, on the ears, or on the sides of the forehead. Newborns with dark coloring may have more lanugo (which is dark and more easily noticed) than infants with fair skin and very light hair, even though they are the same gestational age. The infant receives a score based on the amount of lanugo present on the back, because this is the area where it begins to disappear first (Southgate & Pittard, 2001).

PLANTAR SURFACE

Plantar creases begin to appear at 32 weeks of gestation (Figure 20-26). Although the creases are only red lines near the toes at first, they gradually spread down toward the heel and become deeper. At 37 weeks of gestation, creases cover the anterior two thirds of the sole. By 40 weeks of gestation the entire sole is covered with deep creases. The

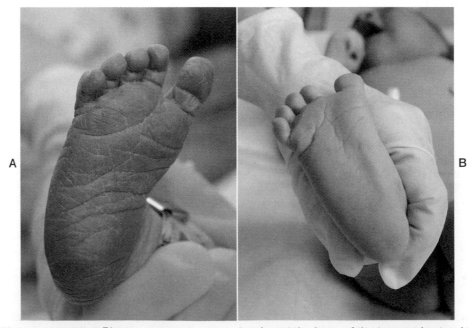

Figure 20-26 ■ Plantar creases begin to develop at the base of the toes and extend to the heel. **A,** The postterm infant has deep creases. **B,** The preterm infant has few creases on the entire foot.

plantar creases must be assessed during the early hours after birth because creases appear more prominent as the infant's skin begins to dry. For the very preterm infant the length of the foot is measured to help determine gestational age.

BREASTS

The nipples, areolae, and size of the breast buds are assessed and scored. In very preterm infants, the structures are not visible. Gradually, they grow larger and the areolae become raised above the chest wall. The breast buds enlarge until they are approximately 1 cm at term. To determine their size, the nurse places a finger on each side and measures the diameter. Use of the thumb and forefinger may cause excess tissue to be drawn together, resulting in an inaccurate score (Figure 20-27).

EYES AND EARS

The eyelids are fused until 26 to 28 weeks of gestation. When the ear is assessed, the incurving and thickness of each pinna are rated (Figure 20-28). At about 33 to 34 weeks of gestation the upper pinnae, which have been flat, begin to curve over. The incurving continues around the ear until it reaches near the earlobe at 39 to 40 weeks' gestation.

The amount of cartilage present in the ears is a more accurate guide to gestational age than the incurving of the pinnae because of individual differences in ear shape. As cartilage is deposited in the pinnae, the ears become stiff and stand away from the head. The ear is folded longitudinally and horizontally to assess the resistance and speed

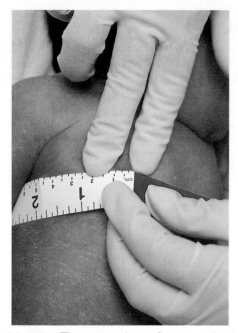

Figure 20-27 ■ The nurse places fingers on both sides of the breast bud and measures the size. In the full-term infant, breast tissue is raised and the nipple is easily distinguished from surrounding skin. (Note the peeling skin.)

with which the ear returns to its original state. In infants less than 32 weeks' gestation, the ear has little cartilage to keep it stiff. When folded, it remains folded over or returns slowly. In the term neonate the ear springs back to its original position immediately.

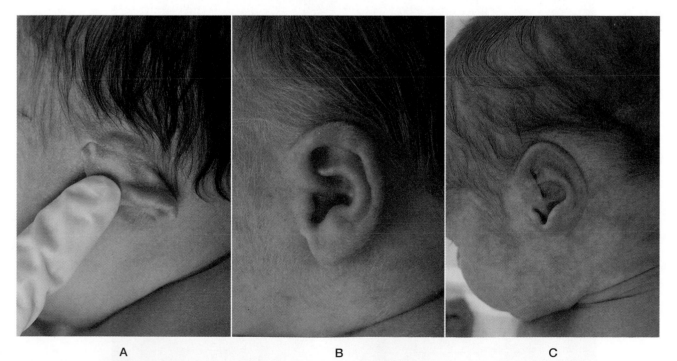

A   B   C

Figure 20-28 ■ Ear maturation. **A,** The nurse folds the ears and notes the quickness with which they return to position. **B,** Ears in the full-term infant are well formed and have instant recoil. **C,** In the preterm infant, ears show less incurving of the pinna and recoil slowly or not at all.

GENITALS

In the female infant the relationship in size of the clitoris, labia minora, and labia majora is noted (Figure 20-29). In the preterm infant the labia majora are small and separated, whereas the clitoris and labia minora are large by comparison. As the infant nears term, the labia majora enlarge until the clitoris and labia minora are completely covered. Because the size of the labia majora is affected by the amount of fat deposited, the infant who is malnourished in utero may have genitalia with an immature appearance.

In the male infant, the location of the testes and the rugae on the scrotum are assessed (Figure 20-30). The testes originate in the abdominal cavity but move down into the inguinal canal at 30 weeks of gestation. By 37 weeks' gestation they are located high in the scrotal sac, and they are generally completely descended by term. Rugae form on the surface of the scrotum beginning at about 36 weeks' and cover the sac by 40 weeks' gestation. Once the testes are completely down into the scrotum, the scrotum appears large and pendulous.

Scoring

As each part of the assessment is performed, the infant's response is matched with the diagrams and explanations on the assessment tool. The total score is compared with the corresponding gestational age. It is important to understand that one or two characteristics alone cannot be used to assign a gestational age. It is the total score of all assessed characteristics that determines the gestational age.

Although slight differences in the scores may be obtained by different examiners, a difference of 2.5 points is necessary to change the gestational age by 1 week. Therefore slight differences in the scores of different examiners are not likely to cause significant differences in the outcome of the examination.

Gestational Age and Infant Size

The appropriateness of the neonate's size for gestational age is determined by plotting the gestational age, weight, length, and head circumference on a graph of intrauterine development (Figure 20-31). This score determines how well the

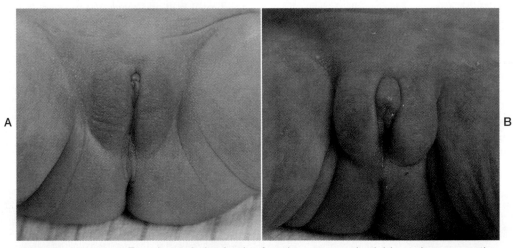

Figure 20-29 ■ Female genitals. As the female matures, the labia majora cover the labia minora and clitoris completely; in the preterm infant these structures are not covered. **A,** Near-term infant. **B,** Preterm infant.

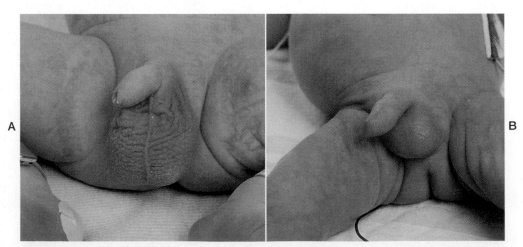

Figure 20-30 ■ Male genitals. **A,** The full-term infant has a pendulous scrotum with deep rugae. **B,** In the preterm infant, the testes may not be descended and rugae are few.

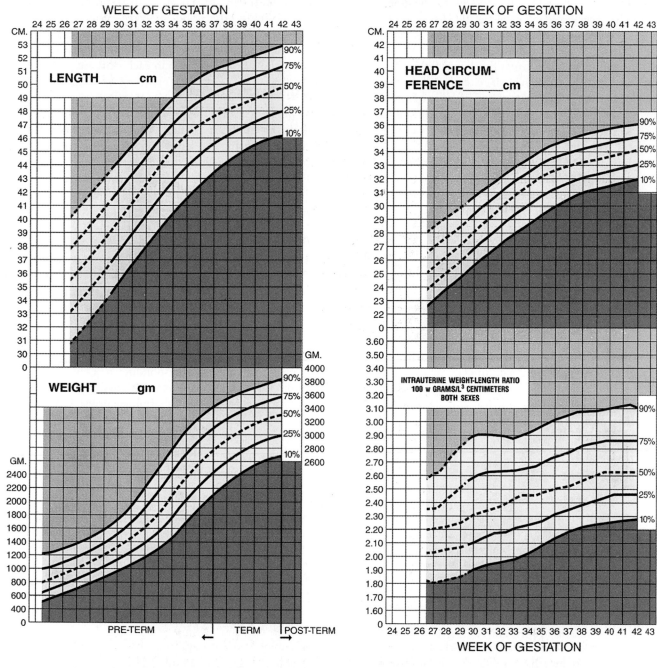

Figure 20-31 ■ Intrauterine growth grids. (Courtesy Bristol-Myers Company, Evansville, Indiana. Modified from Lubchenko, L.C., Hansman, C, & Boyd, E. [1966]. *Pediatrics, 37,* 403; and from Battaglia, F.C., & Lubchenko, L.C. [1967]. *Journal of Pediatrics, 71,* 159.)

infant has grown for the amount of time spent in the uterus. An infant may be small, large, or of appropriate size for gestational age. The infant whose size is appropriate for gestational age falls between the 10th and 90th percentiles on the graph. The large-for-gestational-age (LGA) infant is above the 90th percentile, whereas the small-for-gestational-age (SGA) infant is below the 10th percentile.

Although people sometimes think that the SGA infant is always preterm, SGA infants can also be full term or postterm. Similarly, the LGA infant can be born before term, at term, or beyond term. For example, an infant born at 28 weeks of gestation may have measurements that correspond to the 92nd percentile on the intrauterine growth curve chart. The infant would be LGA even though he or she is preterm. An infant judged to be 43 weeks' gestational age may have measurements that correspond to the 7th percentile on the growth curve. The infant would be SGA.

Further Assessments

When an infant's gestational age or measurements fall outside the expected range, the nurse monitors for complications. Specific complications are common to preterm, postterm, SGA, and LGA infants. For example, pregnancy complications may cause a poorly functioning placenta and an SGA infant. These infants are more prone to hypoglycemia, poor thermoregulation, and respiratory problems.

The most common causes of an LGA infant are diabetes in the mother and very large parents. The nurse monitors these infants especially carefully for hypoglycemia and birth injuries because of the difficulty the large infant's passage through the birth canal.

ASSESSMENT OF BEHAVIOR

Assessment of the infant's behavior helps determine intactness of the central nervous system and provides information about the infant's ability to respond to caretaking activities. Because behavior differs at various times after birth, the nurse should be aware of the periods of reactivity and the six different states of behavior so that nursing care can be adapted appropriately.

Periods of Reactivity

During the first and second periods of reactivity (see Chapter 19), newborns may have elevated pulse and respiratory rates, low temperatures, and excessive respiratory secretions. Careful observation of infants is important during this time, but assessment can usually be done unobtrusively so that parents can continue to enjoy the newborn. During the sleep period between the first and second periods of reactivity, newborns cannot be awakened easily and are not interested in feeding. Infants in the sleep phase have relaxed muscle tone that may affect the score on a gestational age assessment.

Behavioral Changes

Nurses assess the infant's behavior and alert the physician of abnormalities. Assessment includes the six different behavioral states: deep sleep, active sleep, drowsy, quiet alert, active alert, and crying. Movement between states should be smooth and not abrupt. The Brazelton Neonatal Behavioral Assessment Scale often is used when detailed knowledge about the infant is needed. In addition to assessing behavioral states, the scale analyzes other aspects of the newborn's behavior, such as orientation, habituation, self-consoling behaviors, social behaviors, and the appropriateness of the amount of time in each of these activities.

ORIENTATION

The nurse notes the infant's orientation (ability to pay attention) to interesting visual or auditory stimuli. It is most prominent during the quiet alert state. Infants focus their eyes and turn their heads toward a stimulus in an attempt to prolong contact with it. Preterm and ill neonates have less ability to orient to stimuli. Attempts to stimulate these newborns may result in overfatigue.

HABITUATION

The infant's response to a visual, auditory, or tactile stimulus is an important assessment. Generally, the first response of a healthy newborn to an interesting stimulus, such as a brightly colored object or bell, is a period of alertness. If the stimulus is disturbing, like a bright light flashed in the eyes or a pinprick to the foot, the infant startles and attempts to escape by averting the eyes or pulling the foot away.

Infants gradually stop responding to continued noxious stimuli. This gradual habituation allows them to ignore the stimuli and save energy for physiologic needs. Newborns may go into a dull, drowsy state or fall into a deep sleep. Those who seem unresponsive in a bright, noisy nursery may be in a state of habituation. The preterm infant or one with damage to the central nervous system may not be able to habituate.

SELF-CONSOLING ACTIVITIES

Normal newborns are able to console themselves for short periods of time. Self-consoling activities include attempting to bring their hands to the mouth, sucking on their fists, listening to voices, and watching objects in the environment. Infants who are ill, preterm, or exposed to drugs prenatally have less ability to console themselves.

PARENTS' RESPONSE

The parents' growing ability to respond to the infant's behavioral cues should be noted. The nurse can point out the infant's behavioral changes to facilitate bonding and help the parents learn to interpret the infant's cues. The methods that the parents use to meet the infant's needs during different behavior states also are noted.

✓ CHECK YOUR READING

11. When should the first voiding occur? How often do infants void?
12. What is the nurse's responsibility regarding marks on the newborn's skin?
13. Why is the gestational age assessment important?
14. How do the periods of reactivity affect nursing care?

SUMMARY CONCEPTS

- Nurses assess newborns immediately after birth to detect serious abnormalities. If no problems are detected with a quick assessment, a more comprehensive examination is performed.
- Assessment of cardiorespiratory status includes history, airway, color, heart sounds, pulses, and blood pressure.
- Because they are safer and provide accurate measurement, axillary temperatures are preferred to rectal temperatures.
- Molding of the head is normal during birth and may cause the head to appear misshapen. Caput succedaneum (localized swelling from pressure against the cervix) or a cephalhematoma (bleeding between the periosteum and the bone) may be present.
- Measurements are an important way to learn about growth before birth. Abnormal measurements alert the nurse that complications may occur.
- Reflexes are an indication of the health of the central nervous system. Asymmetry or retention of reflexes beyond the time when they should disappear is abnormal.
- Hypoglycemia can cause damage to the brain. Early signs of hypoglycemia include jitteriness, poor muscle tone, respiratory distress, perspiration, low temperature, and poor suck.
- In performing heel sticks for blood glucose measurement, the nurse must choose the site carefully to avoid damage to the bone, nerves, and blood vessels of the heel.
- The initial feeding provides information about the neonate's tolerance to feeding and ability to coordinate sucking, swallowing, and breathing.
- Newborns pass the first stool within 12 to 48 hours of birth. Feeding the infant and inserting a rectal thermometer may stimulate stool passage.
- The newborn's first void occurs within 12 to 24 hours. Infants may void only 1-2 times during the first 2 days and then at least six times daily.
- Marks on the skin should be documented, including location, size, color, elevation, and texture. Because marks can be upsetting, they should be explained to the parents.
- The gestational age assessment provides an estimate of the infant's age from conception. It alerts the nurse to possible complications related to age and size.
- During the first and second periods of reactivity, the infant may have a low temperature, elevated pulse and respirations, and excessive respiratory secretions. Between these periods, the infant is in a deep sleep with relaxed muscle tone and no interest in feeding.

ANSWERS TO CRITICAL THINKING EXERCISE 20-1, p. 483

Failure of the reflexes to fade on schedule may interfere with normal development. For example, the palmar grasp reflex must disappear so that the infant can learn to grasp voluntarily and later to release objects at will. Persistence of the plantar reflex would interfere with walking. Retention of reflexes beyond the age at which they should disappear indicates pathology and should prompt further investigation.

ANSWERS TO CRITICAL THINKING EXERCISE 20-2, p. 491

Begin by expanding your assessment of the facts. First, check through the chart to be sure that no stool is recorded. Did the infant pass meconium at delivery? Check the delivery notes. Ask the mother if she has changed a diaper with stool in it. Instruct her to inform the nurse if she does. Carefully taking a rectal temperature may stimulate peristalsis and passage of meconium and verifies that the anus is patent. However, even with a patent anus, obstruction of the intestine above the anus is possible.

Consider the infant's intake. How often is the infant feeding, and how well are feedings being taken? If the infant has been sleepy and has fed poorly, increase the feedings. Asking the nursing mother to feed more often or offering the neonate extra formula may make the difference.

Alert other caregivers to watch for a stool, and let the mother know that the infant is being watched for stools without alarming her. Although some infants do not have a stool until nearly 48 hours after birth, the primary caregiver may wish to know about the situation at 24 hours.

REFERENCES & READINGS

American Academy of Pediatrics (AAP). (2000). Clinical practice guideline: Early detection of developmental dysplasia of the hip. *Pediatrics, 105*(4), 896-905.

American Academy of Pediatrics (AAP) & American College of Obstetricians and Gynecologists (2002). *Guidelines for perinatal care* (5th ed.). Elk Grove, IL: AAP.

Askin, D.F. (2001). Newborn adaptation to extrauterine life. In K.R. Simpson & P.A. Creehan (Eds.), *Perinatal nursing* (2nd ed., pp. 307-335). Philadelphia: Lippincott Williams & Wilkins.

Ballard, J.L., Khoury, J.C., Wedig, K., Wang, L., Eilers-Walsman, B.L., & Lipp, R. (1991). New Ballard Score, expanded to include extremely premature infants. *Journal of Pediatrics, 19*(3), 417-423.

Berryman, R.E., & Glass, S.M. (2005). Routine care. In P.J. Thureen, J. Deacon, J. Hernandez, & D.M. Hall (Eds.), *Assessment and care of the well newborn* (2nd ed., pp. 198-205). Philadelphia: Saunders.

Blackburn, S.T., (2003). *Maternal, fetal, and neonatal physiology* (2nd ed). Philadelphia: Saunders.

Blackburn, S.T., & Blakewell-Sachs, S. (2003). *Understanding the behavior of term infants*. White Plains, NY: March of Dimes Birth Defects Foundation. Retrieved November 30, 2004, from http://www.marchofdimes.com.

Blake, W.W., & Murray, J.A. (2002). Heat balance. In G.B. Merenstein & S.L. Gardner (Eds.), *Handbook of neonatal intensive care* (5th ed., pp. 102-116). St. Louis: Mosby.

Brodski, D., & Martin, C. (2003). *Neonatology review*. Philadelphia: Hanley & Belfus.

Buschbach, D., & Bordeaux, M.S. (2002). *Newborn physiological and developmental transitions: Integrating key components of perinatal and neonatal assessment*. White Plains, NY: March of Dimes Birth Defects Foundation.

Carlo, W.A., & DiFlore, J.M. (2002). Assessment of pulmonary function. In A.A. Fanaroff & R.J. Martin (Eds.), *Neonatal-perinatal medicine* (Vol. 2, 7th ed., pp. 991-1000). St. Louis: Mosby.

Cheffer, N.D. (2004). Adaptation to extrauterine life and immediate nursing care. In S. Mattson & J.E. Smith (Eds.), *Core curriculum for maternal-newborn nursing* (3rd ed., pp. 421-436). Philadelphia: Saunders.

Cheffer, N.D., & Rannalli, D.A. (2004). Newborn biological/behavioral characteristics and psychosocial adaptations. In S. Mattson & J.E. Smith (Eds.), *Core curriculum for maternal-newborn nursing* (3rd ed., pp. 437-484). Philadelphia: Saunders.

Creehan, P.A. (2001). Newborn physical assessment. In K.R. Simpson & P.A. Creehan (Eds.), *Perinatal nursing* (2nd ed., pp. 513-542). Philadelphia: Lippincott Williams & Wilkins.

D'Harlingue, A.E., & Duran, D.J. (2001). Recognition, stabilization, and transport of the high-risk newborn. In M.H. Klaus & A.A. Fanaroff (Eds.), *Care of the high-risk neonate* (5th ed, pp. 65-99). Philadelphia: Saunders.

Elder, J.S. (2004). Urologic disorders in infants and children. In R.E. Behrman, R.M. Kliegman, & H.B. Jenson (Eds.), *Nelson textbook of pediatrics* (17th ed., pp. 1783-1826). Philadelphia: Saunders.

Furdon, S.A., & Benjamin, K. (2004). Physical assessment of the newborn infant. In *Core curriculum for neonatal intensive care nursing* (3rd ed., pp. 135-172). Philadelphia: Saunders.

Gardner, S.L., Johnson, J.L., & Lubchenco, L.O. (2002). Initial nursery care. In G.B. Merenstein & S.L. Gardner (Eds.), *Handbook of neonatal intensive care* (5th ed., pp. 70-99). St. Louis: Mosby.

Hagedorn, M.I.E., Gardner, S.L., & Abman, S.H. (2002). Respiratory diseases. In G.B. Merenstein & S.L. Gardner (Eds.), *Handbook of neonatal intensive care* (5th ed., pp. 485-497). St. Louis: Mosby.

Hernandez, J.A., Fashaw, L., & Evans, R. (2005). Adaptation to extrauterine life and management during normal and abnormal transition. In P.J. Thureen, J. Deacon, J. Hernandez, & D.M. Hall (Eds.), *Assessment and care of the well newborn* (2nd ed., pp. 83-109). Philadelphia: Saunders.

Howard-Glenn, L. (2000). Adaptation to extrauterine life and immediate nursing care. In *Core curriculum for maternal-newborn nursing* (2nd ed., pp. 346-359). Philadelphia: Saunders.

Kenner, C. (2003). Resuscitation and stabilization of the newborn. In C. Kenner & J.W. Lott (Eds.), *Comprehensive neonatal nursing: A physiologic perspective* (3rd ed., pp. 210-227). Philadelphia: Saunders.

Lissauer, T., & Izatt, S.D. (2002). Physical examination and care of the newborn. In A.A. Fanaroff & R.J. Martin (Eds.), *Neonatal-perinatal medicine* (Vols. 1 and 2, 7th ed., pp. 441-459). St. Louis: Mosby.

Meehan, R.M. (1998). Heelsticks in neonates for capillary blood sampling. *Neonatal Network, 17*(1), 17-24.

Nicholson, J.F., & Pesce, M.A. (2004). Reference ranges for laboratory tests and procedures. In R.E. Behrman, R.M. Kliegman, &

H.B. Jenson (Eds.), *Nelson textbook of pediatrics* (17th ed., pp. 2396-2421). Philadelphia: Saunders.

Sansoucie, D.A., & Cavaliere, T.A. (2003). Newborn and infant assessment. In C. Kenner & J.W. Lott (Eds.), *Comprehensive neonatal nursing: A physiologic perspective* (3rd ed., pp. 308-347). Philadelphia: Saunders.

Sganga, A., Wallace, R., Kiehl, E., Irving, T., & Witter, L. (2000). A comparison of four methods of normal newborn temperature measurement. *MCN: American Journal of Maternal/Child Nursing, 25*(2), 76-79.

Sifuentes, M. (2000). Neonatal examination and nursery visit. In C.D. Berkowitz (Ed.), *Pediatrics: A primary care approach* (2nd ed., pp. 20-23). Philadelphia: Saunders.

Sniderman, S., & Taeusch, H.W. (2005). Initial evaluation: History and physical examination of the newborn. In H.W. Taeusch, R.A. Ballard, & C.A. Gleason (Eds.), *Avery's diseases of the newborn* (8th ed., pp. 301-322). Philadelphia: Saunders.

Southgate, W.M., & Pittard, W.B. (2001). Classification and physical examination of the newborn infant. In M.H. Klaus & A.A. Fanaroff. *Care of the high-risk neonate* (5th ed, pp. 100-129). Philadelphia: Saunders.

Stoll, B.J., & Kliegman, R.M. (2004a). Digestive system disorders. In R.E. Behrman, R.M. Kliegman, & H.B. Jenson (Eds.), *Nelson textbook of pediatrics* (17th ed., pp. 588-599). Philadelphia: Saunders.

Stoll, B.J., & Kliegman, R.M. (2000b). The newborn infant. In R.E. Behrman, R.M. Kliegman, & H.B. Jenson (Eds.). *Nelson textbook of pediatrics* (17th ed., pp. 523-531). Philadelphia: Saunders.

Swinford, R.D., Bonilla-Felix, M., Cerda, R.D., & Portman, R.J. (2002). Neonatal nephrology. In G.B. Merenstein & S.L. Gardner (Eds.), *Handbook of neonatal intensive care* (5th ed., pp. 609-643). St. Louis: Mosby.

Thilo, E.H. (2005). Neonatal jaundice. In P.J. Thureen, J. Deacon, J. Hernandez, & D.M. Hall (Eds.), *Assessment and care of the well newborn* (2nd ed., pp. 245-254). Philadelphia: Saunders.

Thompson, G.H. (2004). The hip. In R.E. Behrman, R.M. Kliegman, & H.B. Jenson (Eds.), *Nelson textbook of pediatrics* (17th ed., pp. 2273-2280). Philadelphia: Saunders.

Townsend, S.F. (2005). Approach to the infant at risk for hypoglycemia. In P.J. Thureen, J. Deacon, J. Hernandez, & D.M. Hall (Eds.), *Assessment and care of the well newborn* (2nd ed., pp. 261-266). Philadelphia: Saunders.

Walker, M., & Creehan, P. (2001). Newborn nutrition. In K.R. Simpson & P.A. Creehan (Eds.), *Perinatal nursing* (2nd ed., pp. 550-574). Philadelphia: Lippincott Williams & Wilkins.

CHAPTER 21

Care of the Normal Newborn

OBJECTIVES

After studying this chapter, you should be able to:

1. Describe the purpose and use of routine prophylactic medications for the normal newborn.
2. Explain the nurse's responsibility in ongoing cardiorespiratory and thermoregulatory assessments and care.
3. Describe collaborative interventions for hypoglycemia.
4. Discuss prevention and parent teaching for jaundice.
5. Explain the risks and benefits of circumcision.
6. Describe the care of circumcised and uncircumcised male infants.
7. Describe ongoing nursing assessments and care of the newborn.
8. Describe methods to protect newborns by proper identification.
9. Explain how nurses can help prevent infant abductions.
10. Describe methods to prevent infections in newborns.
11. Discuss important considerations in parent teaching.
12. Explain the importance of newborn screening tests.

Go to your Student CD-ROM for Review Questions keyed to these Objectives.

The role of the nurse in ongoing assessments and care of the newborn is to help the newborn and parents have a successful transition after birth. The nurse identifies changes in the condition of newborns as they adapt to life outside the uterus, keeps infants safe, and teaches parents how to provide care.

CLINICAL PATHWAYS

Using clinical pathways helps parents and infants to reach the goal of successful transition after childbirth. Birth facilities develop these guides to ensure that all necessary tasks are com-

YORK HEALTH SYSTEM
YORK, PENNSYLVANIA

CLINICAL PATHWAY

NEWBORN

CLINICAL PATH DAY		EXPECTED PATIENT FAMILY OUTCOMES	INTERDISCIPLINARY ASSESSMENT	TESTS	CONSULT
Immediate Newborn Care	Date & Time	☐ Apgar score >7 at 5 min [4] ☐ Maintains axillary temp of 36.5° C to 37.2° C while in radiant warmer or in double blankets [1] ☐ Physiologic parameters WNL [4] ☐ Demonstrates proper latch when breastfeeding [2] ☐ _____	Apgar score 1 & 5 min Transitional newborn assessment q 30 min. Suck reflex _____ _____	Hypoglycemia protocol when indicated _____ _____	_____ _____
Newborn Admission	Date & Time	☐ Maintains axillary temp of 36.5° C to 37.2° C while in radiant warmer or in double blankets [1] ☐ Physiologic parameters WNL [4] ☐ Tolerates initial feeding [2] ☐ Mother's blood type O/Rh − [4] ☐ _____	Weight Temp q 30 min × 4 Multisystem admission assessment Suck reflex _____	Hypoglycemia protocol when indicated _____ _____	_____ _____
0-24 Hours	Date	☐ ☐ ☐ Maintains axillary temp of 36.5° C to 37.2° C independent of external heat source [1] ☐ ☐ ☐ Parents/family verbalize understanding of safety & security measures [6] ☐ ☐ ☐ Physiologic parameters WNL [4] ☐ ☐ ☐ Parent(s)/family & infant demonstrate attachment behaviors [3] ☐ ☐ ☐ Feeding [2] ☐ ☐ ☐ Latch score is 7 or greater for breastfed newborn [2] ☐ ☐ ☐ No jaundice [4] ☐ ☐ ☐ Infant seen by physician within 12 hours [6] ☐ ☐ ☐ Pain score <4	Temp, apical pulse, neuro, cardiac, resp., GI, GU, integ. q shift Parent/infant attachment Positioning and LATCH score of breastfed newborn Freq. and amount of bottle-feeding _____ _____	Hypoglycemia protocol when indicated _____ _____	_____ _____

NAME	INITIALS	NAME	INITIALS

Note: Each patient requires an individual assessment & treatment plan. This Clinical Path is a recommendation for the average patient and requires modification when necessary by the professional staff.

Figure 21-1 ■ An example of a clinical pathway for the newborn from birth through discharge. This form is printed on both sides and is used by all caregivers to plan and document care. (Courtesy Women and Children Services of the York Health System, York, Pennsylvania. Modified with permission.)

pleted to adequately prepare mothers and infants for discharge. The pathways are also used to see that mothers and infants meet criteria for discharge. Figure 21-1 provides one example of a clinical pathway for newborns. Pathways are individualized by each institution based on protocols to meet clients' needs.

EARLY CARE

Early care after birth involves assignment of Apgar scores and assessment and stabilization of the infant as necessary (see discussions of immediate care on pp. 298-299 and infant

Text continued on p. 512.

DOCUMENTATION CODES

Initial = Meets Standard

★ = Exception on pathway identified

C = Chronic problems

N = Not applicable

PATIENT/FAMILY PROBLEMS

1. Potential for altered thermoregulation
2. Potential for feeding intolerance, neonate
3. Potential for ineffective parenting
4. Potential for altered newborn metabolism

5. Potential for infection
6. Safety concerns
7. _____
8. _____

INTERVENTIONS/ACTIVITIES	MEDS	NUTRITION	EDUCATION & DC PLANNING
Clamp cord Dry newborn Radiant warmer or double blanket while being held until temp stable ID bands _____ _____	Neonatal eye prophylaxis & Aquamephyton _____ _____	Determine if bottlefeeding or breastfeeding Assist with initial breastfeeding _____ _____	☐ Initiate safety & security measures with parents/family ☐ Teach breastfeeding mother proper latch ☐ _____
Cord care Admission bath _____ _____	HBIG if indicated _____ _____	Initial feeding: _____ _____	☐ _____ ☐ _____
Cord care Circumcision care when indicated _____ _____ _____	_____ _____	Breast/bottle feed on demand _____ _____	☐☐☐ Reinforce safety and security measures w/parents/family ☐☐☐ Observe & reinforce proper latch and instruct breastfeeding mother/family in alternative positioning ☐ Give and review new pamphlets: –Newborn screening –Car seat –Health insurance for newborns –Preparing formula –Breastfeeding, A Guide for Success ☐☐☐ _____
NAME	**INITIALS**	**NAME**	**INITIALS**
_____	_____	_____	_____
_____	_____	_____	_____
_____	_____	_____	_____

Figure 21-1, cont'd ■ For legend see opposite page.

Continued

CLINICAL PATH DAY		EXPECTED PATIENT/ FAMILY OUTCOMES	INTERDISCIPLINARY ASSESSMENT	TESTS	CONSULT
24-48 Hours	Date	☐ ☐ ☐ Maintains axillary temp of 36.5° C to 37.2° C indep. of external heat source [1] ☐ ☐ ☐ Parent(s)/family & newborn demonstrate attachment behaviors [3] ☐ ☐ ☐ Physiologic parameters WNL [4] ☐ ☐ ☐ Feeding [2] ☐ ☐ ☐ LATCH score 7 or greater for breastfed newborn [2] ☐ ☐ ☐ No jaundice [4] ☐ ☐ ☐ Pain score <4	Temp. apical pulse, cardiac, resp., neuro, GI, GU, integ. q 8 hr Weight Parent(s)/family & infant attachment behaviors LATCH score of breastfed newborn Freq. & amt. of bottle feeding _____ _____	_____ _____	☐ ☐ ☐ Referral made to LC for LATCH score <7 _____ _____ _____
48-72 Hours	Date	☐ ☐ ☐ Maintains axillary temp of 36.5° C to 37.2° C indep. of external heat source [1] ☐ ☐ ☐ Parent(s)/family & newborn demonstrate attachment behaviors [3] ☐ ☐ ☐ Physiologic parameters WNL [4] ☐ ☐ ☐ Feeding [2] ☐ ☐ ☐ LATCH score 7 or greater for breastfed newborn [2] ☐ ☐ ☐ No jaundice [4] ☐ ☐ ☐ Pain score <4	Temp. apical pulse, cardiac, resp., neuro, GI, GU, integ. q 8 hr Weight Parent(s)/family & infant attachment behaviors LATCH score of breastfed newborn Freq. & amt. of bottle feeding _____ _____	_____ _____	☐ ☐ ☐ Referral made to LC for LATCH score <7 _____ _____ _____
Day of Discharge	Date	☐ Maintains axillary temp of 36.5° to 37.2° C indep. of external heat source [1] ☐ Parent(s)/family & newborn demonstrate attachment behaviors and appropriate care of newborn [3] ☐ Physiologic parameters WNL [4] ☐ Circumcision w/o bleeding [5] ☐ Voided × 1 [4] ☐ Stooled × 1 [4] ☐ Bottle feeding ≥$\frac{1}{2}$ oz 6 times/day or LATCH score ≥7 for breastfed newborn [2] ☐ Parent(s)/family verbalize newborn D/C instr [6] ☐ No jaundice [4] ☐ Physician aware of Coombs results ☐ Pain score <4 ☐ Shaken Baby Syndrome papers signed	Temp. apical pulse, cardiac, resp., neuro, GI, GU, integ. q 8 hr Weight Parent(s)/family & infant attachment behaviors LATCH score of breastfed newborn Freq. & amt. of bottle feeding _____ _____	☐ Newborn screening blood tests prior to D/C ☐ Hearing screen prior to D/C _____ _____	☐ Referral made to LC for LATCH score <7 _____ _____

NAME	INITIALS	NAME	INITIALS
_____	_____	_____	_____
_____	_____	_____	_____

Note: Each patient requires an individual assessment & treatment plan. This Clinical Path is a recommendation for the average patient and requires modification when necessary by the professional staff.

Figure 21-1, cont'd ■ An example of a clinical pathway for the newborn from birth through discharge.

TREATMENTS	MEDS	NUTRITION	EDUCATION & DC PLANNING
Cord care Circumcision care when indicated _____ _____ _____	_____ _____	Breast/bottle fed on demand _____ _____	☐ ☐ ☐ Observe return demonst. of breastfeeding mother's use of –alternative positioning –infant's suck, swallow ☐ ☐ ☐ Observe parent(s) providing appropriate newborn care; reinforce ☐ ☐ ☐ _____ _____
Cord care Circumcision care when indicated _____ _____ _____	_____ _____	Breast/bottle fed on demand _____ _____	☐ ☐ ☐ Observe return demonst. of breastfeeding mother's use of –alternative positioning –infant's suck, swallow ☐ ☐ ☐ Observe parent(s) providing appropriate newborn care; reinforce ☐ ☐ ☐ _____ ☐ ☐ ☐ _____ _____
Cord care Circumcision care when indicated Cord clamp removed prior to D/C _____ _____ _____	☐ Hepatitis B vaccine per order _____ _____	NPO for circumcision when indicated Breast/bottle fed on demand _____ _____	☐ Review D/C instructions with parent(s)/family ☐ Shaken Baby Syndrome education reviewed –pamphlet/video ☐ D/C to mother's care _____ _____ _____

Discharge Date	Discharge Time	Discharged To	Accompanied By
_____	_____	_____	☐ W/C ☐ Ambulate

Figure 21-1, cont'd ■ For legend on opposite page.

resuscitation on pp. 800 and 802). Once the infant's condition is stable, prophylactic vitamin K and erythromycin are given.

Administering Vitamin K

Vitamin K is given to neonates because they receive only small amounts of the vitamin from the mother and they cannot synthesize vitamin K in the intestines without bacterial flora (Procedure 21-1 and Drug Guide: Vitamin K_1

[Phytonadione]). This places them at risk for vitamin K–dependent bleeding (vitamin K–deficiency disease, hemorrhagic disease of the newborn) a condition of bleeding in multiple sites that begins after the first 24 hours.

One dose of vitamin K intramuscularly within the first hour after birth prevents bleeding problems until the infant is able to produce it in sufficient amounts. Although oral vitamin K has been used for newborn prophylaxis, it is not

---

PROCEDURE

21-1   Administering Intramuscular Injections to Newborns

PURPOSE: **To place medication into the muscle without injury**

1. Wash the infant's thigh if the bath has not yet been given. *Washing removes blood from the mother that may be present on the infant's skin and prevents its carriage into the infant's tissues during the needle insertion.*
2. Prepare medication for injection. Use a 1-ml syringe with a ⅝-in, 25-gauge needle. Use a filter needle to draw up medications in glass ampules. Remove the filter needle and replace the original sterile needle to give the injection. *A small needle reaches the newborn's muscle but avoids the bone. Use of a filter needle prevents particles of glass from being drawn into the syringe.*
3. Put on gloves. *Gloves protect the nurse from contamination with blood.*
4. Locate the correct site. The best site for intramuscular injections is the infant's vastus lateralis muscle. Divide the area between the greater trochanter of the femur and the knee into thirds. Give the injection in the middle third of the muscle, lateral to the midline of the anterior thigh. *The large vastus lateralis is located away from the sciatic nerve and the femoral artery and vein. The rectus femoris muscle is nearer to these structures and poses more of a danger. (Note: The gluteal muscles are never used until a child has been walking for at least a year. These muscles are poorly developed and dangerously near the sciatic nerve.)*

5. Cleanse the area with an alcohol wipe. *Cleansing removes organisms and prevents infection.*
6. Stabilize the leg firmly while grasping the thigh between the thumb and fingers. *Holding the leg prevents sudden movement by the infant and possible injury.*
7. Insert the needle at a 90-degree angle. *This places the medication into the muscle rather than the subcutaneous tissue.*

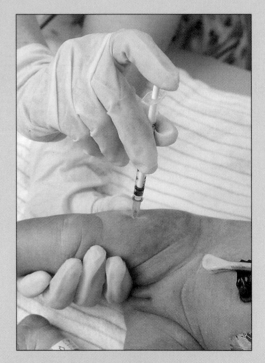

8. Aspirate and inject the medication slowly if no blood returns. If blood returns, withdraw the needle. Discard the medication and syringe and prepare new medication. *Blood return on aspiration indicates that the needle is in a blood vessel. Slow injection reduces discomfort.*
9. Withdraw the needle and apply gentle pressure to the site with an alcohol wipe. *Both reduce discomfort. Massage helps absorption of the medication.*

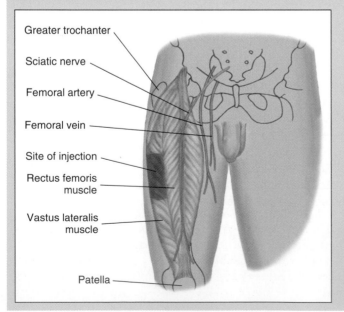

- Greater trochanter
- Sciatic nerve
- Femoral artery
- Femoral vein
- Site of injection
- Rectus femoris muscle
- Vastus lateralis muscle
- Patella

DRUG GUIDE

VITAMIN K₁ (PHYTONADIONE)

Classification: Fat-soluble vitamin, antihemorrhagic.

Other Names: AquaMEPHYTON, Mephyton, Konakion.

Action: Promotes the formation of factors II (prothrombin), VII, IX, and X by the liver for clotting; provides vitamin K, which is not synthesized in the intestines for the first 5 to 8 days after birth because the newborn lacks intestinal flora necessary for vitamin K production.

Indication: Prevention or treatment of vitamin K–dependent bleeding (hemorrhagic disease of the newborn).

Neonatal Dosage and Route: 0.5 to 1 mg (0.25 to 0.5 ml of solution containing 2 mg/ml) given once intramuscularly within 1 hour of birth for prophylaxis (lower dose is given to infants weighing less than 2500 g); higher doses or repeated doses may be used if the mother took anticonvulsants during pregnancy or if the infant shows bleeding tendencies.

Absorption: Readily absorbed after intramuscular injection; effective within 1 to 2 hours; metabolized in the liver.

Adverse Reactions: Erythema, pain, and edema at site of administration; anaphylaxis, hemolysis, or hyperbilirubinemia, especially in a preterm infant or when a large dose is used.

Nursing Considerations: Protect the drug from light until just before administration, as it decomposes and loses potency on exposure to light. Observe all infants for signs of vitamin K deficiency (ecchymoses or bleeding from any site). Check that the newborn has had vitamin K before a circumcision is performed.

recommended at this time because it has not been shown to be as effective as parenteral vitamin K (American Academy of Pediatrics [AAP], 2003).

Providing Eye Treatment

Infants also receive prophylactic treatment to prevent ophthalmia neonatorum in case the mother is infected with gonorrhea (Figure 21-2 and "Drug Guide: Erythromycin Ophthalmic Ointment"). Erythromycin 0.5% (1- to 2-cm ribbon) is most commonly used. Tetracycline 1% ophthalmic ointment or povidone-iodine ophthalmic solution 2.5% may be used also (AAP & American College of Obstetricians and Gynecologists [ACOG], 2002).

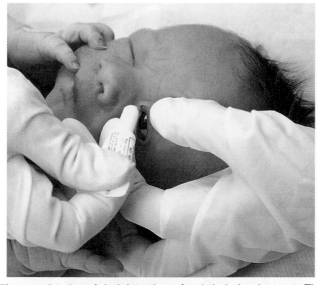

Figure 21-2 ■ Administration of ophthalmic ointment. The nurse gently cleans the eyes of blood or vernix. Then, placing a finger and thumb near the edge of each lid, the nurse gently presses against the periorbital ridges to open the eyes, avoiding pressure on the eye itself. A ribbon of ointment is squeezed into each conjunctival sac.

Because the ointment may temporarily blur the infant's vision, parents may wish to delay treatment for a short time during initial bonding. It may be delayed for as long as an hour after birth without adverse effects.

Some infants develop a mild inflammation a few hours after prophylactic treatment. However, any discharge from the eyes, especially if it is purulent, should alert the nurse to the possibility of infection. A culture may be ordered, and the drainage should be removed with sterile saline and cotton. If the mother is infected, the infant needs additional antibiotics because routine prophylactic treatment may not completely prevent infection.

Application of the Nursing Process
Cardiorespiratory Status

In the early newborn period, problems of transition may include temporary problems in cardiorespiratory status. If identified and managed promptly, most resolve within a short time.

Assessment

Assess the newborn for signs of difficult transition to newborn life. Note the rate and character of the heart rate, pulses, respirations, and breath sounds. Look for signs of respiratory distress, including tachypnea, retractions, flaring of the nares, pallor or cyanosis, grunting, seesaw respirations, and asymmetry of chest movements. Check blood pressure if indicated.

Analysis

Fluid from the lungs must be removed by absorption or drainage from the respiratory passages after birth. This does not happen immediately and may cause a temporary problem during the early hours after birth. The nursing diagnosis "Ineffective Airway Clearance related to excessive secretions in the respiratory passages" addresses this problem.

DRUG GUIDE

ERYTHROMYCIN OPHTHALMIC OINTMENT

Other Name: Ilotycin.

Classification: Antibiotic.

Action: Inhibits protein synthesis in bacteria; bacteriostatic or bactericidal (depending on organism).

Indications: Prophylaxis against the organisms *Neisseria gonorrhoeae* and *Chlamydia trachomatis;* helps prevent ophthalmia neonatorum in infants of mothers infected with gonorrhea and conjunctivitis in infants of mothers infected with *Chlamydia;* prophylaxis against gonorrhea required by law for all infants, whether or not the mother is known to be infected.

Neonatal Dosage and Route: A "ribbon" of 0.5% erythromycin ointment, 1 to 2 cm (0.4 to 0.8 in) long, is applied to the lower conjunctival sac of each eye within 1 hour after birth.

Adverse Reaction: Burning, itching. Irritation may result in chemical conjunctivitis lasting 24 to 48 hours. Ointment may cause temporary blurred vision.

Nursing Considerations: Cleanse the infant's eyes before application, as needed. Hold the tube in a horizontal rather than a vertical position to prevent injury to the eye from sudden movement. Administer from the inner canthus to the outer canthus. Do not touch the tip of the tube to any part of the eye, because this may spread infectious material from one eye to the other. Do not rinse. Ointment may be wiped from outer eye after 1 minute. Observe for irritation. Use a new tube for each infant to prevent spread of infection. Other medications used for prevention of gonorrhea include tetracycline ointment, povidone-iodine, and silver nitrate solution.

Planning

The goals and expected outcomes for this nursing diagnosis are that the newborn will:

- Maintain a patent airway as evidenced by a respiratory rate within the normal range of 30 to 60 breaths per minute
- Show no signs of respiratory distress

Interventions

POSITIONING AND SUCTIONING THE INFANT

Position the infant with the head in a neutral position or to the side. Use the bulb syringe frequently, if necessary, to suction secretions as they drain into the infant's mouth or nose (Procedure 21-2). Suction the mouth first because the infant may gasp when the nose is suctioned, causing aspira-

---

PROCEDURE

21-2   Using a Bulb Syringe

PURPOSE: **To provide an open airway by removing secretions or regurgitated feeding from the infant's mouth and nose**

1. Position the infant's head to the side or hold the infant with the head slightly lower than the rest of the body. *This allows for drainage from the mouth.*
2. Compress the bulb before inserting it into the mouth. *This removes the air from the syringe so that it will suction. (Do not compress the bulb while it is in the infant's mouth or secretions in the bulb will be expelled back into the mouth.)*
3. Gently insert the tip of the syringe into the side of the infant's mouth between the gum and the cheek. Do not insert it straight to the back of the throat. *Inserting the bulb to the back of the throat could stimulate the gag reflex, causing regurgitation and possibly a vagal response that results in bradycardia or apnea.*
4. Release the bulb slowly while it is in the mouth. Remove and empty it by compressing several times before using again. *Releasing the bulb draws secretions into the bulb. Emptying it prepares it for use again.*
5. Suction the nose, only if necessary, after the mouth is suctioned. *Infants often gasp when the nose is suctioned and might aspirate secretions in the mouth if it is not cleared first.*

6. Suction the nose gently and avoid unnecessary suction. *Trauma could cause edema and obstruction of delicate nasal passages. Infants have respiratory difficulty if nasal passages are blocked.*

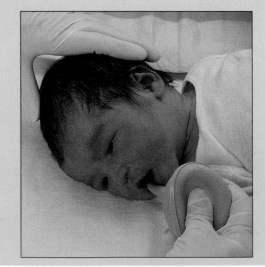

tion of mucus or fluid in the mouth. Then gently suction the nose only if necessary. Suctioning is traumatic to the delicate tissues and may cause edema of the nasal passages.

Keep the bulb syringe in the crib near the infant's head, where it is available if needed quickly. Teach both parents how to use the bulb syringe correctly. Send the syringe home with the infant so that the parents can use it if the infant experiences a problem.

If mechanical suctioning is necessary to remove deeper secretions, choose a small catheter to avoid damaging the tissues of the respiratory tract. Suction for no more than 5 seconds at a time, using minimal negative pressure to avoid trauma, laryngospasm, and bradycardia.

PROVIDING CONTINUING CARE

Continue monitoring the infant for problems throughout the stay at the birth facility. By the second period of reactivity, the infant may be alone with the mother. Although nurses know that regurgitation, gagging, and episodes of cyanosis are normal during this time, these may be very frightening to the mother.

Teach the appropriate responses to the behaviors common to this phase. Remind the mother to use the bulb syringe and call for help if needed. Check frequently with the mother to see if the infant is having difficulty. Assess her ability to use the bulb syringe and her comfort with its use.

Evaluation

The normal newborn has little difficulty clearing the airway after the first few hours of life. (See Nursing Care Plan 21-1.) Goals are met if
- The respiratory rate is between 30 and 60 breaths per minute
- The infant shows no signs of respiratory distress

Application of the Nursing Process
Thermoregulation

Because any neonate may have difficulty with thermoregulation, the nurse must identify problems and intervene to prevent complications related to this vital function.

Assessment

Assess the newborn's temperature shortly after birth and then according to agency policy. Generally the temperature is assessed every half hour until it has been stable for 2 hours. It is checked again at 4 hours and then every 8 hours or according to agency policy. Assess the newborn more often if the temperature is abnormal.

Analysis

Newborns often have temporary difficulty maintaining a stable temperature. Therefore an appropriate nursing diagnosis is "Risk for Ineffective Thermoregulation related to immature compensation for changes in environmental temperature."

Planning

The goal or expected outcome for this diagnosis is that the infant will maintain an axillary temperature within the normal range of 36.5° to 37.5° C (97.7° to 99.5° F).

Interventions
PREVENTING HEAT LOSS

PREPARING THE ENVIRONMENT BEFORE BIRTH. Begin preventive measures before the infant is born. Prepare a neutral thermal environment with a radiant warmer to use during initial assessments. This ensures that excess oxygen and glucose are not used to maintain body temperature. Check the radiant warmer to ensure it is functioning properly. Turn it on early enough that the bed is ready and warm for the newborn. Set the servocontrol between 36° and 36.5° C (96.8° and 97.7° F). This setting regulates the amount of heat produced by the warmer to maintain the infant's skin temperature at the normal level.

PROVIDING IMMEDIATE CARE. Immediately after birth, place the infant on the mother's abdomen to provide warmth from skin-to-skin contact or under the radiant warmer to counteract the cool temperature of the delivery room. Dry the wet infant quickly with warm towels to prevent heat loss by evaporation. Pay particular attention to drying the hair, because the head has a large surface area and hair that remains damp increases heat loss. Remove towels or blankets as soon as they become wet and replace them with dry, warmed linens. Cover the infant's head with a cap when the infant is not under a radiant warmer. Do not use a hat when the infant is under the warmer because it prevents transfer of heat to the infant's head.

When the infant is placed under a radiant warmer, attach a skin probe to the abdomen. The probe allows the warmer to monitor and display the infant's temperature continuously. Check frequently to see that the infant's skin temperature is increasing as expected.

PROVIDING ONGOING PREVENTION. Warm objects that will come in contact with the infant to avoid conduction of heat away from the body. Pad cool surfaces such as scales or circumcision restraint boards before placing infants on them. Warm stethoscopes and clothing before using them. Before touching the infant, run warm water over your hands if they are cold.

To prevent heat loss by radiation, position the newborn's crib or incubator away from walls or windows that are part of the outside of the building in cold weather. These sources of heat loss are easily overlooked when the objects and air around the infant seem warm, but infants may lose heat to objects not in close contact with them. Keep this in mind when positioning cribs in mothers' rooms, which are often short of space. Place the crib between the beds (in a two-bed room) or near the head of the mother's bed and away from windows or doors. Avoid areas with drafts such as near the

NURSING CARE PLAN 21-1   The Normal Newborn

ASSESSMENT: Nicholas, a full-term newborn, was delivered after 18 hours of normal labor. He weighs 3402 g (7 lb, 8 oz) and is 50 cm (20 in) long. His mother, Vicki, is happy and excited about her first baby. Nicholas receives Apgar scores of 8 at 1 minute and 9 at 5 minutes. During the initial assessment, Nicholas has an excessive amount of mucus. His respiratory rate is 62, apical pulse is 164, and breath sounds are slightly moist. He has mild substernal retractions. His color is pink with acrocyanosis.

> **CRITICAL THINKING:** Should the nurse worry about Nicholas, based on the described assessment? What other signs would indicate a serious problem?
>
> **ANSWER:** The infant's condition is not unusual immediately after birth. The nurse should be concerned if Nicholas develops central cyanosis, flaring of the nares, grunting, severe retractions, or further increases in pulse and respiratory rate or if signs do not improve during the first 1 or 2 hours after birth.

NURSING DIAGNOSIS: Ineffective Airway Clearance related to excessive secretions in airways

GOALS/EXPECTED OUTCOMES:

1. Nicholas will maintain a patent airway and have no signs of respiratory distress throughout the birth facility stay as demonstrated by a respiratory rate of 30 to 60 breaths per minute, apical pulse 120 to 160, clear breath sounds, and no cyanosis, retractions, flaring, or grunting.
2. Before discharge, Vicki will demonstrate correct use of the bulb syringe and verbalize when it should be used.

INTERVENTION	RATIONALE
1. Place Nicholas in a side-lying position and observe for the amounts of secretions and any respiratory difficulty.	1. A side-lying position facilitates drainage of secretions from the airways.
2. Use a bulb syringe to suction the mouth, if necessary. If the nose also requires suctioning, suction it gently after suctioning the mouth.	2. Suctioning removes secretions. Suctioning the mouth first prevents aspiration of oral secretions should Nicholas gasp when his nose is suctioned. Suctioning the nose can be traumatic to nasal tissues.
3. Change the infant's position frequently.	3. Position changes promote expansion and drainage of all parts of the lungs.
4. Provide reassurance to Vicki.	4. Suctioning and other care may make the mother think that something is very wrong.
5. Demonstrate and explain use of the bulb syringe to Vicki. Assess her ability and make suggestions as needed during a return demonstration.	5. Demonstration and return demonstration ensure that parents learn correct techniques.
6. Continue to observe Nicholas for signs of respiratory distress. Count pulse and respirations every 30 minutes until they have been stable for 2 hours. Once they are stable, assess vital signs every 8 hours or according to birth facility procedure. Assess more often if there is any sign of abnormality. Observe for other signs of respiratory difficulty, such as cyanosis, retractions, flaring, and grunting.	6. Monitoring should be based on the presence of excessive secretions, ability to cope with mucus, other signs of respiratory difficulty, and changes in the infant's condition.

EVALUATION: Nicholas has clear breath sounds within 3 hours of birth, his apical pulse is 138 to 153, and his respiratory rate is 41 to 53. He has no signs of respiratory difficulty. Vicki uses the bulb syringe to suction Nicholas appropriately.

ASSESSMENT: Nicholas has an axillary temperature that ranges from 36.2° to 36.8° C (97.2° to 98.2° F). Vicki is eager to hold him and frequently unwraps him to admire him. When reminded about the need to keep Nicholas warm, she states, "It seems hot in here to me. Won't he be too warm with so many blankets?"

NURSING DIAGNOSIS: Risk for Ineffective Thermoregulation related to parental lack of knowledge of newborn thermoregulation abilities and needs

GOALS/EXPECTED OUTCOMES:

1. Nicholas will maintain a temperature within the normal range of 36.5° to 37.5° C (97.7° to 99.5° F) axillary throughout his birth facility stay.
2. Vicki will verbalize and practice methods of preventing heat loss by the end of the first day.

NURSING CARE PLAN 21-1 The Normal Newborn—cont'd

INTERVENTION	RATIONALE
1. Explain to Vicki why newborns have problems with thermoregulation.	1. When parents understand the reasons behind precautions they are more likely to practice them.
2. Teach Vicki to keep Nicholas wrapped as much as possible. Show her how to look at him and change his diaper while exposing only small areas of his body at a time.	2. Exposing the skin to the surrounding air increases heat loss by convection and radiation.
3. Teach Vicki to dry Nicholas promptly whenever he is wet, such as during bathing and when changing wet diapers or clothing.	3. Heat loss from evaporation occurs when the infant's skin is wet.
4. Instruct Vicki to keep the infant's crib away from cold walls, windows, or drafts from air conditioners and open doors or windows.	4. Heat loss by radiation and convection occurs from exposure to cold objects or air drafts.
5. Point out commonly used objects that may be cold when they touch Nicholas. Explain the effect of this contact, and suggest methods to warm them before use.	5. Heat can be gained or lost by conduction.
6. Assess the infant's axillary temperature every 30 minutes until it has been stable for 2 hours, or according to birth facility procedure. Report progress to Vicki.	6. Continued assessment shows response to interventions. Keeping the parents aware of the infant's progress involves them in his care.
7. Check the blood glucose if Nicholas becomes jittery or lethargic. If the blood glucose is low, help Vicki breastfeed or use formula if she prefers.	7. Nonshivering thermogenesis results in use of glycogen stores. Infants may show tremors or lethargy as a result of hypoglycemia. Feeding provides calories for heat production. Skin contact with the mother helps warm the infant by conduction.
8. Monitor for tachypnea or other signs of respiratory distress. Suction and apply oxygen if needed.	8. Nonshivering thermogenesis requires use of large amounts of oxygen, increases work of the respiratory system, and may lead to hypoxia.
9. If Nicholas is slow to warm, try placing him (wearing only a diaper) next to Vicki's skin.	9. Placing the infant "skin to skin" with the mother uses conduction to help warm the infant with the mother's body heat.
10. If his temperature is still low or if he has repeated episodes of low temperature, place him in a radiant warmer or an incubator. Alert the physician or nurse practitioner if the problem continues.	10. Radiant heat warms infants and can be adjusted according to their needs. Temperature instability is one sign of infection in newborns. The health care provider may order further tests for continued low temperature.
11. When Nicholas is ready to go into an open crib, warm his clothes before dressing him. Place two warmed blankets, wrapped separately, around him. After he is swaddled, place one or two blankets over him.	11. Warming clothing and blankets keeps Nicholas warm by conduction. Wrapping blankets separately traps air between layers, which acts as an insulating agent.
12. Apply a stockinette or insulated cap over the infant's head.	12. Covering the head decreases heat loss from this large surface area.
13. Remove extra blankets according to the infant's temperature.	13. Overheating increases oxygen and glucose consumption.
14. After transfer to an open crib, monitor the infant's temperature every 30 to 60 minutes until it remains stable.	14. Continued monitoring provides prompt identification of problems infants may have in adjusting to changes in environmental temperature.
15. Teach Vicki how to wrap Nicholas and to expose only small areas of the body at a time when bathing or diapering him. Also teach her how to take an axillary temperature at home.	15. Teaching increases parents' competence in infant care.

EVALUATION: The infant's axillary temperature at 3 hours after delivery is 37° C (98.6° F). Nicholas has no further problems with temperature instability during his birth facility stay. Vicki is conscientious in using correct measures to keep Nicholas warm.

hall door. Keep traffic low around radiant warmers because movement increases air currents.

When assessing or caring for newborns, avoid exposing more of their bodies than necessary. Remove clothing and blankets only from the areas being assessed. Keep the upper part of the body covered when changing diapers. Wrap newborns in blankets, and use a stockinette or insulated hat to prevent heat loss from the large surface area of the head.

RESTORING THERMOREGULATION

If an infant with a previously normal temperature develops a low temperature, institute nursing measures to assist thermoregulation immediately. If the axillary temperature is low, some nurses check the rectal temperature to determine core temperature. However, the process of nonshivering thermogenesis begins before the core temperature becomes abnormal. Core temperature changes indicate that the infant's thermoregulatory resources are exhausted. Nurses must intervene before this happens.

First look for obvious causes for the infant's low temperature. The infant may be unwrapped or wearing wet diapers or clothing. The mother's room may be cold, or the crib may be placed near the air conditioner. These causes can be corrected easily.

A slight drop in temperature may require only the addition of extra clothing. Put a shirt on the infant upside down by placing the legs in the sleeves for added warmth. Use two blankets, each wrapped separately around the infant, to increase insulation of heat by trapping air between the layers. Place another blanket over the infant in the crib and a hat on the infant's head. Heat linens in a warmer before use if added warmth is desired.

A greater drop in temperature requires additional measures. Place the infant under a radiant warmer for a short time. For an infant with a markedly decreased temperature, set the temperature control on the warmer slightly above the infant's temperature to warm the infant slowly. Gradually increase the temperature until the infant's temperature is within the normal range. Warming the infant too rapidly causes complications such as apnea.

PERFORMING EXPANDED ASSESSMENTS

Expanded assessments are necessary whenever temperature is decreased in a newborn. Assess the respiratory rate because nonshivering thermogenesis increases the need for oxygen. Observe for signs of respiratory distress brought on by the additional oxygen requirement.

Because the cold infant uses more glucose to produce heat, test the blood glucose level when the temperature is abnormal. A reading of 40 to 45 mg/dl or lower requires feeding, especially if the infant shows signs of hypoglycemia. Help the mother to breastfeed, or use warmed formula. Warm colostrum or formula and skin contact with the mother help warm the infant.

CRITICAL THINKING ✎ EXERCISE 21-1

You are caring for Nancy Belinsky, who gave birth to a full-term baby boy 6 hours ago. Both mother and baby have been doing well since Andy was born early this morning. As you enter the room after lunch, Nancy says, "Andy's hands and feet are so cold! I've heard that babies have cold hands and feet, but are they always so shaky, too?"

Questions
1. What are the nursing priorities in this situation?
2. What expanded assessments are necessary?
3. What interventions are necessary?
4. How will you respond to Nancy?

Infants who do not respond to these simple measures need additional treatment. Notify the physician or nurse practitioner and keep the infant in an incubator for close observation until the temperature stabilizes. Because low temperature may be a sign of infection, look for other signs that might indicate sepsis.

Evaluation

When a temperature within the normal range has been maintained for several hours, the infant can be considered stable in thermoregulation. Ongoing monitoring of thermoregulation continues throughout the birth facility stay.

✔ CHECK YOUR READING

1. Why are prophylactic medications given to all newborns?
2. How can nurses prevent heat loss in newborns?

Application of the Nursing Process
Hepatic Function

The major early assessments and care of the hepatic system are related to blood glucose levels and bilirubin conjugation.

BLOOD GLUCOSE

Assessment

Assess all infants for risk factors and signs of hypoglycemia (see Chapter 20, p. 488). Perform screening tests for blood glucose according to the signs exhibited and the agency's policy.

Analysis

For infants who have glucose levels below 40 to 45 mg/dl (or the value used by the agency policy), the collaborative problem "Potential Complication: Hypoglycemia" is appropriate.

Planning

Client-centered goals for hypoglycemia are not made because this problem requires collaboration between the nurse and the physician. Planning revolves around the nurse's role, including:
- Assessing for signs of hypoglycemia
- Notifying the physician about signs of hypoglycemia or following routine orders left by the physician for infants with hypoglycemia
- Intervening to minimize hypoglycemia

Interventions
MAINTAINING SAFE GLUCOSE LEVELS

A steady supply of fuel is needed by the brain to prevent permanent damage. To prevent this, follow agency policy and physician orders regarding feeding infants with low glucose levels. A common practice is to feed the newborn if the glucose screening shows a level of 40 to 45 mg/dl or less to prevent further depletion of glucose.

The infant may be fed a small amount of glucose water followed immediately by breast milk or formula. Glucose water alone is not recommended for newborns because the rapid rise in glucose results in increased insulin production, causing a further drop in blood glucose. Milk provides a longer-lasting supply of glucose because of the other nutrients included.

Assist the breastfeeding mother with the first feeding. If she is unable to nurse the infant immediately (because of pain or exhaustion from delivery), feed the infant formula and help her breastfeed at the next feeding. Help formula-feeding mothers with positioning the infant and the bottle.

REPEATING GLUCOSE TESTS

Until glucose levels are stable, closely observe newborns who have shown signs of hypoglycemia. The schedule for retesting varies from one agency to another. It is often performed 30 to 60 minutes after feeding and then before later feedings several times until results are normal. No further testing is performed unless new indications of hypoglycemia develop.

Keep the physician or nurse practitioner aware of the newborn's status. If the blood glucose does not remain at an adequate level, other causative factors are investigated. The infant may be transferred to a nursery for more intensive treatment, including intravenous feedings, until blood glucose is regulated with oral feedings.

PROVIDING OTHER CARE

Watch for signs of other complications. If infants do not have enough glucose, they may experience a drop in temperature that could lead to respiratory distress as oxygen is used for nonshivering thermogenesis. Explain the situation to parents. They will be distressed over the multiple heel sticks their infant must endure. Explain the importance of maintaining adequate blood glucose levels and why the tests and frequent feedings are necessary. Encourage parents to feed the newborn as instructed so that enough glucose is available to meet the infant's needs. Discuss the plans for blood testing and criteria for discontinuing it.

Evaluation

In evaluating collaborative interventions for hypoglycemia, note the infant's response to interventions and the presence or absence of continued signs of hypoglycemia. The blood glucose should remain above 40 to 45 mg/dl.

BILIRUBIN

Because elevated bilirubin levels are common in newborns, be alert to situations that require intervention. Infants who need treatment for hyperbilirubinemia are discussed in Chapter 30. Prevention, however, is an important aspect of care.

Assessment

Assess for jaundice by blanching the infant's skin on the nose or sternum. Determine how far down the body the jaundice extends. When serum bilirubin tests are ordered, compare the results with what is expected for the infant's age and previous results.

Analysis

Hyperbilirubinemia may not occur until after discharge, especially if discharge was early. A nursing diagnosis for this situation is "Risk for Injury related to lack of parental knowledge about hyperbilirubinemia."

Planning

The goals and outcomes for this diagnosis are:
- Parents will identify infants who develop jaundice or whose jaundice worsens when at home.
- Parents will identify methods for preventing or reducing jaundice when at home.

Interventions

During assessment and care of newborns, determine which infants are at increased risk for hyperbilirubinemia (see p. 490). By using extra vigilance in caring for infants at higher risk, nurses can detect jaundice earlier and take measures to decrease it.

Explain the significance of jaundice to parents and show them how to assess for color changes in the skin. Answer parents' questions about blood tests, phototherapy, and other care (see Nursing Care Plan 30-1).

Discuss the importance of adequate feedings to stimulate passage of stools and help prevent high levels of bilirubin in the infant. If a newborn is feeding poorly, determine the reasons and intervene appropriately. Help mothers wake sleepy infants to feed, encourage them to spend extra time with an infant with a poor suck, and explain the appropriate amount to give each feeding. Instruct breastfeeding mothers to nurse within 2 hours after birth and every 2 to 3 hours thereafter. Avoid giving water to jaundiced infants because water does not stimulate stool excretion.

Before discharge, instruct parents to contact their care provider if they see an increase in jaundice or if the infant is not eating every 3 to 4 hours, voiding at least six times daily by the fourth day, and producing at least one stool per day if formula feeding and at least three stools daily if breastfeeding.

Continue to check the infant for jaundice during early home or clinic visits. Use a device to measure transcutaneous bilirubin or end-tidal carbon monoxide to determine the degree of jaundice. Obtain laboratory specimens, according to agency policy, if jaundice is increasing. Reinforce teaching about identification of jaundice and importance of feedings and stooling. Answer questions that have occurred to parents since discharge from the birth facility.

If an infant develops true breast milk jaundice, explain it to the parents. The mother who must discontinue breastfeeding for a day or two will be concerned. Reassure her that her milk is adequate and not harmful to the infant. Help her maintain her milk supply by using a breast pump during the time the infant is taking formula.

Evaluation

With proper nursing observation and parent teaching, infants with hyperbilirubinemia are identified early to allow for appropriate treatment and prevention of injury. Parents are able to discuss signs, prevention, and management of jaundice at home.

✔ CHECK YOUR READING

3. What should the nurse do for infants with signs of hypoglycemia?
4. What are some interventions for preventing jaundice in newborns?

ONGOING ASSESSMENTS AND CARE

A complete assessment is necessary every 8 hours or according to birth facility policy, but the nurse should always watch for signs of change in the newborn's condition (see Appendix C for daily nursing activities for meeting newborn needs). Vital signs are assessed more often if they are abnormal. The infant is weighed once daily, and weight loss or gain is documented.

Providing Skin Care

The skin should be assessed for new marks or changes in old ones. Marks on the scalp may not be obvious if covered by abundant hair. To assess skin turgor, the nurse pinches a small area of skin over the chest or abdomen and notes how quickly it returns to its normal position. The return should be immediate in the normal newborn, with no "tenting." Skin that remains "tented" (raised in the pinched position) is an indication of dehydration.

Bathing

The infant receives a bath to remove blood, amniotic fluid, and excessive vernix as soon after birth as the temperature is stable. Removal of all vernix is unnecessary. The bath is given before the performance of any invasive procedures that might draw organisms on the skin into the infant's subcutaneous tissues or bloodstream. Early bathing decreases exposure to maternal blood and possible bloodborne organisms on the infant's skin, such as hepatitis B and human immunodeficiency virus (HIV). Gloves are worn during all contact with the infant until the bath is completed because of the blood on the infant's skin from birth. After the bath, gloves are necessary only when contact with body fluids or stools is likely. If latex gloves are used, early bathing also decreases exposure to the allergen latex in the gloves.

Studies have shown that infants with stable temperatures and no complications can be bathed within 1 hour of birth with no significant drop in temperature when compared with infants bathed 2 to 6 hours after birth (Behring,

Vezeau, & Fink, 2003; Varda & Behnke, 2000). The temperature at which infants are given the first bath varies according to agency policy. Giving the bath under the radiant warmer helps maintain the infant's temperature. The bath should be performed quickly and the infant thoroughly dried to prevent heat loss by evaporation. The bath may be given by the nurse or by a parent, either in the mother's room or a nursery.

While shampooing the hair the nurse combs through it to remove dried blood. After the bath the infant remains under the radiant warmer until the hair is dry and the temperature returns to the previous level. Combing the hair hastens drying. The infant is dressed and wrapped in two blankets, and a cap is placed on the infant's head before he or she is removed from the radiant warmer. The temperature should be rechecked within an hour to ensure the infant is maintaining thermoregulation adequately.

After the initial bath, the infant may not receive another full bath during the birth facility stay. The skin is cleansed, however, at diaper changes and to remove regurgitated milk. Clear water or a mild soap solution is used according to agency policy.

Parents are taught to give sponge baths until the cord is off and the circumcision is healed. Some authors, however, have found that tub baths for newborns do not increase infection or decrease cord healing and that infants maintain their temperatures better during tub bathing than during sponge bathing (Association of Women's Health, Obstetric and Neonatal Nurses [AWHONN] & National Association of Neonatal Nurses, 2001; Bryanton, Walsh, Barrett, & Gaudet, 2004). Infants should be immersed in enough water to cover the shoulders, and parents should be taught safety precautions. Water temperature should be warm enough (approximately 38° C [100.4° F]) to prevent temperature loss and promote comfort.

Bathing the infant in the presence of the parents allows the nurse to point out infant characteristics in addition to demonstrating the bath procedure. This may be helpful in promoting bonding in the parents (Amy, 2001). Infants receiving tub baths seem more contented and cry less during baths. Mothers of infants who are tub bathed often find the procedure pleasing (Bryanton et al., 2004).

Providing Cord Care

The cord should be checked for bleeding or oozing during the early hours after birth. The cord clamp must be securely fastened with no skin caught in it. Purulent drainage or redness or edema at the base indicates infection. The cord begins to dry shortly after birth. It becomes brownish black within 2 to 3 days and falls off within approximately 10 to 14 days.

Care of the cord varies among agencies. It may be treated with a bactericidal substance such as triple-dye solution, antibiotic ointment, or alcohol, cleaned with a mild soap solution, or allowed to dry naturally. Evidence-based practice guidelines show that none of the treatments commonly used is superior to keeping the cord clean and dry and cleaning with water if soiled. This natural treatment of cords may shorten the time to cord separation and does not lead to increased infections

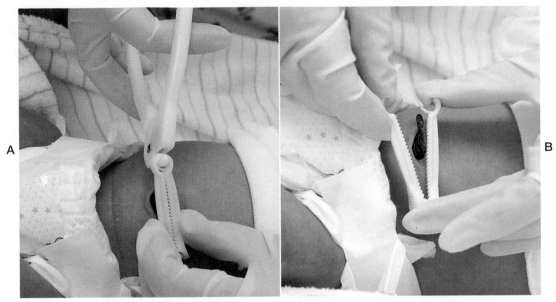

Figure 21-3 ■ The cord clamp is removed when the end of the cord is dry and crisp. The clamp is cut **(A)** and separated **(B)**.

(AWHONN, 2001; Zupan & Garner, 2003). However, it is not clear that all antimicrobial treatment should be discontinued. Although alcohol prolongs cord separation and does not decrease infection, triple dye has been shown to decrease infection. More research is needed on this subject (McConnell, et al., 2004).

Mothers often have concerns about care of the cord, especially in cases of odor or slight bleeding when the cord separates. Parents should be taught that these occurrences are not unusual but that redness at the base of the cord and discharge may indicate infection. If alcohol is used, parents are taught to clean the cord with alcohol at least three times a day until the cord falls off. All parents should be taught to fold the diaper below the cord to keep it dry and free from contamination by urine.

The cord clamp is removed about 24 hours after birth if the end of the cord is dry (Figure 21-3). The base of the cord is still moist, but no danger of bleeding exists if the end is dry and crisp. If the neonate is discharged before the cord is dry enough for the clamp to be removed, it may be tied. In some birth facilities the nurse removes the clamp during the home visit.

Cleansing the Diaper Area

Because contact with body fluids is likely, it is important to wear clean gloves while changing diapers. Meconium is very thick and sticky and can be difficult to remove from the skin. Plain water or mild soap solutions may be used for cleaning the diaper area. Petroleum jelly or baby oil is sometimes used to make cleaning meconium stools easier and to prevent skin irritation. Commercial diaper wipes should be avoided as they may affect skin pH (AWHONN and NANN, 2001).

Assisting with Feedings

The nurse must ensure the infant is eating well and that parents understand their chosen feeding method. This is particularly important for breastfeeding infants (Chapter 22). A

short period of observation at the start of feedings followed by another check during the feedings will help identify any problems that have developed. Assign a LATCH score for breastfeeding mothers and infants and look for changes in the score (see Chapter 22, p. 545).

Positioning the Infant

Parents need to understand how to position infants properly. Infants who are placed in the prone position for sleep have an increased risk for sudden infant death syndrome (SIDS) (see Chapter 23). The AAP recommends that mothers be taught to place infants on the back for sleep, as this position is associated with the lowest rate of SIDS. The side-lying position also reduces the risk, although not as much as the back-lying position (AAP & ACOG, 2002). Parents should also be taught to avoid loose or soft bedding that might interfere with breathing.

Protecting the Infant

Safeguarding the infant is a major role of the nurse. Important ways nurses protect newborns are by (1) ensuring that infants always go to the correct parents, (2) taking precautions to prevent infant abductions, and (3) preventing or recognizing early signs of infection.

IDENTIFYING THE INFANT

A method to identify newborns is instituted at birth to ensure that a mother is never given the wrong infant. This type of mistake could result in interference with bonding, exposure to infections, lack of confidence in the reliability of the staff, and lawsuits.

The most common method of identifying infants is the use of identification bands or bracelets. Two bracelets are placed on the infant, one on the mother, and one on the father or other support person. Information on each band is identical and includes the infant's sex, date and time of

21-3   Identifying Infants

PURPOSE: To ensure that each infant is always given to the correct mother

1. Always identify infants and mothers (or support persons) with identification (ID) bands when reuniting them, even after a brief separation. *This step ensures that infants are given to correct parents.*

2. When taking an infant into a mother's room, unwrap the blankets to expose the ID band on the infant's wrist or ankle. Do *not* rely on memory of the number. *This allows visualization of the band number.*

3. Explain the ID procedure and its purpose to the mother. Show her the imprinted ID number on her band and the matching number on the infant's bands. *This ensures the mother's understanding and cooperation.*

4. Look at the number on the infant's band and ask the mother to read off the ID number on her band. Do *not* re-verse the process by reading the infant's number to the mother. *If the numbers are read to a mother who does not understand, she might indicate that the numbers are correct when they are not.*

5. An alternative procedure is for the nurse to compare the mother's and the infant's bands visually. *If the mother does not speak English or might have difficulty with the process, the nurse can be certain that the infant is identified correctly.*

6. If the infant is to be released to a support person who is wearing an ID band, follow the same ID procedure. *This ensures that the infant is given to the correct support person.*

birth, delivering physician, mother's name, mother's hospital number, and a number imprinted on the plastic band. The imprinted number is used to identify the mother and the infant at any time the infant is brought to the mother after a period of separation, however brief (Procedure 21-3 and Figure 21-4). All staff must follow the facility protocol for identification of infants. In some facilities electronic sensors are used to match the mother's and infant's bands to each other.

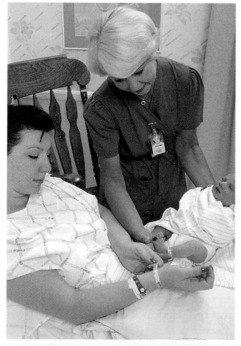

Figure 21-4 ■ The nurse unwraps the infant to compare the infant's identification band with the mother's band. The mother may be asked to read off the identification number on her band as the nurse checks the infant's band, or the nurse may look at both bands together.

Other methods to identify infants include taking footprints of the infant and a fingerprint of the mother or photographs of the infant. Birthmarks or other distinguishing features are carefully documented in the nurses' notes. Cord blood may be used for DNA analysis should there be a later need for identification.

PREVENTING INFANT ABDUCTION

An unfortunate but essential role of the nurse is protecting the infant from abduction (kidnapping). Between 1983 and 2002, 113 infants were abducted from health care facilities (Rabun, 2003). The majority of the abductions (56%) occurred in the mother's room. Abductions also have occurred from the nursery, from the pediatrics unit, and on the hospital grounds.

Newborns are usually abducted by women who are familiar with the birth facility and its routines. Abductors often live near the birth facility. They usually visit more than one agency several times to learn the routines so that they can impersonate birth facility staff to gain access to a newborn. They often know the layout of the facility and the locations of exits well.

The woman is often of childbearing age, overweight, and may want an infant to solidify her relationship with her husband or boyfriend. She may have had a previous pregnancy loss or may be unable to have a child of her own. Although the woman plans the kidnapping, she waits for an appropriate opportunity to take any infant available.

Many precautions are necessary to protect infants from abduction. These include teaching parents how to recognize picture identification badges worn by birth facility personnel. Parents should also be aware of any other identifying measures such as color-coded badges or uniforms for maternity staff. Written and verbal information, including a picture of special identification badges worn by staff, should be given to parents. Parents must be cautioned never to give their infant to anyone who does not have proper identification (Box 21-1).

BOX 21-1 Precautions to Prevent Infant Abductions

All personnel must wear identification that is easily visible at all times. No one without appropriate identification should handle or transport infants.

Enlist parents' help in preventing kidnapping. Teach them to allow only hospital staff with proper identification to take their infants from them.

Teach parents and staff to transport infants only in their cribs and never by carrying them. Question anyone carrying an infant outside the mother's room.

Question anyone with a newborn near an exit or in an unusual part of the facility.

Be suspicious of anyone who does not seem to be visiting a specific mother, asks detailed questions about nursery or discharge routines, asks to hold infants, or behaves in an unusual manner.

Be suspicious of unknown people carrying large bags or packages that could contain an infant.

Respond immediately when an alarm signals that a remote exit has been opened or an infant has been taken into an unauthorized area.

Never leave infants unattended. Teach parents that infants must be observed at all times. Suggest that mothers have the nursing staff take over care of the infant if the mother feels unwell or is napping and no family members are available to watch the infant.

Take infants to mothers one at a time. Never leave an infant in a crib in the hall while the nurse is in a room with another mother. Never leave an infant unsupervised.

When infants are left in mothers' rooms, position the crib away from the doorways, preferably on the side of the mother's bed opposite the door.

If entrances to the maternity unit or nurseries are equipped with locks that open to codes or card keys, protect them from others.

When a parent or family member comes to the nursery to take an infant, always match the infant and adult identification bracelet numbers. Never give an infant to anyone who does not have the correct identification bracelet or other proper identification.

Alert hospital security immediately when any suspicious activity occurs.

Suggest that parents do not place announcements in the paper or signs in their yard that might alert an abductor that a new baby is in the home.

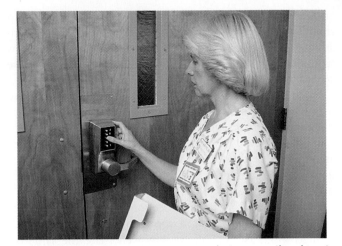

Figure 21-5 ■ The nurse uses a code to open the door to the nursery.

itors to maternity units may be checked in with security guards or other staff members and wear special visitor identification tags.

Remote exits are locked and often equipped with video cameras and alarms. Staff must respond quickly whenever an alarm sounds. Although alarms usually are triggered accidentally, it is always possible that a kidnapper is using a remote exit for a quick getaway.

The nurse should make parents a part of the abduction prevention effort without frightening them. They should be encouraged to feel free to ask for identification at any time and praised when they do. If they feel unsure about anyone asking to remove their baby, they should call the primary nurse or for assistance.

Infant abductions have taken place at parents' homes as well as in birth facilities. Parents should avoid public displays such as yard signs that might inform a kidnapper of the birth. Personal websites should not be easily accessible to the general public and should never include the infant's address.

Additional information about abduction is available for parents and professionals at the National Center for Missing & Exploited Children website, http://www.missingkids.com.

PREVENTING INFECTION

Because the newborn has a limited ability to respond to infection, prevention is of utmost importance throughout the birth facility stay and constitutes a major part of parent teaching.

Many nursing actions help prevent infection. At the beginning of their shift, nurses wash their hands and arms thoroughly, and, in some agencies, use a scrub brush. Throughout the day, handwashing is important before and after any infant is touched. It is essential not to handle one neonate and then another without again washing the hands. Otherwise an infection that develops in one infant could quickly spread to others.

A special disinfectant for cleansing the hands may be used in place of handwashing when the hands are not visibly soiled. Dispensers may be placed in each mother's room and at other locations throughout the unit.

Staff members who are working temporarily on the unit must have a special means of identification that is recognized by parents and other staff members. Temporary identification badges are assigned and monitored each shift so that none can be removed from the premises without alerting the staff.

In some agencies, electronic security systems are used. Although a variety of methods of protecting the infant are available, each makes use of a sensing device on the umbilical clamp or attached to the infant by a bracelet or tag. The sensor activates an alarm if it is near an exit or is cut or removed from the infant. With some systems, all exits lock automatically if an alarm is activated. When such security systems are used, it is essential that staff members are familiar with proper use of the systems. The systems are not designed to replace vigilance by both staff and parents in practicing other measures necessary to prevent abductions.

People entering and leaving maternity units should be observed at all times. Unit doors may be locked and visitors and staff required to knock, press a call signal, or use a card-key or a code on the lock to enter (Figure 21-5). Vis-

The nurse should instruct parents and visitors to wash their hands before touching infants. Parents should be instructed to discourage visitors with colds or other infections from coming in contact with the mother or newborn at the birth facility or during the early weeks at home.

Each infant's supplies should be kept separate from those used for other infants to avoid cross-contamination. Supplies in drawers or cupboards of the crib unit belonging to one infant should be used only for that infant because they are likely to be touched by the nurse while giving care. Using them for another neonate could result in the transfer of infectious organisms.

When the mother has an infection, the physician decides whether it is safe for the newborn to remain with her. Although mothers and infants may well share the same organisms, the infant of a mother who is acutely ill may need to stay in the nursery until the mother is no longer contagious and feels able to perform infant care.

Some birth facilities have a policy governing when separation of mother and newborn is necessary. Often the degree of the mother's fever is one of the determining factors. The separation of mother and infant should be as short as possible, of course, to promote attachment.

Nurses must be vigilant for signs of infection during assessment and care of the infant. These signs are often different from those in the older infant or child and may be subtle (see the discussion of signs of sepsis, p. 814). Instead of a fever, temperature may decrease. The infant may feed poorly or be lethargic. Periods of apnea sometimes occur without obvious cause. Any change in behavior that is unexplained should be recorded and investigated. The same holds true, of course, for the more obvious signs of infection such as drainage from the eyes, cord, or circumcision site.

✔ CHECK YOUR READING

5. How can the nurse prevent a parent from getting the wrong baby?
6. What can nurses and parents do to prevent infant abductions?
7. What is the most important method of preventing infection in newborns?

CIRCUMCISION

Circumcision is the most common surgical procedure of the neonate (Stoll & Kliegman, 2004). It is the removal of the prepuce (foreskin), a fold of skin that covers the glans penis. Although it can be retracted easily for cleaning in the older child, the prepuce usually is not fully retractable until age 3 or older. The prepuce should never be forcibly retracted in any infant because trauma and adhesions can result.

Circumcision is controversial and parents may have questions about whether to choose it for their son. Nurses can help them make an informed choice.

Reasons for Choosing Circumcision

The AAP and ACOG state that although there are potential benefits from the procedure, data are not sufficient to recommend routine neonatal circumcision (AAP & ACOG, 2002). Circumcision may reduce urinary tract infections, which occur in approximately 1% of uncircumcised infants. Cancer of the penis, which is very rare, some sexually transmitted infections, and inflammation of the glans or prepuce occur more frequently in uncircumcised males. However, other factors, such as poor hygiene and risk-taking behavior, are also important causes of these conditions.

Some parents choose circumcision for religious, cultural, or social reasons. Jewish parents may have their infants circumcised on the eighth day after birth as part of a special ceremony. Muslim culture also includes circumcision. Some parents want their son to look like his circumcised father or peers. Others feel circumcision is an expected part of newborn care and some do not realize that they have a choice in the matter.

Parents may be concerned that when the child is older he might develop phimosis, a tightening of the prepuce that prevents its retraction and necessitates circumcision. Although the number of such cases is small, surgery after the newborn period involves hospitalization and anesthesia and can be psychologically disturbing to the young child.

Lack of knowledge about the care of the prepuce leads to some circumcisions. Poor hygiene may increase the risk of infections and other problems. Teaching the parents and child the proper care of the uncircumcised penis can prevent surgery and complications related to inadequate cleanliness.

Reasons for Rejecting Circumcision

Reasons why parents decide against circumcision vary. Some believe that although a few conditions are seen more often in uncircumcised males, the incidence of those conditions is too low to warrant the pain and risk of surgery. Others believe that having the infant circumcised to look like the father or peers is cosmetic surgery and therefore unnecessary. These parents especially object to subjecting their sons to pain during and after the surgery. Circumcision is uncommon in many countries and less often practiced by families from Asian, Hispanic, and Native American cultures.

Parents may be concerned about removing the prepuce, which serves to protect the glans. When unprotected by the prepuce, the glans is more prone to irritation from constant exposure to urine and rubbing against diapers. Many believe that circumcision decreases sexual pleasure later in life because the glans becomes less sensitive.

Complications are unusual but most often include bleeding and infection. Other complications include recurrent phimosis, wound separation, unsatisfactory cosmetic result, urinary retention, meatitis, meatal stenosis, chordee, and inclusion cysts (AAP, 1999). Removal of too much or too little of the prepuce, stenosis or fistulas of the urethra, adhesions, necrosis, or other damage to the glans penis may also occur.

Only healthy newborns should undergo circumcision. The preterm or sick infant should not be circumcised until he is healthy enough to tolerate the procedure. Infants with blood dyscrasias may have excessive bleeding if circumcised. For the repair of anatomic abnormalities of the penis, such as hypospadias or epispadias, an intact prepuce may be needed for use in plastic surgery.

Pain Relief

Pain relief for circumcisions is an important consideration. At one time it was commonly believed that newborns do not feel pain, but it is now known that pain stimuli pass along myelinated pathways by the third trimester of pregnancy (Agarwal, Hagedorn, & Gardner, 2002). Newborns may actually be more sensitive to pain than older children and adults. During circumcision, newborns show changes in vital signs, oxygen saturation levels, and increased cortisol levels, indicating that they feel pain. Infants may show irritability, altered sleep-wake states, and abnormal feeding patterns for up to 22 hours after circumcision without pain medication (Agarwal et al., 2002). Local anesthesia is recommended by the AAP and ACOG (2002). In spite of this, some circumcisions are performed without anesthesia.

Injections of the dorsal penile nerves or as a ring block at the base of the penis with anesthetics such as lidocaine or bupivacaine without epinephrine are safe methods to eliminate pain during circumcision. Complications are uncommon but include hematomas, local skin necrosis, and absorption of the medication into the bloodstream. Eutectic mixture of local anesthetic (EMLA) is a cream that may be applied to anesthetize the skin before the procedure, but it is less effective than anesthetic injection and requires a longer waiting period before it is effective.

Acetaminophen may be given just before the procedure and throughout the first day for postprocedure pain. Infants are likely to show reduced pain responses after the procedure when acetaminophen is given before the circumcision is begun (Malnory, Johnson, & Kirby, 2003). Infants receiving acetaminophen before and after the procedure are more likely to be alert and responsive during postprocedure feedings and have improved mother-infant interaction during this time (Macke, 2001).

Nonpharmacologic pain relief methods include pacifiers, oral sucrose, soothing music, recordings of intrauterine sounds, decreased lights, and talking softly to the infant. All have shown some success in reducing an infant's pain responses to circumcision but are not as effective as anesthetics. They are especially helpful at decreasing the stress of the procedure when combined with regional anesthesia (Geyer et al., 2002). The AAP and ACOG recommend that acetaminophen or other nonpharmacologic methods of pain relief not be used alone but as adjuncts to analgesia during circumcision (AAP & ACOG, 2002).

Methods

The Gomco (Yellen) clamp (Figure 21-6) and the Plastibell (Figure 21-7) are two commonly used devices for performing circumcisions. In both methods the prepuce is first separated from the glans with a probe and incised to expose the

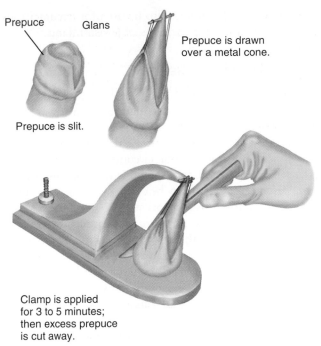

Figure 21-6 ■ Circumcision using the Gomco (Yellen) clamp. The physician pulls the prepuce over a cone-shaped device that rests against the glans. A clamp is placed around the cone and prepuce and is tightened to provide enough pressure to crush the blood vessels. This prevents bleeding when the prepuce is removed after 3 to 5 minutes.

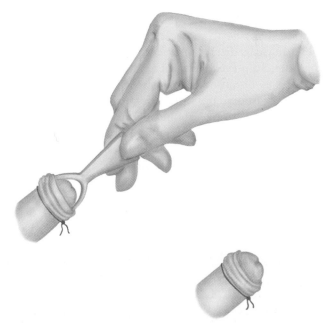

Figure 21-7 ■ Circumcision using the Plastibell. The physician places the Plastibell, a plastic ring, over the glans, draws the prepuce over it, and ties a suture around the prepuce and Plastibell. This prevents bleeding when the excess prepuce is removed. The handle is removed, leaving only the ring in place over the glans. The Plastibell ring falls off in 5 to 8 days.

glans. A Mogan clamp may also be used for circumcisions, especially for ritual circumcisions of Jewish infants.

Nursing Considerations

ASSISTING IN DECISION MAKING

Ideally parents decide about circumcision early in pregnancy on the basis of careful consideration of the risks and benefits. However, this is not always the case. Some parents are not well informed about circumcision. Although the physician is responsible for explaining the risks and benefits to the parents, the nurse may be called on to answer parents' questions or clarify misconceptions.

Although nurses generally teach parents of circumcised infants how to care for the penis, they may not think about providing teaching for parents who decide against circumcision. Proper care of the intact penis should be included in the teaching plan for these parents and should be discussed with parents who are undecided about the procedure as well.

Nurses must be certain that their own biases about circumcision do not interfere with their ability to give objective information to parents. Once the parents come to a decision, the nurse should support it.

PROVIDING CARE DURING CIRCUMCISION

As with any surgical procedure, informed consent is necessary from the parents before a circumcision is performed. The nurse sees that the consent has been signed and informs the physician of any problems that might impair the infant's ability to withstand circumcision. It is especially important to check that the infant has received vitamin K to prevent excessive bleeding. The infant should be stable and at least 12 hours old so he has recovered from the stress of birth.

The nurse gathers equipment and supplies before the procedure. To prevent regurgitation, feedings may be withheld for 2 to 4 hours before the procedure. Because he is restrained in a supine position, regurgitation may cause aspiration. A bulb syringe should be placed nearby in case suction is necessary.

When the physician and equipment are ready, the infant is placed on a circumcision board. This plastic holder is molded to fit the infant's body and has restraints for his arms and legs (Figure 21-8). A blanket is placed under the infant and only the diaper is removed. A drape provides

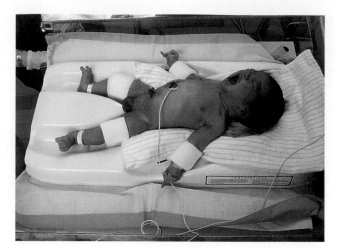

Figure 21-8 ■ The infant is placed on the circumcision board just before the procedure is begun.

warmth and maintains sterility. A heat lamp or radiant warmer helps prevent cold stress.

The nurse should comfort the infant during the procedure. A pacifier, sucrose, talking to the infant, or playing soft music or recordings of intrauterine sounds may help distract the infant from pain.

EVALUATING PAIN

Nurses should evaluate the infant's pain with one of the pain scales available for use with newborns. A commonly used scale is the Neonatal Inventory Pain Scale (NIPS) (Lawrence et al., 1993). This scale measures facial expression, cry, breathing pattern, muscle tone of the extremities, and state of arousal. The infant's pain responses should be measured before, during, and after the procedure.

PROVIDING POSTPROCEDURE CARE

The infant should be removed from the restraints immediately after the circumcision is completed. If a Gomco clamp was used, the nurse uses petroleum gauze strips or squeezes petroleum jelly or antibiotic ointment on the circumcision site to prevent the diaper from sticking to it. A small piece of gauze may be placed over the area. Petroleum jelly should not be used with a Plastibell because it may cause the ring to slip off or be displaced. The diaper is replaced loosely to prevent pressure. The infant should be comforted and returned to his mother, who may be anxious about her son.

PARENTS
WANT TO KNOW   Caring for the Uncircumcised Penis

Wash your son's penis daily and when soiled diapers are changed. Retracting the foreskin is not necessary because it is still attached to the glans, or end of the penis. It will gradually separate from the glans, but it may take 3 or more years for complete separation to occur.

Occasionally, you can gently pull back on the foreskin to see how much separation has occurred. However, *never* force the foreskin to retract. This is painful and may cause bleeding, infections, and adhesions.

As your son gets older and takes over his own care, teach him to wash under the foreskin by gently pulling it back only as far as it retracts easily. This should become a part of his daily bath.

How to Care for the Circumcision Site

Observe the circumcision site at each diaper change. Note the amount of bleeding. Call the physician if more than a few drops of blood are noted during diaper changes the first day or if any bleeding occurs thereafter.

Continue to apply petroleum jelly to the penis with each diaper change for the first 24 hours. If a Plastibell was used, petroleum jelly should not be applied because of possible displacement of the ring.

Keeping the circumcision site clean is important for healing. Squeeze warm water from a clean washcloth over the penis to wash it. Fasten the diaper loosely to prevent rubbing or pressure on the incision site.

Expect a yellow crust to form over the circumcision site. This is a normal part of healing and should not be removed. If a Plastibell was used, the plastic rim will fall off in 5 to 8 days. If it does not fall off by that time, notify your physician. Watch for signs of infection, such as fever or drainage accompanied by a bad odor or pus. *Call your physician if you suspect any abnormalities.* Also call the physician immediately if the plastic rim moves onto the penis. The circumcision site should be fully healed in approximately 10 days.

CRITICAL TO REMEMBER

Signs of Complications after Circumcision

Bleeding more than a few drops with first diaper changes
Failure to urinate
Signs of infection: fever or low temperature, purulent or foul-smelling drainage
Displacement of the Plastibell

The nurse watches carefully for signs of complications after the circumcision. The wound is checked frequently for bleeding during the first few hours after the procedure. If the infant is to be discharged after the circumcision, he should be observed for 1 to 2 hours before release.

If excessive bleeding occurs, pressure is applied to the site. The nurse notifies the physician, who may apply Gelfoam or epinephrine or may suture the small blood vessels. A small amount of blood loss may be significant in an infant, who has a small total blood volume.

Noting the first urination after circumcision is important because edema could cause an obstruction. If the infant goes home before voiding, the mother is instructed to call the physician if the baby does not urinate within 6 to 8 hours.

TEACHING PARENTS

Because circumcision is often performed on the day of discharge, the parents take over care of the site. Each time the site is checked for bleeding, the nurse should show the parents the amount of blood on the diaper to help them understand how much to expect. The normal yellowish exudate that forms over the site should be described and differentiated from purulent drainage. Signs of complications should be discussed fully.

✔ **CHECK YOUR READING**

8. What are the reasons parents decide for or against circumcision?
9. What information do parents need about care of the intact and circumcised penis?

Application of the Nursing Process
Parents' Knowledge of Newborn Care

New mothers often feel unprepared, physically and emotionally, to take over total care of their newborn and themselves. Mothers dealing with exhaustion and physiologic changes from childbirth may have difficulty remembering all the information they are given about care of themselves and their infants. Therefore finding creative teaching methods is especially important. The nurse must use every contact with the parents as an opportunity for further teaching.

Assessment

Assess parents' changing learning needs throughout the birth facility stay. Consider the mother's and infant's physical conditions and any special concerns that the mother may have.

Determine learning needs of experienced mothers. They may be unaware of information that has changed since the birth of the last infant. For example, mothers who have always placed their infants in the prone position for sleep need to know that the supine position is recommended for sleep. They may be unaware of the need for hepatitis B immunization for all infants. Differences in physical requirements or temperament between siblings may cause concern. Parents may need information about helping other children adjust to the newborn.

Assess the father's learning needs and his plans for involvement with infant care. Determine if there are cultural dictates about the father's participation in infant care. In some cultures, the father participates little in the care of the young infant. He may become more involved as the child

---

CRITICAL THINKING ✐ EXERCISE 21-2

A grandmother tells you, "I always put my babies on their tummies to sleep and they did just fine. Some babies get a flat head because they sleep on their back. I don't want that to happen to my grandson." How do you answer her?

gets older. In other families, fathers actively participate in child care, even during the birth facility stay. They often have many questions and are eager to learn about care of their infant.

Analysis

An appropriate nursing diagnosis for the family with learning needs is "Health-Seeking Behavior related to the desire for information about infant care." See Box 21-2 for other nursing diagnoses commonly used for newborns.

Planning

The primary goals and expected outcomes for this diagnosis are that before discharge the parents will:

- Identify their own information needs and seek assistance from nurses to meet those needs
- Correctly demonstrate infant care
- Express confidence in their ability to meet their infant's needs

Interventions

DETERMINING WHO TEACHES

Several different nurses will care for the mother and infant during the time they are in the birth facility. Coordinate the teaching so that all concerns are met. Many facilities use a checklist of major teaching topics to ensure that all important areas are covered (Box 21-3).

BOX 21-2 Common Nursing Diagnoses for Newborns

Family Coping: Potential for Growth
Health-Seeking Behaviors*
Risk for Impaired Parent-Infant Attachment
Risk for Impaired Parenting
Ineffective Airway Clearance*
Risk for Ineffective Thermoregulation*
Risk for Infection
Risk for Injury*

*Nursing diagnoses that are explored in this chapter.

BOX 21-3 Major Teaching Topics

Newborn characteristics and behavior
Use of bulb syringe
Breastfeeding
    Frequency, length, positioning, latch on, supply and demand, supplementing, potential problems
Formula feeding
    Frequency, amount, positioning, avoiding propping, formula preparation
Burping
Cord care
Care of the penis, uncircumcised or circumcised
Holding and positioning
Sleep patterns
Elimination patterns
Bathing and skin care
Clothing
Signs of problems
Taking a temperature
Infant safety
Car seat use

SETTING PRIORITIES

Because of the short time available for teaching, set priorities in determining what to teach. After assessing the parents' learning needs, make a teaching plan with them. Use a topic list to help them point out major concerns regarding infant care to ensure that precious teaching time is spent most effectively. Begin by discussing their most pressing concerns. This enhances further learning by decreasing their anxiety so that they can concentrate on the information. Then, as time allows, proceed to other subjects.

VARYING TEACHING METHODS

Use a variety of teaching methods to increase effectiveness, make the subject more interesting, and increase retention of the material. Use verbal and written methods and demonstrations. Ask the parents to return each demonstration of care skills. Parents often learn best from seeing skills performed correctly and then practicing them while the nurse gives suggestions and makes corrections as needed. Explain the rational for each point made during teaching sessions to increase the likelihood that parents will follow the nurse's instructions.

Discuss information with the mother alone or with her family members, roommate, or a group of mothers. Some women learn better with one-on-one teaching, whereas others benefit from watching and listening to others. Group teaching allows nurses to make more efficient use of time.

Use audiovisual materials, including pamphlets, baby magazines, compact disks (CDs) or videos, and television programs. Highlight the most important areas in written material, watch the programs with the new mother, and clarify information as necessary. This helps reinforce the learning.

Many parents use the Internet to obtain information about child care. Suggest that they look for websites that are accurate, current, and provided by well-known organizations such as health care providers, consumer advocacy groups, or university medical schools. Warn them to be wary of sites with unclear sources of the information or information that seems contrary to generally accepted knowledge. Suggest that they confirm information with their health care provider if they are unsure about it. Commend parents for their interest in obtaining information to increase their parenting skills.

MODELING BEHAVIOR

Modeling by the nurse is an important teaching tool. Mothers watch closely when nurses handle infants. The nurse demonstrates mothering behavior by the way the infant is held and care is given and by talking to the infant. Modeling is particularly important for the mother with no experience in infant care.

Use every opportunity during general care of the infant to point out infant characteristics and behavior states and to model how to calm crying infants. Teach mothers to use progressive consoling interventions such as talking to the infant, touching or folding the infant's arms across the chest, holding, swaddling, and facilitating sucking of the infant's

Techniques for Infant Care

This guide is written in language that the nurse might use when teaching parents about infant care. Adapt the subjects to meet the needs of individual parents.

HANDLING THE INFANT
Head Support

An infant's head is the heaviest part of the body and makes up one fourth of the total body length. Infants are unable to support the head when held in an upright position. You must place your hand behind the infant's head during carrying and positioning. After the first few months of life, babies' muscles become strong enough to support their head.

Positions

Most mothers hold the infant in the cradle position. In the "football" position, support the baby's head in the palm of your hand with the body held along the arm and supported against your side (see Figure 22-4). This position allows one hand to be free when washing the baby's hair or breast-feeding.

The shoulder hold is good for burping the baby. Or sit the baby on your lap and support the head and chest with one hand while gently patting or rubbing the infant's back with the other hand. This allows you to see the baby's face in case of spit-ups.

Always place your baby on the back for sleep, unless your baby's care provider tells you otherwise. This position is recommended by the American Academy of Pediatrics for all infants. It helps prevent sudden infant death syndrome (SIDS), the sudden unexplained death of an infant. The baby should sleep on a firm mattress to avoid suffocation.

Wrapping

Young infants seem more secure when wrapped firmly in a blanket (swaddled), which may feel like the small space of the uterus. Fussy babies often respond well to swaddling. To swaddle the infant, turn down one corner of a blanket and position the baby's head over the edge. Fold one side of the blanket over the body and arm. Bring the lower corner up and fold it over the chest. Then bring the other side around the infant and tuck it underneath snugly.

NORMAL BODY PROCESSES
Breathing

Newborns normally breathe about 30 to 60 times a minute. Their breathing is irregular and may vary from loud to very soft. Sometimes breathing is so quiet that mothers wake babies to be sure that they actually are breathing. Sneezing is normal and not likely to be from a cold unless there are other signs.

Using a Bulb Syringe

Use the bulb syringe if the infant has excessive mucus in the mouth or nose or spits up milk. Be very gentle and use the syringe only if necessary. Squeeze the bulb before you gently insert it into the mouth and aim it to the side of the mouth rather than to the back. Extra mucus is common in the first days of life but is usually not a problem thereafter unless a cold develops. Clean the bulb as necessary with soap and water. Rinse and dry well before using again. Call your physician if the baby's skin becomes blue or the baby stops breathing for more than 15 seconds, has difficulty breathing, or has yellow or green drainage from the nose.

Regulating Temperature

Newborns have difficulty regulating their temperature. If they become cold, they need more calories and more oxygen than when they are warm. A drop in body temperature can be dangerous. Dress your baby as you would like to be dressed. Add a light receiving blanket over the young infant, except in very hot weather.

Using a Thermometer

Check your baby's temperature during illness. Take the temperature under the infant's arm to prevent injury to the rectum. Place the thermometer in the pit of the arm so that the bulb does not stick out the other side of the arm. Hold the arm firmly over the thermometer and read it according to the manufacturer's directions. A digital thermometer is easy to read and takes little time. Call your physician if the baby has a temperature higher than 100° F (37.8° C) or lower than 97.7° F (36.5° C).

Urine Output

Your baby will have at least one or two wet diapers a day during the first day or two and at least six wet diapers a day by the fourth day. Counting the number of wet diapers helps you know if the baby is getting enough milk. *Call your baby's doctor if the baby has no wet diapers for more than 12 hours.*

Stool Output

Breastfed infants pass at least three soft, seedy stools that have a sweet-sour odor and are mustard yellow. Formula-fed infants pass one to several stools each day that are pale yellow to light brown and formed. Babies may appear constipated when they turn red and seem to strain when passing a stool. However, constipated stools are dry with small, hard pieces like marbles. If the movement is soft, you do not need to worry if the baby seems to strain.

Diarrhea

Babies with diarrhea pass an increased number of stools. Because the contents move through the intestines more quickly than normal, diarrhea stools are greener in color and more liquid than usual stools. You may see a water ring, an area in the diaper where the watery stool has been absorbed, sometimes around an area of more solid stool. Call your physician for further instructions if the infant passes more than two diarrhea stools because infants become dehydrated quickly when diarrhea occurs.

Skin Care

A number of normal marks occur on the newborn's skin. A normal newborn rash called *erythema toxicum* resembles small insect bites or pimples. Small whiteheads called *milia* are normal and disappear without treatment. Do not squeeze them or they may become infected and last longer.

Newborns have dry, peeling skin because they were surrounded by water for 9 months and the outer layers of the skin were not shed. After peeling, the baby has soft skin. Lotions or creams are unnecessary and may cause irritation.

Cord

If you have been instructed to let the cord dry naturally, do not put anything on it. Clean it with water alone or with a

Continued

mild soap if it becomes soiled, and keep it dry. Follow the directions of your health care provider regarding use of other substances, such as alcohol, on the cord. Notify your physician if you see bleeding or signs of infection, such as redness, drainage, or a foul odor.

Keep the cord dry by folding the diaper below it so that it is not wet by urine. The cord generally falls off in about 10 to 14 days. It may bleed a few drops when it detaches. Some care providers instruct parents to avoid giving their infant tub baths until the cord is off and the area is well healed, but others allow tub baths. Check with your health care provider.

Diaper Area

Clean the diaper area with each diaper change. For girls, separate the labia (folds) and remove all stool. For boys, wash under the scrotum to help prevent rashes. If the diaper area becomes red, use absorbent diapers, change the diaper more often, and avoid commercial diaper wipes. Leaving the diaper off to expose the area to air is also helpful. If an ointment is needed, petroleum jelly or a barrier-type zinc oxide ointment may be used. If redness persists, ask your baby's doctor for suggestions.

Bathing

Check with your physician regarding tub baths or sponge baths before the cord and circumcision are healed. Because infants are washed as needed after they spit up and with diaper changes, baths are not necessary every day. Fathers often enjoy giving the infant a bath and make this their special time with the baby.

Sponge Baths

Before the bath, gather all the supplies: a container or sink for the warm water, washcloth, towel, baby shampoo, alcohol, cotton or cotton-tipped swabs, and clean clothes. Soap is not necessary for the young infant, but if used, it should be gentle and nonalkaline to protect the natural acids of the infant's skin.

Give the bath in a room that is warm and free of drafts. Bathe the baby on a surface that is safe for the baby and at a comfortable height for you. If you use a counter, pad it with blankets or towels.

Never leave the infant alone on an unprotected surface, even for a minute. Keep one hand on the infant at all times to prevent falls. Taking the phone off the hook during the bath prevents distractions. If you must leave the room, take the baby along or place the baby in the crib.

Before fully undressing the baby use the football position to shampoo the baby's head. Although the fontanel or "soft spot" may seem delicate, it is covered with a tough membrane and is not injured by washing. Pulse movements in the fontanel are normal. Dry the hair well to prevent heat loss.

Keep the baby warm by uncovering only the area you are washing. To prevent chilling, wash and dry one part of the baby's body at a time. Start by washing the face with clear water. Use a separate clean area of the washcloth to wipe each eye. Use a washcloth to clean in and around the ears, where milk may accumulate. Do not use cotton-tipped swabs in the infant's ears or nose, as injury may occur if the baby moves suddenly.

To clean the neck folds, put one hand under the baby's shoulders and lift slightly to cause the head to drop back enough that the creases in the neck can be washed. Clean the diaper area last, using the principle of "clean to least clean." For baby girls, wipe the diaper area from front to back. Wiping back and forth may move stool into the vagina or urethra and cause an infection.

Tub Bath

For a tub bath, use a small plastic tub or a clean sink. Pad the bottom with a towel or foam pad to make it more comfortable and prevent the infant from slipping. Place enough warm water in the tub to cover the baby's shoulders as you hold her or him. Wash the face and hair before placing the baby in the tub. Keeping the baby dressed until after the hair is washed helps prevent chilling.

It may be easier, at first, to lather your hands with soap and water and then lather the infant's body. Immerse the baby in the tub for rinsing. Infants may be frightened when they are first put into the water. To help the baby adjust to this new experience, talk softly and calmly while holding the baby securely.

FEEDING

See Chapter 22 for information on breastfeeding and formula feeding.

BEHAVIOR

Knowing infants' different behavioral states helps you learn about your baby's individual characteristics.

Sleep Phases

During quiet sleep the infant sleeps soundly with quiet breathing and little movement. Your baby will not be disturbed by noises from appliances or other children at this time. In active sleep the baby moves or fusses while still asleep. If your baby sleeps in your room, you may have difficulty sleeping because of the baby's noises and movements. During the drowsy state, the baby is beginning to wake but may go back to sleep if not disturbed. However, if it is time for feeding or other activities, talk softly to help the baby awaken.

Awake Phases

The quiet alert state is the one that parents enjoy most because the infant seems so intent on studying objects and people nearby. This is a good time for infant stimulation and "play time." The quiet alert state lasts only a short time, and infants often need a break from interaction. You can see this if the infant turns the head away, begins to cough, sneeze, hiccough, or spit up, or becomes fussy. These signs show overstimulation. Giving infants a quiet period may allow them to return to the quiet alert state for a short time.

Parents soon learn to recognize the active alert or "fussy" phase in their infant. The infant may be signaling hunger, discomfort, or fatigue. With intervention the baby may move back to the quiet alert state or feed well and then go to sleep. If you do not intervene, the baby soon moves to the crying state.

The baby may use self-consoling measures such as sucking on a hand. However, if these efforts are not effective, parents should comfort the infant quickly. Babies who cry too long may not respond at first to care activities. A few minutes of rocking and holding close may be necessary before the infant settles down.

Socialization

Infants are social beings who enjoy contact with people. They hear voices in the uterus and respond with interest when their parents talk to them after birth. The baby should be part of family life. Use an infant seat or carrier to keep the baby near you and the rest of the family. Infants enjoy watching the human face. Hold your baby close and talk to your baby to provide social stimulation.

Stimulation

- Sounds—Play music of different types to provide auditory stimulation. Infants prefer music that is not too loud.

Music boxes, compact disks (CDs), or a radio can provide a variety of sound.
- Sights—Because babies focus their eyes best at a distance of 7 to 12 inches, items such as mobiles should be placed within this range. Infants especially like black and white geometric figures. They enjoy bright colors early but are not particularly interested in pastels.
- Variety—Place the baby in an infant seat in the kitchen while you prepare meals to stimulate the senses of sight, hearing, and smell. An infant carrier pack provides the stimulation of motion as well.
- Timing—Stimulation is best used during the baby's quiet alert state. Do not try to use stimulation techniques with a fussy infant because it can cause overstimulation. This causes the baby to be irritable and have difficulty going to sleep.

hands or a pacifier. Point out the different behavior states and how to help infants move to a more awake state for feeding. Instruct parents to intervene before infants reach the point of frantic crying.

TEACHING INTERMITTENTLY

Plan teaching in small segments that are interspersed with infant care. Check the parents' understanding frequently. Encourage them to take over various tasks until they are performing all of the infant's routine care.

INCLUDING THE FATHER

Identify fathers who would like to participate in care of their infants but hesitate because of lack of experience. Offer them the same teaching given the inexperienced mother. Give praise liberally to increase confidence and skill when parents practice their new infant care skills.

DOCUMENTING TEACHING

Document all teaching performed and the parent's abilities to carry out infant care. This information shows other nurses what teaching has been completed and what is still needed. It also provides legal proof that teaching was completed before discharge.

PROVIDING FOR FOLLOW-UP CARE

If the mother and infant will be seen by a home or clinic nurse, provide information about unmet learning needs. Reinforcement can then be provided at a time when the mother's memory has improved after the stress of birth.

Provide as much information as possible in written form so that parents can refer to it if they have concerns. Also provide telephone numbers they can call for further help. Offer written information in the parents' primary language, if possible. Even if they speak English as a second language, they may prefer to read in their native language.

Remind parents about timing of follow-up care. Suggest that they call early for an appointment so that the infant can receive care on time.

INCORPORATING CULTURAL CONSIDERATIONS

Take the family's cultural beliefs about child care into consideration when teaching. For example, some Southeast Asian, Hispanic, and Arab women believe colostrum is bad for the baby and wait to begin breastfeeding until the milk comes in when they are home. Asian parents may be uneasy when caregivers are too complimentary about the baby because praise may call attention of the gods to the vulnerable infant (Mattson, 2004). Some Southeast Asians believe the spirit resides in the head and are troubled if someone pats or rubs the head of the newborn. Hmong parents believe that touching the head repeatedly will prevent closure of the fontanels (Moore & Moos, 2003).

However, Hispanic parents may prefer that a person who compliments the infant touch the infant's face or head. Touching the head wards off *mal ojo* or the "evil eye," a sudden unexplained illness that may occur when others admire the infant. The "evil eye" or *najar* is also of concern to women from India who place a black dot on the newborn's forehead to ward it off.

Care of the cord varies in different cultures. Hispanic, Filipino, and black mothers may use a "belly band" or binder over the cord to protect the area or to prevent an umbilical hernia (Mattson, 2004).

Ask the parents who will be helping them care for the baby to determine family members who should be included in the teaching. This varies according to the culture and availability of the traditional caregiver. In addition to the father of the infant, the woman's mother is often the major support person. However, in the Korean culture the husband's mother is the primary caregiver for the infant and the mother in the early weeks to allow the mother to recover from the birth.

If the mother will not be the primary infant caregiver, she may appear uninterested in the nurse's teachings. Nurses must not assume she is not bonding with her infant because she is following the role prescribed by her culture. Sometimes a woman with other children appears to lack knowledge as she tries to assume care of her infant in the birth facility. This lack of knowledge may occur because past care-givers are no longer available and the mother will have to take over infant care herself. These mothers will need more help than is usually given experienced mothers.

Elicit questions during the discussions. However, be aware that women from some cultures will not ask questions. For many Native Americans, asking questions is considered rude (Cesario, 2001). Other women may be too shy or uneasy about their limited English. When questions are not asked, discuss topics that other parents often ask about.

Evaluation

Ongoing evaluation of parents' learning is necessary throughout the birth facility stay and during the follow-up home, clinic, or office visits. Determine whether they feel their questions have been answered and they can demonstrate important aspects of infant care safely and correctly. As they learn more caregiving skills, their confidence should increase as well.

IMMUNIZATION

Hepatitis B is a growing problem in the United States. Immunization for this disease is now included with other routine childhood vaccinations. Infants of mothers with acute or chronic hepatitis B infection (hepatitis B surface antigen [HBsAg] positive) may become infected from exposure to the mother's blood at birth. Infected infants have a 90% chance of becoming chronically infected and a 25% chance of mortality from chronic liver disease during adulthood (Jones, 2002). However, vaccination prevents infection in 95% of exposed infants (AAP & ACOG, 2002).

These infants should receive both the vaccine and hepatitis B immune globulin (HBIG). The immune globulin provides passive immunity to hepatitis to protect infants until they develop their own antibodies and should be given within 12 hours of birth. The vaccine promotes antibody formation to protect infants from further exposure to the disease. (See Drug Guides.)

DRUG GUIDE

HEPATITIS B VACCINE

Classification: Vaccine.

Other Names: Engerix-B, Recombivax HB.

Action: Immunization against hepatitis B infection.

Indications: Prevention of hepatitis B in exposed and unexposed infants.

Neonatal Dosage and Route:
- Recombivax HB: 5 mcg to infant of an infected mother, 2.5 mcg if mother is not infected
- Engerix-B: 10 mcg (whether or not the mother is infected)
   For infants of HBsAg-negative mothers the first dose of vaccine is given by 2 months. The second dose is given at least 4 weeks after the first dose. The third dose is given at least 16 weeks after the first dose and at least 8 weeks after the second dose but not before the infant is 24 weeks old.
   For infants of HBsAg-positive mothers the vaccine is given within 12 hours of birth and at 1 to 2 months and 6 months. Hepatitis B immune globulin (HBIG) is also given within 12 hours of birth at a different site than the vaccine.

The second dose of vaccine is given at age 1 to 2 months, and the last dose is not given before 24 weeks of age.
   If the mother's HBsAg status is unknown, the infant receives the vaccine within 12 hours of birth and the mother is tested. If the HBsAg test is positive, the infant should receive HBIG as soon as possible and no later than 1 week of age. The second dose of vaccine is given at age 1 to 2 months, and the last dose not before 24 weeks of age.
   Give intramuscularly in the anterolateral thigh.

Absorption: Absorbed slowly; not affected by maternal antibodies.

Contraindications: Hypersensitivity to yeast.

Adverse Reactions: Pain or redness at site, fever.

Nursing Considerations: If a vial is used, shake the solution well before preparing. Give vaccine within 12 hours of birth to infants of infected mothers. Do not inject intravenously or intradermally. Bathe infants before the injection to prevent contamination of the injection site with maternal blood on the infant's skin. Obtain parental consent before administering.

DRUG GUIDE

HEPATITIS B IMMUNE GLOBULIN (HBIG)

Classification: Immune globulin.

Other Names: BayHep B, Nabi-HB.

Action: Provides antibodies and passive immunity to hepatitis B.

Indications: Prophylaxis for infants of hepatitis B surface antigen–positive mothers.

Neonatal Dosage and Route: 0.5 ml within 12 hours of birth intramuscularly in the anterolateral thigh; should not be given intravenously.

Absorption: Absorbed slowly.

Contraindications: None known.

Adverse Reactions: Pain and tenderness at the site, urticaria, anaphylaxis.

Nursing Considerations: Do not shake or give intravenously. Bathe infants before the injection to remove blood and prevent contamination of the injection site with maternal blood on the infant's skin. Hepatitis vaccine series should begin within 12 hours of birth. Give injections of vaccine and immune globulin at separate sites.

NEWBORN SCREENING TESTS

Two types of screening tests required in many states are hearing screening and blood tests performed for certain inborn errors of metabolism or other genetic disorders. These tests are performed before discharge from the birth facility.

Hearing Screening

The incidence of hearing loss in infants is estimated to be approximately 1 per 1000 well newborns and 2% to 4% of those with complications requiring intensive care (AAP & ACOG, 2002). Because detection before the age of 3 months greatly improves outcomes, auditory screening of all newborns is recommended by the AAP. A goal of *Healthy People 2010* is to increase the proportion of newborns who are screened for hearing loss by age 1 month, have audiologic evaluation by age 3 months, and are enrolled in appropriate intervention services by age 6 months (U.S. Department of Health and Human Services, 2000).

All states and the District of Columbia require hearing screening of newborns. The screening is performed before discharge from the birth facility, and referrals are made for further testing if the infant shows signs of hearing problems. This allows early intervention that will prevent developmental delays and enable the child to communicate better than if hearing loss is found later in childhood.

Automated acoustic brainstem response (ABR) and evoked otoacoustic emissions (EOAE) are used for screening. Both tests identify moderate and severe hearing losses but may not detect milder hearing losses.

When the ABR test is performed, earphones placed on the infant emit a sound and electrodes record neural activity from the infant's brainstem that occurs in response to the sounds. This shows the function of the ear and the nerves leading to the brain. The EOAE test measures sound waves produced in the infant's inner ear in response to sounds that come through earphones placed on the infant. This test measures hearing to the inner ear but cannot identify a problem with the nerves to the brain.

The nurse ensures that infants receive screening and explains the testing to the parents. An infant who fails the first screening is often retested in the birth facility, sometimes using a different test. Parents of infants referred for further testing after discharge need more explanation and emotional support.

Other Screening Tests

Other screening tests are performed to detect conditions that result from inborn errors of metabolism or other genetic conditions. With early identification and treatment, infants with these conditions may avoid severe mental retardation and other serious problems. The newborn screening tests performed vary among the states and agencies. Some facilities offer all available tests to every infant. Others provide certain tests for all infants and offer others at an extra charge to the parents.

In the United States all states require newborn screening for phenylketonuria (PKU) (see Chapter 30) and hypothyroidism (Lashley, 2002). Each state also requires testing for certain other conditions in which early treatment may prevent or lessen serious consequences such as mental retardation. The conditions tested vary by state. Conditions often included in testing are galactosemia, hemoglobinopathies such as sickle cell disease and thalassemia, and congenital adrenal hyperplasia.

Screening tests are easy and inexpensive. They require a blood sample taken from the infant's heel and are usually performed shortly before discharge. Only one blood sample is needed for all tests. Further testing is necessary to confirm any abnormal test results. Parents may have questions for the nurse about the purpose of the tests. Nurses often refer to the tests as "PKU tests," but they should call them "screening tests" instead to emphasize that a number of conditions are included.

Tests performed within the first 24 hours of life are less sensitive than those performed after 24 hours. Infants tested before 12 to 24 hours of age should have repeat tests at 1 to 2 weeks of age so that disorders are not missed because of early testing (AAP & ACOG, 2002). These tests are performed at a home, clinic, or office visit.

Commonly Screened Conditions

PHENYLKETONURIA

PKU is a genetic condition in which the infant cannot metabolize the amino acid phenylalanine, which is common in protein foods such as milk. Although some phenylalanine is essential to growth, accumulations of it can result in severe mental retardation. Treatment is begun in the first few weeks of life, if possible, to prevent retardation. PKU is treated with a special low-phenylalanine diet, in which the amount of the amino acid is carefully regulated.

CONGENITAL HYPOTHYROIDISM

Congenital hypothyroidism (CH) occurs in 1 in 3600 to 1 in 5000 newborns (Lashley, 2002). It is the most common preventable cause of mental retardation. In CH the thyroid does not produce enough of the hormone thyroxine. Thyroid hormones affect the entire body, and the symptoms in an untreated infant include a large fontanel and tongue, slow reflexes, abdominal distention, lethargy, and feeding problems as well as irreversible brain damage. Infants may have no signs in the early weeks, but early treatment is necessary to prevent mental retardation. Infants are treated with thyroid hormones, and treatment continues throughout life.

GALACTOSEMIA

Absence of the enzyme necessary for the conversion of the milk sugar galactose to glucose causes galactosemia. The condition results in damage to the liver, brain, and eyes and eventually causes death. Treatment includes elimination of milk from the diet and use of milk substitutes. Long-term complications such as delayed growth and neurologic impairment may occur even with treatment.

HEMOGLOBINOPATHIES

Hemoglobinopathies include sickle cell anemia, thalassemia, and other diseases. The diseases are most often found in infants of African, Mediterranean, Indian, or South and Central American background. In sickle cell anemia, erythrocytes may become sickle shaped, resulting in obstruction of blood vessels and erythrocyte destruction. The hemoglobinopathies cause chronic anemias, sepsis, and other serious conditions.

CONGENITAL ADRENAL HYPERPLASIA

The term *congenital adrenal hyperplasia* (CAH) refers to a group of disorders with an enzyme defect that prevents adequate adrenal corticosteroid and aldosterone production and increases production of androgens. Infants may have ambiguous genitalia at birth, or masculinization of female infants. Salt-wasting crisis with low sodium and glucose and high potassium levels may occur within the first week of life. Treatment is with corticosteroids for the rest of the child's life.

OTHER CONDITIONS

Screening may also be performed for maple syrup urine disease, biotinidase deficiency, homocystinuria, cystic fibrosis, and medium chain acyl-CoA dehydrogenase deficiency (MCAD). Each of these conditions can be accurately diagnosed in newborns so that treatment can begin early. Knowing which conditions are included in testing allows the nurse to include appropriate information in parent teaching.

✔ CHECK YOUR READING

10. What are some important considerations in planning parent teaching?
11. What immunizations may be performed at the birth facility and why?
12. Why is it important to perform screening tests on infants as close to discharge as possible? For which infants is retesting important?

DISCHARGE AND NEWBORN FOLLOW-UP CARE

Discharge

Although state and federal legislation allows women and infants to stay in the birth facility for 48 hours after vaginal birth and 96 hours after cesarean birth, some women choose to go home earlier. The time of discharge varies according to the wishes and needs of the mother and newborn and the primary caregivers' assessment of their conditions.

Discharge is considered when term newborns who are appropriate for gestational age have normal physical examination results and show that they are making the transition from fetal to neonatal life without difficulty. Infants should have normal vital signs, have fed successfully at least twice, have passed urine and stool, have no excessive bleeding at the circumcision site for at least 2 hours, and show no significant jaundice in the first 24 hours of life. The mother should demonstrate knowledge, ability, and confidence to provide adequate care of the newborn and should have support available (AAP & ACOG, 2002).

Follow-up Care

Follow-up care after discharge from the birth facility is very important. The AAP recommends that follow-up by a health care professional be provided for all newborns who go home from the birth facility less than 48 hours after birth. This should occur within 48 hours of discharge and can be provided in the home, clinic, or office (AAP & ACOG, 2002).

Follow-up care can be provided in a number of ways. One or more home visits by a nurse are offered as a part of the maternity package in some birth facilities. In other areas, families return to the birth facility, a clinic, or the pediatrician's office to have the newborn checked. Clinics are held in the birth facility in some agencies.

Some birth facilities have "hot lines" or "warm lines" that mothers can call when they have questions about care of their infants or themselves. In many facilities, nurses call mothers during the first few days after discharge to assess the adjustment and health of the mother and baby, clarify information given before discharge, and answer questions. Follow-up care for newborns is discussed further in Chapter 23.

▮▮▮ SUMMARY CONCEPTS

- Prophylaxis against vitamin K–deficiency bleeding (hemorrhagic disease of the newborn) and ophthalmia neonatorum is necessary shortly after birth. It is provided by an injection of vitamin K and use of erythromycin ophthalmic ointment.
- Newborns may need help in clearing the airway. Positioning, suction, and close observation may be necessary.
- Nurses can prevent heat loss in newborns by keeping them dry and covered, avoiding contact between them and cold objects or surfaces, and keeping them away from drafts and outside windows and walls.
- The nurse must identify actual or potential hypoglycemia and intervene appropriately.
- Important interventions for jaundice are to monitor for its occurrence, to be sure that the infant is feeding well, and to explain the condition to the parents.
- The nurse must prevent mistaken identification of infants by checking the mother's and infant's identification bands whenever they have been separated.
- Parents and nurses must work together to prevent infant abductions. Parents must know how to identify hospital staff. Nurses should be alert for suspicious behavior.
- Infection can best be prevented by scrupulous handwashing by staff and all who come in contact with newborns.
- Reasons parents may choose circumcision include decreased incidence of urinary tract infections, penile cancer, phimosis, and some sexually transmitted diseases. Other reasons for circumcision include religious dictates, parental preference, and lack of knowledge about care of the foreskin.

- Parents reject circumcision because of belief that the previously listed conditions are too uncommon to necessitate surgery and pain in infants and concerns about bleeding, infection, phimosis, meatitis, meatal stenosis, urinary retention, chordee, and inclusion cysts.
- Parents with uncircumcised sons should be taught not to retract the foreskin until it becomes separate from the glans later in childhood.
- Parents of circumcised infants should be taught signs of complications and how to care for the area.
- Every nursing contact with parents should be used as an opportunity to teach.
- Screening tests are commonly performed to rule out hearing abnormalities, phenylketonuria, hypothyroidism, galactosemia, and hemoglobinopathies.

ANSWERS TO CRITICAL THINKING EXERCISE 21-1, p. 518

1. Determine whether Andy is showing signs of inadequate thermoregulation, hypoglycemia, or both. Reassure and teach Nancy as assessments and interventions are completed.
2. While taking the infant's temperature, assess for skin temperature, jitteriness, and general behavior. Check the blood glucose level if indicated. Also assess the environment for possible causes of heat loss.
3. If the baby's temperature is slightly low, change any wet linens, double-wrap him, and put a hat on his head. Have Nancy feed him if it is near a feeding time or if the blood glucose is low. Recheck the temperature in 30 minutes. If it is still low, place Andy under a radiant warmer. Notify the physician if Andy continues to have difficulty maintaining temperature. (See Nursing Care Plan 21-1 for other interventions.)
4. Praise Nancy for being so observant of her son. If Andy's temperature is normal and he is not jittery, discuss the fact that peripheral circulation is sluggish in newborns and that their hands and feet tend to be cool. If the "shakiness" is the Moro reflex or normal newborn behavior, discuss the reflex and the immaturity of the central nervous system. Show Nancy how to wrap Andy so he stays warm and the Moro reflex is not elicited. Discuss methods of temperature control, and be sure that Nancy knows how to read a thermometer. Explain all interventions.

ANSWERS TO CRITICAL THINKING EXERCISE 21-2, p. 527

Explain to the grandmother and the parents that although infants have slept on the abdomen without harm, research has shown that infants sleeping in this position have a higher chance of dying of sudden infant death syndrome (SIDS) than those who sleep on the back. To prevent flattening of the head, babies should spend time on the abdomen every day while they are awake. "Tummy time" helps keep the head rounded and helps develop the infant's muscles, as well. Occasionally moving the infant's crib to different positions in the room changes the pressure on the head because an infant is more likely to look toward the door.

REFERENCES & READINGS

Agarwal, R., Hagedorn, M.I.E., & Gardner, S.L. (2002). Pain and pain relief. In G.B. Merenstein & S.L. Gardner (Eds.), *Handbook of neonatal intensive care* (5th ed., pp. 191-218). St. Louis: Mosby.

American Academy of Pediatrics. (2003). Policy Statement: Controversies concerning vitamin K and the newborn. *Pediatrics, 112*(1), 191-192.

American Academy of Pediatrics, Task Force on Newborn and Infant Hearing. (1999). Newborn and Infant Hearing Loss: Detection and Intervention. *Pediatrics, 103*(2), 527-530.

American Academy of Pediatrics and American College of Obstetricians and Gynecologists. (2002). *Guidelines for perinatal care* (5th ed.). Elk Grove, IL: American Academy of Pediatrics.

American Academy of Pediatrics and Canadian Paediatric Society. (2000). Prevention and management of pain and stress in the neonate. *Pediatrics, 105*(2), 454-461.

Amy, E. (2001). Reflections on the interactive newborn bath demonstration. *MCN: American Journal of Maternal/Child Nursing, 26*(6), 320-322.

Association of Women's Health, Obstetric and Neonatal Nurses (AWHONN). (2002). *Policy position statement: National standards for newborn screenings.* Washington, DC: Author.

AWHONN. (2003). *Standards for professional nursing practice in the care of women and newborns* (6th ed.). Washington, DC: Author.

AWHONN and National Association of Neonatal Nurses. (2001). *Evidence-based clinical practice guideline: Neonatal skin care.* Washington, DC: Authors.

Behring, A., Vezeau, T.M., & Fink, R. (2003). Timing of the newborn first bath: A replication. *Neonatal Network, 22*(1), 39-46.

Berryman, R.E., & Glass, S.M. (2005). Routine care. In P.J. Thureen, J. Deacon, J. Hernandez, & D.M. Hall (Eds.), *Assessment and care of the well newborn* (2nd ed., pp. 198-205). Philadelphia: Saunders.

Blackburn, S.T., & Blakewell-Sachs, S. (2003). *Understanding the behavior of term infants.* White Plains, NY: March of Dimes Birth Defects Foundation. Retrieved November 30, 2004, from http://www.marchofdimes.com.

Brennan, R.A. (2003). A nurse-managed universal newborn hearing screen program. *MCN: American Journal of Maternal/Child Nursing, 29*(5), 320-325.

Bryanton, J., Walsh, D., Barrett, M., & Gaudet, D. (2004). Tub bathing versus traditional sponge bathing for the newborn. *Journal of Obstetric, Gynecologic, and Neonatal Nursing, 33*(6), 704-712.

Burns, A.L. (2003). Protecting infants in healthcare facilities from abduction. *Journal of Perinatal and Neonatal Nursing, 17*(2), 139-147.

Buschbach, D., & Bordeaux, M.S. (2002). *Newborn physiological and developmental transitions: integrating key components of perinatal and neonatal assessment.* Washington DC: AWHONN.

Capitulo, K.L., Cox, J.M., & Ianacone, K.L. (2004). Second opinion: Does an electronic infant security system ensure a more secure hospital environment? *MCN: American Journal of Maternal/Child Nursing, 29*(5), 280-281.

Cesario, S.K. (2001). Care of the Native American woman: Strategies for practice, education, and research. *Journal of Obstetric, Gynecologic, and Neonatal Nursing, 30*(1), 13-19.

Cesario, S.K. (2003). Selecting an infant security system. *AWHONN Lifelines, 7*(3), 236-242.

Chagnon, L. (2002). Newborn hearing screening. *AWHONN Lifelines, 6*(5), 398-400.

Cheffer, N.D. (2004). Adaptation to extrauterine life and immediate nursing care. In S. Mattson & J.E. Smith (Eds.), *Core curriculum for maternal-newborn nursing* (3rd ed., pp. 421-436). Philadelphia: Saunders.

Cheffer, N.D., & Rannalli, D.A. (2004). Newborn biological/behavioral characteristics and psychosocial adaptations. In S. Mattson & J.E. Smith (Eds.), *Core curriculum for maternal-newborn nursing* (3rd ed., pp. 437-484). Philadelphia: Saunders.

Gallo, A. (2003). The fifth vital sign: implementation of the neonatal infant pain scale. *Journal of Obstetric, Gynecologic, and Neonatal Nursing, 32*(2), 199-206.

Geyer, J., Ellsbury, D., Kleiber, C., Litwiller, D., Hinton, A., & Yankowitz, J. (2002). An evidence-based multidisciplinary protocol for neonatal circumcision pain management. *Journal of Obstetric, Gynecologic, and Neonatal Nursing, 31*(4), 403-410.

Giger, J.N., & Davidhizar, R. (Eds.) (2004). *Transcultural nursing assessment and intervention* (4th ed.). St. Louis: Mosby.

Greenberg, C.S. (2002). A sugar-coated pacifier reduces procedural pain in newborns. *Pediatric Nursing, 28*(3), 271-277.

Hale, K., & Incao, D. (2002). Infant security education: a multidisciplinary approach. *AWHONN Lifelines, 6*(3), 235-239.

Henry, P.R., Haubold, K., & Dobrykowski, T.M. (2004). Pain in the healthy full-term neonate: Efficacy and safety of interventions. *Newborn and Infant Nursing Reviews, 4*(2), 106-113.

Jones, T.B. (2002). Vaccines in pregnancy. In S.B. Ransom, M.P. Dombrowski, M.I. Evans, & K.A. Ginsburg (Eds.), *Contemporary therapy in obstetrics and gynecology*. Philadelphia: Saunders.

Kaufman, M.W., Clark, J.Y., & Castro, C.L. (2001). Neonatal circumcision: Benefits, risks, and family teaching. *MCN: American Journal of Maternal/Child Nursing, 26*(4), 197-201.

Kraft, N.L. (2003). A pictorial and video guide to circumcision without pain. *Advances in Neonatal Care, 3*(2), 50-64. Retrieved May 31, 2003, from http://www.medscape.com.

Lawrence, J., Alcock, D., McGrath, P., Kay, J., MacMurray, S.B., & Dulberg, C. (1993). The development of a tool to assess neonatal pain. *Neonatal Network, 14*(5), 59-62.

Lashley, F.R. (2002). Newborn screening: New opportunities and new challenges. *Newborn and Infant Nursing Reviews, 2*(4), 228-242.

Lloyd-Puryear, M.A., & Forsman, I. (2002). Newborn screening and genetic testing. *Journal of Obstetric, Gynecologic, and Neonatal Nursing, 31*(2), 200-207.

Macke, J.K. (2001). Analgesia for circumcision: effects on newborn behavior and mother/infant interaction. *Journal of Obstetric, Gynecologic, and Neonatal Nursing, 30*(5), 507-514.

Malnory, M., Johnson, T.S., & Kirby, R.S. (2003). Newborn behavioral and physiological responses to circumcision. *MCN: American Journal of Maternal/Child Nursing, 28*(5), 313-319.

Marlowe, J.A. (2003). *Newborn hearing screening: Testing, follow-up and communication with families*. Washington, DC: AWHONN.

Mattson, S. (2003). Caring for Latino women. *AWHONN Lifelines, 7*(3), 258-260.

Mattson, S. (2004). Ethnocultural considerations in the childbearing period. In S. Mattson & J.E. Smith (Eds.), *Core curriculum for maternal-newborn nursing* (3rd ed., pp. 75-96). Philadelphia: Saunders.

McConnell, T.P., Lee, C.W., Couillard, M., & Sherrill, W.W. (2004). Trends in umbilical cord care: Scientific evidence for practice. *Newborn and Infant Nursing Reviews, 4*(4), 211-222.

Medves, J.M., & O'Brian, B. (2004). The effect of the bather and location of first bath on maintaining thermal stability in newborns. *Journal of Obstetric, Gynecologic, and Neonatal Nursing, 33*(2), 175-182.

Moore, M.L., & Moos, M. (2003). *Cultural competence in the care of childbearing families*. White Plains, NY: March of Dimes Birth Defects Foundation.

Prince, W.L., Horns, K.M., Latta, T.M., & Gerstmann, D.R. (2004). Treatment of neonatal pain without a gold standard: The case for caregiving interventions and sucrose administration. *Neonatal Network, 23*(4), 33-45.

Rabun, J.B. (2003). *For healthcare professionals: Guidelines on prevention of and response to infant abductions*. Alexandria, VA: National Center for Missing & Exploited Children.

Shogan, M.G. (2002). Emergency management plan for newborn abduction. *Journal of Obstetric, Gynecologic, and Neonatal Nursing, 31*(3), 340-346.

Sredl, D. (2003). Myths and facts about pain in neonates. *Neonatal Network, 22*(6), 69-71.

Stoll, B.J. & Kliegman, R.M. (2004). Genitourinary system. In R.E. Behrman, R.M. Kliegman, & H.B. Jenson (Eds.), *Nelson textbook of pediatrics* (17th ed., pp. 608-609). Philadelphia: Saunders.

U.S. Department of Health and Human Services. (2000). *Healthy People 2010 (Conference Edition, in Two Volumes)*. Washington, DC: Author.

Varda, K.E., & Behnke, R.S. (2000). The effect of timing of initial bath on newborn's temperature. *Journal of Obstetric, Gynecologic, and Neonatal Nursing, 29*(1), 24-32.

White, C., Simon, M., & Bryan, A. (2002). Using evidence to educate birthing center staff about infant states, cues, and behaviors. *MCN: American Journal of Maternal/Child Nursing, 27*(5), 294-298.

Whitman-Price, R.A., & Pope, K.A. (2002). Universal newborn hearing screening. *American Journal of Nursing, 102*(11), 71-77.

Zupan, J., & Garner, P. (2003). Topical umbilical cord care at birth (Cochrane Review). *The Cochrane Library*, Issue 1, 2003. Retrieved March 23, 2003, from www.cochrane.org.

Infant Feeding

After studying this chapter, you should be able to:

1. Identify the nutritional and fluid needs of the infant.
2. Compare the composition of breast milk with that of formula.
3. Explain important factors in choosing a method of infant feeding.
4. Explain the physiology of lactation.
5. Describe nursing management of initial and continued breastfeeding.
6. Describe nursing assessments and interventions for common problems in breastfeeding.
7. Describe nursing assessments and interventions in formula feeding.

Go to your Student CD-ROM for Review Questions keyed to these Objectives.

DEFINITIONS

Colostrum Breast fluid secreted during pregnancy and the first week after childbirth.

Engorgement Swelling of the breasts resulting from enlarged lymph glands, increased blood flow, and accumulation of milk when milk begins to be produced.

Foremilk First breast milk received in a feeding.

Hindmilk Breast milk received near the end of a feeding; contains higher fat content than foremilk.

Latch-On Attachment of the infant to the breast.

Let-Down Reflex See *milk-ejection reflex.*

Mastitis Inflammation of the breast, usually caused by infection.

Mature Milk Breast milk that appears after the first 2 weeks of lactation.

Milk-Ejection Reflex Release of milk from the alveoli into the ducts; also known as the *let-down reflex.*

Nonnutritive Sucking Sucking during which no milk flow is obtained.

Nutritive Suckling (Sucking) Steady, rhythmic suckling at the breast or sucking at a bottle to obtain milk.

Oxytocin Hormone produced by the posterior pituitary gland that stimulates uterine contractions and the milk-ejection reflex; also prepared synthetically.

Prolactin Anterior pituitary hormone that promotes growth of breast tissue and stimulates production of milk.

Suckling Giving or taking nourishment from the breast. Sometimes used interchangeably with *sucking,* which refers only to drawing into the mouth with a partial vacuum, as with a bottle or pacifier.

Transitional Milk Breast milk that appears between secretion of colostrum and of mature milk.

Infant feeding is an important part of parenting, and a woman may derive much satisfaction from her perception of success with feeding. Helping her choose and feel comfortable with a feeding method requires knowledge of the infant's nutritional needs and the techniques to meet those needs.

NUTRITIONAL NEEDS OF THE NEWBORN

Calories

The full-term newborn needs 110 to 120 kcal/kg (50 to 55 kcal/lb) of body weight each day. The infant must consume sufficient calories to meet energy needs, prevent use of body stores, and provide for growth.

Breast milk and formulas used for the normal newborn contain 20 kcal/oz. The average newborn weighing 3.4 kg (7.5 lb) requires approximately 570 to 630 ml (19 to 21 oz) of breast milk or formula each day to meet caloric requirements. This is about 45 to 75 ml (1.5 to 2.5 oz) at each feeding for infants who breastfeed every 2 to 3 hours. Formula-fed infants who feed every 3 to 4 hours need approximately 75 to 105 ml (2.5 to 3.5 oz) at each feeding.

During the first 7 to 10 days of life, infants should lose less than 10% of their birth weight (Berryman & Glass, 2005). This loss is a result of normal excretion of extracellular water and meconium and the fact that newborns often consume fewer calories than needed. The cause of weight loss should be identified when it exceeds 7% to ensure that the infant is nursing adequately.

Newborns have a small stomach capacity and may fall asleep before feeding adequately or may sleep through feeding times in the early days. Capacity increases rapidly so that many infants take 60 to 90 ml (2 to 3 oz) by the end of the first week. Infants usually regain the lost weight by approximately 10 days of age. This information should be explained to parents.

Nutrients

Nutrients needed by the newborn are provided by carbohydrates, proteins, and fat in breast milk or formula. Full-term neonates digest simple carbohydrates and proteins well. Fats are less well digested because of the lack of pancreatic lipase in the newborn. Vitamins and minerals are provided by both breast milk and formula.

Water

The newborn needs much larger amounts of fluid in relationship to size than does the adult because infants lose water more easily from the skin, kidneys, and intestines. The

normal newborn needs approximately 40 to 60 ml/kg (18 to 27 ml/lb) during the first 2 days of life and 100 to 150 ml/kg (45 to 68 ml/lb) a day by the end of the first week (Tsang, DeMarini, & Rath, 2003). Breast milk or formula supplies the infant's fluid needs. Additional water is unnecessary.

BREAST MILK AND FORMULA COMPOSITION

Breast Milk

Breast milk is species specific (made for human infants) and offers many advantages compared with formula. The nutrients in breast milk are proportioned appropriately for the neonate and vary to meet the newborn's changing needs. Breast milk provides protection against infection and is easily digested.

CHANGES IN COMPOSITION

The composition of breast milk changes in three phases: colostrum, transitional milk, and mature milk, which vary in makeup to meet the newborn's changing nutritional needs.

COLOSTRUM. The major secretion of the breasts during the first week of lactation is colostrum—a thick, yellow substance. Colostrum is higher in protein, fat-soluble vitamins, and minerals than mature milk but lower in calories, fat, and lactose. It is rich in immunoglobulins, especially secretory immunoglobulin A (IgA), which helps protect the infant's gastrointestinal tract from infection. Colostrum helps establish the normal flora in the intestines, and its laxative effect speeds the passage of meconium.

TRANSITIONAL MILK. Transitional milk appears as the milk changes from colostrum to mature milk. Immunoglobulins and proteins decrease, whereas lactose, fat, and calories increase. The vitamin content is approximately the same as that of mature milk.

MATURE MILK. After the first 2 weeks of lactation, mature milk replaces transitional milk. Because breast milk is bluish and not as thick as colostrum, some mothers think their milk is not "rich" enough for their infants. Nurses should explain the normal appearance of breast milk. Mature milk contains approximately 20 kcal/oz and nutrients sufficient to meet the infant's needs. Unless otherwise stated, discussions of breast milk and its contents refer to mature milk.

NUTRIENTS

The nutrients provided in breast milk are present in the amounts and proportions needed by the human infant.

PROTEIN. The concentrations of amino acids in breast milk are suited to the infant's needs and ability to metabolize them. Breast milk contains a high level of taurine, which is important for bile conjugation and brain development. Tyrosine and phenylalanine are low in breast milk to correspond to the infant's low digestive enzyme levels. The proteins produce a lower solute load (the amount of nitrogenous waste and minerals excreted by the kidneys) for the infant's immature kidneys.

🖋 CRITICAL TO REMEMBER

Daily Calorie and Fluid Needs of the Newborn

Calories
110 to 120 kcal/kg (50 to 55 kcal/lb)

Fluid
40 to 60 ml/kg (18 to 27 ml/lb) for the first 2 days of life
100 to 150 ml/kg (45 to 68 ml/lb) by the end of the first week

Casein and whey are the proteins in milk. Casein forms a large, insoluble curd that is harder to digest than the curd from whey, which is very soft. Breast milk is easily digested because it has a high ratio of whey to casein. Commercial formulas must be adapted to increase the amount of whey so that the curd is more digestible.

The body's immune system recognizes and may react to the protein in cow's milk, making it one of the most common allergens. Because breast milk is species specific, it is unlikely to cause allergies (Biancuzzo, 2003). Although breast milk does not cause allergies, foods the mother has eaten may be allergenic and the antigens may pass into the breast milk (Riordan, 2005a). If the infant reacts to the mother's diet, the offending food should be identified and eliminated.

Breastfeeding prevents absorption of foreign molecules that might precipitate development of allergies and is especially important for infants at high risk for allergic conditions such as eczema and asthma. When there is a significant family history of allergies, mothers can reduce the risk by avoiding highly allergenic foods that might affect the breast milk. These include cow's milk, eggs, fish, peanuts, and tree nuts (American Academy of Pediatrics [AAP], 2000).

CARBOHYDRATE. Lactose is the carbohydrate in breast milk. Its high level in human milk increases the acidity of the intestines, which decreases undesirable bacteria and improves absorption of calcium, phosphorus, and magnesium. Lactose also promotes growth of the normal bacterial flora in the intestines (Biancuzzo, 2003).

FAT. Fat provides 30% to 55% of the calories in breast milk. The fat composition of human milk differs greatly from that of cow's milk. Medium-chain triglycerides form the majority of fat content. Essential fatty acids, such as the long-chain polyunsaturated fatty acids, docosahexaenoic acid (DHA), and arachidonic acid (ARA), that are important for vision and growth of the brain are also present. These fatty acids are added to formulas.

The fat in breast milk is more easily digested by the newborn than that in cow's milk. In addition, the fat in human milk may have antibacterial and antiviral properties. Cholesterol also is higher in breast milk than in cow's milk. The high level of cholesterol may aid in the development of the central nervous system.

The amount of fat in breast milk varies during the feeding and between feedings on the same or different days. Hindmilk, the milk produced at the end of the feeding, contains two to three times the amount of fat as the foremilk, which is produced at the beginning of the feedings (Mitchell, 2003). Hindmilk produces satiety and helps the infant gain weight. Expressed hindmilk is sometimes used to increase caloric intake in preterm infants.

VITAMINS. Vitamin C must be added to commercial formulas to match the levels in human milk, which meet the infant's needs if the mother has an adequate intake.

The vitamin D content of breast milk is low. Infants who are not exposed to the sun and those with dark skin are particularly at risk for insufficient vitamin D. Vitamin D may be inadequate if the mother's diet is poor and she or the infant is not exposed to the sun. Supplementation with 200 international units of vitamin D daily is recommended for all infants (Kleinman, 2004). The infant of a vegan mother may need supplementation with vitamin B_{12} also.

MINERALS. The casein protein in cow's milk interferes with iron absorption. Although iron content in breast milk is lower than in formula, the iron is absorbed five times as well and breastfed infants are rarely deficient in iron (Riordan, 2005a). The increased absorption results from the higher lactose and vitamin C content in breast milk.

The full-term infant who is breastfed exclusively maintains iron stores for the first 6 months of life. The addition of formula or other foods, however, may decrease the absorption of iron, making supplementation necessary. Generally iron is added at 4 to 6 months. Preterm infants need iron supplements earlier. All formula-fed infants should receive formula fortified with iron (AAP & American College of Obstetricians & Gynecologists [ACOG], 2002).

Sodium, calcium, and phosphorus are higher in cow's milk than in human milk. This could cause an excessively high renal solute load if formula is not diluted properly. The amount of fluoride in breast milk is not influenced by the mother's diet. Fluoride supplements may be given starting at 6 months of age to improve dental health.

ENZYMES

Breast milk contains enzymes that aid in digestion. Pancreatic amylase, necessary for digestion of carbohydrates, is low in the newborn but present in breast milk. Breast milk also contains lipase to increase fat digestion.

✔ **CHECK YOUR READING**

1. Why do some newborns lose weight after birth?
2. What are the differences among colostrum, transitional milk, and mature breast milk?
3. How does breast milk compare with commercial formulas?

INFECTION-PREVENTING COMPONENTS

Other factors present in human milk help prevent infection in the newborn. Bifidus factor promotes the growth of *Lactobacillus bifidus,* an important part of the intestinal flora that helps produce an acid environment in the gastrointestinal tract. This protects the infant against infection from common intestinal pathogens.

Leukocytes present in breast milk also help protect against infection. Macrophages are most abundant and secrete lysozyme and lactoferrin. Lysozyme is a bacteriolytic enzyme that acts against gram-positive and enteric bacteria. Lactoferrin is a protein that binds iron in iron-dependent bacteria, such as *Staphylococcus* and *Escherichia coli,* preventing their growth. It also acts against *Candida albicans.* Giving infants supplementary iron may interfere with the effectiveness of lactoferrin.

Immunoglobulins are present in highest amounts in colostrum but also present throughout lactation. Higher levels occur when the infant is born prematurely. Lymphocytes in the milk produce secretory IgA, which helps prevent viral and bacterial invasion of the intestinal mucosa, resulting in fewer intestinal infections in breastfed than in formula-fed infants.

Infants who are breastfed may receive long-term protection against respiratory infections. Even partial breastfeeding results in a decreased incidence not only of respiratory and gastrointestinal infections, but also of ear infections and sudden infant death syndrome (Newton, 2002). Otitis media is half as frequent in breastfeeding infants and less severe if it does occur (Kleinman, 2004).

EFFECT OF MATERNAL DIET

Although the fatty acid content of breast milk is influenced by the mother's diet, malnourished mothers have about the same proportions of protein, carbohydrates, and most minerals as those who are well nourished. Levels of vitamins in breast milk are affected by the mother's intake and stores, however. Breastfeeding women must eat a well-balanced diet to maintain their own health and energy levels (see Chapter 9, p. 193).

Formulas

Commercial formulas are produced to replace or supplement breast milk. Manufacturers adapt commercial formulas to correspond with the components in breast milk as much as possible, although an exact match is impossible. Changes in formula composition are made when a substance in human milk is found to be important enough to add to infant formulas. A variety of formulas that differ in price and ingredients is available.

COW'S MILK

Unmodified cow's milk (whole milk, low-fat milk, or nonfat milk) is not recommended for infants under 12 months of age. Unmodified cow's milk contains too much protein, potassium, and sodium, lacks enough iron and linoleic acid, and may cause gastrointestinal bleeding and anemia. In addition, it causes a higher renal solute load than is appropriate for immature infants (Heird, 2004; Trahms, 2004.)

Modified cow's milk is the source of most commercial formulas. Manufacturers specifically formulate it for infants by reducing protein to decrease renal solute load. Saturated fat is removed and replaced with vegetable fats. Vitamins and other nutrients are added to simulate the contents of breast milk. Formulas with added iron are recommended for all formula-fed infants (AAP & ACOG, 2002).

FORMULAS FOR INFANTS WITH SPECIAL NEEDS

Soy formulas may be given to infants with allergies, galactosemia, or lactase deficiency or whose families are vegetarian. Soy milk is derived from the protein of soybeans and supplemented with amino acids. Examples of soy formulas are ProSobee and Isomil. Some infants allergic to cow's milk are also allergic to soy. Casein hydrolysate formulas are more universally tolerated by infants with allergies. The protein in these modified cow's milk formulas is treated to make them hypoallergenic. The formulas also are used for infants with fat malabsorption. Amino acid–based formulas are available for allergic infants also.

The preterm infant may require a more concentrated formula with more calories in less liquid. Specific nutrients are added for the preterm infant's higher requirements in a more easily digestible form. Human milk fortifiers may be added to breast milk to adapt it to the needs of preterm infants. Lactose-free formula is modified for infants who do not tolerate lactose. Formula low in the amino acid phenylalanine is given to infants with phenylketonuria (PKU), a deficiency in the enzyme to digest phenylalanine found in standard formulas.

CONSIDERATIONS IN CHOOSING A FEEDING METHOD

Many women decide on a feeding method well before the infant's birth. Some may not have questions about which method is best for them until late in pregnancy. Nurses can help mothers decide on a method and gain confidence in feeding their infants.

For women who are undecided, nurses should explain to the mothers the many benefits of breastfeeding for both mother and infant. However, nurses must be sensitive to mothers' feelings about feeding. Although nurses should encourage breastfeeding as the best method of feeding in most circumstances, they should be supportive of the mother's chosen method once a decision is made. The early days of parenting are a very vulnerable time for new mothers, who may feel that their feeding abilities reflect their mothering abilities. The nurse's teaching and encouragement about the chosen feeding method are essential.

Breastfeeding

Breastfeeding offers many advantages (Box 22-1). Recent evidence has shown that not only are certain illnesses decreased during breastfeeding, but the mortality rate is lowered, as well. Children who are breastfed have an approximately 20% lower risk of death between the ages of 28 days and 1 year than children who are never breastfed (Chen & Rogan, 2004). Although breastfeeding was once the major method of feeding, the availability of refrigeration and commercial formulas and the increased incidence of maternal employment has led many mothers to choose formula feeding.

It has been increasingly recognized, however, that formula feeding can never fully equal breastfeeding in terms of providing for the infant's optimal growth and development. Both the AAP and the U.S. Surgeon General recommend breastfeeding. The AAP and the American Dietetic Association recommend that infants receive only breast milk for the first 6 months after birth and that breastfeeding continue after the addition of solid foods until the infant is at least 12 months of age (AAP Work Group on Breastfeeding, 1997; AAP and American College of Obstetricians and Gynecologists, 2002; American Dietetic Association, 2001; Dobson & Murtaugh, 2001).

BOX 22-1 Benefits of Breastfeeding

For the Infant
Breast milk does not cause allergic reactions.
Immunologic properties help prevent infections. The infant may have fewer respiratory, ear, and gastrointestinal infections and less risk for sudden infant death syndrome (SIDS).
Breast milk is species specific: its composition meets the infant's specific nutritional needs.
Nutritional and immunologic properties change according to the infant's needs.
Breast milk is easily digested, with nutrients that are well absorbed.
Protein, fat, and carbohydrate occur in the most suitable proportions.
Improper and potentially dangerous dilution is not possible.
Breast milk is unlikely to be contaminated, decreases growth of bacteria so that it can be unrefrigerated longer than formula, and is not affected by water supply.
Breast milk is less likely to result in overfeeding.
The infant is unlikely to have constipation.

For the Mother
Oxytocin release enhances uterine involution.
The mother loses less blood because of delayed return of menses.
She is more likely to rest while feeding.
She is likely to eat a balanced diet that improves healing.
Frequent, skin-to-skin contact may enhance bonding.
Breastfeeding is convenient: it is always available and does not require preparation of bottles or buying and heating formula.
Breastfeeding is economical: it eliminates cost of formula and bottles and time spent in preparation.
The infant is less likely to be ill, reducing medical care costs.
Traveling is easier: there are no bottles to prepare, carry, refrigerate, and warm.
Breastfeeding may reduce the risk of some cancers.

A goal set by the U.S. Department of Health and Human Services (USDHHS) for the year 2010 is for 75% of all new mothers to breastfeed at the time of birth facility discharge, for at least 50% to be breastfeeding at 6 months, and for 25% at 1 year (USDHHS, 2000). In 2002 70.1% of mothers began to breastfeed their newborns. At 6 months 33.2% of mothers were breastfeeding. At 12 months the rate was 19.7% breastfeeding (Ross Products Division, 2003).

These statistics have shown a gradual increase since 1991. Between 1992 and 2002 the rate of breastfeeding during the hospital stay increased 15.9%. The number of mothers breastfeeding at 3 and 6 months after birth also has increased. This increase has been greatest in mothers who are younger, African-American, Hispanic, enrolled in the Special Supplemental Nutrition Program for Women, Infants, and Children (WIC), and educated at only a grade school level. These groups traditionally have had lower breastfeeding rates (Ross Products Division, 2003).

In an effort to promote breastfeeding, the United Nations Children's Fund (UNICEF) and the World Health Organization (WHO) advocate that birth facilities become certified as baby-friendly hospitals with policies to actively encourage breastfeeding. Guidelines to becoming certified as a baby-friendly hospital emphasize education of staff and parents about breastfeeding, early initiation of breastfeed-

ing, demand feedings, avoidance of formula and pacifiers, and rooming-in.

Formula Feeding

Mothers choose formula feeding for many reasons. Some women are embarrassed by breastfeeding, seeing the breasts only in a sexual context. Many mothers have few relatives or friends who have had breastfeeding experiences. A woman may feel a need to maintain a strict feeding schedule and be uneasy not knowing exactly how much milk the infant takes at each feeding. Her partner or mother may not be supportive of breastfeeding. Occasionally a woman must use formula because she must take medications that might harm the infant. A frequent reason that mothers choose formula feeding instead of breastfeeding is a lack of understanding about the two methods.

Combination Feeding

Some parents prefer a combination of breastfeeding and bottle feeding. Unless medically indicated, it is best to delay giving formula until lactation has been well established at 3 to 4 weeks of age. Giving formula to breastfeeding infants leads to a decrease in breastfeeding frequency and milk production, making successful breastfeeding less likely (AAP & ACOG, 2002). Women who use a combination of breast milk and formula are likely to breastfeed for shorter durations than women who breastfeed exclusively (Chezem, Friesen, & Boettcher, 2003).

If the mother chooses combination feeding, however, the nurse should be supportive so that the infant receives the benefits of breast milk at least part of the time. Either breast milk or formula may be given in the bottle. The mother may give a bottle each day or only occasionally, such as when a baby-sitter is with the infant. This allows the mother to be away from the infant for longer periods of time, yet allows the closeness with the infant that many mothers enjoy and the physical advantages of breastfeeding to continue.

Factors Influencing Choice

Many factors influence a woman's choice of feeding method. These factors must be considered when educating women about their choices.

SUPPORT FROM OTHERS

Family members and friends also may share in the decision-making process. The woman's own mother and the baby's father often are important influences in determining whether women breastfeed. If the woman's mother-in-law will participate in caregiving, her opinion may be important too. The woman with little support or active discouragement from her family probably will have a difficult time nursing. Some women choose not to breastfeed because their partner objects. However, one study of men from African-American, Hispanic, and other cultures found that 81% wanted their infants to be breastfed (Pollock, Bustamante-Forest, & Giarratano, 2002).

Involvement of the father in feedings is important in some families and may be thought possible only if he can give a bottle regularly. Nurses can suggest other ways that fathers can participate in infant care, such as holding and rocking infants. Educating family members about the advantages of breastfeeding and ways to deal with problems may lead to their encouragement of the breastfeeding mother. Support from family also helps prolong the duration of breastfeeding. Women who have less help with household tasks and experience distress in their relationship with their partner are more likely to breastfeed for shorter periods (Sullivan, Leathers, & Kelley, 2004).

Encouragement from the woman's health care provider increases the chance that she will breastfeed. Women are more likely to be breastfeeding at 12 weeks if they receive encouragement from their provider (Taveral et al., 2003). The support the mother receives from the nursing staff plays a significant part in whether she feels comfortable with her choice of feeding method. The woman who does not feel confident in her ability to breastfeed before she leaves the birth facility is less likely to continue breastfeeding if she encounters difficulties at home.

CULTURE

Cultural influences may dictate decisions about the way a mother feeds her infant. For example, many Mormon women believe that breastfeeding is an important part of motherhood. Muslim women often breastfeed for the first 2 years. Immigrants from countries in which breastfeeding is the norm may breastfeed for shorter durations or not at all because they lack the support system they had in their own country. In addition, formula feeding may be seen as a symbol of the new way of life and considered a way to help infants grow larger and become stronger.

Nurses should be particularly watchful for ways to help mothers from other cultures who might wish to breastfeed but fail to do so because of lack of support. Canadian Mohawk mothers were more likely to breastfeed when a woman from their community worked with them and the grandmother in promoting the value of breastfeeding (Banks, 2003).

Rituals may be important to the woman. Women from the Philippines may participate in *lihi*, a ritual of stroking the breasts with papaya leaves and sugar cane stalks to ensure adequate rich milk (Riordan, 2005b).

Some Southeast Asian, Hispanic, and Arab women believe colostrum is bad for the baby and wait to begin breastfeeding until the milk comes in when they are home (Mattson, 2004). They may believe that colostrum is "spoiled" milk because it has been in the breasts for a long time. Women with these beliefs may manually express colostrum and discard it before they begin to breastfeed the infant. Some Korean women believe they should not breastfeed for the first 3 days after birth. Modesty and embarrassment about nursing in front of others and lack of understanding about the value of colostrum may prevent women from nursing in the birth facility. Others may feel breastfeeding is old fashioned (Windsor, 2003). African-American women typically do not breastfeed.

Certain foods are used to increase milk production in some cultures. Examples include broth from blue cornmeal for Navajo Indians, chocolate for women from Guatemala, and anise or sesame seed for Hispanic women (Biancuzzo, 2003).

Some mothers may be amenable to nursing the infant with help while in the birth facility, especially if the antibody and laxative properties of colostrum are explained. Breastfeeding involves a learning process for both mother and infant, which is best started where assistance is available. Nurses can help women learn by offering to help them "practice" breastfeeding at least a few times before discharge. This helps build the woman's confidence and allows for early identification and correction of problems. If the mother is firm in her desire to wait until discharge to begin breastfeeding, nurses can support her by teaching her what she will need to know when she goes home and referring her to sources of help should she need it. Cultural values about feeding, as in other areas of health care, must be respected.

EMPLOYMENT

The need to return to roles outside the home soon after giving birth may cause concern about feeding methods. Returning to work or school is a major cause of discontinuation of breastfeeding by 10 to 12 weeks (Taveral et al., 2003). Assistance from the nurse in providing practical information may help a mother continue breastfeeding after she returns to work or school.

The mother may choose to use a combination of breastfeeding and bottle feeding with either stored breast milk or formula, may plan a short period of breastfeeding before weaning the infant to formula, or may use formula from the beginning. Nurses provide information about options, breastfeeding and working, use of breast pumps, and storage of breast milk. Pamphlets and books for the working breastfeeding mother are particularly helpful.

Women who will be using a breast pump at work should have a clean, private place to pump once or twice during breaks or lunch time. The woman can bring a cooler and ice pack to store the milk. If she pumps a couple of times a day for a week or two before returning to work, she will be adept at using the pump and will have a supply of breast milk for the caregiver to use while she is at work. Frequent breastfeeding during the evenings and weekends will help her maintain her milk supply.

OTHER FACTORS

Other factors also may influence a woman's decision. Her knowledge and past experience with infant feeding are important. Women who are most likely to breastfeed are over age 30, have a college education, and live in the New England or western parts of the United States. Asian, white, and Hispanic women have breastfeeding rates of 80.2%, 73.4%, and 70.7%. Asian women have the highest breastfeeding rates throughout the first year. Those with the lowest breastfeeding rates are African-American, have a grade school education, are under age 20, and live in the southern United States. Although African-American women still have the lowest initiation rates for breastfeeding at 53.9%, they have shown a greater increase in breastfeeding than other groups in recent years (Ross Products Division, 2003).

NORMAL BREASTFEEDING

To be most helpful to lactating mothers, the nurse must have a good understanding of the physiology of lactation. The anatomy and physiology of the breast are discussed in Chapter 4, and breast changes occurring in pregnancy are discussed in full in Chapter 7 (see Figures 4-8 and 7-3).

Breast Changes during Pregnancy

Breast changes begin early in pregnancy. The ducts, lobules, and alveoli develop in response to the hormones estrogen, progesterone, placental lactogen, prolactin, and chorionic gonadotropin. The breasts begin to secrete colostrum by the second trimester, and women who give birth after the sixteenth week of gestation produce colostrum (Walker, 2005). During pregnancy the anterior pituitary secretes high levels of prolactin, the hormone that causes the breasts to produce milk. However, milk production is prevented by estrogen, progesterone, and human placental lactogen, which inhibit breast response to prolactin. Changes such as increase in breast size indicate that the breasts are responding adequately to hormonal stimulation to prepare for lactation. Women who have no breast changes during pregnancy may have more difficulty with lactation.

Milk Production

Milk is produced in the alveoli of the breasts through a complex process by which materials from the mother's bloodstream are reformulated into breast milk. Thus amino acids, glucose, lipids, enzymes, leukocytes, and other materials are used to manufacture the nutrients needed by the infant.

The milk is ejected from the secretory cells of the alveoli into the alveolar lumen by contraction of the myoepithelial cells. From there it travels into the lactiferous ducts, which lead from the alveoli to the nipple. The ducts are compressed during nursing to eject a stream of milk through pores in the nipple.

Hormonal Changes at Birth

PROLACTIN

At birth, loss of progesterone, estrogen, and placental lactogen from the placenta results in increasing levels and effectiveness of prolactin and brings about milk production. The tactile stimulation of suckling and the removal of colostrum or milk causes continued increased levels of prolactin. Prolactin is secreted at highest levels during the night and rises

with suckling. It is high during the early months and then gradually decreases until weaning. Prolactin decreases rapidly after the first few weeks postpartum unless the breast is stimulated and milk is removed by infant suckling or a breast pump (Walker, 2005).

OXYTOCIN

Oxytocin from the posterior pituitary increases in response to nipple stimulation. Oxytocin causes the milk-ejection reflex, commonly known as the *let-down reflex*. The resulting contraction of myoepithelial cells around the alveoli releases milk into the ducts, making it available to the infant. During a feeding, the milk-ejection reflex occurs several times.

When mothers see, hear, or think about their infants, they often have an increase in oxytocin level, bringing about a let-down of milk and causing milk to drip or spurt from the breasts. Pain or lack of relaxation can inhibit oxytocin release. Oxytocin also is responsible for the uterine contractions mothers may feel at the beginning of nursing sessions. These contractions are beneficial because they hasten involution of the uterus (Figure 22-1).

Continued Milk Production

The amount of milk produced depends primarily on adequate stimulation of the breast and removal of the milk by suckling or a breast pump, which causes production of prolactin. Suckling is not essential for the initial production of

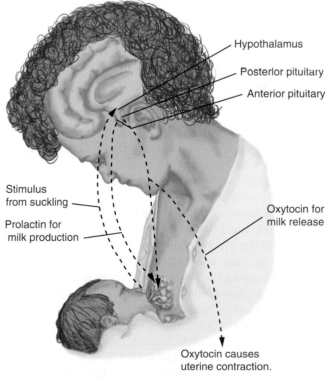

Hypothalamus

Posterior pituitary

Anterior pituitary

Stimulus from suckling

Prolactin for milk production

Oxytocin for milk release

Oxytocin causes uterine contraction.

Figure 22-1 ■ Effect of prolactin and oxytocin on milk production. When the infant begins to suckle at the breast, nerve impulses travel to the hypothalamus, which causes the anterior pituitary to secrete prolactin to increase milk production. Suckling causes the posterior pituitary to secrete oxytocin, producing the let-down reflex, which releases milk from the breast. Oxytocin also results in uterine contractions, which aid in involution.

milk, but it is necessary for continued milk production. This "supply-and-demand" effect continues throughout lactation. Early and frequent suckling may increase prolactin receptors in the breast, making milk production more effective (Riordan, 2005a). Therefore increased demand with more frequent and longer nursing results in more milk available for the infant.

If milk (or colostrum) is not removed from the breasts, the alveoli become very distended. Pressure on the blood vessels reduces blood flow and prevents prolactin from reaching the secretory cells. Lack of nipple stimulation causes release of prolactin inhibiting factor by the hypothalamus, and milk production gradually ceases. The milk in the ducts is absorbed, the alveoli become smaller, and the cells return to a resting state.

Preparation of Breasts for Breastfeeding

Little preparation is needed during pregnancy for breastfeeding. The mother should avoid soap on her nipples because soap removes the natural protective oils secreted by the Montgomery tubercles of the breasts. The use of creams, nipple rolling, pulling, and rubbing to "toughen" nipples does not decrease nipple pain after birth and may cause irritation or uterine contractions from release of oxytocin.

The breasts should be assessed during pregnancy to identify flat or inverted nipples (Figure 22-2). Normally the nipples protrude. Flat nipples appear soft, like the areola, and do not stand erect unless stimulated by rolling them between the fingers. Nipples also may be inverted, or drawn into the breast tissue. Both conditions make it more difficult for infants to latch onto the nipples. Some nipples appear normal but draw inward when the areola is compressed in the infant's mouth. Compressing the areola between the thumb and forefinger determines whether the nipple projects normally or becomes inverted. Nipples that appear inverted at the beginning of pregnancy may be improved near the end.

Women with flat or inverted nipples may find breast shells (also called breast cups) useful (Biancuzzo, 2003). These dome-shaped devices are worn during the last weeks of pregnancy and between feedings after birth. The shells are placed in the bra with the opening over the nipple. They exert slight pressure against the areola and help the nipples protrude. Pumping the breasts for a few minutes before beginning nursing also helps bring the nipples out. Exercises for inverted nipples that involve stretching or manipulation of the nipple or areola (Hoffman technique) are not recommended during pregnancy because they are not effective and may cause uterine contractions.

✔ CHECK YOUR READING

7. What is the effect of suckling on the let-down reflex and milk production?
8. What preparation of the breasts is needed during pregnancy?

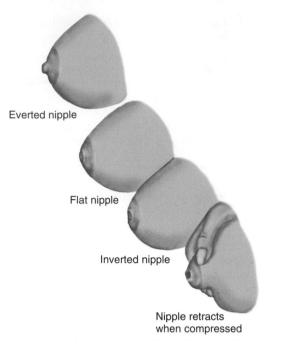

Figure 22-2 ■ Normal everted nipple and other types of nipples that may cause the infant difficulty in latching on. Nipples shown after stimulation.

Everted nipple

Flat nipple

Inverted nipple

Nipple retracts when compressed

Application of the Nursing Process
Breastfeeding

Assessment

Assess both the mother and the infant during the breastfeeding process. Various scoring tools have been developed to assess breastfeeding, but none is completely satisfactory. One method often used is the LATCH breastfeeding assessment tool (Table 22-1).

MATERNAL ASSESSMENT

BREASTS AND NIPPLES. Assess the condition of the breasts and nipples and the mother's knowledge about breastfeeding to determine her need for assistance.

Examine the breasts and nipples during late pregnancy to identify problems that might interfere with feeding. If this assessment did not occur before birth, examine the breasts and nipples before the initial feeding. Assess the protrusion of the nipples to identify flat or inverted nipples.

Ongoing assessments after birth include identification of breast fullness and breast engorgement. Fullness is the swelling of the breasts that may occur early in lactation as a result of increased blood and lymph circulation. It may progress to engorgement if feedings are delayed, too short, or not frequent enough. Palpate the breasts to see if they are soft, filling, or engorged. Soft breasts feel like a cheek. If milk is beginning to come in, the breasts may be slightly firmer, which is charted as "filling." Engorged breasts are hard and tender, with taut, shiny skin. Note any redness, tenderness, and lumps within the breasts.

TABLE 22-1 The LATCH Scoring Tool*

	0	1	2
L Latch	Infant too sleepy or reluctant No sustained latch achieved	After repeated attempts, is able to sustain latch and suck Must hold nipple in infant's mouth Must stimulate infant to suck	Grasps breast Tongue down Lips flanged Rhythmic sucking
A Audible swallowing	None	A few with stimulation	Spontaneous and intermittent <24 hr old Spontaneous and frequent >24 hr old
T Type of nipple	Inverted	Flat	Everted (after stimulation)
C Comfort (breast or nipple)	Engorged Cracked, bleeding, large blisters, or bruises Severe discomfort	Filling Reddened or small blisters or bruises Mild to moderate discomfort	Soft Nontender
H Hold (positioning)	Full assist (staff holds infant at breast)	Minimal assist (e.g., elevate head of bed; place pillows for support) Teach one side; mother does other Staff holds and then mother takes over	No assist from staff Mother able to position or hold infant

Modified from Jensen, D., Wallace, S., & Kelsay, P. (1994). LATCH: A breastfeeding charting system and documentation tool. *Journal of Obstetric, Gynecologic, and Neonatal Nursing,* *23*(1), 27-32. Reprinted with permission of Sage Publications.
*The nurse can use the LATCH scoring system to assess and document the need for assistance with breastfeeding. Each assessment area is scored 0 to 2.

Assess the nipples, which may be red, bruised, blistered, fissured, or bleeding. Ask about nipple tenderness and when it occurs. Evaluate breastfeeding techniques of the mother having problems with her nipples.

KNOWLEDGE. The mother who is breastfeeding for the first time may have many questions and need substantial guidance during her first attempts. The mother who has nursed before has more knowledge but may still have questions about areas she has forgotten or may be unaware of current information that was unavailable when she breastfed her last infant. Lack of adequate knowledge may cause reduction of breast stimulation and prolactin production if mothers do not feed often enough. This can interfere with milk production and cause an early end to breastfeeding.

INFANT FEEDING BEHAVIORS

Before initiating a breastfeeding session, assess an infant's readiness for feeding (Box 22-2). The infant should be awake and hungry. Trying to feed an infant in a deep sleep period is frustrating to both mother and infant. Sucking on the hands, root-

BOX 22-2 Hunger Cues in Infants

Licking movements
Lip smacking
Rooting
Hands to mouth
Sucking on the hands
Increased activity
Crying (a late sign)

ing when the cheek or side of the mouth is touched, smacking the lips, and slight fussiness are common hunger cues. Feeding should begin before crying, which is a late sign of hunger. Crying infants must be calmed before they are ready to feed. Continue to assess for problems throughout the feeding.

Analysis

Women with and without experience often need information to successfully breastfeed. Breastfeeding problems and lack of confidence during the first 1 or 2 days is a good predictor of discontinuation of breastfeeding within the first 2 weeks (Taveral et al., 2003). Nurses can help prevent early weaning by using the nursing diagnosis "Risk for Ineffective Breastfeeding related to lack of understanding of breastfeeding techniques."

Planning

Goals and expected outcomes for this nursing diagnosis are:
- The infant will breastfeed using nutritive suckling for 15 minutes or more on each breast for most feedings before discharge.
- The mother will demonstrate breastfeeding techniques (such as positioning) as taught before discharge.
- The mother will verbalize satisfaction and confidence with the breastfeeding process before discharge.

Interventions

Inexperienced mothers may need detailed teaching. In one study mothers stated that calm reassurance from the nurse was helpful when they felt unsure about breastfeeding. The nurse's concern, patience, presence during feeding sessions, and follow-up after problems were especially appreciated (Hong, Callister, & Schwartz, 2003).

Experienced mothers often need only a review or clarification about techniques they have used previously. Interventions used for the first feeding session are summarized in "Keys to Clinical Practice: Assisting the Inexperienced Breastfeeding Mother" (see Appendix C).

ASSISTING WITH THE FIRST FEEDING

The first feeding should take place within the first hour after birth if both mother and infant are in stable condition. At this time infants are in an alert state, and many begin to nurse at once. Others may nuzzle, lick, or suck intermittently at the breast. Early breastfeeding provides stimulation of prolactin necessary for milk production, improves suckling, and may increase the duration of breastfeeding (Biancuzzo, 2003). Feeding at this time also helps establish early bonding. The mother may be very gratified to see her infant nurse right after birth.

Help the mother move to her side or into Fowler's position. Show her how to hold the breast and explain proper positioning of the infant. This is a short session, and teaching should be repeated at the next feeding for reinforcement. Observe the infant's response to the feeding and watch for signs such as cyanosis or choking, which may indicate the presence of problems. Stay with the mother for a short time during each feeding and check back with her frequently to answer questions that may arise.

TEACHING FEEDING TECHNIQUES

POSITION OF THE MOTHER AND INFANT. Both the mother and the infant must be positioned properly for optimal breastfeeding. Make the mother as comfortable as possible before she begins to nurse. Pain or an awkward posi-

tion may interfere with the let-down reflex and cause her to tire. Prevent interruptions and provide privacy so she can concentrate on learning techniques.

The cradle, football, and cross-cradle holds and the side-lying position are commonly used (Figures 22-3 to 22-6). Use pillows behind the mother's back and to protect an abdominal incision or support her arms. Her shoulders should be relaxed, and she should not be hunched over. Arrange folded blankets or pillows to elevate the infant to the level of the nipple and prevent pulling and tension on the nipple, which would cause it to become sore.

The infant's head and body should directly face the breast with the nose, cheeks, and chin lightly touching the breast. If the infant must turn the head to reach the breast, swallowing is difficult. The neck should be flexed because hyperextension also makes swallowing difficult. The infant's body should be aligned so that the ear, shoulder, and hips are in a straight line.

POSITION OF THE MOTHER'S HANDS. The position of the mother's hands is important. The palmar or C position is most often taught to new mothers. The mother places her thumb on top of the breast with her fingers under the breast. Her little finger is against the chest wall and the other fingers provide support to the breast (Figure 22-7). Her fingers should be behind the areola and her thumb should not press on the breast enough to make the nipple tip upward, or the infant will suck improperly and the nipple may become sore.

Some women use the "scissors hold" or V hold. The woman uses her forefinger and middle finger to support the breast. She must be careful to place her fingers well behind

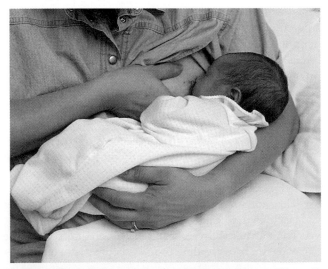

Figure 22-3 ■ For the cradle hold the mother positions the infant's head at or near the antecubital space and level with her nipple, with her arm supporting the infant's body. Her other hand is free to hold the breast. Once the infant is positioned, pillows or blankets can be used to support the mother's arm, which may tire from holding the baby.

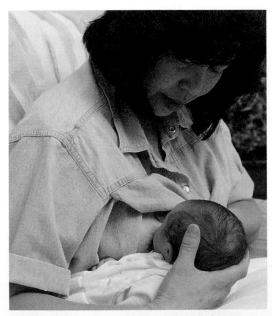

Figure 22-4 ■ For the football hold the mother supports the infant's head in her hand, with the infant's body resting on pillows alongside her hip. This method allows the mother to see the position of the infant's mouth on the breast, helps her control the infant's head, and is especially helpful for mothers with heavy breasts. This hold also avoids pressure against an abdominal incision.

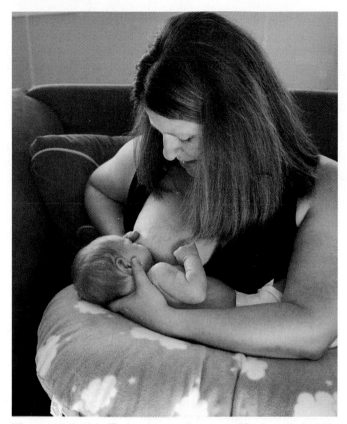

Figure 22-5 ■ The cross-cradle or modified cradle hold is helpful for infants who are preterm or have a fractured clavicle. The mother holds the infant's head in the hand opposite the side on which the infant will feed and supports the infant's body across her lap with her arm. The other hand holds the breast. The mother can guide the infant's head to the breast and see the mouth on the breast during the feeding.

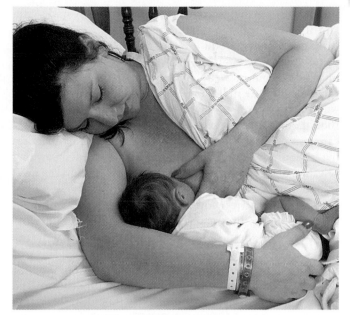

Figure 22-6 ■ The side-lying position avoids pressure on episiotomy or abdominal incisions and allows the mother to rest while feeding. She lies on her side, with her lower arm supporting her head or placed around the infant. A pillow behind her back and between her legs provides comfort. Her upper hand and arm are used to position the infant on the side at nipple level and hold the breast. When the infant's mouth opens to nurse, the mother draws the infant to her to insert the nipple into the mouth. A small blanket or towel can be placed over an abdominal incision to protect it from infant movement.

the areola so her fingers do not slip down the wet areola and interfere with the placement of the infant's mouth.

The mother should support her breast in place for the first few weeks if the weight of it makes it difficult for the infant to hold it in the mouth. As the infant becomes more adept at breastfeeding, the mother will not need to hold the breast.

Although mothers worry about the infant's ability to breathe while nursing, indenting the breast tissue near the infant's nostrils is unnecessary. This might cause improper positioning of the nipple in the infant's mouth, interfere with the grasp of the nipple, or interfere with milk flow. Unless the mother's breasts are very heavy and the infant's nose is buried in the breast, breathing is not occluded. Lifting the infant's hips to a slightly more horizontal position or bringing them closer to the mother is usually sufficient if there appears to be a problem.

LATCH-ON TECHNIQUES. Teach the mother techniques to help the infant latch on to the breast. The infant should be awake and hungry. Talking and cuddling can help a sleepy infant awaken and calm an upset infant.

Eliciting Latch-On. After positioning the infant to face the breast, the mother holds her breast so that the nipple

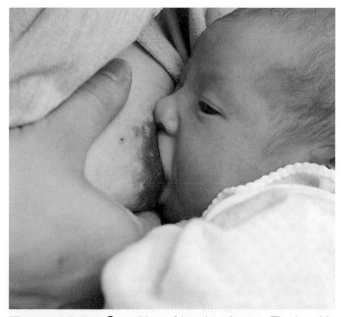

Figure 22-7 ■ C position of hand on breast. The hand is positioned so that the thumb is on top of the breast while the fingers support the breast from below. Note the flaring of the infant's lips.

brushes against the center of the infant's lips. A hungry infant usually opens the mouth, but some need a minute of stroking the area around the mouth. The breast should not be inserted until the infant's mouth is opened widely, or the infant will compress the end of the nipple, causing pain, trauma, and little milk flow. When the mouth opens widely with the tongue down and forward over the gum, the mother should quickly bring the infant close to her so that the infant can latch on to the areola. Suggesting to the mother that during latch-on the infant opens the mouth as though yawning or eating a large sandwich may help her understand the need to wait until the infant's mouth is opened widely.

Position of the Mouth. Assess the position of the infant's mouth on the breast (Figure 22-8). As much of the areola as possible should be in the infant's mouth to allow the nipple to be drawn toward the back of the mouth. This prevents the infant from sucking on the nipple only, which leads to sore nipples and insufficient milk production. The infant's lips should be about 1 to $1\frac{1}{2}$ inches from the nipple base (Lawrence & Lawrence, 2005). This positions the gums over the milk ducts so that milk is released into the infant's mouth when the gums compress them.

Assess the position of the infant's tongue by gently pulling down on the lower lip. The tongue should be under the breast and over the top of the lower gums. The lips should be flared outward. Be sure that the lower lip is not turned in, which may result in a friction burn on the lower side of the nipple.

SUCKLING PATTERN. Teach the mother about the infant's suckling pattern. During nutritive suckling the infant sucks with smooth, continuous movements with only occasional pauses to rest. The infant may swallow after each suck or may suck several times before swallowing. Nonnutritive sucking often occurs when the infant is falling asleep. If a fluttery or choppy motion of the jaw not accompanied

by the sound of swallowing occurs, the mother should remove the infant from the breast because her nipples may become sore. If she thinks that the infant should feed longer, she can try burping and waking the infant before resuming the feeding.

Explain the milk-ejection reflex to the mother. Many mothers learn to recognize a feeling of tingling in the nipples as the let-down occurs. The reflex occurs several times throughout the feeding. She sees the infant begin to swallow more rapidly each time a new let-down brings more rapid expulsion of milk. Milk may drip from the opposite breast when the reflex occurs.

■ Mothers often wonder whether their infants are actually receiving milk from the breast. Point out the sound of swallowing when it occurs. A soft "ka" or "ah" sound indicates the infant is swallowing colostrum or milk.

Short pauses are normal during nursing. Caution mothers not to jiggle the breast in the infant's mouth in an effort to start the suckling again. Moving the breast in the mouth may cause the infant to lose the grasp on the nipple and areola, resulting in "chewing" on the nipple and soreness. If necessary the mother should take the infant off the breast for awakening and then start again.

REMOVAL FROM THE BREAST. Teach the mother to remove the infant from the breast for burping midway in the feeding and whenever suckling becomes nonnutritive. Show her how to avoid trauma to the breast by inserting her finger into the corner of the infant's mouth between the gums to break suction. She then should remove the breast quickly before the infant begins to suck again. Another method is to indent the breast tissue with a finger near the infant's mouth and remove the infant when suction is released.

FREQUENCY OF FEEDINGS. Because breast milk moves through the stomach within 1.5 to 2 hours, infants usually feed every 2 to 3 hours. Frequent feedings are especially important in the early days after birth, while lactation is being established and stomach capacity is small. Explaining that the hormone prolactin, which is responsible for milk production, is released in increased amounts while the infant is suckling helps the mother understand the relationship of frequent feeding to milk supply.

Infants who are fed frequently during the daytime often sleep longer during the night. If possible the infant should be awakened every 3 hours for feeding during the early weeks of life to stimulate milk production (Association of Women's Health, Obstetric & Neonatal Nurses [AWHONN], 2000b). Infants should feed about every 4 hours during the night (Meek, 2002).

Long periods between feedings increase the likelihood of breast engorgement. The resulting decreased stimulation of prolactin may reduce milk supply. Generally, the mother should nurse 8 to 12 times in each 24-hour period.

Some infants may vary the length of feedings and time between each feeding. Several feedings close together (sometimes called "cluster feedings") are followed by a longer interval between feedings. Cluster feedings often occur in the

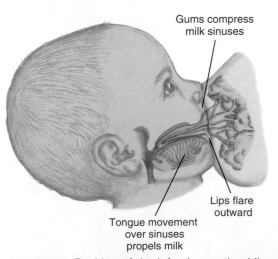

Figure 22-8 ■ Position of the infant's mouth while suckling. When the nipple and areola are properly positioned in the infant's mouth, the gums compress the ducts under the areola. The tongue is between the lower gum and breast. The tongue moves over the breast like a peristaltic wave to bring the milk forward into the infant's mouth. The infant's lips are flared outward.

Gums compress
milk sinuses

Lips flare
outward

Tongue movement
over sinuses
propels milk

late afternoon and early evening (Smith & Riordan, 2005). An infant's frequent need to nurse may cause the mother to think her milk supply is inadequate, when it may be normal. Strict scheduling of infant feedings is unnecessary and leads to frustration for both mother and infant. A mother should take her cues from her infant.

LENGTH OF FEEDINGS. Although early feedings were once limited to only a few minutes per breast in an attempt to prevent sore nipples, improper positioning, rather than time at breast, is the usual cause of nipple trauma. When feedings are too short, infants receive little or no colostrum or milk. It may take as long as 5 minutes for the milk-ejection (let-down) reflex to occur during the early days after birth.

Generally, mothers can allow the infant to set the length of feedings. The infant should suckle vigorously for a period of time. When choppy, nonnutritive suckling without the sound of swallowing occurs, the mother should burp the infant and complete the feeding at the other breast. When the infant is satisfied, the suckling pattern changes and the infant may fall asleep.

Mothers who are uneasy without a specific length of time for feedings can be instructed to start with feedings that last approximately 10 to 15 minutes on each side, or longer if the infant continues to nurse vigorously (AAP & ACOG, 2002).

Although variations in the length of feedings occur, feedings that last less than an average of 20 minutes and occur less than eight times in 24 hours may not be enough (Riordan & Hoover, 2005). Feeding time increases as needed by the infant over the next few days. Teach the mother that longer feedings do not cause nipple tenderness.

Explain the differences between foremilk, the watery first milk that quenches the infant's thirst, and hindmilk, which is richer in fat, is more satisfying, and leads to weight gain. Feeding for too short a time prevents the infant from getting the hindmilk and decreases weight gain.

Switching back and forth between breasts several times during a feeding increases the amount of foremilk the infant receives but decreases the amount of hindmilk. Therefore the mother should continue feeding on the first side as long as the infant nurses vigorously before burping and continuing on the other breast.

PREVENTING PROBLEMS. Women who intend to breastfeed but encounter difficulties that cause them to switch to formula feeding may express guilt and disappointment for months after the experience (Mozingo, Davis, Droppleman, & Merideth, 2000). Nurses can help prevent early problems in several ways.

Teaching. Once women leave the birth facility, they often have no one to advise them about breastfeeding. Help prevent problems after discharge by intensive teaching during the short birth facility stay. Check frequently on the woman as she feeds her infant so she can get her questions answered as she thinks of them. Allow ample time to answer questions.

Include suggestions on how to improve positioning and techniques. Discuss common problems that may occur after discharge and offer solutions. Some facilities hold classes for groups of women during the birth facility stay. If the birth facility provides follow-up telephone calls or home visits, explain the service.

Use breastfeeding pamphlets and videos, and review them with the mother before discharge. Before using pamphlets or videos, evaluate them to be sure that the information is correct and they contain no advertisements for formula.

Formula Gift Packs. Although there is lack of agreement about the effects of formula gift packs given to mothers at discharge, it is likely that having formula available sets up an expectation, at least for some mothers, that formula may be necessary. This is contrary to the message nurses should give to parents about breastfeeding.

Formula Supplementation. Healthy breastfeeding infants are unlikely to need supplements during the hospital stay (AAP & ACOG, 2002). Avoid the use of formula supplementation in the hospital unless there are medical indications. Formula supplementation and initiating feedings after the first hour after birth are associated with early termination of breastfeeding (DiGirolamo, Grummer-Strawn, & Fein, 2001).

Insufficient Milk Supply. One of the major reasons for early weaning to formula is mothers' perception of insufficient milk supply. Women with positive attitudes toward breastfeeding and confidence that they will produce enough milk are less likely to wean early because of perceived lack of enough milk. Explain the normal course of breastfeeding and methods of handling problems to help mothers feel more confident in their abilities.

Teach the mother how to assess swallowing and nutritive suckling. Discuss ways to determine if the infant is receiving enough milk. Suggest that the mother count the number of wet and soiled diapers to help her determine whether the infant is receiving enough milk. Infants should have at least six wet diapers daily by the fourth day and three stools a day after the first few days.

Mothers are not usually encouraged to weigh normal infants at home because it focuses too much attention on weight gain. Intake can also be gauged when the physician or nurse practitioner assesses weight gain at well-baby checkups. Following the initial weight loss after birth, infants generally gain approximately 25 to 30 g (0.88 to 1 oz) each day during the early months of life (Walker & Creehan, 2001). Weight gain generally begins by the fifth day of life. The infant should gain at least 113 to 198 g (4 to 7 oz) per week and at least 480 g (1 lb) per month (Smith & Riordan, 2005).

Common causes of decreased milk supply include formula use, inadequate rest or diet, smoking by the mother or others in the home, and use of caffeine, alcohol, or some medications. Use of oral contraceptives with estrogen decreases milk production. Intervene appropriately if any common causes are present. Although women were once taught to drink large quantities of liquids to maintain milk supply, fluid intake sufficient to satisfy the mother's thirst and to keep her urine light yellow is adequate.

Because the breasts are soft and the mother does not see large amounts of milk, she may believe that none is present. This may lead her to give the infant formula before or after the feeding, decreasing milk production. Teach mothers who need to increase milk supply to feed more often and to use a breast pump after feedings.

Some health care providers give mothers metoclopramide to increase prolactin levels when milk supply is inadequate. However, this drug has side effects such as depression. Domperidone is used in other countries to stimulate milk production but is not available in the United States at this time.

Women who continue to have difficulty with any aspect of breastfeeding should be referred to a lactation consultant. These professionals often are available in the birth facility and can help with the mechanics and psychosocial implications of breastfeeding.

Evaluation

Evaluation of interventions should be continued throughout the birth facility stay. Before discharge the infant should be feeding well at each breast. The woman should demonstrate feeding techniques and voice satisfaction with breastfeeding and confidence in her ability. Satisfaction and confidence are major determinants of whether she continues breastfeeding at home.

✓ CHECK YOUR READING

9. How can the nurse help the mother establish breastfeeding during the initial feeding sessions?
10. What should the nurse teach the mother about frequency and length of feedings?

COMMON BREASTFEEDING CONCERNS

Because mothers may be discharged from the birth facility before problems arise, nurses should teach them how to prevent and treat common difficulties. If the nurse is being consulted about problems that have developed after discharge, she should determine what the mother has done to solve the problem and ask about any complementary or alternative therapies the mother may have tried. The safety of any therapy should be determined.

The mother may have tried teas from fennel, fenugreek, dill, or aniseed to help in milk production, hot parsley compresses for engorgement, and olive oil, yarrow ointment, aloe vera gel, or washing the nipples with marigolds for sore nipples. Because there has not been adequate research on the use of these therapies, she should be referred to the health care provider for information about such substances, as some may be harmful to the mother or baby during lactation (Biancuzzo, 2003; Skidmore-Roth, 2004). Cabbage leaves have been used for engorgement, but most research does not show they are effective. Poultices of grated potato or carrot have also been suggested.

Problems may be divided into those originating with the infant and those involving the mother. (See Nursing Care Plan 22-1.)

Infant Problems

Infant problems generally involve a sleepy infant, suckling difficulties, and complications such as jaundice and prematurity. Crying and fussiness are common problems during the first weeks after birth for all infants (see Chapter 23).

Is My Baby Getting Enough Milk?

Your baby is probably getting enough milk if:
- You hear the baby swallow frequently during feedings. It sounds like a soft "ka" or "ah" sound.
- You see nutritive suckling—a smooth series of sucking and swallowing with occasional rest periods. This is different from short, choppy sucks that occur when the baby is falling asleep and not getting milk. After the first few days you may feel a tingling of your nipples each time a new let-down reflex occurs. This sensation is followed by more nutritive suckling as the infant swallows the increased milk available.
- Your breast is getting softer during the feeding. (However, your breasts do not have to be hard [engorged] for you to have enough milk for the baby.)
- You can see milk in the baby's mouth or dripping from your breast occasionally.
- You feed your baby 8 to 12 times every 24 hours. More milk is produced when you nurse more often. (Keep track, at first, by writing down the time you start each feeding. Once breastfeeding is well established, keeping close track of the time is not necessary; your baby will let you know when it is time for feedings.)
- Your baby has at least one or two wet diapers per day for the first 2 days after birth and at least six wet diapers per day by the fourth day. Disposable diapers are very absorbent, and knowing whether they are wet is sometimes hard. If you are unsure, place a tissue or cotton ball inside the diaper to show even small amounts of urine. Urine should be light yellow, not dark yellow.
- Your baby passes at least three bowel movements per day after the first few days and often more during the first month. The bowel movements are yellow in color by the fourth day.
- Your baby seems satisfied after feedings. Babies remain quietly awake or go to sleep for at least an hour after most feedings. (An occasional fussy time is not unusual and does not mean that the baby is not getting enough to eat.)
- Well-baby checkups show that your baby is gaining weight.

NURSING CARE PLAN 22-1 Breastfeeding an Infant Who Has Complications

ASSESSMENT: Ruth James' son, David, is full term but develops complications at birth and is admitted to the neonatal intensive care unit. Ruth had looked forward to breastfeeding her infant, but David will probably not be able to feed at the breast for a few days. Although Ruth understands the situation, she sounds disappointed and discouraged. She states that she will probably have to use formula after David is better because "it will be too late to start breastfeeding."

NURSING DIAGNOSIS: Interrupted Breastfeeding related to separation from infant secondary to illness

GOALS OR EXPECTED OUTCOMES: Within 2 days Ruth will:
1. Verbalize the importance of breastfeeding her infant and her desire to maintain lactation.
2. Pump her breasts as taught.
3. Breastfeed David successfully when it becomes possible.

INTERVENTIONS	RATIONALE
1. Explore Ruth's perception of the problem and her understanding of the cause for separation and its effect on breastfeeding.	1. Discussion of the problem identifies misconceptions and determines what teaching and support are required.
2. Use therapeutic communication techniques to help Ruth express her feelings of disappointment with the unexpected change in plans.	2. Helping the mother express her feelings and accepting them helps her cope with the situation.
3. Explain to Ruth how valuable breast milk is for her infant and that she can use a breast pump to maintain lactation until David is able to breastfeed.	3. Reinforcing the value of breastfeeding and offering encouragement increase the chance of success.
4. Teach Ruth how to use a breast pump and store her milk. Instruct her to pump her breasts for 15 to 20 minutes every 2 to 3 hours during the day and once or twice at night.	4. Frequent use of a breast pump helps establish lactation by causing release of prolactin and oxytocin so that milk is produced and released from the breasts.
5. Explain prevention and treatment of engorgement.	5. Frequent pumping should prevent engorgement. If it does not, the mother will need assistance in treating it.
6. Feed David breast milk if possible, whether by bottle or gavage. Teach Ruth how to store her milk and prepare it for use for her infant.	6. Breast milk has properties that are especially valuable for the sick infant.
7. Arrange for Ruth to spend as much time with David as possible. Stay with her during the early visits and when she begins to breastfeed to answer her questions and provide support.	7. Bonding occurs more easily if a mother is able to be with her baby. Accompanying a mother during visits with her infant allows the nurse an opportunity to offer support, encouragement, and teaching as needed.
8. When Ruth begins to breastfeed, offer the same teaching given to mothers of well infants. In addition, provide continued support if she has concerns.	8. Women who must delay breastfeeding may be more anxious about the process.
9. Offer praise and realistic encouragement frequently.	9. A mother needs reinforcement of her abilities to increase self-confidence as a mother. Encouragement must be suited to actual circumstances.
10. If Ruth must go home before David is ready for discharge, provide her with information about purchase or rental of a breast pump. Give her containers to bring her milk into the nursery.	10. The mother who must pump her breasts for a longer period of time may find that an electric pump is more efficient.

CRITICAL THINKING: What other interventions might be necessary if Ruth had flat nipples?

ANSWER: Reassure Ruth that she can breastfeed even if her nipples are flat. Teach her to roll her nipples just before David latches on to begin feeding.

EVALUATION: Ruth talks about her determination to provide breast milk for David. She maintains lactation and brings breast milk at each visit. At 5 days of age, David is ready to begin breastfeeding. Ruth is very patient in helping David learn to breastfeed with the nurses' help. David is able to nurse well at each feeding by discharge.

MOTHERS WANT TO KNOW

Solutions to Common Breastfeeding Problems

PROBLEM: SLEEPY INFANT

An infant is sleepy at feeding time or falls asleep shortly after beginning feeding.

Prevention

- Look for signs your baby is ready to wake up, such as movement of the eyes even though the eyelids are closed, small twitches of the face, sucking movements, stretching, and increased movements of the entire body.
- Gently awaken your baby. Talk, gently move the infant's arms and legs, and play with the infant for a short time before beginning the feeding.
- Unwrap the baby's blankets and change the diaper. Swaddling infants by wrapping them tightly with blankets is a calming technique that often helps them sleep. Leave the blanket off as you begin the feeding. Your body and a blanket draped over both of you after your baby begins to nurse will provide adequate warmth.

Solutions

If your baby goes to sleep during the feeding and has fed less than 5 minutes, try the following:

- Rub the baby's hair or cheeks gently, stroke around his or her mouth, or shift the baby's position slightly to see if the infant will wake up.
- Remove the baby from the breast. Rub his or her back to bring up bubbles of air that may cause a sensation of stomach fullness. Rubbing the back also stimulates the central nervous system and arouses the baby.
- Change the diaper.
- Undress the baby (except for the diaper) and place the infant against your skin.
- Express a few drops of colostrum onto the nipple. The baby tastes the colostrum as soon as the nipple is offered and often begins renewed suckling.
- Wash the baby's face gently with a lukewarm washcloth to help the infant wake up.

If your baby cannot be aroused with a few of the gentle techniques listed above, a longer sleep period may be needed. Let the infant sleep another half hour, then begin again. Watch for signs that indicate the baby is in a lighter phase of sleep and can be awakened more easily.

PROBLEM: NIPPLE CONFUSION

An infant who has taken bottles pushes the nipple out of the mouth and sucks poorly during breastfeeding. The infant has become confused about the way to suck from the breast and is using sucking movements used for bottle feeding.

Prevention

- Avoid all bottles and pacifiers unless absolutely necessary. If they are necessary, stop as soon as possible.
- Do not give the baby formula during the night. The extra sleep is not worth the possibility of later feeding difficulties.
- Avoid giving formula at the end of a breastfeeding session because it is unnecessary for healthy newborns. It may cause the infant's stomach to become distended and may result in more "spitting up." Adding formula will cause the infant to wait longer before nursing again, decreasing milk production.

Solution

- Stop all bottle feeding and pacifier use so that the baby gets used to suckling from the breast instead of the bottle. Nurse more often to stimulate milk production and help the baby learn what to do.

LATCH-ON PROBLEM

The infant sucks on the end of the nipple or fails to open his or her mouth widely enough.

Prevention

- Do not insert the breast into the infant's mouth until the infant opens his or her mouth wide with the tongue down and forward. Then bring the baby to the breast.
- Pull down gently on the infant's chin to help the infant open the mouth wider if necessary.
- Be sure that the baby has the nipple at the back of the mouth and 1 to 1½ inches of the areola in the mouth.

Solutions

- Stop the feeding and start again if the infant is sucking on the end of the nipple, you see dimples in the infant's cheeks, or you hear smacking, slurping, or clicking sounds. Short, choppy movement of the jaw means that the infant is going to sleep or has finished feeding.
- If you believe that the infant should nurse longer, awaken the infant and begin again.

PROBLEM: ENGORGEMENT

The mother's breasts are hard and tender from engorgement.

Prevention

- Breastfeed the infant every 2 to 3 hours day and night. Do not give a bottle during the night, as this increases the risk of engorgement. Waiting even 4 hours between feedings may increase the risk of engorgement, but frequent breastfeeding often can prevent it.

SLEEPY INFANT

During the first few days after birth, infants often sleep longer than expected or fall asleep at the breast after feeding for only a short time. They may be tired from the birth process and may not recognize or respond appropriately to hunger. Infants of mothers who received sedation in labor suck at lower rates and pressure and take less milk than infants of unsedated mothers (Heird, 2004). This resolves when the medication effects have worn off.

The nurse should show mothers how to arouse sleepy infants for breastfeeding (see "Mothers Want to Know: Solutions to Common Breastfeeding Problems"). If infants start the feeding fully awake, they are more likely to stay awake to

Solutions

- To reduce edema and nipple pain, apply cold packs to the breasts between feedings. Use commercial cold packs or make inexpensive cold packs from frozen washcloths, packages of frozen vegetables, or clean disposable gloves or plastic bags filled with crushed ice. Cover cold pack with a washcloth before applying it to the skin. A disposable diaper with crushed ice placed between the layers may also be used.
- Just before feedings, take a shower so the heat can stimulate milk flow. Alternatively, apply heat with compresses or a disposable diaper wet with warm water. Apply the diaper over each breast and fasten the tabs to keep it in place and prevent dripping.
- Massage the breasts before and during feedings to stimulate the let-down reflex so the baby can nurse more easily. Massaging the breasts in the shower provides comfort and helps prepare for feeding.
- If the areola are engorged and hard, making it hard for the baby to latch on, express a little milk by hand or with a breast pump. As soon as the areola is soft, begin to feed.
- Feed more often, such as every 1.5 to 2 hours.
- Wear a well-fitting bra for support during the day and at night for comfort.
- Take prescribed pain medication just before feedings, to make you more comfortable.

PROBLEM: SORE NIPPLES

The nipples are sore and may be cracked, blistered, or bleeding.

Prevention

- Position the baby at the breast with enough of the areola in the mouth that the nipple is not compressed between the baby's gums during nursing.
- Avoid engorgement by nursing frequently. Express enough milk to soften the areola if engorgement makes the areola too hard for the infant to grasp.
- Do not use soap on the nipples because it removes the protective oils and causes drying.
- If you use breast pads for leaking milk, remove them when they become wet to prevent irritation of the skin. Avoid pads with plastic linings that retain moisture. Use a handkerchief or pieces of cotton cloth as inexpensive, washable substitutes for commercial breast pads.
- Breast creams may cause sensitivity and irritation. If you choose to use lanolin, use only purified lanolin to protect against allergens. Creams that have to be removed before each feeding may increase soreness.

Solutions

- Begin each feeding with the less sore side first. The hungry baby nurses more vigorously at first, which may be painful. The let-down reflex is started, causing milk to flow more quickly from the second breast. Using warm compresses will also help the milk to flow more quickly.
- Vary the position of the infant during nursing. The area of the nipple directly in line with the infant's nose and chin is most stressed during the feeding.
- Massage the breasts during feedings to enhance milk flow.
- Do not use nipple shields (latex nipples that fit over your own nipples) without help from a lactation consultant. They decrease milk flow, so the baby receives less and milk production is decreased.
- Apply colostrum or breast milk to the nipples after feedings because these have healing properties. Or apply warm water compresses to the nipples.
- Expose the nipples to air between feedings by lowering the flaps of your nursing bra.
- Hydrogel dressings may be helpful in relieving pain and promoting healing. Use according to directions.
- If you have burning, itching, or stabbing pain throughout your breast, look in the baby's mouth for white patches of thrush, a yeast infection that can infect the nipples. Call the health care provider for medication to treat both you and your baby.

PROBLEM: FLAT OR INVERTED NIPPLES

The mother's nipples are flat or inverted, and the baby has difficulty drawing them into his or her mouth.

Prevention

None.

Solutions

- Wearing breast shells in your bra may help make the nipples protrude.
- Just before beginning breastfeeding, apply a cold cloth or roll the nipple between your thumb and forefinger to help it protrude (see Figure 22-12).
- Use a breast pump just before feedings. Put the baby to your breast immediately after the pump causes the nipple to become erect. Once the infant gets the nipple in his or her mouth, the normal suckling process usually causes the nipple to stay erect.
- A nipple shield may be used for a short time with the help of a lactation consultant to help the infant latch onto inverted nipples.

finish the feeding. Pointing out the various behavioral states to the mother helps her develop a greater understanding of her infant and recognize when attempts to feed will be most successful.

When the infant falls asleep during feedings, the nurse should evaluate whether the infant has fed adequately, should be awakened to feed longer, or should be fed again sooner than usual. Emphasizing that wake-up techniques should be gentle is important. The mother should avoid excessively irritating techniques, because breastfeeding should be associated with pleasurable sensations. Infants who continue to be excessively sleepy or nurse poorly need further evaluation. Poor feeding may be an early sign of a complication such as sepsis (see Chapter 30).

NIPPLE CONFUSION

Nipple confusion (or nipple preference) may occur when an infant who has been fed by bottle confuses the tongue movements necessary for bottle feeding with the suckling of breastfeeding. Some infants develop a preference for bottle feeding and refuse to breastfeed. Others use bottle feeding tongue movements that impede breastfeeding.

Movements of the mouth and tongue are different in breastfeeding and bottle feeding. To feed from a bottle, infants must push the tongue over the nipple to slow the flow of milk and prevent choking (Figure 22-9). This can be demonstrated by noting the steady drip of milk when a bottle is held upside down. In bottle feeding, the infant's lips are relaxed because the infant does not need to hold the nipple in place. If the infant uses the same thrusting tongue motion and relaxed lips while nursing, the breast may be pushed out of the mouth.

During breastfeeding, the infant uses suction to hold the nipple in place near the soft palate. The tongue cups around the nipple and areola with the tip over the lower gum. With each compression of the lower jaw, the tongue presses

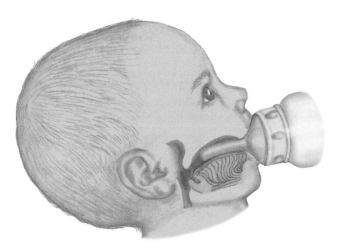

Tongue thrusts forward
to control milk flow

Figure 22-9 ■ During bottle feeding, infants must push the tongue over the nipple to slow the rapid flow of milk.

against the breast like a peristaltic wave, causing the milk to move forward from the ducts and into the infant's mouth.

Nurses should discourage use of formula in normal breastfeeding infants. Formula use reduces breastfeeding time, which decreases prolactin secretion and therefore milk production. Formula takes longer to digest, and the infant is not hungry again for about 4 hours. The increased time between breastfeedings limits breast stimulation and may lead to engorgement.

Pacifier use is controversial. Parents often find them helpful, but pacifier use is associated with suckling problems and an earlier weaning from the breast for some infants (Biancuzzo, 2003). Although some infants can use a pacifier without ensuing problems with breastfeeding, the use of pacifiers should be discouraged at least until the infant is breastfeeding successfully (AWHONN, 2000b).

SUCKLING PROBLEMS

Suckling problems may occur when the nipple is poorly positioned in the infant's mouth. Dimpling of the cheeks and smacking or clicking sounds may indicate that the infant is sucking on the tongue or nipple only. Some infants do not open their mouths widely enough and suck on the end of the nipple. Short, choppy motions of the jaw signal nonnutritive suckling.

Inserting a gloved finger into the infant's mouth helps assess suckling. The peristaltic motion of the tongue should be felt as the infant sucks. The infant who is thrusting the tongue may have become confused by the use of latex nipples, which should be avoided until the problem is resolved. If the infant tends to place the tongue on top of the nipple, inserting a finger in the mouth and pressing the infant's tongue down just before latch-on may be effective. The tongue should be cupped under the breast and should cover the lower gum. Helping the infant open the mouth widely before attachment may improve suckling. More complicated suckling problems may require assistance from a lactation educator or consultant.

✔ **CHECK YOUR READING**

11. What wake-up techniques should the nurse teach the mother of a sleepy infant?
12. How does sucking from a bottle differ from suckling from the breast?

INFANT COMPLICATIONS

Infant complications may be minor and cause minimal interference with breastfeeding or may prevent the infant from breastfeeding for a long period.

JAUNDICE. Jaundice (hyperbilirubinemia) need not interfere with breastfeeding. Even when infants receive phototherapy, they usually can be removed from the lights for feedings. Concern about adequate intake may be more prevalent in caring for the infant with jaundice. Insensible water loss from the skin is increased as a result of the heat and lights used in treatment and could lead to dehydration.

Infants receiving phototherapy should not be given extra water, which may decrease the intake of breast milk. Decreased intestinal motility from insufficient milk intake allows reabsorption of bilirubin through the intestinal wall into the bloodstream, increasing the work of the immature liver. Frequent breastfeeding increases the number of stools, which aids in bilirubin excretion and provides adequate intake of protein and fluid. (Jaundice is discussed in Chapters 19 and 30.)

PREMATURITY. If the preterm infant cannot breastfeed immediately after birth, the mother needs encouragement and instruction about using a breast pump to establish and maintain her milk supply. Breast milk offers immunologic and nutritional benefits and is adapted to preterm needs. It may help prevent or minimize the severity of necrotizing enterocolitis, a serious complication of prematurity. It also helps the mother feel she is providing care for her infant even if she cannot take the infant home with her.

The woman can pump her milk and take it to the nursery for the infant's feedings. The nurse should provide sterile containers for the woman to take home and instruct her in special nursery requirements. In some cases mothers are taught to separate the foremilk from the hindmilk to provide a higher caloric intake for their preterm infants. They may even learn to measure the fat content of the milk so that the milk with the highest fat levels is used (Griffin, Meier, Bradford, Bigger, & Engstrom, 2000).

Some preterm infants or those with breastfeeding problems respond well to the use of supplementary feeding devices. These consist of a container of milk with a small plastic feeding tube attached to the breast. When the infant begins to breastfeed, milk is drawn from both the container and the breast, increasing the infant's intake and motivation to continue suckling. As the infant gains weight and feeding ability increases, use of the device is gradually decreased until it can be discontinued completely.

Women who provide breast milk for their preterm infants may feel something is wrong with their milk when additions such as human milk fortifier are used. They should be reassured that their milk is very important in providing protection against infection and good nutrition but that the infant needs more of some nutrients during the period of very rapid growth.

ILLNESS AND CONGENITAL DEFECTS

Infant illness and congenital defects such as a cleft palate may cause breastfeeding problems. If the mother is not able to nurse the infant at first, she will need assistance to maintain lactation until nursing is possible. Referral to support groups can be particularly helpful. Some groups focus on particular congenital defects, and others focus on breastfeeding infants with special problems.

Maternal Concerns

The most frequent breastfeeding problems of the mother involve concerns about the breasts and nipples. The mother who is ill needs special help to continue breastfeeding. Other common concerns include feeding after multiple births, working, and weaning.

CRITICAL TO REMEMBER

Maternal Signs of Breastfeeding Problems

Hard, tender breasts
Painful, red, cracked, blistered, or bleeding nipples
Flat or inverted nipples
Localized edema or pain in either breast
Fever, generalized aching, or malaise

COMMON BREAST PROBLEMS

Engorgement, nipple trauma, flat or inverted nipples, plugged ducts, and mastitis are common problems involving the breasts.

ENGORGEMENT. Many women have a temporary swelling or fullness of the breasts when the milk begins to "come in" or change from colostrum to transitional breast milk. This usually occurs on the second or third day after birth but may begin earlier in women who have nursed previously. This normal engorgement is the result of accumulation of milk, enlarged lymph glands, and increased blood flow. It should not interfere with breastfeeding.

Engorgement may also be caused by milk retention if feedings are delayed, too short, or infrequent. When this occurs, the breasts become edematous, hard, and tender, making feeding and even movement painful. The areola may become so hard that the infant cannot compress it for nursing. An engorged areola causes the nipple to become flat, making it more difficult for the infant to draw it into the back of the mouth. Engorgement may lead to nipple trauma, mastitis, and even the discontinuation of breastfeeding.

Nurses help prevent engorgement by assisting women to begin breastfeeding early and to feed frequently. Encouraging mothers to breastfeed at night, unless extenuating circumstances are present, ensures that the breasts are emptied regularly. The use of water and formula should be discouraged.

The nurse should teach women with engorgement about application of cold and heat, massage, and breastfeeding techniques. Cold is used after feedings to reduce edema and pain. Heat applied just before feedings increases vasodilation and milk flow. Prolonged heat may increase edema. Massage of the breasts causes release of oxytocin and increases the speed of milk release. This decreases the length of time the infant nurses on painful breasts (Figure 22-10).

A well-fitting bra may be worn both day and night to help support the breasts. The bra should not be uncomfortable or press into the breast tissues. It should be easily opened with one hand for feedings.

If the areola is too engorged for the infant to compress it, the nurse should help the mother express milk by hand or with a breast pump to soften the areola. Nurses should wear gloves if they might come in contact with colostrum or breast milk, as for any other body fluid.

Mothers with engorgement may need medication for discomfort so that they can relax while breastfeeding. Medica-

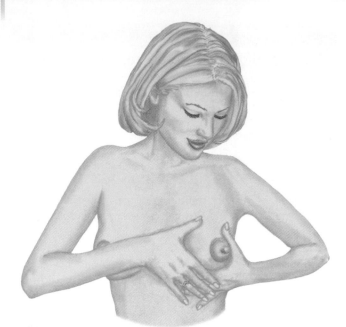

Figure 22-10 ■ To massage the breasts, the mother places her hands against the chest wall with her fingers encircling the breasts. She gently slides her hands forward until the fingers overlap. The position of the hands is rotated to cover all breast tissue. Massaging with the fingertips in a circular motion over all areas of the breast is also helpful.

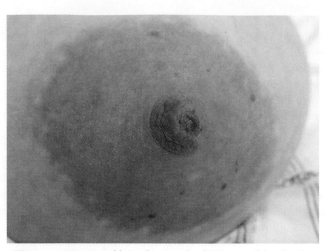

Figure 22-11 ■ Note the cracked area on this nipple.

tions such as acetaminophen, ibuprofen, and other commonly prescribed drugs for postpartum discomfort are considered safe during lactation (AAP, 2001).

NIPPLE PAIN. Nipple pain is common during early breastfeeding. Pain for a minute or less may occur at the be-

ginning of feedings because of tissue stretching and suction on the ductules before they fill with milk. Nipple pain usually peaks at the third to sixth day and resolves soon afterward (Smith & Riordan, 2005). Nipple trauma causes more sustained pain. Traumatized nipples appear red, cracked, blistered, or bleeding (Figure 22-11). Minor nipple trauma can be treated by independent nursing interventions. Redness of breast tissue, purulent drainage, and fever indicate mastitis or breast abscess and require antibiotic treatment (see Chapter 28, p. 749).

Improper positioning or latch-on techniques and exposure to soaps, prolonged moisture from wet breast pads, or irritating creams may cause sore nipples. Using a breast pump too long or with the suction set on high may be traumatic. (See Nursing Care Plan 22-2.)

THERAPEUTIC COMMUNICATIONS

Anxiety about Breastfeeding

Jenny Lavelle gave birth to her second baby, Danny, by cesarean. She tells her nurse, Yvonne Hernandez, that she breastfed her first infant for a week and then switched to bottle feeding because she didn't have enough milk. Danny is a sleepy baby but does nurse at times. Jenny's breasts are engorged, and her nipples are sore.

Jenny: I really wanted to nurse Danny, but I don't know if it's worth the effort. My breasts hurt, and I don't know if he's getting enough milk. I probably should just use the bottle again.

Yvonne: You sound really discouraged! *(Reflecting the feelings expressed.)*

Jenny: When I couldn't nurse my daughter, I was so disappointed. I had this "Mother Earth" view of the kind of mother I was going to be. But the baby wouldn't stop crying, so I went to the bottle.

Yvonne: That must have been hard for you! *(Reflecting the feelings expressed.)*

Jenny: It was awful, and now it looks like I'm going to fail again. Danny won't nurse half the time, and I'm going home this afternoon.

Yvonne: And you're worried about what's going to happen at home. *(Seeking clarification of the mother's concerns.)*

Jenny: What if he won't nurse at home? I don't know what to do!

Yvonne: Breastfeeding isn't always easy. Mothers and babies both have to learn the process, and that takes time and a lot of patience. Danny's hungry now—would you like to try again? I'll stay with you and answer your questions. *(Offering realistic encouragement and assistance in techniques.)*

Jenny: That would be great! Maybe I'll get the hang of this yet!

(By allowing Jenny to express her feelings of discouragement and disappointment before beginning to teach, the nurse learns how important breastfeeding is to Jenny and how best to go about teaching her. Jenny feels accepted even though she is discouraged.)

NURSING CARE PLAN 22-2 Engorged Breasts and Painful Nipples

ASSESSMENT: Sally Portner says during a feeding, "I'm going to give a bottle for the next few feedings. I'm too sore to nurse anymore today." Her breasts are engorged, warm, and tender. Her son, Grady, has difficulty grasping Sally's nipple and areola to feed. Her nipples are everted but red. There are no blisters, fissures, or bleeding. Sally says she has been breastfeeding for about 5 minutes per side every 4 to 4½ hours. She holds Grady lying on his back with his hips and legs lower than the rest of his body during feedings. A few swallowing sounds are heard during nursing.

>*CRITICAL THINKING: Evaluate the information above and assign a LATCH score that can be used in planning care for Sally and Grady. (See Table 22-1.)*
>
>*ANSWER: The LATCH score is 6. One point is given for latch, one for audible swallowing, one for comfort, and one for hold. Two points are given for type of nipple. The focus of teaching will be on improving the areas where only one point is assigned.*

NURSING DIAGNOSIS: Impaired Skin Integrity related to incorrect positioning and engorgement

GOALS OR EXPECTED OUTCOMES: Sally will:
1. Demonstrate correct positioning by the next feeding.
2. Describe prevention and treatment of engorgement and sore nipples within 1 day.
3. Have no engorgement or redness of the nipples within 2 days.

INTERVENTION	RATIONALE
1. Suggest that Sally shower or apply warm compresses (such as clean wet disposable diapers) to her breasts before feeding.	1. Heat dilates blood vessels and milk ducts, encourages the let-down reflex, and relieves pain.
2. Offer Sally ordered medication just before feedings. Be sure that the medication ordered is safe for the infant.	2. Medication relieves pain that could interfere with the let-down reflex, yet only minimal amounts reach breast milk within the feeding time.
3. Demonstrate gentle massage of the breasts before feedings.	3. Massage causes release of oxytocin, resulting in the let-down reflex. The infant gets milk more quickly, reducing nonproductive time on a painful breast.
4. Demonstrate hand expression or use of a breast pump if necessary to soften the areola enough so Grady can grasp it to suckle.	4. If the areola is hard, the infant compresses the nipple rather than the milk ducts because the nipple is not deep enough in the mouth. This causes nipple trauma, inadequate emptying, and decreased milk production.
5. Demonstrate correct positioning of the infant. For the cradle and cross-cradle positions, place Grady on his side so he faces the nipple with his abdomen against Sally.	5. If the infant must turn his head to feed, it interferes with swallowing and causes traction on the nipple.
6. Suggest that Sally use a variety of positions for feeding and demonstrate each.	6. Changing the area of stress on the nipple allows healing of the sore area.
7. Have Sally begin the feeding on the less sore side.	7. The let-down reflex occurs in both breasts at once. Vigorous suckling on the sore side before let-down increases nipple trauma.
8. Assess Grady's mouth position by gently pulling down the lower lip to see that his tongue covers the lower gum. If the lower lip is turned in, gently pull it out so the lips flare. Assess the position of the nipple.	8. The tongue cushions the lower gum compression of the areola. A turned-in lower lip causes a friction rub on the nipple and areola. If the lips are 1 to 1½ inches from the base of the nipple, the nipple should be at the back of infant's mouth.
9. Instruct Sally to wear a well-fitting bra.	9. A bra provides support to painful breasts.
10. Prevent further engorgement by teaching Sally to feed Grady every 2 to 3 hours during the day and at least every 4 hours at night for a total of 8 to 12 feedings per day. She should feed an average of at least 20 minutes of effective suckling per feeding.	10. Frequent feedings empty the breasts, prevent stasis, stimulate milk production, and reduce the risk of mastitis. Adequate length allows time for the let-down reflex, which may be delayed at first, to occur.
11. Teach Sally to apply warm water compresses or colostrum to the sore nipples after feedings. Instruct her to leave the flaps of her nursing bra down between feedings. Ice packs can be used on the breasts after feeding for engorgement.	11. Warm water compresses are soothing. Colostrum has lysosomes and healing properties. Increased air circulation promotes healing. Ice packs help reduce edema of the breast tissue.
12. Teach Sally to avoid creams that must be removed before nursing or to which she may have allergies. If she uses breast pads, suggest that she change them frequently. Tell her to avoid soap on her nipples.	12. Cream removal, allergies, and wet pads increase irritation. Prolonged exposure to wet pads can cause maceration and breakdown of skin. Soap removes protective oils from nipples.

Continued

NURSING CARE PLAN 22-2 Engorged Breasts and Painful Nipples—cont'd

CRITICAL THINKING: *Should Sally use a bottle for the next few feedings?*

ANSWER: *If Sally skips feedings, her engorgement will increase. Grady will not be ready to feed again for 3 to 4 hours after taking formula, increasing the time between breastfeedings. The lack of suckling and engorgement decrease milk production. Using the interventions listed, Sally should be able to breastfeed with less discomfort and prevent further problems.*

EVALUATION: Sally breastfeeds Grady every 2 to 3 hours for approximately 15 minutes per side during the day and every 4 hours at night. She positions Grady correctly and discusses causes and care for sore nipples. When she is seen by the home visit nurse on the day after discharge, her engorgement, nipple redness, and tenderness have resolved. Sally verbalizes methods she will use to prevent further engorgement.

Care. Teaching includes correcting causes of nipple trauma. Helping the mother with proper positioning may be the most important solution. Increasing air flow to the nipples, feeding on the less inflamed side first, and varying positions at each feeding to rotate strain on the nipples also may be helpful. Expressing a small amount of milk to begin the letdown reflex may decrease vigorous suckling on sore nipples.

Studies have not shown that any one comfort measure is significantly more effective than others in treating painful nipples. More research is needed in this area. Warm water compresses may have some effectiveness in reducing pain. Wet tea bags help some mothers but may cause dryness and cracking in others. Application of breast milk to the nipples after feedings may be helpful. Breast milk helps prevent infection and aids in healing because it contains lysozymes.

Ointments are no more effective than other treatments. Women who plan to use lanolin should use only USP modified lanolin that has no pesticides and is hypoallergenic. Many creams have to be removed before feeding and may further irritate sore nipples. Antibiotic creams may be necessary if there is an infection. Hydrogel dressings provide a mechanical barrier and a moist wound environment that helps reduce pain and heal damaged skin. The dressings are removed during feedings and then reapplied (Dodd & Chalmers, 2003). They should not be used if there is an infection (Smith & Riordan, 2005).

Nipple pain that does not respond to correction of latch-on techniques and nursing interventions may be a sign of bacterial or yeast infections. Mothers with vaginal candidiasis may transmit it to the infant during birth. If oral infection with *C. albicans* (thrush) develops in the infant, the mother's nipples may become infected. The infant may have visible white patches in the mouth. The woman has burning, itching, or stabbing pain throughout the breast. The health care provider should be notified, and both mother and infant are treated.

The use of nipple shields–nipples with wide bases that are placed over a mother's own nipple–is controversial. The shields are used by some mothers to decrease pain during feedings or help the baby latch on to inverted nipples. However, shields may interfere with adequate emptying of the breast and markedly reduce the amount of milk the infant receives. Although use of shields should be discouraged in general, they may be used temporarily in some situations to help an infant who cannot latch on to the breast. A lactation consultant should be involved in helping the mother avoid decreasing milk production and wean the baby away from the shield and back to the breast.

FLAT AND INVERTED NIPPLES. Nipple abnormalities should be treated during pregnancy if possible, but interventions can begin after birth if necessary. Use of breast shells can be taught at this time. Nipple rolling just before feeding helps flat nipples become more erect so the infant can grasp them more readily (Figure 22-12). A breast pump used for a few minutes before feedings may help draw out inverted nipples.

✔ CHECK YOUR READING

13. How can the nurse help the mother who has engorged breasts?
14. How should the nurse advise the mother with sore nipples?

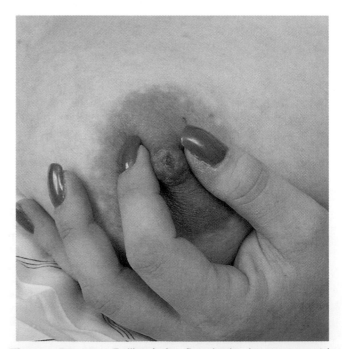

Figure 22-12 ■ Rolling helps flat nipples become erect in preparation for latch-on.

PLUGGED DUCTS. Although the exact cause of occlusion of a lactiferous duct is unknown, engorgement, missed feedings, or a constricting bra may be involved. Localized edema and tenderness are present, and a hard area may be palpated. A tiny, white area may be present on the nipple. Massage of the area followed by heat and continued breastfeeding using varied positions cause the duct to open. The infant should be allowed to nurse for an adequate amount of time after let-down. A plugged duct may progress to mastitis if not treated promptly. Mastitis involves localized pain accompanied by fever, generalized aching, and malaise (see Chapter 28, p. 749).

ILLNESS IN THE MOTHER

When the mother is ill, breastfeeding may have to be postponed temporarily because of the mother's condition or the drugs she receives. When breastfeeding must be stopped, abrupt weaning may lead to mastitis. The mother may be depressed about having to stop her chosen method of feeding. The nurse should help the mother use a breast pump, if she wishes, until she resumes breastfeeding.

DRUG TRANSFER TO BREAST MILK

Most medications taken by the mother cross into the breast milk to some degree, but many pass in very small amounts and are safe for the mother to take during lactation. Some interfere with milk production. Therefore both prescription drugs and over-the-counter drugs should be approved by a physician. Another drug often can be substituted for one that adversely affects the infant. If a mother must take a drug that will be harmful to her infant, she should pump her breasts while she is taking the medication. Once the drug clears her bloodstream, she may resume breastfeeding (see Appendix B). Some drugs may not reach the infant in harmful amounts if taken after a feeding or at night when there is a longer time between feedings.

CONDITIONS IN WHICH BREASTFEEDING SHOULD BE AVOIDED. In some situations, such as a mother's serious illness that can be transmitted to the infant, breastfeeding is contraindicated. Examples are active tuberculosis, human immunodeficiency virus (HIV) infection, and galactosemia. Maternal drug abuse also is usually a contraindication. Mothers with hepatitis A, B, or C may breastfeed. Infants of mothers with hepatitis B should receive hepatitis B immune globulin before breastfeeding. Herpes simplex does not preclude breastfeeding if the mother does not have a lesion on her breast and uses good handwashing (AAP & ACOG, 2002; Biancuzzo, 2003).

PREVIOUS BREAST SURGERY

Women who have had surgery such as breast reduction or augmentation may have difficulty with lactation. The ability to produce and transfer the milk to the nipple depends on the surgical technique used and the amount of tissue involved. Surgery may disrupt the neural pathways, ducts, and blood supply. Some women can breastfeed without problems, and others may be able to do so using a supplemen-

tation device to help build up milk supply when the breasts are able to produce only a small amount of milk.

EMPLOYMENT

Although women who are employed begin to breastfeed in the hospital at a rate similar to unemployed women, they are less likely to still be breastfeeding at 6 months (Ross Products Division, 2003). Help from nurses can assist women to combine working and breastfeeding very well. Because breastfeeding infants have a lower incidence of illnesses than those who are formula fed, nursing mothers are less likely to miss work because their baby is sick. Recognizing this, some employers provide breastfeeding women such services as a place and time to pump, education and support from a lactation consultant, and other assistance to encourage breastfeeding (Ortiz, McGilligan, & Kelly, 2004).

Planning ahead makes the transition from home to work easier. Milk supply can be well established by frequent breastfeeding in the early weeks. A week or two before she returns to work, the mother should use a breast pump once or twice a day to practice pumping her breasts and build up a small supply of frozen breast milk. This avoids the stress of having to learn the technique or worry about having enough milk while adjusting to the work situation.

Most working mothers use a battery-operated or an electric pump once or twice a day during lunch or breaks. Some mothers pump for only a short time (5 minutes) during breaks to relieve engorgement and then pump for a longer time at meal time. The woman needs to find a place where she can pump in privacy. The milk should be refrigerated or placed in an insulated container with ice and can be used for the next day's feeding. Breastfeeding just before leaving for work and again as soon as the mother returns home keeps the time between feedings at a minimum. The infant is breastfed frequently throughout the evening hours and on weekends to build up the milk supply.

Some mothers choose to use formula during work hours but breastfeed when at home. They should prepare for this by gradually eliminating the feedings that occur during work hours and substituting a bottle. Although the total milk supply is diminished, breastfeeding can continue in the mornings and evenings.

MILK EXPRESSION

When milk expression is needed, the nurse helps the mother use hand expression (Figure 22-13) or a breast pump (Figure 22-14). Hand expression can be performed without other equipment but is not as effective as a breast pump. Hand expression or manual pumps are useful for the mother who wants to save breast milk for another feeding or whose areola is so engorged that the infant cannot grasp it.

USE OF A BREAST PUMP

The mother who plans to pump her milk for a prolonged period may prefer using a battery-operated or electric breast pump. Battery-operated pumps are small, portable, and rel-

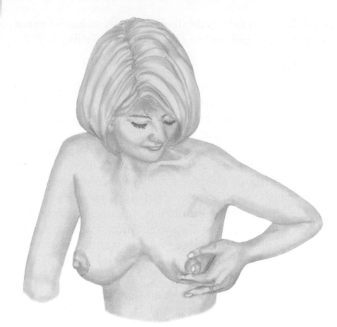

Figure 22-13 ■ To express milk from the breast, the mother places her hand just behind the areola, with the thumb on top and the fingers supporting the breast. The tissue is pressed back against the chest wall, then the fingers and thumb are brought together and toward the nipple. This compresses the ducts and causes milk to flow. The action is repeated to simulate the suckling of the infant. Moving the hands around the areola allows compression of all areas and increases removal of milk from the breast. Compression should be gentle to avoid trauma. Application of heat and massage before expression increases the flow of milk.

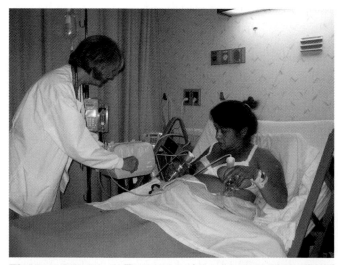

Figure 22-14 ■ The nurse demonstrates methods of pumping breast milk.

atively inexpensive. Large electric pumps can be rented for home use. They are more efficient than hand or battery pumps and are indicated when the mother must pump to maintain her milk supply for a long time. Double pumps that can be used on both breasts at once save time and increase production.

Use of the breast pump should begin within the first 24 hours after birth for the woman who cannot breastfeed her infant. She should pump her breasts as often as the infant would nurse, approximately every 2 to 3 hours during the day and once or twice at night when prolactin levels are elevated. Pumping sessions should last approximately 15 to 20 minutes. A total of eight or more sessions in each 24 hours is best to maintain milk supply.

Massage and application of heat before pumping help initiate the flow of milk. Massage of each quadrant of the breast during pumping may increase the volume of milk obtained at each session. Pumping before or after the first morning feeding often produces the greatest volume. Some women find pumping on one breast while nursing the infant from the other helpful. Relaxation during pumping increases volume, but tension or discomfort may reduce output. The mother should plan enough time for pumping that she does not feel hurried, as that would increase tension and decrease output.

Moistening the breast before attaching the pump improves suction. The amount of suction should be set at a low level in the beginning and gradually increased if necessary. Too much negative pressure traumatizes the breast. If the woman needs to increase her milk supply, pumping more often rather than for longer periods of time is most effective. The pump should be discontinued when the flow of milk stops, because continuing may cause pain and trauma.

Breast pumps should be cleaned according to the manufacturer's instructions after each use. The mother should wash her hands before using the pump and before preparing pumped milk for feeding.

MILK STORAGE

Milk should be stored in clean (sterile for a hospitalized infant) glass or plastic containers with a tight cap. A cap instead of a nipple is used to cover the container during storage because organisms could pass through the hole and contaminate the milk. Rigid plastic containers are easier to use than plastic bottle liners, which may spill or be punctured easily.

The milk can be kept in a refrigerator for 48 hours, if colder than 4° C (39° F). It can be stored in the back of a freezer that is a separate compartment of a refrigerator at −20° C (−4° F), approximately the temperature that keeps ice cream hard, for 3 months. It can be kept in a deep freeze for 6 months (Biancuzzo, 2003). Leukocytes are destroyed by freezing, but most other immunologic properties are preserved. Containers should be labeled with the date so that the oldest is used first.

Milk should be frozen in amounts likely to be used at one feeding. Milk left from one feeding should not be used for another feeding. If necessary, more milk can be defrosted when needed. Warm milk should not be added to frozen milk for storage. Cooled milk can be added to frozen milk if the amount added is less than the amount frozen (La Leche League International, 2003).

Breast milk can be thawed and warmed by holding the container under running water. Cool water should be used first to defrost it, then the milk can be warmed by placing it under warm running water or in a bowl of warm water. It should not be refrozen or heated in a microwave. A microwave heats milk unevenly and may burn the infant because a cool container may have hot spots in the milk. Refrigerated milk should be used as much as possible so that the leukocytes are available for the infant. Thawed breast milk should be gently inverted a few times to mix the foremilk and hindmilk.

BREASTFEEDING AFTER MULTIPLE BIRTHS

Mothers who have more than one newborn have many questions about breastfeeding and need help and support from nurses and family members to be successful. Nursing every 2 to 3 hours to build up the milk supply is important. If the infants are unable to breastfeed, the woman will need help using a breast pump.

If the woman decides to feed two infants simultaneously, she will need help positioning them using the football hold, cradle hold, or a combination of both. She should be encouraged to eat well, get enough rest, and ask for help from family and friends. (See "Mothers Want to Know: Breastfeeding after the Birth of More Than One Infant.")

WEANING

Mothers are sometimes subjected to opinions and pressure from family and friends about weaning. No one "right" time to wean the infant exists. Mothers choose to wean their infants for various reasons. The nurse should provide information so that women can make informed decisions about weaning and should support the woman once her decision is made. Explaining that even a short period of breastfeeding offers her infant many advantages is reassuring.

Mothers may need help in planning a gradual weaning process, if possible. This allows them to avoid engorgement, and infants can get used to a bottle or cup over a period of time. Mothers who are not in a hurry to wean may allow the infant to take the lead. Omitting one breastfeeding session a day and waiting several days or a week before omitting another will allow the mother and infant to adjust to the change more easily.

MOTHERS WANT TO KNOW   Breastfeeding after the Birth of More Than One Infant

ENSURING ADEQUATE MILK PRODUCTION

Because the amount of milk produced depends on the amount of suckling the breasts receive, mothers can produce enough milk for more than one baby. Nursing frequently (every 2 to 3 hours) helps build up the milk supply. Production of milk may be more evenly stimulated if you alternate breasts for each infant, especially if one baby has a weaker suck.

USING A BREAST PUMP

If your infants are not ready for breastfeeding, use a breast pump to build up your milk supply and provide milk for them until they are ready to breastfeed. Use the pump every 2 to 3 hours while you are awake and once or twice during the night. Pump for 15 to 20 minutes during at least 8 pumping sessions daily. Use a double pump to decrease the time spent pumping and increase the production of milk.

If one baby is ready to breastfeed before the other(s), nurse the baby and pump your breasts after each feeding to stimulate milk production. An alternative is to nurse the infant on one breast and use a breast pump on the other at the same time.

FEEDING SIMULTANEOUSLY OR INDIVIDUALLY

You can feed each baby individually or feed two infants at once. Simultaneous nursing shortens feeding times, but both infants must be awake at once. You need help positioning the infants at first. Individual feeding can be done without help and on each infant's own schedule, but a larger portion of your day will be spent feeding. It may be necessary to feed the infants separately at first and begin simultaneous feedings when each infant is nursing well at the breast.

POSITIONING INFANTS FOR SIMULTANEOUS FEEDING

Use a variety of positions for breastfeeding two infants at once. Place pillows under both infants to bring them to the right height and keep them in place. Use pillows under your arms and behind your back so that you are comfortable.

- Football Hold—Place each infant's head on your lap and support each infant's body with pillows alongside your body. Place a hand under each infant's head and bring the infants to the nipples.
- Football and Cradle Hold—Place one infant in a cradle position on pillows across your lap. Place the other in a football position with the body supported on pillows alongside you. Once the infants are in position, help one and then the other latch onto the breast.
- Criss-Cross Hold—Place pillows on your lap and hold each baby in the cradle position. The infants' legs criss-cross over one another.

KEEPING TRACK

Keep track of when and for how long each baby eats, especially if you feed them individually. Record the number of wet diapers and bowel movements each infant has each day. The babies should have at least six wet diapers by the fourth day and at least three bowel movements by the third day with increases thereafter if the infants' intakes are adequate.

You can assign each infant one breast without changing to the opposite breast, if you choose. Mothers often alternate the breast each infant nurses from at each feeding to keep stimulation of the breasts similar. Alternating breasts every 24 hours may be easier to remember.

CARE FOR YOURSELF

Eating well and getting enough rest is important. Ask for help from family and friends. Pamper yourself as much as possible, and leave care of the house and cooking to others if you can. Your major responsibility during this time should be to care for yourself and your new babies!

How to Wean from Breastfeeding

DECIDING WHEN TO WEAN

Breastfeeding has many benefits, and you can continue to breastfeed as long as you are comfortable. Only you can make the decision about when to wean your baby. Before you decide to begin weaning, evaluate the reasons for continuing nursing or beginning weaning.

HOW TO PROCEED

Gradual weaning is best for both you and your baby. Abrupt weaning can lead to engorgement and mastitis for you and can upset your baby. You both need to get used to this change slowly.

- Eliminate one feeding at a time. Replace it with a bottle for the young infant who needs to continue sucking. Infants generally do not drink as much from a cup as they do from a bottle. They may need a bottle to get enough milk to meet their nutritional requirements. The older infant who has learned to use a cup may not need a bottle at all. Use formula instead of cow's milk until the infant is at least 1 year old because formula is more suited to an infant's needs.
- Omit daytime feedings first. Begin with the feeding in which the baby seems least interested, then gradually eliminate others.
- Wait several days before eliminating another feeding. This allows time for your milk production to adjust and the baby to accept the changes.
- Eliminate the baby's favorite feedings last. Many infants are particularly fond of morning and bedtime feedings.
- Expect your infant to want to nurse again when tired, ill, or hurt during the weaning process. This is sometimes called "comfort nursing." A few minutes of nursing may be all that are necessary to comfort the baby.

HOME CARE

Many infants have not breastfed well by the time of discharge from the birth facility, placing them at risk for failure to gain weight, dehydration, and hyperbilirubinemia. Problems with engorgement and sore nipples are more likely to occur after discharge. These families need continued support after discharge.

Guidance for breastfeeding problems can be continued at home by referring the mother to lactation specialists or organizations such as La Leche League, a support group that gives ongoing assistance to breastfeeding mothers. La Leche League chapters are available in most communities and are listed in the telephone book. Support groups also may be provided by the birth facility. Information about appropriate Internet websites, such as the La Leche website at www.lalecheleague.org, can also be provided to parents.

Some birth facilities provide one or two home visits for new mothers by a nurse who can assess both the mother's progress and the infant's progress and intervene appropriately. A home visit allows assessment of the breastfeeding process in the mother's own surroundings and intervention before serious problems develop. The nurse can observe a feeding session and offer suggestions. The mother can ask questions that were not answered during her birth facility stay (Figure 22-15).

Outpatient clinics are a less costly alternative to the home visit and provide care similar to that received during a home visit. "Warm lines" also may be available for mothers to call their birth facilities and talk to nurses about breastfeeding problems. Women with more serious breastfeeding problems need referral to a lactation consultant, a professional educated to deal with more complex situations. Assistance helps prevent infant readmission for dehydration and hyperbilirubinemia.

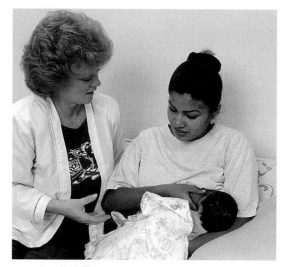

Figure 22-15 ■ The nurse offers suggestions on hand position during the home visit.

✔ **CHECK YOUR READING**

15. What teaching should be included for the mother who plans to work and breastfeed?
16. What types of care may be available after discharge for the breastfeeding mother?

FORMULA FEEDING

Although formula feeding may require less knowledge and skill than breastfeeding, the inexperienced mother often has many questions and may need assistance in learning to use formula correctly. Although breastfeeding is preferable, the nurse should support the woman who has decided to use formula.

Application of the Nursing Process
Formula Feeding

Assessment

Assess both the mother and the infant during the feeding process.

MOTHER'S KNOWLEDGE

Assess the mother's knowledge of bottle feeding. Ask her whether she has fed an infant before and whether she has questions. Observe her technique during the initial and subsequent feedings. Note the way she holds the infant and the bottle, assess her burping technique, and identify areas in which she seems unsure. To determine her understanding of the correct method to prepare formula, ask her to describe the way she will do it at home.

INFANT FEEDING BEHAVIORS

Hungry infants show the same behaviors whether breastfeeding or formula feeding. They may fuss or cry, suck on their hands, and root for the nipple. Waiting until the infant is frantic may result in a feeding taken too fast, with excess swallowing of air or choking. Assess the way the infant sucks during the feeding to identify sucking problems.

Analysis

Because improper formula preparation and feeding techniques could harm the infant, an appropriate nursing diagnosis for the mother using formula feeding is "Risk for Ineffective Health Maintenance related to lack of understanding of formula preparation and feeding techniques."

Planning

The mother will demonstrate correct techniques in holding the infant and bottle during feedings and will describe how to prepare formula and the frequency of feedings.

Interventions

TEACHING ABOUT FORMULA

The mother must learn the type of formula to use and the way to prepare it. Improper preparation can cause problems for the infant. Infection may occur if the milk or water used

---

CRITICAL TO REMEMBER

Formula Dilution

Formulas must be properly diluted to prevent serious illness and to promote weight gain and growth in the infant. It is essential that the label be followed accurately.
- Ready-to-use preparations: Use as is without dilution.
- Concentrated formulas: Dilute with equal parts of water.
- Powdered formulas: Mix one scoop of powder with 2 oz of water.

---

for preparation is contaminated. Emphasize the importance of following the directions on the label when mixing the formula. Improper dilution of the formula may cause undernutrition or imbalances of sodium, which can be dangerous to the infant.

TYPES OF FORMULA. Many types of formula are available, and the physician or nurse practitioner prescribes the type of formula the mother is to use. If milk allergies are prevalent in the family, a soy-based or casein hydrolysate formula may be chosen from the start. Infants should receive iron-fortified formula. Formula may be purchased in three different preparations.

Ready to Use. Ready-to-use formula is available in bottles to which a nipple is added or in cans to be poured directly into a bottle. It should not be diluted. Although expensive, it is practical when there is difficulty in mixing formula or the water supply is in question. An open can should be refrigerated and used within 48 hours.

Concentrated Liquid. Instruct the mother to dilute concentrated liquid formula and be sure that she understands the directions for dilution. Equal parts of concentrated liquid formula and water are mixed in a bottle to provide the amount desired for each feeding. Opened cans should be stored in the refrigerator and used within 48 hours (Walker & Creehan, 2001).

Powdered. Powdered formula is more economical and is particularly useful when a breastfeeding mother plans to give an occasional bottle of formula. Usually one scoop of powder is added to each 2 oz of water in a bottle. Packets with enough powdered formula for one feeding are convenient when away from home. Formula should be well mixed to dissolve the powder and make the solution uniform. Once mixed, the formula should be used immediately or refrigerated for no more than 48 hours.

EQUIPMENT. Many different types of bottles and nipples are available. Mothers may use glass or plastic bottles or a plastic liner that fits into a rigid container. Some nipples are designed to simulate the human nipple to promote jaw development. Selection of type of bottles and nipples depends on individual preference.

PREPARATION. Discuss preparation of formula with the mother. She can prepare a single bottle or a 24-hour supply. If the water supply is safe, sterilization is not necessary for normal newborns. Bottles and nipples can be washed in hot, sudsy water using a brush to clean well, then rinsed, and allowed to air dry. Bottles may be washed in a dishwasher, but nipples tend to deteriorate quickly unless washed by hand. Instruct the mother to wash her hands as well as the top of the can and the can opener (if needed). The formula and water are poured into the bottles, which then are capped. Emphasize that the proportion of water and liquid or powdered formula must be adhered to exactly to prevent illness in the infant.

Explain that if safety of the water supply is questionable, sterilization by aseptic or terminal method is necessary. In both methods all equipment is washed and rinsed well before beginning. In the aseptic method, equipment needed for the procedure is boiled for 5 minutes in a sterilizer or deep pan. Water for diluting the formula is boiled separately. The bottles are assembled using sterilized tongs to avoid contamination by the hands. The formula and boiled water are added, and the bottles are capped and refrigerated until needed.

In the terminal sterilization method, the formula is prepared in the bottles, which are loosely capped. The bottles then are placed in the sterilizer or pan of water, where they are boiled for 25 minutes. After the bottles cool, the caps are tightened and the bottles refrigerated.

EXPLAINING FEEDING TECHNIQUES

POSITIONING. Show the mother how to position the infant in a semi-upright position such as the cradle hold. This allows the mother to hold the infant close in a face-to-face position. The bottle is held with the nipple kept full of formula to prevent excessive swallowing of air (Figure 22-16). Placing the infant in the opposite arm for each feeding provides varied visual stimulation during feedings.

BURPING. For the first few days the infant should be burped or "bubbled" after every half ounce. Gradually, the infant is able to take more milk before burping and should be burped halfway through feeding. Demonstrate placing the infant over the shoulder or in a sitting position with the head supported while patting or rubbing the infant's back (Figure 22-17).

FREQUENCY AND AMOUNT. Instruct the mother to feed the infant every 3 to 4 hours but to avoid rigid scheduling and take her cues from the infant. Explain that the bottle-fed infant takes only $\frac{1}{2}$ to 1 oz per feeding during the first day of life but gradually increases to 2 to 3 oz per feeding by the third to fifth day. An infant who is satisfied often goes to sleep.

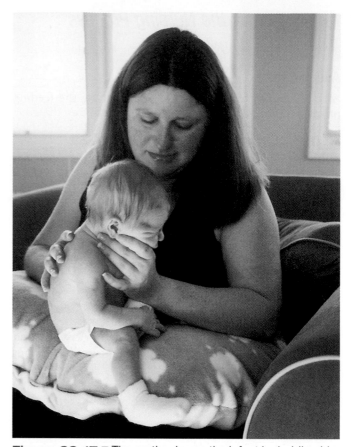

Figure 22-17 ■ The mother burps the infant by holding him in a sitting position. She supports the head and chest with one hand and gently pats the back with the other hand.

CAUTIONS. Caution the mother not to heat formula in a microwave oven because the heating is uneven and may result in some parts of the liquid being very hot even when the outside of the bottle feels only warm. Formula can be heated by placing it in a container of hot water until it is warm. The mother should test the formula temperature by allowing a few drops from the bottle to fall on her inner arm.

Instruct the mother not to prop the bottle. Propping increases the likelihood of choking if regurgitation occurs and eliminates the holding and cuddling that should accompany feeding. Some mothers put an infant to bed with a bottle propped. This not only increases the danger of aspiration but allows milk to stay in the mouth for prolonged periods. The milk may pool in the mouth, promoting growth of bacteria and leading to cavities once the teeth are in. Ear infections also are more common in infants who sleep with a bottle or have a propped bottle.

The mother should not try to coax the infant to finish the bottle at each feeding. This could result in regurgitation and excessive weight gain. She should not save formula from one feeding to the next because of the danger of rapidly growing bacteria. Any formula not used within an hour should be discarded.

INFANT VARIATIONS. Infants vary in their feeding preferences. Some infants drink from the bottle reluctantly.

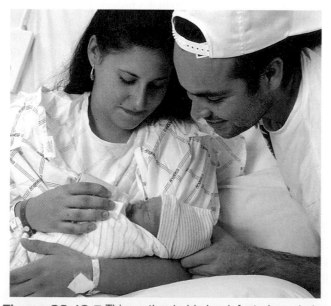

Figure 22-16 ■ This mother holds her infant close during bottle feeding. The bottle is positioned so that the nipple is filled with milk at all times. The father offers encouragement.

Although formula usually is given at room temperature, some infants take heated formula better. The mother of a sleepy infant needs to use the same wake-up techniques discussed for the breastfeeding mother.

Angling the tip of the nipple so that it rubs the palate triggers the suck reflex in most infants. Placing a finger under the chin for support may help some infants suck better. It often takes patience and persistence to find the most effective techniques.

Evaluation

The mother should hold the infant and bottle correctly during feedings. She should be able to describe formula preparation and the amount and frequency of feedings.

✔ CHECK YOUR READING

17. What questions might a mother have about formula feeding?
18. Why should mothers avoid propping bottles?

SUMMARY CONCEPTS

- Full-term infants need 110 to 120 kcal/kg (50 to 55 kcal/lb) daily. They may lose weight in the first few days after birth as a result of insufficient intake and normal loss of extracellular fluid.
- Colostrum is rich in protein, vitamins, minerals, and immunoglobulins. Transitional milk appears between colostrum and mature milk. Mature milk is present after the first 2 weeks of lactation.
- Breast milk has nutrients in proportions required by the newborn and in an easily digested form. Most commercial formulas are cow's milk adapted to simulate human milk.
- Breast milk contains factors that help establish the normal intestinal flora and prevent infection. These include bifidus factor, leukocytes, lysozymes, lactoferrin, and immunoglobulins.
- A variety of commercial formulas is available. They include modified cow's milk formula, soy-based or casein hydrolysate formulas, and formulas for preterm infants or those with special problems.
- Factors that influence the mother's choice of feeding method include knowledge about each method, support from family and friends, cultural influences, and employment.
- Suckling at the breast causes the mother's posterior pituitary to release oxytocin, which triggers the let-down reflex. It also causes the anterior pituitary to release prolactin, which increases milk production.
- The principle of supply and demand applies to breastfeeding. Milk production increases when the infant feeds frequently. When breastfeeding ceases, prolactin is decreased and eventually the alveoli of the breasts atrophy and stop producing milk.
- Flat and inverted nipples should be identified during pregnancy. Creams and methods to toughen the nipples are not necessary.

- The nurse can help the mother establish breastfeeding by initiating early feeding, assisting her to position the infant at the breast, and showing her how to position her hands. The nurse should teach the mother how to help the infant latch onto the breast, assess the position of the mouth on the breast, and remove the infant from the breast.
- The mother should feed the infant 8 to 12 times each day for an average of 10 to 15 minutes of effective suckling on each side, nursing until the infant is satisfied.
- Wake-up techniques for sleepy infants include unwrapping the blankets, talking to the infant, changing the diaper, rubbing the infant's back, and expressing colostrum onto the breast.
- When infants suck from a bottle, they must push the tongue against the nipple to slow the flow of milk. When they suckle at the breast, they position the nipple far into the mouth so that the gums compress the areola as the tongue moves over the breast in a wavelike motion.
- The nurse should help the mother with sore nipples to check the positioning of the infant at the breast. The mother should vary the position of the infant at the breast and apply breast milk and warm-water compresses to the nipples. She should also expose the nipples to air.
- Teaching for the mother who plans to work and breastfeed includes expression of breast milk by hand or pump and proper storage of the milk.
- Mothers who use formula need information about the types of formula available, correct preparation, and feeding techniques.

REFERENCES & READINGS

Adams, C., Berger, R., Conning, P., Cruikshank, L., & Dore, K. (2001). Breastfeeding trends at a community breastfeeding center: An evaluative survey. *Journal of Obstetric, Gynecologic, and Neonatal Nursing, 30*(4), 392-400.

American Academy of Pediatrics (AAP) Committee on Drugs. (2001). The transfer of drugs and other chemicals into human milk. *Pediatrics, 108*(3), 776-789.

American Academy of Pediatrics Committee on Nutrition. (2000). Hypoallergenic infant formulas. *Pediatrics, 106*(2), 346-349.

American Academy of Pediatrics Work Group on Breastfeeding. (1997). Breastfeeding and the use of human milk. *Pediatrics, 100*(6), 1035-1039.

American Academy of Pediatrics & American College of Obstetricians and Gynecologists. (2002). *Guidelines for perinatal care* (5th ed.). Elk Grove Village, IL: AAP.

American Dietetic Association. (2001). Position of the American Dietetic Association: Breaking the barriers to breastfeeding. *Journal of the American Dietetic Association, 101*(10), 1213-1220.

Association of Women's Health, Obstetric, and Neonatal Nurses (AWHONN). (2000a). *Evidence-based clinical practice guideline. Breastfeeding support: Prenatal care through the first year.* Washington, DC: Author. Monograph.

AWHONN. (2000b). *Evidence-based clinical practice guideline: breastfeeding support: prenatal care through the first year. Practice guidelines.* Washington, DC: Author.

AWHONN. (2003). *Standards and guidelines for professional nursing practice in the care of women and newborns* (6th ed.). Washington, DC: Author.

Banks, J.W. (2003). Kanistenhsera teiakotihsnies: a native community rekindles the tradition of breastfeeding. *AWHONN Lifelines, 7*(4), 340-347.

Berryman, R.E., & Glass, S.M. (2005). Routine care. In P.J. Thureen, J. Deacon, J. Hernandez, & D.M. Hall (Eds.), *Assessment and care of the well newborn* (2nd ed., pp. 198-205). Philadelphia: Saunders.

Biancuzzo, M. (2003). *Breastfeeding the newborn: Clinical strategies for nurses* (2nd ed.). St. Louis: Mosby.

Chen, A., & Rogan, W.J. (2004). Breastfeeding and the risk of postneonatal death in the United States. *Pediatrics, 113*(5), e435-e439.

Chezem, J., Friesen, C., & Boettcher, J. (2003). Breastfeeding knowledge, breastfeeding confidence, and infant feeding plans: Effects on actual feeding practice. *Journal of Obstetric, Gynecologic, and Neonatal Nursing, 32*(1), 40-47.

Cobb, M.A.B. (2003). Promoting breastfeeding. *AWHONN Lifelines, 6*(5), 418-423.

Dennis, C.L. (2002). Breastfeeding initiation and duration: a 1990-2000 literature review. *Journal of Obstetric, Gynecologic, and Neonatal Nursing, 31*(1), 12-32.

DiGirolamo, A.M., Grummer-Strawn, L.M., & Fein, S. (2001). Maternity care practices: Implications for breastfeeding. *Birth, 28*(2), 94-100.

Dobson, B., & Murtaugh, M.A. (2001). Position of the American Dietetic Association: Breaking the barriers to breastfeeding. *Journal of the American Dietetic Association, 101*(10), 1213-1220.

Dodd, V., & Chalmers, C. (2004). Comparing the use of hydrogel dressings to lanolin ointment with lactating mothers. *Journal of Obstetric, Gynecologic, and Neonatal Nursing, 32*(4), 486-494.

Dowling, D.A., & Thanattherakul, W. (2001). Nipple confusion, alternative feeding methods, and breastfeeding supplementation: State of the science. *Newborn and Infant Nursing Reviews, 1*(4), 217-223.

Glass, S.M. (2005). Feeding the newborn. In *Assessment and care of the well newborn* (2nd ed., pp 175-197). Philadelphia: Saunders.

Gomez, L.T. (2000). Breastfeeding: Increasing primary adjustment milk supply. *International Journal of Childbirth Education, 15*(1), 29-35.

Griffin, T.L., Meier, P.P., Bradford, L.P., Bigger, H.R., & Engstrom, J.L. (2000). Mothers performing creamatocrit measures in the NICU: Accuracy, reactions, and cost. *Journal of Obstetric, Gynecologic, and Neonatal Nursing, 29*(3), 249-257.

Groer, M.W., Davis, M.W., & Hemphil, J. (2002). Postpartum stress: Current concepts and the possible protective role of breastfeeding. *Journal of Obstetric, Gynecologic, and Neonatal Nursing, 31*(4), 411-417.

Heird, W.C. (2004). The feeding of infants and children. In R.E. Behrman, R.M. Kliegman, & H.B. Jenson (Eds.), *Nelson textbook of pediatrics* (17th ed., pp. 157-167). Philadelphia: Saunders.

Hong, T.M., Callister, L.C., & Schwartz, R. (2003). First-time mothers' views of breastfeeding support from nurses. *MCN: American Journal of Maternal/Child Nursing, 28*(1), 10-15.

Karl, D.J. (2004). Using principles of newborn behavioral state organization to facilitate breastfeeding. *MCN: American Journal of Maternal/Child Nursing, 29*(5), 293-298.

Kleinman, R.E. (Ed.). (2004). *Pediatric nutrition handbook* (5th ed.). Elk Grove Village, IL: AAP.

La Leche League International. (2003). *The womanly art of breastfeeding* (7th ed.). Schaumburg, IL: La Leche League International.

Lawrence, R.A., & Lawrence, R.M. (2005). *Breastfeeding: A guide for the medical profession* (5th ed.). St. Louis: Mosby.

Lawrence, R.M., & Lawrence, R.A. (2004). The breast and the physiology of lactation. In R.K. Creasy & R. Resnik, *Maternal-fetal medicine: Principles and practice* (5th ed., pp. 135-153). Philadelphia: Saunders.

Lowe, N.K. (2004). Health promotion begins at the breast. *Journal of Obstetric, Gynecologic, and Neonatal Nursing, 33*(3), 297.

Mattson, S. (2004). Ethnocultural considerations in the childbearing period. In S. Mattson & J.E. Smith (Eds.), *Core curriculum for maternal-newborn nursing* (3rd ed., pp. 75-95). Philadelphia: Saunders.

Meek, J.Y. (2002). *American Academy of Pediatrics new mother's guide to breastfeeding.* New York: Bantam.

Mitchell, M.K. (2003). Nutrition during infancy. In M.K. Mitchell (Eds.), *Nutrition across the life span* (2nd ed., pp. 209-251). Philadelphia: Saunders.

Mohrbacher, N., & Stock, J. (2003). *The breastfeeding answer book* (3rd ed.). Schaumburg, IL: La Leche League International.

Moore, M.L., & Moos, M. (2003). *Cultural competence in the care of childbearing families.* White Plains, NY: March of Dimes Birth Defects Foundation.

Morin, K.H. (2004). Current thoughts on healthy term infant nutrition. *MCN: American Journal of Maternal/Child Nursing, 29*(5), 312-319.

Mozingo, J.N., Davis, M.W., Droppleman, P.G., & Merideth, A. (2000). "It wasn't working": Women's experiences with short-term breastfeeding. *MCN: American Journal of Maternal/ Child Nursing, 25*(3), 120-126.

Newton, E.R. (2002). Physiology of lactation and breastfeeding. In S.G. Gabbe, J.R. Niebyl, & J.L. Simpson (Eds.), *Obstetrics, normal and problem pregnancies* (4th ed., pp. 105-136). New York: Churchill Livingstone.

Orr, S.S. (2004). Breastfeeding. In S. Mattson & J.E. Smith (Eds.), *Core curriculum for maternal-newborn nursing* (3rd ed., pp. 387-408). Philadelphia: Saunders.

Ortiz, J., McGilligan, K., & Kelly, P. (2004). Duration of breast milk expression among working mothers enrolled in an employer-sponsored lactation program. *Pediatric Nursing, 30*(2), 111-119.

Pollock, C.A., Bustamante-Forest, R., & Giarratano, G. (2002). Men of diverse cultures: Knowledge and attitudes about breastfeeding. *Journal of Obstetric, Gynecologic, and Neonatal Nursing, 31*(6), 673-679.

Riordan, J. (2005a). The biologic specificity of breastmilk. In J. Riordan (Ed.), *Breastfeeding and human lactation* (3rd ed., pp. 97-135). Boston: Jones and Bartlett.

Riordan, J. (2005b). The cultural context of breastfeeding. In J. Riordan (Ed.), *Breastfeeding and human lactation* (3rd ed., pp. 713-728). Boston: Jones and Bartlett.

Riordan, J., & Bocar, D.L. (2005). Breastfeeding education. In J. Riordan (Ed.), *Breastfeeding and human lactation* (3rd ed., pp. 689-712). Boston: Jones and Bartlett.

Riordan, J., & Hoover, L. (2005). Perinatal and intrapartum care. In J. Riordan (Ed.), *Breastfeeding and human lactation* (3rd ed., pp. 185-216). Boston: Jones and Bartlett.

Robinson, L.B. (2003). Olive oil: A natural treatment for sore nipples? *AWHONN Lifelines, 6*(2), 110-112.

Rojjanasrirat, W. (2004). Working women's breastfeeding experiences. *MCN: American Journal of Maternal/Child Nursing, 29*(4), 222-229.

Ross Products Division. (2003). *Breastfeeding trends—2002. Mothers' survey.* Columbus, OH: Ross Products Division, Abbott Laboratories. Retrieved January 3, 2005, from http://ross.com/images/library/bf_trends_2002.pdf.

Santa-Donato, A. (2001). Promoting breastfeeding. *AWHONN Lifelines, 5*(2), 10-12.

Skidmore-Roth, L. (2004). *Mosby's handbook of herbs and natural supplements* (2nd ed). St. Louis: Mosby.

Smith, L.J., & Riordan, J. (2005). Postpartum care. In J. Riordan (Ed.), *Breastfeeding and human lactation* (3rd ed., pp. 217-245). Boston: Jones and Bartlett.

Spicer, K. (2001). What every nurse needs to know about breast pumping: Instructing and supporting mothers of premature infants in the NICU. *Neonatal Network, 20*(4), 35-41.

Sullivan, M.L., Leathers, S.J., & Kelley, M.A. (2004). Family characteristics associated with duration of breastfeeding during early infancy among primiparas. *Journal of Human Lactation, 20*(2), 196-205.

Taveral, E.M., Capra, A.M., Braveman, P.A., Jensvold, N.G., Escobar, G.J., & Lieu, T.A. (2003). Clinician support and psychosocial risk factors associated with breastfeeding discontinuation. *Pediatrics, 112*(1), 108-115.

Tiedje, L.B., Schiffman, R., Omar, M., Wright, J., Buzzitta, C., McCann, A., & Metzger, S. (2002). An ecological approach to breastfeeding. *MCN: American Journal of Maternal/Child Nursing, 27*(3), 154-162.

Trahms, C.M. (2004). Nutrition in infancy. In L.K. Mahan & S. Escott-Stump (Eds.), *Krause's food, nutrition, and diet therapy* (11th ed., pp. 214-233). Philadelphia: Saunders.

Tsang, R.C., DeMarini, S., & Rath, L.L. (2003). Fluids, electrolytes, vitamins, and trace minerals. In C. Kenner, J.W. Lott, & A.A. Flandermeyer (Eds.), *Comprehensive neonatal nursing, a physiologic perspective* (3rd ed., pp. 409-424). Philadelphia: Saunders.

U.S. Department of Health and Human Services. (2000). *Healthy People 2010* (Conference edition, in 2 volumes). Washington, DC: Author.

Walker, M. (2005). Breast pumps and other technologies. In J. Riordan (Ed.), *Breastfeeding and human lactation* (3rd ed., pp. 323-365). Boston: Jones and Bartlett.

Walker, M., & Creehan, P. (2001). Newborn nutrition. In K.R. Simpson & P.A. Creehan (Eds.), *Perinatal nursing* (pp. 550-574). Philadelphia: Lippincott Williams & Wilkins.

Williams, S.R. (2003b). Nutrition during pregnancy and lactation. In S.R. Williams & E.D. Schlenker (Eds.), *Essentials of nutrition and diet therapy* (8th ed., pp. 269-292). St. Louis: Mosby.

Windsor, J.E. (2003). Korean women & breastfeeding. *AWHONN Lifelines, 7*(1), 61-64.

Wight, N.E. (2001). Management of common breastfeeding issues. *Pediatric Clinics of North America, 48*(2), 321-344.

Witt, K.A., & Mihok, M.A. (2003). Lactation and breastfeeding. In M.K. Mitchell (Eds.), *Nutrition across the life span* (2nd ed., pp. 177-206). Philadelphia: Saunders.

Home Care of the Infant

OBJECTIVES

After studying this chapter, you should be able to:

1. Explain why nurses need knowledge about care of the infant during the early weeks after birth.
2. Describe postdischarge nursing care included in home visits, clinic visits, and telephone follow-up.
3. Explain the safety features of infant equipment that parents must consider.
4. Explain methods of resolving common problems involving infant crying and sleep patterns during the early weeks of parenting.
5. Answer common questions that parents might have about care of the young infant.
6. Describe the normal changes in growth and development of the infant during the first 12 weeks of life.
7. Explain the purpose and importance of well-baby checkups and immunizations for infants.
8. List signs that indicate illness in the infant.
9. Discuss current knowledge about sudden infant death syndrome.

Go to your Student CD-ROM for Review Questions keyed to these Objectives.

DEFINITIONS

Extrusion Reflex Automatic nervous system response that causes an infant to push anything solid out of the mouth.

Gastroesophageal Reflux Condition in which stomach contents enter the esophagus and may be aspirated into the lungs.

Hyperbilirubinemia Excessive amount of bilirubin in the blood.

Jaundice Yellow discoloration of the skin and sclera caused by excessive bilirubin in the blood.

Miliaria (Prickly Heat) Rash caused by heat.

Seborrheic Dermatitis (Cradle Cap) Yellowish, crusty area of the scalp.

Strabismus Misalignment or deviation of one or both eyes, normal in newborns.

Sudden Infant Death Syndrome (SIDS) Sudden death of an infant that is unexplained by history, autopsy, or examination of the scene of death.

Thermoregulation Maintenance of body temperature.

Nurses often receive questions from parents about care of infants during the early weeks. This chapter provides information about caring for infants during the first 12 weeks of life. The focus is on teaching parents beyond the usual birth facility discharge teaching, which is included in Chapter 21. Detailed information about ill or older infants can be found in pediatric textbooks.

INFORMATION FOR NEW PARENTS

Needs

The early weeks after birth are often stressful for new parents. The mother is tired from the pregnancy and birth, both parents may be anxious about their new role, and the newborn may be awake much of the night or may behave in unexpected ways. Parents have concerns about ongoing care of the infant and adjustment to parenthood.

Sources of Information

In the birth facility, parents often receive more information about care of the newborn than they can absorb in the short time available. New mothers' physical needs and anxieties often interfere with their ability to learn. This may leave parents inadequately prepared to cope with the multiple demands of early parenting.

Family members, once the primary source of support for new parents, frequently live far away, and parents must rely on friends, health care personnel, child care classes, television, books, and magazines. Many people get information from the Internet. Parents should determine the source of information obtained online, because if it is from nonprofessional sources it may not be accurate. Friends can be important sources of support and information, but their knowledge may be incorrect or outdated. Nurses are ideal sources of assistance in these situations.

CARE AFTER DISCHARGE

Mothers and infants are generally discharged from the birth facility 48 hours after vaginal birth and 96 hours after cesarean birth if there are no complications. Some mothers choose to go home earlier. Infants discharged earlier than 48 hours should have a follow-up visit within 48 hours after they go home (American Academy of Pediatrics [AAP] & the American College of Obstetricians & Gynecologists, 2002). The optimal time of discharge should be based on the individual needs of the woman and her infant.

Various programs have been instituted to provide after-discharge care. They may include nursing contact with the family in the home, in the clinic, or by telephone.

Home Visits

Home visits have been found to be a cost-effective way to avoid hospital admission or emergency department visits for dehydration or jaundice in newborns (Paul, Phillips, Widome, & Hollenbeak, 2004). The home visit is scheduled during the first few days after discharge. This timing allows early assessment and intervention for problems in nutrition, jaundice, newborn adaptation, and maternal-infant interaction. Problems with feeding, weight loss, infection, and jaundice often occur during the early days after discharge. Nurses may visit low-risk mothers and infants or may follow high-risk infants after discharge from the neonatal intensive care nursery (Figures 23-1 to 23-4).

Some community agencies employ paraprofessionals under the supervision of nurses to make visits to families. Paraprofessionals are often women from the community, of the same ethnicity, and able to speak the same language as the family and therefore more likely to be readily accepted. The paraprofessionals receive training to help them provide support and education about pregnancy and parenting. They also identify situations in which referral to the nurse or the health care provider is needed.

Nurses who care for clients in the home setting have a great deal of autonomy. They should be experienced in client care and be able to function independently. Nurses who work in the community should first work in the acute care setting for several years to gain experience and skill in a variety of areas.

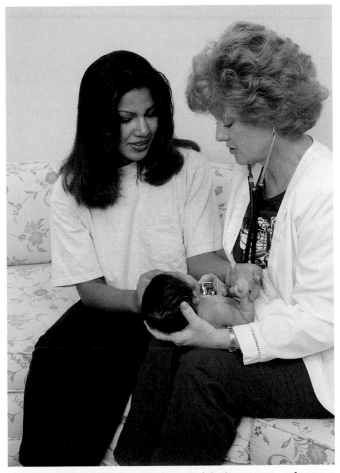

Figure 23-1 ■ During the home visit the nurse performs a complete assessment of the infant. Here she is checking the apical pulse and listening to breath sounds.

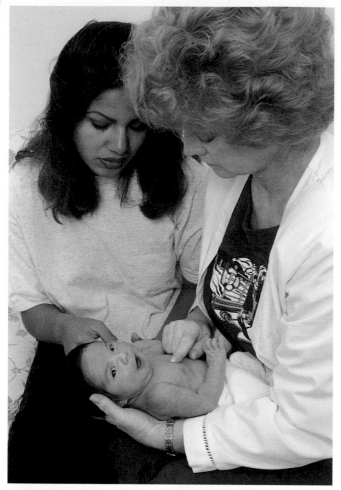

Figure 23-2 ■ Jaundice is especially of concern when infants are discharged early after birth. The nurse shows the mother how to blanch the skin to check for jaundice and discusses what the mother should do if she sees it.

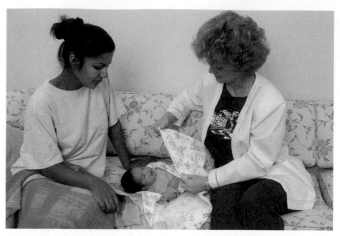

Figure 23-3 ■ The nurse discusses thermoregulation with the mother and demonstrates swaddling.

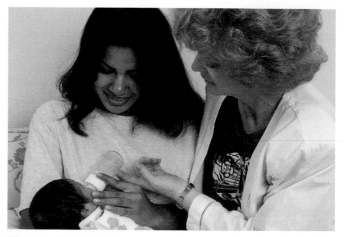

Figure 23-4 ■ The nurse observes a feeding during the visit to assess feeding techniques and provide a chance for parents to ask questions about feeding concerns. This is a good time to assess parent-infant interaction. The infant is weighed to help determine adequacy of intake.

VISITS TO LOW-RISK FAMILIES

During the home visit the nurse performs a physical examination of the mother and infant. The nurse assesses family adaptation to the addition of a new member and the adequacy of the mother's support system. Reinforcement of the teaching that was begun at the birth facility is important. A feeding session should be assessed, especially if the mother is breastfeeding. Blood may be obtained for metabolic screening if the infant went home too early for reliable testing in the birth facility. Safety in the home is often discussed, and questions about infant care and general parenting are answered (Figure 23-5).

Home visits provide reassurance for parents and may increase a woman's confidence and competence in caring for herself and her infant. The visits are especially valuable in recognizing jaundice and intervening before bilirubin levels become dangerously high. When jaundice is found, the nurse can discuss the implications and draw blood for testing bilirubin levels. Appropriate care, including hydration and phototherapy, is discussed as necessary.

Feeding is an area of concern for many parents. Breastfeeding problems are common. When the nurse observes a feeding and helps a woman deal with problems, the infant's intake may increase. Increased intake helps to prevent dehydration and possible hospital readmission and leads to increased excretion of bilirubin, which may prevent a need for phototherapy at home or in the hospital.

VISITS TO FAMILIES WITH HIGH-RISK INFANTS

High-risk infants (see Chapters 29 and 30) often need special care after discharge. Parents may be very anxious about assuming care of an infant who has had a prolonged hospitalization. Many hospitals have programs that enable parents to take over their infant's care gradually before discharge.

A nurse may visit the home before the infant's discharge to help the family plan for accommodating the equipment and the type of care the infant needs. The home is checked for the availability of electricity, heat, and a telephone. If

Expected Newborn/Family Outcomes	Assessments	Interventions	Response
Physical assessment: The newborn assessment is within normal limits.	Vital signs, weight Respiratory status (color, retractions, etc.) Fontanels Skin (rash, jaundice) Cord Circumcision Activity, behavior, crying, sleep patterns Elimination (number of voids and stools in 24 hours)	Complete systematic assessment.	Outcome met. Outcome not met (requires further documentation).
Nutrition: Infant's intake is adequate. LATCH score is over 7 if infant breastfed. (See Chapter 22, p. 545)	Information about previous feedings Behaviors of infant and mother during a feeding	Discuss frequency, length of feedings, and amount (in oz. or time at breast), breastfeeding or bottle feeding techniques, and feeding problems. Provide written educational materials.	Outcomes met. Outcomes not met (requires further documentation). Referral made.
Caregiving: Parents correctly describe infant characteristics and needs and demonstrate care.	Parent's knowledge and performance of infant care	Teach and clarify as necessary. Provide written educational materials.	Outcomes met. Outcomes not met (requires further documentation).
Infant/family relationships: The family demonstrates normal adjustment and attachment behaviors.	Interaction of parents and family members with the infant and each other	Discuss emotional adjustment of all family members, sibling rivalry, postpartum blues or depression. Provide written educational materials.	Outcomes met. Outcomes not met (requires further documentation).
Support system: Parents have an adequate support system.	Interaction of family members, sources of support within and outside the immediate family.	Discuss availability and need for support and resources. Provide written educational materials.	Outcome met. Outcome not met (requires further documentation).
Environment: The home is safe and has adequate facilities and baby equipment and supplies are safe.	Safety and potential hazards in the home; availability of heat, electricity, telephone; sanitation; sleeping arrangements.	Make suggestions for solutions to problems identified. Provide written educational materials.	Outcomes met. Outcomes not met (requires further documentation).

Figure 23-5 ■ An example of a clinical pathway for a home visit by a nurse to the family of a normal newborn.

Continued

Expected Newborn/Family Outcomes	Assessments	Interventions	Response
Need for care: The parents understand the need for well baby follow-up. They recognize signs of infant illness and how to get help. They give any specialized care appropriately and correctly.	Knowledge about well baby check-ups, immunizations, signs of illness, how to take a temperature, where to get care, ability to perform specialized care if needed.	Discuss areas where there is need. Demonstrate temperature taking. Provide written educational materials.	Outcomes met. Outcomes not met (requires further documentation).
Other care: Metabolic screening or other care is received, as ordered.	Need for specimen collection or other care	Collect blood specimens for newborn metabolic screening, give other care (phototherapy, etc.) as ordered. Provide written educational materials.	Outcomes met. Outcomes not met (requires further documentation).
Parent concerns: Parental concerns are addressed and parents verbalize that concerns are alleviated.	Parental concerns	Provide teaching about concerns. Refer to other resources as needed.	Outcome met (document to whom referral made). Outcome not met (requires further documentation).
Referrals: Parents receive necessary referrals.	Need for referrals	Refer to physician, lactation consultant, WIC, community resources, etc. Provide written educational materials.	Outcome met (document to whom referral made). Outcome not met (requires further documentation).

Figure 23-5, cont'd ■ An example of a clinical pathway for a home visit by a nurse to the family of a normal newborn.

the family has a technology-dependent infant, the nurse checks that they have notified the utility companies to ensure that no disruption of services occurs.

After the infant is discharged, nursing visits can help the family maintain the infant's health and decrease the need for rehospitalization. Components of each visit vary according to the infant's needs. The nurse provides assessment of the infant and the parents' caregiving ability in addition to necessary teaching and nursing care.

Medically fragile infants may require home treatment with mechanical ventilation, oxygen therapy, or apnea monitors. Parents may have to perform such nursing skills as tracheostomy care, tube feedings, suctioning, and care of intravenous sites. Mothers often have concerns about feeding the infant, which may differ from feeding a healthy full-term infant. Follow-up telephone calls from nurses between visits help families adapt to the needs of these infants and may also decrease the need for rehospitalization.

The home health nurse may be part of an interdisciplinary team of health care providers working with families in the home. The nurse may help coordinate care by different professionals. Some infants are eligible for home health aides who provide direct care in the home. The aide is supervised by a nurse.

Infants with complications often need more frequent visits to the pediatrician or nurse practitioner or are rehospitalized during the early months after birth. Common problems include respiratory illness, infections (gastroenteritis, sepsis, urinary tract infections, otitis media), and need for surgery. These parents need information on preventive measures and care of the infant with acute illness.

Although parents' greatest concerns involve the infant's health, other problems may exist. Finding a baby-sitter who is qualified to care for an infant on oxygen or who might need resuscitation may be difficult. Siblings often have difficulty adjusting to the needs of the infant and may resent the diversion of the parents' attention. The nurse can make suggestions and put the parents in touch with parent groups that offer practical help in caring for a high-risk infant.

GENERAL CONSIDERATIONS IN HOME VISITS

The nurse making a home visit is a guest of the family and must adapt nursing care usually given in the birth facility to the home setting. The needs of other family members may make care given in the home quite different from care given in the hospital. For example, the examination of the infant may need to wait for a short time while the mother meets the needs of her other small children.

Careful planning before the visit is essential to make the most of the limited time available. Before visiting the nurse calls to schedule the visit at a time convenient for the family and to obtain directions to the home. Setting priorities carefully based on the needs identified by the nurse and the family is important, especially when only one visit is planned. After the home visit the nurse may plan additional visits or provide the family with a telephone number they may call to receive further help if needed.

Communication skills are particularly important when the setting is the home and the client is the family. The nurse must develop rapport with family members quickly and work with them to meet shared goals for the visit. A brief social interaction may be beneficial at the beginning of the visit to develop a trusting relationship. The purpose of the visit should be explained and the family's expectations and desires discussed. Open-ended questions and therapeutic communication techniques help the nurse identify and address the family's needs. Making suggestions in a positive manner is important.

The nurse should be aware of any cultural practices affecting the family's view of care. In patriarchal cultures, the father is the head of the family and teaching should be directed to him and the mother. The elder members of the family also may play a large role in determining essential health care. In some cultures one or both grandmothers are important influences in the care of the mother and infant.

Documentation of the visit is essential. The results of the assessments, teaching, nursing care, referrals, and plans for follow-up should be recorded. Copies of the record usually are sent to the primary caregiver. If problems are identified that need to be discussed with the primary care provider, report is made by telephone.

Outpatient Visits

Outpatient visits may be provided by the birth facility in clinics that are often managed by nurses. The costs may be included in the overall hospital maternity care charges. Assessments and care are essentially the same as those provided for home visits. The advantage of outpatient visits is that the nurse does not have to travel to the home and can see more clients each day, thereby reducing the cost of the service. Assessment of the home setting and family interaction is not possible, however. Clinic visits usually last 30 to 45 minutes. Appointments may be made during the discharge procedure from the birth facility.

In some areas nurses take a van to various neighborhoods to provide nursing care. This allows clients with transportation problems easy access to care. Nurses in the van carry out the same assessment and care of the mother and infant that is provided during clinic visits. Care may begin in the prenatal period and extend through the postpartum period and may include well-child examinations as well.

Telephone Counseling

Telephone counseling can occur during follow-up calls to discharged clients or when parents call "warm lines" for help with problems or questions. Telephone calls are much less expensive than home or clinic visits. The major disadvantage is that the nurse cannot perform an in-person assessment of the mother, baby, or home environment and must rely on the caller to present an accurate picture of the situation.

FOLLOW-UP CALLS

Follow-up calls are placed by nurses in the first few days after discharge. The nurse asks a series of questions to assess the physical condition of the mother and infant and to identify any needs or problems. All mothers may receive calls or only those considered at risk for problems. If problems are discovered, the nurse may schedule another call or a home visit, if available, or refer the woman to her primary care provider.

WARM LINES

Warm lines, also called *help lines,* provide parents with an opportunity to ask a nurse the questions arising from the daily challenges of parenting. They are used for troubling but not emergency situations. The service should be available around the clock to best meet the needs of the callers. Parents often call about infant feeding, breastfeeding concerns, and basic care of the mother and infant. Calls last about 15 to 20 minutes. The nurse answers the caller's questions and assesses for other problems. The nurse may call back later to see if the situation has resolved.

TELEPHONE TECHNIQUES

Nurses caring for clients by telephone must understand telephone counseling techniques. They need special education in telephone communication and triage.

Open-ended questions help the mother describe any problems in her own terms. Examples are shown in the following box.

- "How have you been getting along since you left the hospital?"
- "What kinds of things have happened where you weren't quite sure what to do?"
- "What has been most difficult?"

Telephone triage involves determining the existence of and solution to a serious problem. Callers may not describe the situation accurately. The nurse should help the mother (or caller) describe the major concerns, which may not be those discussed first. "What worries you most?" may help focus on the most important problems. Although most problems discussed are concerns about normal infants, the nurse must be alert for "red flags" that signal serious situations needing immediate referral.

The client should be allowed enough time to avoid feeling hurried. Lay terminology should be used and questions asked to elicit detailed description of the problems. Parents should be reassured that their questions are valued so they don't feel hesitant to ask what they may see as a "silly" question. Such questions often lead to discussion of a problem that might have been missed if the parent had not been encouraged to ask them.

CRITICAL TO REMEMBER

Red Flags of Telephone Triage

- An emergency situation (such as respiratory difficulty, bleeding). Tell the parent to call 911 or take the infant to a hospital emergency department immediately. Call back in 5 minutes to ensure that parents did seek help.
- Illness (fever, dehydration, change in feeding or behavior, unusual rashes).
- Severe feeding problems (infant may become dehydrated or jaundiced or may fail to thrive).
- Problem has been present for longer than usual or usual remedies are ineffective (such as prolonged crying or sleeping, rash is spreading).
- Parent's affect seems inappropriate for situation (extremely emotional with apparently minor situation or unconcerned when situation could be serious).

Note: Callers should be referred to the primary health care provider or the hospital emergency room, if necessary, when a serious problem may be present. Being overcautious is preferable; refer parents to the primary care provider early rather than miss a serious situation.

GUIDELINES AND DOCUMENTATION

When nurses give care by telephone, they must have written protocols and policies that provide guidelines for care. This helps ensure that all who perform this service provide clients with similar information. A list of common questions can be compiled to help nurses obtain appropriate information when parents call about a problem.

Parents should always be told when and how to seek more care if problems are not resolved. If the infant seems ill, referral to the pediatrician or hospital emergency department is most appropriate. The nurse's judgment, based on education, expertise, and experience, determines how helpful the service is to clients.

All calls should be documented so that accurate legal records are available for future reference. The nurse may use a checklist or a simple written description of the call. Documentation should include identifying information for the caller, including address and phone number. The reason for the call, problems described, advice given, and any referrals also should be recorded. In some agencies all calls are audiotaped. A copy of the information is sent to the primary caregiver to provide continuity of care.

CHECK YOUR READING

1. Where do parents obtain information about caring for their infant during the early weeks after birth?
2. What are some ways in which nurses offer follow-up services to new parents?

INFANT EQUIPMENT

Generally parents obtain most of their infant equipment before the infant is born, but nurses may receive questions in the weeks after the birth. Although nurses should never recommend specific brand names of equipment, their guidance about features and safety is helpful.

Safety Considerations

Parents, especially those of limited means, need to understand that few, if any, pieces of equipment are absolutely essential for newborns. Infants sleep in padded dresser drawers and designer cribs with equal comfort. Safety is the most important consideration.

New equipment sold in the United States is generally safe because manufacturers are required to follow certain governmental standards for safety. However, hand-me-down equipment may have been produced before newer requirements were in effect. Older equipment should be checked carefully to ensure that all parts are strong and working properly (Box 23-1).

BOX 23-1 Safety Considerations for Infant Equipment

Cribs
- Crib slats must be no more than 6.7 cm (2 3/8 in) apart so that the infant's head cannot become wedged between them. Remove corner posts that extend more than 1.5 mm (1/16 in) above the end panel to prevent strangulation if clothing catches on them. Plastic teething guards should be firmly attached to side rails. Cribs should not have designs with cutouts in which the infant's head or neck might become wedged.
- Bumper pads prevent the infant from hitting against the side rails. They should fit well around the entire crib and must be anchored to keep them in place so that infants cannot get caught between the side rail and the bumper.
- The crib mattress should fit snugly with less than two fingers able to fit into the space between the mattress and the sides of the crib. More room could allow the infant to become wedged in that space and possibly suffocate. The mattress should be firm. The crib should contain no loose bedding or pillows because they increase the risk of suffocation.
- Crib toys or mobiles should be firmly attached, with no straps or strings within the infant's reach. Mobiles should be removed when the infant can reach them.
- Cribs should be placed away from hanging cords of blinds or drapes, which could become wrapped around an active infant.
- Cribs or playpens with mesh sides should have openings in the mesh smaller than 6.35 mm (1/4 inch).

Other Equipment
- Paint used to refurbish infant equipment should be marked "lead-free" and "safe for children's equipment" to prevent lead poisoning.
- All parts should function properly: crib side rails must be secure, highchair trays must stay firmly in place, latches must remain fastened, etc. The frame and basic construction of all equipment should be sturdy.
- All moving parts should be examined carefully to see whether little fingers could get caught or whether the infant could trigger a catch that would cause the equipment to become unsafe.
- Safety straps for infant seats, swings, changing tables, high chairs, or other equipment must be in good condition. Straps should fit around the infant but not be long enough that the infant could become entangled.
- Automatic swings should have legs that are stable, so that the swing does not have a tendency to tip over. Note how difficult it is to put the infant into the swing and to remove the infant from the swing safely.
- All toys should be examined carefully for parts that can be removed and swallowed. Small toys should have a diameter of less than 3.5 cm (1 3/8 in) to prevent the infant from choking on them.

Car Seats

Car accidents are the greatest cause of death for children in the United States. Approximately half of children killed in car accidents are not restrained (Agran, Anderson, & Winne, 2004). An infant carried by an adult while riding in a car is never safe. A sudden stop or accident could cause the infant to be hurled against the dashboard or crushed by the adult, who would be thrown forward by the force of the impact. Legislation has been passed in Canada and in all 50 states in the United States requiring restraint of infants and young children in car seats when they are riding in automobiles.

Generally laws require that car safety seats be used for children from birth until they are 4 years old and weigh at least 40 pounds. After that time and until they are 8 years old, children should ride in child safety booster seats. Discharge teaching should include information about state car seat laws. In some birth facilities car seats are available for loan or rental. Some facilities include the cost of a car seat in the hospital charges to ensure that all infants leave in a car seat.

The different requirements for car seats may be confusing to parents. Infants who are under 1 year of age and weigh 20 pounds or less must ride in a rear-facing seat. They should recline at approximately a 45-degree angle. Some rear-facing seats are designed for infants under 1 year old who weigh up to 35 pounds.

Infants between 1 and 4 years who weigh 20 to 40 pounds sit in a forward-facing safety seat that allows the child to sit up or recline. Convertible seats are those that meet the needs of both newborns and young children. They are used in a rear-facing position for the infant and turned to face forward for the toddler.

The harness of the car seat should firmly restrain the infant yet be quick and easy to fasten. For the rear-facing infant, shoulder straps should be in the lowest position and at or slightly below the shoulder level (Figure 23-6). In forward-facing seats the straps should be at or slightly above the shoulders. Straps should be snug and should not be twisted. The restraint clip should be placed at mid-chest or axillary level to keep the straps in place on the infant's shoulders.

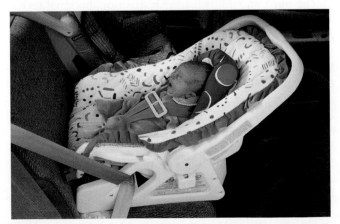

Figure 23-6 ■ A car seat for an infant under 20 pounds should face the rear of the car. Note the clip that holds the straps together for a snug fit.

Blankets should never be placed under the infant or behind the infant's back or head. If a blanket is needed for warmth, it should be placed over the infant after the harness and clip are in place. After the infant is restrained, rolled blankets can be placed at the sides or special bolsters around the head to prevent slouching of the head and increase comfort.

All car seats should be secured by the automobile seat belt to prevent the infant from being thrown forward on impact. Car seats are safest when they are placed in the center back seat of the car. They never should be placed in the front passenger seat in a car with air bags, which can kill or injure the infant when they inflate. Some cars have switches to turn off air bags. If necessary to place a car seat in the front seat, the air bags should be disengaged. Even with the air bags turned off, however, the front seat of the car is not as safe as the back seat for infants and children.

Preterm and small infants may need special adaptations. Blankets or bolsters placed at the head, along the sides, and between the legs may improve the fit. Blankets and bolsters should not be placed under the infant. Some infants have low oxygen levels, bradycardia, or apnea when in a car seat. Facilities often have parents of infants under 37 weeks' gestation or of low birth weight bring their car seat in to the hospital to test the infant's response to being placed in the seat. During testing the infant's vital signs and oxygen level are monitored. Infants who have respiratory compromise in car seats may need to use special seats or beds designed specifically for preterm or low-birth-weight infants (Williams & Martin, 2003).

Most parents believe they are using their car seats correctly. However, according to a National Transportation Safety Board survey, 72.6% of children are incorrectly restrained (Decina & Lococo, 2004). Such misuse of restraint seats could result in injury or death to the child. An incorrectly fastened harness may not restrain the infant in an accident and could cause damage, such as laceration of the liver. If the automobile seat belt is not routed through the correct area of the car seat, the seat may tip or become a flying missile during an accident.

BOX 23-2 Safety Considerations for Infant Car Seats

- Use only car seats that are approved for use in automobiles. Seats designed for use in the home do not provide adequate protection in a car.
- Use car seats that are appropriate for the infant's age and size. Place the seat in the center of the back seat of the car, never where an air bag is installed.
- Follow the manufacturer's directions for fastening the seat in the car and the infant in the car seat. Recheck the restraint straps each time the seat is used.
- Be certain that the straps are tight enough to prevent the infant from getting out of the restraints or turning over in the seat. Infants who turn over can suffocate in the padding of the seat.
- Check to see that the infant cannot become caught with the straps tightly around the neck.
- Use car seats only in an automobile. Do not place them on a soft surface, such as a bed, where they might turn over and suffocate the infant.
- Do not place them on surfaces from which they might fall, such as grocery carts.
- Never leave infants alone in a car, even for a few minutes. They could be kidnapped or injured in an accident involving the car even though it is parked. Cars quickly become very warm, and the infant could become dangerously overheated.

Car seats should be used only according to manufacturer's directions (Box 23-2).

Car seat fitting stations are available in some areas to determine if car seats are used properly and to provide teaching for parents. Further information about proper use of car seats is available on the Internet from sources such as the National Transportation Safety Board, www.ntsb.gov/default.htm.

✔ CHECK YOUR READING

3. What advice can the nurse offer about safety features of equipment used for infants?
4. What should the nurse teach parents about buying and using a car seat?

EARLY PROBLEMS

Infant Crying

Crying is a major parental concern during the early weeks after birth. Crying peaks at approximately 6 weeks of age at up to 3 hours per day. It usually decreases to an hour or less by 3 months (Needlman, 2004). Crying is most frustrating to parents when they cannot find a cause for it. Infants cry for many reasons, including hunger, discomfort, fatigue, overstimulation, and boredom. Parents can often identify the problem based on the type of sound made during crying. Sometimes no specific cause can be determined.

When the cause for crying is not obvious, some parents are afraid that responding may spoil the infant. If the infant stops crying when picked up, their concern may increase. Changing the infant's position may help gas move in the intestines, relieve tired muscles, or distract the infant by changing the scenery, bringing about a temporary cessation of crying.

Infants cannot signal that they have unmet needs in any other way but crying and are not spoiled by parents' meeting of their needs. In fact, their needs must be met in a consistent, warm, prompt manner for the development of trust to occur. Infants of parents who intervene appropriately for crying are less likely to cry excessively as they get older. Infants who are consistently picked up when in distress cry less at 1 year and are less aggressive at 2 years of age (Needlman, 2004). Therefore parents should be taught the importance of consistently and quickly answering infant cries.

Some families develop creative methods for dealing with crying infants. Others benefit from a nurse's suggestions about appropriate techniques to use.

When parents have searched for causes of crying and tried a variety of comfort measures with no success, the infant may need to spend a short time alone. Some infants need to discharge excess tension by crying before going to sleep. Although this is difficult for parents, leaving the infant safely in the crib for 10 to 15 minutes may be enough to allow the infant to fall asleep.

Some parents find that setting a timer is helpful. At the end of the period allowed, they can quietly check to be sure that the infant is all right. Changing the diaper or holding the infant and using soothing techniques before putting the

infant back to bed may be all that is necessary. Talking softly to provide reassurance and patting the infant's back without picking the infant up may also be effective.

Colic

DESCRIPTION

Colic is characterized by irritable crying for no obvious reason for 3 hours or more per day. It usually takes place during the late afternoon or early evening on at least 3 days per week. It occurs in 10% to 20% of all infants, beginning after the first 2 to 3 weeks of life (Grover, 2000a). Although it usually ends about 3 months after birth, some infants continue to have colic until 6 months of age. The infant is in good health, eats well, and gains weight appropriately, despite the daily crying episodes. Both breastfed and formula fed infants have colic.

Infants with colic cry as though in pain, draw their knees onto the abdomen or rigidly extend the legs, and may pass flatus. The crying is intense and may last until the infant falls asleep, exhausted. Because crying causes so much parental distress and may interfere with bonding or be a factor in parenting disorders or child abuse, nurses should find ways to provide support to parents of colicky infants.

Although many theories have been investigated, the cause of colic remains unknown. Allergies to cow's milk or to substances in the breastfeeding mother's diet, abnormal intestinal peristalsis, feeding techniques, parental tension, and exposure to smoking have all been considered. Colic may be a result of immaturity of the gastrointestinal tract or nervous system or a combination of factors. Actual disease states must be ruled out before a diagnosis of colic can be made.

INTERVENTIONS

Nursing interventions include using therapeutic communication to help parents express their frustrations and teaching techniques for coping with the problem. Parents should be encouraged to talk about their feelings and should be reassured that colic does not indicate poor parenting. They often feel inadequate because of their failure to manage the problem and guilty if their frustration develops into anger.

The nurse should explain that it is not abnormal to feel ambivalent or even angry with the infant. Taking time away from infant care to rest and recoup energy needed to cope with the demands of a crying infant is essential. Parents can leave the infant with a baby-sitter for short periods or take turns consoling the infant to provide breaks from the crying.

The techniques listed in "Parents Want to Know: Methods to Relieve Crying in Infants" may alleviate crying from colic temporarily, but generally none gives prolonged relief. The colic holds may be particularly effective for some infants (Figure 23-7). Changing from a cow's milk formula to a caseine hydrolysate formula may help the infant with allergies. Breastfeeding mothers whose diet includes cow's milk, orange juice, peanuts, vegetables in the cabbage family, onions, or chocolate should try eliminating these foods for 5 to 7 days to see if improvement occurs. Chamomile

Methods to Relieve Crying in Infants

TREATING COMMON CAUSES

Hunger—Try feeding the infant if it has been more than ½ hour since the last feeding. A bubble of air may have caused a feeling of fullness too soon during the last feeding. The infant may be experiencing a "growth spurt" and need more frequent feedings for a day or two to provide necessary nutrients for rapid growth.

Air bubbles—Fussy infants may need more frequent burping during and after feedings than other infants. Try burping during crying spells, because the infant may swallow air.

Diapers—Although most infants do not mind wet or soiled diapers, they may become cold or their skin may be irritated when diapers are not changed frequently enough.

Clothing—Check the infant's clothing for anything that could cause discomfort. Look for stiff seams or tags that are scratchy, or elastic on sleeves that is too tight.

Warmth—Be sure that the infant is warm enough, yet not too warm. The abdomen should feel warm even if the hands and feet are slightly cool. Dress the infant as warmly as an adult would want to be dressed, but add a receiving blanket. Infants who are overdressed rarely perspire but often cry because of their discomfort.

Overstimulation—Too many visitors handling the infant or too much noise and commotion in the household may be overstimulating. A quiet environment, rocking, or just being left to work off excess tension alone in the crib for a short time may be necessary.

QUIETING TECHNIQUES

Rocking—The gentle motion of rocking, reminiscent of intrauterine life, is often soothing for infants.

Automatic swings—The continued motion of automatic swings may be helpful. Be sure they move smoothly and are not noisy. Getting the baby into and out of the swing should be easy, to avoid awakening the infant on removal. All parts of the body should be supported. Small infants may need padding with blankets for safety and comfort.

Walking, jiggling, swaying—Sometimes newborns prefer a particular style of motion. Rocking sideways with the infant held in an upright position is helpful for some infants, whereas others prefer vertical rocking. Taking a walk outside with new sights and sounds may provide distraction.

Swaddling—Wrap the infant snugly. This is comforting because infants are used to restricted activity in the uterus. Swaddling is especially helpful during the first few weeks after birth.

Stroller or buggy rides—The motion of a stroller or buggy may be soothing to some infants. The ride can be in or outside the house. A parent can move a stroller back and forth with one foot while doing chores or eating meals. The stroller should allow the infant to lie down rather than sit. Padding may increase comfort.

Car rides—Some infants go to sleep in a moving car. A short ride may put the infant to sleep. The infant may stay asleep when carried into the house.

Music—The sound of a parent singing or humming may be reassuring to the infant. Some newborns respond well to a music box, radio, or compact disc. Music with a steady beat or classical music may be particularly effective. Music should be played softly.

White noise—Background noise sometimes puts infants to sleep by diffusing other noises. A radio set on low, a clock ticking, an indoor fountain, a fan, or the sound of a dishwasher, dryer, or even a vacuum cleaner may be effective. Tapes of sounds heard in utero are available.

Heat—A well-covered warm water bottle placed against the infant's abdomen while you hold the infant may be soothing. (Take care not to burn the infant's skin.) A blanket warmed in the clothes dryer for a few minutes serves the same purpose. Do not use a heating pad. Placing the newborn in an infant seat on top of a dishwasher or clothes dryer provides heat and background noise. Be sure that the infant is well secured and observed, of course.

Bathing—Although older infants love baths, young infants may not yet have reached that stage. However, giving a bath may be a distraction for both parent and infant, and the infant may sleep afterward.

Water—Infants who have been crying may be thirsty. Although extra water is not necessary, some mothers like to give it on occasion. It may help bring up bubbles of air that the infant has swallowed while crying. The breastfed infant's thirst can be alleviated by nursing.

Infant carriers or packs—Front carriers are designed for the young infant and may be especially helpful during crying episodes. A parent's warm body, soothing voice, and gentle swaying motion can often put an infant to sleep. At the same time, the parent can accomplish other tasks. Backpacks should be used only for older infants who are able to support the head well.

Pacifiers—Parents may find pacifiers useful for an irritable infant. The infant may be comforted by sucking even though not hungry.

Position changes—Try varying the infant's position. Laying the infant prone across a parent's lap (or over a warmed blanket) may help expel gas. Try the "colic holds" (see Figure 23-7) to help the infant pass gas. Placing the infant in a supine position and flexing the knees on the abdomen may also help.

Mother's diet—Breastfeeding mothers should review their diet. Some infants react when the mother's diet includes cow's milk, orange juice, foods in the cabbage family, onion, eggs, fish, peanuts, or chocolate. Others react to highly acidic or spicy foods. Caffeine passes into breast milk and can cause wakefulness and irritability. Omit the suspected food for 5 to 7 days, then try it again and watch for irritability after the next feedings to identify the cause of the crying.

Massage—Gentle massage may be soothing for some infants. Massage of the abdomen may help infants with colic.

Smoking—Ask anyone in the home who smokes to do so away from the infant, preferably outside.

THERAPEUTIC COMMUNICATIONS

Coping with Crying

Shannon Gray tells the nurse, Mark Winston, about her daughter, Marina, who has been having crying spells every day lasting 4 hours or longer. Shannon looks tired and worried. Marina, age 4 weeks, eats well, shows good weight gain, and is developing appropriately for her age.

Shannon: It seems like all I do is try to stop Marina's crying. I can't get anything else done.

Mark: You spend a lot of time trying to find ways to comfort her. *(Paraphrasing to encourage the mother to continue.)*

Shannon: I've tried everything! I rock her, walk with her, feed and change her. We go for car rides and put her in her swing, but nothing works for long. She just starts crying again.

Mark: It's so frustrating when nothing seems to work! *(Reflecting mother's feelings shows that the nurse is trying to understand them.)*

Shannon: Sometimes I wonder if I was cut out to be a mother. I never thought it would be like this.

Mark: Being a mother is so much harder than you expected that sometimes you aren't sure you made the right choice. *(Reflecting the content of what the mother said helps her focus and shows acceptance.)*

Shannon: But I really do love her. I just don't know how to help her. I must be a terrible mother (becomes teary).

Mark: Parents often feel guilty when they can't find a way to help an upset baby. And yet, we really don't know all the reasons why babies cry. You've tried very hard to help Marina. Maybe we can work together to think of some other techniques to use. *(Gives reassurance that what the mother is feeling is normal, then offers information and further help.)*

Shannon: I'd love that. It worries me to have Marina so unhappy. What else can I do for her?

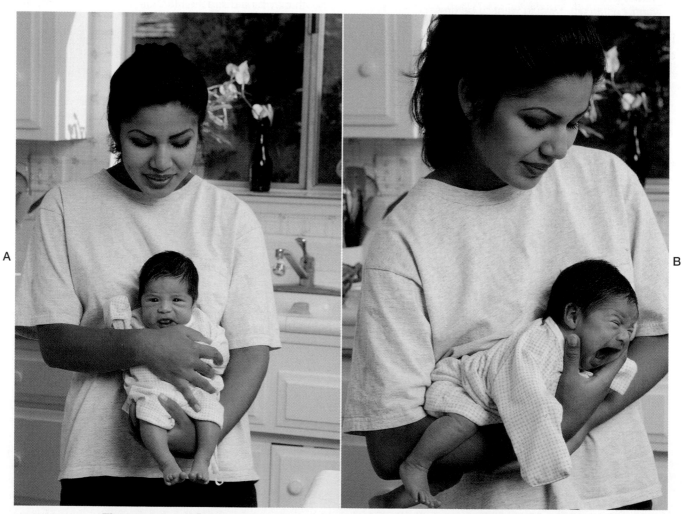

Figure 23-7 ■ Positions for holding an infant with colic. **A,** The mother holds the infant facing forward. One hand creates slight pressure against the abdomen, while the other flexes the legs. This position may help the infant expel flatus. **B,** The prone hold is also effective for some infants. The mother holds the infant in a horizontal position along her arm.

tea is often given to infants, as it has an antispasmotic effect. Any herbs the parents are using should be checked with the health care provider to ensure they are safe.

A quiet environment, calm approach, and fairly regular schedule may help some infants with colic. Increasing the time spent carrying the infant often produces some improvement. Parents should be assured that spoiling does not result from responding to the infant's cries. In severe cases the infant may be given an antiflatulent, sedative, antispasmodic, or antihistamine for a short time.

Shaken Baby Syndrome

One possible result of crying in infants is shaken baby syndrome. Shaken baby syndrome results from shaking an infant vigorously enough to cause the soft tissue of the brain to bounce against the skull. Subdural hemorrhage, retinal hemorrhage or detachment, skeletal fractures, and damage to the spinal cord may result. These may cause severe brain damage or death.

Nurses can help prevent shaken baby syndrome by making parents aware of the danger in shaking infants and by helping them learn methods to cope with infant crying. Birth facilities often include pamphlets and other information on shaken baby syndrome with discharge teaching. Further information on child abuse may be found in pediatrics textbooks.

✔ **CHECK YOUR READING**

5. Why should parents respond to crying without fear of spoiling the infant?
6. How can nurses help parents of crying infants?

Sleep

PARENTS

During the early months after birth, parents often wonder whether they will ever get a full night's sleep again. Because they are so often up during the night, they should try to make up lost sleep at other times. If the mother is not employed, she may be able to sleep during the day when the infant naps. If she is working, parents can alternate responsibility for night or early morning feedings. When mothers are breastfeeding, fathers can change the diaper, bring the infant to the mother for night feedings, and settle the infant back in bed when the feeding is finished. This allows the mother more time to sleep and lets the father share the middle-of-the-night care.

INFANT SLEEP PATTERNS

Although many newborns sleep 17 to 20 hours per day, there is wide variation in the amount of time infants spend sleeping. Infants sleep less deeply than adults and have a higher percentage of lighter, rapid eye movement (REM) sleep. During this type of sleep they sometimes make noises loud enough to wake parents in the same room, and they move about as if awakening. Going to them at this time is likely to wake them, but they may return to deep sleep if left alone.

Infants should be positioned on the back for sleep. The nurse should explain that the prone position has been associated with sudden infant death syndrome (SIDS). No pillows or soft stuffed animals should be allowed in the crib, because they could cause suffocation. Some infants sleep better in an enclosed space and may scoot themselves into a corner of a large crib. The nurse should suggest to parents that they use tightly rolled blankets around the infant to provide a "nest," which feels more like the circumscribed area of the uterus.

POSITIONING AND HEAD SHAPE

Parents may be concerned about abnormalities in head shape that may occur in some infants from sleeping on the back. Flattening of a head (plagiocephaly) that was rounded at birth may result from prolonged lying in the supine position. This can be prevented by placing the infant in the prone position on a firm surface while parents observe during awake periods. Parents should be taught the importance of "tummy time" to help develop the shoulder muscles as well as to prevent a flat area on the head. In addition, placing the infant at alternating ends of the crib often influences the direction of turning the head and distributes pressure more evenly.

SLEEPING THROUGH THE NIGHT

Parents are often confused about when infants should sleep through the night. Newborns are neurologically unable to sleep through the night during the early weeks of life. By 12 weeks of age, many infants sleep at least 5 hours at night and most infants sleep that long by 4 months. By 12 months of age, infants take two naps during the day and sleep about 10 hours at night (Grover, 2000b).

Once infants establish longer sleep patterns, they often awaken at night again when they are teething or ill. Therefore parents can expect to be awakened frequently during the early years. Parents should be taught methods of helping infants achieve longer sleep periods at night.

Concerns of Working Mothers

Although it has been traditional for women who work to have at least 6 weeks of maternity leave, this is not always possible. Some women must return to work as early as 3 weeks after childbirth. The problems of working mothers are different from those of mothers who remain at home. They must find adequate child care, identify methods of managing the household, and try to find enough time and energy to meet the needs of the infant, other family members, and themselves (see Chapter 18, pp. 434-435).

Working mothers should not become so involved in their many responsibilities that they have little time for their own needs. Some mothers regularly schedule time for themselves and for family activities. Many working mothers find that the time they can spend with their infant is particularly precious.

How to Help Infants Sleep through the Night

Allow the infant to cry for a few minutes before responding. The infant may not be completely awake and often returns to sleep if undisturbed. However, once the infant is awake, respond quickly to meet the infant's needs.

Keep night feedings for feeding only. Avoid unnecessary activity, or the infant may learn to think of this as a playtime.

Use a soft light that provides only the amount of light essential for care.

Give night feedings in the infant's room to further avoid stimulation.

Keep sounds subdued. Soft music or humming may help the infant return to sleep, but talking should be kept to a minimum.

Keep night feedings short, and put the infant back to bed immediately.

Change diapers before beginning the feeding to avoid awakening the infant after feeding.

As infants near 12 to 16 weeks, when sleeping through the night is more likely, try patting them on the back instead of feeding. Offer water instead of milk.

Allow infants to fall asleep at bedtime on their own instead of always rocking or feeding the infant. If rocking is used, place the infant into the bed when the infant is drowsy but not fully asleep. This may help infants go back to sleep alone after awakening in the night.

Concerns of Adoptive Parents

Although adoptive parents have not experienced pregnancy and childbirth, they must make adjustments similar to those of biologic parents. In some adoptive situations the parents meet the biologic mother during pregnancy and may even be with her during birth. Other adoptive parents receive a call after months of waiting telling them that their new infant is ready for them. In both cases the lives of the parents change abruptly.

In some agencies, adoptive parents receive the same teaching given to other parents. However, their ability to absorb information may be impaired by the excitement of the situation. Although adoptive mothers have not been pregnant or undergone childbirth, they are still tired from the loss of sleep and sudden changes that they experience. This may be surprising and worrisome to some. They may have many questions that nurses can answer.

Adoptive parents sometimes feel a greater need than biologic parents to be "perfect," and they may feel guilt if they do not meet their own expectations. These parents need reassurance and emotional support as they go through this happy but exhausting change in their lives.

CRITICAL THINKING EXERCISE 23-1

Mary and Skip Reynolds received their adopted daughter, Ashley, 3 days ago. They bring the 6-day-old infant to the pediatrician's office and discuss their concerns with the nurse. They received basic discharge teaching at the hospital where Ashley was born but have many questions about infant care. The last two nights Ashley slept very little, and both parents are exhausted. "We've waited so long to get Ashley," Mary says, "but I'm beginning to wonder if she's all right and if I'll be a good mother."

Questions
1. What are the priorities in this situation?
2. How should the nurse support Mary and Skip?
3. What information should the nurse include in teaching these parents?
4. How should the nurse deal with Ashley's nighttime wakefulness?

COMMON QUESTIONS AND CONCERNS

Dressing and Warmth

A room temperature of about 70° F is warm enough for the infant. The infant should be dressed as the parents would like to be dressed, with a receiving blanket added. The abdomen should be checked to see if the infant is warm enough. The hands and feet may be slightly cooler than the rest of the body but should not be mottled or blue. The infant's head should be kept warm because many thermal skin sensors are located in the scalp. A hat is appropriate if the infant is outside when it is cold or windy.

Stool Patterns

Formula-fed infants generally pass at least one stool each day. Breastfed infants may pass a stool after every feeding or, occasionally in the older infant, only one stool every 2 to 3 days. Infants may get red in the face and appear to be straining when having a bowel movement, but this is normal behavior and does not indicate constipation. Stools that are dry, hard, and marble-like indicate constipation.

Watery stools indicate diarrhea. A watery stool is absorbed into the diaper with little or no solid material left at the surface. A "water ring" remains on the diaper, showing where the liquid was absorbed. Diarrhea stools occur more frequently than the infant's normal stools and are greenish from bile moving quickly through the intestines. Diarrhea can be serious because life-threatening dehydration develops quickly. Infants should be taken to the pediatrician or nurse practitioner for treatment.

Smoking

Many mothers quit smoking before or during pregnancy but may not realize that preventing infant exposure to smoke is just as important after birth as before. Infants exposed to smoke from parents' cigarettes are more likely to develop frequent respiratory problems. Smoking is a risk factor in SIDS. Smoke absorption by infants occurs even when smoking is done in another room. Parents who continue to smoke should do so outside the house and away from the infant.

Eyes

Parents can wipe away small amounts of mucus that accumulate in the corners of the eyes with a damp, clean washcloth, using a separate section for each eye. A large amount of mucus, redness, or excessive tearing indicates an infection or a blocked lacrimal duct. The infant should be seen by the pediatrician or nurse practitioner.

Transient strabismus—misalignment or deviation of one or both eyes—is sometimes called "crossing" of the eyes. Although the condition is normal in newborns, it can be frightening to parents. The nurse should reassure them that it will end after the first few months, when the infant gains control of the small muscles of the eye. It does not indicate that the infant will have later problems. Strabismus that continues after 6 months should be evaluated.

Baths

Sponge and tub bathing are discussed in Chapter 21 (p. 530), as is care of the cord (pp. 529-530) and the circumcision site (p. 527). If the infant is washed well at diaper changes and when milk is regurgitated, bathing the child every day is not necessary. Bathing should be a time for infant stimulation and parent-infant interaction. It can be done at any time of the day that is convenient for parents.

Nails

Nails should be cut straight across with either blunt-ended scissors or clippers. The edges can be carefully smoothed with an emery board. Mothers should not attempt to cut nails too short because this increases the danger of cutting the infant's fingertip. Some mothers prefer to cut nails while the infant is sleeping. Others have someone else hold the hand steady while the mother cuts the nails. Nails grow rapidly and may need trimming twice a week.

Sucking Needs

Parents often have questions about pacifiers and thumb or finger sucking. Nurses should explain that all infants have an urge to suck, although the amount of sucking needed varies with individual infants. Some seem satisfied by feedings, but others suck their hands or a pacifier even when not hungry. Although pacifiers should not be used in breastfeeding infants who are having difficulty with latch-on, they may be helpful to other infants.

Parents may be concerned that sucking a pacifier or thumb will cause the teeth to become maloccluded. The nurse should reassure them that sucking that ends before the secondary teeth begin to erupt is unlikely to cause malocclusion (Berkowitz, 2000). Trying to stop an infant from sucking is difficult and may cause emotional problems if it becomes a major focus.

Some infants increase nonnutritive sucking because the time they spend sucking during feedings is too short. Using bottle nipples with small holes and replacing the nipples every couple of months before they get soft increase the amount of sucking that feedings provide. Breastfed infants should be allowed to continue sucking at the breast long enough to meet basic sucking needs. A short time of sucking after the infant is finished feeding generally satisfies sucking needs and increases production of milk.

When infants use a pacifier, parents should be instructed to examine it often to see if it is in good condition. Cracked, torn, or sticky nipples or nipples that can be pulled away from the shield should be discarded. Pacifiers should be replaced every month or two because they may come apart as they deteriorate and cause aspiration of parts. The shield on the pacifier should be large enough that it will not be pulled into the mouth.

Pacifiers should be kept clean by frequent washing, and parents should buy several so that one is always clean when needed. Pacifiers should never be placed on a string around the infant's neck. The string could become tangled tightly around the neck and cause strangulation. Clips with a short band to attach pacifiers to the infant's clothing without danger are available, or several pacifiers can be placed in the bed for the infant to find.

Some parents find that an advantage to a pacifier is that the infant gives it up more quickly than a thumb or finger because it is not so easily accessible. Parents who resort to the pacifier as the first response when the infant is fussy are likely to reinforce its use and increase dependence on it. Pacifiers used only after other causes of distress are ruled out may be given up sooner. Because the need for nonnutritive sucking begins to diminish between 4 and 6 months of age, pacifier use may begin to decrease at that time with parents' help.

Teething

The timing of tooth eruption varies. The first tooth may appear as early as 3 months or as late as 13 months of age. Generally the two lower central incisors come through the gums at about 6 to 8 months. The average age for eruption of all deciduous teeth is $2\frac{1}{2}$ years.

The actual time when teeth erupt has no relationship to the infant's development in other areas. Parents may think that teething has begun when the infant is about 3 months of age, when the normal increased production of saliva causes drooling. Infants must learn to swallow the extra saliva without drooling.

Some infants show signs of teething for weeks before the first tooth comes through the gums. These signs include excessive salivation, biting, irritability, and decreased feedings. Although slight fever may occur, it should be investigated for other causes. Infants who were sleeping through the night begin to wake again as a result of teething discomfort. A rash around the mouth may result from drooling. The infant's gums may look red and swollen over the area where the tooth will erupt.

Instruct parents that high fevers or other signs of illness are not normal results of teething. Infants may be more susceptible to illness at the time of teething because of poor eating and sleeping. In addition, teething begins at about the time many of the antibodies received in utero are disappearing.

Some teething infants like to bite on hard objects such as teething rings. Some rings can be frozen to soothe inflammation of the gums. Over-the-counter local anesthetics or analgesics, such as acetaminophen, are safe in small amounts for teething discomfort. Alcoholic beverages should never be rubbed on the gums because infants swallow the alcohol.

Common Rashes

DIAPER RASH (DIAPER DERMATITIS)

Diaper rash occurs as a result of prolonged exposure of skin to wetness combined with a chemical reaction between the urine and fecal enzymes that increases skin sensitivity to irritation. A rash is more likely to develop when infants begin to sleep for longer periods and the time between diaper changes increases. Another cause may be sensitivity to commercial disposable washcloths or components of paper diapers.

Treatment of diaper rash is primarily keeping the diaper area clean and dry. The nurse should instruct the parents to change diapers as soon as they are wet or soiled. They should gently wash the perineum with mild soap and warm water but should avoid excessive washing. Removing the diapers and exposing the perineum to warm air helps healing.

Applying a thin layer of a cream such as those with zinc oxide may speed healing and help prevent further outbreaks. The nurse should tell parents not to apply the ointments too thickly because they may be difficult to remove. Ointments contaminated with fecal matter may accumulate in the skin folds and hold bacteria. Low-potency corticosteroid preparations may be necessary for severe cases.

Secondary infection of diaper rash with organisms such as *Candida albicans* or *Staphylococcus* are common. When infection occurs, severe rash, pustules, or crusted areas may be present. The infant should be taken to a pediatrician or nurse practitioner for treatment. Antifungal or antibiotic creams may be necessary for infections.

MILIARIA (PRICKLY HEAT)

Although most common during hot weather, miliaria or prickly heat develops in infants who are too warmly dressed in any weather. It may also occur in infants with a fever. This rash results from occlusion and inflammation of the sweat (eccrine) glands. It has a red base with papules or clear vesicles in the center.

Treatment involves cooling the infant by removing excess clothing or by giving a soothing lukewarm bath. The condition clears quickly with removal of the cause, and ointments or other skin preparations should be avoided. The nurse should discuss the appropriate amount of clothing with parents when infants develop prickly heat.

SEBORRHEIC DERMATITIS (CRADLE CAP)

Cradle cap is a chronic inflammation of the scalp or other areas of the skin characterized by yellow, scaly, oily lesions. It sometimes results when parents do not wash over the anterior fontanel carefully for fear that they will hurt the infant.

Treatment is application of oil or shampoo to the area to help the lesions soften, then removal with a comb before shampooing the head. The nurse should teach parents how to shampoo the scalp and explain that they will not damage the fontanel by normal gentle shampooing. The scalp should be rinsed well to remove all soap, which otherwise may cause irritation. A persistent problem may be treated with hydrocortisone cream or special shampoos.

> ✔ **CHECK YOUR READING**
>
> 7. What are common signs of teething?
> 8. How can parents prevent or treat diaper rash?

NUTRITION DURING THE EARLY WEEKS

Infant feeding is discussed in detail in Chapter 22. This section addresses only the most frequent early concerns parents have about feeding.

Breastfeeding

Breastfeeding mothers should be taught not to set a strict timetable but to feed the infant when signs of hunger are present. This will be more often than if the infant were formula fed, about every 2 to 3 hours. Generally, feedings should last 10 to 15 minutes on each breast (see Chapter 22). As nursing becomes well established, mothers often feed approximately 15 minutes on the first side, then continue on the second side as long as the infant is interested. The feeding concludes when the infant falls asleep or after a short period of nonnutritive suckling.

The total time for each breastfeeding session varies with individual infants and from feeding to feeding. The time may be as short as 20 minutes or as long as 40 minutes. As infants become older, they become more efficient at nursing and obtain all the milk they need in a shorter period.

Mothers may be concerned when an infant suddenly seems fussy and wants to breastfeed much more often than previously. This is frequently a way of increasing milk production for an infant experiencing a growth spurt. Nurses can teach mothers to expect growth spurts at approximately 10 days, 2 weeks, 6 weeks, and 3 months after birth (Grodner, Anderson, & DeYoung, 2004).

Formula Feeding

Mothers using formula may be unsure about how much to feed the infant during the early weeks after birth. Although infants take about $\frac{1}{2}$ to 1 oz at a time during the first day or two of life, this rapidly increases to 2 or 3 oz per feeding within a week. By 12 weeks they usually drink 5 to 6 oz every 3 to 4 hours. Considerable variation is seen among infants, and mothers should be encouraged to adapt to their own infant's needs.

Formula-fed infants generally eat every 3 to 4 hours. Strict schedules are unnecessary, and the mother should feed the infant when signs of hunger appear. Fussiness or crying, rooting, sucking on hands, and eagerly taking the bottle indicate that the infant is hungry.

Mothers should not urge infants to drink all of the formula if they do not seem interested. Infants vary, as adults do, in the amount taken at each meal. Encouraging the infant to complete all feedings places undue emphasis on the feeding and may lead to later feeding problems or obesity.

Water

Both formula and breast milk contain enough water for infants who are eating well. Additional water is not necessary. Some mothers give water to formula-fed infants who are fussy and do not respond to other interventions. Sips of water also can be given to infants with hiccups. Hiccups go away shortly, with or without water, however.

Infants should not be given water with sugar added. Sugar only adds empty calories and accustoms infants to the sweet taste. Honey should never be used for young infants because of the risk of botulism.

Regurgitation

Infants often regurgitate ("spit up") because they may eat more than their stomach can easily hold and because their immature lower esophageal sphincter allows the stomach contents to flow into the esophagus easily. "Wet burps" result when air is trapped under stomach contents. As the air is expelled, a small amount of milk comes with it.

The nurse should teach parents to differentiate normal spitting up from vomiting, which is a sign of illness. Regurgitation may occur frequently, but usually only a small amount at a time. Vomiting may involve the entire feeding, and it is expelled forcefully. Parents should always seek treatment for the infant with projectile vomiting, in which the vomitus is expelled with such force that it travels some distance. This is a sign of pyloric stenosis, which may require surgery, and other serious conditions.

If an infant has frequent regurgitation, parents can elevate the head of the bed or place the infant in a prone position while the infant is awake to help air rise and to decrease regurgitation. Turning the infant to the side promotes drainage of regurgitated fluids and prevents aspiration. Small, more frequent feeding may also help.

Some infants swallow excessive air because they eat very rapidly. Nurses can instruct parents to feed infants before they get too hungry and to stop often for burping. If the hole in a bottle nipple is too small, an infant may swallow air around the nipple. Enlarging the nipple hole slightly with a hot needle may prevent this.

Mild reflux begins within the first few months after birth, peaks at 4 months, and resolves in almost all infants by 12 to 24 months (Orenstein, Peters, Khan, Youssef, & Hussain, 2004). The infant who has excessive regurgitation or vomiting should be referred for follow-up with the pediatrician or nurse practitioner.

Introduction of Solid Foods

Infants do not need solid foods until 4 to 6 months of age. Some mothers introduce solids earlier in the hope that the infant will sleep longer at night. This is seldom successful because the infant receives no more calories from the small amounts of solids taken than from milk. In addition, early introduction of solids may precipitate allergies or cause intestinal upsets because they are incompletely digested. Waiting 4 to 6 months allows time for the infant's ability to produce immune globulin A, which decreases the risk of allergic responses when solids are introduced (Riordan, 2005). When infants start solids, they drink less milk, thus replacing a food that meets their nutrient needs well with a food that is poorly digested.

The extrusion reflex, in which infants push the tongue out against anything that touches it, continues until approximately 4 months of age. This makes feeding a younger infant difficult because the infant pushes almost all of every spoonful out of the mouth. The nurse should explain the problems involved with early introduction of solid foods and encourage parents to wait until the infant is physiologically ready, at 4 to 6 months of age. The concerns that made the parents consider changing the feeding routine should also be discussed.

Weaning

Some mothers decide to wean the infant from the breast to the bottle during the first 12 weeks after birth. Information about weaning is included in Chapter 22, pp. 561-562.

CHECK YOUR READING

9. How much should infants eat during the early weeks after birth?
10. Why should solid foods be avoided until the infant is 4 to 6 months old?

GROWTH AND DEVELOPMENT

Anticipatory Guidance

Parents often have questions about normal patterns of growth and stages of development. Nurses provide anticipatory guidance about these areas to help parents develop realistic expectations about infants' abilities at various ages. This also helps parents prepare for changes they must make to keep the infant's environment safe, especially during the second half of the first year of life, when the infant begins to explore the house alone.

Growth and Developmental Milestones

A brief summary of the changes that can be expected during the infant's first 12 weeks is included here. More in-depth information is included in pediatrics textbooks. The nurse should emphasize to parents that guidelines are only averages, the range of normal is often broad, and individual differences are expected.

During the first 6 months of life, growth proceeds at a predictable rate in normal infants. The weight lost after birth is usually regained by 10 days of age. In the early months the average infant gains at least 480 g (1 lb) and often nearer 907 g (2 lb), grows 3.5 cm (1.4 in), and has an increase in head circumference of 2 cm (0.8 in) each month. The posterior fontanel closes by 2 to 3 months and the anterior fontanel by 12 to 18 months of age. Tears appear 2 to 4 weeks after birth.

The Moro, grasp, tonic neck, and rooting reflexes especially are noticed by parents. The nurse should point out that their gradual disappearance helps prepare the infant to learn new skills, such as voluntary grasping or turning over, which are impossible if the reflexes continue. The infant gradually develops more control of the heavy head and has less bobbing or head lag by the end of the third month.

Infants are social beings. They stare at objects of interest within a range of 8 to 12 inches as newborns and learn to follow objects by turning the head a full 180 degrees during the first 12 weeks of life. A social smile begins as early as 3 to 5 weeks and is well developed by 6 to 8 weeks. Infants make vowel sounds (cooing) by 2 months and begin some consonant sounds (babbling) and may even squeal with delight at 3 months.

Accident Prevention

Knowing what infants can do helps prevent accidents. In the first 3 months after birth, they are totally helpless. Although they can communicate their needs through crying, someone must be available at all times to care for them. Parents must be taught the dangers of leaving the infant on any unprotected surface, even for seconds. In a short time an infant can wiggle from the middle to the edge of a large bed and fall. Crib sides should be raised whenever the infant is in bed. Cribs should be positioned away from hanging cords of blinds or drapes and nothing with strings should be hung on the bed, because these could become wrapped around an active infant and cause strangulation.

Parents should keep one hand on an infant lying on an unprotected surface if they must turn away. Infants should never be left for an instant in even an inch of water because of the danger of drowning. Parents should take the telephone off the hook or take a portable phone with them and ignore the doorbell when bathing the infant. If they must leave the room, parents should take the infant out of the water and with them.

As infants learn to grasp objects with increasing accuracy, parents must be certain that nothing is in the infant's reach that could be swallowed or otherwise cause harm. Help parents to think ahead to the time when the infant will be crawling and walking and make plans for how they will "child-proof" their home.

WELL-BABY CARE

Well-Baby Checkups

Well-baby checkups are an opportunity for the pediatrician or nurse practitioner to assess the infant's growth and development, answer questions about feeding and infant care, observe for abnormalities, and give immunizations. These checkups may be provided by a private practitioner or in a well-baby clinic, where examinations and immunizations are free or at reduced cost. Infants are usually taken to their first well-baby checkup at 2 to 4 weeks of age. They gener-

ally receive well-baby checkups at 2, 4, 6, 9, and 12 months of age.

Well-baby checkups are a good time for mothers to learn about what is normal for their infants in terms of growth and behaviors. Anticipatory guidance is a major part of well-baby visits. Many mothers are reassured to find that such problems as wakefulness at night or changes in feeding habits are normal. Safety is discussed as the parents learn about skills infants will learn soon that might place them in danger.

Immunizations

Nurses often receive questions about the need for immunizations for uncommon diseases, such as diphtheria, that parents have never seen. Parents may consider a condition such as varicella (chickenpox) to be a harmless childhood illness. When they do not understand the need for immunizations, parents may be reluctant to have their infants undergo painful procedures.

The nurse must explain to parents the importance of immunizations, briefly describing the serious illnesses immunizations prevent. Discuss the age at which each immunization is given and when boosters are needed (Table 23-1).

In the United States, national health objectives for the year 2010 include full immunization of at least 90% of children before the age of 3 years. According to the Centers for Disease Control and Prevention 90% or more of children under 3 years had completed the series of *Haemophilus influenzae* (Hib); measles, mumps, and rubella (MMR); polio; and hepatitis B (HepB) vaccines in 2003. The rate was lower for completed immunization against diphtheria, tetanus and pertussis (DTaP) (84.8%), varicella (84.8%), and pneumonia (36.7%) vaccines. These figures are the highest immunization rates to date. However, discrepancies exist among various states and urban areas. Maintaining high levels of immunization is important to prevent the rise of communicable diseases, as has happened in the past when a resurgence of measles occurred in many U.S. communities.

Common reactions to immunizations should also be discussed with the parents. For example, infants may develop a fever and local tenderness, especially after administration of DTaP vaccine. Many care providers suggest that infants receive acetaminophen at the time of the vaccine and every 4 to 6 hours for the first 24 hours to increase comfort.

Because recommendations for immunizations change from time to time, parents should be referred to their pediatrician for the latest information. Another source is the AAP, which offers Internet information for parents as well as professionals. The Internet address is http://www.aap.org.

✔ CHECK YOUR READING

11. How can parents make use of knowledge about infant development to prevent accidents in the first 12 weeks of life?
12. What is the importance of well-baby checkups?
13. Why are immunizations important?

TABLE 23-1 Recommended Immunization Schedule for the First Six Years

Immunization	Age for Original Immunization	Age for Booster
HepB (hepatitis B)	Birth-2 mo, 1-4 mo, 6-18 mo[1,2]	
DTaP (diphtheria, tetanus, and acellular pertussis)	2, 4, 6 mo	15-18 mo[3], 4-6 yr
Hib (*Haemophilus influenzae* type b)	2, 4, 6 mo or 2, 4 mo[4]	12-15 mo
Inactivated poliovirus vaccine	2, 4 mo	6-18 mo, 4-6 yr
MMR (measles, mumps, rubella)	12-15 mo	4-6 yr[5]
Varicella vaccine	12-18 mo or at any time after 12 mo	
Pneumococcal vaccine	2, 4, 6 mo	12-15 mo
Influenza vaccine[6]	Yearly beginning at 6 mo	
Hepatitis A vaccine[7] (if at risk)	24 mo, at least 6 mo later	

From Advisory Committee on Immunization Practices of the Centers for Disease Control and Prevention, the American Academy of Pediatrics Committee on Infectious Diseases, and the American Academy of Family Physicians (2004). *Recommended childhood and adolescent immunization schedule, United States, 2005.* Retrieved January 5, 2005, from http://aap.org.
[1]Hepatitis B (HepB) vaccine: Infants of HBsAg-negative mothers receive the first dose by age 2 months and the second dose at least 4 weeks after the first dose. (Only monovalent HepB can be used at birth. Monovalent or combination vaccine containing HepB can be used for other doses. If combination vaccine is used, the second dose cannot be given before age 6 weeks.) The last dose is given at least 16 weeks after the first dose and at least 8 weeks after the second dose but not before the infant is 24 weeks of age.
[2]Newborns whose mothers are HBsAg-positive should receive hepatitis B immune globulin and the first dose of HepB within 12 hours of birth and at different sites. The second dose of vaccine is given at 1-2 months of age and last dose not before 24 weeks. Four doses may be given if a birth dose is administered. If the mother's HBsAg status is unknown, the infant is vaccinated within 12 hours of birth and hepatitis immune globulin is given as soon as possible (within 1 week) if testing shows the mother is positive. Only monovalent HepB can be used at birth. Monovalent or combination vaccine containing HepB can be used for other doses.
[3]Diphtheria and tetanus toxoids and acellular pertussis (DTaP) vaccine: The fourth dose may be given as early as 12 months of age if 6 months have elapsed since the third dose and if the child is unlikely to return at age 15-18 months.
[4]*Haemophilus influenzae* type b (Hib) conjugate vaccine: The number of doses of Hib depends on the vaccine used.
[5]Measles, mumps, and rubella vaccine (MMR): The second dose of MMR may be given at any time at least 4 weeks after the first dose, if necessary, as long as both doses are given after 12 months of age.
[6]Influenza vaccine: Recommended for children 6-23 months and close contacts of children 0-23 months of age. Also recommended yearly for children with risk factors.
[7]Hepatitis A vaccine: Two doses, at least 6 months apart, are recommended for children at risk.

ILLNESS

Parents have many questions about illness in the infant. They have concerns about how to recognize an illness and when to call the pediatrician or nurse practitioner.

Recognizing Signs

Parents may need help in recognizing signs of illness in infants (Box 23-3). The nurse should explain that any time the infant appears sick or parents believe that something is wrong with the infant, they should call the pediatrician or nurse practitioner. Office staff are usually educated to help parents determine whether the infant is sick enough that he or she should be seen.

Calling the Pediatrician or Nurse Practitioner

When calling the health care provider about an illness, parents should prepare by writing down the information about the illness to avoid forgetting something. They should have the name and telephone number of a pharmacy available in case a prescription drug is needed, and they should be ready to write down instructions (Box 23-4).

Office staff are usually able to answer questions on the telephone about common concerns and simple illnesses. They can help determine if an infant should be brought

---

BOX 23-3 Common Signs of Illness in Infants

- Fever above 37.8° C (100° F) axillary
- Vomiting all of a feeding more than once or twice in a day
- Watery stools or significant increase in number of stools over what is normal for the infant
- Blisters, sores, or rashes that are unusual for the infant
- Unusual changes in behavior: listlessness or sleeping much more than usual, irritability or crying much more than usual
- Coughing, frequent sneezing, runny nose (occasional sneezing is not a problem)
- Pulling or rubbing at the ear, drainage from the ear

BOX 23-4 Calling the Pediatrician or Nurse Practitioner

Write down pertinent information before calling. Have your pharmacy name and telephone number handy, along with a pen and paper to write down instructions.
1. Give the infant's name and age first.
2. Describe the illness or problem.
   a. When did it start?
   b. How often does it occur (e.g., the number of times the infant vomits or passes a stool)?
   c. How does this compare with the infant's normal patterns?
   d. What does it look like (e.g., describe the rash or the color and consistency of the stools)?
3. Describe any fever.
   a. How high is it? (Temperature should be taken by axillary method.)
   b. How long has the fever been present?
   c. Has it been higher than it is now?
4. Describe other signs of illness.
   a. Has eating behavior changed?
   b. Have sleep patterns changed?
5. Describe the infant's behavior.
   a. Does the infant seem sick?
   b. Is the infant irritable, lethargic, acting differently from normal?
6. Describe what has been done so far to treat the condition (e.g., medicines, herbs) and the results.
7. Discuss other relevant information.
   a. Is there a similar illness in family members?
   b. Was the infant treated recently for a similar or different illness?
   c. Does the infant take any other medications?

into the office, but parents should be assertive in asking for an appointment if they believe that one is needed. They have a more complete picture of the infant's condition than can be given over the telephone. Parents should immediately identify emergencies so that the staff can act accordingly. Parents can expect the pediatrician or nurse practitioner to return calls about acute illness as soon as possible and those about other concerns near the end of the day.

Knowing When to Seek Immediate Help

Parents should take the infant to the pediatrician or to an emergency room if signs of dyspnea are present. An infant from birth to 3 months of age should not have a sustained respiratory rate above 60 breaths per minute. If retractions, cyanosis, or extreme pallor is present, parents should get immediate help. If respiratory difficulty occurs suddenly in an infant who is well, the infant may have aspirated a feeding or small object. Parents should call paramedics. Nurses should encourage all parents to take classes in cardiopulmonary resuscitation.

If an infant's respiratory rate is below 30, parents should stimulate the infant and see if the respirations increase and stay within the normal range of 30 to 60 breaths per minute. If the respiratory rate continues to be below normal, the infant should be seen by a pediatrician or nurse practitioner.

Parents should call the pediatrician if the infant is hard to arouse and keep awake. The infant could be semi-comatose and showing signs of central nervous system disease such as meningitis or encephalitis.

Learning about Sudden Infant Death Syndrome

SIDS is the abrupt death of an infant that is unexplained by history, autopsy, or examination of the scene of death. In the United States almost 2300 SIDS deaths occurred in 2002. Although the incidence has decreased, SIDS is the third leading cause of death in infants from birth to 1 year of age and the most common cause of death in infants from 1 month to 1 year of age (Hunt & Hauck, 2004; Kochanek, Murphy, Anderson, & Scott, 2004).

SIDS occurs in apparently healthy infants during sleep and more often in male infants and during cold weather. It peaks in infants who are 2 to 4 months of age. Although the rate is 57.1 deaths per 100,000 live births for all groups in the United States, the rate is 47.1 for white infants and 118.4 for African-American infants (Kochanek et al., 2004). This may be partly a result of the increased prevalence of bed-sharing and use of nonstandard beds (not designed for infants) in this group (Unger et al., 2003). Bed-sharing appears to increase the risk of unexplained death in infants (Thogmartin, Siebert, & Pellan, 2001). Risk of SIDS also is increased when infants sleep in adult beds or sofas (Scheers, Rutherford, & Kemp, 2003). Native American infants also have a higher rate of SIDS. Asian, Pacific Islander, and Hispanic infants have the lowest rate.

There have been many studies, but the cause of SIDS remains unknown. Maternal smoking, young maternal age, late or no prenatal care, prematurity, low birth weight, low socioeconomic status, and maternal drug abuse are some of the factors that have been associated with SIDS. Associations have been found between SIDS and infants sleeping in the prone position, sleeping on a soft surface, overheating, and sleeping in the same bed with another person.

Current recommendations are that a healthy infant be placed in a supine position for sleep because the prone position may increase the risk of upper airway obstruction, rebreathing expired air, and hyperthermia. A national goal for the year 2010 is to reduce the number of SIDS deaths by increasing the number of infants put down to sleep on their backs to at least 70% (U.S. Department of Health and Human Services, 2000).

Although the side-lying position is also associated with a decreased incidence of SIDS, infants who sleep on their side are twice as likely to die from SIDS as those placed on their back for sleep (Hunt & Hauck, 2004). The recommendation for supine positioning for sleep applies to all infants, regardless of their birth weight or gestational age, unless other circumstances necessitate an exception (AAP, 2000).

Nurses should teach parents about proper positioning of their infants for sleep. Although nurses often tell parents about the AAP recommendations for supine position for sleep and may give parents educational material about the position, many nurses position infants in the side-lying position instead of the supine position. It is important for nurses to model this behavior in addition to teaching about it (Bullock, Mickey, Green, & Heine, 2004).

Other modifiable factors that should receive increased parent education are not allowing infants to become overheated or to sleep on a soft surface and avoiding maternal smoking. Objects such as pillows, comforters, quilts, and loose bedding may be hazardous. Blankets should be tucked under the mattress so that they are not likely to cover the infant's face.

It is important that children in child care settings also be placed in a supine position for sleep. Parents should be sure that child care providers are aware of the risk of the prone position and follow the guidelines. Deaths are increased when infants accustomed to sleeping in the supine position are placed prone for sleep. This is more likely to happen when people other than the parents are caring for the infant.

Because parents often have many concerns about SIDS, therapeutic communication techniques may assist them to talk about their fears. They may need reassurance that the chance that any one infant will experience SIDS is small.

✔ **CHECK YOUR READING**

14. When should immediate help be sought for an infant?
15. What should nurses teach parents about SIDS?

SUMMARY CONCEPTS

- Nurses assist parents after discharge by home or clinic visits and telephone calls.
- Careful planning, good communication skills, and knowledge of cultural practices are necessary during home visits.
- Clinic visits include the same assessment and teaching as home visits but do not allow the nurse to assess the home. They are more cost effective, however.
- Telephone calls after discharge from the birth facility are less expensive than home or clinic visits but do not allow the nurse to assess the client or home environment in person.
- All equipment, particularly older, used articles, should be checked by parents for safety.
- Infants younger than 1 year old or weighing less than 20 pounds should use a rear-facing car seat. Older infants need car seats that face forward. All should be placed in the back seat of the car.
- Crying is a major source of concern for parents. They should be reassured that infants are not spoiled by prompt attention to their needs.
- Colic—crying that lasts 3 or more hours—usually occurs in the afternoon or evening and often disappears after 3 months. The cause is unknown, and infants with colic grow and develop appropriately.
- Infants may sleep 5 or more hours at night beginning at about 12 weeks.
- Common signs of teething include drooling, irritability, decreased appetite and sleep, rash, and red and swollen gums. High fever or other signs of illness are not caused by teething.
- Diaper rash may be caused by prolonged exposure to wet or soiled diapers or sensitivity to substances in diapers or disposable wash cloths. It can become infected.
- Both breastfed and formula-fed infants vary in amounts taken at each feeding but average about 1/2 to 1 oz per feeding initially and 5 to 6 oz per feeding at 12 weeks of age.
- Solid foods should be started at 4 to 6 months of age when the extrusion reflex is gone and solids can be digested by infants.
- Well-baby checkups are important for assessment of growth and development, guidance, and immunizations. Immunizations safeguard infants and communities from spread of communicable diseases.
- Parents should learn signs of illness in the infant and when immediate medical care is necessary. They should seek immediate medical attention if infants have respiratory difficulty or are difficult to arouse from sleep.
- The nurse should teach parents about current knowledge about SIDS and the fact that the cause remains unknown. Parents should be taught to place the infant in a supine position for sleep.

ANSWERS TO CRITICAL THINKING EXERCISE 23-1, p. 580

1. The major priorities are to support the parents in their new role and to determine if Ashley is progressing normally.
2. Information should be based on the parent's concerns. Explain normal characteristics and behaviors of the newborn. Determine if Mary and Skip need more information about basic infant care, such as feeding, sleeping, cord care, and signs of illness. Provide frequent opportunities for them to ask questions.
3. Obtain more information about Ashley's sleep patterns. Discuss normal sleep in newborns and methods of helping infants sleep. Offer suggestions for methods of dealing with crying. Help Mary and Skip work out a plan for sharing the burdens and the joys of parenthood.
4. Use therapeutic communication techniques to allow Mary and Skip to express their feelings adequately. If Ashley appears to be progressing normally, emphasize that she is doing well. Point out that the problems they are encountering are quite common for both biologic and adoptive parents.

REFERENCES & READINGS

Agran, P.F., Anderson, C.L., & Winne, D.G. (2004). Violators of a child passenger safety law. *Pediatrics, 114*(1), 109-115.

American Academy of Pediatrics (AAP). (1999). Safe transportation of newborns at hospital discharge. *Pediatrics, 104*(4), 986-987.

American Academy of Pediatrics Committee on Child Abuse and Neglect. (2001). Shaken baby syndrome: rotational cranial injuries—technical report. *Pediatrics 108*(1), 206-210.

American Academy of Pediatrics Task Force on Infant Sleep Position and Sudden Infant Death Syndrome. (2000). Changing concepts of Sudden Infant Death Syndrome: Implications for infant sleeping environment and sleep position. *Pediatrics, 105*(3), 650-656.

American Academy of Pediatrics (AAP) & American College of Obstetricians and Gynecologists (ACOG). (2002). *Guidelines for perinatal care* (5th ed.). Elk Grove, IL: AAP.

Association of Women's Health, Obstetric and Neonatal Nurses (AWHONN). (2000). *Didactic content and clinical skills verification for professional nurse providers of perinatal home care* (2nd ed.). Washington, DC: Author.

AWHONN. (2003). *Standards for professional nursing practice in the care of women and newborns* (6th ed.). Washington, DC: Author.

Berkowitz, C.D. (2000). Thumbsucking and other habits. In C.D. Berkowitz (Ed.), *Pediatrics: A primary care approach* (2nd ed., pp. 127-131). Philadelphia: Saunders.

Blackburn, S.T., & Blakewell-Sachs, S. (2003). *Understanding the behavior of term infants.* White Plains, NY: March of Dimes Birth Defects Foundation. Retrieved November 30, 2004, from http://www.marchofdimes.org.

Bullock, L.F.C., Mickey, K., Green, J., & Heine, A. (2004). Are nurses acting as role models for the prevention of SIDS? *MCN: American Journal of Maternal/Child Nursing, 29*(3), 172-177.

Centers for Disease Control and Prevention. (2004). National, state, and urban area vaccination coverage among children aged 19-35 months, United States, 2003. *MMWR. Morbidity and Mortality Weekly Report, 53*(29), 658-661.

Creehan, P.A. (2001). Sending baby home safely: Developing an infant car seat testing program. *AWHONN Lifelines, 5*(6), 60-70.

Dahlberg, N.F. (2001). Postpartum home care. In K.R. Simpson & P.A. Creehan (Eds.), *AWHONN perinatal nursing* (2nd ed, pp. 643-655). Philadelphia: Lippincott Williams & Wilkins.

Dana, S.N., & Wambach, K.A. (2003). Patient satisfaction with an early discharge home visit program. *Journal of Obstetric, Gynecologic, and Neonatal Nursing, 32*(2), 190-198.

Davis, L.J., Okuboye, S., & Ferguson, S.L. (2000). Healthy people 2010: Examining a decade of maternal and infant health. *AWHONN Lifelines, 4*(3), 26-33.

Decina, L.E., & Lococo, K.H. (2003). *Misuse of child restraints*. National Highway Traffic Safety Administration. Retrieved April 12, 2005 from http://www.nhtsa.dot.gov/people/injury/research/misuse/index.html.

Ellett, M., Schuff, E., & Davis, J.B. (2005). Parental perceptions of the lasting effects of infant colic. *MCN: The American Journal of Maternal/Child Nursing 30*(2), 127-132.

Escobar, G.J., Braveman, P.A., Ackerson, L., Odouli, R., Colman-Phox, K. Capra, A.M., et al. (2001). A randomized comparison of home visits and hospital-based group follow-up visits after early postpartum discharge. *Pediatrics, 108*(3), 719-727.

Gracey, K. (2004). Discharge planning and transition to home care. In M.T. Verklan & M. Walden (Eds.), *Core curriculum for neonatal intensive care nursing* (3rd ed.), Philadelphia: Saunders, pp. 422-434.

Grodner, M., Anderson, S.L., & DeYoung, S. (2004). *Foundations and clinical applications of nutrition: A nursing approach* (3rd ed.). St. Louis: Mosby.

Grover, G. (2000a). Crying and colic. In C.D. Berkowitz (Ed.), *Pediatrics: A primary care approach* (2nd ed., pp. 111-114). Philadelphia: Saunders.

Grover, G. (2000b). Sleep: Normal pattern and common disorders. In C.D. Berkowitz (Ed.), *Pediatrics: A primary care approach* (2nd ed., pp. 39-44). Philadelphia: Saunders.

Hornell, A., Hofvander, Y., & Kylberg, E. (2001). Solids and formula: Association with pattern and duration of breastfeeding. *Pediatrics, 107*(3), e38.

Hunt, C.E., & Hauck, F.R. (2004). Sudden Infant Death Syndrome. In R.E. Behrman, R.M. Kliegman, & H.B. Jenson (Eds.). *Nelson textbook of pediatrics* (17th ed., pp. 1380-1385). Philadelphia: Saunders.

Keppler, A.B., & Simpson, K.R. (2001). Discharge planning. In K.R. Simpson & P.A. Creehan (Eds.), *AWHONN perinatal nursing* (2nd ed, pp. 610-632). Philadelphia: Lippincott Williams & Wilkins.

Kleinman, R.E. (Ed.). (2004). *Pediatric nutrition handbook* (5th ed.). Elk Grove Village, IL: American Academy of Pediatrics.

Kochanek, K.D., Murphy, S.L., Anderson, R.N., & Scott, C. (2004). Deaths: Final data for 2002. *National Vital Statistics Reports, 53*(5). Hyattsville, MD: National Center for Health Statistics.

Logsdon, M.C., & Davis, D.W. (2004). Paraprofessional support for pregnant and parenting women. *MCN: American Journal of Maternal/Child Nursing, 29*(2), 92-99.

Ludington-Hoe, S.M., Cong, X., & Hashemi, F. (2002). Infant crying: Nature, physiologic consequences, and select interventions. *MCN: American Journal of Maternal/Child Nursing, 21*(2), 29-36.

Morin, K.H. (2004a). Current thoughts on healthy term infant nutrition. *MCN: American Journal of Maternal/Child Nursing, 29*(5), 312-319.

Morin, K.H. (2004b). Solids—When and why. *MCN: American Journal of Maternal/Child Nursing, 29*(4), 259.

Needlman, R.D. (2004). The first year. In R.E. Behrman, R.M. Kliegman, & H.B. Jenson (Eds.), *Nelson textbook of pediatrics* (17th ed., pp. 31-38). Philadelphia: Saunders.

National Highway Traffic Safety Administration. *Child passenger safety.* Retrieved January 3, 2005, from http://www.nhtsa.dot.gov/people/injury/childps/.

National Highway Traffic Safety Administration. (2004). *Misuse of child restraints.* Retrieved January 3, 2005, from http://www.nhtsa.dot.gov/people/injury/research/Misuse/images/misusescreen.pdf.

Orenstein, S. Peters, J., Khan, S., Youssef, N., & Hussain, S.Z. (2004). The esophagus. In R.E. Behrman, R.M. Kliegman, & H.B. Jenson (Eds.), *Nelson textbook of pediatrics* (17th ed., pp. 1217-1227). Philadelphia: Saunders.

Paul, I.M., Phillips, T.A., Widome, M.D., & Hollenbeak, C.S. (2004). Cost-effectiveness of postnatal home nursing visits for prevention of hospital care for jaundice and dehydration. *Pediatrics, 114*(4), 1015-1022.

Persing, J., James, H., Swanson, J., & Kattwinkel, J. (2004). Prevention and management of positional skull deformities in infants. *Pediatrics, 112*(1), 199-202.

Riordan, J. (2005). The biologic specificity of breastmilk. In J. Riordan (Ed.), *Breastfeeding and human lactation* (3rd ed., pp. 97-135). Boston: Jones and Bartlett.

Scheers, N.J., Rutherford, G.W., & Kemp, J.S. (2003). Where should infants sleep? A comparison of risk for suffocation of infants sleeping in cribs, adult beds, and other sleeping locations. *Pediatrics 112*(4), 883-889.

Simpson, K.R., & James, D.C. (2005). *Postpartum care.* White Plains, NY: March of Dimes Birth Defects Foundation.

Swenson, D.E. (2001). *Telephone triage for the obstetric patient.* Philadelphia: Saunders.

Thogmartin, J.R., Siebert, C.F., & Pellan, W.A. (2001). Sleep position and bed-sharing in sudden infant deaths: An examination of autopsy findings. *Journal of Pediatrics, 138*(2), 212-217.

Unger, B., Kemp, J.S., Wilkins, D., Psara, R., Ledbetter, T., Graham, M., et al. (2003). Racial disparity and modifiable risk factors among infants dying suddenly and unexpectedly. *Pediatrics, 111*(2), e127-e131.

U.S. Department of Health and Human Services (USDHHS), Public Health Service. (2000). *Healthy People 2010.* Washington, DC: Author.

U.S. Department of Transportation, National Highway Traffic Safety Administration. (2002). *Are you using it right?* Retrieved January 3, 2005, from http://www.nhtsa.dot.gov/people/injury/childps/UsingItRight2002/index.htm.

Williams, L.E., & Martin, J.E. (2003). Car seat challenges: Where are we in implementation of these programs? *Journal of Perinatal and Neonatal Nursing, 17*(2), 158-163.

The Childbearing Family with Special Needs

III

OBJECTIVES

After studying this chapter, you should be able to:

1. Discuss the incidence and identify the factors that contribute to teenage pregnancy.
2. Identify the effects of pregnancy on the adolescent mother, her infant, and her family.
3. Explain the role of the nurse in the prevention and management of teenage pregnancy.
4. Describe the major implications of delayed childbearing in terms of maternal and fetal health.
5. Describe the effects of substance abuse on the mother and the infant.
6. Identify nursing interventions to reduce or minimize the effects of substance abuse in the antepartum, intrapartum, and postpartum periods.
7. Discuss parental responses when an infant is born with congenital anomalies, and identify nursing interventions to assist the parents.
8. Describe parental responses to pregnancy loss, and identify nursing interventions to assist parents through the grieving process.
9. Examine the role of the nurse when the mother relinquishes the infant for adoption.
10. Identify the factors that promote violence against women, and describe the role of the nurse in assessment, prevention, and interventions.

Go to your Student CD-ROM for Review Questions keyed to these Objectives.

DEFINITIONS

Abstinence Syndrome A group of symptoms that occurs when a person who is addicted to a specific drug withdraws or abstains from taking that drug.

Addiction Physical or psychological dependence on a substance such as alcohol, tobacco, or drugs, either legal or illicit.

Alcohol-Related Birth Defect (ARBD) A birth defect that is directly attributed to prenatal exposure to alcohol.

Alcohol-Related Neurodevelopmental Disorder (ARND) Neurologic conditions and delayed development resulting from prenatal exposure to alcohol.

Alcoholism A chronic, progressive, and potentially fatal disease characterized by tolerance for and physical dependency on alcohol, by pathologic organ changes resulting from alcohol abuse, or by both.

Amphetamines Central nervous system stimulants that create a perception of pleasure unrelated to external stimuli.

Crack A highly addictive form of cocaine that has been processed to be smoked.

Egocentrism Interest centered on the self rather than the needs of others.

Fetal Alcohol Syndrome A group of physical and mental disorders of the offspring associated with maternal use of alcohol during pregnancy.

Methadone A synthetic compound with opiate properties; used as an oral substitute for heroin and morphine in the opiate-addicted person.

Neonatal Abstinence Syndrome A cluster of physical signs exhibited by the newborn exposed in utero to maternal use of substances such as heroin. (See also *abstinence syndrome.*)

Opiate Any narcotic containing opium or a derivative of opium.

Prune-Belly Syndrome An absence of abdominal muscles resulting in a flabby, distended, and creased abdomen that may occur in the infant exposed to cocaine in utero.

Withdrawal Syndrome See *abstinence syndrome.*

All families must make major changes as they adapt to pregnancy and childbirth. For some families, however, the changes are particularly difficult. Such families have special needs related to parental age, substance abuse, birth of an infant with congenital abnormalities, perinatal loss, or family violence. Perinatal nurses can make a difference in the lives of these families, particularly in the lives of infants born into them.

ADOLESCENT PREGNANCY

Incidence

Preliminary data for 2003 show a 33% decrease in births to teenagers in the United States since 1991 (Hamilton, Martin, & Sutton, 2004). The incidence has decreased steadily each year to a rate of 41.7 births per 1000 women aged 15 to 19 years. This surpasses the Healthy People 2010 goal of not more than 46 pregnancies per 1000 adolescent girls (U.S. Department of Health and Human Services [USDHHS], 2000).

Adolescent pregnancy remains a problem, however. In 2002, 425,493 adolescents aged 15 to 19 years gave birth in the United States. Within 2 years, 30% to 50% of adolescent mothers have another pregnancy (Hancock, Calhoun, & Hume, 2002) (Figure 24-1). For most of these young women the pregnancy is unplanned and unwanted at conception. In spite of recent decreases the pregnancy and birth rates for teenagers in the United States are higher than those in other developed countries (Alan Guttmacher Institute, 2003).

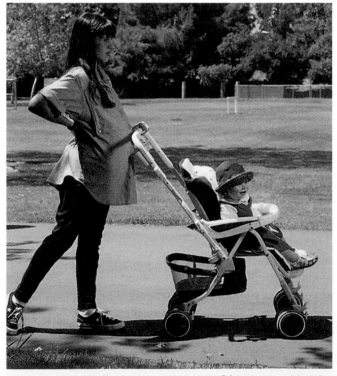

Figure 24-1 ■ Pregnant adolescent. Of teenage girls who become pregnant, 30% to 50% will be pregnant again within 2 years.

Factors Associated with Teenage Pregnancy

Approximately 75% of teen pregnancies are unintended (Davis, 2003). Pregnancy occurs because many adolescents fail to recognize their vulnerability as a result of their sexual activity and believe that pregnancy cannot happen to them. Adolescents tend to have a high rate of sexual activity and low incidence of consistent contraceptive use. Increased abstinence and more effective contraceptive practices have helped bring about recent declines in adolescent pregnancies.

Some adolescents risk pregnancy and parenthood as a means of gaining or maintaining a love relationship. They often see themselves as lacking power in their relationships and defer to their partners' wishes about sex and contraceptive use (Kelly & Morgan-Kidd, 2001; Rickert, Sanghvi, & Wiemann, 2002). Still others see it as a means to gain independence. Other factors that contribute to teenage pregnancy are listed in Box 24-1.

Adolescents who give birth are more likely to have a low income, which may mean they have less access to contraception and abortion. These teenagers may not believe that finishing education and obtaining a good job are possibilities for them and may see little reason to postpone pregnancy (Breedlove & Schorfheide, 2001).

National Health Goals

Teenage pregnancies result in numerous personal, social, and financial problems. The way to achieve further reductions in teen pregnancies is a controversial subject. Part of the controversy centers on the debate over who should provide sex education and how much information should be provided. Some believe that information about sex and contraceptives should be provided only by the family. These people are convinced that providing sex education in schools gives tacit approval to sexual activity among teenagers. Some also believe that teenagers should receive information about abstinence only and should not be taught contraceptive measures.

Conversely, many families advocate early, continuing sex education in public schools. Within this context, ongoing information about prevention of pregnancy and sexually transmissible diseases (STDs) may be combined with other aspects of teenage sexuality, such as personal adjustments, interpersonal associations, and the establishment of values.

BOX 24-1 Factors that Contribute to Teenage Pregnancy

High rate of sexual activity
Lack of accurate information about how to use contraceptives correctly
Limited access to contraceptive devices
Incorrect or lack of use of contraceptives
Fear of reporting sexual activity to parents
Ambivalence toward sexuality; intercourse not "planned"
Feelings of invincibility
Peer pressure to begin sexual activity
Low self-esteem and consequent inability to set limits on sexual activity
Means to attain love or escape present situation
Lack of appropriate role models

Sex Education

Sex education for adolescents should help them identify their own values and beliefs about sexuality, understand ways to set limits on sexual activity, and understand effective measures to prevent pregnancy and STDs when they decide to become sexually active. (See Chapter 31.)

Learning how to set limits on sexual behavior is particularly important for younger teenagers, who may be pressured to become sexually active before they have developed the maturity to deal responsibly with intercourse, contraception, or unplanned pregnancy. They need advice about ways to handle pressure so they can postpone sexual intercourse until they are emotionally and physically ready. Adolescent females need help in learning how to say "not now," "not yet," and "not you."

When providing sex education, nurses must keep in mind that adolescent males and females mature at different rates and are likely to be more comfortable learning in separate groups. In talking with teenagers, nurses should use simple but correct language such as "uterus," "testicles," "penis," and "vagina." Once the meanings of the terms are understood, most teenagers prefer to use them in their discussions.

Options When Pregnancy Occurs

An adolescent who becomes pregnant must choose one of three options: (1) terminate the pregnancy, (2) continue the pregnancy and place the infant for adoption, or (3) keep the infant. Some teenagers choose termination of pregnancy, but this is not an acceptable alternative for other adolescents. Teenagers who might consider termination may not acknowledge the pregnancy until it is too late for abortion.

The choice of abortion or adoption leaves the adolescent with no tangible evidence of her pregnancy and mixed messages from society regarding her decision. Unlike the teenager who decides to keep her infant, these adolescents may receive less assistance about ways to cope with their experiences. They need recognition of the significance of the experience to them and assistance in dealing with their feelings about their decision. (See discussion of relinquishment by adoption, p. 612.)

Few teenagers choose to continue the pregnancy and place the infant for adoption. Those who do may have complicated feelings of grief, relief that a "bad" experience is over, and anger at parents who were unwilling to provide assistance and thus made adoption the only realistic option. For some young women the autonomous decision to relinquish the child "for the child's good" may be an important step toward maturity.

The decision to keep the infant may result from the expectant mother's or her partner's desire for a baby or because of her belief that she could be a better parent than her own mother. Some choose to keep the baby because they are opposed to having an abortion or giving the baby up for adoption.

Socioeconomic Implications

The cost of teenage pregnancy in the United States is estimated to be between $7 billion and $15 billion per year (USDHHS, 2000). Such figures may include funds for Temporary Assistance for Needy Families (TANF), Medicaid, food stamps, and direct payment to care providers. Teenage mothers are more likely than older mothers to be nonwhite, poor, less well educated, and unmarried. Because they are more likely to have larger families at an earlier age, adolescent mothers have more children to feed and clothe on an already inadequate income.

Although the financial cost of teenage pregnancy is enormous, the cost in human terms is often tragic. The developmental tasks of adolescence, such as achieving independence from parents and establishing a lifestyle that is personally satisfying, may be interrupted when a pregnancy increases the need for financial and emotional support from parents (Table 24-1). Instead of becoming independent, they often become more dependent on parents or a boyfriend as a result of pregnancy. Educational goals may be curtailed for some young mothers, limiting employment opportunities and resulting in reliance on the welfare system.

However, positive outcomes from the pregnancy may also occur. For some adolescents, pregnancy motivates a desire to do well in school so they can provide for their infants (Rentschler, 2003). Pregnancy and birth may have a stabilizing effect in adolescents who change past poor lifestyle and become more goal directed than they had previously been (Clemmens, 2003).

Children born into this situation do not escape unscathed. They show a higher incidence of impaired intellectual functioning and poor school adjustment. The negative cycle often is repeated: A large percentage of teenage parents were children of teenage parents. As a result, children of adolescent parents often are among the poorest people in the United States.

Implications for Maternal Health

Pregnancy presents significant problems for the health of adolescent females. They are at increased risk for preeclampsia, anemia, gaining too much or not enough weight, urinary tract infections, and depression (Breedlove, & Schorfheide, 2001). These risks may be lower in adolescents with adequate prenatal care and elimination of other risk factors (Koniak-Griffin & Turner-Pluta, 2001).

Adolescents are often in abusive relationships and should be screened to identify violence so the nurse can help them access available resources. The high incidence of STDs among pregnant teenagers is another concern. Gonorrhea and chlamydial infection are particularly prevalent during these years, and these diseases can be transmitted to the infant and affect the eyes and lungs. STD screening is important during prenatal care.

The reason for the high incidence of complications among teenagers is unclear. It may be related to delayed prenatal care and economic and sociocultural difficulties rather than age. Pregnant adolescents generally begin prenatal care later than

TABLE 24-1 Impact of Pregnancy on the Developmental Tasks of Adolescence

Developmental Task*	Impact of Pregnancy	Nursing Considerations
Achievement of a Stable Identity: How the person sees himself or herself and how the person perceives that others see and accept him or her; peer group approval provides confirmation and is a major component of identity development.	The ability to adapt and respond to stress is a good indicator of identity development, and adolescents who become pregnant before a stable identity is developed may not be able to accept the responsibilities of parenthood and to plan for the future.	Explore the availability of a school-based mothers' program that will provide the peer support that is so important. Emphasize the importance of prenatal classes and the effect of prenatal care on pregnancy. Encourage both parents to attend parenting classes, and describe the expected growth and development of infants. Focus on the infant's need to develop trust and on the parenting behaviors that promote this.
Achievement of Comfort with Body Image: Requires internalization of mature body size, contour, and function.	The adolescent must learn to deal with body changes of pregnancy (increasing size, contour, pigmentation changes, and striae) before she has learned to accept the body changes of puberty. May deny pregnancy or severely restrict calories to avoid gaining weight. May be disgusted with the physical changes of pregnancy that make her look different from her peers.	Allow time for the teenager to verbalize her feelings about the body changes of pregnancy. Emphasize that dieting is harmful to the infant and will not stop the changes in body size and contour. Provide exercises that will help her regain her figure after the birth of the infant.
Acceptance of Sexual Role and Identity: Requires internalization of strong sexual urges and achievement of intimacy with others.	The adolescent may need to achieve an intimate relationship with another and to form an exclusive relationship before ready. The pregnant teenager will also need to cope with changes in relationships with friends. She often has difficulty seeing herself as a sexual being or as a mother.	Allow the teenager to express her feelings about sexuality and about motherhood. Initiate groups designed specifically for adolescents (childbirth education, parenting classes, special groups about nutrition, etc.). This will help her deal with the changing relationships with her peers and move toward a mothering role.
Development of a Personal Value System: Able to consider the rights and feelings of others.	Pregnancy occurs before the adolescent is able to move from following rules to considering the rights and feelings of others and developing ethical standards. She may experience conflict when she must adjust to the responsibilities of premature motherhood.	Initiate a discussion of the teenager's feelings of conflict about her role as mother versus her role as student. Explore her views about motherhood: How does she expect it to change her life? What are her future plans? Present options and assist her to explore her goals.
Preparation for Vocation or Career: Completing educational or vocational goals; youths living in poverty may not have the means or encouragement to accomplish this.	Pregnancy often interrupts school for both parents; this may be a major frustration and it may result in permanent withdrawal from school and limited access to jobs that pay more than the minimum wage.	Discuss the importance of continued education and elicit the teenager's feelings and plans to accomplish this. Determine the amount and availability of support from her parents. Refer her to social services for needed assistance.
Achievement of Independence from Parents: Competent in the social environment and able to function without parental guidance.	Must adjust to the need for continued financial assistance and dependence on parents at a time when achieving independence is a major priority.	Assist the teenager to verbalize her feelings about continued dependence on parents. Discuss the reality of the situation and her need for financial support and help with the care of the infant. Determine the reaction of her parents to the pregnancy and if she will continue to live at home. How much support will they provide? What are the conditions for her remaining in her parents' home with the infant?

*Modified from Mercer, R.T. (1990). *Parents at risk.* New York: Springer.

older women. Some delay seeking care until the third trimester or receive none at all. Delayed prenatal care may result from denial of the pregnancy, lack of knowledge of how to get care, or a negative view of health care providers. Early prenatal care that includes counseling about nutritional needs and close observation for complications is especially important when the expectant mother is very young.

Implications for Fetal-Neonatal Health

Infants of teenage mothers have an increased risk of two major complications: prematurity (birth before the end of the thirty-seventh week of gestation) and low birth weight (less than 2500 g or 5.5 lb). The cause of low birth weight may be intrauterine growth restriction (failure of the fetus to grow at the rate to be expected for the gestational age). This may result from a variety of causes, such as poor placental perfusion, which occurs in preeclampsia, or the underdeveloped vasculature of the uterus in young primigravidas. When placental perfusion is decreased, the newborn may have a low birth weight even if the pregnancy goes to term because transport of nutrients and oxygen to the fetus has been inadequate. Cigarette smoking in young women occurs in 13.4% of those 15 to 17 years and 18.2% of those 18 to 19 years of age (Martin et al., 2003). Smoking by a pregnant adolescent increases the risk that her baby's growth will be restricted or that the infant will be born early.

Prematurity is a major cause of low-birth-weight infants. An infant born before 38 weeks of gestation is more likely to weigh less than 2500 g and has the added risks associated with immature organs. Even infants born at 37 weeks' gestation or more and healthy are more likely to die during the first year of life if they are born to teenaged mothers when compared with those whose mothers are in their twenties (Phipps, Blume, & DeMonner, 2002).

The Teenage Expectant Father

Seven percent of teenaged mothers have partners who are 6 or more years older (Alan Guttmacher Institute, 2003). These men may accept responsibility for the child, or they may become "phantom fathers," who are absent and rarely involved in raising the child. Approximately 64% of adolescent mothers have partners within 2 years of their age (Alan Guttmacher Institute, 2003). The rate of adolescent fatherhood, which has decreased in recent years, was 17.4 per 1000 in 2002 (Martin et al., 2003).

Almost all adolescent expectant fathers indicate that they are not ready for fatherhood, and this attitude does not diminish as the pregnancy progresses. Many are depressed as they grapple with the conflicting roles of adolescence and fatherhood. Although some express interest in learning about childbirth and child care, those who do not want to be fathers are less likely to be supportive. Some do not wish to be involved with the infant, leaving the pregnant girl to seek support elsewhere. Others are involved in some degree during the pregnancy and early years of the child's life, but many become less involved over time (Breedlove & Schorfheide, 2001).

Many teenage expectant fathers are from environments of poverty and lack job skills or educational preparation. Many need job training before they are able to earn enough money to contribute to the support of their children. To help provide financial support, he may have to interrupt his education to find a job.

Impact on Parenting

Adolescent mothers are at risk of becoming nonnurturing parents and having negative parent-infant interactions (Kenner, 2004). Having to focus on an infant at a time when most teenagers are absorbed in their own thoughts and activities may make parenting difficult. The ability to deal with stress plays an important part in mothering skills. Because of their immature coping mechanisms, young adolescents may be unable to separate the stress of other life events from that which occurs when the infant cries and cannot be consoled. They may respond with immature or punitive measures toward the infant when the source of stress is other factors such as social isolation or inadequate financial resources.

Adolescent parents are likely to be surprised and dismayed at how difficult and time consuming parenting can be. Teenage mothers tend to be less sensitive to infant cues. They display fewer instances of mutual gazing, verbal interaction, and touching than do older mothers (American Academy of Pediatrics [AAP], 2001).

Adolescents often have little understanding of the expected growth and development of infants. They may have unrealistic expectations of their children. For instance, they may expect that an infant will sleep through the night or complete toilet training before infants are able to do so. In addition, the infant may be in a neonatal intensive care unit for some time and the mother may have to learn to care for an infant with problems.

Preparing for parenthood is important. Although pregnant adolescents may want to be good mothers, they often do not actively seek information about infant care and development (Rentschler, 2003). The mother's relationship with the father of the baby may affect her parenting abilities. A close and satisfying relationship with the baby's father may increase attachment behaviors in the mother. Therefore the father should be included, when appropriate, in care of the mother and baby. However, many adolescent mothers do not have a good relationship with the father of their baby, which increases their need for support in coping (Clemmens, 2002; Rentschler, 2003).

✔ **CHECK YOUR READING**

1. How does pregnancy affect the developmental tasks of adolescence?
2. What are the major problems associated with teenage pregnancy in terms of maternal and fetal health?

Application of the Nursing Process
The Pregnant Teenager

Assessment

PHYSICAL ASSESSMENT

Assessment of pregnant teenagers is similar to that of older women in many respects. At the initial visit, obtain a thorough health and family history to determine whether conditions such as diabetes or infectious diseases increase the risk for the mother and fetus. Monitor closely for signs of iron-deficiency anemia, preeclampsia, or STDs. Attempt to identify lifestyle behaviors, such as poor nutrition, smoking, alcohol or drug use, or unprotected sex, that could harm the mother or fetus. Screen for physical or sexual abuse, which is elevated in pregnant teenagers (Hancock et al., 2002).

■ Teenagers are sometimes defensive and inconsistent in their responses. Because they may not volunteer information about nutrition, exercise, and the use of alcohol or other drugs, the nurse needs to press for details. The teenager's statement "I eat okay, and I'm pretty active" requires follow-up questions worded to obtain specific information: "What foods do you especially like? What did you eat yesterday?" or "What kind of things do you like to do?"

Structure the interview so that questions can be interspersed in a more general conversation that explores the teenager's likes and concerns. For example, a question such as "Will you be able to continue on the swim team after the baby is born?" may establish rapport and help determine whether the teenager is making plans for the future.

COGNITIVE DEVELOPMENT

Determine the teenager's level of cognitive development and ability to absorb health counseling. The three most important areas of cognitive development are:

1. Egocentrism, which involves the ability to defer personal satisfaction to respond to the needs of the infant: "What will you do when the baby gets sick?" "How will you help the baby get better?"
2. Present-future orientation, which involves the ability to make long-term plans: "What are your plans for finishing high school?" "What will you and the infant need in the first year of the infant's life?"
3. Abstract thinking, which involves identifying cause and effect: "Why is it important to keep clinic appointments?" "Why should condoms be used during sex even though you're pregnant?"

KNOWLEDGE OF INFANT NEEDS

Assess knowledge of infant needs and parenting skills. How does the teenager plan to feed the infant? What will she do when the infant cries? How will she know when the infant is ill and should be taken to a pediatrician? Does she know how much the infant should sleep? What plans have been made to provide for the safety needs of the infant?

FAMILY ASSESSMENT

Begin assessment of the family unit by determining the degree of participation by the father of the infant. The father may deny responsibility for the pregnancy and be totally uninvolved, be married to or plan to marry the expectant mother, or plan to participate in the pregnancy and rearing of the child without marriage.

Assessing the adolescent without the presence of her parents is important, yet it is crucial to determine the availability and amount of family support. Will the pregnant teenager continue to live with her parents? How do her parents feel about the pregnancy? How will they incorporate the mother and her infant into the family?

Families generally respond in one of three ways:

1. A family member (often the adolescent's mother) assumes the mothering role, which the teenager may abdicate willingly.
2. All care and responsibilities are left to the adolescent mother, although shelter and food are provided.
3. The family shares care and responsibilities, which allows the teenager to grow in the mothering role while completing the developmental tasks of adolescence.

It is particularly important to assess the perceptions of the pregnant teenager's mother. How does she feel about becoming a grandmother? Many women feel embarrassed and disgraced. She may feel that she has "failed" as a mother, or she may resent the new cycle of child care in which the pregnancy involves her. Is communication with her daughter open? Is she aware of the difficult role conflict (as adolescent and mother) that her daughter will experience?

If the family is unable or unwilling to provide care for an adolescent with an infant, what other social support can be located?

Analysis

Many adolescents wait until the second or third trimester to seek prenatal care because they either do not realize they are pregnant, continue to deny they are pregnant, or want to hide the pregnancy. They may not know where to get care and may fear the effects of pregnancy on their lives and relationships. In addition, many teenagers have little information about the physiologic demands such as the increased need for nutrients that pregnancy imposes on their bodies. As a result they may have a pattern of sporadic prenatal care and missed appointments (Nursing Care Plan 24-1). One of the most relevant nursing diagnoses is "Risk for Ineffective Health Maintenance related to lack of knowledge of measures to promote health during pregnancy and increased family stress."

Planning

For the nursing diagnosis "Risk for Altered Health Maintenance," the most appropriate goals or outcomes are:

- The expectant mother will obtain all recommended prenatal care and will follow instructions that promote her health and that of the infant throughout pregnancy.
- She will communicate her concerns throughout pregnancy and participate in learning about infant care.
- The family will verbalize emotions and concerns and maintain functional support of the expectant mother and her infant.

Interventions

ELIMINATING BARRIERS TO HEALTH CARE

The two major barriers to health care are (1) scheduling conflicts and (2) negative attitudes of some health care workers. Help the adolescent locate the clinic closest to her that has appointments when she (and her partner, if they wish) are not in school. Provide information about public transportation to that location if necessary. Some clinics are open in the evening or on Saturday. If a scheduling conflict occurs, alternative plans may be necessary.

Pregnant women of all ages state that the negative attitude of some health care workers can discourage them from regularly attending prenatal care. Workers who are rude, insensitive, or condescending discourage families that would benefit most from early, consistent prenatal care.

Nurses can be instrumental in finding ways to overcome negative attitudes and thus encourage pregnant women, including teenagers, to return for needed follow-up care. Recommended strategies include the following:

- Identify pervasive attitudes of the health care team.
- Acknowledge that frustration, stress, and staff burnout are common when health care workers attempt to provide care for families with multiple problems.
- Recognize that health care workers who are parents of teenagers may feel vulnerable and fearful about their own children and may project these feelings onto clients.

NURSING CARE PLAN 24-1 Adolescents' Responses to Pregnancy and Birth

ASSESSMENT: Ann Killian, a 16-year-old white female, visited the neighborhood health clinic during the twentieth week of her pregnancy. She lives with her mother and father, who both work long hours, and a younger sister. Ann sees her boyfriend sporadically but is unsure if he will be involved with the baby. Ann remains in school but verbalizes concern about how she looks: "I'm so fat! How much bigger am I going to get?" "Why is my face so blotchy?" "My feet swell and it looks gross."

NURSING DIAGNOSIS: Disturbed Body Image related to perceived negative effects of pregnancy as evidenced by verbalized concern about appearance

GOALS/EXPECTED OUTCOMES: Ann will:
1. Verbalize her feelings about pregnancy and her perception of herself during each antepartum visit.
2. Make two positive statements about herself during the next antepartum visit.

INTERVENTION	RATIONALE
1. Allow time at each prenatal visit for Ann to express concerns about weight gain and other physiologic changes of pregnancy, such as hyperpigmentation and stretch marks.	1. The adolescent often is ashamed of and uncomfortable with her pregnant body. She feels more comfortable if she is allowed to share these feelings and be reassured that they are a normal part of pregnancy.
2. Initiate interaction about body changes by asking open-ended questions such as "How do you feel about gaining weight because of pregnancy?"	2. Adolescents often are intimidated by health care professionals and may think that their own feelings are not important enough to discuss.
3. Provide anticipatory guidance about normal changes of pregnancy such as the pattern of weight gain during pregnancy and rate of weight loss after childbirth.	3. Most adolescents do not know what to expect during pregnancy, and their fears often are unexpressed. Anticipatory guidance reduces fear and provides information about expected changes.
4. Explain the reason for changes that are most troublesome at each prenatal visit (weight gain, hyperpigmentation, stretch marks, breast changes).	4. Knowing that some changes are temporary and that increasing weight indicates the fetus is growing and developing often is helpful for the adolescent. This may become a source of pride for the young teenager as well as for the older woman.
5. Involve Ann in scheduling follow-up prenatal appointments and other activities related to the birth of the infant (classes, plans for childbirth).	5. Participation in decision making promotes a positive sense of self.
6. Promote positive self-image by praising grooming, posture, and responsible behavior such as keeping prenatal appointments and following recommendations: "You have never missed an appointment, and your baby is growing so well."	6. Positive reinforcement is particularly important to help the adolescent meet the developmental tasks of developing a sense of identity and self-worth.
7. Near the end of pregnancy, discuss postpartum weight loss and exercise planning.	7. Adolescents may expect instant weight loss after delivery. They need information about healthy and realistic measures to lose weight.

EVALUATION: Ann discusses her concerns about how she looks and feels about herself and makes several positive statements about herself at each prenatal visit.

ASSESSMENT: Ann reveals that her father says she has "shamed the family," and she is worried her friends will reject her because she is pregnant. Ann states that she will have to "drop out of everything." She confides, in a trembling voice, that she feels guilty for "putting her family through this."

NURSING DIAGNOSIS: Situational Low Self-Esteem related to feelings of rejection by family and friends as manifested by statements indicating guilt and uncertainty about future support for herself and the infant.

GOALS/EXPECTED OUTCOMES: Ann will:
1. Identify at least two new measures to cope with anxiety by the end of the current antepartum visit.
2. Implement these measures during subsequent antepartum visits.

INTERVENTION	RATIONALE
1. Use therapeutic communication techniques to help Ann express her feelings about her pregnancy and the reactions of significant others.	1. Listening to the adolescent helps her see her feelings as important to others and helps the nurse determine which areas have highest priority for nursing interventions.
2. Help Ann identify what she can do to overcome anxiety about rejection by her family and friends.	2. Planning how to approach the family and friends reduces anxiety.

Continued

NURSING CARE PLAN 24-1 Adolescents' Responses to Pregnancy and Birth—cont'd

INTERVENTION	RATIONALE
a. Role play how Ann can initiate a conversation with friends to discuss activities that they can continue to share.	**a.** Acceptance by the peer group and participation in group activities are major concerns of the adolescent. A change in status within the group is a threat to self-concept that precipitates acute anxiety.
b. Suggest that she talk to family members and acknowledge her feelings of guilt for the unhappiness she is causing and her fear that they will not assist her through the pregnancy and birth.	**b.** Although adolescents strive for independence, family values continue to be a significant influence. Rejection by the family at this time would leave her vulnerable to stress beyond her coping ability.
c. Recommend that she share her feelings with the father of the infant if she continues to see him.	**c.** Expectant fathers may be a source of emotional and financial support.
3. Assist Ann in locating and joining the school-aged mothers' program if available through her school district.	**3.** Teenagers who are either mothers or expectant mothers often replace the pregnant teenager's previous peer group. The shared concerns and activities provide an opportunity for growth.
4. Help Ann to discuss her economic needs and plans for continuing school when the infant is born.	**4.** Beginning to develop plans for the future provides some sense of control over the situation and increases feelings of competency.
5. Point out and praise any positive actions that Ann takes, such as keeping prenatal appointments or eating a balanced diet.	**5.** Sincere praise helps reinforce a positive self-image.

EVALUATION: Ann talks with her family and reports that relationships are somewhat improved. She enters a school-age mother's program and is very pleased. She often makes more positive statements about herself and her life in the future.

ASSESSMENT: Ann has given birth to a 6-lb, 3-oz girl at 38 weeks' gestation. She has decided not to breastfeed because she feels uncomfortable with it and plans to go back to school as soon as possible. Ann will live at home, and her mother has agreed to work part time so that she can care for the infant while Ann is in school. Ann is very concerned about caring for the newborn. Although she participated in infant care classes, she seems unsure how to respond when the infant cries and handles her only during feedings.

NURSING DIAGNOSIS: Risk for Impaired Parenting related to deficient knowledge about the infant's needs and lack of confidence in ability to care for the infant, as evidenced by uncertain responses to infant.

GOALS/EXPECTED OUTCOMES: Ann will:
1. Demonstrate basic infant care (cord care, bathing, burping, feeding, swaddling) by discharge.
2. Verbalize infant needs for gentle, prompt response to crying by the first postpartum day.
3. Demonstrate attachment behaviors (eye contact, gazing, holding, verbal stimulation, and positive comments about the infant) before discharge.

INTERVENTION	RATIONALE
1. Demonstrate infant care on the first postpartum day, and obtain a return demonstration on the second postpartum day.	**1.** Confidence is increased by returning the demonstration of infant care and continued practice in caring for the infant.
2. Model the way to respond when the infant cries, and emphasize the importance of promptness and gentleness.	**2.** Observing how nurses respond to the infant increases the likelihood that adolescents will respond in the same manner. Prompt, gentle responses help the infant develop trust.
3. Emphasize the importance of touch and verbal stimulation, and point out the reciprocal bonding behaviors that the infant exhibits.	**3.** Many teenage parents do not provide adequate tactile and verbal stimulation for their infants, which may decrease the infant's ability to learn. The infant has many behaviors that stimulate mutual attachment between parent and child.
4. Include the grandparents and father of the infant in as many demonstrations as possible.	**4.** When all primary caregivers are included, family cohesiveness and consistency of care are enhanced.
5. Instruct Ann regarding early growth and development of the infant (how often infants need to eat, how much they sleep, what to do when they cry).	**5.** Some teenage parents expect too much too soon from infants and become frustrated when the infant does not respond as expected. Anticipatory guidance may help them have more realistic expectations.
6. Encourage Ann to continue in her school-age mother's program and to attend parenting classes with other teenage mothers.	**6.** Learning along with her peers helps the adolescent increase parenting skills and provides a continuing peer support group.

EVALUATION: Ann responds quickly and gently to infant crying. She gives basic care as she was taught and discusses the infant's expected growth and development. She talks about her daughter in a positive manner.

- Allocate time for staff development, planning programs, and stress reduction.
- Find ways to obtain increased assistance from clerical and support personnel.
- Initiate a scheduling plan that allows health care workers to see the same families whenever possible so that a caring relationship can be established.

APPLYING TEACHING AND LEARNING PRINCIPLES

The lives of adolescents change greatly during pregnancy and even more after the infant is born. They often feel isolated from peers who may not understand the responsibilities of parenthood (Clemmens, 2003). They may no longer be able to participate in activities with their peers because of child care obligations.

Because peers are important to adolescents, arrange for them to participate in small groups with common concerns. Specific needs that might be addressed are the benefits of prenatal care or help in eliminating unhealthful habits such as smoking, drug use, or alcohol consumption. Finding common goals, such as eliminating smoking, may be discussed in groups in which the teens can assist each other to have more healthful pregnancies. As pregnancy progresses, needs and group focus change and preparation for labor and delivery and infant care become priorities.

Repetition is an important method of teaching and clarifying misinformation. Allow ample time for questions and discussions. Although teenagers often do not read or benefit from printed materials to the same degree that older parents do, written material is available that is prepared especially with adolescents in mind. Many teenagers learn well from audiovisual aids. Numerous well-made compact discs (CDs) and videos are available that deal with all aspects of prenatal and infant care.

It is particularly important that the nurse does not sound like a parent when working with adolescents. Refrain from using the words *should* and *ought*, offering unwanted advice, and making decisions for the teenagers. Maintain an open, friendly posture, and convey empathy by using attending behaviors such as eye contact, frequent nodding, and leaning toward the speaker. As with all expectant families, avoid closed posture (arms folded across the chest), finger pointing, and lack of attention to the person speaking. Box 24-2 summarizes additional recommended methods for teaching adolescents.

BOX 24-2 Recommended Methods for Teaching Pregnant Adolescents

Identify and correct barriers to prenatal care.
Communicate with kindness and respect.
Form small groups with like concerns.
Allow ample time for clarification and discussion.
Use audiovisual materials.
Provide information in appropriate language easily understood by teens.
Convey empathetic concern by using nonverbal communication skills.
Include other family members or support persons when appropriate.

COUNSELING

Allow time to counsel teenagers about their specific concerns such as nutrition, stress reduction, and infant care.

NUTRITION. Nutrition counseling is one means of reducing the incidence of low-birth-weight infants. Determine the adolescent's general nutritional status and assess for eating disorders that would reduce caloric intake and possibly affect fetal growth. Emphasize that she is still growing and that her intake must be adequate for her own growth needs as well as those of the fetus. Discuss nutrition during lactation, pointing out the advantages for both mother and baby. Tailor information to the individual adolescent's likes and peer group habits. She often needs instruction in how to make the most nutritious selection from fast-food menus and select and plan for healthy snacks when she is away from home. Nutritional counseling must be socially and culturally appropriate (see Chapter 9).

Refer the adolescent to food stamp providers, the Special Supplemental Nutrition Program for Women, Infants, and Children (WIC), surplus food distributors, and food banks, if necessary, because many teenagers have limited access to food and lack the ability to store or prepare it.

SELF-CARE. Provide the same teaching about self-care that would be given to an older woman (see Chapter 7). In addition, emphasize the importance of using a condom to prevent STDs even though she is pregnant. Counsel the adolescent about lifestyle changes, such as smoking or substance abuse cessation, that will benefit mother and fetus, and refer her to resources to help her with these problems.

STRESS REDUCTION. Stress is an important factor in perinatal outcome, and teenagers are vulnerable to many sources of stress. Identify areas of stress in the adolescent's life. Stress may be related to basic needs such as food, shelter, and health care. Fear of labor and delivery and fear of being single, alone, and unsupported all create stress. Meeting the developmental tasks of adolescence while working on the developmental tasks of pregnancy (overcoming ambivalence, attaining the role of parent) is a major stressor.

A variety of measures may be used to reduce stress, depending on the teenager's age, situation, and available support. Adolescents with chronic life stress may require the concentrated efforts of a social worker to achieve stability. If the pregnancy is a result of rape or incest, social service and law enforcement agencies must become involved to provide protection and assistance.

The pregnant teenager may be concerned that she will no longer be allowed in her school or will lose friends or her job because of the pregnancy. She often experiences stress because she has not told her parents or the father of the infant about the pregnancy. Explore her reluctance to do this and role play the encounter with her to help her work out a plan for breaking the news. Although there is strain on the relationship when the teen first tells her parents, over time her relationship with her parents may become better than it was before the pregnancy if her parents are supportive

(Clemmens, 2003). If appropriate, encourage her to tell the expectant father so that he can work out his role.

ATTACHMENT TO THE FETUS. Because attachment begins during pregnancy, methods of helping the adolescent begin this process are important. Use of ultrasound may increase the expectant mother's awareness of the fetus and facilitate developing attachment. Seeing the fetus move often changes any pregnant woman's perceptions about the fetus. Hearing the fetal heartbeat and feeling the baby move may also increase attachment. Looking at illustrations of the fetus at different gestational ages increases the mother's interest. A heightened awareness of the fetus may make her more likely to follow suggestions that will enhance fetal well-being. Discussion of the fetus as it changes month to month may lead to discussion of the capabilities and needs of the neonate.

INFANT CARE. The priorities for teaching gradually change from maternal to infant needs, with particular emphasis on infant care and normal growth and development. For example, to reduce the worry that many mothers feel when the newborn startles in response to loud noises, explain the reflexes and that the uncoordinated motor responses are normal. Discuss common early developmental changes to help the young mother understand that the infant must learn to sit before walking and must walk before toilet training is possible.

Explain and demonstrate infant cues (using behaviors of the infants in videos or the group as examples) in terms of gaze, vocalization, facial expression, body position, and limb movement. Describe the way that infants use these behaviors to "talk" without words and ways in which parents can use the same behaviors to respond to their infants. Demonstrate how parents can adjust their position, distance, facial expression, voice, and touch to correspond to their infant's cues. Emphasize that eye contact, holding, cuddling, and verbal stimulation are important for the child's development.

Because adolescents tend to have a more rigid and punitive approach to child care, explain that infants develop a sense of trust when their needs are met promptly and gently. In addition, their future development depends on attaining a sense of trust during infancy. Emphasize that crying does not indicate the infant is spoiled but simply that the infant has a need for food, warmth, or comfort and love.

If a support person will be involved in helping care for the infant, include that person in teaching, especially if the support person has little experience with babies. Having a support person learn with her may help the teenager remember the information better.

PROMOTING FAMILY SUPPORT

The pregnant teenager needs encouragement to include her family in her decision making and problem solving. The involvement of her mother, older sister, or other close relative is particularly important in terms of future plans. Discuss topics such as who will care for the infant, whether the teenager will return to school, and what financial assistance is available from the family and the father of the infant.

Adolescent mothers with adequate emotional support are more likely to learn appropriate parenting techniques.

However, involving the family may be inappropriate if they have multiple problems such as substance abuse or family violence. In such situations the teenager should be encouraged to communicate instead with a family friend or other trusted adult.

PROVIDING REFERRALS

Make referrals to national and community resources for pregnant adolescents that are in the most convenient locations. Include well-baby clinics offered by the Public Health Service, assistance programs offered by state social service agencies, and WIC. Programs for school-age mothers are offered by many school districts and provide an opportunity to complete high school education and take much-needed classes in childbearing and parenting. Church and community organizations also may provide needed assistance.

Home visit services throughout the pregnancy and postpartum, if available, help the mother cope with difficulties that occur during the early months. Home visits during pregnancy and the first year help decrease hospitalization of infants and repeat pregnancies (Koniak-Griffin et al., 2003).

Evaluation

Nursing care has been effective if the pregnant adolescent keeps clinic appointments and participates actively in her plan of care, as demonstrated by asking questions, sharing concerns, and adhering to the recommended program of care. She should demonstrate basic knowledge of the infant's needs and care of the infant. Family support should be available, but if it is not, referrals to agencies that can provide assistance should be made.

✔ CHECK YOUR READING

3. What methods are effective for teaching pregnant teenagers?
4. What should prospective teenage parents be taught about infant growth and development?

DELAYED PREGNANCY

An increasing number of women become pregnant relatively late in their reproductive lives. In 2003, more than 574,000 women age 35 years or older gave birth in the United States (Hamilton et al., 2004). Contraceptive techniques available today provide women with freedom to time the births of their first children. Some women may delay childbearing to pursue a career or establish financial security. Furthermore, advances in reproductive medicine increase the chance for infertile women to have children.

Maternal and Fetal Implications

When the mature woman decides to conceive, she may experience a delay in becoming pregnant. This is particularly true after the age of 35 years because of the normal aging of the ovaries and the increased incidence of reproductive tract disorders. For instance, pelvic inflammatory disease can cause pelvic and tubal adhesions that interfere with fertilization and implantation (see Chapter 33).

Once she conceives, the mature woman is at increased risk for complications associated with pregnancy. Possible problems include genetic disorders, conditions related to preexisting medical conditions, and obstetric complications. The increased risk of fetal chromosomal abnormalities with advancing maternal age is well documented. Trisomy 21 (Down syndrome) is the most common example. Genetic abnormalities also increase when the father is over age 40 (Neuman & Graf, 2003).

The most common examples of preexisting diseases that increase maternal or fetal jeopardy are hypertension and diabetes mellitus. Uterine myomas (fibroids) occur with greater frequency in women older than 35 years. Myomas may be associated with postpartum hemorrhage.

Obstetric complications such as preeclampsia, gestational diabetes, placenta previa, vaginal bleeding, preterm labor, dysfunctional labor, and cesarean birth are more frequent in the older gravida. In addition, the risk of a small-for-gestational age infant and risk of multiple birth increase with advanced maternal age (March of Dimes Birth Defects Foundation, 2005). Women who have used fertility treatments to achieve pregnancy are more likely to conceive more than one fetus.

In spite of some increased risk with childbearing after age 35, most women have few problems during their pregnancy and can deliver healthy neonates. Those who do have some complications can often have a successful pregnancy with good medical and nursing care.

Advantages of Delayed Childbirth

Although mature women do have unplanned pregnancies, they are more likely than younger woman to make the decision to have a child after careful thought. They come to the parenting role with a range of personal resources: psychosocial maturity, self-confidence, and a sense of control over their lives (Figure 24-2). They demonstrate high levels of empathy and flexibility in child-rearing attitudes.

In addition, mature primigravidas are capable of solving complex problems and often are adept at maintaining interpersonal relationships. Because they are more likely to be financially secure, they can afford good care for their infants. They are experienced at setting priorities and developing plans. They usually are able to manage stress and will independently seek support and assistance when needed.

Disadvantages of Delayed Childbirth

Mature primiparas need more time to recover from childbirth, and they have less energy than their younger counterparts. They may find child care an exhausting experience for the first few weeks. This is particularly true if they had a cesarean birth or other complications of pregnancy.

Because their friends have teenage children instead of infants, mature primiparas may lack peer support. Many of their friends do not relate to the concerns of a new mother.

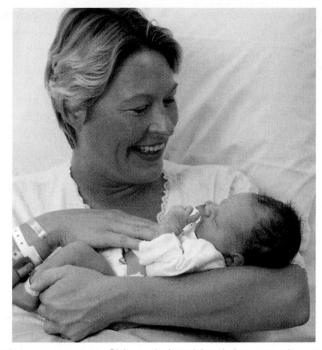

Figure 24-2 ■ Older primigravidas bring maturity and problem-solving skills to the maternal role, but they are at somewhat increased risk for physiologic problems related to pregnancy and birth.

Younger mothers have some of the same concerns, but they often do not share the perspective of older mothers. Family support also may be lacking for the older woman. Her parents are usually in their sixties or seventies and may not be able to assist with child care to the extent that younger grandparents can.

Nursing Considerations

REINFORCING AND CLARIFYING INFORMATION

Because the fetus of a mature gravida is at increased risk for chromosomal anomalies, the woman will be informed about available diagnostic tests. Professionals with special preparation in genetics provide genetic counseling, but all nurses must be prepared to reinforce and clarify the information that has been provided. The tests most often recommended are multiple-marker screening, chorionic villus sampling, amniocentesis, and ultrasonography (see Chapter 10).

The family's beliefs and attitudes about abortion often determine whether to have the recommended tests. The woman who would not consider abortion regardless of the condition of the fetus may refuse diagnostic studies or have them to help prepare for the problems that will occur at birth. Nurses must respect the decision and acknowledge that it may have been difficult to make.

FACILITATING EXPRESSION OF EMOTIONS

Several days or weeks may pass between performance of diagnostic studies and receipt of the results. This is a particularly difficult time for many expectant parents, and nurses often assist the couple to express their concerns and emotions.

■ A broad statement such as "Many couples find it difficult to wait for the results" often will elicit free expression of the parents' feelings. Follow-up questions such as "What concerns you most?" may reveal anxiety about the procedure itself or the possible effects of the procedure on the fetus. Simply acknowledging that it is a stressful time helps the couple cope with their emotions.

Mature gravidas also worry about complications that may affect the fetus or their own health. They are aware that they may not have another opportunity for pregnancy because of their age. They may be concerned about their ability to balance their careers with increased family responsibilities.

PROVIDING PARENTING INFORMATION

Nurses often help the mature primipara prepare for effective parenting by pointing out her individual strengths and advantages. These often include financial security, a stable relationship, and personal maturity. The older mother may have unique needs, however. She often has less energy than younger mothers and must learn to conserve it, particularly during the early weeks after childbirth. Anticipatory guidance about measures that will help conserve energy after childbirth is very useful. These include meal planning and setting realistic housekeeping goals. In addition, many older mothers need to mobilize all available support so that they can reserve their energy for care of the infant.

During the first weeks after childbirth the mother may experience feelings of social isolation, particularly if her friends have children who are much older. If she is accustomed to a great deal of mental stimulation, she may miss it while staying at home. If she elects to return to work, she is likely to experience guilt and grief because she must leave her infant (see Chapter 18). Balancing the needs of the infant and those of what may be a demanding career or occupation may be difficult.

First-time mothers older than age 35 are especially receptive to prenatal classes. These include classes in childbirth education, breastfeeding, and early parenting. When teaching infant care after childbirth, the nurse should allow time for demonstrations and return demonstrations so that the expectant parents feel comfortable with routine care. Older couples are particularly interested in learning how the infant grows and develops and what they can do to provide nurturing care for the infant.

Older gravidas are more likely to seek out information they need from a variety of sources. They ask questions and may interview care providers before choosing one. They often adopt health-promoting activities such as improving nutrition, getting enough rest, and eliminating harmful substances (Viau, Padula, & Eddy, 2002). They are often interested in printed materials that can be used to reinforce teaching.

✔ **CHECK YOUR READING**

5. What special resources do mature primigravidas often have?
6. Why is it important to offer prenatal testing (multiple-marker screening, chorionic villus sampling, amniocentesis) to the mature primigravida?
7. What anticipatory guidance should the nurse provide the older mother for the first weeks at home after childbirth?

SUBSTANCE ABUSE

The use of legal substances such as alcohol and tobacco and illicit drugs such as cocaine, heroin, and marijuana increases the risk of medical complications in the mother and poor birth outcomes in the infant.

Incidence

Approximately 1 in 10 infants is exposed to one or more mood-altering drugs during pregnancy (AAP & American College of Obstetricians and Gynecologists [ACOG], 2002). Although tobacco, alcohol, and marijuana are the most commonly abused drugs, the use of drugs such as cocaine, amphetamines, and heroin has had a major impact on health care for pregnant women and their offspring.

Maternal and Fetal Effects

When the pregnant woman takes a substance by drinking, smoking, snorting, or injecting it, the fetus experiences the same systemic effects as the expectant mother but often more severely. For example, cocaine raises the blood pressure of the woman and fetus and puts both at risk for intracranial bleeding. A drug that causes intoxication in the woman causes it for prolonged periods in the fetus. The fetus is unable to metabolize drugs efficiently and will experience the effects long after they have abated in the woman. Therefore substances taken by the woman can have great impact on the fetus and interfere with normal fetal development and health.

Maternal, fetal, and neonatal effects of commonly abused substances are summarized in Table 24-2.

TOBACCO

Cigarette smoking is the most common form of substance abuse by pregnant women. Although the incidence has declined recently, 11% of women smoke during pregnancy (Hamilton et al., 2004).

The active ingredients of cigarette smoke are nicotine, tar, and harmful gases such as carbon monoxide and cyanide. Nicotine, which causes vasoconstriction, transfers readily across the placenta and reduces placental blood circulation. Carbon monoxide inactivates fetal and maternal hemoglobin. Both substances reduce the amount of oxygen delivered to the fetus. Indirect effects of cigarette smoking include decreased maternal appetite, which results in inadequate intake of calories as well as decreased absorption of some nutrients.

TABLE 24-2 Maternal and Fetal or Neonatal Effects of Commonly Abused Substances

Substance	Maternal Effects	Fetal or Neonatal Effects
Caffeine (coffee, tea, cola, chocolate, cold remedies, analgesics)	Stimulates CNS and cardiac function, causes vasoconstriction and mild diuresis, half-life triples during pregnancy	Crosses placental barrier and stimulates fetus; teratogenic effects are undocumented
Tobacco	Decreased placental perfusion, anemia, PROM, preterm labor, spontaneous abortion	Prematurity, LBW, fetal demise, developmental delays, increased incidence of SIDS, neurologic problems
Alcohol (beer, wine, mixed drinks, after-dinner drinks)	Spontaneous abortion	Fetal demise, IUGR, FAS (facial and cranial anomalies, developmental delay, mental retardation, short attention span), congenital defects
Marijuana ("pot" or "grass")	Often used with other drugs: tobacco, alcohol, cocaine; increased incidence of anemia and inadequate weight gain	Unclear, more study needed, irritability, tremors, sleep problems, sensitivity to light
Cocaine ("crack")	Hyperarousal state, generalized vasoconstriction, hypertension, increased spontaneous abortion, abruptio placentae, preterm labor, cardiovascular complications (stroke, heart attack), seizures, increased STDs	Stillbirth, prematurity, IUGR, irritability, decreased ability to interact with environmental stimuli, poor feeding reflexes, nausea, vomiting, diarrhea, decreased intellectual development; prune-belly syndrome
Sedatives (barbiturates, tranquilizers)	Lethargy, drowsiness, CNS depression, spontaneous abortion, intrauterine growth restriction	Neonatal abstinence syndrome, seizures, delayed lung maturity, possible teratogenic effects
Amphetamines ("speed" or "ice" when processed in crystals to smoke) Methamphetamines ("ecstasy")	Malnutrition, tachycardia, vasoconstriction	Withdrawal symptoms (lethargy, depression), IUGR, fetal death
Narcotics (heroin, methadone, morphine)	Spontaneous abortion, PROM, preterm labor, increased incidence of STDs, HIV exposure, hepatitis, malnutrition	IUGR, perinatal asphyxia, intellectual impairment, neonatal abstinence syndrome, neonatal infections, neonatal death (SIDS, child abuse and neglect)

CNS, Central nervous system; *FAS,* fetal alcohol syndrome; *HIV,* human immunodeficiency virus; *IUGR,* intrauterine growth restriction; *LBW,* low birth weight; *PROM,* premature rupture of membranes; *SIDS,* sudden infant death syndrome; *STDs,* sexually transmissible diseases.

Neonatal consequences of smoking tobacco during pregnancy are intrauterine growth restriction, low birth weight, and prematurity. Smoking during pregnancy also is associated with neurologic and intellectual development problems that affect later school achievement. Problems include hyperactivity, shorter attention spans, and lower reading and spelling scores during the primary grades. Sudden infant death syndrome (SIDS) is twice as frequent in children of smokers (Moran, 2004).

ALCOHOL

Alcohol is the most commonly used drug. An estimated one in seven women of childbearing age report risk drinking (seven or more alcoholic drinks per week or binge drinking, which is five or more drinks on any one occasion). This is a concern because these women may not be aware of a pregnancy yet. Approximately one in 30 women who know they are pregnant reports drinking at that level during pregnancy. Drinking that may be of risk to the fetus occurs in 130,000 pregnant women each year (Centers for Disease Control and Prevention [CDCb], 2004). Binge drinking and six or more drinks a day (3 oz of alcohol) are especially harmful, but drinking in any amount may cause adverse fetal effects. Alcohol is a teratogen, and use during pregnancy may result in fetal alcohol syndrome (FAS), the leading cause of preventable mental retardation (Pitts, 2004).

Alcohol is known to pass easily through the placental barrier, and concentrations found in the fetus are believed to be at least as high as those found in the mother. Alcohol is present in amniotic fluid, which the infant drinks, for prolonged periods. The amount and timing of alcohol intake determines the specific effects on the fetus.

During the first trimester, when the mother often does not know she is pregnant, alcohol may affect cell membranes and alter the organization of tissue, causing structural defects. Throughout pregnancy, alcohol interferes with the transfer of nutrients from the placenta and their metabolism and therefore retards cell growth and division. The central nervous system (CNS) is probably most vulnerable during the third trimester, a time of rapid brain growth.

The teratogenic effects of alcohol are well known. FAS is the leading cause of mental retardation and is the only cause that is preventable (Pitts, 2004). This syndrome is characterized by three clinical features:

1. A recognizable combination of facial features—Facial anomalies include microcephaly, short palpebral fissures (the openings between the eyelids), epicanthal folds, flat midface with a low nasal bridge, indistinct philtrum (groove between the nose and the upper lip), and a thin upper lip (Figure 24-3).
2. Prenatal and postnatal growth restriction—Growth restriction in length, weight, and head circumference is present at birth, and weight is low for height during childhood.
3. CNS impairment—CNS developmental abnormalities including mental retardation or lower intelligence quotient, learning disabilities, high activity level, short attention span, and poor short-term memory may occur.

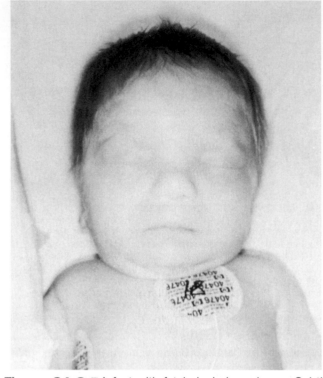

Figure 24-3 ■ Infant with fetal alcohol syndrome. Subtle indicators present are flat midface, indistinct philtrum, and low-set ears. (Courtesy Trish Beachy, Perinatal Program Coordinator, University of Colorado Health Sciences, Denver, Colorado.)

Fetal alcohol effects (FAE) are mild or partial manifestations of FAS, such as low birth weight, developmental delay that may not be obvious for 1 to 2 years, and hyperactivity. *Alcohol-related neurodevelopmental disorder (ARND)* and *alcohol-related birth defects (ARBD)* are other terms used to describe problems caused by prenatal exposure to alcohol. ARND includes problems with judgment, problem solving, and memory, whereas ARBD includes cardiac, skeletal, renal, ocular, and auditory abnormalities. Because the amount of alcohol necessary to cause these problems is unknown, abstaining from drinking alcohol throughout pregnancy is recommended.

MARIJUANA

The active constituent of marijuana is tetrahydrocannabinol (THC), which crosses the placenta and accumulates in the fetus. Marijuana is the most commonly used illicit drug and often is paired with other drugs such as cocaine and alcohol, making it difficult to determine the effects that are solely the result of marijuana use.

Marijuana causes tachycardia and euphoria. An increased incidence of maternal anemia and inadequate maternal weight gain seems to occur with repeated use of marijuana. Clinically the neonate may exhibit hyperirritability, tremors, sleep disruption, and unusual sensitivity to light. Long-term effects of marijuana on the development of the child are unclear.

COCAINE

ACTIONS OF COCAINE. Cocaine, a powerful, short-acting stimulant of the CNS, is the second most commonly used illicit drug during pregnancy after marijuana (Moran, 2004). Cocaine works by blocking the reuptake of the neurotransmitters norepinephrine and dopamine at nerve terminals, producing an excess of circulating catecholamines. The excess neurotransmitters act on the cerebral cortex to produce a hyperarousal state that results in euphoria, physical excitement, reduced fatigue, and a heightened sense of well-being and power. Anorexia, hyperglycemia, hyperthermia, and tachypnea are common side effects.

When the initial euphoria wears off, a period of irritability, fatigue, lethargy, depression, and impatience occurs, which elicits a strong desire for additional cocaine so that the initial feelings can be recaptured. This makes cocaine one of the most addicting drugs of abuse.

Physical effects of cocaine use are related to cardiovascular stimulation and vasoconstriction. The heart rate, systolic blood pressure, and need for oxygen increase. Complications of generalized vasoconstriction include myocardial ischemia or infarction, strokes, and pulmonary, renal, and gastrointestinal problems.

MATERNAL AND FETAL EFFECTS. Many women who use cocaine use additional drugs, such as alcohol, tranquilizers, marijuana, or tobacco, to "come down" from the superarousal state that cocaine produces. This polydrug use makes it difficult to define the precise effect of cocaine use on the fetus. The woman is less likely to seek prenatal care or eat a diet that contains adequate nutrition. Sex may be exchanged for drugs, which places the woman at increased risk for STDs.

Cocaine stimulates uterine contractions, and one of the most common problems attributed to cocaine use during pregnancy is premature delivery. Increased incidence of spontaneous abortion and abruptio placentae also occur because of the cocaine-induced vasoconstriction of placental vessels. Additional complications include spontaneous abortion, preeclampsia, premature rupture of membranes, precipitous delivery, fetal hypoxia, meconium staining, and stillbirth.

Cocaine crosses the placental barrier and causes the same physical stress on the fetus as on the expectant mother. Clearance of the drug by the fetus requires a prolonged period. Fetal effects include tachycardia, decreased variability of the fetal heart rate, fetal overactivity, and intrauterine growth restriction.

NEONATAL EFFECTS. Clinical signs observed in neonates exposed to cocaine in utero include low birth weight, tremors, tachycardia, marked irritability, muscular rigidity, hypertension, and exaggerated startle reflex. Prune-belly syndrome (lack of abdominal muscles) and other congenital defects may occur with use early in pregnancy. Infants are difficult to console and respond poorly to voices or environmental stimuli. They often are poor feeders and have frequent episodes of diarrhea.

Infants may continue to be irritable and have limited interaction with people and objects in their environment. They are at increased risk for SIDS. The long-term behavioral and developmental characteristics of cocaine-exposed infants are unclear but may include learning problems, slower intellectual development, and delayed language and motor development.

AMPHETAMINES AND METHAMPHETAMINES

These drugs produce effects similar to cocaine but are longer acting. Common names include speed, crystal, ice, and ecstasy.

MATERNAL AND FETAL EFFECTS. Amphetamines cause vasoconstriction and hypertension. Effects on the mother and fetus appear similar to those of cocaine. Intrauterine growth restriction and intraventricular hemorrhage may occur. Because these drugs are appetite depressants, infants may not receive required nutrients.

NEONATAL EFFECTS. Infants may have decreased weight and length at birth. Abnormal sleep patterns, agitation, diaphoresis, and vomiting may occur during withdrawal.

OPIOIDS

Opioids include drugs such as morphine, heroin, methadone, meperidine, hydromorphone hydrochloride, propoxyphene, and oxycodone. Heroin is used here as an example of this class of drugs.

Heroin is an illegal opiate derived from morphine and produces severe physical addiction. Like all opiates, heroin is a CNS depressant that produces a feeling of mental dullness, drowsiness, and finally stupor. Addiction is present when discontinuance causes withdrawal symptoms (abstinence syndrome) that are quickly relieved by a dose of the drug.

Women who abuse heroin have poor general health with multiple medical problems associated with their drug abuse and addicted lifestyle. Heroin is an appetite suppressant that also interferes with absorption of nutrients, and many women begin pregnancy malnourished and anemic. Additional problems include a high incidence of STDs, hepatitis, and exposure to human immunodeficiency virus (HIV) from sharing unclean needles.

FETAL EFFECTS. The fetus suffers both direct and indirect effects of heroin use by the expectant mother. The woman's supply of heroin usually is not steady, resulting in episodes of maternal overdose alternating with periods of withdrawal from the drug. This exposes the fetus to intermittent episodes of hypoxia in utero, which increases the risk of prematurity, growth restriction, spontaneous abortion, and stillbirth. Indirect effects result from maternal malnutrition and fetal exposure to STDs.

NEONATAL EFFECTS. Infants born to mothers who are addicted to opiates may have meconium aspiration. They exhibit neonatal abstinence (withdrawal) syndrome, which affects all body systems. Most signs involve the neurologic or gastrointestinal systems. (See Chapter 30, p. 817, for withdrawal signs and management.)

Studies of long-term developmental and learning problems have conflicting results. The lifestyle of parents who are substance abusers is strongly associated with child neglect and abuse, which are major causes of infant death in this population. In addition, infants may have low birth weight and an increased incidence of SIDS.

Diagnosis and Management of Substance Abuse

In addition to undergoing toxicology screening, the pregnant woman who uses illicit drugs must be assessed throughout pregnancy for STDs, hepatitis, and exposure to HIV. Fetal diagnostic tests such as ultrasonography, nonstress tests, and biophysical profiles help pinpoint problems. Nurses monitor weight gain and provide guidance in nutrition at each opportunity to prevent maternal anemia and inadequate weight gain.

Therapeutic management depends on the type of drug used. In the case of opiates such as heroin, withdrawal during pregnancy has been associated with significant fetal stress, fetal seizures, and even fetal death. Pregnant women who use heroin often are placed on an alternative drug such as methadone. Methadone can be taken orally once daily and is long acting, maintaining consistent blood levels, in contrast to the use of heroin, which is short acting and results in wide swings in blood level that can have severe adverse effects on the fetus. Methadone also reduces the risk of infections from contaminated needles and drug-seeking behavior such as prostitution. The woman receives a daily dose of methadone in a drug treatment program and is more likely to receive prenatal care. However, the newborn must withdraw from methadone after birth. Women who use methadone often may use other illicit drugs such as heroin, cocaine, or marijuana.

Treatment is aimed at establishing abstinence and preventing relapse. Outpatient or residential treatment may be used to provide education and individual and group therapy sessions. Peer support groups (such as Narcotics Anonymous, Alcoholics Anonymous, Cocaine Anonymous) are helpful. All members of the health care team must understand that women have extremely positive memories associated with drug use, and therefore relapse is common. Written contracts that focus on abstinence for 1 day at a time often are used to help the patient who has relapsed and experiences feelings of guilt and self-blame.

Various alternative therapies have been tried for treatment of addictions. Research about the various methods has been largely inconclusive. Although no complementary or alternative therapy has been proved to be completely effective, some may be beneficial.

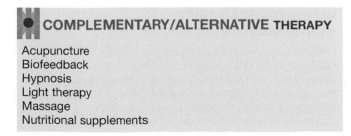

COMPLEMENTARY/ALTERNATIVE THERAPY

Acupuncture
Biofeedback
Hypnosis
Light therapy
Massage
Nutritional supplements

✔ CHECK YOUR READING

8. How does smoking affect the neonate? What are the long-term effects on the child?
9. How does FAS compare with FAE?
10. What are the long-term effects of maternal cocaine use on the child?
11. Why are women who use heroin encouraged to use methadone during pregnancy?

Application of the Nursing Process
Maternal Substance Abuse

ANTEPARTUM PERIOD

Assessment

Polydrug abuse appears to be the most common substance abuse problem among women, and all women must be screened at the first prenatal visit for tobacco, alcohol, and other drug use. Because substance abuse occurs in all populations, the nurse must not make assumptions based on class, race, or economic status.

Certain behaviors are strongly associated with substance abuse: seeking prenatal care late in the pregnancy, failing to keep appointments, and following recommended regimens inconsistently. Poor grooming, inadequate weight gain, or a pattern of weight gain that does not correspond to the stated gestational age may be signs of a lifestyle that includes substance abuse. Intravenous drug users may have fresh needle punctures, thrombosed veins, or signs of cellulitis.

Defensive and hostile behaviors may be overt signs of substance abuse. Women who use drugs have low self-esteem. They are dealing with conflicting issues: the physical or psychological need for the substance, the need to deny that the substance is harming the fetus, and guilt that they may be responsible for harming the fetus. Fear of prosecution for use of illegal drugs may prevent the woman from seeking prenatal care, increasing the risk to the woman and her fetus. In addition, many women with substance abuse problems face discrimination and resentment from health care professionals who direct their frustration at the woman rather than the problem.

Given the powerful deterrents to self-disclosure, extensive history taking provides the best opportunity to determine current and past substance use. The nurse taking the

🖤 CRITICAL TO REMEMBER

Behaviors Associated with Substance Abuse

Seeking prenatal care late in pregnancy
Failure to keep prenatal appointments
Inconsistent follow-through with recommended care
Poor grooming, inadequate weight gain
Needle punctures, thrombosed veins, cellulitis
Defensive or hostile reactions
Anger or apathy regarding pregnancy

health history must exhibit patience, empathy, and tolerance and use a blend of approaches that reinforce concern for the woman and her infant.

MEDICAL HISTORY

Determine whether the woman has medical conditions that are prevalent among women who use drugs, such as depression, seizures, hepatitis, pneumonia, cellulitis, STDs, hypertension, and suicide attempts. Current problems may include insomnia, panic attacks, exhaustion, and heart palpitations.

OBSTETRIC HISTORY

Evaluate for past and current complications of pregnancy. Spontaneous abortions, premature deliveries, abruptio placentae, and stillbirths are associated with substance abuse. Current complications may include STDs, vaginal bleeding, and an inactive or hyperactive fetus. Fundal height may be inconsistent with gestational age, suggesting intrauterine growth restriction.

Investigate emotional responses regarding the pregnancy, such as anger or apathy. These feelings are particularly significant during the latter half of the pregnancy, when the normal feelings of ambivalence are usually resolved. Negative feelings toward the pregnancy may interfere with prenatal compliance with follow-up care.

HISTORY OF SUBSTANCE ABUSE

Obtaining an accurate history of substance abuse is difficult and depends in large part on the way the health care worker approaches the woman. A sincere, nonjudgmental, and empathic approach promotes an open exchange of information.

Investigate all forms of drug use, including cigarettes, over-the-counter drugs, prescribed medications, and alcohol, as well as illicit drugs such as marijuana, amphetamines, cocaine, and heroin. Examine patterns of drug use, which can range from occasional recreational use to weekly binges to daily dependence on a particular drug or group of drugs. (Suggestions for interviewing are shown in Box 24-3.)

Analysis

Some women acknowledge the use of harmful substances but do not fully understand the effects. Other women are aware of the harmful effects but are unable to stop using the substances. A nursing diagnosis that addresses both factors is "Ineffective Health Maintenance related to lack of knowledge of the effects of substance abuse on self and fetus and inability to manage stress without the use of drugs."

Planning

Goals and expected outcomes for this diagnosis are that the woman will:
- Identify the harmful effects of substances on herself and her infant.
- Verbalize feelings related to continued use of harmful substances.
- Identify personal strengths and accept resources offered by the health care delivery system to stop using drugs.

BOX 24-3 Techniques for Interviewing a Woman about Substance Abuse

To determine whether the woman abuses substances:
- Express an accepting and nonjudgmental attitude.
- Explain why it is important to know about substance abuse: "We need to know about anything that might affect you or your baby during the pregnancy."
- Let her know that the questions are asked of all pregnant women.
- Acknowledge that women may be reluctant to disclose information: "I know it's difficult to talk to us about this, but we need to know so that we can give you and your baby the best care possible."
- Begin with questions about over-the-counter or prescription drugs and lead up to use of tobacco, alcohol, and, finally, illicit drugs.
- Demonstrate knowledge of types and forms of drugs commonly used in the community: "Do you see much heroin in your area?" "Do you have friends who are using crack?"

When substance abuse is acknowledged, the important points in the drug history include:
- The type of drug used
- The amount of drug used
- The frequency of use
- The time of last dose

Ask specific questions:
- How often have you taken over-the-counter medications?
- What drugs did you take last month? Were they prescribed?
- How many cigarettes do you smoke on a daily basis? Are there times when you smoke more?
- How many times a week do you drink alcoholic beverages (beer, wine, mixed drinks)?
- How many in a day? Are there times when you have more drinks?
- How often did you use [drug used] before becoming pregnant? How often do you use it now? Do you snort? Smoke crack? Shoot cocaine? How many lines do you use? How long do you stay high?

Interventions

Effective interventions for substance abuse require the combined efforts of nurses, physicians, social workers, and numerous community and federal agencies. Nurses must realize that progress is slow and frustrating. Keep in mind that the major priority is to protect the fetus and the expectant mother from the harmful effects of drugs.

EXAMINING ATTITUDES

When working with substance-abusing pregnant women, nurses must identify and acknowledge their own knowledge level, feelings and prejudices. They may have limited knowledge about perinatal substance abuse and negative attitudes toward mothers who abuse substances. Nurses may be angry at the woman who not only engages in self-destructive behavior but also may be inflicting harm on an innocent victim. Maintaining feelings of empathy or concern without becoming judgmental or even unknowingly punitive to the pregnant woman may be difficult. Nurses also may feel helpless, incompetent, and discouraged when the pregnant woman continues to abuse drugs despite the best efforts of the health care team.

Inservice education, professional consultation, and peer support are all helpful when working with pregnant women who abuse drugs. These processes can allow opportunities for discussion and sharing of feelings, problems, and particularly troublesome treatment issues.

PREVENTING SUBSTANCE ABUSE

Campaign to prevent substance abuse throughout the community. Provide accurate information in terms that clients can easily understand. Use posters, diagrams, pamphlets, and other visual aids to describe the effects of tobacco, alcohol, and other drugs on the fetus. Post visual aids in schools, supermarkets, shopping centers, and other areas where women of childbearing age will be exposed to them.

Focus on the benefits of remaining drug free, which include a decrease in maternal and neonatal complications. For example, the effects of smoking tobacco are potentially dose related and cumulative, and nurses need to encourage and support cessation at any point during pregnancy.

COMMUNICATING WITH THE WOMAN

Ask the expectant mother about stressors in her life that may be contributing to the pattern of substance abuse. Additional stressors may include inadequate housing, economic predicaments, intimate partner violence (IPV), and emotional or physical illness.

Be honest at all times while displaying a patient, nonjudgmental attitude as well as genuine interest and concern. This is especially important when the woman relapses into substance-abusing patterns. Allow her to express guilt, and reassure her that abstinence is possible and she can and must begin again.

Discuss how the woman's life will change after the birth. Help her to make realistic plans for care of the baby. Include support persons if possible.

HELPING THE WOMAN IDENTIFY STRENGTHS

Assist the substance-abusing pregnant woman in identifying personal strengths because she generally has a poor self-image. Acknowledge her actions when she abstains from drugs or alcohol for even a short time. Praise for maintaining an adequate weight gain and attending prenatal classes may increase self-esteem and compliance with the recommended regimen of care.

PROVIDING ONGOING CARE

At each antepartum visit, consider the current status of substance use, social service needs, education needs, and compliance with treatment referrals. In particular, address current drug use because women may change their pattern of drug use during pregnancy. For instance, they may stop using cocaine but may increase their use of marijuana or alcohol.

Verify compliance with recommended treatment regimens such as antepartum clinics and chemical-dependence referral programs. Coordinate care among various service providers such as group therapy and prenatal classes. Establish communication with all agencies that provide care, and facilitate communication that helps the woman with a chaotic lifestyle meet treatment objectives.

Provide continuing prenatal education about the anatomy and physiology of pregnancy and consequences of prenatal substance abuse. Describe the way the newborn benefits when the mother abstains from using drugs including tobacco and alcohol. Praise any attempts at abstinence and encourage the expectant mother to try again if she relapses.

Maternal attachment to the fetus may help her to reduce or eliminate her substance use. Assess signs of increasing attachment at each visit. Fetal movement often increases the woman's awareness of the fetus and may lead to a discussion about her plans for the infant and changes in her life that have occurred and will occur.

When women take drugs during pregnancy, child welfare services may be involved to ensure the safety of the infant after discharge. The infant may become a ward of the courts, and the mother may need to show she is in rehabilitation before being allowed to take the infant home with her. Use therapeutic communication techniques to help the mother express her feelings about this loss. Help her to make plans for making changes that will allow her to be with her infant.

Evaluation

Interventions have been successful if the expectant mother identifies the harmful effects of substance abuse on herself and on the fetus, discusses her strengths and her feelings about continued use of substances, and is receptive to assistance to stop using drugs.

INTRAPARTUM PERIOD

Assessment

COCAINE

Nurses who work in labor and delivery units must become skilled at identifying drug-induced signs and symptoms. Signs associated with frequent or recent use of crack cocaine include profuse sweating, hypertension, and irregular respirations combined with a lethargic response to labor and apparent lack of interest in the necessary interventions. Additional signs include dilated pupils, increased body temperature, and sudden onset of severely painful contractions. Fetal signs often include tachycardia and excessive fetal activity. Fetal bradycardia and late decelerations may occur.

Emotional signs of recent cocaine use may include angry, caustic, or abusive reactions to those attempting to provide care. Emotional lability and paranoia are signs of cocaine intoxication.

HEROIN

Typically, the pregnant woman addicted to heroin comes to the labor and delivery unit intoxicated from a recent drug administration. When the effects of the drug begin to wear off, withdrawal symptoms may be observed. These include

---

yawning, diaphoresis, rhinorrhea, restlessness, and excessive tearing of the eyes.

Analysis

One of the most relevant nursing diagnoses during the intrapartal period is "Risk for Injury related to physiologic and psychological effects of recent drug use."

Planning

The major goal or expected outcome for this nursing diagnosis is that the woman and the fetus will remain free from injury during labor and childbirth.

Interventions

PREVENTING INJURY

When a laboring woman has recently used a substance such as cocaine, the nurse must intervene to meet the needs of the woman and the fetus for safety, oxygen, and comfort.

ADMITTING PROCEDURE. Two nurses may be needed to admit the woman into the labor unit and to persuade her to assume a safe position. One nurse helps the woman into bed, initiates electronic fetal monitoring, and begins administration of oxygen, as needed. The other nurse acts as communicator.

Because the woman who has recently used a drug may have difficulty following directions, she should hear only one voice telling her what to do. The second nurse states firmly what is happening and exactly what the woman must do: "Lie on your left side." "This helps us watch how the baby is doing." "This gives you more oxygen." This nurse maintains eye contact with the woman while giving her instructions.

SETTING LIMITS. Realizing the importance of setting limits is critical to protect the safety of the mother and the fetus. For instance, the mother cannot smoke. The nurse may say, "It's difficult not to smoke, but there is real danger to everyone if you smoke when oxygen is being used." The mother who must remain in bed may become agitated. The nurse may say, "I know it's hard to stay in bed, but we can't take good care of the baby when you walk." If walking is safe for the woman, the nurse must set limits about where she can walk (in the labor room, not to the cafeteria).

INITIATING SEIZURE PRECAUTIONS. The laboring woman who recently used cocaine is at risk for hypertensive crisis and must be protected from injury in case of seizures. Seizure precautions are as follows:

- Keep the bed in a low, locked position.
- Pad side rails and keep them up at all times.
- Make sure suction equipment functions properly to prevent aspiration.
- Reduce environmental stimuli (lights, noise) as much as possible.

MAINTAINING EFFECTIVE COMMUNICATION

Establishing a therapeutic pattern of communication is essential. Avoid confrontation. Instead, acknowledge feelings: "I know you hurt, and I know how frightened you are. I'll do everything I can to make you comfortable." When the

---

CRITICAL TO REMEMBER

Signs of Recent Cocaine Use

Diaphoresis, high blood pressure, irregular respirations
Dilated pupils, increased body temperature
Sudden onset of severely painful contractions
Fetal tachycardia, excessive fetal activity
Angry, caustic, abusive reactions and paranoia

woman is abusive, be careful not to take the abuse personally or react in a nontherapeutic manner.

Examine your own feelings when women are abusive and acknowledge when anger is getting in the way of providing care. Another nurse may need to assume care of the woman for a time to allow some relief from unrelenting abusive comments.

PROVIDING PAIN CONTROL

Pain control for women who are substance abusers poses a difficult problem because it is often impossible to determine the type or combination of drugs that were used before admission. If pain medication can be administered safely, do not withhold it under the false assumption that the woman does not need it or that medication will contribute to addiction. Include nonpharmacologic comfort measures such as sacral pressure, back rubs, a cool cloth on the head, and continual support and encouragement as for any other woman in labor.

PREVENTING HEROIN WITHDRAWAL

To prevent or stabilize heroin withdrawal during labor, administer methadone intramuscularly as ordered if the woman is nauseated or vomiting. Give methadone to the woman who usually receives methadone at chemical-dependence centers if she did not receive her daily dose. It is essential to avoid use of drugs such as butorphanol (Stadol) in opiate-dependent women because acute withdrawal signs and symptoms will occur in the woman and the fetus.

Evaluation

Both the expectant mother and the fetus may have experienced harmful effects of drugs throughout pregnancy. However, the interventions for this nursing diagnosis can be considered effective if neither the woman nor the fetus sustains additional injury during labor and childbirth.

POSTPARTUM PERIOD

During the postpartum period, nursing care is focused on helping the mother with bonding, infant care, and planning to provide care of herself and the infant after discharge. Encourage the woman to continue her efforts to stop taking substances. Assess for signs of recent drug use and continue to assess the vital signs and level of consciousness of the mother.

Observe the mother-infant interaction so that bonding and attachment can be promoted. This is a major concern at this time (see Chapter 30). Encourage the woman to continue her efforts to stop taking substances. Women who stop or reduce use during pregnancy may return to using at previous levels after pregnancy and need support to continue abstinence.

✔ CHECK YOUR READING

12. What prenatal behaviors indicate substance abuse?
13. What signs and symptoms indicate recent cocaine use?
14. How does nursing care differ during the intrapartum period when the woman has recently taken cocaine?

BIRTH OF AN INFANT WITH CONGENITAL ANOMALIES

Even when everything goes according to plan, childbirth is a time of stress for parents. Their anxiety about the condition of the infant is obvious as they carefully trace the features and count the fingers and toes of their newborn. When the infant is not perfect but is born with anomalies, the parents often are overwhelmed with feelings of shock and grief. Because nurses are with the parents more than other members of the perinatal team, they have an opportunity to help the family adjust and cope with their feelings.

Factors Influencing Emotional Responses of Parents

TIMING AND MANNER OF BEING TOLD

At one time, common practice was to remove the infant from the delivery area before parents could see the congenital anomaly. Parents were told about the anomalies at a later time, often after the physician had prepared them for disturbing news. This practice changed, however, with the discovery that parents experienced less stress if they were told at once and permitted to hold their baby if the physical status of the infant allowed (Figure 24-4). The manner of presenting information also changed. Physicians and nurses became aware of the importance of helping the parents accept and bond with the newborn.

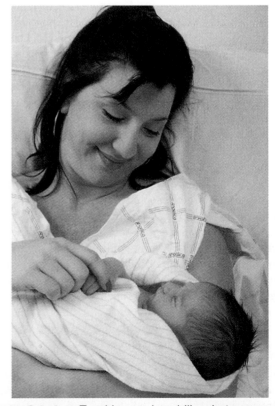

Figure 24-4 ■ Touching and cuddling between parents and the infant with a congenital anomaly foster attachment and help resolve the grieving process.

PRIOR KNOWLEDGE OF THE DEFECT

Although ultrasonography does not identify all fetal anomalies, many parents become aware of congenital anomalies during ultrasound examinations during pregnancy. These parents may not demonstrate the shock and disbelief at the birth that is seen in parents who are unprepared. Their reactions should not be interpreted to mean that they do not experience grief but rather that they have completed some of the early stages of grieving before the birth. Their grief is real and profound, even though it is expressed differently.

One couple was aware from 18 weeks' gestation that the fetus had hydrocephalus and protrusion of brain tissue from the skull. The mother elected to carry the fetus to term so that the infant would have "every chance at life." When the infant died within minutes after birth, the parents calmly held their child and called the infant by the name they had selected several weeks previously. The only overt signs of grief were silent tears and a request to see their clergyman.

TYPE OF DEFECT

Although any defect in a newborn produces feelings of extreme concern and anxiety, certain defects are associated with long-term parenting problems. Accepting an infant with facial or genital anomalies is particularly difficult for the family and community. The face is visible to everyone, and parents are fearful about whether the child will be accepted. If the defect is cleft lip and palate, the parents are extremely concerned about surgical repair. Common questions include "When can it be done?" "Will the child look normal?" "Will the child sound normal?" "Will the scars be obvious?" Parents often are anxious about how grandparents and siblings will accept the child. With time and support, parents often work out unique methods to help the family develop strong feelings of attachment.

One father, profoundly disturbed about the birth of a daughter with a cleft lip and palate and extremely concerned about the way his 6-year-old daughter would respond to the infant, took control of the situation. He carefully presented the infant to her sister and pointed out that the baby was small and had special problems. She would need the love of her big sister to overcome them. The 6-year-old held the infant and promised to help care for her.

Gender is at the core of a person's identity, and any defect of the genitals, however slight or correctable, arouses deep concern in both parents. Some anomalies such as hypospadias (opening of the urethra on the underside of the penis) are repaired in early childhood. Other genital anomalies such as ambiguous genitalia (when assignment of gender is in doubt) cause extreme concern in the family and affect such basic issues as what to name the infant, how to dress the infant, and how to respond to questions about the infant's sex.

IRREPARABLE DEFECT

Although the initial impact of any defect is profound disappointment and concern, when the defect is irreparable the parents must grapple with the knowledge that the infant will have a lifelong disability. Examples of irreparable defects include Down syndrome, microcephaly, and amelia (absence of an entire extremity).

Grief and Mourning

Grief describes the emotional response to loss. Mourning is the process of going through the phases of grief until the loss can be accepted and resolved. Birth of an infant with an anomaly evokes a grief response, and the family must mourn the loss of the perfect infant they imagined during pregnancy. Early emotions include denial, anger, and guilt.

Denial and disbelief are the initial reactions of most parents to the birth of an infant with a congenital defect. "This can't be true." "How could this happen?" Anger often is a pervasive response and may take the form of fault-finding or resentment. Anger may be directed toward the family, the medical personnel, or the self, but it is seldom directed toward the infant. Guilt may be expressed as a question of responsibility for the defect: "I shouldn't have worked so much while I was pregnant."

Other emotions include fear, which may be expressed as concern about what must be done in the immediate or distant future (surgical procedures, complicated care, the infant's potential for a normal life). Sadness and depression, manifested by crying, withdrawal from relationships, lack of energy, inability to sleep, and decreased appetite, may precede acceptance and resolution. Gradually—often after a prolonged time—the feelings of sadness abate and the family is able to accept the loss and resolve its grief.

✔ CHECK YOUR READING

15. When should parents be told that the infant has anomalies?
16. What types of defects most affect parenting?
17. How can the reaction of parents to birth anomalies be described?

Nursing Considerations

ASSISTING WITH THE GRIEVING PROCESS

Parents must grieve the loss of the perfect infant they expected before they can form an attachment with this newborn. Nurses can help by remaining with the parents through the initial phase of shock and disbelief and maintaining an atmosphere that encourages them to express their feelings. One way to do this is to listen carefully to what the parents say and respond by reflecting the content and feelings that they express.

For example, the mother of an infant girl with cleft palate says, "How could this happen? I should have gone to the doctor earlier." A helpful response might be, "It sounds like you feel responsible for this problem. Actually, we don't know what causes cleft palate, but let's talk about how you are feeling." This offers reassurance but keeps the interaction open to explore the underlying feelings of guilt that the mother may be expressing.

Grief responses vary among individuals, and cultural and religious beliefs affect the expression of grief. People in some groups express grief openly by crying, becoming angry or seeking comfort from a support group. Members of other cultures (such as Chinese, Japanese, and Native American) do not. They may appear stoic and may not reveal the depths of their grief. In some cultures (such as Latino), it is acceptable for women, but not for men, to show their grief in public.

PROMOTING BONDING AND ATTACHMENT

A priority nursing intervention is to promote bonding and attachment, which may be disrupted when parents who expected a perfect infant give birth to an infant with an abnormality. The process often begins when the nurse communicates acceptance of the infant.

- To promote bonding the nurse handles the newborn gently and presents the infant as something precious. Parents are particularly sensitive to facial expressions of shock or distress. Many nurses emphasize the normal aspects of the infant's body: "She's so alert, and she has beautiful eyes." Perhaps it is most important to help the parents hold their infant as soon as possible. Touching and cuddling are essential to caring.

PROVIDING ACCURATE INFORMATION

Nurses who work in perinatal settings are responsible for becoming informed about follow-up treatment and timing of surgical procedures for common anomalies so they can clarify and reinforce information provided by the physician. This involves discussing the plan of care with the physician as well as researching the nursing care that will be required. Parents develop trust in the health care team when consistent information is presented clearly and explained fully.

If possible, one primary nurse or a team of nurses should work with the family throughout the hospital stay. The nurse should assess the parents' understanding of the condition and the treatment plan. Simple diagrams, pictures, or videos about the defect and the effects of treatment may be helpful. Parents often need to have information repeated frequently because it is difficult for them to take in all they are told at this time of intense emotions.

FACILITATING COMMUNICATION

Nurses are sometimes fearful of being asked questions they are unable to answer, or they fear they will say the wrong thing.

- The most helpful course of action is to answer questions as honestly as possible. If unsure of information, say so: "I'm not sure about that, but I'll find out for you." In addition to answers, parents need kindness, support, and genuine concern.

It is crucial that family members communicate with one another as well as with the health professionals. Information and empathy should be offered consistently to both parents. Fathers should be included in all discussions, demon-strations, and care of the infant. Without this the father cannot be expected to support his partner, explain the infant's condition to relatives and friends, or begin to deal with his own shock and sadness.

The nurse should assess the mother for signs of postpartum depression (see Chapter 28). The support person should be made aware of the mother's increased risk for prolonged depression, and the differences among normal "baby blues," normal grieving, and postpartum depression should be explained.

PLANNING FOR DISCHARGE

Teach the parents special feeding, holding, and positioning techniques needed for care of their infant. For example, parents may need to learn ways to feed an infant with cleft palate. Early participation in infant care fosters feelings of attachment and responsibility for the infant. They should also know what type of follow-up care with the heath care provider is necessary and what other services may be needed.

Provide other anticipatory guidance that may help prevent problems when the infant is discharged to home care. The reaction and behavior of siblings depend on their ages and abilities to understand the needs of the infant. Young children, who often are jealous of the attention and care that the infant requires, may regress to infantile behaviors such as bed wetting and thumb sucking. Remind parents that this indicates a need for attention rather than naughtiness.

Although grandparents can be a great source of strength and support, they also may have difficulty adjusting to the infant with an abnormality. When appropriate and if the parents indicate their willingness, include grandparents when teaching the special care the infant will need.

PROVIDING REFERRALS

Initiate referrals to national and community resources, as needed. In addition to a referral to the social worker in the hospital, parents also may benefit from information about the National Easter Seal Society for Crippled Children, the March of Dimes Birth Defects Foundation, or the disabled children's services of the public health department. In addition, organizations such as the Shriners provide funds for the care of children. Support groups vary among communities, and perinatal nurses may wish to make a list of the names, addresses, and telephone numbers of these organizations.

✔ CHECK YOUR READING

18. How do nurses promote bonding and attachment in families who have an infant with congenital anomalies?
19. What should be included in discharge planning for the family of an infant with congenital anomalies?

PREGNANCY LOSS

Perinatal death can occur at any time. Early spontaneous abortion, ectopic pregnancy, fetal demise during the latter half of pregnancy, stillbirth, or neonatal death when the infant survives for a few days or weeks can be equally devastating for the parents, who may experience profound sadness and grief.

Because many people do not consider perinatal loss to be on the same level as the loss of an older child or adult, parents experiencing perinatal death often feel alone in their grief. In addition, friends and family members often are hesitant to discuss the loss for fear of saying the wrong thing. They may be uncomfortable with the topic and change the subject when parents want to talk.

Early Pregnancy Loss

Early pregnancy loss from spontaneous abortion or ectopic pregnancy may precipitate intense grief by the parents. The parents may not yet have told family and friends about the pregnancy. Those who do know may minimize the grief that occurs at this time. Comments such as "You shouldn't have any problems getting pregnant again" discount the feelings of the mother and father.

When ectopic pregnancy is the reason for the loss, the woman has to deal with the loss of the pregnancy and the loss or damage of a fallopian tube. Health care workers mean well when they say, "You still have one fallopian tube left; you'll get pregnant again," but this does not acknowledge to the mother that a child has been lost. Ectopic pregnancy is more frequent in women over 35, increasing the impact if the woman has experienced infertility problems.

Concurrent Death and Survival in Multifetal Pregnancy

Parents experience conflicting and complex feelings of joy and grief when one or more infants in a multifetal pregnancy live and one or more infants in the same gestation die. Contrary to common belief, parents do not grieve less for the dead infant because of the joy they experience in the living child. They experience an acute sense of loss despite having a surviving infant, and they grieve no less for the infant who was lost.

For parents experiencing both survival and death of an infant, the grieving process may be more complicated. They may have fears about the health of the surviving infant, especially if the infant is preterm or ill. They may be unable to grieve for the dead child because of their concerns and responsibilities for the surviving child. They also may experience problems with attachment to the surviving infant because of grieving and fear that they will lose that infant too. In addition, they may receive less support from others than parents who have lost the only child in a single gestation.

Parents who experience the death of one infant and the survival of another need the same interventions as those offered for parents who lose the only child in a single gestation. These interventions include allowing the parents to hold the dead infant and gathering mementos. In addition, nurses must be prepared to confirm the cause of death, if known, and the health status of the surviving infant.

Previous Pregnancy Loss

Women who have experienced previous pregnancy losses often have a sense of reliving the anguish in the next pregnancy. They may have higher levels of anxiety and lower levels of attachment during subsequent pregnancies, especially until they pass the point at which the loss occurred or they deliver a normal baby (Van & Meleis, 2003). Waiting to attach to the fetus may be a protective effort to prevent the pain of another loss. However, for some women, passing the time in pregnancy when the loss occurred does not decrease the anxiety. Signs of depression are more likely to be present (Armstrong, 2004).

Having other, healthy children does not reduce the degree of anxiety during a pregnancy that follows a perinatal loss. Parents may not tell others about the new pregnancy and may not tell others who do not already know about the loss of the previous pregnancy.

Women may want more frequent contact with the health care provider throughout the pregnancy to reassure themselves that all is going well (Cote-Arsenault, 2003). These mothers are also at risk for having a preterm or low-birth-weight infant in pregnancies that follow perinatal loss (Heinonen & Kirkinen, 2000). Therefore they should be counseled about obtaining early prenatal care and will need extra emotional support if they become pregnant again.

Application of the Nursing Process
Pregnancy Loss

Assessment

Nursing assessment of the family that has experienced the loss of a fetus or infant requires a great deal of sensitivity. In the case of infant death, collect as much information as possible before meeting the woman and her family for the first time so that hurtful mistakes can be avoided. Knowing the child's sex, weight, length, and gestational age and whether any abnormalities were noted will help the nurse communicate effectively.

Many perinatal units design a sticker or symbol to place on the door, chart, and Kardex so that all staff who come in contact with the family, including auxiliary, housekeeping, and laboratory personnel, will be alerted that the infant has not survived. Designs include a flower, fallen leaf, teardrop, or rainbow. This visual symbol diminishes the chance that an uninformed person will make inadvertent comments that cause the family pain.

Nurses often are unsure about how to interact with a family that has experienced the loss of an infant. It is helpful to acknowledge the situation and clarify the nurse's role at once: "I'm Bette Turner, and I'll be your nurse today. I'm so sorry for your loss. Let me know if there is any way I can be of help." This is not an appropriate time for self-disclosure or for false reassurance. Keep the focus on the family's response and their ability to support one another.

Initial grief responses are similar to those expressed by parents of infants with anomalies. Crying and expressions of anger often occur during the woman's stay in the birth facility. Guilt is often an underlying feeling as the parents search for a reason for their infant's death. Nurses who provide home care or make follow-up telephone calls must be aware of subtle cues of grief, such as sighing, excessive sleeping, apathy, poor hygiene, and loss of appetite. These signs are especially important when assessing members of cultural groups that do not display grief publicly. In addition, nurses must observe for signs of postpartum depression.

Evaluate the availability of a support system that includes family members or clergy. If appropriate, ask whether a spiritual adviser would offer comfort. Many religions emphasize the acceptance of God's will and the immortality of the soul, and hearing these beliefs affirmed may help the family cope with the grief that they are experiencing.

Include the father in the assessment, too, because fathers often do not receive the support they need. Many fathers feel a need to appear strong so that they can support their partners. As a result they often hold back their own feelings of grief and pain and are sometimes perceived as needing less support than mothers. In addition, fathers often grieve differently than mothers.

Analysis

Several nursing diagnoses could be used when a family experiences perinatal death. "Risk for Dysfunctional Grieving or Risk for Ineffective Coping" may apply. Because perinatal loss affects the whole family, the nursing diagnosis "Interrupted Family Process related to grief over newborn (or fetal) death" is discussed here.

Planning

Goals and expected outcomes for this diagnosis are that the parents will:

- Acknowledge their grief and express the meaning of the loss.
- Share their grief with significant others.
- Provide support to each family member.

Interventions

ACKNOWLEDGING THE INFANT

For many years the common belief was that when an infant was stillborn or died shortly after birth, the less parents knew of the infant, the less they would grieve. The infant often was whisked away so that the parents never saw their newborn. Relatives often disposed of the clothes and infant equipment before the mother returned home, and the parents were left with very few memories of the infant's birth.

The response to perinatal death changed as nurses discovered that the most helpful interventions for grieving parents were those that acknowledged the rights of the baby. These include the following rights:

- To be recognized as a person who was born and died
- To be named

- To be seen, touched, and held by the family
- To have life-ending acknowledged
- To be put to rest with dignity (Primeau & Lamb, 1995)

PRESENTING THE INFANT TO THE PARENTS. The way in which the infant is presented to the parents is extremely important because these are the memories they will retain. Parents should be prepared for the appearance of the infant, especially if maceration (peeling) of the skin is present or there are disfigured areas. If necessary, wash the infant and apply baby lotion or powder. Wrap the infant in a soft, warm blanket. If possible, bring the parents and infant together while the infant is still warm and soft. Keeping the infant in a warmed incubator may be necessary if some time elapses before the parents have contact with the infant. If this is not possible, tell the parents that the skin may feel cool. Allow parents to keep the infant as long as they wish, and make them feel free to unwrap the infant if they wish.

Many nurses are concerned about the way to present the stillborn infant with severe deformities. Explain the defect briefly and gently. Wrap the infant to expose the most normal aspects. When the infant has deformities of the head and face, wrap the infant with the blanket draped loosely over the most severely affected areas so that the parents do not see those areas first.

It is not advisable, however, to try to hide the defects completely. Allow parents to progress at their own speed in inspecting the infant. Parents may examine the abnormality or choose to leave the infant wrapped. They may quietly discuss positive features of the infant: "He has your ears." "Look at the long fingers."

Allow as much privacy and time as the parents and other family members need to be together. Remain sensitive to cues that members of the family want to talk or prefer silence. Keeping up a flow of conversation is not necessary. A sympathetic smile or a gentle touch of the hand suffices. It is all right to ask "Do you want to talk?" Then, listening quietly and reflecting the mother or father's feelings are all that are required. Allow the parents to be alone if they wish, and check every so often to see if they need assistance.

Offer the parents the opportunity to bathe or dress the infant, if they wish. Assist them during this care. Performing such activities as holding, bathing, and dressing allow the mother and father the only chance they will have to parent the infant.

PREPARING A MEMORY PACKET. Mourning requires memories. Nurses have explored measures that help the family create memories of the infant so that the existence of the child is confirmed and the parents can complete the grieving process.

Most parents treasure a memory packet that includes a photograph, handprints or footprints, a birth identification band with the date and time of birth, the crib card with the infant's name, weight, and length, tape measure and blanket used for the baby, and if possible, a lock of hair. Some hospitals buy commercial remembrance materials to give parents. The packets or boxes may contain clothing for the baby to wear and provide a place to put baby items.

Give the parents pictures of the infant to help them remember the baby's features and assist them through the grieving process. Some parents and grandparents want pictures taken of themselves with the infant. Keep the memory packet on file if the parents do not wish to take it home because they may want to have it at a later time. Many couples feel these concrete forms of remembrance are invaluable in helping them remember the baby as a person who really existed when they have no other signs of that life.

Some families may not want pictures taken of the infant. Taking pictures after death may not be culturally acceptable for Native American, Eskimo, Amish, Hindu, and Muslim families (Kavanaugh & Wheeler, 2003). If possible, take pictures of the infant before death occurs. Autopsies also may not be permitted in some cultures.

ASSISTING WITH OTHER NEEDS. If the family includes other children, help the parents plan how to tell them about the death of the expected infant. Give them information about sibling responses and needs based on the ages of their other children. Provide the parents with written information about perinatal loss, grieving, and children's responses to death. It is important that parents explain the cause of the death in understandable terms because some children will blame themselves. Parents can take written material home for later reading when they are less overwhelmed with immediate concerns.

Offer to call clergy for them and discuss plans for a funeral or memorial service, if they wish. A baptism or blessing can also be performed, if parents wish.

Discuss the normal grieving process and explain the steps of grieving and that a considerable amount of time is involved. Describe common reactions that family members and friends might have, and mention that some may minimize the loss or urge them to have another baby in a misguided attempt to offer comfort. Let them know that grandparents also go through grief because of the loss as well as the pain their children must endure.

FOLLOW-UP CARE

Parents may find that friends and relatives expect them to recover quickly from perinatal loss and cannot understand their continued grief. Because parents experience grief and go through the process in different ways, they may not understand each other's responses. Mothers who want to talk about the loss repeatedly may have partners who deal with their grief by being stoic and brooding or by focusing their energy on work. Emphasize the individuality of grief and that no single method or duration of grieving is right for everyone.

Couples usually want to know the cause of death of their infant. An autopsy may be recommended even if the cause of death is obvious. This gives parents the most accurate diagnosis for risk of recurrence in a future pregnancy. In some cases the cause may never be found. Referral for genetic counseling may be appropriate for some parents who are concerned about the risk of a repeated tragedy. Future pregnancies will be stressful, and the woman will need closer follow-up than usual to identify any possible problems as soon as possible. The anxiety may continue in the neonatal period, and parents may need education and emotional support during this time.

PROVIDING REFERRALS

Some birth agencies offer ongoing support groups. Telephone calls made during the first week, 1 to 2 weeks later, at the time of the postpartum checkup, and at the 1-year anniversary are helpful. Home visits may be made by agency staff, and cards may be sent to help parents with their grief. A bereavement counselor may be available. The greatest help often comes from contact with persons who have experienced a similar loss, and a variety of support groups have been formed.

Refer parents to organizations designed to help parents cope with loss of a child. These include Resolve Through Sharing, AMEND (Aiding Mothers and Fathers Experiencing Neonatal Death), SHARE (Source of Help in Airing and Resolving Experiences), and HAND (Helping After Neonatal Death). Some women join Internet perinatal loss support groups. Such groups may be particularly helpful after the immediate period surrounding the death. Extended family and friends may no longer be as supportive at this time and do not realize the length of time involved in grieving. Gaining a feeling of control over their lives and being able to make decisions gradually develop as the parents move toward healing (Kavanaugh & Wheeler, 2003).

Evaluation

Nursing care has been successful if the family members share their feelings of loss and grief, communicate them to significant others, and are supportive of one another.

✔ **CHECK YOUR READING**

20. How should the stillborn infant be presented to the parents? Why?
21. What is a memory packet, and what should it include?

RELINQUISHMENT FOR ADOPTION

Some women carry a pregnancy to term and then relinquish the newborn to the care of another family for adoption. The decision to place the infant for adoption is a painful one that can produce long-lasting feelings of ambivalence and chronic sorrow. On the one hand, the expectant mother may be satisfied that the infant is going into a stable home where the child is wanted and will receive excellent care. On the other hand, the social pressures against giving up one's child are often intense.

The process of adoption is relatively simple for the expectant mother. Each state and many organized churches have adoption agencies. In addition, private adoptions are available. In private adoptions an attorney acts as the intermediary between the expectant woman and the couple wanting to adopt the infant. The adoptive family usually agrees to pay the medical expenses of the woman, and sometimes a supportive relationship is established between the expectant mother and adoptive family.

The relationship between the birth mother and the adoptive parents varies greatly. The adoptive parents may be unknown to the birth mother, or she may have chosen them after interviewing many candidates. Some adoptive mothers participate in the birth and act as coach or support person during the birth. The birth mother may never see the infant again or may keep in contact with and participate in the child's life.

Nurses are sometimes unsure of how to communicate with the woman who is relinquishing her infant. First, the nursing staff who come in contact with the woman must be informed of her decision to place the infant for adoption. This information prevents inadvertent comments that could cause distress. Second, nurses must remember that adoption is *an act of love, not one of abandonment* because the woman relinquishes the newborn to a family that is better able to provide financial and emotional support.

Nurses also must be prepared to respect any special wishes that the mother may have about the birth. Many mothers make plans for the degree of their involvement with the infant and with the adoptive parents. For instance, most birth mothers want to know all about the infant—how big he or she is, how healthy, how beautiful. Encourage them to see and hold the newborn and give the baby a name. Prepare them for the appearance of the baby before they see the infant. Many parents take photographs or save mementos such as the birth identification band or crib card. Such actions provide memories of the infant and help the mother through the grieving process that may accompany relinquishment of the child.

■ The nurse should try to establish rapport and a trusting relationship with the birth mother. It is helpful to acknowledge the situation at the initial contact with the woman: "Hello, my name is Claire, and I'll be your nurse today. I understand the adoptive family is coming this morning. How can I help you get ready?" This is much more helpful than providing care without reference to an event that is of utmost concern to the mother. It also provides an opening for her to express feelings that may include strong attachment and love for the infant, ambivalence about her decision, and profound sadness.

Therapeutic communication techniques such as reflecting, paraphrasing, and summarizing are useful to help the mother explore her feelings. Although the mother has chosen to relinquish her baby, the grief she experiences may be similar to loss by death. Her grief may not be shared with family and friends, who may not understand her feelings. The nurse should acknowledge the feelings the mother may have, avoid offering advice, and remain nonjudgmental.

Nurses also teach adoptive families how to care for the newborn and what to expect in terms of growth and development. Teaching requires that adequate time and a private place be provided. This family benefits from all the teaching that is provided for other new parents. They may be anxious, and demonstrations as well as return demonstrations are appropriate.

✓ **CHECK YOUR READING**

22. What is meant by the phrase "adoption is an act of love"?
23. What are the nurse's responsibilities to the adoptive parents?

INTIMATE PARTNER VIOLENCE

According to the CDC approximately 5.3 million incidents of intimate partner abuse occur each year to women over the age of 18 years in the United States (CDC, 2003). Approximately 1.5 million women face IPV each year, and one in every four women has been physically assaulted or raped by an intimate partner at some point in her life (Tjaden & Thoennes, 2000). The costs in terms of medical and mental health expenses and lost productivity exceed $5.8 billion yearly (CDC, 2003). Adolescents as well as older women are victims of IPV. Although some studies show an increased incidence in economically disadvantaged groups, IPV is seen at all socioeconomic levels.

Pregnancy may offer some protection for some women who were previously abused by their partners. However, IPV may start or increase in frequency and severity during pregnancy and the postpartum period (Toohey, 2000). It has been recognized as a risk to the health of both mothers and infants (Figure 24-5). The incidence during pregnancy varies between 1% and 20% and is more frequent (with the possible exception of preeclampsia) than any major medical condition screened for during the prenatal period (AAP & ACOG, 2002).

Physical abuse during pregnancy may result in spontaneous abortion, abruptio placentae, premature labor, low birth weight, and fetal death. Some factors that may be pre-

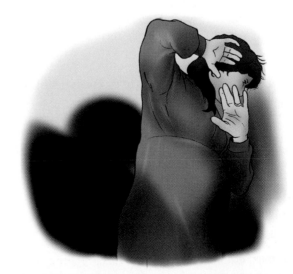

Figure 24-5 ■ The woman who is abused by her partner lives with an ever-present risk of violence. Because an abused woman may not seek help, all women should be asked about abuse whenever they receive health care.

dictors of abuse during pregnancy include depression, lack of contraceptive use, stressful life events, and lack of faith in God or a higher power (Dunn & Oths, 2004). Substance abuse by both the woman and her partner is often associated with IPV (El-Bassel et al., 2003).

Physical abuse may involve threats, slapping, and pushing. It also may escalate to punching, kicking, and beating that results in internal injury, wounds from weapons, or death. Sexual abuse, including rape, often is part of physical abuse, with almost half the abused women reporting being forced into sex by their male partners.

Physical violence occurs within the context of continuous mental abuse, threats, and coercion. As a result, women feel shame, loss of self-respect, and powerlessness. They often are isolated from sources of help and support. They are more likely to experience depression and lower self-esteem and have a greater need for health and community services than other women (Peterson, Gazmararian, & Clark, 2001).

In addition, physical abuse of the mother may be an indication of what life holds for the unborn child. In over 50% of homes in which domestic violence occurs, the children also are injured (Toohey, 2000). In the majority of cases the man who batters the woman also batters the children, and some women who are victims physically abuse their children. Children who witness abuse of their mother often react with sleep problems, regression, aggression or other behavioral disturbances, and difficulty in school (Lemmey, McFarlane, Wilson, & Malecha, 2001). Adults who abuse others often were abused as children.

Factors That Promote Violence

Family violence occurs in cultures in which roles are gender based and little value is placed on the woman's role. Men hold the power, and women are viewed as less worthy of respect than men. In these cultures, strength and aggression, the ability to "show her who is boss," are considered attractive and desirable in males.

In many cultures, women are seen as having less worth than men. Women earn less than men in the job market, and they often are victimized by marriage. For example, women who hold full-time jobs continue to carry the major responsibilities for housekeeping and child care. They may remain in unhealthy relationships because they are financially dependent on their partners. If they divorce, women often become single parents with a standard of living much lower than that of their former husbands.

The woman's role in her own culture is important. For example, many Hispanic women believe they must be submissive to the male and must sacrifice for their families because it is their duty to keep the family together. They may not have the education to be able to access help or obtain a job to provide a means of support if they should leave their partners. If the woman is an illegal immigrant, she is less likely to seek help from authorities for fear of being deported (de Mendoza, 2001). When asking women who do not speak English about IPV, it is essential that family members or friends not be used as translators.

Stereotyping males as powerful and females as weak and without value has a profound effect on the self-esteem of women. Many women internalize these messages and come to believe that they are less worthy than their partners and that they are the cause of their own punishment. They accept the implication from society that women who are battered or raped "got what they deserved."

The woman may come to accept her partner's statements that she is the cause of the violence. She may minimize the abuse or indicate to others that it is unusual. Women often feel a need to help the abuser and hope that the partner will change and the abuse will end. As the relationship becomes more and more abusive, the woman may begin to look for help.

Although alcohol often is stated as a cause of violence against women, chemical dependence and domestic violence are two separate problems. Chemical dependence is a disease of addiction, but abuse is a learned behavior that can be unlearned. Violence may become more severe or bizarre when alcohol or drugs are involved, however.

See Table 24-3 for a summary of the myths and realities of violence against women.

TABLE 24-3 Myths and Realities of Violence Against Women

Myths	Realities
The battered-woman syndrome affects only a small percentage of the population.	Battering is the single major cause of injury to women. Approximately 1.5 million women are battered each year by their partners.
Violence against women occurs only in lower socioeconomic classes and minority groups.	Violence occurs in families from all social, economic, educational, racial, and religious backgrounds.
The problem is really "partner abuse," couples who assault each other.	Approximately 95% of serious assaults are male against female. Violence against women is about control and power.
Alcohol and drugs cause abusive behavior.	Substance abuse and violence against women are two separate problems. Substance abuse is a disease, but violence is a learned behavior that can be unlearned.
The abuser is "out of control."	He is not out of control. Instead, he is making a decision, because he chooses who, when, and where he abuses.
The woman "got what she deserved."	No one deserves to be beaten. No one has the right to beat another person. Violent behavior is the responsibility of the violent person.
Women "like it," or they would leave.	Women are threatened with severe punishment or death if they attempt to leave. Many have no resources and are isolated, and they and their children are dependent on the abuser.
Couples counseling is a good recommendation for abusive relationships.	Couples counseling is not only ineffective for the couple, but also can be dangerous for the abused woman.

Characteristics of the Abuser

Physical abuse concerns power, and it is only one of many tactics that abusive men use to control their partners. Other tactics include isolation, intimidation, and threats. Extreme jealousy and possessiveness are typical of the abuser. An abusive man often attempts to control every aspect of the woman's life, such as where she goes, to whom she speaks, and what she wears. He controls access to money and transportation and may force the woman to account for every moment spent away from him.

The abusive man often has a low tolerance for frustration and poor impulse control. He does not perceive his violent behavior as a problem and often denies responsibility for the violence by blaming the woman. Most abusive men come from homes in which they witnessed the abuse of their mothers or were themselves abused as children. Although many abusive men have alcohol problems that contribute to the abuse, many men without alcohol problems also batter their partners.

Cycle of Violence

Although IPV may be random, there is often a pattern. The violence occurs in a cycle that consists of three phases: (1) a tension-building phase, (2) a battering incident, and (3) a "honeymoon phase." Being aware of the behaviors that accompany each phase will enable the nurse to counsel the woman (Figure 24-6).

Effects of Battering

Abuse during pregnancy is correlated with health problems for the mother and infant. These women are likely to have multiple injury sites, particularly of the abdomen, face, and breasts. They are likely to start prenatal care in the third trimester and to have health problems such as STDs (Winn, Records, & Rice 2003). They may miss appointments because the abuser will not let them leave the house or because they wish to hide signs of recent injury. Low weight gain, anemia, and use of alcohol and illicit drugs are increased in women experiencing IPV. Infants born to women with IPV have a higher risk of prematurity, low birth weight, and neonatal death (Lipsky, Holt, Easterling, & Critchlow, 2003).

Nurse's Role in Prevention of Abuse

Nurses can do a great deal to prevent physical abuse. First, they must examine their beliefs to determine whether they accept the prevailing attitude that blames the victim: "Why was she wearing that?" "She shouldn't have flirted with someone else." "Why does she stay with him?" Second, nurses can consciously practice in ways that empower women and make it clear that the woman owns her body and has the right to decide how it should be treated. Nurses must use language that indicates the woman is an active partner in her care: "You understand your body; what do you think?" "How did your body respond when you tried that?"

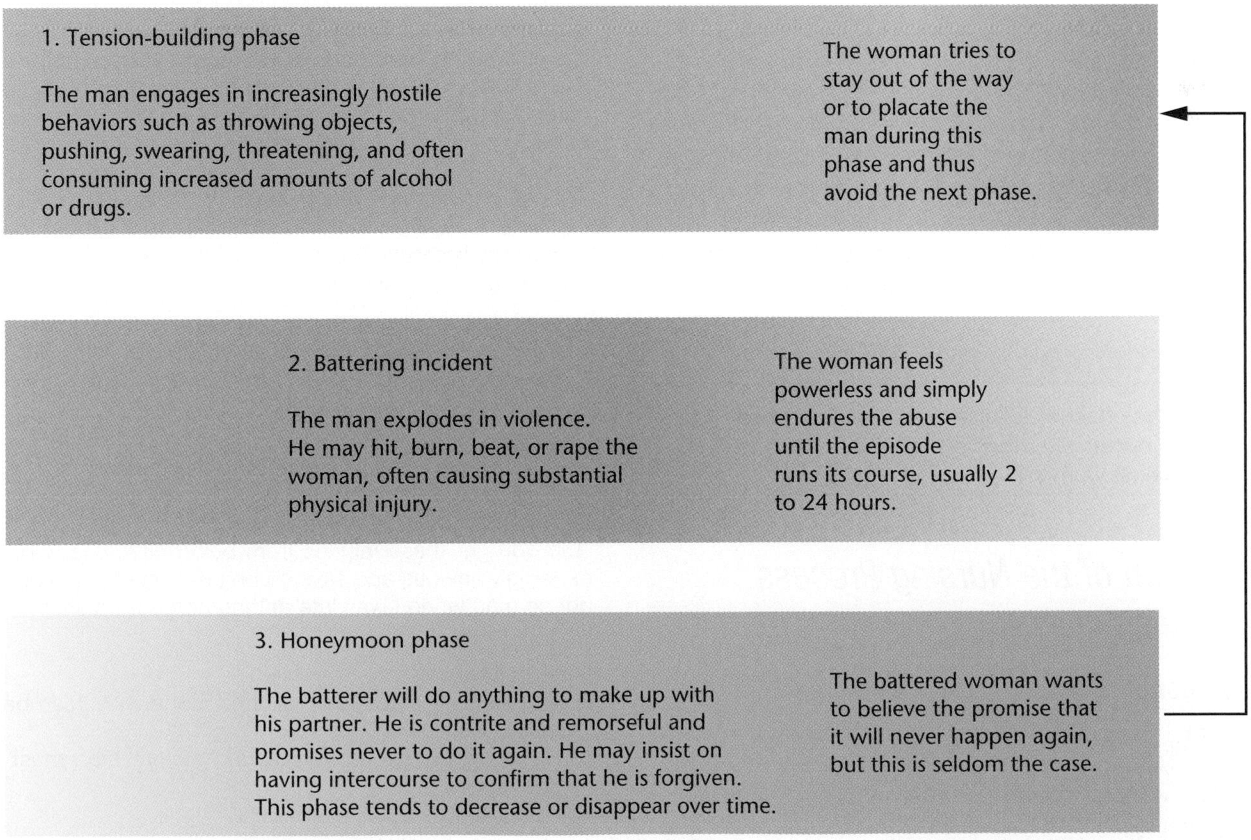

1. Tension-building phase

The man engages in increasingly hostile behaviors such as throwing objects, pushing, swearing, threatening, and often consuming increased amounts of alcohol or drugs.

The woman tries to stay out of the way or to placate the man during this phase and thus avoid the next phase.

2. Battering incident

The man explodes in violence. He may hit, burn, beat, or rape the woman, often causing substantial physical injury.

The woman feels powerless and simply endures the abuse until the episode runs its course, usually 2 to 24 hours.

3. Honeymoon phase

The batterer will do anything to make up with his partner. He is contrite and remorseful and promises never to do it again. He may insist on having intercourse to confirm that he is forgiven. This phase tends to decrease or disappear over time.

The battered woman wants to believe the promise that it will never happen again, but this is seldom the case.

Figure 24-6 ■ Types of behaviors that are evident in each step of the cycle of violence.

During examinations, nurses can introduce aspects of care that increase the woman's control over the situation. For example, make sure that the woman is seated and clothed when meeting the physician or nurse practitioner who is to examine her instead of being unclothed and in a lithotomy position. Nurses can place the examination table so that the woman's head, not her genitalia, meets the examiner's eye when he or she enters the room. When the woman is positioned for the examination, the table can be raised 45 degrees so that she has an opportunity to make eye contact with the examiner.

School nurses are in an excellent position to influence the way teenagers define gender roles: "Real men don't beat up women." "Girls don't have to put up with verbal or physical abuse from anyone." "Use a condom; it's not cool to give someone you care about STDs or an unwanted pregnancy."

Nurses should be familiar with national resources that are designed to provide health care workers with technical assistance, training materials, posters, bibliographies, and relevant articles. The sources listed here provide information but are not crisis lines.

- National Domestic Violence Hotline
  1-800-799-7233
  www.ndvh.org
- National Clearinghouse for the Defense of Battered Women
  215-351-0010
- National Coalition against Domestic Violence
  303-839-1852
  www.ncadv.org
- National Resource Center on Domestic Violence
  1-800-537-2238
  www.nrcdv.org

The National Domestic Violence Hotline (1-800-799-SAFE) offers information on crisis assistance throughout the United States. Their website, www.ndvh.org, is another source of information. Women who are being abused should be warned not to access Internet sources of information about abuse at home because their partners may be able to determine recently used Internet sites.

✔ CHECK YOUR READING

24. What is the effect of pregnancy on battering behavior?
25. How can nurses alter their practice to help prevent violence against women?

Application of the Nursing Process
The Battered Woman

Assessment

Victims of IPV can be found in every prenatal clinic and every obstetrician's or nurse-midwife's office. Unfortunately, few women identify themselves as such, and many remain unrecognized. Because of the prevalence of IPV dur-

ing pregnancy, it is recommended that every woman be screened for physical abuse at each contact. When they are first approached, women may deny that abuse has occurred. Women should be asked about IPV once during each trimester, at admission to the hospital, and again at the postpartum checkup. Asking, and especially asking more than once, may lead the woman to seek help at a later time.

Nurses often are unsure of the way to approach the issue of suspected abuse. Women may seek care during the "honeymoon phase" of the violence cycle. During this phase the man often is overly solicitous ("hovering husband syndrome") and eager to explain any injuries that the woman exhibits. *Introducing the subject of violence in the presence of the man who may be responsible for it places the woman in danger. Separating the woman from the man for the interview is absolutely essential.* It is also important that no other adults or children be present.

When a private, secure place has been found, the nurse can explain that many women experience abuse. For example, "Because abuse is very common and can affect the woman's health, it is the policy at this agency to ask all women about abusive situations." This lets the woman know that she is not being singled out for questioning. Screening questions often include:

- Have you been threatened, hit, slapped, kicked, choked, or otherwise physically hurt by anyone within the last year?

CRITICAL THINKING ❓ EXERCISE 24-1

Joan Piszarek, a 28-year-old primigravida, is admitted to the labor and delivery unit with contractions at 34 weeks' gestation. The right side of her face is swollen, old bruises that look like fingerprints are found on her upper arms, and a large bruised area is apparent on her abdomen. She is accompanied by her husband, who is very solicitous. He verbalizes concern about her labor status and remains close beside her at all times. Joan appears lethargic and avoids eye contact with the nurse who is admitting her. She states that she fainted at home and hurt herself when she fell against the bathtub. The nurse accepts the explanation and asks no further questions.

Questions
1. What assumptions has the nurse made?
2. What should make the nurse question whether the injuries resulted from falling?

At the change of shifts, Joan is assigned to a new nurse. The nurse waits for a time when Joan's husband is out of the room and she can be alone with Joan. The nurse asks, "Did you get these injuries from being hit?" Joan appears extremely anxious and says, "Don't say anything to him! He got so mad when I was late getting home from shopping. It was my fault."

Questions
3. Why did the nurse wait for time alone with Joan before asking questions?
4. How should the nurse respond? What bias must she guard against?
5. How can Joan be protected?

- Has this happened since you have been pregnant?
- Within the last year, has anyone forced you to have sexual activities?
- Are you ever afraid of anyone?

A "yes" answer should prompt questions about who hurt the woman and the frequency and kinds of abuse. If a woman has old or new signs that might be from abuse, ask questions such as "Did someone hurt you?" and "Did you receive these injuries from being hit?"

The abused woman often appears hesitant, embarrassed, or evasive. She may speak in a low tone of voice, be unable to look the nurse in the eye, and appear guilty, ashamed, jumpy, or frightened. Her affect may be flattened and inappropriate for the situation. Reassure the woman that her privacy will be protected and confidentiality will be absolute. Document all information in the chart.

Asking women about abuse frequently during the pregnancy and when they come for other health care is essential. Women often deny the abuse when first approached. The woman who is not ready to seek help when she is first asked may be ready at a later time, however.

Provide written information about abuse in areas such as restrooms, where it will not be seen by the partner. Pamphlets or cards listing general community resources including a few devoted to domestic violence may be acceptable for her to take with her. Laminate cards of phone numbers that can be hidden in a shoe may also be used. A small piece of paper with phone numbers can also be rolled and placed in an empty tampon container in her purse. The availability of such material signifies that health care professionals are interested and the woman can discuss her problems safely.

Evaluate and document all signs of injury, both past and present. This includes areas of welts, bruising, swelling, lacerations, burns, and scars. Injuries are most commonly noted on the face, breasts, abdomen, and genitalia. Many women have new or old fractures. These usually are fractures of the face, nose, ribs, or arms. A photograph or a drawing may be used to show areas of injury. These may be important for future legal action.

If sexual abuse has occurred, a gynecologic examination is necessary because trauma to the labia, vagina, cervix, or anus often is present. Types of forced sex may include vaginal intercourse, anal intercourse, and insertion of objects into the vagina and anus.

Be particularly alert for nonverbal cues that indicate that abuse has occurred. Facial grimacing or a slow, unsteady gait may indicate pain. Vomiting or abdominal tenderness may indicate internal injury. A flat affect (absence of facial response) is indicative of women who mentally withdraw from the situation to protect themselves from the horror and humiliation they experience during an abusive episode. Keep in mind that the woman may fear for her life because abusive episodes tend to escalate. Open-ended questions help prompt full disclosure and the expression of feelings. Record direct quotes of what the woman says about her experience.

Analysis

A variety of nursing diagnoses may be appropriate depending on the assessment data collected. The most meaningful diagnosis may be "Fear related to possibility of severe injury to self and/or children during unpredictable cycles of violence." (See Box 24-4.)

Planning

The abused woman may have difficulty developing a long-term plan of care without a great deal of specialized assistance. She often is unwilling to leave the abusive situation, and nurses must focus on working with the woman to plan short-term goals that will protect her from future injury.

For realistic, short-term goals and expected outcomes, the woman will:

- Acknowledge the physical assaults.
- Develop a specific plan of action to implement when the abusive cycle begins.
- Identify community resources that provide protection for her and her children.

CRITICAL TO REMEMBER

Cues Indicating Violence against Women

Nonverbal—Facial grimacing, slow and unsteady gait, vomiting, abdominal tenderness, absence of facial response

Injuries—Welts, bruises, swelling, lacerations, burns, vaginal or rectal bleeding; evidence of old or new fractures of the nose, face, ribs, or arms

Vague somatic complaints—Anxiety, depression, panic attacks, sleeplessness, anorexia

Discrepancy between history and type of injuries—Wounds that do not match woman's story; multiple bruises in various stages of healing; bruising on the arms (which she may have raised to protect herself); old, untreated wounds

---

BOX 24-4 Common Nursing Diagnoses for Families with Special Needs

Anxiety
Disturbed Body Image*
Chronic Sorrow
Decisional Conflict
Interrupted Family Processes
Fear*
Grieving*
Health-Seeking Behaviors
Impaired Social Interaction
Ineffective Coping
Ineffective Health Maintenance*
Powerlessness
Risk for Impaired Parenting*
Risk for Delayed Growth and Development
Risk for Injury*
Risk for Spiritual Distress
Situational Low Self-Esteem*

*Nursing diagnoses discussed in this chapter.

Interventions

DEVELOPING A PERSONAL SAFETY PLAN

Ask the woman what she does to decrease or avoid violence from her partner. Help her to find other options to add to those she has used.

Help the woman make concrete plans to protect her safety and the safety of her children. For example, if the woman insists on returning to the shared home, describe the cycle of behavior that culminates in physical abuse and instruct her in factors that precipitate a violent episode. Discuss the use of alcohol or other drugs and behaviors that indicate that the level of frustration and anger is increasing to the point where the danger is escalating.

Assist her to:

- Locate the nearest shelter or safe house and make specific plans to go there once the cycle of violence begins.
- Identify the safest, quickest routes out of the home.
- Hide extra keys to the car and house, money, personal information (social security numbers, birth certificates, drivers license, bank account numbers, insurance policy numbers), and personal necessities.
- Devise a code word, and prearrange with someone to call the police when the word is used.
- Memorize the telephone number of the shelter or hotline, because time often is a crucial element in the decision to leave. An easy number to remember is the one for the National Domestic Violence Hotline (1-800-799-SAFE), which provides immediate crisis intervention assistance in the caller's community.
- Review the safety plan frequently, because leaving the batterer is one of the most dangerous times.

AFFIRMING SHE IS NOT TO BLAME

The abused woman often believes that she is responsible for the abuse. Let her know that no one deserves to be hit for any reason. The one who hit her is the person responsible. She did not provoke it or cause it, and she could not have prevented it. Nurses often are responsible for teaching basic family processes such as:

- Violence is not normal.
- Violence usually is repeated and escalates.
- Battering is against the law.
- Battered women have alternatives.

She also needs nonjudgmental acceptance and recognition of the difficulties involved in making changes in her situation. Praise her for any actions she takes, even if they are only minor steps toward making her life safer. Reassure her that she is doing the right thing for herself and her children when she seeks help and makes plans for escape.

PROVIDING REFERRALS

When contact with the battered woman is short term, many interventions are outside the scope of nursing practice. Refer the family to community agencies such as the local police department, legal services, community shelters, counseling services, and social service agencies. Include mental health referrals, if necessary, for depression or counseling. Document that referrals were made and whether the woman accepted them.

It is essential to accept the decisions of the battered woman and acknowledge that she is on her own timetable. She may not contact the police, go to a shelter, or take any actions at the time they are recommended. Therefore listening to her, believing her, and providing information about resources may be the only help the nurse can provide until the woman is ready to do more.

Do not become negative or pass judgment on the partner of an abused woman. She often is tied to the man by both economic and emotional bonds and may become defensive if her partner is criticized. Tell her that resources are available for her partner but he must first admit abuse and seek assistance before help can be offered. To initiate referrals for the partner before he asks for help will increase the danger to the woman if her partner feels he has been betrayed.

Evaluation

The plan of care can be judged successful if the woman acknowledges the violent episodes in the home, makes concrete plans to protect herself and her children from future injury, and makes plans to use the community resources available to her.

✓ CHECK YOUR READING

26. What major cues indicate that a woman has been physically abused?
27. How can nurses intervene to help women protect their safety if they choose to remain in a home situation with a partner who physically abuses them?

SUMMARY CONCEPTS

- Teenage pregnancy is a major health problem in the United States. Adolescents need to receive accurate information about contraceptives and ways to set limits on sexual behavior.
- Adolescent pregnancy imposes serious physiologic risks that result in a higher incidence of complications for the mother and fetus. These include preeclampsia, anemia, insufficient or excessive weight gain, urinary tract infections, and depression for the mother and prematurity and low birth weight for the infant.
- Teenage pregnancy interrupts the developmental tasks of adolescence and may result in childbirth before the parents are capable of providing a nurturing home for the infant without a great deal of assistance.
- The mature primigravida often has financial and emotional resources that younger women do not have. She may experience anxiety, however, about recommended antepartum testing and her ability to parent effectively.
- Multidrug substance abuse is a widespread problem that can have devastating fetal and neonatal effects, which may persist and become long-term developmental problems for the child.

- The lifestyle associated with illicit drug abuse includes inadequate nutrition, inadequate prenatal care, and increased incidence of sexually transmissible diseases. It necessitates interdisciplinary interventions to prevent injury to the expectant mother and fetus.
- The birth of an infant with congenital anomalies produces strong emotions of shock and grief in the family. It calls for a sensitive response from the health care team to help the family grieve for the loss of the perfect or "fantasy" infant and form an attachment to the newborn.
- Pregnancy loss at any stage produces grief that must be acknowledged and expressed before it can be resolved. Nurses realize that mourning requires memories, and they intervene to arrange unlimited contact between the family and the stillborn infant and gather a memento packet for the family.
- Nursing care for the mother who is placing her infant for adoption is based on the knowledge that relinquishment (adoption) is an act of love, not abandonment.
- Multiple factors are associated with violence against women, which is deliberate, severe, and generally repeated in a predictable cycle that often causes severe physical harm (or death) to the woman.
- All perinatal nurses come into contact with abused women who require assistance to protect themselves and their children from serious injury.

ANSWERS TO CRITICAL THINKING EXERCISE 24-1, p. 616

1. The nurse may have assumed that the husband's behavior indicated concern for his wife. Instead, it may have been a manifestation of "hovering husband syndrome," which occurs in the honeymoon phase of the cycle of violence.
2. Facial injury, signs of previous bruising that resemble "grab marks," and abdominal bruising. Joan's story of falling and hurting herself is not congruent with the location of abdominal injury and injuries on her arms. Joan's lethargy and avoidance of eye contact also suggest that she is afraid.
3. The nurse should not question Joan's explanation of the injury in the presence of the husband, because this can increase the danger of escalating violence when the mother and infant are discharged.
4. The nurse should respond, "No one deserves to be hurt; it's not your fault. There are resources to help you." Nurses must examine their own thinking to be certain that they do not accept a common bias that physical abuse is deserved by the victim.
5. Joan needs information about protecting herself and the coming infant from future harm. This is not, however, the appropriate time to give her this information. The nurse must inform the physician and the postpartum staff of the problem, and she must make the necessary referrals to the hospital's social service department for follow-up.

REFERENCES & READINGS

Alan Guttmacher Institute. (2003). *Facts in brief: Teenagers' sexual and reproductive health.* Retrieved January 5, 2005, from http://agi-usa.org/pubs/fb_teens.html.

Alexander, K.V. (2001). "The one thing you can never take away": Perinatal bereavement photographs. *MCN: American Journal of Maternal/Child Nursing, 26*(3), 123-127.

American Academy of Pediatrics. (2001). Care of adolescent parents and their children. *Pediatrics, 107*(2), 429-434.

American Academy of Pediatrics, Committee on Substance Abuse & Committee on Children with Disabilities. (2000). Fetal alcohol syndrome and alcohol-related neurodevelopmental disorders. *Pediatrics, 106*(2), 358-361.

American Academy of Pediatrics & American College of Obstetricians and Gynecologists. (2002). *Guidelines for perinatal care* (5th ed.). Washington, DC: Author.

Anderson, C. (2002). Battered and pregnant: A nursing challenge. *MCN: American Journal of Maternal/Child Nursing, 6*(2), 95-99.

Andres, R.L. (2004). Effects of therapeutic, diagnostic, and environmental agents and exposure to social and illicit drugs. In R.K. Creasy & R. Resnik (Eds.), *Maternal-fetal medicine: Principles and practice* (5th ed., pp. 281-314). Philadelphia: Saunders.

Armstrong, D.S. (2004). Impact of prior perinatal loss on subsequent pregnancies. *Journal of Obstetric, Gynecologic, and Neonatal Nursing, 33*(6), 765-773.

Askin, D.F., & Diel-Jones, B. (2001). Cocaine: Effects of in utero exposure on the fetus and neonate. *Journal of Perinatal and Neonatal Nursing, 14*(4), 83-102.

Breedlove, G.K., & Schorfheide, A.M. (2001). *Adolescent pregnancy* (2nd ed.) White Plains, NY: March of Dimes Birth Defects Foundation.

Capitulo, K.L. (2004). Perinatal grief online. *MCN: American Journal of Maternal/Child Nursing, 29*(5), 305-311.

Centers for Disease Control and Prevention. (2003). *Costs of intimate partner violence against women in the United States.* Retrieved January 10, 2005, from http://www.cdc.gov/ncipc/pub-res/ipv_cost/03_incidence.htm.

Centers for Disease Control and Prevention. (2004a). *Intimate partner violence: Fact sheet.* Retrieved January 10, 2005, from http://www.cdc.gov/ncipc/factsheets/ipvfacts.htm.

Centers for Disease Control and Prevention. (2004b). *Preventing alcohol-exposed pregnancies.* Retrieved January 8, 2005, from http://www.cdc.gov/ncbddd/fas/fasprev.htm.

Clemmens, D. (2001). The relationship between social support and adolescent mothers' interactions with their infants: a meta-analysis. *Journal of Obstetric, Gynecologic, and Neonatal Nursing, 30*(4), 410-420.

Clemmens, D. (2003). Adolescent motherhood: A metasynthesis of qualitative studies. *MCN: American Journal of Maternal/Child Nursing, 28*(2), 93-99.

Cocey, C.D. (2004). Screening for violence in pregnancy. *AWHONN Lifelines, 7*(6), 495-497.

Cote-Arsenault, D. (2003). The influence of perinatal loss on anxiety in multigravidas. *Journal of Obstetric, Gynecologic, and Neonatal Nursing, 32*(5), 623-629.

Cunningham, F.G., Leveno, K.J., Bloom, S.L., Hauth, J.C., Gilstrap, L.C., & Wenstrom, K.D. (2005). *Williams obstetrics* (22nd ed.). New York: McGraw-Hill.

Davis, A.H. (2003). Pediatric and adolescent gynecology. In J.R. Scott, R.S. Gibbs, B.Y. Karlan, & A.F. Haney (Eds.), *Danforth's obstetrics and gynecology* (9th ed., pp. 529-540). Philadelphia: Lippincott Williams & Wilkins.

Delaney-Black, V., Covington, C.Y., Dhar, S., & Sokol, R.J. (2000). Illicit substance abuse during pregnancy. In S.B. Ransom, M.P. Dombrowski, S.G. McNeeley, K.S. Moghissi, & A.R. Munkarah (Eds.), *Practical strategies in obstetrics and gynecology* (pp. 390-402). Philadelphia: Saunders.

Dunn, L.L., & Oths, K.S. (2004). Prenatal predictors of intimate partner abuse. *Journal of Obstetric, Gynecologic, and Neonatal Nursing, 33*(1), 54-63.

deLisser, R., & Trimmer, T. (2001). Teen talk: An intervention for pregnant and parenting adolescents. *AWHONN Lifelines, 5*(4), 36-41.

de Mendoza, V.B. (2001). Culturally appropriate care for pregnant Latina women who are victims of domestic violence. *Journal of Obstetric, Gynecologic, and Neonatal Nursing, 30*(6), 579-588.

Easterwook, B. (2004). Silent lullabies: Helping parents cope with early pregnancy loss. *AWHONN Lifelines, 8*(4), 356-360.

El-Bassel, N., Gilbert, L., Witte, S., Wu, E., Gaeta, T., Schilling, R., & Wada, T. (2003). Intimate partner violence and substance abuse among minority women receiving care from an inner-city emergency department. *Women's Health Issues, 13*(1), 16-22.

Eustace, L.W., Kang, D., & Coombs, D. (2003). Fetal alcohol syndrome: A growing concern for health care professionals. *Journal of Obstetric, Gynecologic, and Neonatal Nursing, 32*(2), 215-221.

Fike, D.L. (2003). Assessment and management of the substance-exposed newborn and infant. In C. Kenner & J.W. Lott (Eds.), *Comprehensive neonatal nursing: A physiologic perspective* (3rd ed., pp. 773-802). Philadelphia: Saunders.

Gardner, S.L., Hauser, P., & Merenstein, G.B. (2002). Grief and perinatal loss. In G.B. Merenstein & S.L. Gardner (Eds.), *Handbook of neonatal intensive care* (5th ed., pp. 754-786). St. Louis: Mosby.

Gazmararian, J.A., Petersen, R., Spitz, A.M., Goodwin, M.M., Salzman, L.E., & Marks, J.S. (2000). Violence and reproductive health: Current knowledge and future research. *Maternal and Child Health Journal, 4*(2), 79-84.

Gemma, P.B., & Arnold, J. (2002). *Loss and grieving in pregnancy and the first year of life: A caring resource for nurses.* White Plains, NY: March of Dimes Birth Defects Foundation.

Gileber, E. (2004). Labor and delivery at risk. In S. Mattson & J.E. Smith (Eds.), *Core curriculum for maternal newborn nursing* (3rd ed., pp. 818-849). Philadelphia: Saunders.

Greene, C.M., & Goodman, M.H. (2003). Neonatal abstinence syndrome: Strategies for care of the drug-exposed infant. *Neonatal Network, 22*(4), 15-25.

Haggerty, L.A., & Goodman, L.A. (2003). Stages of change-based nursing interventions for victims of interpersonal violence. *Journal of Obstetric, Gynecologic, & Neonatal Nursing 32*(1), 68-75.

Hamilton, B.E., Martin, J.A., & Sutton, P.D. (2004). Births: Preliminary data for 2003. *National Vital Statistics Reports, 53*(9). Hyattsville, MD: National Center for Health Statistics.

Hancock, E.G., Calhoun, B.C., & Hume, R.F. (2002). Adolescent pregnancy: Improving outcomes through focused multidisciplinary obstetric care. In S.B. Ransom, M.P. Dombrowski, M.I. Evans, & K.A. Ginsburg (Eds.), *Contemporary therapy in obstetrics and gynecology* (pp. 152-155). Philadelphia: Saunders.

Heinonen, S., & Kirkinen, P. (2000). Pregnancy outcome after previous stillbirth resulting from causes other than maternal conditions and fetal abnormalities. *Birth, 27*(1), 33-37.

Higgins, L.P., & Hawkins, J.W. (2005). Screening for abuse during pregnancy: Implementing a multisite program. *MCN: The American Journal of Maternal/Child Nursing, 30*(2), 109-114.

Jansen, J.L. (2003). A bereavement model for the intensive care nursery. *Neonatal Network, 22*(3), 17-23.

Kavanaugh, K., & Wheeler, S.R. (2003). When a baby dies: Caring for bereaved families. In C. Kenner, J.W. Lott, & A.A. Flandermeyer (Eds.), *Comprehensive neonatal nursing: A physiologic perspective* (3rd ed., pp. 108-126). Philadelphia: Saunders.

Kelly, P.J., & Morgan-Kidd, J. (2001). Social influences on the sexual behaviors of adolescent girls in at-risk circumstances. *Journal of Obstetric, Gynecologic, and Neonatal Nursing, 30*(5), 481-489.

Kenner, C. (2004). Families in crisis. In M.T. Verklan & M. Walden (Eds.), *Core curriculum for neonatal intensive care nursing* (3rd ed., pp. 392-409). Philadelphia: Saunders.

Koniak-Griffin, D., Anderson, N.L.R., Verzemnieks, I., & Brecht, M. (2003). A public health nursing early intervention program for adolescent mothers: Outcomes from pregnancy through 6 weeks postpartum. *Nursing Research, 49*(3), 130-138.

Koniak-Griffin, D., & Turner-Pluta, C. (2001). Health risks and psychosocial outcomes of early childbearing: A review of the literature. *Journal of Perinatal and Neonatal Nursing 15*(2), 1-17.

Kowalski, K. (2001). Perinatal loss and bereavement. In K.R. Simpson & P.A. Creehan (Eds.), *Perinatal nursing* (pp. 476-491). Philadelphia: Lippincott Williams & Wilkins.

Lemmey, D., McFarlane, J., Wilson, P., & Malecha, A. (2001). Intimate partner violence: Mothers' perspectives of effects on their children. *MCN: American Journal of Maternal/Child Nursing, 26*(2), 98-103.

Lipsky, S., Holt, V.L., Easterling, T.R., & Critchlow, C.W. (2003). Impact of police-reported intimate partner violence during pregnancy on birth outcomes. *Obstetrics & Gynecology, 102*(3), 557-564.

Marcellus, L. (2002). Care of substance-exposed infants: The current state of practice in Canadian hospitals. *Journal of Perinatal and Neonatal Nursing, 16*(3), 51-68.

March of Dimes Birth Defects Foundation. (2005). *Pregnancy after 35.* Retrieved January 7, 2005, from http://www.marchofdimes.com.

Martin, J.A., Hamilton, B.E., Sutton, P.D., Ventura, S.J., Menacker, F., & Munson, M.L. (2003). Births: Final data for 2002. *National Vital Statistics Reports, 52*(10). Hyattsville, MD: National Center for Health Statistics.

Mattson, S. (2004). Intimate partner violence. In S. Mattson & J.E. Smith (Eds.), *Core curriculum for maternal-newborn nursing* (3rd ed., pp. 537-553). Philadelphia: Saunders.

McComish, F.F., Greenberg, R., & Shewmaker, K. (2002). Contemporary options in substance abuse treatment for women. In S.B. Ransom, M.P. Dombrowski, M.I. Evans, & K.A. Ginsburg (Eds.), *Contemporary therapy in obstetrics and gynecology* (pp. 387-395). Philadelphia: Saunders.

McFarlane, J., Parker, B., & Cross, B. (2001). *Abuse during pregnancy: A protocol for prevention and interventions* (2nd ed.). White Plains, NY: March of Dimes Birth Defects Foundation.

Montgomery, K.S. (2003a). Health promotion for pregnant adolescents. *AWHONN Lifelines, 7*(5), 432-444.

Montgomery, K.S. (2003b). Nursing care for pregnant adolescents. *Journal of Obstetric, Gynecologic, and Neonatal Nursing, 32*(2), 249-257.

Moran, B.A. (2004). Substance abuse in pregnancy. In S. Mattson & J.E. Smith (Eds.), *Core curriculum for maternal-newborn nursing* (3rd ed., pp. 750-770). Philadelphia: Saunders.

Neuman, M., & Graf, C. (2003). Pregnant after age 35: Are these women at high risk? *AWHONN Lifelines, 7*(5), 422-430.

Peterson, R., Gazmararian, J., & Clark, K.A. (2001). Partner violence: Implications for health and community settings. *Women's Health Issues, 11*(2), 116-125.

Phipps, M.G., Blume, J.D., & DeMonner, S.M. (2002). Young maternal age associated with increased risk of neonatal death. *Obstetrics & Gynecology, 100*(3), 481-486.

Pitts, K. (2004). Perinatal substance abuse. In M.T. Verklan & M. Walden (Eds.), *Core curriculum for neonatal intensive care nursing* (3rd ed., pp. 46-79). Philadelphia: Saunders.

Plichta, S.B., & Falik, M. (2001). Prevalence of violence and implications for women's health. *Women's Health Issues, 11*(3), 244-258.

Primeau, M.R., & Lamb, J.M. (1995). When a baby dies: Rights of the baby and parents. *Journal of Obstetric, Gynecologic, and Neonatal Nursing, 24*(3), 206-208.

Renker, P.R. (2002). "Keep a blank face. I need to tell you what has been happening to me." *MCN: American Journal of Maternal/Child Nursing, 27*(2), 109-116.

Renker, P.R. (2003). Keeping safe: Teenagers' strategies for dealing with perinatal violence. *Journal of Obstetric, Gynecologic, and Neonatal Nursing, 32*(1), 58-6788.

Rentschler, D.D. (2003). Pregnant adolescents' perspectives of pregnancy. *MCN: American Journal of Maternal/Child Nursing, 28*(6), 377-383.

Rickert, V.I., Sanghvi, R., & Wiemann, C.M. (2002). Is lack of sexual assertiveness among adolescent and young adult women a cause for concern? *Perspectives on Sexual and Reproductive Health, 34*(4), 178-183.

Rillstone, P., & Hutchinson, S.A. (2001). Managing the reemergence of anguish: Pregnancy after a loss due to anomalies. *Journal of Obstetric, Gynecologic, and Neonatal Nursing, 30*(3), 291-298.

Samuelsson, M., Radestad, I., & Segesten, K. (2001). A waste of life: Fathers' experience of losing a child before birth. *Birth, 28*(2), 124-130.

Savage, C., Wray, J., Ritchey, P.N., Sommers, M., Dyehouse, J., & Fulmer, M. (2003). Current screening instruments related to alcohol consumption in pregnancy and a proposed alternative method. *Journal of Obstetric, Gynecologic, and Neonatal Nursing, 32*(4), 437-446.

Seimer, B.S. (2004). Intimate violence in adolescent relationships. *MCN: American Journal of Maternal/Child Nursing, 29*(2), 117-121.

Shuzman, E. (2003). Facing stillbirth or neonatal death: Providing culturally appropriate care for Jewish families. *AWHONN Lifelines, 7*(6), 537-543.

Simpson, K.R., & James, D.C. (2005). *Postpartum Care.* White Plains, NY: March of Dimes Birth Defects Foundation.

Smith, J.E. (2004). Age-related concerns. In S. Mattson & J.E. Smith (Eds.), *Core curriculum for maternal-newborn nursing* (3rd ed., pp. 147-160). Philadelphia: Saunders.

Tillett, J., & Osborne, K. (2001). Substance abuse by pregnant women: Legal and ethical concerns. *Journal of Perinatal and Neonatal Nursing, 14*(4), 1-11.

Tjaden, P., & Thoennes, N. (2000). *Full report of the prevalence, incidence, and consequences of violence against women: Findings from the National Violence Against Women Survey, research report.* Washington, DC: National Institute of Justice & Centers for Disease Control and Prevention.

Toohey, J.S. (2000). Battered women. In E.J. Quilligan & F.P. Zuspan (Eds.), *Current therapy in obstetrics and gynecology* (5th ed., pp. 453-456). Philadelphia: Saunders.

Upham, M., & Medoff-Cooper, B. (2004). What are the responses and needs of mothers of infants diagnosed with congenital heart disease? *MCN: American Journal of Maternal/Child Nursing, 30*(1), 24-29.

U.S. Department of Health and Human Services. (2000). *Healthy People 2010* (Conference ed). Washington, DC: Author.

Van, P., & Meleis, A.I. (2003). Coping after grief after involuntary pregnancy loss: Perspectives of African American women. *Journal of Obstetric, Gynecologic, and Neonatal Nursing, 32*(1), 28-39.

Viau, P.A., Padula, C.A., & Eddy, B. (2002). An exploration of health concerns and health-promotion behaviors in pregnant women over age 35. *MCN: American Journal of Maternal/Child Nursing, 27*(6), 328-334.

Watts, N. (2004). Screening for domestic violence: A team approach for maternal/newborn nurses. *AWHONN Lifelines, 8*(3), 211-219.

Winn, N., Records, K., & Rice, M. (2003). The relationship between abuse, sexually transmitted diseases, and group B Streptococcus. *MCN: American Journal of Maternal/Child Nursing, 28*(2), 106-110.

Complications of Pregnancy

DEFINITIONS

Abortion Pregnancy that ends before 20 weeks' gestation, either spontaneously or electively. *Miscarriage* is a lay term for a spontaneous abortion that is frequently used by professionals.

Abruptio Placentae Premature separation of a normally implanted placenta.

Antiphospholipid Antibodies Autoimmune antibodies that are directed against phospholipids in cell membranes. It is associated with recurrent spontaneous abortion, fetal loss, and severe preeclampsia.

Bicornuate (Bicornate) Uterus Malformed uterus having two horns.

Cerclage Encircling the cervix with suture to prevent recurrent spontaneous abortion caused by early cervical dilation.

Dilation and Curettage (D&C) Stretching the cervical os to permit suctioning or scraping of the walls of the uterus. The procedure is performed in abortion, to obtain samples of uterine lining tissue for laboratory examination, and during the postpartum period to remove retained fragments of placenta.

Dilation and Evacuation (D&E) Wide cervical dilation followed by mechanical destruction and removal of fetal parts from the uterus. After complete removal of the fetus, a vacuum curet is used to remove the placenta and remaining products of conception.

Eclampsia Form of hypertension of pregnancy complicated by generalized (grand mal) seizures.

Ectopic Pregnancy Implantation of a fertilized ovum in any area other than the uterus; the most common site is the fallopian tube.

Erythroblastosis Fetalis Agglutination and hemolysis of fetal erythrocytes resulting from incompatibility between maternal and fetal blood. In most cases the fetus is Rh-positive and the mother is Rh-negative.

Gestational Trophoblastic Disease Spectrum of diseases that includes both benign hydatidiform mole and gestational trophoblastic tumors, such as invasive moles and choriocarcinoma.

Hydatidiform Mole Abnormal pregnancy resulting from proliferation of chorionic villi that give rise to multiple cysts and rapid growth of the uterus.

Hypovolemic Shock Acute peripheral circulatory failure resulting from loss of circulating blood volume.

Kernicterus Staining of brain tissue caused by accumulation of unconjugated bilirubin in the brain. Bilirubin encephalopathy is the brain damage that results from these deposits.

Laparoscopy Insertion of an illuminated tube into the abdominal cavity to visualize contents, locate bleeding, and perform surgical procedures.

Linear Salpingostomy Incision along the length of a fallopian tube to remove an ectopic pregnancy and preserve the tube.

Maceration Discoloration and softening of tissues and eventual disintegration of a fetus that is retained in the uterus after its death.

Perinatologist Physician who specializes in the care of the mother, fetus, and infant during the perinatal period (from about the twentieth week of pregnancy to 4 weeks after childbirth).

Preeclampsia A hypertensive disorder of pregnancy characterized by hypertension and proteinuria.

Salpingectomy Surgical removal of a fallopian tube.

Vacuum Curettage (Vacuum Aspiration) Removal of the uterine contents by application of a vacuum through a hollow curet or cannula introduced into the uterus.

Vasoconstriction Narrowing of the lumen of blood vessels.

Although childbearing is a normal process, numerous maternal and fetal adaptations must occur in an orderly sequence. If problems develop in these physiologic processes, complications may arise that threaten the well-being of the expectant mother, the fetus, or both. A nurse-midwife or family physician may manage some mild conditions, or the woman may be referred to an obstetrician or a perinatologist for management of severe complications.

Nurses who work at a primary care site or perinatal center frequently fill the role of case manager or coordinator of services provided for the woman. Often the nurse is the only consistent provider involved in the woman's care and therefore is the person on whom the woman relies to guide her through the system.

Conditions that complicate pregnancy are divided into two broad categories: (1) those that are related to pregnancy and are not seen at other times and (2) those that could occur at any time but when they occur concurrently with pregnancy may complicate its course. Concurrent conditions that affect pregnancy are covered in Chapter 26.

The most common pregnancy-related complications are hemorrhagic conditions that occur in early pregnancy, hemorrhagic complications of the placenta in late pregnancy, hyperemesis gravidarum (HEG), hypertensive disorders of pregnancy, and blood incompatibilities.

HEMORRHAGIC CONDITIONS OF EARLY PREGNANCY

The three most common causes of hemorrhage during the first half of pregnancy are abortion, ectopic pregnancy, and gestational trophoblastic disease.

Abortion

Abortion is the loss of pregnancy before the fetus is viable, or capable of living outside the uterus. The medical consensus today is that a fetus of less than 20 weeks' gestation or one weighing less than 500 g is not viable. Ending of pregnancy before this time is considered an abortion. Abortion may be either spontaneous or induced. *Abortion* is an accepted medical term for either a spontaneous or induced ending of pregnancy, although the lay term *miscarriage* is becoming an accepted medical term to denote spontaneous abortion. Induced abortion is described in Chapter 33.

SPONTANEOUS ABORTION

Spontaneous abortion is a termination of pregnancy without action taken by the woman or another person.

INCIDENCE AND ETIOLOGY. Determining the exact incidence of spontaneous abortion is difficult because many unrecognized losses occur in early pregnancy, but it averages about 15% to 20% with any pregnancy. The incidence of spontaneous abortion increases with parental age. The incidence is 12% for women younger than 20 years, rising to 26% for women older than 40 years. Paternal age younger than 20 years is associated with a spontaneous abortion rate of 12%, rising to 20% for fathers older than 40 years. Most spontaneous abortions occur in the first 12 weeks of pregnancy, with the rate declining rapidly thereafter (Cunningham et al., 2001).

The most common cause of spontaneous abortion is severe congenital abnormalities that are often incompatible with life. Chromosomal abnormalities account for about 50% to 60% of early spontaneous abortions. Additional causes include maternal infections such as syphilis, listeriosis, toxoplasmosis, brucellosis, rubella, and cytomegalic inclusion disease. Intraabdominal infections also increase the risk. Maternal endocrine disorders such as hypothyroidism and abnormalities of the reproductive organs have also been implicated. Still other women who have repeated early pregnancy losses appear to have immunologic factors that play a role in their higher-than-expected spontaneous abortion incidence. Anatomic defects of the uterus or cervix may contribute to pregnancy loss at any gestational age (Branch & Scott, 2003; Cunningham et al., 2001).

Spontaneous abortion is divided into six subgroups: threatened, inevitable, incomplete, complete, missed, and recurrent. Figure 25-1 illustrates threatened, inevitable, and incomplete abortion.

THREATENED ABORTION

Clinical Manifestations. The first sign of threatened abortion is vaginal bleeding, which is rather common during early pregnancy. One third of pregnant women experi-

Threatened abortion

Inevitable abortion

Incomplete abortion

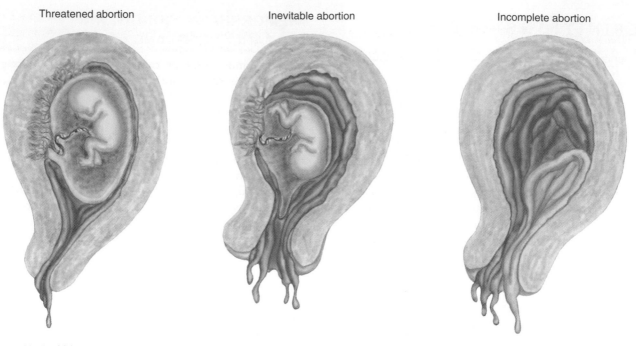

Vaginal bleeding occurs.

Membranes rupture and cervix dilates.

Some products of conception have been expelled, but some remain.

Figure 25-1 ■ Three types of spontaneous abortion, also called *miscarriage.*

ence "spotting" or bleeding in early pregnancy, and up to 50% of these pregnancies end in spontaneous abortion. Pregnancies complicated by early bleeding that do not end with a spontaneous abortion are more likely to have further complications during late pregnancy such as prematurity, a small-for-gestational age infant, abnormal presentation, or perinatal asphyxia (Branch & Scott, 2003; Cunningham, et al., 2001; Lu & Hobel, 2004).

Vaginal bleeding may be followed by rhythmic uterine cramping, persistent backache, or feelings of pelvic pressure. These symptoms increase the chance that the threatened abortion will progress to inevitable abortion.

Therapeutic Management. Bleeding during the first half of pregnancy should be considered a threatened abortion, and women must be advised to notify their physician or nurse-midwife if brownish or red vaginal bleeding is noted. When a woman reports bleeding in early pregnancy, the nurse obtains a detailed history that includes length of gestation (or first day of her last menstrual period) and the onset, duration, and amount of vaginal bleeding. Any accompanying discomfort, such as cramping, backache, or abdominal pain also is noted. Ultrasound examination helps to verify if the embryo or fetus is present and alive and the approximate gestational age. Determining if the woman's chorionic gonadotropin (β-hCG) levels are normal for the estimated gestational age provides added information about whether the pregnancy is likely to continue.

Vaginal ultrasound examination is performed to determine whether a fetus is present and, if so, whether it is alive. Maternal serum β-hCG and progesterone levels provide added information about the viability of the pregnancy.

No evidence exists to support physical activity restrictions to stop spontaneous abortion. The woman may be advised to limit sexual activity until bleeding has ceased. The woman is instructed to count the number of perineal pads used and to note the quantity and color of blood on the pads. She should also look for evidence of tissue passage, which would indicate progression beyond a threatened abortion.

Bleeding episodes are frightening, and psychological support is important. The woman often wonders whether her actions may have contributed to the situation and is anxious about her own condition and that of the fetus. The nurse should offer accurate information and avoid false reassurance, because the woman may lose her pregnancy despite every precaution.

INEVITABLE ABORTION

Clinical Manifestations. Abortion is usually inevitable (that is, it cannot be stopped) when membranes rupture and the cervix dilates. Rupture of membranes generally is experienced as a loss of fluid from the vagina and subsequent uterine contractions and active bleeding. If complete evacuation of the products of conception does not occur spontaneously, excessive bleeding or infection can occur.

Therapeutic Management. Natural expulsion of uterine contents is common in inevitable abortion. Vacuum curettage is used to clean out the uterus if the natural process is ineffective or incomplete. If the pregnancy is more advanced or if bleeding is excessive, a dilation and curettage (D&C) may be needed. Intravenous (IV) sedation or other anesthesia provides pain management for the procedure.

INCOMPLETE ABORTION

Clinical Manifestations. Incomplete abortion occurs when some but not all of the products of conception are expelled from the uterus. The major manifestations are active uterine bleeding and severe abdominal cramping. The cervix is open, and fetal and placental tissue is passed. The products of conception may have been expelled from the uterus but remain in the vagina because of their small size, often no larger than a ping-pong ball if the gestation is very early.

Therapeutic Management. The retained tissue prevents the uterus from contracting firmly, thereby allowing profuse bleeding from uterine blood vessels. Initial treatment should focus on stabilizing the woman cardiovascularly. A blood specimen is drawn for blood type and screen or cross-match, and an IV line is inserted for fluid replacement. When the woman's condition is stable, a D&C usually is performed to remove the remaining tissue. This procedure may be followed by IV administration of oxytocin (Pitocin) or intramuscular administration of methylergonovine (Methergine) to contract the uterus and control bleeding.

A D&C may not be performed if the pregnancy has advanced beyond 14 weeks because of the danger of excessive bleeding. In this case, oxytocin or prostaglandin is administered to stimulate uterine contractions until all products of conception (fetus, membranes, placenta, and amniotic fluid) are expelled.

COMPLETE ABORTION

Clinical Manifestations. Complete abortion occurs when all products of conception are expelled from the uterus. After passage of all products of conception, uterine contractions and bleeding subside and the cervix closes. The uterus feels smaller than the length of gestation would suggest. The symptoms of pregnancy are no longer present, and the pregnancy test becomes negative as hormone levels fall.

Therapeutic Management. Once complete abortion is confirmed, no additional intervention is required unless excessive bleeding or infection develops. The woman should be advised to rest and to watch for further bleeding, pain, or fever. She should not have intercourse until after a follow-up visit with her health care provider. Contraception is discussed at the follow-up visit if she wishes to prevent pregnancy.

MISSED ABORTION

Clinical Manifestations. Missed abortion occurs when the fetus dies during the first half of pregnancy but is retained in the uterus. When the fetus dies, the early symptoms of pregnancy (nausea, breast tenderness, urinary frequency) disappear. The uterus stops growing and decreases in size, reflecting the absorption of amniotic fluid and maceration of the fetus. Vaginal bleeding of a red or brownish color may or may not occur.

Therapeutic Management. An ultrasound examination confirms fetal death by identifying a gestational sac or fetus that is too small for the presumed gestational age. No fetal heart activity can be found. Pregnancy tests for hCG should show a decline in placental hormone production.

In most cases, the woman would expel the contents of the uterus spontaneously, but this is emotionally difficult once she knows her fetus is not living. Therefore her uterus usually is emptied by the most appropriate method for the size when the diagnosis of missed abortion is made. For a first-trimester missed abortion, a D&C can usually be done. If the missed abortion occurs during the second trimester, when the fetus is larger, a D&E may be done or vaginal prostaglandin E_2 (PGE_2) or misoprostol (Cytotec) may be needed to induce uterine contractions that expel the fetus.

Two major complications of missed abortion are infection and disseminated intravascular coagulation (DIC). If signs exist of uterine infection, such as elevation in temperature, vaginal discharge with a foul odor, or abdominal pain, evacuation of the uterus will be delayed until cultures are obtained and antimicrobial therapy is initiated.

RECURRENT SPONTANEOUS ABORTION

Clinical Manifestations. Recurrent spontaneous abortion usually is defined as three or more spontaneous abortions, although some authorities now use two or more pregnancy losses as the definition. The primary causes of recurrent abortion are believed to be genetic or chromosomal abnormalities and anomalies of the reproductive tract, such as bicornuate uterus or incompetent cervix. Additional causes include an inadequate luteal phase with insufficient secretion of progesterone and immunologic factors that involve increased sharing of human leukocyte antigens by the sperm and ovum of the man and woman who conceived. The theory is that because of this sharing the woman's immunologic system is not stimulated to produce blocking antibodies that protect the embryo from maternal immune cells or other damaging antibodies. Systemic diseases such as lupus erythematosus and diabetes mellitus have been implicated in recurrent abortions. Reproductive infections and some sexually transmitted diseases are also associated with recurrent abortions.

Therapeutic Management. The first step in management of recurrent spontaneous abortion is a thorough examination of the reproductive system to determine whether anatomic defects are the cause. If the cervix and uterus are normal, the woman and her partner are usually referred for genetic screening to identify chromosomal factors that would increase the possibility of recurrent abortions.

Additional therapeutic management of recurrent pregnancy loss depends on the cause. For instance, treatment may involve assisting the woman to develop a regimen to maintain normal blood glucose if diabetes mellitus is a factor. Supplemental hormones may be given if her progesterone or other hormone levels are lower than normal. Additional therapeutic management of recurrent pregnancy loss depends on the cause. For example, antimicrobials are prescribed for the woman with infection, or hormone-related drugs may be prescribed if imbalance preventing normal fetal implantation and support is found.

Recurrent spontaneous abortion may be caused by cervical incompetence, an anatomic defect that results in painless dilation of the cervix in the second trimester. In this situation the cervix may be sutured to keep it from opening in a cerclage procedure. The cerclage is most likely to be successful if done before much cervical dilation or bulging of the membranes through the cervix has occurred. Sutures may be removed near term in preparation for vaginal delivery, or they may be left in place if a cesarean birth is planned. Prophylactic antimicrobials are ordered if the woman is at increased risk for infection.

Rh immune globulin (RhoGAM) is given to the unsensitized $Rh_o(D)$-negative woman to prevent development of anti-Rh antibodies (see p. 654). A microdose (50 mcg) is given to the woman whose fetus is less than 13 weeks' gestational age at the time of the abortion.

NURSING CONSIDERATIONS. Nurses must consider the psychological needs of the woman experiencing spontaneous abortion. Vaginal bleeding is frightening, and waiting and watching are often difficult (although possibly the only treatment recommended). Many women and their families feel an acute sense of loss and grief with spontaneous abortion. Grief often includes feelings of guilt and speculation about whether the woman could have done something to prevent the loss. Nurses may help by emphasizing that abortions usually occur as the result of factors or abnormalities that could not be avoided.

Anger, disappointment, and sadness are commonly experienced emotions, although the intensity of the feelings may vary. For many people the fetus has not yet taken on specific physical characteristics, but they grieve for their fantasies of the unseen, unborn child. The couple may want to express their feelings of sadness but may feel that family, friends, and often health personnel are uncomfortable or unable to provide emotional support after early pregnancy loss.

Recognizing the meaning of the loss to each woman and her significant others is important. Nurses must listen carefully to what the woman says and observe how she behaves. Nurses must convey acceptance of the feelings expressed or demonstrated. A couple should remain together as much as possible. Providing information and simple brief explanations of what has occurred and what will be done facilitates the family's ability to grieve.

The family should realize that grief may last from 6 months to a year, or even longer. Family support, knowledge of the grief process, spiritual counselors, and the support of other bereaved couples may provide needed assistance during this time. Chapter 24 provides additional information about pregnancy loss and grief.

DISSEMINATED INTRAVASCULAR COAGULATION

DIC, also called *consumptive coagulopathy*, is a life-threatening defect in coagulation that may occur with several complications of pregnancy. DIC is not limited to obstetric conditions. While anticoagulation is occurring, inappropriate coagulation also is occurring in the microcirculation. The second result of DIC is that tiny clots form in the tiny blood vessels, blocking blood flow to the organs and causing ischemia.

Something in one of these disease processes initiates clotting mechanisms inappropriately. The first result is a con-

sumption of plasma factors including platelets, fibrinogen, prothrombin, factor V, and factor VIII. When these plasma factors are consumed, the circulating blood is then deficient in clotting factors and unable to clot. Fibrin degradation products accumulate and further interfere with coagulation.

Diseases that cause DIC fall into three major groups:

- Infusion of tissue thromboplastin into the circulation, which consumes, or "uses up," other clotting factors such as fibrinogen and platelets. Abruptio placentae and prolonged retention of a dead fetus cause this because the placenta is a rich source of thromboplastin.
- Conditions characterized by endothelial damage. Severe preeclampsia and the HELLP syndrome (p. 653) are characterized by endothelial damage.
- Nonspecific effects of some diseases. Diseases such as maternal sepsis or amniotic fluid embolism (see Chapter 27) are in this category.

DIC allows excess bleeding to occur from any vulnerable area, such as IV sites, incisions, or the gums or nose, and from expected sites such as the site of placental attachment during the postpartum period.

Laboratory studies help establish a diagnosis. Fibrinogen and platelets usually are decreased, prothrombin time (PT) and activated partial thromboplastin time (aPTT) may be prolonged, and fibrin degradation products, the most sensitive measurement, are increased. A newer test, the D-dimer study, which normally has negative results, confirms fibrin split products (FSP) and is presumptive for DIC when results are positive.

The priority in treatment of DIC is to correct the cause. In the case of a missed abortion, delivery of the fetus and placenta ends production of thromboplastin, which is fueling the process. Blood replacement products, such as whole blood, packed red blood cells, and cryoprecipitate, are administered as needed to maintain the circulating volume and to transport oxygen to body cells.

NURSING CONSIDERATIONS

When caring for a woman who has any of the disorders that increase her risk for having DIC, the nurse should observe for bleeding from unexpected sites. Sites for IV insertion or lab work, nosebleeds, or spontaneous bruising may be early indicators of DIC and should be reported. Also, if her coagulation studies are severely abnormal, an epidural block may be contraindicated because of possible bleeding into the spinal canal, so other types of labor pain management should be anticipated.

✓ CHECK YOUR READING

1. What are the signs of threatened abortion, and how do they differ from those of inevitable abortion?
2. What are the major causes of recurrent spontaneous abortion?
3. How can nurses intervene for the grief families experience as a result of early pregnancy loss?
4. What is DIC?

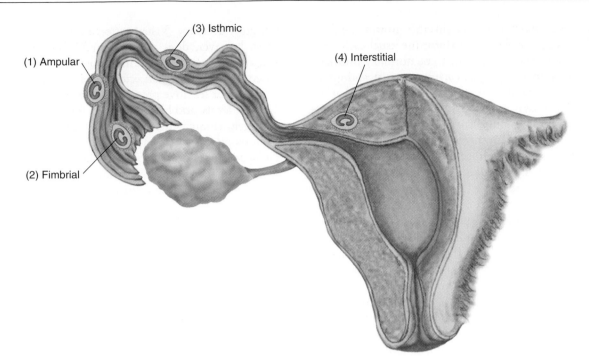

Figure 25-2 ■ Sites of tubal ectopic pregnancy. Numbers indicate the order of prevalence.

Ectopic Pregnancy

Ectopic pregnancy is an implantation of a fertilized ovum in an area outside the uterine cavity. Although implantation can occur in the abdomen or cervix, more than 98% of ectopic pregnancies are in the fallopian tube (Heard & Buster, 2003). Figure 25-2 illustrates common sites of ectopic implantation.

Ectopic pregnancy has been called "a disaster of reproduction" for two reasons:

- It remains a significant cause of maternal death from hemorrhage.
- It reduces the woman's chance of subsequent pregnancies because of damage or destruction of a fallopian tube.

INCIDENCE AND ETIOLOGY

Ectopic pregnancies have increased in the United States since 1970 from a rate of 4.5 per 1000 pregnancies to 19.7 per 1000 pregnancies. The increase in incidence is attributed to the growing number of women of childbearing age who experience scarring of the fallopian tubes because of pelvic infection, inflammation, or surgery. Additionally, sensitive tests that identify pregnancy earlier and transvaginal ultrasound allow diagnosis of some pregnancies within the fallopian tube that previously might have resolved spontaneously before diagnosis (Heard & Buster, 2003).

Pelvic infection often is caused by *Chlamydia* or *Neisseria gonorrhoeae*. A failed tubal ligation, even if undergone many years before, and a history of previous ectopic pregnancy also increase the risk for an ectopic pregnancy that implants in the fallopian tube. Greater incidences of ectopic pregnancies occur in women who conceived with assisted reproduction, most likely related to the tubal factors

that contributed to infertility. Contraception such as intrauterine contraceptive devices or low-dose progesterone agents is associated with increased risk of ectopic pregnancy (Cunningham et al., 2001; Heard & Buster, 2003).

Additional causes of ectopic pregnancy are delayed or premature ovulation, with the tendency of the fertilized ovum to implant before arrival in the uterus, and altered tubal motility in response to changes in estrogen and progesterone levels. Multiple induced abortions increase the risk for tubal pregnancy, possibly because of salpingitis (infection of the fallopian tube) that has occurred after induced abortion (Box 25-1). Regardless of the cause of tubal pregnancy, the effect is that transport of the fertilized ovum through the fallopian tube is hampered.

CLINICAL MANIFESTATIONS

The classic signs of ectopic pregnancy include the following:

- Missed menstrual period
- Abdominal pain
- Vaginal "spotting"

More subtle signs and symptoms depend on the site of implantation. If implantation occurs in the distal end of the

---

BOX 25-1 Risk Factors for Ectopic Pregnancy

History of sexually transmitted diseases (gonorrhea, chlamydial infection)
History of pelvic inflammatory disease
History of previous ectopic pregnancies
Failed tubal ligation
Intrauterine device
Multiple induced abortions
Maternal age older than 35 years
Some assisted reproductive techniques such as gamete intrafallopian transfer (GIFT)

fallopian tube, which can contain the growing embryo longer, the woman may at first exhibit the usual early signs of pregnancy and consider herself to be normally pregnant. Several weeks into the pregnancy, intermittent abdominal pain and small amounts of vaginal bleeding occur that initially could be mistaken for threatened abortion. Because routine ultrasound examination in early pregnancy is common, however, it is not unusual to diagnose an ectopic pregnancy before onset of symptoms.

If implantation has occurred in the proximal end of the fallopian tube, rupture of the tube may occur within 2 to 3 weeks of the missed period because the tube is narrow in this area. Symptoms include sudden, severe pain in one of the lower quadrants of the abdomen as the tube tears open and the embryo is expelled into the pelvic cavity, often with profuse hemorrhage. Radiating pain under the scapula may indicate bleeding into the abdomen caused by phrenic nerve irritation. Hypovolemic shock is a major concern because systemic signs of shock may be rapid and extensive without external bleeding.

DIAGNOSIS

The combined use of transvaginal ultrasound examination (see Chapter 10) and determination of the beta subunit of human chorionic gonadotropin (β-hCG) are helpful in early detection of ectopic pregnancy. An abnormal pregnancy is suspected if hCG is present but at lower levels than expected. If a gestational sac cannot be visualized when hCG is present, a diagnosis of ectopic pregnancy may be made

with great accuracy. Visualization of an intrauterine pregnancy, however, does not absolutely rule out an ectopic pregnancy. A woman may have an intrauterine pregnancy and concurrently have an ectopic pregnancy.

The use of sensitive pregnancy tests, maternal serum progesterone levels, and high-resolution transvaginal ultrasound has largely eliminated invasive tests for ectopic pregnancy. Laparoscopy (examination of the peritoneal cavity by means of a laparoscope) occasionally may be necessary to diagnose rupture of an ectopic pregnancy. A characteristic bluish swelling within the tube is the most common finding.

THERAPEUTIC MANAGEMENT

Management of tubal pregnancy depends on whether the tube is intact or ruptured. Medical management may be possible if the tube is unruptured. The goal of medical management is to preserve the tube and improve the chance of future fertility. The chemotherapeutic agent methotrexate (a folic acid antagonist) is used to inhibit cell division in the developing embryo.

Surgical management of a tubal pregnancy that is unruptured may involve a linear salpingostomy to salvage the tube (Figure 25-3). Linear salpingostomy also may be attempted if the tube is ruptured but damage to the tube is minimal. Salvaging the tube is particularly important to women concerned about future fertility.

When ectopic pregnancy results in rupture of the fallopian tube, the goal of therapeutic management is to control the bleeding and prevent hypovolemic shock. When the

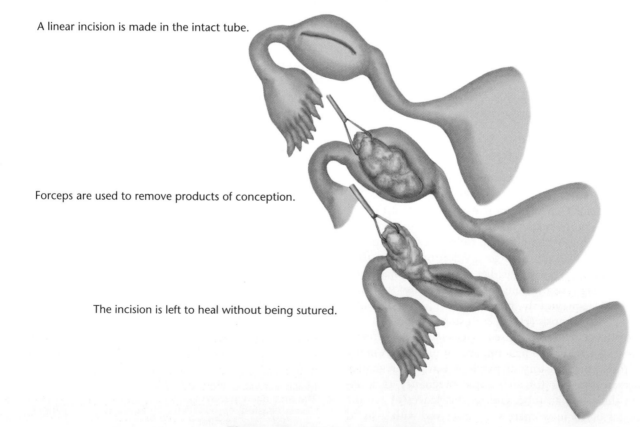

A linear incision is made in the intact tube.

Forceps are used to remove products of conception.

The incision is left to heal without being sutured.

Figure 25-3 ■ Linear salpingostomy.

woman's cardiovascular status is stable, removal of the tube (salpingectomy) with ligation of bleeding vessels may be required. With early diagnosis and medical management, salpingectomy has become uncommon in the treatment of ectopic pregnancy.

Rh immune globulin is given to appropriate Rh$_o$(D)-negative women.

NURSING CONSIDERATIONS

Nursing care focuses on prevention or early identification of hypovolemic shock, pain control, and psychological support for the woman who experiences ectopic pregnancy. Nurses monitor the woman for decreasing hematocrit levels and pain that would indicate a ruptured ectopic pregnancy. Nurses administer analgesics and evaluate their effectiveness so that pain can be controlled.

If methotrexate is used, the nurse must explain adverse side effects, such as nausea and vomiting, and the importance of communicating to the health care team any physical changes. Transient abdominal pain during methotrexate therapy occurs, probably because of expulsion of the products of conception from the tube (Heard & Buster, 2003). The woman must also be instructed to refrain from drinking alcohol, which decreases effectiveness, ingesting vitamins that contain folic acid, and having sexual intercourse until hCG is not detectable. If the treatment is successful, this hormone disappears from plasma within 2 to 4 weeks. Maintaining follow-up appointments is essential to identify whether the hCG titer becomes negative and remains negative. Continued presence of hCG in the serum requires follow-up to identify whether the ectopic pregnancy is still present (Cunningham et al., 2001)

The woman and her family will need psychological support to resolve intense emotions that may include anger, grief, guilt, and self-blame. The woman also may be anxious about her ability to become pregnant in the future. Because ectopic pregnancy may occur when a woman had an assisted reproductive technique, she may be more anxious about when she might become pregnant again and if similar risks exist for another pregnancy. The nurses should clarify the physician's explanation and use therapeutic communication techniques that assist the woman to deal with her anxiety.

Gestational Trophoblastic Disease (Hydatidiform Mole)

Hydatidiform mole is one form of gestational trophoblastic disease that occurs when the trophoblasts (peripheral cells that attach the fertilized ovum to the uterine wall) develop abnormally. As a result of the abnormal growth, the placenta, but not the fetal part of the pregnancy, develops. The condition is characterized by proliferation and edema of the chorionic villi. The fluid-filled villi form grapelike clusters of tissue that can rapidly grow large enough to fill the uterus to the size of an advanced pregnancy (Figure 25-4). The mole may be complete with no fetus present, or partial, in which fetal tissue or membranes are present.

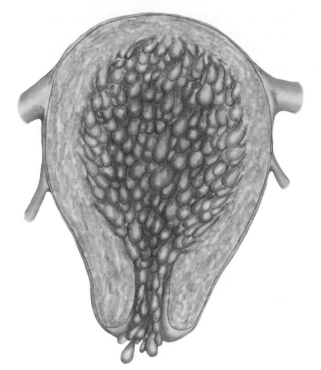

Figure 25-4 ■ Gestational trophoblastic disease, also called *hydatidiform mole.*

INCIDENCE AND ETIOLOGY

In the United States and Europe, the incidence of hydatidiform mole is 1 in every 1500 to 2000 pregnancies. The rate is higher in Asian countries, reported as 1 in every 120 pregnancies. Age is a factor, with the frequency of molar pregnancies highest at both ends of reproductive life. Women who have had one molar pregnancy have four to five times the risk to have another in a subsequent pregnancy (Berman & Di Saia, & Tiwari, 2004; Li & Karlan, 2003). Persistent gestational trophoblastic disease may undergo malignant change (choriocarcinoma) and may metastasize to distant sites such as the lung, vagina, liver, and brain.

Complete mole is thought to occur when the ovum is fertilized by a sperm that duplicates its own chromosomes while the maternal chromosomes in the ovum are inactivated. In a partial mole, the maternal contribution is usually present but the paternal contribution is doubled, and therefore the karyotype is triploid (69,XXY or 69,XYY). If a fetus is identified with the partial mole, it is grossly abnormal because of the abnormal chromosomal makeup.

CLINICAL MANIFESTATIONS

Routine use of ultrasound allows earlier diagnosis of hydatidiform mole, usually before the more severe manifestations of the disorder develop. Possible signs and symptoms of molar pregnancy include the following:

- Elevated levels of hCG
- Characteristic ultrasonographic pattern that shows the vesicles and the absence of a fetal sac or fetal heart activity in a complete molar pregnancy

630 **PART V** Families at Risk during the Childbearing Period

- A uterus that is larger than one would expect based on the duration of the pregnancy
- Vaginal bleeding, which varies from dark-brown spotting to profuse hemorrhage
- Excessive nausea and vomiting (HEG), which may be related to high levels of hCG from the proliferating trophoblasts
- Early development of preeclampsia, which is rarely diagnosed before 24 weeks in an otherwise normal pregnancy

DIAGNOSIS

Measurement of the hCG levels detects the abnormally high levels of the hormone before treatment. Following treatment, hCG levels are measured to determine if they fall and then disappear.

In addition to the characteristic pattern showing the vesicles, ultrasound examination allows a differential diagnosis to be made between two types of molar pregnancies: (1) a partial mole that includes some fetal tissue and membranes and (2) a complete mole that is composed only of enlarged villi but contains no fetal tissue or membranes.

THERAPEUTIC MANAGEMENT

Medical management includes two phases: (1) evacuation of the trophoblastic tissue of the mole and (2) continuous follow-up of the woman to detect malignant changes of any remaining trophoblastic tissue. At the same time the woman is treated for any other problems such as preeclampsia or HEG.

Before evacuation, chest radiography, computed tomography (CT), or magnetic resonance imaging (MRI) may be performed to detect metastatic disease. A complete blood count, laboratory assessment of coagulation status, and blood type and screen or cross-match are also necessary in case a transfusion is needed.

The mole usually is removed by vacuum aspiration followed by curettage. After tissue removal, IV oxytocin is given to contract the uterus. Avoiding uterine stimulation with oxytocin before evacuation is important. Uterine contractions can cause trophoblastic tissue to be pulled into large venous sinusoids in the uterus, resulting in embolization of the tissue and respiratory distress (Berman & Di Saia, & Tiwari, 2004). The tissue obtained is sent for laboratory evaluation. Although a hydatidiform mole is usually a benign process, choriocarcinoma may occur.

Follow-up is critical to detect changes suggestive of trophoblastic malignancy. Follow-up protocol involves evaluation of serum hCG levels every 1 to 2 weeks until undetectable. The test is then repeated every 1 to 2 months for a year. A persistent or rising hCG level suggests continued gestational trophoblastic disease. Pregnancy must be avoided during the 1-year follow-up because it would obscure the evidence of choriocarcinoma. Oral contraceptives are the preferred birth control method (Berman & Di Saia, & Tiwari, 2004).

NURSING CONSIDERATIONS

Bleeding and infection are the early possible complications after a molar pregnancy. The nurse should observe the vital signs for an elevated temperature and pulse and observe vaginal bleeding for excessive amount or foul odor.

Women who have had a hydatidiform mole experience emotions similar to those of women who have had any other type of pregnancy loss. In addition, they may be anxious about follow-up evaluations, the possibility of malignant change, and the need to delay pregnancy for at least a year.

✓ CHECK YOUR READING

5. Why is ectopic pregnancy sometimes called a "disaster of reproduction"?
6. Why is the incidence of ectopic pregnancy increasing in the United States? How is ectopic pregnancy treated?
7. What is a hydatidiform mole, and why are two phases of treatment necessary?

Application of the Nursing Process
Hemorrhagic Conditions of Early Pregnancy

Regardless of the cause of early antepartum bleeding, nurses play a vital role in its management. Nurses are responsible for monitoring the condition of the pregnant woman and for collaborating with the physician to provide treatment.

Assessment

Confirmation of pregnancy and length of gestation are important initial data to obtain. Physical assessment focuses on determining the amount of bleeding and the description, location, and severity of pain. Estimate the amount of vaginal bleeding by examining linen and peripads. If necessary, make a more accurate estimation by weighing the linen and peripads (1 g weight equals 1 ml volume).

■ When asking a woman how much blood she lost at home, ask her to compare the amount lost with a common measure such as a tablespoon or a cup. Ask also how long the bleeding episode lasted and what was done to control the bleeding.

Bleeding may be accompanied by pain. Uterine cramping usually accompanies spontaneous abortion; deep, severe pelvic pain is associated with ruptured ectopic pregnancy. Remember that in ruptured ectopic pregnancy, bleeding may be concealed and pain could be the only symptom.

The woman's vital signs and urine output give a clue to her cardiovascular status. A rising pulse and respiratory rate and falling urine output are associated with hypovolemia. The blood pressure usually falls late in hypovolemic shock. Check laboratory values for hemoglobin and hematocrit and report abnormal values to the health care provider. Check laboratory values for coagulation factors to identify

CRITICAL THINKING 🖋 EXERCISE 25-1

All women who have experienced prenatal bleeding and invasive procedures are at increased risk for infection.

Question
What common assumptions do nurses make about those who are at risk for developing infections?

added risks for hemorrhage. Identify women who are Rh-negative so that they can receive Rh₀(D) immune globulin.

Because abortion or hydatidiform mole may be associated with infections, assess the woman for fever, elevated pulse, malaise, and prolonged or malodorous vaginal discharge. Determine the family's knowledge of needed follow-up care and how to prevent complications such as infection.

Analysis

A variety of collaborative problems or nursing diagnoses should be considered in the woman who has a bleeding disorder of early pregnancy. Collaborative problems such as bleeding and potential for infection are present. Current diagnostic techniques often permit early diagnosis before hemorrhage occurs. A nursing diagnosis that would apply to these early pregnancy disorders is Deficient Knowledge: diagnostic and therapeutic procedures, signs and symptoms of additional complications, dietary measures to prevent infection or reduction in therapeutic drug levels, and importance of follow-up care.

Planning

Goals or expected outcomes for this nursing diagnosis are that the woman will:

- Verbalize understanding of diagnostic and therapeutic procedures
- Verbalize measures to prevent infection
- Verbalize signs of infection to report to the health care provider
- Maintain follow-up care

Interventions

PROVIDING INFORMATION ABOUT TESTS AND PROCEDURES

Women and their families experience less anxiety if they understand what is happening. Explain planned diagnostic procedures, such as transvaginal or transabdominal ultrasonography (see Chapter 10). Include the purpose of the tests, how long they will take, and whether the procedures cause discomfort. Briefly describe the reasons for blood tests such as hCG, hemoglobin, hematocrit, or coagulation factors. Explain that diagnostic and therapeutic measures sometimes must be performed quickly to prevent excessive blood loss. If surgical intervention is necessary, reinforce explanations of the anesthesia professional about planned anesthesia. Obtain needed consents before procedures.

TEACHING MEASURES TO PREVENT INFECTION

The risk for infection is greatest during the first 72 hours after spontaneous abortion or operative procedures. Personal hygiene should include daily showers and careful hand washing before and after changing perineal pads. Perineal pads, applied in a front-to-back direction, should be used instead of tampons until bleeding has subsided. The woman should consult with the health care provider about safe timing of resuming intercourse.

PROVIDING DIETARY INFORMATION

Nutrition and adequate fluid intake help maintain the body's defense against infection, and the nurse must promote an adequate and culturally sensitive diet. The woman who has a hemorrhagic complication is also at risk for infection. She needs foods that are high in iron to increase hemoglobin and hematocrit values. These foods include liver, red meat, spinach, egg yolks, carrots, and raisins (Anderson, 2004; Shabert, 2004). Foods high in vitamin C include citrus fruits, broccoli, strawberries, cantaloupe, cabbage, and green peppers. Adequate fluid intake (2500 ml per day) promotes hydration after bleeding episodes and maintains digestive processes.

Iron supplementation also frequently is prescribed, and the woman may require information on how to lessen the gastrointestinal upset that many people experience when iron is administered. Less gastric upset is experienced when iron is taken with meals. Iron supplements having a slow release may also be better tolerated. A diet high in fiber and fluid helps reduce the commonly associated constipation.

TEACHING SIGNS OF INFECTION TO REPORT

Ensure that the woman has a thermometer and knows how to use it. Tell her to take her temperature every 8 hours for the first 3 days at home. Teach the woman to seek medical help if her temperature rises above 38° C (100.4° F) or as her physician instructs. She also should report other signs of infection, even if she does not have a fever, such as vaginal discharge with foul odor, pelvic tenderness, or persistent general malaise.

REINFORCING FOLLOW-UP CARE

A variety of follow-up procedures such as repeat ultrasonic examinations or serum hCG levels may be necessary for women with gestational trophoblastic disease such as hydatidiform mole. Immunologic or genetic testing and counseling may be advised for couples having recurrent abortions. All couples who have had a pregnancy loss should be seen and counseled.

At this time acknowledge their grief, which often manifests as anger. Many women have guilt feelings that must be recognized. They often need repeated reassurance that the loss was not a result of anything they did or anything they neglected.

Women who do not desire pregnancy right away will need contraception. Reliable contraception for at least 1 year also will be essential for women who have had a molar pregnancy. Teach the woman how to use the prescribed contraceptive method correctly to enhance effectiveness (see Chapter 31).

Evaluation
Interventions are judged successful and the goals and expected outcomes are met if the woman does the following:
- Verbalizes understanding of diagnostic and therapeutic procedures
- Verbalize measures to prevent infection
- Verbalizes signs of infection that should be reported to a health care professional
- Helps develop and participate in a plan of follow-up care

HEMORRHAGIC CONDITIONS OF LATE PREGNANCY
After 20 weeks of pregnancy the two major causes of hemorrhage are the disorders of the placenta called *placenta previa* and *abruptio placentae*. Abruptio placentae may be further complicated by DIC, which was discussed earlier.

Placenta Previa
Placenta previa is an implantation of the placenta in the lower uterus. As a result the placenta is closer to the internal cervical os than the presenting part (usually the head) of the fetus. The three classifications of placenta previa (total, partial, and marginal) depend on how much of the internal cervical os is covered by the placenta (Figure 25-5). High-resolution ultrasound allows measurement of the distance between the internal cervical os and the lower border of the placenta:
- Marginal (sometimes called *low-lying*): Placenta is implanted in the lower uterus, but its lower border is more than 3 cm from the internal cervical os.

- Partial: Lower border of the placenta is within 3 cm of the internal cervical os but does not completely cover the os.
- Total: Placenta completely covers internal cervical os.

Marginal placenta previa is common in early ultrasound examinations and often appears to move upward and away from the internal cervical os *(placental migration)* as the fetus grows and the upper uterus develops more than the lower uterus. Only about 10% of placenta previas diagnosed in the second trimester remain a previa at term (Clark, 2004).

INCIDENCE AND ETIOLOGY
In the United States the incidence of placenta previa averages 1 in 200 births. It is more common in women who have had previous placenta previa, cesarean birth, or pregnancy termination and in older women. The multipara is more likely to have placenta previa than the nullipara. African or Asian ethnicity also increases the risk. Cigarette smoking and cocaine use are personal habits that add to a woman's risk for a previa.

CLINICAL MANIFESTATIONS
The classic sign of placenta previa is the sudden onset of painless uterine bleeding in the last half of pregnancy. However, many cases of placenta previa are diagnosed by ultrasound examination before any bleeding occurs. Bleeding results from tearing of the placental villi from the uterine wall, resulting in exposure of uterine vessels. Bleeding is painless because it does not occur in a closed cavity and does not cause pressure on adjacent tissue. It may be scanty or profuse, and it may cease spontaneously, only to recur later.

Bleeding may not occur until labor starts, when cervical changes disrupt placental attachment. The admitting nurse may be unsure whether the bleeding is just heavy "bloody show" or a sign of a placenta previa, particularly if the woman had no prenatal care.

If any doubt exists, the nurse never performs a vaginal examination or takes any action that would stimulate uterine activity. Digital examination of the cervical os when a placenta previa is present can cause additional placental separation or tear the placenta itself, causing severe hemorrhage and extreme risk to the fetus. Until the location and position of the placenta are verified by ultrasonography, no manual examinations should be performed, and administration of oxytocin should be postponed to prevent strong contractions that could result in sudden placental separation and rapid hemorrhage.

THERAPEUTIC MANAGEMENT
When the diagnosis of placenta previa is confirmed, medical interventions are based on the condition of the expectant mother and fetus. The woman is evaluated to determine the amount of hemorrhage, and electronic fetal monitoring is initiated to evaluate the fetus. Fetal gestational age is a third consideration.

Options for management include conservative management if the mother's cardiovascular status is stable and the

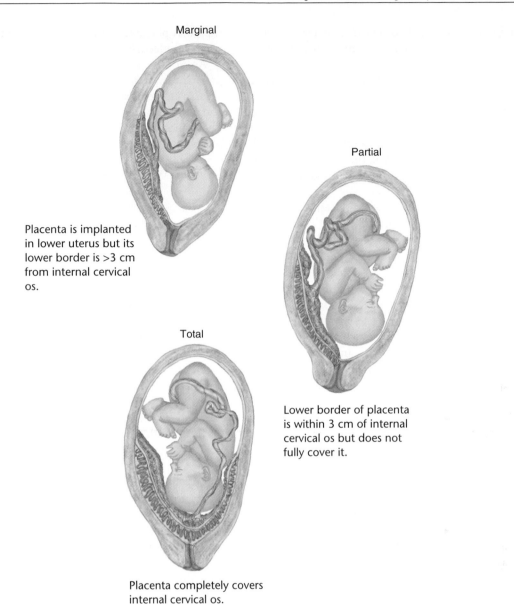

Marginal

Placenta is implanted in lower uterus but its lower border is >3 cm from internal cervical os.

Partial

Lower border of placenta is within 3 cm of internal cervical os but does not fully cover it.

Total

Placenta completely covers internal cervical os.

Figure 25-5 ■ The three classifications of placenta previa.

fetus is immature and has a reassuring status by ultrasound examination and monitoring. Delaying birth may increase birth weight and maturity and administration of corticosteroids to the mother speeds maturation of the fetal lungs. Antepartal units are often designed to consider the woman's needs for physical and occupational therapy and for diversion as well as care for her pregnancy complication. Conservative management may take place in the home or hospital.

HOME CARE. Criteria for home care include the following (Clark, 2004):

- No evidence of active bleeding is present.
- The woman is able to maintain bed rest at home.
- Home is a reasonable distance from the hospital.
- Emergency systems are available for immediate transport to the hospital 24 hours a day.

Nurses are often responsible for helping the woman and family understand the physician's plan of care. Nurses help the woman and family develop a workable plan for home care that may include strict bed rest except for going to the bathroom, the presence of another adult to manage the home and be present if an emergency arises, and a procedure to follow if heavy bleeding begins. Teaching also includes emphasizing the importance of (1) assessing color and amount of vaginal discharge or bleeding, especially after each urination or bowel movement, (2) assessing fetal activity (kick counts) daily (see Chapter 10), (3) assessing uterine activity at prescribed intervals, and (4) refraining from sexual intercourse to prevent disruption of the placenta. Home care nurses may be responsible for making daily phone contact to assess the woman's perception of uterine activity (cramping, regular or sporadic contractions), bleeding, fetal activity, and adherence to the prescribed treatment plan. In addition, they may make home visits for comprehensive maternal-fetal assessments with portable equipment, such as nonstress tests. The woman and her family are instructed to report a decrease in fetal movement or an increase in uterine contractions or vaginal bleeding.

Nurses should provide specific, accurate information about the condition of the fetus. For example, parents are reassured when they hear that the fetal heart rate is within the expected range and daily kick counts are reassuring. Nurses also may need to help the family understand the physician's plan of care. For instance, the nurse may explain why a cesarean birth is necessary and why blood transfusion may be required.

INPATIENT CARE. Women with placenta previa are admitted to the antepartum unit if they do not meet the criteria for home care or if they require additional care to meet the goal of greater fetal maturity. When the expectant mother is confined to the hospital, nursing assessments focus on determining whether she experiences bleeding episodes or signs of preterm labor. Periodic electronic fetal monitoring is necessary to determine whether there are fetal heart activity changes in association with fetal compromise. A significant change in fetal heart activity, an episode of vaginal bleeding, or signs of preterm labor should be reported immediately to the physician.

At times conservative management is not an option. For instance, delivery is scheduled if the fetus is older than 36 weeks' gestation and the lungs are mature. Immediate delivery may be necessary regardless of fetal immaturity if bleeding is excessive, the woman demonstrates signs of hypovolemia, or signs of fetal compromise are present. If cesarean birth is necessary, nurses must prepare the expectant mother for surgery. See Box 16-1 for a summary of care for the woman having cesarean birth.

The preoperative procedures are often performed quickly if the woman is hemorrhaging, and the family may be anxious about the condition of the fetus and the expectant mother. Nurses must use whatever time is available to keep the family informed.

■ During the rapid preparations for surgery the nurse can reassure both the woman and the family by briefly describing the necessary preparations: "I'm sorry we have to rush, but we need to start the IV in case she needs extra fluids." "Do you have questions I might answer as we prepare for the cesarean?"

Abruptio Placentae

Separation of a normally implanted placenta before the fetus is born (called *abruptio placentae, placental abruption,* or *premature separation of the placenta*) occurs in cases of bleeding and formation of a hematoma (clot) on the maternal side of the placenta. As the clot expands, further separation occurs. Hemorrhage may be apparent (vaginal bleeding) or concealed. The severity of the complication depends on the amount of bleeding and the size of the hematoma. If bleeding continues, the hematoma expands and obliterates intervillous spaces. Fetal vessels are disrupted as placental separation occurs, resulting in fetal and maternal bleeding.

Abruptio placentae is a dangerous condition for both the pregnant woman and the fetus. The major dangers for the woman are hemorrhage and consequent hypovolemic shock and clotting abnormalities (see discussion of DIC, p. 626). The major dangers for the fetus are asphyxia, excessive blood loss, and prematurity.

INCIDENCE AND ETIOLOGY

Published incidence of abruptio placentae varies but is about 0.5% to 1%. Placental abruption extensive enough to cause the death of the fetus has declined to about 1 in 830 deliveries but accounts for 10% to 15% of perinatal deaths (Cunningham et al., 2001; Kay, 2003).

The cause is unknown; however, several factors that increase the risk have been identified. Maternal use of cocaine, which causes vasoconstriction in the endometrial arteries, is a leading cause of abruptio placentae. Other risk factors include maternal hypertension, maternal cigarette smoking, multigravida status, short umbilical cord, abdominal trauma, premature rupture of the membranes, and history of previous premature separation of the placenta. Maternal age is also associated with abruptio placentae, probably associated with a larger number of births for each mother (Clark, 2004; Cunningham et al., 2001).

CLINICAL MANIFESTATIONS

Although evidence of abruptio placentae may be quickly evident, it is not always a dramatic or acute event. Five classic signs and symptoms of abruptio placentae include:

■ Bleeding, which may be evident vaginally or may be concealed behind the placenta

■ Uterine tenderness that may be localized at the site of the abruption

■ Uterine irritability with frequent low-intensity contractions and poor relaxation between contractions

■ Abdominal or low back pain that may be described as aching or dull

■ High uterine resting tone identified with use of an intrauterine pressure catheter

Additional signs include hypovolemic shock, fetal distress, and fetal death. Many women have a normal blood pressure, however, because the blood loss masks an undiagnosed hypertensive disorder (Clark, 2004).

Cases of abruptio placentae are divided into two main types: (1) those in which hemorrhage is concealed and (2) those in which hemorrhage is apparent. In either type the placental abruption may be complete or partial. In cases of concealed hemorrhage the bleeding occurs behind the placenta but the margins remain intact, causing formation of a hematoma. The hemorrhage is apparent when bleeding separates or dissects the membranes from the endometrium and blood flows out through the vagina. Figure 25-6 illustrates abruptio placentae with external and concealed bleeding. Apparent bleeding does not always correspond to the actual amount of blood lost, and signs

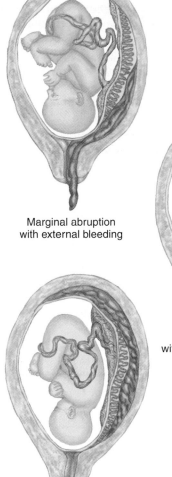

Marginal abruption
with external bleeding

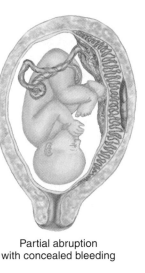

Partial abruption
with concealed bleeding

Complete abruption
with concealed bleeding

Figure 25-6 ■ Types of abruptio placentae.

of shock (tachycardia, hypotension, pale color, and cold, clammy skin) may be present when little or no external bleeding occurs.

Abdominal pain is also related to the type of separation. It may be sudden and severe when bleeding occurs into the myometrium (uterine muscle) or is intermittent and difficult to distinguish from labor contractions. The uterus may become exceedingly firm (boardlike) and tender, making palpation of the fetus difficult. Ultrasound examination is helpful to rule out placenta previa as the cause of bleeding, but it cannot be used to diagnose abruptio placentae reliably because the separation and bleeding may not be obvious on ultrasonography.

THERAPEUTIC MANAGEMENT

Any woman who exhibits signs of abruptio placentae should be hospitalized and evaluated at once. Evaluation focuses on the cardiovascular status of the expectant mother and the condition of the fetus. If the condition is

mild and the fetus is immature and shows no signs of distress, conservative management may be initiated. This includes bed rest and may include administration of tocolytic medications to decrease uterine activity. Conservative management is rare, however, owing to the great risks of fetal death and maternal hemorrhage associated with abruptio placentae.

Immediate delivery of the fetus is necessary if signs of fetal compromise exist or if the expectant mother exhibits signs of excessive bleeding, either obvious or concealed. Intensive monitoring of both the woman and the fetus is essential because rapid deterioration of either can occur. Blood products for replacement should be available, and two large-bore IV lines should be started for replacement of fluid and blood.

Women who have experienced abdominal trauma are at increased risk for abruptio placentae. They may be monitored for 24 hours after significant trauma such as a motor vehicle accident, even if they are not having any signs of bleeding, because it may take this long for an abruptio placentae to develop. If they are not having contractions after the trauma and the fetal heart rate pattern is reassuring, monitoring for 4 to 6 hours may be sufficient (Clark, 2004).

NURSING CONSIDERATIONS

Abruptio placentae is frightening for a woman. She experiences severe pain and is aware of the danger to herself and to the fetus. She must be carefully assessed for signs of concealed hemorrhage.

If immediate cesarean delivery is necessary, the woman may feel powerless as the health care team hurriedly prepares her for surgery. If at all possible in the time available, nurses must explain anticipated procedures to the woman and her family to reduce their feelings of fear and anxiety.

Excessive bleeding and fetal hypoxia are always major concerns with abruptio placentae, and nurses are responsible for continuous monitoring of both the expectant mother and the fetus so that problems can be detected early before the condition of the woman or the fetus deteriorates.

CRITICAL **TO REMEMBER**

Signs of Concealed Hemorrhage in Abruptio Placentae

Increase in fundal height
Hard, boardlike abdomen
High uterine baseline tone on electronic monitoring strip when an intrauterine pressure catheter is used
Persistent abdominal pain
Systemic signs of early hemorrhage (tachycardia [maternal and fetal], tachypnea, falling blood pressure, falling urine output, restlessness)
Persistent late deceleration in fetal heart rate or decreasing baseline variability; absence of accelerations
Slight or absent vaginal bleeding

8. What are the signs and symptoms of placenta previa? How is it managed in the home?
9. What are the signs and symptoms of abruptio placentae?
10. What are the major dangers to the expectant mother and the fetus during the placental abruption?

Application of the Nursing Process
Hemorrhagic Conditions of Late Pregnancy

Assessment

For hemorrhagic conditions of late pregnancy, some nursing assessments should be performed immediately and others can be deferred until initial interventions have been taken to stabilize the cardiovascular status of the woman. Many nursing assessments are concurrent with medical assessments and include:

- Amount and nature of bleeding (time of onset, estimated blood loss before admission to hospital, and description of tissue or clots passed): Peripads and underpads should be saved as needed to accurately estimate blood loss.
- Pain (type [constant, intermittent, sharp, dull, severe]; onset [sudden, gradual]; and location [generalized over abdomen, localized in back]): Is uterine tenderness present with gentle palpation? Is the tenderness localized?
- Maternal vital signs: Are these within normal limits, or is hypotension, tachycardia, or both present? A normal blood pressure may be misleading in a woman with abruptio placentae because she may have been hypertensive before the blood loss caused her blood pressure to fall to normal or hypotensive levels.
- Condition of the fetus: An electronic fetal monitor determines fetal heart rate, presence of accelerations, and fetal response to uterine activity. The presence of late decelerations or poor variability is of particular concern.
- Uterine contractions: Application of an external monitor determines frequency and duration of contractions. An intrauterine pressure catheter can identify hypertonic contractions and an increased resting tone associated with abruptio placentae. Palpation can identify that the uterus does not relax fully between contractions. Thick abdominal fat reduces the ability to identify poor uterine relaxation by external means.
- Obstetric history (gravida, para, previous abortions, preterm infants, previous pregnancy outcomes). Does the history include previous abruptio placentae?
- Length of gestation (date of last menstrual period, fundal height, correlation of fundal height with estimated gestation): If bleeding occurs into the myometrium, the fundus enlarges as bleeding progresses. A piece of tape can mark the top of the fundus at a given time, and then the nurse can observe and report increasing fundal size, which indicates that bleeding into uterine muscles is occurring.
- Laboratory data (complete blood count and blood type and screen, coagulation studies): Laboratory data are obtained to prepare for transfusions if necessary and to determine whether signs of DIC are developing. Type and Rh factor identify possible need for Rh immune globulin (RhoGAM). Other tests may be done serially to identify whether the abruptio is stable or worsening. The Kleihauer-Betke (K-B) test identifies fetal blood cells in the maternal circulation and is usually done after a traumatic event such as a motor vehicle accident. Coagulation studies include fibrinogen, FSP, PT and PTT, and D-dimer.

Despite the emphasis on physical assessment, the emotional response of the mother and her partner must also be addressed. They will most likely be anxious, fearful, confused, and overwhelmed by the activity. They may have little knowledge of expected medical management and may not realize that the fetus will need to be delivered as quickly as possible and that a surgical procedure is necessary. They may fear for the life of the woman and the fetus.

Analysis

Nursing diagnoses vary, depending on the cause and severity of the bleeding. The most commonly used nursing diagnoses for antepartum bleeding appear in Nursing Care Plan 25-1. The most dangerous potential complication is hypovolemic shock, which jeopardizes the life of the mother as well as the fetus.

Planning

The nurse cannot independently manage hypovolemic shock but must confer with physicians for medical orders for treatment. Planning should reflect the nurse's responsibility to:

- Monitor for signs of hypovolemic shock
- Consult with the physician if signs of hypovolemic shock are observed
- Perform actions to minimize the effects of hypovolemic shock

Interventions

MONITORING FOR SIGNS OF HYPOVOLEMIC SHOCK

Assess for any sign of developing hypovolemic shock. The body attempts to compensate for decreased blood volume and to maintain oxygenation of essential organs by increasing the rate and effort of the heart and lungs and by shunting blood from less essential organs, such as the skin and the extremities, to more essential organs, such as the brain and the kidneys. This compensatory mechanism results in the early signs and symptoms of hypovolemic shock:

- Fetal tachycardia (often the first sign of either maternal or fetal hypovolemia)
- Maternal tachycardia, diminished peripheral pulses

NURSING CARE PLAN 25-1 Antepartum Bleeding

ASSESSMENT: Beth Dixon, a 28-year-old gravida 2, para 1, is admitted to the antepartum unit at 32 weeks' gestation after an episode of vaginal bleeding resulting from total placenta previa. Vital signs are stable, and fetal heart rate is 140 to 150 beats per minute with no nonreassuring signs. Beth and her husband Bob appear anxious about the condition of the fetus and the plan of care. Beth is particularly worried about her 5-year-old son, who is at home with a neighbor.

NURSING DIAGNOSIS: Anxiety related to unknown effects of bleeding and lack of knowledge of predicted course of management

> **CRITICAL THINKING:** *Although this diagnosis is correct, what are priority nursing actions for Beth? Why?*
>
> **ANSWER:** *To monitor the condition of the fetus and to observe Beth for vaginal bleeding or change in vital signs. These priorities are based on a hierarchy of needs; physiologic needs and the need for safety must be ensured before psychological needs are fully addressed.*

GOALS/EXPECTED OUTCOMES: The couple will:
1. Verbalize expected routines and projected management by the end of the first day after admission.
2. Express less anxiety after the course of management is explained.

INTERVENTION	RATIONALE
1. Remain with the couple and acknowledge the emotions that they exhibit: "I know this is unexpected, and you must have many questions. Perhaps I can answer some of them."	1. The nurse's presence and empathetic understanding are therapeutic tools to prepare the family to cope with the unexpected situation.
2. Determine the couple's level of understanding of the situation and the projected management: "Tell me what you've been told to expect."	2. This allows the nurse to reinforce the physician's explanations and to notify the physician if additional explanations are necessary.
3. Provide the couple with factual information about projected management. a. Explain that Beth will need to remain in the hospital so that her condition and the condition of the fetus can be watched closely. b. Explain why a cesarean birth is necessary this time even though she delivered vaginally before. c. Provide information about hospital routines (meals, visiting hours) and any fetal surveillance techniques (such as frequent ultrasound exams and biophysical profiles).	3. Patient education has proved to be an effective measure for preventing and reducing anxiety. Knowledge reduces fear of the unknown and reinforces medical explanations of care.
4. Explain corticosteroid therapy ordered to speed fetal lung maturation.	4. Knowing that corticosteroids can speed fetal lung maturity may reduce anxiety if a preterm birth must occur.
5. Ask Beth and her family if they would like to talk with a nurse from the special care nursery.	5. Continued bleeding or nonreassuring fetal factors may necessitate a preterm delivery.
6. Allow Beth and her family to participate in the routine as much as possible. This may mean scheduling nursing care around times when Bob and their son can visit.	6. Many women feel a sense of powerlessness when their activities are limited and a course of treatment is prescribed without consultation.

EVALUATION: The interventions are considered successful if Beth and Bob demonstrate knowledge of the projected management and why it is necessary and verbalize reduced anxiety.

ASSESSMENT: Beth continues to have episodes of light vaginal bleeding, although none has been so heavy as to demand immediate delivery. Her doctor wants the fetus to mature at least 2 more weeks if possible. Beth cries frequently, telling the nurse, "I miss my son so much. He just started kindergarten and he is so shy. I feel useless and he really needs me now. It's hard on Bob, too; he has to do everything."

NURSING DIAGNOSIS: Situational Low Self-Esteem related to temporary inability to provide care for family

GOALS/EXPECTED OUTCOMES: Beth will:
1. Identify positive aspects of self during hospitalization
2. Identify ways of providing comfort and affection for her son during the hospital stay

INTERVENTION	RATIONALE
1. Encourage Beth to express her concerns about the need for hospitalization: "What bothers you most about being away from home?"	1. Major concerns may not be identified or may be misunderstood unless the woman clarifies them.

Continued

NURSING CARE PLAN 25-1 Antepartum Bleeding—cont'd

INTERVENTION	RATIONALE
2. After acknowledging feelings, encourage examination of the need for hospitalization and its consequences: it provides time for the fetus to mature.	2. This identifies positive aspects of the situation and her important role. It helps Beth understand that her role in fetal maturity extends beyond the corticosteroid therapy given to mature the fetal lungs if birth must occur before 34 weeks.
3. Explore reality of Beth's self-appraisal ("I feel useless") by assisting her to investigate ways to provide nurturing care for her son while she is hospitalized: a. Keep in close touch by telephone (wake-up, goodnight, and after-school calls). b. Make small handmade items such as bookmarks, games, needlework. c. Explain in simple, nonfrightening terms why she must stay in the hospital. d. Offer reassurances of continued love.	3. Daily involvement in the life of the child helps reduce feelings of isolation and failure to meet obligations to her family.
4. Assist Beth to involve her son in plans for the newborn. He might benefit from sibling classes or playtime with the mother that involves caring for newborn-sized dolls.	4. Involving siblings provides goals for combined family interaction that increases feelings of self-worth. Young children often benefit from understanding that they can benefit their new sibling's life.

EVALUATION: Beth is able to make positive comments about the importance of rest to the health of the new baby, and she initiates numerous activities that permit her to continue close, comforting contact with her child during the period of hospitalization.

- Normal or slightly decreased blood pressure
- Increased respiratory rate
- Cool, pale skin and mucous membranes

The compensatory mechanism fails if hypovolemic shock progresses and insufficient blood exists to perfuse the brain, heart, and kidneys. Later signs of hypovolemic shock include the following:

- Falling blood pressure
- Pallor; skin becomes cold and clammy
- Urine output less than 30 ml/hr
- Restlessness, agitation, decreased mentation

MONITORING THE FETUS

Use continuous electronic fetal monitoring so that signs of fetal compromise, such as decreasing baseline variability or late decelerations, can be seen (see Chapter 14). If nonreassuring patterns are seen, contact the physician at once because the fetus often shows signs of compromise before maternal signs of hypovolemia are obvious. Give the physician

CRITICAL TO REMEMBER

Signs and Symptoms of Hypovolemic Shock Caused by Blood Loss

Increased pulse rate, falling blood pressure, increased respiratory rate
Weak, diminished, or "thready" peripheral pulses
Cool, moist skin, pallor, or cyanosis (late sign)
Decreased (<30 ml/hr) or absent urinary output
Decreased hemoglobin, hematocrit levels
Change in mental status (restlessness, agitation, difficulty concentrating)

a report on new laboratory data that suggest an increasing degree of placental abruption, such as rising K-B levels after abdominal trauma.

PROMOTING TISSUE OXYGENATION

To promote oxygenation of tissues:

- Place the woman in a lateral position, with the head of the bed flat to increase cardiac return and thus to increase circulation and oxygenation of the placenta and other vital organs.
- Limit maternal activity to decrease the tissue demand for oxygen.
- Provide simple explanations, reassurance, and emotional support to the woman to reduce anxiety, which increases the metabolic demand for oxygen.

COLLABORATING WITH THE PHYSICIAN FOR FLUID REPLACEMENT

To replace fluids:

- Insert IV lines according to hospital protocol; usually two lines that use large-gauge catheters (16- to 18-gauge) are recommended so that blood can be administered quickly if necessary.
- Administer fluids for replacement as directed by the physician to maintain a urinary output of at least 30 ml/hr.

PREPARING THE WOMAN FOR SURGERY

Quick preparation of the woman for cesarean delivery may be necessary. The nurse is responsible for the following:

- Validating that preoperative permits have been correctly signed

- Validating that essential laboratory work has been done
- Surgical preparation and insertion of an indwelling urinary catheter
- Administering nonparticulate antacid or other medications as ordered by the anesthesia provider
- Providing information and appropriate reassurance to the family
- Notifying the newborn resuscitation team
- Assessing bleeding (before and after birth) from the vagina as well as from any surgical sites or puncture wounds (epidural or IV sites) so that uncontrolled bleeding or bleeding from unexpected sites, which may indicate DIC, can be reported to the physician for prompt medical management

PROVIDING EMOTIONAL SUPPORT

Once the safety of the woman and the fetus is ensured, nursing interventions promote comfort and provide emotional support. Explain what is causing the discomfort, and reassure the woman that pain relief measures will be initiated as soon as possible without causing harm to the fetus. Although offering false reassurance about the condition of the fetus is unwise, remain with the woman and provide accurate and timely information. Find time to explain what is going on to the woman and her family. They can feel overwhelmed by all the activity.

Evaluation

Although client-centered goals are not developed for collaborative problems, the nurse collects and compares data with established norms and judges whether the data are within normal limits. For hypovolemic shock, the maternal vital signs remain within normal limits and the fetal heart demonstrates no signs of compromise, such as abnormal rate, late decelerations, or decreasing baseline variability.

HYPEREMESIS GRAVIDARUM

HEG is persistent, uncontrollable vomiting that begins before the twentieth week of pregnancy. HEG may continue throughout pregnancy, although its severity usually lessens. Unlike morning sickness, which is self-limited and causes no serious complications, HEG can have serious consequences. It can lead to loss of 5% or more of prepregnancy weight, dehydration, ketosis, acid-base imbalance, and electrolyte imbalance (both sodium and potassium are lost from gastric fluids). Metabolic alkalosis may develop because large amounts of hydrochloric acid are lost in the vomitus. Deficiency of vitamin K may cause coagulation disorders, and thiamine deficiency can cause encephalopathy.

Etiology

The cause of HEG is not known, but the condition is more common among unmarried white women, during first pregnancies, and in multifetal pregnancies. Other possible causes include possible allergy to fetal proteins. Elevated levels of pregnancy-related hormones, such as estrogen and hCG, are considered a possible cause, as is maternal thyroid dysfunction. More recently, an association with the organism that causes peptic ulcer disease, *Helicobacter pylori,* has been identified. Psychological factors may interact with the nausea and vomiting that occurs during early pregnancy to worsen it (Buckwalter & Simpson, 2002; Cunningham et al., 2001; Gilbert & Harmon, 2003; Scott & Abu-Hamda, 2004; Weyermann et al., 2003).

Therapeutic Management

The physician will exclude other causes for persistent nausea and vomiting, such as cholecystitis or peptic ulcer disease, before diagnosing hyperemesis. Laboratory studies include determining the hemoglobin and hematocrit, which may be elevated as a result of dehydration, which results in hemoconcentration. Electrolyte studies may reveal reduced sodium, potassium, and chloride. Elevated creatinine levels indicate renal dysfunction.

Treatment occurs primarily in the home, where the woman first attempts to control the nausea with methods that are used for morning sickness (see Chapter 7). In addition, some physicians prescribe vitamins, such as pyridoxine (vitamin B_6), that may provide some relief. A daily vitamin and mineral supplement may be recommended.

Drug therapy may be required if the vomiting becomes severe. Drugs prescribed may include the following:

- Promethazine (Phenergan)
- Diphenhydramine (Benadryl)
- Histamine-receptor antagonists such as famotidine (Pepcid) or ranitidine (Zantac)
- Gastric acid inhibitors such as esomeprazole (Nexium) or omeprazole (Prilosec)
- Metoclopramide (Reglan)
- Ondansetron (Zofran)

The steroid methylprednisolone has recently been found to reduce the nausea and vomiting. Metoclopramide can be given with a subcutaneous infusion pump to provide continuous therapy at home. If drugs are required, a single drug is first prescribed in the lowest effective dose to minimize fetal effects. The benefit of the drug at controlling the adverse effects of the intractable vomiting is balanced against any fetal risk from the drugs (Magee, Mazzotta & Koren, 2002; Modigliani, 2000; Steinlauf, Magee, & Traube, 2004).

If simpler methods are unsuccessful and weight loss or electrolyte imbalance persists, IV fluid and electrolyte replacement or total parenteral nutrition may be necessary. In some women, IV fluid replacement improves the nausea and vomiting quickly. The woman usually can be managed at home with periodic home nursing visits if she must have total parenteral nutrition. Periodic brief hospitalizations may be needed until the hyperemesis problem lessens.

Nursing Considerations

Because management frequently occurs in the home, nurses are often responsible for assessing and intervening for the woman with HEG. Physical assessment begins with determining the intake and output. Intake includes IV fluids and parenteral nutrition, as well as oral nutrition, which is allowed once vomiting is controlled. Output includes the amount and character of emesis and urinary output. As a rule of thumb, the normal urinary output is about 1 ml/kg/hr (1 ml/2.2 lb/hr). A record of bowel elimination also provides significant information about oral nutrition because a woman's intake may have been so minimal that many days have passed since her last normal bowel movement.

Laboratory data may be evaluated to determine fluid and metabolic status. Elevated levels of hemoglobin and hematocrit may occur as a result of dehydration, which results in hemoconcentration. Concentrations of sodium, potassium, and chloride may be reduced, resulting in hypokalemia and alkalosis.

The woman weighs herself daily, first thing in the morning and in similar clothing each day. Her urine is tested for ketones. Weight loss and the presence of ketones in the urine suggest that fat stores and protein are being metabolized to meet energy needs.

Signs of dehydration include decreased fluid intake (less than 2000 ml/day), decreased urinary output, increased urine specific gravity (more than 1.025), dry skin or dry mucous membranes, and nonelastic skin turgor.

Nursing interventions focus on reducing nausea and vomiting, maintaining nutrition and fluid balance, and providing emotional support.

REDUCING NAUSEA AND VOMITING

When food is offered to the woman, portions should be small so that the amount does not appear overwhelming. Food should be attractively presented, and foods with strong odors should be eliminated from the diet because food smells often incite nausea. Low-fat foods and easily digested carbohydrates, such as fruit, breads, cereals, rice, and pasta, provide important nutrients and help prevent low blood sugar, which can cause nausea. Soups and other liquids should be taken between meals to avoid distending the stomach and triggering vomiting. Sitting upright after meals reduces gastric reflux.

MAINTAINING NUTRITION AND FLUID BALANCE

Women with nausea and vomiting should eat every 2 to 3 hours. Salting food helps replace chloride lost when hydrochloric acid is vomited. Eating potassium- and magnesium-rich foods and fluids should be encouraged when the woman can do so, because stores of these nutrients are likely to be depleted and magnesium deficiency can exacerbate nausea. Potassium is found in fruits, vegetables, and meat. Sources of magnesium include seeds, nuts, legumes, and green vegetables.

IV fluids and total parenteral nutrition are administered as directed by the physician. IV fluid containing potassium is often ordered until the low serum level returns to normal. Small oral feedings of clear liquids are started when nausea and vomiting subside. When oral fluids and adequate food intake are tolerated, parenteral nutrition is gradually discontinued. Continued inability to tolerate oral feedings or con-

tinued episodes of vomiting should be reported to the physician so that continued parenteral fluids and nutrition can be prescribed.

PROVIDING EMOTIONAL SUPPORT

The woman with HEG needs the opportunity to express how it feels to be pregnant and to live with constant nausea. The woman, and possibly her significant other, may have been surprised by the pregnancy and may not have accepted it. Helping the woman express reluctance to accept the pregnancy and identify her sources of support may reduce nausea, although its intensity may remain higher than in most women.

Often a curious lack of sympathy and support exists for these women, however. Nurses must use critical thinking to examine their own biases so that they can provide comfort and support. Case conferences or inservice educational programs may be necessary to overcome preset beliefs and to establish a level of care that meets the needs of the woman.

CHECK YOUR READING

11. How do "morning sickness" and HEG compare in terms of onset, duration, and effect on the client?
12. What are the nursing goals in therapeutic management of HEG?
13. Why is critical thinking particularly important in the care of the woman with HEG?

HYPERTENSIVE DISORDERS OF PREGNANCY

Terminology used to describe hypertension in pregnancy is not always uniform. Four categories of hypertensive disorders occurring during pregnancy were identified by a group working within the National Heart, Lung, & Blood Institute of the National Institutes of Health for the United States (2001). Hypertension of pregnancy and chronic hypertension that is present when not pregnant can coexist (Table 25-1).

- *Preeclampsia:* A systolic blood pressure of ≥ 140 mm Hg or diastolic blood pressure of ≥ 90 mm Hg occurring after 20 weeks of pregnancy that is accompanied by significant proteinuria (> 0.3 g in a 24-hour urine collection, which usually correlates with a random urine dipstick evaluation of $\geq 1+$). Edema, although common in preeclampsia, is now considered to be nonspecific because it occurs in many pregnancies not complicated by hypertension.
- *Eclampsia:* Progression of preeclampsia to generalized seizures that cannot be attributed to other causes. Seizures may occur postpartum.
- *Gestational hypertension:* Blood pressure elevation after 20 weeks of pregnancy that is not accompanied by proteinuria. Gestational hypertension must be considered a working diagnosis because it may progress to preeclampsia. If gestational hypertension persists after birth, chronic hypertension is diagnosed.

TABLE 25-1 Classifications of Hypertension in Pregnancy

Classification	Comments
Preeclampsia	Systolic blood pressure ≥140 mm Hg or diastolic blood pressure ≥ 90 mm Hg that develops after 20 weeks of pregnancy and is accompanied by proteinuria >0.3 g in a 24-hr urine collection (random urine dipstick is usually ≥1+).
Eclampsia	Progression of preeclampsia to generalized seizures that cannot be attributed to other causes.
Gestational hypertension	Systolic blood pressure ≥140 mm Hg or diastolic blood pressure ≥90 mm Hg that develops after 20 weeks of pregnancy, but without significant proteinuria (negative or trace on a random urine dipstick).
Chronic hypertension	Systolic blood pressure ≥140 mm Hg or diastolic blood pressure ≥90 mm Hg that was known to exist before pregnancy or develops before 20 weeks of gestation. Also diagnosed if the hypertension does not resolve during the postpartum period.
Preeclampsia superimposed on chronic hypertension	Development of new-onset proteinuria >0.3 g in a 24-hr collection in a woman who has chronic hypertension. In a woman who had proteinuria before 20 weeks, preeclampsia should be suspected if the woman has a sudden increase in proteinuria from her baseline levels, a sudden increase in blood pressure when it had been previously well controlled, development of thrombocytopenia (platelets <100,000/mm³), or abnormal elevations of liver enzymes (AST or ALT).

ALT, Alanine aminotransferase (formerly SGPT); *AST,* aspartate aminotransferase (formerly SGOT).

■ *Chronic hypertension:* The elevated blood pressure was known to exist before pregnancy. Unrecognized chronic hypertension may not be diagnosed until well after the end of pregnancy when the blood pressure remains high.

Preeclampsia

Preeclampsia is a condition in which hypertension develops during the last half of pregnancy in a woman who previously had normal blood pressure. In addition to hypertension, renal involvement may cause proteinuria. Many women also experience generalized edema. The only known cure is delivery of the fetus. Maternal and fetal morbidity can be minimized if preeclampsia is detected early and managed carefully.

INCIDENCE AND RISK FACTORS

Preeclampsia is relatively common, affecting 8% of all pregnancies (American Academy of Pediatrics & American College of Obstetricians and Gynecologists, 2002). It is a major cause of perinatal death, and it often is associated with intrauterine fetal growth restriction (IUGR).

Although the cause of preeclampsia is not understood, several factors are known to increase a woman's risk. Many risk factors may be interrelated such as overweight and prepregnancy diabetes.

Women with an increased risk for developing preeclampsia are those having their first baby. Women who are over 35, are African-American, or have a positive family history have a greater risk, as do women with a multifetal pregnancy or preexisting vascular disease. African-Americans were once thought to have the highest risk, but newer research shows a higher rate in American Indian women, possibly related to their tendency toward youth, anemia, poor nutrition, and late prenatal care. Low socioeconomic status was once thought to be a risk factor, but the true contribution of socioeconomic status is not certain because of the impact of other factors such as age, parity, race, and family history. Women who have eclampsia are more likely to be of low socioeconomic status.

Less well–known risk factors include both genetic and immunologic factors. The presence of the angiotensinogen gene T235 greatly increases the woman's sensitivity to angiotensin, a powerful vasoconstrictor that could lead to hypertension. Also, a woman is more likely to have preeclampsia if her mother or sister also had the disorder. Antiphospholipid syndrome (APS) is also strongly associated with the development of preeclampsia. The syndrome results from the development of antiphospholipid antibodies (aPL). These antibodies are directed against phospholipids that are widely distributed in cell membranes. The clinical picture of APS includes thrombosis, recurrent fetal loss, IUGR, and a higher incidence of preeclampsia (Lockwood & Silver, 2004). Box 25-2 summarizes major known risk factors for the development of preeclampsia.

The father's contribution to the pregnancy also appears to play a role in development of preeclampsia. Women who had prior pregnancies without hypertension are more likely to have preeclampsia if the expectant father previously fathered a pregnancy in another woman who had the disorder.

BOX 25-2 Risk Factors for Pregnancy-Related Hypertension

First pregnancy
Age >35 years
Anemia
Family history of pregnancy-induced hypertension
Chronic hypertension or preexisting vascular disease
Chronic renal disease
Obesity
Diabetes mellitus
Antiphospholipid syndrome
Multifetal pregnancy
Angiotensin gene T235
Mother or sister who had preeclampsia

From Poole, J.H., Sosa, M.E., Freda, M.C., Kendrick, J.M., Luppi, C.J., Krening, C.F., & Dauphinee, J.D. (2001). High-risk pregnancy. In K.R. Simpson & P.A. Creehan (Eds.), *AWHONN perinatal nursing* (2nd ed., pp. 173-296). Philadelphia: Lippincott Williams & Wilkins; Martin, J.A., Hamilton, B.E., Sutton, P.D., Ventura, S.J., Menacker, F., & Munson, M.L. (2003). Births: Final data for 2002. *National Vital Statistics Reports, 52*(10). Hyattsville, MD: National Center for Health Statistics, 2003. Retrieved December 19, 2004, from www.cdc.gov/nchs/data/nvsr52/nvsr52_10.pdf; Roberts, J.M. (2004). Pregnancy-related hypertension. In R.K. Creasy, R. Resnik, & J.D. Iams (Eds.), *Maternal-fetal medicine* (5th ed., pp. 859-899). Philadelphia: Saunders.

PATHOPHYSIOLOGY

Preeclampsia is a result of generalized vasospasm. The underlying cause of the vasospasm remains a mystery, although some of the pathophysiologic processes are known. In normal pregnancy, vascular volume and cardiac output increase significantly. Despite these increases, blood pressure does not rise in normal pregnancy. This is probably because pregnant women develop resistance to the effects of vasoconstrictors, such as angiotensin II. Peripheral vascular resistance decreases because of the effects of certain vasodilators, such as prostacyclin (PGI_2), PGE, and endothelium-derived relaxing factor (EDRF).

In preeclampsia, however, peripheral vascular resistance increases because some women are sensitive to angiotensin II. They also may have a decrease in vasodilators. For instance, the ratio of thromboxane (TXA_2) to PGI_2 increases. TXA_2, produced by kidney and trophoblastic tissue, causes vasoconstriction and platelet aggregation (clumping). PGI_2, produced by placental tissue and endothelial cells, causes vasodilation and inhibits platelet aggregation.

Vasospasm decreases the diameter of blood vessels, which results in endothelial cell damage and decreased EDRF. Vasoconstriction also results in impeded blood flow and elevated blood pressure. As a result, circulation to all body organs, including the kidneys, liver, brain, and placenta, is decreased. The following changes are most significant:

- Decreased renal perfusion reduces the glomerular filtration rate. Blood urea nitrogen, creatinine, and uric acid levels begin to rise.
- Reduced renal blood flow results in glomerular damage, allowing protein to leak across the glomerular membrane, which is normally impermeable to large protein molecules.
- Loss of protein reduces colloid osmotic pressure and allows fluid to shift to interstitial spaces. This may result in edema and a reduction in intravascular volume, which causes increased viscosity of the blood and a rise in hematocrit. In response to reduced intravascular volume, additional angiotensin II and aldosterone trigger the retention of both sodium and water. Generalized edema may occur.
- Decreased circulation to the liver impairs function and leads to hepatic edema and subcapsular hemorrhage, which can result in hemorrhagic necrosis. This is manifested by elevation of liver enzymes in maternal serum.
- Vasoconstriction of cerebral vessels leads to pressure-induced rupture of thin-walled capillaries, resulting in small cerebral hemorrhages. Symptoms of arterial vasospasm include headache and visual disturbances, such as blurred vision, "spots" before the eyes, and hyperactive deep tendon reflexes.
- Decreased colloid oncotic pressure can lead to pulmonary capillary leak that results in pulmonary edema. Dyspnea is the primary symptom.
- Decreased placental circulation results in infarctions that increase the risk for abruptio placentae and DIC.

In addition, the fetus is likely to experience intrauterine growth restriction and persistent hypoxemia and acidosis when maternal blood flow through the placenta is reduced. Figure 25-7 summarizes the pathologic processes of preeclampsia.

PREVENTIVE MEASURES

PRENATAL CARE. Proper prenatal care with attention to pattern of weight gain and monitoring of blood pressure and urinary protein may minimize maternal and fetal morbidity and mortality by allowing early detection of the problem.

Past attempts at prevention have included low-dose aspirin, calcium and magnesium supplements, and fish oil supplements. These measures have not proved to be beneficial for the general population, however.

More recent research assessed the benefits of antioxidant therapy with 1000 mg of vitamin C and 15 mg of vitamin E starting at 22 weeks. Although the results were promising, safety and effectiveness of antioxidant supplementation for the general population require further study (National Institutes of Health, 2001).

CLINICAL MANIFESTATIONS OF PREECLAMPSIA

CLASSIC SIGNS. The first indication of preeclampsia is usually hypertension. Blood pressure measurements vary with the woman's position, so the blood pressure should be measured uniformly at each office visit. Blood pressure should be measured with the woman seated and her arm supported, and the cuff size should be appropriate for the size of her arm. The diastolic pressure should be recorded at Korotkoff phase V, disappearance of sound (National High Blood Pressure Education Program Working Group on High Blood Pressure in Pregnancy, 2000). Hospitalizing the woman for serial observations of her blood pressure may identify true elevations from those induced by anxiety.

Proteinuria can be identified by using a clean-catch specimen to prevent contamination of the specimen by vaginal secretions or blood. Women with a urinary tract infection often have erythrocytes and leukocytes in the urine, which would elevate urine protein in the absence of preeclampsia.

ADDITIONAL SIGNS. Careful assessment may reveal additional signs associated with preeclampsia. For instance, when the retina is examined, vascular constriction and narrowing of the small arteries are obvious in most women with preeclampsia. The vasoconstriction that can be seen in the retina is occurring throughout the body. Deep tendon reflexes may be very brisk (hyperreflexia) suggesting cerebral irritability secondary to decreased brain circulation and edema.

Laboratory studies may identify liver, renal, and hepatic dysfunction if preeclampsia is severe. Coagulation may be impaired, as evidenced by a fall in platelets, which are often in the high normal range in a woman without preeclampsia. See also the discussion of DIC, p. 626.

Although it is a nonspecific sign that may have many causes, generalized edema often occurs with preeclampsia,

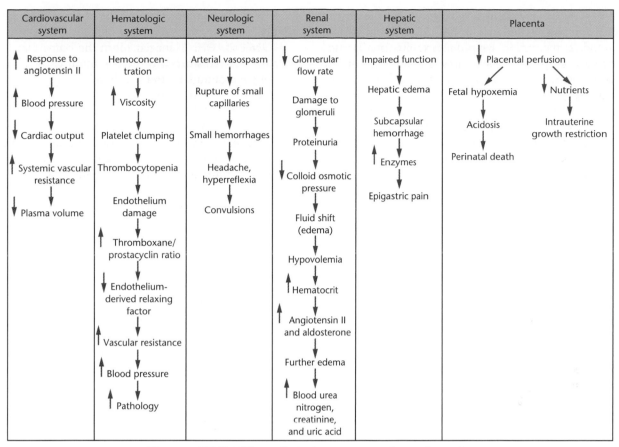

Cardiovascular system	Hematologic system	Neurologic system	Renal system	Hepatic system	Placenta
↑ Response to angiotensin II	Hemoconcentration	Arterial vasospasm	↓ Glomerular flow rate	Impaired function	↓ Placental perfusion
↑ Blood pressure	↑ Viscosity	Rupture of small capillaries	Damage to glomeruli	Hepatic edema	Fetal hypoxemia / Nutrients
↓ Cardiac output	Platelet clumping	Small hemorrhages	Proteinuria	Subcapsular hemorrhage	Acidosis / Intrauterine growth restriction
↑ Systemic vascular resistance	Thrombocytopenia	Headache, hyperreflexia	↓ Colloid osmotic pressure	↑ Enzymes	Perinatal death
↓ Plasma volume	Endothelium damage	Convulsions	Fluid shift (edema)	Epigastric pain	
	↑ Thromboxane/ prostacyclin ratio		Hypovolemia		
	↓ Endothelium-derived relaxing factor		↑ Hematocrit		
	↑ Vascular resistance		↑ Angiotensin II and aldosterone		
	↑ Blood pressure		Further edema		
	↑ Pathology		↑ Blood urea nitrogen, creatinine, and uric acid		

Figure 25-7 ■ The pathologic processes of preeclampsia.

and it may be severe. Edema may first manifest as a rapid weight gain caused by fluid retention. Edema may be present in the lower legs, which is common in pregnancy, and in the hands and face (Figure 25-8). Edema may be so massive that the woman's appearance is distorted. Edema may not, however, be present in all women who develop preeclampsia, and it may be severe in women who do not have the disorder. Pulmonary edema is also more common in women with massive edema from any cause, including drug therapy such as that given to stop preterm labor.

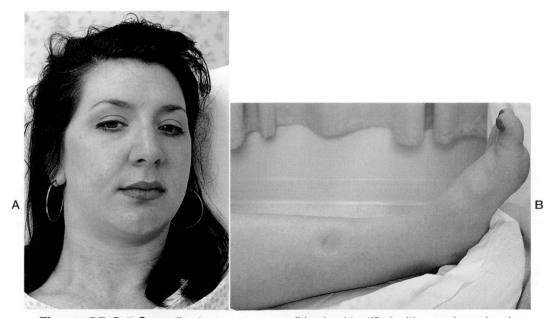

Figure 25-8 ■ Generalized edema is a possible sign identified with preeclampsia, although it may occur in normal pregnancy or in a pregnancy complicated by another disorder. **A,** Facial edema may be subtle. **B,** Pitting edema of the lower leg.

SYMPTOMS. Preeclampsia is dangerous for the woman and fetus for two reasons: (1) it can develop and worsen rapidly, and (2) the earliest symptoms are often not noticed by the woman. By the time she notices symptoms, the disease may have progressed to an advanced state with loss of valuable treatment time.

Certain symptoms, such as continuous headache, drowsiness, or mental confusion, indicate poor cerebral perfusion and may be precursors of seizures. Visual disturbances, such as blurred or double vision or spots before the eyes, indicate arterial spasms and edema in the retina. Numbness or tingling of the hands or feet occurs when nerves are compressed by retained fluid. Some symptoms, such as epigastric pain or "upset stomach," are particularly ominous because they indicate distention of the hepatic capsule and often warn that a seizure is imminent. Decreased urinary output indicates poor perfusion of the kidneys and may precede acute renal failure.

THERAPEUTIC MANAGEMENT OF MILD PREECLAMPSIA

The only cure for preeclampsia is delivery of the baby. However, the decision about delivery will be based on the severity of the hypertensive disorder and the degree of fetal maturity. If the fetus is less than 34 weeks of gestation, steroids to accelerate fetal lung maturity will be given and an attempt made to delay birth for 48 hours. However, if the maternal or fetal condition deteriorates, the infant will be delivered, regardless of fetal age or administration of steroids. Vaginal birth is preferred because of the multisystem impairments.

Preeclampsia is categorized as either mild or severe, depending on the presenting signs and symptoms (Table 25-2). However, an apparently mild condition can become severe in a very short time because the disease may progress rapidly.

HOME CARE. Management in the home may be possible for selected women if the condition is mild and they are not good candidates to have their labor induced, usually because of fetal immaturity. The woman must be in stable condition with a reassuring fetal status. She must be willing to adhere to a prescribed treatment plan that includes bed rest or reduced activity, home blood pressure monitoring, and follow-up visits to the physician every 3 to 4 days. The woman on home care should be taught how to check her blood pressure and the symptoms to report that suggest worsening preeclampsia, such as visual disturbance, severe headache, or epigastric pain. Symptoms that suggest a nonreassuring fetal status should also be taught, such as reduced fetal movement. If the woman is hospitalized with mild preeclampsia, the following assessments for home care are adapted for her inpatient care.

Activity Restrictions. The mother should rest frequently although full bed rest is not required for mild preeclampsia. A lateral position for at least $1\frac{1}{2}$ hr/day decreases pressure on the vena cava, thereby increasing cardiac return and circulatory volume and thus improving perfusion of the woman's vital organs and the placenta.

Blood Pressure. If monitoring of blood pressure is prescribed, the family must be taught to use electronic blood pressure equipment, readily available in drug, grocery, and discount stores. Blood pressure should be checked in the same arm and in the same position two to four times each day. A large cuff should be used for a woman with a large upper arm.

Weight. The woman should weigh herself each morning, preferably on the same scale and in clothing of similar weight.

TABLE 25-2 Mild Versus Severe Preeclampsia

Parameter Evaluated	Mild	Severe
Systolic blood pressure	≥140 but <160 mm Hg	≥160 mm Hg (two readings, 6 hours apart, while on bed rest)
Diastolic blood pressure	≥90 but <110 mm Hg	≥110 mm Hg
Proteinuria (24-hr specimen is preferred to eliminate hour-to-hour variations)	≥0.3 g but <2 g in 24-hr specimen (1+ on random dipstick)	≥5 g in 24-hr specimen (3+ or higher on random dipstick sample)
Creatinine, serum (renal function)	Normal	Elevated (>1.2 mg/dl)
Platelets	Normal	Decreased (<100,000 cells/mm³)
Liver enzymes (alanine aminotransferase [ALT] or aspartate aminotransferase [AST])	Normal or minimal increase in levels	Elevated levels
Urine output	Normal	Oliguria common, often <500 ml/day
Severe, unrelenting headache not attributable to other cause; mental confusion (cerebral edema)	Absent	Often present
Persistent right upper quadrant or epigastric pain or pain penetrating to the back (distention of the liver capsule); nausea and vomiting	Absent	May be present and often precedes seizure
Visual disturbances (spots or "sparkles"; temporary blindness; photophobia)	Absent to minimal	Common
Pulmonary edema; heart failure; cyanosis	Absent	May be present
Fetal growth restriction	Normal growth	Growth restriction; reduced amniotic fluid volume

From American Academy of Pediatrics & American College of Obstetricians and Gynecologists. (2002). *Guidelines for perinatal care* (5th ed.). Elk Grove, IL: Author; National High Blood Pressure Education Program Working Group on High Blood Pressure in Pregnancy. (2000). Report of the national high blood pressure education program working group on high blood pressure in pregnancy. *American Journal of Obstetrics and Gynecology, 183*(1), S1-S22.

Urinalysis. A urine dipstick test for protein, using the first voided midstream specimen, should be performed daily. The physician may request that she test at other times also.

Fetal Assessment. Because vasoconstriction can reduce placental flow, the woman will have increased fetal assessments to observe for evidence of fetal compromise. Fetal compromise can be evidenced by reduced fetal movement noted by the mother ("kick counts"), a nonreactive nonstress test, reduced amniotic fluid on ultrasound examination, or a biophysical profile score of 6 or lower. See Chapter 10 for discussion of fetal surveillance methods.

Diet. The diet should have ample protein and calories. Sodium and fluid should not be limited (Castro, 2004). The woman should be taught symptoms that indicate worsening of the preeclampsia and to report these at once. Indications of disease progression or fetal deterioration necessitate admission to the hospital.

INPATIENT MANAGEMENT OF SEVERE PREECLAMPSIA

Preeclampsia is severe if the systolic blood pressure is ≥ 160 mm Hg or the diastolic blood pressure is ≥ 110 mm Hg or if evidence of multisystem involvement is present (see Table 25-2). Delivery is usually necessary, even if the gestation is less than 34 weeks, because of disease severity. A decreased volume of amniotic fluid is considered significant because it suggests reduced placental blood flow, even if the blood pressures are not high.

ANTEPARTUM MANAGEMENT. Goals of management are to improve placental blood flow and fetal oxygenation and to prevent seizures and other maternal complications such as stroke as the woman's condition is stabilized before delivery.

BED REST. The woman is kept on bed rest in the lateral position, and her environment is kept quiet. External stimuli (lights, noise) that might precipitate a seizure should be reduced.

ANTIHYPERTENSIVE MEDICATIONS. If the woman's systolic blood pressure is ≥ 160 mm Hg or her diastolic blood pressure is ≥ 110 mm Hg, the risk for stroke or congestive heart failure is higher. Hydralazine (Apresoline) is often used because of its record of safety. Hydralazine's major advantage over other antihypertensives is that it is a vasodilator that increases cardiac output and blood flow to the placenta. Other antihypertensive medications such as nifedipine (a calcium channel blocker) or labetalol (a beta-adrenergic blocker) may be used. Caution is essential when antihypertensive medications are given to the woman receiving magnesium sulfate because hypotension may result, reducing placental perfusion.

ANTICONVULSANT MEDICATIONS. In the United States, magnesium sulfate is the drug most commonly given to prevent seizures. Phenytoin (Dilantin, Diphenylan) is sometimes used. Magnesium acts as a central nervous system (CNS) depressant by blocking neuromuscular transmission and decreasing the amount of acetylcholine liberated. Magnesium is not an antihypertensive medication, but it relaxes smooth muscle and therefore reduces vasoconstriction. Decreased vasoconstriction promotes circulation to the mother's vital organs and increases placental circulation, so some reduction in the blood pressure may occur. Increased circulation to the maternal kidneys leads to diuresis, as interstitial fluid is shifted into the vascular compartment and excreted.

Magnesium is usually administered by IV infusion, providing immediate onset of action without the discomfort associated with intramuscular administration. IV magnesium is administered via a secondary ("piggyback") line so that the medication can be discontinued at any time while the primary line remains open and functional.

Although magnesium sulfate is not risk-free, the major advantage of magnesium is its long record of safety for mother and baby while preventing maternal convulsions (Roberts, 2004). Fetal magnesium levels are nearly identical

---

DRUG GUIDE

HYDRALAZINE

Classification: Antihypertensive.

Action: Relaxes arterial smooth muscle to reduce blood pressure.

Indications: Used in preeclampsia when blood pressure is elevated to a degree that might be associated with intracranial bleeding.

Dosage and Route: Obstetric uses in pregnancy-induced hypertension: Intravenous doses: 5 to 10 mg may be administered as often as every 15 to 20 minutes if necessary. Duration of action is 3 to 8 hours (American College of Obstetrics and Gynecologists [ACOG], 2002; Roberts, 2004).

Absorption: Widely distributed, crosses the placenta; enters breast milk in minimal concentrations.

Excretion: Metabolized and excreted by the liver.

Contraindications and Precautions: Contraindicated in coronary artery disease, cerebrovascular disease, and hypersensitivity to hydralazine. Used cautiously in pregnancy; pregnancy category C.

Adverse Reactions: Headache, dizziness, drowsiness, hypotension that can interfere with uterine blood flow, epigastric pain, which may be confused with worsening preeclampsia.

Nursing Implications: Obstetric clients are hospitalized before initiation of antihypertensive medications. Blood pressure and pulse must be monitored every 2 to 3 minutes for 30 minutes after initial dose and periodically throughout the course of therapy. Therapy is repeated only when diastolic pressure exceeds limits set by physician or facility protocol, usually ≥105-110 mm Hg (ACOG, 2002; Roberts, 2004).

to those of the expectant mother. As a result, the fetal monitor tracing may show decreased fetal heart rate variability. No cumulative effect occurs, however, because the fetal kidneys excrete magnesium effectively.

The therapeutic serum level for magnesium is 4 to 8 mg/dl. Adverse reactions to magnesium sulfate usually occur if the serum level becomes too high. The most important is CNS depression, including depression of the respiratory center. Magnesium is excreted solely by the kidneys, and the reduced urine output that often occurs in preeclampsia allows magnesium to accumulate to toxic levels in the woman. Assessment of serum levels, deep tendon reflexes (Procedure 25-1), and respiratory rate and oxygen saturation can identify CNS depression before it progresses to respiratory depression or cardiac dysfunction. Monitoring urine output, usually with an indwelling catheter, identifies oliguria that may allow magnesium to accumulate and reach excessive levels. Policies related to care of the woman with hypertension and magnesium administration, such as specific assessments and lab studies, provide an organized framework for medical and nursing care.

INTRAPARTUM MANAGEMENT. Most seizures occur during labor or the first 24 hours after birth. The fetus and the expectant mother must be monitored continuously to detect signs of decreased fetal oxygenation and imminent seizures. The woman should be kept in a lateral position to promote circulation through the placenta, and efforts should focus on controlling pain that may cause agitation and precipitate seizures.

Oxytocin to stimulate uterine contractions and magnesium sulfate to prevent seizures are often administered simultaneously during labor when a woman has preeclampsia. The woman will have two secondary infusions in addition to her primary infusion line, one for oxytocin and one for magnesium. Infusion pumps should be used to ensure that the medications and fluids are administered at the prescribed rate, and equipment and IV lines should be checked carefully for correct placement and function.

Narcotic analgesics or epidural analgesia may be administered to provide comfort and to reduce painful stimuli that could precipitate a seizure. However, some women with severe preeclampsia have coagulation abnormalities that may contraindicate use of epidural analgesia.

Continuous electronic fetal monitoring identifies changes in fetal heart rate patterns that suggest compromise (see Chapter 14). Late decelerations, associated with reduced placental perfusion, or decreased variability, associated with reduced placental perfusion or magnesium use, is more likely to occur, but any other nonreassuring pattern may occur as well. Interventions are tailored to the nonreassuring fetal heart pattern identified, such as maternal oxygen administration, stopping the oxytocin infusion, and increases in the IV fluid rates.

A pediatrician, neonatologist, or neonatal nurse practitioner must be available to care for the newborn at birth. A resuscitation team is called to the delivery if needed.

POSTPARTUM MANAGEMENT. After birth, careful assessment of the mother's blood loss and signs of shock are essential because the hypovolemia caused by preeclampsia may be aggravated by blood loss during the delivery. Assessments for signs and symptoms of preeclampsia must be continued for at least 48 hours, and magnesium with its associated care usually is continued to prevent seizures for at least 24 hours.

DRUG GUIDE

MAGNESIUM SULFATE

Classification: Miscellaneous anticonvulsant.

Action: Decreases acetylcholine released by motor nerve impulses, thereby blocking neuromuscular transmission. Depresses the central nervous system (CNS) to act as an anticonvulsant; also decreases frequency and intensity of uterine contractions. Produces flushing and sweating because of decreased peripheral blood pressure.

Indications: Prevention and control of seizures in severe preeclampsia. Prevention of uterine contractions in preterm labor.

Dosage and Route: A common intravenous (IV) administration protocol for preeclampsia includes a loading dose and a continuous infusion using a controlled infusion pump. The loading dose is 4 to 6 g of magnesium sulfate administered in 100 ml of IV fluid over 15 to 20 minutes. The continuing infusion to maintain control is 2 g/hr. Doses are individualized as needed. Deep intramuscular injection is acceptable but is painful. A primary IV infusion with no medication is maintained if the magnesium must be discontinued.

Magnesium sulfate may also be administered in a similar dose profile to stop preterm labor contractions.

Absorption: Immediate onset after IV administration.

Excretion: Excreted by the kidneys.

Contraindications and Precautions: Contraindicated in persons with myocardial damage, heart block, myasthenia gravis, or impaired renal function. Magnesium toxicity, possibly related to incomplete renal drug excretion, may be evidenced by thirst, mental confusion, or a decrease in reflexes.

Adverse Reactions: Result from magnesium overdose and include flushing, sweating, hypotension, depressed deep tendon reflexes, and CNS depression, including respiratory depression.

Nursing Implications: Monitor blood pressure closely during administration. Assess client for respiratory rate above 12 breaths per minute, presence of deep tendon reflexes, and urinary output greater than 30 ml/hr before administering magnesium. Place resuscitation equipment (suction, oxygen) in the room. Keep calcium gluconate, which acts as an antidote to magnesium, in the room, along with syringes and needles.

25-1   Assessing Deep Tendon Reflexes

PURPOSE: **To identify exaggerated reflexes (hyperreflexia) or diminished reflexes (hyporeflexia)**

You will need a reflex hammer to best assess both the brachial and the patellar reflexes.

Support the woman's arm and instruct her to let it go limp while it is being held so that the arm is totally relaxed and slightly flexed as you assess the brachial reflex. If you have difficulty identifying the correct tendon to tap, have the woman flex and extend her arm until you can feel it moving beneath your thumb. Have her fully relax her arm after you identify the tendon.

Place your thumb over the woman's tendon, as illustrated, to allow you to feel as well as see the tendon response when the tendon is tapped. Strike the thumb with the small end of the triangular reflex hammer. The normal response is slight flexion of the forearm.

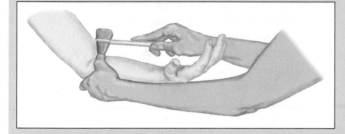

The patellar, or "knee-jerk," reflex can be assessed with the woman in two positions, sitting or lying. When the woman is sitting, allow her lower legs to dangle freely to flex the knee and stretch the tendons. If her patellar tendon is difficult to identify, have her flex and extend her lower legs slightly until you palpate the tendon. Strike the tendon directly with the reflex hammer just below the patella. The patellar reflex is less reliable if the woman has had epidural analgesia, and upper extremity reflexes should be assessed.

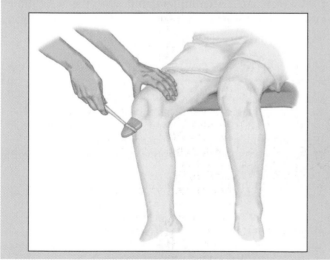

When the woman is supine, the weight of her leg must be supported to flex the knee and stretch the tendons. An accurate response requires that the limb be relaxed and the tendon partially stretched. Strike the partially stretched tendons just below the patella. Slight extension of the leg or a brief twitch of the quadriceps muscle of the thigh is the expected response.

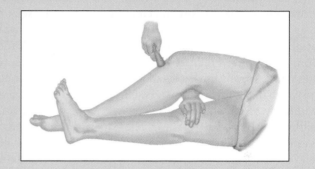

For assessment of clonus, the woman's lower leg should be supported, as illustrated, and the foot well dorsiflexed to stretch the tendon. Hold the flexion. If no clonus is present, no movement will be felt. When clonus (indicating hyperreflexia) is present, rapid rhythmic tapping motions of the foot are present.

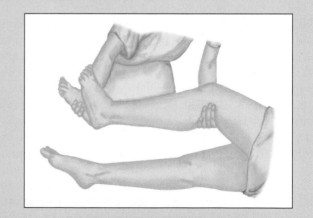

DEEP TENDON REFLEX RATING SCALE*

0	Reflex absent
+1	Reflex present, hypoactive
+2	Normal reflex
+3	Brisker than average reflex
+4	Hyperactive reflex; clonus may also be present

*The rating scales of some facilities omit the plus signs.

Signs that the woman is recovering from preeclampsia include the following:

- Urinary output of 4 to 6 L/day, which causes a rapid reduction in edema and rapid weight loss
- Decreased protein in the urine
- Return of blood pressure to normal, usually within 2 weeks

THERAPEUTIC MANAGEMENT OF ECLAMPSIA

Eclampsia is a potentially preventable extension of severe preeclampsia marked by one or more generalized seizures, at times occurring before the woman goes to the hospital. Early identification of preeclampsia in a pregnant woman allows intervention before the condition reaches the seizure stage in most cases. Generalized seizures usually start with facial twitching, followed by rigidity of the body. Tonic-clonic movements then begin and last for about 1 minute. Breathing stops during a seizure but resumes with a long, noisy inhalation. The woman is temporarily in a coma and is unlikely to remember the seizure when she resumes consciousness. Transient fetal heart rate patterns may be nonreassuring, such as bradycardia, loss of variability, or late decelerations. Fetal tachycardia may occur as the fetus compensates for the period of maternal apnea during the seizures. Eclampsia may occur during pregnancy or in the intrapartum or postpartum period.

Magnesium sulfate is the drug of choice to control eclamptic seizures. Other anticonvulsants or sedatives are not routinely given.

The woman's blood volume is often severely reduced in eclampsia, increasing the risk for poor placental perfusion. Fluid shifts from her intravascular space to the interstitial space, including the lungs, causing pulmonary edema and possibly heart failure as forward blood flow from the maternal heart is impeded. Renal blood flow is severely reduced, with oliguria (<30 ml/hr urine output) and possible renal failure. Cerebral hemorrhage may accompany eclampsia because of the high blood pressure and coagulation deficits. The woman's lungs should be auscultated at regular intervals, usually hourly. A pulse oximeter provides continuous readings of oxygen saturation. Furosemide (Lasix) may be administered if pulmonary edema develops. Oxygen by facemask at 8 to 10 L/min improves maternal and fetal oxygenation. Digitalis may be needed to strengthen contraction of the heart if circulatory failure results. Urine output should be assessed hourly; if output drops below 30 ml/hr, renal failure should be suspected.

Because eclampsia stimulates uterine irritability, the woman should be monitored carefully for ruptured membranes, signs of labor, or abruptio placentae. While the woman is unresponsive, she should be kept on her side to prevent aspiration and to improve placental circulation. The side rails should be padded and raised to prevent an injury from a fall. When vital signs have stabilized, delivery of the fetus is considered.

Aspiration of gastric contents is a leading cause of maternal morbidity after an eclamptic seizure. Equipment to suction the woman's airway should be immediately available. After initial stabilization the nurse should anticipate orders for chest radiography and arterial blood gas determination to identify aspiration.

Magnesium may be given intravenously to control the seizures. A sedative such as phenobarbital or diazepam is used only if magnesium fails to bring the seizures under control. Sedatives should not be given if birth is expected within 2 hours because of their depressant effects on the fetus.

Pulmonary edema, circulatory or renal failure, and intracranial hemorrhage are additional complications that may occur with severe preeclampsia or eclampsia. The woman's lungs should be auscultated frequently, and furosemide (Lasix) may be administered if pulmonary edema develops. Digitalis may be needed to strengthen heart function if circulatory failure results. Urine output should be assessed hourly. Urine output below 30 ml/hr may indicate renal failure.

The combination of hemolysis, elevated liver enzymes, and low platelets (HELLP syndrome) is associated with severe preeclampsia. DIC is an added complication of unexpected bleeding that may occur with coagulation abnormalities of severe preeclampsia or eclampsia. Lab studies are performed at frequent intervals to identify both falling and recovering coagulation values as well as identifying hemolysis and elevated liver enzymes.

The woman should be monitored for ruptured membranes, signs of labor, and abruptio placentae because eclampsia stimulates uterine irritability. While the woman is postictal (the unresponsive state after a seizure), she should be kept on her side to prevent aspiration and improve placental circulation. The side rails should be raised to prevent a fall and possible injury. After maternal and fetal conditions are stabilized, the fetus usually is delivered, either by induction of labor if the woman's cervix is favorable or by cesarean birth if she is farther from term.

Aspiration may cause maternal morbidity after an eclamptic seizure. After initial stabilization the nurse should expect orders for chest radiographs and arterial blood gases to identify whether aspiration has occurred.

✓ CHECK YOUR READING

14. What are the effects of vasospasm on the fetus?
15. What are the signs and symptoms of preeclampsia? Why is reduced activity one part of management?
16. What is the effect of vasospasm on the brain?
17. What are the effects of magnesium sulfate, including the primary adverse effect?
18. What are the major complications of eclampsia?

Application of the Nursing Process
Preeclampsia

Assessment

Nursing assessment is one of the most important components of successful management of preeclampsia. Careful assessment is the only way to determine whether the condition is responding to medical management or whether the disease is worsening. A one-to-one nurse-patient ratio is needed for the woman with severe pregnancy-induced hypertension.

Weigh the woman on admission and daily. Check vital signs and auscultate the chest at least every 4 hours for moist breath sounds that indicate pulmonary edema. Assess the location and severity of edema at least every 4 hours. Table 25-3 provides a guideline to describe edema. Insert an indwelling catheter to measure hourly urine output. Check the urine for protein every 4 hours. Apply an external electronic fetal monitor to identify changes in fetal heart rate, variability, or nonreassuring patterns. Consider maternal medications and their relationship to the fetal monitoring pattern.

Check reflexes such as brachial, radial, and patellar reflexes for hyperreflexia, which indicates cerebral irritability. Determine if clonus is present with hyperactive reflexes by dorsiflexing the woman's foot sharply and then releasing it while her knee is held in a flexed position. Clonus (rapidly alternating muscle contraction and relaxation) may occur when reflexes are hyperactive. If clonus is present, it should be reported to the physician. Procedure 25-1 illustrates how to assess and rate deep tendon reflexes.

Question the woman carefully about symptoms she may be experiencing, such as headache, visual disturbances, epigastric pain, nausea or vomiting, or a sudden increase in edema.

■ Detailed questions are usually needed to identify important symptoms. Ask targeted questions, such as "Do you have a headache? Describe it for me." "Do you have any pain in the abdomen? Show me where it is and describe it." "Do you see spots before your eyes? Flashes of light?" "Do you have double vision?" "Is your vision blurred?" "Does the light bother you?" "I see you have removed your rings. Did you do that because your hands were swollen? When did that happen?"

ASSESSMENTS FOR MAGNESIUM TOXICITY

Obstetric units have protocols that address routine assessments when magnesium is being administered and their frequency. Reflexes may be slightly hypotonic but should not be absent at therapeutic levels of magnesium. Absent reflexes suggest CNS depression that precedes respiratory depression if magnesium levels are too high. Determining the respiratory rate and oxygen saturations by pulse oximetry identifies the adequacy of maternal respirations. Checking urine output identifies oliguria (<30 ml/hr) that may result in magnesium toxicity as the drug accumulates. Assess the woman's level of consciousness (alert, drowsy [expected], confused, oriented). Table 25-4 summarizes nursing assessments and their implications.

PSYCHOSOCIAL ASSESSMENT

The development of preeclampsia places added stress on the childbearing family. The woman may be on reduced activity at home if the condition is mild and her gestation is early. She may be hospitalized, complicating child care. This creates anxiety about the condition of the fetus and that of the expectant mother. Many families do not understand the seriousness of the disease. After all, the woman often feels well after its onset, especially if her preeclampsia does not advance rapidly. The possibility that a preterm birth may be

TABLE 25-3 Assessment of Edema

Characteristics	Grade
Minimal edema of lower extremities	+1
Marked edema of lower extremities	+2
Edema of lower extremities, face, hands, and sacral area	+3
Generalized massive edema that includes ascites (accumulation of fluid in peritoneal cavity)	+4

TABLE 25-4 Nursing Assessments for Preeclampsia and Magnesium Toxicity

Assessment	Implications
Daily weight	Provides estimate of fluid retention.
Blood pressure	To determine worsening condition, response to treatment, or both.
Respiratory rate, pulse oximeter readings	Drug therapy (magnesium sulfate) causes respiratory depression, and drug should be withheld and the physician notified if respiratory rate is <12/min or as specified by hospital policy. Pulse oximeter readings 95% or greater.
Breath sounds	To identify sounds of excess moisture in lungs associated with pulmonary edema.
Deep tendon reflexes	Hyperreflexia indicates increased cerebral irritability and edema; hyporeflexia is associated with magnesium excess.
Edema	For estimation of interstitial fluid.
Urinary output	Output of at least 30 ml/hr indicates adequate perfusion of the kidneys (25 ml/hr is used by some authorities). Magnesium levels may become toxic if urinary output is inadequate.
Urine protein	Normal protein in a random dipstick urine sample is negative or trace. Higher protein levels suggest greater leaking of protein secondary to glomerular damage with worsening preeclampsia. A 24-hour urine sample is most accurate for quantitative urine protein level.
Level of consciousness	Drowsiness or dulled sensorium indicates therapeutic effects of magnesium; no responsive behavior or muscle weakness is associated with magnesium excess.
Headache, epigastric pain, visual problems	These symptoms indicate increasing severity of the condition caused by cerebral edema, vasospasm of cerebral vessels, and liver edema. Eclampsia may develop quickly.
Fetal heart rate and baseline variability	Rate should be between 110 and 160 beats per minute in a term fetus. Decreasing baseline variability may be caused by therapeutic magnesium level or by inadequate placental perfusion.
Laboratory data	Elevated serum creatinine, elevated liver enzymes, or decreased platelets (thrombocytopenia) are significant signs of increasing severity of disease. Serum magnesium levels should be in the therapeutic range designated by the physician.

necessary to reduce harm to mother and infant adds to the family's concerns about the outcome.

Explore how the family will function while the expectant mother is hospitalized. Determine how the woman is adapting to the "sick role" and the necessity of being dependent on others instead of functioning in her primary role. Ask how much support is available and who is willing to participate. Determine if referrals to manage loss of in-

come are needed. Finally, determine the priority concerns of the family.

Analysis

Analysis of the data collected can lead to both nursing diagnoses (see Nursing Care Plan 25-2) and collaborative problems for potential complications. Both physician-prescribed and nurse-prescribed interventions are used to minimize the com-

---

NURSING CARE PLAN 25-2 Preeclampsia

ASSESSMENT: Julie Frost, a 16-year-old primigravida, is seen in the prenatal clinic at 30 weeks of gestation. Her blood pressure is 136/90, and there is some edema of the lower legs and trace proteinuria. She is given instructions about home care for pregnancy-induced hypertension. The regimen includes bed rest; frequent monitoring of blood pressure, weight, and urine; and doing fetal "kick counts." Julie is told she must return to the clinic in a week. She states that she feels fine and doesn't want to miss school. She says that she doesn't see the reason for bed rest.

NURSING DIAGNOSIS: Impaired Adjustment related to lack of knowledge of health status and the need for a change in lifestyle

GOALS/EXPECTED OUTCOMES: Julie will:
1. Verbalize the benefits of the recommended regimen by the end of the first prenatal appointment.
2. Comply with the recommended care for the next week.
3. Keep prenatal appointments.

INTERVENTION	RATIONALE
1. Allow Julie to verbalize her feelings about the recommended regimen: "What concerns you most about missing school?" Acknowledge her feelings as important: "It must be difficult to think of falling behind in your schoolwork. It isn't any fun to miss all the after-school activities or time with your friends."	1. When feelings are identified and acknowledged as important, anxiety decreases and teaching and learning can begin.
2. Identify family support that is likely to improve compliance with the recommended regimen of bed rest and home care.	2. Compliance with the regimen is impossible without family assistance, which includes assistance with activities of daily living and necessary assessments.
3. Describe in general terms the pathophysiologic processes that affect Julie and her fetus.	3. Expectant mothers are usually motivated to comply with a therapeutic regimen that will benefit the fetus.
4. Explain that Julie may feel well even when the condition worsens and that she must be observed for signs and symptoms at home and at the clinic.	4. The expectant mother does not notice hypertension and proteinuria. Although edema is not always present in hypertensive complications during pregnancy, clients may not be aware that it may also be associated with other disorders.
5. Instruct Julie to call the clinic if she notices headache, double vision, or spots before her eyes.	5. These signs indicate rapid progression of the disease and the prompt necessity for additional management.
6. Collaborate with Julie to arrange for contact with her boyfriend or selected friends and to arrange for ongoing home-bound classes.	6. Such an agreement will allow a schedule to provide peer support but allow for prolonged periods of quiet. Home-bound classes alleviate the concern that she is falling behind with schoolwork.

EVALUATION: Despite following the recommended regimen of bed rest with the help of her mother and sister and keeping prenatal appointments, Julie's condition worsens. She develops a rise in blood pressure and a rapid gain in weight, indicating generalized edema, at 32 weeks.

ASSESSMENT: Julie is admitted to the hospital at 32 weeks of gestation with a blood pressure of 160/110, heart rate of 92, and respiratory rate of 22 per minute. There is 2+ proteinuria and marked edema of the hands and face as well as her lower extremities. Fetal heart rate is 136 with average variability. An intravenous infusion of magnesium sulfate is started, seizure precautions are initiated, and environmental stimuli are reduced. Julie is agitated and verbalizes concern that the procedures are going to hurt her or the fetus. She frequently asks, "How sick am I?" "Is the baby going to be okay?" Her hands are perspiring, and they shake when she reaches for a tissue.

NURSING DIAGNOSIS: Anxiety related to hospitalization and concern about her health and the health of the fetus

plication. Potential complications for the woman with preeclampsia are eclamptic seizures and magnesium toxicity.

Planning

Client-centered goals are inappropriate for the potential complications of eclamptic seizures and magnesium toxicity because the nurse cannot independently manage these conditions but must confer with physicians and use established protocols for treatment. For seizures, planning should reflect the nurse's responsibility to do the following:

- Perform actions that minimize the risk of seizures and prevent injury if seizures do occur
- Monitor for signs of impending seizures
- Consult with the physician if signs of impending seizures are observed
- Support the family of the woman with eclampsia

NURSING CARE PLAN 25-2 Preeclampsia—cont'd

GOALS/EXPECTED OUTCOMES: Julie will:
1. Verbalize her concerns and describe the benefits of the treatment while her family is present
2. Manifest less anxiety (agitation, physiologic signs such as tremors, tachycardia, and perspiration)

INTERVENTION	RATIONALE

1. Initiate measures to reduce anxiety:
  a. Provide positive reassurance that a solution for anxiety can be found: "I can see you are really worried, and I will try to answer all your questions."
  b. Allow Julie to cry, get angry, or express any feeling that is present.
  c. Encourage a discussion of feelings: "Tell me more about how you feel."
  d. Reflect observations: "I see you wringing your hands; do you want to talk about it?"
  e. Convey empathy and positive regard; use nonverbal behavior, including touch, when appropriate.
	1. Anxiety is an ominous feeling of tension resulting from a physical or emotional threat to the self. It is a global, often unnamed sense of doom, a feeling of helplessness, isolation, and insecurity. Anxiety needs to be ventilated and then addressed by conveying that the person is not alone and will be protected.

2. Provide information about hospital routines and procedures when Julie's anxiety has diminished enough for learning to take place:
  a. Be very specific about procedures, such as fetal monitoring, assessment of deep tendon reflexes, taking of vital signs, and care specific for magnesium sulfate therapy. Explain the reasons for these procedures, who will perform them, and how long they will be continued after birth.
  b. Focus on Julie's present concerns; she is not able to be future oriented at this time.
  c. Speak slowly and calmly, give very short directions, and do not ask Julie to make decisions: "Turn on your side." "Breathe slowly."
  d. Allow a friend or family member to remain with Julie, and instruct the person about the need for a low-stimulus environment.
	2. Knowledge of procedures to be performed and the purpose of these procedures provides a sense of control that reduces anxiety. Perception is somewhat narrowed when anxiety is high; therefore brief instructions are easier for the anxious person to understand than long explanations.

EVALUATION: Julie discusses her feelings with the nurse and with her sister. She feels in control of anxiety, as manifested by fewer signs of agitation and fewer physiologic signs (tachycardia, tachypnea) and by the ability to use relaxation techniques.

CRITICAL THINKING:
1. What two potential complications cause the greatest concern for nurses who care for Julie?
2. Why do nurses not develop goals for these problems?
3. What are the nurses' responsibilities for these complications?

ANSWERS
1. The most common complications that cause the greatest concern are magnesium toxicity and generalized seizures.
2. These are collaborative problems that require collaboration with physicians for management. The nurse does not independently manage magnesium toxicity or seizures.
3. The nurse must monitor for signs of these conditions, administer prescribed medications, observe and report Julie's response to the medications, and collaborate with the physicians to lessen the chance that these complications will occur.

The following steps are necessary in cases of magnesium toxicity:

- Monitor for signs of magnesium toxicity.
- Consult with the physician if signs of magnesium toxicity are observed.
- Perform actions that reduce the possibility of magnesium toxicity.

Interventions

INTERVENTIONS FOR SEIZURES

MONITORING FOR SIGNS OF IMPENDING SEIZURES. Signs of impending seizures include the following:

- Hyperreflexia, possibly accompanied by clonus
- Increasing signs of cerebral irritability (headache, visual disturbances)
- Epigastric or right upper quadrant pain, nausea, or vomiting

None of these signs is a predictor of imminent seizure. Nurses must be alert for subtle changes and be prepared for seizures in all women with preeclampsia.

INITIATING PREVENTIVE MEASURES. In the presence of cerebral irritability, generalized seizures may be precipitated by excessive visual or auditory stimuli. Nurses should reduce external stimuli by doing the following:

- Admitting the woman to a private room in the *quietest* section of the unit and keeping the door to the room closed. Intense nursing observation is needed regardless of the specific room location that is available.
- Padding the door to reduce noise when the door must be opened and closed.
- Keeping lights low and noise to a minimum. This may include blocking incoming telephone calls and turning the noises of the electronic monitors (fetal monitor, pulse oximeter, IV pump) as low as possible.
- Grouping nursing assessments and care to allow the woman periods of undisturbed quiet.
- Moving carefully and calmly around the room and avoiding bumping into the bed or startling the woman.
- Collaborating with the woman and her family to restrict visitors.

PREVENTING SEIZURE-RELATED INJURY. Hard side rails should be padded and the bed kept in the lowest position with the wheels locked to prevent trauma during a seizure.

Oxygen and suction equipment should be assembled and ready to use to suction secretions and to provide oxygen if it is not already being administered. Check equipment and connections at the beginning of each shift because sufficient time for setup will not exist if seizures occur.

A preeclampsia tray or box should be in the room. Typical contents include a medium plastic airway, an Ambu bag with mask, an ophthalmoscope, a tourniquet, a reflex hammer, and syringes and needles. Medications that should be on hand include magnesium sulfate, sodium bicarbonate, heparin, epinephrine, phenytoin, and calcium gluconate.

PROTECTING THE WOMAN AND FETUS DURING A SEIZURE. Nurses must protect the woman and the fetus during a seizure. The nurse's primary responsibilities are the following:

- Remain with the woman and press the emergency bell for assistance.
- If she is not on her side already, attempt to turn the woman onto her side when the tonic phase begins. A side-lying position permits greater circulation through the placenta and may prevent aspiration.
- Note the time and sequence of the seizure. Eclampsia is marked by a tonic-clonic seizure that may be preceded by facial twitching that lasts for a few seconds. A tonic contraction of the entire body is followed by the clonic phase, which may last about a minute.
- Insert an airway after the seizure, and suction the woman's mouth and nose to prevent aspiration. Administer oxygen by mask at 8 to 10 L/min to increase oxygenation of the placenta and all maternal body organs.
- Notify the physician that a seizure has occurred. This is an obstetric emergency that is associated with cerebral hemorrhage, abruptio placentae, severe fetal hypoxia, and death.
- Administer medications and prepare for additional medical interventions as directed by the physician.

PROVIDING INFORMATION AND SUPPORT FOR THE FAMILY. Explain to the family what has happened without minimizing the seriousness of the situation. A generalized seizure is frightening for anyone who witnesses it, and the family often is reassured when the nurse explains that the seizure lasts for only a few minutes and that the woman will be unconscious, then drowsy for some time afterward. Acknowledge that the seizure indicates worsening of the condition and that it will be necessary for the physician to determine future management, which may include delivery of the infant as soon as possible. Vaginal birth is preferred if the maternal and fetal conditions permit because of abnormalities in the coagulation and other body systems.

INTERVENTIONS FOR MAGNESIUM TOXICITY

MONITORING FOR SIGNS OF MAGNESIUM TOXICITY. Magnesium excess depresses the entire CNS, including the brainstem, which controls respirations and cardiac function, and the cerebrum, which controls memory, mental processes, and speech. Carbon dioxide accumulates if the respiratory rate is reduced, leading to respiratory acidosis and further CNS depression, which could culminate in respiratory arrest.

Signs of magnesium toxicity include the following:

- Respiratory rate of less than 12 breaths per minute (hospitals may specify a rate of less than 14 breaths per minute)
- Maternal pulse oximeter reading lower than 95%

- Absence of deep tendon reflexes
- Sweating, flushing
- Altered sensorium (confused, lethargic, slurred speech, drowsy, disoriented)
- Hypotension
- Serum magnesium above the therapeutic range of 4 to 8 mg/dl

RESPONDING TO SIGNS OF MAGNESIUM TOXICITY. Discontinue magnesium if the respiratory rate is below 12 breaths per minute, a low pulse oximeter level (<95%) persists, or deep tendon reflexes are absent. Additional magnesium will make the condition worse. Notify the physician of the woman's condition for additional orders. If the urinary output falls below 30 ml/hr, the physician is notified so that the drug's administration can be adjusted to maintain a therapeutic range.

Calcium opposes the effects of magnesium at the neuromuscular junction, and it should be readily available whenever magnesium is administered. Magnesium toxicity can be reversed by IV administration of 1 g (10 ml of 10% solution) calcium gluconate at 1 ml/min.

Evaluation

Collect and compare data with established norms and then judge whether the data are within normal limits. For seizures, interventions are judged to be successful if

- Reflexes remain within normal limits (+1 to +3)
- The woman is free of visual disturbances, headache, and epigastric or right upper quadrant pain
- The woman remains free of seizures or free of preventable injury if a seizure occurs

For magnesium toxicity, determine whether respiratory rates remain at least 12 breaths per minute, deep tendon reflexes are present and not hyperactive, and maternal plasma levels of magnesium do not exceed the therapeutic range of 4 to 8 mg/dl.

✔ **CHECK YOUR READING**

19. What nursing assessments should be made for the woman with preeclampsia? Why?
20. What measures may be initiated to prevent or manage seizures?
21. How can injury during seizure be prevented?
22. What are the signs of magnesium toxicity? How should it be managed?

HEMOLYSIS, ELEVATED LIVER ENZYMES, AND LOW PLATELETS (HELLP) SYNDROME

The acronym *HELLP* (hemolysis, elevated liver enzymes, low platelets) refers to a life-threatening occurrence that complicates about 10% of pregnancies. Half of the women affected with HELLP also have severe preeclampsia, although hypertension may be absent. As in preeclampsia,

HELLP syndrome may occur during the postpartum period (Abramovici, Mattar, & Sibai, 2000; Moldenhauer & Sibai, 2003).

Hemolysis is believed to occur as a result of the fragmentation and distortion of erythrocytes during passage through small damaged blood vessels. Liver enzyme levels increase when hepatic blood flow is obstructed by fibrin deposits. Hyperbilirubinemia and jaundice may occur as a result of liver impairment. Low platelet levels are caused by vascular damage resulting from vasospasm; platelets aggregate at sites of damage, resulting in thrombocytopenia, which increases the risk for bleeding, usually in the liver.

The prominent symptom of the HELLP syndrome is pain in the right upper quadrant, the lower right chest, or the midepigastric area. There may also be tenderness because of liver distention. Additional signs and symptoms include nausea, vomiting, and severe edema. It is important to avoid traumatizing the liver by abdominal palpation and to use care in transporting the woman. A sudden increase in intraabdominal pressure, including a seizure, could lead to rupture of a subcapsular hematoma, resulting in internal bleeding and hypovolemic shock. Hepatic rupture can lead to fetal and maternal mortality (August, 2004; Moldenhauer & Sibai, 2003; Riely & Fallon, 2004).

Women with the HELLP syndrome should be managed in a setting with intensive care facilities available. Treatment includes magnesium sulfate to control seizures and hydralazine to control the blood pressure. Fluid replacement is managed to avoid worsening the woman's reduced intravascular volume without giving her too much, which could cause pulmonary edema or ascites. Cervical ripening with labor induction usually is done if the gestation is at least 34 weeks. Delivery may be delayed if the gestation is less than 34 weeks and the woman's condition is stable to give steroids a chance to stimulate fetal lung maturation (Landon, 2004). After delivery, most women begin recovering within 72 hours.

CHRONIC HYPERTENSION

A diagnosis of chronic hypertension is made whenever evidence suggests that hypertension preceded the pregnancy or when a woman is hypertensive before 20 weeks' gestation. Chronic hypertension is seen most often in older women, in those who are obese, and in those with diabetes. Heredity, including race, plays a role in the development of chronic hypertension, which is more common in African-Americans at any age than in people of other races (National Center for Health Statistics, 2004). Late childbearing and rising obesity rates will no doubt fuel an increase in hypertension. Chronic hypertension is usually essential, or primary. However, it may be secondary to another problem, such as renal disease or an autoimmune disorder (Cunningham et al., 2001; Moldenhauer & Sibai, 2003).

Because of the natural fall in blood pressure during early pregnancy, the woman's blood pressure may appear normal when she enters prenatal care. If she already is taking an antihypertensive drug, she usually continues this drug unless her blood pressure becomes low because of the vasodilators of pregnancy. If she is not on an antihypertensive drug, she may be placed on one if her diastolic pressure is consistently above 90 mm Hg.

The most common maternal hazard is the development of preeclampsia, which occurs in 20% of pregnant women with chronic hypertension. New-onset proteinuria or a significant rise in preexisting proteinuria identifies the development of superimposed preeclampsia. The rise in blood pressure with preeclampsia is likely to be greater in these women (Cunningham et al., 2001; National High Blood Pressure Education Program Working Group on High Blood Pressure in Pregnancy, 2000; Roberts, 2004).

A dietitian should be consulted about the appropriate diet and weight gain, because many of these women are obese and they frequently have diabetes. Adequate intake of protein helps counteract the protein lost in urine. A reduced salt intake may be advised, unlike recommendations for the woman with preeclampsia alone. More frequent prenatal visits will be needed. Regular fetal surveillance by biophysical profile and kick counts (see Chapter 10) is the usual method for identification of poor growth patterns or signs that are nonreassuring, such as a falling amount of amniotic fluid.

Antihypertensive medications must be chosen carefully because they may reduce placental blood flow. Antihypertensive medication should be initiated if the diastolic pressure remains higher than 100 mm Hg in early pregnancy (Roberts, 2004). Methyldopa (Aldomet) is the drug of choice because of its record of safety and effectiveness in pregnancy. β-Blockers and calcium channel blockers may also be used if methyldopa is not effective, but their record of safety in pregnancy is less well established. Angiotensin-converting enzyme (ACE) inhibitors are not recommended in pregnancy but may be used in the postpartum period. Hydralazine is a vasodilator reserved for hypertensive crisis. Diuretics are avoided if possible because they may shrink the blood volume, which may already be reduced if preeclampsia exists with the chronic hypertension. If regular diuretics are needed, thiazides are considered safe for pregnancy.

✔ CHECK YOUR READING

23. What is the unabbreviated form of the term *HELLP*? What are the prominent signs and symptoms of this syndrome? Why should the liver not be palpated?
24. Compare preeclampsia with chronic hypertension in terms of onset and treatment.

INCOMPATIBILITY BETWEEN MATERNAL AND FETAL BLOOD

Rh Incompatibility

Rhesus (Rh) factor incompatibility during pregnancy is possible only when two specific circumstances coexist: (1) the expectant mother is Rh-negative, and (2) the fetus is Rh-positive. For such a circumstance to occur, the father of the fetus must be Rh-positive. Rh incompatibility is a problem that affects the fetus; it causes no harm to the expectant mother.

Rh-negative blood is an autosomal recessive trait, and a person must inherit the same gene from both parents to be Rh-negative. Approximately 15% of the white population in the United States is Rh-negative. The incidence is lower in the African-American and Asian populations.

PATHOPHYSIOLOGY

People who are Rh-positive have the Rh antigen on their red blood cells, whereas people who are Rh-negative do not have the antigen. When blood from a person who is Rh-positive enters the bloodstream of a person who is Rh-negative, the body reacts as it would to any foreign substance: it develops antibodies to destroy the invading antigen. To destroy the Rh antigen, which exists as part of the red blood cell, the entire red blood cell must be destroyed. Exposure of the Rh-negative male or female to Rh-positive blood may occur unrelated to a pregnancy, such as emergency blood transfusion Rh-negative blood. Destruction of Rh-positive cells occurs in the Rh-negative person after they have become sensitized to the Rh-positive antigens.

Theoretically, fetal and maternal blood do not mix during pregnancy. In reality, small placental accidents occur that allow a drop or two of fetal blood to enter the maternal circulation and initiate the production of antibodies to destroy the Rh-positive blood. Sensitization also can occur during a spontaneous or elective abortion or during antepartal procedures such as amniocentesis and chorionic villus sampling (Figure 25-9). A rapid immune response against Rh-positive blood occurs with an extensive fetal-maternal hemorrhage in complications like placenta previa or abruptio placentae (p. 634) or with an uncomplicated birth.

Most exposure of maternal blood to fetal blood occurs during the third stage of labor, when active exchange of fetal and maternal blood may occur from damaged placental vessels. In this case the woman's first child is not usually affected because antibodies are formed after the birth of the infant. Subsequent Rh-positive fetuses may be affected, however, unless the mother receives $Rh_o(D)$ immune globulin (RhoGAM) to prevent antibody formation after the birth of each Rh-positive infant.

FETAL AND NEONATAL IMPLICATIONS

If antibodies to the Rh factor are present in the expectant mother's blood, they cross the placenta and destroy fetal erythrocytes. The fetus becomes deficient in red blood cells, which are needed to transport oxygen to fetal tissue. As fetal red blood cells are destroyed, fetal bilirubin levels increase (icterus gravis), which can lead to neurologic disease (kernicterus, leading to bilirubin encephalopathy). This hemolytic process results in rapid production of erythroblasts (immature red blood cells), which cannot carry oxygen. The entire syndrome is termed *erythroblastosis fetalis*. The fetus may become so anemic that generalized fetal edema (hydrops fetalis) results and can end in fetal congestive heart failure.

Management of the infant born with erythroblastosis fetalis is discussed in Chapter 30.

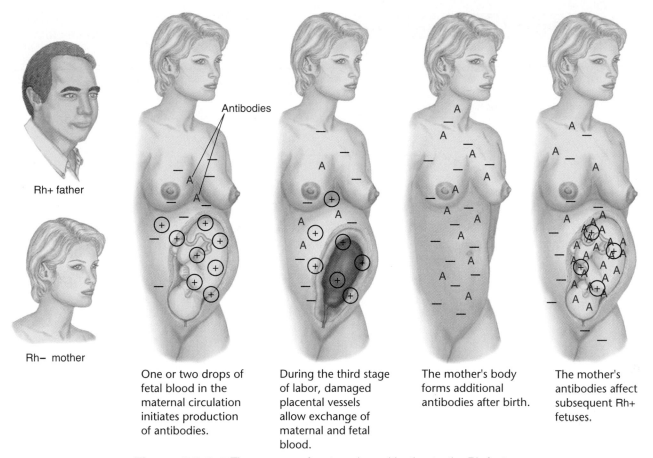

| Rh+ father | | | | |

Antibodies

Rh− mother

One or two drops of fetal blood in the maternal circulation initiates production of antibodies.

During the third stage of labor, damaged placental vessels allow exchange of maternal and fetal blood.

The mother's body forms additional antibodies after birth.

The mother's antibodies affect subsequent Rh+ fetuses.

Figure 25-9 ■ The process of maternal sensitization to the Rh factor.

CRITICAL TO REMEMBER

Treatment for Rh-Negative Women

All unsensitized Rh-negative women should receive $Rh_o(D)$ immune globulin (RhoGAM) after abortion, ectopic pregnancy, chorionic villus sampling, amniocentesis, or birth of an Rh-positive infant. RhoGAM prevents the development of Rh antibodies that would result in destruction of fetal erythrocytes in subsequent pregnancies.

PRENATAL ASSESSMENT AND MANAGEMENT

Women should have a blood test to determine blood type and Rh factor at the initial prenatal visit. Rh-negative women should have an indirect Coombs' test to determine whether they are sensitized (have developed antibodies) as a result of previous exposure to Rh-positive blood. If the indirect Coombs' test is negative, it is repeated at 28 weeks of gestation to identify if they have developed subsequent sensitization.

$Rh_o(D)$ immune globulin (such as RhoGAM) is administered to the unsensitized Rh-negative woman at 28 weeks of gestation to prevent sensitization, which may occur from small leaks of fetal blood across the placenta. $Rh_o(D)$ immune globulin is a commercial preparation of passive antibodies against Rh factor. It effectively prevents the formation of active antibodies against Rh-positive erythrocytes if a small amount of fetal Rh-positive blood enters the circulation of the Rh-negative mother during the remainder of the pregnancy. $Rh_o(D)$ immune globulin is repeated after birth if the woman delivers an Rh-positive infant.

If the indirect Coombs' test result is positive, indicating maternal sensitization and the presence of antibodies, it is repeated at frequent intervals throughout the pregnancy to determine whether the antibody titer is rising. An increase in titer indicates that the process is continuing and that the fetus will be in jeopardy.

Amniocentesis may be performed to determine the Rh factor of the fetus and to evaluate change in the optical density (ΔOD) of amniotic fluid. If the fluid optical density remains low, it may indicate that the fetus is Rh-negative or that the fetus is Rh-positive but in no jeopardy. DNA analysis allows determination of the Rh factor of the fetus from amniotic fluid cells with high accuracy, reducing uncertainty when other testing results fall in the borderline zone. For example, if the optical density is slightly elevated but DNA testing shows the fetus to be Rh-negative, amniocentesis can eliminate the need to test further for Rh-related problems.

The optical density reflects the amount of bilirubin, the residue of red blood cell destruction, which is present in the amniotic fluid. If the fluid optical density remains low, it may indicate that the fetus is Rh-positive but in no jeopardy. An elevated optical density suggests fetal jeopardy.

Ultrasound examination also is used to evaluate the condition of the fetus. Generalized fetal edema, ascites, enlarged heart, or hydramnios indicates serious fetal compromise. A cordocentesis may be performed to evaluate the

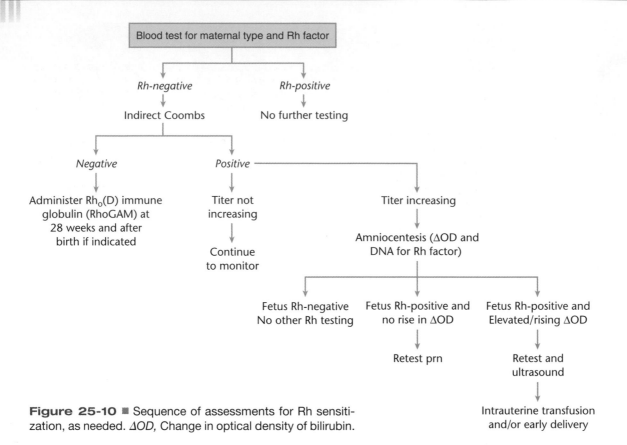

Figure 25-10 ■ Sequence of assessments for Rh sensitization, as needed. *ΔOD,* Change in optical density of bilirubin.

fetal hematocrit, and an intrauterine transfusion may follow if the preterm fetus is anemic (Figure 25-10).

POSTPARTUM MANAGEMENT

If the mother is Rh-negative, umbilical cord blood is taken at delivery to determine blood type, Rh factor, and antibody titer (direct Coombs' test) of the newborn. Rh-negative, unsensitized mothers who give birth to Rh-positive infants are given an intramuscular injection of $Rh_o(D)$ immune globulin (RhoGAM) within 72 hours after delivery. If RhoGAM is given to the mother in the first 72 hours after delivery of an Rh-positive infant, Rh antigens present in her blood are destroyed before she forms antibodies to the Rh factor. If the infant is Rh-negative, Rh antibody formation does not occur and RhoGAM is not necessary.

Families often are concerned about the fetus, and nurses must be sensitive to cues that indicate that the family is anxious and must be able to offer honest reassurance. This is especially important if the expectant mother is sensitized and fetal testing is necessary throughout pregnancy (Box 25-3).

BOX 25-3 Nursing Diagnoses for the Woman with a Complication of Pregnancy

Anxiety*
Deficient Diversional Activity
Fear
Impaired Adjustment*
Deficient Knowledge*
Risk for Dysfunctional Family Processes
Risk for Infection
Situational Low Self-Esteem*

*Nursing diagnoses explored in this chapter.

During labor the nurse must carefully label the tube of cord blood obtained for analysis of the newborn's blood type and Rh factor. During the postpartum period, nurses are responsible for follow-up to determine whether RhoGAM is necessary and for administering the injection within the prescribed time.

ABO Incompatibility

ABO incompatibility occurs when the mother is blood type O and the fetus is blood type A, B, or AB. Types A, B, and AB blood contain a protein component (antigen) that is not present in type O blood.

People with type O blood develop anti-A or anti-B antibodies naturally as a result of exposure to antigens in the foods that they eat or to infection by gram-negative bacteria. As a result, some women with blood type O have developed high serum anti-A and anti-B antibody titers before pregnancy. The antibodies may be either IgG or IgM. When the woman becomes pregnant, the IgG antibodies cross the placental barrier and cause hemolysis of fetal red blood cells. Although the first fetus can be affected, ABO incompatibility is less severe than Rh incompatibility because the primary antibodies of the ABO system are IgM, which do not readily cross the placenta.

No specific prenatal care is needed; however, the nurse must be aware of the possibility of ABO incompatibility. During the delivery, cord blood is taken to determine the blood type of the newborn and the antibody titer (direct Coombs' test). The newborn is carefully screened for jaundice, which indicates hyperbilirubinemia. See Chapter 30 for medical and nursing management of hyperbilirubinemia in newborns.

DRUG GUIDE

RH₀(D) IMMUNE GLOBULIN (RHOGAM, HYPRHOD, GAMULIN RH)

Classification: Concentrated immunoglobulins directed toward the red blood cell antigen Rh₀(D).

Action: Prevents production of anti-Rh₀(D) antibodies in Rh-negative women who have been exposed to Rh-positive blood by suppressing the immune reaction of the Rh-negative woman to the antigen in Rh-positive blood; prevents antibody response and thereby prevents hemolytic disease of the newborn in future Rh-positive pregnancies. Used for both males and females who are Rh-negative but exposed to Rh-positive blood or for immune thrombocytopenic purpura (ITP).

Indications (Pregnancy Related): Administered to Rh-negative women who have been exposed to Rh-positive blood by

1. Delivering an Rh-positive infant
2. Aborting an Rh-positive fetus
3. Undergoing chorionic villus sampling, amniocentesis, or intraabdominal trauma while carrying an Rh-positive fetus
4. Receiving inadvertent transfusion of Rh-positive blood

Dosage and Route: One *standard* dose (300 mcg) administered intramuscularly:

1. At 28 weeks of pregnancy and within 72 hours of delivery
2. Within 72 hours after termination of a pregnancy of 13 weeks or more of gestation

One *microdose* (50 mcg) within 72 hours after the termination of a pregnancy of less than 13 weeks' gestation.

RBCs, Red blood cells.

Dose is calculated based on the volume of fetal-maternal hemorrhage or Rh-positive blood administered in transfusion accidents. A standard dose will protect against 30 ml of Rh-positive whole blood or 15 ml of packed RBCs (Weiner & Buhimschi, 2004).

Absorption: Well absorbed from intramuscular sites.

Excretion: Metabolism and excretion unknown.

Contraindications and Precautions: Women who are Rh-positive or women previously sensitized to Rh₀(D) should not receive Rh₀(D) immune globulin. It is used cautiously for women with previous hypersensitivity reactions to immune globulins.

Adverse Reactions: Local pain at intramuscular site, fever, or both.

Nursing Implications: Type and antibody screen of the mother's blood and cord blood type of the newborn must be performed to determine the need for the medication. The mother must be Rh-negative and negative for Rh antibodies. The newborn must be Rh-positive. If the fetal blood type after termination of pregnancy is uncertain, the medication should be administered. The newborn may have a weakly positive antibody test if the woman received Rh₀(D) immune globulin during pregnancy. The drug is administered to the mother, not the infant. The deltoid muscle is recommended for intramuscular administration.

About Rh Incompatibility

What does it mean to be Rh-negative?
Those who are Rh-negative lack a substance that is present in the red blood cells of those who are Rh-positive.

How can the expectant mother be Rh-negative and the fetus be Rh-positive?
The fetus can inherit the Rh-positive factor from the father.

What does sensitization *mean?*
Sensitization means that the Rh-negative person has been exposed to Rh-positive blood and has developed antibodies against the Rh factor.

Do the antibodies harm the woman?
No, because she does not have the Rh factor.

Do Rh-positive men always father Rh-positive children?
No. Rh-positive men who have an Rh-positive gene and an Rh-negative gene can father Rh-negative children.

Why is Rh₀(D) immune globulin (RhoGAM) necessary during pregnancy and after childbirth?
RhoGAM prevents the development of Rh antibodies in the mother, which might be harmful to subsequent fetuses who are Rh-positive. Administering Rh₀(D) immune globulin during pregnancy to the mother who delivers an Rh-positive infant is not harmful to the baby.

Why will the next fetus be jeopardized if RhoGAM is not administered?
If RhoGAM is not administered when a baby is Rh-positive, the expectant mother may develop antibodies that cross the placental barrier and affect the next Rh-positive fetus.

✔ CHECK YOUR READING

25. Why do unsensitized Rh-negative expectant mothers receive Rh₀(D) immune globulin during pregnancy and after an abortion, amniocentesis, and childbirth?
26. What are the effects on the fetus of maternal Rh sensitization?
27. Why is the first fetus sometimes affected if ABO incompatibility occurs? Why are the effects of ABO incompatibility milder than those of Rh-sensitization?

SUMMARY CONCEPTS

- Spontaneous abortion is one of the leading causes of pregnancy loss. Treatment is aimed at preventing complications, such as hypovolemic shock and infection, and providing emotional support for grieving.
- The incidence of ectopic pregnancy is increasing in the United States as a result of pelvic inflammation associated with sexually transmissible diseases. The goals of therapeutic management are to prevent severe hemorrhage and to preserve the fallopian tube so that future fertility is retained.

- Management of gestational trophoblastic disease (hydatidiform mole) involves two phases: (1) evacuation of the molar pregnancy, and (2) continued follow-up for 1 year to detect malignant changes in the remaining trophoblastic tissue.
- Disorders of the placenta (placenta previa and abruptio placentae) are responsible for hemorrhagic conditions of the last half of pregnancy. Either condition may result in maternal hemorrhage and fetal or maternal death.
- Disseminated intravascular coagulation is a life-threatening complication of missed abortion, abruptio placentae, and severe hypertension, in which procoagulation and anticoagulation factors are simultaneously activated. DIC may occur with problems unrelated to pregnancy.
- The cause of hyperemesis gravidarum remains unclear, but the goals of management are to prevent dehydration, malnutrition, excess weight loss, and electrolyte imbalance. Emotional support is an important responsibility of nurses, in addition to physical care.
- Classifications of hypertension during pregnancy include preeclampsia, eclampsia, gestational hypertension, chronic (preexisting or persistent) hypertension, and preeclampsia superimposed over existing chronic hypertension. The underlying process is generalized vasospasm, which decreases circulation to all organs of the body, including the placenta. Major maternal organs affected include the liver, kidneys, and brain.
- Treatment of preeclampsia includes reduced activity, reduction of environmental stimuli, and administration of medications to prevent generalized seizures.
- Magnesium sulfate, used to prevent preeclampsia from progressing to eclamptic seizures, may have adverse effects. The most serious of these is central nervous system depression, which includes depression of the respiratory center. Adverse effects such as respiratory depression or absent deep tendon reflexes are more likely to occur if the blood level of magnesium rises over the therapeutic range.
- Nurses monitor the woman with preeclampsia to determine the effectiveness of medical therapy and to identify signs that the condition is worsening, such as increasing hyperreflexia. Nurses also control external stimuli and initiate measures to protect her in case of eclamptic seizures.
- Women who have chronic hypertension are at increased risk for preeclampsia and should be monitored for worsening hypertension, proteinuria, or generalized edema. Antihypertensive medication should be continued or initiated if diastolic blood pressure is consistently higher than 100 mm Hg.
- Rh incompatibility can occur if an Rh-negative woman conceives a child who is Rh-positive. As a result of exposure to the Rh-positive antigen, maternal antibodies may develop that cause hemolysis of fetal Rh-positive red blood cells in subsequent pregnancies.
- Administration of $Rh_o(D)$ immune globulin (RhoGAM) prevents production of anti-Rh antibodies, thereby preventing destruction of Rh-positive red blood cells in subsequent pregnancies.
- ABO incompatibility usually occurs when the mother has type O blood and naturally occurring anti-A and anti-B antibodies, which cause hemolysis if the fetus's blood is not type O. ABO incompatibility may result in hyperbilirubinemia of the infant, but it usually presents no serious threat to the health of the child.

ANSWERS TO CRITICAL THINKING EXERCISE 25-1, p. 631

Nurses often assume that patients know how to use a thermometer and that they know the signs of infection. Many nurses assume that patients realize the connection between blood loss and the tendency to develop infection. As a result, nurses may not emphasize the need for a diet that is high in nutrients that increase hemoglobin and hematocrit (iron and vitamin C). Nurses also may assume incorrectly that women know foods that contain these nutrients.

ANSWERS TO CRITICAL THINKING EXERCISE 25-2, p. 632

1. Many people wrongly assume that early pregnancy loss does not produce the grieving that accompanies loss at a later stage. Telling Alice that she is lucky ignores her feelings and invalidates any grief she feels.
2. The nurse also mistakenly assumes that little cause for grief exists over the loss of this pregnancy if later children are possible. However, a unique relationship exists between Alice and this fetus. Alice may experience an emotional upheaval when this special relationship comes to an abrupt end. Another pregnancy is not guaranteed.
3. It would be beneficial if Helen examined her assumptions before having the interaction with Alice. She might then allow Alice to express her feelings and acknowledge the grief that she is feeling.

REFERENCES & READINGS

Abramovici, D., Mattar, F., & Sibai, B. (2000). Hypertensive disorders in pregnancy. In S.B. Ransom, M.P. Dombrowski, S.G. McNeeley, K.S. Moghissi, & A.R. Munkarah (Eds.), *Practical strategies in obstetrics and gynecology* (pp. 380-389). Philadelphia: Saunders.

American Academy of Pediatrics & American College of Obstetricians and Gynecologists. (2002). *Guidelines for perinatal care* (5th ed.). Elk Grove Village, IL: Authors.

American College of Obstetricians & Gynecologists. (2001). *Chronic hypertension in pregnancy*, Practice Bulletin No. 29. Washington, DC: Author.

American College of Obstetricians & Gynecologists. (2002). *Diagnosis and management of preeclampsia and eclampsia*, Practice Bulletin No. 33. Washington, DC: Author.

Anderson, J.J.B. (2004). Minerals. In L.K. Mahan & S. Escott-Stump (Eds.), *Krause's food, nutrition, and diet therapy* (11th ed., pp. 120-163). Philadelphia: Saunders.

August, P. (2004). Hypertensive disorders in pregnancy. In G.N. Burrow, T.P. Duffy, & J.A. Copel (Eds.), *Medical complications during pregnancy* (6th ed., pp. 43-67). Philadelphia: Saunders.

Berek, J.S. (2004). Gestational trophoblastic neoplasm. In N.F. Hacker, J.G. Moore, & J.C. Gambone (Eds.), *Essentials of obstetrics and gynecology* (4th ed., pp. 486-494). Philadelphia: Saunders.

Berman, M.L., Di Saia, P.J., & Tiwari, K.S. (2004). Pelvic malignancies, gestational trophoblastic neoplasia, and nonpelvic malignancies. In R.K. Creasy, R. Resnik, & J.D. Iams (Eds.), *Maternal-fetal medicine: Principles and practice* (5th ed., pp. 1213-1242). Philadelphia: Saunders.

Blackburn, S.T. (2003). *Maternal, fetal, and neonatal physiology: A clinical perspective*. Philadelphia: Saunders.

Branch, D.W., & Scott, J.R. (2003). Early pregnancy loss. In J.R. Scott, R.S. Gibbs, B.Y. Karlan, & A.F. Haney (Eds.), *Danforth's obstetrics and gynecology* (9th ed., pp. 75-87). Philadelphia: Lippincott Williams & Wilkins.

Buckwalter, J.G., & Simpson, S.W. (2002). Psychological factors in the etiology and treatment of severe nausea and vomiting of pregnancy. *American Journal of Obstetrics & Gynecology, 186*(5), S210-S214.

Carolan, M. (2003). The graying of the obstetric population: Implications for the older mother. *Journal of Obstetric, Gynecologic, and Neonatal Nursing, 32*(1), 19-27.

Carpenito-Moyet, L.J. (2004). *Handbook of nursing diagnosis* (10th ed.). Philadelphia: Lippincott Williams & Wilkins.

Castro, L.C. (2004). Hypertensive disorders of pregnancy. In N.F. Hacker, J.G. Moore, & J.C. Gambone (Eds.), *Essentials of obstetrics and gynecology* (4th ed., pp. 197-207). Philadelphia: Saunders.

Clark, S.L. (2003). Critical care obstetrics. In J.R. Scott, R.S. Gibbs, B.Y. Karlan, & A.F. Haney (Eds.), *Danforth's obstetrics and gynecology* (9th ed., pp. 89-103). Philadelphia: Lippincott Williams & Wilkins.

Clark, S.L. (2004). Placenta previa and abruptio placentae. In R.K. Creasy, R. Resnik, & J.D. Iams (Eds.), *Maternal-fetal medicine* (5th ed., pp. 707-722). Philadelphia: Saunders.

Cunningham, F.G., Gant, N.F., Leveno, K.J., Gilstrap, L.C., Hauth, J.C., & Wenstrom, K.D. (2001). *Williams obstetrics* (21st ed.). Norwalk, CT: Appleton & Lange.

Gilbert, E.S., & Harmon, J.S. (2003). *Manual of high risk pregnancy & delivery*. St. Louis: Mosby.

Hayashi, R.H., & Hayashi, R.H. (2004). Obstetric hemorrhage and puerperal sepsis. In N.F. Hacker, J.G. Moore, & J.C. Gambone (Eds.), *Essentials of obstetrics and gynecology* (3rd ed., pp. 146-158). Philadelphia: Saunders.

Heard, M.J., & Buster, J.E. (2003). Ectopic pregnancy. In J.R. Scott, R.S. Gibbs, B.Y. Karlan, & A.F. Haney (Eds.), *Danforth's obstetrics and gynecology* (9th ed., pp. 89-103). Philadelphia: Lippincott Williams & Wilkins.

Hill, J.A. (2004). Recurrent pregnancy loss. In R.K. Creasy, R. Resnik, & J.D. Iams (Eds.), *Maternal-fetal medicine: Principles and practice* (5th ed., pp. 579-601). Philadelphia: Saunders.

Iams, J.D. (2004). Abnormal cervical competence. In R.K. Creasy, R. Resnik, & J.D. Iams (Eds.), *Maternal-fetal medicine: Principles and practice* (5th ed., pp. 603-622). Philadelphia: Saunders.

Kay, H.H. (2003). Placenta previa and abruption. In J.R. Scott, R.S. Gibbs, B.Y. Karlan, & A.F. Haney (Eds.), *Danforth's obstetrics and gynecology* (9th ed., pp. 365-379). Philadelphia: Lippincott Williams & Wilkins.

Kilpatrick, S.J., & Laros, R.K. (2004). Maternal hematologic disorders. In R.K. Creasy, R. Resnik, & J.D. Iams (Eds.), *Maternal-fetal medicine: Principles and practice* (5th ed., pp. 975-1004). Philadelphia: Saunders.

Landon, M.B. (2004). Disease of the liver, biliary system, and pancreas. In R.K. Creasy, R. Resnik, & J.D. Iams (Eds.), *Maternal-fetal medicine* (5th ed., pp. 1127-1145). Philadelphia: Saunders.

Laros, R.K. (2004). Thromboembolic disease. In R.K. Creasy, R. Resnik, & J.D. Iams (Eds.), *Maternal-fetal medicine: Principles and practice* (5th ed., pp. 845-857). Philadelphia: Saunders.

Li, A.J., & Karlan, B.Y. (2003). Gestational trophoblastic neoplasms. In J.R. Scott, R.S. Gibbs, B.Y. Karlan, & A.F. Haney (Eds.), *Danforth's obstetrics and gynecology* (9th ed., pp. 1019-1030). Philadelphia: Lippincott Williams & Wilkins.

Lockwood, C.J., & Silver, R. (2004). Thrombophilias in pregnancy. In R.K. Creasy, R. Resnik, & J.D. Iams (Eds.), *Maternal-fetal medicine: Principles and practice* (5th ed., pp. 1005-1021). Philadelphia: Saunders.

Lu, M.C., & Hobel, C.J. (2004). Antepartum care. In N.F. Hacker, J.G. Moore, & J.C. Gambone (Eds.), *Essentials of obstetrics and gynecology* (4th ed., pp. 83-103). Philadelphia: Saunders.

Magee, L.A., Mazzotta, P., & Koren, G. (2002). Evidence-based view of safety and effectiveness of pharmacologic therapy for nausea and vomiting of pregnancy (NVP). *American Journal of Obstetrics & Gynecology, 186*(Suppl. 5), S256-S261.

Modigliani, R.M. (2000). Gastrointestinal and pancreatic diseases. In W.M. Barron, M.D. Lindheimer, & J.M. Davison (Eds.), *Medical disorders during pregnancy* (3rd ed., pp. 257-271). St. Louis: Mosby.

Moise, K.J. (2004). Hemolytic disease of the fetus and newborn. In R.K. Creasy, R. Resnik, & J.D. Iams (Eds.), *Maternal-fetal medicine: Principles and practice* (5th ed., pp. 315-355). Philadelphia: Saunders.

Moldenhauer, J.S., & Sibai, B.M. (2003). Hypertensive disorders of pregnancy. In J.R. Scott, R.S. Gibbs, B.Y. Karlan, & A.F. Haney (Eds.), *Danforth's obstetrics and gynecology* (9th ed., pp. 257-271). Philadelphia: Lippincott Williams & Wilkins.

Moore, T.R. (2004). Diabetes in pregnancy. In R.K. Creasy, R. Resnik, & J.D. Iams (Eds.), *Maternal-fetal medicine: Principles and practice* (5th ed., pp. 1023-1061). Philadelphia: Saunders.

National Center for Health Statistics. (2004). *Health, United States, 2004, with Chartbook on Trends in the Health of Americans*. Hyattsville, MD: Author.

National High Blood Pressure Education Program Working Group on High Blood Pressure in Pregnancy. (2000). Report of the national high blood pressure education program working group on high blood pressure in pregnancy. *American Journal of Obstetrics and Gynecology, 183*(1), S1-S22.

National Institutes of Health, National Heart, Lung, and Blood Institute. (2001). *Report of the working group on research on hypertension during pregnancy*. Retrieved January 14, 2005, from www.nhlbi.nih.gov/resources/hyperten_preg/index.html.

Nelson, A.L., DeUgarte, C.M., & Gambone, J.C. (2004). Ectopic pregnancy. In N.F. Hacker, J.G. Moore, & J.C. Gambone (Eds.), *Essentials of obstetrics and gynecology* (4th ed., pp. 325-333). Philadelphia: Saunders.

Nick, J.M. (2004). Deep tendon reflexes, magnesium, and calcium: Assessments and implications. *Journal of Obstetric, Gynecologic, and Neonatal Nursing, 33*(2), 221-230.

Nick, J.M. (2003). Deep tendon reflexes: The what, why, where, and how of tapping. *Journal of Obstetric, Gynecologic, and Neonatal Nursing, 32*(3), pp. 297-306. [See also Erratum article printed in the fourth issue (*JOGNN, 32*(4)).]

Peters, R.M., & Flack, J.M. (2004). Hypertensive disorders of pregnancy. *Journal of Obstetric, Gynecologic, and Neonatal Nursing, 33*(2), 209-220.

Poole, J.H., Sosa, M.E., Freda, M.C., Kendrick, J.M., Luppi, C.J., Krening, C.F., & Dauphinee, J.D. (2001). High-risk pregnancy. In K.R. Simpson & P.A. Creehan (Eds.), *AWHONN perinatal nursing* (2nd ed., pp. 173-296). Philadelphia: Lippincott Williams & Wilkins.

Riely, C.A., & Fallon, H.J. (2004). Liver diseases. In G.N. Burrow, T.P. Duffy, & J.A. Copel (Eds.), *Medical complications during pregnancy* (6th ed., pp. 279-304). Philadelphia: Saunders.

Roberts, J.M. (2004). Pregnancy-related hypertension. In R.K. Creasy, R. Resnik, & J.D. Iams (Eds.), *Maternal-fetal medicine: Principles and practice* (5th ed., pp. 859-899). Philadelphia: Saunders.

Scott, L.D., & Abu-Hamda, E. (2004). Gastrointestinal disease in pregnancy. In R.K. Creasy, R. Resnik, & J.D. Iams (Eds.), *Maternal-fetal medicine: Principles and practice* (5th ed., pp. 1109-1126). Philadelphia: Saunders.

Shabert, J.K. (2004). Nutrition during pregnancy and lactation. In L.K. Mahan & S. Escott-Stump (Eds.), *Krause's food, nutrition, and diet therapy* (11th ed., pp. 182-213). Philadelphia: Saunders.

Simpson, K.R., & Knox, G.E. (2004). Obstetrical accidents involving intravenous magnesium sulfate: Recommendations to promote patient safety. *MCN: American Journal of Maternal/Child Nursing, 29*(3), 161-169.

Steinlauf, A.F., Chang, P.K., & Traube, M. (2004). Gastrointestinal complications. In J.W. Burrow, T.P. Duffy, & J.A. Copel (Eds.), *Medical complications during pregnancy* (6th ed., pp. 259-277). Philadelphia: Saunders.

Weiner, C.P., & Buhimschi, C. (2004). *Drugs for pregnant and lactating women*. New York: Churchill Livingstone.

Weyermann, M., Brenner, H., Adler, G., Yasar, Z., Handke-Veseley, A., Grab, D., et al. (2003). *Helicobacter pylori* infection and the occurrence and severity of gastrointestinal symptoms during pregnancy. *American Journal of Obstetrics & Gynecology, 189*(2), 526-531.

Concurrent Disorders during Pregnancy

OBJECTIVES

After studying this chapter, you should be able to:

1. Describe the effects of pregnancy on fuel metabolism.
2. Discuss the effects and management of preexisting diabetes mellitus during pregnancy.
3. Explain the effects and management of gestational diabetes mellitus.
4. Describe the major effects of pregnancy on the woman who has heart disease, and identify the goals of therapy.
5. Explain the maternal and fetal effects of specific anemias and the required management during pregnancy.
6. Identify the effects, management, and nursing considerations of specific preexisting conditions discussed in this chapter.
7. Identify the major causes of trauma during pregnancy, and describe therapeutic management.
8. Discuss the maternal, fetal, and neonatal effects of the most common infections that may occur during pregnancy.

Go to your Student CD-ROM for Review Questions keyed to these Objectives.

DEFINITIONS

Caudal Regression Syndrome A malformation that results when the sacrum, lumbar spine, and lower extremities fail to develop.

Congenital Anomaly Abnormal intrauterine development of an organ or structure.

Congestive Heart Failure Condition resulting from failure of the heart to maintain adequate circulation; characterized by weakness, dyspnea, and edema in body parts that are lower than the heart.

Diabetes Mellitus A disorder of carbohydrate metabolism caused by a relative or complete lack of insulin secretion; characterized by glycosuria (glucose in the urine) and hyperglycemia.

Diabetogenic Refers to a condition such as pregnancy that produces the effects of diabetes mellitus.

Dystocia Difficult or prolonged labor; often associated with abnormal uterine activity and cephalopelvic disproportion.

Gluconeogenesis Formation of glycogen by the liver from noncarbohydrate sources such as amino and fatty acids.

Hydramnios Excess volume of amniotic fluid (more than 2000 ml at term). Also called *polyhydramnios*.

Ketosis Accumulation of ketone bodies (metabolic products) in the blood; frequently associated with acidosis.

Lipogenic Substance such as insulin that stimulates the production of fat.

Macrosomia Unusually large fetal size; infant birth weight more than 4000 g.

Marfan Syndrome A hereditary condition that involves weakness in connective tissue, bones, and muscles; the vascular system is affected, particularly the aorta.

Osmotic Diuresis Secretion and passage of large amounts of urine as a result of increased osmotic pressure that can result from hyperglycemia.

Polydipsia Excessive thirst.

Polyphagia Excessive ingestion of food.

Polyuria Excessive excretion of urine.

Seroconversion Change in a blood test result from negative to positive, indicating the development of antibodies in response to infection or immunization.

Pregnancy affects the care of women with a medical condition in two ways. First, pregnancy may alter the course of the disease. Second, the disease or its treatment may have unwanted effects on the pregnancy. Antepartum care must be adapted to include increased surveillance of the mother and fetus. Also, some disorders that are mild or even subclinical in the pregnant woman can produce massive damage to the fetus. This chapter describes some common disorders that can cause significant fetal jeopardy.

DIABETES MELLITUS

Pathophysiology

ETIOLOGY

Diabetes mellitus is a complex disorder of carbohydrate metabolism caused primarily by a partial or complete lack of insulin secretion by the beta cells of the pancreas. Some cells, such as those in skeletal and cardiac muscles and adipose tissue, rely on insulin to carry glucose across the cell membranes. Without insulin, glucose accumulates in the blood, resulting in hyperglycemia. The body attempts to dilute the glucose load by any means possible. The first strategy is to increase thirst (polydipsia), a classic symptom of diabetes mellitus. Next, fluid from the intracellular spaces is drawn into the vascular bed, resulting in dehydration at the cellular level but fluid volume excess in the vascular compartment. The kidneys attempt to excrete large volumes of this fluid and the heavy solute load of glucose (osmotic diuresis). This excretion produces the second hallmark of diabetes, polyuria, as well as glycosuria (glucose in the urine). Without glucose the cells starve, so weight loss occurs even though the person ingests large amounts of food (polyphagia).

Because the body cannot metabolize glucose, it begins to metabolize protein and fat to meet energy needs. Metabolism of protein produces a negative nitrogen balance, and the metabolism of fat results in the buildup of ketone bodies (such as acetone, acetoacetic acid, or β-hydroxybutyric acid) or ketosis (accumulation of acids in the body).

If the disease is not well controlled, serious complications may occur. Hypoglycemia or hyperglycemia can result if the amount of insulin does not match the diet. Fluctuating periods of hyperglycemia and hypoglycemia damage small blood vessels throughout the body. This damage can cause serious impairment, especially in the kidneys, eyes, and heart.

EFFECT OF PREGNANCY ON FUEL METABOLISM

To understand the relationship between diabetes mellitus and pregnancy, an understanding of the way pregnancy and diabetes alter the metabolism of food is necessary.

EARLY PREGNANCY. Metabolic changes can be divided into those that occur early in pregnancy (from 1 to 20 weeks' gestation) and those that occur late in pregnancy (from 20 to 40 weeks' gestation). During early pregnancy, maternal metabolic rates and energy needs change little. During this time, however, insulin release in response to serum glucose levels accelerates. As a result, significant hypoglycemia may occur, particularly in women who experience the nausea, vomiting, and anorexia that often occur during the first weeks of pregnancy.

In an uncomplicated pregnancy, the availability of glucose and insulin, a lipogenic substance, favors the development and storage of fat during the first half of pregnancy. Accumulation of fat prepares the mother for the rise in energy use by the growing fetus during the second half of pregnancy.

LATE PREGNANCY. During the second half of pregnancy, when fetal growth accelerates, placental hormones rise sharply. These hormones, particularly estrogen, progesterone, and human placental lactogen (hPL), create resistance to insulin in maternal cells. This resistance allows an abundant supply of glucose to be available for the fetus. However, the hormones have a diabetogenic effect in that they may leave the woman with insufficient insulin and episodes of hyperglycemia.

For most women, insulin resistance is not a problem. The pancreas responds by simply increasing the production of insulin. If the pancreas is unable to respond adequately, the woman will have periods of hyperglycemia.

The fetus continually draws nutrients such as glucose and amino acids from maternal blood during late pregnancy. The result is an earlier-than-normal switch from carbohydrate metabolism to gluconeogenesis (formation of glycogen from noncarbohydrate sources such as proteins and fat). Because the fetus uses many of the amino acids, the process becomes predominantly one of fat utilization. This process produces high levels of free fatty acids that further inhibit the uptake and oxidation of glucose, therefore preserving glucose for use by the central nervous system (CNS) and fetal needs. These metabolic changes are similar to those occurring during "accelerated starvation," when fat is metabolized to meet many of the body's energy needs.

Classification

Diabetes that exists before pregnancy is classified as type 1 (insulin deficient) or type 2 (insulin resistant, with a relative deficiency of insulin to metabolize carbohydrate) according to whether the client requires the administration of insulin to prevent ketoacidosis. A third type is one in which any degree of glucose intolerance has its onset or first recognition during pregnancy. The onset of glucose intolerance during pregnancy is termed *gestational diabetes mellitus* (GDM).

An additional classification of diabetes is sometimes used for descriptive purposes. The White classification describes the age at onset of diabetes, its duration based on the woman's current age, and vascular complications, such as retinopathy, that are present. GDM descriptions in White's classification include A-1 (diet controlled) and A-2 (diet and insulin controlled). Another classification for diabetes during pregnancy lists complications that may be found with type 1 or type 2 diabetes (retinopathy, nephropathy, and/or coronary artery disease) and whether GDM is controlled by diet alone or also requires insulin to supplement diet control (Gambone, Moore, & Koos, 2004; Kenshole, 2004).

Incidence

The pregnant woman may have preexisting diabetes (type 1 or type 2), or she may develop GDM during the course of pregnancy. Diabetes mellitus is a common medical condition complicating pregnancy. About 7% of all pregnancies are affected by GDM, but the range varies from 1% to 14% among different groups of pregnant women (American College of Obstetricians & Gynecologists [ACOG], 2001; American Diabetes Association [ADA], 2004). (See Box 26-1 for additional characteristics of the three types of diabetes.) One of every 200 pregnant women has preexisting diabetes. Between 2% and 5% of pregnant women will develop gestational diabetes (March of Dimes Birth Defects Foundation, 2004).

Preexisting Diabetes Mellitus

MATERNAL EFFECTS

The course of pregnancy for women with diabetes mellitus has improved greatly as a result of new treatments and more effective methods of fetal surveillance. However, the incidence of complications affecting the mother and fetus remains higher than that experienced by nondiabetic women.

Diabetes can adversely affect a pregnant woman and her developing baby in several ways. During the first trimester, when major fetal organs are developing, the effects of the abnormal metabolic environment, such as hypoglycemia, hyperglycemia, and ketosis, may lead to increased incidence of spontaneous abortion or major fetal malformations. Preeclampsia is two to three times more likely to develop if the woman has preexisting diabetes (Cunningham et al., 2001). The development of ketoacidosis is a threat to women with type 1 diabetes and is most often precipitated by infection or missed insulin doses. In addition, ketoacidosis may develop in these women at lower thresholds of hyperglycemia than those seen in nonpregnant individuals.

BOX 26-1 Classification of Diabetes Mellitus

Type 1, Insulin-Dependent
Onset in childhood or young adulthood. Involves autoimmune destruction of pancreatic beta cells by autoimmune activity. Prone to ketosis. Usually lean body mass.

Type 2, Non–Insulin-Dependent
Usual onset after 40 years. Associated with obesity. Increasing insulin resistance. Ketosis less likely to occur than in type 1 diabetes mellitus.

Gestational
Onset of glucose intolerance first diagnosed during pregnancy. Exogenous insulin may or may not be needed.

Data from American Diabetes Association. (2004). Position statement: Gestational diabetes mellitus. *Diabetes Care, 27*(Suppl. 1), S88-S90; American Diabetes Association. (2005). Position statement: Standards of medical care in diabetes. *Diabetes Care, 28*(Suppl. 1), S4-S36; Kenshole, A.B. (2004). Diabetes in pregnancy. In G.N. Burrow, T.P. Duffy, & J.A. Copel (Eds.), *Medical complications during pregnancy* (6th ed., pp. 15-42). Philadelphia: Saunders; and Moore, T.R. (2004). Diabetes in pregnancy. In R.K. Creasy, R. Resnik, & J.D. Iams (Eds.), *Maternal-newborn medicine: Principles and practice* (5th ed., pp. 1023-1061). Philadelphia: Saunders.

Untreated ketoacidosis can progress to fetal and maternal death. Urinary tract infections are more common, possibly because of glucose in the urine, which provides a nutrient-rich medium for bacterial growth.

Other effects include hydramnios, which may result from fetal hyperglycemia and consequent fetal diuresis, and premature rupture of membranes, which may be caused by overdistention of the uterus by hydramnios or a large fetus. Problems that arise during labor and childbirth if the fetus has macrosomia (weighs more than 4000 g, or 8.8 lb) may include a difficult labor, shoulder dystocia (delayed or difficult birth of fetal shoulders after the head is born), and consequent injury to the birth canal or the infant. Large fetal size also increases the likelihood that a cesarean birth will be necessary and the risk of postpartum hemorrhage (Table 26-1).

FETAL EFFECTS

Fetal and neonatal effects of preexisting diabetes depend on the timing and severity of maternal hyperglycemia and the degree of vascular impairment that has occurred.

CONGENITAL MALFORMATION. The most common major congenital malformations associated with preexisting diabetes are neural tube defects, caudal regression syndrome, and cardiac defects. The risk for a major congenital malformation is two to six times higher than that of the general population. The incidence correlates directly with the degree of maternal hyperglycemia during the first trimester. Fewer malformations occur if the woman is able to maintain a normal blood glucose level before conception and throughout early pregnancy (Gambone, Moore, & Koos, 2004; Kenshole, 2004).

VARIATIONS IN FETAL SIZE. Fetal growth is related to maternal vascular integrity. In women without vascular impairment, glucose and oxygen are easily transported to the fetus; if the woman is hyperglycemic, so is the fetus. Although maternal insulin does not cross the placental barrier, the fetus produces insulin by the tenth week of gestation. Fetal macrosomia results when elevated levels of blood glucose stimulate excessive production of fetal insulin, which acts as a powerful growth hormone. This is a major neonatal effect with consequent increase in cesarean birth or birth injury from shoulder dystocia.

Conversely, if vascular impairment occurs, placental perfusion may be decreased. Vascular impairment may be caused by complications of the diabetes, such as vasoconstriction, which occurs in preeclampsia. Impaired placental perfusion decreases supplies of glucose and oxygen delivered to the fetus. As a result, the infant is likely to be small for gestational age. This condition is called *intrauterine growth restriction* (IUGR). Amniotic fluid may be reduced (oligohydramnios) as the fetus conserves oxygen for the heart and brain.

NEONATAL EFFECTS

The four major neonatal complications of preexisting diabetes are hypoglycemia, hypocalcemia, hyperbilirubinemia, and respiratory distress syndrome. Maintaining normal ma-

TABLE 26-1 Major Effects of Diabetes Mellitus on Pregnancy

Effect	Probable Cause
Increased Maternal Risks	
Hypertension; preeclampsia	Unknown but increased even without renal or vascular impairment
Urinary tract infections	Increased bacterial growth in nutrient-rich urine
Ketoacidosis (risk for mother and fetus)	Uncontrolled hyperglycemia or infection; most common in women with type 1 diabetes
Labor dystocia; cesarean birth; uterine atony with hemorrhage after birth	Hydramnios secondary to fetal osmotic diuresis caused by hyperglycemia; uterus is overstretched
Birth injury to maternal tissues (hematoma, lacerations)	Fetal macrosomia causing difficult birth
Increased Fetal and Neonatal Risks	
Congenital anomalies	Maternal hyperglycemia during organ formation in first trimester
Perinatal death	Poor placental perfusion because of maternal vascular impairment, primarily in woman with type 1 diabetes
Macrosomia (>4000 g)	Fetal hyperglycemia stimulating production of insulin to metabolize carbohydrates; excess nutrients transported to fetus
Intrauterine fetal growth restriction	Maternal vascular impairment
Preterm labor; premature rupture of membranes; preterm birth	Overdistention of uterus caused by hydramnios and large fetal size at preterm gestation
Birth injury	Large fetal size; shoulder dystocia or other difficult delivery
Hypoglycemia	Neonatal hyperinsulinemia after birth when maternal glucose is no longer available (but insulin production remains high)
Polycythemia	Fetal hypoxemia stimulating erythrocyte production
Hyperbilirubinemia	Breakdown of excessive red blood cells after birth
Hypocalcemia	Transfer of calcium abruptly stopped at birth, reduced fetal parathyroid function
Respiratory distress syndrome	Delayed maturation of fetal lungs; inadequate production of pulmonary surfactant; slowed absorption of fetal lung fluid

ternal levels of glucose reduces the incidence and severity of neonatal complications.

HYPOGLYCEMIA. The neonate is at higher risk for hypoglycemia because fetal insulin production was accelerated during pregnancy to metabolize excessive glucose received from the mother. The constant stimulation of hyperglycemia leads to hyperplasia and hypertrophy of the islets of Langerhans in the fetal pancreas. When the maternal glucose supply is abruptly withdrawn at birth, the level of neonatal insulin exceeds the available glucose, and hypoglycemia develops rapidly.

HYPOCALCEMIA. During the last half of pregnancy, large amounts of calcium are transported across the placenta from the mother to the fetus. At the time of birth, this transfer is abruptly stopped, leading to a dramatic decrease in total and ionized calcium. Hypocalcemia, defined as 7 mg/dl or less, most often occurs within the first 3 days of life. It is associated with preterm birth and perinatal asphyxia, which are more likely to occur with poor maternal glycemic control.

HYPERBILIRUBINEMIA. The fetus who experiences recurrent hypoxia compensates by production of additional erythrocytes to carry oxygen supplied by the mother. After birth the excess erythrocytes are broken down, releasing large amounts of bilirubin into the neonate's circulation. Prematurity, more likely in the woman with poor glycemic control, further reduces the infant's ability to metabolize and excrete excess bilirubin.

RESPIRATORY DISTRESS SYNDROME. Fetal hyperinsulinemia retards cortisol production, which is necessary for synthesis of surfactant needed to keep the new-

born's alveoli open after birth, thereby increasing the risk for respiratory distress syndrome. Reduced lung fluid clearance and delayed thinning of lung connective tissue may also play a part, although other authorities believe that gestational age is the primary determinant of whether an infant will have respiratory distress syndrome (Cunningham et al., 2001; Roberts, 2004). Respiratory distress syndrome is more likely to occur if the mother's glycemic control is poor, because wide fluctuations in her insulin and glucose levels have slowed lung maturation. Tests of fetal lung maturity, such as the lecithin/sphingomyelin (L/S) ratio and presence of phosphatidylglycerol (PG), will be done before elective delivery of the fetus by induction or scheduled cesarean if questions about maturity exist. (See Chapter 10 for additional information about tests of fetal lung maturity and Chapter 30 for information about care of the infant of a diabetic mother.)

Complications in a mother and her fetus and newborn can be reduced if the mother maintains normal and stable blood glucose levels. The objective of the team providing treatment is to devise a plan that allows the woman to maintain a level as close to normal as possible (Nursing Care Plan 26-1).

✓ CHECK YOUR READING

1. What effects do the hormones of pregnancy have on maternal glucose metabolism?
2. What are the maternal effects of type 1 diabetes mellitus? What are possible fetal and neonatal effects?
3. How do insulin needs vary from the first trimester through the postpartum period?

NURSING CARE PLAN 26-1 Pregnancy and Diabetes Mellitus

ASSESSMENT: Kathy Ringold is a 24-year-old primigravida at 9 weeks' gestation. She was diagnosed with type 1 diabetes mellitus 6 years ago. She has been on a daily regimen of insulin and is comfortable with insulin administration and blood glucose monitoring. She is experiencing daily nausea and vomiting. Kathy states that she is concerned because she is not eating as much as before becoming pregnant. She also reveals that she had sometimes "binged" on food before becoming pregnant and didn't always monitor blood glucose as often as directed. She does not see why her blood glucose has to be watched so carefully.

NURSING DIAGNOSIS: Risk for Ineffective Health Maintenance related to knowledge deficit of the effects of pregnancy on diabetes control

GOALS/EXPECTED OUTCOMES: Kathy will:
1. Describe predicted changes in insulin needs throughout pregnancy
2. Follow prescribed schedule of blood glucose monitoring, insulin administration, diet, and exercise
3. Describe the importance of frequent fetal surveillance and follow the prescribed schedule

INTERVENTION	RATIONALE
1. Reduce barriers to learning: a. Allow Kathy to express emotions and concerns before teaching. b. Examine her beliefs and past experiences related to diabetes. c. Assess readiness to learn, based on interest, attention, and participation in scheduled learning sessions.	1. Motivation and readiness to learn are essential if permanent learning is to occur. Kathy will learn only if she sees the value of the information.
2. Instruct Kathy about the predicted changes in diabetes management during pregnancy: a. Explain the importance of blood glucose testing; Kathy will need less insulin because of the nausea and vomiting occurring in the first trimester. b. Emphasize that she will probably need more insulin as the second and third trimesters progress because of the effects of the placental hormones. Insulin requirements usually fall immediately after birth but will reach longer-term levels after the immediate postdelivery period. c. Describe the importance of following the prescribed diet and exercise regimen to maintain normal blood glucose levels.	2. Behaviors change when learning occurs. Understanding how insulin needs change throughout pregnancy, labor, and the postpartum period increases the likelihood that Kathy will follow the recommended regimen.
3. Inform Kathy about specific fetal surveillance techniques recommended during pregnancy (serial nonstress tests, contraction stress tests, biophysical profiles, kick counts, ultrasound examinations), and explain the importance of the tests. Reinforce or clarify medical explanations.	3. Some frequently ordered tests are time consuming and expensive, and others are simple. The woman is more likely to comply if she understands the importance of monitoring the fetal condition at frequent intervals.
4. Allow time for Kathy to focus on her feelings and concerns at each teaching session; offer praise and encouragement for her adherence to the prescribed regimen.	4. Motivation to comply with the regimen is strengthened by praise and the awareness that the woman's feelings are important.
5. Explain in simple, positive terms the advantages to the fetus of maintaining a normal maternal blood glucose level. These advantages include an optimal pattern of growth, the increased likelihood that the baby will be born near term, and fewer complications associated with prematurity.	5. Understanding that the fetus benefits when maternal glucose levels are normal reduces anxiety and increases the likelihood that the mother will comply with recommended treatment.
6. Review the recommended plan for diet and exercise during pregnancy, and determine whether Kathy knows the importance of these factors in her care.	6. Maintenance of normal blood glucose depends on coordinating the amount of food, insulin, and exercise. If any of these factors is altered, the others must also be altered to prevent hypoglycemia or hyperglycemia.

EVALUATION: Kathy verbalizes her understanding of changing insulin needs and the importance of glucose monitoring. She states that she feels in better control of the diabetes and plans to comply with the recommended schedule of fetal surveillance, diet, and exercise.

NURSING CARE PLAN 26-1 Pregnancy and Diabetes Mellitus—cont'd

ASSESSMENT: At 32 weeks' gestation, Kathy's blood glucose is consistently above the desired level, and twice-weekly biophysical profiles with nonstress testing are prescribed. The nonstress tests are reactive, indicating no present fetal compromise. Other portions of the biophysical profile (see Chapter 10) are also reassuring about fetal growth and placental function. Kathy, however, verbalizes anxiety about the condition of the fetus and asks when it will be safe for the baby to be born.

NURSING DIAGNOSIS: Anxiety related to perceived threat to the health of the fetus, including his expected gestation when born

GOALS/EXPECTED OUTCOMES: Kathy will:
1. Relate her perception of the condition of the fetus and the significance of the fetal evaluations as the tests are performed
2. Describe her concerns about the timing of the delivery at the conclusion of the next fetal evaluation session

INTERVENTION	RATIONALE
1. Ask Kathy to describe her concern about the fetus and to clarify her feelings.	1. Kathy's concerns must be identified and clarified so that misconceptions do not occur.
2. Explain that a reactive nonstress test indicates that the fetal heart rate accelerates whenever the fetus moves, a good sign that the fetus is not in immediate jeopardy. Reinforce medical explanations of how other parts of the biophysical profile are also reassuring of fetal well-being. Frequency of testing will be changed if a need is identified.	2. Reassurance that the fetus is not in jeopardy and that the tests will detect early signs if a problem develops reduces anxiety about the fetal condition.
3. Ask Kathy how she feels about the labor and delivery; determine whether she is taking childbirth education classes and whether she has selected her coach.	3. It is normal for women to become concerned about the birth process and how they will cope with labor during the last few weeks of pregnancy. Medical professionals should not neglect the need for normal pregnancy care for women with high-risk pregnancies.
4. Help Kathy locate a childbirth education class if she has not done so previously and suggest that she and her coach begin classes.	4. Knowledge learned at childbirth classes may reduce the anxiety about the birth processes.
5. Acknowledge that the prospect of labor and delivery causes many women some anxiety, even when the infant is not at risk.	5. Knowledge that her feelings are common to most women may provide some relief from anxiety.

EVALUATION: Kathy says she is reassured by explanations regarding the tests for fetal well-being but is concerned about how she will do in labor. She initiates plans to attend a childbirth education class with her sister as the coach.

ADDITIONAL NURSING DIAGNOSES TO CONSIDER:
Readiness for enhanced family coping
Risk for Injury

MATERNAL ASSESSMENT

Whenever a pregnant woman with preexisting diabetes initiates prenatal care, a thorough evaluation of her health status must be completed. This evaluation includes history, physical examination, and laboratory tests.

HISTORY. A detailed history should include the onset and management of the diabetic condition. How long has she had the disease? How does she maintain normal blood glucose? Is she familiar with ways to monitor blood glucose and administer insulin? The degree of glycemic control before pregnancy is of particular interest. Effective management depends on her adherence to a plan of care. Therefore her knowledge of how diabetes affects pregnancy and pregnancy affects diabetes must be determined. The support person's knowledge also must be assessed, and specific learning needs should be identified. In addition, the woman's emotional status should be assessed to determine how she is coping with pregnancy superimposed on preexisting diabetes.

All women with diabetes should be seen by a qualified nurse educator for an individualized assessment to ensure that they can monitor their blood glucose accurately. Accurate readings depend on performing the test correctly and at the times recommended by her health care team. In addition to home monitoring of blood glucose, the nurse must observe the woman's skill in mixing and administering insulin, using a sliding scale for added insulin, or using an insulin pump if the drug will be given that way. Most pregnant women who need a hypoglycemic agent take insulin rather than an oral agent, even if the oral agent was effective in the woman with type 2 diabetes. An occasional woman refuses to take injectable medication for blood glucose control. Adverse fetal effects of oral agents have not been confirmed, but discontinuing their use during pregnancy is currently recommended.

PHYSICAL EXAMINATION. In addition to routine prenatal examination (see Chapter 7), specific efforts should be made to assess the effects of diabetes. A baseline electrocardiogram (ECG) should be obtained to determine cardiovascular status. Evaluation for retinopathy should be performed, with referral to an ophthalmologist if necessary. The woman's weight and blood pressure must be monitored because of the increased risk for preeclampsia. Fundal height should be measured, noting any abnormal increase in size that may indicate macrosomia or hydramnios, which may occur as a result of diuresis by the hyperglycemic fetus. Fundal height less than expected for the gestation may indicate fetal growth restriction or sometimes intrauterine death.

LABORATORY TESTS. In addition to routine prenatal laboratory examinations (see Chapter 7), baseline renal function should be assessed with a 24-hour urine collection for total protein excretion and creatinine clearance. A random urine sample should be checked at each prenatal visit for possible urinary tract infections, which are common in women with diabetes. Urine also should be checked using a dipstick for the presence of glucose, ketones, protein. Thyroid function tests should be performed in the woman with preexisting diabetes because of her risk for coexisting thyroid disease.

Glycemic control should be evaluated on the basis of glycosylated hemoglobin. With prolonged hyperglycemia a percentage of hemoglobin will remain saturated with glucose for the life of the red blood cell. The glycosylated hemoglobin assay (HbA_{1c}) is an accurate measurement of the average glucose concentrations during the preceding 2 to 3 months. Unlike tests that reflect the amount of glucose in the plasma at that moment, the HbA_{1c} is not affected by recent intake or restriction of food.

FETAL SURVEILLANCE

Because of the increased risk for congenital anomalies or fetal death, surveillance should begin early for women with preexisting diabetes. Testing for anomalies includes triple marker screening (or multiple marker screening) to identify possible neural tube or other open defects and for possible chromosome abnormalities. Testing also includes performing ultrasonography and fetal echocardiography at 20 to 22 weeks to determine the integrity of the fetal body and cardiac structure (ACOG, 2001; Cunningham et al., 2001; Moore, 2004).

During the third trimester, the goal of fetal surveillance is to identify markers that suggest a worsening intrauterine environment with a higher probability of fetal death. Surveillance may include maternal assessment of fetal movement ("kick counts"), biophysical profiles, nonstress tests, and contraction stress tests. Ultrasonography is also used to document fetal growth rates. Doppler velocimetry may be recommended if vascular complications exist or if hypertension develops. See Chapter 10 for a description of fetal surveillance methods.

THERAPEUTIC MANAGEMENT

The goals of therapeutic management for a pregnant woman with diabetes are to (1) maintain normal blood glucose levels, (2) facilitate the birth of a healthy baby, and (3) avoid accelerated impairment of blood vessels and other major organs. To achieve this outcome, an intensive, team approach to care is required.

Members of the team often include a diabetologist, who assists in regulation of maternal blood glucose; an obstetrician, who monitors the mother and fetus and determines the optimal time for birth; a dietitian, who provides a balanced meal plan; and a diabetes educator, often a nurse, who provides ongoing education and support. The team is completed by a neonatologist, who will care for the newborn; the family physician; and the pediatrician, who will provide ongoing care for the infant and mother. A maternal-fetal medicine specialist and support staff may be added if multiple fetal surveillance procedures are needed.

PRECONCEPTION CARE. Ideally the team approach should begin before conception. Both prospective parents should participate in care sessions to learn more about the following issues (Blackburn, 2003; Moore, 2004):

- Establishing the optimal time for pregnancy based on maintenance of normal maternal blood glucose levels so that the risk of major fetal malformations can be reduced.
- Identifying whether complications of diabetes exist in other body systems. Examples of these complications include hypertension, retinopathy, neuropathy, and thyroid dysfunction.
- Identifying whether obesity is a factor in management of diabetes.
- Determining the current degree of glycemic control and providing information about maintenance of normal blood glucose levels throughout the pregnancy (this is particularly important if excellent control has not been achieved before conception); helping the woman identify ways to incorporate the need for tight glycemic control into her personal and family life.
- Providing instruction, if necessary, in the use of home glucose monitoring techniques and insulin administration for women who have previously taken oral hypoglycemic drugs or those who have taken insulin by injections that are less frequent than needed during pregnancy.
- Taking a daily prenatal vitamin that includes 400 mcg (0.4 mg) of folic acid to reduce the risk for neural tube defects in the fetus. Ideally, 400 mcg folic acid intake by supplements or food intake is the ideal for all women of childbearing age. If the woman has had a previous child with a neural tube defect, the recommendation is to take a larger dose (4 mg) from 3 months before conception through the first trimester.

DIET. Diet recommendations are individualized during a diabetic pregnancy. The average recommended caloric intake for the pregnant diabetic woman of normal weight is

30 kcal/kg/day. Approximately 40% to 45% of the calories should be from carbohydrates, 12% to 20% from protein (about 60 g), and up to 40% from fat. Caloric intake should be distributed among three meals and two or more snacks. The bedtime snack should include a complex carbohydrate and protein. Women who are overweight or underweight usually have lower or higher caloric goals.

SELF-MONITORING OF BLOOD GLUCOSE. The best frequency for self-monitoring of glucose of capillary blood has not yet been established. One common testing regimen requires obtaining fasting and 2-hour postprandial levels. Another includes testing six times per day: a fasting capillary glucose, 1 to 2 hours after breakfast, before and after lunch, before dinner, and at bedtime. One study found that the postprandial levels were most effective at predicting fetal macrosomia and other adverse outcomes (ACOG, 2001; Kenshole, 2004; Moore, 2004). In addition to regular monitoring, the woman should also perform a glucose test whenever she experiences symptoms of hypoglycemia. The woman should record all test results on a log sheet for review by the health care provider at each visit. Instruments for self-monitoring of blood glucose usually have a memory to provide accurate recall of times and glucose levels.

INSULIN THERAPY. The need to maintain rigorous control of maternal metabolism during pregnancy requires more frequent doses of insulin than usual. Most treatment regimens rely on three daily injections, with a combination of short-acting (regular) insulin and intermediate-acting (NPH) insulin given before breakfast, regular insulin before dinner, and NPH insulin at bedtime. Lispro and aspart (Humalog and NovoLog, respectively) insulins act rapidly and should be injected just before a meal. The rapid-acting insulins have been shown to control postprandial hyperglycemia with less between-meal hypoglycemia (Moore, 2004). Because placental hormones cause insulin needs to change throughout pregnancy, insulin coverage will need to be adjusted as pregnancy progresses.

First Trimester. Insulin needs generally decline during the first trimester because the secretion of placental hormones antagonistic to insulin remains low. The woman also may experience nausea, vomiting, and anorexia, resulting in decreased intake of food, and therefore requires less insulin. In addition, the fetus receives its share of glucose, which reduces maternal plasma glucose levels and decreases the need for maternal insulin.

Second and Third Trimesters. Insulin needs increase markedly during the second and third trimesters when placental hormones, which initiate maternal resistance to the effects of insulin, reach their peak. In addition, the nausea of early pregnancy usually resolves and the diet includes additional calories per day to meet the increased metabolic demands of pregnancy.

During Labor. Maintenance of tight maternal glucose control during birth is desirable to reduce neonatal hypoglycemia. Continuous infusion of a regular or lispro insulin solution combined with a separate intravenous solution containing glucose, such as 5% dextrose in Ringer's lactate, allows titration to maintain blood glucose levels between 80 and 110 mg/dl. The insulin solution is raised, lowered, or discontinued to maintain euglycemia based on hourly capillary blood glucose levels. If blood glucose levels remain too high, the insulin infusion is adjusted and the primary intravenous infusion is changed to one without glucose.

Women with type 2 or gestational diabetes that has been controlled by diet during pregnancy can usually maintain normal glucose levels during labor if glucose-bearing intravenous solutions are avoided (Cunningham et al., 2001; Moore, 2004).

Postpartum. Insulin needs should decline rapidly after the delivery of the placenta and abrupt cessation of placental hormones. However, blood glucose levels should be monitored at least four times daily so that the insulin dose can be adjusted to meet individual needs. Women with type 1 diabetes usually return to their prepregnancy dosages. Women with type 2 diabetes are monitored, and insulin is ordered only if needed.

TIMING OF DELIVERY. If possible the pregnancy should be allowed to progress to 38 weeks to allow fetal lungs to mature, reducing the risk for neonatal respiratory distress syndrome. With evidence of fetal compromise, such as nonreassuring biophysical profile or reduced amniotic fluid, delivery may be required. If delivery before 38 weeks is needed for nonemergency reasons, amniocentesis to determine fetal lung maturity is often performed, because lung maturation may be slower than in nondiabetic pregnancies.

Gestational Diabetes Mellitus

RISK FACTORS

GDM is a carbohydrate intolerance of variable severity that develops or is first recognized during pregnancy. Some women diagnosed with gestational diabetes may actually have unrecognized type 2 diabetes. GDM is an added risk factor that a woman will develop type 2 diabetes later in life. Factors such as obesity, inactivity, abnormal cholesterol levels, vascular disease, or family members with type 2 diabetes further increase a woman's risk to develop type 2 diabetes outside pregnancy.

Diagnosis begins with the taking of the history to identify the woman at risk to develop gestational diabetes. Factors known to increase the risk include:

- Overweight (BMI of ≥26-29) or obesity (BMI >29)
- Chronic hypertension
- Maternal age older than 25 years
- Family history of diabetes in close relatives
- Previous birth of a large infant (>4000 g)
- Previous birth of an infant with unexplained congenital anomalies
- Previous unexplained fetal death
- Gestational diabetes in previous pregnancy
- Multifetal pregnancy
- Fasting serum glucose ≥140 mg/dl or random serum glucose >200 mg/dl

Women with any of these factors should be screened for gestational diabetes at the first prenatal visit (ACOG, 2001; ADA, 2004; Moore, 2004).

IDENTIFYING GESTATIONAL DIABETES MELLITUS

All pregnant women should be screened by identification of a history or risk factors that are consistent for GDM or by blood glucose testing. Low-risk women include those with no risk factors. A woman at low risk for GDM must have all of the following characteristics: she is younger than 25 years of age; is of normal weight; has no known first-degree relatives with diabetes; is not a member of an ethnic group in which diabetes is prevalent; and has not had a pregnancy with a poor obstetric outcome.

SCREENING

GLUCOSE CHALLENGE TEST. A common screening test is the glucose challenge test (GCT), administered between 24 and 28 weeks. An oral glucose tolerance test (OGTT) may be used as the initial test if a woman is at high risk for GDM but is more likely to be used as a diagnostic test when abnormally high GCT results occur.

Fasting is not necessary for a GCT, and the woman is not required to follow any pretest dietary instructions. The woman should ingest 50 g of oral glucose solution. One hour later a blood sample is taken. If the blood glucose concentration is 140 mg/dl or greater, a 3-hour oral glucose tolerance test is recommended. Some practitioners use a lower cutoff of 130 or 135 mg/dl to identify more women at risk (ACOG, 2001; ADA, 2004; Moore, 2004).

ORAL GLUCOSE TOLERANCE TEST. The OGTT is the gold standard for diagnosing diabetes, but it is a more complicated test. The woman must fast from midnight on the day of the test. After a fasting plasma glucose level is determined, the woman should ingest 100 g of oral glucose solution. Plasma glucose levels are then determined at 1, 2, and 3 hours. Gestational diabetes is the diagnosis if the fasting blood glucose level is abnormal or if two or more of the following values occur on the OGTT (ACOG, 2001; ADA, 2004):

- Fasting, greater than 95 mg/dl
- 1 hour, greater than 180 mg/dl
- 2 hours, greater than 155 mg/dl
- 3 hours, greater than 140 mg/dl

MATERNAL, FETAL, AND NEONATAL EFFECTS

With a few important exceptions, the effects of gestational diabetes are similar to those associated with preexisting diabetes. The exceptions are that gestational diabetes is not associated with an increased risk for maternal ketoacidosis or spontaneous abortion. Because gestational diabetes develops after the first trimester, the critical period of major fetal organ development (organogenesis), it usually is not associated with an increase in major congenital malformations. Nevertheless, poorly controlled gestational diabetes, characterized by maternal hyperglycemia during the third trimester, is associated with increased neonatal morbidity

and mortality. The major fetal complications are macrosomia, leading to birth injuries or necessitating cesarean birth, and neonatal hypoglycemia. Other problems such as hypocalcemia, hyperbilirubinemia, and respiratory distress also may occur. (See Table 26-1 for a summary of maternal, fetal, and neonatal effects of diabetes mellitus and their probable causes.)

THERAPEUTIC MANAGEMENT

DIET. Ideally a registered dietitian or diabetes educator determines the dietary needs of the woman with GDM. The diet should provide the calories and nutrients needed for maternal and fetal health, result in euglycemia, avoid ketosis, and promote appropriate weight gain. Calories should be distributed in a way similar to that for preexisting diabetes. Simple sugars found in concentrated sweets should be eliminated from the diet. Based on a nonobese prepregnancy weight, an average of 30 kcal/kg/day is recommended. Calorie restriction to 25 kcal/kg each day may be recommended for the obese woman. The obese woman may be prescribed a diet with a smaller percentage of carbohydrates than the woman of normal weight to limit hyperglycemia. Carbohydrates should be adequate to prevent ketosis in all women. Calories should be divided among three meals and at least three snacks (ACOG, 2001; Franz, 2004; Moore, 2004).

EXERCISE. Research results have been mixed about whether exercise reduces the need for insulin in the woman with GDM. Nevertheless, exercise and an active lifestyle can improve cardiorespiratory fitness. A graduated physical exercise program should be recommended by a physician who takes into account each woman's risk factors, but exercise has been shown to be safe for women with GDM (ACOG, 2001; ADA, 2004; Kenshole, 2004).

BLOOD GLUCOSE MONITORING. Blood glucose levels should be evaluated to determine whether levels are normal. A common method is measurement of fasting blood sugar (no food for the previous 4 hours) and postprandial blood sugar (2 hours after each meal). If fasting capillary blood glucose levels repeatedly exceed 95 mg/dl or postprandial values exceed 120 mg/dl, insulin is begun. Additional tests for glucose levels may be performed as needed.

FETAL SURVEILLANCE. Testing to identify fetal compromise may begin as early as 28 weeks' gestation if the woman has poor glycemic control or by 34 weeks' gestation in lower-risk women with gestational diabetes. The surveillance testing often includes "kick counts," ultrasonography for fetal growth and amniotic fluid volume, biophysical profile, nonstress test, contraction stress test, or amniocentesis for fetal lung maturity (Moore, 2004).

NURSING CONSIDERATIONS

The care of a pregnant woman with diabetes mellitus focuses primarily on maintaining normal blood glucose. As stated earlier, this maintenance involves a rather rigid schedule of controlling the diet, blood glucose tests, administration of insulin, and regular fetal surveillance. Some women respond calmly to the intense medical supervision. Others respond with anxiety, fear, denial, or anger and may feel inadequate or unable to control the diabetes to the degree expected by the health care team. These feelings may not be shared spontaneously, but they may affect the woman's ability to achieve the desired outcomes. Also, nurses should remember to provide for normal pregnancy care in addition to monitoring the pregnant woman's diabetes.

INCREASING EFFECTIVE COMMUNICATION. A woman often does not volunteer information about her feelings and concerns, especially if she has negative feelings about her care. In addition, the woman and the nurse both may be unaware of misunderstandings or conflicts regarding the plan of care. Nurses must ask specifically about the feelings and concerns the woman and her family have about the pregnancy.

> Broad opening questions such as "What are your major concerns?" and "How do you feel about the plan of care?" are helpful. These should be followed by more specific questions such as "How do you feel about the fetal testing?" and "What would you like to change about the diet?" The woman's comments can provide valuable information about her emotional response to the care plan. One woman remarked, "I can tell you one thing, I don't feel like a person. I feel like an incubator, a faulty incubator." Another woman, who had a difficult time achieving the desired blood glucose level, said, "I feel as though my whole life has been taken over by diabetes. I'm tired of feeling like a sick person."

The nurse must be an active listener and allow time for the woman and her family to express concerns and feelings. The nurse must convey acceptance of both negative feelings and positive feelings that are expressed. Many women are re-

CRITICAL THINKING EXERCISE 26-1

Marcia Mahoney, a 28-year-old primigravida, is diagnosed with gestational diabetes in her thirtieth week of pregnancy. The health care team provides her with a diet and exercise regimen and tells her that she will need weekly tests to monitor her condition and that of the fetus. Although Marcia accepts the information without comment, she does not keep the next scheduled appointment.

Questions
1. What assumptions has the health care team made?
2. What could the team have done to ensure that Marcia would adhere to the recommendations?

Marcia is located and agrees to return to the clinic for follow-up care. She states she does not "see what all the fuss is about." She understands she may have a large baby, but states that she was a 10-pound baby and did just fine. She wonders if the weekly tests are necessary and if they could harm the baby.

Questions
3. How can the nurse respond to Marcia's comments about having a large baby without frightening her?
4. How can the nurse explain the need for weekly biophysical profiles?

assured to hear that their feelings of stress or anger are normal and learn that the health care team understands those feelings. Sharing of emotions will help her avoid or diminish unnecessary guilt, anxiety, and frustration and therefore promote positive feelings about her ability to participate successfully in her plan of care.

Most women benefit from praise when diabetic control is well maintained. They feel competent and trusted by the health care team and are motivated to continue their efforts.

PROVIDING OPPORTUNITIES FOR CONTROL. Allowing the woman to make as many decisions as possible increases her sense of being in control. For instance, she can select foods from the exchange list that provide the necessary nutrients but still allow her some choice. A dietitian should be consulted if the list does not include food she likes or that suit her ethnic or cultural preferences. A regular schedule of exercise and sleep that helps keep the blood glucose level under control is important. The woman can develop the best schedule for rest and exercise that suits her lifestyle. Nurses should allow as much flexibility as possible when scheduling stressful events such as fetal monitoring tests and amniocentesis.

Some women resent being "treated as though ill" even though their diabetic control is excellent. These women may be capable of making more decisions regarding their care during pregnancy, but they need the support of an understanding team to do this.

PROVIDING NORMAL PREGNANCY CARE. Some women express a need for more attention to the normal aspects of their pregnancies. This can be overlooked because of the intense focus on preventing complications that might occur as a result of diabetes. Women with diabetes also experience the discomforts that nondiabetic women experience during pregnancy, such as morning sickness, fatigue, backache, and difficulty sleeping. The nurse caring for women with diabetes should provide education and counseling regarding normal pregnancy.

✔ CHECK YOUR READING

4. What is the importance of glycosylated hemoglobin (HbA_{1c}) in monitoring diabetes mellitus?
5. How does GDM compare with type 1 diabetes mellitus in terms of onset and treatment?
6. What is the difference between a GCT and oral glucose tolerance test?
7. How do the maternal, fetal, and neonatal effects of gestational diabetes differ from those of preexisting diabetes?

Application of the Nursing Process
The Pregnant Woman with Diabetes Mellitus

Assessment

Determine how well the woman understands the prescribed management and how the family plans to carry out the recommended regimen. She may be newly diagnosed and have no experience in the necessary skills and procedures. On the other hand, the woman who had diabetes before becoming pregnant may be skilled in monitoring glucose and administering insulin. However, the woman with preexisting diabetes may have no knowledge of how diabetes can affect pregnancy or how pregnancy can affect diabetes. She may have been using premixed insulin exclusively and now must begin mixing insulins of different types.

To determine whether her techniques are accurate, ask the mother to demonstrate how she monitors blood glucose and observe as she mixes and injects insulins. Verify that she and her family are aware of the need to select appropriate sites and injection techniques that prevent insulin leakage.

Although diet is prescribed by a dietitian or diabetes educator, the nurse should assess how well the family understands the diet. Determine whether special problems with food preferences or availability of recommended foods exist. Diet recommendations include a target number of calories, plus targets for grams of carbohydrate, protein, and fat to meet calorie needs. Any of several methods to count and exchange foods may be used. One method uses exchange lists, in which the listed foods all have about the same number of grams of carbohydrate, protein, and fat. Therefore one food from the list may be substituted, or exchanged, for another in the same list. Another method uses carbohydrate counting, in which foods on the starch, fruit, or milk list supply about 15 g of carbohydrate, or one carbohydrate choice. The diet plan would prescribe the number of carbohydrate choices for each meal and snack. Insulin is often adjusted according to the carbohydrate count for each meal or snack.

Identify special needs related to food preferences, culturally prescribed foods, or the availability of recommended foods. It may be necessary to review the exchange list and ask the woman how she plans to substitute and exchange foods to obtain the prescribed number of foods from each list.

Identify the woman's knowledge of potential complications, such as hypoglycemia and hyperglycemia, so that she and her family can be provided with pertinent information to avoid and treat it.

Determine her knowledge of fetal surveillance techniques and her response to the need for frequent tests. Some women are highly motivated to continue the treatment regimen when test results indicate the fetus is thriving. Other women find the frequent testing stressful and inconvenient.

Analysis

One of the most common nursing diagnoses is Risk for (or actual) Ineffective Health Maintenance related to knowledge deficit of specific measures to maintain normal blood glucose levels; signs, symptoms, and management of hypoglycemia and hyperglycemia; and recommended fetal surveillance procedures.

Planning

Goals and expected outcomes for this nursing diagnosis are that the woman and her family will:

- Demonstrate competence in home glucose monitoring and administration of insulin before home management is initiated.

- Describe a plan for meeting dietary recommendations that fits family lifestyle and food preferences.
- Identify signs and symptoms of hypoglycemia and hyperglycemia and the management required for each.
- Verbalize knowledge of fetal surveillance procedures and keep scheduled appointments for testing.

Interventions

Although management of diabetes mellitus during pregnancy is a team effort, the nurse's major responsibility is to provide accurate information about the recommended therapeutic regimen and offer consistent support for the woman's efforts to comply with the recommendations. It may be necessary to demonstrate specific skills that the woman and her support person must master and to review and reinforce information from other members of the health care team.

TEACHING SELF-CARE SKILLS

Demonstrations and return demonstrations are the most effective ways to teach and evaluate psychomotor skills. The woman (and her family) must learn to use a meter and obtain a small sample of blood to test for glucose determination and to mix and inject insulin. Both procedures are invasive and cause mild discomfort, which may make the woman reluctant to start. Mixing insulins accurately or using a sliding scale may be intimidating at first. Using food exchanges is often unfamiliar to the woman who is newly diagnosed, but it is critical to glucose control. Acknowledge these feelings before teaching begins.

HOME BLOOD GLUCOSE MONITORING. Spring-loaded lancets make home blood glucose monitoring easier. The side of the fingertip is less sensitive than the pad, reducing discomfort. Teach the woman to cleanse the area with warm water before obtaining a sample, to prevent infection. The first drop of blood is wiped away, and the second drop is used to place blood on the meter's strip. Each home monitoring kit contains specific instructions for use of the meter and the type of reagent strip or cartridge that should be used. Teach the woman how to record glucose values in a handwritten log. Glucose monitors have a memory option that allows previous readings to be viewed.

INSULIN ADMINISTRATION. Two types of insulin usually are prescribed: intermediate-acting and short-acting (regular) insulin. Teach the woman the differences in onset, peak, and duration of action of each type of insulin. She usually needs to learn how to accurately mix the two insulins in the same syringe to avoid two separate injections for a mixed dose of the two types.

Insulin is administered subcutaneously. Common sites include the upper thighs, abdomen, and upper arms. Aseptic technique is recommended to prevent infection. Because the pregnant woman is injecting insulin frequently, emphasize these precautions:

- To prevent hypoglycemia, a meal should be eaten 30 minutes after insulin is injected, or within 15 minutes if lispro insulin is used.

- The angle of injection is usually 90 degrees unless the woman is very thin, in which case the insulin is injected at a lesser angle.
- The needle should be inserted quickly to minimize discomfort.
- The tissue pinch, if used, is released after inserting the needle and before injecting insulin because pressure from the pinch can promote insulin leakage from the subcutaneous tissue.
- Aspirating when injecting into subcutaneous tissue is not necessary.
- Insulin is injected slowly (over 2 to 4 seconds) to allow tissue expansion and minimize pressure, which can cause insulin leakage.
- The needle is withdrawn quickly to minimize the formation of a track that might permit insulin to leak out.

Emphasize the importance of administering the correct dose at the correct time. Teach the woman and her family the function of insulin and the importance of following the directions of her physician with regard to coordinating meals with the administration of insulin.

CONTINUOUS SUBCUTANEOUS INSULIN INFUSION. Many women who have preexisting diabetes use continuous subcutaneous insulin infusion and wish to continue with this method during pregnancy. The use of programmable insulin infusion pumps allows tailoring of insulin administration to the woman's individual lifestyle. Prompt, emergency counseling and assistance must be available 24 hours a day to deal with unexpected problems such as pump malfunction.

TEACHING DIETARY MANAGEMENT

Although a dietitian prescribes the recommended diet, the nurse must be aware of the general requirements and sensitive to the expectant mother's dietary habits and preferences. Often, reviewing and clarifying how exchange lists are used to plan meals and snacks are necessary. Encourage the patient to avoid simple sugars (candy, cake, cookies), which raise the blood glucose levels quickly but may result in wide swings between high and low glucose levels.

It may be necessary to help the woman select foods that are high in nutrients but low in cost or meet cultural or religious constraints. Animal protein is especially expensive, and alternative sources of protein (beans, peas, corn, grains) can be substituted to meet some of the protein needs as well as provide high-quality carbohydrate and fiber.

Allow the expectant mother to verbalize her frustrations or problems with the diet, and collaborate with the dietitian if she has a particular problem.

RECOGNIZING AND CORRECTING HYPOGLYCEMIA AND HYPERGLYCEMIA

Every woman and her family must be aware of the signs and symptoms that indicate abnormal blood glucose levels. Hypoglycemia and hyperglycemia pose a threat to the mother and fetus if they are not identified and corrected quickly.

HYPOGLYCEMIA. Treat hypoglycemia at once to prevent damage to the brain, which is dependent on glucose.

CRITICAL TO REMEMBER

Signs and Symptoms of Maternal Hypoglycemia

- Shakiness (tremors)
- Sweating
- Pallor; cold, clammy skin
- Disorientation; irritability
- Headache
- Hunger
- Blurred vision

CRITICAL TO REMEMBER

Signs and Symptoms of Maternal Hyperglycemia

- Fatigue
- Flushed, hot skin
- Dry mouth; excessive thirst
- Frequent urination
- Rapid, deep respirations; odor of acetone on the breath
- Drowsiness; headache
- Depressed reflexes

The woman should take 15 g of carbohydrate if she can swallow. Examples of foods that supply this are 3 or 4 glucose tablets (depending on their carbohydrate quantity), ½ cup of fruit juice or regular soft drink, six saltine crackers, or 1 tablespoon of sugar or honey (Franz, 2004). Large quantities of high-carbohydrate foods such as candy will increase the blood glucose excessively, making a sudden fall in the level more likely. The woman should retest 15 minutes after the carbohydrate intake and repeat the treatment if her blood glucose level remains below 70 mg/dl. If it is more than 1 hour until the next meal or snack, the woman should add an additional 15 g of carbohydrate, such as one serving of fruit (Franz, 2004).

Teach family members how to inject glucagon in the event that the woman cannot swallow or retain food. Notify the physician at once. Intravenous glucose will be administered if she is hospitalized. If untreated, hypoglycemia can progress to convulsions and death.

To prevent hypoglycemia, instruct the woman to have meals at a fixed time each day and to plan snacks at 10 AM, 3 PM, and bedtime. Suggest that she carry glucose tablets or some crackers with her.

HYPERGLYCEMIA. Because infection is the most common cause of hyperglycemia, pregnant women must be instructed to notify the physician whenever they have an infection of any type.

If untreated, hyperglycemia can lead to ketoacidosis, coma, and maternal and fetal death. If signs and symptoms occur, notify the physician at once so that treatment can be initiated. Hospitalization often is necessary for monitoring blood glucose levels and intravenous administration of insulin and treatment of any underlying infection.

EXPLAINING PROCEDURES, TESTS, AND PLAN OF CARE

Explain the schedule and the reasons for frequent checkups and necessary tests. Encourage the woman and her family to ask questions if any part of the schedule is confusing. This is particularly important for women who are aware that their prenatal care differs significantly from that of their nondiabetic friends. Knowing that the tests provide information about the condition of the mother and fetus reduces frustration and anxiety. Explain why more frequent antepartum surveillance testing is needed when diabetes complicates pregnancy. The woman needs to know that her diabetic care will require more time and effort than it did before pregnancy but that this care greatly improves her likelihood of having a healthy infant.

Evaluation

After procedures, tests, and plan of care have been explained, evaluation should ensure that:

- The woman and at least one support person can demonstrate competence in home glucose monitoring and administration of insulin.
- The woman can describe a satisfactory plan for meeting her individual dietary requirements.
- The woman and at least one support person can list the signs and symptoms of hypoglycemia and hyperglycemia and describe the initial management of these conditions.
- The woman can verbalize knowledge of the reason for fetal surveillance procedures and keeps appointments for tests.

CARDIAC DISEASE

Alterations in cardiovascular function are necessary in pregnancy to meet additional maternal metabolic demands and the needs of the fetus. Plasma volume, venous return, and cardiac output all increase. Heart rate and stroke volume, the components of cardiac output, increase during pregnancy. The heart rate gradually rises above the baseline during the third trimester. However, increases in stroke volume are primarily responsible for the overall rise in cardiac output during early pregnancy.

A normal heart can adapt to the changes so that pregnancy and birth are tolerated without difficulty. For women with preexisting or underlying heart disease, however, the changes can impose an additional burden on an already compromised heart, which may result in cardiac decompensation and congestive heart failure.

Incidence and Classification

Heart disease complicates about 1% of pregnancies (Cunningham et al., 2001). Pregnancy may unmask a previously asymptomatic heart condition, or it may aggravate known heart disease.

The two major categories of heart disease are rheumatic heart disease and congenital heart disease in the mother. Although rheumatic fever is uncommon in the United States, it is prevalent in less-developed countries, which may be the countries of origin for immigrant women seeking health care in the United States. Women with congenital heart disease are more likely to survive to reproductive age, adding cardiac risk to their pregnancy in some cases. A third category, mitral valve prolapse, is a common but benign condition that usually does not cause problems during pregnancy. Myocardial infarction and conduction defects also may occur in women of childbearing age, although these conditions are most common in older adults.

RHEUMATIC HEART DISEASE

A remarkable decline in rheumatic heart disease has occurred in North America and Western Europe as a result of early treatment of streptococcal pharyngitis ("strep throat") in childhood, which often precedes the onset of rheumatic fever. Even one bout of rheumatic fever may cause scarring of the valves in the heart. This results in narrowing (stenosis) of the openings between the chambers of the heart.

The mitral valve is the most common site of stenosis. Mitral stenosis obstructs the free flow of blood from the left atrium to the left ventricle. The left atrium becomes dilated. As a result, pressure in the left atrium, pulmonary veins, and pulmonary capillaries is chronically elevated. This elevation may lead to pulmonary hypertension, pulmonary edema, or congestive heart failure. The first warnings of heart failure include persistent rales at the base of the lungs, dyspnea on exertion, cough, and hemoptysis. Progressive edema and tachycardia are additional signs of heart failure.

CONGENITAL HEART DISEASE

Congenital heart defects can be grouped into those that cause a left-to-right shunt and those resulting in a right-to-left shunt. Defects that produce left-to-right shunting include atrial and ventricular septal defects and patent ductus arteriosus. In contrast, right-to-left shunting occurs when a cyanotic heart defect such as tetralogy of Fallot is present. Right-to-left shunting also may occur through a septal defect or patent ductus arteriosus when pulmonary vascular resistance exceeds peripheral vascular resistance and pulmonary hypertension (Eisenmenger syndrome) occurs. The fetus is more likely to inherit congenital defects, although the risk varies with different maternal defects.

LEFT-TO-RIGHT SHUNT

Atrial Septal Defect. Atrial septal defect often is first discovered in women of childbearing age because symptoms are absent or vague. This defect produces a left-to-right shunt because pressure in the left side of the heart is higher than in the right side. Pregnancy is well tolerated by patients with an uncomplicated atrial septal defect, and no specific treatment is recommended. Bacterial endocarditis is rare, and prophylactic antibiotics are not required (Setaro & Caulin-Glaser, 2004). Pulmonary hypertension occasionally develops because the additional blood that moves to the right side of the heart is transported to the lungs through the pulmonary artery.

Ventricular Septal Defect. Although ventricular septal defects are more common than atrial septal defects at birth, they usually are detected and corrected before childbearing age. Most women with ventricular septal defects who become pregnant are asymptomatic, but fatigue or symptoms of pulmonary congestion occur occasionally.

Pregnancy is well tolerated with small to moderate left-to-right shunts (Cunningham et al., 2001). However, pregnancy occasionally precipitates heart failure or a dysrhythmia, either of which is managed as in nonpregnant patients. Bacterial endocarditis is common with unrepaired defects, and antibacterial prophylaxis is recommended.

Patent Ductus Arteriosus. The communicating shunt between the pulmonary artery and aorta is usually discovered and treated in childhood. If the condition is untreated, the physiologic effects are related to size. If small this lesion, like septal defects, may be well tolerated during pregnancy unless complicated by pulmonary hypertension. The patent ductus arteriosus tends to become infected, so antibiotic prophylaxis is recommended, particularly at the time of labor.

RIGHT-TO-LEFT SHUNT

Tetralogy of Fallot. The primary cause of right-to-left shunting is tetralogy of Fallot, a combination of four defects (ventricular septal defect, pulmonary valve stenosis, right ventricular hypertrophy, and displacement of the aorta toward the right ventricle). Untreated patients with tetralogy of Fallot have obvious symptoms of heart disease that include (1) cyanosis; (2) clubbing of the fingers, indicating proliferation of capillaries to transport blood to the extremities; and (3) inability to tolerate activity.

Women who have undergone repair and in whom cyanosis did not reappear may do well during pregnancy. With uncorrected tetralogy of Fallot, maternal mortality approaches 10% (Blanchard & Shabetai, 2004; Cunningham et al., 2001).

Eisenmenger Syndrome. Eisenmenger syndrome is a cyanotic heart condition that develops when pulmonary resistance equals or exceeds systemic resistance to blood flow and a right-to-left shunt develops. Tissue hypoxia occurs as deoxygenated blood that should go to the lungs is pushed into the systemic circulation. Several underlying congenital defects may underlie the equalization of pressures within the ventricles, such as a large ventricular septal defect or a large patent ductus arteriosus. Operative closure of these defects must be done as soon as possible in defects that may cause Eisenmenger syndrome. A late surgical correction often results in the patient's death. If she survives delayed surgery, pregnancy may carry a 50% maternal mortality risk, usually from right ventricular failure (Blanchard & Shabetai, 2004).

MITRAL VALVE PROLAPSE

Mitral valve prolapse is one of the most common cardiac conditions among the general population. The incidence among otherwise normal young women is as high as 15%, but community-based studies have shown the incidence to be far lower, at 2% to 3% (Cunningham et al., 2001; Setaro & Caulin-Glaser, 2004). Although the condition appears to be inherited, it may be associated with a variety of other cardiac disorders such as atrial septal defects and Marfan's syndrome. In mitral valve prolapse, the leaflets of the mitral valve prolapse into the left atrium during ventricular contraction.

Mitral valve prolapse is considered a benign condition, and most women with mitral valve prolapse are asymptomatic and tolerate pregnancy well. Some women experience dysrhythmias or chest pain. Some physicians consider mitral valve prolapse to be a significant risk factor for bacterial endocarditis and administer prophylactic antibiotics before and during labor and delivery. β-Blockers, such as atenolol or metoprolol, may be given for chest pain or dysrhythmias.

PERIPARTUM AND POSTPARTUM CARDIOMYOPATHY

Cardiomyopathy in the peripartum or postpartum period is a rare condition exclusively associated with pregnancy. Women with the condition have no underlying heart disease, but symptoms of cardiac decompensation appear during the last weeks of pregnancy or from 2 to 20 weeks postpartum. The symptoms are those of congestive heart failure: dyspnea, edema, weakness, chest pain, and heart palpitations. Cardiomyopathy may suddenly appear in a woman who has been healthy. An abrupt downhill course in which the woman can be saved only with cardiac transplantation may occur in about 20% of women. About 50% of other women with cardiomyopathy may have a partial recovery with persistent congestive heart failure or other cardiac dysfunction. The remaining women may show recovery. Peripartum cardiomyopathy often recurs with subsequent pregnancies, particularly in women who did not have complete recovery of their left ventricular function. The woman should be informed of this risk (Blanchard & Shabetai, 2004; Cunningham, 2001; Setaro & Caulin-Glaser, 2004).

Anticoagulation with low-molecular-weight heparin is typical to prevent clot formation during pregnancy when coagulation factors are higher. Other medical therapy includes fluid restriction to reduce pulmonary edema and treatment of congestive heart failure and other pathologies associated with cardiomyopathy.

Diagnosis and Classification

Early recognition of underlying heart disease is essential, and careful assessment for specific signs and symptoms of heart disease is part of every initial prenatal visit. Signs and symptoms include dyspnea, syncope (fainting) with exertion, hemoptysis, paroxysmal nocturnal dyspnea, and chest pain with exertion. Additional signs that confirm the diagnosis are (1) cyanosis; (2) clubbing; (3) diastolic, presystolic, or continuous heart murmur; (4) cardiac enlargement; (5) a loud, harsh systolic murmur associated with a thrill; and (6) serious dysrhythmias (Blanchard & Shabetai, 2004).

Diagnosis of heart disease may be made from clinical signs and symptoms and physical examination. It often is confirmed by chest radiograph, electrocardiography, or echocardiography.

Once the diagnosis is made, the severity of the disease can be determined by the client's ability to endure physical activity. A clinical classification based on the effect of exercise on the heart has been developed by the New York Heart Association (Box 26-2).

Therapeutic Management

Therapeutic management care of the pregnant woman who has a heart disorder is discussed in this segment. Management may include interventions that are not advised in most pregnancies, such as maintaining a low-sodium diet. The nurse should consult a medical-surgical nursing textbook for additional information that pertains to medical and nursing care for cardiac conditions.

CLASS I OR II HEART DISEASE

All pregnant women with heart disease should do the following:

- Limit physical activity so that demand does not exceed the functional capacity of the heart. In other words, the woman should remain free of symptoms of cardiac stress, such as dyspnea, chest pain, and tachycardia.
- Avoid excessive weight gain, which increases demands on the heart. A diet adequate in protein, calories, and sodium is necessary. A low-sodium diet may be advised to avoid congestive heart failure.
- Prevent anemia, which decreases the oxygen-carrying capacity of the blood and results in a compensatory increase in heart rate that a diseased heart may be unable to tolerate. Most anemia is prevented by administration of iron and folic acid.
- Prevent infection. Immunizations for influenza and pneumonia are available. Prevention may include administration of prophylactic antibiotics. As with other people, a pregnant woman with cardiac disease should be advised to avoid contact with those who may be ill during times when upper respiratory infections are prevalent, such as winter months.

- Undergo careful assessment for the development of congestive heart failure, pulmonary edema, and cardiac dysrhythmias. Characteristics of heart failure may include persistent basilar rales, often accompanied by a cough during the night as the woman tries to sleep, sudden inability to carry out usual activities, dyspnea, cough, hemoptysis, increasing edema, and tachycardia.

CLASS III OR IV HEART DISEASE

The primary goal of management is to prevent cardiac decompensation and development of congestive heart failure. Also, every effort is made to protect the fetus from hypoxia and IUGR, which can occur if placental perfusion is inadequate. In addition to the precautions listed for classes I and II heart disease, the woman may require bed rest, especially during the last trimester, because she has little reserve to tolerate rising metabolic demands. Reduced activity increases the risk for thrombus formation and will require prophylaxis such as elastic compression stockings or a serial or boot compression device. Prophylactic anticoagulation may be needed.

DRUG THERAPY

ANTICOAGULANTS. During pregnancy, clotting factors normally increase and thrombolytic activity decreases. These changes predispose the pregnant woman to thrombus formation. Superimposed cardiac problems such as mitral valve stenosis may require anticoagulant therapy during pregnancy. Warfarin (Coumadin) is associated with fetal malformations and should be restricted throughout pregnancy. Subcutaneous heparin, which does not cross the placental barrier, is an effective alternative anticoagulant for most women. Careful monitoring of the partial thromboplastin time, activated partial thromboplastin time, and platelet count is essential to achieve effective, safe anticoagulation. Enoxaparin (Lovenox), a low-molecular-weight heparin, may be used instead of standard heparin because it requires less-frequent monitoring for bleeding complications. Enoxaparin and heparin are not interchangeable. Both are given subcutaneously, but only heparin may be given intravenously.

ANTIDYSRHYTHMICS. Use of medications for heart disease during pregnancy must balance benefits to the mother against possible harm to the fetus. Another consideration is that maternal heart failure itself is harmful to the fetus. In addition to controlling the dysrhythmias, β-blockers and calcium channel blockers may be used to control maternal hypertension. Digoxin, adenosine, and calcium channel blockers appear to be safe. β-Blockers have been associated with neonatal respiratory depression, sustained bradycardia, and hypoglycemia when administered late in pregnancy or just before delivery but may be needed in selected cases. The β-blockers atenolol and metoprolol may be preferred because they do not cause the uterine stimulation that other drugs of this class may cause (Blanchard & Shabetai, 2004; Cunningham et al., 2001; Setaro & Caulin-Glaser, 2004).

ANTIINFECTIVES. Antiinfective agents for endocarditis are chosen based on the infecting agent. Gram-positive staphylococcus infections are common in intravenous drug users, and the mortality is high. Maternal gonorrhea infection may cause acute, rapidly developing endocarditis. A woman with an increased risk for bacterial endocarditis may receive prophylactic antibiotics at delivery, such as amoxicillin, penicillin, ampicillin, and gentamicin. Ceftriaxone or vancomycin also may be given for acute endocarditis.

DRUGS FOR HEART FAILURE. Diuretics may be needed when congestive heart failure is uncontrolled by restriction of activity and sodium intake. Careful monitoring of electrolytes and water balance is necessary to avoid excessively reducing maternal blood volume with resulting adverse effects on the fetus. Experience is greatest with furosemide and thiazide diuretics. Fetal growth retardation has been associated with furosemide, and neonatal jaundice, thrombocytopenia, anemia, and hypoglycemia have been associated with thiazide diuretics (Blanchard & Shabetai, 2004; Moore, 2004). β-Blockers, angiotensin-converting enzyme (ACE) inhibitors, or angiotensin receptor blockers, and digoxin also may be used if beneficial for treatment of pregnancy-associated heart failure.

INTRAPARTUM MANAGEMENT

Every effort is made to minimize the effects of labor on the cardiovascular system. For example, with every contraction, 300 to 500 ml of blood is shifted from the uterus and placenta into the central circulation. This extra fluid causes a sharp rise in cardiac workload. Therefore careful management of intravenous fluid administration is essential to prevent fluid overload. The woman should be positioned on her side, with her head and shoulders elevated. Oxygen is administered to increase the blood oxygen saturation and is monitored by pulse oximetry. Discomfort should be reduced to a minimum, but the use of an epidural block is sometimes controversial because of its potential hemodynamic effects (see Chapter 16). The environment is kept as quiet and calm as possible to decrease anxiety, which can cause tachycardia.

The fetus is monitored electronically, and signs of fetal compromise as well as maternal signs of cardiac decompensation (tachycardia, rapid respirations, moist rales, and exhaustion) should be reported immediately to the physician.

A vaginal delivery is recommended for a woman with heart disease unless there are specific indications for cesarean birth. Vacuum extraction or outlet forceps are often used to minimize the mother's use of the Valsalva maneuver when pushing and to shorten the second stage of labor.

Cesarean delivery may be chosen to limit prolonged labor, which can add to the hemodynamic stress for the woman with cardiac disease. Although it is a common obstetric procedure, the woman and her physician must consider the added stress of major surgery on the heart. Expected blood loss is higher in a cesarean than in a vaginal birth. General anesthesia may be required if epidural anesthesia is not an option, leading to operative airway management by an anesthesiologist.

The fourth stage of labor is associated with special risks. After delivery of the placenta, about 500 ml of blood is added to the intravascular volume. To minimize the risks of overloading the heart, abrupt positional changes should be avoided. Moreover, the uterus should not be massaged to expedite separation of the placenta. Careful assessment for signs of circulatory overload, such as a bounding pulse, distended neck and peripheral veins, and moist rales in the lungs, is performed throughout labor and the postpartum.

POSTPARTUM MANAGEMENT

Women who have shown no evidence of distress during pregnancy, labor, and childbirth may have cardiac decompensation during the postpartum period. The relief of vena caval compression and autotransfusion of blood from the uterus after placental delivery abruptly increases the blood returning to the right side of the heart.

The woman also must be observed closely for signs of infection, hemorrhage, and thromboembolism. These conditions can act together to precipitate postpartum heart failure in women with underlying heart disease. The woman is vulnerable postpartum, as interstitial fluid is mobilized into the vascular space for elimination. Continue to observe for signs of congestive heart failure. Observe urine output, because inadequate urine output may reflect the heart's inability to circulate blood adequately to the kidneys. If the mother cannot assume the care of her infant, nurses should make every effort to promote contact between the mother, her significant others, and the infant.

Breastfeeding imposes extra demands on the mother's heart, and whether it is advised is individualized. If no evidence of cardiac compromise during labor and the early postpartum period exists, breastfeeding usually is not contraindicated.

Application of the Nursing Process
The Pregnant Woman with Heart Disease

Assessment

Begin with a review of the woman's medical record to determine the functional classification assigned (see Box 26-2). Assess the woman at each prenatal appointment to determine how pregnancy affects the functional capacity of the heart.

- Take vital signs and compare them with preconception levels. Note any changes since the last prenatal appointment.
- Assess the level of fatigue and any changes in fatigue since the last prenatal appointment. This is especially important when fluid volume peaks and the chance of cardiac decompensation is greatest (18 to 32 weeks' gestation).
- Observe for signs or symptoms of congestive heart failure.
- Note additional factors that may increase the workload of the heart (anemia, infections, anxiety, lack of adequate support to manage the activities of daily living).

CRITICAL TO REMEMBER

Signs and Symptoms of Congestive Heart Failure

- Cough (frequent, productive, hemoptysis)
- Progressive dyspnea with exertion
- Orthopnea
- Pitting edema of legs and feet or generalized edema of face, hands, or sacral area
- Palpitations of heart
- Progressive fatigue or syncope with exertion
- Moist rales in lower lobes, indicating pulmonary edema

- Weigh the client and compare the desired and actual patterns of weight gain to detect excessive weight gain or fluid retention.
- Assess the woman's knowledge of the prescribed regimen of care and her ability to comply with it.

Analysis

The pregnant woman with a cardiac defect may be unable to tolerate activity to the same degree as before pregnancy because of the stress imposed on the cardiovascular system. Arriving at the nursing diagnosis "Activity Intolerance related to insufficient knowledge of measures that reduce cardiac stress" is a priority.

Planning

Goals and outcomes are as follows:
- The woman (and her family) will identify factors that increase cardiac workload.
- The woman (and family) will describe measures that promote adaptation to activity restrictions.

Interventions

Prenatal nursing care focuses on teaching the woman and her family about the possible effects of the disease on their lives. This teaching may include specific instructions about factors increasing the workload of the heart and measures promoting adaptation to restrictions in activity. Teaching may also reinforce or clarify the physician's instructions.

TEACHING ABOUT INCREASED CARDIAC WORKLOAD

EXCESSIVE WEIGHT GAIN AND ANEMIA. Excessive weight gain and anemia increase the workload of the heart just as they do in the nonpregnant state and should be avoided. A well-balanced diet that contains approximately 2200 calories is recommended, with adequate high-quality protein. Emphasize the importance of taking any prescribed iron supplements to prevent anemia and reduce the risk of tachycardia. Folic acid should be taken from before conception to avoid anemia and reduce the risk for neural tube defects in the fetus.

EXERTION. Instruct the woman to modify approaches to activities to regulate energy expenditures and reduce cardiac workload. For example, she might take rest periods dur-

ing the day and for an hour after meals. If possible, she should sit rather than stand when performing activities. She should rest every few minutes when performing an activity that increases the heart rate to allow the heart time to recover. Emphasize that she should stop an activity if she experiences dyspnea, chest pain, or tachycardia.

EXPOSURE. Instruct the woman to avoid unnecessary exposure to environmental extremes. She should dress warmly during cold weather and create a barrier to cold temperatures by wearing layers of clothing. She must become aware that exertion in hot, humid weather or during extreme cold weather places additional demands on the heart and should be avoided.

EMOTIONAL STRESS. Help the woman to identify areas of stress in her life, if applicable, and explain the effects of emotional stress on the cardiovascular system (increased blood pressure, heart rate, and respiratory rate). Discuss various methods for stress management, such as meditation, progressive relaxation of muscles, and biofeedback. Teach that cigarette smoking and use of illicit drugs such as cocaine and amphetamines greatly increase stress on the heart.

HELPING THE FAMILY ACCEPT RESTRICTIONS ON ACTIVITY

Assist family members to accept the need for activity restriction. The amount of activity that can be tolerated depends on the severity of the disease. However, all women with heart disease require 8 to 10 hours of sleep each night, with periods of morning and afternoon rest. For some women, bed rest with bathroom privileges is necessary during the last half of pregnancy, and this may create special problems for the family. Nurses often help family members plan ways to meet their needs while the expectant mother remains on bed rest. See the Nursing Care Plan for Preterm Labor (Chapter 27) for additional interventions when a prolonged period of bed rest is required.

PROVIDING POSTPARTUM CARE

After childbirth the mother may be unable to assume care of the newborn, especially after a prolonged period of bed rest. However, every effort should be made to promote contact between the mother and baby. Many nurses assess the baby and perform the necessary newborn care at the bedside, then allow the mother ample time to hold the infant. The father and other family members should be included in the care of the infant whenever possible.

The decision about breastfeeding will be individualized according to the mother's condition and its demands on her energy. She should be encouraged to feed the infant whenever possible to promote maternal-infant attachment, even if she feeds formula. Consult with physicians, and make referrals as necessary for follow-up care, which may include home care by a nurse or nursing assistant. Be certain that the family understands the signs and symptoms of cardiac complications and when to notify the physician that problems have developed.

Evaluation

The ability to identify the factors increasing cardiac workload offers reassurance that the woman and her family will initiate measures promoting adaptation to restricted activity.

✓ CHECK YOUR READING

8. How do the cardiovascular changes of pregnancy affect the condition of the woman who has a cardiac defect?
9. What are the two major categories of heart disease? What is the functional classification of heart disease?
10. What are the primary goals for management of heart disease in terms of diet, activity, and weight gain?
11. Why must the administration of fluids, both oral and intravenous, be monitored closely during labor?
12. Why is the fourth stage of labor particularly dangerous for the woman with heart disease?

ANEMIAS

Anemia is a condition in which a decline in circulating red blood cell mass occurs, which reduces the capacity to carry oxygen to the vital organs of the mother or fetus. During pregnancy and the puerperium, anemia is defined as a hemoglobin concentration of less than 11 g/dl in the first and third trimesters and less than 10.5 g/dl in the second trimester (Cunningham et al., 2001; Kilpatrick & Laros, 2004).

Anemia is one of the most common problems of pregnancy. An estimated 20% to 60% of women will be anemic at some time during pregnancy (Kilpatrick & Laros, 2004). The incidence varies according to geographic location and socioeconomic group. Anemia may be caused by a variety of factors including nutrition, hemolysis, and blood loss. The most common types of anemia observed during pregnancy include iron-deficiency anemia, folic acid–deficiency anemia, sickle cell disease, and thalassemia.

Iron-Deficiency Anemia

The total iron requirement for a typical pregnancy with a single fetus is approximately 1000 mg (Cunningham et al., 2001). Unfortunately, most women do not have iron stores that equal this amount. Furthermore, meeting pregnancy needs by diet alone is difficult, although iron is present in many foods. The primary sources are meat, fish, chicken, liver, and green leafy vegetables.

MATERNAL EFFECTS

Signs and symptoms of iron-deficiency anemia include pallor, fatigue, lethargy, and headache. Clinical findings also may include inflammations of the lips and tongue. Pica (consuming nonfood substances such as clay, dirt, ice, and starch) also is a sign of iron-deficiency anemia (Kilpatrick & Laros, 2004). Laboratory findings for iron-deficiency anemia include red blood cells that are microcytic (small) and hypochromic (pale). The plasma iron and serum ferritin are low, whereas the total iron-binding capacity is higher than normal. Women who have multifetal pregnancies or bleeding complications are more likely to be anemic during pregnancy.

FETAL AND NEONATAL EFFECTS

All effects of maternal iron-deficiency anemia on the fetus and neonate are unclear. In general, even with significant maternal iron deficiency, the fetus will receive adequate stores at a cost to the mother. If the mother is severely anemic, the fetus may have reduced red cell volume, hemoglobin, and iron stores. Profound maternal anemia can reduce fetal oxygen supply (Kilpatrick & Laros, 2004).

THERAPEUTIC MANAGEMENT

Iron replacement is easily achieved in most patients with administration of ferrous sulfate, 320 mg, one to three times per day. Giving the iron with a citrus drink or 500 mg of ascorbic acid is believed to improve iron absorption from the gastrointestinal tract. Many women experience less gastrointestinal discomfort if iron is taken with meals, although doing so reduces absorption somewhat. Therapy often is continued for about 6 months after the anemia has been corrected. Parenteral therapy may be needed if the woman cannot take oral preparations.

Folic Acid-Deficiency (Megaloblastic) Anemia

Folic acid, which functions as a coenzyme in the synthesis of deoxyribonucleic acid (DNA), is essential for cell duplication and fetal and placental growth. It also is an essential nutrient for the formation of red blood cells.

MATERNAL EFFECTS

Maternal needs for folic acid double during pregnancy in response to the demand for greater production of erythrocytes and fetal and placental growth. A deficiency in folic acid results in a reduction in the rate of DNA synthesis and mitotic activity of individual cells, resulting in the presence of large, immature erythrocytes (megaloblasts). Folate deficiency is the primary cause of megaloblastic anemia during pregnancy.

Nonnutritional factors that contribute to folic acid deficiency include hemolytic anemias with increased red blood cell turnover, some medications such as phenytoin (Dilantin), and malabsorption entities. Folic acid deficiency often is present in association with iron-deficiency anemia.

FETAL AND NEONATAL EFFECTS

Folate deficiency is associated with increased risk of spontaneous abortion, abruptio placentae, and fetal anomalies. A known association exists between folic acid deficiency and an increase in neural tube defects.

THERAPEUTIC MANAGEMENT

The recommended daily allowance for folic acid doubles during pregnancy, and some women have difficulty ingesting the amount needed even though it does occur widely in foods. The best sources of folic acid are liver, kidney beans, lima beans, and fresh, dark-green, leafy vegetables (see Table 9-5). Folic acid often is destroyed in cooking. As a result of the awareness of the association between folic acid deficiency and neural tube defects, it is now recommended that all women of childbearing age take 400 mcg (0.4 mg) of folic acid daily to reduce this risk. This supplementation should be increased to 600 mcg (0.6 mg) when pregnancy is confirmed. Women who have had a previous child with a neural tube defect should take 4 mg of folic acid for 1 month before and during the first trimester of pregnancy (American Academy of Pediatrics [AAP] & ACOG, 2002; Blackburn, 2003).

Most prenatal vitamins contain 1 mg of folate to ensure sufficient intake. Higher doses of folate may be ordered according to individual needs.

✓ CHECK YOUR READING

13. Why is supplemental iron needed by most women who are pregnant?
14. What are the neonatal effects of iron-deficiency anemia?
15. What are the fetal and neonatal effects of folic acid deficiency?

Sickle Cell Anemia

Sickle cell anemia is an autosomal recessive genetic disorder. It occurs when the gene for the production of hemoglobin S is inherited from both parents. The defect in the hemoglobin causes erythrocytes to become shaped like a sickle, or crescent, under certain conditions. Low oxygen concentration usually causes the sickling, with acidosis and dehydration worsening the process. At first the erythrocytes regain their normal shape, but eventually they remain permanently sickled. Because of their distorted shape, the erythrocytes cannot pass through small arteries and capillaries and tend to clump together and occlude the blood vessel.

The disease is characterized by chronic anemia, increased susceptibility to infection, and periodic episodes of obstruction of blood vessels by the abnormally shaped erythrocytes. Sickle cell disease occurs most often in people who have ancestors from sub-Saharan Africa, South America, Cuba, Central America, Saudi Arabia, India, and Mediterranean countries. About 1 in 500 African-American and 1 in 1000 to 1400 Hispanic births in the United States will result in an infant with sickle cell anemia. Sickle cell anemia affects 72,000 people in the United States. More than 2 million U.S. residents are carriers of the sickle cell trait and may pass the gene on to their children even though they are not affected (Ashley-Koch, Yang, & Olney, 2000; National Institutes of Health: National Heart, Lung, and Blood Institute, 2002; Sickle Cell Disease Association of America, 2004).

MATERNAL EFFECTS

Pregnancy may exacerbate sickle cell anemia and bring on *sickle cell crisis*. This broad term includes several different conditions, particularly temporary cessation of bone marrow function, hemolytic crisis with massive erythrocyte destruction resulting in jaundice, and severe pain caused by infarctions located in the joints and the major organs. In addition, expectant mothers with sickle cell anemia are prone to pyelonephritis, bone infection, and heart disease.

FETAL AND NEONATAL EFFECTS

The fetus is prone to serious complications including prematurity and IUGR. The incidence of fetal death is particularly high in the presence of maternal sickle cell crisis.

THERAPEUTIC MANAGEMENT

Women with sickle cell anemia should seek preconception or early prenatal care and be informed of the maternal and fetal risks associated with the pregnancy. Frequent evaluations of hemoglobin, complete blood count, serum iron, total iron-binding capacity, and serum folate are necessary to determine the degree of anemia and iron and folic acid stores. Testing is performed for infections, such as hepatitis, human immunodeficiency virus (HIV), tuberculosis, and sexually transmitted infections. Hepatitis B and varicella vaccine may be given to the noninfected woman who is not immune to the infections. Urinalysis, with culture and sensitivity if indicated, identifies both clinical and subclinical urinary tract infections that should be treated.

Fetal surveillance studies (ultrasonography, nonstress tests, and biophysical profiles) assess fetal growth and development and placental function. Exchange transfusions or prophylactic transfusions may be used to increase the amount of normal hemoglobin in the mother's circulation and to reduce severe anemia. Risks of prophylactic transfusions are comparable to risks if the woman does not have sickle cell disease. She may have a transfusion reaction to the transfused blood and is likely to develop higher levels of antibodies to cells in the transfused blood. Finding compatible blood for later transfusion might be more difficult (Cunningham et al., 2001; Kilpatrick & Laros, 2004; National Institutes of Health: National Heart, Lung, and Blood Institute, 2002).

The goal of nursing management is to help the pregnant woman maintain a healthy status and avoid hospitalization. Women must be encouraged to keep all prenatal care appointments, usually every other week and more frequently if needed. Topics in prenatal education include the need for (1) adequate hydration to prevent sickling, (2) adequate nutrition to meet metabolic needs, (3) folic acid supplementation for erythrocyte production, (4) rest periods throughout the day, (5) good hygiene practices and the avoidance of persons with infectious illnesses, and (6) prompt treatment for fever or other signs of infection.

Nurses must be alert for signs of sickle cell crisis. The most common indications are pain in the abdomen, chest, vertebrae, joints, or extremities; pallor; and signs of cardiac failure. Nurses also must provide comfort measures such as repositioning, good skin care, assisting with ambulation and movement in bed, and assisting the woman to splint the abdomen with a pillow when she must cough or breathe deeply.

Nurses must remember that pain is not always related to the sickling crisis but could be related to a complication of pregnancy. Women with sickle cell disease also can have ectopic pregnancy, abruptio placentae, appendicitis, and other painful complications not related to their blood disorder.

Intrapartum care focuses on preventing the development of sickle cell crisis. Oxygen is administered continuously, and fluids should be administered to prevent dehydration because hypoxemia and dehydration as well as exertion, infection, and acidosis stimulate the sickling process. Packed red blood cells may be administered to women who have a hematocrit lower than 20%.

Thalassemia

Like sickle-cell anemia, thalassemia is a genetic disorder that involves the abnormal synthesis of alpha or beta chains of hemoglobin. This abnormal synthesis leads to alterations in the red blood cell membrane and decreased life span of red blood cells. Thalassemia is named and classified by the type of chain that is abnormal. Beta-thalassemia is most frequently encountered in the United States, often in those of Mediterranean, Middle Eastern, and Asian descent.

Beta-thalassemia minor refers to the heterozygous form that results from the inheritance of one abnormal gene from either parent. *Beta-thalassemia major* refers to inheritance of the gene from both parents (homozygous form). Females with beta-thalassemia major (Cooley's anemia) usually die in young adulthood. Those females who survive are often sterile (Cunningham et al., 2001; Kilpatrick & Laros, 2004).

MATERNAL EFFECTS

Women with beta-thalassemia minor often are mildly anemic but otherwise healthy. Laboratory values normally associated with beta-thalassemia minor indicate a mild hypochromic and microcytic anemia. Large amounts of iron usually are not given despite the anemia because persons with beta-thalassemia absorb and store iron in their bodies excessively and must take a chelating agent to rid the excess (Duffy, 2004; Kotter & Osguthorpe, 2005; Quirolo & Vichinsky, 2004).

FETAL AND NEONATAL EFFECTS

Controversy exists regarding whether this disorder is associated with increased fetal or neonatal morbidity. There appears to be no increase in prematurity, low-birth-weight infants, or abnormal size for gestation. The fetus may inherit the serious problem of beta-thalassemia major.

THERAPEUTIC MANAGEMENT

No specific therapy for beta-thalassemia minor during pregnancy exists. Generally, the outcomes for the mother and fetus are satisfactory (Cunningham et al., 2001). Infections, which depress production of red blood cells and accelerate erythrocyte destruction, should be identified and treated promptly.

✔ CHECK YOUR READING

16. What are the maternal effects of sickle cell disease?
17. How is sickle cell disease treated during pregnancy?
18. Why is iron supplementation often not recommended for women with thalassemia?

MEDICAL CONDITIONS

Women with a preexisting medical condition should be aware of the effects that pregnancy will have on their conditions as well as the impact of their medical conditions on pregnancy outcome. Some conditions that complicate pregnancy are discussed in this section. (See Table 26-2.)

Immune-Complex Diseases
SYSTEMIC LUPUS ERYTHEMATOSUS

Systemic lupus erythematosus (SLE) is a chronic, inflammatory, autoimmune disease that can affect any organ or system in the body. Although the cause is unknown, an imbalance appears to exist between immune response and tolerance of specific antigens in which the body produces antibodies to its own cells and tissue. Signs and symptoms result from inflammation of multiple organ systems, especially the joints, skin, kidneys, and nervous system. The most common signs and symptoms are joint pain, photosensitivity, and a characteristic "butterfly rash" on the face, which may be less apparent because of the pigmentation changes of pregnancy. The disease is marked by episodes of exacerbation (flares), when the symptoms become worse, and quiescence, when the symptoms recede.

The disease tends to affect young women but may occur in any age group. Females are affected more than 10 times as often as men. The incidence is approximately 1 per 1000 persons. It is more common in women of African, Hispanic, Asian, and Native American descent (Lupus Foundation of America, 2003).

Because pregnancy can worsen SLE, the woman must be carefully observed for signs that the disease has progressed. Renal complications, often evidenced by proteinuria or cellular casts in the urine, pose a special risk. Women with a history of kidney problems should be advised to seek the advice of a physician before becoming pregnant. Pregnancy is most likely to have a favorable outcome in the woman whose disease is under good control at the beginning and who does not have renal involvement. However, flares or disorders such as preeclampsia are more likely to occur during pregnancy and early postpartum.

SLE is associated with increased incidences of abortion and fetal death during the first trimester. After the first trimester the prognosis for a live birth is higher if no active disease exists. Newborn risks include preterm birth, often resulting from preterm rupture of the membranes, and growth restriction. The most serious potential complication for the neonate is a congenital heart block, which usually is permanent and will require a pacemaker (Hankins & Suarez, 2004; Laskin, 2004).

TABLE 26-2   Other Conditions and Their Effect on Pregnancy

Condition	Maternal-Fetal Effects	Nursing Considerations
Appendicitis Inflammation of the appendix, often with fever. The most common nongynecologic surgical emergency during pregnancy.	Is difficult to diagnose during pregnancy. Early symptoms mimic common conditions of pregnancy. Ultrasonography may help rule out other diagnoses such as ectopic pregnancy.	When reasonable doubt exists that the patient has appendicitis, the appendix should be removed to prevent rupture and consequent complications. The location often is altered by the growing uterus.
Asthma An obstructive lung disease caused by airway inflammation. Characterized by dyspnea, cough, wheezing. Course in pregnancy is variable.	Effective therapy and avoidance of severe attacks are associated with a good pregnancy outcome. Medications used are well tolerated in pregnancy and appear to be safe for the fetus. Breastfeeding is safe for the newborn and may reduce the risk for allergies.	Early use of antiinflammatory agents such as inhaled corticosteroids (e.g., beclomethasone) may prevent severe attacks. Cromolyn sodium and nedocromil sodium are effective but require more time to become effective than inhaled corticosteroids. Bronchodilators such as theophylline and inhaled beta-agonists may be required.
Glucose-6-Phosphate Dehydrogenase Deficiency Female-linked genetic disorder that predisposes to lysis of red blood cells when exposed to oxidizing drugs (salicylates, acetaminophen, phenacetin, and some sulfa drugs) and ingestion of fava beans in some people.	Is not affected by pregnancy unless complicated by anemia. Iron and folic acid supplementation is recommended. Newborn males have a higher incidence of severe jaundice.	Advise client of risks and suggest she consult with her health care provider for recommended list of drugs for minor discomforts.
Hyperthyroidism An overactive, enlarged thyroid gland that is difficult to diagnose and manage during pregnancy because the normal changes of pregnancy increase the metabolic rate and mimic hyperthyroidism. Graves' disease is the most common cause during pregnancy. Treatment ideally begins before pregnancy.	Increased incidence of hypertension such as preeclampsia and postpartum hemorrhage if not well controlled during pregnancy. Treatment is complicated by the presence of the fetus, which may be jeopardized by surgery or antithyroid medications. Propylthiouracil has limited placental transfer and is widely used during pregnancy to control thyroid function. Additional drugs such as iodides and beta blockers may be needed, particularly in a thyroid crisis.	Be aware of the major signs that should be reported. These include a resting pulse rate greater than 100/min, loss of weight or failure to gain weight in spite of normal intake of food, heat intolerance, and abnormal protrusion of the eyes (exophthalmos).
Hypothyroidism Characterized by inadequate thyroid secretion; confirmed by an elevated level of thyroid-stimulating hormone and low levels of triiodothyronine and thyroxine.	Women with hypothyroidism have a higher incidence of preeclampsia, abruptio placentae, and low-birth-weight or stillborn infants. If the expectant mother is untreated, there is an increased risk of neonatal goiter and congenital hypothyroidism; severity of symptoms depends on time of onset and severity of the deprivation but may include neurologic deficits. Treatment is with levothyroxine.	Suspect neonatal hypothyroidism when the infant is large for gestational age, with respiratory and feeding difficulties, rough and dry skin, and an umbilical hernia.
Maternal Phenylketonuria (PKU) Inherited single-gene recessive defect leading to an inability to metabolize essential amino acid phenylalanine, resulting in high serum levels of phenylalanine. Irreparable mental retardation occurs if the pregnant woman is not treated early with a diet that provides adequate protein but restricts phenylalanine.	The woman must be on a low-phenylalanine diet before conception and pregnancy. If not, the fetal risk for microcephaly, mental retardation, heart defects, and intrauterine growth restriction increases.	The child either will be a carrier of the gene or will inherit the disease, depending on the presence of the gene in the father of the child. Special low-phenylalanine foods are expensive, but they may be obtained through the state's Supplemental Nutrition Program for Women, Infants, and Children (WIC) or Medicaid or may be covered by insurance.

ANTIPHOSPHOLIPID SYNDROME

Antiphospholipid syndrome (APS) is an autoimmune condition characterized by the production of antiphospholipid antibodies combined with certain clinical features. The most specific clinical features include arterial and venous thrombosis, decreased platelets, and pregnancy loss. Pregnancy complications that are more common with APS include early-onset preeclampsia, IUGR, fetal loss, and preterm birth. Stroke related to arterial thrombosis may occur.

Although the syndrome occurs most often in women with other underlying autoimmune diseases such as SLE, it also is diagnosed in women with no other recognizable autoimmune disease.

Women with APS should be informed of the potential maternal and obstetric problems, including a possible risk of stroke. They should be assessed for evidence of anemia, thrombocytopenia, and underlying renal disease. Some physicians believe that treatment with heparin may be warranted on the basis of increased risk for thrombosis, even in women with no previous clotting problems. Combinations of low-dose aspirin and subcutaneous heparin sometimes are recommended.

RHEUMATOID ARTHRITIS

Rheumatoid arthritis is a chronic inflammatory disease that usually affects the synovial (hinged) joints. Although the cause is unknown, an autoimmune mechanism is suspected. It is strongly associated with rheumatoid factor, an autoantibody present in 75% to 80% of patients with inflammatory rheumatoid arthritis. It occurs in 1% to 2% of the population and affects females two to four times more frequently than males (Hankins & Suarez, 2004; Laskin, 2004).

Marked improvement in symptoms of rheumatoid arthritis often occurs during pregnancy. The exact reason is unclear, but improvement is reported to parallel the rise in pregnancy-specific protein, which suppresses inflammatory reactions. Hormonal factors also have been suggested. For instance, increased levels of cortisol, estrogen, and progesterone may be beneficial in suppressing the immune response. Unfortunately, a relapse (postpartum flare) occurs within 6 weeks to 6 months after birth.

In contrast to SLE, the risk of abortion does not increase in women with rheumatoid arthritis. Usually, obstetric problems do not occur at delivery unless the hips or cervical spine are significantly deteriorated (Hankins & Suarez, 2004; Laskin, 2004).

HASHIMOTO'S THYROIDITIS

Hashimoto's thyroiditis, characterized by antithyroid antibodies, causes most cases of hypothyroidism in women. Maternal hypothyroidism during pregnancy can adversely affect the child's mental development. Thyroid-stimulating hormone (TSH) should be tested before or in early pregnancy, and hypothyroidism corrected.

Neurologic Disorders

SEIZURE DISORDERS

Seizures are the most common form of epilepsy, which is a recurrent disorder of cerebral function. Epilepsy occurs in 0.3% to 0.6% of pregnant women. Seizures may occur during pregnancy even though the woman has been seizure free for many years. Seizures that occur only during pregnancy have also been reported (Aminoff, 2004).

The effect of pregnancy on the course of epilepsy is variable and unpredictable. The frequency of seizures may increase, decrease, or remain the same. In general, the longer the woman has been seizure free before pregnancy, the less likely she is to develop seizures during pregnancy. Those with partial (focal) seizures are more likely to have an increased frequency. Vomiting, reduced gastric motility, use of gastrointestinal medications, and weight gain affect the absorption and distribution of anticonvulsant drugs. Serum levels of anticonvulsants may rise, fall, or remain the same during pregnancy.

Women with epilepsy have a higher-than-normal incidence of stillbirth, and some studies have shown a higher incidence of preterm labor. Maternal bleeding may occur because of a deficiency of clotting factors associated with anticonvulsant drugs such as hydantoins (Dilantin) and phenobarbital. Anticonvulsant drugs also compete with folate for absorption, which may result in folate deficiency. Most anticonvulsants are pregnancy category C or D. (See Appendix B for additional drugs and possible adverse effects on the fetus.) Interactions between anticonvulsant drugs and other medications must be considered by the physician and pharmacist, because dose changes or selection of valid alternative drugs may be needed. Effects of anticonvulsants and over-the-counter drugs must be considered as well.

A major concern is the teratogenic effects of anticonvulsant drugs. A specific syndrome known as *fetal hydantoin syndrome* has been described that includes craniofacial abnormalities, limb reduction defects, growth restriction, mental retardation, and cardiac anomalies. Other anticonvulsants such as trimethadione, paramethadione, and carbamazepine also are associated with malformation syndromes. The teratogenic effects of phenobarbital are difficult to assess because it often is combined with other drugs. Newer anticonvulsants, such as levetiracetam, have fewer data accumulated related to fetal effects.

Health professionals should recommend that the woman consult a neurologist before conception. The goal of treatment is to prevent generalized (formerly called *grand mal*) seizures and also reduce the adverse effects of anticonvulsant medications on the fetus. The family must be made aware of the risks involved when anticonvulsant drugs must be used. They also should realize that treatment cannot be stopped during pregnancy unless the woman has been seizure free for a prolonged time. Generalized seizures result in fetal hypoxia and acidosis and therefore pose a serious problem for the fetus.

BELL'S PALSY

Bell's palsy is a sudden unilateral neuropathy of the seventh cranial (facial) nerve that causes facial paralysis with weakness of the forehead and lower face. No cause for the neuropathy is often identified, although inflammation or viral infection of the facial nerve are possible causes. It is three times more common during pregnancy and generally occurs in the third trimester. Although the reason for the increase during pregnancy is unknown, one theory suggests that estrogen-induced edema puts pressure on the facial nerve, making the pregnant woman more vulnerable to the disease. Pregnancy does not affect recovery rate, and nearly 90% of women will recover function within a few weeks to months (Aminoff, 2004).

The face feels stiff and pulled to one side. Maternal attempts to close the eye on the affected side may be difficult or impossible. Difficulty with eating or fine facial movements may occur. The ability to taste also may be disturbed.

Treatment is controversial. Some physicians prescribe steroids within the first few days. Supportive care includes patching the eye and applying ointment or eye drops to prevent dryness or injury to the exposed cornea. Facial massage may be helpful, and the woman should be cautioned to chew carefully since she could easily bite the inside of her mouth or her tongue. Psychological support is necessary to assist the woman and her family deal with anxiety they naturally feel when sudden paralysis of the face occurs. They must be reassured that the condition is temporary for the majority of women who have Bell's palsy.

✔ **CHECK YOUR READING**

19. What are the maternal and fetal effects of SLE?
20. In what ways does pregnancy affect rheumatoid arthritis?
21. How can Hashimoto's thyroiditis affect the newborn?
22. What is the major concern about administering anticonvulsant drugs for the woman with epilepsy?
23. What is the recommended supportive care for those with Bell's palsy?

TRAUMA IN PREGNANCY

Blunt Force Injuries

Automobile accidents cause most blunt force injuries to the pregnant woman. Maternal deaths are most often caused by head injury or intraabdominal hemorrhage. Fetal death may be secondary to maternal death or may follow sudden premature separation of the placenta or rupture of the uterus. Pelvic fracture is a commonly reported nonfatal injury in automobile accidents, falls, and domestic violence. Neurologic deficits may be identified in the newborn who recovers after maternal injury, but cause and effect are difficult to establish because of the time interval between the trauma and postbirth outcomes for the child.

During the first trimester, the fetus is protected from external forces by the bony pelvis, amniotic fluid, and soft tissue surrounding the pelvis. Later in pregnancy, the fetal compartment extends beyond the bony pelvis, and as a result the fetus is more vulnerable to blunt force injury. Fetal growth brings the fetus nearer the uterine walls, and the thickness of the walls lessens. Amniotic fluid volume proportionate to fetal size decreases as the fetus grows, reducing the fluid cushion surrounding the fetus. Fetal injury may include skull fracture and intracranial hemorrhage. In addition, disruption of uteroplacental blood flow because of premature separation of the placenta can result in fetal anoxia.

Use of seatbelt restraints significantly improves maternal and fetal outcomes in automobile accidents. Current recommendations are that the pregnant woman wear three-point restraint seatbelts during automobile travel, with the lap belt under her protruding abdomen.

Penetrating Injuries

Gunshot and knife wounds are the most common penetrating injuries and may be associated with assaults or suicide attempts. Mortality rates from penetrating wounds in the pregnant woman are less than those in nonpregnant women because the uterus acts as a shield for the abdominal structure. The fetus fares poorly, with high injury and mortality rates (Gonik & Foley, 2004).

Therapeutic Management

Initial management of trauma in pregnancy is similar to that in the nonpregnant state. Primary goals are evaluation and stabilization of maternal injuries. Basic rules are applied to resuscitation, including establishing ventilation and arrest of hemorrhage. During attempted resuscitation, however, prolonged supine positioning should be avoided so that compression of the large blood vessels can be minimized. Lateral displacement of the uterus can be accomplished by placing a wedge along the right side of the woman. In addition, the need for large amounts of fluid replacement should be anticipated. After resuscitation, evaluation is continued for neurologic injuries, fractures, bleeding sites, and internal injuries. Exploratory abdominal surgery may be necessary to identify and control internal bleeding. The uterus and fetus must also be evaluated for injuries. Kleihauer-Betke (K-B) testing is done at intervals to identify if fetal blood has entered the maternal circulation. K-B tests that show a growing percentage of fetal erythrocytes in maternal blood suggest disruption of the placenta, although the test alone is not diagnostic. Rh immune globulin (RhoGAM) will be given if a fetal-maternal hemorrhage is identified in the $Rh_o(D)$-negative mother.

Electronic fetal monitoring may reflect the condition of the mother as well as that of the fetus. For example, although the mother is stable, electronic monitoring may detect signs of early maternal hypovolemia or premature separation of the placenta, such as uterine contractions, fetal tachycardia, and late decelerations. The duration of fetal monitoring varies according to the severity of the trauma. Ultrasonography provides additional information about the fetal condition. Antibiotics and tetanus immunization are given when indicated.

The need for cesarean delivery of a live fetus depends on several factors, including the age of the fetus, fetal condition, and extent of uterine injury. Because placental abruption usually develops soon after trauma, electronic monitoring is begun as soon as possible. It is continued as long as signs of uterine contractions, vaginal bleeding, uterine tenderness, and ruptured membranes are present.

INFECTIONS DURING PREGNANCY

A number of different infections can adversely affect the health of the fetus, mother, or both when acquired during pregnancy. Some infections are mild or even subclinical in the mother yet may cause severe birth defects or death of the fetus. Other infections may have adverse effects by increasing the risk for other pregnancy complications such as preterm labor. Some infections are transmitted primarily or exclusively by sexual means, whereas others may be transmitted in this way but also by other avenues.

The wide variety of infections affecting pregnancy care are divided into those caused by viruses and those caused by other organisms. Table 26-3 presents nursing considerations related to major sexually transmitted diseases and vaginal infections. Also, Table 26-3 summarizes urinary tract infections and their effect on pregnancy. (See also Chapter 33 for information about infection in the nonpregnant woman.)

Viral Infections

Pregnancy does not worsen the effects of most viral infections in the woman. Although viral infections may be mild or even asymptomatic in adults, fetal and neonatal consequences can be catastrophic. Maternal infection with cytomegalovirus (CMV), rubella, varicella-zoster virus, herpes simplex, hepatitis B, and HIV have the greatest potential for harm to the fetus or newborn.

CYTOMEGALOVIRUS

CMV, a member of the herpesvirus group, is widespread and eventually infects most humans. CMV has been isolated from urine, saliva, blood, cervical mucus, semen, breast milk, and stool. Transmission may occur from contamination with any of these fluids, although close personal contact is required. The highest rate of infection occurs between the ages of 15 and 35 years, so the possibility of CMV infection occurring during pregnancy is high if the woman has not had a primary CMV infection.

Daycare centers are a common place for transmission of CMV among children, especially toddlers, because they often share objects contaminated with saliva. Mothers of and caregivers for young children who attend a daycare center should be aware that a child might acquire an infection in the center and transmit it to those who are at risk for a primary infection. As puberty approaches, behaviors such as kissing, sexual intercourse, and other close contact again in-

crease the possibility that CMV infection will be transmitted to a female who may be pregnant (Gibbs, Sweet, & Duff, 2004; Landry, 2004).

After primary infection the virus becomes latent, but like other herpesvirus infections, periodic reactivation and shedding of the virus may occur. Primary infection is more likely to cross the placenta, infecting the fetus, than is a reactivation infection. Seroconversion and a rise in the specific IgM antibody titer can detect a primary infection that has occurred within the past 4 to 8 months. Isolation of the virus in culture identifies infection but does not distinguish whether the infection is primary or recurrent (Gibbs et al., 2004; Landry, 2004). However, most infections are asymptomatic, so they may not be suspected during pregnancy and testing may not be done. Diagnosis of neonatal infection is by urine culture.

FETAL AND NEONATAL EFFECTS. If a woman develops a primary CMV infection during pregnancy, her fetus has a 40% to 50% chance of being infected. Of infected fetuses, 5% to 18% are symptomatic at birth, having problems such as enlarged spleen and liver, CNS abnormalities, jaundice, chorioretinitis, hearing loss, and IUGR. Another 10% to 15% will develop manifestations within the first 2 years of life (Gibbs et al., 2004).

THERAPEUTIC MANAGEMENT. No effective therapy is currently available for the treatment of congenital infection. Ultrasound scanning may identify manifestations of the infection, such as cranial abnormalities or growth restriction. Antiviral agents, such as ganciclovir and foscarnet, may be used for severe infections, but these drugs are toxic and only temporarily suppress shedding of the virus. Primary prevention, such as emphasizing handwashing (especially to women who care for small children), warning of the risks imposed by having several sexual partners, and transfusing only CMV-free blood, is most effective (Gibbs et al., 2004).

RUBELLA

Rubella is caused by a virus transmitted from person to person by droplets or through direct contact with articles contaminated with nasopharyngeal secretions. Rubella is a mild disease. Major symptoms include fever, general malaise, and a characteristic maculopapular rash that begins on the face and migrates over the body. Although the overall incidence has declined since rubella vaccine became available, up to 20% of adults in the United States remain susceptible (Gibbs et al., 2004).

FETAL AND NEONATAL EFFECTS. Rubella virus from the mother can cross the placental barrier and infect the fetus at any time during pregnancy. The greatest risk to the fetus occurs during the first trimester, when fetal organs are developing. If maternal infection occurs during this time, approximately one third of these cases will result in spontaneous abortions and the surviving fetuses may be seriously compromised. Deafness, mental retardation, cataracts, cardiac defects, IUGR, and microcephaly are the most common fetal complications. In addition, infants

TABLE 26-3 Sexually Transmitted Diseases and Urinary Tract and Vaginal Infections: Impact on Pregnancy

Maternal, Fetal, and Neonatal Effects	Nursing Considerations
Sexually Transmitted Diseases	
Syphilis (Causative Organism: Spirochete Treponema pallidum)	
If untreated, the infection may cross the placenta to the fetus and result in spontaneous abortion, a stillborn infant, premature labor and birth, or congenital syphilis. Major signs of congenital syphilis are enlarged liver and spleen, skin lesions, rashes, osteitis, pneumonia, and hepatitis.	Penicillin is the primary treatment to cure the disease in both the woman and fetus. Women who are allergic are desensitized and then treated.*
Gonorrhea (Causative Organism: Bacterium Neisseria gonorrhoeae)	
Not transmitted via the placenta; vertical transmission from mother to newborn during birth may cause ophthalmia neonatorum. Endocervicitis and weakness of the fetal membranes increase the risk for premature rupture of membranes and preterm labor. Chlamydia infection is likely to accompany the gonorrhea infection.	Ceftriaxone or cefixime plus amoxicillin or azithromycin are now recommended for penicillin-resistant organisms because 20%-50% of women with gonorrhea will also have chlamydial infection.*† The partner must also be treated to prevent reinfection. Infants are treated with an ophthalmic antibiotic such as ceftriaxone at birth to prevent ophthalmia neonatorum.
Chlamydial Infection (Causative Organism: Bacterium Chlamydia trachomatis)	
Chlamydial infection is the most common sexually transmitted disease in the United States. The fetus may be infected during birth and may suffer neonatal conjunctivitis or pneumonitis. Conjunctivitis is prevented by erythromycin ophthalmic ointment. *Chlamydia* may also be responsible for premature rupture of membranes, premature labor, and chorioamnionitis.	Education is particularly important because *Chlamydia* infection is the most common sexually transmitted disease in the United States and infection is usually asymptomatic. Both partners should be treated to prevent recurrent infection. As with all sexually transmitted diseases, the use of condoms decreases the risk for infection. Erythromycin or amoxicillin is the recommended treatment. Azithromycin is an alternate treatment.†
Trichomoniasis (Causative Organism: Protozoan Trichomonas vaginalis)	
Common cause of vaginitis in 10%-50% of pregnant women. Associated with premature rupture of membranes and postpartum endometritis.†	Metronidazole (Flagyl) may be given to the pregnant woman as a 2-g single oral dose. Consistent association between fetal abnormalities or injury and metronidazole use has not been upheld.†
Condyloma Acuminatum (Causative Organism: Human Papillomavirus)	
Transmission of condyloma acuminatum, also called *venereal* or *genital warts,* may occur during vaginal birth and is associated with the development of epithelial tumors of the mucous membranes of the larynx in children. Pregnancy can cause proliferation of lesions, which are associated with cervical dysplasia and cancer.	The common choices for nonpregnant therapy (podophyllin, podofilox, imiquimod) are not recommended during pregnancy. Excision of the maternal lesions by cryotherapy or cautery may be done.†
Vaginal Infections	
Candidiasis (Causative Organism: Yeast Candida albicans)	
Oral candidiasis (thrush) may develop in newborns if infection is present at birth. Thrush is treated with application of nystatin (Mycostatin) over the surfaces of the oral cavity four times a day for several days. Characteristic "cottage cheese" vaginal discharge with vulvar pruritus, burning, and dyspareunia. Vulva may be red, tender, and edematous.	Candidiasis (sometimes called *Monilia vaginitis*) is a persistent problem for many women during pregnancy. Maternal treatment choices include miconazole, clotrimazole, and fluconazole.†

*Centers for Disease Control and Prevention. (2002b). Sexually transmitted diseases treatment guidelines, 2002. *MMWR. Morbidity and Mortality Weekly Report, 51*(RR-6). Retrieved February 20, 2005, from www.cdc.gov/STD/treatment/rr5106.pdf.

†Gibbs, R.S., Sweet, R.L., & Duff, W.P. (2004). Maternal and fetal infectious diseases. In R.K. Creasy, R. Resnik, & J.D. Iams (Eds.), *Maternal-fetal medicine: Principles and practice* (5th ed., pp. 741-801). Philadelphia: Saunders.

‡Formerly called *nonspecific vaginitis* or *Gardnerella vaginitis.*

born to mothers who had rubella during pregnancy shed the virus for many months and therefore pose a threat to other infants and susceptible adults who come in contact with them.

THERAPEUTIC MANAGEMENT. Prevention is the only effective protection for the fetus. A Healthy People 2010 objective is to reduce the number of congenital rubella syndrome cases to zero through immunization of susceptible individuals. Women who are immune do not become infected, so determining the immune status of all women of childbearing age is critical. Immune status assays such as the enzyme-linked immunosorbent assay (ELISA) have replaced many older serologic tests such as hemagglutination inhibition (HAI) to determine rubella immunity. Immunity or nonimmune status can be identified by the following results of the ELISA and HAI tests:

- ELISA test: Immunity is indicated by a level of >10 international units/ml, but a level of <7 international units/ml indicates that a person has no immunity to rubella.
- HAI titer: Immunity is clearly indicated by a titer >1:20, but a level <1:8 indicates that a person has no immunity to rubella.

Women who are not immune should be vaccinated before they become pregnant, and they should be advised not to become pregnant for 28 days after vaccination because of the possible risk to the fetus from the live-virus vaccine. Many women are vaccinated during the postpartum period so that they will be immune before becoming pregnant

TABLE 26-3 Sexually Transmitted Diseases and Urinary Tract and Vaginal Infections: Impact on Pregnancy—cont'd

Maternal, Fetal, and Neonatal Effects	Nursing Considerations
Bacterial Vaginosis‡ (Causative Organism: Gardnerella vaginalis) No known fetal effects. May be associated with postpartum endometritis; has been associated with preterm birth. Marked by a major shift in vaginal flora from the normal predominance of lactobacilli to a predominance of anaerobic bacteria. Causes profuse, malodorous, "fishy" vaginal discharge, itching, and burning.	Metronidazole (oral therapy or intravaginal gel) or clindamycin intravaginal cream may be used in the pregnant woman.
Urinary Tract Infections *Asymptomatic Bacteriuria (Causative Organisms: Escherichia coli, Klebsiella, Proteus)* Ascending bacterial infection can result in cystitis or pyelonephritis in later pregnancy if condition remains untreated.	Recovery of a urinary pathogen from a midstream, clean-catch urine specimen is defined as 100,000 colony-forming units (CFUs) per milliliter of urine. Rapid, less-expensive office tests to identify the infection may also be used. Treatment for asymptomatic bacteriuria may include treatment for pathogens that also cause symptomatic cystitis.
Cystitis (Causative Organisms: E. coli, Klebsiella, Proteus) Signs and symptoms include dysuria, frequency, urgency, and suprapubic tenderness. Ascending infection may lead to pyelonephritis.	Antibiotics used for both asymptomatic bacteriuria and cystitis include amoxicillin, sulfisoxazole, trimethoprim-sulfamethoxazole, nitrofurantoin, and third-generation cephalosporins such as cefixime or cefpodoxime. Emphasize importance of reporting signs of urinary tract infection. Stress the importance of taking all the medication prescribed even if the symptoms abate. Provide information about hygiene measures.
Acute Pyelonephritis (Causative Organisms: E. coli, Klebsiella, Proteus) Increased risk for preterm labor and premature delivery. Maternal complications include a high fever, septic shock, and adult respiratory distress syndrome.	Inform women with asymptomatic bacteriuria or cystitis of signs and symptoms, such as sudden onset of fever (temperature often higher than 39° C [102.2° F]), chills, flank pain or tenderness, nausea, and vomiting, so that treatment can begin promptly. Skin cooling equipment may be used to lower her temperature below 38° C (100.4° F), reducing possible compromise of fetal oxygen level. Woman may be hospitalized for intravenous administration of antibiotics. Common combinations include ampicillin or a cephalosporin plus an aminoglycoside. Serum levels of aminoglycosides are often measured to ensure an adequate dose without its reaching a toxic level.

again. In most facilities, women of childbearing age must read and sign a document indicating that they understand the risks to the fetus if they become pregnant within 28 days. (See Chapter 17 for the drug guide for rubella vaccine.)

VARICELLA-ZOSTER VIRUS

Varicella infection (chickenpox) is caused by varicella-zoster virus, a herpesvirus that is transmitted by direct contact or through the respiratory tract. After the primary varicella infection, the virus can become latent in nerve ganglia. If the varicella virus is reactivated, herpes zoster (shingles) results. Maternal complications of acute varicella infection may include preterm labor, encephalitis, and varicella pneumonia, which is the most serious complication associated with varicella-zoster virus. Over 90% of nonimmune people will have varicella before reaching reproductive age. Varicella immunization has resulted in a marked decrease in children's varicella, well before they reach reproductive age.

FETAL AND NEONATAL EFFECTS. Fetal and neonatal effects depend on the time of maternal infection. If the infection occurs during the first trimester, the fetus has a small risk for congenital varicella syndrome (0.4%). The greatest risk for development of congenital varicella syndrome occurs from 13 to 20 weeks of pregnancy (2% of

births). Clinical findings include limb hypoplasia, cutaneous scars, chorioretinitis, cataracts, microcephaly, and IUGR. In later pregnancy, transplacental passage of maternal antibodies usually protects the fetus (Gibbs et al., 2004; Landry, 2004).

However, the infant who is infected during the perinatal period (5 days before through 2 days after birth) will not have the benefit of maternal antibodies. Four days before birth is not sufficient time for the mother to develop antibodies to varicella and pass them to the fetus. A varicella infection occurring in the fetus or infant just before or after birth would not be inactivated by antibodies, leaving the infant at risk for life-threatening neonatal varicella infection (Centers for Disease Control and Prevention [CDC], 2001b; Gibbs et al., 2004; Landry, 2004).

THERAPEUTIC MANAGEMENT. Immune testing may be recommended for pregnant women who are presumed to be susceptible. Varicella-zoster immune globulin (VZIG) should be administered to women who have been exposed and whose fetuses are at high risk for the congenital rubella syndrome (Gibbs et al., 2004; Landry, 2004). Those infected with varicella during pregnancy should be instructed to report pulmonary symptoms immediately. Hospitalization, fetal surveillance, full respiratory support, and hemodynamic monitoring should be available for women diagnosed with varicella pneumonia because it may become severe in a short time. Acyclovir is the primary drug used to treat varicella pneumonia.

For infants born to mothers infected with varicella during the perinatal period, immunization with VZIG as soon as possible but within 96 hours of birth provides passive immunity against varicella. Women and infants with varicella are highly contagious and should be placed in strict isolation. Only staff members known to be immune to varicella should come in contact with these clients.

Adult immunization is recommended for nonpregnant adults who have no evidence of having had varicella or documentation of the immunization. A pregnant woman should not be immunized, but members of her household may be immunized because the vaccine is not transmissible from one person to another. If the vaccine is given to a female of childbearing age, it is important to teach her to avoid pregnancy for 1 month after each of the two injections, which are given 4 to 8 weeks apart. Nonimmune healthcare workers should be immunized (CDC, 2001b; CDC, 2004; Gibbs et al., 2004).

HERPES SIMPLEX VIRUS

Genital herpes is one of the most common sexually transmitted diseases in the herpes simplex virus (HSV) group. It may be caused by HSV type 1 or 2. Most infections of genital herpes are caused by type 2. Type 1, which is more common in the mouth and upper body, also may infect the genital area. HSV infection occurs as a result of direct contact of the skin or mucous membrane with an active lesion. Lesions form at the site of contact and begin as a group of painful papules that progress rapidly to become vesicles, shallow ulcers, pustules, and crusts. The woman sheds the virus until the lesions are healed. The virus then migrates along the sensory nerves to reside in the sensory ganglion, and the disease enters a latent phase. It can be reactivated later as a recurrent infection. Many women infected with HSV do not have signs and symptoms of infection. A woman may shed the virus without knowing she has it (Gibbs et al., 2004; Landry, 2004).

Vertical transmission (from mother to infant) generally occurs in one of two ways: (1) after rupture of membranes, when the virus ascends from active lesions; or (2) during birth, when the fetus comes into contact with infectious genital secretions or the fetal skin is punctured, such as with a fetal scalp electrode.

Diagnosis usually is based on clinical signs and symptoms. Definitive diagnosis requires culture of the virus from an active lesion, and results may take as long as 5 days. Newer tests based on genetic analysis (polymerase chain reaction [PCR]) are becoming more available for detection of HSV and other infections.

FETAL AND NEONATAL EFFECTS. Complications of pregnancy from a recurrent infection are rare. However, if primary infection occurs during pregnancy, the rates of spontaneous abortions, IUGR, and preterm labor increase. Neonatal herpes infection is uncommon but potentially devastating. The neonate may have infection that is limited to skin lesions or systemic (disseminated). Symptoms usually appear within the first week, and the disease progresses rapidly. The likelihood of death or serious sequelae for infants who have systemic herpes infection is about 50%. The risk of neonatal infection is greatest if the mother has a primary (rather than recurrent) infection during the perinatal period. This is most likely because the amount of virus shed is higher during a primary infection than subsequent ones (Gibbs et al., 2004; Landry, 2004).

THERAPEUTIC MANAGEMENT. No known cure for herpes infection exists, although antiviral chemotherapy (acyclovir) is prescribed to reduce symptoms and shorten the duration of the lesions. Acyclovir may be given during late pregnancy to a woman with a recurrent outbreak to reduce the possibility that she will have active lesions at the time of birth.

THERAPEUTIC COMMUNICATIONS

Concern about Confidentiality

Mary Smith, who had a cesarean delivery the previous day because of two active herpes lesions in her vaginal and labial areas, appears anxious and uncomfortable during the morning assessment by nurse Eileen Sinclair.

Mary: Why does everyone wear gloves when they come near me?

Eileen: You wonder why we wear gloves when we care for you? *(Reflecting content)*

Mary: Well, it bothers me that you think I am so contagious.

Eileen: You seem to think we wear gloves because you have a herpes outbreak. *(Clarifying content and feeling since glove use is now standard for infection control in many settings)*

Mary: Yes, why else would it be necessary?

Eileen: We wear gloves when we care for all patients whenever we might come into contact with body fluids so we don't transmit infection from one person to another. I'm sorry you thought it was only because of your infection. *(Providing information and conveying empathy)*

Mary: I'm just so touchy about having my family find out I have herpes.

Eileen: You don't want your family to know why you had a cesarean? *(Clarifying and reflecting feelings)*

Mary: Yes, I'm so embarrassed. I wish they didn't have to know.

Eileen: They will know only if you tell them. We do everything possible to protect your privacy. I'd like to come back in a few minutes and we can talk more about how you feel. *(Offering reassurance about Mary's privacy and giving her the option to express her feelings more completely at a later time)*

For women with a history of genital herpes, vaginal delivery is allowed if there are no genital lesions at the time of labor. Cesarean birth is recommended for women with active lesions in the genital area, whether recurrent or primary, at the time of labor. Use of fetal scalp electrodes, which cause a break in the skin, is acceptable if there are no active lesions (AAP & ACOG, 2002).

Expectant mothers need information about effective ways to deal with the emotional and physical effects of herpes. Many women are concerned about privacy and do not want family members to know why cesarean birth is necessary. These women must be assured that their wishes will be respected. Women may need an opportunity to discuss their feelings of shame, anger, or anxiety about possible effects of the virus on their infant.

After delivery, isolation of the mother from her infant is not necessary if direct contact with lesions is avoided and mothers use careful handwashing techniques. Mothers may breastfeed if there are no lesions on the breasts. The infant is observed for signs of infection, including temperature instability, lethargy, poor sucking reflex, jaundice, seizures, and herpetic lesions. Acyclovir therapy is prescribed for neonatal infection. (See Chapter 33 for care of herpes in nonpregnant women.)

✔ CHECK YOUR READING

24. What are the fetal and neonatal effects of CMV infection?
25. Why is rubella infection most dangerous in the first trimester?
26. How can rubella be prevented?
27. How are infants born to mothers with varicella treated?
28. How does vertical transmission of the herpes virus occur?

PARVOVIRUS B19

Erythema infectiosum (also called *fifth disease*), caused by human parvovirus B19, is an acute, communicable disease characterized by a highly distinctive rash. The rash starts on the face with a "slapped-cheeks" appearance, followed by a generalized maculopapular rash. Other symptoms include fever, malaise, and joint pain. Erythema infectiosum is more common among children and often occurs in community epidemics. The prognosis is usually excellent. However, if the disease occurs in pregnancy, potential fetal and neonatal effects exist. Parvovirus titers can be done if exposure during pregnancy is suspected to determine whether the mother is immune.

FETAL AND NEONATAL EFFECTS. When infection occurs during pregnancy, fetal death can result, usually from failure of fetal red blood cell production, followed by severe fetal anemia, hydrops (generalized edema), and heart failure. Maternal serum alpha-fetoprotein (MSAFP) is sometimes elevated when fetal hydrops is present. Serial ultrasonography can also be performed to detect hydrops. Intrauterine transfusion is an option to treat severe fetal anemia if it does not spontaneously resolve. The risk to the fetus is greatest when the mother is infected in the first 20 weeks of pregnancy. The affected infant is examined for any defect, and the child is assessed regularly for several years to identify delayed complications such as persistent infection because of low levels of viral replication.

THERAPEUTIC MANAGEMENT. No specific treatment exists. Starch baths may help reduce pruritus, and analgesics may be necessary to relieve mild joint pain.

HEPATITIS B

Hepatitis B is one of six currently recognized serotypes of hepatitis: A, B, C, D, E, and G. Hepatitis A accounts for about one third of cases in the United States. Hepatitis A is rarely transmitted perinatally, and supportive care is usually sufficient. Hepatitis B accounts for 40% to 45% of cases in the United States and can be transmitted to the infant perinatally before the mother develops clinical symptoms. Hepatitis C may go undiagnosed until the woman develops chronic liver disease that often requires liver transplantation. The incidence of hepatitis C in pregnant women is 1% to 5% (Landon, 2004; Riely & Fallon, 2004).

Hepatitis B is caused by a virus that is transmitted via blood, saliva, vaginal secretions, semen, or breast milk and readily crosses the placental barrier. The disease is prevalent in certain population groups, such as Africans, Asians, Southeast Asian immigrants, Native Americans, Eskimos, and intravenous drug users. Symptoms may include vomiting, abdominal pain, jaundice, fever, rash, and painful joints. Fortunately, most infected adolescents and adults recover within 6 months and acquire long-lasting immunity.

Chronic hepatitis B develops in 10% of infected adults, who can continue to transmit the disease to others. Persons with chronic hepatitis B also are at greater risk for chronic liver disease, cirrhosis of the liver, and primary hepatocellular carcinoma.

FETAL AND NEONATAL EFFECTS. The incidence of prematurity, low birth weight, and neonatal death increases when the mother has hepatitis B infection during pregnancy. Infants born to mothers who have hepatitis B during pregnancy or who are chronic carriers of hepatitis B surface antigen (HBsAg) are at risk for the development of acute infection at birth. Chronic hepatitis B infection develops in about 90% of infected newborns. The infected infant also is more likely to have chronic liver disease (Landon, 2004; Riely & Fallon, 2004).

THERAPEUTIC MANAGEMENT. Hepatitis B is a preventable infection. Simple hygiene measures such as safe sex and the use of standard precautions with body fluids provide primary prevention. Hepatitis B vaccines are available as a series of three intramuscular injections into the deltoid for adults, with the second and third doses given 1 and 6 months after the first. Vaccination is recommended for any population at risk, including nurses and other healthcare workers who frequently come in contact with body fluids.

All pregnant women should be screened for HBsAg. Women at high risk for hepatitis should be rescreened in the third trimester if the initial screen is negative. Household members and sexual contacts should be tested and offered vaccination if they are not immune. No specific treatment exists for acute hepatitis B. Recommended supportive treatment includes bed rest and a high-protein, low-fat diet.

Infection of the newborn whose mother is known to be HBsAg-positive usually can be prevented by administration of hepatitis B immune globulin (H-BIG, Hep-B-Gammagee), followed by hepatitis B vaccine (Recombivax-HB, Engerix-B) within 12 hours of birth. The newborn must be carefully bathed before any injections are given to prevent infections from skin surface contamination with the virus. The vaccination should be repeated at 1 to 2 months and 6 months of age. Breastfeeding is considered safe as long as the newborn has been vaccinated (AAP & ACOG, 2002). (See Chapter 21 for the drug guide for hepatitis B vaccine in the newborn.)

HUMAN IMMUNODEFICIENCY VIRUS

Acquired immunodeficiency syndrome (AIDS) is a breakdown in the immune function caused by the retrovirus HIV. The infected person develops opportunistic infections or malignancies that ultimately are fatal. The time from infection with HIV to development of AIDS is approximately 10 years with current antiretroviral therapy, although the interval may be much longer for some individuals. Transmission of HIV infection is predominantly through three modes: (1) sexual exposure to genital secretions of an infected person, (2) parenteral exposure to infected blood or tissue, and (3) perinatal exposure of an infant to infected maternal secretions through birth (vertical transmission). Heterosexual transmission causes about two thirds of female infections, and infection by blood or tissue exposure occurs in about one fourth of the cases. Infection of the infant varies with the severity of maternal infection and the time and extent of retrovirus transmission to the infant. The continuing occurrence of HIV infections of infants demonstrates the importance of identifying and treating maternal infections during pregnancy to reduce the risks of infant infections (AAP & ACOG, 2002; CDC, 2001a; Minkoff, 2004).

After rapid increases in cases of HIV infections during the early years of the epidemic in the United States, deaths from AIDS have declined as a result of more effective combination antiretroviral therapies. However, many new cases are among women, African Americans, and Latinos. Heterosexual spread is now the major mode of transmission, although HIV was largely confined to gay men in the early years of the epidemic. The AIDS epidemic in women living in the United States is most pronounced in African-American and Hispanic women, who account for 78% of current cases. More female cases now occur in the southern United States. Infected women more often have heterosexual relationships than homosexual relationships that can have caused their infection (Minkoff, 2004).

PATHOPHYSIOLOGY. Like other retroviruses, HIV integrates its viral genetic makeup into the genetic makeup of the cell when infecting it. This results in an abnormal cell that cannot perform its functions properly. At the same time, this cell replicates and produces more viruses that invade more cells. The disease worsens as more cells cease to function, and at the same time a greater number of viruses are produced. The principal mechanism whereby HIV leads to immunodeficiency is through its destructive effect on cells that provide and regulate immunity. CD4+ T lymphocytes, or helper T cells, play a key role in organizing the body's immune response to help immune functions. CD8 lymphocytes are T-suppressor cells that limit excessive immune responses that might attack the person's body tissues. Helper CD4+ T lymphocytes make up about 75% of these two types of lymphocytes in a healthy person.

When HIV infection invades body cells, the ratio of CD4+ T lymphocytes to CD8 lymphocytes decreases. As the number of CD4+ T lymphocytes declines, the immune response declines and opportunistic infections are able to overwhelm the HIV-positive person. A CD4+ T-lymphocyte total count of less than 200 cells/mm^3 confirms the diagnosis of AIDS. Greater accuracy of testing includes the ratio of CD4 to CD8 T lymphocytes (>1 is normal) and determining specific antigens on the CD4+ T lymphocytes. CD4+ counts help determine how a person who develops infection should be treated. If the CD4+ level is within normal values, the infection is less likely to be an opportunistic infection seen in AIDS and treatment can be routine (Guyton & Hall, 2000; Landry, 2004; Pagana & Pagana, 2005).

The clinical course of HIV infection follows fairly predictable stages:

- An early or acute stage occurs several weeks after HIV exposure. Flulike symptoms may develop and last a few weeks. Antibodies to HIV (seroconversion) generally appear within a few months, but delays of more than a year have been reported occasionally.
- A middle or asymptomatic period of minor or no clinical problems follows. This period is characterized by continuous low-level viral replication and CD4 cell loss.
- A transitional period of symptomatic disease follows.
- A late or crisis period of symptomatic disease follows, which consists of opportunistic infections lasting months or years.

During stages 1 and 2 the infected person is said to be HIV-positive. During stages 3 and 4, the immune system no longer offers adequate protection, and opportunistic diseases occur. The person is then said to have AIDS, regardless of the CD4 counts.

FETAL AND NEONATAL EFFECTS. An infant born to an HIV-positive mother who did not have antiretroviral treatment during pregnancy has a higher risk of becoming infected. The infant's risk is greatest if the mother has a high level of the HIV virus infecting her body. Typically, the newborn is asymptomatic at birth, but signs usually become obvious during the first year of life. The most common early signs are enlargement of the liver and spleen, lymphadenopathy, failure to thrive, persistent thrush, and extensive seborrheic dermatitis (cradle cap). Infants frequently experience chronic bacterial infections such as meningitis, pneumonia, osteomyelitis, septic arthritis, and septicemia.

CRITICAL TO REMEMBER

Facts about HIV

- After initial exposure, there is a period of 3 to 12 months before seroconversion. The person is considered infectious during this time.
- There is a long period of time, averaging 11 years, from HIV infection to development of AIDS, varying with whether the person receives treatment.
- A person infected with HIV can pass the virus to another person, even if he or she does not have symptoms.
- There is not yet a cure for the HIV infection or AIDS. Medications are available to slow replication of the virus and delay onset of opportunistic diseases.
- Zidovudine should be part of the medication regimen for a pregnant woman to reduce the transmission to her fetus. The newborn also should receive zidovudine after birth.
- HIV is transmitted by sexual contact with an infected person, by contact with infected body fluids, and through the placenta from mother to fetus.

AIDS, Acquired immunodeficiency syndrome; *HIV,* human immunodeficiency virus.

PREVENTION. Prevention remains the only way to control HIV infection. Sexual transmission can be avoided by several methods. Abstinence would render a person safe from all sexually transmissible diseases including HIV. However, for many people, sexual expression adds to the quality of life, and many are not willing to practice abstinence. Transmission of HIV also can be prevented if infected persons do not have intercourse with susceptible persons. If intercourse does occur, barrier methods such as latex condoms reduce contact with infectious secretions. A condom offers protection from transmission through cunnilingus or fellatio (oral sex).

Intravenous drug users who refuse rehabilitative treatment must be taught to wash the equipment with water, soap, and bleach before each use to reduce transmission of the virus through a soiled needle.

MEDICAL MANAGEMENT. No cure exists for HIV infection at this time, but several medications are beneficial in extending the person's lifespan after infection. To reduce vertical transmission of the virus to the infant, zidovudine (ZDV) is recommended for pregnant women who are HIV-positive. Additional drugs are used for greatest treatment effectiveness for the woman, but ZDV is included because of the drug's effectiveness in reducing HIV transmission to the fetus. Other drugs used for HIV therapy include nucleotide analogs, nucleoside analogs, reverse transcriptase inhibitors, and protease inhibitors. A medical-surgical nursing text should be consulted for greater detail about these drugs in the treatment of HIV infection. Guidelines for the latest treatments from the National Institutes of Health for both pregnant and nonpregnant patients may be found at www.aidsinfo.nih.gov.

The AIDS epidemic in women living in the United States is most pronounced in African-American and Hispanic women, who account for 78% of current cases. More female cases now occur in the southern United States. Infected women more often have heterosexual relationships than homosexual relationships that could have caused their infection, and as many of half the infections are acquired by women in their teens or 20s, increasing the risk that the infant will be infected (Minkoff, 2004).

The following situations and conditions must be considered when maternal ZDV therapy is prescribed:
- Whether the mother has had any antiretroviral therapy during pregnancy, including ZDV, and when it began
- Whether the mother had prenatal care, and when she started
- Fetal gestational age
- Whether the membranes have ruptured, and how long they have been ruptured

The healthcare team may encounter the pregnant woman with HIV infection in many situations; several guidelines exist for administration of ZDV to protect the infant. ZDV appears to be safe for the infant. A slight anemia appears to be the main adverse effect. Examples of ZDV administration include
- Antepartum: Oral ZDV to the mother beginning after 14 weeks to 34 weeks' gestation:
  - 100 mg ZDV orally 5 times daily
  - Alternative adult dose regimens for oral ZDV include 200 mg TID or 300 mg BID
- Intrapartum:
  - Intravenous ZDV starting 3 hours before delivery: Loading dose 2 mg/kg over 1 hour followed by 1 mg/kg/hr until delivery
  - Delivery by cesarean at 38 weeks to avoid transmission to the infant by onset of labor and ruptured membranes
  - Vaginal delivery may be attempted because of maternal refusal of cesarean birth, rapid labor progress at the time of admission, or membranes that have been ruptured for more than 4 hours; invasive procedures such as internal monitoring devices should be avoided if possible
- ZDV oral syrup to the newborn for 6 weeks, beginning 8 to 12 hours after birth
  - 2 mg/kg of body weight every 6 hours
- ZDV should be offered to the woman and her newborn if she had no or late prenatal care because it may reduce perinatal transmission after 34 weeks' gestation

NURSING CONSIDERATIONS. Learning of HIV infection during pregnancy can have a devastating and immobilizing effect on the entire family. A nursing diagnosis of "Anticipatory Grieving related to multiple losses that include shortened life expectancy and possible death of the infant" should be considered. Initially, crisis intervention may be necessary to help the family cope.

Nurses frequently must determine what the family perceives as the most pressing needs and worries. Some of the most common fears are loss of control, loss of support and love, social isolation, and loss of privacy. The nurse's response may involve finding ways for the woman to retain control while she is physically able and assisting her to select those in her family who will provide continued love and emotional support. Reassuring the woman that her right to privacy will not be violated is necessary.

Nurses can help the woman maintain the highest possible level of wellness. Adequate, high-quality nutrition decreases the risk of opportunistic infections and promotes vitality. A daily regimen should include sufficient rest and activity. Avoiding large crowds, travel to areas with poor sanitation, and exposure to infected individuals is important. Meticulous skin care is essential, especially during recurrent herpes infections.

The HIV virus has been found in breast milk. Although breast milk is usually ideal for an infant, artificial formulas for infant feeding are available in developed nations that may be not be available in the poor countries of our world. Therefore breast milk may be safer for an infant in these underdeveloped nations because infants have greater risks for other infections from artificial formulas or other sources even if the mother has HIV. In developed countries the woman should know that breastfeeding is contraindicated but that she can provide all other care for her infant.

The mother almost certainly will experience a great deal of anxiety about whether the infant will be HIV-positive. Nurses need to respond honestly that testing will be required but that most infants do not get the virus if the medication regimen is followed carefully. In addition, nurses must reinforce information about medications that both slow the progression of the disease for the mother and decrease the incidence of vertical transmission.

✓ CHECK YOUR READING

29. What are the fetal and neonatal effects of parvovirus B19 infection?
30. How is hepatitis B virus transmitted? How are newborns treated?
31. How can HIV infection be prevented?
32. What is the medical management for HIV infection?

Nonviral Infections

TOXOPLASMOSIS

Toxoplasmosis is a protozoan infection caused by *Toxoplasma gondii*. Infection is transmitted through organisms in raw and undercooked meat, through contact with infected cat feces, and across the placental barrier to the fetus if the expectant mother acquires the infection during pregnancy.

Toxoplasmosis often is subclinical. The woman may experience a few days of fatigue, muscle pains, and swollen glands but be unaware of the disease. If the infection is suspected, diagnosis can be confirmed by positive results of serologic tests, which include indirect fluorescent antibody tests for IgG and IgM. Immune-compromised persons, such as transplant patients or those infected with HIV, are more likely to have severe toxoplasmosis infection.

FETAL AND NEONATAL EFFECTS. Although toxoplasmosis may go unnoticed in the pregnant woman, it may cause abortion or result in the birth of a liveborn infant with the disease. About 40% of infants born to mothers who had an acute primary infection during pregnancy acquire congenital toxoplasmosis. About 50% of affected infants may be asymptomatic at birth, but others have serious effects such as low birth weight, enlarged liver and spleen, jaundice, and anemia or coagulation disorders. Severe complications may develop several years after birth and include chorioretinitis that leads to blindness; deafness; seizures; hydrocephalus; and microcephaly (Gibbs et al., 2004; Savoia, 2004).

THERAPEUTIC MANAGEMENT. All pregnant women should be advised to do the following:

- Cook meat thoroughly, particularly pork, beef, and lamb.
- Avoid touching mucous membranes of the mouth and eyes while handling raw meat.
- Wash all kitchen surfaces that come into contact with uncooked meat.
- Wash the hands thoroughly after handling raw meat.
- Avoid uncooked eggs and unpasteurized milk.
- Wash fruits and vegetables before consumption.
- Avoid contact with materials that are possibly contaminated with cat feces (such as cat litter boxes, sandboxes, garden soil).

Maternal treatment of toxoplasmosis during pregnancy is essential to reduce the risk for congenital infection. Sulfonamides can be used alone but are less effective than combination therapy. Spiramycin is successfully used in Europe for maternal toxoplasmosis and may be used according to specific guidelines within the United States (Gibbs et al., 2004).

GROUP B STREPTOCOCCUS INFECTION

Group B streptococcus (GBS) is a leading cause of life-threatening perinatal infections in the United States. The gram-positive bacterium colonizes the rectum, vagina, cervix, and urethra of pregnant and nonpregnant women. Approximately 10% to 30% of pregnant women are colonized with GBS in the vaginal or rectal area, but isolating the organism is often possible only intermittently. Often these women are asymptomatic, although symptomatic maternal infections can occur. These infections include urinary tract infection, chorioamnionitis, and metritis. Most women respond quickly to antimicrobial therapy. However, potentially fatal maternal complications such as meningitis, fasciitis, and intraabdominal abscess can occur if the mother is infected at the time of birth (AAP, 2002; CDC, 2002a).

FETAL AND NEONATAL EFFECTS. Early-onset newborn GBS disease occurs during the first week after birth, often within 48 hours. Women who have GBS in the rectovaginal area at the time of birth have a 60% chance of transmitting the organism to the newborn, and about 1% to 2% of these infants will develop early-onset GBS disease. Sepsis, pneumonia, and meningitis are the primary infections in early-onset GBS disease. Late-onset GBS disease occurs after the first week of life, and meningitis is the most common clinical manifestation. Permanent neurologic consequences are more likely in infants who survive meningeal infections (AAP & ACOG, 2002; Gibbs et al., 2004; Savoia, 2004). (See Chapter 30 for additional information about manifestations and recommended management of neonatal sepsis.)

THERAPEUTIC MANAGEMENT. Health care providers have difficulty identifying pregnant women who are asymptomatic GBS carriers because the duration of carrier status is unpredictable. Prenatal screening cultures may not identify the woman who will be a GBS carrier at the time of membrane rupture or onset of labor. Optimal identification of the GBS carrier status is obtained by vaginal and rectal culture between 35 and 37 weeks' gestation. Penicillin is the first-line agent for antibiotic treatment of the infected woman during birth. Ampicillin is an acceptable alternative. Patients who have clindamycin- and erythromycin-resistant GBS infections are more often observed than during the past.

Additional recommendations based on CDC guidelines in 2002 include the following:

- Routine intrapartum antibiotic prophylaxis treatment for GBS infection is not required for the woman having a planned cesarean birth if labor or membrane rupture did not precede her planned cesarean birth.
- A woman whose GBS culture is not known at the time of birth is managed according to her risk. Newborn GBS infection risk is higher if the pregnancy is shorter than 37 weeks, membrane rupture has persisted 18 hours or more, or temperature is higher than 38° C (>100.4° F).
- A mother who previously gave birth to an infant with GBS disease or who had bacterial infection with GBS during pregnancy should receive antibiotic prophylaxis at birth.

TUBERCULOSIS

Tuberculosis results from infection with *Mycobacterium tuberculosis*. It is transmitted by aerosolized droplets of liquid containing the bacterium, which are inhaled by a noninfected individual and taken into the lung. Initially, most individuals are asymptomatic. Women at risk should be screened for tuberculosis when obtaining prenatal care if they are not already known to be positive. This screening involves an intradermal injection of mycobacterial protein (purified protein derivative, or PPD). If the reaction is positive or the woman is already known to have a positive reaction, her abdomen should be protected by a lead shield while a radiograph is taken of her chest, preferably after the first trimester. Diagnosis is confirmed by isolating and identifying the bacterium in the sputum.

Signs and symptoms include general malaise, fatigue, loss of appetite, weight loss, and fever. Symptoms occur in the late afternoon and evening and are accompanied by night sweats. As the disease progresses, a chronic cough develops and a mucopurulent sputum is produced.

Tuberculosis is associated with poverty, malnutrition, and HIV infection. Worldwide, it is responsible for more deaths than any other communicable disease. The incidence is increasing in inner-city areas and among homeless persons. It is also prevalent among immigrants from Southeast Asia and Central and South America.

FETAL AND NEONATAL EFFECTS. Although perinatal infection is uncommon, it may be acquired as a result of the fetus swallowing or aspirating infected amniotic fluid. Diagnosis is made by finding the bacilli in gastric aspirate of the neonate or placental tissue. Signs of congenital tuberculosis include failure to thrive, lethargy, respiratory distress, fever, and enlargement of the spleen, liver, and lymph nodes. If the mother remains untreated, the newborn is at high risk for acquiring tuberculosis by inhalation of infectious respiratory droplets from the mother.

THERAPEUTIC MANAGEMENT. Treatment of tuberculosis is based on two principles. First, more than one drug must be used to prevent growth of resistant organisms. Second, treatment must continue for a prolonged period of time. The preferred treatment for pregnant women is isoniazid, rifampin, and pyrazinamide every day for 9 months. Ethambutol is added unless resistance to these three drugs is unlikely. Treatment drugs may be altered based on the sensitivity of the organism. Pyridoxine (vitamin B_6) should be given with isoniazid to prevent fetal neurotoxicity and because pregnancy itself increases the demand for this vitamin. Short-course therapy is now preferred, meaning that after the first 1 to 2 months of therapy, an alternative to daily therapy is twice-weekly therapy. Directly-observed therapy is preferred, in which a responsible person observes the woman taking the medication at each dose to increase compliance and completion of the full regimen and reduce the emergence of drug-resistant organisms (AAP & ACOG, 2002; Mandel & Weinberger, 2004).

Management of the infant born to a mother with tuberculosis involves preventing the disease and treating infection early. If the mother's sputum is free of organisms, the infant does not need to be isolated from the mother. Breastfeeding is safe in most cases, but antituberculosis drugs are secreted in breast milk. If the infant is also taking the medications, drug serum levels may reach excessive levels and breastfeeding might be contraindicated. Disease prevention focuses on teaching the mother and family how the disease is transmitted so that they can protect the infant and other family members from airborne organisms. The infant should be skin tested at birth and may be started on preventive isoniazid therapy. Skin testing is repeated at 3 months. Isoniazid is usually continued until the mother's tuberculosis has been inactive for at least 3 months. Infant tuberculosis medication may stop if the mother and family members are well treated and show no additional disease. If the skin test result shows conversion to positive, a full course of drug therapy should be given (Mandel & Weinberger, 2004).

✓ CHECK YOUR READING

33. How can toxoplasmosis be prevented?
34. What are the risk factors for colonization of the newborn with GBS during the intrapartum period? How is colonization prevented?
35. How is tuberculosis treated in the mother? How is it diagnosed and treated in the newborn?

Application of the Nursing Process
The Pregnant Woman with Tuberculosis

Assessment

Question each pregnant woman about signs or symptoms of tuberculosis. These include fever, night sweats, fatigue, weight loss, and cough. Ask whether the cough is productive and the sputum is purulent. Administer and read a PPD skin test as directed. Identify factors that increase the risk of tuberculosis, such as poverty, homelessness, recent immigration from an area that has a high incidence of tuberculosis, and HIV infection. Determine whether a family member or close friend has a history of tuberculosis.

If a woman has tuberculosis, determine the amount of knowledge she has about the disease. For example, does she know the ways in which the disease is transmitted, the importance of completing the lengthy course of prescribed medications, and the major side effects of medications? Does she know about drug resistance in tuberculosis, particularly if she does not adhere to the drug regimen? Ask about stressors in her life that increase the risk that she will not adhere to therapy, such as lack of support from a significant other, substance abuse, unstable living conditions, and other factors.

Analysis

To achieve a cure, the woman with tuberculosis must adhere to a prolonged treatment regimen that has significant side effects. In addition, women with tuberculosis often have many other stressors in their lives, including poverty, uncertain housing, and other infections such as HIV. The most relevant nursing diagnosis for this woman might be "Ineffective Individual Management of Therapeutic Regimen related to lack of knowledge of disease process and expected course of treatment."

Planning

Goals and expected outcomes for this nursing diagnosis are that:

- The woman and at least one other responsible person will verbalize information about the mode of transmission of tuberculosis, importance of medications, duration of treatment, and possible side effects of antituberculosis medications
- The woman will adhere to the prescribed treatment plan

Interventions
PROVIDING INFORMATION

1. Teach about the ways in which tuberculosis is transmitted to decrease the chance of transmission:
   - Isolating infants and other persons from persons who have infectious sputum is essential.
   - Covering the mouth when coughing, sneezing, and laughing helps prevent the organisms from entering the air.
   - Washing the hands carefully after any contact with body substances or soiled tissues decreases exposure to others.
2. Furnish reassuring information about pregnancy and tuberculosis:
   - Tuberculosis usually does not affect the course of pregnancy, type of delivery (vaginal, or cesarean), or birth weight of newborns.
   - Congenital tuberculosis infection of the newborn is rare.
   - Skin testing of the mother does not have adverse fetal effects.
   - Commonly used antituberculosis medications are in pregnancy risk category B or C (see Appendix B).
   - Tuberculosis may be cured or arrested if medication is taken as prescribed.
3. Teach the woman and another responsible person about correct administration of medications:
   - Take medication at the same time each day.
   - Rifampin and isoniazid are best taken on an empty stomach (1 hour before or 2 hours after a meal). Isoniazid can be given with meals, but doing so will delay absorption. Ethambutol should be given with food.
   - Do not skip medications or double up on missed doses.
   - Avoid the use of alcohol, which increases the risk of liver toxicity.
   - Avoid antacids containing aluminum because they impair absorption of isoniazid.
4. Educate the woman and another responsible person about expected or potential side effects:
   - Oral contraceptives are less effective when a woman is taking rifampin.
   - Body fluids such as urine, saliva, and tears may become a characteristic red-orange when taking rifampin. Soft contact lenses may be stained.
   - Nausea, heartburn, diarrhea, and flatulence are fairly common side effects. Rifampin may cause drowsiness.
   - Symptoms of hepatitis (jaundice, anorexia, excessive fatigue) should be reported to the physician.
5. Teach the necessity of continuing medication after symptoms have disappeared to eradicate the organism and avoid development of drug-resistant organisms. The total duration of therapy varies with medications that are prescribed.
6. Emphasize the importance of keeping follow-up appointments.

BOX 26-3 **Common Nursing Diagnoses for Women Who Have Medical Complications of Pregnancy**

Activity Intolerance*
Anticipatory Grieving*
Anxiety*
Fatigue
Fear
Health-Seeking Behaviors
Ineffective Individual Management of Therapeutic Regimen*
Risk for Interrupted Family Processes
Risk for Impaired Parenting
Risk for Ineffective Health Maintenance*
Risk for Infection
Risk for Injury

*Nursing diagnoses explored in this chapter.

PROVIDING SUPPORT

Respiratory isolation may be necessary if the woman's sputum still contains organisms, and a new mother may be separated from her newborn. The nursing staff must provide emotional support and counseling so that the mother can deal with the anxiety and frustration she may feel because she is not allowed to care for the infant. Language barriers and cultural implications also should be addressed. Referral to social services may be necessary to arrange temporary care of the newborn outside the home until the infant and mother have received adequate treatment (Box 26-3).

Evaluation

Goals or outcomes are met if the following occur:

- The woman and another responsible person demonstrate knowledge of the mode of transmission, verbalize the importance of taking medications as prescribed, and describe possible side effects of antituberculosis medications.
- The woman adheres to the treatment regimen as directed.

SUMMARY CONCEPTS

- The release of insulin accelerates during early pregnancy, which may result in episodes of maternal hypoglycemia. The availability of glucose and insulin favors the development and storage of fat that the mother will need later.
- Placental hormones, which reach their peak during the second and third trimesters, create resistance to insulin in maternal cells and precipitate increases in insulin needs throughout the rest of pregnancy.
- Diabetes is classified according to onset (before or during pregnancy) and whether the woman requires the administration of insulin to prevent ketoacidosis.
- Type 1 diabetes mellitus adversely affects the mother in a variety of ways during pregnancy, including increasing the risk of hypertension, urinary tract infections, and ketosis.

- Because maternal hyperglycemia during the first trimester increases the risk for congenital anomalies in the fetus, a major goal of management is to establish normal blood glucose levels before pregnancy occurs.
- Fetal growth depends on the condition of maternal blood vessels. If no vascular impairment occurs, placental perfusion is adequate and the infant is likely to be large (macrosomia). If vascular impairment does occur, placental perfusion may be reduced and the fetus may have intrauterine growth restriction.
- In addition to having an increased risk for congenital anomalies, the infant of a diabetic mother has an increased risk for hypoglycemia, hypocalcemia, hyperbilirubinemia, and respiratory distress syndrome.
- Maternal adverse effects of gestational diabetes include increased urinary tract infections, hydramnios, premature rupture of membranes, and the development of hypertension.
- Gestational diabetes increases the risk for fetal macrosomia and neonatal hypoglycemia.
- Gestational diabetes usually can be treated by diet and exercise. However, insulin may be administered if blood glucose levels remain high.
- Cardiovascular changes occurring in normal pregnancy impose an additional burden that may result in cardiac decompensation if the expectant mother has preexisting heart disease.
- The primary goal of management of the pregnant woman with heart disease is to prevent the development of congestive heart failure. This may be done by restricting activity, limiting weight gain, and preventing anemia and infection so that cardiac demand does not exceed cardiac reserves.
- Intrapartum and postpartum management of heart disease focuses on preventing fluid overload, which can cause a sharp rise in cardiac effort.
- Iron supplementation often is needed during pregnancy because most women do not have sufficient iron stores to meet the demands of pregnancy with diet alone.
- Folic acid deficiency is associated with increased risk of spontaneous abortion, abruptio placentae, and fetal anomalies such as neural tube defects. Folic acid supplementation of 400 mcg (0.4 mg) daily is recommended for all women of childbearing age to reduce the risk for neural tube defects.
- Sickle cell disease often is worsened by pregnancy, and a primary goal is to prevent sickle cell crisis during pregnancy.
- Laboratory values for thalassemia are similar to those of iron deficiency. However, administration of iron is risky because increased iron absorption and storage makes the woman susceptible to iron overload.
- Although the woman with systemic lupus erythematosus can have a normal pregnancy and give birth to a normal newborn, the pregnancy must be treated as high risk because of the increased incidence of abortion, fetal death

during the first trimester, and possible exacerbation of the disease.

- Antiphospholipid syndrome (an autoimmune disorder) is a cluster of clinical entities that includes increased risk for thrombosis, fetal loss, and the presence of antiphospholipid antibodies.

- Marked improvement in rheumatoid arthritis often occurs during pregnancy, possibly as a result of pregnancy-specific hormone and hormonal factors. However, most women relapse soon after childbirth.

- Management of epilepsy is complicated because of the teratogenic effects of anticonvulsant medications coupled with the importance of preventing seizures.

- Although Bell's palsy usually is temporary, the woman may be anxious. Supportive care and emotional support are essential.

- Motor vehicle accidents are a major cause of blunt force trauma that may result in premature separation of the placenta, hemorrhage, fractures, and internal injuries. Penetrating injuries caused by knife or gunshot wounds are particularly dangerous for the fetus.

- Treatment of trauma in the pregnant woman is similar to that in a nonpregnant woman. Cardiopulmonary resuscitation and controlling bleeding are the priorities. Careful evaluation of the uterus and fetus also are essential after even minor trauma.

- Viral infections that occur during pregnancy can be transmitted to the fetus in two ways: across the placental barrier or by exposure to organisms during birth. Although they may be mild or even subclinical in the mother, viral infections can have serious effects for the fetus.

- The health care team is responsible for teaching how infectious diseases can be prevented and that early treatment also may reduce fetal and neonatal exposure to infections.

- Human immunodeficiency virus is a retrovirus that invades the CD4+ subset of T lymphocytes and destroys them, producing acquired immunodeficiency syndrome, which allows opportunistic infections to overwhelm the immune system.

- Pregnant women who are HIV-positive experience anxiety, fear, and grief as they contemplate potential losses resulting from the disease. Nurses must provide emotional support, information, and counseling, which will help the woman cope with her emotions and retain control of her care for as long as possible.

- Nonviral infections such as toxoplasmosis, group B streptococcus infection, and tuberculosis can be prevented or treated.

ANSWERS TO CRITICAL THINKING EXERCISE 26-1, p. 669

1. The team may have assumed that Marcia knew the maternal and fetal effects of gestational diabetes and the importance of following the plan of care.

2. The team could have explained the reasons for the recommended plan and allowed adequate time to answer all questions. Emphasizing why it is necessary to monitor the condition of the fetus is particularly important because mothers usually are motivated to do whatever they can to ensure the health of the fetus.

3. The nurse should acknowledge Marcia's belief. "I realize that we haven't made our concerns clear to you. Let me explain why it is important for you and for your baby to be watched carefully during these last weeks." The nurse must then provide clear, simple explanations and allow time to answer questions.

4. The nurse must acknowledge that weekly fetal surveillance tests are time consuming but emphasize that they provide valuable information about the well-being of the baby. Usually the information is reassuring, but additional tests can be performed if questions exist.

REFERENCES & READINGS

American Academy of Pediatrics & American College of Obstetricians and Gynecologists (ACOG). (2002). *Guidelines for perinatal care* (5th ed.). Elk Grove Village, IL: Authors.

American College of Obstetricians and Gynecologists. (1999a). *Management of herpes in pregnancy*, Practice Bulletin No. 8. Washington, DC: Author.

American College of Obstetricians and Gynecologists. (2001). *Gestational diabetes*, Practice Bulletin No. 30. Washington, DC: Author.

American Diabetes Association. (2004). Position statement: Gestational diabetes mellitus. *Diabetes Care, 27*(Suppl. 1), S88-S90.

American Diabetes Association. (2005). Position statement: Standards of medical care in diabetes. *Diabetes Care, 28*(Suppl. 1), S4-S36.

Aminoff, M.J. (2004). Neurologic disorders. In R.K. Creasy, R. Resnik, & J.D. Iams (Eds.), *Maternal-fetal medicine: Principles and practice* (5th ed., pp. 1165-1191). Philadelphia: Saunders.

Anderson, S.L. (2004). Diabetes mellitus. In S.R. Williams & E.D. Schlenker (Eds.), *Essentials of nutrition and diet therapy* (8th ed., pp. 493-518). St. Louis: Mosby.

Ashley-Koch, A., Yang, Q., & Olney, R.S. (2000). Human genome epidemiology (HuGE) reviews. *American Journal of Epidemiology, 151*(9), 839-845.

Beckman, C.A. (2002). Women's perceptions of their asthma during pregnancy. *MCN: American Journal of Maternal/Child Nursing, 27*(2), 98-102.

Blackburn, S.T. (2003). *Maternal, fetal, and neonatal physiology: A clinical perspective*. Philadelphia: Saunders.

Blair, M. (2005). Management of clients with acquired immunodeficiency syndrome. In J.M. Black & J.H. Hawks (Eds.), *Medical-surgical nursing: Clinical management for positive outcomes* (7th ed., pp. 2375-2399). Philadelphia: Saunders.

Blanchard, D.G., & Shabetai, R. (2004). Cardiac diseases. In R.K. Creasy, R. Resnik, & J.D. Iams (Eds.), *Maternal-newborn medicine: Principles and practice* (5th ed., pp. 815-843). Philadelphia: Saunders.

Burton, J., & Reyes, M. (2001). Breathe in, breathe out: Controlling asthma during pregnancy. *AWHONN Lifelines, 5*(1), 24-30.

Centers for Disease Control and Prevention. (2001a). Revised guidelines for HIV counseling, testing, and referral. *MMWR. Morbidity and Mortality Weekly Report, 50*(RR19), November 9, 2001. Retrieved April 8, 2005, from www.cdc.gov/mmwr/pdf/rr/rr5019.pdf. Retrieval data 4/8/05.

Centers for Disease Control and Prevention. (2001b). *Varicella vaccine (chickenpox)*. Retrieved February 13, 2005, from www.cdc.gov/nip/vaccine/varicella/default.htm.

Centers for Disease Control and Prevention. National Center for Infectious Diseases. (2002a). Prevention of perinatal group B streptococcal disease: Revised guidelines from CDC. *MMWR. Morbidity and Mortality Weekly Report, 55*(RR11). Retrieved April 8, 2005, from www.phppo.cdc.gov/nltn/pdf/2005/6_MMWRBstrep.pdf.

Centers for Disease Control and Prevention. (2002b). Sexually transmitted diseases treatment guidelines, 2002. *MMWR. Morbidity and Mortality Weekly Report, 51*(RR6). Retrieved February 20, 2005, from www.cdc.gov/STD/treatment/rr5106.pdf.

Centers for Disease Control and Prevention. (2004). Recommended adult immunization schedule: United States, October 2004-September, 2005. Retrieved February 12, 2005, from www.cdc.gov/nip/vaccine/varicella/default.htm.

Centers for Disease Control and Prevention. National Center for Infectious Diseases. (2005). Parvovirus B19 infection and pregnancy. Retrieved April 9, 2005, from http://www.cdc.gov/ncidod.

Cunningham, F.G., Gant, N.F., Leveno, K.J., Gilstrap, L.C., Hauth, J.C., & Wenstrom, K.D. (2001). *Williams obstetrics* (21st ed.). Norwalk, CT: Appleton & Lange.

Damato, E.G., & Winnen, C.W. (2002). Cytomegalovirus infection: Perinatal implications. *Journal of Obstetric, Gynecologic, and Neonatal Nursing, 31*(1), 86-92.

Davison, J.M., & Lindheimer, M.D. (2004). Renal disorders. In R.K. Creasy, R. Resnik, & J.D. Iams (Eds.), *Maternal-newborn medicine: Principles and practice* (5th ed., pp. 901-923). Philadelphia: Saunders.

Donahue, D.B. (2002). Diagnosis and treatment of herpes simplex infection during pregnancy. *Journal of Obstetric, Gynecologic, and Neonatal Nursing, 31*(1), 99-106.

Donaldson, J.O., & Duffy, T.P. (2004). Neurologic complications. In G.N. Burrow, T.P. Duffy, & J.A. Copel (Eds.), *Medical complications during pregnancy* (6th ed., pp. 69-86). Philadelphia: Saunders.

Duffy, T.P. (2004). Hematologic aspects of pregnancy. In G.N. Burrow, T.P. Duffy, & J.A. Copel (Eds.), *Medical complications during pregnancy* (6th ed., pp. 69-86). Philadelphia: Saunders.

Fanaroff, A.A., Martin, R.J., & Rodriguez, R.J. (2004). Identification and management of problems in the high-risk neonate. In R.K. Creasy, R. Resnik, & J.D. Iams (Eds.), *Maternal-newborn medicine: Principles and practice* (5th ed., pp. 1263-1301). Philadelphia: Saunders.

Farrell, M. (2003). Improving the care of women with gestational diabetes. *MCN: American Journal of Maternal/Child Nursing, 28*(5), 301-305.

Franz, M.J. (2004). Medical nutrition therapy for diabetes mellitus and hypoglycemia of nondiabetic origin. In L.K. Mahan & S. Escott-Stump (Eds.), *Krause's food, nutrition, and diet therapy* (11th ed., pp. 792-837). Philadelphia: Saunders.

Gambone, J.C., Moore, J.G., & Koos, B.J. (2004). Common medical and surgical conditions complicating pregnancy. In N.F. Hacker, J.G. Moore, & J.C. Gambone (Eds.), *Essentials of obstetrics and gynecology* (4th ed., pp. 216-246). Philadelphia: Saunders.

Gibbs, R.S., Sweet, R.L., & Duff, W.P. (2004). Maternal and fetal infectious disorders. In R.K. Creasy, R. Resnik, & J.D. Iams (Eds.), *Maternal-fetal medicine* (5th ed., pp. 741-801). Philadelphia: Saunders.

Golden, L.H., & Burrow, G.N. (2004). Thyroid disease in pregnancy. In G.N. Burrow, T.P. Duffy, & J.A. Copel (Eds.), *Medical complications during pregnancy* (6th ed., pp. 131-161). Philadelphia: Saunders.

Gonik, B., & Foley, M.R. (2004). Intensive care monitoring of the critically ill pregnant patient. In R.K. Creasy, R. Resnik, & J.D. Iams (Eds.), *Maternal-newborn medicine: Principles and practice* (5th ed., pp. 925-951). Philadelphia: Saunders.

Guyton, A.C., & Hall, J.E. (2000). *Textbook of medical physiology* (10th ed.). Philadelphia: Saunders.

Hadden, R. (2004). What nurses need to know: Hepatitis C and pregnancy. *AWHONN Lifelines, 8*(3), 224-231.

Hankins, G.D.V., & Suarez, V.R. (2004). Rheumatologic and connective tissue disorders. In R.K. Creasy, R. Resnik, & J.D. Iams (Eds.), *Maternal-newborn medicine: Principles and practice* (5th ed., pp. 1147-1163). Philadelphia: Saunders.

Houry, D., & Abbott, J.T. (2004). Emergency management of the obstetric patient. In G.N. Burrow, T.P. Duffy, & J.A. Copel (Eds.), *Medical complications during pregnancy* (6th ed., pp. 235-245). Philadelphia: Saunders.

Jackson, D.J., Chopra, M., Witten, C., & Sengwana, M.J. (2003). HIV and infant feeding: Issues in developed and developing countries. *Journal of Obstetric, Gynecologic, and Neonatal Nursing, 32*(1), 117-127.

Katz, A. (2003). The evolving art of caring for pregnant women with HIV infection. *Journal of Obstetric, Gynecologic, and Neonatal Nursing, 32*(1), 102-108.

Kenshole, A.B. (2004). Diabetes and pregnancy. In G.N. Burrow, T.P. Duffy, & J.A. Copel (Eds.), *Medical complications during pregnancy* (6th ed., pp. 15-42). Philadelphia: Saunders.

Kilpatrick, S.J., & Laros, R.K. (2004). Maternal hematologic disorders. In R.K. Creasy, R. Resnik, & J.D. Iams (Eds.), *Maternal-newborn medicine: Principles and practice* (5th ed., pp. 975-1004). Philadelphia: Saunders.

Kotter, M., & Osguthorpe, S. (2005). Alterations in oxygen transport. In L.C. Copstead & J.L. Banasik (Eds.), *Pathophysiology: Biological and behavioral perspectives* (3rd ed., pp. 318-362). Philadelphia: Saunders.

Landon, M.B. (2004). Diseases of the liver, biliary system, and pancreas. In R.K. Creasy, R. Resnik, & J.D. Iams (Eds.), *Maternal-newborn medicine: Principles and practice* (5th ed., pp. 1127-1145). Philadelphia: Saunders.

Landry, M.L. (2004). Viral infections. In G.N. Burrow, T.P. Duffy, & J.A. Copel (Eds.), *Medical complications during pregnancy* (6th ed., pp. 347-373). Philadelphia: Saunders.

Laskin, C.A. (2004). Pregnancy and the rheumatic diseases. In G.N. Burrow, T.P. Duffy, & J.A. Copel (Eds.), *Medical complications during pregnancy* (6th ed., pp. 429-449). Philadelphia: Saunders.

Lupus Foundation of America. (2003). *Lupus fact sheet.* Retrieved February 5, 2005, from www.lupus.org/education.

Mandel, J., & Weinberger, S.E. (2004). Pulmonary diseases. In G.N. Burrow, T.P. Duffy, & J.A. Copel (Eds.), *Medical complications during pregnancy* (6th ed., pp. 375-414). Philadelphia: Saunders.

March of Dimes Birth Defects Foundation. (2004). *Fact sheet: Diabetes in pregnancy.* Fact sheet 09-601-00. Retrieved January 26, 2005, from www.modimes.org.

McCarter, D. (2002). Parvovirus B19 in pregnancy. *Journal of Obstetric, Gynecologic, and Neonatal Nursing, 31*(1), 107-112.

Minkoff, H.L. (2004). Human immunodeficiency virus. In R.K. Creasy, R. Resnik, & J.D. Iams (Eds.), *Maternal-fetal medicine: Principles and practice* (5th ed., pp. 803-814). Philadelphia: Saunders.

Monga, M. (2004). Maternal cardiovascular and renal adaptation to pregnancy. In R.K. Creasy, R. Resnik, & J.D. Iams (Eds.), *Maternal-newborn medicine: Principles and practice* (5th ed., pp. 111-120). Philadelphia: Saunders.

Moore, T.R. (2004). Diabetes in pregnancy. In R.K. Creasy, R. Resnik, & J.D. Iams (Eds.), *Maternal-newborn medicine: Principles and practice* (5th ed., pp. 1023-1061). Philadelphia: Saunders.

Morgan, K.L. (2004). Management of UTIs during pregnancy. *MCN: American Journal of Maternal/Child Nursing, 29*(4), 254-258.

Nader, S. (2004). Thyroid disease and pregnancy. In R.K. Creasy, R. Resnik, & J.D. Iams (Eds.), *Maternal-newborn medicine: Principles and practice* (5th ed., pp. 1063-1081). Philadelphia: Saunders.

National Institutes of Health: National Heart, Lung, and Blood Institute. (2002). *The management of sickle cell disease* (NIH Publication No. 02-2117). Retrieved February 5, 2005, from www.nhlbi.nih.gov/health/prof/blood/sickle/sc_mngt.pdf.

Pagana, K.D., & Pagana, T.J. (2005). *Diagnostic and laboratory test reference.* St. Louis, MO: Elsevier.

Perinatal HIV Guidelines Working Group. (2004). Recommendations for use of antiretroviral drugs in pregnant HIV-1–infected women for maternal health and interventions to reduce perinatal HIV-1 transmission in the United States. Retrieved February 19, 2005, from www.aidsinfo.nih.gov.

Quirolo, K., & Vichinsky, E. (2004). Hemoglobin disorders. In R.E. Behrman, R.M. Kliegman, & H.B. Jenson (Eds.), *Nelson textbook of pediatrics* (17th ed., pp. 1623-1634). Philadelphia: Saunders.

Riely, C.A., & Fallon, H.J. (2004). Liver diseases. In G.N. Burrow, T.P. Duffy, & J.A. Copel (Eds.), *Medical complications during pregnancy* (6th ed., pp. 279-304). Philadelphia: Saunders.

Roberts, J.M. (2004). Pregnancy-related hypertension. In R.K. Creasy, R. Resnik, & J.D. Iams (Eds.), *Maternal-fetal medicine: Principles and practice* (5th ed., pp. 859-899). Philadelphia: Saunders.

Savoia, M.C. (2004). Bacterial, fungal, and parasitic disease. In G.N. Burrow, T.P. Duffey, & J.A. Copel (Eds.), *Medical complications during pregnancy* (6th ed., pp. 305-345). Philadelphia: Saunders.

Scott, L.D., & Abu-Hamda, E. (2004). Gastrointestinal disease in pregnancy. In R.K. Creasy, R. Resnik, & J.D. Iams (Eds.), *Maternal-newborn medicine: Principles and practice* (5th ed., pp. 1023-1061). Philadelphia: Saunders.

Setaro, J.F., Caulin-Glaser, T., & (2004). Pregnancy and cardiovascular disease. In G.N. Burrow, T.P. Duffy, & J.A. Copel (Eds.), *Medical complications during pregnancy* (6th ed., pp. 103-129). Philadelphia: Saunders.

Shames, K.H., & Youngkin, E.Q. (2002). The thyroid dance: Nursing approaches to autoimmune low thyroid. *AWHONN Lifelines, 6*(1), 52-59.

Sickle Cell Disease Association of America. (2004). *Break the sickle cycle.* Retrieved February 5, 2005, from www.sicklecelldisease.org.

Silver, R.M., Peltier, M.R., & Branch, D.W. (2004). The immunology of pregnancy. In R.K. Creasy, R. Resnik, & J.D. Iams (Eds.), *Maternal-newborn medicine: Principles and practice* (5th ed., pp. 89-109). Philadelphia: Saunders.

Stopler, T. (2004). Medical nutrition therapy for anemia. In L.K. Mahan & S. Escott-Stump (Eds.), *Krause's food, nutrition, and diet therapy* (11th ed., pp. 838-859). Philadelphia: Saunders.

Tiller, C.M. (2002). Chlamydia during pregnancy: Implications and impact on perinatal and neonatal outcomes. *Journal of Obstetric, Gynecologic, and Neonatal Nursing, 31*(1), 93-98.

U.S. Department of Health and Human Services. (2004). Recommended adult immunization schedule, United States 2004-2005. Retrieved April 9, 2005, from www.cdc.gov/nip/recs/adult-schedule.pdf.

Whitty, J.E., & Dombrowski, M.P. (2004). Respiratory diseases in pregnancy. In R.K. Creasy, R. Resnik, & J.D. Iams (Eds.), *Maternal-fetal medicine: Principles and practice* (5th ed., pp. 953-974). Philadelphia: Saunders.

CHAPTER 27

Intrapartum Complications

OBJECTIVES

After studying this chapter, you should be able to:

1. Explain abnormalities that may result in dysfunctional labor.
2. Describe maternal and fetal risks associated with premature rupture of the membranes.
3. Analyze factors that increase a woman's risk for preterm labor.
4. Explain maternal and fetal problems that may occur if pregnancy persists beyond 42 weeks.
5. Describe the intrapartum emergencies discussed in this chapter.
6. Explain therapeutic management of each intrapartum complication.
7. Apply the nursing process to care of women with intrapartum complications and care of their families.

Go to your Student CD-ROM for Review Questions keyed to these Objectives.

DEFINITIONS

Abruptio Placentae Premature separation of a normally implanted placenta.

Amniocentesis Transabdominal puncture of the amniotic sac to obtain a sample of amniotic fluid that contains fetal cells and biochemical substances for laboratory analysis.

Amniotic Fluid Embolism An embolism in which amniotic fluid with its particulate matter is drawn into the pregnant woman's circulation, lodging in her lungs.

Anaphylactoid Syndrome A disorder in which amniotic fluid with its particulate matter enters the pregnant woman's circulation, lodging in her lungs. Previously called *amniotic fluid embolism*.

Cephalopelvic Disproportion Condition in which fetal head is too large to fit through the maternal pelvis at birth. Also called *fetopelvic disproportion*.

Cerclage Encircling of the cervix with suture to prevent recurrent spontaneous abortion caused by early cervical dilation.

Chorioamnionitis Inflammation of the amniotic sac (fetal membranes); usually caused by bacterial or viral infection. Also called *amnionitis*.

Dystocia Difficult or prolonged labor; often associated with abnormal uterine activity and cephalopelvic disproportion.

Hydramnios Excessive volume of amniotic fluid (more than 2000 ml at term). Also called *polyhydramnios*.

Hypertonic Labor Dysfunction Ineffective labor characterized by erratic and poorly coordinated contractions. Uterine resting tone is higher than normal.

Hypotonic Labor Dysfunction Ineffective labor characterized by weak, infrequent, and brief but coordinated uterine contractions. Uterine resting tone is normal.

Macrosomia Unusually large fetal size; infant birth weight more than 4000 g (8.8 lb).

Multifetal Pregnancy A pregnancy in which the woman is carrying two or more fetuses. Also called *multiple gestation*.

Occult Prolapse See *Prolapsed Cord*.

Oligohydramnios Abnormally small volume of amniotic fluid (less than 500 ml at term).

Placenta Accreta A placenta that is abnormally adherent to the uterine muscle. If the condition is more advanced, it is called *placenta increta* (the placenta extends into the uterine muscle) or *placenta percreta* (the placenta extends through the uterine muscle).

Placenta Previa Abnormal implantation of the placenta in the lower uterus, at or very near the cervical os.

Precipitate Birth A birth that occurs without a trained attendant present.

Precipitate Labor An intense, unusually short labor (less than 3 hours).

DEFINITIONS—cont'd

Preterm Labor Onset of labor after 20 weeks and before the beginning of the thirty-eighth week of gestation.

Prolapsed Cord Displacement of the umbilical cord in front of or beside the fetal presenting part. An occult prolapse is one that is suspected on the basis of fetal heart rate patterns; the umbilical cord cannot be palpated or seen.

Shoulder Dystocia Delayed or difficult birth of the fetal shoulders after the head is born.

Tocolytic A drug that inhibits uterine contractions.

Uterine Inversion Turning of the uterus inside out after birth of the fetus.

Uterine Resting Tone Degree of uterine muscle tension when the woman is not in labor or during the interval between labor contractions.

Uterine Rupture A tear in the wall of the uterus.

For most women, birth is a normal process free of major complications. However, complications sometimes make childbearing hazardous for the woman or her baby. The nurse's challenge is to identify the complications promptly and provide effective care for such mothers while nurturing the entire family at this significant time of life.

The complications addressed in this chapter are often interrelated. For example, a dysfunctional labor is likely to be prolonged, and the woman is more vulnerable to infection, psychological distress, and fetal compromise. Also, women who have complications are more likely to need interventions such as lengthy hospitalization before birth or cesarean birth. The nurse should provide nursing care that relates to all problems experienced by the woman.

DYSFUNCTIONAL LABOR

Normal labor is characterized by progress. Dysfunctional labor is one that does not result in normal progress of cervical effacement, dilation, and fetal descent. *Dystocia* is a general term that describes any difficult labor or birth. A dysfunctional labor may result from problems with the powers of labor, the passenger, the passage, the psyche, or a combination of these. Dysfunctional labor often is prolonged but may be unusually short and intense.

An operative birth (assisted with a vacuum extractor or forceps, or cesarean birth) may be needed if dysfunctional labor does not resolve or fetal or maternal compromise occurs. Signs of possible compromise include persistent nonreassuring fetal heart rate (FHR) patterns (see Chapter 14), fetal acidosis, and meconium passage. Maternal exhaustion or infection may occur, especially with long labors. Nursing measures that enhance progress and maternal comfort and promote fetal well-being also are discussed in this chapter.

Problems of the Powers

The powers of labor may not be adequate to expel the fetus because of ineffective contractions or ineffective maternal pushing efforts.

INEFFECTIVE CONTRACTIONS

Effective uterine activity is characterized by coordinated contractions that are strong and numerous enough to propel the fetus past the resistance of the woman's bony pelvis and soft tissues. It is not possible to say how frequent, long, or strong labor contractions must be. One woman's labor may progress with contractions that would be inadequate for another woman. Possible causes of ineffective contractions include the following:

- Maternal fatigue
- Maternal inactivity
- Fluid and electrolyte imbalance
- Hypoglycemia
- Excessive analgesia or anesthesia
- Maternal catecholamines secreted in response to stress or pain
- Disproportion between the maternal pelvis and fetal presenting part
- Uterine overdistention such as with multiple gestation or hydramnios

Two patterns of ineffective uterine contractions are hypotonic and hypertonic dysfunction. Hypotonic dysfunction is more common than hypertonic dysfunction. Characteristics and management of each are different, but either results in poor labor progress if it persists (Table 27-1).

HYPOTONIC DYSFUNCTION. Hypotonic contractions are coordinated but too weak to be effective. They are infrequent and brief and can be indented easily with fingertip pressure at the peak.

Hypotonic dysfunction usually occurs during the active phase of labor, when progress normally quickens. Active phase usually begins at about 4 cm of cervical dilation. Uterine overdistention is associated with hypotonic dysfunction because the stretched uterine muscle contracts poorly.

The woman may be fairly comfortable because her contractions are weak. However, she often is frustrated because labor slows at a time when she expects to be making more rapid progress. Hypotonic dysfunction is tiring simply because it adds to labor's duration. Fetal hypoxia is not usually seen with hypotonic labor.

Management depends on the cause. Many women respond to simple measures. Providing intravenous (IV) or oral fluids corrects maternal fluid and electrolyte imbalances or hypoglycemia. Maternal position changes, particularly different upright positions, favor fetal descent and promote effective contractions. The woman who moves about actively typically has better labor progress and is more comfortable than the woman who remains in one position. Pain management techniques such as epidural block may have outcomes that reduce contraction effectiveness, requiring interventions specific to that factor.

TABLE 27-1 Patterns of Labor Dysfunction

Hypotonic Dysfunction	Hypertonic Dysfunction
Contractions Coordinated but weak. Become less frequent and shorter in duration. Easily indented at peak. Woman may have minimal discomfort because the contractions are weak.	Uncoordinated, irregular. Short and of poor intensity, but painful and cramplike.
Uterine Resting Tone Not elevated.	Higher than normal. Important to distinguish from abruptio placentae, which has similar characteristics (see p. 634).
Phase of Labor Active. Typically occurs after 4-cm dilation. More common than hypertonic dysfunction.	Latent. Usually occurs before 4-cm dilation. Less common than hypotonic dysfunction.
Therapeutic Management Amniotomy (may increase the risk of infection). Oxytocin augmentation. Cesarean birth if no progress.	Correct cause if it can be identified. Light sedation to promote rest. Hydration. Tocolytics to reduce high uterine tone and promote placental perfusion.
Nursing Care Interventions related to amniotomy and oxytocin augmentation. Encourage position changes. An abdominal binder may help direct the fetus toward the mother's pelvis if her abdominal wall is very lax. Ambulation if no contraindication and if acceptable to the woman. Emotional support: Allow her to express feelings of discouragement. Explain measures taken to increase effectiveness of contractions. Include her partner or family in emotional support measures because they may have anxiety that will heighten the woman's anxiety.	Promote uterine blood flow: side-lying position. Promote rest, general comfort, and relaxation. Pain relief. Emotional support: Accept the reality of the woman's pain and frustration. Reassure her that she is not being childish. Explain reason for measures to break abnormal labor patterns and their goals or expected results. Allow her to express her feelings during and after labor. Include partner or family (see hypotonic labor dysfunction).

The nurse should use therapeutic communication to help the woman identify anxieties or beliefs about labor and its progress. Identifying her anxieties is the first step to managing them effectively so that the stress response does not slow her labor. For example, the nurse might ask, "What do you think is making your labor slow?" or "How do you feel that your labor is going?"

Many women need measures such as amniotomy and oxytocin infusion to promote labor progress. The birth attendant evaluates the woman's labor to confirm that she is having hypotonic active labor rather than a prolonged latent phase of labor or false labor. The latent phase of labor occurs within the first 3 cm of cervical dilation. The maternal pelvis and fetal presentation and position are assessed to identify abnormalities. Interventions to reduce undesired maternal effects of a prolonged latent phase such as exhaustion or infection is a goal. However, the birth attendant must consider the possibility that a woman is in false labor rather than a prolonged latent phase when choosing interventions to correct labor progress.

Amniotomy or augmentation, usually with oxytocin, may be used to stimulate a labor that slows after it is established. The risks of amniotomy are umbilical cord prolapse, infection, and abruptio placentae. Reduced placental perfusion caused by excessive uterine contractions is the most common risk of oxytocin labor augmentation.

HYPERTONIC DYSFUNCTION. Hypertonic dysfunction of labor is less common than hypotonic dysfunction. Contractions are uncoordinated and erratic in their frequency, duration, and intensity. The contractions are painful but ineffective. Hypertonic dysfunction usually occurs during the latent phase of labor.

Although each contraction varies in its intensity, the uterine resting tone between contractions is higher than normal, reducing uterine blood flow. This uterine ischemia decreases fetal oxygen supply and causes the woman to have almost constant cramping pain. Because high uterine resting tone and constant pain also are seen in abruptio placentae, this complication should be considered as well.

The mother becomes very tired because of nearly constant discomfort. She may lose confidence in her ability to give birth and cope with labor. She often thinks, "If it hurts this much so early, I must be a real baby about pain." Frustration and anxiety further reduce her pain tolerance and interfere with the normal processes of labor. The nurse should accept her frustration and discomfort. Cervical dilation should not be equated with the amount of pain a woman "should" experience.

Management of hypertonic labor depends on the cause. Relief of pain is the primary intervention to promote a normal labor pattern. Warm showers and baths promote relaxation and rest, often allowing a normal labor pattern to ensue. Systemic analgesics or, occasionally, low-dose epidural analgesia may be required to achieve this purpose.

Oxytocin is not usually given because it can intensify the already high uterine resting tone. However, very low doses of oxytocin sometimes are given to promote coordinated uterine contractions. Tocolytic drugs may be ordered to reduce uterine resting tone and improve placental blood flow. The decision to order uterine stimulant or relaxant drugs is very individualized, based on each woman's labor pattern.

INEFFECTIVE MATERNAL PUSHING

A reflexive urge to push with contractions usually occurs as the fetal presenting part reaches the pelvic floor during second-stage labor. However, ineffective pushing may result from the following:

- Use of incorrect pushing techniques and positions
- Fear of injury because of pain and tearing sensations felt by the mother when she pushes
- Decreased or absent urge to push
- Maternal exhaustion
- Analgesia or anesthesia that suppresses the woman's urge to push
- Psychological unreadiness to "let go" of her baby

Management focuses on correcting causes contributing to ineffective pushing. If maternal and fetal vital signs are normal, no maximum allowable duration for the second stage exists. Each woman is evaluated individually by her birth attendant to determine whether labor should be ended with an operative delivery or can continue safely (see Chapter 16).

Nursing care to promote effective pushing helps the mother make each effort more productive. Most women, even women who have had epidural analgesia, can detect the urge to push with today's techniques. The practice of *laboring down* or *delayed pushing*—encouraging the woman to wait until she feels the reflexive urge to push—has been shown to have a lower incidence of adverse effects than pushing immediately on full cervical dilation (Mayberry et al., 2000). (See Chapter 13 for more information about the evidence-based nursing practice of laboring down.)

Upright positions such as squatting add gravity to the woman's pushing efforts. Semi-sitting, side-lying, and pushing while sitting on the toilet are other options. If she prefers to lie in bed on her side, she should pull her upper leg toward her chest with each push. Leaning forward while in a sitting or squatting position maintains the best alignment of the fetal head with the pelvis.

The woman who fears injury because of the sensations she feels when pushing may respond to accurate information about the process of fetal descent. If she understands that sensations of tearing often accompany fetal descent but her tissues can expand to accommodate the baby, she may be more willing to push with contractions.

Epidural analgesia for labor uses a mixture of a local anesthetic agent and an epidural opioid analgesic to provide pain control without the major loss of sensation that is likely if local anesthetic is used alone. However, if a woman cannot feel the urge to push at all or cannot feel it strongly after the fetus has descended, she can be coached to push with each contraction.

The woman who is exhausted may push more effectively if she is encouraged to rest and push only when she feels the urge, or she may push with every other contraction. Giving oral or IV fluids as ordered provides energy for the strenuous work of second-stage labor. Reassuring her about fetal well-being and the fact that she has no absolute deadline to meet helps her work with her body's efforts most effectively. This reassurance also helps the woman who may be emotionally readying herself to "let go" of her fetus in exchange for a newborn as she labors.

Problems with the Passenger

Fetal problems associated with dysfunctional labor are related to the following:

- Fetal size
- Fetal presentation or position
- Multifetal pregnancy
- Fetal anomalies

These variations may cause mechanical problems and contribute to ineffective contractions.

FETAL SIZE

MACROSOMIA. The macrosomic infant weighs more than 4000 g (8.8 lb) or more at birth. The head may be so large that it cannot mold enough to adapt to the pelvis. Even if the head makes it through the pelvis, the shoulders may be too large to pass. Uterine distention by the large fetus reduces contraction strength during and after birth.

Size is relative, however. The woman with a small or abnormally shaped pelvis may not be able to deliver an average-sized or small infant. The woman with a large pelvis may easily give birth to an infant heavier than 4000 g.

SHOULDER DYSTOCIA. Delayed or difficult birth of the shoulders may occur as they become impacted above the maternal symphysis pubis. After the head is born, it retracts against the perineum, much like a turtle's head drawing into its shell ("turtle sign"). Shoulder dystocia is more likely to occur when the fetus is large or the mother has diabetes, but many cases occur in pregnancies with no identifiable risk factors. Labor may be long, but shoulder dystocia may occur after a normal labor (American College of Obstetricians and Gynecologists [ACOG], 2002; Bashore & Hayashi, 2004).

Shoulder dystocia is an urgent situation because the umbilical cord can be compressed between the fetal body and maternal pelvis. Although the infant's head is out of the vaginal canal, the chest is inside, preventing respirations. Any of several methods may be used to quickly relieve the impacted fetal shoulders (Figure 27-1). Fundal pressure should be avoided so that the shoulders are not pushed even harder against the symphysis. The infant's clavicles should be checked for crepitus, deformity, and bruising, each of which suggests fracture. Documentation of all care is essential, including a clear description if suprapubic pressure was used to avoid confusion with fundal pressure in any subsequent legal action (Simpson & Knox, 2001).

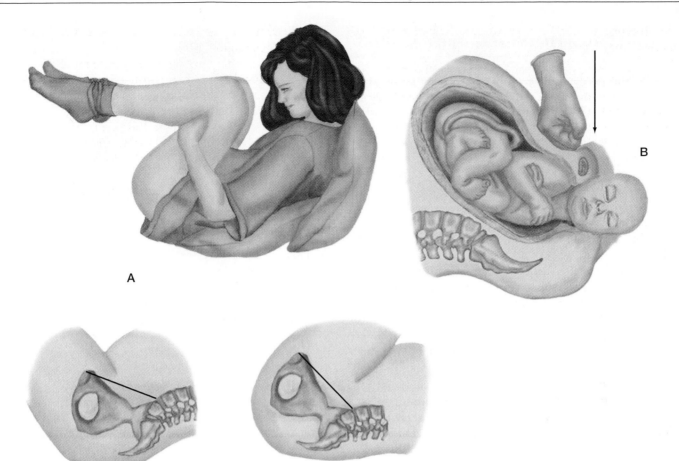

Figure 27-1 ■ Methods that may be used to relieve shoulder dystocia. **A,** McRobert's maneuver. The woman flexes her thighs sharply against her abdomen, which straightens the pelvic curve somewhat. A supported squat has a similar effect and adds gravity to her pushing efforts. **B,** Suprapubic pressure by an assistant pushes the fetal anterior shoulder downward to displace it from above the mother's symphysis pubis. Fundal pressure should not be used because it will push the anterior shoulder even more firmly against the mother's symphysis.

ABNORMAL FETAL PRESENTATION OR POSITION

An unfavorable fetal presentation or position may interfere with cervical dilation or fetal descent.

ROTATION ABNORMALITIES. Persistence of the fetus in the occiput posterior or occiput transverse position can contribute to dysfunctional labor. These positions prevent the mechanisms of labor (cardinal movements) from occurring normally. Most fetuses that begin labor in an occiput posterior position rotate spontaneously to an occiput anterior position, promoting normal extension and expulsion of the head. The fetus may not rotate or may partly rotate and remain in an occiput transverse position. Although many women cannot readily deliver a fetus in the occiput posterior position, the woman with a large pelvis compared with the fetal size may be able to do so.

Labor usually is longer and more uncomfortable when the fetus remains in the occiput posterior or occiput transverse position. Intense back or leg pain that may be poorly relieved with analgesia makes coping with labor difficult for the woman. "Back labor" aptly describes the sensations a woman feels when her fetus is in an occiput posterior position. Some women who had a fetus in the occiput posterior position during labor continue to feel more back or coccyx pain during the postpartum period.

Maternal position changes promote fetal head rotation to an occiput anterior position and descent (see Figure 13-5). Examples are as follows:

- Hands and knees—Rocking the pelvis back and forth while on hands and knees encourages rotation. The woman's knees should be slightly behind her hips in this position.
- Side-lying (on the opposite side of the fetal occiput).
- Lunge—The mother places one foot on a chair with her foot and knee pointed to that side. She lunges sideways repeatedly for 5 seconds at a time during a contraction. The lunge also can be done in a kneeling position. The nurse or her partner must secure the chair and help the woman balance.
- Squatting (for second-stage labor); sitting on a slightly underinflated birth ball gives a similar effect
- Sitting, kneeling, or standing while leaning forward

CRITICAL THINKING ⟨?⟩ EXERCISE 27-1

A woman having her first baby has been in labor for several hours. Her nurse-midwife performs a vaginal examination and says that the cervix is 6 cm dilated and completely effaced, with the fetus in right occiput posterior position. The mother is having persistent back pain that worsens during contractions.

Questions
How should the nurse interpret this information? Should the nurse take any specific action based on the nurse-midwife's examination?

Using a birthing ball—a large plastic ball capable of supporting an adult's weight—helps support the woman when in the hands-and-knees position. She can also sit on it and gain many of the benefits of squatting. In addition, the woman tends to move her hips back and forth, favoring fetal descent.

Upright maternal positions promote descent, which usually is accompanied by fetal head rotation. The first two maternal positions promote rotation because the mother's abdomen is dependent in relation to her spine. In the hands-and-knees position the convex surface of the fetal back tends to rotate toward the convex anterior uterus, similar to nesting two spoons (Figure 27-2). A side-lying position has a similar effect, although not quite as pronounced. These positions decrease the mother's discomfort by reducing fetal head pressure on her sacrum.

The lunge widens the side of the pelvis toward which the woman lunges. If the fetal position is known, she lunges toward the side where the occiput is located (Figure 27-3). If the fetal position is not known, the woman can lunge toward the side that gives her greater comfort.

All variations of the squatting position aid rotation and fetal descent by straightening the pelvic curve and enlarging the pelvic outlet. They add gravity to the force of maternal pushing.

If spontaneous rotation does not occur, the physician may assist rotation and descent of the head with forceps. The vacuum extractor cannot always be applied to the fetal head when it remains in an occiput posterior position. However, some styles of vacuum extractors may be used for minor degrees of malrotation because the fetal head tends to rotate as

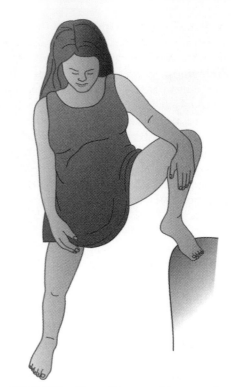

Figure 27-3 ■ The "lunge" to one side promotes rotation of the fetal occiput from a posterior position to an anterior one.

it descends with downward traction. Cesarean birth may be needed if these methods are unsuccessful or cannot be used.

DEFLEXION ABNORMALITIES. The poorly flexed fetal head presents a larger diameter to the pelvis than if flexed with the chin on the chest (see Figure 12-8). In the vertex presentation the head diameter is smallest. In the military and brow presentations the head diameter is larger. In the face presentation the head diameter is similar to that of the vertex presentation but the maternal pelvis can be traversed only if the fetal chin (mentum) is anterior.

BREECH PRESENTATION. Cervical dilation and effacement often are slower when the fetus is in a breech presentation because the buttocks or feet do not form a smooth, round dilating wedge like the head. The greatest fetal risk is that the head—the largest fetal part—is last to be born. By the time the lower body is born, the umbilical cord is well into the pelvis and may be compressed. The shoulders, arms, and head must be delivered quickly so that the infant can breathe.

A breech presentation is common well before term, but only 3% to 4% of term fetuses remain in this presentation. Adverse outcomes for infants that remain in a breech presentation may relate to causes other than their mode of birth:

- Fetal injury with a difficult vaginal birth
- Prolapsed umbilical cord
- Low birth weight because of preterm gestation, multifetal pregnancy, or intrauterine growth restriction
- Fetal anomalies such as hydrocephalus
- Complications secondary to placenta previa or cesarean birth

External cephalic version (ECV) may be attempted to change the fetus in a breech presentation or transverse lie to

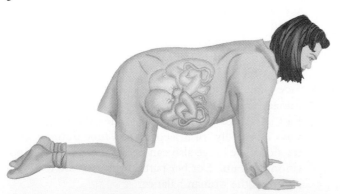

Figure 27-2 ■ A hands-and-knees position helps this fetus rotate from a left occiput posterior (LOP) position to an occiput anterior position.

a cephalic presentation (see Chapter 16). If the fetus remains in the abnormal presentation, cesarean birth usually is performed to avoid complications of a difficult vaginal birth. Birth for the nulliparous woman with a fetus in a breech presentation is almost always cesarean. The fetus remaining in a transverse lie is delivered by cesarean.

However, a cesarean is not clearly beneficial for every woman with a fetus in a breech presentation. The physician may offer a trial of labor when the fetus is in a breech presentation in the following cases (Bowes & Thorpe, 2004):

- The maternal pelvis is of normal size and shape.
- The estimated fetal weight is 2000 to 3800 g (4.4 to 8.4 lb).
- The fetus is in either a frank or a complete breech presentation (see Chapter 12).
- The fetal head is well flexed.

Some women are admitted in advanced labor with the fetus in a breech presentation, so birth attendants and intrapartum nurses must be prepared to care for the woman having either a planned or an unexpected vaginal breech birth. (Figure 27-4 illustrates the mechanisms of vaginal birth for an infant in a breech presentation.)

MULTIFETAL PREGNANCY

Multifetal pregnancy may result in dysfunctional labor because of uterine overdistention, which contributes to hypotonic dysfunction, and abnormal presentation of one or both fetuses (Figure 27-5). In addition, the potential for fetal hypoxia during labor is greater because the mother must supply oxygen and nutrients to more than one fetus. She also is at greater risk for postpartum hemorrhage resulting from uterine atony because of uterine overdistention.

Because of these problems, cesarean birth is more common for a woman with a multifetal pregnancy. If three or more fetuses are involved, the birth is almost always cesarean. The physician considers fetal viability, fetal presentations, maternal pelvic size, and presence of other complications such as preeclampsia or chronic hypertension.

Each twin's FHR is monitored during labor. When in bed the woman should remain in a lateral position to promote adequate placental blood flow. After vaginal birth of the first twin, assessment of the second twin's FHR continues until birth, which usually occurs within about 30 minutes. Birth of the second twin is faster in a cesarean than in a vaginal birth.

The delivery staff must be prepared for the care and possible resuscitation of multiple infants. Radiant warmers, resuscitation equipment, medications, blankets, hats, and identification materials must be prepared for each infant. One or more neonatal nurses, a neonatal nurse-practitioner, and a pediatrician or a neonatologist should be available to care for each infant. One nurse should be free to care for the mother.

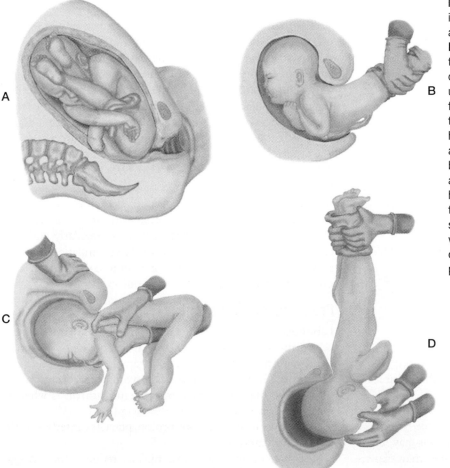

A

B

C

D

Figure 27-4 ■ Sequence for vaginal birth in a frank breech presentation. **A,** Descent and internal rotation of the fetal body. **B,** Internal rotation complete; extension of the fetal back and neck as the trunk slips under the symphysis pubis. The birth attendant uses a towel for traction when grasping the fetal legs. **C,** After the birth of the shoulders, the attendant maintains flexion of the fetal head by using the fingers of the left hand to apply pressure to the lower face. The fetal body straddles the attendant's left arm. An assistant provides suprapubic pressure to help keep the fetal head well flexed. **D,** After the fetal head is brought under the symphysis pubis, an assistant grasps the fetal legs with a towel for traction while the attendant delivers the face and head over the mother's perineum.

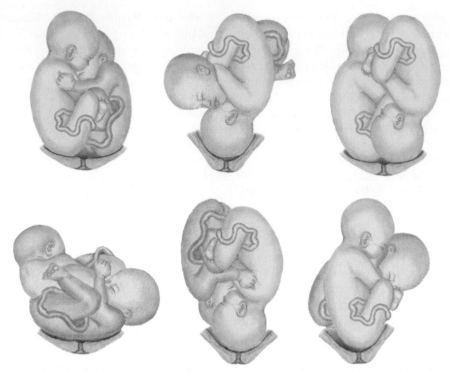

Figure 27-5 ■ Twins can present in any combination of presentations and positions.

FETAL ANOMALIES

Fetal anomalies such as hydrocephalus or a large fetal tumor may prevent normal descent of the fetus. Abnormal presentations such as breech or transverse lie also are associated with fetal anomalies. These abnormalities often are discovered by ultrasound examination before labor. A cesarean birth is scheduled if vaginal birth is not possible or inadvisable.

✓ CHECK YOUR READING

1. How does hypotonic labor dysfunction differ from hypertonic labor in terms of the most common labor phase when it becomes evident? Uterine contractions? Presence of pain? Therapeutic management?
2. How can maternal position changes favor rotation of the fetus from an occiput transverse or occiput posterior position to an occiput anterior position?
3. Why does a cesarean birth not eliminate all adverse outcomes for infants in a breech presentation?
4. How does preparation for the birth of multiple infants (vaginal or cesarean) differ from preparation for a single infant's birth?

Problems with the Passage

Dysfunctional labor may occur because of variations in the maternal bony pelvis or soft-tissue problems that inhibit fetal descent.

PELVIS

A small (contracted) or abnormally shaped pelvis may retard labor and obstruct fetal passage. The woman may experience poor contractions, slow dilation, slow fetal descent,

and a long labor. The danger of uterine rupture is greater with thinning of the lower uterine segment, especially if contractions remain strong.

Four basic pelvic shapes exist, each with different implications for labor and birth (Figure 27-6). Most women do not have a pure pelvic shape but instead have mixed characteristics from two or more types. Different racial characteristics of the woman and her fetus may enhance labor and vaginal birth because they create a good fit between the two. Different racial characteristics may also result in a less-than-ideal fit between the pelvis and the passenger, however.

MATERNAL SOFT-TISSUE OBSTRUCTIONS

During labor a full bladder is a common soft-tissue obstruction. Bladder distention reduces available space in the pelvis and intensifies maternal discomfort. The woman should be assessed for bladder distention regularly and encouraged to void every 1 to 2 hours. Catheterization may be needed if she cannot urinate or if epidural analgesia depresses her urge to void.

Problems of the Psyche

Labor is a stressful event for most women. However, a perceived threat caused by pain, fear, nonsupport, or personal situation can result in excessive maternal stress and interfere with normal labor progress. The woman's perception of stress more than the actual existence of a threat is what is most important.

Responses to excessive or prolonged stress interfere with labor in several ways:
- Increased glucose consumption reduces the energy supply available to the contracting uterus.

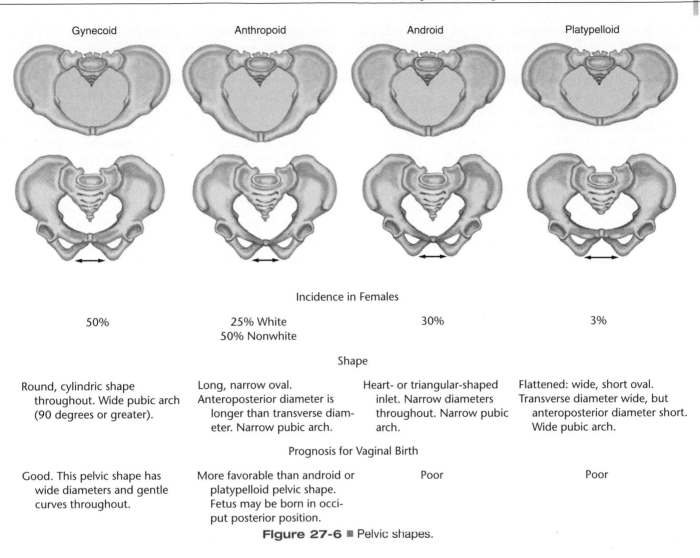

Gynecoid	Anthropoid	Android	Platypelloid
Incidence in Females			
50%	25% White 50% Nonwhite	30%	3%
Shape			
Round, cylindric shape throughout. Wide pubic arch (90 degrees or greater).	Long, narrow oval. Anteroposterior diameter is longer than transverse diameter. Narrow pubic arch.	Heart- or triangular-shaped inlet. Narrow diameters throughout. Narrow pubic arch.	Flattened: wide, short oval. Transverse diameter wide, but anteroposterior diameter short. Wide pubic arch.
Prognosis for Vaginal Birth			
Good. This pelvic shape has wide diameters and gentle curves throughout.	More favorable than android or platypelloid pelvic shape. Fetus may be born in occiput posterior position.	Poor	Poor

Figure 27-6 ■ Pelvic shapes.

- Secretion of catecholamines (epinephrine and nor-epinephrine) by the adrenal glands stimulates uterine beta receptors, which inhibit uterine contractions (an action similar to that of tocolytic drugs such as terbutaline).
- Adrenal secretion of catecholamines diverts blood supply from the uterus and placenta to skeletal muscle.
- Labor contractions and maternal pushing efforts are less effective because these powers are working against the resistance of tense abdominal and pelvic muscles.
- Pain perception is increased and pain tolerance is decreased, which further increase maternal anxiety and stress.

Assisting the woman to relax helps her body work more effectively with the forces of labor. General nursing measures involve the following:

- Establishing a trusting relationship with the woman and her significant other
- Making the environment comfortable by adjusting temperature and light
- Promoting physical comfort such as cleanliness
- Providing accurate information
- Implementing nonpharmacologic and pharmacologic pain management

Chapter 15 describes specific methods to encourage relaxation and promote comfort.

CHECK YOUR READING

5. Why should the nurse observe the laboring woman's bladder frequently?
6. Why is psychological support during labor important for effective physiologic function?

Abnormal Labor Duration

An unusually long or short labor may result in maternal, fetal, or neonatal problems.

PROLONGED LABOR

Prolonged labor results from problems with any of the factors in the birth process. After the woman reaches the active phase of labor, cervical dilation should proceed at a minimum rate of 1.2 cm per hour in the nullipara and 1.5 cm per hour in the parous woman. The fetal presenting part is expected to descend at a minimal rate of 1 cm per hour in the nullipara and 2 cm per hour in the parous woman (Bashore & Hayashi, 2004; Bowes & Thorpe, 2004). If previous births were by cesarean before much cervical dilation occurred, the criteria that apply to a nullipara may be applied.

Possible maternal and fetal problems in prolonged labor include the following:

- Maternal infection, intrapartum or postpartum
- Neonatal infection, which may be severe or fatal
- Maternal exhaustion
- Higher levels of anxiety and fear during a subsequent labor

Maternal and neonatal infections are more likely if the membranes have been ruptured for a prolonged time because organisms ascend from the vagina. The mother is more likely to have an intrapartum infection, postpartum infection, or both.

Nursing measures for the woman who has prolonged labor include promotion of comfort, conservation of energy, emotional support, position changes that favor normal progress, and assessments for infection. Nursing care for the fetus includes observation for signs of intrauterine infection and compromised fetal oxygenation (see Chapter 14).

PRECIPITATE LABOR

Precipitate labor is one in which birth occurs within 3 hours of its onset. Intense contractions often begin abruptly rather than gradually increasing in frequency, duration, and intensity, as typical of most labors.

Precipitate labor is not the same as a precipitate birth. A precipitate birth occurs after a labor of any length, in or out of the hospital or birth center, when a trained attendant is not present to assist. However, a woman in precipitate labor also may have a precipitate birth. If the physician or nurse-midwife will not arrive in time for the baby's birth, the nurse should wear gloves and simply support the infant's body as it emerges. If the maternal pelvis is adequate and the soft tissues yield easily to fetal descent, little maternal injury is likely. However, if the soft tissues are firm and resist stretching, trauma (uterine rupture, cervical lacerations, and hematoma) of the vagina or vulva may occur.

The mother or her fetus or newborn may be affected by several conditions that can be associated with precipitate labor. These conditions may include abruptio placentae, fetal meconium, maternal cocaine use (also may be associated with abruptio placentae), postpartum hemorrhage, or low Apgar scores for the infant (Clark, 2003; Cunningham et al., 2001). The fetus may suffer direct trauma such as intracranial hemorrhage or nerve damage during a precipitate labor. The fetus may become hypoxic because intense contractions with a short relaxation period reduce time available for gas exchange in the placenta. Nonreassuring electronic fetal monitoring patterns may include bradycardia and late decelerations.

Priority nursing care of the woman in precipitate labor includes promotion of fetal oxygenation and maternal comfort. A side-lying position enhances placental blood flow and reduces the effects of aortocaval compression. An added benefit of the side-lying position is to slow the rapid

fetal descent and minimize perineal tears. Additional measures to enhance fetal oxygenation include administering oxygen to the mother and maintaining adequate blood volume with nonadditive IV fluids. If oxytocin is being used when rapid-fire contractions begin, it should be stopped. A tocolytic drug may be ordered.

Promoting comfort is difficult in a precipitate labor because intense contractions give the woman little time to prepare and use coping skills such as breathing techniques. Pharmacologic measures such as analgesics or epidural block may not be useful if rapid labor progress does not allow time for them to become effective. Also, possible newborn respiratory depression must be considered if opioid analgesia is given near birth. The nurse helps the woman focus on techniques to cope with pain, one contraction at a time. The nurse must remain with her to provide support and assist with an emergency birth if it occurs.

✔ CHECK YOUR READING

7. During the active phase of labor, what is the minimal dilation and fetal descent rate expected for a nulliparous woman? For the parous woman?
8. What is the priority nursing care for a woman in prolonged labor?
9. What are the maternal and fetal risks when labor is unusually short?

Application of the Nursing Process
Dysfunctional Labor

Several nursing diagnoses and collaborative problems may be appropriate when caring for a woman having dysfunctional labor. The potential complication of fetal compromise should be part of all intrapartum management (see Chapter 14). Pain management is especially important to women in dysfunctional labor because they may find that their coping skills are inadequate or difficult to use because of fatigue. Anxiety or fear often is higher with abnormal labor, which limits the woman's ability to cope with labor. Anxiety or fear may reduce the effectiveness of pain medications or regional block analgesia. Maternal or newborn injury may become apparent after the birth.

In addition to these problems, nursing care is directed toward two other nursing diagnoses: possible intrauterine infection and maternal exhaustion.

INTRAUTERINE INFECTION
Assessment

Infection can occur with both normal labors and dysfunctional labors. Assess the FHR and maternal vital signs for evidence of infection:

- Fetal tachycardia (>160 beats per minute [bpm] for a term fetus); a rising baseline FHR often is the first sign of intrauterine infection.

- Maternal temperature; assess every 2 to 4 hours in normal labor and every 2 hours after membranes rupture; assess hourly if elevated (38° C, or 100.4° F) or other signs of infection are present.
- Maternal pulse, respirations, and blood pressure; assess at least hourly to identify tachycardia or tachypnea, which often accompanies temperature elevation.

Assess amniotic fluid for normal clear color and mild odor. Small flecks of white vernix are normal in amniotic fluid. Yellow or cloudy fluid or fluid with a foul or strong odor suggests infection. The strong odor may be noted before birth or afterward on the infant's skin.

Analysis

For the woman without signs of infection but with risk factors, the nursing diagnosis selected is "Risk for Infection related to presence of favorable conditions for development." The nurse may specify the specific conditions that may cause infection when choosing this nursing diagnosis.

Planning

Goals and expected outcomes relate to detecting the onset of infection:

- Maternal temperature will remain below 38° C (100.4° F).
- The FHR will remain near the baseline and below 160 bpm.
- The amniotic fluid will remain clear and without a foul or strong odor.

Interventions

REDUCING THE RISK FOR INFECTION

Nurses should wash their hands before and after each contact with the woman and her infant to reduce transmission of organisms. Limit vaginal examinations to reduce transmission of vaginal organisms into the uterine cavity, and maintain aseptic technique during essential vaginal examinations. The intrapartum nurse learns to estimate a woman's progress with few vaginal examinations. For example, increased bloody show and heightened anxiety may occur when the cervix is about 6 cm dilated. The woman may become irritable and lose control at about 8 cm dilation if she does not have epidural block analgesia.

Keep underpads as dry as possible to reduce the moist, warm environment that favors bacterial growth. Periodically clean excess secretions from the vaginal area in a front-to-back direction to limit fecal contamination and promote the mother's comfort. Use personal protective equipment to avoid contact with body secretions.

IDENTIFYING INFECTION

Assess the woman and fetus for signs of infection. Increase the frequency of assessments if labor is prolonged, if other risk factors are present, or if any signs of infection are found. If signs of infection are noted, report them to the birth at-

---

tendant for definitive treatment. Note the time at which the membranes ruptured to identify prolonged rupture, which adds to the risk for infection.

The birth attendant may collect specimens from the uterine cavity or placenta for culture to identify infectious organisms and determine antibiotic sensitivity. Aerobic and anaerobic culture specimens may be collected in containers specifically made for these two types of organisms. Follow directions on the container for proper handling and prevention of contamination with extraneous organisms, which would result in inaccurate results. Transport specimens to the laboratory promptly, because living organisms are required for culture and sensitivity study.

Inform the newborn nursery staff if signs of infection are noted or increased maternal risk factors exist. Specimens of infant secretions also may be obtained for testing.

The infant may receive prophylactic antibiotics to prevent neonatal sepsis (see p. 813). If results of infant cultures indicate that no infection is present, the antibiotic usually is discontinued. Culture and sensitivity testing may reveal an infection and indicate that a different antibiotic would be more effective.

Evaluation

If the goals and expected outcomes are achieved,

- The woman's temperature remains below 38° C (100.4° F).
- The amniotic fluid has no abnormal characteristics that are typical of infection (cloudiness, yellow color, foul or strong odor).
- The FHR remains within the expected range, not showing tachycardia, whether sudden or gradual in onset.

Even if the woman has no signs of intrapartum infection, she remains at higher risk for postpartum infection and should be observed for signs and symptoms of infection.

MATERNAL EXHAUSTION

Assessment

Many women begin labor with a sleep deficit because of fetal movement, frequent urination, and shortness of breath associated with advanced pregnancy. As labor drags on, the mother's reserves are further depleted. Even with epidural analgesia, a long labor drains the mother's energy. Also, some women do not choose or cannot take epidurals.

Therefore the labor nurse must be prepared to deal with this problem.

Assess the mother for signs of excessive fatigue:

- Verbal expression of tiredness, fatigue, or exhaustion
- Verbal expression of frustration with a prolonged, unproductive labor ("I can't go on any longer. Why doesn't the doctor just take the baby?")
- Ineffectiveness of or inability to use coping techniques (such as patterned breathing) that she previously used effectively
- Changes in her pulse, respiration, and blood pressure (increased or decreased)

Analysis

The intense energy demands of a dysfunctional labor may exceed a woman's physical and psychological ability to meet them. For this reason, "Activity Intolerance related to depletion of maternal energy reserves" is an appropriate nursing diagnosis.

Planning

Contractions must continue for labor to progress. Two realistic goals or expected outcomes are that the woman will do the following:

- Rest between contractions with her muscles relaxed
- Use coping skills such as breathing and relaxation techniques

Interventions

CONSERVING MATERNAL ENERGY

Reduce factors that interfere with the woman's ability to relax. Lower the light level, and turn off overhead lights. Reduce noise by closing the door or using soft music, water sounds, or other comforting sounds. Maintain a comfortable maternal temperature with blankets or a fan. If not contraindicated, a warm shower or bath is soothing.

Position the woman to encourage comfort, promote fetal descent, and enhance fetal oxygenation. Support her with pillows to reduce muscle strain and added fatigue. Help her change positions regularly (about every 30 minutes) to reduce muscle tension from constant pressure.

A soothing back rub reduces muscle tension and therefore decreases fatigue. Firm sacral pressure and use of some maternal positions discussed in the section on fetal occiput posterior positions may reduce back pain. Using the birthing ball can relax and support her in some positions. Warmth to her back can reduce back pain. (See Chapters 13 and 15 for added comfort measures.)

Maintain IV fluids at the rate ordered to provide fluid, electrolytes, and occasionally glucose. Assess intake and output to identify dehydration, which may accompany prolonged labor. Dehydration also may cause maternal fever. If not contraindicated, provide juice, lollipops, frozen juice bars, or other clear liquids, as ordered by the physician or nurse-midwife, to moisten the woman's mouth and replenish her energy.

PROMOTING COPING SKILLS

When position changes or medical therapies are used to enhance labor, explain their purpose and expected benefits. Encourage the woman to visualize her baby passing downward smoothly through her pelvis as a result of her efforts. Provide her with mental images that allow her to "see" herself giving birth.

Generous praise and encouragement of the woman's use of skills such as breathing techniques motivate her to continue them even when she is discouraged. As with any laboring woman, tell her when she is making progress. Tell her that fetal heart rates and patterns are reassuring if this is true. Knowing that her efforts are having the desired results and her fetus is doing well gives the woman courage to continue.

EVALUATION

Goals are met if the woman does the following:

- Rests and relaxes between contractions. If she is unable to relax, discuss analgesia options with her. Inability to relax between contractions is associated with pain beyond the woman's tolerance.
- Continues to demonstrate adequate use of learned skills to cope with labor.

In addition, solicit the woman's perceptions of her ability to relax and cope with labor.

PREMATURE RUPTURE OF THE MEMBRANES

Rupture of the amniotic sac before onset of true labor is called *premature rupture of the membranes* (PROM). A precise term, *preterm premature rupture of the membranes* (PPROM, sometimes abbreviated as pPROM), refers to the rupture of membranes earlier than the end of the thirty-seventh week of gestation, with or without contractions. PPROM is associated with preterm labor and birth.

Etiology

Several conditions are associated with PROM, but the exact cause often remains unclear. Conditions associated with preterm ruptured membranes include the following:

- Infections of the vagina or cervix, such as chlamydia, gonorrhea, group B streptococcal infection, and *Gardnerella vaginalis* infection (bacterial vaginosis)
- Chorioamnionitis, which may be associated with group B streptococci, *Neisseria gonorrhoeae*, *Listeria monocytogenes*, or species such as *Mycoplasma*, *Bacteroides*, and *Ureaplasma* in the amniotic fluid
- Incompetent cervix or short cervical length (≤25 mm by transvaginal ultrasonography)
- Fetal abnormalities or malpresentation
- Hydramnios
- Amniotic sac with a weak structure
- Recent procedures such as amniocentesis or cerclage
- Recent sexual intercourse

- Nutritional deficiencies
- Previous preterm birth related to PPROM
- Positive fetal fibronectin results (see p. 713)

Complications

Both mother and newborn are at risk for infection during the intrapartum and postpartum periods. Chorioamnionitis can be both a cause and a result of PROM. Organisms that cause chorioamnionitis weaken the amniotic membrane, leading to the rupture. The mother is at higher risk for postpartum infection, and the newborn is vulnerable to neonatal sepsis.

Chorioamnionitis, characterized by maternal fever and uterine tenderness, is most likely to precede preterm birth in the infant born before 34 weeks' gestation. Preterm infants with the lowest maturity, such as 24 weeks' gestation, have higher risk for the infection than preterm infants who are even a few weeks more mature (Rao & Andersen, 2003). The exact time at which infection occurs cannot be predicted for either term or preterm infants. Frequent performance of digital examination of the cervix increases the risk for term or preterm infants. If chorioamnionitis does not precede PROM, it is more likely to occur if a long time elapses between membrane rupture and birth because vaginal organisms can readily enter the uterus. The risk for chorioamnionitis is known to increase after 24 hours.

Membranes that rupture before term may form a seal, stopping the fluid leak and allowing the amniotic fluid cushion to become reestablished. However, membranes may continue to leak, prolonging the loss of the amniotic fluid cushion (oligohydramnios) for the fetus. Umbilical cord compression, reduced lung volume, and deformities resulting from compression may occur, particularly if rupture occurs near the age of fetal viability, about 23 weeks' gestation, possibly extending the duration of amniotic fluid loss.

If preterm birth occurs, the infant is more likely to have respiratory distress syndrome (RDS) and complications related to prematurity. The hazards of prematurity are greatest before 34 weeks' gestation, especially if the woman did not receive steroids to accelerate fetal lung maturation before birth (see p. 718).

Therapeutic Management

Management of PROM depends on the gestation and whether evidence of infection or other fetal or maternal compromise exists. For a woman at or near term (36 weeks' or more gestation), PROM may herald the imminent onset of true labor. Often the cervix is soft, with some dilation and effacement. If the fetus is immature or the woman's cervix is not soft and favorable for labor induction, therapeutic management is more complex. The risk of infection or prematurity for the fetus and newborn is weighed against the hazards of labor induction or cesarean birth.

DETERMINING TRUE MEMBRANE RUPTURE

The first step is to determine whether the membranes are truly ruptured. Urinary incontinence, increased vaginal discharge, or loss of the mucus plug can make a woman think that her membranes have ruptured when they have not. A digital vaginal examination is avoided, particularly if the gestation is preterm and no evidence of labor exists. Instead, the physician or nurse-midwife performs a sterile speculum examination to look for a pool of fluid near the cervix and estimate cervical dilation and effacement. A Nitrazine or fern test may be done on the fluid to verify that the liquid is amniotic fluid. Tests to assess fetal lung maturity and identify infection are often performed, as well. A transvaginal ultrasound examination may be performed to measure cervical length. A short (25 mm) cervix is more likely to continue effacement and dilation even if the gestation is far from term.

GESTATION NEAR TERM. If the woman is at or near term and her cervix is soft, labor may be induced if it does not begin spontaneously. This will usually be done if the gestation is at least 36 weeks because the infant is unlikely to have severe problems associated with prematurity. Walking often helps stimulate the contractions of early labor as long as the woman takes adequate fluids and rests periodically. Labor is usually induced within 12 to 24 hours if contractions do not begin. Prostaglandin inserts such as Cervidil or Prepidil may assist cervical softening if needed before induction (see Chapter 16).

PRETERM GESTATION. If the gestation is preterm, the physician weighs the risks of maternal-fetal infection against the newborn's risk for complications of prematurity. Many variables must be considered by the physician and patient to determine the best course of management. Medical management changes as fetal maturation and conditions of the mother and fetus change with the continuation of pregnancy.

The cervix usually is not favorable for induction far from term. Factors such as gestational age, amount of amniotic fluid remaining, fetal lung maturity, and any signs of fetal compromise are considered. A cerclage may have been placed earlier in the pregnancy to prevent premature cervical dilation. If infection is not already present, the physician must consider whether leaving the cerclage in place is likely to increase the risk for infection.

Between 32 and 35 weeks' gestation the physician may test for fetal lung maturity using a sample from the amniotic fluid pooled in the vagina or from an amniocentesis. The L/S ratio, which measures the ratio of lecithin to sphingomyelin in amniotic fluid, is most reliable if collected by amniocentesis, reducing contamination with blood. A 2:1 L/S ratio indicates that the fetal lungs are likely to be mature. Another test may indicate the presence (mature) or absence (immature) of phosphatidylglycerol (PG), but this test has limited usefulness because it remains negative in many women until late in pregnancy. The surfactant/albumin (S/A) assay of amniotic fluid has become common because it is rapid, reliable, and less expensive compared with other tests for fetal lung maturity. An S/A assay greater than 50 is usually predictive of fetal lung maturity (Hobel, 2004; Mercer, 2004).

At the time of amniocentesis, cultures for infecting organisms and glucose levels (which are low in infection) usually are done. If these tests show infection or the fetal lungs are mature, delivery usually is done by induction or cesarean. Antibiotics are given to the mother, including prophylactically if no infection exists.

If no evidence of infection exists and the fetal lungs are immature, the woman usually is observed for infection or onset of labor in the hospital. Daily nonstress tests are performed to watch for FHR nonreactivity, which often occurs with intraamniotic infection. Biophysical profiles, in which sonographic evaluation is added to the nonstress test, may be done one or more times per week (see Chapter 10). Fetal lung maturity testing will be done periodically, and delivery will occur when the fetal lungs are mature unless other complications require delivery before fetal lung maturity. Antibiotics are given during labor. An amnioinfusion (see Chapter 14) may be done prophylactically to reduce cord compression during labor (Garite, 2004).

With very early gestations, management is more complex. Steroids given to the mother accelerate fetal lung maturity, and antibiotics reduce the risk of intrauterine infection, possibly extending pregnancy. Before 25 weeks' gestation, the likelihood of having a newborn who does well is lower. For the women whose membranes rupture at these very early gestations, home care may be offered to spare them extended hospitalization (Garite, 2004).

MATERNAL ANTIBIOTICS

Maternal antibiotics are usually prescribed for premature membrane rupture because of the increased likelihood that an infection caused or further complicated the rupture for both mother and fetus or newborn. Antibiotics may stop the infection that caused or will occur with the rupture, thereby delaying the onset of labor and allowing the fetus to mature. Drugs to stop infection if early membrane rupture occurs may include ampicillin, gentamicin, erythromycin, clindamycin, a cephalosporin antibiotic, and piperacillin. Infection with group B streptococci is also treated if indicated (see Chapter 26). Guidelines for drugs to correct infection associated with early membrane rupture vary with culture and sensitivity test results, other maternal laboratory results, or changes in the drugs most currently recommended for this purpose.

Nursing Considerations

The woman may be hospitalized until birth, and a long stay may be anticipated if her membranes ruptured very early, such as at 23 weeks. The nurse observes for signs of infection along with the onset of labor and provides appropriate teaching. Care includes the following:

- Take her vital signs and the FHR every 4 hours, reporting any temperature above 38° C (100.4° F) or as her caregiver directs. A rise in the baseline of the FHR is a common indicator of infection.
- Note a foul or strong odor or cloudy or yellow appearance to the vaginal drainage.
- Teach her to avoid breast stimulation with preterm gestation because it causes release of oxytocin from the posterior pituitary and therefore stimulates contrac-

tions. Breast stimulation can occur during a shower, from not wearing a bra, or during sexual activity.
- Avoid insertion of anything into the vagina to reduce the risk for carrying organisms into the area of the cervix. This includes vaginal examinations, vaginal suppositories, and vaginal intercourse. Additionally, seminal fluid contains prostaglandins, a potent stimulant of uterine contractions.
- Maintain any activity restrictions recommended.
- Note uterine contractions and report an increase in their frequency or intensity or a change in character.
- Teach the mother to observe fetal activity (kick counts) and report a decrease in the usual activity of the fetus.

Also see p. 719 for additional care of the woman with preterm labor.

✔ CHECK YOUR READING

10. How does PROM differ from PPROM?
11. What is the relationship of infection to PROM?
12. What is the usual therapeutic management of PROM if the woman is at or near term? What if the gestation is preterm?
13. What are the nursing considerations for a woman with PPROM?

PRETERM LABOR

Preterm labor begins after the twentieth week but before the end of the thirty-seventh week of pregnancy. Preterm labor may result in the birth of an infant who is ill equipped for extrauterine life. The classification of preterm and low-birthweight (less than 2500 g) infants is second only to that of infants with birth defects in the top 10 causes of infant mortality in the United States (Kochanek, Murphy, Anderson, & Scott, 2004).

Associated Factors

- Just as all causes of labor's onset at term are not known, the causes of preterm labor are not fully known. Over half of the women who have preterm labor and birth do not show known risk. Maternal medical conditions may include infections of the urinary tract, reproductive organs, or systemic organs; dental disorder (periodontal disease); preexisting or gestational diabetes; connective tissue disorders; chronic hypertension; and drug abuse
- Conceptions assisted by assisted reproductive technology, including conceptions resulting in a single fetal gestation rather than a multifetal gestation
- Present and past obstetric conditions, such as unusually short cervical length, multifetal gestation, preterm membrane rupture, preeclampsia, and bleeding disorders that involve the woman, fetus, or placental implantation area
- Fetal conditions such as growth retardation, inadequate amniotic fluid volume, and chromosome abnormalities and other birth defects

TABLE 27-2 Maternal Risk Factors for Preterm Labor

Medical History	Obstetric History	Present Pregnancy	Lifestyle and Demographics
Low weight for height Obesity Uterine or cervical anomalies, uterine fibroids History of cone biopsy Diethylstilbestrol (DES) exposure as a fetus Chronic illness (e.g., cardiac disorder, renal disorder, diabetes, clotting disorders, anemia, hypertension) Periodontal disease	Previous preterm labor Previous preterm birth Previous first-trimester abortions (more than two) Previous second-trimester abortion History of previous pregnancy losses (two or more) Incompetent cervix Cervical length 25 mm (2.5 cm) or less at midtrimester of pregnancy Number of embryos implanted (assisted reproductive techniques [ART])	Uterine distention (e.g., multifetal pregnancy, hydramnios) Abdominal surgery during pregnancy Uterine irritability Uterine bleeding Dehydration Infection Anemia Incompetent cervix Preeclampsia Preterm premature rupture of membranes (PPROM) Fetal or placental abnormalities	Little or no prenatal care Poor nutrition Age <18 yr or >40 yr Low educational level Low socioeconomic status Smoking >10 cigarettes daily Nonwhite Employment with long hours and/or long standing Chronic physical or psychological stress Intimate partner violence Substance abuse

- Social and environmental factors such as inadequate or absent prenatal or dental care, maternal domestic violence episodes, maternal smoking, and housing deficiency such as homelessness
- Demographic factors such as race and age of the parents, financial stability, and the number and birth intervals of the woman's other children

See Table 27-2 for more detail about each of these factors. However, many women who have preterm labor and birth have no obvious risk factors.

Signs and Symptoms

Signs and symptoms of early preterm labor are more subtle than those of labor at term and often occur in normal pregnancies as well. The woman may be only vaguely aware that something seems different, or she may not detect that anything is amiss. Only when preterm labor reaches the active phase is it likely to have characteristics typical of term labor. Symptoms vary among women, but common ones are as follows:

- Uterine contractions that may or may not be painful (the woman may not feel contractions at all)
- A sensation that the baby is frequently "balling up"
- Cramps similar to menstrual cramps
- Constant low backache; irregular or intermittent low back pain
- Sensation of pelvic pressure or a feeling that the baby is pushing down
- Pain, discomfort, or pressure in the vagina or thighs
- Change or increase in vaginal discharge (increased, watery, "spotting," bleeding)
- Abdominal cramps with or without diarrhea
- A sense of "just feeling bad" or "coming down with something"

Preventing Preterm Birth

COMMUNITY EDUCATION

Preterm birth can impose substantial physical, emotional, and financial burdens on the child, family, and society. Ideally, nursing strategies to prevent preterm birth begin before conception, with community education. Topics may include the following:

- Duration of normal pregnancy
- Consequences of preterm birth
- Role of early and regular prenatal care, including dental care, in preventing preterm birth
- Conditions that increase risk for preterm birth
- Signs and symptoms of preterm labor
- Consequences of preterm birth for mother, baby, and family members

Women who are aware of the consequences of preterm birth may be more likely to take action to prevent it. If they recognize that they have risk factors, they may seek prenatal care earlier in pregnancy than they otherwise might. Recognizing that onset of labor in early gestation has subtle signs and symptoms compared with labor near term make the woman aware that she should seek care promptly rather than waiting for more definite signs of labor.

DURING PREGNANCY

During pregnancy, measures to prevent preterm birth include the following:

- Reducing barriers and improving access to early prenatal care for all women
- Assessing for risk factors to permit changes, if possible
- Promoting adequate nutrition
- Promoting smoking cessation
- Educating women and their partners about the subtle signs and symptoms of preterm labor and ways in which they differ from normal pregnancy changes
- Empowering women and their partners to take an active approach in seeking care if they have signs and symptoms of preterm labor

IMPROVING ACCESS TO CARE. Improving access to prenatal care must be customized for the community. What works in one area may be inappropriate for another. Difficult access is a serious problem for women who rely on public clinics for their care. Long waits, fragmented care, language barriers, and insensitivity of caregivers discourage women from obtaining care. Expanding the number of caregivers by using advanced-practice nurses, such as certified nurse-midwives and nurse practitioners, can reduce waits for care significantly. Nurses can help coordinate various aspects of care to limit the number of different appointments a woman needs to obtain complete care.

IDENTIFYING RISK FACTORS. Identification of risk factors may allow reduction or elimination of these factors. Women should be rescreened regularly to identify new risks that emerge as pregnancy progresses. Women with high-risk factors benefit from care such as more frequent prenatal care appointments, reinforcement of the symptoms of preterm labor, telephone contacts, and added assessments of fetal growth and health.

Some risk factors can be reduced or eliminated if the woman changes her lifestyle. Many women have stopped smoking or using drugs to benefit their babies, changes that may have been difficult for them. A woman may need to rest more or stop working, which may be difficult or impossible for many. Nurses and social workers can help the woman reduce her risks as much as possible by helping her identify realistic sources of support.

The role of subclinical infection in PPROM and preterm labor is becoming better known. Screening at the appropriate times for pathogenic organisms in the urine, vagina, and cervix identifies women who may benefit from antibiotic therapy.

PROMOTING ADEQUATE NUTRITION. An adequate maternal diet contributes positively to the length of gestation and the infant's birth weight. The mother's height should be measured at the first prenatal visit, and her weight should be taken at each visit to evaluate adequacy of weight gain. Every pregnant woman should be offered culturally sensitive dietary counseling. The Special Supplemental Nutrition Program for Women, Infants, and Children (WIC) is available to supplement the diet of some low-income women. Anemia can be corrected with appropriate supplements. (See Chapter 9 for additional information about nutrition and pregnancy, including nutrition related to cultural practices and vegetarianism.)

EDUCATING WOMEN AND THEIR PARTNERS ABOUT PRETERM LABOR. All pregnant women and their partners should be taught about symptoms of preterm labor, because half of preterm births occur in women with no identified risk factors. Interpreters who are culturally acceptable to the woman and printed materials in her primary language should be used if needed. Diagrams should supplement the words of any language for women of limited reading skills.

The nurse should verify the woman's understanding by seeking feedback, such as having her restate the signs and symptoms of preterm labor and the appropriate responses to them.

EMPOWERING WOMEN AND THEIR PARTNERS. Delaying birth depends critically on early identification of preterm labor. Women should be encouraged to seek treatment promptly if they suspect preterm labor. The woman must communicate her concerns clearly when she arrives at the clinic or hospital. She should tell the triage person that she should be checked for labor, regardless of the subtlety of the symptoms. Caregivers must not make the woman feel foolish if she reports signs and symptoms that could be preterm labor but turn out to be a false alarm. Otherwise she may not seek care for recurrent episodes when she truly is in labor, and the opportunity to delay preterm birth may be lost.

The nurse might suggest that a woman who is seeking care for possible preterm labor say, "I'm not due for 8 more weeks, but I think I may be in labor. I need to be seen right away or I might have a premature baby."

Therapeutic Management

Management focuses on identifying those at risk for preterm birth, identifying preterm labor early, delaying birth, and accelerating fetal lung maturity if preterm birth is likely. Onset of changes that lead to preterm labor and birth may be subtle. The woman may not perceive any changes in her pregnancy.

PREDICTING PRETERM BIRTH

Because treatment for preterm labor has been less than satisfactory at preventing preterm birth, research has focused on predicting which women will deliver early. Better identification of these women would allow more intensive treatment, ideally before preterm labor or rupture of membranes occurs. Also, many signs and symptoms of preterm labor occur in women who deliver at term, possibly exposing them to unneeded treatment. The key is to identify which women with the symptoms are really at risk for preterm birth and treat those women intensively while continuing regular prenatal care for women with these symptoms as a variant of normal pregnancy symptoms. A good screening test would provide quick results and would be inexpensive, usable for all pregnant women, noninvasive, and highly specific for the condition. No screening test meeting these criteria is available to screen for preterm labor yet. For this reason many evaluations may be used in an attempt to determine the best medical management for a woman.

The results of a major preterm prediction study looked at multiple factors and found that their relevance to preterm birth interrelated according to the mother's parity and obstetric history. In this study the factors most strongly associated with predicting preterm birth included (1) a short cervical length of ≤25 mm (1 inch), (2) a previous preterm birth caused by PPROM, and (3) a positive fetal fibronectin (fFN) screening result (Mercer et al., 2000).

CERVICAL LENGTH. A short cervix (≤25 mm), measured by transvaginal ultrasound, may allow vaginal organisms easier access to the uterus, where they weaken the membranes and cause premature rupture. Alternately, the shortened cervix may reflect structural changes caused by an intrauterine infection or uterine contractions. The woman may have no symptoms of infection or pressure against the cervix (ACOG, 2001; Iams & Creasy, 2004; Mercer et al., 2000).

PPROM IN A PREVIOUS BIRTH. Some women may have a predisposition to weak amniotic membrane structure that predates the actual leaking of fluid (Mercer et al., 2000). This predisposition seems to repeat in subsequent pregnancies.

FETAL FIBRONECTIN. A protein present in fetal tissues, fFN is normally found in the cervical and vaginal secretions until 16 to 20 weeks' gestation and again at or near term. If it appears too early, it suggests that labor may begin early, similar to the way cardiac enzymes rise in the person with a myocardial infarction. Maternal or fetal infections may be present if the fFN test result is positive during midpregnancy. The fFN test is a better test for excluding preterm labor than establishing that preterm labor has started. The fFN test may help the physician make a better judgment about whether the woman's symptoms are true preterm labor that should be treated aggressively or a variant of normal pregnancy symptoms that can be managed more conservatively. To reduce false-positive results from the fFN test, the test must be collected before significant vaginal manipulation from examination. Cervical examination, recent sexual intercourse, and vaginal bleeding can result in a false-positive test result when preterm labor is not truly present (ACOG, 2001; Guinn & Gibbs, 2003; Iams & Creasy, 2004).

INFECTIONS. Infections often increase the risk for preterm membrane rupture or birth, even if the woman does not initially have clinical signs or symptoms with the preterm labor. A urinary tract infection is common with preterm labor, so catheterized or midstream urine is often obtained for urinalysis and for culture and sensitivity testing. Tests for other infections associated with preterm birth risk include those that often are found if membranes rupture prematurely (see discussion of premature rupture of the membranes on p. 708).

Blood peak and trough levels of indicated antibiotics, such as gentamicin, ensure that the woman is receiving a therapeutic level (peak) of the drug. Determining if the drug blood level is excessive just before the next dose (a high trough level) is important to prevent possible damage to mother or baby with some drugs. Testing for peak and trough drug levels allows the dose to be adjusted appropriately for the drug.

A woman with an infection that is not always related to pregnancy may seek care. Relevant testing may relate to acute gastrointestinal or respiratory infections that affect pregnant women as well as other people of both sexes. More serious maternal infections may require cultures of maternal blood or respiratory or other secretions to determine the ideal treatment. Maternal pneumonia, although rare during pregnancy, increases the risk for fetal or maternal death as well as increasing the risk that a woman will give birth to a living preterm infant. Other poor health conditions during pregnancy, such as crowded living conditions or a chronic condition such as asthma, may increase a woman's risk for pneumonia as well.

IDENTIFYING PRETERM LABOR

The reason to predict risk for preterm birth or to identify preterm labor early is to delay birth, thereby promoting further fetal maturation.

FREQUENT PRENATAL VISITS. Women at risk for preterm labor should have more frequent prenatal visits, at which time they are checked for evidence of preterm labor and their ability to follow preventive therapy, in addition to their regular prenatal checkup. They should be assessed for development of new risk factors with each visit. Gentle cervical examinations are done if indicated by other signs or symptoms. A transvaginal ultrasound examination may identify the shortened, thinned cervix that often precedes onset of labor in the asymptomatic woman. Infections can be identified and treated promptly before rupture of membranes or onset of labor occurs.

STOPPING PRETERM LABOR

Once the diagnosis of preterm labor is made, management focuses on stopping uterine activity before the point of no return, usually after about 3 cm dilation. Preterm delivery may be inevitable, but steroid therapy promotes earlier fetal lung maturation. Particularly for very early gestations, such as 25 weeks, treatment may add enough time for the steroids to be effective. Even one more day of fetal maturation may make a great difference in the outcome for the very premature infant.

INITIAL MEASURES. The physician initially determines whether any maternal or fetal conditions contraindicate continuing the pregnancy. Examples of these conditions include:

- Preeclampsia or eclampsia; persistent hypertension from any cause
- Significant or prolonged maternal alterations, such as hypovolemia, hypoxemia, or acid-base imbalance
- Serious infection, including chorioamnionitis or maternal infection such as maternal pyelonephritis
- FHR monitoring data showing inability to correct signs that are nonreassuring for the gestation of the fetus

Initial measures to stop preterm labor include identifying and treating infections, identifying other causes of preterm labor that may be treatable, and reducing activity. Hydration with IV fluids may be chosen if maternal dehydration is a factor. Excess fluid hydration increases the risk for pulmonary edema if some drugs also are used to stop preterm labor such as magnesium sulfate.

IDENTIFYING AND TREATING INFECTIONS. Infection, both systemic and local, has a strong association with preterm birth and premature rupture of the membranes. However, it may be unclear whether various microorganisms found at diagnosis of preterm labor are significant if the membranes remain intact. Blood studies identify signs of infection and also conditions such as anemia that are associated with preterm labor or affect its management. Common studies include a complete blood count with differential white blood cell analysis and cultures for group B streptococcus, chlamydia, gonorrhea, or other suspected infections. Amniocentesis may be done to obtain amniotic fluid for culture if chorioamnionitis is suspected because this infection would contraindicate stopping preterm labor.

Fetal lung maturity testing will likely be done on an amniotic fluid specimen as well. Urinalysis with culture and sensitivity testing may be done to determine if treatment is indicated (Iams & Creasy, 2004).

If infection is suspected, it is treated with the antiinfective agent or agents expected to be effective before completion of cultures, which requires a minimum of 24 to 48 hours. If cultures show that a different drug would be best, the medication is changed. The value of treating acute infections, such as pyelonephritis, is clear for improved maternal and fetal outcomes. Broad-spectrum antibiotics, such as ampicillin, penicillin, and an aminoglycoside, may be chosen for chorioamnionitis because multiple types of bacteria may be found in the infected amniotic fluid. Anaerobic organisms may also cause infection in a woman who requires a cesarean birth, and antibiotics such as clindamycin or metronidazole may be prescribed (American Academy of Pediatrics [AAP] & ACOG, 2002; Iams & Creasy, 2004).

IDENTIFYING OTHER CAUSES FOR PRETERM CONTRACTIONS. The woman with polyhydramnios, identified by ultrasonography, may have more contractions because her uterus is stretched more than normal. Therapeutic amniocentesis to remove some amniotic fluid can reduce uterine irritability. Multifetal gestations also can be identified by ultrasonography if not previously diagnosed. These mothers may benefit from improved nutrition, stress reduction, assistance with household care, and other interventions.

LIMITING ACTIVITY. Activity limitation, usually by relaxing in a side-lying or semi-sitting position, increases placental blood flow and reduces fetal pressure on the cervix. However, lengthy and substantial activity restriction (e.g., complete bed rest) has not been shown to prolong pregnancy significantly. As in other persons, activity restriction also is associated with serious maternal side effects, some of which develop within as few as 24 hours. Adverse effects of activity restriction during pregnancy may include:

- Muscle weakness, including aching; muscle atrophy and bone loss
- Diuresis as the body tries to reduce the normally higher fluid level of pregnancy
- Poor nutrition as a result of appetite loss, lower intake, and increased indigestion; weight loss or inadequate weight gain
- Orthostatic hypotension caused by the change in blood pressure regulation by baroreceptors
- Psychological effects, such as increased stress about separation from her family, anxiety about the pregnancy's outcome, depression; boredom from a decreased activity level and less contact with other people; concerns about finances if her job was essential to her family
- Sleep changes as depression increases or usual activities that direct her sleep-wake cycles are not present

Because of problems and lack of benefits for most women, limited and individualized activity reductions are now prescribed if preterm birth risk is higher. Changes may be relatively simple, such as a change in work hours or duties or finding ways to help the woman meet the needs for her other children, such as transportation to school or other activities. Several rest periods may be prescribed for home care when the woman's risk status is lower. Positions for rest may include a semi-sitting position with the feet and legs elevated. If she is lying down for rest, a mother's frequent change of the side-lying position reduces discomfort from the pressure of remaining on one side for a prolonged time. Frequent position changes are also beneficial to women who require hospitalization for their preterm labor.

Women hospitalized for care of preterm labor may have a greater activity restriction. Because of IV hydration and drug therapy, bed rest is common during initial care. Ambulating to the bathroom may be contraindicated because of maternal sedative effects from a drug that depresses uterine activity, such as magnesium sulfate (also given for preeclampsia; see Chapter 25). The woman usually has a Foley catheter for the precise urine output assessment needed with administration of magnesium or other drugs. If labor is successfully stopped, the woman may be able to walk to the restroom for voiding and bowel movements. If she remains hospitalized for longer-term care, she may sit in a chair periodically or take occasional short trips to another area in a wheelchair pushed by a family member or friend.

Services such as physical therapy are often prescribed to help the woman maintain muscle strength and coordination and to reduce muscle aching, fatigue, and bone loss. Recreational therapy helps the woman identify activities that are suited to temporary treatment limitations, help relieve boredom, and often help her find friends with similar interests. Occupational therapy helps a woman cope with temporary lifestyle changes. Complementary therapy may be offered to reduce stressors, enhancing the woman's physical care. Social work helps identify how needs such as financial or child care assistance and housing may be met. Issues such as illicit drug use by the mother and safety of other children in the family are often coordinated by a social worker. Consultations with a psychologist may be appropriate to help the woman and her family to identify and cope with the additional stressors imposed by therapy intended to reduce the additional problems that occur with preterm birth. Although preterm birth may occur, the severity of its effects on the infant may be reduced if even a few days are gained in the duration of pregnancy.

HYDRATING THE WOMAN. Hydration to stop preterm contractions has not been shown to be beneficial for all women. High-volume IV infusions may cause maternal respiratory distress if a drug such as magnesium sulfate to decrease uterine contractions is being administered because the drug may also reduce the respiratory rate, even if a woman has a normal blood pressure level.

However, dehydration may contribute to uterine irritability for some women. This is often the case in those who have had an infection such as an acute gastrointestinal infection in which loss of fluid through diarrhea may exceed the nauseated woman's ability to drink water or other fluids. Infections with maternal fever (temperature of 38° C [100.4° F]) sometimes reduce the woman's fluid ingestion. IV fluids are ordered according to their expected benefit, such as administration of magnesium sulfate drug therapy to stop preterm labor or initiation of an antibiotic.

TOCOLYTICS. The advantage of tocolytic drug therapy to reduce preterm birth is not clear. Tocolysis is most likely ordered if preterm labor occurs before the thirty-fourth week of gestation because the infant's risk for respiratory and other complications of prematurity is high if the infant is born during this time. Delay of preterm birth with tocolysis may provide time to give maternal corticosteroids to reduce respiratory distress in the newborn or time for transfer of the mother to a facility with a neonatal intensive care unit that is appropriate for the gestation of her fetus at the time of birth. Tocolysis is most likely to be effective if the cervix is less than 3 cm dilated.

Because tocolytic drugs have significant side effects the decision about whether to treat for preterm labor is individualized, based on risk factors, cervical dilation, and other signs and symptoms. If the cervix is between 2 and 3 cm dilated, the physician may recheck the cervix for further dilation or effacement after 1 or 2 hours. Electronic fetal monitoring helps identify uterine contractions or irritability and establish fetal status. A fFN test also will be done to determine whether the woman is likely to be in preterm labor. Ultrasound imaging provides information that may be useful to determine fetal age, adequacy of placental supply, and status of the cervix. Tests for infection are done if indicated.

Most tocolytic drugs are used primarily for conditions other than preterm labor and therefore have effects on body systems other than the reproductive system. The lowest possible dose that inhibits contractions is used. Four types of drugs are used for tocolysis: (1) beta-adrenergics, (2) magnesium sulfate, (3) prostaglandin synthesis inhibitors, and (4) calcium antagonists. (Table 27-3 summarizes doses and routes of administration for each of these drugs.)

Beta-Adrenergic Drugs. Although ritodrine (Yutopar) is the only beta-adrenergic currently approved by the U.S. Food and Drug Administration (FDA) for tocolysis, it is infrequently used because of significant side effects and minimal increase in the length of pregnancy. Terbutaline (Brethine), considered investigational for treatment of preterm labor, is the more widely used beta-adrenergic for tocolysis because of lower cost, longer duration of action between doses, and the ability to promptly administer a dose by the subcutaneous rather than the oral route if needed (AAP & ACOG, 2002; Guinn & Gibbs, 2003).

The main side effects of beta-adrenergic drugs involve the cardiorespiratory system. Maternal and fetal tachycardia are common. Other maternal side effects may include decreased blood pressure, wide pulse pressure, dysrhythmias, myocardial ischemia, chest pain, and pulmonary edema. Metabolic changes include hyperglycemia and hypokalemia. Headaches, tremors, and restlessness are other side effects, with headaches often becoming less severe as the woman becomes accustomed to the drug. Propranolol,

an agent that blocks beta-adrenergic drugs, should be available to reverse severe adverse effects.

A beta-adrenergic, such as terbutaline, may be given by the IV, subcutaneous, or oral route. Subcutaneous terbutaline may be given with a continuous, low-dose infusion pump. The subcutaneous pump for terbutaline allows the physician to order a baseline infusion rate plus greater doses at specific intervals for a bolus dose. Time intervals and doses for the bolus doses may be individualized to permit most efficient and safe reduction of contraction frequency.

Tolerance may develop when terbutaline is given, resulting in recurrent frequent contractions. Magnesium sulfate may be substituted to allow terbutaline to be eliminated from a woman's system while reducing contraction frequency. Terbutaline may be resumed or another tocolytic drug may be prescribed if indicated after contractions slow to acceptable frequency and intensity.

The nurse should assess a woman's apical heart rate and lung sounds before administering each intermittent dose of terbutaline for preterm labor. Addition of these maternal assessments to scheduled maternal vital signs and FHR is often adequate when a woman receives terbutaline by subcutaneous infusion pump. A maternal heart rate over 120 bpm or respiratory findings such as "wet" lung sounds or a more rapid rate, possibly accompanied by shortness of breath, suggest drug toxicity that may be a reason to discontinue terbutaline. Nonreassuring maternal and fetal assessments should be promptly reported to the physician. (See the Drug Guide for nursing care related to terbutaline tocolysis.)

Magnesium Sulfate. Magnesium sulfate is used in management of pregnancy-associated hypertension to prevent seizures (see the drug guide on p. 646). Because of its added effect of quieting uterine activity, it often is used to inhibit preterm labor. Magnesium sulfate therapy has a well-established record of safety during pregnancy. When given to suppress preterm labor, magnesium sulfate has similar side effects as those seen in its use to prevent seizures related to hypertension such as lethargy and sedation.

Magnesium sulfate for tocolysis is given intravenously using a similar protocol to that for hypertension during pregnancy. The loading dose, given in 15 to 20 minutes, is 4 to 6 g. The maintenance dose of magnesium sulfate ranges from 1 to 4 g/hr to stop preterm labor, often a broader range than when the drug is used for preeclampsia. The magnesium sulfate infusion is continued for 12 to 24 hours, when uterine contractions number no more than four to six per hour. The magnesium sulfate infusion is then reduced. Continuing magnesium sulfate therapy for a total of 48 hours may be chosen so the mother can receive the full course of corticosteroids to speed fetal lung maturation. When magnesium sulfate is discontinued, the woman may be changed to a medication such as terbutaline to maintain tocolysis.

Common hospital criteria for continuation of magnesium sulfate therapy include the following:

- Urine output of at least 30 ml per hour
- Presence of deep tendon reflexes
- At least 12 respirations per minute

TABLE 27-3 Drugs Used In Preterm Labor

Drug Name and Purpose	Common Dose Regimens*	Side or Adverse Effects
Terbutaline (beta-adrenergic for tocolysis)	See "Drug Guide: Terbutaline" (p. 717). *Intravenous (IV):* Begin at 0.01-0.05 mg/min. Increase by 0.01-mg/min increments every 10-30 min until contraction frequency is six or fewer per hour or significant side effects develop. Maximum dose guideline, 0.08 mg/min. When contraction frequency is no higher than four to six per hour, maintain the infusion for 1 hr; then reduce rate at 20-min intervals to reach the minimum maintenance dose, which may be continued for 12 hr after contractions stop or stabilize at acceptable maximum levels. *Subcutaneous (SC):* 0.25 mg q3-4h (maximum dose interval may be q6h, depending on client response). By SC infusion pump: continuous low dose baseline infusion plus intermittent bolus doses of 0.25 mg at times of greatest uterine activity. *Oral (PO):* 2.5-5 mg q2-4h. Hold for maternal pulse >120/min.	Cardiovascular: Maternal and fetal tachycardia, palpitations, cardiac dysrhythmias, chest pain, wide pulse pressure. Respiratory: Dyspnea, chest discomfort, pulmonary edema. Central nervous system: Tremors, restlessness, weakness, dizziness, headache. Metabolic: Hyperglycemia, hypokalemia. Gastrointestinal: Nausea, vomiting, reduced bowel motility Skin: Flushing, diaphoresis. Infection at injection site for subcutaneous infusion pump.
Magnesium sulfate (use as tocolytic)	*IV:* Loading dose, 4-6 g in 15-20 min. Maintenance dose for tocolysis, 1-4 g/hr. When contraction frequency is no higher than four to six per hour, maintain infusion rate for 12-24 hr; then reduce rate. An oral drug may be ordered to continue tocolysis after magnesium sulfate is stopped for this purpose.	Side and adverse effects are dose-related, occurring at higher maternal serum levels. Depression of deep tendon reflexes, which should be present, although less active. Respiratory or cardiac depression if serum levels are high; greatest risk is in woman with poor urine elimination of drug. Less serious side effects: Lethargy, weakness, visual blurring, headache, sensation of heat, nausea, vomiting, constipation. Fetal-neonatal effects: Reduced fetal heart rate (FHR) variability, hypotonia.
Indomethacin (Indocin); sulindac (Clinoril) (prostaglandin synthesis inhibitors)	Loading dose: up to 100 mg (rectal) or 50 mg (oral). Rectal preparation usually prepared by birth facility's pharmacy. Maintenance dose: 25-50 mg orally q6h. Ideal duration of treatment has not been established. Ultrasound examinations and fetal echocardiography help determine if maternal indomethacin has adverse effects on the fetus.	Epigastric pain, nausea, gastrointestinal bleeding. Asthma in aspirin-sensitive woman. Increased blood pressure in hypertensive woman. Fetus: Adverse fetal effects may include constriction of the ductus arteriosus, particularly if the mother receives indomethacin for more than 48-72 hr and the gestation is earlier than 32 weeks. Impairs fetal renal function, which may reduce the volume of amniotic fluid and result in cord compression.
Nifedipine (Procardia); nicardipine (Cardene) (calcium channel blockers for tocolysis)	Oral loading dose of 10-20 mg. Continued oral therapy: 10-20 mg q4-6h. Duration of calcium channel blocking drug for tocolysis has not been established.	Maternal flushing, dizziness, headache, nausea. Transient maternal tachycardia. Mild hypotension. Modest increases in blood glucose levels.

Data from American Academy of Pediatrics & American College of Obstetricians and Gynecologists. (2002). *Guidelines for perinatal care* (5th ed.). Elk Grove Village, IL, and Washington, DC: Authors; Blackburn, S.T. (2003). *Maternal, fetal, and neonatal physiology: A clinical perspective.* Philadelphia: Saunders; Goldenberg, R.L. (2002). The management of preterm labor. *Obstetrics & Gynecology, 100*(5 Pt. 1), 1020-1037; Iams, J.D., & Creasy, R.K. (2004). Preterm labor and delivery. In R.K. Creasy & R. Resnik (Eds.), *Maternal-fetal medicine: Principles and practice* (5th ed., pp. 498-531). Philadelphia: Saunders.
*Doses and frequency of administration are examples; actual protocols vary.

In addition, the nurse should check heart and lung sounds with hourly vital signs because fluid overload and electrolyte imbalances can lead to pulmonary edema or cardiac dysrhythmias. Oxygen saturations are often included with the hourly vital signs and other assessments. Bowel sounds are checked when therapy begins and every 4 to 8 hours because the smooth muscle in the intestinal tract may be relaxed just as the uterus is relaxed. Serum magnesium level measurements guide maintenance of therapeutic levels. Electronic fetal monitoring identifies drug effects on the fetus, such as reduced variability, that are common in preterm labor and with magnesium sulfate therapy.

Calcium gluconate (10%) should be available to reverse magnesium toxicity and prevent respiratory arrest if serum levels become high. Excess serum levels of magnesium are less likely when the drug is given for preterm labor because the woman's renal function is usually normal. However, the nurse must remain alert for this complication of magnesium sulfate therapy.

DRUG GUIDE

TERBUTALINE (BRETHINE)

Classification: Beta-adrenergic agent.

Action: Stimulates beta-adrenergic receptors of the sympathetic nervous system. Action results primarily in bronchodilation and inhibition of uterine muscle activity. Increases pulse rate and widens pulse pressure.

Indications: Stop preterm labor. Reduce or stop hypertonic labor contractions, whether natural or stimulated. Tolerance and loss of tocolytic effect occur with prolonged use.

Dosage and Route: *Intravenous (IV) infusion:* Begin at the ordered rate of approximately 0.01-0.05 mg/min. Increase rate if needed to stop contractions by 0.01 mg/min at 10- to 30-min intervals until contractions stop (maximum of 0.08 mg/min). The infusion rate is not increased or may be decreased if the maternal pulse rate remains over 120 beats per minute (bpm) or systolic blood pressure falls below 80-90 mm Hg. Maintain this dose for at least 1 hour; then reduce the rate at 20-min intervals to reach minimum maintenance dose. Continue maintenance dose for 12 hr or as ordered after contractions stop.

Subcutaneous (SC) (most common parenteral route): Intermittent injections, 0.25 mg, q3-4h. A subcutaneous programmed infusion pump may be used for low-dose continuous (baseline) drug infusion plus intermittent bolus doses of approximately 0.25 mg at times of greatest uterine activity. The subcutaneous pump is typically placed and its programming for continuous and bolus doses verified before the intermittent IV terbutaline line is removed.

Oral: 2.5-5 mg q2-4h.

When changing from IV to oral therapy, give oral dose 30 min before discontinuing IV infusion.

Absorption:
1. *IV:* Prompt; duration about 2 hr
2. *SC:* 6-15 min; duration 1½-4 hr
3. *Oral:* 1-2 hr; duration 4-8 hr

Excretion: Metabolized in the liver. Excreted in urine.

Contraindications: Hypersensitivity. Contraindicated before 20 weeks' gestation and if continuing the pregnancy is hazardous to the mother or fetus, as in fetal distress, premature rupture of membranes, hemorrhage, chorioamnionitis, and intrauterine fetal death. Contraindicated in conditions that may be adversely affected by beta-adrenergic agents (uncontrolled diabetes, hyperthyroidism, bronchial asthma treated with other beta-adrenergic agents or steroids, cardiac dysrhythmias, hypovolemia, uncontrolled hypertension).

Precautions: Terbutaline is not approved by the Food and Drug Administration (FDA) for inhibiting uterine activity, although it is widely used for this purpose. Research has been mixed regarding the drug effects of terbutaline for this purpose, but its lower risk for adverse side effects combined with some efficacy has maintained terbutaline's use as a tocolytic.

Adverse Reactions:
1. *Cardiovascular:* Maternal and fetal tachycardia, palpitations, cardiac dysrhythmias, chest pain, wide pulse pressure
2. *Respiratory:* Dyspnea, chest discomfort
3. *Central nervous system:* Tremors, restlessness, weakness, dizziness, headache
4. *Metabolic:* Hypokalemia, hyperglycemia
5. *Gastrointestinal:* Nausea, vomiting, reduced bowel motility
6. *Skin:* Flushing, diaphoresis

Nursing Considerations: Diagnostic studies that may be ordered related to terbutaline therapy: electrocardiogram, blood glucose, electrolytes, and urinalysis. Explain common side effects that are usually well tolerated, such as palpitations, tremors, restlessness, weakness, and headache. Assess fetal heart rate (FHR), usually with continuous electronic fetal monitoring when the drug is initiated, recording rate and patterns at recommended intervals and with IV dose increases. Assess maternal pulse, respirations, and blood pressure on same schedule as for FHR. Maintain adequate IV or oral hydration. Encourage the woman to empty her bladder every 2 hr. Notify the physician for significant or unacceptable side effects (maternal heart rate >120 bpm, respirations >24/min, dyspnea, pulmonary edema, systolic blood pressure <80-90 mm Hg, FHR >160 bpm, chest pain). Report continuing or recurrent uterine activity. Teach signs and symptoms of recurrent preterm labor and follow-up medical care after discharge.

Prostaglandin Synthesis Inhibitors. Because prostaglandins stimulate uterine contractions, drugs can be used to inhibit their synthesis. Indomethacin (Indocin) is the drug in this class that is most often used for tocolysis.

The main fetal and neonatal side effects are constriction of the ductus arteriosus, pulmonary hypertension, and oligohydramnios. These effects are unlikely if treatment is no longer than 48 to 72 hours and the gestation is less than 32 weeks. The drug's effect in reducing the amount of amniotic fluid makes indomethacin useful for normalizing the volume if hydramnios is present. The amniotic fluid volume usually returns to its previous level when indomethacin treatment is discontinued. Regular ultrasound examinations and fetal echocardiography help determine if indomethacin is having adverse effects on the infant. Assessment of the infant after birth for other complications, such as pulmonary hypertension or intracranial hemorrhage, may be done related to the duration of maternal indomethacin intake, gestation, and the probability that delivery occurs less than 24 hours after the drug is discontinued (Guinn & Gibbs, 2003; Iams & Creasy, 2004).

The nurse should observe the woman for side effects such as nausea, heartburn, vomiting, and rash. Because indomethacin can prolong bleeding time, the nurse observes for abnormal bleeding such as prolonged bleeding after injections and bruising with no apparent cause. The antiinflammatory effect of indomethacin can mask infection because fever may not be present. Checking the height of the fundus at the beginning of therapy and daily thereafter helps identify reduced amniotic fluid. Decreased fetal movements and absent FHR accelerations with fetal movement may occur if the fetal condition deteriorates.

Calcium Antagonists. Nifedipine (Adelat, Procardia) is a calcium channel blocker usually given for problems such as hypertension. Calcium is essential for muscle contraction in smooth muscles such as the uterus, so blocking calcium reduces the muscular contraction. Flushing of the skin, headache, and a transient increase in the maternal and fetal heart rates are common side effects. Because nifedipine is a vasodilator, the woman may have postural hypotension (Guinn & Gibbs, 2003; Iams & Creasy, 2004).

The nurse should observe for side effects of nifedipine and report a maternal pulse greater than 110. The woman should be assisted when sitting or standing and should do so gradually to reduce the effects of postural hypotension.

ACCELERATING FETAL LUNG MATURITY

The physician may order corticosteroids to speed fetal lung maturation if birth before 34 weeks seems inevitable. Steroid therapy may reduce the incidence and severity of RDS and intraventricular hemorrhage (IVH) in the preterm infant (AAP & ACOG, 2002; Iams & Creasy, 2004). Administering the steroid as late as 37 weeks' gestation may be chosen if fetal lung maturity studies demonstrate immature lungs later than 34 weeks. Betamethasone (Celestone) or dexamethasone (Decadron) may be used for this purpose.

Corticosteroids are indicated if the woman is between 24 and 34 weeks' gestation because of the high incidence of problems such as RDS that affect infants of this age. Delay of preterm birth for 24 hours after a woman begins corticosteroid therapy provides the greatest benefit in reducing critical problems associated with prematurity. Evidence also shows that a fetus born sooner than 24 hours after the mother begins taking the corticosteroid may have some maturation benefits of the drug. Therefore one benefit of tocolytic drugs to the woman at risk for preterm birth is to prolong labor enough that her fetus may receive benefits of the corticosteroid drug given. Benefits of corticosteroids to the preterm infant are known to last for 7 days after the drug is initiated, although they may last longer. Repeating the corticosteroid therapy 7 days after the prior dose is not now recommended but is being studied for possible benefits (AAP & ACOG, 2002; ACOG, 2001; Iams & Creasy, 2004; National Institutes of Health, 2000).

Current recommendations for corticosteroids for threatened preterm birth are:

- Betamethasone 12 mg: two doses (intramuscular [IM]), 24 hours apart
- Dexamethasone 6 mg: four doses (IM), 12 hours apart

The woman may have a temporary increase in her leukocytes or glucose intolerance while she receives betamethasone or dexamethasone. An increase in the insulin dose may be required for both the woman with gestational diabetes and the woman whose diabetes is present when she is not pregnant. Nervousness and insomnia are common but temporary maternal side effects.

Vital signs should be assessed to identify fever and elevated pulse that may indicate infection associated with steroid administration. Lung sounds should be assessed with vital signs because corticosteroids can cause sodium retention with accompanying fluid retention and pulmonary edema. The nurse should observe for and teach the woman about signs of pulmonary edema. The woman is taught to report any chest pain or heaviness or any difficulty breathing, because these symptoms could indicate pulmonary edema or possibly pneumonia. Pain and burning with urination are symptoms of urinary tract infection that is common in pregnancy even when steroids are not given.

DRUG GUIDE

BETAMETHASONE, DEXAMETHASONE

Classification: Corticosteroids.

Indications: Acceleration of fetal lung maturity to reduce the incidence and severity of respiratory distress syndrome (RDS). Studies suggest that antenatal steroids can also reduce the incidence of intraventricular hemorrhage (IVH) and neonatal death in the preterm infant. Greatest benefits accrue if at least 24 hours elapse between the initial dose and birth of the preterm infant, but the drug is indicated if birth is not imminent.

Dosage and Route:
Betamethasone: 12 mg intramuscularly (IM) for two doses, 24 hr apart.
Dexamethasone: 6 mg IM q12h for four doses.

Absorption: Rapid and complete after intramuscular administration.

Excretion: Metabolized in the liver. Excreted in urine.

Contraindications: Active infection, such as chorioamnionitis, is a relative contraindication, although further study is needed. The National Institutes of Health recommend use of corticosteroids for the woman who has preterm rupture of the membranes (24-32 weeks' gestation), but the American College of Obstetricians and Gynecologists has not yet endorsed this recommendation.

Precautions: Possible infection. Pregnancies complicated by diabetes.

Adverse Reactions: Few, owing to the short-term use of the drug. Pulmonary edema is possible secondary to sodium and fluid retention.

Nursing Considerations: Explain the potential benefits of corticosteroid administration for the preterm neonate. Explain that the drug cannot prevent or lessen the severity of all complications of prematurity. If the woman is diabetic, explain that more frequent blood glucose determinations are common because these levels are often elevated. Assess lung sounds. Report chest pain, heaviness, or dyspnea.

14. What symptoms of preterm labor should be taught to women at risk?
15. Why is it important to identify preterm labor early?
16. What four classifications of drugs may be used to stop preterm labor contractions?
17. What is the purpose of giving corticosteroids to a woman who is in preterm labor at 27 weeks' gestation? Why is it important that birth be delayed at least 24 hours?

Application of the Nursing Process
Preterm Labor

Nursing care for the woman experiencing preterm labor often includes interventions related to tocolytic, corticosteroid, or antibiotic drug therapy. If labor cannot be halted, care is similar to that for other laboring women, with additional care to prepare for a preterm infant's needs at birth. Support for anticipatory grieving may be needed if the infant is very immature and expected to die.

Nursing care when an extremely preterm infant (20 to 24 weeks' gestation) is expected to be born can be heavily laden with ethical and legal issues. For example, if labor cannot be halted, should fetal monitoring be used if the infant's survival is unlikely? If no intervention is done for a nonreassuring pattern, it can distress parents and caregivers alike. Plus, less information is known about fetal monitor patterns at very early gestations compared with gestations nearer term. On the other hand, knowledge of how the immature fetus responds to labor helps the neonatologist make better decisions about how to treat the infant after birth. In addition, ultrasound estimates have greater uncertainty for dating gestation in the woman who had no previous prenatal care. A fetus whose gestation was presumed to be 23 weeks before birth may be assessed at 26 weeks' gestation after birth and suited to more intense treatment than expected.

Much of the general nursing care for a woman having preterm labor also applies to women experiencing other types of high-risk pregnancies. Women may need multiple hospitalizations that occur in the middle of the night, disrupting sleep and family routines. Other women may have attended a routine prenatal visit and be shocked to discover that they may be in preterm labor. These women often have some activity restriction and may have to stop working if the best outcome for their pregnancy is to be achieved. Therefore this section focuses on the family's psychosocial concerns, management of home care, and the woman's boredom.

PSYCHOSOCIAL CONCERNS
Assessment

The entire family is affected by stressors associated with a high-risk pregnancy. Assess how the woman and her family usually cope with crisis situations and how they are coping with this one. Identify their greatest concerns to prioritize care. For example, the nurse might say, "This development in your pregnancy must have been a shock." Other questions the nurse might ask include "How are you handling things?" "In what ways do you usually handle crisis situations in your family?" and "What concerns you the most right now?" Rather than asking questions in a rapid-fire manner, the nurse must give the woman time to answer assessment questions, because stress has narrowed her focus.

The woman or her family may have physical, emotional, and cognitive impairments because of the unexpected problems. Physical signs of emotional distress, such as tremulousness, palpitations, and restlessness, also are side effects of beta-adrenergic drugs and corticosteroids. The woman may express fear, helplessness, or disbelief. She may be irritable and tearful. Her ability to concentrate may be impaired at a time when she needs to absorb new information.

Her partner often feels at loose ends. He struggles to keep the household running if she must be inactive. Young children pick up on their parents' anxiety and may misbehave or regress. They may feel abandoned if they must be temporarily placed with relatives or friends.

The woman often must curtail or stop working, straining family finances. If she does not have sick time or other benefits, the family sustains an abrupt drop in income at a time when medical expenses are mounting. The woman's career may not progress as expected if she must be off work for a prolonged time. A woman may be transferred to a distant hospital having a better capacity to care for her and her preterm baby. A distant transfer to a higher-level maternity care facility makes it more difficult for the woman to receive support from friends, family, or support groups.

Overlaid on the sudden change in lifestyle is the family's concern for their baby's well-being. A woman may feel pulled in many directions by the needs of all her children—those already born and the fetus she is trying to mature. She may be concerned about the effects of drug therapy on the fetus and her own body.

Analysis

Unexpected development of complications during pregnancy can prevent a woman and her family from using their normal coping mechanisms. Therefore the nursing diagnosis selected for the woman and family is "Anxiety related to uncertain outcome of the pregnancy, disruption of relationships with family and friends, and financial concerns."

Planning

The outcome of any pregnancy is never certain, especially when the pregnancy is a high-risk one. Goals and expected outcomes should focus on the family's ability to cope with the crisis of preterm labor. Appropriate outcomes include the following:

- The family will identify one or more constructive methods to cope with this temporary disruption in their lives.

Interventions

PROVIDING INFORMATION

Knowledge decreases anxiety and fear related to the unknown. Include appropriate family members so that they are more likely to be supportive. Appropriate family members may include the woman's partner, mother or mother-in-law, adult siblings, and others, which may vary with her culture. Determine the extent of the woman's knowledge about preterm birth and the specific therapy recommended. Determine what information the parents need about problems that a preterm infant may face. Use this opportunity to correct misinformation and reinforce accurate information.

Initially, the woman for whom activity restriction is prescribed may be highly motivated to maintain the restrictions. Because contractions often diminish, even if for only a short time, she may become restless. She may feel that there is now no need for any restriction, such as how far she can ambulate. Explain what is currently known about the benefits of activity restriction for her pregnancy complication and assure her that recommendations to restrict her activity often lessen as her pregnancy progresses. Initiate consultations from caregivers such as physical, occupational, and recreational therapists, social workers, and other professionals who might benefit the woman.

The Sidelines national support network (www.sidelines.org) is an online network of local groups across the country for women experiencing high-risk pregnancy, including the risk for preterm birth. The site has information for women "sidelined" by pregnancy complications, including articles, information about reimbursement from insurance, and contact via e-mail with others who have been "sidelined" (Nursing Care Plan 27-1).

PROMOTING EXPRESSION OF CONCERNS

Encourage the woman and her family to express their concerns. Begin by exploring common concerns of women with problem pregnancies. For example, say, "Most women are

---

NURSING CARE PLAN 27-1 Preterm Labor

ASSESSMENT: Rhonda Ellis is a 28-year-old gravida 4, para 3. Her children were born at 40 weeks, 28 weeks, and 32 weeks of gestation. Her children are 7 and 4 years and 18 months old. She has mild cramping and pelvic pressure at 28 weeks and comes to the hospital right away. Her cervix is dilated 1 to 2 cm and is beginning to efface. She responds to intravenous (IV) magnesium sulfate to stop her contractions. The physician also orders betamethasone 12 mg intramuscularly (IM) for two doses, 24 hours apart. After her contractions stop, Rhonda is started on oral terbutaline to maintain tocolysis and will be discharged home in 48 hours if no recurrent symptoms develop.

NURSING DIAGNOSIS: Impaired Home Maintenance related to activity restrictions and family demands.

GOAL/EXPECTED OUTCOME: By hospital discharge, Rhonda will:
1. Relate ways that she can maintain prescribed activity restrictions.

INTERVENTION	RATIONALE
1. Assess what support systems are available and financially feasible to help Rhonda with child care and transportation, such as daycare, "mother's day out" programs at churches, family, and friends.	1. Responsibilities for other children may impede a woman's ability to maintain activity limits. Coordination among several resources helps provide all-day coverage for child care.
2. Encourage Rhonda to lower her standards for home management temporarily: a. Eat nourishing take-out or fast food. b. Set priorities regarding household tasks that must be done. c. Let her children do tasks that are within their abilities. d. Make lists of tasks for different people who ask to help her. Encourage her to consider the talents, resources, and obligations of volunteers.	2. Many usual roles must be reallocated during this time. Having alternative arrangements increases the chance that the woman can maintain therapy. Considering the strengths and personal obligations of those who volunteer to help her increases the satisfaction of both Rhonda and her family as well as the satisfaction of those who help.
3. Encourage Rhonda to accept help from others. Remind her that this situation is temporary and that she may be able to help someone else at another time.	3. If a woman feels that she can help others at another time, she may be more willing to accept help when she needs it.

EVALUATION: Rhonda identifies three friends in addition to her mother-in-law who may be able to help with child care. She says she cannot afford to continue sending her children to their daycare center if she is not working. She feels that if her children are cared for, her husband can handle the other home management needs.

worried when they must stop working. How has this affected your family?" An open question gives the woman and her family a chance to express their feelings so that they can take the next step: identifying constructive methods to cope with the situation. Collaboration with a social worker may identify financial or other community resources available. Ask her if she would like a visit from a chaplain.

TEACHING WHAT MAY OCCUR DURING A PRETERM BIRTH

Because preterm birth often occurs despite all interventions, a pregnant woman and her partner should be prepared for this possibility. If the hospital has a neonatal intensive care unit, a nurse often visits the parents to explain what might occur if their baby is born early. One or both parents may tour the unit to see the equipment and care given to preterm infants. Often, just seeing the infants in the neonatal intensive care unit motivates a woman to maintain recommended therapy even though she is tired of doing so.

In hospitals with neonatal intensive care units, one or more neonatal nurses, a neonatal nurse-practitioner, a neonatologist, or a combination of these are present at birth to care for the infant. The woman who has planned to give birth in a hospital without a neonatal intensive care unit may be transferred to a facility with this type of unit before the birth to allow immediate care and stabilization of her newborn. The infant also may be transferred after birth if there is no time to transfer the woman before birth or the infant has more problems than were anticipated. Hospitalization of the mother, infant, or both at a distant location adds to the stress on the family and can impair the attachment process.

Evaluation

The goal or expected outcome for this nursing diagnosis is achieved if the woman and her family can identify one or more constructive methods to deal with their anxiety. If a high-risk pregnancy situation is prolonged or the family has

---

NURSING CARE PLAN 27-1 Preterm Labor—cont'd

ASSESSMENT: At 31 weeks' gestation, Rhonda again experiences preterm labor and goes to the hospital. Her cervix is dilated 2 to 3 cm and is 75% effaced (about 0.5 cm long). Her contractions occur every 6 to 7 minutes, and last about 20 to 30 seconds each. The physician again orders a magnesium sulfate infusion. Because of a research study being conducted at several facilities, the physician also discusses the risks and possible benefits of repeating the betamethasone injections. The physician explains that preterm birth may be delayed but will probably occur within the next 24 to 48 hours. Rhonda begins crying and says, "I did what I was supposed to do and now I'm still going to have another preemie! It will be weeks before I can be a real mother!"

NURSING DIAGNOSIS: Anticipatory Grieving related to loss of expected birth experience.

GOAL/EXPECTED OUTCOME: Rhonda will:
1. Express her feelings about the loss of her expected birth at term.

INTERVENTION	RATIONALE
1. Sit down and spend time with Rhonda. Use therapeutic communication to encourage her to express her feelings.	1. Unhurried time allows expression of feelings, which is the first step in dealing with the anticipated loss.
2. When she has expressed her frustration about this development in her pregnancy, explain that much remains unknown about why labor begins, whether at term, preterm, or postterm.	2. If a woman knows that professionals do not have all the answers but must make recommendations based on what is known or appears to work for an individual woman, she may be more accepting of the inevitability of preterm birth.
3. Explain that Rhonda's efforts have paid off because she has gained 3 valuable weeks of gestation for her baby. In addition, the drug betamethasone may reduce the chance that her preterm newborn will have the usual degree of common respiratory problems if born at that gestation.	3. Knowing that her self-care has benefits, although not the hoped-for term birth, reduces the sense of failure that she may feel.

Making a decision about whether she should repeat the betamethasone for the baby adds to the decisions she must make very soon. |

EVALUATION: Rhonda cries and expresses her frustration about the developments in her pregnancy. She says that she knew she was more likely to have another preterm infant but hoped that this time would be different. As the day goes by, Rhonda gradually begins expressing feelings that she did do something positive for this baby. Because contractions have not diminished but have become more intense, she plans to deal with the probable preterm birth. She has elected not to take additional betamethasone because it is apparent that birth will likely occur in less than 24 hours.

ADDITIONAL NURSING DIAGNOSES TO CONSIDER:
Health-Seeking Behaviors
Readiness for Enhanced Family Coping
Interrupted Family Processes
Ineffective Health Maintenance
Compromised or disabled individual or family coping
Readiness for enhanced individual or family coping

difficulty adapting constructively to the situation, a nursing diagnosis of "Interrupted Family Processes" may be more appropriate.

MANAGEMENT OF HOME CARE

Assessment

Despite their uncertain value in the treatment of preterm labor, activity restrictions continue to be widely prescribed. If the membranes are not ruptured, the woman may be managed at home rather than in the hospital, particularly if a longer course is anticipated. Therefore the nurse should expect that part of the care of women with high-risk pregnancies, including a risk for preterm birth, often occurs in the home. Many daily household activities are probably managed by the woman. When she is disabled, even briefly and in her home, the usual roles of family members are disrupted.

Determine the level of activity prescribed by the physician and identify the role of each family member. A good way to do this is to have the woman describe a usual day before any activity restrictions. Determine the number and ages of children in the home.

Evaluate the home itself, either by visual inspection or questions to the family. Does the home have more than one level? If it is an apartment, is it upstairs or downstairs? Determine whether a telephone is available for emergency contact.

Evaluate the family's resources and their willingness to use them. Ask whether family members and friends in the area are available to help. Explore local support groups such as churches and mother-to-mother networks that the family might contact for assistance. Ask if the family has a computer that may be a resource for support organizations such as Sidelines. Determine whether insurance covers assistance such as homemaker services.

Analysis

The diagnosis chosen is "Impaired Home Maintenance related to change in usual roles and responsibilities."

Planning

Two goals or expected outcomes are appropriate for this nursing diagnosis:

- Short-term goal—The family will identify methods for management of daily household routines.
- Long-term goal—The woman will be able to maintain the prescribed levels of activity and drug therapy.

Interventions

The pregnancy threatened by preterm labor or other complications that require activity restriction is a self-limiting situation, making temporary adjustments somewhat easier. Needed changes in home routines may be brief but sometimes extend over several weeks. Even if the restriction consists only of added rest periods during the day, the woman still is unable to fulfill all her usual roles. For the woman who is prescribed more restricted activity, the disruptions are greater.

CARING FOR CHILDREN

The woman who has children has different concerns than the woman who does not. Toddlers and preschoolers rarely understand why their mother does not play with them as usual. If they already are in daycare, this can continue if the family can afford it. They may temporarily live with a relative or friend. Toddlers may feel that their parents have abandoned them if they are sent away, although this may be the only realistic solution if no one except the mother is available to supervise them.

School-age children can understand the situation better and often are quite helpful. They may assist with care of other children, but they should not be put into the role of an adult. They may resent responsibility that is excessive for their age. School-age children often enjoy learning new facts about their mother's pregnancy and tests the baby may need.

Adolescents may welcome their parents' trust but also resent the intrusion on independent activities with their peers. Teenagers who drive can be very helpful in taking younger siblings to school and other activities. They may be enlisted for grocery shopping and meal preparation. If resentment flares, a reminder that the situation is temporary and they are valuable contributors to the health of the new baby may defuse the situation.

MAINTAINING THE HOUSEHOLD

The first step to home maintenance during this time may be for the woman to lower her standards of housekeeping. Things may not be as clean or organized as she would like. The partner may take over some household tasks, but these may compete with responsibilities outside the home. Talk to the woman about ignoring chores that are not performed exactly as she wants and tell her to remember that it is temporary.

Advise the woman to have a list of tasks ready when friends and family ask, "Can I do anything to help?" If they offer to bring a meal or do laundry, encourage her to accept. Remind her that people who offer to help mean it and that she may be able to return the favor to someone else. Homemaker services may be an option to help the family deal with the woman's temporary disability.

Transportation of school-aged children may be a concern. If no family or friends are available, the school nurse or Parent-Teacher Association (PTA) may help find someone willing to take the children to school each day.

Evaluation

Goals and expected outcomes with a short term help the nurse and patient, often including the family, identify resolution of their immediate needs. Longer-term outcomes may be evaluated over a series of days or weeks as the prescribed therapy for the complicated pregnancy changes.

- The short-term goal is met if the family can identify ways to manage minimal household care.
- The long-term goal is met if the woman can maintain the prescribed therapy.

BOREDOM

Assessment

If activity is restricted, determine what skills the woman has for coping with boredom. Although bedrest to prolong gestation is often brief because of the questionable benefits and known problems, some reduction in activity is prescribed. The nurse should consider helping the woman choose appropriate activities, whether she is at home or hospitalized.

Ask about a usual day to identify activities that are still appropriate within the restrictions prescribed. Ask about hobbies, present and past. What type of leisure activities does the woman enjoy? Which activities are available or possible? Does she have more than one resting place to still give her a change of scenery and surrounding activity?

Assess her personality. Is she calm and composed, taking whatever comes with serenity? Or does she need to be busy most of the time? No matter how motivated, the woman who finds inactivity tiresome will find even limited activity restriction difficult to maintain.

Analysis

The nursing diagnosis is "Deficient Diversional Activity related to lack of knowledge about appropriate activities for her pregnancy restrictions."

Planning

A possible goal or expected outcome is that the woman will:

- Pursue (with help of others) appropriate activities to relieve boredom while maintaining recommended activity limits.

Interventions

IDENTIFYING APPROPRIATE ACTIVITIES

Determine the woman's understanding about needed activity restrictions to identify misunderstandings and reinforce correct information. Help her identify which usual activities are reasonable and which ones should not be done and why. If she understands the rationale, she may be more willing to maintain restrictions.

Some women continue work activities such as paperwork or phone calls that can be accomplished with minimal physical exertion. Workplace deadlines can increase stress, even at home. However, the feeling of usefulness gained by such activities may be beneficial because it reduces some financial concerns.

Computer connections can be used for work activities in some jobs and may also provide support from other women with similar problems or entertainment such as games played with other users. Internet sites, if carefully chosen, may provide health information about what she might expect with diagnostic tests and treatment for preterm labor, care of her baby in the special care nursery setting, providing breast milk for her preterm newborn, and comfort measures that have been effective for others in her situation.

Help the woman identify appropriate activities to stay busy and productive. These may include household activities that can be done at rest, volunteer activities such as phone calls, and leisure activities such as puzzles, games, and hand needlework. Instructions for hobbies such as knitting are often available online. Help the woman identify someone who can obtain the necessary supplies for her. This might be a good time to reactivate an old (quiet) hobby or read books that she has previously delayed until "later."

The woman can participate in some activities with her children while she is in bed. She can read to them and play board or card games. Encourage her to help the children with their homework and stimulate their development with thought-provoking discussions.

CHANGING THE PHYSICAL SURROUNDINGS

Encourage the woman to identify at least two areas where she can maintain her prescribed rest. This gives her a change of scene and helps her feel more a part of the family activities. Each area should include pillows, blankets, and a clipboard with writing materials. An adjustable ironing board can provide a movable table for her things, and a shoe bag helps keep supplies organized and at hand. Ideally, the telephone is within reach or cordless and she has a television with a remote control unit.

Evaluation

The goal is met over time if the woman actually pursues only appropriate activities.

PROLONGED PREGNANCY

A prolonged pregnancy is one that lasts longer than 42 weeks. Most women who receive prenatal care today do not reach 42 weeks before their labor is induced if they have accurate due dates. Many apparent cases of prolonged pregnancy are actually miscalculations of the estimated date of delivery (EDD) because the woman has had irregular menstrual periods or forgotten the date of her last normal menstrual period.

Complications

The main physical risk in prolonged pregnancy is to the fetus or newborn. Insufficiency of the placental function secondary to aging and infarction reduces transfer of oxygen and nutrients to the fetus and removal of waste. Because the fetus with placental insufficiency has less reserve to tolerate uterine contractions, signs of fetal compromise, such as late decelerations and decreased variability, may develop during labor. In addition, reduced amniotic fluid volume (oligohydramnios) that often accompanies placental insufficiency can result in umbilical cord compression. Meconium in the amniotic fluid may cause respiratory distress in the newborn if it is aspirated before or during birth. The infant may have late growth retardation and appear to have lost weight, with a normal-sized head and thin body.

Many postterm fetuses do not suffer from placental insufficiency and may continue growing. If the fetus becomes large, the woman and fetus then may have complications related to dysfunctional labor, inadequate postpartum uterine contraction to control bleeding, and injury if the birth is traumatic.

Psychologically, the woman often feels as though her pregnancy will never end. The added fatigue imposed by a pregnancy that extends significantly beyond her due date diminishes her resources for tolerating the added stress and anxiety about labor and birth.

Therapeutic Management

If the woman has no prenatal care until late in pregnancy, therapeutic management begins by determining her gestation as accurately as possible. Several markers used to pinpoint gestation, such as ultrasound examination, fundal height measurements, dates of quickening, and first identification of fetal heart tones with a nonamplified fetoscope or Doppler, may be lost if a woman begins prenatal care very late. Also, the woman may have forgotten the date of her last menstrual period or may have irregular menstrual cycles.

Another factor in management decisions is whether the fetus is thriving in the uterus. If antepartum tests such as a biophysical profile indicate that the fetus is doing well, the birth attendant can take a more conservative approach than if the placental function is diminished and can allow labor to begin naturally.

If the gestation appears to be truly postterm and no fetal urgency to deliver quickly exists, management depends on whether the cervix is favorable for induction of labor. If so, induction is usually begun. If the cervix is not favorable, the caregiver often uses a cervical ripening procedure (see Chapter 16) to soften the cervix. The cervical ripening also would be done if the fetal signs were nonreassuring and delivery was needed but the cervix was not favorable (unless the fetal situation was sufficiently nonreassuring that a cesarean was indicated).

Nursing Considerations

Nursing care for the woman with a prolonged pregnancy is tied to the medical management. The nurse's role may include the following:

- Teaching about procedures such as antepartum testing or induction of labor
- Support for her psychological and physical fatigue
- Nursing care related to specific procedures such as induction of labor

INTRAPARTUM EMERGENCIES

Placental Abnormalities

Women with placental abnormalities may experience hemorrhage during the antepartum or intrapartum period. Placenta previa is sometimes associated with an abnormally adherent placenta (placenta accreta). Placenta accreta may cause immediate or delayed hemorrhage immediately after birth because the placenta does not separate cleanly, often leaving small fragments that prevent full uterine contraction. More extreme degrees of abnormal adherence occur when the placenta penetrates the uterine muscle itself (placenta increta) or even all the way through the uterus (placenta percreta). All or only part of the placenta may be involved. A hysterectomy often is required if a large portion of the placenta is abnormally adherent.

Prolapsed Umbilical Cord

A prolapsed umbilical cord slips downward after the membranes rupture, subjecting it to compression between the fetus and pelvis (Figure 27-7). It may slip down immediately with the fluid gush or long after the membranes rupture. Interruption in blood flow through the cord interferes with fetal oxygenation and is potentially fatal.

CAUSES

Prolapse of the umbilical cord is more likely when the fit is poor between the fetal presenting part and the maternal pelvis. When the fit is good, the fetus fills up the pelvis, leaving little room for the cord to slip down. Although prolapse of the cord is possible during any labor, it is more likely if these conditions are present:

- A fetus that remains at a high station
- A very small fetus
- Breech presentations (the footling breech is more likely to be complicated by a prolapsed cord because the feet and legs are small and do not fill the pelvis well)
- Transverse lie
- Hydramnios (often associated with abnormal presentations; also, the unusually large amount of fluid exerts more pressure to push the cord out)

SIGNS OF PROLAPSE

Prolapse may be complete, with the cord visible at the vaginal opening. A prolapsed cord may not be visible but may be palpated on vaginal examination as it pulsates synchronously with the fetal heart. An occult prolapse of the cord is one in which the cord slips alongside the fetal head or shoulders. The prolapse cannot be palpated or seen but is suspected because of changes in the FHR, such as sustained bradycardia or variable decelerations.

CRITICAL TO REMEMBER

Factors That Increase a Woman's Risk for a Prolapsed Umbilical Cord

Ruptured membranes *and*
- The fetal presenting part at a high station
- A fetus that poorly fits the pelvic inlet because of small size or abnormal presentation
- Excessive volume of amniotic fluid (hydramnios)

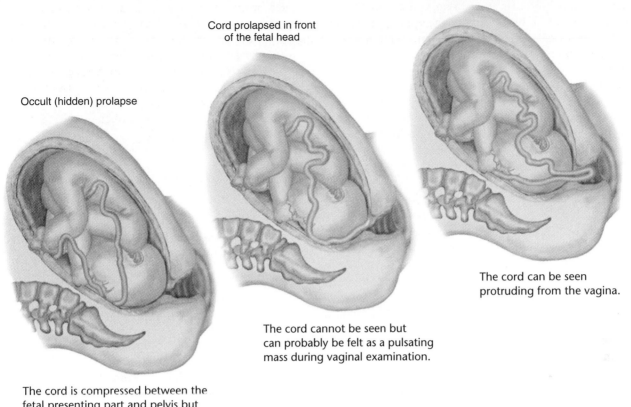

Occult (hidden) prolapse

Cord prolapsed in front
of the fetal head

Complete cord prolapse

The cord can be seen
protruding from the vagina.

The cord cannot be seen but
can probably be felt as a pulsating
mass during vaginal examination.

The cord is compressed between the
fetal presenting part and pelvis but
cannot be seen or felt during vaginal
examination.

Figure 27-7 ■ Variations of prolapsed umbilical cord.

Therapeutic Management

Medical and nursing management often overlap, as they do in many emergency situations. Either the nurse or the birth attendant may be the first to discover umbilical cord prolapse. Birth is almost always cesarean unless vaginal delivery can be accomplished more quickly and less traumatically. If fetal death has already occurred, management will focus on the best care for the mother based on other complications.

When cord prolapse occurs, the priority is to relieve pressure on the cord to improve blood flow through it until delivery. None of these interventions should delay the promptest possible delivery of a living fetus. Push the call light to summon help. Others should call the physician and prepare for birth while the nurse caring for the woman relieves pressure on the cord, if the physician or nurse-midwife is not doing so. Neonatal nurses and a pediatrician or neonatologist should be notified, and the staff should prepare for neonatal resuscitation.

Prompt actions reduce cord compression and increase fetal oxygenation:

1. Position the woman's hips higher than her head to shift the fetal presenting part toward her diaphragm. Any of these methods (Figure 27-8) may be used:
   a. Knee-chest position
   b. Trendelenburg position
   c. Hips elevated with pillows, with side-lying position maintained
2. If elevation of the maternal hips does not result in an upward shift of the fetus to relieve cord compression, vaginal elevation of the presenting part using a sterile gloved hand may be required. Maintain this position until the physician orders it stopped, usually just before cesarean delivery, while minimizing added cord compression from the hand.
3. Avoid or minimize manual palpation or handling of the cord, because possible cord vessel vasospasm or trauma may further reduce umbilical blood flow to and from the fetus.
4. Ultrasound examination may be used to confirm presence of fetal heart activity before cesarean delivery.

While preparing for surgery, give oxygen at 8 to 10 L/min by facemask to increase maternal blood oxygen saturation, making more available for the fetus.

Other actions may be used to enhance fetal oxygenation, but prompt delivery is the priority. A tocolytic drug such as terbutaline inhibits contractions, increasing placental blood flow and reducing intermittent pressure of the fetus against the pelvis and cord. Warm, saline-moistened towels retard cooling and drying of the cord. If the cord is protruding from the vagina, no attempt should be made to replace it because doing so could traumatize and further reduce blood

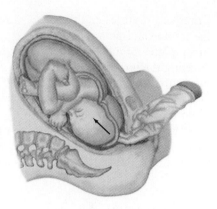

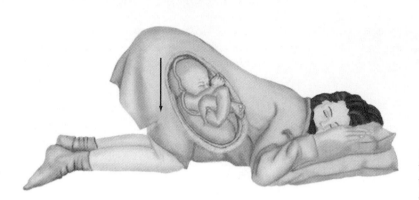

A gloved hand in the vagina pushes the fetus upward and off the cord.

Knee-chest position uses gravity to shift the fetus out of the pelvis. The woman's thighs should be at right angles to the bed and her chest flat on the bed.

The woman's hips are elevated with two pillows; this is often combined with the Trendelenburg (head down) position.

Figure 27-8 ■ Measures that may be used to relieve pressure on a prolapsed umbilical cord until delivery can take place.

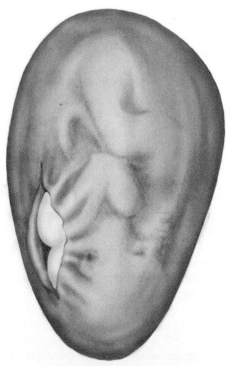

Figure 27-9 ■ Uterine rupture in the lower uterine segment.

flow through the cord. Manipulating the cord can induce umbilical artery spasm, which would reduce blood flow between the fetus and placenta.

Prognosis for the woman is good because the only additional risks are those associated with cesarean birth. Prognosis for the infant depends on how long and how severely blood flow through the cord has been impaired. With prompt recognition and corrective actions, the infant usually does well.

NURSING CONSIDERATIONS

In addition to taking prompt corrective actions, the nurse must consider the woman's anxiety. The nurse must remain calm while working quickly during this time and acknowledge the woman's anxiety. Explanations must be simple because anxiety interferes with the woman's ability to comprehend them. Her partner and family should be included as much as possible.

Uterine Rupture

Sometimes a tear in the wall of the uterus occurs because the uterus cannot withstand the pressure against it (Figure 27-9). Uterine rupture may occur at home rather than in the hospital. Uterine rupture may precede labor's onset. Three variations of uterine rupture exist:

- Complete rupture—A direct communication between the uterine and peritoneal cavities
- Incomplete rupture—A rupture into the peritoneum covering the uterus or into the broad ligament but not the peritoneal cavity
- Dehiscence—A partial separation of an old uterine scar. Little or no bleeding may occur. No signs or symptoms may exist, and the rupture ("window") may be found incidentally during a subsequent cesarean birth or other abdominal surgery.

CAUSES

Although uterine rupture is rare, dehiscence is not unusual. Uterine rupture is associated with previous uterine surgery such as cesarean birth or surgery to remove fibroids. The risk for rupture in a woman who has had a prior cesarean birth depends on the type of uterine incision. The risk for rupture is greater in the woman with a classic incision (vertical into the upper uterine segment) than the woman with a low transverse incision. For this reason, vaginal birth after cesarean is not recommended for women who have had a previous classic cesarean birth.

Rupture of the unscarred uterus is more likely for women of high parity with a thin uterine wall, women sustaining blunt abdominal trauma, and women having intense contractions, especially if fetopelvic disproportion is present. Excessively strong contractions (hypertonic) may cause the intrauterine pressure to exceed the tensile strength of the uterine wall. If the fetus cannot be expelled downward through the pelvis, contractions may push it through the lower uterine segment. Intense contractions are more likely to occur when uterine stimulants such as oxytocin and misoprostol are administered for induction or augmentation of labor, but they also may occur spontaneously.

SIGNS AND SYMPTOMS

Dehiscence does not have symptoms initially and may not interfere with labor or vaginal delivery if the area is small. However, labor progress may stop because the open area prevents efficient expulsion of the fetus. Intrauterine pressures may have little change during contractions. A larger area of dehiscence may cause abdominal pain that persists despite analgesia.

Manifestations of uterine rupture vary with the degree of rupture and may mimic other complications. Possible signs and symptoms of uterine rupture are as follows:
- Abdominal pain and tenderness—The pain may not be severe; it may occur suddenly at the peak of a contraction. The woman may describe a feeling that something "gave way" or "ripped."
- Chest pain, pain between the scapulae, or pain on inspiration—Pain occurs because of the irritation of blood below the woman's diaphragm.
- Hypovolemic shock caused by hemorrhage—Falling blood pressure, tachycardia, tachypnea, pallor, cool and clammy skin, and anxiety. Signs of shock may not occur until after birth. The fall in blood pressure is often a late sign of hemorrhage.

- Signs associated with impaired fetal oxygenation, such as late decelerations, reduced variability, tachycardia, and bradycardia
- Absent fetal heart sounds with a large disruption of the placenta; absent fetal heart activity by ultrasound examination
- Cessation of uterine contractions
- Palpation of the fetus outside the uterus (usually occurs only with a large, complete rupture). The fetus is likely to be dead.

If the rupture is incomplete, blood loss is slower and signs of shock, chest pain, or intrascapular pain may be delayed. Complete rupture results in massive blood loss. Signs of shock and pain develop quickly. External bleeding may not be impressive, however, because most blood is lost into the peritoneal cavity. The fetus often dies in complete rupture because the placental blood supply is disrupted.

THERAPEUTIC MANAGEMENT

Initial management is to stabilize the woman and fetus and perform cesarean delivery. If the rupture is small and the woman wants other children, it may be repaired. A woman with a large uterine rupture requires hysterectomy. Blood is replaced as needed.

NURSING CONSIDERATIONS

The nurse must be aware of women who are at increased risk for uterine rupture and must stay alert for the signs and symptoms. Administer uterine stimulant drugs cautiously to reduce the likelihood of excessive contractions. The nurse must keep in mind that hypertonic contractions also can occur spontaneously. Notify the birth attendant if hypertonic contractions occur. A tocolytic drug may be needed to reduce excessive contractions.

Uterine rupture may not be detected before birth. If postpartum bleeding is excessive and the fundus is firm, injury to the birth canal, including uterine rupture, is possible. Bleeding may be concealed if the ruptured area bleeds into the broad ligament. In this case, signs of hypovolemic shock are likely to develop quickly.

✔ CHECK YOUR READING

18. What are three risks to the fetus or neonate when pregnancy lasts longer than 42 weeks?
19. What is the immediate management if prolapse of the umbilical cord occurs?
20. How can contractions stimulated with drugs such as oxytocin or misoprostol increase the risk for uterine rupture?

Uterine Inversion

An inversion occurs when the uterus completely or partly turns inside out, usually during the third stage of labor. Such an event is uncommon but potentially fatal.

CAUSES

Often, no single cause is identified. Predisposing factors are as follows:

- Pulling on the umbilical cord before the placenta detaches from the uterine wall
- Fundal pressure during birth
- Fundal pressure on an incompletely contracted uterus after birth
- Increased intraabdominal pressure
- An abnormally adherent placenta
- Congenital weakness of the uterine wall
- Fundal placenta implantation

SIGNS AND SYMPTOMS

The birth attendant notes that either the uterus is absent from the abdomen or a depression in the fundal area is present. The interior of the uterus may be seen through the cervix or protruding into the vagina. Massive hemorrhage, shock, and pain quickly become evident. The woman has severe pelvic pain.

MANAGEMENT

Quick action by nursing and medical personnel is required to reduce maternal morbidity and mortality. The birth attendant tries to replace the uterus through the vagina into a normal position. If that is not possible, laparotomy with replacement is done. Hysterectomy may be required.

Two IV lines are established to allow rapid fluid and blood replacement. A tocolytic drug or general anesthesia usually is needed to relax the uterus enough to replace it. After the uterus is replaced and the placenta removed, oxytocin is given to contract the uterus and control blood loss. Oxytocin is not given until the uterus is repositioned, to avoid trapping the inverted fundus in the cervix.

NURSING CONSIDERATIONS

Nursing care during the emergency supplements that provided by other staff members. Postpartum nursing care is directed toward observing and maintaining maternal blood volume and correcting shock. The woman may be transferred to the intensive care unit.

Assess the uterine fundus for firmness, height, and deviation from the midline. Assess vital signs every 15 minutes or more frequently until stable, then according to recovery room routine. Observe for tachycardia and a falling blood pressure, which are associated with shock. Remember that the fall in blood pressure is often a late sign of hemorrhagic shock. A cardiac monitor identifies dysrhythmias, which may occur with shock, and a pulse oximeter provides information about oxygenation. Invasive hemodynamic monitoring with central venous pressure and arterial lines is common to directly evaluate functions such as heart rate, venous and arterial pressures, circulation to the lungs, venous functions, and other tests that may be needed.

An indwelling catheter often is inserted to observe fluid balance and keep the bladder empty so that the uterus can contract well. Assess the catheter for patency, and record intake and output. Urine output should be at least 30 ml per hour. A fall in urine output may indicate hypovolemia or an obstructed catheter.

The woman is allowed nothing by mouth until her condition is stable. She usually can receive fluids and progress to solid foods quickly because uterine inversion does not usually recur in the current postpartum period. It may recur in a future pregnancy if conditions favor its development.

Anaphylactoid Syndrome

Pregnancy-related anaphylactoid syndrome, often called *amniotic fluid embolism,* occurs when amniotic fluid is drawn into the maternal circulation and carried to the woman's lungs. Fetal particulate matter (skin cells, vernix, hair, and meconium) in the fluid obstructs pulmonary vessels. Failure of the right ventricle occurs early and can lead to hypoxemia. Left ventricular failure follows. Abrupt respiratory distress, depressed cardiac function, and circulatory collapse may occur rapidly. Disseminated intravascular coagulation (see Chapter 25) is likely because thromboplastin-rich amniotic fluid interferes with normal blood clotting. This infrequent disorder is often fatal, possibly having a 50% maternal death rate during the acute episode. Survivors may have neurologic deficits (Clark, 2004; Gonik & Foley, 2004).

Although this disorder has been called *amniotic fluid embolism,* the newer name of *anaphylactoid syndrome* is preferred because of findings related to other complications. Other maternal conditions that are not characterized by leaking of amniotic fluids into her circulation include septic shock, preeclampsia, and cardiac disease. Other complications may be associated with this disorder but are not fully known (Gonik & Foley, 2004).

Therapeutic management of a pregnancy-related anaphylactoid syndrome is primarily medical and includes the following (Clark, 2003; Gonik & Foley, 2004):

- Cardiopulmonary resuscitation and support
- Oxygen with mechanical ventilation
- Fluid volume expansion; blood transfusion as indicated
- Hemodynamic monitoring to guide therapeutic interventions
- Vasopressor therapy
- Blood component therapy such as fibrinogen, packed red blood cells, platelets, fresh frozen plasma to correct coagulation defects

The mother's well-being takes precedence in cases of anaphylactoid syndrome. If she is in full cardiac arrest, her survival is unlikely and the fetus may be delivered to improve survival odds for the baby (Clark, 2003).

TRAUMA

Most trauma during pregnancy occurs because of accidents, assault, or suicide. Battering is a significant cause of maternal-fetal trauma during pregnancy. (The social and emotional issues of battering are addressed in Chapter 24.) Trauma may be blunt, such as that sustained in an automobile accident, or penetrating, such as gunshot and knife wounds. Burns and electrical injuries also may occur.

Although injury may not be fatal, infant neurologic deficits may be found after birth. Direct fetal trauma, such as skull fracture or intracranial hemorrhage, may occur from pelvic fracture, penetrating wounds, or blunt trauma. Indirect causes of fetal injury or death include abruptio placentae and disruption of the placental blood flow secondary to maternal hypovolemia or uterine rupture. The most common cause of fetal death is death of the mother.

The anatomic and physiologic changes of pregnancy make trauma care unique. During early pregnancy, the uterus is surrounded by the pelvis and is well protected from direct damage. As the uterus grows, it protrudes and becomes a large target for trauma. At the same time, it acts as a shield for other maternal organs such as the kidneys, often protecting them from direct trauma.

Normal alterations of pregnancy can affect the maternal and fetal outcomes after traumatic injury and can affect the interpretation of diagnostic studies that may be done. Pregnant women have a greater blood volume than nonpregnant women, which gives them a cushion against blood loss. However, the fetus may suffer if the woman hemorrhages because maternal blood is diverted from the placenta to increase her blood volume. Fetal hypoxia, acidosis, and death may then occur.

Maternal fibrinogen levels are higher during pregnancy (300 to 600 mg/dl). A decrease to lower levels is associated with abruptio placentae and may indicate that disseminated intravascular coagulation is developing.

MANAGEMENT

Care of the pregnant trauma victim first focuses on injuries that threaten her life. Management of the fetus depends on whether the fetus is living and on the gestational age. The fetus may be delivered by cesarean birth if it is mature enough to survive and if the maternal or fetal condition is likely to be improved by prompt delivery. The fetus that is dead or too immature to survive is not usually delivered unless delivery will improve the mother's outcome.

NURSING CONSIDERATIONS

Nursing care of the pregnant trauma victim also focuses first on maternal and then on fetal stabilization. A wedge is placed under one side of the mother to tip her uterus away from her major blood vessels. "Tipping" her to displace the uterus may prevent supine hypotension and further hemodynamic instability, also improving placental blood flow. Vital signs are taken as needed, based on the woman's condition. Vital signs and urine output (at least 30 ml/hr) provide information about the adequacy of her blood volume. Bloody urine suggests bladder or renal damage. Other nursing care is directed toward specific injuries and implementation of medical care.

Signs suggesting abruptio placentae (vaginal bleeding with uterine pain and tenderness) should be reported because this complication may occur with abdominal trauma.

The uterine height may also increase as the uterus fills with blood. Tachycardia usually precedes a fall in blood pressure. Fetal tachycardia or cessation of the FHR is likely to occur in more extensive uterine trauma or maternal hemorrhage. Fetal hemorrhage may occur with trauma to the placenta or the umbilical cord.

Once the woman's condition is stable, nursing care intensifies for the fetus. External monitoring is appropriate if the fetus has reached a viable gestational age. Preterm labor may occur but may not be recognized if the woman is unconscious or if pain from injuries overshadows discomfort from contractions. Recurrent restlessness or moaning may accompany contractions. *The nurse should palpate the woman's uterus for contractions periodically because they may not be evident on the fetal monitoring strip, especially if the fetus is small.*

✔ CHECK YOUR READING

21. What are the primary complications of a uterine inversion? How are they managed?
22. What are important nursing considerations for each kind of intrapartum emergency: Prolapsed umbilical cord? Uterine rupture? Uterine inversion? Amniotic fluid embolism?
23. What kinds of fetal injury may occur with maternal trauma during pregnancy?

Application of the Nursing Process
Intrapartum Emergencies

Nursing care of the woman with an intrapartum emergency overlaps with care in other situations discussed elsewhere. Much of the nursing care is collaborative and supports medical management. Parents may suffer loss if the fetus dies or the mother loses her ability to bear future children, as may occur with uterine rupture. One problem expected in any emergency situation is the emotional distress of the woman and her family.

Assessment

When an emergency occurs, the woman and her family have little time to absorb what has happened, simply because of its suddenness. In umbilical cord prolapse, for example, labor often has been uneventful up to that point. Suddenly, nurses place the woman in a strange position, apply oxygen, and pull her toward the operating room. The staff is clearly excited as well.

Under such circumstances, the woman and her family have a very narrow focus. They are obviously apprehensive and feel out of control. The woman or her partner may be immobilized by fear.

Analysis

The nursing diagnosis is "Anxiety related to unexpected occurrences because of the sudden development of complications." This diagnosis is expected to differ from the anxiety associated with preterm labor because the onset is acute. The anxiety also may lessen more quickly because the emergency is sometimes resolved quickly. Grief because of mother and baby may also occur, however.

Planning

The focus of a goal is very narrow in an emergency situation. Two appropriate goals, during and after the emergency, are that the woman and her family will do the following:

- Indicate an understanding of emergency procedures
- Express their feelings about the complication

Interventions

Although little time for discussion exists, explain honestly and simply what is occurring. To reduce fear and anxiety of the unknown, tell the woman what is happening and why. Include her partner and family if appropriate. Provide continued reassurance and support to the woman because her partner often must be excluded from the emergency or operating room when an emergency occurs.

The infant born in an emergency situation may need resuscitation or other supportive measures. Nurses and a neonatal nurse-practitioner or pediatrician from the neonatal intensive care unit, if available, usually are present at the birth to attend the infant. A neonatologist also may be present. Explain to the family who the other professionals are and their roles. If possible, explain what is being done to care for the baby.

After the emergency, give the woman and her family a chance to ask questions. The ability to absorb new knowledge during periods of severe anxiety is very limited. Adequate explanations afterward help them understand and assimilate the experience (Box 27-1).

■ Although the nurse is usually anxious in an emergency situation, keeping a calm attitude is important. The woman and her family quickly pick up on the staff's anxiety, and consequently their anxiety escalates. Remain with the woman to reduce fears of abandonment. If possible, hold her hand. Speak in a low, calm voice. The nurses involved should take time to talk out anxieties with colleagues after the emergency situation is over, as well.

BOX 27-1   **Nursing Diagnoses to Consider When Caring for Women with Intrapartum Complications**

Activity intolerance*
Anticipatory Grieving*
Anxiety*
Compromised or disabled individual or family coping
Readiness for enhanced individual or family coping
Deficient Diversional Activity*
Health-Seeking Behaviors*
Impaired Home Maintenance*
Interrupted Family Processes
Ineffective Health Maintenance
Powerlessness
Risk for infection*

*Nursing diagnoses explored in this chapter.

Evaluation

Evaluation of the goals is probably impossible until the emergency is over and the woman's physical condition stabilizes. Goals for this nursing diagnosis are achieved if the woman and her family do the following:

- Indicate that they understand the problem and the rationale for emergency procedures.
- Express, over several days, their feelings about what has occurred.

SUMMARY CONCEPTS

- Dysfunctional labor may occur because of abnormalities in the powers, the passenger, the passage, or the psyche. Combinations of abnormalities are common.
- Nursing care in dysfunctional labor focuses on prevention or prompt identification and action to correct additional complications such as fetal hypoxia, infection, injury to the mother or fetus, and postpartum hemorrhage.
- Premature rupture of the membranes is associated with infection as both a cause and a complication.
- The early indications of preterm labor are often vague. Prompt identification of preterm labor enables the most effective therapy to delay preterm birth.
- Nursing care for the woman at risk for a preterm birth before 34 weeks' gestation focuses on helping her delay birth long enough to provide time for fetal lung maturation with corticosteroids, allow transfer to a facility that has neonatal intensive care, or reach a gestation at which the infant's problems with immaturity are minimal.
- The main risk in prolonged pregnancy is reduced placental function. This may compromise the fetus during labor and result in meconium aspiration in the neonate. Dysfunctional labor may occur if a fetus continues growing during the prolonged pregnancy.
- The key intervention for umbilical cord prolapse is to relieve pressure on the umbilical cord and to expedite delivery.
- Be aware of women at risk for uterine rupture, and observe for signs and symptoms such as signs of shock, abdominal pain, a sense of tearing, chest pain, pain between the scapulae, abnormal fetal heart rate patterns, cessation of contractions, and palpation of the fetus outside the uterus. However, lesser degrees of uterine rupture or dehiscence may have minimal symptoms.
- Uterine inversion can be accompanied by massive blood loss and shock. Recovery care promotes uterine contraction and maintenance of adequate circulating volume.
- Anaphylactoid syndrome (formerly *amniotic fluid embolism*) is more likely to occur when labor is intense and the membranes have ruptured. The true causes of anaphylactoid syndrome are not known, because it is uncommon.
- The uterus is protected by the maternal pelvis during early pregnancy. As the uterus enlarges and ascends out of the pelvis, it is more vulnerable to trauma from direct impact. The fetus may be injured by disruption of the placenta, direct trauma, or either fetal or maternal hemorrhage.

ANSWERS TO CRITICAL THINKING EXERCISE 27-1, p. 702

When the fetus is in one of the occiput posterior positions, back pain is usually persistent because the fetal head presses on the mother's sacrum with each contraction, often called "back labor." Additionally, the fetal head has to rotate internally through a wider arc to ultimately reach an occiput anterior position for birth. This process prolongs labor in most women.

The nurse should take actions to make the woman more comfortable and promote rotation of the fetal head to an occiput anterior position. The nurse should encourage the woman to change positions regularly. Positions that cause her uterus to fall forward reduce pressure on her sacrum and straighten the pelvic curve somewhat to encourage fetal rotation. Examples of these are leaning forward while sitting, kneeling, or standing and a hands-and-knees position. Lunging toward her right side provides slightly more room on that side of her pelvis. If she wants to lie in bed, a left side-lying position favors fetal rotation toward an occiput anterior position. Analgesia may be helpful.

REFERENCES & READINGS

American Academy of Pediatrics and American College of Obstetricians and Gynecologists (ACOG). (2002). *Guidelines for perinatal care* (5th ed). Elk Grove, IL: Authors.

American College of Obstetricians and Gynecologists. (2000). *Operative vaginal delivery,* Practice Bulletin No. 17. Washington, DC: Author.

American College of Obstetricians and Gynecologists. (2001). *Assessment of risk factors for preterm birth,* Practice Bulletin No. 31. Washington, DC: Author.

American College of Obstetricians and Gynecologists. (2002). *Shoulder dystocia,* Practice Bulletin No. 40. Washington, DC: Author.

American College of Obstetricians and Gynecologists. (2003a). *Dystocia and augmentation of labor,* Practice Bulletin No. 49. Washington, DC: Author.

American College of Obstetricians and Gynecologists. (2003b). *Management of preterm labor,* Practice Bulletin No. 43. Washington, DC: Author.

Bashore, R.A., & Hayashi, R.H. (2004). Uterine contractility and dystocia. In N.F. Hacker, J.G. Moore, & J.C. Gambone (Eds.), *Essentials of obstetrics and gynecology* (4th ed., pp. 159-166). Philadelphia: Saunders.

Bernhardt, J., & Dorman, K. (2004). Preterm birth risk assessment tools: Exploring fetal fibronectin and cervical length for validating risk. *AWHONN Lifelines,* 8(1), 38-44.

Bowes, W.A., & Thorpe, J.M. (2004). Clinical aspects of normal and abnormal labor. In R.K. Creasy, R. Resnick, & J.D. Iams (Eds.), *Maternal-fetal medicine: Principles and practice* (5th ed., pp. 671-705). Philadelphia: Saunders.

Cesario, S.K. (2004). Reevaluation of Friedman's labor curve: A pilot study. *Journal of Obstetric, Gynecologic, and Neonatal Nursing,* 33(6), 713-722.

Clark, S.L. (2003). Critical care obstetrics. In J.R. Scott, R.S. Gibbs, B.Y. Karlan, & A.F. Haney (Eds.), *Danforth's obstetrics and gynecology* (9th ed., pp. 461-475). Philadelphia: Lippincott Williams & Wilkins.

Clark, S.L. (2004). Placenta previa and abruptio placentae. In R.K. Creasy, R. Resnik, & J.D. Iams (Eds.), *Maternal-fetal medicine: Principles and practice* (5th ed., pp. 707-722). Philadelphia: Saunders.

Cruikshank, D.P. (2003). Breech, other malpresentations and umbilical cord complications. In J.R. Scott, R.S. Gibbs, B.Y. Karlan, & A.F. Haney (Eds.), *Danforth's obstetrics and gynecology* (9th ed., pp. 381-395). Philadelphia: Lippincott Williams & Wilkins.

Cunningham, F.G., Gant, N.F., Leveno, K.J., Gilstrap, L.C., Hauth, J.C., & Wenstrom, K.D. (2001) *Williams obstetrics* (21st ed.). New York: McGraw-Hill.

Dudley, D.J. (2003). Complications of labor. In J.R. Scott, R.S. Gibbs, B.Y. Karlan, & A.F. Haney (Eds.), *Danforth's obstetrics and gynecology* (9th ed., pp. 397-417). Philadelphia: Lippincott Williams & Wilkins.

Gahart, B.L., & Nazareno, A.R. (2005). *2005 intravenous medications.* St. Louis: Mosby.

Garite, T.J. (2004). Premature rupture of the membranes. In R.K. Creasy, R. Resnick, & J.D. Iams (Eds.), *Maternal-fetal medicine: Principles and practice* (5th ed., pp. 723-739). Philadelphia: Saunders.

Goldenberg, R.L. (2002). The management of preterm labor. *Obstetrics & Gynecology,* 100(5 Pt 1), 1020-1037.

Gonik, B., & Foley, M.R. (2004). Intensive care monitoring of the critically ill pregnant patient. In R.K. Creasy, R. Resnick, & J.D. Iams (Eds.), *Maternal-fetal medicine: Principles and practice* (5th ed., pp. 925-951). Philadelphia: Saunders.

Guinn, D.A., & Gibbs, R.S. (2003). Preterm labor and delivery. In J.R. Scott, R.S. Gibbs, B.Y. Karlan, & A.F. Haney (Eds), *Danforth's obstetrics and gynecology* (9th ed., pp. 173-190). Philadelphia: Lippincott Williams & Wilkins.

Hamilton, B.E., Martin, J.A., Sutton, P.D. (2004). Births: Preliminary data for 2003. Retrieved March 2, 2005, from www.cdc.gov/nchs/data/nvsr/nvsr53/nvsr53_09.pdf.

Hobel, C.J. (2004). Obstetric complications: Preterm labor, PROM, IUGR, postterm pregnancy, and IUFD. In N.F. Hacker, J.G. Moore, & J.C. Gambone (Eds.), *Essentials of obstetrics and gynecology* (4th ed., pp. 167-182). Philadelphia: Saunders.

Hoebel, C.J., & Chang, A.B. (2004). Normal labor, delivery, and postpartum care: Anatomic considerations, obstetric analgesia and anesthesia, and resuscitation of the newborn. In N.F. Hacker, J.G. Moore, & J.C. Gambone (Eds.), *Essentials of obstetrics and gynecology* (4th ed., pp. 104-135). Philadelphia: Saunders.

Houry, D., & Abbott, J.T. (2004). Emergency management of the obstetric patient. In G.N. Burrow, T.P. Duffy, & J.A. Copel (Eds.), *Medical complications of pregnancy* (6th ed., pp. 235-245). Philadelphia: Saunders.

Iams, J.D. (2004). Abnormal cervical competence. In R.K. Creasy, R. Resnick, & J.D. Iams (Eds.), *Maternal-fetal medicine: Principles and practice* (5th ed., pp. 623-661). Philadelphia: Saunders.

Iams, J.D., & Creasy, R.K. (2004). Preterm labor and delivery. In R.K. Creasy, R. Resnick, & J.D. Iams (Eds.), *Maternal-fetal medicine: Principles and practice* (5th ed., pp. 623-661). Philadelphia: Saunders.

Kendrick, J.M., & Simpson, K.R. (2001). Childbirth. In K.R. Simpson & P.A. Creehan (Eds.), *AWHONN perinatal nursing* (2nd ed., pp. 298-377). Philadelphia: Lippincott Williams & Wilkins.

Kochanek, K.D., Murphy, S.L., Anderson, R.N., & Scott, C. (2004). Deaths: Final data for 2002. *National Vital Statistics Reports* 53(5). Hyattsville, MD: National Center for Health Statistics. Retrieved March 2, 2005, from www.cdc.gov/nchs/data/nvsr/nvsr53/nvsr53_05.pdf.

Malone, F.D., & D'Alton, M.E. (2004). Multiple gestation: Clinical characteristics and management. In R.K. Creasy, R. Resnick, & J.D. Iams (Eds.), *Maternal-fetal medicine: Principles and practice* (5th ed., pp. 513-536). Philadelphia: Saunders.

Mayberry, L.J., Wood, S.H., Strange, L.B., Lee, L., Heisler, D.R., & Nielsen-Smith, K. (2000). *Second stage labor management: Promotion of evidence-based practice and a collaborative approach to patient care.* Washington, DC: Association of Women's Health, Obstetric and Neonatal Nurses.

Mercer, B.M. (2004). Assessment and induction of fetal pulmonary maturity. In R.K. Creasy, R. Resnick, & J.D. Iams (Eds.), *Maternal-fetal medicine: Principles and practice* (5th ed., pp. 451-463). Philadelphia: Saunders.

Mercer, B.M., Goldenberg, R.L., Meis, P.J., Moawad, A.H., Shellhaas, C., Das, A., et al. (2000). The Preterm Prediction Study: Prediction of preterm premature rupture of membranes through clinical findings and ancillary testing. *Obstetrics & Gynecology, 183*(3), 738-745.

Moore, T.R. (2004). Multifetal gestation and malpresentation. In N.F. Hacker, J.G. Moore, & J.C. Gambone (Eds.), *Essentials of obstetrics and gynecology* (4th ed., pp. 183-196). Philadelphia: Saunders.

Moos, M.K. (2004). Understanding prematurity: Sorting fact from fiction. *AWHONN Lifelines, 8*(1), 32-37.

National Institutes of Health. (2000). Antenatal corticosteroids revisited: Repeat statement. *NIH Consensus Statement, 17*(2). Retrieved Feb. 2, 2004, from http://consensus.nih.gov/cons/112/112_statement.pdf.

Poole, J., Burke, M.E., Freda, M.C., Kendrick, J.M., Luppi, C.J., Krening, C.F., Dauphinee, J.D., & Sosa, M.E.B. (2001). High-risk pregnancy. In K.R. Simpson & P.A. Creehan (Eds.), *AWHONN perinatal nursing* (2nd ed., pp. 173-296). Philadelphia: Lippincott Williams & Wilkins.

Rao, P., & Andersen, H.F. (2003). Outcome of preterm premature rupture of membranes: A contemporary perspective. *American Journal of Obstetrics & Gynecology, 189*(6), S171.

Resnik, J.L., & Resnik, R. (2004). Post-term pregnancy. In R.K. Creasy, R. Resnick, & J.D. Iams (Eds.), *Maternal-fetal medicine: Principles and practice* (5th ed., pp. 663-669). Philadelphia: Saunders.

Ruiz, R.J., Fullerton, J., & Brown, C.E.L. (2004). The utility of fFN for the prediction of preterm birth in twin gestations. *Journal of Obstetric, Gynecologic, and Neonatal Nursing, 33*(4), 446-454.

Salmon, B., & Bruick-Sorge, C. (2003). Pneumonia in pregnant women: Exploring this high risk complication and its links to preterm labor. *AWHONN Lifelines, 7*(1), 48-52.

Simpson, K.R., & Knox, G.E. (2001). Fundal pressure during the second stage of labor. *MCN: American Journal of Maternal/Child Nursing, 26*(2), 64-70.

Stringer, M., Miesnik, S.R., Brown, L., Martz, A.H., & Marcones, G. (2004). Nursing care of the patient with preterm premature rupture of membranes. *MCN: American Journal of Maternal/Child Nursing, 29*(3), 144-150.

Wener, M.E., & Lavigne, S.E. (2004). Can periodontal disease lead to premature delivery? *AWHONN Lifelines, 8*(5), 422-431.

Postpartum Maternal Complications

OBJECTIVES

After studying this chapter, you should be able to:

1. Describe postpartum hemorrhage in terms of predisposing factors, causes, clinical signs, and therapeutic management.
2. Explain major causes, clinical signs, and therapeutic management of subinvolution.
3. Describe three major thromboembolic disorders (superficial venous thrombosis, deep vein thrombosis, pulmonary embolism) in terms of predisposing factors, causes, clinical signs, and therapeutic management.
4. Discuss puerperal infection in terms of location, predisposing factors, causes, signs and symptoms, and therapeutic management.
5. Describe two major affective disorders (postpartum depression and psychosis).
6. Describe the role of the nurse in the management of women who have a postpartum complication.

Go to your Student CD-ROM for Review Questions keyed to these Objectives.

DEFINITIONS

Atony Absence or lack of usual muscle tone.

Dilation and Curettage (D&C) Stretching of the cervical os to permit suctioning or scraping of the walls of the uterus. The procedure is performed in abortion, to obtain samples of uterine lining tissue for laboratory examination, and during the postpartum period to remove retained fragments of placental tissue.

Embolus A mass which may be composed of a thrombus (blood clot) or amniotic fluid released into the bloodstream to cause obstruction of pulmonary vessels.

Hematoma Localized collection of blood in a space or tissue.

Hydramnios Excess volume of amniotic fluid (more than 2000 ml at term). Also called *polyhydramnios*.

Hypovolemia Abnormally decreased volume of circulating fluid in the body.

Hypovolemic Shock Acute peripheral circulatory failure resulting from loss of circulating blood volume.

Placenta Accreta A placenta that is abnormally adherent to the uterus. If the condition is more advanced, it is called *placenta increta* (the placenta extends into the uterine muscle) or *placenta percreta* (the placenta extends through the uterine muscle).

Psychosis Mental state in which a person's ability to recognize reality, communicate, and relate to others is impaired.

Subinvolution A slower-than-expected return of the uterus to its nonpregnancy size after childbirth.

Thrombus Collection of blood factors, primarily platelets and fibrin, that may cause vascular obstruction.

Pregnancy and childbirth are natural functions that most women recover from without complication. However, nurses must be aware of problems that may occur and their effect on the family. The most common physiologic complications are hemorrhage, thromboembolic disorders, and infection. Complications that are psychogenic in origin include postpartum depression (PPD) and postpartum psychosis.

POSTPARTUM HEMORRHAGE

Postpartum hemorrhage has been defined as blood loss of more than 500 ml after vaginal birth or 1000 ml after cesarean birth. Estimating blood loss is difficult, especially when bleeding is brisk or when hemorrhage is concealed. Furthermore, blood loss during childbirth is frequently underestimated and constitutes only about half the actual loss (Cunningham et al., 2005). A more measurable definition of hemorrhage is a decrease in hematocrit of 10 percent or more since admission or a need for a blood transfusion (American College of Obstetricians, 1998). Hemorrhage in the first 24 hours after childbirth is called *early postpartum hemorrhage*. When it occurs after 24 hours, it is called *late postpartum hemorrhage*.

Postpartum hemorrhage complicates approximately 5% of deliveries (Katz & Wolfe, 2002). Hemorrhage, along with pulmonary embolism, infection, and hypertensive disorders, is a leading cause of maternal morbidity and mortality.

Early Postpartum Hemorrhage

Early postpartum hemorrhage is most common during the first hour after delivery (Simpson & James, 2005). The two major causes of early postpartum hemorrhage are uterine atony and trauma to the birth canal during labor and delivery. Hematomas and retention of placental fragments are other causes. Abnormalities of the third stage of labor, such as placenta accreta (abnormal adherence of the placenta to the uterine wall) and inversion of the uterus, are described in Chapter 27. Disseminated intravascular coagulation (DIC) is discussed in Chapter 25.

UTERINE ATONY

Uterine atony causes 75% to 85% of cases of early hemorrhage (Higgins, 2004). *Atony* refers to lack of muscle tone that results in failure of the uterine muscle fibers to contract firmly around blood vessels when the placenta separates. The relaxed muscles allow rapid bleeding from the endometrial arteries at the placental site. Bleeding continues until the uterine muscle fibers contract to stop the flow of blood. Figure 28-1 illustrates the effect of uterine contraction on the size of the placental site and the amount of bleeding that occurs.

PREDISPOSING FACTORS. Knowledge of factors that increase the risk of uterine atony can be used to anticipate and therefore reduce excessive bleeding. Overdistention of the uterus from any cause (multiple gestations, a large infant, hydramnios) makes it more difficult for the uterus to contract with enough firmness to prevent excessive bleeding. Multiparity results in muscle fibers that have been stretched repeatedly, and these flaccid muscle fibers may not remain contracted after birth.

Intrapartum factors include contractions that were barely effective, resulting in prolonged labor, or contractions that were excessively vigorous, which may have resulted in precipitate labor. Labor that was induced or that was aug-

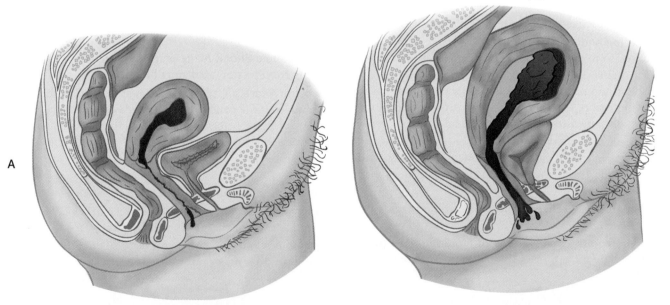

A

Contracted uterus

B

Uterine atony
Uterus remains inadequately contracted

Figure 28-1 ■ A, When the uterus remains contracted, the placental site is smaller, so bleeding is minimal. **B,** If uterine muscles fail to contract around the endometrial arteries at the placental site, hemorrhage occurs.

Overdistention of the uterus (multiple gestations, large infant, hydramnios)
Multiparity (five or more)
Precipitate labor or delivery
Prolonged labor
Use of forceps or vacuum extractor
Cesarean birth
Manual removal of the placenta
Previous postpartum hemorrhage
Placenta previa or accreta
Drugs: oxytocin, prostaglandins, tocolytics, or magnesium sulfate
General anesthesia
Chorioamnionitis
Clotting disorders
Previous postpartum hemorrhage or uterine surgery
Disseminated intravascular coagulation

mented with oxytocin is more likely to be followed by post-delivery uterine atony and hemorrhage. Retention of a large segment of the placenta does not allow the uterus to contract firmly and therefore can result in uterine atony. DIC also may be the cause of postpartum hemorrhage. Box 28-1 summarizes predisposing factors.

CLINICAL SIGNS. Major signs of uterine atony include:

- A uterine fundus that is difficult to locate
- A soft or "boggy" feel when the fundus is located
- A uterus that becomes firm as it is massaged but loses its tone when massage is stopped
- A fundus that is located above the expected level, which is at or near the umbilicus
- Excessive lochia, especially if it is bright red
- Excessive clots expelled

For the first 24 hours after birth the uterus should feel like a firmly contracted ball roughly the size of a large grapefruit. It should be located easily at about the level of the umbilicus. Lochia should be dark red and moderate in amount. If a peripad is saturated in an hour, a large amount of blood is considered to have been lost, and saturation in 15 minutes represents an excessive loss of blood in the early postpartum period (Scoggin, 2004). The nurse must realize that although bleeding may be profuse and dramatic, a constant steady trickle is just as dangerous (see Chapter 17 for assessment of the uterus and lochia).

THERAPEUTIC MANAGEMENT. Nurses are with the mother during the hours after childbirth and are responsible for assessments and initial management of uterine atony. If the uterus is not firmly contracted, the first intervention is to massage the fundus until it is firm and to express clots that may have accumulated in the uterus. One hand is placed just above the symphysis pubis to support the lower uterine segment while the other hand gently but firmly massages the fundus in a circular motion. Figure 28-2 illustrates correct hand placement for fundal massage.

Clots that may have accumulated in the uterine cavity interfere with the ability of the uterus to contract effectively. They are expressed by applying firm but gentle pressure on the fundus in the direction of the vagina. It is critical that the uterus is contracted firmly before clots are expressed. *Pushing on an uncontracted uterus could invert the uterus and cause massive hemorrhage and rapid shock.*

If the uterus does not remain contracted as a result of uterine massage or if the fundus is displaced, the problem may be a distended bladder. A full bladder lifts the uterus, moving it up and to the side, preventing effective contraction of the uterine muscles. The nurse should assist the

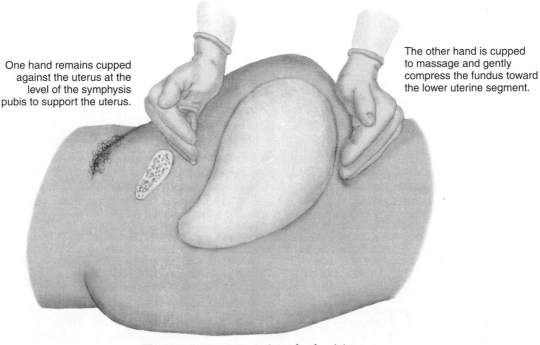

One hand remains cupped against the uterus at the level of the symphysis pubis to support the uterus.

The other hand is cupped to massage and gently compress the fundus toward the lower uterine segment.

Figure 28-2 ■ Technique for fundal massage.

mother to urinate or catheterize her, if necessary, to correct uterine atony caused by bladder distension.

Pharmacologic measures also may be necessary to maintain firm contraction of the uterus. A rapid intravenous infusion of dilute oxytocin (Pitocin) often increases uterine tone and controls bleeding (see "Drug Guide: Oxytocin," p. 370). Methylergonovine (Methergine) may be given intramuscularly but elevates blood pressure and should not be given to a woman who is hypertensive (see "Drug Guide: Methylergonovine"). Analogues of prostaglandin $F_{2\alpha}$ ($PGF_{2\alpha}$) (carboprost tromethamine, Hemabate, Prostin) are often given intramuscularly or into the uterine muscle if oxytocin is ineffective in controlling uterine atony (Hayashi & Gambone, 2004). (See "Drug Guide: Carboprost Tromethamine.") Misoprostol (Cytotec) is a less expensive drug that also may be used to control bleeding.

If uterine massage and pharmacologic measures are ineffective in stopping uterine bleeding, the physician or nurse-midwife may use bimanual compression of the uterus to stop the bleeding. In this procedure, one hand is inserted into the vagina and the other compresses the uterus through the abdominal wall (Figure 28-3). The woman may need to return to the delivery area for exploration of the uterine cavity and removal of placental fragments that interfere with uterine contraction.

Ligation of the uterine or hypogastric artery or embolization (occlusion) of pelvic arteries may be necessary if other measures are not effective. Hysterectomy is a last resort to save the life of a woman with uncontrollable postpartum hemorrhage.

Hemorrhage requires prompt replacement of intravascular fluid volume. Lactated Ringer's solution, normal saline,

DRUG GUIDE

METHYLERGONOVINE (METHERGINE)

Classification: Oxytocic.

Action: Stimulates sustained contraction of the uterus and causes arterial vasoconstriction.

Indications: Used for the prevention and treatment of postpartum or postabortion hemorrhage caused by uterine atony or subinvolution.

Dosage and Route: Usual dosage is 0.2 mg intramuscularly (IM) every 2 to 4 hours for a maximum of five doses. Change to the oral route 0.2 mg every 6 to 8 hours for a maximum of 7 days. Intravenous use not recommended; use in life-threatening emergency only; may cause severe hypertension.

Absorption: Well absorbed after oral or intramuscular route.

Excretion: Metabolized by the liver, excreted in the feces and urine.

Contraindications and Precautions: Methylergonovine should never be used during pregnancy or to induce labor. Do not use IM if the mother is hypersensitive to ergot. Contraindicated for women with hypertension, severe hepatic or renal disease, coronary artery disease, peripheral vascular disease, hypocalcemia, or sepsis or before the fourth stage of labor.

Adverse Reactions: Nausea, vomiting, uterine cramping, hypertension, dizziness, headache, dyspnea, chest pain, palpitations, peripheral ischemia, and uterine and gastrointestinal cramping.

Nursing Considerations: Before administering the medication, assess the blood pressure. Follow facility protocol if medication must be withheld (usually if the reading is 136/90). Caution the mother to avoid smoking, because nicotine constricts blood vessels. Remind her to report any adverse reactions.

DRUG GUIDE

CARBOPROST TROMETHAMINE (HEMABATE, PROSTIN/15M)

Classification: Prostaglandin, oxytocic.

Action: Stimulates contraction of the uterus.

Indications: Used for the treatment of postpartum hemorrhage caused by uterine atony. Also used for abortion.

Dosage and Route: Postpartum hemorrhage: 250 micrograms intramuscularly. May repeat at 15- to 90-minute intervals for up to eight doses.

Absorption: Metabolized by the liver and by enzymes in the lungs.

Excretion: Primarily excreted in urine.

Contraindications and Precautions: Contraindicated for women with hypersensitivity to carboprost or other prostaglandins; acute pelvic inflammatory disease; cardiac, pulmonary, renal, or hepatic disease. Use caution if the woman has a history of asthma, hypotension or hypertension, anemia, jaundice, diabetes, epilepsy.

Adverse Reactions and Side Effects: Excessive dose may cause tetanic contraction and laceration or uterine rupture. May cause uterine hypertonus if used with oxytocin. Nausea, vomiting, diarrhea (frequent), fever, chills, facial flushing, headache, hypertension or hypotension.

Nursing Considerations: Should be refrigerated. Give via deep intramuscular injection and aspirate carefully to avoid intravenous injection. Rotate sites if repeated. Monitor vital signs. Administer antiemetics and antidiarrheals as ordered.

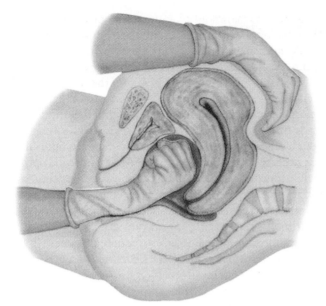

Figure 28-3 ■ Bimanual compression. One hand is inserted in the vagina, and the other compresses the uterus through the abdominal wall.

or other plasma extenders, whole blood, or packed cells may be used. Enough fluid should be given to maintain a urine flow of at least 30 ml and preferably 60 ml/hr (Cunningham et al., 2005). The nurse often is responsible for obtaining properly typed and cross-matched blood and, if they are not already present, inserting large-bore intravenous (IV) lines that are capable of carrying whole blood.

TRAUMA

Trauma to the birth canal is the second most common cause of early postpartum hemorrhage. Trauma can include vaginal, cervical, or perineal lacerations as well as hematomas.

PREDISPOSING FACTORS. Many of the same factors that increase the risk of uterine atony increase the risk of soft-tissue trauma during childbirth. For example, trauma to the birth canal is more likely to occur if the infant is large or if labor and delivery occur rapidly. Induction and augmentation of labor and use of assistive devices, such as a vacuum extractor, increase the risk of tissue trauma.

LACERATIONS. The perineum, vagina, and cervix and the area around the urethral meatus are the most common sites for lacerations. Cervical lacerations occur frequently when the cervix dilates rapidly during the first stage of labor. Lacerations of the vagina, perineum, and periurethral area usually occur during the second stage of labor, when the fetal head descends rapidly or when assistive devices such as forceps or a vacuum extractor are used to assist in delivery of the fetal head.

Lacerations of the birth canal should always be suspected if excessive uterine bleeding continues when the fundus is contracted firmly and is at the expected location. Bleeding from lacerations of the genital tract often is bright red, in contrast to the darker red color of lochia. Bleeding may be heavy or may appear to be minor, but a steady trickle (dribble or oozing) of blood continues.

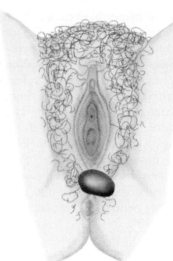

Figure 28-4 ■ A vulvar hematoma is caused by rapid bleeding into soft tissue, and it causes severe pain and feelings of pressure.

HEMATOMAS. Hematomas occur when there is bleeding into loose connective tissue while overlying tissue remains intact. Hematomas develop as a result of blood vessel injury in spontaneous deliveries and deliveries in which forceps or vacuum extractors are used. Hematomas may be found in vulvar, vaginal, and retroperitoneal areas.

The rapid bleeding into soft tissue may cause a visible vulvar hematoma, a discolored bulging mass that is sensitive to touch (Figure 28-4). Hematomas in the vagina or retroperitoneal areas cannot be seen. Hematomas produce deep, severe, unrelieved pain and feelings of pressure. Formation of a hematoma also should be suspected if the mother demonstrates systemic signs of concealed blood loss, such as falling blood pressure or tachycardia, when the fundus is firm and lochia is within normal limits.

THERAPEUTIC MANAGEMENT. When postpartum hemorrhage is caused by trauma of the birth canal, surgical repair often is necessary. Visualizing lacerations of the vagina or cervix is difficult, and it is necessary to return the mother to the delivery area, where surgical lights are available. She is placed in a lithotomy position and carefully draped. Surgical asepsis is required while the laceration is being visualized and repaired.

Small hematomas usually reabsorb naturally, but large hematomas may require incision, evacuation of the clots, and location of the bleeding vessel so that it can be ligated.

Late Postpartum Hemorrhage

The most common causes of late postpartum hemorrhage are subinvolution (delayed return of the uterus to its nonpregnant size and consistency) and fragments of placenta that remain attached to the myometrium when the placenta is delivered. Clots form around the retained fragments, and excessive bleeding can occur when the clots slough away several days after delivery.

Late postpartum hemorrhage caused by retained placental fragments is generally preventable. The nurse-midwife or physician carefully inspects the placenta to determine whether it is intact. If a portion of the placenta is missing, the health care provider can manually explore the uterus, locate the missing fragments, and remove them soon after delivery of the placenta.

Late postpartum hemorrhage, which typically occurs without warning at 7 to 14 days after delivery, can be dangerous for the unsuspecting mother. Families must be taught how to assess the fundus and the normal duration of lochia. They must be instructed to notify their health care provider if bleeding persists or becomes unusually heavy.

PREDISPOSING FACTORS

Attempts to deliver the placenta before it separates from the uterine wall, manual removal of the placenta, and placenta accreta are the primary predisposing factors for retention of placental fragments.

THERAPEUTIC MANAGEMENT

Initial treatment for late postpartum hemorrhage is directed toward control of the excessive bleeding. Oxytocin, methylergonovine, and prostaglandins are the most commonly used pharmacologic measures. Placental fragments often are dislodged and swept out of the uterus by the bleeding, and if the bleeding subsides when oxytocin is administered, no other treatment is necessary. Sonography can identify placental fragments that remain in the uterus. If bleeding continues or recurs, dilation and curettage may be necessary to remove fragments. Broad-spectrum antibiotics also may be given if postpartum infection is suspected because of uterine tenderness, foul-smelling lochia, or fever.

Application of the Nursing Process
Excessive Bleeding

Assessment

The initial postpartum assessment includes a chart review to determine whether any factors such as prolonged labor, birth of a large infant, or use of assistive devices increase the risk for the woman to bleed excessively.

✔ CHECK YOUR READING

1. Why does the nurse examine the mother's prenatal record and her labor and delivery record?
2. Why is a mother who has given birth to twins at increased risk for postpartum hemorrhage?
3. Can the nurse be positive that bleeding is controlled when the fundus is firm and the lochia is moderate? Why or why not?
4. How is uterine atony treated?
5. How are hematomas treated?

UTERINE ATONY

Priority assessments for uterine atony include those of the fundus, bladder, lochia, vital signs, and skin temperature and color. Assess the consistency and the location of the uterine fundus. The fundus should be firmly contracted, at or near the level of the umbilicus, and midline. If the uterus is not firmly contracted, the fundus feels soft (boggy) and bleeding from the placental site is rapid and continuous. If the fundus is above the level of the umbilicus and displaced, a full bladder may be the cause of excessive bleeding. A full bladder lifts the uterus and impedes contraction, which allows excessive bleeding. The accumulation of clots also expands the uterus, making contraction difficult and resulting in continued bleeding. (See Procedure 17-1 [p. 410] for complete information about assessing the fundus.)

When inspecting for blood loss, always ask the woman to turn on her side because blood that pools under her is not visible when checking pads from the front. Large amounts of blood could be collecting undetected underneath her. Although bleeding may be profuse and dramatic, a continuing steady trickle may lead to significant blood loss that becomes increasingly life threatening.

Estimating the volume of lochia is difficult by visual examination of peripads. More accurate information is obtained by weighing peripads and bed liners before and after use and subtracting the difference. One gram (weight) equals approximately 1 ml (volume).

Measure vital signs at least every 15 minutes to detect trends, such as tachycardia or a decrease in pulse pressure (difference between systolic and diastolic blood pressure), that may reveal a deteriorating status in a woman with significant blood loss. Initially the body compensates for excessive bleeding by constricting the peripheral blood vessels and shunting blood to vital organs. This can be misleading because the vital signs may remain normal although the woman is becoming hypovolemic.

The skin should be warm and dry, mucous membranes of the lips and mouth should be pink, and capillary return should occur within 3 seconds when the nails are blanched. These signs confirm adequate circulating volume to perfuse the peripheral tissue.

TRAUMA

If the fundus is firm but bleeding is excessive, the cause may be lacerations of the cervix or birth canal. Inspect the perineum to determine whether a laceration is visible in that area. Lacerations of the cervix or vagina are not visible, but bleeding in the presence of a firmly contracted uterus suggests a laceration. This sign warrants examination of the vaginal walls and the cervix by the health care provider.

Assess comfort level. If the mother complains of deep, severe pelvic or rectal pain or if vital signs or skin changes suggest hemorrhage but excessive bleeding is not obvious, the cause may be concealed bleeding and the formation of a hematoma. Examine the vulva for bulging masses or dis-

TABLE 28-1 Nursing Assessments for Postpartum Hemorrhage

Assessments	Abnormal Signs and Symptoms	Nursing Implications
Chart review	Presence of predisposing factors	Perform more frequent evaluations.
Fundus	Soft, boggy, displaced	Massage, express clots, assist to void or catheterize, notify primary health care provider if measures are ineffective.
Lochia	Bleeding (steady trickle or profuse flow); heavy: saturation of more than 1 pad per hour; exccessive: more than 1 pad in 15 min)	Assess for trauma, save and weigh pads so estimation of blood loss will be more accurate. Notify health care provider.
Vital signs	Tachycardia, decreasing pulse pressure, falling blood pressure	Report signs of excessive blood loss.
Comfort level	Severe pelvic or rectal pain	Signs of hematoma, usually perineal or vaginal; examine vulva for masses or discoloration, report findings.
Skin	Cool, damp, pale	Signs of hypovolemia; vigilant assessment and management by entire health care team is necessary.

coloration of the skin. However, a hematoma developing in the vagina or in the retroperitoneal area will not be obvious when the vulva is examined. Table 28-1 summarizes assessments, abnormal signs and symptoms, and nursing implications.

Analysis

Certain signs and symptoms, such as uterine atony that does not respond to massage, excessive lochia, pelvic or rectal pain, or changes in vital signs, may be the earliest signs of postpartum hemorrhage. Postpartum hemorrhage is a potential complication that requires the efforts of the health care team to control the hemorrhage and prevent further complications such as hypovolemic shock.

Planning

Client-centered goals are inappropriate for this potential complication because the nurse cannot manage postpartum hemorrhage independently but must confer with the physician or nurse-midwife for medical orders to treat the condition. Planning should reflect the nurse's responsibility to:

- Monitor for signs of postpartum hemorrhage
- Perform actions to minimize postpartum hemorrhage and prevent hypovolemic shock
- Consult with the health care provider if signs of postpartum hemorrhage are observed

Interventions

PREVENTING HEMORRHAGE

Every nurse should be aware of factors that put the new mother at risk for postpartum hemorrhage. This knowledge alerts the nurse to be particularly vigilant in monitoring these women so that excessive bleeding can be anticipated and minimized.

When predisposing factors are present, initiate frequent assessments. Many hospitals and birth centers have a standard of care that calls for assessments every 15 minutes during the first hour after delivery, every 30 minutes for the next 2 hours, and hourly for the next 4 hours. This may not be adequate for the woman at known risk for postpartum hem-

CRITICAL TO REMEMBER

Signs of Postpartum Hemorrhage

An uncontracted uterus
Large gush or slow, steady trickle or ooze of blood from the vagina
Saturation of more than one peripad per hour
Severe, unrelieved perineal or rectal pain
Tachycardia

orrhage, however, because bleeding occurs rapidly. A delay in assessment may result in a great deal of blood loss.

COLLABORATING WITH THE HEALTH CARE PROVIDER

When excessive bleeding is suspected, begin uterine massage. Weigh blood-soaked pads and linens to determine the amount of blood loss. If massage is not effective in controlling bleeding promptly, notify the physician or nurse-midwife. Save any tissue or clots passed.

In some facilities, protocols permit nurses to initiate specific laboratory studies, such as hemoglobin and hematocrit levels and typing and cross-matching of blood, so that blood is available should transfusions be necessary. Other laboratory studies that may be ordered include platelet counts, prothrombin time, activated partial thromboplastin time, fibrinogen, fibrin degradation products, and fibrin split products. Many protocols also allow the nurse to start IV fluids or increase the flow rate of an existing IV while the health care provider is being informed of the mother's condition. These actions do not substitute for notifying the health care provider, but they do allow nurses to make initial interventions quickly.

Keep the woman on bed rest to increase venous return and maintain cardiac output. The Trendelenburg position may interfere with cardiac function and is not advised. Continue assessments, call for assistance, and save all pads, linen savers, and linen so that an accurate estimation of blood loss can be made. Assistance is necessary, because one nurse must continue to massage the uncontracted uterus and perform and record assessments while the other notifies the health care provider of the mother's condition.

When notifying the provider, document the time and content of each communication. For example, "1300: Dr. X notified of difficulty maintaining uterine contraction and continued excessive bleeding. Requested Dr. X to see client. Orders received."

Administer medications and fluids ordered by the health care provider and evaluate their effect. For example, add the prescribed amount of oxytocin to the IV solution and infuse the solution at the prescribed rate. When large amounts of oxytocin are used, listen to breath sounds to identify signs of fluid overload (Bowes & Thorp, 2004). Evaluate the effect of the medication on the uterus, and relay this information to the health care provider. Physicians and nurse-midwives depend on the nurse for accurate information, and they base medical management on information relayed by the nurse.

If measures fail to control bleeding, notify the health care provider so that additional procedures can be initiated. These may include preparation for operative intervention (surgical preparation, consent signed for operative procedure, or confirmation that blood replacement is available).

PROVIDING SUPPORT FOR THE FAMILY

The unusual activity of the hospital staff may make the mother and her family anxious. Be alert to their nonverbal cues, and when they appear frightened acknowledge their feelings. Keeping the family informed is one of the most effective ways of reducing anxiety.

■ Acknowledge the anxiety and provide simple appropriate explanations of the activity. "I know all this activity must be frightening. She is bleeding a little more than we would like and we are doing several things at once."

POSTHEMORRHAGE CARE

After the hemorrhage is controlled, continue to assess the woman frequently for a resumption of bleeding. The woman may be anemic and fatigued. Allow rest periods and organize work to help her conserve energy. Because the woman may experience orthostatic hypotension, assist her in getting out of bed after dangling her legs and assess for dizziness and low blood pressure. Encourage intake of foods high in iron.

Evaluation

Although client-centered goals are not developed for potential complications (collaborative problems), the nurse collects and compares data with established norms and judges whether the data are within normal limits. If problems arise, the nurse acts to minimize hemorrhage and notifies the health care provider.

HYPOVOLEMIC SHOCK

During and after giving birth, the woman can tolerate blood loss that approaches the volume of blood added during pregnancy (approximately 1500-2000 ml) (Cunningham et

---

CRITICAL THINKING EXERCISE 28-1

Dolores Navarra, a 26-year-old gravida 4, para 3, has a rapid labor and delivers a baby boy weighing 4000 g (8 lb, 12 oz). Two hours later, she is transferred to postpartum. At the initial postpartum assessment, Dolores' fundus is firm, at the level of the umbilicus. Lochia is heavy, with occasional small clots expressed. Vital signs are unchanged from prenatal norms.

Questions
1. Do any "red flags" suggest a potential problem or complication? What actions should the nurse take?
2. The nurse observes that the fundus is soft and lochia is excessive. What are the priority interventions? Why?
3. Within an hour the fundus becomes "boggy" again and is located 3 cm above the umbilicus and displaced to the right. What is the priority nursing action? Why?
4. Dolores voids 500 ml. The fundus is difficult to locate, however, and lochia is excessive. What is the next nursing action? Why?

---

al., 2005). A woman who was anemic before birth has less reserve than a mother with normal blood values. When more than this reserve is lost, hypovolemic shock can ensue. Hypovolemia endangers vital organs by depriving them of oxygen. The brain, heart, and kidneys are especially vulnerable to hypoxia and may suffer damage in a brief period.

How the Body Compensates for Hypovolemia

Recognition of hypovolemic shock may be delayed because the body activates compensatory mechanisms that mask the severity of the problem. Carotid and aortic baroreceptors are stimulated to constrict peripheral blood vessels. This shunts blood to the central circulation and away from less essential organs, such as the skin and extremities. The skin becomes pale and cold, but cardiac output and perfusion of vital organs are maintained.

In addition, the adrenal glands release catecholamines, which compensate for decreased blood volume by promoting vasoconstriction in nonessential organs, increasing the heart rate, and raising the blood pressure. As a result, blood pressure remains normal initially, although a decrease in pulse pressure may be noted. The tachycardia that develops is an early sign of compensation for excessive blood loss.

As shock worsens, the compensatory mechanisms fail and physiologic insults spiral. Inadequate organ perfusion and decreased cellular oxygen for metabolism result in a buildup of lactic acid and the development of metabolic acidosis. Decreased serum pH (acidosis) results in vasodilation, which further increases bleeding.

Eventually, circulating volume becomes insufficient to perfuse cardiac and brain tissue. Cellular death occurs as a result of anoxia, and the mother dies.

Clinical Signs and Symptoms

Tachycardia is one of the earliest signs of hypovolemic shock, and even gradual increases in the pulse rate should be noted. A decrease in blood pressure and narrowing of pulse pressure occurs when the circulating volume of blood is sufficiently decreased. The respiratory rate increases as the woman becomes more anxious and attempts to take in more oxygen to overcome the need that is created when hemoglobin is inadequate to transport oxygen adequately.

Skin changes also provide early cues. Vasoconstriction in the skin causes it to become pale and cool to the touch. As hemorrhage worsens, the skin changes become more obvious; pallor increases, and the skin becomes cold and clammy.

As shock progresses, changes also occur in the central nervous system. The mother becomes anxious, then confused, and finally lethargic when blood loss totals 30% to 40% of the total blood volume. Urine output also decreases from more than 30 ml/hr in early shock to less than 5 ml/hr when more than 40% of the blood is lost. Eventually, urine output stops.

Therapeutic Management

The goals of therapy are to control bleeding and prevent hypovolemic shock from becoming irreversible. A second IV line should be inserted with a large-bore (16- to 18-gauge) catheter capable of carrying whole blood. Central intravenous catheters may be placed. Sufficient fluid volume is infused to produce a urinary output of at least 30 ml/hr. At the same time, the health care team makes every effort to locate the source of bleeding and to stop the loss of blood. Interventions may include uterine packing; ligation of the uterine, ovarian, or hypogastric artery; or hysterectomy.

Nursing Considerations

One person should be assigned to evaluate and record vital signs. Blood pressure and pulse should be assessed every 3 to 5 minutes. The location and consistency of the fundus, amount of lochia, skin temperature and color, and capillary return also are assessed. A pulse oximeter should be applied to determine oxygen saturation of the blood. Nurses often follow facility protocols that allow them to draw blood for hemoglobin, hematocrit, clotting studies, and type and cross-match.

A urinary catheter should be inserted so that hourly urinary output can be measured. The catheter is also necessary if a surgical procedure to control the hemorrhage is required. Oxygen may be needed to increase the saturation of fewer red blood cells. It should be administered by tight face mask at 8 to 10 L/min or as directed by the health care provider.

Nurses are also responsible for administering fluids, whole blood, and medications as directed and for reporting their effectiveness. In addition, nurses must make every effort to provide information and emotional support to the woman and her family.

Home Care

Nurses who work in home care or nurse-managed postpartum clinics must be aware that women who have had postpartum hemorrhage are subject to a variety of complications. In general, they are exhausted, and it may take weeks for them to feel well again. Anemia often results, and a course

of iron therapy may be prescribed to restore hemoglobin level. Activity may be restricted until strength returns. Some women need extra assistance with housework and care of the new infant. Exhaustion may interfere with bonding and attachment. Because extensive blood loss increases the risk of postpartum infection, the woman and her family must be taught to observe for specific signs and symptoms.

SUBINVOLUTION OF THE UTERUS

Subinvolution refers to a slower-than-expected return of the uterus to its nonpregnant size after childbirth. Normally the uterus descends at the rate of about 1 cm or one fingerbreadth per day. By 10 days, it is no longer palpable above the symphysis pubis. The endometrial lining has sloughed off as part of the lochia, and the site of placental attachment is well healed by 6 weeks after childbirth if involution progresses as expected.

The most common causes of subinvolution are retained placental fragments and pelvic infection. Signs of subinvolution include prolonged discharge of lochia, irregular or excessive uterine bleeding, and sometimes profuse hemorrhage. Pelvic pain or feelings of pelvic heaviness, backache, fatigue, and persistent malaise are reported by many women. On bimanual examination the uterus feels larger and softer than normal for that time of the puerperium.

Therapeutic Management

Treatment is tailored to correct the cause of subinvolution. Methylergonovine maleate (Methergine) given for 24 to 48 hours provides long, sustained contraction of the uterus. Infection responds to antimicrobial therapy.

Nursing Considerations

In most cases subinvolution is not obvious until the mother has returned home after childbirth. For this reason, nurses must teach the mother and her family how to assess for the condition and how to recognize its occurrence.

The nurse should demonstrate how to locate and palpate the fundus and how to estimate fundal height in relation to the umbilicus. The uterus should become smaller each day (by approximately one fingerbreadth). The nurse also explains the progressive changes from lochia rubra, to lochia serosa, and then to lochia alba (see Chapter 17).

The mother is instructed to report any deviation from the expected pattern or duration of lochia. A foul odor often indicates uterine infection, for which treatment must be sought. Additional signs include pelvic or fundal pain, backache, and feelings of pelvic pressure or fullness.

✔ CHECK YOUR READING

6. Why is it sometimes difficult to recognize that the woman is becoming hypovolemic?
7. What are the major signs of subinvolution?
8. What is the nurse's primary responsibility in the management of subinvolution?

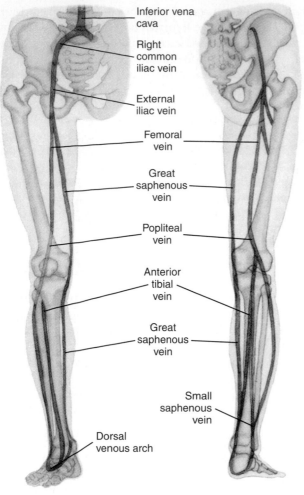

Inferior vena cava

Right common iliac vein

External iliac vein

Femoral vein

Great saphenous vein

Popliteal vein

Anterior tibial vein

Great saphenous vein

Small saphenous vein

Dorsal venous arch

Figure 28-5 ■ The venous system of the leg is affected when deep venous thrombosis occurs.

THROMBOEMBOLIC DISORDERS

The three most common thromboembolic disorders encountered during pregnancy and the postpartum period are superficial venous thrombosis, deep venous thrombosis (DVT), and occasionally, pulmonary embolism. Superficial venous thrombosis generally involves the saphenous venous system and is confined to the lower leg. DVT can involve veins from the foot to the iliofemoral region. It is a major concern because it predisposes to pulmonary embolism. Pulmonary embolism is a potentially fatal complication that occurs when the pulmonary artery is obstructed by a blood clot that was swept into circulation from a vein or by amniotic fluid. Figure 28-5 illustrates the venous system of the leg.

Incidence and Etiology

The incidence of thromboembolic disease in pregnancy and the puerperium is 0.5 to 3 per 1000 divided equally between pregnancy and postpartum (Laros, 2004). It remains a major cause of maternal death in the United States.

A thrombus is a collection of blood factors, primarily platelets and fibrin, on a vessel wall. Thrombi can form when-ever the flow of blood is impeded. Once started, the thrombus can enlarge with successive layering of platelets, fibrin, and blood cells as the blood flows past the clot. Thrombus formation is often associated with an inflammatory process in the vessel wall, which is termed *thrombophlebitis.*

The three major causes of thrombosis are venous stasis, hypercoagulable blood, and injury to the endothelial surface (the innermost layer) of the blood vessel. Two of these conditions—venous stasis and hypercoagulable blood—are present in all pregnancies.

VENOUS STASIS

During pregnancy, compression of the large vessels of the legs and pelvis by the enlarging uterus causes venous stasis. Stasis is most pronounced when the pregnant woman stands for prolonged periods of time. It results in dilated vessels and the potential for continued pooling of blood postpartum. Relative inactivity during pregnancy and activity restriction resulting from pregnancy complications lead to venous pooling and stasis of blood in the lower extremities. Prolonged time in stirrups for delivery and repair of the episiotomy also may promote venous stasis and increase the risk of thrombus formation.

HYPERCOAGULATION

Pregnancy also is characterized by changes in the coagulation and fibrinolytic systems that persist into the postpartum period. During pregnancy the levels of many coagulation factors are elevated. In addition, the fibrinolytic system (plasminogen activator and antithrombin III), which causes clots to disintegrate (lyse), is suppressed. The net result is that factors that promote clot formation are increased to prevent maternal hemorrhage and factors that prevent clot formation are decreased, resulting in a higher risk for thrombus formation during pregnancy and the postpartum period.

BLOOD VESSEL INJURY

Injury to the endothelium of the blood vessel may occur during vaginal or cesarean birth and could trigger a pelvic vein thrombosis. Thrombosis is nine times more likely to occur if the birth was cesarean (Laros, 2004).

ADDITIONAL PREDISPOSING FACTORS

Certain factors create additional risk for some women. These factors include varicose veins, obesity, a history of thrombophlebitis, use of oral contraceptives before pregnancy, and smoking. Women older than 35 years or who have had more than three pregnancies are also at increased risk (Box 28-2).

Superficial Venous Thrombosis

CLINICAL SIGNS AND SYMPTOMS

Superficial thrombophlebitis usually is associated with varicose veins and limited to the calf area. It can also occur in the arms as a result of intravenous therapy. Thrombosis of superficial veins is accompanied by signs and symptoms of inflammation. Signs and symptoms include swelling of the involved extremity as well as redness, tenderness, and warmth. An enlarged, hardened, cordlike vein may be palpated. The woman may experience pain when she walks, but some women have no signs at all.

THERAPEUTIC MANAGEMENT

Treatment includes analgesics, rest, and elastic support. Elevation of the lower extremity improves venous return. Warm packs may be applied to the affected area to promote healing. Anticoagulants or antiinflammatory agents are not needed unless the condition persists. After a period of bed rest the woman may ambulate gradually if symptoms have disappeared. She should avoid standing for long periods and should continue to wear support hose to help prevent venous stasis and a subsequent episode of superficial thrombosis. There is little chance of pulmonary embolism if the thrombosis remains in the superficial veins of the lower leg.

Deep Venous Thrombosis

In DVT signs and symptoms may be absent or diffuse. Those that occur are caused by an inflammatory process and obstruction of venous return. Swelling of the leg (more than 2 cm larger than the opposite leg), erythema, heat, tenderness, and pedal edema are the most common signs.

It is commonly believed that a positive Homans' sign (presence of pain behind the knee when the foot is dorsiflexed) is an indicator of DVT in postpartum women. Homans' sign has proved to be of little value in the diagnosis, however, because pain may also be caused by a strained muscle or contusion and the sign may be absent in many women who have a venous thrombosis.

Reflex arterial spasms may cause the leg to become pale and cool to the touch with decreased peripheral pulses. Additional symptoms may include pain on ambulation, chills, general malaise, and stiffness of the affected leg.

DIAGNOSIS

Ultrasonography with vein compression and Doppler flow analysis is most commonly used to detect alterations in blood flow diagnostic of DVT (McPhedran, 2004). Magnetic resonance imaging (MRI) may be used for pelvic veins. Impedance plethysmography, which measures changes in venous blood volume and flow, is less often used. Venography is an accurate method for diagnosing DVT but may cause pain, anaphylaxis, and radiation exposure (Clarke-Pearson, 2000).

THERAPEUTIC MANAGEMENT

PREVENTING THROMBUS FORMATION. Women who have had a previous DVT or pulmonary embolism are at risk for another. These women and others at high risk may be placed on prophylactic heparin, which does not cross the placenta. Standard unfractionated heparin (UH) or a low-molecular-weight heparin (LMWH) such as enoxaparin (Lovenox) may be used. LMWH is longer acting and can be given less frequently and with less laboratory testing but is more expensive than UH. Heparin is discontinued during labor and birth and resumed 4 to 12 hours after childbirth (Bobrowski & Dzieczkowski, 2002).

Risks of thrombus development during birth can be reduced by placing the woman's legs in stirrups that are padded to prevent prolonged pressure against the popliteal angle during the second stage of labor. If possible, the time in stirrups or footrests should be no more than 1 hour.

To prevent thrombus formation after birth, all new mothers are encouraged to ambulate frequently and as early as possible. Ambulation prevents stasis of blood in the legs and decreases the likelihood of thrombus formation.

If the woman is unable to ambulate, range-of-motion and gentle leg exercises, such as flexing and straightening the knee and raising one leg at a time, should begin within 8 hours after childbirth. In addition, the mother should not use pillows under her knees or the knee gatch on the bed. These devices may cause sharp flexion at the knees and pressure against the popliteal space, leading to pooling of blood in the lower extremities.

Antiembolism stockings or sequential compression devices are used for mothers with varicose veins, a history of thrombosis, or a cesarean birth. The stockings should be applied before the mother gets out of bed to prevent venous congestion, which begins as soon as she stands. It is important that she understands the correct way to put on the antiembolism stockings. Improperly applied stockings can roll or bunch and slow venous return from the legs.

Before discharge from the birth facility, the mother should be taught about lifestyle changes that can improve peripheral circulation. This includes avoiding clothing that is constricting around the legs and prolonged sitting. If sitting for long periods is necessary, walking for a short time hourly or moving her feet and legs frequently will help prevent circulatory stasis.

INITIAL TREATMENT. Initial treatment when a DVT has occurred includes:

- Bed rest, with the affected leg elevated to decrease interstitial swelling and to promote venous return from that leg.
- Gradual ambulation, which is allowed when symptoms have disappeared. Sitting with the legs dependent should be avoided.

- Anticoagulant therapy is begun with a continuous infusion of intravenous UH or subcutaneous LMWH to prevent extension of the thrombus by delaying the clotting time of the blood. The activated partial thromboplastin time (aPTT) should be monitored, and the heparin dose should be adjusted to maintain a therapeutic level of 1.5 to 2.5 times control (Laros, 2004). If LMWH is used, less frequent laboratory monitoring in necessary. Antifactor Xa levels may be obtained when LMWH is used.
- Analgesics, as necessary, to control pain.
- Antibiotic therapy, if necessary, to prevent or control infection.
- Continuous, moist heat for relief of pain and increased circulation.

SUBSEQUENT TREATMENT. The long-term management of DVT depends on whether the woman is pregnant or in the postpartum period. The pregnant woman at risk may receive heparin until labor and delivery and be restarted 4 to 12 hours after birth. Warfarin is contraindicated during pregnancy because of teratogenic effects and the risk of fetal hemorrhage. It is used only in women with prosthetic heart valves and contraindications to use of heparin. Heparin is safe in pregnancy because it does not cross the placenta.

During the postpartum period, heparin can be changed to warfarin (Coumadin) therapy and may be continued for 6 weeks to as long as 4 to 6 months (Laros, 2004). Prothrombin time and the international normalized ratio (INR) are used to monitor coagulation time when warfarin is used. The INR corrects for variations in the potency of the thromboplastins used by different laboratories. An appropriate level for treatment of DVT is 2 to 3 (Bobrowski & Dzieczkowski, 2002; Laros, 2004).

✓ CHECK YOUR READING

9. Why is the risk of thrombus formation increased in pregnancy and in the postpartum period?
10. What are the signs and symptoms of superficial venous thrombosis?
11. How does the long-term treatment for DVT in the pregnant woman differ from that in the woman who is in the postpartum period?
12. Why is bed rest prescribed for the woman with DVT?

Application of the Nursing Process
The Mother with Deep Venous Thrombosis

Assessment

Assessment focuses on determining the status of the venous thrombosis. Palpate the pedal pulses to determine whether they are absent, diminished, or easily palpable and equally strong on both sides. Inspect the affected leg for unusual warmth or redness, which indicates inflammation, or for unusual coolness or cyanosis, which indicates venous obstruction. Assess the affected and unaffected leg for size and color and compare the circumference to obtain an estimation of the edema that may be present in the affected leg.

Determine the degree of discomfort present. Pain is caused by tissue hypoxia, and increasing pain indicates progressive obstruction.

Evaluate the laboratory reports of clotting studies. In addition to activated partial thromboplastin time, whole-blood partial thromboplastin time and platelets may be evaluated when heparin is used. Thrombocytopenia is a concern when heparin is administered for a prolonged time. The INR is evaluated when the anticoagulant for the postpartum woman is changed to warfarin. Anti-factor Xa may be monitored when LMWH is used.

Analysis

The treatment of DVT includes the administration of anticoagulants for a prolonged time. An appropriate nursing diagnosis for this situation is "Risk for Injury from hemorrhage related to lack of understanding of anticoagulant therapy precautions."

Planning

Goals and expected outcomes for this diagnosis are that the woman will:
- Remain free of injury from anticoagulant therapy
- Verbalize precautions necessary when taking anticoagulants
- Plan for changes necessary as a result of anticoagulant therapy

Interventions

MONITORING FOR SIGNS OF BLEEDING

At least twice a day, inspect the mother for the appearance of bruising or petechiae. Instruct her to report signs of any bleeding: bruises, bloody nose, blood in urine or stools, bleeding gums, or increased vaginal bleeding. Be alert for signs of hemorrhage, such as tachycardia, falling blood pressure, or other signs of shock that may indicate internal bleeding.

Observe for excessive or bright red lochia. If the uterus is boggy, the cause is uterine atony. Massage the uterus and express clots. If the fundus is firm, bleeding may be from trauma or anticoagulant therapy. In either case the physician should be notified.

Unless frank hemorrhage is present, the usual treatment for excessive anticoagulation is temporary discontinuation of the anticoagulant. Protamine sulfate, which is the antidote for UH and is partially effective against LMWH, should be available. The antidote for warfarin is vitamin K.

EXPLAINING CONTINUED THERAPY

Instruct the woman in measures to prevent excessive anticoagulation. Carefully explain the treatment regimen, including the schedule of medication and possible side effects, such as unexplained fever, unusual fatigue, or sore throat (signs of agranulocytosis or diminished number of neutrophils). Help her devise a method for remembering to take the medication as directed, for example, marking a calendar each time the drug is taken. Caution her not to "double up" if a dose is missed. If necessary, teach her and another family member how to inject heparin or enoxaparin.

Because oral anticoagulants are associated with many clinically significant drug interactions, emphasize the importance of keeping the health care provider informed about any medications the mother takes. Caution the woman that common over-the-counter medications, such as aspirin and nonsteroidal antiinflammatory drugs, increase the risk of hemorrhage.

Explain the need for repeated laboratory testing to regulate the dose of the anticoagulant. Emphasize the importance of careful attention to dosage changes to keep the blood levels at the appropriate levels.

Instruct the woman to avoid eating large amounts of vitamin K–containing foods, such as broccoli, cabbage, lettuce, spinach, and lentils. The woman should use effective contraception as long as she is taking warfarin because the drug can cause fetal defects.

Suggest that the mother use a soft toothbrush and floss her teeth gently to prevent bleeding from the gums. An electric toothbrush may be too vigorous and may cause bleeding. She should postpone dental appointments until the therapy is completed. A depilatory to remove unwanted hair is safer than a razor during anticoagulant therapy.

 COMPLEMENTARY/ALTERNATIVE THERAPY

Many herbs affect the effectiveness of anticoagulants, and the woman should check with her health care provider before using them. Examples of herbs that increase the risk of bleeding include ginko biloba, garlic, and feverfew. Examples of herbs that decrease the effect of anticoagulants include chamomile, goldenseal, and St. John's wort.

Remind the new mother not to go barefoot and to avoid activities that could cause injury. Caution her against the use of alcohol, which inhibits the metabolism of oral anticoagulants. Also emphasize the importance of reporting unusual bleeding.

HELPING THE FAMILY ADAPT TO HOME CARE

In addition to the assessments, physical care, and teaching described above, nurses often must help the family adapt to home care. Assess the family structure and function to determine how prepared the family is to cope with the mother's illness. How many children are in the family? What are their ages? Who is usually the primary caregiver? Are family members or friends available to provide care while the mother is confined to bed or on limited activity? Who helps the family in times of need?

If the father is not present, determine who else will be available to support the mother during the subsequent weeks. Help the family develop a plan of care that includes temporary assistance by members of the extended family.

Note interactions between the mother and the newborn and between the father and the newborn. Although the health of the mother is of primary importance, care must be taken that the attachment process between her and the infant progresses normally.

Evaluation

- The mother demonstrates no signs of unusual bleeding or other side effects of the medication.
- The woman discusses precautions she has taken to prevent hemorrhage.
- Necessary changes have been made in the home.

Pulmonary Embolism

PATHOPHYSIOLOGY

Pulmonary embolism is a serious complication of DVT and a leading cause of maternal mortality. It occurs when fragments of a blood clot dislodge or amniotic fluid and its debris are carried to the lungs. The embolus occludes a vessel and partially or completely obstructs the flow of blood into the lungs. If pulmonary circulation is severely compromised, death may occur within a few minutes. If the embolus is small, adequate pulmonary circulation may be maintained until treatment can be initiated.

CLINICAL SIGNS AND SYMPTOMS

Clinical signs and symptoms depend on how much the flow of blood is obstructed. Dyspnea; sudden, sharp chest pain; tachycardia; syncope; tachypnea; pulmonary rales; cough; and hemoptysis are the most common. Pulse oximetry shows low oxygen saturation. Arterial blood gas determinations show decreased partial pressure of oxygen, and chest radiography reveals areas of atelectasis and pleural effusion. A ventilation-perfusion scan shows areas of the lung that are ventilated but not perfused because of the blockage.

THERAPEUTIC MANAGEMENT

Treatment of pulmonary embolism is aimed at dissolving the clot and maintaining pulmonary circulation. Oxygen is used to decrease hypoxia, and narcotic analgesics are used to reduce pain and apprehension. The woman is kept on bed rest, with the head of the bed slightly elevated to reduce dyspnea. Intensive care, support of ventilation, and other measures depend on her pulmonary status. Pulse oximetry should be initiated, and arterial blood gases should be evaluated. Emergency medications, such as dopamine, may be used to support falling blood pressure. Thrombolytic drugs, such as streptokinase or urokinase, may be used for life-threatening pulmonary emboli but are associated with high fever and bleeding. Embolectomy (surgical removal of the embolus) may be attempted if no time exists to allow the clot to dissolve. Heparin therapy is initiated and is continued throughout pregnancy if the embolism occurs at that time. Therapy may be continued for months after delivery to prevent further emboli.

NURSING CONSIDERATIONS

MONITOR FOR SIGNS. When caring for a woman with DVT, nurses must be aware of the danger of pulmonary embolism and focus the assessment for early signs and symptoms. This includes frequent assessment of respiratory rate and auscultation of breath sounds. Abnormalities, such as diminished or unequal breath sounds, or coughing should be reported immediately to the health care provider. Additional signs that require immediate attention include air hunger, dyspnea, tachycardia, pallor, and cyanosis.

FACILITATE OXYGENATION. Oxygen should be administered at 8 to 10 L/min by tight face mask. The nurse should remain with the mother to allay fear and apprehension. The head of the bed should be raised to facilitate breathing, and the woman should be kept warm. Narcotic analgesics, such as morphine, may be used to relieve pain.

SEEK ASSISTANCE. The woman's condition is precarious until the clot is lysed or until it adheres to the pulmonary artery wall and is reabsorbed. The primary nurse should call for assistance to initiate interventions. These include IV administration of heparin, continuous assessment of vital signs, and administration of emergency drugs that may be needed. The woman who has pulmonary embolism requires critical care nursing skills and is transferred to an intensive care unit.

✔ **CHECK YOUR READING**

13. What additional nursing assessments are necessary when the mother is receiving anticoagulants?
14. In addition to assessment, physical care, and teaching, what are the home care nurse's responsibilities?

PUERPERAL INFECTION

Puerperal infection is a term used to describe bacterial infections after childbirth. Infection occurs in 3% of all women who have had vaginal births and is 5 to 10 times more fre-

quent in those who have had cesarean births (Gibbs, Sweet, & Duff, 2004). Until the advent of antibiotics, puerperal infection resulting in death was not uncommon. Even today, it is one of the leading causes of maternal deaths.

The most common postpartum infections are metritis, wound infections, urinary tract infections, mastitis, and septic pelvic thrombophlebitis.

Definition

The definition of puerperal infection is a fever of 38° C (100.4° F) or higher after the first 24 hours and occurring on at least 2 days during the first 10 days after childbirth. Although a slight elevation of temperature may occur during the first 24 hours because of dehydration or the exertion of labor, any mother with fever should be assessed for other signs of infection.

Effect of Normal Anatomy and Physiology on Infection

To understand the seriousness of infection of the reproductive tract, consider the anatomy of the region. Every part of the reproductive tract is connected to every other part, and organisms can move from the vagina, through the cervix, into the uterus, and through the fallopian tubes to infect the ovaries and the peritoneal cavity. The entire reproductive tract is particularly well supplied with blood vessels during pregnancy and after childbirth. Bacteria that invade or are picked up by the blood vessels or lymphatics can carry the infection to the rest of the body, which can result in life-threatening septicemia.

The normal physiologic changes of childbirth increase the risk of infection. During labor the acidity of the vagina is reduced by the amniotic fluid, blood, and lochia, which are alkaline. An alkaline environment encourages growth of bacteria.

Necrosis of the endometrial lining and the presence of lochia provide a favorable environment for the growth of anaerobic bacteria. Many small lacerations, some microscopic, occur in the endometrium, cervix, and vagina during birth and allow bacteria to enter the tissue. Although the uterine interior is not sterile until 3 to 4 weeks after childbirth, infection does not develop in most women. This is partly because of the presence of granulocytes in the lochia and endometrium that prevent infection. Scrupulous aseptic technique during labor and birth and careful handwashing during the postpartum period are also major preventive factors.

Other Risk Factors

Other factors may predispose a woman to infection (Table 28-2). Cesarean birth is a major predisposing factor. This is because of the tissue trauma that occurs in surgery, the incision that provides an entrance for bacteria, the possibility of contamination during surgery, and the foreign bodies such as sutures that can promote infection. In addition, women who must have a surgical delivery because of a problem that develops during labor may have other risk fac-

TABLE 28-2 Risk Factors for Puerperal Infection

Risk Factor	Reason
History of previous infections (urinary tract infection, mastitis, thrombophlebitis)	May be more vulnerable to infectious process
Colonization of lower genital tract by pathogenic organisms	Infections usually caused by several microbes that have ascended to the uterus from the lower genital tract
Cesarean birth	Increased portals of infection
Trauma	Provides entrance for bacteria and makes tissues more susceptible
Prolonged rupture of membranes	Removes barrier of amniotic membranes and allows access by organisms to interior of uterus
Prolonged labor	Increases number of vaginal examinations; allows time for bacteria to multiply
Catheterization	Could introduce organisms into bladder
Excessive number of vaginal examinations	Increases chance that organisms from vagina or outside source are carried into the uterus
Retained placental fragments	Provide growth medium for bacteria and may interfere with flow of lochia
Hemorrhage	Loss of infection-fighting components of blood
Poor general health (excessive fatigue, anemia, frequent minor illnesses)	Increases vulnerability to infections and complications of labor
Poor nutrition (decreased protein, vitamin C)	Less able to repair tissue and defend against infection
Poor hygiene	Excessive exposure to pathogens
Medical conditions, such as diabetes mellitus	Decreases ability to defend against infections of any kind; diabetes increases glucose in urine
Low socioeconomic status	More likely to have poor nutrition and inadequate prenatal care

tors, such as prolonged labor, that raise the chances of infection. Colonization of the vagina with virulent organisms, such as group B streptococcus, *Chlamydia trachomatis*, *Mycoplasma hominis*, and *Gardnerella vaginalis*, also predisposes to the development of infection after childbirth.

Any trauma to maternal tissues increases the hazard of infection. Trauma may occur with rapid delivery, birth of a large infant, use of a vacuum extractor or forceps, or the need for manual delivery of the placenta as well as lacerations and episiotomies. Catheterization during labor increases the chance of introduction of organisms into the bladder and adds to the trauma of the urinary tract that occurs during normal childbirth.

When prolonged rupture of membranes occurs during labor, organisms from the vagina are more likely to ascend into the uterine cavity. This is especially true if more than 24 hours pass before delivery. A long labor or the performance of many vaginal examinations during labor increases the danger of infection. Each vaginal examination increases the possibility of contamination from gloves or from organisms in the vagina that are pushed through the open cervix. Use of a fetal scalp electrode or intrauterine pressure catheter has the same effect. If part of the placenta remains inside the uterus after delivery, the tissue becomes necrotic and provides a good place for bacteria to grow.

Additional factors include postpartum hemorrhage, which causes loss of some of the infection-fighting components of the blood, such as leukocytes, and leaves the mother in a weakened condition. Prenatal conditions (poor nutrition, anemia) interfere with the mother's ability to resist infection. Lack of knowledge of hygiene or lack of access to facilities that permit adequate hygiene increases the risk of postpartum infection.

✔ CHECK YOUR READING

15. Why is the woman who had an assisted birth or cesarean birth at increased risk for postpartum infection?
16. Why do the normal physiologic changes of childbearing make a mother especially susceptible to infection of the reproductive system?
17. Why is infection more likely to develop in a mother who had prolonged labor?

Specific Infections

ENDOMETRITIS

Endometritis is infection of the endometrium of the uterus. If the infection involves the muscle and inner lining of the uterus, it is endomyometritis. If the surrounding tissues are also involved, endoparametritis is present. Together these infections are often called *metritis*. Uterine infection occurs after 1% to 3% of vaginal births, 15% to 20% of unexpected cesarean births, and 5% to 10% of elective cesareans before the onset of labor (Gibbs et al., 2004).

ETIOLOGY. Endometritis is usually caused by organisms that are normal inhabitants of the vagina and cervix. Most infections are polymicrobial, with both aerobic and anaerobic organisms involved. Organisms most often found include group B streptococci, enterococci, *Escherichia coli*, *Klebsiella pneumoniae*, *Proteus*, *Bacteroides*, and *Prevotella*. *C. trachomatis* is not a cause of early infection but is associated with late-onset infections (Gibbs et al., 2004).

CLINICAL SIGNS AND SYMPTOMS. The mother with severe endometritis looks sick. She presents a different picture from the typical happy new mother. The major signs and symptoms are fever, chills, malaise, lethargy, anorexia, abdominal pain and cramping, uterine tenderness, and purulent, foul-smelling lochia. Additional signs include tachycardia and subinvolution. In most cases the signs and symptoms occur within the first 24 to 48 hours after delivery (Gibbs et al., 2004). When the causative organisms are group A beta-hemolytic or group B streptococci, however, the lochia may be scant and odorless and the woman may exhibit no signs except fever.

Laboratory data may confirm the diagnosis. The results of a complete blood count may show an elevation of leukocytes. Leukocytes are normally elevated during labor and for a short time afterward, however. Leukocytosis after the first day that is not decreasing should prompt further evaluation.

Specimens may be taken from the blood, endocervix, and uterine cavity for cultures. A catheterized urine specimen may also be obtained. The antibiotic sensitivity from these cultures may be used to determine the appropriate second-line antibiotic therapy in case the broad-spectrum therapy is unsuccessful in halting the infection.

THERAPEUTIC MANAGEMENT. IV administration of antibiotics is the initial treatment for metritis. The goal of this therapy is to confine the infectious process to the uterus and to prevent spread of the infection throughout the body. Broad-spectrum antibiotics such as clindamycin plus gentamicin are often used. Other drugs include ampicillin, cephalosporins, and metronidazole. Antibiotics are continued until the woman has been afebrile for 48 hours.

Improvement in clinical signs usually occurs within 48 to 72 hours. If they persist, additional investigation is needed to determine the cause and precise location. Oral antibiotics are usually unnecessary after completion of an IV course of treatment. Other drugs include antipyretics for fever and oxytocics such as methylergonovine to increase drainage of lochia and promote involution.

Many physicians give prophylactic antibiotics intravenously, orally, or both for any woman who is having a cesarean birth or who is particularly at risk for infection. A single dose given during surgery after cord clamping may be sufficient if there are no signs of infection present (Savoia, 2004). Prophylaxis lowers the incidence of endometritis and wound infection.

COMPLICATIONS. If the infection spreads outside the uterine cavity, it may affect the fallopian tubes (salpingitis) or the ovaries (oophoritis), which could result in sterility. Peritonitis (inflammation of the membrane lining the walls of the abdominal and pelvic cavities) may occur and lead to formation of a pelvic abscess. In addition, the risk of pelvic thrombophlebitis is increased when pathogenic bacteria enter the bloodstream during episodes of metritis. Figure 28-6 illustrates complications of metritis.

Signs and symptoms that the infection is spreading may be similar to those of metritis but more severe. Fever and abdominal pain will be particularly pronounced. Peritonitis may result in paralytic ileus and a distended, boardlike abdomen with absent bowel sounds.

NURSING CONSIDERATIONS. The mother with metritis should be placed in a Fowler's position to promote

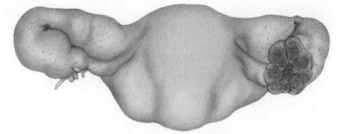

Salpingitis: Infection in fallopian tubes causes them to become enlarged, hyperemic, and tender.

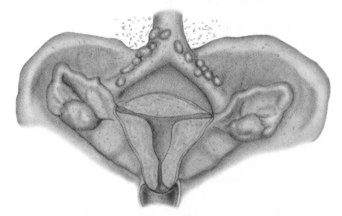

Peritonitis: Infection spreads through the lymphatics to the peritoneum; a pelvic abscess may form.

Figure 28-6 ■ Areas of spread of uterine infection.

drainage of lochia. She should be medicated as needed for abdominal pain or cramping, which may be severe. The nurse should observe the mother for signs of improvement or new signs and symptoms, such as nausea and vomiting, abdominal distention, absent bowel sounds, and severe abdominal pain. Comfort measures include warm blankets, cool compresses, cold or warm drinks, or use of a heating pad.

Teaching incorporates signs and symptoms of worsening condition, side effects of therapy, and the importance of adhering to the treatment plan and follow-up care. If the woman is so sick that she must be separated from her infant, a nursing diagnosis of "Risk for Impaired Parenting related to separation from infant" should be considered. If the mother is breastfeeding, she will need help to pump her breasts to establish and maintain lactation.

WOUND INFECTION

Wound infections are common types of puerperal infection because any break in the skin or mucous membrane provides a portal of entry for bacteria. The most common sites are cesarean surgical incisions. Episiotomies and lacerations are infected less often (Figure 28-7). *Staphylococcus aureus* is the cause of 25% to 30% of wound infections (Bowes & Thorp, 2004).

CLINICAL SIGNS AND SYMPTOMS. Signs of wound infection are edema, warmth, redness, tenderness, and pain. The edges of the wound may pull apart, and seropurulent drainage may be present. If the wound remains untreated,

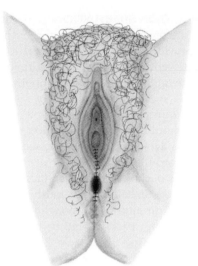

Figure 28-7 ■ Any break in the skin, such as the episiotomy site, provides a portal of entry for bacteria and can result in localized infection.

generalized signs of infection, such as fever and malaise, may develop, as well. As with other puerperal infections, cultures may reveal mixed aerobic and anaerobic bacteria.

THERAPEUTIC MANAGEMENT. An incision and drainage of the affected area may be necessary. Broad-spectrum antibiotics may be ordered until a report of the organism is returned. Analgesics are often necessary, and warm compresses or sitz baths may be used to provide comfort and to promote healing by increasing circulation to the area.

NURSING CONSIDERATIONS. Wound infections are painful and annoying to the mother out of proportion to their size. Perineal infections cause discomfort during many activities, such as walking, sitting, or defecating, and are particularly troublesome because they are not expected by the new mother.

Wound infections may require readmission to the hospital or home health care visits. The woman requires reassurance and supportive care. Comfort measures might include sitz baths, warm compresses, and frequent perineal care. She should be taught to wipe from front to back and to change perineal pads frequently. Good handwashing techniques are emphasized. Adequate fluid intake and diet are important. Activity may be modified depending on the site, severity, and treatment of the wound infection.

The infant is not routinely isolated from the mother with a wound infection, but she must be advised how to protect her infant from contact with contaminated articles such as dressings. Anticipatory guidance should include teaching side effects of medications, signs of worsening condition, and self-care measures.

✔ **CHECK YOUR READING**

18. What are the signs and symptoms of metritis? How is it usually treated?
19. What are the most common sites for wound infections?
20. How does the nurse assess for wound infection?

URINARY TRACT INFECTIONS

ETIOLOGY. During childbirth the bladder and urethra are traumatized by pressure from the descending fetus. Insertion of a catheter, with its risk of infection, occurs at least once during many labors. After childbirth the bladder and urethra are hypotonic, with urinary stasis and retention common problems. Residual urine and reflux of urine may occur during voiding.

Women who had bacteria in the urine during pregnancy are at greatly increased risk for pyelonephritis, which may result in preterm labor. Asymptomatic bacteriuria may be discovered during urine screens in 2% to 11% of pregnant women (Savoia, 2004). Urinary tract infections are usually caused by coliform bacteria, such as *E. coli.*

CLINICAL SIGNS AND SYMPTOMS. Symptoms typically begin on the first or second postpartum day. They include dysuria (a burning pain on urination), urgent and frequent urination, and suprapubic pain. A low-grade fever is sometimes the only symptom. In some women an upper urinary tract infection, such as pyelonephritis, may develop the third or fourth day, with chills, spiking fever, costovertebral angle tenderness, flank pain, and nausea and vomiting. This infection of the kidney pelvis may result in permanent damage to the kidney if not promptly treated.

THERAPEUTIC MANAGEMENT. Most urinary tract infections can be treated on an outpatient basis. Asymptomatic bacteriuria treated during pregnancy reduces the incidence of pyelonephritis. Pyelonephritis during pregnancy may require hydration and IV administration of broad-spectrum antibiotics. In addition, the woman should be observed for signs of preterm labor. If the postpartum woman is not severely ill, she can be treated with IV antibiotics at home. Antibiotics that are safe for use during lactation are given if the mother is breastfeeding.

NURSING CONSIDERATIONS. The woman with a urinary tract infection must be instructed to take the medication for the entire time it is prescribed and not to stop when symptoms abate. In addition, she must drink at least 2500 to 3000 ml of fluid each day to help dilute the bacterial count and flush the infection from the bladder. Acidification of the urine inhibits multiplication of bacteria, and drinks that acidify urine, such as apricot, plum, prune, and cranberry juices, are frequently recommended. Carbonated drinks should be avoided because they increase urine alkalinity.

Teaching should also include measures to prevent urinary tract infections, such as proper perineal care, increasing fluid intake, and urinating frequently.

MASTITIS

Mastitis, an infection of the lactating breast, occurs most often after the second and third weeks postpartum, although it may develop at any time during breastfeeding. Approximately 5% of lactating women are affected (Gibbs et al., 2004). It usually affects only one breast.

ETIOLOGY. Mastitis is often caused by *S. aureus.* The bacteria are most often carried on the hands of the mother or agency staff or in the mouth of the newborn. The organism may enter through an injured area of the nipple, such as a crack or blister, although only redness may be present or no obvious signs of injury are apparent. Soreness of a nipple may result in insufficient emptying of the breast during breastfeeding.

Engorgement and stasis of milk frequently precede mastitis. This may occur when a feeding is skipped, when the infant begins to sleep through the night, or when breastfeeding is suddenly stopped. Constriction of the breasts by a bra that is too tight may interfere with emptying of all the ducts and may lead to infection. The mother who is fatigued or stressed or who has other health problems that might lower her immune system is also at increased risk for mastitis.

CLINICAL SIGNS AND SYMPTOMS. At first, the mother may think that she has the flu because of fatigue and aching muscles. Symptoms progress to include fever of 38.4° C (101.1° F) or higher, chills, malaise, and headache. Mastitis is characterized by a localized area of pain, redness, and inflammation. A hard, tender area may be palpated (Figure 28-8). Untreated mastitis may progress to breast abscess.

THERAPEUTIC MANAGEMENT. Antibiotic therapy and continued emptying of the breast by breastfeeding or breast pump constitute the first line of treatment. With early antibiotic treatment, mastitis usually resolves within 24 to 48 hours. Women who develop a breast abscess are treated with surgical drainage and antibiotics.

Supportive measures include moist heat or ice packs, breast support, bed rest, and analgesics. The mother should continue to breastfeed from both breasts. If the affected breast is too sore, she can pump the breast gently. Regular emptying of the breast is important in preventing abscess formation. If an abscess forms and ruptures into the ducts, breastfeeding should be discontinued and a mechanical pump used to empty the breast. Milk obtained from that breast should be discarded.

NURSING CONSIDERATIONS. Because mastitis rarely occurs before discharge from the birth facility, the nurse must provide adequate information for prevention. Measures to prevent mastitis include positioning the infant correctly and avoiding trauma to the nipples and milk stasis. The mother should breastfeed every 2 to 3 hours and should avoid formula supplements and nipple shields. Nursing pads should be changed as soon as they are wet. She should also avoid continuous pressure on the breasts from tight bras or infant carriers.

Once mastitis occurs, nursing measures are aimed at increasing comfort and helping the mother maintain lactation. Moist heat promotes comfort and increases circulation. A shower or hot packs should be used before feeding or pumping the breasts. Cold packs can be used between feedings to reduce edema. The woman should complete the entire course of antibiotics to prevent recurrence or a breast abscess.

One way to apply heat or cold to the breast is to use a disposable diaper moistened with warm water or with crushed ice between the layers. The thickness helps to maintain the temperature, and the plastic cover prevents dripping.

The breast should be completely emptied at each feeding to prevent stasis of milk, which can result in an abscess. If the mother is too sore to breastfeed on the affected side or if she must take antibiotics that are contraindicated during lactation, she should be shown how to express the milk or use a pump to empty the breasts.

Breastfeeding or pumping every 1.5 to 2 hours makes the mother more comfortable and prevents stasis. Starting the feeding on the unaffected side causes the milk-ejection reflex to occur in the painful breast and makes the process more efficient. Massage over the affected area before and during the feeding helps to ensure complete emptying.

The mother should stay in bed during the acute phase of her illness. Her fluid intake should be 2500 to 3000 ml per day. Analgesics may be required to relieve discomfort.

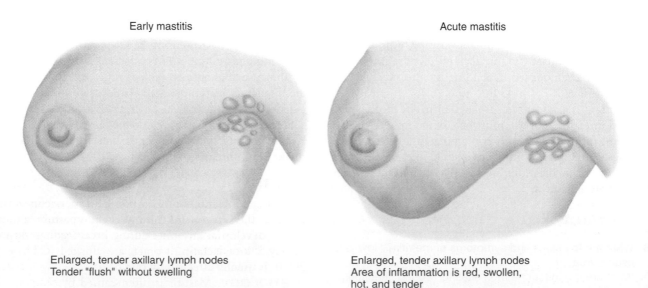

Early mastitis

Acute mastitis

Enlarged, tender axillary lymph nodes
Tender "flush" without swelling

Enlarged, tender axillary lymph nodes
Area of inflammation is red, swollen, hot, and tender

Figure 28-8 ■ Mastitis typically occurs after 2 to 3 weeks following birth in the breast of a woman who breastfeeds.

The mother with mastitis is likely to be very discouraged. Some mothers decide to stop breastfeeding because of the discomfort involved. The nursing diagnosis "Interrupted Breastfeeding related to discomfort, infectious process, or effects of therapy" may be appropriate. Weaning during an episode of mastitis may increase engorgement and stasis, leading to abscess formation or recurrent infection. The mother may need much encouragement, and she will need help in arranging care for other children or with other responsibilities so that she can remain in bed.

SEPTIC PELVIC THROMBOPHLEBITIS

Septic pelvic thrombophlebitis is the least common of the puerperal infections. It usually is not seen until 2 to 4 days after childbirth. It occurs when infection spreads along the venous system and thrombophlebitis develops. It develops more often in women with wound infection and usually involves the ovarian, uterine, or hypogastric veins.

CLINICAL SIGNS AND SYMPTOMS. The primary symptom is pain in the groin, abdomen, or flank. Also present may be fever, tachycardia, gastrointestinal distress, and decreased bowel sounds. Spiking fever that does not respond to antibiotics may be the only sign in a woman who appears well otherwise. Laboratory data may be used to exclude other diagnoses and usually include complete blood count with differential, blood chemistries, coagulation studies, and blood cultures. Computed tomography (CT) or MRI may be performed.

THERAPEUTIC MANAGEMENT. Readmission to the hospital is usually necessary. Primary treatment includes IV antibiotics and anticoagulation therapy with IV heparin. Supportive care is similar to that for DVT and includes monitoring for safe levels of anticoagulation therapy and for signs and symptoms of pulmonary embolism.

Application of the Nursing Process
Infection

Assessment

Although all women are observed for indications of infection as part of routine nursing assessments, the nurse must practice increased vigilance for mothers who are at increased risk of infection.

Pay particular attention to signs that may be expected in infection, such as fever; tachycardia; pain; or unusual amount, color, or odor of lochia. Generalized symptoms of malaise and muscle aching may also be significant. Examine all wounds each shift for signs of localized infection, such as redness, edema, tenderness, discharge, or pulling apart of incisions or sutured lacerations. Ask the mother if she has difficulty emptying her bladder or discomfort related to urination.

Assess the mother's knowledge of hygiene practices that prevent infections, such as proper handwashing, perineal care, and handling of perineal pads. Evaluate her knowledge of breastfeeding and any problems that might result in breast engorgement and stasis of milk in the ducts. Examine

the nipples for signs of injury that might provide a portal of entry for organisms.

Analysis

Because all women are at risk for infection after childbirth, most facilities have developed standards of practice that protect postpartum women from infection, and individual nursing care plans are usually not necessary. When predisposing factors increase the likelihood of infection, however, routine assessments and care must be modified and preventive measures intensified. In this case the most relevant nursing diagnosis is "Risk for Infection related to the presence of significant risk factors."

Planning

The goals and expected outcomes for this nursing diagnosis are that the mother will:
- Remain free of signs of infection during the postpartum period
- Describe methods to prevent infection
- List signs of infection that should be reported immediately

Interventions
PREVENTING INFECTION

PROMOTING HYGIENE. Nursing responsibilities for the woman at risk for puerperal infection focus on prevention of initial infection. Preventive measures include aseptic technique for all invasive procedures and meticulous attention to handwashing. Handwashing is important for the nursing staff and the mother. She should wash her hands before and after changing pads or touching the perineum. Instruct her on care of the perineum and episiotomy site (see Chapter 17). Make sure that she can demonstrate cleansing methods before she is discharged.

PREVENTING URINARY STASIS. An adequate intake of fluids (at least 2500 to 3000 ml/day) is important for preventing stasis of urine. Encourage the woman to empty her bladder at least every 2 to 3 hours during the day.

NURSING CARE PLAN 28-1 Postpartum Infection

ASSESSMENT: Lisa Pyle, a thin, pale, 16-year-old primipara, is admitted to the postpartum unit after a cesarean birth because of fetal distress. Her membranes were ruptured for 14 hours, and she was in labor for 16 hours before the birth. She was catheterized twice during labor, with insertion of an indwelling catheter shortly before her surgery. She plans to breastfeed her infant.

> **CRITICAL THINKING:** *What data indicate that Lisa is at increased risk for infection? What additional data should be obtained?*
>
> **ANSWER:** *Factors that increase the risk for metritis include a cesarean birth and rupture of membranes 14 hours before the surgery was performed. Catheterization increases the risk for urinary tract infection. Additional necessary data to better evaluate the risks for infection include estimated blood loss and prenatal conditions such as anemia or other infections.*

NURSING DIAGNOSIS: Risk for Infection related to presence of favorable conditions for infections

GOALS/EXPECTED OUTCOMES: Before discharge Lisa will:
1. Demonstrate no signs of infection
2. Discuss methods she will use to prevent infections
3. List signs of infection she will report to her health care provider

INTERVENTION	RATIONALE
1. Assess vital signs every 4 hours.	1. Temperature above 38° C (100.4° F) or tachycardia suggests an infectious process and should be reported.
2. Observe the surgical incision for redness, tenderness, edema, drainage, and approximation and note the odor of lochia every 4 hours. Determine character of urine and whether Lisa experiences frequency, urgency or pain with urination after the catheter is removed.	2. Redness, pain, or edema of the incision suggests wound infection. Drainage could be bleeding or a sign of infection. Separation also can indicate infection. Foul odor of lochia suggests endometrial infection. Frequency, urgency, or painful urination may indicate urinary tract infection.

3. Instruct Lisa in hygienic practices to prevent infection:
  a. Careful handwashing before and after perineal care
 	
  b. Perineal cleansing after elimination
  c. Changing peripads frequently
 	
  d. Wiping the perineum from front to back
	3. Good hygiene helps prevent infection.
	  a. Handwashing is the most important defense against infection and its spread.
	  b. Perineal cleansing helps prevent growth of bacteria.
	  c. Frequent pad changes remove accumulated lochia, an excellent culture medium for bacteria.
	  d. Wiping from front to back prevents fecal contamination of the vagina.

4. Initiate measures to reduce the risk of urinary tract infection.
  a. Provide fluids of Lisa's choice when she is able to take them, and emphasize the importance of drinking 2500 to 3000 ml/day.
  b. Monitor bladder distention to prevent overfilling. Teach Lisa the importance of emptying her bladder every 2 to 3 hours during the first days after childbirth.
  c. Use methods to promote bladder emptying, such as running water in the shower or sink, pouring warm water over the perineum, and providing pain medication as needed.
	4. Adequate hydration and frequent emptying of the bladder help prevent stasis of urine, which increases the risk of urinary tract infection. Relief of pain may allow the mother to relax enough to void. The sound of running water may stimulate the urge to void.

5. Assist Lisa with breastfeeding. Explain the reasons for proper positioning and frequent adequate feedings.	5. Poor positioning and short, infrequent feedings may cause nipple trauma, engorgement, and incomplete emptying of the breasts, leading to mastitis.
6. Offer and encourage Lisa to eat well-balanced meals when she progresses to a regular diet. Emphasize the importance of a diet high in protein and vitamin C.	6. Adequate protein and vitamin C are necessary for healing damaged tissues.
7. Teach Lisa signs of infection that she should report to her health care provider. Include fever, chills, dysuria, increased incisional tenderness or drainage, lochia with a foul odor, or pain and redness of the breast.	7. Prompt recognition and reporting of signs of infection ensures early treatment and reduces further complications.

EVALUATION: Lisa is free of signs and symptoms of infection throughout her hospital stay and at her postpartum checkup. She verbalizes measures she will take to reduce her risk of infection when she is discharged from the hospital. She is able to list signs of infection that requires treatment.

Measure the first two voidings after delivery or removal of an indwelling catheter, and assess the bladder and fundus to be certain the bladder is empty. Instruct her to report any signs of urinary tract infection immediately so that early treatment can be initiated.

Use appropriate measures to promote bladder emptying if she has difficulty. Drinking hot fluids, such as tea, helps some mothers void. Running water or having the mother blow bubbles in a glass of water uses the sound of water to stimulate the urge to urinate. Pouring warm water over the perineum or having the mother void in a sitz bath or shower may help relax the urinary sphincter. Administration of analgesics may help her relax enough to urinate.

TEACHING BREASTFEEDING TECHNIQUES. Mothers often need assistance in establishing an effective pattern of breastfeeding that results in complete emptying of the breasts at each feeding and that reduces the risk of nipple trauma (see Chapter 22).

PROVIDING INFORMATION. Advise mothers to obtain adequate rest and sufficient food of high nutritive value to replenish their energy and prevent infection. If necessary, identify foods high in protein and vitamin C, necessary for repair of damaged tissue. Whole-grain breads, cereals, or pasta; cheese; eggs; poultry; fish; and red meat are some of the best sources of protein. This is particularly important if the mother is breastfeeding.

Obtaining adequate rest is a problem for many mothers. Nursing interventions focus on helping them plan a schedule that allows them to rest while the infant sleeps and to identify family members or friends who are available to provide support and assistance.

TEACHING SIGNS AND SYMPTOMS THAT SHOULD BE REPORTED

Because many women are discharged 24 to 48 hours after childbirth, they must be taught signs and symptoms of infection that should be reported to their health care provider. These include fever, chills, dysuria, and redness and tenderness of a wound. Malodorous lochia or discharge from a wound as well as prolonged lochial discharge also should be reported.

Evaluation

The interventions can be judged to be successful if the mother:
- Shows no signs of infection
- Explains methods she will use to prevent infection
- Lists signs and symptoms that she should report to her health care provider

If infection occurs, the problem is no longer amenable to independent nursing actions but becomes a collaborative problem requiring medical and nursing interventions.

✔ CHECK YOUR READING

21. What measures can the woman take to decrease the risk of urinary tract infection? How does the treatment for cystitis differ from that for pyelonephritis?
22. How may mastitis be prevented?

AFFECTIVE DISORDERS

Affective (mood) disorders are disturbances in function, affect, or thought processes that can affect the family after childbirth as severely as physiologic problems. They include postpartum blues, postpartum depression (PPD), and postpartum psychosis. Postpartum blues is discussed in Chapter 18. PPD and postpartum psychosis are more serious disorders that disrupt the family and require intervention to resolve.

Postpartum Depression

INCIDENCE

PPD is the most common affective disorder of the postpartum period. It occurs in 15% to 20% of women (Hayashi & Zettelmaier, 2000). Women of all ethnic groups and educational levels are affected. Many investigators believe that PPD is underdiagnosed and underreported. It usually develops during the first 3 weeks to 3 months but may occur at any time during the first year postpartum.

PREDICTORS OF POSTPARTUM DEPRESSION

The cause of PPD is unknown, but it is probably a result of a combination of biologic, psychosocial, and situational stressors. It is more likely to occur in primigravidas. The strongest predictor is depression during pregnancy or previous PPD (Epperson & Czarkowski, 2004). Other factors that are believed to increase the risk include:
- Hormonal fluctuations that follow childbirth
- Medical problems during pregnancy or after birth, such as preeclampsia, preexisting diabetes mellitus, anemia, or postpartum thyroid dysfunction
- Personal or family history of depression, mental illness, or alcoholism
- Personality characteristics, such as immaturity and low self-esteem
- Marital dysfunction or difficult relationship with the significant other, resulting in lack of support
- Anger or ambivalence about the pregnancy
- Feelings of isolation, lack of social support, or support that does not meet the mother's needs
- Fatigue, sleep deprivation
- Financial worries
- Birth of an infant with illness or anomalies
- Multifetal pregnancy
- Chronic stressors

CLINICAL SIGNS AND SYMPTOMS

The woman experiencing PPD shows less interest in her surroundings and a loss of her usual emotional response toward her family. Even though she cares for the infant in a loving manner, she is unable to feel pleasure or love. She sees the infant as demanding and herself as inept at mothering. The woman may have intense feelings of unworthiness, guilt, and shame, and she often expresses a sense of loss of self. Generalized fatigue, irritability, complaints of ill health, and difficulty in concentrating and making decisions are also present. She often has little interest in food, may have weight changes, and experiences sleep disturbances. She describes panic attacks and relentless obsessive thinking, and thoughts of suicide may occur.

PPD is differentiated from the normal labile emotions of pregnancy and the postpartum period by the number, intensity, and persistence of symptoms. A majority of the symptoms are intensely and consistently present for at least a 2-week period. These are not mood swings but a persistent depressed state.

IMPACT ON THE FAMILY

PPD has an impact on the entire family. It creates strain on each member's usual methods of coping and often causes difficulties in relationships. Stressors tend to be magnified, and, as a result, family members may decrease their interactions with the depressed mother at a time when she needs support the most. Communication is impaired because she gradually withdraws from contact with others. The decreased libido commonly associated with depression may also affect her relationship with her significant other.

Partners of depressed women report many changes in their lives after the birth. These include a sense of loss of the partner and the relationship they had known previously, feelings of loss of control, anger, and frustration. Fathers may take on household chores and child care duties that the depressed mother is unable to manage. They may be suffering from depression along with their partners (Meighan, Davis, Thomas, & Droppleman, 2000).

Depressed mothers interact differently with their infants than do women who are not depressed. They appear tense, are more irritable, and feel less competent as mothers. They may not pick up on the infant's cues or smiles and may therefore fail to meet the infant's needs and to enjoy the positive feedback (Beck, 1995). Infants of depressed mothers tend to be fussier, to be more discontented, and to make fewer positive facial expressions (Beck, 1999). Major depression interferes with the normal mother-child relationship and places the infant at risk for later cognitive and behavioral problems (Needlman, 2004).

THERAPEUTIC MANAGEMENT

Depression responds best to a combination of psychotherapy, social support, and medication. Psychotherapy may be helpful to assist the woman to cope with changes in her life. The partner and immediate family must be included in counseling sessions so they can develop an understanding of what the woman feels and needs.

Antidepressants are often used for PPD and may be continued for 6 months or more. Selective serotonin reuptake inhibitors are commonly prescribed medications. They have few side effects and have been used safely in breastfeeding mothers (Wisner, Parry, & Piontek, 2002). Other drugs include tricyclic antidepressants and hormones. Medication may be continued for 6 months or more. Electroconvulsive therapy may also be necessary.

If the woman wants to continue breastfeeding, medications safe for use during lactation should be used because this may enhance the bonding process. The breastfeeding infant should be monitored carefully by the pediatrician for signs of adverse reactions to medications (Burt et al., 2001).

Application of the Nursing Process
Postpartum Depression

Assessment

Early identification of depression or women at risk for depression allows intervention that may reduce the duration and damaging effects of depression. Although early treatment of PPD is important, women often do not seek treatment. They may deny the extent of their depression, be embarrassed to tell anyone about it, or believe it is part of the normal adjustment to new parenthood. Some may fear that the baby will be taken away if their feelings are discovered.

All women should be assessed for depression during pregnancy, at the birth facility, and during follow-up visits. The woman should be reassessed at each contact with health care providers. New mothers bring their infants to the pediatrician's office frequently during the early months after childbirth. This is an ideal setting in which to include assessment of the new mother's emotional state and provide referrals if necessary.

Assessment tools such as the Postpartum Depression Predictors Inventory are often used to identify depressed mothers (Beck, 2002a). This inventory identifies prenatal depression, life stress, social support, prenatal anxiety, satisfaction with marital relationship, depression history, self-esteem, unwanted or unplanned pregnancy, marital status, socioeconomic status, child care stress, infant temperament, and maternity blues as factors that may foretell the likelihood that a woman will develop PPD. Another screening tool for assessment of risk factors or actual depression is the Postpartum Depression Screening Scale, which may be used to determine which mothers should be referred for further help (Beck & Gable, 2000).

A brief screening can also be performed without a specific tool. Assessing for excessive fatigue in the first 2 weeks after childbirth may help identify women who will later develop PPD and enable them to get early treatment (Bozoky & Corwin, 2002). Simply asking women if they are often sad or depressed and if they have felt a loss of pleasure or interest in things they once enjoyed may identify depression without further screening. Asking also shows interest and acceptance of their feelings and opens the door for further discussion.

Observe for subjective symptoms, such as apathy, lack of interest or energy, anorexia, or sleeplessness. Ask the mother about her feelings. The mother's verbalizations of failure, sadness, loneliness, anxiety, or vague confusion are important cues. Focus on the frequency, duration, and intensity of the woman's feelings to determine their severity.

Assess for objective data, such as crying, poor personal hygiene, or inability to follow directions or to concentrate. If mothers show signs that may indicate depression, ask them about their feelings and let them know depression is common after childbirth.

Determine whether family support is available. Single mothers or mothers with an absent or unavailable support system may feel increasingly isolated, leading to stress that they are unable to manage. Inappropriate expressions of blame or anger toward the partner and unmet expectations of the baby or the parenting role are sometimes present.

Analysis

A likely nursing diagnosis, particularly if predisposing factors are present, is "Risk for Ineffective Coping related to depression in response to stressors associated with childbirth and parenting."

Planning

To achieve the goals and expected outcomes for this nursing diagnosis, the new mother will:

- Verbalize feelings with the health care provider and significant other throughout the postpartum period
- Discuss her own strengths
- Identify resources that are available during the postpartum period

Interventions

DEMONSTRATING CARING

Conveying a caring attitude is one nursing strategy to help mothers decrease their emotional distress and to guide them in regaining their well-being during the postpartum period. Acknowledge that something is wrong and that the woman seems depressed. Spend time with her and explain that the condition is not her fault. It is an illness that can be treated, and it will end.

PROVIDING ANTICIPATORY GUIDANCE

Some mothers, particularly young mothers, are unprepared for the rapid change in lifestyle that follows the birth of an infant. During the prenatal period, initiate a discussion with all new mothers to provide anticipatory guidance about the early weeks at home. Discuss the need for frequent contact with other adults so that the mother does not become isolated. Emphasize the need for continued communication with the partner or with a close friend who is available to provide support when loneliness or anxiety becomes a problem. Explain the importance of adequate rest and nutrition for maintaining energy and a feeling of health and well-being. Teach mothers the signs of PPD and when they should seek help.

HELPING THE MOTHER VERBALIZE FEELINGS

Because women are expected to be happy after giving birth, many women do not discuss their feelings with others. They are ashamed and feel there is a social stigma to admitting to depression at any time and especially after giving birth. If they do discuss their feelings, their friends or even health care workers may trivialize the problem by making comments such as, "You'll get over it. After all, you have a beautiful baby." Women and their families minimize depression because they cannot find the exact cause.

Recommend that although some of her feelings may seem "unreasonable" (anger, guilt, shame), the woman should acknowledge negative feelings to herself and insist that others recognize them too. Discuss the realities of parenting and the fact that it may be exhausting. It may be helpful to rehearse some of the situations that may occur, such as a fussy baby or being home alone and feeling lonely, as a means to develop perspective and to find solutions.

ENHANCING SENSITIVITY TO INFANT CUES

Point out infant cues and explain their meaning. Model behavior to show the mother how to respond to the infant's cues. Suggest measures that may enhance her sensitivity to cues, such as kangaroo care. Kangaroo care (skin-to-skin) also may increase bonding and may help the woman feel better about herself and her ability to care for the infant (Dombrowski, Anderson, Santori, & Burkhammer, 2001). Measures to help the mother relax may help improve her mood and her response to her infant.

Assess the infant to see that he or she is progressing normally. Depressed mothers may not give the care and nurturing needed. Determine the infant's weight gain or loss and observe the mother's response to the infant's crying. If the mother is breastfeeding, make suggestions to help her continue as it may increase her feelings of closeness with the infant. If she is taking medication, be sure it is one that is recommended for use during lactation.

HELPING FAMILY MEMBERS

Include the father in discussions about depression, before and after the birth. Acknowledge his feelings as well as those of the mother. Stress his role in helping his partner and other family members. Offer practical suggestions of ways he can help manage the changes in their lives. Explain the impact of PPD on each family member. Emphasize the importance of the mother's taking medications as ordered. Discuss signs that the mother is getting worse and when to call the health care provider.

■ COMPLEMENTARY/ALTERNATIVE THERAPY

Music
Relaxation therapy
Massage and aromatherapy using jasmine, sandalwood, or rose oil
Reflexology
Yoga
Caution: St. John's wort is often used as an over-the-counter remedy to treat depression. It has not been proved to be safe for use by lactating women, however.

DISCUSSING OPTIONS AND RESOURCES

Ask the new mother about stressors in her life that may be contributing to her feelings of depression. Help her plan ways to reduce common areas of stress.

Assist the mother and her partner in identifying people who are available to provide support. Suggest that she explain her anticipated needs to those people before the development of symptoms. In addition, provide her with telephone numbers of PPD support groups in the area. Internet sources are helpful for some families. Examples are Postpartum Support International (www.postpartum.net) and Depression After Delivery (www.depressionafterdelivery.com).

Evaluation

The interventions have been successful if the mother:

- Talks about her feelings to staff and family members
- Identifies her personal strengths
- Discusses community and family resources and makes plans to use them

Postpartum Psychosis

Postpartum psychosis is a rare condition that causes psychiatric admission for 2 in 1000 postpartum women (Hayashi & Zettelmaier, 2000). It generally surfaces within 3 months of delivery. Women who have one episode of postpartum psychosis have an increased risk of having another episode. A history of bipolar disorder is also an important risk factor.

Symptoms of postpartum psychosis include sleep disturbances, confusion, agitation, irritability, hallucinations, delusions, and the possibility that the mother may kill herself or the infant (Simpson & James, 2005). Other signs and symptoms include tearfulness, preoccupation with guilt, feelings of worthlessness, lack of appetite, and an inordinate concern with the baby's health. Delusions about the infant's being dead or defective are common, and hallucinations may be present.

Assessment and management of postpartum psychosis are beyond the scope of maternity nurses, and mothers who experience this condition must be referred to specialists for comprehensive therapy. Women with signs of postpartum

---

> **BOX 28-3** Common Nursing Diagnoses for the Woman with a Postpartum Complication
>
> Activity Intolerance
> Fatigue
> Interrupted Breastfeeding*
> Pain
> Risk for Impaired Parenting
> Risk for Ineffective Coping*
> Risk for Injury*
> Risk for Infection*

*Nursing diagnoses discussed in this chapter.

---

psychosis need immediate medical attention, and hospitalization is usually necessary.

Antidepressants and antipsychotic drugs are used as appropriate. Women who have bipolar disease may be treated with lithium or carbamazepine. Lithium is not recommended during pregnancy, but it may be used if the benefit outweighs the risk. It is resumed in the postpartum period if the mother is not breastfeeding. Women who have depressive symptoms must be assessed for suicidal potential and treated according to the severity of the threat.

✔ CHECK YOUR READING

23. What are the symptoms of PPD, and how does it differ from postpartum "blues"?
24. How can nurses intervene for PPD?
25. What is the therapeutic management for postpartum psychosis?

SUMMARY CONCEPTS

- Postpartum hemorrhage sometimes can be anticipated and prevented by careful examination of antepartum and intrapartum factors that predispose to excessive bleeding.
- Overstretching of the muscle fibers during pregnancy and repeated stretching during past pregnancies predispose to uterine atony and excessive uterine bleeding.
- Soft tissue trauma (lacerations, hematomas) also can cause rapid loss of blood even when the uterus is firmly contracted.
- Initial management of uterine atony focuses on measures to contract the uterus and provide fluid replacement.
- Management of trauma of the reproductive tract involves locating the trauma and repairing it before excessive blood loss occurs.
- Compensatory mechanisms maintain the blood pressure so that vital organs receive adequate oxygen. When compensatory mechanisms fail, hypovolemic shock follows.
- The process of uterine involution is delayed (subinvolution) when placental fragments are retained or when the inner lining of the uterus is infected (metritis).
- Subinvolution of the uterus develops after the mother goes home. The nurse teaches the family the process of normal involution and the signs and symptoms that should be reported to the health care provider.
- Venous stasis that occurs during pregnancy, increased levels of coagulation factors, and decreased thrombolytic

---

CRITICAL THINKING ❓ EXERCISE 28-2

Aricella Nunez, a 23-year-old multipara, gave birth several days ago to her second baby. It is obvious to the nurse making a telephone follow-up call after discharge that Aricella is crying. She says, "I don't know what's wrong with me! I can barely get out of bed in the morning and I'm worn out just trying to take care of the kids." The nurse responds, "Oh, that's just the 'baby blues'. Just look at those beautiful babies and you'll feel better."

Questions
1. Has the nurse made any assumptions?
2. Is the nurse's response helpful for Aricella? Why or why not?
3. What would be a more therapeutic response?
4. What additional action should the nurse take?

factors that persist into the postpartum period increase the risk of thrombus formation during the puerperium.

- Treatment for deep venous thrombosis includes anticoagulants, analgesics, and bed rest with the affected leg elevated.
- Nurses who administer anticoagulant therapy assess the mother to determine whether her clotting time is within the recommended therapeutic range so that overmedication with anticoagulants does not result in bleeding from unusual sites.
- Pulmonary embolism occurs when a clot is dislodged from the vein, or amniotic fluid debris is carried by the blood to a pulmonary vessel, which may be completely or partially occluded.
- The risk of infection is increased with childbearing because there is open access to bacteria from the vagina through the fallopian tubes and into the peritoneal cavity. Increased blood supply to the pelvis and the alkalinization of the vagina by the amniotic fluid further increase the risk of metritis.
- Any break in the skin or mucous membranes during childbirth provides a portal of entry for pathogenic organisms and increases the risk of puerperal infection. Nurses must assess women with an incision or laceration for signs of localized wound infections.
- Urinary stasis and trauma to the urinary tract increase the risk of urinary tract infection. Nurses must initiate measures to prevent urinary stasis.
- Nurses must provide information about the importance of completely emptying the breasts at each feeding and about measures to avoid nipple trauma to prevent mastitis.
- Postpartum depression is a disabling affective disorder that affects the entire family. Nurses help the woman acknowledge her feelings and assist her in identifying measures that will help her cope with the condition.

ANSWERS TO CRITICAL THINKING EXERCISE 28-1, p. 740

1. Her history of multiparity, birth of a large infant, and rapid labor and delivery indicate that Dolores is at risk for postpartum hemorrhage. The nurse will increase the frequency of her assessments of the fundus, lochia, vital signs, and skin temperature and color.
2. Massage the fundus and express clots that may have accumulated in the uterus. Massage stimulates uterine contractions that compress torn myometrial blood vessels and stop excessive bleeding. Continued assessment of the fundus and lochia is imperative to determine whether the uterus relaxes again, leading to resumption of bleeding.
3. Assist Dolores to void, because a distended bladder lifts the uterus, making contraction more difficult and resulting in excessive bleeding.
4. Continue to massage the fundus and turn on the call light to ask a colleague for help. Ask that another nurse notify the health care provider because excessive bleeding requires the combined efforts of primary health care providers and nurses to prevent postpartum hemorrhage. Start IV fluids or increase the flow rate of an existing IV according to hospital policy.

ANSWERS TO CRITICAL THINKING EXERCISE 28-2, p. 756

1. The nurse assumed that Aricella's feelings are the transient, self-limiting moods of depression that come and go in most women who give birth. The nurse fails to obtain additional data that may indicate whether Aricella is experiencing postpartum depression that requires additional therapy.
2. The nurse's response is not helpful because it minimizes the feelings Aricella has expressed and it offers no measures for dealing with them.
3. It would be more therapeutic for the nurse to acknowledge the feelings and ask follow-up questions that allow Aricella to express her feelings fully.
4. The nurse must convey genuine interest and caring. She can do this best by
   a. Indicating awareness that something may be wrong
   b. Sharing as much time as Aricella needs to express her feelings
   c. Providing hope by reassuring Aricella that this condition is not her fault and that it can be cured
   d. Making appropriate referrals to provide as much continuity of care as possible

REFERENCES & READINGS

American Academy of Pediatrics & American College of Obstetricians and Gynecologists. (2002). *Guidelines for perinatal care* (5th ed.). Elk Grove Village, IL: Authors.

American College of Obstetricians. (1998). *Postpartum hemorrhage* (Educational Bulletin, 243). Washington, DC: ACOG.

Beck, C.T. (1995). The effects of postpartum depression on maternal-infant interaction: A meta-analysis. *Nursing Research, 44*(5), 298-304.

Beck, C.T. (1999). *Postpartum depression: Case studies, research, and nursing care.* Washington, DC: Association of Women's Health, Obstetric & Neonatal Nurses.

Beck, C.T. (2002a). Revision of the Postpartum Depression Predictors Inventory. *Journal of Obstetric, Gynecologic, and Neonatal Nursing, 31*(4), 394-402.

Beck, C.T. (2002b). Theoretical perspectives of postpartum depression and their treatment implications. *MCN: American Journal of Maternal/Child Nursing, 27*(5), 282-287.

Beck, C.T., & Gable, R.K. (2000). Postpartum Depression Screening Scale: Development and psychometric testing. *Nursing Research, 49*(5), 272-282.

Beck, C.T., & Gable, R.K. (2001). Further validation of the Postpartum Depression Screening Scale. *Nursing Research, 50*(3), 155-164.

Beeber, L., (2002). The pinks and the blues. *American Journal of Nursing, 102*(11), 91-96.

Benedetti, T.J. (2002). Obstetric hemorrhage. In S.G. Gabbe, J.R. Niebyl, & J.L. Simpson (Eds.), *Obstetrics: Normal and problem pregnancies* (4th ed., pp. 503-538). New York: Churchill Livingstone.

Bobrowski, R.A., & Dzieczkowski, J.S. (2002). Anticoagulation. In S.B. Ransom, M.P. Dombrowski, M.I. Evans, & K.A. Ginsburg (Eds.), *Contemporary therapy in obstetrics and gynecology* (pp. 142-146). Philadelphia: Saunders.

Bowes, W.A., & Thorp, J.M. (2004). Clinical aspects of normal and abnormal labor. In R.K. Creasy, R. Resnik, & J.D. Iams (Eds.), *Maternal-fetal medicine: Principles and practice* (5th ed., pp. 671-706). Philadelphia: Saunders.

Bozoky, I., & Corwin, E.J. (2002). Fatigue as a predictor of postpartum depression. *Journal of Obstetric, Gynecologic, and Neonatal Nursing, 31*(4), 436-443.

Brumfield, C.G., Hauth, J.C., & Andrews, W.W. (2000). Puerperal infection after cesarean delivery: Evaluation of a standardized protocol. *American Journal of Obstetrics & Gynecology 182*(5), 1147-1151.

Burt, V.K., Suri, R., Altshuler, L., Stowe, Z., Hendrick, V.C., & Muntean, E. (2001). The use of psychotropic medications during breastfeeding. *American Journal of Psychiatry, 158*(7), 1001-1009.

Clarke-Pearson, D.L. (2000). Venous thromboembolic disease in pregnancy. In E.J. Quilligan & F.P. Zuspan (Eds.), *Current therapy in obstetrics and gynecology* (5th ed., pp. 368-371). Philadelphia: Saunders.

Clemmens, D., Driscoll, J.W., & Beck, C.T. (2004). Postpartum depression as profiled through the postpartum depression screening scale. *MCN: American Journal of Maternal/Child Nursing, 29*(3), 180-185.

Coleman-Brochu, S. (2004). Deep vein thrombosis in pregnancy. *MCN: American Journal of Maternal/Child Nursing, 29*(3), 186-192.

Cunningham, F.G., Leveno, K.J., Bloom, S.L., Hauth, J.C., Gilstrap, L.C., & Wenstrom, K.D. (2005). *Williams obstetrics* (22nd ed.). New York: McGraw-Hill.

Dietch, K.V., & Bunney, B. (2002). The "silent" disease: Diagnosing and treating depression in women. *AWHONN Lifelines, 6*(2), 140-145.

Dombrowski, M.A.S., Anderson, G.C., Santori, C., & Burkhammer, M. (2001). Kangaroo (skin-to-skin) care with a postpartum woman who felt depressed. *MCN: American Journal of Maternal/Child Nursing, 26*(4), 214-216.

Duff, P. (2002). Maternal and perinatal infection. In S.G. Gabbe, J.R. Niebyl, & J.L. Simpson (Eds.), *Obstetrics: Normal and problem pregnancies* (4th ed., pp. 1293-1345). New York: Churchill Livingstone.

Epperson, C.N., & Czarkowski, K. (2004). Psychiatric complications. In G.N. Burrow, T.P. Duffy, & J.A. Copel (Eds.), *Medical complications during pregnancy* (6th ed., pp. 595-513). Philadelphia: Saunders.

Faro, S. (2002). Postpartum endometritis. In S.B. Ransom, M.P. Dombrowski, M.I. Evans, & K.A. Ginsburg (Eds.), *Contemporary therapy obstetrics and gynecology* (pp. 181-183). Philadelphia: Saunders.

Gambone, J.C., Moore, J.G., & Koos, B.J. (2004). Common medical and surgical conditions complicating pregnancy. In N.F. Hacker & J.G. Moore (Eds.), *Essentials of obstetrics and gynecology* (4th ed., pp. 216-246). Philadelphia: Saunders.

Gibbs, R.S., Sweet, R.L., & Duff, P. (2004). Maternal and fetal infectious disorders. In R.K. Creasy, R. Resnik, & J.D. Iams (Eds.), *Maternal-fetal medicine: Principles and practice* (5th ed., pp. 741-801). Philadelphia: Saunders.

Goodman, J.H. (2004). Postpartum depression beyond the early postpartum period. *Journal of Obstetric, Gynecologic, and Neonatal Nursing, 33*(4), 410-420.

Hanna, B., Jarman, H., Savage, S., & Layton, K. (2004). The early detection of postpartum depression: Midwives and nurses trial a checklist. *Journal of Obstetric, Gynecologic, and Neonatal Nursing, 33*(2), 191-197.

Hauth, J.C. (2000). Postpartum hemorrhage. In E.J. Quilligan & F.P. Zuspan (Eds.), *Current therapy in obstetrics and gynecology* (5th ed., pp. 317-320). Philadelphia: Saunders.

Hayashi, R.H., & Gambone, J.C. (2004). Postpartum hemorrhage and puerperal sepsis. In N.F. Hacker & J.G. Moore (Eds.), *Essentials of obstetrics and gynecology* (4th ed., pp. 146-158). Philadelphia: Saunders.

Hayashi, R.H., & Zettelmaier, M.A. (2000). Postpartum management. In S.B. Ransom, M.P. Dombrowski, S.G. McNeeley, K.S. Moghissi, & A.R. Munkarah (Eds.), *Practical strategies in obstetrics and gynecology* (pp. 321-325). Philadelphia: Saunders.

Higgins, P.G. (2004). Postpartum complications. In S. Mattson & J.E. Smith (Eds.), *Core curriculum for maternal-newborn nursing* (3rd ed.), pp. 850-870.

Jesse, D.E., & Graham, M. (2005). Are you often sad or depressed? *MCN: American Journal of Maternal/Child Nursing, 30*(1), 40-45.

Katz, V.L., & Wolfe, H.M. (2002). Selective arterial embolization in the management of obstetric hemorrhage. In S.B. Ransom, M.P. Dombrowski, M.I. Evans, & K.A. Ginsburg (Eds.), *Contemporary therapy obstetrics and gynecology* (pp. 165-169). Philadelphia: Saunders.

Kennedy, H.P., Beck, C.T., & Driscoll, J.W. (2002). A light in the fog: Caring for women with postpartum depression. *Journal of Midwifery & Women's Health, 47*(5), 318-330.

Laros, R.K. (2004). Thromboembolic disease. In R.K. Creasy, R. Resnik, & J.D. Iams (Eds.), *Maternal-fetal medicine: Principles and practice* (5th ed., pp. 845-857). Philadelphia: Saunders.

MacMullen, N.J., Dulksi, L.A., & Meagher, B. (2005). Red alert: Perinatal hemorrhage. *MCN: American Journal of Maternal/Child Nursing, 30*(1), 46-51.

Maley, B. (2002). Out of the blue: creating a postpartum depression support group. *AWHONN Lifelines, 6*(1), 62-65.

McPhedran, P. (2004). Venous thromboembolism during pregnancy. In G.N. Burrow, T.P. Duffy, & J.A. Copel (Eds.), *Medical complications during pregnancy* (6th ed., pp. 87-101). Philadelphia: Saunders.

Meighan, M., Davis, M.W., Thomas, S.P., & Droppleman, P.G. (2000). Living with postpartum depression: The father's experience. *MCN: American Journal of Maternal/Child Nursing, 24*(4), 202-208.

Needlman, R.D. (2004). The first year. In R.E. Behrman, R.M. Kliegman, & H.B. Jenson (Eds.), *Nelson textbook of pediatrics* (17th ed., pp. 31-38). Philadelphia: Saunders.

Parry, B.L. (2004). Management of depression and psychoses during pregnancy and the puerperium. In R.K. Creasy, R. Resnik, & J.D. Iams (Eds.), *Maternal-fetal medicine: Principles and practice* (5th ed., pp. 1193-1200). Philadelphia: Saunders.

Rickert, V.I., Wiemann, C.M., & Berenson, A.B. (2000). Ethnic differences in depressive symptomatology among young women. *Obstetrics & Gynecology, 95*(1), 55-60.

Riordan, J. (2005a). Breast-related problems. In *Breastfeeding and human lactation* (3rd ed., pp. 247-275). Boston: Jones and Bartlett.

Riordan, J. (2005b). Women's health and breastfeeding. In *Breastfeeding and human lactation* (3rd ed., pp. 459-486). Boston: Jones and Bartlett.

Rouse, D.J., & St. John, E. (2003). Normal labor, delivery, newborn care, and postpartum. In J.R. Scott, R.S. Gibbs, B.Y. Karlan, & A.F. Haney (Eds.), *Danforth's obstetrics and gynecology* (9th ed, pp. 35-56). Philadelphia: Lippincott Williams & Wilkins.

Savoia, M.C. (2004). Bacterial, fungal, and parasitic disease during pregnancy. In G.N. Burrow, T.P. Duffy, & J.A. Copel (Eds.), *Medical complications during pregnancy* (6th ed., pp. 305-345). Philadelphia: Saunders.

Scoggin, J. (2004). Physical and psychological changes. In S. Mattson & J.E. Smith (Eds.), *Core curriculum for maternal-newborn nursing* (3rd ed., 371-386). Philadelphia: Lippincott Williams & Wilkins.

Simpson, K.R., & James, D.C. (2005). *Postpartum care*. White Plains, NY: March of Dimes Birth Defects Foundation.

Summers, A.L., & Logsdon, M.C. (2005). Web sites for postpartum depression. *MCN: The American Journal of Maternal/Child Nursing, 30*(2), 88-96.

Ugarriza, D.N. (2002). Postpartum depression women's explanation of depression. *Journal of Nursing Scholarship, 34*(3), 227-334.

Vieira, T. (2003). When joy becomes grief: Screening tools for postpartum depression. *AWHONN Lifelines, 6*(6), 507-513.

Wisner, K.L., Parry, B.L., & Piontek, C.M. (2002). Postpartum depression. *New England Journal of Medicine, 347*(3), 194-199.

Wroblewski, M., & Tallon, D. (2004). Implementing a comprehensive postpartum depression support program. *AWHONN Lifelines, 8*(3), 248-252.

High-Risk Newborn: Complications Associated with Gestational Age and Development

OBJECTIVES

After studying this chapter, you should be able to:

1. List risk factors that may lead to complications of gestational age and development in the newborn.
2. Explain the special problems of the preterm infant.
3. Identify common nursing diagnoses for preterm infants, and explain the nursing care for each.
4. Describe the complications that may result from premature birth.
5. Describe the characteristics and problems of the infant with postmaturity syndrome.
6. Explain the effects of intrauterine growth restriction.
7. Compare the problems of the large-for-gestational-age infant with those of the small-for-gestational-age infant.

Go to your Student CD-ROM for Review Questions keyed to these Objectives.

DEFINITIONS

Apneic Spells Cessation of breathing for more than 20 seconds or accompanied by cyanosis or bradycardia.

Bronchopulmonary Dysplasia Chronic pulmonary condition in which damage to the infant's lungs requires prolonged dependence on supplemental oxygen.

Compliance Stretchability or elasticity of the lungs and thorax that allows distention without resistance during respirations.

Containment A method of increasing comfort in infants by swaddling or other means to keep the extremities in a flexed position near the body.

Corrected Age Gestational age that a preterm infant would be if still in utero. Also may be called *developmental age;* the chronologic age minus the number of weeks the infant was born prematurely.

Enteral Feeding Nutrients supplied to the gastrointestinal tract orally or by feeding tube.

Extremely Low-Birth-Weight Infant An infant weighing 1000 g (2 lb, 3 oz) or less at birth.

Intrauterine Growth Restriction Failure of a fetus to grow as expected for gestational age.

Large-for-Gestational-Age Infant An infant whose size is above the 90th percentile for gestational age.

Low-Birth-Weight Infant An infant weighing less than 2500 g (5 lb, 8 oz) at birth.

Macrosomia Infant birth weight more than 4000 g.

Minimal Enteral Nutrition Very small feedings designed to help the gastrointestinal tract mature. Also called *trophic feedings.*

Necrotizing Enterocolitis Serious inflammatory condition of the intestines.

DEFINITIONS—cont'd

Noncompliance Resistance of the lungs and thorax to distention with air during respirations.

Parenteral Nutrition Intravenous infusion of all nutrients known to be needed for metabolism and growth.

Periventricular-Intraventricular Hemorrhage Bleeding around and into the ventricles of the brain.

Postmaturity Syndrome Condition in which a postterm infant shows characteristics indicative of poor placental functioning before birth.

Postterm Infant An infant born after 42 weeks of gestation.

Preterm Infant An infant born before the beginning of the thirty-eighth week of gestation. Also called *premature infant.*

Pulse Oximetry Method of determining the level of blood oxygen saturation by sensors attached to the skin.

Respiratory Distress Syndrome Condition caused by insufficient production of surfactant in the lungs; results in atelectasis (collapse of the lung alveoli), hypoxemia (decreased oxygen [O_2]), and hypercapnia (increased [CO_2]).

Retinopathy of Prematurity Condition in which damage to blood vessels often associated with oxygen use may cause decreased vision or blindness.

Small-for-Gestational-Age Infant An infant whose size is below the 10th percentile for gestational age.

Transcutaneous Oxygen Monitoring Method of continuous noninvasive measurement of oxygen in the blood by transducers attached to the skin.

Very-Low-Birth-Weight Infant An infant weighing 1500 g (3 lb, 5 oz) or less at birth.

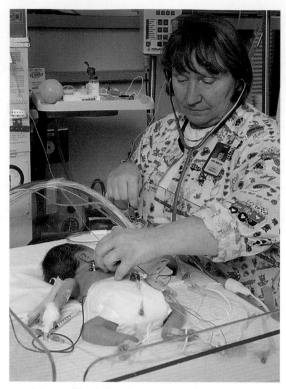

Figure 29-1 ■ The infant in a neonatal intensive care unit is cared for by nurses with highly specialized skills.

Maternity nurses identify and care for the immediate needs of neonates with complications until they are transferred to the neonatal intensive care unit (NICU). Nurses also provide information and emotional care for parents. Neonatal intensive care nursing is a specialty. Nurses who work in this setting need additional education and experience to prepare them for this role.

CARE OF HIGH-RISK NEWBORNS

Approximately 9% of all newborns are sick enough at birth to require intensive care (Stoll & Kliegman, 2004b). Nurses care for minor illness in the mother-baby unit or the normal newborn nursery, but more serious problems require care in specialized nurseries, which are designed for that purpose (Figure 29-1).

Multidisciplinary Approach

The care of infants with problems at birth often necessitates collaboration among many different professionals. In the hospital setting such professionals may include nurses, nurse practitioners, physicians with different specialties, respiratory therapists, laboratory personnel, and pharmacists. Care from social workers, physical therapists, feeding specialists, occupational therapists, and infant development experts may begin during the hospital stay and continue after the infant is discharged. Nurses often must coordinate this care and explain or clarify it for parents.

Case Management and Clinical Pathways

Neonates with complications may remain in the NICU for many days at a cost of thousands of dollars each day. Methods to reduce the length of stay and cost of hospitalization include case management and clinical pathways.

The case manager is a nurse who follows infants from admission to discharge to identify or prevent situations that would interfere with progression toward discharge. Clinical pathways are guidelines developed collaboratively by members of all disciplines to ensure that discharge can occur as soon as possible. They list the care infants will need along a timeline and the expected outcomes of that care. Different pathways are created to meet the needs of different types of situations, such as various complications of prematurity. Figure 29-2 is an example of a clinical pathway used for infants in the NICU.

PRETERM INFANTS

Preterm infants (also called *premature infants*) are born before the beginning of the thirty-eighth week of gestation. A gestational age assessment of a preterm infant's size and development may show that the infant is small, appropriate, or large for the amount of time spent in the uterus. Most preterm infants are appropriate for their gestational age.

The word *preterm* is sometimes confused with the term *low birth weight* (LBW), which refers to infants weighing 2500 g (5 lb, 8 oz) or less at birth and of any gestational age. Very-low-birth-weight (VLBW) infants weigh 1500 g (3 lb, 5 oz) or less at birth. Extremely low-birth-weight (ELBW) infants weigh 1000 g (2 lb, 3 oz) or less at birth. Although most of these infants are preterm, others are full term and have failed to grow normally while in the uterus, a condition called *intrauterine growth restriction* (IUGR).

Incidence and Etiology

SCOPE OF PROBLEM

Advances in technology have resulted in survival at much lower birth weights than ever before. Although advances have allowed very small infants to survive, the rate of preterm births is not decreasing. In 2003 12.3% of all births were preterm, 7.9% were of low-birth-weight infants, and 1.4% were of very-low-birth-weight infants (Hamilton, Martin, & Sutton, 2004). These figures show a slight increase in preterm and low-birth-weight infants over the previous year. In terms of medical expense, lost potential, and suffering of infants and their parents, preterm birth is extremely costly.

Disorders related to short gestation and low birth weight are the second leading cause of infant mortality. Only congenital anomalies cause more infant deaths. Infant mortality and morbidity increase as gestational age decreases.

Care of very preterm infants raises ethical questions concerning the benefit of saving them at great expense versus the risk that they may have serious, permanent disabilities and little chance to live normal lives. The incidence of problems such as blindness, hearing loss, developmental retardation, and cerebral palsy increases as the gestational age decreases.

CAUSES

The exact causes of preterm birth are not known, but all risk factors in pregnancy are potential causes of complications for the newborn. Problems during pregnancy may lead to preterm birth, and complications may occur during labor or delivery that result in decreased oxygenation of the fetus or trauma during delivery. Multifetal pregnancy is an increasing cause of early birth because of infertility treatment to achieve pregnancy.

PREVENTION

Prevention of preterm birth is best accomplished by provision of adequate prenatal care for every pregnant woman to identify and treat risk factors as early as possible. Teaching women signs of preterm labor will help them seek care when halting labor is still a possibility (see Chapter 27).

Characteristics of Preterm Infants

Characteristics of preterm infants vary by gestational age. For example, the appearance and problems of infants born at 34 weeks' gestation are different from those of infants born at 26 weeks' gestation. Some characteristics, however, are common to all preterm infants.

APPEARANCE

Preterm infants often appear frail and weak, and they have underdeveloped flexor muscles and muscle tone. Their extremities are limp and offer little or no resistance when moved. Premature newborns typically lie in an extended position (see Figure 20-20). The head of the normal preterm infant is large in comparison with the rest of the body.

Preterm infants lack subcutaneous or white fat, which makes their thin skin appear red and translucent, with blood vessels clearly visible. The nipples and areola may be barely perceptible, but vernix caseosa and lanugo may be abundant. Plantar creases are absent in infants of less than 32 weeks' gestation (see Figure 20-26).

The pinna of the ear are flat and soft and contain little cartilage (see Figure 20-28). In the female infant the clitoris and labia minora appear large and are not covered by the small, separated labia majora. The male infant may have undescended testes, with a small, smooth scrotal sac (see Figures 20-29 and 20-30).

BEHAVIOR

The behavior of preterm infants varies according to gestational age. It often differs from that of full-term infants because of the stress of having to adjust to extrauterine life before they are ready. They may have little excess energy for maintaining muscle tone and poor development of flexion. Premature newborns are easily exhausted from noise and routine activities. Their responses are varied, including lowered oxygenation levels and behavior changes. Their cries may be feeble.

Assessment and Care of Common Problems

Because preterm infants are "unfinished" in their growth and development, they are prone to problems affecting all systems and body processes. Some of the most common problems are discussed here. Problems with environmental stress, nutrition, and parenting are discussed in the section on application of the nursing process.

PROBLEMS WITH RESPIRATION

Problems of the respiratory system are a major concern because preterm newborns must go through the same processes as the full-term infant to begin breathing but with less-mature lungs. The presence of surfactant in adequate amounts is of primary importance. Surfactant reduces surface tension in the alveoli and prevents their collapse with expiration. Infants born before surfactant production is ad-

YORK HEALTH SYSTEM
YORK, PENNSYLVANIA

NICU CLINICAL PATHWAY

Gest. age _____ wks. Birthweight _____ gms. DOB _____

Admitting diagnosis _____

Family Care Team Members _____

Mother's/Father's names _____

Phone No. (home) _____ alternative _____

CODES:

Initials = Completed
N = Not applicable
D = Deferred
* = See progress notes

PROBLEM LIST:

1. Altered Pulmonary Status
2. Altered Nutritional Status
3. Altered Skin Integrity
4. Parental Knowledge Deficit
5. Thermoregulation
6. Immunological Impairment
7. Altered Parenting
8. Altered Cardiovascular Status
9. Altered Neuro Status
10. Altered Metabolic Status

	PHASE 1: ADMISSION/CRITICAL	PHASE 2: CONVALESCENT	PHASE 3: DISCHARGE

**PSYCHOSOCIAL/
DISCHARGE
PLANNING**
	☐ Orient parents to NICU environment, visitation & handwashing policies, provide phone numbers
	☐ Provide NICU booklet
	☐ Review equipment in use
	☐ Discuss disease process and plan of care
	☐ Review Family Care Team
	☐ Assess family learning needs, family structure and support systems
	☐ Social Services consult completed
	☐ Encourage verbalization of fears/concerns
	☐ Document parental interaction/teaching
	☐ Provide Support Group information
	☐ Informed of Lactation Consultant Support
	
	EXPECTED OUTCOME:
	Prob #4: Parents verbalize understanding of disease process and plan of care
	
	_____ OUTCOME MET
		☐ Provide Support Group information
		☐ Parents introduced to Developmental F/U Services (i.e., Growth & Development, Early Intervention)
		☐ Discharge Booklet given
		☐ Discuss/demonstrate infant care techniques
		☐ Parents safely perform/verbalize understanding of:
		  ☐ axillary temp & normal range ☐ eye/oral care
		  ☐ diapering/elimination patterns ☐ nail care ☐ cord care
		  ☐ bath (sponge/tub) & skin care ☐ umbilicus care ☐ bulb syringe
		  ☐ feeding techniques
		    ☐ duration/amount ☐ scheduled/demand ☐ positioning
		    ☐ burping ☐ formula preparation
		  ☐ vitamin administration ☐ appropriate clothing/weather
		  ☐ visitors/outings ☐ sleep/wake cycles
		  ☐ temperament/disposition
		  ☐ stress management ☐ "Back to Sleep" positioning
		  ☐ s/s of illness/when to call the M.D. ☐ safety
		☐ Assess home readiness
		☐ has car seat/provide loaner information
		  car seat safety reviewed
		☐ has adequate supplies (i.e., diapers, clothing, formula)
		☐ discuss rooming in ☐ circ consent signed
		☐ CPR class scheduled ☐ CPR class completed/reviewed
		☐ Begin teaching specialized care
		  ☐ gastrostomy feeds ☐ home O₂ ☐ ostomy care ☐ trachea care
		  ☐ other: _____
		
		EXPECTED OUTCOME:
		Prob #4: Parents safely perform/verbalize understanding of infant care techniques.
		
		_____ OUTCOME MET
			☐ Review Discharge Booklet
			☐ Age appropriate vaccinations given
			☐ Vitamins relabeled
			☐ prescriptions filled prior to D/C
			☐ Circ completed
			☐ Circ care reviewed
			☐ Car seat check passed
			☐ Rooming-in scheduled _____
			☐ Review s/s of illness
			☐ Specialized instruction completed
			  ☐ monitor training completed
			  ☐ home O₂ training completed
			  ☐ F/U home care arranged
			  ☐ Other: _____
			☐ Ongoing Social Service intervention
			☐ Home visits scheduled
			  ☐ Lactation consultant
			  ☐ Nursing
			☐ Pediatrician/follow-up physician identified
			
			EXPECTED OUTCOME:
			Prob #4: discharged to home
			
			_____ OUTCOME MET

	PHASE 1: ADMISSION/CRITICAL	PHASE 2: CONVALESCENT	PHASE 3: DISCHARGE
CARDIOVASCULAR Indocin / Lasix 1. ___ 2. ___ 3. ___ 4. ___	☐ Assess CV status, auscultate for murmur/PDA ☐ VS q 1°, H.O. q 8° ☐ VS q 2°, H.O. q 4° when stable ☐ Continuous B/P monitoring via UAC or PAL ☐ Cuff B/P when stable ☐ Echocardiogram as ordered **EXPECTED OUTCOME:** Prob #8: Hemodynamically stable without evidence of PDA OUTCOME MET ___	☐ Assess CV status ☐ VS as ordered ☐ Cuff B/P q shift ☐ F/U echo as ordered **EXPECTED OUTCOME:** Prob #8: Hemodynamically stable with B/P in normal range OUTCOME MET ___	☐ Assess CV status ☐ VS a̅c̅ ☐ Cuff B/P daily **EXPECTED OUTCOME:** Prob #8: Discharged with VS WNL OUTCOME MET ___
RESPIRATORY surfactant administered 1. ___ 2. ___ 3. ___ 4. ___	☐ Assess respiratory status ☐ Pulse oximetry within prescribed range ☐ Noted @ bedside ☐ Mechanical ventilation ☐ Suction to pre-measured depth ☐ ETT placement depth @ bedside ☐ CXR as ordered ☐ G + 3 as ordered ☐ CPT as ordered ☐ Aerosol therapy as ordered ☐ TCOM as ordered ☐ Meds started ☐ Caffeine ☐ Aminophylline ☐ Albuterol ☐ Vancenase ☐ Decadron ☐ Other: ___ **EXPECTED OUTCOME:** Prob #1: Extubated OUTCOME MET ___	☐ Assess respiratory status ☐ Pulse oximetry within prescribed range ☐ Noted @ bedside ☐ NCPAP ☐ TCOM as ordered ☐ CXR as ordered ☐ CPT as ordered ☐ Aerosol therapy as ordered ☐ G + 3 as ordered ☐ Wean to NC as tolerated ☐ Meds continued ☐ Caffeine ☐ Aminophylline ☐ Albuterol ☐ Decadron ☐ Vancenase ☐ Monitor training scheduled ☐ Completed ☐ Pneumogram done **EXPECTED OUTCOME:** Prob #1: CPAP D/C'd OUTCOME MET ___	☐ Assess respiratory status ☐ Maintain oximetry while on O₂ ☐ Discharge Meds ___ ___ ___ **EXPECTED OUTCOME:** Prob #1: Nasal Cannula D/C'd OUTCOME MET ___
THERMOREGULATION INTEG.	☐ Minimize insensible H₂O loss ☐ Initiate skin care guidelines **EXPECTED OUTCOME:** Prob #5: Transferred to isolette OUTCOME MET ___	☐ Wean isolette as tolerated ☐ Maintain skin care guidelines **EXPECTED OUTCOME:** Prob #5: Temp stable out of heat OUTCOME MET ___	☐ Maintain skin care guidelines **EXPECTED OUTCOME:** Prob #5: Maintains temp in open crib OUTCOME MET ___

Note: Each patient requires an individual assessment & treatment plan. This clinical path is a recommendation for the average patient which requires modification when necessary by the professional staff.

Figure 29-2 ■ An example of a clinical pathway for infants in an NICU. The pathway is adapted to meet the needs of each individual infant. *CPT*, Chest physiotherapy; *CXR*, chest x-ray; *ETT*, endotracheal tube; *HAL/lipids*, hyperalimentation; *H.O.*, hands-on; *NCPAP*, nasal continuous positive airway pressure; *NGT*, nasogastric tube; *OGT*, orogastric tube; *PDA*, patent ductus arteriosus; *TCB*, transcutaneous bilirubinometer; *TCOM*, transcutaneous oxygen monitor; *TPN*, total parenteral nutrition. (Courtesy Women and Children Services of the York Health System, York, Pennsylvania. Modified with permission.) *Continued.*

YORK HEALTH SYSTEM
YORK, PENNSYLVANIA

NICU CLINICAL PATHWAY

	PHASE 1: ADMISSION/CRITICAL	PHASE 2: CONVALESCENT	PHASE 3: DISCHARGE
FLUIDS, ELECTROLYTES, NUTRITION Extended metabolic screen drawn Date _____ Repeated _____	☐ Assess abdomen for bowel sounds, distention, tenderness ☐ Assess fluid/hydration status ☐ IV fluids as ordered ☐ Blood glucose as ordered ☐ TPN, lipids as ordered ☐ NPO ☐ OGT/NGT change q 72° ☐ Trophic feeds initiated ☐ Advance to full OG feeds as tolerated ☐ Lactation consultation ☐ Breastfeeding Care Plan initiated ☐ Pumping started within 24 hrs ☐ Breast milk storage reviewed ☐ Received NICU Breastfeeding Information Folder **EXPECTED OUTCOME:** Prob #2: HAL/lipids D/C'd _____ OUTCOME MET _____ Prob #2: Returned to birthweight _____ OUTCOME MET _____ Prob #4: Mother verbalized/demonstrated understanding of pumping frequency, storage & cleaning _____ OUTCOME MET _____	☐ Assess abdomen for bowel sounds, distention, tenderness ☐ Assess fluid/hydration status ☐ IV fluids as ordered ☐ C/S as ordered ☐ Advance to breast/nipple feeds as tolerated ☐ Lactation consultation assessment ☐ Reports maintaining milk supply **EXPECTED OUTCOME:** Prob #2: Weight gain pattern achieved _____ OUTCOME MET _____ Prob #2: Nippling/breastfeeding all feeds _____ OUTCOME MET _____ Prob #4: Breastfeeding support/education continued _____ OUTCOME MET _____	☐ Assess abdomen for bowel sounds, distention, tenderness ☐ Lactation consultation assessment ☐ Discharge Breastfeeding Care Plan reviewed **EXPECTED OUTCOME:** Prob #2: Ad lib feeds with overall weight _____ OUTCOME MET _____ Prob #4: Verbalizes understanding of Discharge Breastfeeding Care Plan _____ OUTCOME MET _____
HEME/BILI Vitamin K given _____ Type & cross as ordered _____ Transfusion Dates: _____ _____ _____	☐ Assess for S/S jaundice ☐ TCB as ordered ☐ Phototherapy as ordered ☐ Serum bili as ordered ☐ Assess for S/S of anemia ☐ CBC, IT, retic as ordered **EXPECTED OUTCOME:** Prob #10: Phototherapy discontinued _____ OUTCOME MET _____	☐ Assess for S/S jaundice ☐ TCB as ordered ☐ Serum bili as ordered ☐ Assess for S/S anemia ☐ CBC, IT, retic as ordered **EXPECTED OUTCOME:** Prob #10: Jaundice resolved _____ OUTCOME MET _____	☐ Assess for S/S anemia **EXPECTED OUTCOME:** Prob #4: Discharged with stable HCT _____ OUTCOME MET _____

	PHASE 1: ADMISSION/CRITICAL	PHASE 2: CONVALESCENT	PHASE 3: DISCHARGE
NEURO	☐ Assess neuro status ☐ Assess for & document seizure activity ☐ Head sono as ordered **EXPECTED OUTCOME:** Prob #9: Free of seizure activity OUTCOME MET ___	☐ Assess neuro status ☐ Assess for & document seizure activity ☐ Algo as ordered ☐ Eye exam as ordered ☐ F/U head sono as ordered **EXPECTED OUTCOME:** Prob #9: Hearing & eyes evaluated OUTCOME MET ___	☐ Late sono as ordered ___ ☐ F/U referrals made ___ **EXPECTED OUTCOME:** Prob #9: Appropriate referrals for F/U will be made OUTCOME MET ___

INFECTIOUS DISEASE	☐ Assess for S/S of infection
	☐ Blood culture as ordered
	☐ Antibiotics as ordered
	☐ Warmer changed after swamping D/C'd
	
	EXPECTED OUTCOME:
	Prob #6: D/C Amp/Gent if blood cultures negative
	
	OUTCOME MET ___
		☐ Assess for S/S nosocomial infection
		☐ Blood cx as ordered
		☐ Antibiotics as ordered
		
		EXPECTED OUTCOME:
		Prob #6: Free of signs and symptoms of infection
		
		OUTCOME MET ___
			☐ Med assessment for Synargis
			  ☐ Synargis given
			  ☐ RSV education reviewed
			
			EXPECTED OUTCOME:
			Prob #6: Age appropriate vaccination administered
			
			OUTCOME MET ___
			
			Prob #4: Parents verbalize understanding of RSV prophylaxis
			
			OUTCOME MET ___

DEVELOPMENTALLY SENSITIVE CARE	☐ Maintain minimal stimulation, ↑ noise & light, cluster care
	☐ Position flexed using H₂O beds, rolls, nesting, etc.
	☐ Offer non-nutritive sucking
	☐ Provide comfort measures such as swaddling, music, position changes
	☐ Provide opportunities for touching, holding as tolerated
	☐ Kangaroo care as tolerated
	☐ Pain scale reviewed q shift
	
	EXPECTED OUTCOME:
	Prob #4: Developmentally sensitive care techniques implemented
	
	OUTCOME MET ___
	
	Prob #9: Infant's comfort maximized as demonstrated by minimal pain scores
	
	OUTCOME MET ___
		☐ Provide as appropriate:
		  ☐ Visual stimulation ☐ NSS ☐ Soft music
		  ☐ Swaddling ☐ holding, rocking
		  ☐ Social interaction ☐ Kangaroo care
		☐ Cluster care, enforce undisturbed time-out periods
		☐ Position flexed ☐ OT/PT as ordered
		☐ Infant massage as tolerated ☐ Pain scale reviewed pm
		
		EXPECTED OUTCOME:
		Prob #4: Parents verbalize understanding and demonstrate developmentally sensitive care techniques
		
		OUTCOME MET ___
		
		Prob #9: Infant cues indicative of comfort
		
		OUTCOME MET ___
			☐ Referral to Growth & Development Clinic
			☐ Referral to Early Intervention
			☐ Pain assessment prn
			
			EXPECTED OUTCOME:
			Prob #4: Appropriate discharge referrals and appointments made
			
			OUTCOME MET ___
			
			Prob #9: Pain assessment zero
			
			OUTCOME MET ___

Figure 29-2, cont'd ■ For legend, see p. 763.

Note: Each patient requires an individual assessment & treatment plan. This clinical path is a recommendation for the average patient which requires modification when necessary by the professional staff.

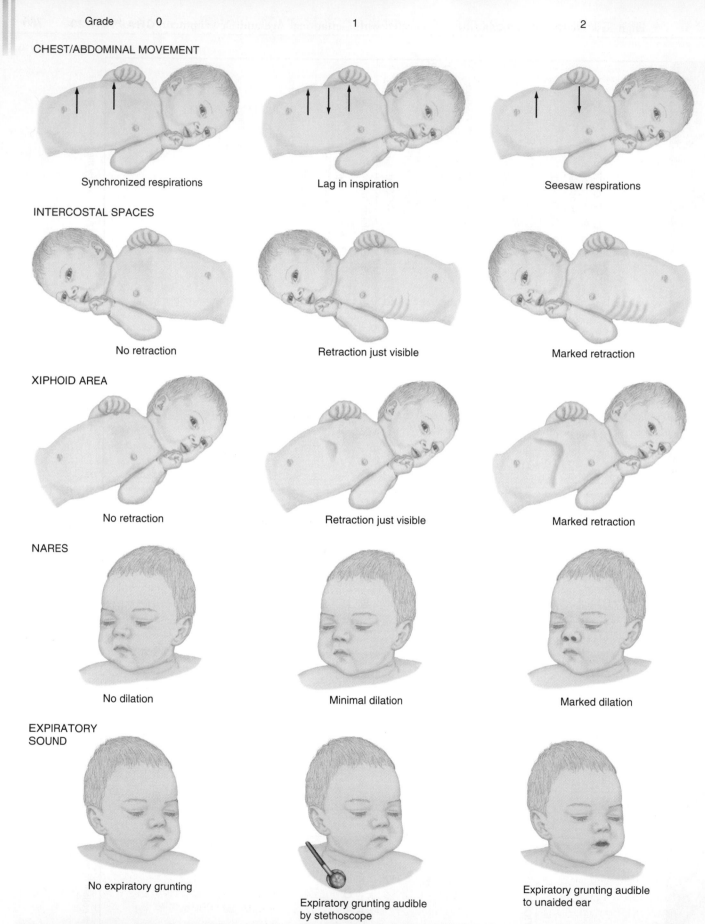

Figure 29-3 ■ Assessment of respiratory distress. The Silverman-Andersen index is used to score the infant's degree of respiratory difficulty. The score for individual criteria matches the grade, with a total possible score of 10 indicating severe distress. (Modified with permission of the American Academy of Pediatrics; from Silverman, W., & Andersen, D. [1956]. A cold clinical trial of effects of water mist on obstructive respiratory signs, death rate and necropsy findings among premature infants, *Pediatrics,* 17, 4.)

equate develop respiratory distress syndrome (RDS) (p. 789). In addition, preterm infants have a poorly developed cough reflex and narrow respiratory passages, which increase the risk for respiratory difficulty.

ASSESSMENT. The infant's respiratory status must be observed constantly. The lungs are assessed for adventitious breath sounds or areas of absent breath sounds. The Silverman-Andersen index is a useful tool for evaluating the degree of respiratory distress (Figure 29-3).

The nurse differentiates periodic breathing from apneic spells. Periodic breathing is the cessation of breathing for 5 to 10 seconds without other changes. It may be followed by 10- to 15-second periods of rapid respirations (Hagedorn, Gardner, & Abman, 2002). Changes in color or heart rate do not occur. Although periodic breathing sometimes occurs in term infants, preterm infants experience it more often.

Apneic spells generally last more than 20 seconds and are accompanied by cyanosis and bradycardia (Hagedorn et al., 2002). Apnea lasting a shorter time with heart rate or color changes also is a concern. Apneic spells are common in preterm infants, increasing in incidence with lower gestational age. Apnea without an identified cause in a preterm infant is called *apnea of prematurity* and generally improves as the infant matures. Medications such as aminophylline, theophylline, and caffeine may be necessary. Spells may occur along with periodic breathing, and the infant may require gentle stimulation or bag and mask ventilation. Apnea should be investigated because it may be related to other causes.

The nurse observes the effort required for breathing and the location and severity of retractions. Retractions are particularly noticeable in preterm infants, whose weak chest wall is drawn in with each inspiration. The excessive compliance (elasticity) of the chest cage during retractions occurs because the bones of the chest wall are very pliable. This may interfere with full expansion of the lungs.

Grunting may be an early sign of RDS. It closes the glottis and increases the pressure within the alveoli. This keeps the alveoli partially open during expiration and increases the amount of oxygen absorbed.

NURSING INTERVENTIONS. Interventions focus on collaborating with other team members such as the respiratory therapist to manage technical equipment and facilitate removal of secretions.

Working with Respiratory Equipment. An oxygen hood is often used for infants who are able to breathe alone but need extra oxygen. The hood is a plastic dome that fits over the infant's head or head and upper body. The infant breathes the higher levels of oxygen within the hood, and the device does not interfere with access to the rest of the infant's body for care (Figure 29-4).

Oxygen also may be given by nasal cannula to the infant who breathes well alone. After discharge, many preterm infants continue to receive oxygen via nasal cannula at home. Oxygen must be humidified to prevent insensible water loss and drying of the delicate mucous membranes. It is warmed to maintain body temperature.

Continuous positive airway pressure (CPAP) may be necessary to keep the alveoli open and improve expansion of

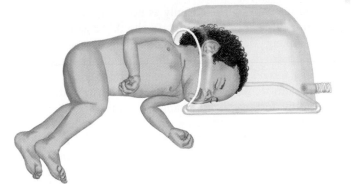

Figure 29-4 ■ The oxygen hood is one way of delivering oxygen to an infant who can breathe unassisted.

the lungs. It can be delivered with nasal prongs or an endotracheal tube. The infant may need conventional mechanical ventilation, or high-frequency ventilation may be used to provide very fast, frequent respirations with less pressure and volume. This helps decrease injury to the tissue from pressure (barotrauma) and volume (volutrauma) compared with other methods.

When oxygen is administered, the level of oxygen in the infant's blood must be monitored. Arterial blood may be drawn for testing oxygen levels. Pulse oximetry or transcutaneous monitoring also may be used. These methods are less invasive and provide continuous information about oxygen partial pressure (PO_2) levels through sensors attached to the skin.

The nurse must observe the infant's increasing or decreasing dependence on breathing assistance and need for oxygen. The infant's response to activity that may increase oxygen need, such as handling, feeding, and linen changes, may require changes in settings on equipment to meet the infant's needs. Oxygen flow is increased when suctioning is necessary.

Positioning the Infant. Frequent position changes help drain air passages and prevent stasis of secretions. The side-lying and prone positions facilitate drainage of respiratory secretions and regurgitated feedings. The prone position is not recommended for normal newborn infants because it is associated with an increased incidence of sudden infant death syndrome (SIDS). In the preterm infant, however, the prone position increases oxygenation and lung compliance and decreases energy expenditure (Lefrak-Okikawa & Lund, 2001). This should be explained to parents. The supine position should be used for sleep when infants have recovered enough to tolerate it. By changing to the supine position as soon as possible before discharge, infants will become used to sleeping on the back.

Infants should be repositioned every 2 to 3 hours when other care is given to help dependent areas of the lungs drain into the main bronchi. Frequent position changes help air passages drain and prevent stasis of secretions.

Suctioning Secretions. The weak or absent cough reflex and very small air passages make the preterm infant's airways susceptible to obstruction by mucus. The nurse checks suction equipment at the beginning of each shift to ensure it is available and functioning properly.

The infant is suctioned only as necessary when the need becomes apparent. Suction always should be gentle to avoid traumatizing the delicate mucous membranes. Trauma could cause edema, which could further decrease the size of the air passages and lead to more respiratory difficulty.

In addition, suctioning decreases oxygenation during the procedure and may cause changes in heart rate, blood pressure and cerebral blood flow and provides an entry for organisms. Increased oxygen should be provided before and after each suction attempt. The mouth is suctioned before the nose because stimulation of the nares causes reflex inspiration that could cause aspiration of fluids in the infant's mouth (Hagedorn et al., 2002).

Maintaining Hydration. Adequate hydration is essential to keep secretions thin so that they can be removed by drainage or suction. If infants become dehydrated, secretions will become thick and viscous and could obstruct tiny air passages. Fluid intake should be increased (within the limits of the overall treatment plan ordered by the physician) if secretions seem to indicate even minimal dehydration.

✓ CHECK YOUR READING

1. How does the appearance of a preterm infant differ from that of a full-term infant?
2. What factors contribute to respiratory problems in preterm infants?
3. What nursing responsibilities relate to care of preterm respiratory problems?

PROBLEMS WITH THERMOREGULATION

Although heat loss can be a problem for full-term infants, it is even more significant in preterm infants. The skin is thin with blood vessels near the surface, and little subcutaneous white fat is present to serve as insulation. As a result, heat loss is rapid. The shorter time in the uterus allows less brown fat to accumulate before birth, impairing the preterm infant's ability to produce heat by nonshivering thermogenesis.

Preterm infants have a larger head and greater body surface area in proportion to size than full-term infants. Although full-term infants maintain heat by flexion of the extremities, the limp, extended body of preterm newborns exposes a greater surface area to the air for heat loss. The temperature control center of the brain of preterm infants is less mature and may be further impaired by asphyxia. These conditions all contribute to heat loss.

Complications from heat loss, such as hypoglycemia and respiratory problems, are more likely to develop in preterm infants. This limits the glucose and oxygen available to increase metabolism as a method of heat production. Vasoconstriction, which occurs when body temperature drops, may lead to metabolic acidosis, pulmonary vasoconstriction, interference with production of surfactant, and more respiratory difficulty.

ASSESSMENT. The infant's temperature is monitored continuously by a skin probe on the infant's abdomen, which is attached to the heat control mechanism of the radiant warmer or incubator. The abdominal skin temperature is usually maintained at 36° to 36.5° C (96.8° to 97.7° F). The infant's temperature as shown on the monitor should be recorded every 30 to 60 minutes initially and every 3 to 4 hours when the infant is stable. The nurse should assess the axillary temperature every 4 to 8 hours and compare it with the heat control reading to ensure that the machinery is functioning properly.

The axillary temperature for a preterm infant should remain between 36.3° and 36.9° C (97.3° and 98.4° F), slightly lower than the temperature for full-term infants (Blake & Murray, 2002). If the infant has accumulated brown fat, a normal axillary temperature when the monitor shows a decreased skin temperature may indicate that brown fat in the axillary space is being used to maintain the infant's core temperature.

Indications of inadequate thermoregulation include poor feeding or intolerance to feedings in an infant who previously had little difficulty, lethargy, irritability, poor muscle tone, cool skin temperature, and mottled skin (Figure 29-5). Hypoglycemia and respiratory distress may be the first signs that the infant's temperature is low. Because temperature instability may be an early sign of infection, the nurse should assess for other evidence that infection may be present. A decrease in weight gain or weight loss may occur over time.

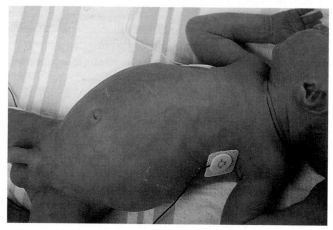

Figure 29-5 ■ This preterm infant has mildly mottled skin and slight abdominal distention and retractions.

⚕ CRITICAL TO REMEMBER

Signs of Inadequate Thermoregulation

Axillary temperature <36.3° C or >36.9° C (<97.3° or >98.4° F)
Abdominal skin temperature <36° C or >36.5° C (<96.8° or >97.7° F)
Change in feeding behavior
Lethargy
Irritability
Weak cry or suck
Decreased muscle tone
Cool skin temperature
Mottled skin
Signs of hypoglycemia
Signs of respiratory difficulty
Poor weight gain

NURSING INTERVENTIONS. Maintenance of heat in preterm infants involves the same basic nursing care principles as for the full-term infant (see Chapter 21). These principles must be adapted to meet the needs of the preterm infant, however.

Maintaining a Neutral Thermal Environment. A neutral thermal environment is especially important to prevent the need for increased oxygen to maintain the infant's body temperature. Radiant warmers or incubators are used until infants can maintain normal body temperature alone. Charts are available that indicate the appropriate temperature setting to maintain a neutral thermal environment according to the infant's size and maturity. Because they lose more heat and produce heat less effectively, smaller, less-mature infants need more warmth to maintain body heat than larger or older preterm infants.

Infants needing many procedures are usually placed under the open radiant warmer to make it easier to see them and work with equipment. However, air currents around an unclothed infant can cause heat loss by convection despite the heat generated by the warmer. Doors near the warmer should be closed and traffic kept to a minimum to decrease convective heat loss. The infant should receive only warmed oxygen because thermal receptors in the face are very sensitive to cold. Cold oxygen could quickly lead to cold stress.

Equipment and caregivers should not come between the infant and the heat source, preventing heat from reaching the infant. A transparent plastic blanket over the infant allows heat from the warmer to pass across to the infant. The blanket decreases convective heat loss from exposure to drafts as well as insensible and evaporative water loss. At the same time, it maintains visibility of the infant's body parts.

Incubators are used for infants who do not need to be under radiant warmers. Warmed air is circulated inside the incubator to provide heat. Humidity should also be added to decrease insensible water loss.

When infants are in incubators, the nurse should keep portholes and doors closed as much as possible. A significant amount of heat is lost each time the incubator is opened, and it may take as long as an hour for the temperature to reach the original level (Chandra & Baumgart, 2005). Infants removed from the incubator for procedures or holding should be wrapped in heated blankets with head coverings. Incubator doors should be closed while the infant is outside to retain heat inside.

Infants should be placed under a radiant warmer or on a surface padded with warm blankets for procedures that cannot be performed inside the incubator. A heat lamp provides an alternative source of heat.

Although temperature regulation in preterm infants is usually provided in incubators until infants can maintain their own temperature, warmth can also be provided by holding by the parents. Adequate temperature is maintained in stable infants during kangaroo care (KC) (p. 786) or even when infants are swaddled and held close to the parent's body (Mellien, 2001).

Although temperature loss is the most common concern, overheating also is a problem for preterm infants. Over-heating may occur when heating devices such as radiant warmers are set too high or the skin probe is inadvertently removed. Overheating leads to an increase in the metabolic rate, with increased oxygen and glucose needs, and insensible water losses. Alarms to detect high or low temperature should be turned on at all times.

WEANING TO AN OPEN CRIB. Preparation of infants for moving to an open crib should begin early. When they are stable, infants can be dressed in a shirt, diaper, and hat while in the incubator. Clothing conserves heat and helps infants adjust to a different temperature on the face than the rest of the body. Infants who weigh about 1500 g (3 lb, 7 oz), have a consistent weight gain for 5 days, and are tolerating feedings can begin gradual weaning from external heat (Blake & Murray, 2002).

Each NICU has its own protocol for the weaning process. The incubator temperature usually is decreased gradually. It is raised if the infant's temperature falls below the normal range. If the temperature remains stable, the process can continue the next day.

When infants are ready for transfer to an open crib they should be double-wrapped with warm blankets at first to help insulate body heat. The temperature is assessed at gradually increasing intervals until the infant is on a routine schedule. A blanket is added for a low temperature, but if the temperature does not rise to normal, infants are returned to the incubator.

Nurses should observe infants carefully during the first few days after transfer to an open crib. Signs that may indicate inadequate thermoregulation include decreased weight gain, poor feeding, or increased requirement for oxygen.

PROBLEMS WITH FLUID AND ELECTROLYTE BALANCE

Preterm infants lose fluid very easily, and the loss increases with the degree of prematurity. Their thin skin has little protective subcutaneous white fat and a greater water content, and it is more permeable than the skin of term infants. The large surface area in proportion to body weight and lack of flexion further increase transepidermal water losses. Radiant warmers and the heat from phototherapy lights cause even more fluid loss through the skin. Radiant warmers heighten insensible water losses enough to result in a 40% to 50% increase in fluid needs (Blake & Murray, 2002).

Water loss also occurs through the respiratory and gastrointestinal tracts. The rapid respiratory rate and use of oxygen can increase fluid loss from the lungs. Loose stools will lead to rapid dehydration.

Development of the kidneys is not complete until approximately 35 weeks of gestation. The ability of the kidneys to concentrate or dilute urine is poor before that time, causing a fragile balance between dehydration and overhydration. Great variation in fluid needs occurs, depending on many variables such as the infant's size, gestational age, insensible water loss from radiant warmers or phototherapy, and medical needs. The fluid needs of preterm infants range from 80 to 120 ml/kg on the first day to 90 to 140 ml/kg/day on the second and third days of life and may reach 100 to

175 ml/kg each day by the end of the first week. Very-low-birth-weight and extremely low-birth-weight infants may need more fluid. Normal urinary output is 2 to 5 ml/kg per hour (Berry, Adcock, & Starbuck, 2002).

Regulation of electrolytes by the kidneys also is a problem. Common electrolyte imbalances include excess calcium and too little or too much sodium or potassium. Preterm infants need higher intakes of sodium because the kidneys do not reabsorb it well. If they receive too much sodium, however, they may be unable to increase sodium excretion adequately and are susceptible to sodium and water overload.

ASSESSMENT. The nurse must be alert for fluid overload or deficit. The infant's intake and output by all routes is carefully calculated. Parenteral, feeding tube, and oral fluids are included when intake is measured. Output from regurgitation, drainage tubes, stools, and urine should be measured. The nurse also must keep track of the amount of blood taken for laboratory tests, because the loss can be substantial and the infant cannot make new blood fast enough.

Urinary Output. There are several methods for measuring urinary output. Plastic bags that adhere to the perineum are not suitable for the preterm infant because they may damage the fragile skin. Weighing diapers is less harmful to the infant. The weight of dry diapers is subtracted from the weight of wet diapers to determine the amount of urine excreted. One gram is equivalent to 1 ml of urine. However, humidification may add moisture to the diaper and a radiant warmer may cause evaporation of urine on the diaper. When precise measurement is essential, diapers can be fastened instead of being placed open under the infant.

Specific gravity should be checked to determine if urine is more concentrated or dilute than expected. Urine is collected by placing cotton balls at the perineum. The specific gravity should range between 1.002 and 1.010 (Berry et al., 2002).

Weight. Changes in the infant's weight can give an indication of fluid gain or loss, especially if the changes are sudden and greater than would be expected. The undressed infant should be weighed at the same time each day with the same scale. Very small infants often are placed in a bed with a scale so that they do not have to be disturbed for daily weighing. They may be weighed twice a day to monitor their fluid status more closely.

Signs of Dehydration or Overhydration. The nurse should observe for signs that indicate the infant has received too little or too much fluid. Early signs of dehydration include decreased urine output (<2 ml/hr) and increased specific gravity. Weight loss may exceed that expected for the infant's age and general condition. Dry skin or mucous membranes, sunken anterior fontanelle, and poor tissue turgor are late signs. Changes in the blood include increased sodium, protein, and hematocrit levels resulting from decreased plasma volume.

Signs of overhydration include increased output of urine (>5 ml/hr) with a below-normal specific gravity. Edema and weight gain occur from retention of fluids. Bulging

---

CRITICAL TO REMEMBER

Signs of Fluid Imbalance in the Newborn

Dehydration
Urine output <2 ml/kg/hr
Urine specific gravity >1.010
Weight loss greater than expected
Dry skin and mucous membranes
Sunken anterior fontanelle
Poor tissue turgor
Blood: elevated sodium, protein, and hematocrit levels
Hypotension

Overhydration
Urine output >5 ml/kg/hr
Urine specific gravity <1.002
Edema
Weight gain greater than expected
Bulging fontanels
Blood: decreased sodium, protein, and hematocrit levels
Moist breath sounds
Difficulty breathing

---

fontanels, moist breath sounds, and decreased blood sodium, protein, and hematocrit levels also are present. Complications of excess fluid may include patent ductus arteriosus and congestive heart failure.

NURSING INTERVENTIONS. The nurse must carefully regulate intravenous (IV) fluids using infusion control devices that administer 1 ml/hr or less to help prevent fluid volume overload. IV medications should be diluted in as little fluid as is consistent with safe administration of the drug and be included when intake is measured. Starting IV lines on infants with poor veins is a lengthy, difficult procedure. Infants must be restrained as necessary to prevent dislodging of the catheter. If they infiltrate, some solutions will cause extensive damage as a result of tissue sloughing.

IV sites should be assessed at least every hour for signs of infiltration. Many infants have central venous catheters or umbilical lines that must be assessed for infection and position changes. Small blood transfusions may be necessary to replace blood drawn for frequent laboratory tests.

PROBLEMS WITH THE SKIN

Preterm infants have fragile, permeable, easily damaged skin. They often have endotracheal tubes, IV lines, electrodes, and other equipment that must be maintained in place, but standard adhesive tape should not be used because it can be very damaging to the skin. Removal of adhesive tape may strip the epidermal layer of the skin, causing pain and increasing transepidermal water loss and the risk of infection. Alcohol, povidone-iodine, and other preparations used to disinfect the skin before invasive procedures can be damaging to fragile skin and may be absorbed.

ASSESSMENT. The nurse should frequently assess the condition of the infant's skin and note any changes. The infant's response to products used for cleansing and disinfection should be noted.

NURSING INTERVENTIONS. Care of the skin is a subject of much research. Evidence-based practice guidelines for care of the neonate's skin have been developed and endorsed by the Association of Women's Health, Obstetric and Neonatal Nurses (AWHONN) and the National Association of Neonatal Nurses (NANN) (Lund et al., 2001).

Tape should be used as little as possible. Backing tape with cotton, waiting more than 24 hours to remove it, and using gauze wraps decrease skin damage. Tape that is specially prepared to be less traumatic on removal is available. Semipermeable dressings and products that use pectin or hydrogel adhesive are less disruptive to the skin surface. They can be removed with water or mineral oil.

The nurse should avoid the use of chemicals that can injure the skin or may be absorbed through it. If these solutions are used, sterile saline or water can be used to remove them and minimize damage. Alcohol should not be used (AWHONN, 2001).

Bathing preterm infants is not necessary on a daily basis and should be performed only as needed. Bathing can disrupt the chemistry of the skin and may be stressful. Soap should be avoided during the first week for infants less than 32 weeks' gestational age. If there are areas of skin breakdown, sterile water is safest for cleansing (AWHONN, 2001).

Stable preterm infants without umbilical catheters may be immersed in water for bathing if there are no contraindications. After the bath the infant should be wrapped in warm towels and not dressed until thoroughly dry, about 10 minutes. If the infant is dressed too soon, the clothing will be damp and will increase heat loss.

Humidity in incubators should be regulated to reduce the drying effects of heat. Preservative-free petrolatum-based emollients may be used to protect the skin and to help reduce fissures in dry skin. Emollients also help decrease transepidermal water loss and may be used under phototherapy. The infant's skin should be observed for signs of infection. Transparent adhesive dressings may be placed on uninfected wounds and excoriations but should not be removed daily because the adhesive can further injure the skin (AWHONN, 2001).

Infants and their equipment should be positioned to avoid undue pressure on the skin. Frequent position changes are important but should be based on the infant's ability to tolerate changes. Devices such as mattresses filled with water, air, or gel are available to help distribute weight to prevent pressure areas.

PROBLEMS WITH INFECTION

The incidence of infection in preterm infants is 3 to 10 times greater than that in full-term newborns (Stoll, 2004). Many preterm infants have one or more episodes of sepsis during their hospital stay. They have several risk factors for infections. A maternal infection may have caused labor to begin prematurely and exposed the infant to the same infection. The infant may not have received adequate passive immunity from the transfer of immunoglobulin G from the mother that takes place during the third trimester. In addition, the preterm infant's immune response to infection is less mature than that of the full-term newborn.

Preterm infants often are exposed to situations that may cause infection. In addition to their fragile skin, they are subject to invasive procedures such as insertion of IV lines and drawing of blood specimens. A prolonged stay in the hospital increases the likelihood of acquiring an infection from multiple exposures to organisms.

ASSESSMENT. The nurse should be alert for signs of infection at all times (see Chapter 30, p. 814).

NURSING INTERVENTIONS. Handwashing is one of the most important aspects of preventing infections. Nursing care involves scrupulous cleanliness and maintenance of the infant's skin integrity. Even normal flora on the hands of caretakers may cause sepsis. Therefore parents and staff members should thoroughly wash their hands and arms before handling infants. Exposure to family and staff members who have contagious diseases should be prevented.

Early signs of infections should be identified and reported so that treatment may begin immediately. The nurse carefully notes the infant's response to treatment as some organisms become resistant to antibiotics. Other nursing care for infection is discussed in Chapter 30.

PROBLEMS WITH PAIN

Infants in the NICU undergo many painful procedures and treatments, such as intubation, heel sticks, chest tube placement, and venipuncture each day. Younger and sicker infants tend to need more interventions and suffer more pain-producing procedures than older, less-ill infants. Caregivers once thought that newborns, particularly preterm infants, were neurologically too immature to feel pain. Pain stimuli are now recognized to cause physiologic and behavioral changes in infants as early as 20 weeks' gestation (Walden, 2004). The long-term effects of pain in the neonate are not yet fully understood. The American Academy of Pediatrics (AAP) and the Canadian Paediatric Society recommend that environmental, nonpharmacologic, and pharmacologic interventions be used to prevent, reduce, or eliminate pain in neonates (AAP & Canadian Paediatric Society, 2000).

Preterm infants may be even more sensitive to pain than older infants. Their pain may be greater and last longer than that of older children or adults (Evans, 2001). Pain can have numerous untoward effects. For example, increases in intracranial pressure resulting from pain may elevate the risk for intraventricular hemorrhage. Release of catecholamines and cortisol as a result of pain leads to increases or decreases in heart and respiratory rate, elevated blood sugar, higher metabolic rate, and greater need for oxygen (Blackburn, 2003a). In addition, infants repeatedly exposed to pain may respond to touch or other nonpainful stimuli as though they were in pain (Agarwal, Hagedorn, & Gardner, 2002).

ASSESSMENT. Because pain is the fifth vital sign, pain assessment is performed whenever vital signs are taken. In addition, the nurse must assess the infant for pain level and response to potentially painful stimuli, as well as response to pharmacologic and nonpharmacologic interventions.

NANN has developed guidelines for the assessment and management of pain in newborns (NANN, 2000). Recommendations include use of a pain scale to assess infant pain.

Assessment tools are available to evaluate physiological and behavioral responses to pain in term and preterm infants. Some, such as the Premature Infant Pain Profile (PIPP) are designed for preterm infants. Such tools assess gestational age and behavior states, heart rate, oxygen saturation rate, brow bulge, eye squeeze, and nasolabial furrow (lines from the edge of the nostrils to beyond the corners of the mouth) to assign a pain score.

Physiologic responses to pain include changes in heart rate and respirations, increased blood pressure, and decreased oxygen saturation. However, physiologic changes may be unpredictable and cannot be used alone to assess pain.

Behavioral changes include high-pitched, intense, harsh crying. In infants who are intubated or too weak to cry, a "cry face" is seen, with a facial expression of crying without the sound of a cry. Some preterm infants are too weak or overwhelmed by repeated or prolonged pain to show behavioral responses even though they are experiencing pain. Therefore, an infant's lack of response to a situation that is likely to cause pain should not be perceived as absence of pain.

Parents often spend many hours with their preterm infants in the NICU setting. The nurse should involve them in assessing the infant's pain and encourage them to share their evaluation of the infant's response to relief measures. They may have questions the nurse can answer about the effects of pain and the measures used to treat it.

NURSING INTERVENTIONS. Nurses should prepare infants for potentially painful procedures by waking them slowly and gently and using containment. Containment simulates the enclosed space of the uterus, prevents excessive and disorganized motor activity, and is comforting to infants. It involves keeping the extremities in a flexed position near the body by swaddling with blankets or use of nesting or positioning devices. Facilitated tucking is a method of

---

CRITICAL TO REMEMBER

Common Signs of Pain in Infants

High-pitched, intense, harsh cry
Whimpering, moaning
"Cry face"
Eyes squeezed shut
Mouth open
Grimacing
Furrowing or bulging of the brow
Tense, rigid muscles or flaccid muscle tone
Rigidity or flailing of extremities
Color changes: red, dusky, pale
Heart rate and respiratory changes, apnea
Increased blood pressure
Decreased oxygen saturation
Sleep-wake pattern changes

---

swaddling using the nurse's hands to hold the infant's extremities flexed, in the midline, and close to the body. The infant is in the supine or side-lying position with at least one of the infant's hands near the mouth for sucking.

Handling before a painful procedure should be minimized, if possible. Positioning for procedures can be uncomfortable and upsetting. Other care should be performed at another time to allow the infant to rest after the procedure. If several things must be done together, the least noxious should be performed first.

Comfort measures help the infant cope with short-term, mild pain and reduce agitation. Nonnutritive sucking with a pacifier is helpful but is effective only as long as the infant continues to suck. A single dose of sucrose placed in the infant's mouth or on a pacifier shortly before a painful stimulus increases pain relief. Sucrose may not be appropriate for very young preterm infants, however. Talking softly, restraining the extremities to prevent flailing, and holding and rocking are other common methods of pain relief. Measures should be adapted according to the infant's responses.

Comfort measures alone are not enough for moderate to severe pain. The nurse should discuss the infant's pain with the primary care provider to ensure that medications are available for long-term and more severe pain. Opioids such as morphine and fentanyl can be tolerated by preterm infants. Nonnarcotic analgesics such as acetaminophen may also be used.

Sedatives are sometimes used for agitation in sick newborns or to potentiate the effects of analgesics. They are not effective for pain, however, and should not be used in place of analgesics. They may be inappropriate for preterm infants. Regional or general anesthesia is used during surgery.

The nurse gives ordered medications before painful procedures and when the infant demonstrates pain signs. The infant's response is carefully noted to determine the need to increase or decrease the dosage. Analgesics may be given continuously or on an as-needed basis.

✔ **CHECK YOUR READING**

4. How do nurses help infants adjust to the cooler environment of an open crib?
5. How does the nurse keep track of an infant's intake and output?
6. What special problems related to fluid balance, infections, and pain occur in preterm infants?
7. What nonpharmacologic measures can nurses use to alleviate pain in infants?

Application of the Nursing Process
The Preterm Infant

Preterm infants commonly have difficulty with stress from the NICU environment and inability to obtain adequate nutrition. Their parents may have difficulty with bonding.

ENVIRONMENTALLY CAUSED STRESS

In the past, preterm infants were frequently exposed to bright lights and a noisy environment. The recommended hourly maximum level of background and transient noise is 50 decibels with a transient maximum level of 70 decibels. However, higher levels of noise may occur in NICUs (Consensus Committee to Establish Recommended Standards for Newborn ICU Design, 2002).

Sounds of alarms, ventilators, incubators, doors, and people can create a noise level that increases the risk for hearing loss and other complications. In addition, stimulation of any kind can cause increased energy expenditure by the preterm infant. Noise and routine but disturbing handling and nursing interventions often are accompanied by changes in heart rate and respirations, oxygen saturation levels, and behavior states.

Although touch is generally thought to be comforting to infants, it often is associated with painful events for preterm infants. This can cause infants to develop touch aversion, a negative response to touch of any kind. Preterm infants undergo multiple assessments and treatments that may cause frequent interruptions of sleep and interfere with the development of normal sleep-wake cycles. Energy that must be directed toward coping with an overstimulating and stressful environment may be unavailable for normal growth and development.

Assessment

Assess the amount of noise to which the infant is exposed. Determine how often interruptions occur and how the infant responds to different types of care.

Assess the infant's ability to tolerate activity and noise. Overstimulation results in changes in oxygenation and behavior. Behavioral indications of stress, also called *avoidance cues* or *avoidance behavior,* show the infant is seeking to escape the noxious stimuli. Observe for these signs and determine what situations cause them to occur or increase.

Analysis

A nursing diagnosis appropriate for preterm infants having difficulty enduring the multiple stimuli in their environment is "Risk for Disorganized Infant Behavior related to stress from an overstimulating environment." Use of this nursing diagnosis can help the nurse plan ways to increase the infant's ability to tolerate interventions.

Planning

The goals or expected outcomes for this nursing diagnosis are that the infant will:
- Show decreasing signs of overstimulation during routine activity as evidenced by fewer respiratory and behavioral changes during handling and increased periods of relaxed behavior or sleep
- Gradually show an ability to withstand more activity before signs of overstimulation occur

Interventions

Interventions are focused on providing developmentally supportive nursing care that meets the preterm infant's ability to tolerate stimulation. Developmental care keeps stressors in the environment to a minimum based on the infant's physiologic and behavioral responses.

SCHEDULING CARE

Schedule periods of undisturbed rest throughout the day to allow the infant to recover from treatments. Avoid waking the infant during the short quiet sleep phase. If the infant must be awakened for care, try to do it during an active period of sleep when the infant can be more easily aroused using quiet talking and gentle touch.

Avoid disturbing rest by arranging routine care to correspond with the infant's awake periods. Decrease the frequency of taking vital signs and performing other routine care as soon as possible. Even the handling involved in routine sponge bathing may cause stress in small infants. Routine daily baths are unnecessary and should be avoided. Instead baths should be given every few days with careful attention to the infant's response.

Cluster or group care activities so that several routine tasks are performed at one time to allow for more rest between interruptions. However, be alert to the infant's signs of stress, such as changes in oxygen saturation or vital signs. Too many activities may be more than the infant can tolerate without rest. Provide short rest periods or "time out" periods for recovery within grouped activities or during long or painful procedures if the infant shows signs of overstimulation.

An important nursing responsibility is managing the infant's care by coordinating activities of different health care workers. For example, many different tests often are needed, and the nurse must see that they are done properly while protecting the infant from overstimulation.

CRITICAL TO REMEMBER

Signs of Overstimulation in Preterm Infants

Oxygenation Changes
Increase or decrease in pulse and respiratory rate
Cyanosis, pallor, or mottling
Flaring nares
Decreased oxygen saturation levels

Behavior Changes
Stiff, extended arms and legs
Fisting of the hands or splaying of the fingers
Alert, worried expression
Turning away from eye contact (gaze aversion)
Hiccuping
Regurgitation
Fatigue
Coughing
Yawning

REDUCING STIMULI

Keep noise around the infant as low as possible. Place incubators away from traffic and congestion of people, and avoid talking near the incubator. Use incubator covers to help lower sound inside the incubator. Set alarms on low volume and respond quickly when they sound. Open and close portholes and doors on incubators and cupboards quietly. Do not place objects on top of the incubator or use it as a writing surface because it increases the noise inside. Teach parents and others to avoid tapping on the incubator.

Lights that are on 24 hours a day in the nursery may interfere with the development of sleep cycles. Position the incubator so that the infant is not facing bright lights, and drape a blanket or commercial incubator cover over the back and end to decrease light and noise further. Use a dimmer switch to vary the intensity of lights as needed. Place infants in a prone position to help them avoid looking at ceiling lights.

PROMOTING REST

When possible, schedule "quiet periods" when lights and noise in the unit are kept to a minimum to promote rest. Rest periods should be at least an hour in length to allow preterm infants to complete a sleep cycle (Gardner & Goldson, 2002). Scheduled naps when infants are disturbed as little as possible may help increase sleep, decrease waking, and lead to longer uninterrupted sleep. They may be associated with decreased periods of apnea and increased weight gain for some infants. A daytime and evening nap and two naps during the night will help the infant begin to differentiate between day and night sleeping patterns. Lights should be lowered at night to help development of circadian rhythms.

Contain the infant's arms and legs to promote flexion and reduce energy loss from flailing extremities. Containment also promotes quieting and improves physiologic stability. Provide a "nest" with rolled blankets or commercial nesting or positioning devices placed around the infant for boundaries. Use the prone position to increase flexion and quiet sleep periods. For the side-lying and supine positions, arrange the infant's arms and legs in a flexed position, with the hands near midline to allow hand-to-mouth activity and sucking.

PROMOTING MOTOR DEVELOPMENT

Preterm infants may have musculoskeletal and developmental problems from prolonged immobilization and the effects of gravity on their immature neuromuscular system. Because the extensor muscles mature before the flexor muscles, the infant tends to remain in an extended, "frog-leg" position. Shoulder retraction, abduction and external rotation of the lower extremities, and lateral flexion of the arms may result.

When possible, position the infant in a side-lying or prone position with the extremities flexed and the hands placed near the mouth to allow the infant to suck the hands for comfort. The prone position also facilitates breathing and development of head control. Swaddling, when appropriate, may help keep the infant in a contained position. Turn the infant every 2 hours, and use blankets, rolls, and positioning devices to maintain flexion.

INDIVIDUALIZING CARE

Although each NICU nurse is competent in caring for preterm infants, each one has a slightly different style in approaching infants. When possible, the same nurse should care for the infant each day. This allows the nurse to learn the infant's unique behavior and response to stress and allows the infant to get accustomed to the nurse's individual caregiving pattern. A team of several nurses may be assigned to each infant to allow consistent caregiving even when the primary nurse is not working. Infant care can be individualized to meet the infant's needs better if fewer nurses are involved in each infant's care.

The ability to tolerate stress varies with each infant. Adapt general care according to the infant's ability to tolerate it. Determine the infant's response to various stimuli, particularly those that cause adverse responses. Even positive stimuli such as talking quietly to the infant can cause overstimulation at times. Use these measures judiciously and according to the infant's tolerance level.

Infants often require extra energy to adjust to changes in care. Observe how well they tolerate changes such as moving from assisted to more independent breathing or introduction of new feeding methods. Increase rest periods during these times.

COMMUNICATING INFANTS' NEEDS

Use the nursing care plan, Kardex, and shift reports to inform other caregivers of techniques that are especially effective for certain infants. Tape notes at the bedside as reminders of needs unique to each infant. Doing so also alerts the parents to the methods nurses use to help the infant. Explain all techniques to the parents, and solicit their suggestions.

Evaluation

As a result of interventions, the infant displays signs of overstimulation less often and shows an increasing tolerance to stimuli before signs appear.

NUTRITION

The need for adequate nutrition in the preterm newborn is especially acute because the infant is born before full accumulation of nutrient stores and digestive capacity is achieved. The problem increases with decreasing gestational age.

Full-term newborns have reservoirs of calcium, iron, and other nutrients, but these are lacking in preterm infants. Fat stores are minimal or absent, and glucose reserves are used soon after birth. Nutrients are needed not only to promote growth but to prevent injury to the brain. Hypoglycemia is a major concern because of the lack of glucose and fat reserves. Low blood glucose develops very quickly and must be prevented or treated quickly.

Preterm infants need approximately 105 to 130 kcal/kg/day (Kleinman, 2004). This amount varies according to activity, illness, and other factors that may affect caloric need. Preterm infants need more protein, iron, calcium, and phosphorus. The average healthy preterm infant should gain approximately 15 to 20 g/kg/day (Anderson, Johnson, Townsend, & Hay 2002).

The gastrointestinal tract of preterm infants does not absorb nutrients as well as that of full-term infants. Although they digest protein well, preterm infants have insufficient bile acids and pancreatic lipase to absorb fat adequately. They have some lactase deficiency but digest glucose and sucrose adequately. Their smaller stomach capacity limits the volume preterm infants can tolerate at each feeding. They need more of many nutrients per kilogram than do full-term infants and supplementation is necessary.

Assessment

Changes in feedings often are made according to the nurse's assessment of an infant's adjustment to feedings, readiness for change, and signs indicating complications.

FEEDING TOLERANCE

Assess how well the infant tolerates feedings, whether by feeding catheter or nipple. Aspirate the stomach contents to measure the residual amount in the stomach every 2 to 4 hours before tube feedings. This procedure helps determine whether the stomach is emptying and prevents overdistention. If the residual measures more than 2 to 4 ml/kg or the equivalent of the volume given over an hour for continuous feeding, the amount is too much (Anderson et al., 2002). An excessive residual indicates that the amount or type of formula or the flow rate may need changing. It also may be an early sign of a complication such as obstruction, ileus, necrotizing enterocolitis (NEC), or sepsis and should be reported to the physician.

Practice varies regarding whether to replace gastric residuals (Wyckoff, McGrath, Griffin, Malan, & White-Traut, 2003). Unless they are bloody, have large amounts of mucus, or are otherwise abnormal, residuals are often replaced to prevent loss of electrolytes. The next feeding may be reduced by the amount of the residual. If residuals are not replaced, observe carefully for signs of electrolyte imbalance.

Vomiting or frequent regurgitation may indicate that the feedings are too large. Vomitus containing bile may be a sign of intestinal obstruction and may require surgery. Diarrhea may be caused by rapid advancement of the feeding or intolerance to the type of formula.

Observe for signs of intestinal complications, such as visible loops of bowel. Obtain objective data about abdominal distention by using a tape to measure abdominal girth every 4 hours. Place the tape at the level of the umbilicus, and record the placement on the nursing care plan to ensure consistency. Stools may be tested for occult blood and for reducing substance, which indicates malabsorption of carbohydrates. Report signs of feeding intolerance to the health care provider because they may be early indications of complications.

READINESS FOR NIPPLE FEEDING

Preterm infants often are fed parenterally or by gavage (feeding tube) initially to conserve energy for growth and basic functioning. During feedings, watch for signs that nipple feeding may soon be possible, such as rooting, respiratory rate below 60, and an increasing ability to tolerate holding and handling. Although sucking on the gavage tube, a finger, or a pacifier may be a sign of readiness, it is not enough. Infants must also have an intact gag reflex or they are more likely to aspirate feedings. Note whether the infant gags on the catheter or a gloved finger inserted into the mouth.

The ability to feed orally and gain weight are important milestones as they are often among the criteria for discharge from the hospital. Coordination of sucking, swallowing, and breathing is a complex task for infants. Preterm infants do not have the well-developed buccal sucking pads in the cheeks that term infants use to form a seal around the nipple for efficient sucking. The jaw is less stable and the infant tires easily during oral feedings. The gag reflex, which helps prevent aspiration, may function poorly. The infant's respiratory status, other problems, and distractions in the environment can greatly affect feeding ability.

Oral feedings often are begun when the infant reaches 32 to 34 weeks' corrected gestational age (Kleinman, 2004). At this time many healthy preterm infants are able to coordinate sucking with swallowing and breathing and have a functional gag reflex. In addition, infants must have enough energy to feed orally without compromising oxygenation. Very weak infants expend too much oxygen, glucose, and energy when sucking and must continue to receive gavage feedings.

When the infant begins to feed by nipple, assess coordination of suck, swallow, and breathing and observe for aspi-

---

CRITICAL TO REMEMBER

Signs of Readiness to Nipple

Signs of Readiness for Nipple Feedings
Rooting
Sucking on gavage tube, finger, or pacifier
Ability to tolerate holding
Respiratory rate <60 breaths per minute
Presence of gag reflex

Signs of Nonreadiness for Nipple Feedings
Respiratory rate >60 breaths per minute
No rooting or sucking
Absence of gag reflex
Excessive gastric residuals

Adverse Signs during Nipple Feedings
Tachycardia
Bradycardia
Increased respiratory rate
Markedly decreased oxygen saturation level
Cyanosis
Apnea
Coughing
Gagging
Falling asleep early in feeding
Feeding time beyond 20 to 30 minutes

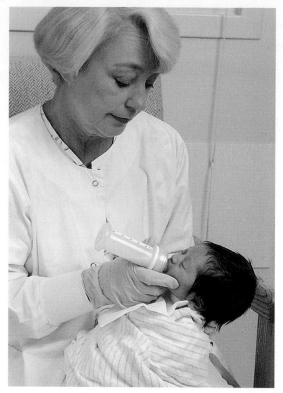

Figure 29-6 ■ The nurse positions her hands to provide cheek and jaw support for feeding this preterm infant.

ration. Frequent choking, gagging, or cyanosis during feedings may indicate that the infant is unable to coordinate sucking, swallowing, and breathing well enough for nipple feeding. Some infants are so weak that the usual signs of aspiration are minimal or absent.

Assess the respiratory rate before and during feedings (Figure 29-6). When the respiratory rate is more than 60 breaths per minute before feedings, gavage feed to prevent aspiration. An increased respiratory rate, tachycardia, bradycardia, color changes, decreased oxygen saturation levels, or excessive fatigue demonstrates that the effort of nipple feeding requires too much energy for the infant.

Analysis

When the infant's nutritional needs are met by parenteral methods, the nursing care is mainly collaborative. However, once the infant is able to take formula by nipple or breastfeed, many nursing interventions are involved. They address the nursing diagnosis "Risk for Imbalanced Nutrition: Less Than Body Requirements related to uncoordinated suck and swallow and fatigue during feedings."

Planning

Goals or expected outcomes for an individual infant with this nursing diagnosis take into consideration the specific needs of that infant. The infant will:

- Consume adequate amounts of breast milk or formula to meet nutrient needs for age and weight
- Gain weight as appropriate for age, generally 15 to 20 g/kg/day

The actual amount of feedings and weight gain will vary according to the infant's gestational age and other conditions. Discuss what is appropriate for a particular infant with the health care provider.

Interventions

ADMINISTERING PARENTERAL NUTRITION

The nurse manages the administration of parenteral nutrition, which may be necessary for very immature infants because of respiratory problems, limited gastric capacity, and reduced peristalsis. Parenteral nutrition is the IV infusion of solutions containing the major nutrients known to be needed for metabolism and growth. It provides calories, amino acids, fatty acids, vitamins, and minerals in amounts adapted to the specific needs of infants. It is continued, in decreasing amounts, until the infant is able to tolerate full enteral feedings.

ADMINISTERING ENTERAL FEEDINGS

Enteral feedings (feeding into the gastrointestinal tract, orally or by feeding tube) are usually begun within the first few days, if possible, because they may improve intestinal hormone production and promote intestinal growth and maturity. Bowel sounds should be present, there should be no significant abdominal distention, and infants should be in relatively stable condition (Evans & Thureen, 2001).

The first feedings are minimal enteral nutrition (also called *trophic feedings*) administered by gavage with only a few milliliters of breast milk or formula given at a time. This helps prime the gastrointestinal tract and promotes maturation and gastric hormone and enzyme production and increases gastrointestinal motility, mineral absorption, later feeding tolerance, and weight gain (Anderson et al., 2002; Schanler, 2005). Human milk is preferred if it is available. Feedings are gradually increased according to the infant's tolerance.

Preterm infants need special formulas or fortified breast milk. These formulas are adapted to meet the need for easily digestible, concentrated nutrients in a smaller volume of fluid. Preterm infants may need 24 kcal/oz (instead of 20 kcal/oz used for the full-term infant) to meet their requirements. Formulas contain added calcium, phosphorus, and vitamins needed by the preterm infant, and other components may be added to meet the needs of individual infants. Breast milk fortifiers add needed nutrients to breast milk to make it more concentrated. Very small infants may begin with half-strength breast milk or formula, and the amount and strength are gradually increased.

ADMINISTERING GAVAGE FEEDINGS

Gavage feedings usually are started before oral feedings for preterm infants (Procedure 29-1). A small, semi-soft catheter may be inserted through the mouth or nose every 2 to 3 hours for intermittent (bolus) feedings. An indwelling catheter may also be used to provide for intermittent or continuous feedings. Indwelling catheters are left in place for 1 to 3 days and then replaced, although some can be left in place as long as a month (McGrath, 2004b).

29-1   Administering Gavage Feeding

PURPOSE: Used for infants who are unable to take the full feeding by nipple; may be used alone or along with nipple feedings

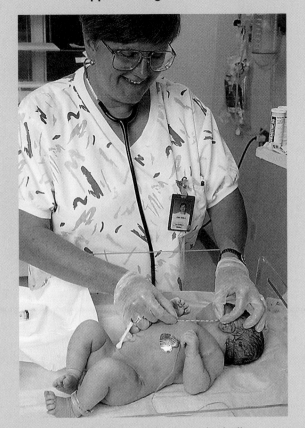

1. Wash hands. Gather equipment, including gavage catheter of proper size (3.5, 5, or 8 French, depending on size of the infant), measured container, and 20-ml syringe. Warm breast milk or formula to room or body temperature. Check the chart to determine how previous feedings were tolerated. Add fortifier to breast milk if necessary. *Having all materials ready helps the procedure go smoothly and avoids disturbing the infant or delaying feedings. Cold milk could interfere with thermoregulation. Information about previous feedings will help meet the infant's needs.*

2. Don gloves. If the infant has a tendency to regurgitate when moved after feedings, position him or her on the right side or prone. If parents are present, they may hold the infant in their arms once the catheter is inserted or may hold the hands if the infant cannot be held. *Positioning uses gravity to help avoid reflux of milk into the trachea and promotes emptying of the stomach. Feeding is important to parents, and helping increases their sense of involvement.*

3. Determine the length of catheter to insert. For orogastric insertion, measure from the mouth to the ear to the xiphoid process. For nasogastric feedings, measure from the infant's nose to the earlobe and to the end of the xiphoid process and add 1 cm or measure from the ear to the nose and then to the midpoint between the xiphoid process and the umbilicus. Mark the catheter at the proper point with a piece of tape or indelible ink. If the tube is to be indwelling, check every 4 to 8 hours to see that the mark or tape remains in the same place. *The measured distance is equal to the distance from the mouth or nose to the stomach. Mark on the catheter shows if the tube has moved out of place.*

4. Give the infant a pacifier. Moisten the tip of the catheter. While holding the infant's head steady, gently insert the catheter through the mouth or nose to the point marked. Remove the catheter immediately if persistent coughing, choking, cyanosis, apnea, or bradycardia occurs. *Nonnutritive sucking helps the tube pass more easily. Moistening the tip provides lubrication. Signs may indicate that the catheter is entering the trachea instead of the esophagus. Stimulation of the vagus nerve may cause bradycardia or apnea.*

5. Check for placement when the catheter is first placed, before beginning bolus feedings, and at least once a shift for continuous feedings.

    a. Insert 1 to 2 ml of air through the tube while listening over the stomach with a stethoscope. Gently draw back on the plunger to withdraw the inserted air. Hearing air enter the stomach may show the catheter is in place but is not as accurate as pH testing of gastric aspirate. Withdrawing the inserted air provides more room for feeding and helps prevent regurgitation.

    b. Attach a syringe to the catheter and gently aspirate stomach contents. Move or rotate the catheter slightly if the plunger does not withdraw easily. Check the pH of the aspirate to be sure it is gastric contents. *Aspirating stomach contents provides further proof that the feeding catheter is in the proper place. Use of force could traumatize the stomach lining if the end of the catheter is resting against it. Moving the catheter may draw it away from the stomach lining. pH shows if the aspirate is stomach contents.*

6. Secure the catheter in place with an adhesive dressing. *Securing ensures the catheter will remain inserted to the proper length during the procedure.*

7. Withdraw stomach contents. Observe amount, color, and consistency of the aspirate. During continuous feedings, check the gastric residual every 2 to 4 hours. Do not feed the infant if the aspirate is abnormal. Report abnormal appearance or amount of stomach contents. *Stomach contents that are red or dark brown may indicate blood. If the aspirate is green with bile or brown with feces, intestinal obstruction may have occurred. An excessive amount may mean that the infant is receiving too much or that stomach emptying is delayed. The residual should not be more than the hourly volume or 2 to 4 ml/kg.*

Continued

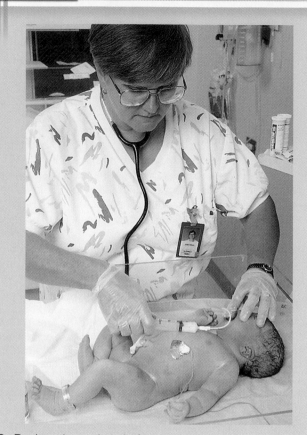

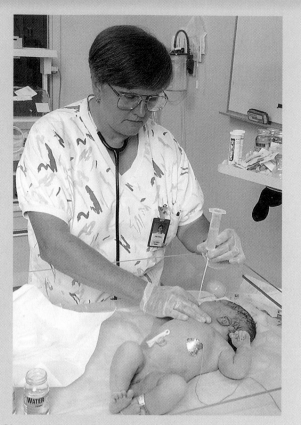

8. Replace the aspirate before beginning the feeding or discard according to agency policy. If it is replaced, subtract the amount of gastric residual from the amount of milk to be given. *Replacement of aspirate prevents loss of electrolytes. Overdistention of the stomach is avoided by subtracting the residual from the feeding to be given.*

9. Remove the plunger and attach the syringe to the feeding tube. Pour the correct amount of solution into the syringe. Attach to a feeding pump that will regulate the amount of flow. *A gravity flow or regulation of the flow by a pump causes less trauma and prevents filling the stomach too fast.*

10. If using gravity flow, raise or lower the syringe to increase or decrease the rate of flow so that the feeding moves slowly into the stomach over 15 to 30 minutes. *The higher the syringe, the faster the flow of solution and the greater the pressure. Feedings should be given slowly to prevent sudden distention or trauma from pressure.*

11. For continuous feedings, place no more than a 2- to 4-hour supply of milk in a feeding bag or syringe. Set the pump to deliver the correct rate of flow. Change the equipment every 4 hours or according to hospital policy. *Limiting the amount and changing equipment prevents excessive growth of bacteria in the milk or tubing. Infusion pumps deliver the feeding at a constant, measured rate.*

12. Give the infant a pacifier during the feeding. *The pacifier stimulates the sucking reflex, helps prepare the infant for nippling, is comforting, and helps the infant associate sucking with feeding.*

13. For intermittent feedings with a catheter that remains in place, clear the catheter with air or sterile water according to agency policy and close off the end when the feeding is completed. *This prevents clogging of the tubing. Closing the end prevents formula from coming back through the catheter.*

14. When the catheter is to be withdrawn, pinch the catheter and remove it quickly. *Pinching prevents drops of milk from entering the trachea as the catheter is removed, and quick removal decreases irritation.*

15. Burp the infant, and position on the right side or prone, with the head of the bed elevated 35 to 45 degrees. If movement tends to cause regurgitation, omit burping. Allow the infant to remain on the right side or prone. *Air is swallowed around the catheter and can cause the infant to regurgitate and aspirate. Position helps prevent reflux of feeding into the esophagus and promotes emptying of the stomach by gravity. If regurgitation occurs, the milk will flow out of the mouth.*

16. Record time, amount, and characteristics of gastric residual, type and amount of feeding given, and how the infant tolerated it. *Documentation allows monitoring of infant's ability to tolerate feedings and meet nutritional needs.*

Inserting the catheter at each feeding may be more traumatic than leaving it in place. Frequent oral placement may cause vomiting or increase infant aversion to oral stimuli, which may lead to difficulty with oral feedings later. Vagal stimulation during insertion may cause apnea and bradycardia. Nasal placement avoids aversive oral stimulation but may increase airway resistance by interfering with air flow through the infant's small nasal passages.

Intermittent bolus feedings provide a more normal feeding pattern with periodic stimulation of gastric hormones and enzymes. Continuous feedings may be better for very small infants, those with severe respiratory problems, and infants who have large residuals with bolus feedings. However, continuous feedings carry a higher risk of aspiration because the infant is not attended at all times during the feeding. In addition, bacteria counts in the milk or formula may become too high, and fats tend to adhere to the tubing during continuous feeding.

Feedings are gradually increased according to the infant's tolerance. Carefully observe the infant's response at each feeding to determine when the feeding type or amount can be changed. Parenteral nutrition continues until the infant is able to take adequate enteral feedings.

Pacifiers are often used during gavage feedings. Preterm infants have been exposed to aversive oral stimulation, such as intubation and suctioning. As a result, they may react negatively to any additional oral stimulation, which interferes with feedings. Allowing the infant to use a pacifier during gavage feedings provides positive oral stimulation and helps associate the comfortable feeling of fullness with sucking. Nonnutritive sucking also increases later success in oral feedings, decreases behavior changes during feedings, and helps bring the infant to an alert awake state, which improves feeding success.

ADMINISTERING ORAL FEEDINGS

The first nipple feedings may consist of only a few milliliters once a day and may be completed by gavage. Placing the gavage catheter before beginning oral feedings helps prevent regurgitation stimulated by passing the catheter. Gradually increase the amount and frequency of oral feedings until the infant feeds by breast or bottle once a shift, then every second or third feeding, and eventually every feeding.

PREPARING FOR FEEDINGS. Provide for maintenance of heat during feeding times. When infants have stable temperature maintenance, wrap them in warm blankets and hold them for feedings. If thermoregulation is a problem, use a heat lamp over the infant or feed the infant in the radiant warmer or incubator.

Nipple feedings involve a greater expenditure of energy by the infant than gavage feedings. Allow for a period of rest before and after feedings. Use of a pacifier before feedings helps bring preterm infants to an alert state that enhances oral feeding success. Infants may be fed according to a feeding schedule, such as every 3 hours, or when they demonstrate hunger cues such as sucking on fingers or crying. Infants who receive cue-based feedings may sleep better and may be able to attain full nipple feedings earlier than infants who receive scheduled feedings (McCain & Gartside, 2002).

CHOOSING A NIPPLE

A variety of nipples for neonates is available. Soft, high-flow nipples ("preemie" nipples) are more pliable than regular nipples and require less energy for sucking. However, they often deliver milk too rapidly, cause choking, and interfere with breathing between sucking bursts. Low-flow nipples (standard nipples) are firmer and deliver the milk more slowly so the infant can control it more easily. These nipples are used more often than high-flow nipples. Nipples are available in several sizes for infants with a very small mouth.

Nursing interventions for bottle feeding the preterm infant are presented in Nursing Care Plan 29-1.

FACILITATING BREASTFEEDING

More than 50% of mothers who try breastfeeding their preterm infants change to formula feeding before the infant is discharged (Wyckoff et al., 2003). To prevent breastfeeding failure, offer support and encouragement to mothers who would like to breastfeed. Contributing her milk helps the mother realize she has something important to offer at a time when she may feel that she can do little to help her baby.

Explain the many advantages breastfeeding offers. The immunologic benefits of breast milk are particularly important to the preterm infant who did not receive passive immunity during fetal life. Nutrients in breast milk are more easily digested, and it provides antimicrobial components, enzymes, hormones, and growth factors important for preterm infants. Although milk from mothers of preterm infants is higher in protein, calories, and electrolytes during the early weeks, it may be necessary to add special fortifiers to meet total nutrient needs.

Breast milk may increase feeding tolerance, reduce infections and later allergies, enhance neurologic development, and help prevent NEC. In addition, breastfeeding may be less stressful than bottle feeding for some preterm infants. Oxygenation levels often are higher during breastfeeding because the infant can regulate breathing and suckling better than with bottle feeding. In addition, the mother's body temperature helps keep the infant warm.

The mother who plans to breastfeed needs help with maintaining lactation until the infant is mature enough to nurse. Teach her how to use a breast pump and help her begin within 24 hours of the birth. Provide her with sterile containers in which to store her milk. Tell her to place her milk in a refrigerator if the infant will receive it within

CRITICAL THINKING ❓ EXERCISE 29-1

What are the major differences between formula feeding a preterm infant and formula feeding a full-term infant?

NURSING CARE PLAN 29-1 The Preterm Infant

ASSESSMENT: Giovanni was born at 31 weeks' gestation and now weighs 1800 g (4 lb). He breathes on his own with oxygen by hood. Giovanni needs many treatments throughout the day. He demonstrates pallor and increased respiratory rate when tired. Noises often cause a drop in oxygen saturation. When held or disturbed for care, Giovanni may stiffen and extend his arms with the fingers splayed. He sleeps most of the time when he is undisturbed.

NURSING DIAGNOSIS: Activity Intolerance related to weakness, fatigue, and possible overstimulation

GOALS/EXPECTED OUTCOMES: Giovanni will:
1. Show fewer signs of overstimulation (increased respirations, pallor, decreased oxygen saturation level, stiffening of arms and legs, or splaying of fingers) as a result of normal activity
2. Increase tolerance to activity gradually as demonstrated by fewer signs of fatigue or stress

INTERVENTION	RATIONALE
1. Arrange to provide routine care during Giovanni's natural awake periods, whenever possible.	1. Preterm infants need undisturbed sleep to promote growth.
2. Schedule periods of uninterrupted rest, especially before and after energy-draining activities.	2. Infants tolerate activities best when they begin in a rested state and are allowed to recover from them before other activities are necessary.
3. Experiment with grouping care to determine the number and combination of care activities that Giovanni tolerates best.	3. Flexible nursing care allows individualization to meet the infant's needs. Grouping accomplishes more tasks at once so that longer rest periods are possible between tasks. However, too many activities are too fatiguing.
4. Determine the infant's stress level before beginning care activities. Reassess carefully during each period of care and again after care to evaluate the infant's response.	4. Careful assessment allows the nurse to individualize nursing care to the changing needs of the infant.
5. Assess carefully to determine what activities bring about signs of overstimulation and fatigue: changes in color, respirations, or pulse; stiff, extended extremities; worried, hyperalert expression. Stop and allow short rest periods, if possible.	5. Careful observation allows the nurse to be sensitive to the infant's ability to tolerate care.
6. Reduce the noise level around Giovanni. Avoid unnecessary talking, open and close doors softly, and keep alarm volumes low.	6. Noise may be overstimulating and may result in increased oxygen need.
7. Reduce nonessential lighting. Turn Giovanni's bed facing away from bright lights. Place him prone and partially cover the incubator over Giovanni's head to keep out light but allow him to be seen.	7. Continuous lighting interferes with the infant's sleep. Reducing light in the infant's face will increase rest.
8. Use blanket rolls or positioning devices to form "boundaries" around Giovanni and keep his extremities flexed.	8. Enclosed space promotes rest and comfort because it is similar to the small space of the uterus. Positioning devices prevent the infant from bumping against the hard walls of the bed.
9. Collaborate with parents and other nurses to determine what works best in decreasing fatigue and stimulation for Giovanni. Use shift report, the nursing care plan, the Kardex, and signs taped on the bed to provide this information to others.	9. All caregivers should have information available to help meet the infant's needs consistently.
10. Explain Giovanni's needs for rest and low stimulation to his parents. Suggest ways that they can interact appropriately to meet his needs, and point out signs that he is receiving too much stimulation. Ask for their input.	10. Parents who are informed can care for the infant appropriately and feel that they are members of the team and parenting their child by learning his needs.

CRITICAL THINKING: Who else besides the primary nurse needs to know about methods to maintain appropriate stimuli in Giovanni's environment?

ANSWER: Everyone involved in caring for Giovanni—other nurses, physicians, respiratory therapists, and other members of the health care team, as well as parents—need to know about the plan for appropriate stimuli so that everyone will follow the same methods for developmental care.

EVALUATION: Giovanni gradually shows increased ability to tolerate progressive activity with fewer episodes of overstimulation. His respirations and oxygen saturation levels remain stable, and he rarely stiffens his arms and legs during activity.

NURSING CARE PLAN 29-1   The Preterm Infant—cont'd

ASSESSMENT: Two or three times a day Giovanni receives feedings by nipple supplemented by gavage when he becomes too tired. The feeding plan is for him to receive 120 kcal/kg/day to meet his needs. He has occasional episodes of increased respirations or short cyanotic spells when fed. He sometimes takes only half the feeding before falling asleep and must receive the rest by gavage. Giovanni's mother has decided to formula feed.

NURSING DIAGNOSIS: Ineffective Infant Feeding Pattern related to muscle weakness and fatigue during feedings.

GOALS/EXPECTED OUTCOMES: Giovanni will:
1. Take approximately 216 kcal/day to meet his needs at a weight of 1800 g
2. Gain approximately 27 to 36 g (15 to 20 g/kg) daily
3. Complete nipple feedings without signs of excessive fatigue (such as increased respiratory rate or falling asleep during feeding)

INTERVENTION	RATIONALE
1. Schedule rest periods before and after nipple feedings. Feed the infant when he begins to show feeding cues but before he begins to cry with hunger.	1. Nippling consumes a great deal of energy. Rest helps prevent excessive fatigue that might prevent the infant from completing the feeding. Crying increases energy use.
2. Use a pacifier before feedings.	2. Nonnutritive sucking helps alert the infant to prepare him for feeding.
3. Gather equipment. Use a feeding container (such as a Volutrol) on which each milliliter is marked. Place the container in warm water to heat the milk to room or body temperature. Do not use a microwave oven to warm.	3. Having all equipment ready prevents wasted motion and ensures that infant is fed without interruption. Exact measurement of the amount taken is important to ensure that infants receive required nutrients. Some infants will take slightly warmed milk better. Microwaving provides uneven heating of formula and may cause the infant to be burned.
4. Determine the type of nipple that works best for Giovanni. Choose between various sizes and consistencies.	4. The correct nipple will deliver milk at a rate the infant can manage without choking or expending more energy than necessary.
5. Wrap Giovanni in warmed blankets with his extremities flexed and at the midline. Place a hat on his head. Choose an area of the nursery where distractions will be minimal.	5. A hat and blankets help maintain temperature. The position is calming and decreases disorganized behavior. Distractions can interfere with feeding.
6. Position Giovanni at a 45- to 60-degree angle. Support the head and neck in a neutral position. If necessary, place a finger on each cheek and one under the jaw at the base of the tongue midway between the chin and the throat. Provide gentle pressure.	6. A flexed, upright position decreases the flow of formula. The finger position may increase sucking efficiency and jaw stability. It should be used only for infants having difficulty with latching or sealing the lips around the nipple.
7. Allow the infant to set the pace of the feeding. Feed slowly, and allow the infant to rest when he stops sucking.	7. Slow feeding is necessary because of the infant's decreased energy. Preterm infants need rest periods during feedings because they have difficulty regulating their breathing while feeding.
8. Do not move the nipple around in his mouth to force Giovanni to resume feeding before he is ready. Burp the infant frequently by rubbing his back while he is in an upright position.	8. Twisting, jiggling, pumping, or otherwise moving the nipple forces the infant to take more formula when he needs to rest. Preterm infants may swallow more air than full-term infants because sucking is less efficient.
9. Observe for coughing, gagging, cyanosis, apnea, and changes in heart rate, respirations, and oxygen saturation. Stop the feeding and evaluate the infant's ability to continue.	9. These signs show difficulty coordinating sucking, swallowing, and breathing, and possible aspiration. Some infants have prolonged sucking bursts without stopping to breathe and need to have the nipple removed so they will rest and resume breathing. Feeding requires more oxygen intake.
10. Tip the bottle down to stop the flow if the infant is drinking too fast or having difficulty with pacing or coordination.	10. Allows the infant to rest yet avoids removing the nipple from the mouth if the infant has difficulty latching again.
11. Reduce external stimuli during feedings if the infant shows signs of overstimulation.	11. Too many stimuli may exhaust the infant and prevent optimal feeding behaviors.
12. Assess for signs of overfatigue: falling asleep during feedings, feedings lasting more than 20 to 30 minutes, increased respirations, decreased oxygen saturation.	12. Feedings may require more energy than the infant has available. Infants who are overfatigued are more likely to aspirate. Calories may be used for energy for feeding instead of for growth.
13. Finish the feeding by gavage if necessary.	13. Completing the feeding by gavage conserves energy, prevents aspiration, and ensures that the infant receives the desired nutrient intake.

Continued

NURSING CARE PLAN 29-1 The Preterm Infant—cont'd

INTERVENTION	RATIONALE
14. Position Giovanni on the right side or prone with his head elevated approximately 30 degrees after feeding.	14. The right-side position and elevation of the head allow gravity to help empty the stomach and fluids to drain if the infant regurgitates.
15. Involve parents in the feedings as soon as possible. Teach them to assess feeding cues and Giovanni's response to feedings. Help them learn the infant's usual pattern of sucking, swallowing, and breathing and to watch for changes such as milk dribbling out of the infant's mouth or breathing irregularities that indicate a need to stop the feeding temporarily.	15. Feeding allows parents to participate in the infant's care. Their comfort with feedings and learning about the infant's responses will help them prepare for discharge.

EVALUATION: Giovanni consumes an average of 220 calories a day and gains an average of 31 g daily. He gradually takes more of his feeding by nipple and rarely needs gavage feeding to finish it. His respiratory rate remains under 60 breaths per minute, and he stays awake for the entire feeding.

24 hours or a freezer if it will be more than 24 hours before it is given to the infant (Lemons, 2001). If fortifiers will be added to the milk, explain the higher needs of the preterm infant so that the mother does not think something is wrong with her milk or that it is inadequate.

Ongoing support for the mother is important. Encourage her in her efforts in feeding, which may be difficult at first. Remind her that even full-term infants must learn how to breastfeed. Relaxation needed for feeding is difficult in the busy NICU. Provide as much privacy as possible, using a separate room or screens. Help the mother feel comfortable holding the tiny infant and any attached equipment such as monitor leads.

Adapt breastfeeding teaching to the needs of a very small infant. Show the mother how to use the cross-cradle hold, which is very effective for small infants (see Figure 22-5). The mother holds her breast with the hand on the same side, pressing slightly back and downward behind the areola to make the nipple prominent. She holds the infant's head in the other hand with the infant across her body and supported by her arm. This allows the mother to see the infant's face well during latching on and throughout the feeding.

A supplemental nursing system, a device that holds expressed breast milk in a bag with a small catheter attached to the mother's nipple, may be used to help infants receive more milk with less effort during early feedings. Other methods to increase the amount of milk received include supplementation with gavage or cup feedings. These methods avoid bottle feeding and may increase the length and success of breastfeeding.

Make the same observations of the infant during breastfeeding as during bottle feeding. Signs of fatigue, bradycardia, tachypnea, or apnea may show lack of readiness for breastfeeding. Be sure that the infant stays warm. The mother's body heat will help maintain the infant's temperature during feedings. Kangaroo care (p. 786) often can be combined with breastfeeding.

MAKING ONGOING ASSESSMENTS

Continuously assess the infant's responses to all feeding methods. Watch for signs of distress, especially when feedings are first initiated. These may include changes in heart or respiratory rate, decreased oxygen saturation, color changes, gagging, choking, and fatigue. Record the amount of breast milk or formula the infant takes by gavage or bottle feeding and compare it with the amount needed to meet nutrient needs for the infant's age and weight. Because accurate estimation of milk intake is difficult during breastfeeding, infants may be weighed on an electronic scale before and after feedings. Both weights should be taken with the infant wearing the same clothing and before the diaper is changed after the feeding. This allows supplementary gavage feeding amounts to be calculated based on the infant's oral intake of breast milk.

Note the infant's response to other stimuli during feeding. Some infants respond well to being talked to and rocked during feedings. Others become distracted by any noise, motion, or nearby activities.

Weigh the infant daily at the same time with the same scale. Record the length and head circumference each week. Plot measurements on a growth chart for preterm infants to see whether changes are within expected ranges. Weight increase not accompanied by increased length may be caused by edema and may be a sign of a complication such as congestive heart failure.

Observe changes in the infant's ability to take feedings. The suck and swallow coordination should gradually improve with maturity and practice. As the infant becomes more mature, less energy should be expended during the feeding sessions. The infant will take the feedings more quickly and show fewer signs of fatigue, such as falling asleep during feedings.

Evaluation

If the goals have been met, the infant will consume adequate amounts of formula or breast milk to meet nutrient needs for age and weight and will gain weight as appropriate for age.

8. What can the nurse do for the infant at risk for stress from overstimulation?
9. How does the nurse assess feeding tolerance?
10. Why should the nurse allow the infant to set the pace of feedings instead of urging continuous sucking?
11. How can the nurse help the mother who wants to breastfeed her preterm infant?

PARENTING

The birth of a preterm infant is generally unexpected and always emotionally traumatic to parents. Infants are often hurried to the NICU shortly after birth. Later, when parents see the infant attached to an array of machines, they may have difficulty developing feelings of attachment to a tiny baby who looks so different from what they expected.

At first, parents cannot hold or feed the infant or offer any of the usual care that parents expect to give their infants. The infant may not be capable of common newborn behaviors such as making eye contact and grasping the parent's finger. When the infant's appearance and behavior are different from the parents' expectations, attachment may be delayed (Bialoskurski, Cox, & Hayes, 2000). Interference in the attachment process increases vulnerability for parents in establishing a nurturing relationship with the infant (Kenner, 2004).

The extended hospitalization of the preterm infant results in separation of the parents from their newborn, produces emotional trauma, and disrupts family life. Parents must relinquish the role of primary caregiver during their infant's hospitalization. They may feel they are in the nurse's way and may state they do not feel like parents at all. Loss of the parental role is a major stressor for these parents.

Being unable to participate fully in the infant's care for a prolonged period also interferes with the parents' ability to learn their baby's unique characteristics such as the way the infant responds to stress and the methods of consolation that work best. Separation and inability to assume the parenting role delay the development of the parent-infant relationship and may impair the parents' bonding.

In addition, parents worry about the infant's condition and outcome. They need help in understanding the infant's condition and what is expected to occur throughout the hospital stay. Nurses must evaluate the progress of attachment and assist parents to feel important in caring for their infant.

Assessment

Assess for signs of parental attachment on the first and subsequent visits to the NICU nursery. Expect parents to be fearful at first but more able to focus on the infant as they get over the initial shock of preterm birth. Assess for common behaviors that show normal progression of attachment. These include talking about the infant in positive terms, making eye contact, pointing out physical characteristics, naming the infant, and calling the infant by name. Parents should ask questions about the infant. When they are able to hold and participate in the

Signs That Bonding May Be Delayed

Using negative terms to describe the infant
Discussing the infant in impersonal or technical terms
Failing to give the infant a name or to use the name
Visiting or calling infrequently or not at all
Decreasing the number and length of visits
Showing interest in other infants equal to that in their own infant
Refusing offers to hold and learn to care for the infant
Showing a decrease in or lack of eye contact
Spending less time talking to or smiling at the infant

care of the infant, observe for gradual increase in comfort and skill. The parents should smile and talk to the infant and verbalize increasing confidence in their caretaking abilities.

Watch for signs that bonding is not occurring as expected. These include failure to perform usual attachment behaviors or a decrease in behaviors that were previously present. Parents who seem as interested in other infants in the NICU as in their own infant or talk about the infant in an impersonal way may be having difficulty. Note how often the parents make visits or calls to the NICU and changes that may indicate a need for support. Determine whether other stressors exist in the parents' lives that may interfere with their ability to visit and attach to the infant. The financial need to return to work, lack of transportation, or the need to care for other children may prevent parents from visiting as often as they would like.

Analysis

Whenever parents and infants must be separated because of hospitalization during the newborn period, a risk for disruption of the attachment process exists. The nursing diagnosis that fits this concern is "Risk for Impaired Parent-Infant Attachment related to separation of parents from infant and lack of understanding about the preterm infant's condition and characteristics."

Planning

The goals or expected outcomes for this nursing diagnosis are that the parents will:

- Demonstrate bonding behaviors, including visiting frequently and interacting as appropriate for the infant's condition throughout the hospital stay
- Verbalize understanding of the preterm infant's condition and characteristics within 2 days
- Express gradually increasing comfort in caring for the infant throughout the hospital stay

Interventions

MAKING ADVANCE PREPARATIONS

Preparing for threatening situations such as preterm birth helps parents cope with the actual event. Parents at higher risk for a preterm birth should visit the NICU before delivery. If the mother is confined to bed, arrange for a nurse from the NICU to visit her so that she feels a link with the nursery and can ask questions. The father or another support person should have a tour of the nursery so that he will know where to go and can discuss the nursery environment with the mother.

Parents have many questions before the birth, which should be answered truthfully but in an encouraging manner. Questions about how the infant will be cared for and about the prognosis are common. The nurse can help the parents get the information they desire and clarify it as necessary.

ASSISTING PARENTS AT BIRTH

After the birth, allow the parents to see and touch the newborn in the delivery room, even if only for a few moments, so that they have a realistic idea of the infant's appearance and condition. This helps the bonding process that began in pregnancy to continue.

If possible, allow the father or primary support person to watch the initial care in the NICU. Explain what is happening and why. This attention allows him to see the intensive efforts made on behalf of his infant, increases his confidence in the staff, and enables him to give the mother a full description later. Support the father and mother by using therapeutic communication techniques during this difficult time.

If the infant must be transported to another facility, ask the transport team to visit the mother just before they leave,

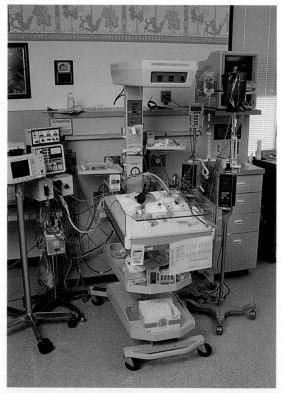

Figure 29-7 ■ An infant in the NICU is surrounded by highly technologic equipment. This can be very frightening to parents at first. Preparation of parents before they visit is an important nursing responsibility.

if possible. The visit helps her feel connected to her infant and the staff providing care. Leaving photographs with the mother is another way of helping her bond even though the infant is not with her.

SUPPORTING PARENTS DURING EARLY VISITS

Take the mother to the NICU nursery as soon as she is able. If she is too ill to be with her infant, bring her photographs of the infant and the NICU. Before parents first visit the infant, prepare them for what they will see. Describe the equipment and its purposes, the various attachments to the infant, and the sounds of alarms (Figure 29-7). Explain how the infant will look and behave. Box 29-1 provides specific steps that the nurse can follow to help parents become familiar with the NICU setting.

At first, stay with the parents during visits. When they are comfortable, allow them time alone with the infant so that they can interact in private. Answer questions and explain changes in the infant's condition and treatment. Parents may not know what questions to ask at first or may be too overwhelmed to ask questions. In this situation, discuss questions that are common to parents when they first visit the NICU nursery. Use therapeutic communication as the parents cope with feelings of grief, guilt, and emotional turmoil.

BOX 29-1 **Introducing Parents to the NICU Setting**

Before Parents Visit the NICU

Describe the NICU environment. Include the noise of alarms, the busyness of the staff, and the number of people and sick infants.

Show parents photographs of the infant. This helps prepare them, but it is not as overwhelming as seeing the infant in person.

Describe the infant. Include the size, lack of fat, breathing, and weak cry.

Explain that no sound of crying can be heard if the infant is intubated. Include some personal aspects: "He's a real fighter" or "She makes the funniest faces during her feedings."

Describe the equipment. Include ventilators, intravenous lines, and monitors. Explain how they look and how they are attached to the infant. Keep the explanations simple, without technical details.

When Parents Visit the NICU

Help parents perform thorough handwashing and explain the purpose and importance.

Stay with the parents during their visit. Having a familiar person nearby will help them feel more comfortable while they adjust to this unfamiliar environment.

Introduce them to their infant's nurse. Ask the NICU nurse to explain some of the care being provided for the infant.

Provide parents with written information about the NICU so that they can take it home with them to read later. This usually includes visiting hours, telephone updates about the infant, availability of classes on infant care, and support groups.

Tell the parents that they will receive instruction on how to care for their infant in time. Encourage them to visit the infant as much as possible. Emphasize how important they are to their infant.

Offer realistic encouragement based on the infant's condition.

Provide an opportunity for the parents to express their concerns and feelings and ask questions.

NICU, Neonatal intensive care unit.

Parents should touch the infant as soon as possible, because touching helps promote the development of attachment. They may be hesitant initially because of fear that they will interfere with equipment. The smaller the infant, the more reluctant parents may be. Some parents may hesitate to touch because they are afraid of becoming attached to an infant whom they may lose. They need sensitive support from the nurse until they are ready to progress in their relationship with the infant.

Show parents how to touch in ways appropriate for the infant, such as holding the infant's hand through the portholes of the incubator or touching the small areas of skin not encumbered by equipment. Explain to parents that handling is kept to a minimum for physiologically unstable infants because it is too stressful to them. As the infant becomes more stable and mature, help parents learn various kinds of touch and determine which ones work best with their infant. This helps parents feel more a part of the infant's plan of care.

Help the parents to hold the baby as soon as possible. Parents often look forward to the opportunity to hold the baby as a positive sign of the infant's condition. Yet it may be frightening, too, especially if the infant is attached to various kinds of equipment. Help the parents find a comfortable position for themselves and the infant and point out positive responses from the infant. Parents often find holding the infant very satisfying.

Nurses often concentrate on the mother in providing support and pay less attention to the father. However, fathers, too, must deal with the shock of having a preterm infant in the NICU. They must get to know the infant as a separate person with special needs and learn how to take care of the infant. In addition, fathers have work responsibilities, are expected to provide support for the mother, and may take on other family responsibilities as the mother focuses on care of the newborn. Fathers may spend less time in the NICU because they are at work, but may have many questions and concerns. If their time for visiting is limited, they may be less comfortable with caregiving activities than the mother.

PROVIDING INFORMATION

An important nursing role is providing information to parents. In one study 71% of parents believed nurses were the best source of information (Brazy, Anderson, Becker, & Becker, 2001). Encourage parents to ask questions about all aspects of their infant's condition and care. Although some mothers are not hesitant to ask questions, other mothers of NICU infants are fearful about asking for explanations because they are afraid that they might be seen as "difficult" parents and that this might jeopardize the infant's care (Hurst, 2001). Let parents know their questions are welcomed and do everything possible to obtain answers when they ask.

Explain the equipment used to care for the infant. Interpret the information obtained from monitors and the meaning of alarms. Clarify all nursing care, its purpose, and the expected response. Point out ways in which preterm infants are similar to and different from full-term infants to help parents develop a realistic understanding of the infant's capabilities.

Offer realistic reassurance about the infant's condition. This means emphasizing positive aspects yet being truthful in all communication with the parents. If the parents have misconceptions or did not understand a physician's explanations, explain or ask the physician to go over specific information again. Translate medical terms into words the parents can understand. Repeat explanations, especially at first. Because of their emotional distress, parents often are unable to fully comprehend or remember what is said to them.

THERAPEUTIC COMMUNICATIONS

Reassuring Parents during Visits to the NICU

Ann Gibson gave birth to a preterm infant, Molly, at 30 weeks' gestation. Ann is visiting the NICU for the first time the day after the birth. The nurse, Lee Wills, has talked to her about what to expect and stays with her during the visit.

Ann: Oh, she looks so tiny! I saw her for only a minute after she was born, and I didn't really get a good look. How can she ever survive when she's so small and covered with tubes?

Lee: So far, Molly's doing very well. Her vital signs are stable, and she's holding her own. But it's frightening when she looks so small and vulnerable, isn't it? *(Offering realistic reassurance and reflecting Ann's fearful feelings. Using infant's name to promote bonding.)*

Ann: I stayed in bed like they told me to do. I thought she wouldn't be born so soon if I stayed in bed.

Lee: It must have been a shock, especially when you tried so hard to prevent it. *(Reflecting feelings and acknowledging that Ann did what she could to prevent early birth.)*

Ann: Now she's so tiny and so sick! She looks very different from what I expected.

Lee: Molly's small, but babies her size grow very quickly. Would you like to touch her? *(Offering realistic reassurance and attempting to bring Ann closer to her infant.)*

Ann: Oh, I might hurt her. Maybe I should wait until she's bigger.

Lee: Even tiny babies like to have their mothers touch their skin and talk to them. She listened to your voice all through your pregnancy, so it's familiar to her. Why don't you talk softly to her while I work with her? And I can tell you about all this equipment and what we are doing for Molly. *(Emphasizing the mother's importance, involving her in care being given, and offering information about the infant's equipment and care.)*

NICU, Neonatal intensive care unit.

CRITICAL THINKING *?* **EXERCISE 29-2**

A woman delivered a 29-week preterm infant 3 days ago. She comes to see her baby infant each day, but refuses to touch the infant, in spite of frequent offers from the nurses.

Questions
1. What might explain her behavior?
2. How might the nurse help her?

Use an interpreter if the parents do not understand English. Offer written information in the language of the parents about NICU policies and procedures. Explanations about visiting hours, who can visit, routines for handwashing, and the role of parents can be reinforced in writing so they are available for later reading by overwhelmed parents.

INSTITUTING KANGAROO CARE

Begin Kangaroo care (KC) as soon as possible, if the parents are willing. KC is a method of providing skin-to-skin contact between preterm infants and their parents. The infant, wearing only a diaper and hat, is placed upright under the mother's clothes between her breasts. A blanket is added over the mother and infant (Figure 29-8). Mothers may breastfeed if they wish and if the infant is able. Fathers are encouraged to participate in KC also (Figure 29-9).

Explain the advantages of KC to parents, and elicit their participation. This method of care has been found safe for stable infants, even if intubated or of very low birth weight. It provides an opportunity for parents to participate in the infant's care and increases parental attachment. KC provides developmental care that is so important for the preterm infant. It is associated with improved infant growth and decreased length of hospital stay (Byers, 2003).

The upright position of the infant against the parent's chest makes breathing easier during KC. The containment

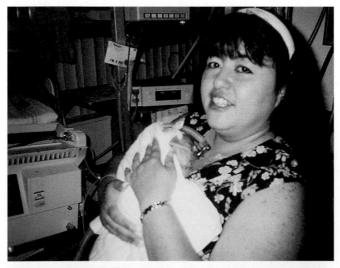

Figure 29-8 ■ This mother has her 27-week-gestation preterm infant tucked under her clothes against her skin as she gives kangaroo care. Such care enhances bonding and has many other benefits for infants and parents.

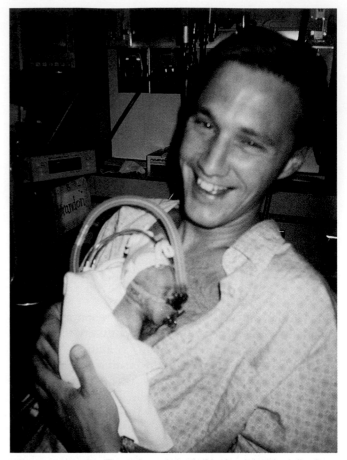

Figure 29-9 ■ Even though he is intubated, this 1-lb, 8-oz preterm infant goes to sleep against his father's chest.

of the extremities decreases purposeless movements that use valuable oxygen and calories. Breastfeeding is facilitated, and the infant has more alert periods and increased deep sleep. The contact with the parent's skin maintains the infant's body temperature. Parents often are gratified to see how they are able to cause these positive responses in their infants. Because of this, KC helps increase parent-infant attachment and feelings of confidence in caring for the infant (Gardner & Goldson, 2002).

KC also provides gentle stimulation. This includes tactile stimulation against the parent's skin, auditory stimulation as the infant listens to the parent's heartbeat and voice, and the vestibular stimulation of moving with the parent's breathing or rocking (Carrier, 2004). The infant became used to these sensations before birth, and they may be relaxing after birth (Ludington-Hoe, Anderson, Swinth, Thompson, & Hadeed, 2004).

When a mother is interested in providing KC, provide privacy. Assist her in transferring the infant from the bed, managing the various attachments, and making the infant comfortable. Check to see that the mother is comfortable, also. Explain that infants often set off alarms because of changes in vital signs or oxygenation during the transfer process, but that they become stable again once settled. Offer fathers the opportunity to hold the infant skin to skin, too.

FACILITATING INTERACTION

Parents may feel rejected by the infant's lack of the expected response or by negative responses during interactions. Explain to them that infants born at less than 34 weeks of gestation may not be able to cope with socialization. The talking, smiling, and eye contact so effective with full-term infants may be too stimulating for very young or sick preterm infants. Suggest forms of touch and interaction based on the individual infant's capacity. Quiet holding may be better until the infant is able to tolerate more stimulation.

Help parents understand the infant's behavior and cues. Teach them signs of overstimulation to help them adapt their interaction to meet the infant's needs. Let them know that stress signs like gaze aversion help protect the infant from overstimulation and the infant should be allowed a short rest period without added stimuli.

Discuss methods to avoid too much stimulation and ways to calm the infant. If several types of stimulation (such as rocking, eye contact, and talking) cause signs of distress, suggest they stop one or more activities until the infant has had a period of rest. Show them how to position the infant with the hands near the mouth so that the infant can suck on them as a self-comforting measure. As the infant matures, show parents signs that the infant is ready for more interaction and suggest appropriate types of stimulation.

Point out small signs of improvement and even minor strengths. Talk about normal preterm characteristics and point out individual traits that make this infant different from all others. The way the infant eats, how the infant reacts to sounds, or even how the infant seems to get tangled in the monitor leads may help parents feel closer to their newborn and understand the infant's uniqueness.

Involve the parents in care of the infant as soon as possible (Figure 29-10). As the parents become familiar with the NICU setting and equipment, more involvement will help them gain a sense of control. At first, plan to change the linens in the incubator or radiant warmer when the parents are there so that they can hold their infant, even if for only a few moments. As the infant's condition improves, parents can develop skill in caring for the tiny infant by changing diapers, feeding, and bathing.

Include other family members by allowing them to visit with the parents (Figure 29-11). Being able to see the infant in the hospital setting allows family members to provide more realistic emotional support while the infant is hospitalized. Involve family members in learning how to feed and care for the infant if they will be helping the parents after discharge.

INCREASING PARENTAL DECISION MAKING

Parents need to be given the role of partners with the NICU staff to provide an environment that is best for the infant. As parents get to know the infant better they become experts on the infant's response to various situations and caregiving activities. Their expertise should be recognized and taken into consideration in planning infant care.

Give parents the information they need to take an active part in decisions made about the infant's treatment plan. This will increase their feelings of control over a situation in which many parents feel they have little power. As parents become more knowledgeable and participate more in the caregiving, seek their input about how the infant is progressing and practices that seem to work best.

Look for opportunities to praise parenting abilities. Point out positive ways the infant responds to the parents' touch and caregiving. Model methods to respond to behavioral cues and acknowledge parents when they respond to the infant's signals appropriately. Listen to their ideas about what works best for the infant, and incorporate them if at all possible.

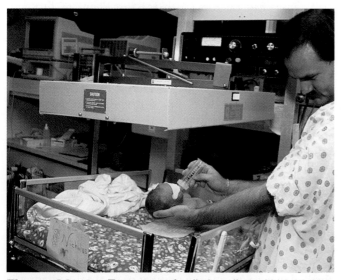

Figure 29-10 ■ To promote family bonding with the infant, parents are involved as much as possible in the care of their infant. This father bottle feeds his infant while the baby is in a radiant warmer.

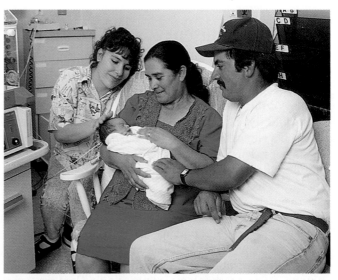

Figure 29-11 ■ The parents look on while the grandmother holds the infant in the NICU.

ALLEVIATING CONCERNS

Invite parents to call the NICU at any time for information about their infant. This helps allay worry when parents wake up at night and wonder how the infant is doing. Phone calls are especially beneficial for parents unable to visit the infant because of distance or other reasons.

Parents also need support from others besides nursing staff. Put them in touch with parents of other preterm infants and refer them to parent groups. Talking with those who have faced the same problems can be very comforting. They can compare notes and get practical suggestions from an experienced parent's point of view. It is important to take language and culture into consideration during this process. Some agencies pair parents with a "buddy" who has had a similar experience and is from the same culture.

Cultural practices should be incorporated into the care of the infant. Determine who in the family will make the decisions and who will be managing the infant's care. It may be one parent, both together, or another person in the family. In some cultures the father makes decisions and the grandmother is the major caregiver instead of the mother. In these cases, it is essential that the right persons be included in appropriate teaching.

HELPING WITH ONGOING PROBLEMS

Parents may be unprepared for the inconsistent progress that infants often make after surviving the risks of the early days. They expect steady progress once the infant can breathe alone and take feedings. However, complications such as NEC or sepsis can cause major setbacks at this time. To cope with a new and unexpected crisis parents need extensive support from the nurse. Use therapeutic communication techniques such as reflecting feelings to help them express and cope with their extreme disappointment. Give information about the infant's changing condition and what to expect in the days ahead.

PREPARING FOR DISCHARGE

In the past, preterm infants have often been discharged at about the time of their expected birth. However, infants are now frequently sent home before 40 weeks' corrected age. Because of this early discharge, it is important that parents understand the expected hospital course and estimated discharge. If a clinical pathway is being used for the infant, give them a copy. They can chart the infant's achievement of major milestones in development and changes in care as the infant moves toward discharge. This timeline helps them prepare themselves and their home to provide the special care that their infant may need after discharge.

After the critical period in the early days after birth, healthy preterm infants become more stable. They still require specialized nursing care and hospitalization but gradually need fewer technologic interventions. They are sometimes called "growers" at this time. Parent participation in the infant's care should increase at this time in preparation for discharge.

Begin early to teach parents and other caregivers any special procedures that the infant will need after discharge. Show them how to manage treatments and medications. Observe the parents as they perform care until they are comfortable and can do it safely. Provide hints to make the care easier, and praise their efforts.

Help parents learn what is normal for their infant and how to recognize and respond to abnormal signs. Some hospitals have parents spend a night or two in a special "parent room," where they take over full 24-hour care of the infant. This provides an opportunity to practice complete care of the infant in an environment in which help is available if needed and increases parents' confidence that they can care for the infant alone.

Help the parents determine what adaptations they will need to make at home before discharge. Utility companies should be notified if the infant is considered medically fragile to ensure that the family receives priority service in cases of power failure. Arrange home nursing services, purchase of supplies, and delivery of special equipment before discharge.

Discuss what to expect with regard to care of the infant after discharge. Infants may require oxygen, suctioning, or tube feedings, which parents will have to learn to perform. Some infants have complex treatments such as apnea monitors or even home mechanical ventilation. Many infants need feedings every 3 hours, day and night, to help them gain the 20 to 40 g a day expected after discharge (Sifuentes, 2000). Feedings may be time consuming, and parental fatigue resulting from interruptions of sleep may be more than the parents expected.

Infants are used to the noises of a nursery 24 hours a day and may not sleep well at first in a quiet home environment. Suggest parents play soft music and use a night light for the first week. They should gradually eliminate these aids to avoid conditioning the infant to their use. Visitors and noise or activity may be too much for the infant at first and should be limited.

Explore with parents what kind of help they might need to meet the everyday requirements of the infant and the rest of the family. Help them identify where they might find assistance from family and friends. Refer the parents to a family support group, if available, so that they can learn from the experiences of other parents and receive encouragement and emotional support for the problems they will encounter. Many hospitals offer these groups, which often are facilitated by nurses and social workers.

Help parents form realistic expectations of the infant. For example, they should know that the infant will accomplish developmental tasks, such as crawling and walking, later than full-term infants. Parents should base expectations on the infant's developmental or corrected age rather than chronologic age. Developmental age is the chronologic age minus the number of weeks the infant was born early.

Assist the parents in planning how to integrate the new infant into the family. Meeting the needs of their other children, in addition to the new responsibilities of caring for the preterm infant, is a major source of worry. Listen to their concerns about other children, and encourage siblings to visit, if possible. Caution parents that siblings with infections should not visit the infant, who cannot fight off infections well. Help parents explain to the other children what they will see when they visit the infant. Siblings should touch or hold the infant, if possible, to help them bond. Taking photographs of the siblings with the infant will help them remember the visit.

Before discharge, infants are often evaluated for apnea or bradycardia in the car seat the parents will use (see p. 575). Proper positioning with blanket rolls may be necessary because the infants may slump over, which interferes with chest expansion. Some infants need car beds to allow them to ride in a recumbent position.

Evaluation

Goals are met if parents visit often and interact appropriately with the infant, express their understanding of and comfort with the infant's needs, and take an increasingly active role in the care of the infant.

✔ **CHECK YOUR READING**

12. How can the nurse help parents be comfortable with their preterm infant?
13. How should the nurse prepare parents for the discharge of their preterm infant?

COMMON COMPLICATIONS OF PRETERM INFANTS

The preterm infant is at risk for a number of complications that increase as the infant's gestational age and birth weight decrease. Some complications that occur in full-term and preterm infants, such as hyperbilirubinemia and patent ductus arteriosus, are discussed in Chapter 30. Complications most often associated with preterm birth are discussed in this section. Further information about each condition can be found in pediatric texts.

Respiratory Distress Syndrome

Respiratory distress syndrome (RDS) occurs most often in preterm infants and increases as the gestational age decreases. Approximately 60% of infants born at less than 28 weeks' gestation, but fewer than 30% of those born at 28 to 34 weeks' gestation and less than 5% of those born after 34 weeks, develop the condition (American Lung Association, 2004).

RDS also occurs in birth asphyxia, birth by cesarean, and infants of diabetic mothers because these conditions interfere with surfactant production. The syndrome is less frequent, however, when chronic fetal stress, such as in heroin addiction, preeclampsia, IUGR, and prolonged rupture of membranes causes the lungs to mature more quickly (Stoll & Kliegman, 2004a; McGrath, 2004a).

PATHOPHYSIOLOGY

RDS is caused by insufficient production of surfactant, a phospholipid that lines the alveoli. Surfactant is first produced in the alveoli at 22 weeks of gestation. By 34 to 36 weeks, production of surfactant is usually mature enough to enable the infant to breathe normally outside the uterus (Hagedorn et al., 2002).

Surfactant decreases surface tension to allow the alveoli to remain open when air is exhaled. It must be continuously produced as it is used. When too little surfactant is present, the alveoli collapse each time the infant exhales. The lungs become noncompliant, or "stiff," and resist expansion. Noncompliant lungs require a much higher negative pressure for the alveoli to open each time the infant inhales. This results in severe retractions with each breath because the chest wall is very compliant. The weak muscles of the chest wall are drawn inward, placing pressure on the lungs that further interferes with expansion. Seesaw respirations may also occur.

As fewer alveoli expand, atelectasis and hypoxia occur. This causes pulmonary vasoconstriction and decreased blood flow to the lungs because of the high resistance within the pulmonary blood vessels, resulting in persistent pulmonary hypertension (see Chapter 30, p. 805). There may be a return to fetal circulation patterns, with opening of the ductus arteriosus. Acidosis and alveolar necrosis further complicate the condition by interfering with surfactant synthesis. Hyaline membranes, consisting of debris from necrotic cells in fibrous material, line the distal airways.

Tests of amniotic fluid can detect lecithin, sphingomyelin, phosphatidylglycerol, and phosphatidylinositol, which are components of surfactant. These tests can predict whether the fetal lungs are mature enough that survival outside of the uterus is possible (see Chapter 10, p. 210). The incidence and severity of RDS may be reduced by giving the mother corticosteroids before birth (see Chapter 27, p. 718).

MANIFESTATIONS

Signs of RDS begin within the first hours after birth and if not treated with surfactant become worse until they peak at 2 to 3 days, then begin to improve (Rodriguez, Martin, & Fanaroff, 2002). They include tachypnea, tachycardia, nasal flaring, xiphoid and intercostal retractions, and cyanosis. Audible grunting on expiration is characteristic. It results from air moving past a partially closed glottis, which helps maintain lung expansion, gas exchange during exhalation, and functional residual capacity. Breath sounds may be decreased, and rales may be present.

Acidosis develops as a result of hypoxemia. Blood gases show increased carbon dioxide levels and decreased oxygen. Chest radiographs show the "ground glass" reticulogranular appearance of the lungs that is characteristic of RDS. Areas of atelectasis are present.

THERAPEUTIC MANAGEMENT

Surfactant replacement therapy is used prophylactically to prevent RDS or as "rescue" treatment once RDS has occurred. It is instilled into the infant's trachea during stabilization immediately after birth or as soon as signs of RDS become apparent. Improvement in breathing occurs in minutes. Doses are repeated if necessary. Infants treated with surfactant have higher survival rates, although the incidence of bronchopulmonary dysplasia (BPD) is unchanged (Fanaroff, Martin, & Rodriguez, 2004).

Other treatment is supportive, including mechanical ventilation or CPAP, correction of the acidosis, IV fluids, and care of other complications. Low temperature and glucose may occur and should be treated immediately.

NURSING CONSIDERATIONS

The nurse observes for signs of developing RDS at birth and during the early hours after the delivery. Changes in the infant's condition are constantly assessed. For example, diuresis occurs with improvement in the disease. Changes in ventilator settings may be necessary as the infant's ability to oxygenate increases. Observation for signs of common complications such as patent ductus arteriosus and BPD is important. The nurse must monitor the results of laboratory tests for abnormalities in blood gases and acid-base balance. Early signs of sepsis must be identified and reported. Other care is similar to general care for the preterm infant.

Bronchopulmonary Dysplasia

BPD, also known as *chronic lung disease,* is a chronic condition occurring most often in infants weighing less than 1500 g at birth. It is associated with a mortality rate of 10% to 25%. Infants generally continue to require oxygen, positive pressure ventilation, or continuous positive airway pressure (CPAP) at 36 weeks' postmenstrual age (Banks-Randall & Ballard, 2005).

PATHOPHYSIOLOGY

BPD results from a combination of factors. High levels of oxygen, oxygen-free radicals, and high positive-pressure ventilation that damage bronchial epithelium and interfere with alveolar development are major factors in the condition. The result is inflammation, atelectasis, edema, and airway hyperreactivity with loss of cilia, thickening of the walls of the alveoli, and fibrotic changes.

MANIFESTATIONS

The major sign of BPD is an increased need for ventilation or an inability to be weaned from the ventilation and oxygen. Other signs include tachycardia, tachypnea, retractions, rales, wheezing, respiratory acidosis, increased secretions, bronchospasm, and characteristic changes in the lungs on chest radiographs. Pulmonary edema may occur.

THERAPEUTIC MANAGEMENT

Prevention includes use of maternal steroids to reduce prematurity and RDS, minimizing exposure to oxygen and pressure with ventilation as much as possible, avoidance of fluid overload, and increased nutrition. Treatment is supportive, with gradual decreases in the amount of oxygen, bronchodilators, and antibiotics as necessary. Diuretics are given and fluids are restricted, as infants are prone to fluid overload. Increased calories and protein are important. Corticosteroids are not recommended; they are associated with impairment of growth, neurodevelopmental problems, and gastrointestinal bleeding (AAP & American College of Obstetricians & Gynecologists [ACOG], 2002). The infant may go home on long-term oxygen therapy, and some need frequent rehospitalization because of respiratory infections.

Periventricular-Intraventricular Hemorrhage

Periventricular-intraventricular hemorrhage (PIVH) occurs most often in infants of less than 32 weeks' gestation or those who weigh less than 1500 g (Blackburn, 2003b). The first few days of life are the most common times for hemorrhage to occur.

PATHOPHYSIOLOGY

PIVH results from rupture of the fragile blood vessels in the germinal matrix, located around the ventricles of the brain. It is most often associated with hypoxic injury to the vessels, increased or decreased blood pressure, and increased or fluctuating cerebral blood flow. Rapid blood volume expansion, hypercarbia, anemia, and hypoglycemia are other causes.

Hemorrhage is graded 1 through 4, according to the amount of bleeding. Grade 1 is a very small bleed at the germinal matrix, producing few if any clinical changes. Grade 2 hemorrhage extends into the lateral ventricles, and grade 3 causes distention of ventricles. Grade 4 hemorrhage causes ventricular dilation and extends into surrounding brain tissue. Those with grade 4 hemorrhage have a poor survival rate.

Although fewer complications and less mortality occurs with grade 1 and 2 hemorrhages, infants with grade 3 and 4 hemorrhages may have neurologic abnormalities and developmental delays. The degree of neurologic deficits may not always correlate with the amount of hemorrhage, however. The mortality rate for infants with PIVH ranges from 5% to 15% for infants with mild to moderate bleeding and 50% for those with severe hemorrhage (Papile, 2002).

MANIFESTATIONS

Signs of PIVH are determined by the severity of the hemorrhage. They may include lethargy, poor muscle tone, deterioration of respiratory status with cyanosis or apnea, drop in hematocrit level, decreased reflexes, full or bulging fontanelle, and seizures. Subtle aberrations of eye position or movement may occur.

THERAPEUTIC MANAGEMENT

Because most hemorrhages take place in the first week, ultrasonography is performed on preterm infants at risk for PIVH after that time. If bleeding is found, serial ultrasonography may be performed to determine progression of the problem.

Treatment is supportive and focuses on maintaining respiratory function and dealing with other complications. Hydrocephalus may develop from blockage of cerebrospinal fluid flow. Lumbar taps or a ventriculoperitoneal shunt (catheter leading from the ventricles of the brain to the peritoneal cavity) may be necessary to drain the fluid.

NURSING CONSIDERATIONS

Many aspects of care may increase cerebral blood flow and blood pressure. These include mechanical ventilation, suctioning, and excessive handling. Even crying may produce changes in cerebral blood flow. Therefore the nurse must be alert for early signs of PIVH. Nursing care includes daily measurement of the head circumference and observation for changes in neurologic status, which may be subtle. Handling is kept to a minimum, and environmental stressors are reduced as much as possible. Developmental care has been found helpful in preventing or minimizing the problem.

Parents need assistance to cope with the diagnosis and their concerns regarding long-term implications. They should learn how to assess for signs of increasing intracranial pressure from hydrocephalus and understand that follow-up care may include periodic ultrasound examinations.

Retinopathy of Prematurity

Retinopathy of prematurity (ROP), previously known as *retrolental fibroplasia,* may result in visual impairment or blindness in preterm infants. It occurs more often in premature infants of less than 28 weeks' gestation or weighing 1500 g or less.

PATHOPHYSIOLOGY

ROP is caused by damage to immature blood vessels in the retina. The exact cause of the damage is unknown, but one cause may be high levels of oxygen. However, ROP develops in some infants who never received supplementary oxygen. Prolonged ventilation, acidosis, sepsis, and shock have all been associated with ROP (AAP & ACOG, 2002).

In ROP, immature blood vessels in the retina of the eye are injured. After a period of time new vessels proliferate, extending throughout the retina and into the vitreous of the eye in some infants. Fluid leakage and hemorrhages from the fragile vessels may cause scarring, traction on the retina, and retinal detachment. However, the progress of pathology stops in more than 90% of infants and there is little visual loss (Olitsky & Nelson, 2004).

THERAPEUTIC MANAGEMENT

Infants born at less than 28 weeks' gestation or weighing 1500 g or less should be screened 4 to 6 weeks after birth or at 31 to 33 weeks' postmenstrual age to detect changes of the eye. Infants weighing 1500 g to 2000 g with complications may also need screening (AAP & ACOG, 2002). Laser photocoagulation surgery is used most often for infants whose ROP is advancing. Cryotherapy is used less frequently to destroy the proliferating blood vessels. Reattachment of the retina also may be necessary.

NURSING CONSIDERATIONS

The nurse should check the pulse oximetry readings frequently for any infant receiving oxygen. Parents should be informed about ophthalmologic tests and receive an explanation of the results. Eye examinations can be very stressful to the infant, and swaddling and rest periods should be provided as appropriate. Mydriatic eye drops given to dilate the eyes may cause tachycardia, restlessness and feeding intolerance. If surgery is performed, the eye is assessed for drainage. Ice packs may be used for edema, and pain medication should be given. Support for parents is essential throughout the examinations and especially if damage to the eye is found.

Necrotizing Enterocolitis

Necrotizing enterocolitis (NEC) is a serious inflammatory condition of the intestinal tract that may lead to cellular death of areas of intestinal mucosa. The mortality rate is 25% to 30%, and 25% of survivors have long-term gastrointestinal problems (Berseth & Poenaru, 2005). The ileum and proximal colon are the areas most often affected.

PATHOPHYSIOLOGY

Although the exact causes are unknown, immaturity of the intestines may be a major factor in preterm infants. In addition, NEC may be caused by interference with blood supply to the intestinal mucosa. During asphyxia, blood is diverted from the gastrointestinal tract to the brain, heart, and kidneys. Sepsis, polycythemia, umbilical vessel catheterization, and maternal cocaine use are other causes of decrease in intestinal blood flow. The resulting ischemia causes death of some mucosa cells and further injury by intestinal digestive enzymes. This makes the area more susceptible to invasion with bacteria.

The incidence of NEC is much higher after infants have received feedings. Although minimal enteric feedings are thought to increase maturation of the intestines, feedings that are too early or increasing the feedings too fast may cause NEC. When infants are fed, bacteria proliferate and gas-forming organisms may invade the intestinal wall. Eventually, necrosis, perforation, and peritonitis may occur. Breast milk, which contains immunoglobulins, leukocytes, and antibacterial agents, may have a preventive effect on the development of NEC.

MANIFESTATIONS

Signs include increased abdominal girth caused by distention, increased gastric residuals, decreased or absent bowel sounds, loops of bowel seen through the abdominal wall, vomiting, bile-stained residuals or emesis, abdominal tenderness, signs of infection, and occult blood in the stools. Respiratory difficulty may occur because of pressure from the distended abdomen on the diaphragm. Apnea, bradycardia, temperature instability, lethargy, hypotension, and shock also may be present. On radiographs, there may be loops of bowel dilated with air. The presence of air within the intestinal wall is characteristic of the condition. Free air in the peritoneum indicates that perforation has occurred, although perforation may occur without the sign.

THERAPEUTIC MANAGEMENT

Treatment includes antibiotics, discontinuation of oral feedings, continuous or intermittent gastric suction, and use of parenteral nutrition to rest the intestines. Surgery may be necessary if perforation or continued lack of improvement occurs. The necrotic area is removed, and an ostomy may be performed. Infants who have had large areas of bowel removed may develop short bowel syndrome with malabsorption and malnutrition.

NURSING CONSIDERATIONS

Nurses should encourage interested mothers to provide breast milk for their infants because NEC is less likely to occur in breastfed infants. Early recognition of signs of NEC is essential to decrease mortality. Because nurses are constantly observing the infant, they often are able to detect the early, subtle signs that lead to prompt diagnosis. If one or more signs are noted, the nurse withholds the next feeding and notifies the physician.

Abdominal girth is measured, and IV fluids and parenteral nutrition must be managed. Intake and output are important, as third-space fluid loss occurs when fluid moves from the intravascular spaces to the extracellular spaces. The infant should be positioned on the side to minimize the effects of pressure on the diaphragm from the distended intestines. During recovery, the nurse must observe for signs of feeding intolerance when feedings are resumed. Scar tissue may cause partial or complete bowel obstruction.

POSTTERM INFANTS

Postterm infants are those who are born after the forty-second week of gestation. Their longer-than-normal gestation places them at risk for a number of complications.

Scope of the Problem

Approximately 12% of all pregnancies are considered postterm (Stoll & Kliegman, 2004b). In most cases the fetus continues to be well supported by the placenta and is of normal size or is large for gestational age, if the placenta continues to function well (Resnik & Resnik, 2004). Some postterm fetuses grow to more than 4000 g (8 lb, 13 oz), placing them at risk for birth injuries or cesarean birth.

In other cases, placental functioning decreases when pregnancy is prolonged. If placental insufficiency is present, decreased amniotic fluid volume (oligohydramnios) and compression of the umbilical cord may occur. The fetus may not receive the appropriate amount of oxygen and nutrients and may be small for gestational age. This condition results in hypoxia and malnourishment in the fetus and is called *postmaturity syndrome.*

When labor begins, poor oxygen reserves may cause fetal compromise. The fetus may pass meconium as a result of hypoxia before or during labor, increasing the risk of meconium passage and possible aspiration at delivery (Chapter 30). They are also at higher risk for asphyxia than other infants. Postterm infants have a higher perinatal mortality rate than infants born at term.

Assessment

Most infants will be normal at birth. If the infant is large, the nurse should observe for injury and hypoglycemia. However, signs of distress may occur during labor, and the nurse should observe the fetal monitor carefully for late or variable decelerations. When the amniotic membranes rupture, the fluid may be stained with meconium. Respiratory difficulties may occur at birth. The cord, skin, and nails may be stained, indicating that meconium was present for some time.

The infant with postmaturity syndrome is unusually alert and wide-eyed and has a worried look. The infant may be thin with loose skin and little subcutaneous fat. There is little or no lanugo and vernix caseosa, but the infant has abundant hair on the head and long nails. The skin is wrinkled, cracked, and peeling (Figure 29-12).

Postterm infants should be assessed for hypoglycemia because of rapid use of glycogen stores. If loss of subcutaneous fat has occurred, the infant is at risk for low temperature. The skin may be like parchment with peeling, sloughing, and even maceration. The umbilical cord is thin with little Wharton's jelly. Vernix and lanugo are sparse or absent, and fingernails are long.

Therapeutic Management

Therapeutic management focuses on prevention and symptomatic treatment. Expectant mothers who are "overdue" are scheduled for tests of placental functioning, and labor is induced if signs of placental deterioration are discovered during fetal diagnostic testing. If the fetus cannot tolerate labor, a cesarean birth is necessary. Apgar scores less than 7 are more likely in postterm infants. In cases of asphyxia or meconium aspiration, respiratory support is needed at birth (Chapter 30, pp. 800 and 801).

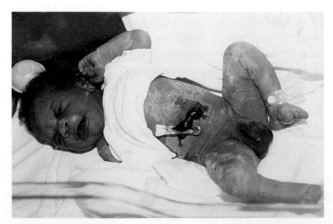

Figure 29-12 ■ The postmature infant has no vernix and dry, cracked, peeling skin.

Nursing Considerations

The nurse's role is primarily one of prevention of complications, where possible, and monitoring of changes in status. During labor and delivery, the nurse responds appropriately to fetal heart rate decelerations, prepares for and assists in emergency delivery, and cares for respiratory problems at birth. Initial assessments should include a thorough assessment for injuries if the infant is large.

Signs of postmaturity syndrome in infants are noted during the initial assessment. Respiratory problems may necessitate continued assessment and care. Infants with any indications of postmaturity should be tested for hypoglycemia soon after birth and again an hour later. They need early and more frequent feedings to help compensate for the period of poor nutrition in utero.

Temperature regulation may be poor because fat stores were used for nourishment in utero. Using extra blankets, assessing temperature frequently, and teaching parents about prevention of cold stress may be necessary throughout the hospital stay. Polycythemia, resulting from hypoxia before birth, increases the risk of hyperbilirubinemia.

SMALL-FOR-GESTATIONAL-AGE INFANTS

Small-for-gestational-age (SGA) infants are those who fall below the 10th percentile in size on growth charts. They have failed to grow in utero as expected and have IUGR. Some infants who do not meet the definition for SGA may have IUGR and fail to grow to full potential in utero for a variety of reasons. However, the terms *SGA* and *IUGR* often are used interchangeably.

Infants who are SGA may be preterm, full-term, or postterm. Infant mortality and morbidity increase steadily as growth restriction increases. Approximately one third of all low-birth-weight (LBW) infants are full term but SGA (Stoll & Kliegman, 2004b).

Causes

Many risk factors may cause an infant to be SGA. Congenital malformations, chromosomal anomalies, and fetal infections from rubella or cytomegalovirus may cause IUGR. Poor placental function resulting from aging, small size, separation, or malformation may interfere with fetal growth. Illness in the expectant mother, such as preeclampsia or severe diabetes, restricts uteroplacental blood flow and decreases fetal growth. Smoking, drug or alcohol abuse, and severe maternal malnutrition also impair fetal growth.

Scope of the Problem

Infants affected with IUGR have higher perinatal morbidity and mortality rates than infants who are not growth restricted. Full-term infants who are SGA are subject to many of the same complications as those who are preterm or postterm. Specific complications and their severity depend on the cause and degree of growth restriction. Infants with congenital defects also have problems at birth associated with the anomaly. Drug-exposed infants may have the added complication of drug withdrawal. SGA infants are more likely to experience fetal distress and asphyxia. Problems tend to be greatest in infants who are preterm in addition to being SGA.

Low Apgar scores, meconium aspiration, and polycythemia are increased in the SGA infant. Hypoglycemia is common because of inadequate storage of glycogen in the liver. Although muscle tone enables the SGA infant to maintain better flexion than the preterm infant, SGA infants are prone to inadequate thermoregulation because subcutaneous white fat and brown fat stores have been used to survive in utero. If hypoglycemia develops, inadequate glucose is available for increased metabolism to produce heat, increasing the problem.

Characteristics

The appearance of the SGA infant varies according to whether the cause of growth restriction began early or late in the pregnancy. Variation occurs because growth restriction affects the weight first. If it continues, the length and then the head size eventually will be affected.

Symmetric growth restriction involves the entire body. It may be caused by congenital anomalies or exposure to infections or drugs early in pregnancy. Although the infant's weight, length, and head circumference are all below the 10th percentile, the body is proportionate and appears normally developed for size. The total number of cells as well as the cell size decrease, and the infant may have long-term complications. These infants often are small throughout their lives.

Asymmetric restriction is caused by complications that begin after 28 weeks of gestation and result in placental insufficiency, such as preeclampsia. In asymmetric restriction, the head is normal in size but seems large for the rest of the body. Brain growth and heart size are normal, but other organs may be small in size. The length is generally normal, but the weight is below the 10th percentile for gestational age. The abdominal circumference is decreased because the liver is smaller than normal. The infant appears long and thin. The loose skin has longitudinal thigh creases from loss of subcutaneous fat. The infant has sparse hair, a thin cord, dry skin, and the wide-eyed look associated with intrauterine hypoxia. Infants have a normal number of cells, but the cell size is decreased (Resnik & Creasy, 2004). These infants may "catch up" in growth, particularly in the first year, if they are adequately nourished after birth.

Therapeutic Management

Therapeutic management is focused on prevention with good prenatal care to identify and treat problems early. When growth restriction cannot be prevented, ultrasound examination may permit early discovery of the condition. Serial nonstress tests and biophysical profiles help determine if the infant should be delivered early, and preparation can be made for the expected complications at birth. Problems during and after birth are treated as they occur. They may include asphyxia, meconium aspiration, hypoglycemia, and polycythemia (Resnik & Creasy, 2004).

Nursing Considerations

Because the causes of growth restriction are so varied, care of the SGA infant must be adapted to meet the specific problems that the infant demonstrates. When signs of growth restriction are present, the nurse must observe for complications that commonly accompany it. The general appearance and measurements will give an indication of the type of growth restriction that has occurred. Measurements of the head, chest, length, and weight are below normal in the infant with symmetric growth restriction. If the restriction is asymmetric, the head circumference and length will be normal and the abdominal circumference and weight will be low.

The nurse should assess for hypoglycemia, especially in asymmetric, growth-restricted infants. The brain of the infant is normal and needs large amounts of glucose, but the liver is small and has inadequate stores of glycogen. Caloric needs are higher than for a normal infant, making early and more frequent feedings important. Temperature regulation and respiratory support are added nursing concerns. Observation for jaundice is important in infants with polycythemia because a large amount of bilirubin may be released when the red blood cells break down.

LARGE-FOR-GESTATIONAL AGE INFANTS

Large-for-gestational age (LGA) infants are those who are above the 90th percentile on intrauterine growth charts. They may weigh more than 4000 g (8 lb, 13 oz) and are usually born at term, although they may be preterm or postterm. The preterm LGA infant may be mistaken for full-term but has the same problems as other preterm infants.

Causes

Infants who are LGA may be born to multiparas, large parents, and certain ethnic groups known to have large infants. Diabetes in the mother may also cause increased size, as may erythroblastosis fetalis (see Chapter 30).

Scope of the Problem

The LGA infant is more likely to go through a longer labor, have injury during birth, or need a cesarean birth. Shoulder dystocia may occur because the shoulders are too large to fit through the pelvis. Fractures of the clavicle or skull, damage to the brachial plexus or facial or phrenic nerves, cephalhematoma, and bruising occur more often in these infants than those of normal size. Congenital heart defects and a higher mortality rate also are more common (Stoll & Kliegman, 2004b).

Therapeutic Management

Therapeutic management is based on identification of macrosomia (large size) during pregnancy by measurements of fundal height and ultrasound examination. Delivery prob-

---

BOX 29-2 Common Nursing Diagnoses for Preterm Infants
Activity Intolerance*
Ineffective Airway Clearance
Ineffective Infant Feeding Pattern*
Ineffective Thermoregulation
Interrupted Family Processes
Pain
Risk for Delayed Growth and Development
Risk for Disorganized Infant Behavior*
Risk for Imbalanced Nutrition: Less Than Body Requirements*
Risk for Impaired Parent-Infant Attachment*
Risk for Impaired Parenting
Risk for Caregiver Role Strain
Risk for Imbalanced Fluid Volume
Risk for Impaired Skin Integrity
Risk for Infection

*Nursing diagnoses explored in this chapter.

lems may lead to use of vacuum extraction, forceps, or cesarean birth. Specific treatment involves identification and treatment of birth injuries and complications as they arise.

Nursing Considerations

The nurse assists in a difficult delivery or cesarean birth resulting from dystocias when the infant is LGA. After birth the infant is carefully assessed for injuries or other complications such as hypoglycemia (p. 488) or polycythemia (p. 816). Common nursing diagnoses used for infants at risk are listed in Box 29-2.

✓ CHECK YOUR READING

14. What is the typical appearance of the infant with postmaturity syndrome?
15. What special problems might a postmature infant have?
16. How are symmetric and asymmetric IUGR different?
17. What problems may occur in infants who are LGA?

SUMMARY CONCEPTS

- Preterm infants differ in appearance from full-term infants. Some differences include small size, limp posture, red skin, abundant vernix and lanugo, and immature ears and genitals.
- The lungs of preterm infants may lack adequate surfactant, which may cause the lungs to be noncompliant, increasing the amount of energy necessary for breathing and leading to atelectasis.
- Other factors that may increase respiratory problems are poor cough reflex, narrow respiratory passages, and weak muscles.
- Preterm infants should be positioned on the side or prone to increase drainage of respiratory secretions. The prone position decreases breathing effort because respiratory muscles are used efficiently.
- Preterm infants are prone to cold stress because they have thin skin with blood vessels near the surface, little subcutaneous white fat or brown fat, a large surface area, a limp position, and an immature temperature control center.

- Maintaining a neutral thermal environment at all times for infants is important. The nurse should prevent air drafts, use warmed oxygen, and keep incubator doors and portholes closed. After being taken out of heating devices, the infant should be wrapped in warmed blankets and should wear a hat.
- Preterm infants are subject to increased insensible water losses and have difficulty maintaining fluid balance. Their kidneys do not concentrate or dilute urine as well as those of full-term infants. Intake and output must be carefully measured.
- The fragile skin of a preterm infant is easily damaged. Adhesives or chemicals that could injure the skin should be avoided. Special products designed to prevent injury to the skin should be used.
- Preterm infants are subject to infections because they lack passive antibodies from the mother, have an immature immune system, have fragile skin, and are subjected to many invasive procedures.
- The nurse must watch carefully for signs of pain and use comfort measures, containment, pacifiers, sucrose, and medications to alleviate it.
- Infants demonstrate that they are receiving too much stimulation by changes in oxygenation and behavior. The nurse should schedule care to allow rest periods, keep noise to a minimum, and teach parents ways to interact with the infant appropriately.
- Preterm infants lack nutrient stores and need more nutrients but do not absorb them well. They lack coordination in sucking and swallowing and fatigue easily.
- Signs indicating an infant may be ready for nipple feeding include rooting, sucking on a gavage catheter or pacifier, presence of gag reflex, and respiratory rate below 60 breaths per minute.
- The nurse should teach mothers who wish to breastfeed their preterm infants how to use a breast pump and store breast milk. Nurses provide privacy, give support and encouragement, explain the infant's behavior, and answer questions about breastfeeding.
- Nurses can increase parents' comfort with their preterm infant by providing information about the infant's condition and characteristics, the neonatal intensive care unit, equipment, and care. Spending time with parents during visits, offering therapeutic communication and realistic encouragement, and involving parents in care of the infant also help bonding.
- Preparation for discharge should be started early in the infant's hospital stay. This allows parents to gradually learn about and take on increasing responsibility in the care of the infant until they are comfortable with complete care.
- Common complications of preterm birth are respiratory distress syndrome, bronchopulmonary dysplasia, periventricular-intraventricular hemorrhage, retinopathy of prematurity, and necrotizing enterocolitis.
- Infants with postmaturity syndrome may appear thin with loose skin folds, cracked peeling skin, and meconium staining. They appear worried. They may have respiratory difficulties at birth and suffer hypoglycemia and inadequate temperature regulation.
- Infants with intrauterine growth restriction may be small for gestational age at birth. In symmetric growth restriction, the infant is proportionately small; in asymmetric growth restriction, the head and usually the length are normal and the body is thin.
- Large-for-gestational-age infants may have birth injuries such as fractures, nerve damage, or bruising as a result of their size. They may have hypoglycemia or polycythemia.

ANSWERS TO CRITICAL THINKING EXERCISE 29-1, p. 779

Compared with the full-term infant, the preterm infant may need more frequent feedings with special formula in smaller amounts. The preterm infant will take longer to feed, might need gavage feedings before introduction of a bottle, and is more prone to complications in feeding. See Nursing Care Plan 29-1 for interventions appropriate for bottle feeding the preterm infant.

ANSWERS TO CRITICAL THINKING EXERCISE 29-2, p. 786

1. The mother may be intimidated by the equipment and fear she might break it or cause it to malfunction if she touches it. If alarms sound frequently, she may be especially uneasy. She may be frightened of the infant's small size and afraid she might cause harm by touching her baby. She may be experiencing anticipatory grieving because her infant may not survive. She may also be too overwhelmed to be able to participate in touching her infant at this time and may need more time.
2. To assist the mother, the nurse can use therapeutic communication techniques to help her express her feelings and fears. The purpose of equipment and reasons for alarms should be explained. Involving the mother in small tasks, such as handing the nurse a blanket or holding a bottle of formula, may help her feel more a part of her baby's care. The nurse should continue to suggest that the mother touch the baby and to suggest ways it might be appropriate. For example, the nurse might ask the mother to hold the infant's hand during minor procedures to comfort the infant.

REFERENCES & READINGS

Agarwal, R., Hagedorn, M.I.E., & Gardner, S.L. (2002). Pain and pain relief. In G.B. Merenstein & S.L. Gardner (Eds.), *Handbook of neonatal intensive care* (5th ed., pp. 191-218). St. Louis: Mosby.

Altimier, L.B. (2003). Management of the NICU environment. In C. Kenner & J.W. Lott (Eds.), *Comprehensive neonatal nursing: A physiologic perspective* (3rd ed., pp. 229-235). Philadelphia: Saunders.

American Academy of Pediatrics & American College of Obstetricians and Gynecologists. (2002). *Guidelines for perinatal care* (5th ed.). Elk Grove Village, IL, and Washington, DC: Authors.

American Academy of Pediatrics & American Pain Society. (2001). The assessment and management of acute pain in infants, children, and adolescents. *Pediatrics, 108*(3), 793-797.

American Academy of Pediatrics and Canadian Paediatric Society. (2000). Prevention and management of pain and stress in the neonate. *Pediatrics, 105*(2), 454-461.

American Lung Association. (2004). *Respiratory distress syndrome of the newborn fact sheet.* Retrieved January 22, 2005, from http://www.lungusa.org.

Anderson, D.M. (2002). Feeding the ill or preterm infant. *Neonatal Network, 21*(7), 7-14.

Anderson, G.C., Chiu, S., Dombrowski, M.A., Swinth, J.Y., Albert, J.M., & Wada, N. (2003). Mother-newborn contact in a randomized trial of kangaroo (skin-to-skin) care. *Journal of Obstetric, Gynecologic, and Neonatal Nursing, 32*(5), 604-611.

Anderson, M.S., Johnson, C.B., Townsend, S.F., & Hay, W.W. (2002). Enteral nutrition. In G.B. Merenstein & S.L. Gardner (Eds.), *Handbook of neonatal intensive care* (5th ed., pp. 314-340). St. Louis: Mosby.

Asklin, D.F., & Diehl-Jones, W. (2004). Ophthalmologic and auditory disorders. In M.T. Verklan & M. Walden (Eds.), *Core curriculum for neonatal intensive care nursing* (3rd ed., pp. 913-932). Philadelphia: Saunders.

Association of Women's Health, Obstetric and Neonatal Nurses (AWHONN). (2001). *Evidence-based clinical practice guideline: Neonatal skin care.* Washington, DC: Author.

Bakewell-Sachs, S. (2004). Nutritional management. In M.T. Verklan & M. Walden (Eds.), *Core curriculum for neonatal intensive care nursing* (3rd ed., pp. 205-235). Philadelphia: Saunders.

Bakewell-Sachs, S., & Blackburn, S. (2001). *Discharge and follow-up of the high-risk preterm infant.* White Plains, NY: March of Dimes Birth Defects Foundation.

Banks-Randall, B.A., & Ballard, R.A. (2005). Bronchopulmonary dysplasia. In H.W. Taeusch, R.A. Ballard, & C.A. Gleason (Eds.), *Avery's diseases of the newborn* (8th ed., pp. 723-736). Philadelphia: Saunders.

Beacham, P.S. (2004). Behavioral and physiological indicators of procedural and postoperative pain in high-risk infants. *Journal of Obstetric, Gynecologic, and Neonatal Nursing, 33*(2), 246-255.

Beachy, J.M. (2003). Premature infant massage in the NICU. *Neonatal Network, 22*(3), 39-45.

Berry, D.D., Adcock, E.W., & Starbuck, A. (2002). Fluid and electrolyte management. In G.B. Merenstein & S.L. Gardner (Eds.), *Handbook of neonatal intensive care* (5th ed., pp. 283-297). St. Louis: Mosby.

Berseth, C.L., & Poenaru, D. (2005). Necrotizing enterocolitis and short bowel syndrome. In H.W. Taeusch, R.A. Ballard, & C.A. Gleason (Eds.), *Avery's diseases of the newborn* (8th ed., pp. 1123-1133). Philadelphia: Saunders.

Biancuzzo, M. (2003). *Breastfeeding the newborn: Clinical strategies for nurses* (2nd ed.). St. Louis: Mosby.

Bialoskurski, M., Cox, C.L., & Hayes, J. (2000). The nature of attachment in a neonatal intensive care unit. *Journal of Perinatal & Neonatal Nursing, 13*(1), 66-77.

Blackburn, S.T., (2003a). *Maternal, fetal, and neonatal physiology* (2nd ed). Philadelphia: Saunders.

Blackburn, S.T. (2003b). Assessment and management of neonatal neurobehavioral development. In C. Kenner & J.W. Lott (Eds.), *Comprehensive neonatal nursing: A physiologic perspective* (3rd ed., pp. 624-660). Philadelphia: Saunders.

Blake, W.W., & Murray, J.A. (2002). Heat balance. In G.B. Merenstein & S.L. Gardner (Eds.), *Handbook of neonatal intensive care* (5th ed., pp. 102-116). St. Louis: Mosby.

Bracht, M., Kandankery, A., Nodwell, S., & Stade, B. (2002). Cultural differences and parental responses to the preterm infant at risk: Strategies for supporting families. *Neonatal Network, 21*(6), 31-38.

Brazy, J.E., Anderson, B.M.H., Becker, P., & Becker, M. (2001). How parents of premature infants gather information and obtain support. *Neonatal Network, 20*(2), 41-48.

Bremmer, P., Byers, J.F., & Kiehl, E. (2003). Noise and the premature infant: Physiological effects and practice implications. *Journal of Obstetric, Gynecologic, and Neonatal Nursing, 32*(4), 447-454.

Bruns, D.A., & McCollum, J.A. (2002). Partnerships between mothers and professionals in the NICU: Caregiving, information exchange, and relationships. *Neonatal Network, 21*(7), 15-23.

Byers, J.F. (2003). Components of developmental care and the evidence for their use in the NICU. *MCN: American Journal of Maternal/Child Nursing, 28*(1), 174-181.

Byers, J.F., & Thornley, K. (2004). Cueing into infant pain. *MCN: American Journal of Maternal/Child Nursing, 29*(2), 84-89.

Carrier, C.T. (2004). Developmental support. In M.T. Verklan & M. Walden (Eds.), *Core curriculum for neonatal intensive care nursing* (3rd ed., pp. 236-264). Philadelphia: Saunders.

Chandra, S., & Baumgart, S. (2005). Temperature regulation of the premature infant. In H.W. Taeusch, R.A. Ballard, & C.A. Gleason (Eds.), *Avery's diseases of the newborn* (8th ed., pp. 364-371). Philadelphia: Saunders.

Cifuentes, J., Segars, A.H., & Carlo, W.A. (2003). Respiratory system management. In C. Kenner & J.W. Lott (Eds.), *Comprehensive neonatal nursing: A physiologic perspective* (3rd ed., pp. 348-362). Philadelphia: Saunders.

Colon, E.J. (2001). Culturally congruent care in the NICU. *AWHONN Lifelines, 5*(5), 60-64.

Consensus Committee to Establish Recommended Standards for Newborn ICU Design. (2002). *Recommended standards for newborn ICU design.* Retrieved January 19, 2005, from http://www.nd.edu/kkolberg/DesignStandards.htm.

Creehan, P.A. (2001). Sending baby home safely: Developing an infant car seat testing program. *AWHONN Lifelines, 5*(6), 60-70.

DiMaggio, T.J., & Gibbons, M.A.E. (2005). Neonatal pain management in the 21st century. In H.W. Taeusch, R.A. Ballard, & C.A. Gleason (Eds.), *Avery's diseases of the newborn* (8th ed., pp. 438-446). Philadelphia: Saunders.

Engler, A.J., Ludington-Hoe, S.M., Cusson, R.M., Adams, R., Bahnsen, M., Brumbaugh, E., et al. (2002). Kangaroo care: National survey of practice, knowledge, barriers, and perceptions. *MCN: American Journal of Maternal/Child Nursing, 27*(3), 146-153.

Evans, J.C. (2001). Physiology of acute pain in preterm infants. *Newborn and Infant Nursing Reviews, 1*(2), 75-84.

Evans, R.A., & Thureen, P.J. (2001). Early feeding strategies in preterm and critically ill neonates. *Neonatal Network, 20*(7), 7-18.

Fanaroff, A.A., Martin, R.J., & Rodriguez, R.J. (2004). Identification and management of the high-risk neonate. In R.K. Creasy & R. Resnik (Eds.), *Maternal-fetal medicine: Principles and practice* (5th ed., pp. 1263-1301). Philadelphia: Saunders.

Franck, L.S., Bernal, H., & Gale, G. (2002). Infant holding policies and practices in neonatal units. *Neonatal Network, 21*(2), 13-20.

Gardner, S.L., & Goldson, E. (2002). The neonate and the environment: Impact on development. In G.B. Merenstein & S.L. Gardner (Eds.), *Handbook of neonatal intensive care* (5th ed., pp. 219-282). St. Louis: Mosby.

Gardner, S.L., Snell, B.J., & Lawrence, R.A. (2002). Breastfeeding the infant with special needs. In G.B. Merenstein & S.L. Gardner (Eds.), *Handbook of neonatal intensive care* (5th ed., pp. 376-418). St. Louis: Mosby.

Gates, L.V., McGrath, J.M., & Jorgensen, K.M. (2004). Family issues/professional-parent partnerships. In C. Kenner & J.M. McGrath (Eds.), *Developmental care of newborns and infants: A guide for health professionals* (pp. 343-357). St. Louis: Mosby.

Gracey, K. (2004). Discharge planning and transition to home care. In M.T. Verklan & M. Walden (Eds.), *Core curriculum for neonatal intensive care nursing* (3rd ed., pp. 422-434). Philadelphia: Saunders.

Grow, J.L., & Schumacher, R.E. (2003). Breastfeeding and premature or sick infants. In S.M. Donn (Ed.), *Michigan manual of neonatal intensive care* (3rd ed., pp. 164-175). Philadelphia: Hanley & Belfus.

Hagedorn, M.I., Gardner, S.L., & Abman, S.H. (2002). Respiratory diseases. In G.B. Merenstein & S.L. Gardner (Eds.), *Handbook of neonatal intensive care* (5th ed., pp. 485-575). St. Louis: Mosby.

Hall, W.A., Shearer, K., Mogan, J., & Berkowitz, J. (2002). Weighing preterm infants before and after breastfeeding: Does it increase maternal confidence and competence? *MCN: American Journal of Maternal/Child Nursing, 27*(6), 318-327.

Hamilton, B.E., Martin, J.A., & Sutton, P.D. (2004). Births: Preliminary data for 2003. *National Vital Statistics Reports, 53*(9). Hyattsville, MD: National Center for Health Statistics.

Han-Markey, T., & Schumacher, R.E. (2003). Enteral nutrition. In S.M. Donn (Ed.), *Michigan manual of neonatal intensive care* (3rd ed., pp. 146-163). Philadelphia: Hanley & Belfus.

Holditch-Davis, D., Blackburn, S.T., & VandenBerg, K. (2003). Newborn and infant neurobehavioral development. In C. Kenner & J.W. Lott (Eds.), *Comprehensive neonatal nursing: A physiologic perspective* (3rd ed., pp. 236-284). Philadelphia: Saunders.

Horton, K.K. (2005). Pathophysiology and current management of necrotizing enterocolitis. *Neonatal Network, 24*(1), 37-46.

Hummel, P. (2003). Parenting the high-risk infant. *Newborn and Infant Nursing Reviews, 3*(3), 88-92.

Hurst, I. (2001). Mothers' strategies to meet their needs in the newborn intensive care nursery. *Journal of Perinatal and Neonatal Nursing, 15*(2), 65-82.

Hurst, N.M., & Meier, P.P. (2005). Breastfeeding the preterm infant. In J. Riordan. *Breastfeeding and human lactation* (3rd ed., pp. 367-408.). Sudbury, MA: Jones and Bartlett.

Kenner, C. (2004). Families in crisis. In M.T. Verklan & M. Walden (Eds.), *Core curriculum for neonatal intensive care nursing* (3rd ed., pp. 392-410). Philadelphia: Saunders.

Kenner, C., Bagwell, G.A., & Torok, L.S. (2003). Transition to home. In C. Kenner & J.W. Lott (Eds.), *Comprehensive neonatal nursing: A physiologic perspective* (3rd ed., pp. 893-901). Philadelphia: Saunders.

Klaus, M.H., & Kennell, J.H. (2002). Care of the mother, father, and infant. In A.A. Fanaroff & R.J. Martin (Eds.), *Neonatal-perinatal medicine: Diseases of the fetus and infant* (7th ed., pp. 563-577). St. Louis: Mosby.

Kledzik, T. (2005). Holding the very low birth weight infant: skin-to-skin techniques. *Neonatal Network, 24*(1), 7-14.

Kleinman, R.E. (Ed.). (2004). *Pediatric nutrition handbook* (5th ed.). Elk Grove Village, IL: American Academy of Pediatrics.

Kliegman, R.M., & Das, U.G. (2002). Intrauterine growth retardation. In A.A. Fanaroff & R.J. Martin (Eds.), *Neonatal-perinatal medicine: Diseases of the fetus and infant* (7th ed., pp. 228-262). St. Louis: Mosby.

LeBlanc, M.H. (2002). The physical environment. In A.A. Fanaroff & R.J. Martin. (Eds.), *Neonatal-perinatal medicine: Diseases of the fetus and infant* (7th ed., pp. 512-529). St. Louis: Mosby.

Lefrak, L., & Lund, C.H. (2001). Nursing practice in the neonatal intensive care unit. In M.H. Klaus & A.A. Fanaroff (Eds.), *Care of the high-risk neonate* (5th ed., pp. 223-242). Philadelphia: Saunders.

Lemons, P.K. (2001). Breast milk and the hospitalized infant: Guidelines for practice. *Neonatal Network, 20*(7), 47-52.

Levy, G.D., Woolston, D.J., & Browne, J.V. (2003). Mean noise amounts in level II vs level III neonatal intensive care units. *Neonatal Network, 22*(2), 33-38.

Loo, K.K., Espinosa, M., Tyler, R., & Howard, J.(2003). Using knowledge to cope with stress in the NICU: How parents integrate learning to read the physiologic and behavioral cues of the infant. *Neonatal Network, 20*(1), 31-37.

Ludington-Hoe, S.M., Anderson, G.C., Swinth, J., Thompson, C., & Hadeed, A.J. (2004). Randomized controlled trial of kangaroo care: Cardiorespiratory and thermal effects on healthy preterm infants. *Neonatal Network, 23*(3), 39-48.

Ludington-Hoe, S.M., Ferreira, C., Swinth, J., & Ceccardi, J.J. (2003). Safe criteria and procedure for kangaroo care with intubated preterm infants. *Journal of Obstetric, Gynecologic, and Neonatal Nursing, 32*(5), 579-588.

Lund, C.H., Kuller, J., Lane, A.T., Lott, J.W., Raines, D.A., & Thomas, K.K. (2001). Neonatal skin care: Evaluation of the AWHONN/NANN research-based practice project on knowledge and skin care practices. *Journal of Obstetric, Gynecologic, & Neonatal Nursing 30*(1), 30-39.

Lynam, L., & Verklan, M.T. (2004). Neurologic disorders. In M.T. Verklan & M. Walden (Eds.), *Core curriculum for neonatal intensive care nursing* (3rd ed., pp. 821-857). Philadelphia: Saunders.

Maguire, D.P. (2004). Care of the extremely low birth weight infant. In M.T. Verklan & M. Walden (Eds.), *Core curriculum for neonatal intensive care nursing* (3rd ed., pp. 472-484). Philadelphia: Saunders.

McCain, G.C. (2003). An evidence-based guideline for introducing oral feeding to healthy preterm infants. *Neonatal Network, 22*(5), 45-50.

McCain, G.C., & Gartside, P.S. (2002). Behavioral responses of preterm infants to a standard-care and semi-demand feeding protocol. *Newborn and Infant Nursing Reviews, 2*(3), 187-193.

McGrath, J.M. (2004a). Identification of the sick newborn. In S. Mattson & J.E. Smith (Eds.), *Core curriculum for maternal-newborn nursing* (3rd ed., pp. 497-533). Philadelphia: Saunders.

McGrath, J.M. (2004b). Feeding. In C. Kenner & J.M. McGrath (Eds.), *Developmental care of newborns and infants: A guide for health professionals* (pp. 321-342). St. Louis: Mosby.

Mellien, A.C. (2001). Incubators versus mothers' arms: Body temperature conservation in very-low-birth-weight premature infants. *Journal of Obstetric, Gynecologic, and Neonatal Nursing, 30*(2), 157-164.

Melnyk, B.M., Feinstein, N.F., & Fairbanks, E. (2002). Effectiveness of informational/behavioral interventions with parents of low birth weight (LBW) premature infants: An evidence base to guide clinical practice. *Pediatric Nursing, 28*(5), 511-516.

Merchant, J.R., Worwa, C., Porter, S., Coleman, J.M., & deRegnier, R.O. (2001). Respiratory instability of term and near-term healthy newborn infants in car safety seats. *Pediatrics, 108*(3), 647-652.

Monterosso, L., Kristjanson, L., & Cole, J. (2002). Neuromotor development and the physiologic effects of positioning in very low birth weight infants. *Journal of Obstetric, Gynecologic, and Neonatal Nursing, 31*(2), 138-146.

National Association of Neonatal Nurses. (2001). *Infant and family-centered developmental care guideline for practice.* Glenview, IL: Author.

Neu, M. (2004). Kangaroo care: Is it for everyone? *Neonatal Network, 23*(5), 47-54.

Noerr, B. (2004). Thermoregulation. In S. Mattson & J.E. Smith (Eds.), *Core curriculum for maternal-newborn nursing* (3rd ed., pp. 125-134). Philadelphia: Saunders.

Nystrom, K., & Axelsson, K. (2002). Mothers' experience of being separated from their newborns. *Journal of Obstetric, Gynecologic, and Neonatal Nursing, 31*(3), 275-282.

Olitsky, S.E., & Nelson, L.B. (2004). Disorders of the eye. In R.E. Behrman, R.M. Kliegman, & H.B. Jenson (Eds.), *Nelson textbook of pediatrics* (17th ed., pp. 2083-2126). Philadelphia: Saunders.

Paige, P.L., & Carney, P.R. (2002). Neurologic disorders. In G.B. Merenstein & S.L. Gardner (Eds.), *Handbook of neonatal intensive care* (5th ed., pp. 644-678). St. Louis: Mosby.

Papile, L. (2002). Intracranial hemorrhage. In A.A. Fanaroff & R.J. Martin (Eds.), *Neonatal-perinatal medicine: Diseases of the fetus and infant* (7th ed., pp. 879-887). St. Louis: Mosby.

Pohlman, S. (2004). Father's role in NICU care: Evidence-based practice. In C. Kenner & J.M. McGrath (Eds.), *Developmental care of newborns and infants: A guide for health professionals* (pp. 359-372). St. Louis: Mosby.

Premji, S.S. (2005). Enteral feeding for high-risk neonates: a digest for nurses into putative risks and benefits to ensure safe and confortable care. *Journal of Perinatal Neonatal Nursing, 119*(1), 59-71.

Prince, W.L., Horns, K.M., Latta, T.M., & Gerstmann, D.R. (2004). Treatment of neonatal pain without a gold standard: The case for caregiving interventions and sucrose administration. *Neonatal Network, 23*(4), 33-45.

Putman, M. (2004). Risks associated with gestational age and birth weight. In S. Mattson & J. E. Smith (Eds.), *Core curriculum for maternal-newborn nursing* (3rd ed., pp. 465-496). Philadelphia: Saunders.

Resnik, J.L., & Resnik, R. (2004). Post-term pregnancy. In R.K. Creasy & R. Resnik (Eds.), *Maternal-fetal medicine: Principles and practice* (5th ed., pp. 663-669). Philadelphia: Saunders.

Resnik, R., & Creasy, R.K. (2004). Intrauterine growth restriction. In R.K. Creasy & R. Resnik (Eds.), *Maternal-fetal medicine: Principles and practice* (5th ed., pp. 495-512). Philadelphia: Saunders.

Rodriguez, R.J., Martin, R.J., & Fanaroff, A.A. (2002). Respiratory distress syndrome and its management. In A.A. Fanaroff & R.J. Martin (Eds.), *Neonatal-perinatal medicine: Diseases of the fetus and infant* (7th ed., pp. 1001-1011). St. Louis: Mosby.

Schanler, R.J. (2005). Enteral nutrition for the high-risk neonate. In H.W. Taeusch, R.A. Ballard, & C.A. Gleason (Eds.), *Avery's diseases of the newborn* (8th ed., pp. 1043-1060). Philadelphia: Saunders.

Siegel, R., Gardner, S.L., & Merenstein, G.B. (2002). Families in crisis: Theoretic and practical considerations. In G.B. Merenstein & S.L. Gardner (Eds.), *Handbook of neonatal intensive care* (5th ed., pp. 725-753). St. Louis: Mosby.

Sifuentes, M. (2000). Well child care for preterm infants. In C.D. Berkowitz (Ed.), *Pediatrics: A primary care approach* (2nd ed, pp. 84-88). Philadelphia: Saunders.

Southgate, W.M., & Pittard, W.B. (2001). Classification and physical examination of the newborn infant. In Klaus, M.H., & Fanaroff, A.A. (Eds.), *Care of the high-risk neonate* (5th ed, pp. 100-129). Philadelphia: Saunders.

Spatz, D.L. (2004). Ten steps for promoting and protecting breastfeeding for vulnerable infants. *Journal of Perinatal Neonatal Nursing, 18*(4), 385-396.

Sredl, D. (2003). Myths and facts about pain in neonates. *Neonatal Network, 22*(6), 69-71.

Stoll, B.J. (2004). Infections of the neonatal infant. In R.E. Behrman, R.M. Kliegman, & A.M. Arvin (Eds.), *Nelson textbook of pediatrics* (17th ed., pp. 623-640). Philadelphia: Saunders.

Stoll, B.J., & Kliegman, R.M. (2004a). Respiratory tract disorders. In R.E. Behrman, R.M. Kliegman, & H.B. Jenson (Eds.), *Nelson textbook of pediatrics* (17th ed., pp. 573-588). Philadelphia: Saunders.

Stoll, B.J., & Kliegman, R.M. (2004b). The high-risk infant. In R.E. Behrman, R.M. Kliegman, & H.B. Jenson (Eds.), *Nelson textbook of pediatrics* (17th ed., pp. 547-559). Philadelphia: Saunders.

Swartz, M.K. (2005). Parenting preterm infants: A metasynthesis. *MCN: American Journal of Maternal/Child Nursing 30*(2), 115-120.

Townsend, S.F. (2005). The large-for-gestational-age and the small-for-gestational-age infant. In P.J. Thureen, J. Deacon, J.A. Hernandez, & D.M. Hall (Eds.), *Assessment and care of the well newborn*. St. Louis: Saunders.

Trahms, C.M. (2004). Nutrition for low-birth-weight infants. In L.K. Mahan & S. Escott-Stump (Eds.), *Krause's food, nutrition, and diet therapy* (11th ed., pp. 234-258). Philadelphia: Saunders.

Turnage-Carrier, C.S. (2004). Caregiving and the environment. In C. Kenner & J.M. McGrath (Eds.), *Developmental care of newborns and infants: A guide for health professionals* (pp. 271-297). St. Louis: Mosby.

Updegrove, K. (2004). Necrotizing enterocolitis: The evidence for use of human milk in prevention and treatment. *Journal of Human Lactation, 20*(3), 335-339.

Walden, M. (2001). *Pain assessment and management: Guideline for practice*. Glenview, IL: National Association of Neonatal Nurses.

Walden, M. (2004). Pain assessment and management. In M.T. Verklan & M. Walden (Eds.), *Core curriculum for neonatal intensive care nursing* (3rd ed., pp. 375-391). Philadelphia: Saunders.

Walden, M., & Franck, L.S. (2003). Identification, management, and prevention of newborn/infant pain. In C. Kenner & J.W. Lott (Eds.), *Comprehensive neonatal nursing: A physiologic perspective* (3rd ed., pp. 844-856). Philadelphia: Saunders.

Walden, M., & Jorgensen, K.M. (2004). Pain management. In C. Kenner & J.M. McGrath (Eds.), *Developmental care of newborns and infants: A guide for health professionals* (pp. 197-222). St. Louis: Mosby.

Watson, R. (2004). Gastrointestinal disorders. In M.T. Verklan & M. Walden (Eds.), *Core curriculum for neonatal intensive care nursing* (3rd ed., pp. 643-932). Philadelphia: Saunders.

Welty, S., Hansen, T.N., & Corbet, A. (2005). Respiratory distress in the premature infant. In H.W. Taeusch, R.A. Ballard, & C.A. Gleason (Eds.), *Avery's diseases of the newborn* (8th ed., pp. 687-703). Philadelphia: Saunders.

White-Traut, R.C., Berbaum, M.L., Lessen, B., McFarlin, B., & Cardenas, L. (2005). Feeding readiness in preterm infants. *MCN: American Journal of Maternal/Child Nursing, 30*(1), 52-59.

Wyckoff, M.M., McGrath, J.M., Griffin, T., Malan, J., & White-Traut, R. (2003). Nutrition: Physiologic basis of metabolism and management of enteral and parenteral nutrition. In C. Kenner & J.W. Lott (Eds.), *Comprehensive neonatal nursing: A physiologic perspective* (3rd ed., pp. 425-447). Philadelphia: Saunders.

Zukowsky, L. (2004). Respiratory distress. In M.T. Verklan & M. Walden (Eds.), *Core curriculum for neonatal intensive care nursing* (3rd ed., pp. 487-523). Philadelphia: Saunders.

High-Risk Newborn: Acquired and Congenital Conditions

OBJECTIVES

After studying this chapter, you should be able to:

1. Describe the steps involved in neonatal resuscitation.
2. Explain common respiratory problems in the newborn.
3. Explain the causes and significance of pathologic jaundice.
4. Describe the nursing care of the infant with pathologic jaundice.
5. Describe causes of neonatal infections and nursing care for infants with infections.
6. Explain the effect of maternal diabetes on the newborn and the implications for nursing care.
7. Describe the effect of maternal substance abuse on the newborn and the nursing care needed.
8. Describe common congenital anomalies.

Go to your Student CD-ROM for Review Questions keyed to these Objectives.

DEFINITIONS

Asphyxia Insufficient oxygen and excess carbon dioxide in the blood and tissues.

Bilirubin Encephalopathy Acute neurologic condition resulting from deposits of unconjugated bilirubin in the brain tissue (kernicterus).

Bilirubin-Induced Neurologic Dysfunction Permanent brain damage resulting from kernicterus.

Erythroblastosis Fetalis Agglutination and hemolysis of fetal erythrocytes caused by incompatibility between the maternal and fetal blood types, such as when the fetus is Rh-positive and the mother is Rh-negative.

Esophageal Atresia Condition in which the esophagus is separated from the stomach and ends in a blind pouch.

Gastroschisis Protrusion of the intestines through a defect in the abdominal wall. The intestines are not covered by a peritoneal sac or skin.

Hydrops Fetalis Heart failure and generalized edema in the fetus secondary to severe anemia resulting from destruction of erythrocytes.

Kernicterus Staining of brain tissue caused by accumulation of unconjugated bilirubin in the brain.

Meconium Aspiration Syndrome Obstruction and air trapping caused by meconium in the infant's lungs, which may lead to severe respiratory distress.

Meningocele Protrusion of the meninges through a defect in the vertebrae; a form of neural tube defect.

Myelomeningocele Protrusion of the meninges and spinal cord through a defect in the vertebrae; a form of neural tube defect.

Neonatal Abstinence Syndrome A cluster of physical signs exhibited by the newborn who was exposed in utero to maternal use of substances such as heroin.

Omphalocele Protrusion of the intestines into the base of the umbilical cord. The intestines are covered by a peritoneal sac.

Persistent Pulmonary Hypertension Vasoconstriction of the infant's pulmonary vessels after birth; may result in right-to-left shunting of blood flow through the ductus arteriosus, the foramen ovale, or both.

Spina Bifida Defective closure of the bony spine that encloses the spinal cord; a type of neural tube defect.

Tracheoesophageal Fistula Abnormal connection between the esophagus and trachea.

Transient Tachypnea of the Newborn Condition of rapid respirations caused by inadequate absorption of fetal lung fluid.

In addition to the high-risk conditions related to gestational age discussed in Chapter 29, the newborn at risk may have acquired or congenital complications. Acquired conditions may be associated with prenatal complications or may occur at birth or shortly thereafter.

RESPIRATORY COMPLICATIONS

Respiratory distress is one of the most common problems of the neonate. It may be caused by asphyxia before or during birth, disease of the respiratory system, and other conditions that affect the infant's ability to breathe. The nurse is responsible for identification and evaluation of respiratory status at birth and throughout the hospital stay.

Asphyxia

Asphyxia is a lack of oxygen and increase of carbon dioxide in the blood. It may occur in utero, at birth, or later and results in ischemia to major organs. The causes of asphyxia may involve maternal, placental, or fetal factors. Maternal factors include complications such as hypertension, infection, and drug use. Asphyxia in utero may be caused by placental conditions such as placenta previa, abruptio placentae, or postmaturity. Cord problems, infection, premature birth, and multifetal gestation are among the fetal causes of asphyxia.

Lack of oxygen to the cells leads to anaerobic metabolism and the production of lactic acid. Metabolic acidosis develops when available bicarbonate is no longer able to buffer the accumulating acids. Respiratory acidosis occurs as carbon dioxide accumulates. A high partial pressure of carbon dioxide occurs in arterial blood ($PaCO_2$), and the partial pressure of oxygen (PO_2), pH, and bicarbonate are low.

Vasoconstriction caused by low oxygen decreases blood flow to all organs except the brain, myocardium, and adrenal glands. The ductus arteriosus and foramen ovale may remain open because of the low oxygen in the blood, high resistance to blood flow through constricted pulmonary vessels, and elevated pressure on the right side of the heart. Therefore, even circulating blood remains low in oxygen. Progress toward brain damage and death is rapid unless intervention is prompt.

Problems may continue if the infant survives. Pulmonary ischemia interferes with the ability to produce surfactant, increasing the risk of respiratory distress syndrome (RDS). Intrauterine stress may lead to passage of meconium and meconium aspiration syndrome (MAS).

MANIFESTATIONS

When asphyxia begins after birth, rapid respirations are followed by cessation of respirations (primary apnea) and a rapid fall in heart rate. Stimulation, alone or with oxygen, may restart respirations. If asphyxia continues without intervention, gasping respirations may resume weakly until the infant enters a period of secondary apnea. In secondary apnea, the oxygen levels in the blood continue to decrease,

the infant loses consciousness, and stimulation is ineffective. Resuscitative measures must be initiated immediately to prevent permanent damage to the brain or death. Asphyxia seen at birth may be a continuation of asphyxia that began before or during birth. Therefore it is essential to begin resuscitation without delay.

INFANTS AT RISK

Whenever complications occur during pregnancy, labor, or birth, the infant may be at risk for asphyxia. In addition, if the expectant mother receives narcotics for analgesia shortly before birth, the infant may be too depressed at birth to breathe spontaneously. Naloxone (Narcan) may be given to these infants (see drug guide).

NEONATAL RESUSCITATION

Although 90% of newborns have no difficulty with breathing at birth, approximately 10% require some help to begin respirations and 1% require extensive resuscitative measures (Kattwinkel, 2000). Therefore all personnel involved in deliveries should know how to perform resuscitative measures. Courses in neonatal resuscitation are usually required of all staff members working with newborns, and many agencies expect these skills to be updated annually. (See Procedure 30-1.)

The recommendations for neonatal resuscitation are reviewed periodically, and changes are made so that the practice is evidence based. The next revisions should be published in spring 2006. Possible changes include using less than 100% oxygen in some situations and changes in inflation pressures and times and medication dosages (Zaichkin & Simon, 2004).

Nurses must be prepared for situations in which asphyxia may develop. Equipment should be readily available and functioning properly at all times so that there is no delay in starting resuscitation. Nurses begin resuscitation measures as necessary and assist the physician with intubation, insertion of umbilical vein catheters, and administration of medications. Some nurses and neonatal nurse practitioners are taught to intubate infants in emergency situations.

Once the infant is stabilized, the nurse continues to assess for changes. Infants with asphyxia often have other complications. Communication with the parents is a vital nursing function. They will be confused and frightened and will need explanation and realistic reassurance. Parents often need continued support after the crisis to talk about their fears and concerns.

Transient Tachypnea of the Newborn (Retained Lung Fluid)

Infants who experience transient tachypnea of the newborn (TTN) develop rapid respirations soon after birth. The condition, which resolves within a few days, is also called *retained lung fluid and respiratory distress syndrome, type II*. Risk factors include cesarean birth without labor, asphyxia,

DRUG GUIDE

NALOXONE HYDROCHLORIDE (NARCAN)

Classification: Opioid antagonist.

Action: Reverses central nervous system and respiratory depression caused by narcotics (opiates). Competes with narcotics at receptor sites.

Indications: Severe respiratory depression when the mother has received narcotics within 4 hours of delivery.

Dosage and Route: Available in 0.4 mg/ml and 1 mg/ml. Dose is 0.1 mg/kg. Given intravenously, intramuscularly, subcutaneously, or into an endotracheal tube. Intravenous and endotracheal routes are preferred during resuscitation.

Absorption: Well absorbed by all routes. Onset of action is 1 to 2 minutes if given intravenously.

Excretion: Metabolized by the liver and excreted by the kidneys.

Contraindications and Precautions: Duration of effect is 45 to 60 minutes. The dose may need to be repeated because the opiate may have a longer half-life than naloxone. If given to an infant of a mother addicted to opiates, it will cause withdrawal and may cause seizures. Resuscitative measures should be used as necessary.

Nursing Considerations: Note the strength of the medication available when calculating the dose. Prepare the syringe before birth by drawing up more than is needed. After birth, the excess is removed from the syringe and the amount given is determined according to the estimate of the infant's weight. Inject rapidly. Monitor for response, and be prepared to give repeated doses if necessary.

Common Dosages of Naloxone Hydrochloride (Narcan): Dosage must be calculated based on weight (0.1 mg/kg). The amount for various weights is given below for *two different drug concentrations.*

Infant's Weight	Total Dose	Drug Concentration 0.4 mg/ml	Drug Concentration 1 mg/ml
1 kg (2 lb, 3 oz)	0.1 mg	0.25 ml	0.1 ml
2 kg (4 lb, 7 oz)	0.2 mg	0.50 ml	0.2 ml
3 kg (6 lb, 10 oz)	0.3 mg	0.75 ml	0.3 ml
4 kg (8 lb, 13 oz)	0.4 mg	1 ml	0.4 ml

precipitous or breech delivery, macrosomia, and maternal analgesia, bleeding, or diabetes. Mild immaturity of surfactant production also may be a factor. Infants are usually full term or near term, although some may be preterm.

CAUSE

Although the exact cause of TTN is unknown, it is thought to result from excess fluid in the lungs or a delay in absorption of fetal lung fluid by the pulmonary capillaries and lymph vessels, or both. Aspiration of amniotic fluid during gasping in utero may also be involved. This leads to decreased lung compliance and air trapping and brings about signs similar to RDS. Lack of chest compression in cesarean births has little effect because much of the removal of fetal lung fluid takes place before and during labor (Blackburn, 2002).

MANIFESTATIONS

In TTN, respirations as high as 120 per minute develop within hours of birth. Grunting, retractions, nasal flaring, and mild cyanosis also are present. Chest radiography shows hyperinflation, streaking radiating from the hilum of the lungs showing interstitial fluid along the bronchovascular spaces, and presence of fluid in the fissures between the lobes and in the pleural space. There may be mild cardiac enlargement. The condition is self-limiting and usually lasts from 1 to 5 days.

THERAPEUTIC MANAGEMENT

Treatment is supportive and may include oxygen if cyanosis is present. Gavage feeding may be necessary while the respiratory rate is high to prevent aspiration and conserve energy. Because the signs are similar to RDS and sepsis, the infant is observed for those complications. Antibiotics may be given until sepsis is ruled out.

NURSING CONSIDERATIONS

The nurse may be the first person to see signs of TTN, especially if they are not apparent at birth. After identifying signs, the nurse notifies the appropriate provider and carries out treatment. General nursing care is similar to that of the respiratory care of the preterm infant (see Chapter 29).

✔ CHECK YOUR READING

1. Why shouldn't an Apgar score be given before resuscitation is begun?
2. What is the role of the nurse in care of the infant with asphyxia?
3. How is TTN different from RDS?

Meconium Aspiration Syndrome

Meconium staining of amniotic fluid occurs in 10% to 15% of births, and 5% of those infants develop meconium aspiration syndrome (MAS) (Stoll & Kliegman, 2004c). The condition occurs most often in postterm infants who have decreased amniotic fluid and are prone to cord compression. It also occurs in term infants who have suffered intrauterine asphyxia. Infants may be small for gestational age (SGA). Meconium passage is rare before 36 weeks' gestation. MAS results in obstruction of the airways, pneumonitis, and air trapping. It may lead to persistent pulmonary hypertension of the newborn (PPHN) (Figure 30-1).

30-1 Performing Resuscitation in the Newly Born

PURPOSE: **To ensure adequate oxygenation of the neonate with asphyxia**

Note: Although this procedure is described in steps, several steps may be performed at the same time. Resuscitation is performed as an integrated process rather than in individual steps. Because two people often are working together, more than one step can be performed at one time.

1. Place the infant under a preheated radiant warmer immediately. *Prevention of cold stress is important to prevent increased oxygen need.*

2. Position the infant with the neck in a neutral or slightly extended ("sniffing") position. Avoid hyperextension or flexion of the neck. Place a small, folded blanket under the shoulders. *Proper positioning will help maintain an open airway. Hyperextension or flexion may obstruct the airway.*

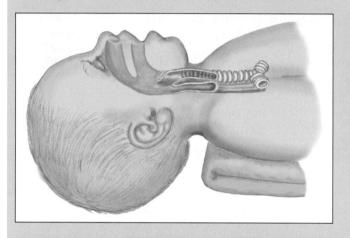

3. Suction the mouth and then the nose. Endotracheal intubation may be necessary to clear the airway if meconium is present. *Suctioning removes mucus from the airways. Infants often gasp when the nose is suctioned and may aspirate secretions from the mouth into the lungs. An endotracheal tube may be inserted at this time or later, if necessary, to provide an open airway.*

4. Dry and stimulate the infant if necessary. (Drying is often performed simultaneously with the previous steps.) Gently rub the infant's back or body, or flick or slap the soles of the feet. If two people are present, one can dry the infant while the other positions and suctions (unless meconium is present and stimulation should be avoided until after suctioning). If the baby does not respond adequately, additional stimulation may be needed. *Drying helps prevent cold stress and increased oxygen need. The tactile stimulation of drying the infant and suctioning the mouth and nose may cause spontaneous respirations. Stimulation should be gentle to avoid injury.*

5. If no response occurs after stimulating once or twice, stop and initiate immediate resuscitation. Do not delay resuscitation to continue stimulating or until the Apgar scores are determined. *Resuscitation becomes more difficult the longer it is delayed. Apgar scores at 1, 5, and 10 minutes can be determined during the resuscitation process without interrupting it.*

6. Remove wet linens and reposition the head as necessary. *Removal of wet linens prevents heat loss. Repositioning may be necessary because the infant has been moved.*

7. Give 100% oxygen if the infant is breathing but cyanotic. Hold the oxygen mask or tubing close to the infant's nose (called "blow-by" oxygen). *Oxygen will help relieve cyanosis and prevent damage to vital tissues. Holding the source close to the nose helps provide 100% oxygen rather than diluting it by combining it with room air.*

8. Evaluate the respirations, heart rate, and color. Use a stethoscope or feel the pulsations at the base of the cord. Count for 6 seconds and multiply by 10 to obtain the heart rate per minute. Positioning, clearing the airway, drying, stimulating, and providing oxygen should take no more than 30 seconds. *Evaluation determines whether further resuscitation is necessary. Immediate resuscitation is necessary to prevent hypoxic brain damage.*

9. Begin positive-pressure ventilation with an appropriately sized bag and mask if the infant fails to breathe spontaneously with initial stimulation, if the infant has gasping respirations, or if the heart rate is 100 beats per minute or less when respirations have begun. The mask should fit well, covering the chin, mouth, and nose but not the eyes. *Positive-pressure ventilation ensures oxygen entry into the lungs. An appropriately sized mask allows a seal to prevent oxygen from escaping around the sides.*

10. Attach the bag to an oxygen source with 100% oxygen. Place the mask snugly over the infant's nose and mouth. Squeeze the bag gently to force air into the infant's lungs. Use a bag with a manometer to show the amount of pressure being used and a flow-control valve that can be adjusted to control the pressure delivered to the infant, or use a bag with a pressure release valve that releases if the pressure is high enough to cause lung damage. The initial breaths require pressures of 30 to 40 cm H_2O to inflate the lungs. Less pressure is used for subsequent breaths but varies with the infant's condition. *Great care must be taken to use a pressure that is high enough to inflate the lungs without causing damage from overinflation. More pressure is needed for the first breaths and diseased lungs.*

11. If bag-and-mask ventilation is necessary for more than a few minutes, insert a feeding tube through the mouth

30-1 Performing Resuscitation in the Newly Born—cont'd

to the stomach and leave it open to the air. *The orogastric tube allows air that may enter the stomach to escape through the tube.*

12. Observe the rise and fall of the chest during ventilation. If the chest does not move, suction secretions and reposition the head and the mask. Ventilate the infant at a rate of 40 to 60 breaths per minute until the infant is breathing spontaneously and the heart rate is above 100 beats per minute. *The airway must not be occluded by positioning or secretions.*

13. If the heart rate is less than 60 beats per minute after 30 seconds of effective assisted ventilation, a second person should begin chest compressions while the first continues to ventilate the infant. *Adequate ventilation causes improvement of bradycardia in most infants. Evaluation of the infant's status determines whether ventilation can be discontinued or chest compressions must be added for the infant to survive.*

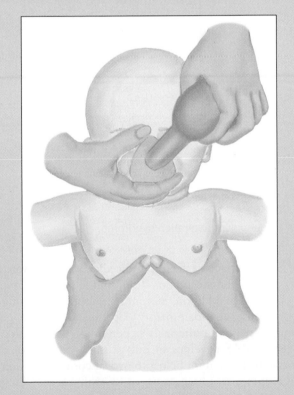

14. Compress the chest by placing the hands around the infant's chest with the fingers under the back to provide support and the thumbs over the lower third of the sternum (just below an imaginary line between the nipples and above the xiphoid process). An alternate method is to use two fingers of one hand to compress the chest, with the other hand under the back to provide support. *Correct hand position compresses the heart but avoids or minimizes injury to the liver or spleen, fractures of the ribs, and pneumothorax. The alternative method may be necessary to allow access to umbilical vessels or for people with small hands.*

15. Compress the sternum to a depth of approximately one third of the anterior-posterior diameter of the chest and sufficient to cause a palpable pulse. Do not remove the fingers from the chest between compressions. *The size of the infant determines the depth of compressions to avoid injury. The fingers should remain in contact with the chest at all times to prevent the need to repeatedly reposition them.*

16. Use three compressions followed by one ventilation for a combined rate of compressions and ventilations of 120 each minute. This is 90 compressions and 30 ventilations each minute. Pause for $\frac{1}{2}$ second after every third compression for ventilation. *Simultaneous compression and ventilation may interfere with adequate ventilation. The short pause allows air to enter the lungs.*

17. Check the heart rate after approximately 30 seconds. If it is 60 beats per minute or more, discontinue compressions but continue ventilation until the heart rate is above 100 beats per minute and spontaneous breathing begins. If the heart rate is less than 60 beats per minute after 30 seconds of effective assisted ventilation and compressions, epinephrine will be necessary. Endotracheal intubation may be performed at this point if not performed previously. *Periodic evaluation is necessary to ensure that treatment is appropriate to the infant's status. Endotracheal intubation may be used to ensure an adequate airway. Medications may be necessary to stimulate the heart.*

18. Prepare medications, if necessary. Epinephrine and naloxone may be given through an umbilical vein catheter or endotracheal tube. Intravenous volume expanders may include normal saline, Ringers lactate, or type O-negative red blood cells. Sodium bicarbonate is given intravenously only after prolonged arrest and with effective ventilation. *Epinephrine stimulates the heart. Naloxone counteracts the effects of opioids given to the mother in labor. Volume expanders may be used for fluid or blood loss. Sodium bicarbonate corrects acidosis after prolonged asphyxia that does not respond to other treatment.*

Data from Kattwinkel, J. (Ed.). (2000). *Textbook of neonatal resuscitation* (4th ed.) Elk Grove, IL: American Academy of Pediatrics and American Heart Association.

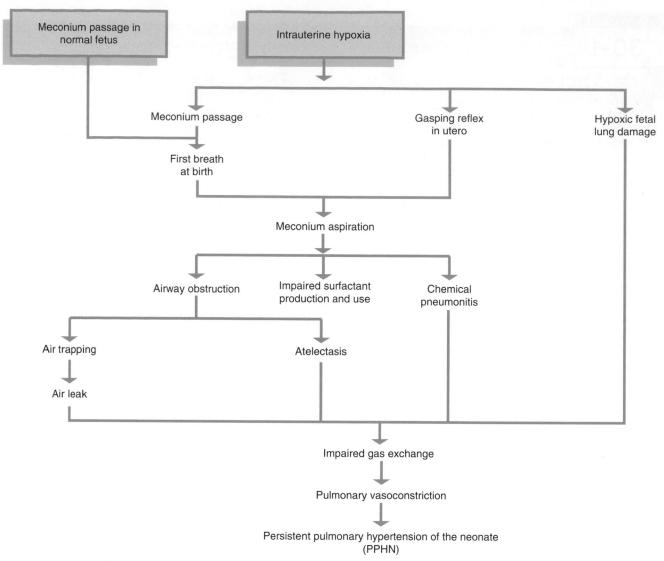

Figure 30-1 ■ Flow chart showing the effects of meconium aspiration syndrome.

CAUSES

Although the normal fetus may pass meconium, MAS is most often seen when hypoxia causes increased peristalsis of the intestine and relaxation of the anal sphincter before or during labor. MAS develops when meconium in the amniotic fluid enters the lungs during fetal life or at birth. It may be drawn into the lungs if gasping movements occur in utero as a result of asphyxia and acidosis, or the meconium in the upper airways may be pulled deep into the respiratory passages when the infant takes the first breaths after birth.

Obstruction of the airways may be complete or partial. Atelectasis may result if small airways are completely obstructed. In partial obstruction, air can enter but not escape from the alveoli. During inhalation, the bronchioles expand slightly as air flows into them past the meconium. During exhalation, the passages constrict and meconium blocks the passage of air out of the lungs.

This ball-valve mechanism results in air trapping. The overdistended alveoli may develop an air leak, with escape of air into the pleural cavity (pneumothorax) or mediastinum (pneumomediastinum). Surfactant production may be im-

paired, and surfactant that is produced may be inactivated by fatty acids in the meconium. The result is increased respiratory distress. In addition, meconium is irritating to lung tissue and causes an inflammatory reaction and chemical pneumonitis. Persistent pulmonary hypertension may result.

Severe MAS develops in only a small number of newborns with meconium below the vocal cords. The addition of meconium to a lung damaged by asphyxia may increase the severity of the condition. Damage from asphyxia interferes with clearing of lung fluid and surfactant production and causes pulmonary vasoconstriction that can result in return to fetal circulation.

MANIFESTATIONS

If meconium in the amniotic fluid is light, respiratory problems usually do not develop. However, thick meconium may cause serious respiratory pathology. Signs of mild to severe respiratory distress are present at birth, with tachypnea, cyanosis, retractions, nasal flaring, grunting, rales, rhonchi, and in severe cases, a barrel-shaped chest from hyperinflation. Radiography shows patchy areas of atelectasis and hyperexpansion from air trapping. The infant's nails, skin, and umbilical cord may be stained a yellow-green color.

THERAPEUTIC MANAGEMENT

When thick meconium is noted in the amniotic fluid during labor, an amnioinfusion may be performed. This involves infusing normal saline into the uterus to prevent cord compression and to dilute thick meconium in the amniotic fluid.

At birth the airway must be cleared, especially if meconium is thick. The infant's mouth and pharynx are suctioned using wall suction as soon as the head is delivered and before delivery of the rest of the body. This helps prevent drawing the meconium from the upper air passages deep into the lungs during the infant's first breath.

In depressed infants an endotracheal tube is inserted for suctioning immediately after birth. If the infant is vigorous with a heart rate over 100, spontaneous respirations, and good muscle tone, intubation is not necessary (Miller, Fanaroff, & Martin, 2002).

Infants may need only warmed, humidified oxygen, or extensive respiratory support with a ventilator may be required. High-frequency ventilation or nitric oxide therapy may be used. Ongoing management consists of supportive care to meet the problems presented.

Infants with severe MAS who do not respond to conventional treatment may benefit from extracorporeal membrane oxygenation (ECMO). ECMO, which is available in some hospitals, oxygenates the blood while bypassing the lungs, much like heart-lung machines used during heart surgery. It allows the infant's lungs to rest temporarily and recover.

NURSING CONSIDERATIONS

When meconium is noted in the amniotic fluid during labor, the nurse notifies the primary caregiver of the amount of meconium present so that delivery care can be adapted as necessary. The nurse ensures that equipment such as oxygen and suction is functioning properly and assists with care at delivery. After the infant's birth, nursing care is adapted to the problems presented. Although meconium is sterile, lung damage promotes the growth of bacteria. Infants should be closely observed for infection, which may further complicate the condition.

Persistent Pulmonary Hypertension of the Newborn

Persistent pulmonary hypertension (PPHN) is a condition in which the vascular resistance of the lungs does not decrease after birth and normal changes to neonatal circulation are impaired. For this reason, the condition also is called *persistent fetal circulation.*

CAUSES

The cause of PPHN may be abnormal lung development, hypoxia, or maternal use of nonsteroidal antiinflammatory agents or aspirin, or it may develop for unknown reasons. Pulmonary blood vessels may be underdeveloped, or hypertrophy of the smooth muscles may be present. This narrows the lumen of the vessels, increasing resistance (Ballard, Hansen, &

Corbet, 2005). The condition is often associated with hypoxemia and acidosis from conditions such as asphyxia, meconium aspiration, RDS, sepsis (such as with group B streptococcus), polycythemia, and diaphragmatic hernia.

Inadequate oxygenation results in vasoconstriction, instead of the normal dilation, of the pulmonary artery and small pulmonary vessels and produces increased resistance in the lungs. It also causes relaxation, instead of constriction, of the ductus arteriosus. The elevated pulmonary vascular resistance causes a rise in pressure on the right side of the heart. This results in a right-to-left shunting of unoxygenated blood that flows through the patent foramen ovale and ductus arteriosus and bypasses the lungs, as occurs during fetal circulation. Metabolic acidosis causes more pulmonary vasoconstriction, making the condition even worse.

MANIFESTATIONS

Infants with PPHN are usually near term, term, or postterm and develop signs within the first 12 hours after birth. Tachypnea, respiratory distress, and progressive cyanosis often become worse with handling. Oxygen saturation and partial pressure of oxygen in arterial blood (PaO_2) are decreased and acidosis is present. Partial pressure of carbon dioxide (PCO_2) may be normal or elevated. Other signs may result from associated conditions.

THERAPEUTIC MANAGEMENT

Management involves treating the underlying cause of poor oxygenation and relieving pulmonary vasoconstriction. Arterial pH may be increased with respiratory and drug therapy to cause pulmonary vasodilation. Sedation, high-frequency ventilation, and surfactant therapy may be necessary. Inhaled nitric oxide may be given to dilate pulmonary vessels. ECMO therapy may be used if conventional therapies are unsuccessful.

NURSING CONSIDERATIONS

Nursing care is similar to care of other infants with severe respiratory disease. Because infants become hypoxic with activity and other stimuli, handling and noise are kept to a minimum. Cold stress increases the metabolic rate and need for oxygen and causes additional pulmonary vasoconstriction. Therefore the nurse should pay particular attention to maintaining the infant's temperature in the normal range.

✔ CHECK YOUR READING

4. Which infants are most likely to have meconium staining of the amniotic fluid?
5. Why is there resistance of blood flow into the lungs in PPHN?

HYPERBILIRUBINEMIA (PATHOLOGIC JAUNDICE)

Jaundice is a common concern in caring for neonates. Conjugation of bilirubin and physiologic jaundice are discussed in Chapter 19, pp. 460-462, and Chapter 20, p. 489. This discussion focuses on pathologic jaundice.

When the total serum bilirubin (TSB) reaches 5 mg/dl, jaundice is visible in the face. TSB includes both direct (conjugated) and indirect (unconjugated) bilirubin. Jaundice moves down the body as the bilirubin level rises (Stoll & Kliegman, 2004a). Jaundice is considered pathologic when it appears in the first 24 hours after birth; TSB rises by more than 0.2 mg/dl/hr or 5 mg/dl/day or is above the 95th percentile for the infant's age in hours; direct bilirubin is above 1.5 to 2 mg/dl; or jaundice continues beyond 2 weeks in a full-term infant (Madan, MacMahon, & Stevenson, 2005). Some authors also include a TSB concentration higher than 12 mg/dl in a full-term infant or 10 to 14 mg/dl in a preterm infant (Stoll & Kliegman, 2004a).

Pathologic jaundice is a concern because it may lead to kernicterus. In this condition, bilirubin deposits cause yellowish staining of the brain, especially the basal ganglia, cerebellum, and hippocampus. The condition may result in acute bilirubin encephalopathy, which may be reversible in the early stages. However, it may progress to bilirubin-induced neurologic dysfunction and cause permanent damage to the brain.

Although kernicterus is rare today because of improved treatment measures, the mortality rate among affected infants is approximately 50% (Madan, MacMahon, & Stevenson, 2005). Those who survive may suffer from cerebral palsy, mental retardation, hearing loss, or more subtle long-term neurologic and developmental problems. The exact level at which bilirubin encephalopathy develops is not known. Causes and other factors must be considered in each case.

Causes

The most common cause of pathologic jaundice is hemolytic disease of the newborn caused by incompatibility between the blood of the mother and that of the fetus. The best known cause is Rh incompatibility, in which the Rh-negative mother forms antibodies when blood from an Rh-positive fetus enters her circulation (see Chapter 25). Antibodies may have developed during a previous pregnancy or after injury, abortion, amniocentesis, or a transfusion of Rh-positive blood. The antibodies cross the placenta, attach to fetal red blood cells, and destroy them. Excessive hemolysis causes erythroblastosis fetalis.

Infants with erythroblastosis fetalis are anemic from destruction of red blood cells. However, jaundice usually does not develop until soon after birth because bilirubin crosses the placenta and is excreted by the mother. Severely affected infants may develop hydrops fetalis, a severe anemia that results in heart failure and generalized edema. Use of $Rh_o(D)$ immune globulin (RhIG) such as RhoGAM to prevent the mother from forming antibodies against Rh-positive blood has greatly decreased the incidence of erythroblastosis fetalis.

ABO incompatibility also causes pathologic jaundice. Mothers with type O blood have natural antibodies to type A or B blood. The antibodies cross the placenta and cause hemolysis of fetal red blood cells. However, the destruction is much less severe than with Rh incompatibility and causes

milder signs. This is because many of the antibodies are immunoglobulin M, which does not cross the placenta. In addition, fetal red blood cells have fewer sites where the antibodies can bind than adult erythrocytes have (Cunningham et al., 2001).

Other causes of pathologic jaundice include infection, hypothyroidism, glucuronyl transferase deficiency, polycythemia, glucose-6-phosphate dehydrogenase deficiency, and biliary atresia. Infants of diabetic mothers are more likely to develop pathologic jaundice, especially if they have macrosomia. It is more likely to occur in infants who have suffered hypoxia or respiratory acidosis, which impairs the blood-brain barrier and allows unconjugated bilirubin to enter the brain. Any condition that causes destruction of erythrocytes or impairment of the liver may result in pathologic bilirubin levels.

Therapeutic Management

The focus of therapeutic management is prevention of kernicterus. The cause is determined by history and diagnostic tests to identify infections or blood abnormalities. During pregnancy an Rh-negative expectant mother will have blood drawn for an indirect Coombs test to identify the presence of antibodies against fetal blood. If the test is positive, amniocentesis may be performed to determine the fetal Rh factor and the degree of hyperbilirubinemia.

When an infant is jaundiced, the infant's blood type and a direct Coombs test are performed on the cord blood. A positive Coombs test indicates that antibodies from the mother have attached to the infant's red blood cells. Serum bilirubin levels are followed closely for changes that indicate that treatment should be initiated or changed. There are charts available to help determine the appropriate response to rising TSB according to the infant's age in hours. For example, phototherapy may be considered if the TSB exceeds the 95th percentile for the infant's age. This is approximately 8 mg/dl at 24 hours, 13 mg/dl at 48 hours, and 16 mg/dl at 72 hours (Thilo, 2005). The health care provider weighs the bilirubin level with other factors such as gestational age and presence of other risk factors to determine if therapy is appropriate for an individual infant.

Because visual inspection for jaundice may be inaccurate and drawing blood for TSB is painful and expensive, other noninvasive tests may be used. Reflectance photometers are hand-held devices that allow screening of transcutaneous bilirubin. When the sensor on the device is placed against the forehead or sternum, the amount of bilirubin in the tissues is measured. This provides an estimate of the TSB.

End-tidal carbon monoxide concentration is a test to measure the amount of carbon monoxide in the infant's breath. Carbon monoxide produced along with bilirubin when red blood cells break down is excreted by the lungs. Therefore, a high level of CO in expired air indicates a hemolytic process causing increased production of bilirubin and helps predict infants who are at risk for excessively high bilirubin levels. The test is noninvasive (Madan, MacMahon,

& Stevenson, 2005; Reiser, 2001; Stevenson, Vreman, Wong, & Contag, 2001).

PHOTOTHERAPY

Approximately 10% of newborns in the United States receive phototherapy (Frank, Cooper, & Merenstein, 2002). It is the most common treatment of jaundice and involves placing the infant under special fluorescent lights. During phototherapy, bilirubin in the skin absorbs the light and changes into water-soluble photoisomers, the most important of which is lumirubin. These products do not require conjugation by the liver and can be excreted in the bile and urine. Because bilirubin encephalopathy develops in preterm infants at lower bilirubin levels than in full-term infants, phototherapy is begun at lower levels for them.

Phototherapy can be delivered in several ways. A halogen spotlight may be used alone or with other lamps. More commonly a bank of fluorescent lamps or "bili" lights is placed over the infant. A newer overhead device that uses high intensity gallium nitrate light-emitting diodes (LEDs) to provide the light source for phototherapy is also available.

During phototherapy an incubator or radiant warmer is used to provide warmth because the infant wears only a diaper to ensure maximal exposure of the skin to the lights. Patches cover the infant's eyes to protect them from the constant light. The lights are placed above the incubator at a distance determined by the type of bulb used (usually 12 to 30 inches) (Figure 30-2). More than one bank of lights may be used if the TSB is high. Blood is drawn frequently to monitor the TSB and determine the effectiveness of treatment and when it can be discontinued.

A fiberoptic phototherapy blanket that is placed against the infant's skin is another option. The infant can be swaddled with the blanket and does not need patches over the eyes. Use of the blanket allows the parents to hold the infant, or the infant may be taken to the mother's room, causing less interference with bonding. It is also less frightening to the parents. However, because a smaller surface area is in contact with the blanket than the surface area affected by light, the blanket may not be as effective. The blanket may be used under an infant with phototherapy lights placed above to increase the effectiveness.

Side effects of phototherapy include frequent, loose, green stools that result from increased bile flow and peristalsis. This causes more rapid excretion of the bilirubin but may be damaging to the skin and result in fluid loss. Lactose-free formula may help decrease the diarrhea some infants experience.

An erythematous macular skin rash also may occur. African-American infants may experience a tanning effect from the light. Bronze baby syndrome, a transient grayish-brown discoloration of the skin and urine, may occur in infants with cholestatic jaundice (elevated direct serum bilirubin) with impairment of liver function. The color changes and rash disappear gradually when phototherapy is completed.

A rebound TSB increase of 1 to 2 mg/dl is normal after the infant has completed phototherapy (Watson, 2004). Therefore the TSB level should be monitored to ensure the level is not excessively high. Explain to parents that the infant may have an elevation in bilirubin after phototherapy ends and that the health care provider may order additional blood tests after discharge.

Home phototherapy is a way to avoid prolonged hospitalization, separation from parents, and interference with breastfeeding. Parents using phototherapy at home need extensive teaching on managing the equipment and caring for the infant. Home visits by nurses are important to help ensure that the infant is making adequate progress and that the parents understand how to provide care.

EXCHANGE TRANSFUSIONS

Exchange transfusions are seldom necessary but are performed when phototherapy cannot reduce dangerously high bilirubin levels quickly enough. This treatment removes maternal antibodies, unconjugated bilirubin, and antibody-coated (sensitized) red blood cells. It provides fresh albumen with binding sites for bilirubin and corrects severe anemia. When an immediate transfusion is needed for Rh incompatibility, type O, Rh-negative blood is used so that circulating antibodies will not destroy the erythrocytes. If time allows, Rh-negative blood of the infant's blood type should be used.

PROCEDURE. During the exchange transfusion, blood is removed from the infant and replaced with an equal amount of donor blood in small portions. Because the donor blood mixes with the infant's blood, approximately twice the infant's blood volume is usually administered. Normal blood volume is 85 to 100 ml/kg in a full-term infant and 110 ml/kg in a preterm infant (Sniderman

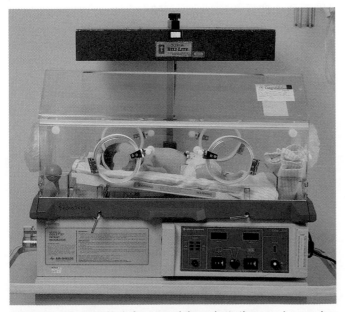

Figure 30-2 ■ An infant receiving phototherapy is wearing eye patches to protect the eyes.

PARENTS
WANT TO KNOW

Home Care for the Infant Receiving Phototherapy

Dress your baby in only a diaper to expose as much skin as possible to the phototherapy lights. You may have to keep the room temperature higher than usual to keep the baby warm. Change your baby's position about every 2 hours so that the light reaches all areas of the body.

Position the phototherapy or "bili" light at the proper distance from your baby according to the manufacturer's directions. Placing it too close to the infant could result in fever or burns. Placing it too far away will make the treatment ineffective.

Close the baby's eyes, and place patches over the eyes before placing the infant under the lights. Check frequently to see that the patches remain in place. They must cover the eyes but not press on the nose because they can interfere with breathing. The patches should not press against the eyes.

The infant may be removed from phototherapy for feedings, diaper changes, and other general care but should remain under the lights most of the time to decrease the jaundice as fast as possible. Hold and cuddle your infant during the time the baby is not under the lights. When the baby is under the lights, you can talk to her or him. The sound of your voice will be comforting.

If you are using a fiberoptic blanket, keep it next to the baby's skin at all times. Be sure the baby does not wiggle off the blanket. You may wrap the baby with receiving blankets over the "bili" blanket and hold the baby for feedings and other activities. It is not necessary to cover the infant's eyes if the blanket alone is used.

Check your baby's temperature under the arm before every feeding. The temperature should remain between 97.7° and 99.5° F. If it is abnormal, verify whether the heat in the room is too low or high or the "bili" light source is positioned incorrectly. Use warm blankets when you remove the baby from the warmth of phototherapy. Call your physician if the baby has a temperature of less than 97.7° F or above 100° F.

Feed your baby every 2 to 3 hours. It is important for the infant to eat well while receiving phototherapy, which causes the baby to lose fluid from the skin and have loose stools. This could cause dehydration. The infant needs protein, which helps eliminate the bilirubin that causes the jaundice. Do not give your baby water because it is less effective than milk in helping to reduce the jaundice.

Count your baby's wet diapers and stools. If there are less than 6 wet diapers a day or the urine appears dark, increase the feedings. Keep a journal of the baby's temperature, feedings (time and amount), wet and dirty diapers, color and consistency of stools, and amount of time spent out of phototherapy.

Keep all appointments for examinations or blood tests so that the baby's progress can be evaluated by your health care provider. Take your journal with you when you go to see your pediatrician. Also take a list of your questions so you can ask them during the examination.

Call the pediatrician, nurse practitioner, or home care nurse if you have questions about care, if the baby has a fever or appears sick to you, if the mouth seems dry, or if the urine is dark or less than normal.

& Taeusch, 2005). At the end of the transfusion, approximately 85% to 90% of the infant's red blood cells will have been replaced.

The bilirubin level after transfusion is about 50% of the preexchange level (Madan, MacMahon, & Stevenson, 2005). When the level in the blood decreases, bilirubin from the tissues moves into the plasma. This may increase the blood level to 60% or more of the original level (Frank, Cooper, & Merenstein, 2002). This rebound elevation of bilirubin may necessitate repeat transfusions, but phototherapy is generally adequate to resolve it.

COMPLICATIONS. Many complications may occur from exchange transfusion, including electrolyte imbalances, acidosis, infection, hypoglycemia, cardiac arrhythmias, necrotizing enterocolitis, bleeding, thrombosis, and embolism. Samples of blood are analyzed before and after the exchange with a complete blood count, bilirubin and calcium levels, and other tests as needed.

ROLE OF THE NURSE. The nurse's role during exchange transfusion is to prepare equipment, assess the infant during and after the procedure, and keep accurate records. A cardiac monitor is attached to the infant, and warmth is provided by a radiant heater. The nurse also must clarify any misunderstandings that the parents may have about the treatment and help allay their anxiety.

Application of the Nursing Process
Hyperbilirubinemia

Although collaborative care of the infant with jaundice is an important part of the nurse's role, several nursing diagnoses are appropriate. "Risk for Injury" is discussed in this section. The diagnoses "Risk for Imbalanced Fluid Volume" and "Impaired Skin Integrity" are discussed in Nursing Care Plan 30-1.

Assessment

Assess the level of jaundice at least every 8 hours by blanching the skin (pressing the skin over a bony prominence) to see the color in the area before the blood returns. Evaluate the skin color in good light with phototherapy lights turned off, because they distort the infant's color. Visual assessment of infants with dark skin is less accurate. Assess the color of the conjunctiva of the eyes, the palate, and the mucous membranes of the mouth for these infants. Determine the areas of the body affected by jaundice, and document carefully to use for comparison during future assessment. Jaundice begins at the head and moves down the body as the bilirubin level rises. Monitor laboratory TSB for change, especially because visualization of jaundice is a subjective assessment and the color in the skin may be affected by phototherapy.

NURSING CARE PLAN 30-1 The Infant with Jaundice

ASSESSMENT: Holly, a 3-day-old, full-term infant born by cesarean, is jaundiced secondary to ABO incompatibility and is receiving phototherapy. She weighs 3.2 kg (7 lb, 1 oz), and her mucous membranes appear slightly dry. Skin turgor is good with quick recoil, and the anterior fontanel is flat. Urine appears slightly dark in color. Holly had three loose green stools with no water ring on this shift. She is a sleepy infant who takes formula poorly. Valerie, her mother, appears tired and frustrated with the infant's slow eating behavior.

NURSING DIAGNOSIS: Risk for Imbalanced Fluid Volume related to inadequate oral intake to meet needs of increased insensible water loss and frequent loose stools.

GOALS/EXPECTED OUTCOMES: Within 24 hours Holly will:
1. Take at least 318 to 480 ml of fluid per day (100 to 150 ml/kg/day or 45 to 68 ml/lb/day) to meet normal needs
2. Show adequate hydration (moist mucous membranes, elastic skin turgor, flat fontanels, pale yellow urine, and at least six wet diapers a day)

INTERVENTION	RATIONALE
1. Instruct Valerie to feed Holly every 2 to 3 hours. Feed Holly in the nursery at night or when Valerie needs rest, if she prefers.	1. Adequate intake of formula is necessary to meet the infant's nutrient and fluid requirements and ensure excretion of bilirubin in the stools. The mother's need for rest must be met without interfering with the infant's needs.
2. Explain to Valerie that Holly needs frequent feedings to help her pass stools that contain the bilirubin causing her jaundice.	2. The mother's understanding of the reasons will increase her willingness to work with the infant.
3. Observe Valerie feeding Holly and offer suggestions as needed. Show her how to waken the infant by unwrapping and gentle stimulation. Try warming the formula slightly or inserting a finger to elicit the suck reflex before feedings.	3. Observation of feedings may identify problems and interventions that work for this situation. A wide-awake infant is more likely to feed well. Some infants prefer warm milk. Nonnutritive sucking may help the infant suck effectively during feedings.
4. Tell the parents about the need for frequent feeding to provide added fluid, protein, and other nutrients.	4. Infants receiving phototherapy have a greater than normal insensible water loss. Albumin (protein) is necessary to carry bilirubin to the liver for conjugation. Heightened intestinal motility decreases absorption of nutrients.
5. Avoid offering water or dextrose water. Use formula instead.	5. Water supplements may decrease the intake of formula and its necessary nutrients. Formula increases motility of intestines and expedites excretion of bilirubin in stools, but water does not have the same effect.
6. If water loss appears excessive, weigh all diapers and check the specific gravity of the urine. Urine output should be 1 to 3 ml/kg/hr, which for Holly is a total of 76.8 to 230.4 ml daily. Specific gravity should be 1.001 to 1.020 for full-term infants.	6. Weighing the diapers will identify inadequate output and dehydration early. The wet diaper weight in grams minus the weight of the dry diaper equals the milliliters of urine.
7. Use therapeutic communication techniques to help Valerie vent her frustrations. Offer praise for her attempts to feed Holly.	7. Helping the mother cope with her feelings helps her meet the infant's needs. Feeding difficulties often interfere with the mother's view of herself as a "good" mother. Praise increases her sense of adequacy.

EVALUATION: Holly drinks a total of 450 ml (15 oz) of formula during 24 hours. Valerie is able to wake Holly, who begins to suck more vigorously. Holly's mucous membranes are moist, and she has 10 diapers with pale yellow urine during the 24 hours.

ASSESSMENT: Holly's diaper area is slightly red and irritated from her frequent loose stools.

NURSING DIAGNOSIS: Impaired Skin Integrity related to frequent loose stools.

GOALS/EXPECTED OUTCOME: Holly's skin will return to normal within 2 days without further signs of irritation or breakdown.

INTERVENTION	RATIONALE
1. Check diapers every hour. Gently cleanse the diaper area with soap and water after each stool.	1. Extended exposure of the skin to stool and urine may cause skin breakdown. Thorough cleansing removes irritating substances from the skin.
2. Expose the entire diaper area to air for short periods when the phototherapy light is off. Place a diaper under Holly to catch urine and stools.	2. Exposure to air dries the area and aids healing.

NURSING CARE PLAN 30-1   The Infant with Jaundice—cont'd

3. Avoid lotions or wipes containing alcohol and powders. Apply ointments, if prescribed, and cover with the diaper.

3. Alcohol changes the pH of the skin and may irritate. Powder may promote bacterial and *Candida albicans* growth. If ointments are used, the area should be covered to prevent the risk of burns from the phototherapy lights.

4. Explain the reason for loose stools and methods of treatment of the skin irritation to Valerie.

4. The mother may need help to understand that the condition is not the result of poor care. She should learn how to care for diaper rash at home.

EVALUATION: Holly's diaper area returns to normal within 1.5 days.

Assess for risk factors that might further increase bilirubin levels. Note temperature fluctuations, hypoglycemia, and infection. Determine the infant's oral intake and number of stools.

Analysis

Nurses can do many things to prevent situations that might cause further rises in TSB. They also must protect the infant from injury from the light during phototherapy. Therefore an appropriate nursing diagnosis is "Risk for Injury related to preventable causes of further elevation of bilirubin or damage to the skin or eyes secondary to phototherapy."

Planning

The goal or expected outcome for this nursing diagnosis is that the infant will avoid injury resulting from increased bilirubin or exposure of the skin or eyes to phototherapy lights.

Interventions

Interventions are designed to prevent situations that might cause injury to the infant from rising bilirubin levels or effects of treatment.

MAINTAINING A NEUTRAL THERMAL ENVIRONMENT

Prevent situations, such as cold stress or hypoglycemia, that could result in increased fatty acids in the blood caused by acidosis, thereby decreasing the availability of albumin-binding sites for unconjugated bilirubin. Prevent cold stress at birth and during all care by maintaining the infant in a neutral thermal environment. Check the infant's axillary temperature every 2 to 4 hours to identify an early decrease before it becomes a problem. Dress the infant in warmed clothes and blankets on removal from phototherapy lights.

Prevent elevation of the infant's temperature from exposure to the heat of the "bili" lights. Use a skin probe when the infant is in an incubator or radiant warmer to maintain the appropriate environmental temperature, and monitor settings to be sure they are correct for the infant's needs. Position the lights according to the manufacturer's guidelines to prevent overheating or burning the skin.

PROVIDING OPTIMAL NUTRITION

Ensure that the infant receives feedings every 2 to 3 hours, whether by breast or bottle. Breastfeeding should not be stopped because the infant is receiving phototherapy. Frequent feedings prevent hypoglycemia, provide protein to maintain the albumin level in the blood, and promote gastrointestinal motility and prompt emptying of bilirubin from the bowel. Avoid offering water because the infant may take less milk, which is more effective in removing bilirubin from the intestines. If breastfeeding must be supplemented, use formula instead of water.

PROTECTING THE EYES

Provide patches to protect the eyes from possible retinal damage from the phototherapy lights. Close the infant's eyes before placing the patches to avoid abrasions to the cornea. Check the position of the patches at least every hour. Infants often wiggle enough to push the patches above or below the eyes, leaving them exposed. The edges of the patches can dig into the eyes or compress the nose and interfere with breathing. Observe for skin irritation around or under the patches at least every 4 hours. Explain to parents that it is normal for the yellow color under the patches to be deeper than in areas that have been exposed to the lights.

ENHANCING RESPONSE TO THERAPY

Position the lights the proper distance away from the infant. Lights that are too close may burn the skin. Lights too far away from the infant will not be effective in reducing jaundice. Halogen lights must be placed farther away from the infant than fluorescent lights to prevent burning. Follow the manufacturer's instructions about light placement. Although phototherapy increases insensible water loss from the skin, avoid the use of creams or lotions on the infant's skin as they might cause burning.

CRITICAL THINKING ✒ EXERCISE 30-1

Why is it important to remove the patches from the eyes each time the infant is taken from phototherapy for feeding or when parents visit?

Use a light meter to check the level of irradiance (energy output) to be sure the apparatus is functioning appropriately and to determine if the bulbs need to be replaced. Check laboratory reports of TSB to determine the effectiveness of treatment and when it can be discontinued.

Expose as much skin as possible to the light. Remove all of the infant's clothing except a diaper. Turn the infant frequently to expose all areas and prevent irritation of the skin from lack of position change. If a fiberoptic blanket is used, check the position of the blanket frequently. Infants sometimes need to be repositioned so that the blanket remains in contact with the skin.

DETECTING COMPLICATIONS

Observe for other complications. Although bilirubin encephalopathy is rare today, monitor for signs that indicate its presence. These include lethargy, increased muscle tone of extensor muscles, decreased or absent Moro reflex, poor feeding, high-pitched cry, irritability, opisthotonos, and seizures. Note the presence of rashes or changes in the color of the skin. Inform parents that they are not harmful and will disappear when phototherapy is discontinued.

TEACHING PARENTS

Explain care to parents, who may be frightened to see their infant in an incubator with the eyes covered. Explaining the causes of jaundice and the purpose of phototherapy will decrease their worry. In addition, they will be more willing to hold their baby for only short times during feeding so that the therapy is not unduly interrupted.

When the infant is discharged, give parents written and verbal information about assessing for jaundice and when to call the health care provider. Emphasize the need to keep follow-up visits so that any increases in jaundice or other problems can be identified and treated early.

Evaluation

No signs of injury should be present. The eyes will not have been exposed to the phototherapy lights, and the skin should not be harmed. Laboratory reports should show a steady decrease of serum bilirubin.

✔ CHECK YOUR READING

6. How can kernicterus be prevented?
7. How can the nurse help reduce bilirubin levels in infants receiving phototherapy?

INFECTION

The nurse must be constantly alert for signs of infection in newborns. As many as 10% of infants have infections in the first month of life. Bacterial infection of the newborn affects 1 to 4 in every 1000 live births (Stoll, 2004). Infection is a major cause of death during the neonatal period.

TRANSMISSION OF INFECTION

Newborns can acquire infections before, during, or after birth. Vertical infection is acquired before or during birth from the mother. Organisms such as those causing rubella, cytomegalovirus infection, syphilis, and toxoplasmosis may pass across the placenta and cause infection during pregnancy. During labor and birth, organisms in the vagina such as group B streptococci, herpesvirus, and hepatitis B virus may enter the uterus after rupture of membranes or infect the infant during passage through the birth canal.

Horizontal infection occurs after birth from contact with hospital staff members or contaminated equipment (nosocomial or hospital-acquired infections) or with family members. An example is staphylococcal infections. Some common infections and their effects on the neonate are listed in Table 30-1. Other infections are discussed in Chapter 26, p. 683.

SEPSIS NEONATORUM

Infection that occurs during or after birth may result in sepsis neonatorum, systemic infection from bacteria in the bloodstream. Newborns are particularly susceptible to sepsis because their immune system is immature and they react more slowly to invasion by organisms. Full-term and especially preterm infants have fewer antibodies and are unable to localize infection as well as older children. This inability allows the infection to spread easily from one organ to another. In addition, the blood-brain barrier is less effective in keeping out organisms, and central nervous system infection may result.

CAUSES

The most common causative agents of neonatal sepsis currently are group B streptococci and *Escherichia coli*. Other organisms that may be involved include coagulase-negative staphylococci (such as *Staphylococcus epidermidis*), *Staphylococcus aureus*, *Haemophilus influenzae*, and *Listeria monocytogenes*. Coagulase-negative staphylococci and *Candida albicans* are the most common causes of nosocomial infection in low-birth-weight infants in the hospital.

Sepsis may be divided into early onset and late onset according to when signs of disease begin. Early-onset sepsis is usually acquired before or during birth, often from complications of labor such as prolonged rupture of membranes or labor and chorioamnionitis. It generally begins within the first 5 days, with the majority of infants showing signs within 12 hours (Polin, Parravicini, Regan, & Taeusch, 2005). It progresses more rapidly than late onset-sepsis and has a mortality rate of 15% to 20%. Although multisystem involvement occurs, pneumonia is most common and may be fatal (Edwards, 2002). Meningitis may also occur.

Late-onset sepsis generally develops after the first week of life. It is acquired during or after birth, before or after hospital discharge. It usually is a more localized infection, such as meningitis, and serious long-term effects are common. The mortality rate is 5% (Edwards, 2002).

TABLE 30-1 Common Infections In the Newborn*

Transmission	Effect on Newborn	Nursing Considerations
Viral Infections		
Cytomegalovirus Transplacental, during birth, in breast milk.	Most infants asymptomatic at birth. LBW, IUGR, enlarged liver and spleen, jaundice, mental retardation, hearing loss, purpura, blindness, and seizures. May have no signs for months or years.	May shed virus in saliva and urine for months or years. No effective drug therapy.
Hepatitis B Usually during birth through contact with maternal blood. Also transplacental and in breast milk.	Asymptomatic at birth. LBW, prematurity. Most become chronic carriers. Risk of later liver cancer.	Wash well to remove all blood before skin is punctured for any reason. After cleaning, administer hepatitis B immune globulin and hepatitis B vaccine to prevent infection.
Herpes Usually during birth through infected vagina or ascending infection after rupture of membranes. Transplacental rarely. Transmission highest with primary infection.	Clusters of vesicles, temperature instability, lethargy; poor suck, seizures, encephalitis, jaundice, purpura. Death or severe neurologic impairment is high with disseminated infection.	Contact precautions. Obtain lesion specimens for culture. High mortality and morbidity rate if untreated. Antiviral drug therapy improves outcome.
Human Immunodeficiency Virus and Acquired Immunodeficiency Syndrome Transplacental, during birth from infected blood and secretions, or from breast milk. Transmission rate is greatly decreased if mother takes antiretroviral drugs during pregnancy and birth.	Asymptomatic at birth, signs usually apparent at 4 to 12 months. Enlarged liver and spleen, lymphadenopathy, failure to thrive, pneumonia, persistent *Candida* and bacterial infections.	Diagnosis may be delayed because of maternal antibodies. Some early tests available. Wash early and before skin is punctured to remove blood. Treat with antiretroviral drugs and prophylaxis against other infections. Advise against breastfeeding.
Rubella Transplacental	Asymptomatic or IUGR, cataracts, cardiac defects, deafness, mental retardation. Damage greatest if infected in first trimester.	Contact precautions. Infant may shed virus for months after birth. Diagnosed by presence of antibody. No treatment.
Varicella Zoster Virus (Chickenpox) Transplacental	Congenital varicella syndrome (skin scarring, IUGR, limb hypoplasia, CNS involvement), rash, eye damage, death. Damage greatest before the twentieth week of gestation.	Immune globulin for pregnant woman exposed in pregnancy or for infants of mothers infected just before or after delivery. Airborne isolation precautions for infants with lesions.
Other Infections		
Group B Streptococcal Infection During birth or ascending after rupture of membranes.	Sudden onset of respiratory distress in infant usually well at birth, pneumonia, shock, meningitis. May have early or late onset.	Early identification essential to prevent death. Treatment of infected mothers during labor has decreased neonatal infection. IV antibiotics given to infected infants.
Gonorrhea Usually during birth.	Conjunctivitis (ophthalmia neonatorum), with red, edematous lids and purulent eye drainage. May result in blindness if untreated.	All infants receive prophylactic treatment. Erythromycin eye ointment is most common. Infected infants are treated with more antibiotics.
Chlamydial Infection During birth.	Conjunctivitis, pneumonia, otitis media.	Erythromycin or tetracycline eye ointment for prevention of conjunctivitis. Infection treated with more antibiotics.
Candidiasis During birth.	White patches in mouth (thrush) that bleed if removed. Rash on perineum. May be systemic.	Administer antifungal drops or cream and teach parents how to administer them. Assess mother for vaginal or breast infection. IV antibiotics for systemic infection.
Toxoplasmosis Transplacental	Asymptomatic, or LBW, thrombocytopenia, enlarged liver and spleen, jaundice, anemia, seizures, microcephaly, hydrocephalus, chorioretinitis. Signs may not develop for years.	Consider in infants with IUGR. Confirmed by serum tests. Treatment: spiramycin during pregnancy, pyrimethamine, sulfadiazine, folinic acid, and steroids.
Syphilis Transplacental	Asymptomatic or enlarged liver and spleen, jaundice, lymphadenopathy anemia, rhinitis, pink or copper-colored peeling rash, pneumonitis, osteochondritis, CNS involvement.	Diagnosed by blood and cerebrospinal fluid testing. Administer penicillin as ordered.

CNS, Central nervous system; *IUGR*, intrauterine growth restriction; *IV*, intravenous; *LBW*, low birth weight.
*Standard precautions for infection control apply to all patients and are not listed above.

THERAPEUTIC MANAGEMENT

DIAGNOSTIC TESTING. Neonatal sepsis may be confused with other illnesses. For example, group B streptococcal pneumonia has the same initial symptoms as RDS. Diagnostic testing helps identify sepsis and the organisms responsible.

A complete blood count with differential may show decreased total neutrophils, increased bands (a form of immature neutrophils), an increased ratio of immature neutrophils to total neutrophils, and decreased platelets. Elevated leukocytes are normal in newborns and are not helpful in diagnosing infection. Presence of elevated immunoglobulin M levels in cord blood or shortly after birth indicates that infection was acquired in utero because this immunoglobulin does not cross the placenta. It often indicates transplacental infection.

The C-reactive protein (CRP), a sign of an inflammatory process, may be elevated after the first 8 to 12 hours of infection. Serial CRP measurements may be performed to detect changes that show effectiveness of treatment. Cultures of the blood, urine, any skin lesions, and cerebral spinal fluid are obtained. Cultures of the nasopharynx, umbilical cord, and gastric aspirate usually show colonization with organisms but not infection. Chest radiography helps differentiate between respiratory distress syndrome (RDS) and sepsis. Blood glucose levels should be checked because they may be unstable (high or low) in sepsis.

TREATMENT. Broad-spectrum antibiotics are given intravenously until culture and sensitivity results are available. Continued antibiotic therapy is based on culture results. Commonly used antibiotics for early-onset infection include ampicillin and an aminoglycoside such as gentamicin. If the organism is *Staphylococcus,* a cephalosporin, such as cefotaxime, and methicillin, nafcillin, or vancomycin are often used (Edwards, 2002). Intravenous (IV) immunoglobulins are being studied for use in preterm infants.

Other care is supportive to meet the infant's specific needs. The infant may require oxygen or mechanical ventilation. Fluid balance maintenance and monitoring of the blood pressure and hourly urine output are important. Shock, hypoglycemia or hyperglycemia, electrolyte imbalances, and problems in temperature regulation are potential complications.

NURSING CONSIDERATIONS

ASSESSMENT

Risk Factors. The nurse should identify infants at risk for infection. Infants of mothers who have rupture of membranes longer than 18 hours are more likely to become infected (Stoll, 2004). Other risk factors for sepsis include prolonged or precipitous labor, signs of infection before or during labor, and foul-smelling or meconium-stained amniotic fluid. The nurse needs to identify women known to have group B streptococcus and those who show signs of infection so they can be treated with antibiotics during labor to reduce risk to the infant.

Nosocomial (hospital-acquired) infections occur more often in infants who require the specialized care of the neonatal intensive care unit (NICU). These infants have complications or conditions such as prematurity that make them more susceptible to infection. The risk of infection increases as gestational age and birth weight decrease. Preterm infants have not received maternal antibodies to help protect them from infection. In addition, they sometimes spend prolonged periods of time in the NICU, where they are exposed to many invasive procedures such as use of IV catheters and endotracheal tubes that increase their risk of infection. NICU patients may develop abnormal flora that may be carried by personnel from one infant to another and may be resistant to usual drug therapy (Saiman, 2002).

Signs of Infection. In the newborn, signs of infection are not as specific or obvious as those in the older infant or child. Instead, they tend to be subtle and could indicate other conditions. Temperature instability may occur. Respiratory problems are common, and changes may occur in feeding habits or behavior. Other than the parent, the nurse is the only person who spends a significant amount of time with the infant and is in a position to identify the early, subtle changes in behavior that may indicate sepsis. Experienced nurses may have a feeling that the infant is not doing well even before specific signs of infection are present. When this occurs, the nurse expands the assessment and watches carefully for the development of other signs. Early identification and treatment are important because infants can develop septic shock with little warning.

NURSING INTERVENTIONS

Preventing Infection. Although it is not always possible to prevent infection, every effort should be made. Handwashing is the most important aspect of infection prevention. The nurse should practice and teach parents to practice careful handwashing or use of alcohol-based hand disinfectants before and after touching any infant. Equipment must be disinfected according to protocols. Meticulous sterile technique must be used during invasive procedures.

Transmission of infection to other infants in the nursery must be prevented. This is accomplished with the same techniques used to prevent cross-contamination between normal infants (such as handwashing, separation of supplies, and standard precautions for infection control). They must be conscientiously performed by all who come in contact with the infant. Parents should be taught about infection control measures so that they can help protect their infants too.

Placing the infant in an incubator provides a physical separation between infected and well infants, similar to placing adults in isolation in private rooms. In addition, the nurse can observe the infant in an incubator more easily.

Providing Antibiotics. The nurse is responsible for obtaining or helping obtain specimens for laboratory analysis and checking that other tests ordered by the physician are completed. Laboratory tests will help determine the type of antibiotics given and for how long.

Because the signs of sepsis are nonspecific and the disease can be fatal, physicians may order antibiotics before an

CRITICAL TO REMEMBER

Signs of Sepsis in the Newborn

General Signs
Temperature instability (low or fever)
Nurse's feeling that infant is not doing well
Rash

Respiratory Signs
Tachypnea
Respiratory distress (nasal flaring, retractions, grunting)
Apnea

Cardiovascular Signs
Color changes (cyanosis, pallor, mottling)
Tachycardia
Hypotension
Decreased peripheral perfusion

Gastrointestinal Signs
Decreased oral intake
Vomiting
Excessive gastric residuals
Diarrhea
Abdominal distention
Hypoglycemia or hyperglycemia

Neurologic Signs
Decreased or increased muscle tone
Lethargy
Jitteriness
Irritability
Bulging fontanel

Signs That May Indicate Advanced Infection
Jaundice
Evidence of hemorrhage (petechiae, purpura, pulmonary
   bleeding)
Anemia
Enlarged liver and spleen
Respiratory failure
Shock
Seizures

---

actual diagnosis is made for infants who are at high risk or show early signs. Broad-spectrum antibiotics are given intravenously until culture and sensitivity results are available. Continued antibiotic therapy is based on the organisms that are positive on culture. The nurse must be knowledgeable about the specific antibiotics used and possible side effects.

The nurse starts IV fluids and ensures that medications are administered on time. If more than one antibiotic is ordered, the timing of administration must be coordinated to increase effectiveness. Laboratory analysis of peak and trough levels may be ordered to measure blood levels of the medications at times when they are expected to be at the highest and lowest points. This requires planning with the laboratory so that blood is drawn at the correct time in relation to medication administration. Changes in dosage are based on test results. Antibiotics usually are continued for 10 to 14 days for sepsis and 21 days for meningitis.

Providing Other Supportive Care. Infants may be critically ill and need intensive nursing care. Care includes giving oxygen or other respiratory support as needed. Fluid balance maintenance, monitoring of vital signs, and hourly urine output measurements are important. Gavage feeding may be necessary if the infant is unable to take oral feedings.

Infants with sepsis may have additional problems. They may be premature or have other transplacentally acquired infections. In addition, the nurse must be alert for signs of other complications such as disseminated intravascular coagulation.

Supporting Parents. Nurses provide support to parents of newborns with sepsis and help them understand their infant's illness and treatment. The infant with sepsis often appears healthy at birth but suddenly becomes critically ill. Parents experience feelings of shock, fear, and disappointment when their apparently healthy newborn is suddenly moved to the intensive care nursery. Or the preterm infant they thought was making progress may suddenly develop a life-threatening illness. Parents benefit from a chance to talk about their feelings with an understanding nurse who can explain the infant's treatment and care. Keeping the parents informed of the infant's changes in condition and involving them in care are essential.

INFANT OF A DIABETIC MOTHER

Scope of the Problem

The infant of a diabetic mother (IDM) faces many risks that depend on the type of diabetes the mother has and how well it is controlled. Congenital anomalies are three times more likely in infants of mothers with pregestational diabetes if hyperglycemia is present during the early weeks of pregnancy when fetal organs are formed (Stoll & Kliegman, 2004b). Cardiac, urinary tract, and gastrointestinal anomalies, neural tube defects, and caudal regression syndrome are most frequent. Cardiomegaly is common and may lead to heart failure. The incidence of anomalies is less if blood glucose levels remain within normal limits, especially before conception and in the early weeks of gestation.

Infants of mothers with long-term diabetes and vascular changes may be SGA because decreased placental blood flow causes intrauterine growth restriction. Hypertension occurs more often in diabetic women and further compromises uteroplacental blood flow.

Macrosomia (birth weight over 4000 g [8.8 lb or 8 lb, 13 oz]) occurs in approximately one third of IDMs, even with good control of maternal glucose (Fanaroff, Martin, & Rodriguez, 2004). When the mother is hyperglycemic, large amounts of amino acids, free fatty acids, and glucose are transferred to the fetus. Insulin does not cross the placenta because the molecules are too large. The excessive glucose received by the fetus causes the fetal pancreas to secrete large amounts of insulin and leads to hypertrophy of the islet cells. Hypoglycemia may occur after birth when the supply of glucose from the mother is no longer available but the infant's high insulin level continues.

Insulin also acts as a growth hormone. The accelerated protein synthesis and the deposit of fat and glycogen in fe-

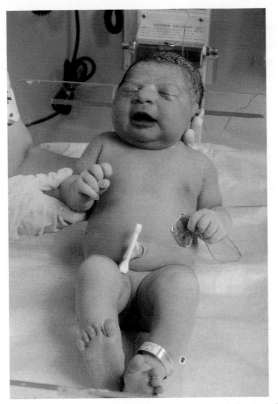

Figure 30-3 ■ Macrosomia is common in infants of diabetic mothers.

tal tissues result in macrosomia (Figure 30-3). Macrosomic infants are at risk for trauma during birth, including fracture of the clavicles, cephalhematoma, facial palsy, subdural hemorrhage, and brachial plexus injury. Strict control of the mother's blood glucose during the second and third trimesters reduces the incidence of macrosomia.

The IDM has a higher risk of asphyxia and RDS. RDS occurs because increased levels of insulin interfere with the production of surfactant. Maintaining strict control of the diabetes and allowing the pregnancy to progress to full term reduces the incidence of RDS.

Other complications for which the IDM is at risk include hypocalcemia (p. 816) as a result of decreased parathyroid hormone production, especially when the mother's diabetes was poorly controlled. Magnesium levels may also be low. Polycythemia (p. 816) may occur because hyperglycemia stimulates production of erythropoietin and red blood cells. In addition, IDMs are more likely to be born prematurely and four times more likely to be admitted to an NICU than infants whose mothers are not diabetic (Chmait & Moore, 2005).

Characteristics of Infants of Diabetic Mothers

The macrosomic IDM is different from other large-for-gestational age (LGA) infants. The infant's size results from fat deposits and hypertrophy of the liver, adrenals, and heart. All organs except the brain are larger than normal. The length and head size are generally within the normal range for gestational age. Other LGA infants do not have enlargement of the organs and tend to be long, with large heads to match the rest of their bodies. Infants of diabetic mothers have a characteristic appearance. The face is round, the skin is often red (plethoric), and the body is obese. The infant has poor muscle tone at rest but becomes irritable and may have tremors when disturbed. The SGA IDM is similar to infants who are SGA from other causes but is more likely to have congenital anomalies.

Therapeutic Management

Therapeutic management includes controlling the mother's diabetes throughout the pregnancy to decrease complications in the fetus and newborn (see Chapter 26). If the infant is large, there may be shoulder dystocia or cephalopelvic disproportion and a cesarean birth may be required. Immediate care of respiratory problems and continued observation for complications determine treatment.

Nursing Considerations

ASSESSMENT

The IDM is assessed for signs of complications, trauma, and congenital anomalies at delivery and during the early hours after birth. Respiratory problems may be apparent at birth or may develop later. The initial assessment may reveal injuries. For example, an infant who cries when an arm is moved or fails to move an arm may have a fractured clavicle or nerve damage.

Hypoglycemia occurs in 25% to 50% of infants of mothers with pregestational diabetes and 15% to 25% of those with gestational diabetes (Stoll & Kliegman, 2004b). It may be present without observable signs.

The most frequent sign of low glucose is jitteriness or tremors. Diaphoresis is uncommon in newborns but may occur with hypoglycemia. Rapid respirations, low temperature, and poor muscle tone also are common (Chapter 20, p. 488). Because these signs are not specific for hypoglycemia, the nurse must be alert for other complications, particularly if signs continue after feeding.

NURSING INTERVENTIONS

The nurse monitors glucose levels according to hospital policy. An example is screening every hour for 4 hours after birth and then every 4 hours twice or until the results are normal. Glucose levels of less than 40 to 45 mg/dl measured with bedside glucose screening should be reported and verified by laboratory analysis. Glucose levels reach the lowest point at 1 to 3 hours after birth and begin to improve by 4 to 6 hours (Stoll & Kliegman, 2004b).

CRITICAL THINKING *?* EXERCISE **30-2**

Although 5% or 10% dextrose water was often used for the first feeding for infants with low blood glucose in the past, using breast milk or formula is now more common. What is the rationale for this?

Infants should be fed early to prevent hypoglycemia and immediately if low blood glucose occurs, to prevent further decreases in glucose. In some agencies the infant is given a very small amount of 10% dextrose (2 ml/kg), which is followed with 5 ml/kg of breast milk or formula. Giving larger amounts of dextrose is likely to stimulate increased insulin production and cause a rebound hypoglycemia. Gavage feeding may be used if the infant does not suck well or the respirations are high. Some infants need IV glucose to maintain balance and prevent injury to the brain.

The nurse must be alert for signs of other complications that occur in IDMs. Signs of RDS or other respiratory complications may develop. Cold stress, which increases the need for oxygen and glucose, could increase respiratory problems and exacerbate hypoglycemia. Infants with polycythemia need adequate hydration to prevent sluggish blood flow and ischemia to vital organs. Hypocalcemia may be suspected if continued tremors occur and the blood glucose is normal.

Providing support to parents is important. They may not understand why their infant, who appears fat and healthy to them, needs close observation and frequent blood tests. The mother may have had a difficult pregnancy and may feel guilty, even if she followed a program of good diabetic control. Ample opportunity for discussion of feelings and information about the care of the infant is important.

✔ CHECK YOUR READING

8. What is the difference between vertical and horizontal transmission of infection?
9. What is the role of the nurse in caring for the infant with sepsis?
10. Why are IDMs more likely to develop macrosomia?
11. Why are IDMs at risk for hypoglycemia after birth?

POLYCYTHEMIA

In polycythemia, infants have a hemoglobin above 22 g/dl and a hematocrit higher than 65% during the first week of life. The increased viscosity of the blood causes resistance to blood flow. Organ damage from ischemia and microthrombi, pulmonary hypertension, renal vein thrombosis, necrotizing enterocolitis, and congestive heart failure may result. Polycythemia also may result in hyperbilirubinemia as the excessive red blood cells break down after birth.

Causes

Polycythemia may occur when poor intrauterine oxygenation causes the fetus to produce more erythrocytes than normal to compensate. It is more common in infants who have intrauterine growth restriction or postmaturity or are LGA or SGA and in infants of mothers who smoke or have preeclampsia or diabetes. Delayed cord clamping or a transfusion from one twin to another may also cause the condition. The incidence in infants of diabetic mothers is 15% to 30% (Wallerstedt & Clokey, 2004).

Therapeutic Management

Treatment is primarily supportive but may include partial exchange transfusion. Blood is replaced with normal saline or albumin to decrease the total number of red blood cells.

Nursing Considerations

Infants may be plethoric (ruddy or dark red) but have no other signs, or they may have lethargy, jitteriness, cyanosis, respiratory distress, feeding problems, hypoglycemia, or hypocalcemia. Monitoring of bilirubin levels is important if jaundice occurs as blood cells break down. Infants must be hydrated adequately to prevent dehydration that would increase sluggish blood flow and ischemia to vital organs. If an exchange transfusion is performed, the nurse assists and watches for complications.

HYPOCALCEMIA

Hypocalcemia is a total serum calcium concentration of less than 7 mg/dl. It is divided into early onset (in the first 72 hours of age) and late onset (at about 5 to 10 days of age).

Causes

Early-onset hypocalcemia occurs most often in IDMs, infants with asphyxia, premature infants, and low-birth-weight infants. Late hypocalcemia is caused by maternal hyperparathyroidism or vitamin D deficiency, high phosphate formula, low magnesium levels, and congenital hypoparathyroidism. Other causes of hypocalcemia include alkalosis, administration of bicarbonate or citrate-preserved blood, furosemide therapy, and renal disease.

Therapeutic Management

Laboratory testing of serum calcium determines the presence of the problem. Oral or IV calcium gluconate is given if feeding alone does not raise the calcium level. A cardiac monitor is necessary when IV calcium is given, because bradycardia can occur.

Nursing Considerations

The nurse must be alert for signs of hypocalcemia, including irritability, tremors, poor feeding, high-pitched cry, tachycardia, apnea, muscle twitching, seizures, and electrocardiographic changes. Hypocalcemia often is asymptomatic.

Oral calcium should be given with feedings because it may cause gastric irritation. IV calcium should be administered slowly and stopped immediately if bradycardia or arrhythmia develops. The IV site should be assessed frequently because infiltration can cause necrosis and ulceration.

PRENATAL DRUG EXPOSURE

Substance abuse affects the fetus at any time during pregnancy. Most drugs readily cross the placenta and cause a variety of problems. Abuse during the first 2 months of pregnancy may cause congenital anomalies. Later abuse may interfere with development or functioning of organs already formed. Abuse of more than one substance is common, making it difficult to determine which substance led to individual effects.

The effects of substance abuse on pregnancy, the fetus, and the neonate are discussed in Chapter 24. This section includes nursing care for infants with neonatal abstinence syndrome (NAS), the disorder in which neonates demonstrate signs of drug withdrawal.

Identification of Drug-Exposed Infants

Maternal substance abuse may be identified before an infant is born, but many infants are born to women whose substance use is not known to the health professionals caring for them during labor and delivery. A history of no or minimal prenatal care or the mother's behavior during labor may cause nurses to suspect substance abuse. Placental abruption may occur after cocaine use. When there is any reason to suspect drug use, the infant is observed closely for signs of prenatal drug exposure.

NAS occurs in infants who have suffered prenatal opiate exposure sufficient to cause withdrawal signs after birth. The syndrome is also seen in some infants exposed to other drugs such as codeine, tranquilizers, and sedatives. Infants with prenatal cocaine exposure may have signs similar to NAS such as irritability and poor sucking patterns, but these are thought to be caused by toxicity of the drug. These effects are not severe enough to require medication (Weiner & Finnegan, 2002).

CRITICAL TO REMEMBER

Signs of Intrauterine Drug Exposure*

Behavioral Signs
Irritability
Jitteriness, tremors, seizures
Muscular rigidity, increased muscle tone
Restless, excessive activity
Exaggerated Moro reflex
Prolonged high-pitched cry
Difficult to console
Poor sleeping patterns
Yawning

Signs Relating to Feeding
Uncoordinated sucking and swallowing
Frequent regurgitation or vomiting
Diarrhea

Respiratory Signs
Nasal stuffiness, sneezing
Tachypnea, apnea

Other Signs
Hypertension
Fever
Diaphoresis
Excoriation
Mottling

*Some infants with prenatal drug exposure will have no abnormal signs at all, or signs may be delayed.

Signs of drug exposure usually begin during the first 48 to 72 hours after birth for opiates, 2 to 3 days for cocaine, and within 3 to 12 hours for alcohol. The time of onset may vary according to the time and amount of the mother's last dose, the length of her addiction, and the gestational age of the infant. Polydrug use is common, and signs differ according to the drug or combination of drugs. Signs often include neurologic and gastrointestinal abnormalities. Some infants with prenatal drug exposure show no abnormal signs or do not show signs until after the first week.

Infants with NAS may be irritable and have hyperactive muscle tone and a high-pitched cry. Although they have tremors, the blood glucose level is normal. They appear hungry and suck vigorously on their fists but have poor coordination of suck and swallow. Frequent regurgitation, vomiting, and diarrhea are common. Infants are restless, and their excessive activity coupled with poor feeding ability result in failure to gain weight. Seizures may occur.

Various scoring systems are available to determine the number, frequency, and severity of behaviors that indicate NAS. The score is used when considering whether drug therapy to alleviate withdrawal signs is needed and to determine dosage. Behaviors are generally scored every 2 to 4 hours until low scores are obtained.

Congenital anomalies and other effects of prenatal drug exposure may be apparent at birth. Many of these infants are SGA. They also may be preterm and suffer from related complications. Infants are more likely to have respiratory problems at birth, jaundice, or sudden infant death syndrome. Specific problems may vary by the drug involved. For example, infants exposed to heroin are more likely to have retained lung fluid and meconium aspiration but less likely to develop RDS. Infants exposed to cocaine are more likely to be premature and to develop necrotizing enterocolitis (Fike, 2003). Infants with fetal alcohol syndrome have a characteristic appearance (see Figure 24-3).

When drug exposure is suspected, a urine specimen is collected from the infant for analysis. Drugs or their metabolites are present in the newborn's urine for various lengths of time after the mother has used them. Some drugs last several days because of the infant's difficulty in excreting them, whereas others disappear very soon. For example, urine tests detect marijuana use for the previous 5 days, cocaine use for 3 days, and heroin use for 2 days. Therefore, it is important to obtain the first urine output from the infant, if possible (Procedure 30-2). Meconium also may be tested because it is more sensitive at detecting drug use over a longer period. However, meconium testing is more expensive and not available at all facilities.

Therapeutic Management

Because many signs of drug exposure are similar to those for other conditions, testing may be performed to rule out other causes. Sepsis, hypoglycemia, hypocalcemia, and neurologic disorders are possible causes for the infant's prob-

PROCEDURE

30-2 Applying a Pediatric Urine Collection Bag

PURPOSE: **To collect a nonsterile urine specimen from an infant**

1. Wash and dry the genitalia. Apply tincture of benzoin according to hospital policy. Allow to dry until "tacky." *Removal of gross contaminants prevents contamination of the specimen. The bag adheres to a clean, dry surface best. Tincture of benzoin increases adherence of the bag to the skin.*

2. Remove the paper covering on the posterior adhesive tabs of the bag first. To apply to female infants, stretch the perineum (skin between the rectum and the vagina). Fold the bag in half and apply smoothly over the perineum, extending the tabs to the side. For male infants, place the penis and scrotum (if small) inside the bag and apply the posterior adhesive tabs to the perineum. If the scrotum will not fit in the bag easily, apply the tabs smoothly over the scrotum. *Covering the perineum with the posterior tabs first helps ensure smooth fit at this area, where leakage of urine may occur in the female infant especially, and prevents contamination with feces. Care in application prevents losing the specimen.*

3. Remove the paper covering on the anterior adhesive tabs, and apply to cover the genitalia. Be sure that there

are no wrinkles in the tabs. *Wrinkles allow openings for urine to leak out of the bag.*

4. Cut a slit in the diaper and gently pull the bag through the slit. Apply the diaper loosely. *Cutting a slit in the diaper allows visualization of the bag. Placing the diaper too tightly over the bag might pull against the adhesive, causing trauma to the skin and providing an opening through which the specimen is lost.*

5. Check the bag for urine frequently and remove it as soon as urine is present. Transfer the urine to a specimen cup by removing the tab over the hole in the bottom and pouring. The specimen also can be aspirated with a syringe after cleaning the puncture site with alcohol. *Ensures removal of the bag before urine loosens the adhesive. Prepares the specimen to be sent to the laboratory for analysis.*

6. Clean the genitalia, and observe for irritation. *Removes urine and adhesive from the skin.*

7. Label the specimen and transport to the lab or refrigerate if necessary. Record in the infant's chart. *Ensures proper disposition of the specimen.*

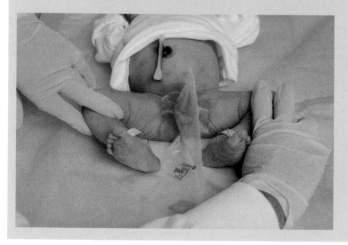
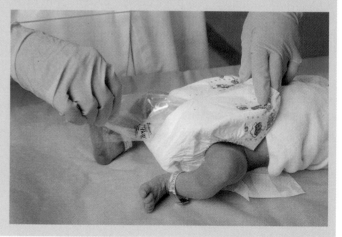

lems. In addition, the infant may have been exposed to infections from the mother, such as hepatitis or sexually transmitted diseases.

Therapeutic management includes dealing with the complications common to drug-exposed infants during and after birth. Respiratory problems and those related to prematurity are treated as for other infants. Drug therapy may be necessary for approximately 50% to 60% of these infants, who have vomiting, diarrhea, marked irritability, and high scores on abstinence scales (Weiner & Finnegan, 2002). Medications commonly used include oral morphine, tincture of opium, methadone, phenobarbital, and benzodiazepines. Medication dosage is gradually tapered until the infant no longer needs it. Although these drugs help relieve the signs of withdrawal, all have side effects that may be undesirable.

Because the infant's suck and swallow are uncoordinated, gavage or IV feeding may be required. Some infants need more than the normal caloric requirements because of their excessive activity. The specific calories needed for each infant will be prescribed by the health care provider. Involvement by social services in and out of the hospital is important to deal with the long-term effects of the drugs, placement of the infant after hospitalization, and follow-up of the mother or other caretaker to help provide for the infant's needs.

Nursing Considerations

The infant who has been exposed to drugs prenatally needs special care to cope with drug withdrawal. Care is focused on feeding, rest, and, if possible, enhancing parental attachment (Nursing Care Plan 30-2).

NURSING CARE PLAN 30-2 The Drug-Exposed Infant

Tracy was born at 38 weeks' gestation to Gloria, who was on a methadone maintenance program. However, Gloria admitted using heroin several times in the last weeks of her pregnancy.

ASSESSMENT: Tracy weighs 2240 g (4 lb, 15 oz) and is small for gestational age. She is jittery, becomes agitated easily, and has a poor suck and swallow. Tracy regurgitates her feedings frequently. She has been fed by gavage but is now taking formula feedings orally. The prescribed caloric intake for Tracy is 300 kcal/day.

NURSING DIAGNOSIS: Ineffective Infant Feeding Patterns related to abnormal coordination of suck and swallow and excessive activity

GOALS/EXPECTED OUTCOMES: Tracy will:
1. Take and retain 300 kcal daily
2. Gain 25 to 30 g (0.88 to 1 oz) each day

INTERVENTION	RATIONALE
1. Prepare Tracy's formula near feeding times so it is ready as soon as she begins to waken.	1. Drug-exposed infants often move from sleeping to an agitated state very quickly. This makes feeding more difficult.
2. Swaddle Tracy with her extremities in a flexed position during feeding.	2. Infants become more agitated if they are allowed to startle. Swaddling provides a sense of security and prevents excessive movement.
3. Try warming the formula slightly before feeding.	3. Some infants take warmed formula more readily.
4. Use chin and cheek support with the chin tucked downward during the feedings as needed.	4. Chin and cheek support increases sucking strength and increases intake. Tucking the chin prevents the infant from pushing the head back and improves swallowing.
5. Feed slowly in an upright position with frequent stops for burping Tracy. If frantic sucking continues when the feeding is stopped, use a pacifier to soothe her.	5. The upright position and frequent burping while keeping the infant calm help prevent regurgitation.
6. Place Tracy on her right side with her head elevated 30 to 45 degrees or in a prone position after feedings. Keep the environment as nonstimulating as possible after feedings.	6. Positioning uses gravity to promote gastric emptying and helps prevent aspiration during regurgitation. Quiet surroundings promote sleep and weight gain and decrease agitation.

EVALUATION: Tracy's intake averages between 275 and 325 calories each day. She gains about 25 g (0.88 oz) daily.

ASSESSMENT: Tracy sleeps less than an hour after feedings. When she awakens, her high-pitched cry and agitation begin immediately. She wiggles out of her blankets, and her activity elicits the Moro reflex, which leads to more agitation. She is irritable and does not respond to care activities as quickly as other infants.

NURSING DIAGNOSIS: Disturbed Sleep Pattern related to agitation from own activity and irritability

GOALS/EXPECTED OUTCOMES: Tracy will:
1. Sleep for periods of 2 hours or more after feedings within 3 days
2. Decrease crying by at least 1 hour a day within the first week

INTERVENTION	RATIONALE
1. Place Tracy's crib in the quietest corner of the nursery, away from areas where alarms sound frequently. Silence alarms quickly.	1. Drug-exposed infants are easily overstimulated by noise and activity.
2. Keep lights turned down as much as possible. Partially cover the head end of the crib with a blanket to decrease light.	2. Lowered lighting provides a more restful environment.
3. Keep Tracy tightly swaddled in a flexed position during sleep and feedings.	3. The drug-exposed infant's own movements can cause startling, awakening, and agitation.
4. Use a pacifier, and position her hands near her mouth.	4. Nonnutritive sucking may have a calming effect on the infant. Positioning the hands near the mouth allows the infant to self-comfort by sucking.
5. Try using slow rhythmic vertical or horizontal rocking when Tracy is upset.	5. Rhythmic rocking may increase rest, decrease agitation, and help infants move more smoothly from one behavior state to another.
6. Use a front infant carrier or walk around holding Tracy during her awake periods.	6. An infant carrier provides the same effect as swaddling. In addition, it provides warmth and a rocking motion from the caretaker's body that may be soothing.

Continued

NURSING CARE PLAN 30-2 The Drug-Exposed Infant—cont'd

7. Provide firm touch to Tracy's chest, back, or soles of the feet.
8. Stop all activity if Tracy shows signs of increased stress.

9. Organize nursing care so that Tracy is not disturbed unnecessarily, especially when sleeping. Provide care when Tracy is awake for feedings if possible.

7. Firm touch is often soothing.
8. Providing a time-out in response to stress signs allows the infant to rest.

9. Drug-exposed infants have difficulty going back to sleep if awakened. Providing care at feeding times clusters care to allow longer undisturbed periods.

EVALUATION: Tracy gradually lengthens her sleep periods to 2 hours and decreases crying episodes within the first week.

ASSESSMENT: Gloria visits Tracy sporadically. She seems hesitant when she comes into the nursery and afraid to touch or care for Tracy. She asks, "Why does she cry so much?" When the nurse helps her hold Tracy, Gloria states, "I don't think she likes me."

NURSING DIAGNOSIS: Impaired Parenting related to lack of understanding of the infant's characteristics and how to relate to an irritable infant.

GOALS/EXPECTED OUTCOMES: Gloria will:
1. Visit at least every other day
2. Participate in Tracy's care by holding and feeding her
3. Make positive statements about her daughter

INTERVENTION	RATIONALE
1. Show acceptance of Gloria when she comes to visit Tracy. Greet her and provide her with an update on Tracy's progress.	1. A mother is more likely to visit her infant if she feels accepted by staff. The more she visits, the more she is likely to learn to parent her infant.
2. Assist Gloria to hold and feed Tracy. Explain nursing actions such as placing the crib in a secluded corner and covering the top. Offer kangaroo care.	2. Participating in care of the infant helps the mother get to know her infant and how to care for the infant more quickly. Kangaroo care can help the mother feel closer to her infant.
3. Demonstrate and explain comfort measures. Show her how to place a rolled blanket or positioning device around the infant to provide a feeling of security and help promote sleep.	3. When the mother learns ways to comfort her infant, the positive response from the infant may increase bonding.
4. Explain the behavioral characteristics of infants who are drug exposed. Explain that Tracy's stiff body posture, failure to "mold" to the mother's body, and excessive activity are normal at this time for her. Point out signs such as gaze aversion and increase in irritability that show Tracy is overstimulated. Explain that the high pitched cry is common.	4. Understanding that the infant's behavior is part of the infant's problem and is not caused by the mother's handling of her is reassuring to the mother.
5. Model ways of interacting with Tracy and calming her when she becomes agitated. Point out signs that Tracy is ready to interact. Suggest only one stimulus at a time, such as talking softly without rocking.	5. The mother learns appropriate interaction when she sees it performed by the nurse. Infants may need short time-outs before they are ready for more stimulation. Decreasing the number of stimuli may be more effective.
6. Point out positive points about Tracy, such as her long eyelashes or delicate fingers. Discuss signs that show that Tracy is making progress.	6. The mother needs help to focus on positive aspects of the infant as well as the problems.
7. Explain the routine care of a newborn. Spread teaching out over Gloria's visits.	7. The mother needs to learn the usual care of any newborn as well as the infant's special needs.
8. Give praise and encouragement frequently as Gloria works with Tracy.	8. The mother needs positive reinforcement and help to feel that she is capable of mothering her infant.
9. Use therapeutic communication techniques to help Gloria discuss her feelings as she cares for Tracy.	9. Mothers often find it frustrating to care for the drug-exposed infant. Helping them vent their feelings may increase their ability to cope with the infant's special needs.
10. Discuss sources of support from family members or friends. Refer her to support groups in the community.	10. Ongoing support is necessary for the woman with addiction problems. Support for the mother will help her care more effectively for her infant.
11. If Gloria will have custody of Tracy, help her make plans for discharge. Discuss ongoing problems and concerns such as continued withdrawal signs and sudden infant death syndrome (SIDS).	11. Preparation for discharge must be made well in advance. Infants will have ongoing problems that will continue in the home setting. Infants exposed to heroin have an increased incidence of SIDS.

EVALUATION: Gloria begins to visit more often, coming four to five times a week. She participates in care, begins to talk about her "pretty little girl," and discusses her plans for when she can regain custody and take Tracy home with her.

FEEDING

Feeding can be difficult and time consuming. The poor suck and swallow coordination of drug-exposed infants interferes with caloric intake, yet their excessive activity increases their caloric needs.

ASSESSMENT. The nurse should assess the infant's ability to coordinate sucking and swallowing with breathing. Infants often suck frantically on their fists or a nipple but are unable to coordinate feeding behaviors well. Changes in the frequency and amount of regurgitation, vomiting, or the length of time it takes infants to finish feedings should be noted.

NURSING INTERVENTIONS. Gavage feedings may be necessary to conserve the infant's energy and prevent aspiration if the infant is excessively agitated, is unable to suck and swallow adequately, or has rapid respirations. When oral feedings begin, infants may need chin and cheek support to help them suck more efficiently. Formula with 24 calories or more per ounce instead of the usual 20 calories per ounce may be used because the infant's excessive activity, poor sleeping, vomiting, and diarrhea increase the caloric need. More frequent feedings may be needed, as well.

Distractions during feedings can be prevented by choosing a quiet, low-activity area of the nursery for feedings. Infants should be swaddled to prevent the startling that occurs when drug-exposed infants are handled. Stimuli such as rocking and talking should be kept to a minimum during feedings. After feedings, infants should be positioned on the right side with the head of the bed elevated 30 to 45 degrees. Some infants respond better to a prone position. If possible, the infant should be positioned in a supine position for sleep.

REST

The excessive activity and poor sleep patterns of drug-exposed neonates interfere with their ability to rest.

ASSESSMENT. The infant's muscle tone, tremors, and tendency for excessive activity with and without being disturbed should be assessed. The degree of tremors and stimuli that increase or decrease irritability are important. The nurse also keeps track of the number of hours that the infant sleeps after each feeding.

NURSING INTERVENTIONS. Stimulation of the drug-exposed infant should be kept to a minimum, especially at first when the infant is excessively irritable. The number of different types of stimulation should be kept to a minimum and adapted to each infant's needs. Noise and bright lights are reduced as much as possible. If the infant shows signs of overstimulation, all activity should be stopped briefly to allow a rest. Swaddling or placing the excessively agitated infant in a dark, quiet room may be necessary. As the infant shows the ability to withstand stimulation, new types can be gradually added, one at a time. Some infants respond well to soft music, which has the added advantage of masking other environmental sounds.

The nurse should organize nursing care to reduce handling and disturbances. Care should be clustered to avoid unnecessary interruptions, yet rest periods should be allowed if signs of stress occur. A calm approach and slow, smooth movements during care help avoid startling the infant. Swaddling the infant in a flexed position helps prevent startling and agitation. Nonnutritive sucking also helps quiet the infant.

Skin abrasions from excessive activity and rubbing of the face, elbows, and knees may increase discomfort and agitation. Diaper rash from frequent diarrhea also may occur. Skin breakdown should be prevented if possible and treated promptly if it occurs. Placing the infant in a prone position promotes better sleep for some infants.

BONDING

When an infant tests positive for drugs, child protective services may become involved. The infant may not be released to the mother until her ability to care for her infant safely has been assessed by social services or a court. She may be required to enter a drug rehabilitation program before she can obtain custody of the infant. After hospital discharge, infants must be cared for by family members approved by the court or in a foster home. The mother will most likely gain custody of the infant eventually if she complies with court-ordered treatment, and attachment to the infant should be encouraged.

ASSESSMENT. The frequency of her visits and her response to the infant may give an indication of the mother's apparent interest in the infant. Although some substance-abusing mothers are uninterested in their infants, for others the infant provides a reason to attempt to overcome their addiction. Bonding behaviors such as calling the infant by name and smiling at the infant should be noted.

NURSING INTERVENTIONS. Child neglect, child abuse, and failure to respond to infant signals and cues are associated with alcohol and drug abuse. Because the mother may become the infant's primary caretaker, it is essential that nurses do whatever they can to enhance mother-infant bonding. Helping the mother feel welcome when she visits the infant provides a challenge. It is sometimes easy to be judgmental and difficult to be accepting when the mother's behavior has been harmful to her infant. Yet a friendly approach will make the mother more likely to visit the infant and accept teaching from the nurse.

The nurse can promote bonding by encouraging mothers to participate actively in infant care during visits. Including the mother will help her feel that the nurses trust her to care for the infant and may increase her confidence. This may help increase her determination to go through recovery to regain her newborn.

The mother's participation also provides a chance to assess her infant care skills and areas in which further discussion of the newborn's needs will be helpful. In addition, it gives the nurse an opportunity to demonstrate parenting skills. Many mothers who use drugs have not had good parenting role models and do not know what to do. Frequent positive feedback about the mother's participation is also important.

The mother needs the same teaching given to all new parents, as well as special techniques necessary to meet the needs of drug-exposed infants. The nurse should teach her about her newborn's special characteristics and help her take on more of the infant's care as she demonstrates readiness. For example, she will need to learn the way to swaddle the infant in a flexed position to prevent excessive startles and tremors.

Parents of a drug-exposed infant need to know that they may experience feelings of rejection, frustration, and even hostility. These feelings are likely to occur when the infant stiffens while being held, cries after being fed, or looks away. Parents also must know that drug-exposed infants are easily stressed because of the decreased stability of their central nervous systems. Emphasize that the infant needs gentle handling. Also explain that crying indicates a need, not a spoiled infant.

Infants are often comforted when they are snugly swaddled with their hands brought to midline. These infants cannot tolerate simultaneous visual and tactile stimulation. Some infants are consoled with slow, rhythmic, vertical or horizontal rocking movements. Placing them in a front pack as the nurse or mother moves around may also be comforting.

The mother needs to learn that infants are easily overstimulated and how to comfort them. Signs of overstimulation in drug-exposed infants have some similarities with those for the preterm infant. In addition, some infants cannot tolerate more than brief periods of interaction. They may not make eye contact, or they may avert their eyes after 30 to 60 seconds of social interaction. Cuddling and soothing to console the infant may not elicit the same response in these infants as in other infants. The nurse should teach the mother that the infant responds poorly to everyone so that she does not think that only she is being rejected.

Cocaine, amphetamines, heroin, and other drugs pass into breast milk. Trying to breastfeed an infant with poorly developed feeding skills may be too much stress for the mother who is trying to recover from addiction. Therefore mothers who are likely to continue drug use after delivery should be discouraged from breastfeeding. In some situations, however, breastfeeding may be acceptable. Women taking methadone may be allowed to breastfeed if they are not taking other drugs that are contraindicated (AAP, Committee on Drugs, 2001). If the woman has a strong desire to breastfeed, the nurse should consult the health care provider.

The nurse can provide information and referral to any special programs available to help parents learn special stimulation techniques appropriate for drug-exposed infants. Some withdrawal signs may continue for 2 to 6 months, and the mother needs to know how to deal with them (Weiner & Finnegan, 2002). If the mother is unable or not allowed to care for the newborn, the same interventions can be used to help the person who will take over care of the infant on hospital discharge.

✓ CHECK YOUR READING

12. How can the nurse deal with the inability to rest in infants with prenatal exposure to drugs?
13. How can the nurse promote bonding when there has been prenatal drug abuse?

PHENYLKETONURIA

Phenylketonuria (PKU) is a genetic disorder that causes central nervous system damage from toxic levels of the amino acid phenylalanine in the blood. In the United States all newborns are screened for this condition before or shortly after discharge from the birth facility. The incidence in the United States is 1 in 10,000 to 25,000 live births (Glass, 2005).

Causes

PKU is caused by a deficiency of the liver enzyme phenylalanine hydroxylase, which is necessary to convert phenylalanine to tyrosine for use. It is an autosomal recessive disorder.

Therapeutic Management

Positive screening tests are followed by further evaluation. Treatment is a low-phenylalanine diet that must be continued throughout life. The infant receives a special formula low in phenylalanine, and low protein foods are introduced when solids begin. The diet is primarily fruits, vegetables, and starches with a phenylalanine-free protein supplement given to provide sufficient protein for growth. Small amounts of phenylalanine are allowed because it is a neces-

---

PARENTS WANT TO KNOW   Measures to Prevent Frantic Crying in a Drug-Exposed Infant

Swaddle the infant with the hands brought to the midline and secured.

Provide a pacifier.

Slowly and smoothly rock in a vertical or horizontal motion with the infant upright.

Coo softly and gently.

Place the infant over your shoulder and gently stroke the back.

Keep the room fairly dark because some infants are particularly sensitive to light.

Avoid simultaneous auditory and visual stimuli.

Curtail stimulation if infant shows signs of stress (yawning, sneezing, jerky movements, or spitting up).

sary amino acid. Early and continued treatment are necessary to prevent mental retardation.

Nursing Considerations

The nurse should be sure that all newborns are screened for PKU at the appropriate time. Screening performed before 24 to 48 hours of age should be repeated because the infant may not have consumed enough protein for the test to be accurate.

Signs of untreated disease begin at about 3 months, with feeding difficulties, vomiting, hypertonia, and irritability. The infant has eczema and a musty odor of the urine. Older children have eczema, hypertonia, hyperactive behavior, mental retardation, seizures, and hypopigmentation of the hair, skin, and irises.

The nurse assists parents in regulating the diet to meet the infant's changing phenylalanine needs. Parents may need to talk about their feelings regarding the difficulty of following the diet for their children. They can be reassured that good control helps promote normal infant growth and development.

CONGENITAL ANOMALIES

Approximately 2% to 3% of newborns have major congenital anomalies at birth. These defects are responsible for approximately 20% of all perinatal deaths (Lott, 2003). They are the leading cause of deaths in the first year of life. Some infants have more than one anomaly, which may be part of a syndrome or result from unrelated causes. Although congenital anomalies generally are treated in the pediatric setting, they usually are identified soon after birth. Common congenital anomalies are noted in Table 30-2. Congenital cardiac conditions are discussed in this section. (See a pediatric nursing textbook for more detailed information.)

CONGENITAL CARDIAC DEFECTS

Approximately 0.5% to 0.8% of newborns have congenital heart defects (Bernstein, 2004). Congenital heart defects are a major cause of death in the first year. Genetics, teratogens, maternal diabetes, and rubella are known to be possible factors. The heart forms by the sixth week of gestation, and problems in development during this period may be associated with anomalies of other structures as well.

Classification of Cardiac Defects

Cardiac defects are generally categorized according to whether cyanosis results from the defect and by the pattern of blood flow. Some of the most common defects are illustrated in Figure 30-4.

ACYANOTIC DEFECTS

In acyanotic conditions an obstruction of blood flow from the left side of the heart or a defect that causes increased flow of blood to the lungs occurs. Both increase the work of the heart. In addition, congestion in the lungs may eventually cause increased resistance of the pulmonary vessels and pulmonary hypertension. Infants are prone to respiratory infections because of the pulmonary congestion and increased work of the heart and lungs. Growth is slowed, and the infant fatigues easily. The heart may fail from overwork. Patent ductus arteriosus is an example of this group.

CYANOTIC DEFECTS

In cyanotic defects, blood flow to the lungs decreases, venous and oxygenated blood are mixed in the general systemic circulation, or both, decreasing the oxygen carried to the tissues and resulting in cyanosis. When venous blood from the right side of the heart flows through an abnormal opening to the left side of the heart, it is called a *right-to-left shunt*. Although the heart and lungs work harder, adequate oxygenation may be impossible, resulting in hypoxia of the major organs. Infants usually have serious problems from birth. The infant grows poorly, has frequent infections, and is easily fatigued. Heart failure may be an early complication. Transposition of the great vessels is an example of a cyanotic heart defect.

The presence of cyanosis depends on the severity and combination of defects and the child's ability to compensate. Some infants with cyanotic heart disease may be pink, and some with acyanotic heart defects may develop cyanosis. Because of this potential change in classification, further classification by blood flow is helpful.

DEFECTS WITH INCREASED PULMONARY BLOOD FLOW

These heart defects allow blood to flow from the higher pressure of the left side of the heart to the right side or from the aorta to the pulmonary artery. This increases blood flow to the lungs and is called a *left-to-right shunt*. It causes some oxygenated blood to be sent to the lungs instead of to the rest of the body, increasing the work of the right side of the heart. Examples are ventricular septal defects and patent ductus arteriosus.

DEFECTS WITH OBSTRUCTION OF BLOOD FLOW

In defects with obstruction of blood flow, a decrease in the blood flow through a vessel or valve occurs because of stenosis (narrowing). This adds to the work of the heart, causes hypertrophy of the heart or major blood vessels, and may lead to heart failure. Coarctation of the aorta fits into this classification.

DEFECTS WITH DECREASED PULMONARY BLOOD FLOW

An impairment in the flow of blood from the right side of the heart to the lungs, combined with abnormal openings between pulmonary and systemic circulations, occurs in defects with decreased pulmonary blood flow. An example is tetralogy of Fallot.

MIXED DEFECTS

Mixed defects allow survival only if a mixing of venous and oxygenated blood in the heart occurs. There is increased blood flow to the lungs and a mixture of venous and oxygenated blood in the systemic circulation. Transposition of the great vessels is a mixed defect.

TABLE 30-2 Common Congenital Anomalies

Gastrointestinal Tract
Cleft Lip and Palate
These are among the most common congenital anomalies, and they occur together or separately, on one or both sides. *Lip:* minor notching of the lip or complete separation through the lip and into floor of nose. *Palate:* only the soft palate or division of entire hard and soft palate. Both genetic and environmental factors are included in the causes.

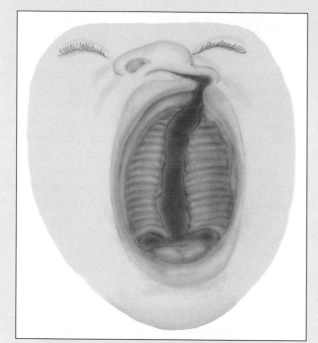

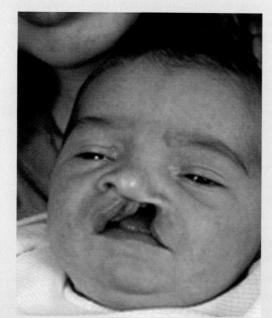

ASSESSMENT
Severe clefts are obvious at birth.
Palpate the hard and soft palate of all neonates during initial assessment.

THERAPEUTIC MANAGEMENT
Lip surgery is generally performed by 3 months to enhance appearance and parental bonding. Further surgery may be needed at 4 to 5 years.

Palate repair surgery is done in stages, depending on the degree, usually beginning before 1 year to minimize speech problems.
Long-term follow-up is necessary for orthodontia, speech therapy, and treatment of possible hearing problems.

NURSING CONSIDERATIONS
The degree of cleft determines the approach to feeding.
Experiment to find methods that works best for individual infants. Try:
1. Breastfeeding (soft breast tissue fills in the cleft of the lip)
2. Soft preemie nipples directed away from a cleft palate
3. Nipples with enlarged hole
4. Compressible bottles
5. Special longer nipples
6. Nipples with extensions to cover the cleft

Feed the infant in an upright position because milk enters nasal passages through the palate, causing an increased tendency to aspirate.
Feed slowly with frequent stops to burp because infants tend to swallow excessive air.
Wash away milk curds with water after feeding.
Help parents deal with their disappointment over the infant with an obvious anomaly. Show them before and after pictures of plastic surgery.
Reinforce the physician's explanation of plans for surgery.
Teach parents feeding techniques. Let them observe at first, then take over gradually. Discuss positioning the infant upright during feedings and on the side after feedings to prevent aspiration.
Prevent infections. Infants are especially susceptible to respiratory and ear infections, which can delay surgery. Ear infections may lead to hearing loss.
Emphasize the need for long-term follow-up. Refer to agencies that help with the expense of long-term care and to support groups for help and emotional support from other parents.

Esophageal Atresia and Tracheoesophageal Fistula
The esophagus is most commonly divided into two unconnected segments (atresia) with a blind pouch at the proximal end. The distal end is connected to the trachea, resulting in tracheoesophageal fistula (TEF). The cause is a failure of normal development during the fourth week of pregnancy. Common variations of the condition are shown in the figure.

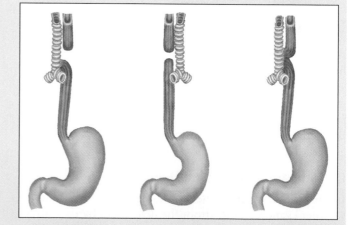

ASSESSMENT
Watch for TEF when polyhydramnios occurs because the excessive fluid may be caused by fetal inability to swallow amniotic fluid.
Other defects occur in 50% of infants with TEF.
Signs vary by the type of defect.
Suspect TEF in infants with excessive frothy drooling and needing suction more often than usual, when regurgitation occurs from secretions that pool in a blind pouch, and when a catheter will not pass into the stomach.

TABLE 30-2 Common Congenital Anomalies—cont'd

If the upper esophagus connects with the trachea, feedings enter the lungs and cause immediate coughing, choking, and cyanosis.

If the fistula is between the distal esophagus and the trachea, the stomach becomes distended with air from the trachea. Gastric secretions are aspirated into the lungs, causing a severe inflammatory reaction.

THERAPEUTIC MANAGEMENT
Diagnosis is confirmed by symptoms and radiography.
Continuous suction should be used for the upper pouch, and a gastrostomy performed. Surgery may be in stages to allow growth.
Long-term follow-up is needed for esophageal reflux and dilation of strictures that form at the surgical site.

NURSING CONSIDERATIONS
Observe all infants carefully during the first feeding for respiratory difficulty or other signs.
Prevent aspiration by maintaining the infant in a semi-upright position to prevent reflux of gastric fluids.
Maintain suction equipment.
Care after surgery involves low pressure ventilation, chest tubes, parenteral nutrition, and gastrostomy feedings.
Omphalocele and Gastroschisis
These anomalies are both caused by congenital defects in the abdominal wall. In omphalocele, the intestines protrude into the base of the umbilical cord. Other anomalies often occur with omphalocele.
Gastroschisis is a defect to the side of the abdomen, next to and not involving the cord. The intestines protrude through the defect and float freely in the amniotic fluid.

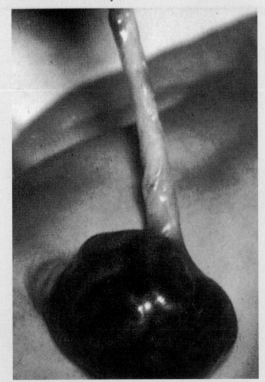

ASSESSMENT
Diagnosis is made by elevated alpha-fetoprotein and prenatal ultrasound and is obvious at birth.

THERAPEUTIC MANAGEMENT
A gastric tube is placed to decrease air in the stomach. Gastric suction, parenteral nutrition, and antibiotics are necessary.
Surgery is performed as soon as the infant is stable. A Silastic silo (pouch) may be used to replace the intestines gradually over 7 to 10 days to prevent pressure on the other organs.

NURSING CONSIDERATIONS
Cover the intestines with sterile saline dressings covered with plastic or place the infant's torso into a sterile plastic bag immediately after birth to reduce heat and water loss.
Prevent infection and trauma.
Position to avoid pressure on the intestines.
Diaphragmatic Hernia
The diaphragm fails to fuse during the eighth to tenth weeks of gestation. A large or small part of the abdominal contents moves into the chest cavity, usually on the left side.
If the herniation is large enough, the lungs may fail to develop (hypoplastic lungs). When gas fills the bowel, further pressure on the heart and lungs results.

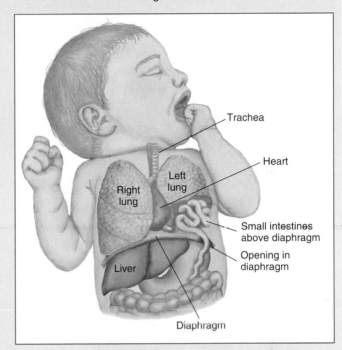

ASSESSMENT
Mild to severe respiratory distress may occur at birth, with breath sounds diminished or absent over the affected area, and barrel chest. The heartbeat may be displaced to the right.
The abdomen may be scaphoid (concave).
The condition may be diagnosed prenatally by ultrasound or by radiography after birth.

THERAPEUTIC MANAGEMENT
An endotracheal tube is placed for ventilation and a gastric tube for decompression of the stomach.
Surgery to replace the intestines and repair the defect is performed when the infant is stable.
Extracorporeal membrane oxygenation (ECMO) may be used.
Fetal surgery has been performed.

NURSING CONSIDERATIONS
Position the infant on the affected side to allow the unaffected lung to expand. Elevate the head to decrease pressure on the heart and lungs. Assist with ventilation, and monitor respiratory status.
Continue to monitor respiratory status after surgery to determine whether lung function will be adequate.

Central Nervous System
Neural Tube Defects
Forms of spina bifida are the most common central nervous system defects.
Folic acid supplements in pregnancy may help prevent neural tube defects.

Continued

TABLE 30-2 Common Congenital Anomalies—cont'd

Spina bifida occulta is failure of the vertebral arch to close, usually without other anomalies. It is seen by a dimple on the back, which may have a tuft of hair over it.

Meningocele is protrusion of meninges and spinal fluid through the spina bifida, covered by skin or thin membrane. Because the spinal cord is not involved, paralysis does not occur.

Myelomeningocele is protrusion of a membrane-covered sac through the spina bifida. The sac contains meninges, nerve roots, spinal cord, and spinal fluid. The degree of paralysis depends on the location of the defect. The infant may also have hydrocephalus, or it may develop after surgery.

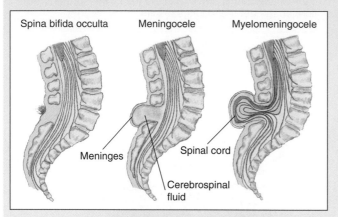

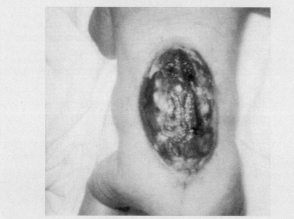

ASSESSMENT
Prenatal diagnosis by elevated alpha-fetoprotein or ultrasound.
Note the position and covering of the defect at birth.
Observe movement below the defect to determine the degree of paralysis.
Examine for a relaxed anus and dribbling of stool and urine.
Check for other anomalies.

THERAPEUTIC MANAGEMENT
Surgery is performed for meningocele and myelomeningocele as soon as possible.

A shunt is placed to divert cerebrospinal fluid if hydrocephalus develops.
Antibiotics are given to prevent infection.
Long-term follow-up is necessary, with physical therapy and other care as needed.

NURSING CONSIDERATIONS
Place the infant's torso in a sterile plastic bag or cover the defect with a sterile saline dressing and plastic to prevent drying.
Handle the infant carefully, and position prone or to the side to prevent trauma to the sac.
Observe for signs of infection. Keep free of contamination from urine and feces.
Inspect the sac for intactness before surgery. Monitor for signs of infection.
Every shift, check for increasing head circumference, bulging fontanels, separation of sutures, intermittent apnea, and other signs of increased intracranial pressure to identify early hydrocephalus.
Fetal surgery has been performed.
The mother should take increased folic acid before and during future pregnancy to help prevent recurrence.

Congenital Hydrocephalus
This is a problem with absorption or obstruction to flow of cerebral spinal fluid in the ventricles of the brain causing compression of the brain and enlargement of the head.

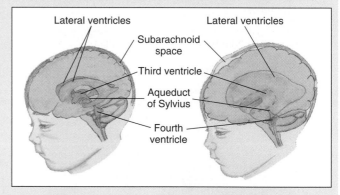

ASSESSMENT
The fontanel is full or bulging, and sutures may be separated.
The head is enlarged, especially in the frontal area.
The setting-sun sign is apparent (sclera visible above the pupils of the eyes).

THERAPEUTIC MANAGEMENT
Surgery, most often with a ventriculoperitoneal shunt to drain fluid into the peritoneal cavity.

NURSING CONSIDERATIONS
Measure head circumference daily.
Prevent pressure areas.
Observe for signs of infection and intracranial pressure.
Teach parents how to care for the shunt and observe for signs of increased intracranial pressure.

Manifestations

Congenital heart defects may present obvious signs at birth or may not become apparent until later, when changes from fetal to neonatal circulation are completed. Some infants have no difficulty for months or years, but others experience early heart failure. The most common indications of cardiac problems are cyanosis, heart murmurs, tachycardia, and tachypnea.

CYANOSIS

Cyanosis is a major sign of cardiac anomaly when it is not a result of respiratory disease. If the cyanosis is caused by a right-to-left shunt, giving oxygen will not improve the infant's color. Cyanosis increases with crying, feeding, or other activity. Pallor, mottling, or a gray color may be present in infants who do not have cyanosis.

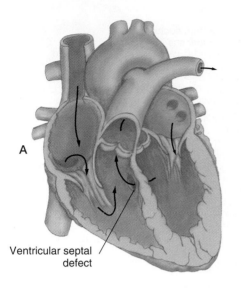

Ventricular septal defect is the most common type of congenital heart defect. It occurs alone or with other defects. The opening in the septum ranges from the size of a pin to very large. Many small defects close spontaneously. When the pressure in the left ventricle increases after birth, oxygenated blood is shunted through a large ventricular septal defect into the right ventricle and then recirculated to the lungs (a left-to-right shunt). Increased pulmonary resistance may cause pulmonary hypertension, hypertrophy of the right ventricle, and heart failure. Surgery is necessary for a large ventricular septal defect and increasing symptoms.

Patent ductus arteriosus is a failure of the ductus arteriosus to close after birth. Blood flows from the higher pressure of the aorta to the pulmonary artery and the lungs (left-to-right shunt). It is most common in the preterm infant. Symptoms vary from none to early congestive heart failure. Prostaglandins cause vasodilation and may interfere with closure of the ductus arteriosus. Indomethacin, a prostaglandin inhibitor, may be effective in causing closure. Surgical ligation is used when necessary. Devices to close the defect nonsurgically are also used.

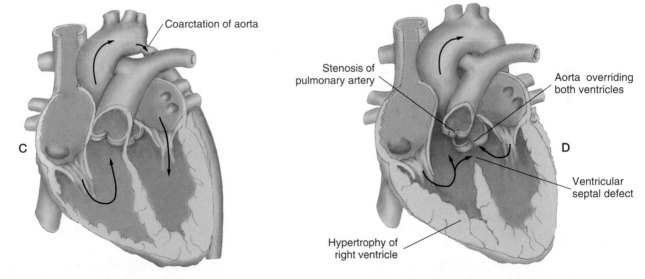

In coarctation of the aorta, blood flow is impeded through a constricted area of the aorta near the ductus arteriosus, increasing pressure behind the defect. The blood pressure is higher in the upper extremities than in the lower extremities. Carotid, brachial, and radial pulses are bounding, but pulses in the legs are weak or absent. The increased pressure in the left ventricle causes hypertrophy from the added workload. Congestive heart failure may result.

Tetralogy of Fallot has four characteristics: a ventricular septal defect, aorta positioned over the ventricular defect, pulmonary stenosis, and hypertrophy of the right ventricle. Cyanosis occurs if venous blood from the right ventricle flows through the septal defect and into the overriding aorta and blood flow to the lungs is diminished because of the narrowed pulmonary valve. The amount of right-to-left shunting and cyanosis varies according to the degree and position of each defect.

Figure 30-4 ■ Common congenital heart defects. **A,** Ventricular septal defect. **B,** Patent ductus arteriosus. **C,** Coarctation of the aorta. **D,** Tetralogy of Fallot.

Continued

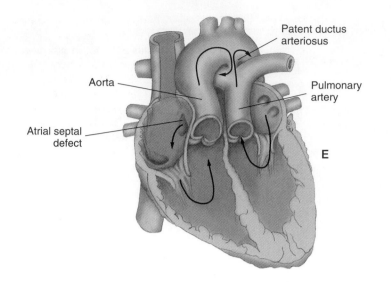

Aorta

Patent ductus arteriosus

Pulmonary artery

Atrial septal defect

E

In transposition of the great arteries, the positions of the aorta and the pulmonary artery are reversed. The aorta carries venous blood from the right ventricle back to the general circulation. The pulmonary artery returns oxygenated blood from the left ventricle to the lungs. Unless there is another source for mixing oxygenated and venous blood, the infant cannot survive. A septal defect, open foramen ovale, or patent ductus arteriosus may be present. Prostaglandins may be given to keep the ductus open, and surgical correction is performed.

Figure 30-4, cont'd ■ **E,** Transposition of the great arteries.

HEART MURMURS

Murmurs may sound like clicks, machinery, rumbling, swishing, or other muffled noises. It takes much practice to detect heart murmurs accurately. Although many infants have a temporary murmur until the fetal structures are closed, all abnormal sounds must be referred to the physician.

TACHYCARDIA AND TACHYPNEA

Tachycardia and tachypnea may occur anytime the heart and lungs must work harder to provide sufficient oxygen to the body. Therefore they are present in both respiratory conditions and cardiac conditions. They increase in congestive heart failure.

OTHER SIGNS

Fatigue may interfere with the infant's ability to eat. Infants may feed slowly and take small amounts. They may fall asleep before the feeding is finished because of the effort required for sucking. As a result, weight gain may be slow. Although diaphoresis is uncommon in the newborn, it may appear during feedings in the infant with a heart defect.

Therapeutic Management

Therapeutic management involves diagnosis of the specific defect and supportive and surgical treatment as indicated. Various tests such as echocardiograms and cardiac catheterizations confirm the diagnosis. The decision for surgery depends on the status of the infant and whether surgery can be delayed safely. Palliative surgery may be performed to partially correct a defect or make another defect to allow

> ### CRITICAL TO REMEMBER
> #### Common Signs of Cardiac Anomalies
> Cyanosis increasing with crying
> Pallor
> Murmurs
> Tachycardia
> Tachypnea
> Dyspnea
> Choking spells
> Poor intake, falling asleep during feedings
> Diaphoresis

greater amounts of oxygenated blood to get to the systemic circulation.

Oxygen and drugs such as digitalis, diuretics, potassium supplements, and sedatives may be prescribed for the infant. Prostaglandins may be given to prevent the ductus arteriosus from closing in those cases in which keeping it open will increase the flow of oxygenated blood to the infant's body.

Nursing Considerations

Nursing care is focused on assessing for changes in condition and reducing the infant's need for oxygen. The need for rest is especially important, and the infant's response to all activity is assessed. Infants with rapid respirations are at risk for aspiration and may need feeding by gavage. Oxygen may be increased during feedings or other exertion, but only enough oxygen to maintain saturation levels adequately

BOX **30-1** Common Nursing Diagnoses for Families of Newborns with Complications

Anxiety
Compromised Family Coping
Disorganized Infant Behavior
Disturbed Sleep Patterns*
Imbalanced Nutrition: Less Than Body Requirements
Impaired Parenting*
Impaired Skin Integrity*
Ineffective Coping
Ineffective Infant Feeding Pattern*
Ineffective Thermoregulation
Interrupted Family Processes
Risk for Imbalanced Fluid Volume*
Risk for Impaired Parent-Infant Attachment
Risk for Injury*

*Nursing diagnoses discussed in this chapter.

should be used. Frequent rest periods are provided by clustering small amounts of nursing care

Feedings with increased calories may be used to promote nutrition and weight gain. Accurate intake and output measurement is necessary. Maintaining a neutral thermal environment is important to avoid increasing oxygen need.

Support of the parents and education about the infant's condition and expected treatment are essential. The nurse uses drawings to help parents understand the defect and plans for surgery. The parents are taught techniques for accurate administration of medications because the range between the therapeutic and toxic dosage of the drugs is narrow. Parents may be referred to support groups for families of children with heart anomalies.

✔ CHECK YOUR READING

14. How are heart defects classified?

SUMMARY CONCEPTS

- Asphyxia before or during birth may cause apnea, acidosis, pulmonary hypertension, and possible death. Neonatal resuscitation must be initiated immediately.
- Nurses must identify conditions that increase the risk of asphyxia, begin resuscitation promptly, and assist other members of the team during treatment. Continued follow-up of the infant and parental support are important.
- In transient tachypnea of the newborn, respiratory difficulty in full-term or preterm infants is caused by failure of fetal lung fluid to be absorbed completely. It usually resolves spontaneously with supportive care.
- Meconium in amniotic fluid enters the lungs before birth during gasping movements or is drawn in during the first breaths after birth, causing obstruction, air trapping, and inflammation.
- The nurse's role in meconium aspiration is to notify caregivers when meconium is discovered, prepare equipment, perform amnioinfusion if ordered, assist with intubation if necessary, and observe for further respiratory difficulty, infection, and other problems.

- Pathologic jaundice appears in the first 24 hours of life or lasts longer than 2 weeks. It occurs when total bilirubin is above 12 mg/dl in full-term infants or 10 to 14 mg/dl in preterm infants; when it rises more than 0.2 mg/dl/hr or 5 mg/dl in 24 hours; or when bilirubin is above the 95th percentile for the infant's age. Pathologic jaundice may result in damage to the brain from kernicterus.
- The nurse's role in phototherapy is to decrease situations such as cold stress or hypoglycemia that might further elevate bilirubin levels, see that lights are used properly, protect the eyes, observe for excessive fluid loss or skin impairment, ensure adequate oral intake, and teach parents.
- Infection can be transmitted to the neonate from the mother during pregnancy or birth or from family members or agency staff after birth.
- Infection in neonates is a problem because their immune system is immature, infection spreads easily, and the blood-brain barrier is less effective.
- The infant of a diabetic mother may have congenital anomalies, may be large (macrosomia) or small for gestational age, and may suffer from respiratory distress syndrome, hypoglycemia, hypocalcemia, and polycythemia.
- Nursing responsibilities in caring for the infant of a diabetic mother include early identification and follow-up of complications, monitoring of blood glucose levels, ensuring early and adequate feedings, and support of parents.
- Infants with prenatal exposure to drugs may have congenital defects and behavioral and feeding abnormalities. They may have difficulty relating to others and may fail to gain weight.
- Nursing care for infants with neonatal abstinence syndrome includes decreasing stimuli from lights, noise, and handling; increasing feeding abilities; and fostering the mother's attachment to and ability to care for her infant.
- In cyanotic heart defects, unoxygenated blood flows into the systemic circulation, producing cyanosis. In acyanotic heart defects, impairment of blood flow or flow of oxygenated blood into the pulmonary system occurs. Defects may increase or decrease blood to the lungs.

ANSWERS TO CRITICAL THINKING EXERCISE 30-1, p. 810

Patches hide the eye area, and an irritation or infection might not be noticed immediately. The warm, dark, moist area under the patches provides a good breeding ground for organisms to grow. Removal of the patches at feedings allows inspection for signs of infection such as redness, edema, and drainage. Removal also allows a time of visual sensory stimulation for the infant. Parental visits should be coordinated with feedings if possible so parents can see the infant's whole face while they visit. This will help the infant appear more normal to them and enhances attachment.

ANSWERS TO CRITICAL THINKING EXERCISE 30-2, p. 815

Giving infants fluids with high levels of glucose will correct the immediate problem of hypoglycemia but also will stimulate the production of additional insulin. This causes a rebound hypoglycemia. Giving glucose in a form that will be metabolized more slowly provides longer normal glucose levels. If dextrose water is given, it should be followed within an hour by colostrum or formula.

REFERENCES & READINGS

American Academy of Pediatrics, Committee on Drugs. (2001). Transfer of drugs and other chemicals into human milk. *Pediatrics, 108*(3), 776-789.

American Academy of Pediatrics, Subcommittee on Hyperbilirubinemia. (2004). Clinical practice guideline: Management of hyperbilirubinemia in the newborn infant 35 or more weeks of gestation. *Pediatrics, 114*(1), 297-316.

American Academy of Pediatrics & American College of Obstetricians and Gynecologists. (2002). *Guidelines for perinatal care* (5th ed.). Elk Grove, IL: American Academy of Pediatrics.

Armentrout, D. (2004). Glucose management. In M.T. Verklan & M. Walden (Eds.), *Core curriculum for neonatal intensive care nursing* (3rd ed., pp. 192-204). Philadelphia: Saunders.

Askin, D.F. (2002). Complications in the transition from fetal to neonatal life. *Journal of Obstetric, Gynecologic, and Neonatal Nursing, 31*(3), 318-327.

Askin, D.F. (2004). Intrauterine infections. *Neonatal Network, 23*(5), 23-30.

Association of Women's Health, Obstetric and Neonatal Nurses. (2003). *Standards for professional nursing practice in the care of women and newborns* (6th ed.). Washington, DC: Author.

Ballard, J.L. (2002). Treatment of neonatal abstinence syndrome with breast milk containing methadone. *Journal of Perinatal and Neonatal Nursing, 15*(4), 76-85.

Ballard, R.A., Hansen, T.N., & Corbet, A. (2005). Respiratory failure in the term infant. In H.W. Taeusch, R.A. Ballard, & C.A. Gleason (Eds.), *Avery's diseases of the newborn* (8th ed., pp. 705-722). Philadelphia: Saunders.

Berkowitz, C.D. (Ed.). (2000). Infants of substance abusing mothers. In *Pediatrics: A primary care approach* (2nd ed., pp. 486-489). Philadelphia: Saunders.

Bernstein, D. (2004). Epidemiology and genetic basis of congenital heart disease. In R.E. Behrman, R.M. Kliegman, & H.B. Jenson (Eds.). *Nelson textbook of pediatrics* (17th ed., pp. 1499-1502). Philadelphia: Saunders.

Blackburn, S.T. (2003). *Maternal, fetal, and neonatal physiology: A clinical perspective* (2nd ed.). Philadelphia: Saunders.

Blackwell, J.T. (2003). Management of hyperbilirubinemia in the healthy term newborn. *Journal of the American Academy of Nurse Practitioners, 15*(5), 194-198.

Bloom, R.S. (2002). Delivery room resuscitation of the newborn. In A.A. Fanaroff & R.J. Martin (Eds.), *Neonatal-perinatal medicine* (Vol. 1, 7th ed., pp. 416-439). St. Louis: Mosby.

Botham, S. (2004). Perinatal substance abuse. In M.T. Verklan & M. Walden (Ed.), *Core curriculum for neonatal intensive care nursing* (3rd ed., pp. 46-79). Philadelphia: Saunders.

Chmait, R., & Moore, T.R. (2005). Endocrine disorders in pregnancy. In H.W. Taeusch, R.A. Ballard, & C.A. Gleason (Eds.), *Avery's diseases of the newborn* (8th ed., pp. 71-86). Philadelphia: Saunders.

Cifuentes, J., Segars, A.H., & Carlo, W.A. (2003). Respiratory system management. In C. Kenner & J.W. Lott (Eds.), *Comprehensive neonatal nursing: A physiologic perspective* (3rd ed., pp. 348-362). Philadelphia: Saunders.

Contributors and Reviewers for the Neonatal Resuscitation Guidelines. (2000). International guidelines for neonatal resuscitation: An excerpt from the guidelines 2000 for cardiopulmonary resuscitation and emergency cardiovascular care–International consensus on science. *Pediatrics, 106*(3), e29.

Cunningham, F.G., Gant, N.F., Leveno, K.J., Gilstrap, L.C., Hauth, J.C., & Wenstrom, K.D. (2001). *Williams obstetrics* (21st ed.). New York: McGraw-Hill.

Edwards, M.S. (2002). Postnatal bacterial infections. In A.A. Fanaroff & R.J. Martin (Eds.), *Neonatal-perinatal medicine: Diseases of the fetus and infant* (7th ed., pp. 706-749). St. Louis: Mosby.

Fanaroff, A.A., Martin, R.J., & Rodriguez, R.J. (2004). Identification and management of the high-risk neonate. In R.K. Creasy & R. Resnik (Eds.), *Maternal-fetal medicine: Principles and practice* (5th ed., pp. 1263-1301). Philadelphia: Saunders.

Fike, D.L. (2003). Assessment and management of the substance-exposed newborn and infant. In C. Kenner, J.W. Lott, & A.A. Flandermeyer (Eds.), *Comprehensive neonatal nursing: A physiologic perspective* (3rd ed., pp. 773-802). Philadelphia: Saunders.

Ford, L. (2004). Group B streptococcus: Re-examining the practice of routine swabs for newborns. *AWHONN Lifelines, 8*(2), 102-103.

Frank, C.G., Cooper, S.C., & Merenstein, G.B. (2002). Jaundice. In G.B. Merenstein & S.L. Gardner (Eds.), *Handbook of neonatal intensive care* (5th ed., pp. 443-461). St. Louis: Mosby.

Gagnon, A.J., Wagnorn, K., Jones, M.A., & Yang, H. (2001). Indicators nurses employ in deciding to test for hyperbilirubinemia. *Journal of Obstetric, Gynecologic, and Neonatal Nursing, 30*(6), 626-633.

Glass, S.M. (2005). Genetic screening. In P.J. Thureen, J. Deacon, J.A. Hernandez, & D.M. Hall (Eds.), *Assessment and care of the well newborn* (pp. 206-218). St. Louis: Saunders.

Greene, C.M., & Goodman, M.H. (2003). Neonatal abstinence syndrome: Strategies for care of the drug-exposed infant. *Neonatal Network, 22*(4), 15-25.

Hagedorn, M.I., Gardner, S.L., & Abman, S.H. (2002). Respiratory diseases. In G.B. Merenstein & S.L. Gardner (Eds.), *Handbook of neonatal intensive care* (5th ed., pp. 485-475). St. Louis: Mosby.

Halamek, L.P., & Stevenson, D.K. (2002). Neonatal jaundice and liver disease. In A.A. Fanaroff & R.J. Martin (Eds.), *Neonatal-perinatal medicine: Diseases of the fetus and infant* (7th ed., pp. 1309-1350). St. Louis: Elsevier.

Hernandez, J.A., Fashaw, L., & Evans, R. (2005). Adaptation to extrauterine life and management during normal and abnormal transition. In P.J. Thureen, J.Deacon, J.A. Hernandez, & D.M. Hall (Eds.), *Assessment and care of the well newborn* (pp. 83-109). St. Louis: Saunders.

Horns, K.M. (2004). Immunology and infectious disease. In M.T. Verklan & M. Walden (Eds.), *Core curriculum for neonatal intensive care nursing* (3rd ed., pp. 759-793). Philadelphia: Saunders.

Johnson, W.L. (2000). Infant of a diabetic mother. In S. Mattson & J.E. Smith (Eds.), *Core curriculum for maternal-newborn nursing* (2nd ed., pp. 730-743). Philadelphia: Saunders.

Jones, C.W. (2001). Gestational diabetes and its impact on the neonate. *Neonatal Network, 20*(6), 17-23.

Juretschke, L.J. (2005). Kernicterus: Still a concern. *Neonatal Network 24*(2), 7-19.

Kattwinkel, J., American Academy of Pediatrics, & American Heart Association. (2000). *Textbook of neonatal resuscitation* (4th ed.). Elk Grove, IL: American Academy of Pediatrics & American Heart Association.

Kenner, C. (2003). Resuscitation and stabilization of the newborn. In C. Kenner & J.W. Lott (Eds.), *Comprehensive neonatal nursing: A physiologic perspective* (3rd ed., pp. 210-227). Philadelphia: Saunders.

Kenner, C. (2004). Families in crisis. In M.T. Verklan & M. Walden (Eds.), *Core curriculum for neonatal intensive care nursing* (3rd ed., pp. 392-409). Philadelphia: Saunders.

Lott, J.W. (2003). Fetal development: Environmental influences and critical periods. In C. Kenner, J.W. Lott, & A.A. Flandermeyer (Eds.), *Comprehensive neonatal nursing, a physiologic perspective* (3rd ed., pp. 151-172). Philadelphia: Saunders.

Lott, J.W., & Kenner, C. (2003). Assessment and management of immunologic dysfunction. In C. Kenner, J.W. Lott, & A.A. Flandermeyer (Eds.), *Comprehensive neonatal nursing, a physiologic perspective* (3rd ed., pp. 550-579). Philadelphia: Saunders.

Madan, A., MacMahon, J.R., & Stevenson, D.K. (2005). Neonatal hyperbilirubinemia. In H.W. Taeusch, R.A. Ballard, & C.A. Gleason (Eds.), *Avery's diseases of the newborn* (8th ed., pp. 1226-1256). Philadelphia: Saunders.

Maisels, M.J. (2001). Neonatal hyperbilirubinemia. In M.H. Klaus & A.A. Fanaroff (Eds.), *Care of the high-risk neonate* (5th ed., pp. 324-362). Philadelphia: Saunders.

Marcellus, L. (2002). Care of substance-exposed infants: The current state of practice in Canadian Hospitals. *Journal of Perinatal and Neonatal Nursing, 16*(3), 51-68.

Marcellus, L. (2004). Foster families who care for infants with prenatal drug exposure: Support during the transition from NICU to home. *Neonatal Network, 23*(6), 33-41.

Martin, R.J., Sosenko, I., & Bancalari, E. (2001). Respiratory problems. In M.H. Klaus & A.A. Fanaroff (Eds.), *Care of the high-risk neonate* (5th ed., pp. 243-276). Philadelphia: Saunders.

Martinez, A., Partridge, J.C., & Taeusch, H.W. (2005). Perinatal substance abuse. In H.W. Taeusch, R.A. Ballard, & C.A. Gleason (Eds.), *Avery's diseases of the newborn* (8th ed., pp. 106-126). Philadelphia: Saunders.

McGrath, J.M. (2004). Identification of the sick newborn. In S. Mattson & J.E. Smith (Eds.), *Core curriculum for maternal-newborn nursing* (3rd ed., pp. 497-533). Philadelphia: Saunders.

Merenstein, G.B., Adams, K., & Weisman, L.E. (2002). Infection in the neonate. In G.B. Merenstein & S.L. Gardner (Eds.), *Handbook of neonatal intensive care* (5th ed., pp. 462-484). St. Louis: Mosby.

Merill, J.D., & Ballard, R.A. (2005). Resuscitation in the delivery room. In H.W. Taeusch, R.A. Ballard, & C.A. Gleason (Eds.), *Avery's diseases of the newborn* (8th ed., pp. 349-363). Philadelphia: Saunders.

Miller, M.J., Fanaroff, A.A., & Martin, R.J. (2002). Respiratory disorders in preterm and term infants. In A.A. Fanaroff & R.J. Martin (Eds.), *Neonatal-perinatal medicine diseases of the fetus and infant* (7th ed., pp. 1025-1049). St. Louis: Mosby.

Montoya, K.D., & Washington, R.L. (2002). Cardiovascular diseases and surgical interventions. In G.B. Merenstein & S.L. Gardner (Eds.), *Handbook of neonatal intensive care* (5th ed., pp. 576-608). St. Louis: Mosby.

Moran, B.A. (2004). Substance abuse in pregnancy. In S. Mattson & J.E. Smith (Eds.), *Core curriculum for maternal-newborn nursing* (3rd ed., pp. 750-770). Philadelphia: Saunders.

Nash, P. (2001). Common neonatal complications. In K.R. Simpson & P.A. Creehan (Eds.), *AWHONN's perinatal nursing* (2nd ed., pp. 575-598). Philadelphia: Lippincott Williams & Wilkins.

National Association of Neonatal Nurses. (2003). *Position statement: Prevention of bilirubin encephalopathy and kernicterus in newborns.* Glenview, IL: Author

Pappas, B.E., & Walker, B. (2004). Neonatal delivery room resuscitation. In M.T. Verklan & M. Walden (Eds.), *Core curriculum for neonatal intensive care nursing* (3rd ed., pp. 102-121). Philadelphia: Saunders.

Pitts, K. (2004). Perinatal substance abuse. In M.T. Verklan & M. Walden (Eds.), *Core curriculum for neonatal intensive care nursing* (3rd ed., pp. 46-77). Philadelphia: Saunders.

Polak, J.D., Ringler, N., & Daugherty, B. (2004). Unit based procedures: Impact on the incidence of nosocomial infections in the newborn intensive care unit. *Newborn and Infant Nursing Reviews, 4*(1), 38-45.

Polin, R.A., Parravicini, E., Regan, J.A., & Taeusch, H.W. (2005). Bacterial sepsis and meningitis. In H.W. Taeusch, R.A. Ballard, & C.A. Gleason (Eds.), *Avery's diseases of the newborn* (8th ed., pp. 551-577). Philadelphia: Saunders.

Reiser, D.J. (2001). *Hyperbilirubinemia: Identification and management in healthy term and near term newborns.* White Plains, NY: March of Dimes Birth Defects Foundation.

Rodriguez, R.J., Martin, R.J., & Fanaroff, A.A. (2002). Respiratory distress syndrome and its management. In A.A. Fanaroff & R.J. Martin (Eds.), *Neonatal-perinatal medicine diseases of the fetus and infant* (7th ed., pp. 1001-1011). St. Louis: Mosby.

Rubarth, L.B. (2003). The lived experience of nurses caring for newborns with sepsis. *Journal of Obstetric, Gynecologic, and Neonatal Nursing, 32*(3), 348-356.

Saddowski, S.L. (2004). Cardiovascular conditions. In M.T. Verklan & M. Walden (Eds.), *Core curriculum for neonatal intensive care nursing* (3rd ed., pp. 584-642). Philadelphia: Saunders.

Saiman, L. (2002). Risk factors for hospital-acquired infections in the neonatal intensive care unit. *Seminars in Perinatology, 26*(5), 315-321.

Schwoebel, A., Bhutani, V.K., & Johnston, L. (2004). Kernicterus: A "never-event" in healthy term and near term newborns. *Newborn and Infant Nursing Reviews, 4*(4), 201-210.

Shaw, N.M. (2003). Assessment and management of the hematological system. In C. Kenner & J.W. Lott (Eds.), *Comprehensive neonatal nursing: A physiologic perspective* (3rd ed., pp. 580-623). Philadelphia: Saunders.

Siegel, R., Gardner, S.L., & Merenstein, G.B. (2002). Families in crisis: Theoretic and practical considerations. In G.B. Merenstein & S.L. Gardner (Eds.), *Handbook of neonatal intensive care* (5th ed., pp. 725-753). St. Louis: Mosby.

Sniderman, S., & Taeusch, H.W. (2005). Initial evaluation: History and physical examination of the newborn In H.W. Taeusch, R.A. Ballard, & C.A. Gleason (Eds.), *Avery's diseases of the newborn* (8th ed., pp. 301-322). Philadelphia: Saunders.

Steffensrud, S. (2004). Hyperbilirubinemia in term and near-term infants: Kernicterus on the rise? *Newborn and Infant Nursing Reviews, 4*(4), 191-200.

Stevenson, D.K., Vreman, H.J., Wong, R.J., & Contag, C.H. (2001). Carbon monoxide and bilirubin production in neonates. *Seminars in Perinatology, 25*(2), 85-93.

Stoll, B.J. (2004). Infections of the neonatal infant. In R.E. Behrman, R.M. Kliegman, & H.B. Jenson (Eds.), *Nelson textbook of pediatrics* (17th ed., pp. 623-640). Philadelphia: Saunders.

Stoll, B.J., & Kliegman, R.M. (2004a). Digestive system disorders. In R.E. Behrman, R.M. Kliegman, & H.B. Jenson (Eds.), *Nelson textbook of pediatrics* (17th ed., pp. 588-599). Philadelphia: Saunders.

Stoll, B.J., & Kliegman, R.M. (2004b). The endocrine system. In R.E. Behrman, R.M. Kliegman, & H.B. Jenson (Eds.), *Nelson textbook of pediatrics* (17th ed., pp. 613-616). Philadelphia: Saunders.

Stoll, B.J., & Kliegman, R.M. (2004c). Respiratory tract disorders. In R.E. Behrman, R.M. Kliegman, & H.B. Jenson (Eds.), *Nelson textbook of pediatrics* (17th ed., pp. 573-588). Philadelphia: Saunders.

Thilo, E.H. (2005). Neonatal jaundice. In P.J. Thureen, J. Deacon, J. Hernandez, & D.M. Hall (Eds.), *Assessment and care of the well newborn* (2nd ed., pp. 245-254). Philadelphia: Saunders.

Vreman, H.J., Wong, R.J., & Stevenson, D.K. (2004). Phototherapy: Current methods and future directions. *Seminars in Perinatology, 28*(5), 326-333.

Wallerstedt, C., & Clokey, D.E. (2004). Endocrine and metabolic disorders. In S. Mattson & J.E. Smith (Eds.), *Core curriculum for maternal-newborn nursing* (3rd ed., pp. 660-702). Philadelphia: Saunders.

Watson, R. (2004). Gastrointestinal disorders. In M.T. Verklan & M. Walden (Eds.), *Core curriculum for neonatal intensive care nursing* (3rd ed., pp. 643-702). Philadelphia: Saunders.

Weiner, S.M., & Finnegan, L.P. (2002). Drug withdrawal in the neonate. In G.B. Merenstein & S.L. Gardner (Eds.), *Handbook of neonatal intensive care* (5th ed., pp. 163-178). St. Louis: Mosby.

Welty, S., Hansen, T.N., & Corbet, A. (2005). Respiratory distress in the premature infant. In H.W. Taeusch, R.A. Ballard, & C.A. Gleason (Eds.), *Avery's diseases of the newborn* (8th ed., pp. 687-703). Philadelphia: Saunders.

Wilbourne, P., Wallerstedt, C., Dorato, V., & Curet, L.B. (2000). Clinical management of methadone dependence during pregnancy. *Journal of Perinatal and Neonatal Nursing, 14*(4), 26-45.

Zaichkin, J., & Simon, W.M. (2004). NRP 2006: How revised guidelines develop. *Neonatal Network, 23*(5), 37-40.

Zukowsky. L. (2004). Respiratory distress. In M.T. Verklan & M. Walden (Eds.), *Core curriculum for neonatal intensive care nursing* (3rd ed., pp. 487-523). Philadelphia: Saunders.

Family Planning

After studying this chapter, you should be able to:

1. Describe the role of the nurse in helping couples choose contraceptive methods.
2. Compare and contrast contraceptive methods in terms of safety, effectiveness, convenience, education needed to use, interference with spontaneity, availability, expense, and preference.
3. Explain why informed consent is important for contraception.
4. Compare and contrast contraceptive needs of adolescent and perimenopausal women.
5. Explain the mechanism of action of each method of family planning available: sterilization, hormonal contraceptives, intrauterine contraceptives, barrier method, and natural family planning.
6. Describe education needed for effective use of each contraceptive method.

Go to your Student CD-ROM for Review Questions keyed to these Objectives.

DEFINITIONS

Basal Body Temperature Body temperature at rest.

Cervical Cap A small cuplike device placed over the cervix to prevent sperm from entering, thus preventing pregnancy.

Coitus Sexual union between a male and a female.

Coitus Interruptus Withdrawal of the penis from the vagina before ejaculation.

Condom Latex, polyurethane, or natural membrane sheath covering the penis or lining the vagina to prevent sperm from entering the cervix and prevent infection.

Contraception Prevention of pregnancy.

Contraceptive Vaginal Ring Flexible ring releasing small amounts of estrogen and progesterone to prevent pregnancy.

Diaphragm A latex dome that covers the cervix and prevents entrance of sperm; must be used with a spermicide to be effective.

Female Sterilization Cutting or mechanically occluding the fallopian tubes to prevent passage of ova or sperm, thus preventing pregnancy. May also be called *tubal ligation*.

Intrauterine Contraceptive A mechanical device inserted into the uterus to prevent pregnancy; also called *intrauterine device* (IUD).

Libido Sexual desire.

Mittelschmerz Low abdominal pain that occurs at ovulation.

Natural Family Planning Method of predicting ovulation based on normal changes in a woman's body.

Oral Contraceptive Drug that inhibits ovulation; contains progestins alone or in combination with estrogen.

Progestin Any natural or synthetic form of progesterone.

Semen Spermatozoa with their nourishing and protective fluid, discharged at ejaculation.

Sexually Transmitted (or Transmissible) Disease (STD) A disease that is passed to others primarily through sexual contact. Also called *sexually transmissible (or transmitted) infection* (STI).

Spermicide A chemical that kills sperm.

Spinnbarkeit Clear, slippery, stretchy quality of cervical mucus during ovulation.

Transdermal Contraceptive Patch Adhesive patch containing estrogen and progestin, which are absorbed through the skin to prevent pregnancy.

Vasectomy Cutting or occluding the vas deferens to prevent passage of sperm, thus preventing pregnancy.

Family planning involves choosing if and when to have children. It includes contraception—the prevention of pregnancy—as well as methods to achieve pregnancy. Chapter 32 describes methods used by couples having difficulty attaining pregnancy. This chapter focuses on techniques used to avoid pregnancy.

If both partners are fertile, approximately 90% of women will conceive within 1 year if they do not use contraception (Cunningham et al., 2005). Therefore those who wish to control the timing of pregnancies cannot leave contraception to chance.

A Healthy People 2010 goal is to increase the number of pregnancies that are intended to 70% (U.S. Department of Health and Human Services, 2000). At this time nearly half of all pregnancies are unintended. Unintended pregnancies are those that are unwanted or mistimed. Mistimed pregnancies are those that occur in women who want to become pregnant at some time in the future but not at the time the pregnancy occurs (Moos, 2003).

Unintended pregnancies may cause a major disruption of the woman's life. They may result in economic hardship, interference with educational or career plans, health problems, and other disruptions in the lives of women and their families.

Because most contraceptive methods available must be practiced by women, women often choose the type of contraception used. In the United States 98% of sexually experienced women have used contraception at some time. Some method of contraception is used by 89% of all women at risk for pregnancy who do not want to become pregnant (Mosher, Martinez, Chandra, Abma, & Willson, 2004). During a woman's reproductive lifetime, her needs for contraception change.

Most women use a variety of methods before they reach menopause. Because the average woman in the United States bears only two children, she must make contraceptive decisions for more than 35 years. Many of those years occur after she has borne the number of children she would like to have and the desire to avoid further pregnancies is high.

INFORMATION ABOUT CONTRACEPTION

Common Sources

Women often obtain information about contraception from friends, relatives, newspapers, magazines, and the Internet. They seek answers to practical questions about comfort, partners' responses, and problems encountered. The information they receive may be incomplete or incorrect when their source is not a qualified health care professional, however.

Women frequently turn to nurses in clinics, physicians' offices, birth settings, and even social settings for accurate information about family planning. Some women are more comfortable asking a nurse about contraception than a physician, particularly when they are unsure about what technique would be best for them.

Role of the Nurse

The nurse's role in family planning is that of counselor and educator. To fulfill this role, nurses need current, correct information about contraceptive methods. Almost half of unintended pregnancies occur in women who are using a contraceptive method but use it incorrectly or inconsistently or have a contraceptive failure (Garcia & Huggins, 2002). This would occur less often if women had adequate ongoing education about their chosen method. The initial teaching that accompanies selection of the contraceptive technique may be insufficient to meet the woman's needs. Reinforcing teaching and providing an opportunity to ask questions after initial use can help ensure that the woman is using her method correctly.

Nurses must feel comfortable discussing contraception and be sensitive to the woman's concerns and feelings. In discussing family planning, the woman's preferences take precedence. Nurses must be careful not to introduce their own biases toward or against specific methods. The nurse's personal experiences and choices regarding contraception are not pertinent. The focus of counseling must be the needs and feelings of the woman and her partner (Figure 31-1).

Many women who do not wish to become pregnant do not use any contraception during the month before they become pregnant (Peterson, Gazmararian, Clark, & Green, 2001). Women are more likely to use contraception if they have received counseling that is directed to their own needs instead of general information about contraception (Weisman, Maccannon, Henderson, Shortridge, & Orso, 2002). Therefore the nurse must provide individualized family planning information to women in every situation in which it would be appropriate. For example, nurses working in maternity settings should discuss family planning with women after birth to provide an opportunity to clarify misinformation and answer questions. Then the woman will be ready to discuss contraception further with her primary caregiver, if necessary.

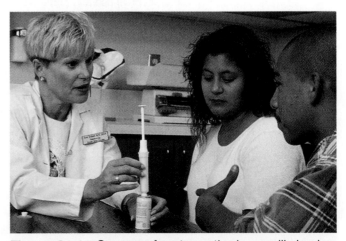

Figure 31-1 ■ Success of contraception is more likely when both the woman and her partner are involved in discussions. The nurse demonstrates filling a foam applicator.

TABLE **31-1** Advantages and Disadvantages of the Most Common Contraceptive Methods

Method	Advantages	Disadvantages
Sterilization	Ends concern about contraception. Female sterilization performed right after childbirth or between pregnancies. Vasectomy performed in the physician's office with local anesthesia. Low long-term cost.	No protection against STDs. Reversal is difficult, expensive, and potentially unsuccessful. Potential complications as in any surgery. Vasectomy requires another contraceptive method until semen is free of sperm. Expensive initially.
Progestin injections (Depo-Provera)	Unrelated to coitus. Avoids need for daily use. May cause eventual amenorrhea.	No protection against STDs. Must remember to repeat every 12 weeks. May decrease bone density. Side effects similar to other progestin contraceptives.
Oral contraceptives	See Table 31-4.	See Table 31-4.
Transdermal contraceptive patch	Unrelated to coitus. Requires application only weekly. Regulates menstrual cycles.	No protection against STDs. Requires prescription. Must apply on the right day. Less effective for women over 90 kg (198 lb). May cause skin irritation. Other side effects similar to those of oral contraceptives.
Vaginal contraceptive ring	Unrelated to coitus. In place for 3 weeks at a time. No fitting required.	No protection against STDs. Requires prescription. Must remember when to remove and when to insert. Side effects include expulsion, vaginitis, vaginal discomfort, and others similar to those of oral contraceptives.
Intrauterine device or intrauterine system	Unrelated to coitus. In place at all times. Low long-term cost.	No protection against STDs. High initial cost. Can be expelled without the woman's knowledge; must check for strings. Potential side effects or complications: menorrhagia, infection, ectopic pregnancy, abortion, perforation.
Barrier All methods	Avoid use of systemic hormones. Offer some protection against STDs.	Most coitus related (must be used just before coitus). May interfere with sensation. Contraindicated for allergies to components of spermicide or latex.
Chemical (spermicides)	Quick and easy. No prescription needed. Inexpensive per single use.	Films and suppositories must melt to be effective. Effective for only 1 hr. May be messy. New application needed for repeated intercourse.
Condoms	Quick and easy. No prescription needed. Best protection available for STDs. Low cost per single use. Can be carried discreetly. Vaginal condoms increase women's control over contraceptive use and protection from STDs.	Must be checked for expiration date and holes. Can break or slip off. Can be used only once. Vaginal condom may seem unattractive.
Diaphragm	Can be inserted several hours before coitus.	Initially expensive. Requires health care provider to fit. Requires education on proper use. Difficult to insert or remove for some women. Added spermicide necessary for repeat coitus. Possibility of toxic shock or bladder infection. Should be checked for fit annually and after birth, abortion, or weight change of 10 lb or more.
Cervical cap	Smaller than a diaphragm and may fit women who cannot wear a diaphragm. No pressure against bladder. Less noticeable than diaphragm. Can remain in place 48 hr (24 hr for Lea's Shield).	Initially expensive. Requires health care provider to fit. Requires education on proper use. Possibility of toxic shock. Added spermicide necessary for repeat coitus.
Natural family planning All methods	Inexpensive. No drugs or hormones. Help woman learn about her body. Can be combined with barrier methods to increase effectiveness. Acceptable in most religions. May be used to help achieve pregnancy.	No protection from STDs. Requires high motivation and extensive education. Abstinence necessary for large part of each cycle. High risk of pregnancy from error. Many factors may change ovulation time.

STD, Sexually transmissible disease.

Counseling about contraception should include the following information:

- Types of contraception available
- Risks and benefits of each
- How to ensure proper use of each method
- What to do if an error is made
- Emergency contraception (EC)
- Backup methods and when they should be used
- What to do if the woman wants to change methods
- Questions and concerns

CONSIDERATIONS WHEN CHOOSING A CONTRACEPTIVE METHOD

The perfect contraceptive method does not exist. Each has advantages and disadvantages (Table 31-1). Women change contraceptive methods as circumstances in their lives change and in response to dissatisfaction with side effects or other traits of their contraceptive. They may try several before finding one that is satisfactory. Thirty percent of married women and 61% of unmarried women switch contraceptive methods within 2 years (Grady, Billy, & Kepinger, 2002). Some women have an interval of using no contraception before beginning a new method, even though they do not wish to become pregnant.

The most popular methods of contraception in the United States are oral contraception, female sterilization, and condoms (National Center for Health Statistics, 2005). However, the most popular methods may not be right for every woman. The nurse can help women weigh factors involved in choosing a family planning method. Careful consideration of all factors can help a woman choose the method that best meets her needs and that she will continue to use. (Table 31-2).

TABLE 31-2 Discontinuation of Various Types of Contraception

Method	Women Who Discontinue Use at 1 Year (%)
Intrauterine devices	
LNG-IUS (Mirena)	19
Copper T 380A (ParaGard)	22
Depo-Provera	44
Oral contraceptives	32
Contraceptive patch	32
Vaginal ring	32
Condoms	
Male	47
Female	51
Diaphragm	43
Spermicides, gel, foam, films, suppositories (used alone)	58
Natural family planning (all types)	49
Withdrawal	57

Data from Trussell, J. (2004). The essentials of contraception: Efficacy, safety, and personal considerations. In R.A. Hatcher, J. Trussell, F. Stewart, A.L. Nelson, W. Cates, F. Guest, & D. Kowal. *Contraceptive technology* (18th ed., pp. 221-252). New York: Ardent Media.

Safety

The safety of the method is a primary consideration. Medical conditions may make some methods unsafe for certain women. For example, oral contraceptives (OCs) should not be used by women who have had thrombophlebitis or strokes because the hormones used may cause these conditions to recur. The diaphragm and cervical cap are unsafe for women with a history of toxic shock syndrome, a possible complication of these methods.

Protection from Sexually Transmissible Diseases

No contraceptive (other than abstinence practiced perfectly) is 100% effective in preventing sexually transmissible diseases (STDs). The risk for exposure to STDs should be considered in counseling women about contraceptive choices. The male condom offers the best protection available. It should be used whenever there is a risk that one partner may have an STD, even when another form of contraception is practiced.

Effectiveness

The importance of avoiding pregnancy must be considered when choosing a contraceptive method. A woman may wish to put off pregnancy for a time but may not care if pregnancy occurs earlier. Other women may be extremely upset about an accidental pregnancy because it would affect their health or have a major impact on their financial stability.

Effectiveness is determined by how often the method prevents pregnancy or fails to prevent pregnancy (Table 31-3). Effectiveness rates reflect two different types of contraceptive failure:

1. The ideal, perfect, or theoretic effectiveness rate refers to perfect use of the method with every act of intercourse. Failures are caused by a problem with the method itself rather than with the use of the method.
2. The typical, actual, or user effectiveness rate is taken from studies of occurrence of pregnancy in real people using the method. Failure is presumably the result of incorrect or inconsistent use of the technique. Failures are most often caused by not using the method for every act of intercourse.

The difference between the two rates of effectiveness shows how forgiving a method is—that is, how likely pregnancy is to occur if use is occasionally imperfect. For example, in 100 women using OCs in 1 year, perfect use results in 0.3 pregnancies but typical use results in 8 pregnancies. The typical failure rate is more meaningful when counseling women and their partners. When comparing different methods, the same method of analysis must be used.

Effectiveness rates are listed as the number of women in 100 women per year who avoid unintended pregnancies. Although a typical effectiveness rate of 88% for a method might seem fairly good, it means that 12 of every 100 women using that method experience unintended pregnancies each year. For women who feel that a one-in-eight yearly risk for pregnancy is too great, a more effective method should be chosen.

TABLE 31-3 Comparison of Pregnancy Rates among Common Contraceptive Methods

Method	Pregnancy Rate: Actual or Typical Use (%)
Sterilization	
Vasectomy	0.15
Tubal ligation	0.5
Intrauterine devices	
Copper T 380A (ParaGard)	0.8
LNG-IUS (Mirena)	0.1
Depo-Provera	3
Transdermal contraceptive patch	8
Vaginal contraceptive ring	8
Oral contraceptives	8
Condoms	
Male	15
Female	21
Diaphragm with spermicide	16
Sponge	
Nulliparous women	16
Parous women	32
Natural family planning (all types)	25
Coitus interruptus (withdrawal)	27
Spermicides, gel, foam, films, suppositories (used alone)	29
No contraceptive use	85

Data from Trussell, J. (2004). The essentials of contraception: Efficacy, safety, and personal considerations. In R.A. Hatcher, J. Trussell, F. Stewart, A.L. Nelson, W. Cates, F. Guest, & D. Kowal. *Contraceptive technology* (18th ed., pp. 221-252). New York: Ardent Media.

Effectiveness varies according to accuracy of use. It drops greatly when the user does not understand how to use the method. The failure rate commonly decreases after the first year of use because experience with the method leads to more accurate use. Combining two less-reliable methods, such as a condom and a spermicide, increases effectiveness.

Other factors that affect the number of unintended pregnancies that occur with contraceptive use include frequency of intercourse and age of the woman. Women who have more frequent intercourse have more opportunities for failing to use the contraceptive correctly. Both frequency of intercourse and fertility tend to decline with age.

Acceptability

The effectiveness of the method must be balanced against the acceptability of the method to the couple. Surgical sterilization is an extremely effective method but is unacceptable to couples planning to have children at a later time. Side effects or religious objections may cause some women to choose less-effective methods.

A contraceptive such as spermicide that seems "messy" may be considered unacceptable because it is unattractive. Spermicide may drip from the vagina and decrease satisfaction for both the woman and the man. Less spermicide may decrease dripping but increase the risk for pregnancy. Teenagers who are not comfortable with their bodies may be unlikely to be accepting of methods that involve inserting a device into the vagina.

Convenience

Convenience is another important factor in choosing a contraceptive method. If the woman perceives her contraceptive as difficult to use, time consuming, or too much "bother," she is unlikely to use it consistently unless her level of motivation is very high. The education she receives about the method may affect her perception of its difficulty. Women who are knowledgeable about their family planning method are less likely to feel that the contraceptive is difficult to use.

Methods that require less-frequent use are likely to lead to better compliance than those that must be used daily or with each intercourse. Spotting between periods, common with some methods, may be viewed as very inconvenient by many women.

Education Needed

Women may fail to use contraception because they do not understand their risk for pregnancy. They may not be familiar with the variety of methods available to prevent pregnancy or the risks and benefits of different types of contraceptives. Some methods of contraception, such as condoms, involve very little education, whereas others depend on one or more teaching sessions to ensure adequate knowledge. Natural family planning methods rely on extensive education about body changes that denote ovulation. Women using these methods need rather sophisticated information to practice them successfully.

Benefits

Some methods have special benefits that should be discussed with the woman. OCs have many beneficial side effects such as improvement of acne and decreased bleeding with periods. Natural family planning methods offer freedom from exposure to hormones.

Side Effects

Many methods of contraception have side effects that women may dislike. Side effects must be explained clearly when discussing the advantages and disadvantages of each method. When women know what to expect, they often are more willing to tolerate side effects, especially if they know that the effect does not indicate a health risk. This may help them continue an effective contraceptive method instead of discontinuing it and using no method or a less-effective one.

Interference with Spontaneity

Contraceptive methods such as barrier methods, withdrawal, and periodic abstinence that require skill and motivation near the time of intercourse have the highest failure rates (Flynn, Clark, & Hume, 2002). Coitus-related contraceptive methods such as spermicides and barrier methods must be used just before sexual intercourse. They must be readily available and interrupt lovemaking, increasing the chance that the method will not be used. Some couples remedy this by including placement of the contraceptive device, such as a condom, as a part of foreplay. Others prefer methods such as OCs or intrauterine devices (IUDs) that do not interrupt sexual activity.

Availability

Condoms and spermicides are readily available without prescriptions. They can be purchased anonymously at any time without a trip to a health care provider. This may be important to an adolescent who wants to hide her sexual activity or to women who are embarrassed to discuss contraception with a health care provider.

Expense

The cost of family-planning methods is important. Less-effective contraceptives are often chosen by some couples to save money or until they can afford a more expensive method. Some methods may be less expensive but more likely to result in pregnancy, which costs more than the yearly expense of any contraceptive method.

The cost of family planning methods per use can be compared with long-term expense. The price of condoms or spermicides is relatively low, but frequent use makes them expensive over a period of years. Couples may find them economical for occasional sexual intercourse or until they can afford a more expensive method. Methods that depend on periodic visits to a nurse practitioner or physician are more costly than over-the-counter methods. However, the visits provide an opportunity for teaching that may enhance contraceptive effectiveness, as well as other health teaching and screening for health problems. Long-term contraceptives such as IUDs are very cost-effective over a 5-year period because they prevent pregnancy so well.

Publicly funded family planning clinics may provide free or low-cost contraceptives, as well as counseling about all contraceptive methods and follow-up services. However, women who attend these clinics may have a long wait to see a different health care provider at each visit.

Insurance coverage for contraception is variable. Many insurance companies pay for the more common prescription contraceptives. Some states have mandated that contraceptives be covered if other prescription drugs are included (Sonfield, Benson, & Frost, 2004). Sterilization is often covered. Organizations such as the Association of Women's Health, Obstetric and Neonatal Nurses support legislation to increase contraceptive insurance coverage for women.

Approximately half of women needing contraception in the United States have a low income and need help in obtaining family planning services (Alan Guttmacher Institute, 2003). These women often rely on family planning services provided by Medicaid, but these services may be in jeopardy when there are budget changes.

Preference

The woman usually makes the final decision about her contraceptive method, and her satisfaction with her choice is crucial. Consistent use of any method depends on whether it meets the needs of the woman and her partner. If the woman feels pressured to choose a certain method or if the chosen method fails to live up to her expectations, use is likely to be inconsistent. The opinion of the woman's partner and her friends also may influence what method she chooses.

Some women are uncomfortable with their bodies and embarrassed by methods that involve touching the vagina. Inserting a vaginal contraceptive ring or performing a daily assessment of cervical mucus may be unacceptable to them.

Religious and Personal Beliefs

Religious or other personal beliefs also affect the choice of contraceptives. Roman Catholics may not believe in the use of any contraceptives other than natural family planning methods.

Culture

Culture may also influence the method chosen. Some cultures place a high value on large families and especially on male children. A woman may have more pregnancies than she might otherwise desire in an effort to have sons. Asian and Hispanic women are often very modest and do not talk about sexuality with others. They need to feel very comfortable with the nurse before talking about sexual matters. Taking time to establish rapport before discussing intimate subjects is important.

Although there is much diversity within each group, many Hispanic adolescents engage in risk-taking behavior such as beginning to have sex at an early age, having multiple partners, and having unprotected intercourse (Villarruel & Rodriguez, 2003). First generation Mexican-American women have different values than many women born in the United States and engage in less risky sexual behavior (Kelly & Morgan-Kidd, 2001). Emphasizing the importance of a Hispanic woman's health to her family may be an effective way to encourage family planning and well-woman care because of the high importance of the family in this culture.

Some women may cling to less-effective methods even though others are available. In one study, over a third of Turkish women used coitus interruptus (withdrawal) for contraception although 45% used more modern methods (Aytekin, Pala, Irgil, & Aytekin, 2001). Use of contraceptives in a group may vary because of special needs. African-American women are more likely than other groups to use condoms (Upchurch, Kusunoki, Simon, & Doty, 2003). This may be true because of the high incidence of STDs in this group.

Other Considerations

There are other factors women consider when choosing a contraceptive. The length of time before another pregnancy is desired will determine if a long-acting contraceptive is appropriate. Breastfeeding women must choose a method that will not harm the baby or reduce milk production. The risk for acquiring an STD is important. If it is high, condoms should be used alone or with another, more effective, method of preventing pregnancy.

Informed Consent

Because some methods have potentially dangerous side effects, it is necessary that a woman sign an informed consent form to show that she received and understands information about risks and benefits. For example, written consent may be obtained from women choosing surgical sterilization, OCs, hormone injections, and IUDs. Of course, regardless of whether a consent form is used, every woman should receive information about the chosen contraceptive method and its proper use, its risks and benefits, and alternative methods available.

✔ CHECK YOUR READING

1. Why do women usually choose the method of contraception that a couple uses?
2. What is the role of the nurse in helping women with contraceptive choices and use?
3. What are some important considerations in choosing a contraceptive technique?
4. Which contraceptive methods may require that the woman sign an informed consent form?

ADOLESCENTS

In 2003, 46.7% of high school students reported that they had been sexually active. The incidence of those who were sexually experienced increased from 32% in the ninth grade to 61.6% in the twelfth grade. Thirty-seven percent reported that they had not used a condom at last intercourse (Grunbaum et al., 2004).

The rate of adolescent pregnancies has diminished in recent years. (See Chapter 24 for information about adolescent pregnancy.) Preliminary data for 2003 show a pregnancy incidence of 41.7 births per 1000 women aged 15 to 19 years (Hamilton, Martin, & Sutton, 2004). This exceeds a U.S. Healthy People 2010 goal of reducing pregnancies in women aged 15 to 17 to no more than 46 per 1000 adolescents from the 1995 baseline of 72 per 1000 in this age group (U.S. Department of Health and Human Services, 2000).

The reduction of teen pregnancy has largely been accomplished by more effective use of contraception and by adolescents who are abstinent for longer periods than in the past. The major impact of pregnancy on the lives of teenagers makes continued work on finding methods to enhance adolescent contraception extremely important.

Adolescent Knowledge

Many adolescents have little knowledge about their own anatomy and physiology, including how and when conception occurs. They are likely to learn about contraception from other teenagers, who often pass on incorrect information. Even adolescents who have been pregnant often are misinformed about contraceptive techniques, and they may become pregnant again because of lack of information about family planning. In addition, adolescent mothers are more likely to use nonhormonal, less-effective methods like condoms and to use them less consistently than sexually active adolescents who have never been pregnant (Paukku, Quan, Darney, & Raine, 2003).

MISINFORMATION

Misinformation and erroneous beliefs cause adolescents to use ineffective methods of contraception or no method at all. Some teenagers think they cannot become pregnant the first time they have intercourse. Others believe they must have an orgasm, or must have been menstruating a certain length of time. However, pregnancy can result from any intercourse near the time of ovulation. Although many adolescents have anovulatory menstrual cycles during the early months after menarche, they cannot depend on failure to ovulate to prevent pregnancy because some will ovulate before their first menses.

Teenagers and older women may douche (insert a solution into the vagina) after intercourse to prevent pregnancy. Douching is ineffective, however, because sperm may enter the cervix soon after ejaculation. Coitus interruptus (withdrawal) is another unreliable method used by teenagers. It requires more control over timing of ejaculation than most adolescent boys have. Semen spilled near the vagina can enter and cause pregnancy, even without penetration by the penis.

RISK-TAKING BEHAVIOR

Adolescents often have a feeling of invincibility. They are more likely than adults to take risks in sexual activity because they believe that their chances of becoming pregnant are small. They often do not plan intercourse and therefore are not prepared with contraceptives. They are more likely to engage in risk-taking behavior than older women, and this may lead to STDs and pregnancy.

Some adolescents are ambivalent about becoming pregnant. Although they do not plan to become pregnant they do not have a firm commitment to avoid pregnancy during their teenage years. Because of this ambivalence, they are inconsistent in using contraception. Discussing how pregnancy may affect them will help determine their true feelings about it (Stevens-Simon, Beach, & Klerman, 2001).

In spite of these factors, 79% of adolescents use a method of contraception (usually a male condom) at their first premarital intercourse (Mosher et al., 2004). This indicates an increased knowledge and acceptance of the value of contraception and protection from STDs.

Counseling Adolescents

Approximately 75% of teens are interested in talking about contraception and STDs by the age of 15 (Speroff & Darney, 2001). Nurses who counsel adolescents about sexuality must be sensitive to the feelings, concerns, and needs of the teenager. They must be prepared to be accepting of the teenager regardless of personal feelings about adolescent sexuality.

For an adolescent to seek information about contraception, she must admit that she is and plans to continue to be sexually active. The teenager may be afraid to ask about contraception because she does not want anyone to know she is sexually active or she fears she will be lectured about her behavior. Her need for secrecy may cause her to miss appointments for family planning. The nurse must be adept at determining the adolescent's needs and reassure her that her visits are confidential and will not be shared with others.

Opportunities to provide counseling must not be missed. Adolescent visits to a health care provider for well-woman checkups or treatment of minor illnesses provide such opportunities. Another chance for counseling occurs when a young woman seeks a pregnancy test. If the test result is negative, she can be asked about her desire to become pregnant. The nurse can assess the adolescent's use of contraception and the adequacy of her knowledge and can provide information as appropriate.

Although nurses should encourage adolescents to discuss contraception with their parents, many teenagers will forgo contraception rather than talk to their parents about it. In one study only 45% of adolescent girls had told their mothers about their visits to a clinic to obtain contraception. They were more likely to tell their partner or a friend (Harper, Callegari, Raine, Blum, & Darney, 2004). Therefore they need other reliable sources of information. Schools have helped increase birth control use among adolescents by offering information about family planning and prevention of STDs.

Contraceptive services also are available on some school campuses. School nurses and classroom discussions supply information about abstinence as well as contraception. Encouragement to delay becoming sexually active and discussion of the effect pregnancy might have and ways to remain abstinent are included.

Family planning clinics in most states may provide information and supplies to minors without parental permission. Some family planning clinics are designed to meet the special needs of teenagers. They may be open after school, during the evenings, and on weekends and have staff who are especially skilled in working with adolescents.

Because adolescent girls frequently fear the pelvic examination, it may be postponed until a later time. Pelvic examinations are not needed for a healthy adolescent girl to begin using contraceptives such as condoms or hormonal contraceptives such as OCs (Hatcher & Nelson, 2004). Current recommendations from the American Cancer Society (ACS) are that yearly Papanicolaou (Pap) tests should begin within 3 years of first vaginal intercourse or by age 21, whichever is first (ACS, 2005). Laboratory blood screening may be postponed until a second visit. During the first visit the teenager receives information about contraceptive techniques. Taking this extra time to explain different methods helps allay the common concern of adolescents about potential adverse health effects of contraceptives. It also helps the teenager to feel comfortable in the clinic setting.

Because of her youth and possible lack of knowledge about anatomy and physiology, the adolescent often needs more extensive teaching than the older woman. Liberal use of audiovisual materials such as pictures, anatomic models, and samples of various methods helps the teenager understand the information more easily. Giving her a patch, vaginal ring, and condom to manipulate or showing her the packet of pills she will be using are important aids.

Using understandable terminology is especially important when teaching adolescents. The nurse must know street terms for body parts and sexual intercourse because they may be the only words with which the teenager is familiar.

Adolescents have higher failure rates with all methods of contraception (Speroff & Darney, 2001). They are most successful when they choose contraceptive methods that are easy to use and seem unrelated to coitus. Many teenagers choose oral or injectable contraceptives. These methods are safe, seem unrelated to sex, and are not difficult or messy. In addition, OCs increase bone density and can decrease acne (Cunningham et al., 2005). Menstrual cramps are reduced, and periods are more regular.

Adolescent girls may be inconsistent in taking pills every day, however. They are more likely to discontinue any method for minor side effects such as nausea or spotting. Their concerns should be taken seriously, and attempts should be made to alleviate side effects. Otherwise, adolescents are likely to stop using the method, with pregnancy a possible result. They should understand all aspects of management of their contraceptive method and when a backup method is necessary.

Adolescents may use condoms alone to prevent pregnancy and STDs, especially at the beginning of a relationship or with casual partners. With long-term partners, they may switch from condoms to hormonal methods if they are concerned about pregnancy prevention. Increased use of hormonal methods is associated with decreased use of condoms for many adolescents. Some use condoms, with or without hormonal methods, only if they also have casual partners or if they are very concerned about both pregnancy and STDs (Ott, Adler, Millstein, Tschann, & Ellen, 2002).

Condom use should be encouraged to help prevent STDs, even when another contraceptive method is used (Figure 31-2). Discussing perceived barriers to using condoms helps dispel misconceptions about them. Many young women are uneasy about asking a partner to use a condom. Discussing ways to negotiate condom use with a partner can be particularly helpful. Adolescent males often are more concerned about avoiding pregnancy than STDs. They may not want to use a condom if they know their part-

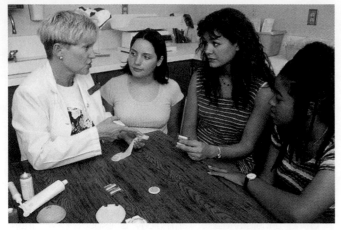

Figure 31-2 ■ Although many adolescents choose oral contraceptives, the nurse emphasizes the need to use condoms for protection against sexually transmissible diseases. Demonstrating with actual contraceptives increases understanding.

CRITICAL THINKING ⸮ EXERCISE 31-1

A 15-year-old girl approaches the nurse with questions about contraception. She says she does not want to become pregnant, but her boyfriend does not want to use condoms. She says she is too embarrassed to go to see a physician for other contraceptive methods because she is afraid of the examination.

Questions
1. How should the nurse begin the discussion?
2. What should the nurse tell her about visiting a health care provider for contraception?
3. What should the nurse discuss about condom use?

ner is using another contraceptive method. Teaching should include signs of STDs and what to do if they should occur.

PERIMENOPAUSAL WOMEN

Perimenopausal women may continue to ovulate as long as they have regular menstrual periods, and some ovulate even when indications of menopause are present. Therefore, contraceptive counseling is important for these women. However, women over 40 are less likely to receive counseling about contraception even though they are more at risk for an unintended pregnancy than women in their 30s (Weisman et al., 2002).

The mature woman who does not smoke and has no other contraindications can use any method of contraception. Low-dose OCs may be used in nonsmokers to provide contraception and help regulate the irregular bleeding that often occurs during the perimenopausal time. Perimenopausal women should have regular physical examinations to identify any conditions that would necessitate a change in contraceptive method. Many couples who do not plan to have more children choose sterilization.

✔ CHECK YOUR READING

5. What are some erroneous beliefs about contraception commonly held by adolescents?
6. Why might teenagers be hesitant to seek contraceptive information?
7. How can the nurse increase effectiveness in teaching adolescents about contraception?
8. What considerations are necessary in contraception for perimenopausal women?

METHODS OF CONTRACEPTION

Sterilization

Sterilization is an extremely popular method of contraception for couples who have completed their families. Although it is expensive at the time of surgery, sterilization ends all further contraceptive costs. It should always be considered a permanent end to fertility because reversal surgery is difficult, expensive, not always successful, and often not covered by insurance.

Couples considering sterilization need counseling to ensure that they understand all aspects of the procedure. When surgery is planned for immediately after childbirth, the decision should be made well before labor begins. Future marriage, divorce, or death of a child may cause couples to regret their decision. Younger age, an unstable marriage, or a situation in which the decision is made at a time of financial crisis or related to a pregnancy increases the incidence of later regret. Most women do not regret their decision 5 years after male or female sterilization. Those who do are more likely to have been in conflict with their partner about sterilization before the procedure (Jamieson et al., 2002).

Complications of sterilization are those of any surgery, including hemorrhage, infection, and anesthesia complications. Although pregnancy is rare, the possibility of failure should be discussed. Pregnancies occurring after female sterilization are more likely to be ectopic.

FEMALE STERILIZATION

Female sterilization (also called tubal ligation) is the second leading method of contraception and is used by 10.3 million women in the United States (Mosher et al., 2004). The surgery involves cutting or mechanically occluding the fallopian tubes and can be performed at any time. It is easiest during cesarean birth or in the first 48 hours after vaginal birth when the fundus is located near the umbilicus and the fallopian tubes are directly below the abdominal wall. Interval sterilization, not associated with childbirth, is generally performed as outpatient surgery. General anesthesia is most common, but regional or local anesthesia may be used.

The procedure is usually performed in one of three ways. In the first method, a minilaparotomy incision is made near the umbilicus in the postpartum period or just above the symphysis pubis for interval sterilization. In the second method, surgery is performed through a laparoscope inserted through a small incision. The third method is performed during other surgery, generally along with cesarean birth, when a woman is sure that she wants the procedure regardless of the outcome of the birth. The fallopian tubes may be occluded by removing a section and tying the ends, or by using clips, bands, or rings or destroying a portion of the tubes with electrocoagulation.

After sterilization the woman should rest for 24 hours and should not lift heavy objects for a week. Mild analgesics may be needed for pain. Intercourse is avoided for a week. The woman should call the health care provider if she has a fever, fainting, severe pain, or bleeding or discharge from the incision (Pollack, Carignan, & Jacobstein, 2004).

A nonsurgical method of female sterilization is the vaginal insertion of a tiny coil (Essure) through the cervix and into each fallopian tube. The tubes become permanently blocked during the next 3 months as tissue grows into the inserts. During this time another contraceptive method is used. The procedure can be performed in the physician's office. A hysterosalpingogram is performed at the end of 3 months to ensure the tubes are completely blocked.

VASECTOMY

Vasectomy, the male sterilization procedure, involves making a small incision or puncture in the scrotum to lift out the vas deferens, which carries sperm from the testes to the penis. Ligation and removal of a section of the vas or cautery may be used. After vasectomy, semen no longer contains sperm.

Although performed less frequently than female sterilization, vasectomy is a very popular method of contraception. It involves lower morbidity rates than tubal ligation, and because it can be performed in a physician's office under local anesthesia, it is less expensive as well. After surgery the man rests for 48 hours, applies ice to the area, uses a scrotal support for 2 days, and takes a mild analgesic, if necessary. Strenuous activity should be avoided for a week to prevent bleeding. The health care provider should be notified of a fever, severe pain, bleeding or discharge at the site, swelling more than twice the normal size, or a painful nodule.

Intercourse may be resumed in 2 to 3 days, but the man is not sterile at that time. The couple should understand that complete sterilization does not occur until sperm are no longer present in the semen, which may be 3 months or more. The man should submit semen specimens for analysis until two specimens show no sperm present.

Hormonal Contraceptives

Hormonal contraceptives alter the normal hormone fluctuations of the menstrual cycle. Hormones may be delivered by implant, injection, patch or vaginal ring or may be taken orally.

HORMONE IMPLANT

The progestin implant (Norplant), consisting of six flexible capsules inserted subcutaneously into the upper inner arm under local anesthesia, is no longer available in the United States.

A single-rod progestin implant (Implanon), is expected to receive U.S. Food and Drug Administration (FDA) approval and be marketed shortly. The implant is 4 cm (1.6 in) long and releases progestin continuously to provide 3 years of contraception. It acts to inhibit ovulation and thicken cervical mucus. During clinical trials there were no pregnancies in women using the method. Side effects include irregular menstrual bleeding and bleeding between periods, as with other progestin-only contraceptives. When the rod is removed, fertility returns immediately.

HORMONE INJECTIONS

Depo-Provera (medroxyprogesterone acetate, or DMPA) is an injectable progestin that prevents ovulation for 12 weeks. It is convenient, contains no estrogen, and has a failure rate of only 3%. Action and side effects are similar to those of other progestin contraceptives. Menstrual irregularities are the major reason for discontinuation. Although spotting and breakthrough bleeding are common, amenorrhea occurs in 30% to 50% of women at 1 year and increases with longer use (Hatcher, 2004). Weight gain may approximate 1.8 kg (4 lb) per year for some women. Other side effects include headaches, nervousness, decreased libido, breast discomfort, and depression.

There has been recent concern about a decrease in bone density in adolescents and with prolonged use (Hatcher, 2004). It is now suggested that Depo-Provera not be used in adolescents or in other women for longer than 2 years unless no other suitable method is available. More studies are necessary regarding the long-term effects of Depo-Provera. A warning to this effect has been issued by the FDA. Women should get adequate amounts of calcium and vitamin D in their diets or by supplements and increase their weight-bearing exercise while using Depo-Provera.

Depo-Provera is given by deep intramuscular injection. The site should not be massaged after injection because this accelerates absorption and decreases the period of effectiveness. The injection is best given within 5 days of the menstrual period. If given later in the cycle, an additional form of contraception should be used for the first week. A backup method of contraception is used if the woman is more than 1 week late returning for a subsequent injection, and a pregnancy test is recommended.

Women who should not use other hormone contraceptives generally should avoid Depo-Provera as well. For breastfeeding women, it often is started 6 weeks after delivery, when lactation is well established. There are no adverse effects on production of breast milk (Weiner & Buhimschi, 2004). Fertility returns in approximately 10 to 18 months (Kaunitz, 2001).

ORAL CONTRACEPTIVES

OCs are the leading contraceptive method in the United States and are used by approximately 11.6 million women (Mosher et al., 2004). They are available as combination OCs, which contain both estrogen and progestin, and "minipills," which contain only progestin. Both types have much lower hormone levels than the original OCs, and therefore the risk for long-term side effects is decreased. If OCs are used perfectly, three women in 1000 become pregnant in the first year. The failure rate is 8% for the typical user (Hatcher & Nelson, 2004).

COMBINATION. Estrogen and progestin combinations are the most common OCs. The major action of combination OCs is to cause thickening of the cervical mucus, which prevents sperm from entering the upper genital tract. OCs also block the luteinizing hormone surge from the pituitary, which inhibits maturation of the follicle and ovulation. (See Chapter 4 for information about the menstrual cycle.) In addition, capacitation of sperm is impaired, tubal motility is slowed, and the endometrium becomes less hospitable to implantation.

Most combination OCs are available in packets of 21 or 28 tablets. With 21-tablet packets, the woman takes one pill daily for 3 weeks, then stops for a week, during which time menstruation occurs. Packets of 28 tablets include 21 active tablets and seven tablets made of an inert substance that the woman takes during the fourth week. The extra pills avoid disrupting the everyday routine of taking pills. In addition, a formulation with 84 active pills and seven placebo tablets (Seasonale) is available for women who want fewer menstrual periods. This allows women to have only four periods a year.

Monophasic or multiphasic dosages are available. Monophasic pills have an estrogen and progestin content that remains constant throughout the cycle. With multiphasic pills the estrogen dose may be constant or increased in the later part of the cycle. The progestin dose is low at the beginning and is increased later. This helps reduce side effects. Because the dosage changes throughout the phases, women must take the pills in the proper order to maintain effectiveness.

PROGESTIN ONLY. OCs that contain progestin without estrogen are called *minipills*. Minipills are taken daily with no hormone-free days. They are less effective at inhibiting ovulation but cause thickening of the cervical mucus to prevent penetration by sperm. They also make the endometrial lining unfavorable for implantation. These pills avoid side effects and risk factors associated with estrogen and are useful for women who cannot take estrogen. Another method of contraception should be used during the first cycle.

If the woman misses any pills or does not take them at the same time each day, her chances of pregnancy increase. If any minipills are missed, the woman should continue to use the pills but should use an additional method of contraception for the rest of the cycle. However, instructions vary, and the woman should check with her health care provider about what to do if she misses a pill. Breakthrough bleeding and higher risk for pregnancy have made these OCs less popular than the combination OCs. Amenorrhea occurs in some women.

BENEFITS, RISKS, AND CAUTIONS. When OCs are chosen, the balance between the benefits and the risks must be weighed for each individual (Table 31-4). The method has many benefits in addition to safe, reliable contraception. Benefits include the reduction of heavy menstrual bleeding, dysmenorrhea, and anemia. For young women with acne, OCs may be very helpful. Some formulations reduce premenstrual syndrome and improve bone density. Cycle control to provide regular periods and minimal bleeding are important to many women.

Women often believe the risks of OCs are higher than they are. Although there are risks in using OCs, women should know that the chances of complications and death are higher during pregnancy and childbirth than in women using OCs except for women of any age who smoke 25 or

TABLE 31-4 Potential Benefits, Disadvantages, and Risks of Oral Contraceptives

Benefits	Disadvantages	Risks*
Unrelated to coitus	Must be taken every day at near same time, especially minipills	No protection against STDs
Highly effective contraception		May increase risk of cervical cancer
Reduces ovarian and endometrial cancer	Side effects may include:	Increased incidence of:
Protection continues for years after use	Breakthrough bleeding	Deep and superficial vein
Regulates menstrual cycles and reduces	Nausea	thrombosis
cramping, menstrual blood loss, and	Headache	Pulmonary embolism
associated anemia	Breast tenderness	Myocardial infarction
Return to fertility usually within 3 months	Weight gain	Stroke
when ended (up to 6 months for some)	Melasma	Hypertension
Decreased incidence of:	Mood swings	Migraines
Benign breast disease		Chlamydial infection
Ovarian cysts		Benign liver tumors
Pelvic inflammatory disease		Gallbladder disease
Ectopic pregnancy		Higher risks in women who smoke
Improves:		
Acne		
Endometriosis		
Many premenstrual symptoms		
Dysmenorrhea		
Bleeding from fibroids (leiomyomas)		
Bone mass (combined OCs only)		
Polycystic ovary syndrome		
Hirsutism (excessive hair growth)		

OC, Oral contraceptive; *STD*, sexually transmissible disease.

*Incidence of many risks is significantly reduced with low-dose OCs presently used. Avoiding OC use in women who smoke or have other risk factors lowers risk for cardiovascular disease significantly.

more cigarettes daily (Trussell, 2004). Women over age 35 who smoke more than 15 cigarettes a day and women over age 40 who smoke at all should not use estrogen-containing contraceptives (Hatcher & Nelson, 2004).

OCs were once thought unsafe for older women, but studies show that women in good health who do not smoke can continue to take low-dose OCs until menopause (Speroff & Darney, 2001; Sieber, Barbouche, & Fagan, 2003; Hatcher & Nelson, 2004). Smoking significantly increases the incidence of complications for women of all ages. Other risk factors include hypertension, high cholesterol levels, obesity, and diabetes with vascular involvement. Diabetics with no complications who have had the condition for less than 20 years and are otherwise in good health may use OCs if their condition is adequately supervised.

Many risks were associated with the higher doses of hormones used in the original OCs but are less of a problem with current OCs. Hazards are decreased by careful screening for risk factors in each woman. OCs provide no protection against STDs and may increase susceptibility to chlamydia. A woman should be advised to use condoms and spermicide if her partner may be infected.

SIDE EFFECTS. Approximately 32% of women who do not wish to become pregnant discontinue OCs within a year, usually because of side effects. Most side effects are minor and include signs and symptoms often seen in pregnancy. Using a different formulation of hormones may reduce some side effects. For example, decreasing the amount of estrogen helps relieve nausea and breast tenderness. Other side effects include weight gain or loss, fluid retention, amenorrhea, and melasma. Side effects often decrease after the first few months of use and are less frequent in low-dose OCs.

CRITICAL TO REMEMBER

Cautions in Using Oral Contraceptives

Oral contraceptives should not be used by women with a history of any of the following:

- Thrombophlebitis and thromboembolic disorders
- Cerebrovascular or cardiovascular diseases
- Any estrogen-dependent cancer or breast cancer
- Benign or malignant liver tumors
- Hypertension (unless well controlled by medication)
- Migraines with focal aura
- Diabetes with vascular involvement or of more than 20 years' duration

Oral contraceptives should not be used by women who currently have any of the following:

- Any of the previously listed conditions
- Impaired liver function
- Suspected or known pregnancy
- Undiagnosed vaginal bleeding
- Heavy cigarette smoking (more than 15 per day in women older than 35 years or any smoking over age 40; any use of cigarettes is discouraged and should be evaluated individually)
- Major surgery requiring prolonged immobilization

ORAL CONTRACEPTIVE INITIATION AND PATTERN

Methods of beginning OC use include taking the first pill on the day the pills are prescribed, beginning on the first day of the next menstrual period, and beginning on the first Sunday after the first day of menses. If a woman begins the pill pack on a Sunday, she may avoid having a period on the weekend. Unless the first pill is taken on the first day of her period, the woman should use a backup contraceptive for 7 days.

A variety of patterns of pill use may also be used. The woman may take active pills for 21 days and no pills or placebo pills for the next 7 days. Some providers suggest taking the first OC on the first day of menses each month, shortening the time of no hormones. Some women prefer extended cycles in which menses is delayed for a few days for special occasions or for a longer time. These women take two or more pill packs without taking the placebo pills for several packs or indefinitely. An OC designed to provide 84 days of active pills and seven placebo pills allows women to have menses only four times a year. Although they have fewer periods, women using extended cycle methods may have more spotting (Hatcher & Nelson, 2004).

TEACHING. Many unintended pregnancies result from failure to follow instructions about OCs correctly. However, education about proper use greatly increases their effectiveness. Teaching should be extensive when the woman begins to use the hormones. Follow-up is necessary to ensure that her questions and unanticipated problems are resolved. Because the instructions can be complicated, they should be written clearly and simply in her own language, if she can read.

Side effects are the most common reason for discontinuing OCs. The nurse should listen carefully to women's concerns about side effects and help them find methods of relief. When women discontinue OCs because they are unhappy with the side effects, they may not use another contraceptive or may use one that is less effective and become pregnant as a result. Women should be instructed that they need a backup contraceptive method readily available in case they decide to stop taking their OCs.

It is essential that nurses be honest about the side effects that should be expected with all contraceptives. Teaching about side effects that are temporary may help the woman endure them until they are no longer present. Women should know that spotting is a common side effect of many hormonal contraceptive methods, particularly at the beginning. Over time, amenorrhea may develop. If changes in bleeding patterns or irregularity are unacceptable to the woman, she should choose another contraceptive method.

Blood Hormone Levels. Maintaining a constant blood hormone level is important for effectiveness, especially with the minipills. Therefore the woman must take the pills at the same time each day. Many women make them a part of their bedtime routine, and others take their OCs with a meal to avoid nausea. Breakthrough bleeding is more likely when a significant time variation occurs between doses.

Unless they begin the pills on the first day of menses, women should use another contraceptive method during the first week of the first cycle until the blood hormone levels are established (Hatcher & Nelson, 2004). Women also should understand that some pills must be taken in a certain order and that changing the order will decrease the effectiveness of the method.

Illness may affect the blood hormone levels. A woman who experiences severe vomiting or diarrhea should use a backup method of contraception for 7 days as the hormones may not have been properly absorbed (Speroff & Darney, 2001).

Missed Doses. Instructions for the woman who misses one or more doses should be provided. Women who frequently miss OCs should be counseled about other contraceptive methods that might be more effective for them.

The woman should follow instructions from her provider if she misses doses of her OC. Instructions may vary according to the type of OC she uses, the number of doses missed, and the time in the cycle the OC is missed. Different health care providers may use different regimens. An example of instructions is provided in the box "Women Want to Know: What to Do if an Oral Contraceptive Dose Is Missed."

If a woman misses a period and thinks she may be pregnant because she missed one or more doses, she should stop taking the pills and get a sensitive pregnancy test immediately. Using another contraceptive method during this time is essential. Although association with fetal anomalies has not been established, continued use of OCs during pregnancy is not advisable.

Postpartum and Lactation. Because of their increased risk for thrombosis, postpartum women who are not breastfeeding should wait at least 3 to 4 weeks to begin OCs (Hatcher & Nelson, 2004). Combination OCs reduce milk production in lactating women, and very small amounts may be transferred to the milk. Many experts recommend that combined OCs not be used during lactation (Kennedy & Trussell, 2004). Progestin-only contraceptives may be a better choice if a woman wishes to use a hormonal contraceptive because they do not affect milk production. They are often started 6 weeks after birth.

Other Medications. OCs may interact with other medications, and the effectiveness of each may be changed. Anticonvulsants such as phenobarbital, phenytoin, topiramate, carbamazepine, oxcarbazepine, felbamate, and primidone decrease the effectiveness of OCs. The antituberculosis drug rifampin and the antifungal drug griseofulvin are other examples. St. John's Wort, which some women take for depression, interferes with OC effectiveness. Interactions between OCs and antiretroviral drugs are also possible. However, the antibiotics amoxicillin and tetracycline do not reduce OC effectiveness. Because of this variety of interactions, the woman should always tell any health care provider prescribing medications for her about other drugs she is taking.

Follow-Up. The woman who takes OCs should have a yearly breast examination and blood pressure measurement.

WOMEN WANT TO KNOW — What to Do if an Oral Contraceptive Dose Is Missed

The following provides one example of information given to women who miss contraceptive pills. Talk with your nurse practitioner, nurse-midwife, or physician for specific information suited to your needs.

GENERAL

If less than 24 hours have elapsed since the time the OC should have been taken, take the pill and take the rest of the pack as usual. If 24 hours or more have elapsed, follow these instructions.

COMBINED ORAL CONTRACEPTIVES
One Pill Missed

- Take two pills as soon as possible.
- Continue the pack as usual.
- Use another contraceptive method for 7 days, or consider using emergency contraception if unprotected sexual intercourse occurred.

Two to Four Pills Missed

- If the missed pills were from the first week of a new pack, take two pills as soon as possible. Finish the pack. Use backup contraception, or consider emergency contraception if unprotected sexual intercourse occurred.
- If the missed pills were from the second week of a new pack, take two pills as soon as possible. Finish the pack. Backup contraception is not necessary but may be used if desired.
- If the missed pills were from the third week of the pack, start a new pack of pills. Backup contraception is not necessary.

Five Pills Missed

- If five active pills are missed at any time, take two pills. Then start a new pack. Use backup contraception, and consider emergency contraception.

Inactive Pills Missed between Days 21 and 28

- Throw away pills missed, and continue to take the rest as scheduled. Contraception will not be affected.
- Begin a new packet of pills on the same day as usual.

PROGESTIN-ONLY ORAL CONTRACEPTIVES (MINIPILLS)
- Check with your health care provider.

Data from Hatcher, R.A., & Nelson, A. (2004). Combined hormonal contraceptive methods. In R.A. Hatcher, J. Trussell, F. Stewart, Nelson, A.L., Cates, W., Guest, F., & Kowal, D. *Contraceptive technology* (18th ed., pp. 391-460). New York: Ardent Media.
OC, Oral contraceptive.

TABLE 31-5 Aches*: Warning Signs of Oral Contraceptive Complications

	Warning Sign	Possible Complication
A	Abdominal pain (severe)	Benign liver tumor, gallbladder disease
C	Chest pain, dyspnea, hemoptysis	Pulmonary emboli or myocardial infarction
H	Severe headache, weakness or numbness of extremities, hypertension	Stroke, migraine with neurologic problems
E	Eye problems (visual changes such as blurred or double vision or visual loss, speech disturbance)	Stroke
S	Severe leg pain or swelling (calf or thigh)	Deep vein thrombosis

Data from Hatcher, R.A., & Nelson, A. (2004). Combined hormonal contraceptive methods. In R.A. Hatcher, J. Trussell, F. Stewart, Nelson, A.L., Cates, W., Guest, F., & Kowal, D. *Contraceptive technology* (18th ed., pp. 391-460). New York: Ardent Media.
*The acronym *ACHES* can be used to help women remember warning signs that may indicate complications when using oral contraceptives. Other signs include jaundice, a breast lump, and depression. The woman should contact her health care provider if any of these signs develops.

Current recommendations for Papanicolaou (Pap) tests are within 3 years of beginning vaginal intercourse but not later than age 21, then yearly for regular Pap tests or every 2 years for liquid-based tests. After the woman reaches age 30, screening may be every 2 to 3 years if there have been three previous normal tests (ACS, 2005).

During the follow-up visit, the woman's ability to remember to take a pill every day should be evaluated. Other methods should be discussed if this is a problem or if she wants to change methods. Return of fertility usually occurs within 2 to 3 months after the pills are discontinued for women who wish to become pregnant. A woman should wait until her menstrual cycle is reestablished before conceiving so that she can date the beginning of her pregnancy more accurately. She should be advised to take folic acid for several months to help prevent neural tube defects.

The woman should report any signs of adverse reaction immediately. Use of the acronym *ACHES* may help the woman remember signs that may indicate complications (Table 31-5). Other adverse reactions include severe mood changes, depression, and jaundice.

TRANSDERMAL CONTRACEPTIVE PATCH

The contraceptive patch (Ortho Evra) releases small amounts of estrogen and progestin to suppress ovulation and make cervical mucus thick. It also regulates menstrual cycles. The contraceptive patch is as effective as OCs and may be more effective because it is used once a week instead of daily (Hatcher & Nelson, 2004). A nonhormonal contraceptive should be used during the first week of use, unless the patch is started on the first day of the menstrual period.

The patch is applied to clean, dry skin on the abdomen; upper torso excluding the breasts; buttock; or upper outer arm. Areas where clothing such as straps or waistbands may rub the patch should be not be used. The woman should avoid using oils or lotions in the area. The patch should not be placed on irritated or sunburned skin or areas of eczema or rashes. Adherence to the skin is good even in the shower or when exercising or swimming. The patch should not be cut or altered, and no more than one patch should be worn at a time.

A new patch is applied to a different site weekly on the same day of the week for 3 weeks and worn continuously for 7 days. Then the woman goes without a patch for one week.

During the patch-free week, she has a period. After 7 patch-free days, the woman applies a new patch and begins the cycle again.

Side effects include breakthrough bleeding, especially during the first two cycles, breast tenderness, headaches, and skin reactions. Other side effects and risks are similar to combination OCs. The patch has been found to be less effective in women who weigh more than 90 kg (198 lb) (Zieman, et al., 2002).

Because the patch must be applied only once a week, it may be easier than OCs for women who have difficulty remembering to take a pill every day. However, it is visible on the skin, which may be a problem for adolescents who do not want their contraceptive use known by others.

CONTRACEPTIVE VAGINAL RING

Women using the contraceptive ring (NuvaRing) insert a soft flexible vinyl ring into the vagina and leave it in place for 3 weeks. The ring, which measures 5 cm (2 in) in diameter and is 0.3 cm ($\frac{1}{8}$ in) thick, releases small amounts of progestin and estrogen continuously to prevent ovulation. The woman removes the ring at the end of the third week, and bleeding occurs. A new ring is inserted to begin the next cycle a week after the old ring was removed. Although a prescription is required, no fitting or particular placement in the vagina is necessary. There is no need to think about contraception except twice a month when the ring is being placed or removed.

The device should be inserted high into the vagina against the vaginal wall. It should be placed during the first 5 days of the menstrual cycle, even if the woman is still bleeding. A backup method is necessary for 7 days if the woman was not using a hormonal method during the previous cycle.

Women must be comfortable inserting the device into the vagina. Placement and removal are quick and easy. Allowing a woman to try placing the ring in the provider's office where help is available often increases comfort. For the woman who doesn't want her contraceptive use known by others, the fact that the ring is not visible to others is appealing.

The most common side effect is headache. Other side effects include nausea, breast tenderness, vaginitis, expulsion, or vaginal discharge or discomfort. Although some women or their partners feel the ring during intercourse, it is generally not a problem. Women who should not use hormonal contraceptives should not use the vaginal ring.

The ring may be removed for up to 3 hours without loss of effectiveness. If a longer time elapses, a backup method is necessary for 7 days. The rate of spotting or bleeding between periods is lower than with other hormonal methods.

EMERGENCY CONTRACEPTION

EC is often called the "morning-after pill." It is a method to prevent pregnancy after unprotected intercourse. It may be used after contraceptive failure, such as a condom breaking during intercourse. It also may be used after rape or in other situations in which contraceptives were used incorrectly or not at all.

Many women are unaware of the availability of EC. Information about it and how to obtain it should be included any time education about contraception is offered to women, in case they might later wish to use it. Information about where EC can be obtained is available on the Internet at http://www.NOT-2-LATE.com, or the woman can call 1-888-NOT-2-LATE. Women who require EC should receive counseling about their regular contraceptive method. They may not understand how to use their method correctly or may wish information about other, more effective options.

EC involves taking two tablets that contain a high dose of progestin (Plan B). The first tablet should be taken as soon as possible after unprotected intercourse. The second tablet may be taken at the same time as the first or within 12 hours. There is no increase in side effects if both tablets are taken together. The effectiveness is greatest if EC is used within 72 hours of intercourse, but it may also be used as long as 120 hours later. Plan B reduces the risk for pregnancy by 89% (Stewart, Trussell, & Van Look, 2004).

Combined OCs may also be used in larger-than-usual doses to prevent pregnancy. The number of tablets varies according to the specific OC used. Because of the short time frame during which EC is effective, some health care providers give women prescriptions to use if necessary at a later date. In some states, pharmacists are allowed to provide EC without a prescription.

Treatment with combined OCs reduces the risk for pregnancy as much as 75%. The high hormone levels prevent or delay ovulation, thicken cervical mucus, and alter sperm transport to prevent fertilization. The treatment is ineffective if implantation has already occurred, and it does not harm a developing fetus (Stewart, Trussell, & Van Look, 2004).

Combined OC treatment should not be used in women who have contraindications to its use. High doses of progestin-only contraceptives may be preferable for these women. Antiemetics may be prescribed to treat the side effects of nausea and vomiting, which are more severe with combination tablets. They may be started an hour before the woman takes the first dose of EC.

Insertion of the copper T 380A IUD within 5 days of intercourse also may be used and provides 99% effectiveness. It has the added advantage of providing long-term (10 years') protection from pregnancy for those who choose this method.

Mifepristone may also be used for EC. The drug inhibits ovulation and prevents endometrial development. Unlike the other drugs used for postcoital contraception, mifepristone will disrupt an existing pregnancy. Because it is also used for medical induced abortion, some women will prefer to use another method.

✔ CHECK YOUR READING

9. What factors should a couple consider in deciding which method of sterilization to use?
10. What is the mechanism of action of hormonal contraceptives?
11. What side effect is most likely to cause some women to discontinue use of some hormonal contraceptives?
12. What do women taking OCs need to know about this contraceptive method?
13. How soon after unprotected intercourse should EC be used?

Intrauterine Devices

IUDs are inserted into the uterus to provide continuous pregnancy prevention. The Copper T 380A (ParaGard) (Figure 31-3) and the levonorgestrel intrauterine system (LNG-IUS or Mirena) are both shaped like the letter T. The failure rate for ParaGard is 0.8% and it is 0.1% for Mirena. Mirena is more effective than any other contraceptive method, including sterilization.

Although safety was a concern with early models, IUDs are considered very safe at this time. They are often inserted at the 6-week postpartum checkup and are safe for use dur-

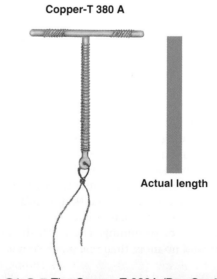

Copper-T 380 A

Actual length

Figure 31-3 ■ The Copper T 380A (ParaGard) intrauterine device (IUD). Currently, IUDs are considered a very safe method for preventing pregnancy.

ing lactation. IUDs are expensive at the time of insertion but have a low long-term cost.

Once they are inserted, IUDs provide long-term, continuous contraception without the need to take pills, have injections, or perform other tasks before or during intercourse. They are appropriate for many women who cannot use other hormonal contraception and can be inserted at any time the woman is not pregnant. Fertility returns promptly when the device is removed.

ACTION

The mechanism of action for IUDs is a sterile inflammatory response resulting in a spermicidal intrauterine environment (Speroff & Darney, 2001). Very few sperm reach the fallopian tubes. The ParaGard IUD is covered with copper that changes the uterine and tubal fluids to impair sperm function. It remains effective for 10 years.

Progestin is continuously released from the LNG-IUS, Mirena, which must be replaced in 5 years. The progestin thickens cervical mucus, inhibits sperm function and survival, and causes the endometrium to react against foreign bodies (Grimes, 2004). Only a small amount of progestin is absorbed systemically, leading to lower blood levels than for users of other progestin-containing contraceptives.

SIDE EFFECTS

Side effects include cramping and bleeding with insertion. Menorrhagia (increased bleeding during menstruation) is a common reason for removal of the copper device. Irregular periods with light bleeding or spotting may occur during the early months with Mirena but may be followed by amenorrhea (Grimes, 2004). Ibuprofen may relieve bleeding and cramping, and some women need iron for anemia.

Complications include perforation of the uterus at the time of insertion. Expulsion occurs in 2% to 10% of users. Although the rate of ectopic pregnancies in IUD users is much less than in women not using contraceptives, pregnancies that do occur are more likely to be ectopic or result in spontaneous abortion or preterm birth. Nulliparous women and those with recent or recurrent pelvic infections, a history of ectopic pregnancy, bleeding disorders, or abnormalities of the uterus should choose another contraceptive method.

There is a small risk for infection at the time of insertion and during the following few weeks. After that, risk for infection is low. There is no data on whether the risk for upper genital tract infection is higher in women with STDs and IUDs than in those with STDs who are not using IUDs. To be safe, only women in mutually monogamous relationships and at low risk for STDs should use IUDs.

TEACHING

Teaching the woman about side effects and to check for the presence of the plastic strings or "tail" extending from the IUD into the vagina is important. The woman should feel for the strings once a week during the first 4 weeks of use, then monthly after menses, and if she has signs of expulsion

(cramping or unexpected bleeding). If the strings are longer or shorter than they were previously, she should see her health care provider. Signs of infection such as unusual vaginal pain, discharge, or itching, low pelvic pain, and fever should prompt a call to the health care provider. Any signs of pregnancy should be reported to rule out ectopic pregnancy and remove the device if pregnancy has occurred. The woman should return yearly for a Pap smear and to check for anemia if menses are heavy.

Barrier Methods

Barrier methods of contraception involve chemicals or devices that prevent sperm from entering the cervix. The method may kill the sperm or place a temporary partition between the penis and cervix. All barrier methods are coitus related and may interfere with spontaneity. They avoid use of systemic hormones, however, and provide some protection from STDs. Infection with human papillomavirus, an STD, may increase the risk for cervical cancer. Therefore use of barrier contraceptives may lower the incidence of cervical cancer.

CHEMICAL BARRIERS

Chemicals that kill sperm are called *spermicides* and come in many forms. Creams and gels are generally used with mechanical barriers such as the diaphragm or cervical cap. Foams, foaming tablets, suppositories, and vaginal film may be used alone or with another contraceptive measure. They are inserted deep into the vagina so that they are in contact with the cervix just before sexual intercourse. Vaginal films and suppositories must melt before they become effective, which takes approximately 15 minutes. They are effective for about 1 hour and should be reapplied if more than an hour elapses or intercourse is repeated. Women should avoid douching for at least 6 hours after intercourse and should add more spermicide if coitus is repeated.

Spermicides are readily available without a prescription, inexpensive per use, and easy to use. Using spermicides with condoms increases lubrication, which decreases the risk for condom breakage. This is an advantage, especially during lactation or in menopausal women when vaginal secretions are decreased. When spermicides are used alone, the failure rate is 29%. Effectiveness is increased when spermicides are used with a mechanical barrier method.

Some women and their partners believe that spermicides are messy and interfere with sensation during intercourse. Spermicides do not protect against STDs and should not be used for that purpose. Frequent use (more than twice a day) or sensitivity to the products may cause genital irritation, which could increase susceptibility to infection and human immunodeficiency virus (HIV).

MECHANICAL BARRIERS

Mechanical barriers are devices placed over the penis or cervix to prevent passage of sperm into the uterus. They include the condom, sponge, diaphragm, and cervical cap.

What Is the Proper Way to Use Condoms?

Although condoms are easy to use, proper use increases their effectiveness.

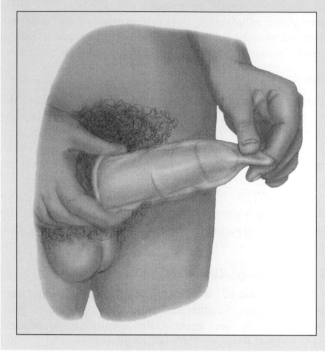

- Condoms are available in a variety of colors, textures, and materials, but those made of latex are most effective. Others may help protect against pregnancy but not against STDs.
- Check the expiration dates on packages, because condoms may deteriorate after 5 years. Open the package carefully and check the condom to see that it is not torn or damaged before using it.
- Lubrication may increase comfort for the woman and reduce the risk of breakage. Use a water-soluble lubricant or a spermicide because oil-based products (such as petroleum jelly or baby oil) cause deterioration of latex condoms.
- Always apply the condom before there is any contact of the penis with the vagina because sperm may be present in preejaculatory fluid.
- Squeeze the air out of the tip of the condom, and leave ½ inch of space at the tip as the condom is rolled onto the erect penis. This allows a place for sperm to collect and helps prevent breakage.
- Withdraw the penis from the vagina while it is still erect, and hold the condom in place so it does not slip off and no semen spills into the vagina.
- Use a new condom each time intercourse is repeated.

MALE CONDOM. Condoms, the only male contraceptive device currently available, are the third most popular method of contraception in the United States and are used by 9 million women and their partners. Condoms are the method most often used for first intercourse (Mosher et al., 2004). They cover the penis to prevent sperm from entering the vagina. Condoms are most often made of latex and may be lubricated. Couples allergic to latex may use condoms made from polyurethane, other synthetic materials, or natural membrane. Polyurethane condoms are thinner than latex but may require lubrication to avoid breakage. Natural-membrane condoms do not prevent passage of viruses and do not provide protection from STDs caused by viruses. Latex condoms provide the best protection available (other than abstinence) against STDs. For this reason, condoms should be used during any possible exposure to an STD, even if another contraceptive technique is practiced or if the woman is pregnant.

Condoms are readily available and inexpensive and can be carried inconspicuously by the man or the woman. The typical failure rate of 15% can be decreased greatly by combining condom use with another method such as a vaginal spermicide. Reservoir tips and water-based lubricants help prevent breakage, which occurs about 2% of the time.

Because condoms must be applied just before intercourse, some couples object to the interference with spontaneity. Others feel that condoms interfere with sensation. People who are allergic to latex should avoid the use of latex condoms because severe reactions are possible. Condoms may be affected by vaginal medications, and they should not be used concurrently.

FEMALE CONDOM. The female condom (also called a *vaginal pouch*) is a polyurethane sheath inserted into the vagina. A flexible ring fits over the cervix like a diaphragm, and another ring extends outside the vagina to partially cover the perineum (Figure 31-4). The female condom is the first contraceptive device that allows a woman some protection from STDs without relying on the male condom.

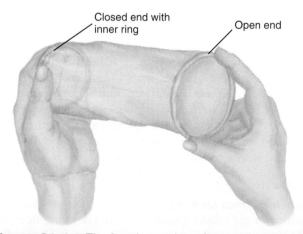

Closed end with inner ring   Open end

Figure 31-4 ■ The female condom. A woman can protect herself from sexually transmissible diseases without relying on use of the male condom.

The female condom is less effective than the male condom, with a typical failure rate of approximately 21%. Many women object to it on esthetic grounds. Use of the female condom is more likely if the woman has training in how to use it and can practice on a pelvic model (Van Devanter et al., 2002). Some women use the female condom some of the time and the male condom at other times (Macaluso et al., 2000). Male and female condoms should not be used together, however, as they may adhere to each other.

SPONGE. The contraceptive sponge is made of soft polyurethane that contains spermicide. It traps and absorbs semen and the spermicide nonoxynol-9 kills sperm. The sponge provides contraception for 24 hours without the need for added spermicide for repeated intercourse. It does not require a prescription, is easy to use, and can be inserted just before intercourse or hours before intercourse is expected.

To use the sponge, the woman should wash her hands and wet the sponge with water, squeezing it until it becomes sudsy. The sponge is folded with the concave ("dimple") area inside and the loop on the outside of the fold. It is then inserted into the vagina and released so the "dimple" covers the cervix. It should remain in place for at least 6 hours after intercourse. It is removed by inserting a finger into the loop and pulling slowly.

The sponge should not be left in the vagina for more than 30 hours. Prolonged use or use during menstruation increases the risk of toxic shock syndrome (see Chapter 33). It should not be used by women with a history of toxic shock syndrome and does not protect against STDs. The sponge may cause irritation or be difficult to remove for some women.

DIAPHRAGM. The diaphragm is a latex dome surrounded by a spring or coil. The woman places spermicidal cream or gel into the dome and around the rim, then inserts it over the cervix. When folded, some models arch to form a half-moon shape, which assists in proper placement.

Because it covers the cervix, the diaphragm prevents passage of sperm while holding spermicide in place for additional protection. The typical failure rate is 16%. Diaphragms must be fitted by a health care provider. The woman should be checked for size changes yearly, after a weight gain or loss of more than 10 lb, and after each pregnancy or abortion. The diaphragm should be replaced every 2 years. The correct size may not be available for all women.

To eliminate interference with spontaneity, some women insert the diaphragm hours in advance when intercourse is possible. Pressure on the urethra may cause irritation and urinary tract infections. The presence of allergies to latex or a history of toxic shock syndrome precludes use. The diaphragm may be damaged by oil-based lubricants and some medications used for vaginal infections.

CERVICAL CAP. The Prentif cervical cap, which has been used for some time, is no longer available. However, a new cap, FemCap, is available. The woman inserts the silicone cap over the cervix after placing spermicide on both sides. Because it is smaller than the diaphragm, the cervical cap does not cause pressure on the bladder. It can remain in place for 48 hours, and more spermicide is needed if intercourse is repeated. It should not be removed for 6 hours after the last intercourse. Insertion and removal are similar to those for the diaphragm, but there is a loop to assist in removal. It should not be used during menses or in women with a history of toxic shock syndrome. Cap sizes are based on whether the woman has had past pregnancies and births. It should be replaced after 2 years or after pregnancy.

LEA'S SHIELD. This device is made of silicone with a central valve and a loop to allow easy removal. It is filled with spermicide like a diaphragm or cap. A prescription is required. The shield must remain in place for 8 hours after last intercourse but not longer than 24 hours, and more spermicide should be added for repeated intercourse.

Natural Family Planning Methods

Natural family planning methods, also called *fertility awareness* or *periodic abstinence methods,* use physiologic cues to predict ovulation and avoid coitus when conditions are favorable for fertilization. They also help women who wish to become pregnant (see Chapter 32). The methods are based on knowledge that the ovum may be fertilized for approximately 24 hours and that most sperm survive no more than 24 hours in the female genital tract (although some sperm may live up to 5 days) (Guyton & Hall, 2000).

Natural family planning helps women learn about how their bodies change throughout the menstrual cycle. It is acceptable to most religious groups and avoids the use of drugs, chemicals, and devices. However, couples must be highly motivated because they must abstain from intercourse during as much as half the menstrual cycle. Natural family planning methods may be very effective, with failure rates ranging from 2% to 5% if used perfectly, but have a typical failure rate of 25%. The method is very unforgiving, and errors in predicting ovulation may lead to intercourse during the fertile time with a high risk for pregnancy. Some women use the method to determine when they are fertile and use a barrier contraceptive at that time.

CALENDAR

The calendar method is based on the timing of ovulation approximately 14 days before the onset of menses. To determine the range in cycle length, the woman keeps track of her cycles for 6 months and uses it to estimate when ovulation will occur (Table 31-6). The couple must abstain or use a barrier method during the days calculated to be fertile. The calendar method is unreliable because many factors such as illness or stress can affect the time of ovulation.

STANDARD DAYS METHOD

This method uses a string of beads that is color coded to help keep track of the days of each cycle. It is designed for women with cycles that vary from 26 to 32 days and is ineffective for women whose cycles are shorter or longer. Days 8 through 19 are considered the fertile days.

How to Use a Diaphragm

Follow instructions carefully when using your diaphragm. Skill at insertion and removal increases with practice.

- Plan to insert the diaphragm up to several hours before intercourse. Empty your bladder before insertion.
- Spread about a teaspoon of spermicidal cream or gel inside the dome and around the rim.

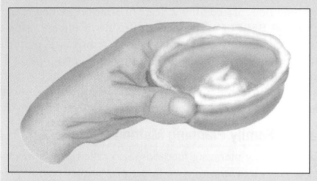

- Insert the diaphragm into the vagina with the spermicide toward the cervix. A squatting position or placing one foot on a chair makes insertion easier.

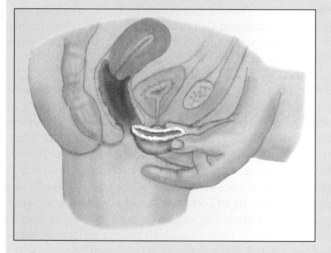

- Be sure that the front rim fits behind your pubic bone and that you can feel the cervix through the center of the diaphragm.

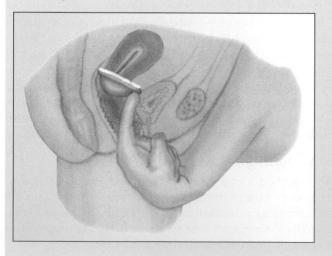

- If more than 6 hours pass between the insertion and intercourse or if you have intercourse again, insert more spermicide into the vagina without removing the diaphragm.
- Leave the diaphragm in place at least 6 hours after the last intercourse. Take it out the next morning. Leaving it in place more than 24 hours increases the risk of infection.
- Douching with the diaphragm in place is unnecessary and lessens effectiveness.
- To remove the diaphragm, assume a squatting position and bear down. Hook a finger around the front rim to break the suction, and pull down.

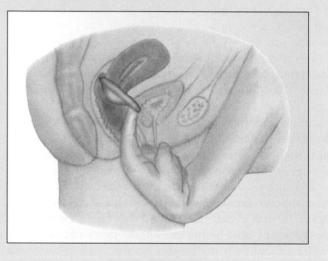

- Wash the diaphragm with mild soap and dry well after each use. Inspect it for small holes by holding it up to a light or filling it with water. If you find a hole, use another contraceptive method and go to your health care provider for a new diaphragm.

TABLE 31-6 Natural Family Planning Methods

Method and Failure Rate (Perfect Use)	Application	Comments
Calendar—9%	Subtract 18 days from shortest cycle and 11 days from longest cycle to determine fertile period.	Example: 28-32 day cycle = fertile between days 10 and 21 (28 − 18 = 10; 32 − 11 = 21).
Standard days method	Intercourse is allowed only on days 1-7 and 20 to the end of the cycle. Use a barrier method or abstain on days 8-19.	Ineffective if the cycle length is shorter than 26 days or longer than 32 days.
Basal body temperature	See Procedure 32-1, p. 863.	Avoid intercourse until the third day after temperature rise. Unreliable if used alone. Affected by illness, lack of sleep, stress.
Cervical mucus (ovulation or Billings)—3%	Assess mucus at vaginal orifice daily. Avoid intercourse during menses and from the time of thick, sticky mucus until 4 days after last day of clear, slippery, stretchy mucus.	Intercourse is allowed only every other day, as semen interferes with assessment of mucus. See Procedure 32-1.
Symptothermal—2%	Combine all above methods and assess weight gain, libido, bloating, and mittelschmerz.	Requires much education and motivation.

BASAL BODY TEMPERATURE

In the basal body temperature method, the woman charts her oral temperature each morning before getting out of bed or increasing her activity, which would cause her temperature to rise (see Procedure 32-1, p. 863). Some women have a slight temperature drop just before ovulation. With ovulation the temperature rises 0.2° to 0.4° C (0.4° to 0.8° F) and remains higher throughout the rest of the cycle because of progesterone. The woman is no longer fertile after the temperature rise. Used alone, this method is not reliable because temperature changes are very small and the rise in temperature indicates that ovulation has already occurred. Intercourse the day before the temperature rise may well result in pregnancy.

CERVICAL MUCUS

Also called the *ovulation* or *Billings* method, the cervical mucous technique is based on changes in cervical secretions caused by rising estrogen levels during the follicular phase of the menstrual cycle. The woman assesses the cervical mucus by wiping it from the vaginal orifice with tissue each day (see Procedure 32-1, p. 864). To prevent pregnancy, couples must avoid intercourse from the time clear stretchy mucus is first present to 4 days after the end of the slippery mucus.

SYMPTOTHERMAL METHOD

The symptothermal method combines the calendar, basal body temperature, and cervical mucus methods. In addition, symptoms that occur near ovulation, such as weight gain, abdominal bloating, mittelschmerz (pain on ovulation), and increased libido, are noted. This increases awareness of when ovulation occurs and increases effectiveness.

✓ CHECK YOUR READING

14. What education is important for women choosing an IUD?
15. How do barrier methods of contraception work?
16. What are the advantages and disadvantages of natural family planning methods?

Abstinence

Abstinence is avoidance of sexual intercourse and any activity that may allow sperm to enter the vagina. Although it is the only completely effective method of preventing pregnancy and STDs, abstinence requires perfect use to be effective. Depending on the time within the menstrual cycle it occurs, intercourse without the use of a contraceptive has up to an 85% chance of resulting in pregnancy. Most women are not abstinent for all of their reproductive lives but many practice abstinence at various intervals. Some women practice abstinence part of the time, but have other methods available to use if they decide to become sexually active. Periodic abstinence is also practiced by women using the natural family planning methods.

Nurses should support women who choose to be abstinent. Sexual education programs in schools often include information on ways to maintain abstinence. Adolescents especially need assistance to define their values and learn practical methods of reaching their goal of abstinence. Role playing often is used to help them work through situations in which they might have difficulty maintaining abstinence.

Abstinence has no cost, avoids the use of hormones, and has no side effects or medical risks. It must be practiced perfectly to avoid risking pregnancy or STDs, however. Therefore women should know where to get information about other contraceptive methods should they decide to become sexually active at a later time.

Least Reliable Methods of Contraception

The following methods of contraception are not considered reliable. However, they are used by women who lack information about their risks and other options or who do not wish to use other methods for medical or personal reasons. The nurse needs to be familiar with these methods to help women understand the risks involved.

BREASTFEEDING

Breastfeeding inhibits ovulation because suckling and prolactin interfere with secretion of gonadotropin-releasing hormone and luteinizing hormone. During lactation the ovarian response to follicle-stimulating hormone and luteinizing hormone may be altered. The frequency, intensity, and duration of suckling are very important in inhibiting ovulation.

Women who breastfeed completely with no supplements during the night as well as the day may avoid ovulation and resumption of menstrual cycles. However, use of formula or solid foods decreases the frequency and duration of breastfeeding, increases the length of time between feedings, and reduces night feedings. This may lead to ovulation and a return of menses. The menstrual cycle generally resumes by 6 months, even if the woman is fully breastfeeding. Another method of contraception should be used at 6 months or before that time if menses has resumed or supplementary feedings are used.

COITUS INTERRUPTUS

Also called *withdrawal,* coitus interruptus is the removal of the penis from the vagina before ejaculation. It has a failure rate of 27%. The method requires great control by the man and may be unsatisfying for both partners. Even a man who wishes to use the method may misjudge the timing and withdraw too late. Sperm spilled on the vulva may enter the vagina and cause pregnancy.

Application of the Nursing Process
Choosing a Contraceptive Method

Contraceptive failure often occurs because women lack knowledge about how to use their contraceptive methods correctly or choose methods unsuited to their needs. When contraception fails, the woman is exposed to the physical, psychological, and social consequences of unintended pregnancy. Lack of understanding also may expose her to unnecessary side effects, possible complications, or STDs.

Assessment

Because contraception is a very private matter, approach it in a sensitive manner. Perform the assessment in a quiet area where interruptions are unlikely, and keep voices low to increase the woman's comfort. Assure the woman that her confidentiality will be maintained.

INTRODUCING THE SUBJECT

In the postpartum setting, introduce the subject by asking the woman whether she plans to have more children. Most women indicate a desire to wait a period of time before the next pregnancy. Ask, "What method of family planning are you thinking about using now?" or "How did you feel about the method you used before pregnancy?" These questions may identify problems that the woman has had with contraception in the past.

Introduce the topic during well-woman checkups by asking about the woman's current contraceptive method and her satisfaction. In other settings a woman may make some reference to her contraceptive method. The nurse can respond by asking, "How do you like using (name method)?"

This shows the nurse is interested if the woman wishes to pursue the topic.

DETERMINING THE WOMAN'S UNDERSTANDING

Determine the woman's understanding of her contraceptive technique. For example, ask when she inserts her contraceptive ring, where she places her patch, or what time of day she takes her OC. The woman should know how to use her technique effectively and what to do in special circumstances, such as when she misses an OC pill. Explore any misinformation, concerns, or problems that she may have with regard to effectiveness, technique, or common side effects of the method.

ASSESSING THE WOMAN'S SATISFACTION

Assess the woman's satisfaction with her contraceptive. Women may be unsure about their method in the early months until they gain comfort from repetitive use. Satisfaction and effectiveness increase with greater familiarity with the method. Side effects also affect satisfaction. They may be severe enough to cause the woman to consider another method, or they may be relieved by simple techniques. A discussion of side effects may also identify more serious complications that necessitate referral for treatment.

ASSESSING APPROPRIATE CHOICES

If the woman is considering a change in contraceptive method, assess factors that would help determine the best method for her. Include a history of medical conditions that might eliminate certain methods, childbearing history, cultural and religious beliefs, and intensity of desire to prevent pregnancy. The woman's ability to understand and follow complicated directions is important as well.

The couple's relationship is important in terms of contraceptive choice and protection against STDs. If the relationship is mutually monogamous and neither partner is infected, STDs are not a risk. If there is a possibility that either member of the couple has more than one partner, protection against STDs with a barrier method is essential, even if the woman uses another type of contraceptive.

Frequency of coitus may help determine the best choice of contraception. For occasional sexual intercourse, a barrier method may be most satisfactory. If intercourse is frequent, the woman may desire a method that is always in place, such as an IUD or a hormone implant. Explore her past experience with other methods, what she considers important, and her individual preferences. The woman who wants to avoid hormones that have a systemic effect is not a candidate for OCs. Ask about beliefs and values that might eliminate certain choices.

Analysis

Lack of knowledge about family planning is common and can lead to physical, psychological, and social complications in a woman's life. A nursing diagnosis that addresses this problem is "Risk for Ineffective Health Maintenance related to lack of understanding about contraceptive methods chosen and available."

Planning

Goals and expected outcomes for this diagnosis are that the woman will:

- Correctly describe how to use her contraceptive method, including solving common problems
- Describe common side effects, indications of complications, and correct follow-up
- Report that she and her partner are satisfied with their contraceptive method or explore choosing another method

Interventions

Interventions involve follow-up of problems that may interfere with the woman's ability to maintain health and teaching about contraceptive techniques.

INCREASING UNDERSTANDING OF THE CHOSEN METHOD

Fill in gaps in the woman's knowledge about the way her contraceptive method works, its effectiveness, advantages and disadvantages, common side effects and complications, and when to seek help. Use demonstrations and return demonstrations for using the method (such as inserting a vaginal ring or checking for IUD strings). Give suggestions for managing side effects and common problems.

TEACHING ABOUT OTHER METHODS

Provide information about other forms of contraceptives, if the woman wishes. Compare other methods with the one the woman is using. Discuss aspects most important to the individual woman and her lifestyle. If the woman expresses interest in one or two other methods, discuss their characteristics. Include benefits, disadvantages, and risks of each method so that she can make an informed choice. She may wish to have written information to take home to discuss with her partner before making a final decision. If a prescription or fitting is needed for a new method, discuss what may happen during the visit.

PROTECTING AGAINST SEXUALLY TRANSMISSIBLE DISEASES

Address defense against STDs, particularly if the woman is using a method that does not provide protection. This is a delicate subject. A way to approach it might be to say, "The method you are using is very effective against pregnancy but does not protect you against diseases like HIV you might catch from a partner. If there is any chance that you or your partner might have sex with more than one person or that your partner might have an infection, you should protect yourself by using condoms along with your regular contraception."

INCLUDING THE WOMAN'S PARTNER

Invite the woman to include her partner in discussions, if possible. He may influence the woman's choice of contraception and whether she actually uses it and uses it correctly. If the partner understands the proper method of use, he may be more cooperative and willing to help ensure contraceptive success.

ONGOING TEACHING

If the woman chooses a new contraceptive method, instruct her to call if she has any questions or difficulties. Suggest that she visit again in 1 to 2 months to discuss her satisfaction with her method. Make a note in the chart to discuss contraception at her next visit, even if it is for another reason.

Evaluation

The woman should accurately describe all aspects of her contraceptive method, including ways to solve common problems and when to seek help for side effects or complications. At later visits, evaluate continued understanding, compliance with proper use, and satisfaction with the method. The woman who wishes to change her contraceptive method should describe other contraceptives available and how they should be used. She should choose a new method and, if necessary, visit a health care provider for further discussion, examination, fitting, or prescription.

SUMMARY CONCEPTS

- The average woman must consider use of contraception for as many as 35 years of her life.
- The nurse helps women with family planning by providing current, accurate information about contraception and assisting them to find methods that best meet their needs.
- Because some methods have potential for serious complications, an informed consent form may be necessary.
- Adolescents may lack knowledge about their own bodies, conception, and methods of contraception. Risk-taking behaviors are common.
- Because teenagers often do not wish to talk to their parents about contraception, they need alternative sources of information and counseling.
- The most successful methods of contraception for adolescents are often those unrelated to coitus. They need information about methods from a nurse with an accepting attitude.
- The healthy perimenopausal woman with no complications or risk factors such as smoking can use any method of contraception safely.
- Sterilization offers permanent contraception. A tubal ligation can be performed soon after birth or at any time. Vasectomy is less expensive and can be performed in an office, using local anesthesia. Although surgery to reverse sterilization is possible, it is expensive and not always successful.
- Hormonal contraceptives include oral contraceptives, hormone injections, patches, and vaginal rings. Hormonal contraceptives inhibit ovulation and make the cervical mucus unreceptive to sperm. Side effects and complications make these unsuitable for some women.
- Intrauterine devices are very effective and safe in women with no risk for sexually transmissible diseases. Women must check for the device's strings each month and know when to seek medical treatment.

- Barrier methods may be chemical or mechanical. They kill or prevent sperm from entering the cervix and provide some protection against sexually transmissible diseases.
- Natural family planning methods involve avoidance of coitus when physiologic cues suggest that ovulation is likely. Women need high motivation and extensive education about their bodies to be successful with these methods.

ANSWERS TO CRITICAL THINKING EXERCISE 31-1, p. 840

1. Find a private place to talk without interruption. Use therapeutic communication techniques to explore her feelings further. Help her think through the ways in which a pregnancy might change her life and how she would feel about those changes.
2. Explore what the teenager feels would be most embarrassing about seeing a physician. Would a female nurse practitioner, midwife, or physician be more acceptable? Discuss what happens when a woman is examined during a visit for contraceptive counseling. Let her know that a pelvic examination may not be necessary if she is not having any problems and that the provider may prescribe contraceptives without an examination on the first visit. Discuss common contraceptive methods and determine her understanding and feelings about them.
3. Discuss negotiation skills for condom use, because condoms are important for prevention of STDs as well as pregnancy. Try role playing, with the adolescent acting in the role of her partner and the nurse taking the role of the adolescent.

REFERENCES & READINGS

Abma, J.C., Martinez, G.M., Mosher, W.D., & Dawson, B.S. (2002). Teenagers in the United States: Sexual activity, contraceptive use, and childbearing, 2002. National Center for Health Statistics. *Vital Health Statistics, 23*(24), 2004.

Alan Guttmacher Institute. (2000). *Issue brief: Medicaid—A critical source of support for family planning in the United States.* Retrieved May 24, 2004, from http://www.agi-usa.org/.

Alan Guttmacher Institute (2003). *The Guttmacher report: Preventing unintended pregnancy—The need and the means.* Retrieved May 5, 2004, from http://www.agi-usa.org/.

American Cancer Society. (2005). *Cancer facts and figures 2005.* Atlanta: American Cancer Society.

Aytekin, N.T., Pala, K., Irgil, E., & Aytekin, H. (2001). Family planning choices and some characteristics of coitus interruptus users in Gemlik, Turkey. *Women's Health Issues, 11*(5), 442-447.

Cunningham, F.G., Leveno, K.J., Bloom, S.L., Hauth, J.C., Gilstrap, L.C., & Wenstrom, K.D. (2005). *Williams obstetrics* (22nd ed.). New York: McGraw-Hill.

Dardano, K., & Burkman, R.T. (2002). The contraceptive and non-contraceptive health benefits of oral contraceptives: An update. In S.B. Ransom, M.P. Donbrowski, M.I. Evans, & K.A. Ginsburg (Eds.), *Contemporary therapy in obstetrics and gynecology* (pp. 349-353). Philadelphia: Saunders.

Davidson, M.R. (2003). Contraception update: The latest hormonal options. (2003). *Clinician Reviews, 13*(6), 53-59.

Davis, A.H. (2003). Pediatric and adolescent gynecology. In J.R. Scott, R.S. Gibbs, B.Y. Karlan, A.F. Haney (Eds.), *Danforth's obstetrics and gynecology* (9th ed., pp. 529-540). Philadelphia: Lippincott.

Dieben, T.O.M., Roumen, F.J.M.E., & Apter, D. (2002). Efficacy, cycle control, and user acceptability of a novel combined contraceptive vaginal ring. *Obstetrics & Gynecology, 100*(3), 585-593.

English, A., & Ford, C.A. (2004). The HIPAA privacy rule and adolescents: Legal questions and clinical challenges. *Perspectives on Sexual and Reproductive Health, 35*(2), 80-86.

Flynn, D.M., Clark, J.B., & Hume, R.F. (2002). Unintended pregnancy. In S.B. Ransom, M.P. Donbrowski, M.I. Evans, & K.A. Ginsburg (Eds.), *Contemporary therapy in obstetrics and gynecology* (pp. 157-163). Philadelphia: Saunders.

Garcia, F.A.R., & Huggins, G.R. (2002). Emergent postcoital contraception. In S.B. Ransom, M.P. Donbrowski, M.I. Evans, & K.A. Ginsburg (Eds.), *Contemporary therapy in obstetrics and gynecology* (pp. 359-361). Philadelphia: Saunders.

Gold, C., Nardontonia, T., & Condon, M.C. (2004). Gynecological wellness and illness. In M.C. Condon (Ed.), *Women's health: Body, mind, spirit* (pp. 319-364). Upper Saddle River, NJ: Prentice-Hall.

Grady, W.R., Billy, J.O.G., & Kepinger, D.H. (2002). Contraceptive method switching in the United States. *Perspectives on Sexual and Reproductive Health, 34*(3), 135-145.

Grimes, D.A. (2004). Intrauterine devices (IUDs). In R.A. Hatcher, J. Trussell, F. Stewart, A.L. Nelson, W. Cates, F. Guest, & D. Kowal, *Contraceptive technology* (18th ed., pp. 495-530). New York: Ardent Media.

Grunbaum, J.A., Kann, L., Kinchen, S., Ross, J., Hawkins, J., Lowry, R., et al. (2004). Youth risk behavior surveillance—United States, 2003. *MMWR. Morbidity and Mortality Weekly Report, 53*(SS02), 1-96.

Guyton, A.C., & Hall, J.E. (2000). *Textbook of medical physiology* (10th ed.). Philadelphia: Saunders.

Hamilton, B.E., Martin, J.A., & Sutton, P.D. (2004). Births: Preliminary data for 2003, *National vital statistics reports, 53*(9). Hyattsville, MD: National Center for Health Statistics.

Harper, C., Callegari, L., Raine, T., Blum, M., & Darney, P. (2004). Adolescent clinic visits for contraception: Support from mothers, male partners, and friends. *Perspectives on Sexual and Reproductive Health, 36*(1), 20-26.

Hatcher, R.A. (2004). Depo-Provera injections, implants, and progestin-only pills (minipills). In R.A. Hatcher, J. Trussell, F. Stewart, A.L. Nelson, W. Cates, F. Guest, & D. Kowal. *Contraceptive technology* (18th ed., pp. 461-494). New York: Ardent Media.

Hatcher, R.A., & Nelson, A. (2004). Combined hormonal contraceptive methods. In R.A. Hatcher, J. Trussell, F. Stewart, Nelson, A.L., Cates, W., Guest, F., & Kowal, D. *Contraceptive technology* (18th ed, pp. 391-460). New York: Ardent Media.

Holt, V.L., Cushing-Haugen, K.L., & Daling, J.R. (2002). Body weight and risk of oral contraceptive failure. *Obstetrics & Gynecology, 99*(5), 820-827.

Hutti, M.H., (2003). New and emerging contraceptive methods. *AWHONN Lifelines, 7*(1), 34-39.

Jamieson, D.J., Kaufman, S.C., Costello, C., Hillis, S.D., Marchbanks, P.A., & Peterson, H.B. (2002). A comparison of women's regret after vasectomy versus tubal sterilization. *Obstetrics & Gynecology, 99*(6), 1073-1079.

Jones, M.E., Bond, M.L., Garnner, S.H., & Hernandez, M.C. (2002). A call to action: Acculturation level and family-planning patterns of Hispanic immigrant women. *MCN: American Journal of Maternal/Child Nursing, 27*(1), 26-32.

Kartoz, C.R. (2004). New options for teen pregnancy. *MCN: American Journal of Maternal/Child Nursing, 29*(1), 30-35.

Katz, A. (2003). "Where I come from, we don't talk about that": Exploring sexuality among Blacks, Asians, and Hispanics. *AWHONN Lifelines, 6*(6), 533-536.

Kaunitz, A. (2001). Choosing an injectable contraceptive. *Contemporary OB/GYN, 46*(6), 29-48.

Kelly, P.J., & Morgan-Kidd, J. (2001). Social influences on the sexual behaviors of adolescent girls in at-risk circumstances.

Journal of Obstetric, Gynecologic, and Neonatal Nursing, 30(5), 481-489.

Kennedy, K.I. (2005). Fertility, sexuality, & contraception during lactation. In J. Riordan (Ed.), *Breastfeeding and human lactation* (3rd ed., pp. 621-651). Boston: Jones and Bartlett.

Kridli, S.A. (2002). Health beliefs and practices among Arab women. *MCN: American Journal of Maternal/Child Nursing, 27*(3), 178-182.

Lindberg, C.E. (2003). Emergency contraception for prevention of adolescent pregnancy. *MCN: American Journal of Maternal/Child Nursing, 28*(3), 199-204.

Link, D.G. (2004). Family planning. In S. Mattson & J.E. Smith (Eds.), *Core curriculum for maternal-newborn nursing* (3rd ed., pp. 409-418). Philadelphia: Saunders.

Macaluso, M., Demand, M., Artz, L., Fleenor, M., Robey, L., Kelaghan, J., et al. (2000). Female condom use among women at high risk of sexually transmitted disease. *Family Planning Perspectives, 32*(3), 138-144.

Moos, M.K. (2003). Unintended pregnancies: A call for nursing action. *MCN: American Journal of Maternal/Child Nursing, 28*(1), 24-30.

Mosher, W.D., Martinez, G.M., Chandra, A., Abma, J.C., & Willson, S.J. (2004). Use of contraception and use of family planning services in the United States, 1982-2002. *Advance data from vital and health statistics.* No. 350. Hyattsville, MD: National Center for Health Statistics.

National Center for Health Statistics. (2005). QuickStats: Primary contraceptive methods among women aged 15-44 years–United States, 2002. Retrieved Feb. 17, 2005, from http://www.cdc.gov/mmwr.

Ott, M.A., Adler, N.E., Millstein, S.G., Tschann, J.M., & Ellen, J.M. (2002). The trade-off between hormonal contraceptives and condoms among adolescents. *Perspectives on Sexual and Reproductive Health, 34*(1), 6-14.

Paukku, M., Quan, J., Darney, P., & Raine, T. (2003). Adolescents' contraceptive use and pregnancy history. Is there a pattern? *Obstetrics & Gynecology, 101*(3), 534-538.

Peterson, H., Curtis, K.M., Meirik, O., d'Arcangues, C. (2003). Contraception. In J.R. Scott, R.S. Gibbs, B.Y. Karlan, & A.F. Haney (Eds.), *Danforth's obstetrics and gynecology* (9th ed., pp. 541-559). Philadelphia: Lippincott Williams & Wilkins.

Peterson, R., Gazmararian, J.A., Clark, K.A., & Green, D.C. (2001). How contraceptive use patterns differ by pregnancy intention: Implications for counseling. *Women's Health Issues, 11*(5), 427-435.

Pollack, A.E., Carignan, C.S., & Jacobstein, R. (2004). Female and male sterilization. In R.A. Hatcher, J. Trussell, F. Stewart, A.L. Nelson, W. Cates, F. Guest, & D. Kowal. *Contraceptive technology* (18th ed., pp. 531-573). New York: Ardent Media.

Schnare, S.M. (2002). Progestin contraceptives. *Journal of Midwifery & Women's Health, 47*(3), 157-166.

Siebert, C., Barbouche, E., & Fagan, J. (2003). Prescribing oral contraceptives for women older than 35 years of age. (Electronic version.) *Annals of Internal Medicine, 138*(1), 54-64.

Simpson, K.R., & James, D.C. (2005). *Postpartum care.* White Plains, NY: March of Dimes Birth Defects Foundation.

Sonfield, A., Benson, R., & Frost, J.J. (2004). U.S. insurance coverage of contraceptives and the impact of contraceptive coverage mandates, 2002. *Perspectives on Sexual and Reproductive Health, 365*(2), 72-79.

Speroff, L., & Darney, P.D. (2001). *A clinical guide for contraception* (3rd ed.). Philadelphia: Lippincott Williams & Wilkins.

Stevens-Simon, C., Beach, R.K., & Klerman, L.V. (2001). To be rather than not to be–that is the problem with the questions we ask adolescents about their childbearing intentions. *Archives of Pediatric Adolescent Medicine, 155,* 1298-1300.

Stewart, F., Trussell, J., & Van Look, P.F.A. (2004). Emergency contraception. In R.A. Hatcher, J. Trussell, F. Stewart, A.L. Nelson, W. Cates, F. Guest, & D. Kowal. *Contraceptive technology* (18th ed., pp. 279-303). New York: Ardent Media.

Tinkle, M., Reifsnider, E., & Ransom, S.P. (2002). A quality assurance problem: Why women quit using Depo-Provera. *AWHONN Lifelines, 5*(6), 36-41.

Trussell, J. (2004). The essentials of contraception: Efficacy, safety, and personal considerations. In R.A. Hatcher, J. Trussell, F. Stewart, A.L. Nelson, W. Cates, F. Guest, & D. Kowal. *Contraceptive technology* (18th ed., pp. 221-252). New York: Ardent Media.

Trussell, J., Brown, S., Hogue, C. (2004). Adolescent sexual behavior, pregnancy, and childbearing. In R.A. Hatcher, J. Trussell, F. Stewart, A.L. Nelson, W. Cates, F. Guest, & D. Kowal. *Contraceptive technology* (18th ed., pp. 701-744). New York: Ardent Media.

Tufts, K.A., & Chung, C. (2003). Prescribing oral contraceptives: Focusing on each woman as an individual case. *AWHONN Lifelines, 7*(4), 332-338.

Upchurch, D.M., Kusunoki, Y., Simon, P., & Doty, M.M. (2003). Sexual behavior and condom practices among Los Angeles women. *Women's Health Issues, 13*(1), 8-15.

U.S. Department of Health and Human Services. (2000). *Healthy People 2010: Healthy People 2010* (Conference edition, in 2 volumes). Washington, DC.

Van Devanter, N., Gonzales, V., Merzel, C., Parikh, N., Celantano, D., & Greenberg, J. (2002). Effect of an STD-HIV behavioral intervention on women's use of the female condom. *American Journal of Public Health, 92*(1), 109-115.

VandeVusse, L., Hanson, L., Fehring, R.J., Newman, A., & Fox, J. (2003). Couples' views of the effects of natural family planning on marital dynamics. *Journal of Nursing Scholarship, 35*(2), 171-176.

Villarruel, A.M., & Rodriguez, D. (2003). Beyond stereotypes: Promoting safer sex behaviors among Latino adolescents. *Journal of Obstetric, Gynecologic, and Neonatal Nursing, 32*(2), 258-263.

Weiner, C.P. & Buhimschi, C. (2004). *Drugs for pregnant and lactating women.* New York: Churchill Livingstone.

Weisman, C.S., Maccannon, D.S., Henderson, J.T., Shortridge, E., & Orso, C.L. (2002). Contraceptive counseling in managed care: Preventing unintended pregnancy in adults. *Women's Health Issues, 12*(2), 79-95.

Zieman, M., Guillebaud, J., Weisberg, E. Shangold, G.A., Fisher A.C., & Creasy, G.W. (2002). Contraceptive efficacy and cycle control with the Ortho Evra/Evra transdermal system: The analysis of pooled data. *Fertility and Sterility, 77*(2 Suppl. 2), S13-S18.

After studying this chapter, you should be able to:

1. Describe settings in which the nurse may encounter couples with infertility problems.
2. Explain factors that can impair a couple's ability to conceive.
3. Explain factors that may cause repeated pregnancy losses.
4. Specify evaluations that may be performed when a couple seeks help for infertility.
5. Explain the use of procedures and treatments that may aid a couple's ability to conceive and carry the fetus to viability.
6. Analyze ways in which infertility can affect a couple and other family members.
7. Summarize the nurse's role in caring for couples experiencing problems with fertility.

Go to your Student CD-ROM for Review Questions keyed to these Objectives.

DEFINITIONS

Anovulatory (or Anovular) Relating to menstrual cycles that occur without ovulation.

Assisted Reproductive Techniques Medical, surgical, laboratory, and micromanipulation techniques used with ova and sperm to improve chances of conception.

Azoospermia Absence of sperm in semen.

Basal Body Temperature Body temperature at rest.

Climacteric Endocrine, body, and psychic changes occurring at the end of a woman's reproductive period. Also informally called *menopause*.

Endometriosis Presence of endometrial tissue (uterine lining) outside the uterine cavity.

Erectile Dysfunction Consistent inability of a man to achieve or maintain an erection of the penis that is sufficiently rigid to permit successful sexual intercourse. Also called *impotence*.

Ferning (or Fern Test) The microscopic fernlike appearance of dried cervical mucus that is most apparent at the time of ovulation.

Gametogenesis Development and maturation of the sperm and ova.

Gestational Surrogate A woman who carries the embryo of an infertile couple and relinquishes the child to the couple after birth.

Impotence See *erectile dysfunction*.

Incompetent Cervix Inability of the cervix to remain closed long enough during pregnancy for the fetus to reach a maturity sufficient to survive.

Infertility Inability of a couple to conceive after 1 year of regular intercourse (two to three times weekly) without using contraception; also, the involuntary inability to conceive and produce viable offspring when the couple chooses. Primary infertility occurs in a couple who has never conceived; secondary infertility occurs in a couple who has conceived at least once before.

Oligospermia A decreased number of sperm in semen, usually considered to be under 20 million per milliliter.

Retrograde Ejaculation Discharge of semen into the bladder rather than from the end of the penis.

Semen Spermatozoa with their nourishing and protective fluid; discharged at ejaculation.

Spinnbarkheit Clear, slippery, stretchy quality of cervical mucus during ovulation.

Sterility Total inability to conceive.

Surrogate Mother A fertile woman who is inseminated with the purpose of conceiving and relinquishing a child to an infertile couple.

Varicocele Abnormal dilation or varicosity of veins in the spermatic cord.

Infertility nursing is a specialty, but general practice nurses also meet couples who are seeking help or have had treatment for infertility in varied settings. The nurse's own friends and family members often turn to the nurse as a source of information when they have problems conceiving. Nurses working in the perioperative area may care for these couples during diagnostic or therapeutic surgery. Nurses in urology settings often see men who are being evaluated or treated for infertility. In the emergency department, nurses may care for women who are having a spontaneous loss of a hard-won pregnancy.

Nurses in antepartum, intrapartum, and postpartum settings often encounter women with high-risk pregnancies or couples who have a new baby after infertility therapy. In addition, parenthood after infertility is not always easy, and nurses in pediatric and psychosocial settings may counsel families about parenting and changes in their personal relationships.

EXTENT OF INFERTILITY

The extent of infertility depends on its definition. Infertility is not an absolute condition but is a reduced ability to conceive. *Infertility* is strictly defined as the inability to conceive after 1 year of unprotected, regular sexual intercourse. A more workable definition does not specify a time limit but recognizes that infertility is any involuntary inability to conceive when desired. The definition is commonly expanded to include couples who conceive but repeatedly lose a pregnancy (pregnancy wastage) before the fetus is old enough to survive. Couples with primary infertility have never conceived. Couples with secondary infertility may have conceived before but are unable to conceive again.

About 10% to 20% of couples cannot have a baby when they desire. In 1995 the most recent U.S. data, about 9 million women had used infertility services because they could not have a baby when desired. Slightly more women, or 9.3 million, were currently in infertility therapy at the time of the national survey (Abma, Chandra, Mosher, Peterson, & Piccinino, 1997; American Society for Reproductive Medicine [ASRM], 2004). Current national statistics may be higher, because those who have been unable conceive or carry their offspring may try the newer therapies. Couples who delay childbearing until their mid to late 30s or later feel pressured by the approaching end of the woman's reproductive years. To older couples, delay in achieving pregnancy or having a living baby is more significant than for young couples, who have more time to pursue pregnancy and make treatment decisions. As new methods of diagnosis and treatment emerge, couples who once accepted childlessness may enter infertility therapy or resume therapy they abandoned. Also, some women want to have a child without a male partner and may be served by infertility services.

FACTORS CONTRIBUTING TO INFERTILITY

Conception depends not only on normal reproductive function in each partner but also on a sensitive interaction between the partners. For some couples, identification and treatment of infertility are simple, but others require complex evaluation and treatment. Factors in the United States and United Kingdom that have increased demand for infertility care include the following (Balen & Jacobs 2003):

- Age at which the woman attempts to conceive has risen, increasing the possibility that she will need infertility therapy.
- Male fertility has declined, reducing the chance that the man will father children without therapy.
- Expectations of successful results of infertility therapy have risen.

Because some factors contributing to infertility remain unknown, treatment of an identified problem does not always lead to a successful pregnancy. For example, it may be likely that a couple will be infertile because of problems in either or both partners, yet the couple nevertheless has several children. About 20% of infertile couples have no identified problem, yet some never conceive despite having undergone all available treatments.

Factors in the Man

The test of a man's fertility is his ability to initiate pregnancy in a fertile woman. Few absolute criteria exist to distinguish normal from abnormal male fertility, although an adequate number of sperm having normal structure and function must be deposited near the woman's cervix. Problems may exist with the sperm, erection or ejaculation of semen, or the seminal fluid that carries the sperm into the woman's reproductive tract.

ABNORMALITIES OF THE SPERM

Many factors can impair the number, structure, or function of sperm. Some conditions are temporary, such as an acute illness. Other conditions are permanent, such as a genetic disorder. A single or several findings may be abnormal. Further complicating evaluation of a man's fertility are the normal daily variations in semen.

Evaluation of the semen may reveal that the man has azoospermia or oligospermia. The average number of sperm released at ejaculation has a wide range of normal, 40 to 250 million (Blackburn, 2003). Twenty million sperm with normal motility per milliliter of semen is probably the minimum number adequate for unassisted fertilization (Guyton & Hall, 2000; Jones & DeCherney, 2003b).

A sufficient number of normal sperm must move in a purposeful direction to reach the ovum in the fallopian tube. Semen analysis is used to evaluate whether the quantities and qualities of sperm and the seminal fluid are likely to result in successful conception, assuming that the woman's studies are normal. Abnormal sperm structure or movement may reduce fertility, regardless of the actual number of sperm (Figure 32-1). Inflammatory processes in the man's reproductive organs may cause the sperm to clump, inhibiting their motility and fertilizing ability. Other sperm may have a normal appearance but may not be able to penetrate the ovum.

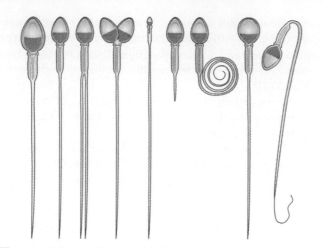

Figure 32-1 ■ Abnormal infertile sperm compared with a normal sperm on the left. (From Guyton, A.C., & Hall, J.E. [2000]. *Textbook of medical physiology* [10th ed., p. 920]. Philadelphia: Saunders.)

Factors that can impair the number and function of the sperm include the following:

- Abnormal hormonal stimulation of sperm production
- Acute or chronic illness such as mumps, cirrhosis, or renal failure
- Infections of the genital tract
- Anatomic abnormalities such as a varicocele or obstruction of the ducts that carry sperm to the penis
- Exposure to toxins such as lead, pesticides, or other chemicals
- Therapeutic treatments such as antineoplastic drugs or radiation for cancer
- Excessive alcohol intake
- Use of illicit drugs such as marijuana or cocaine
- An elevated scrotal temperature resulting from febrile illness, repeated use of saunas or hot tubs, or sitting for prolonged periods of time
- Immunologic factors, produced by the man against his own sperm (autoantibodies) or by the woman, causing the sperm to clump or be unable to penetrate the ovum

ABNORMAL ERECTIONS

Abnormal erections reduce the man's ability to deposit sperm-bearing seminal fluid in the woman's upper vagina. Erections are influenced by physical and psychological factors. Central nervous system dysfunction, which may be caused by drugs, psychiatric disturbance, or chronic illness, can interfere with erections. Surgery and disorders affecting the spinal cord or autonomic nervous system also may disrupt normal erections. Peripheral vascular disease reduces the amount of blood entering the penis and thereby reduces the ability to maintain an erection. Drugs such as antihypertensives or antidepressants may reduce the erection or shorten its duration.

ABNORMAL EJACULATION

Abnormal ejaculation prevents deposition of the sperm in the ideal place to achieve pregnancy. Retrograde ejaculation is the release of semen backward into the bladder rather than forward through the tip of the penis. Conditions that may cause retrograde ejaculation are diabetes, neurologic disorders, surgery that impairs function of the sympathetic nerves, and drugs such as antihypertensives and psychotropics. Men who have suffered spinal cord injury may retain the ability to ejaculate, depending on the level of cord damage.

Anatomic abnormalities such as hypospadias (urethral opening on the underside of the penis) may cause deposition of semen near the vaginal outlet rather than near the cervix.

Excessive alcohol intake or use of illicit drugs can adversely affect ejaculation as well as sperm number and function. Ejaculation may be slow, absent, or retrograde when a man takes drugs that affect neurologic coordination of this event. Premature ejaculation is usually related to psychological disorders such as performance anxiety or unresolved conflicts.

ABNORMALITIES OF SEMINAL FLUID

The seminal fluid nourishes, protects, and carries sperm into the vagina until they enter the cervix. Only sperm enter the cervix; the seminal fluid remains in the vagina. Semen coagulates immediately after ejaculation but liquefies within 30 minutes, permitting forward movement of sperm. Seminal fluid that remains thick traps the sperm, impeding their movement into the cervix. The pH of seminal fluid is slightly alkaline to protect the sperm from the acidic secretions of the vagina. Adequate fructose, citric acid, and other nutrients must be present to provide energy for the sperm.

The specific abnormality found in the seminal fluid suggests the cause of the abnormality, such as obstruction or infection in a specific area of the genital tract. Seminal fluid that is abnormal in amount, consistency, or chemical composition suggests obstruction, inflammation, or infection. The presence of large numbers of leukocytes suggests infection.

✓ CHECK YOUR READING

1. How is infertility defined? What is the difference between primary and secondary infertility?
2. What are normal characteristics of sperm and the seminal fluid that carries sperm into the woman's vagina?
3. What problems in the man can occur with erection? With ejaculation of semen?
4. What can cause abnormalities in the sperm, ejaculation, and seminal fluid?

Factors in the Woman

A woman's fertility depends on the following:

- Regular production of normal ova
- An open path from her cervix to the fallopian tube to permit fertilization and movement of the embryo into the uterus for implantation
- A uterine endometrium that supports the pregnancy after implantation

See Chapter 4 for a complete discussion of the interrelated factors that contribute to normal female fertility.

DISORDERS OF OVULATION

Normal ovulation depends on delicately timed and balanced secretions from the hypothalamus and pituitary and an ovarian response to mature and release an ovum. The hypothalamus secretes gonadotropin-releasing hormone (GnRH) beginning even before the obvious changes of puberty. GnRH stimulates the pituitary to release follicle-stimulating hormone (FSH) and luteinizing hormone (LH). FSH stimulates maturation of several follicles in the ovary. As the follicles mature, the ovary secretes estrogen to thicken the endometrium. About 24 to 36 hours before ovulation, a marked increase of LH occurs, which stimulates final maturation and release of one ovum from its follicle. The other follicles regress permanently. The collapsed follicle from which the ovum was released, now called a *corpus luteum*, produces progesterone and estrogen, which further prepare the endometrium for implantation and nourishment of the fertilized ovum.

Ovulation can be disrupted by many factors, including the following:

- A dysfunction in the hypothalamus or pituitary gland that alters the secretion of GnRH, FSH, and LH
- Failure of the ovaries to respond to FSH and LH stimulation, preventing maturation and release of the ovum

Disruption of hormone secretion or the ovarian response to hormone secretion can be caused by many factors such as cranial tumors, stress, obesity, anorexia, systemic disease, and abnormalities in the ovaries or other endocrine glands. As a woman approaches the end of her reproductive life, she ovulates and menstruates more erratically. Thus her fertility naturally declines with age, falling dramatically after age 40. An occasional woman may be infertile at a younger age because of premature ovarian failure, also known as *early menopause*.

A woman does not produce new oocytes after her birth. Her existing oocytes therefore are vulnerable to aging and to cumulative toxic effects from therapeutic drugs, social or abused drugs, and environmental agents until the end of her reproductive life. Examples of factors that may impair normal ovulation include cancer chemotherapeutic agents, excessive alcohol intake, and cigarette smoking.

Women with ovulation disorders often have abnormal menses because hormone levels do not permit normal development and shedding of the endometrium. The woman may have absent, scant, or heavy menstrual periods. However, other women may have no menstrual disorders and the inability to conceive may be their only complaint.

ABNORMALITIES OF THE FALLOPIAN TUBES

At least one open fallopian tube is needed for natural conception and implantation to occur (Figure 32-2). Tubal obstruction may occur because of scarring and adhesions after reproductive tract infections. Infections such as chlamydia, gonorrhea, and other sexually transmissible diseases (STDs) are responsible for many cases of infertility from tubal obstruction. Prevention or prompt treatment and eradication of pelvic infections can reduce the incidence of fallopian tube damage.

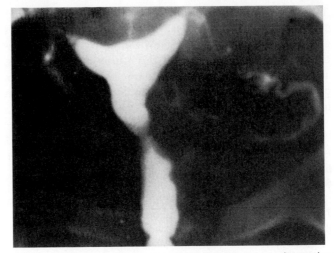

Figure 32-2 ■ A hysterosalpingogram can determine whether fallopian tubes are patent. When tubes are open, as in this photograph, contrast medium that was injected through the cervix spills out of the fallopian tubes into the peritoneal cavity. (From Hacker, N.F., Moore, J.G., & Gambone, J.C. [2004]. *Essentials of obstetrics and gynecology* [4th ed., p. 418A]. Philadelphia: Saunders.)

Endometriosis may cause tubal adhesions, painful menstrual periods, and painful intercourse. Small lesions are unlikely to affect tubal function, but large lesions can distort tubal anatomy and lead to infertility.

Tubal obstruction also may occur if adhesions develop after pelvic surgery, ruptured appendix, peritonitis, or ovarian cysts. In addition, the fallopian tubes and other reproductive organs may have congenital anomalies that disrupt normal function.

The conditions that cause obstruction also may interfere with normal motility within the fallopian tube. Poor movement of the fimbriated (distal) end of the tube may prevent the pickup of the ovum from the ovarian surface after ovulation. Abnormal action of the cilia within the tube prevents normal transport of the ovum toward the uterine cavity.

Depending on the extent and location of the blockage, fallopian tube obstructions can prevent fertilization of the ovum or lead to an ectopic pregnancy. Complete tubal occlusion prevents fertilizing sperm from reaching the ovum, and the woman will be sterile without the use of advanced techniques such as in vitro fertilization (IVF). Partial obstruction may result in a tubal ectopic pregnancy because sperm can reach the ovum to fertilize it but the embryo cannot reach the uterine cavity to implant.

ABNORMALITIES OF THE CERVIX

Estrogen levels from the ovary peak twice during the menstrual cycle, once before ovulation and again about 1 week after ovulation. The first peak occurs about 2 days before ovulation and causes the woman's cervix to dilate slightly and produce a clear, thin, slippery mucus that is similar to egg white in consistency. This mucus facilitates passage of sperm into the uterus and capacitation to prepare one sperm for fertilization. Low estrogen levels prevent development of this mucus and are usually associated with anovulation.

Polyps or scarring from past surgical procedures such as cauterization or conization may obstruct the woman's cervix. Abnormal cervical mucus caused by estrogen deficiency, surgical destruction of the mucus-secreting glands, and cervical damage secondary to infection or other factors prevent normal capacitation and movement of the sperm into the uterus and fallopian tubes for fertilization.

✔ CHECK YOUR READING

5. What factors can result in abnormal ovulation?
6. Why does a woman with ovulation problems often have abnormal menstrual periods?
7. What are some causes of fallopian tube obstruction?
8. How do abnormalities of cervical mucus contribute to infertility?

Repeated Pregnancy Loss

Couples who repeatedly lose pregnancies have the same result as those unable to conceive: no living child after conception. Repeated losses may result from abnormalities in the fetus or placenta or from maternal factors.

ABNORMALITIES OF THE FETAL CHROMOSOMES

Errors in the fetal chromosomes may result in spontaneous abortion, usually in the first trimester. Chromosome abnormalities often severely disrupt development, and the embryo or fetus cannot survive to live birth. Maternal age–associated chromosome abnormalities in the ova increase spontaneous abortions and decrease live births in women who conceive.

Most chromosome abnormalities are sporadic, occurring randomly. Others occur because one parent has a balanced chromosome translocation that is passed on to the offspring. The parent with the balanced translocation has a normal total amount of chromosome material, but the chromosome material is rearranged. When the chromosomes are divided during gametogenesis, the resulting sperm or ovum may receive too much or too little chromosome material, or it may receive a balanced translocation like the parent. The sperm or ovum also may receive a normal chromosome complement with no translocation. (See Chapter 5 for more information about chromosome abnormalities that may affect fertility.)

ABNORMALITIES OF THE CERVIX OR UTERUS

Stenosis or congenital malformations of the cervix or uterine cavity may cause repeated loss of a normal embryo or fetus (Figure 32-3). These malformations may prevent normal implantation of the fertilized ovum or normal prenatal growth of the placenta or fetus. Others may increase the risk for miscarriage or birth before the fetus is viable.

Women who were exposed prenatally to diethylstilbestrol (DES), a synthetic estrogen, are more likely to have uterine malformations or an incompetent cervix. Cervical or uterine abnormalities also may occur after surgery or trauma from a previous birth. Painless and premature cervical dilation, often early in the second trimester, is characteristic in the woman with an incompetent cervix. Uterine malformations occur in many forms and may result in early spontaneous abortion

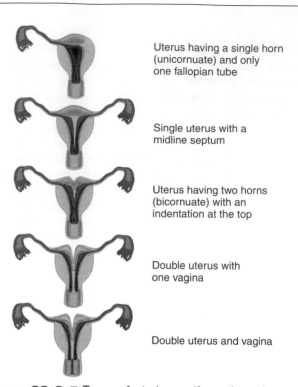

Uterus having a single horn (unicornuate) and only one fallopian tube

Single uterus with a midline septum

Uterus having two horns (bicornuate) with an indentation at the top

Double uterus with one vagina

Double uterus and vagina

Figure 32-3 ■ Types of uterine malformations that may cause infertility or repeated pregnancy loss.

(miscarriage) or preterm labor. A few women (<0.05%) developed adenocarcinoma. DES use was discontinued in the early 1970s because of these risks. A small number of women, now in their mid to late 30s, may be affected by DES when trying to conceive and carry a baby. Most exposed women are past their childbearing years, but the risks of DES must be considered when evaluating them for gynecologic problems.

Uterine myomas (benign tumors of the uterine muscle) and adhesions inside the uterine cavity may cause repeated fetal losses. These problems can alter the blood supply to the developing fetus or cause uterine irritability that results in preterm labor and birth.

ENDOCRINE ABNORMALITIES

Inadequate progesterone secretion by the corpus luteum (luteal phase defect) prevents normal implantation and establishment of the placenta. The embryo may not implant, or it may implant poorly. In other cases, the corpus luteum may develop and function properly but the woman's endometrium may not respond to its progesterone secretion.

Hypothyroidism and hyperthyroidism may be associated with the inability to conceive and with recurrent pregnancy loss. Poorly controlled diabetes can result in repeated pregnancy loss and many other complications of pregnancy because of its effects on maternal blood glucose levels and the vascular system (see Chapter 26).

IMMUNOLOGIC FACTORS

Immunologic factors are implicated in some cases of recurrent pregnancy loss, although not all are established conclusively. The embryo has antigens different from those of the mother and ordinarily would be rejected like any other foreign tissue. However, the mother's body normally blocks this rejection response and tolerates the developing baby. Some women's bodies respond inappropriately to the embryo, rejecting it as any other foreign tissue. These women often have recurrent spontaneous abortions.

Women with autoimmune disease such as systemic lupus erythematosus (SLE) are more likely to experience fetal loss. Pregnancy loss in these women appears related to thrombosis or other damage in placental blood vessels. Women with SLE often have other complications during pregnancy, such as exacerbation of their symptoms, fetal heart block, nonreassuring fetal status on antepartum tests or labor monitoring, and fetal death.

ENVIRONMENTAL AGENTS

Some environmental agents have a well-established relationship to impairment of fertility and pregnancy loss. Others are believed to be damaging but do not show a conclusive link to pregnancy loss. In addition, the amount of exposure (dose) relates to the pregnancy outcome in most cases. For example, radiation exposure in the form of a chest radiograph is unlikely to have an adverse effect on pregnancy, whereas the larger doses used for cancer therapy might be toxic.

Examples of established toxins are ionizing radiation, alcohol, and isotretinoin (Accutane). Suspected or known toxins are numerous—for example, cigarette smoke, anesthetic gas, chemicals such as organic solvents or pesticides, and lead and mercury in occupational settings. These agents may be directly toxic to the embryo or fetus, causing its death, or they may interfere with the normal placental function necessary to sustain the pregnancy.

INFECTIONS

Infections of the reproductive tract are associated with general complications of pregnancy, and they also may be related to early pregnancy losses. These infections often are asymptomatic, making their diagnosis and link to pregnancy loss difficult to establish. Chapter 26 provides greater details about significant infections affecting pregnancy.

✔ CHECK YOUR READING

9. How can anatomic abnormalities of a woman's uterus or cervix cause her to lose a normal pregnancy?
10. What endocrine factors can cause repeated pregnancy loss?
11. What known immunologic factors may cause loss of a normal fetus?

EVALUATION OF INFERTILITY

Devine (2003) has likened the infertility evaluation to reading a mystery novel, moving from the simpler evaluations to the more complex ones. Couples are often in a hurry for definitive therapy, but a thorough assessment of their problem is essential for effective and financially sound treatment. Some tests, such as semen evaluation, must be repeated sequentially for an accurate picture. The prolonged evaluation process is frustrating to many couples, especially those who are anxious for a child before the end of the woman's reproductive years. In addition, the usefulness and well-accepted normal values are not yet established for some tests, and other diagnostic tests are investigational. Despite many examinations and tests, infertility remains unexplained in 10% to 20% of couples who seek care (ASRM, 2004; Devine, 2003).

Infertility specialists use the history, physical examinations, and diagnostic testing to identify the best course of treatment. The proposed treatments will consider the couple's ages, especially the woman's, and the results of their histories, physical examinations, and diagnostic testing. Therapy may require a series of steps rather than a single treatment.

Numerous professionals may be involved in evaluation and care of infertile couples: nurses, physicians specializing in reproductive medicine, gynecologists, urologists, microsurgeons, embryologists, and ultrasonographers. In addition, general and specialized laboratory facilities may provide diagnostic services. Psychological counseling may be offered to help the couple deal with personal issues such as the probability of success with therapy or their anticipated ages when their child reaches adulthood. Nurses working in infertility clinics often coordinate communication among the many providers and help the couple negotiate the maze of evaluation and treatment.

Preconception Counseling

Couples may be offered preconception counseling to help them evaluate their risk for birth defects and perhaps reduce their risk for bearing a child with a serious birth defect. Many women seeking infertility care are older than 35, an age at which having an infant with a chromosome defect increases (see Chapter 5). A thorough history and physical examination of both members of the couple, including their family histories, may identify increased risk for having a child with a single-gene defect. Counseling can help the woman understand *before conception* the importance of an adequate diet and avoidance of teratogens that can harm the developing fetus before she knows she is pregnant.

History and Physical Examination

A thorough history and physical examination of each partner can help identify the appropriate diagnostic tests and therapy and identify risks for birth defects in the couple's offspring.

HISTORY

The partners' general health history is reviewed to determine problems that affect their general health and fertility. A reproductive history including the following also is taken:

- The woman's menstrual pattern, including age at onset, length of cycle, and characteristics of menstrual periods (frequency, regularity, duration, amount of flow, pain)
- Any pregnancies, complications, and their outcomes

- Contraception methods, past and present
- Previous fertility of the man or woman with other partners
- Pattern of intercourse in relation to the woman's menstrual cycles
- Length of time the couple has had intercourse without using contraception
- Exposure to potential toxins; prescribed and over-the-counter medications
- Family history of multiple pregnancy losses, birth defects, or mental retardation
- Home tests the couple has used, such as basal body temperature or over-the-counter ovulation predictor kits
- Past surgeries, pelvic inflammatory disease, STDs, abnormal Pap tests and treatment

The past medical history, including childhood illnesses and surgery, and a history of exposure to toxins may give clues about the cause of infertility. The couple's past and present occupations may identify toxin exposure, stresses, or other adverse influences on reproduction. Investigation of their usual frequency and timing of intercourse may identify the need for a change to promote conception at the time of ovulation.

PHYSICAL EXAMINATION

Couples who seek help for infertility are usually healthy. However, a thorough physical examination of each partner may identify endocrine disturbances, cranial tumors, or un-diagnosed chronic disease. Examination of the reproductive organs may reveal structural defects, infection, cysts, or other abnormalities. Chromosomal analysis may be performed for couples experiencing repeated pregnancy loss that is not explained by other factors.

Diagnostic Tests

Each couple's evaluation is individualized, but, based on the history and physical examinations, testing generally proceeds from the tests that are simple, least invasive, and less expensive to the more complex and expensive diagnostics expected to pinpoint the problem. Simple evaluations are done simultaneously, but more complex tests are delayed until their need is established.

Common tests for early infertility evaluation include the following:

- Basal body temperature (Procedure 32-1) or, more commonly, ovulation predictor kits
- Hormone evaluations such as estrogen, progesterone, LH, FSH, and thyroid function
- Ultrasound
- Hysterosalpingogram
- Endometrial biopsy
- Semen analysis

Table 32-1 describes diagnostic tests that may be offered to an infertile couple and the nursing care associated with each.

INFERTILE COUPLES

WANT TO KNOW

What Is Infertility Treatment Like?

GENERAL

Both members of the couple are evaluated systematically to identify the most time- and cost-effective therapy.

Simpler evaluations and therapies are done before more complex efforts are undertaken.

A complete medical history is taken and physical examination performed for each partner.

The ages of the partners, particularly the woman's, are considered. Evaluations and therapy proceed more quickly if the woman is in her mid 30s or older.

Costs may be partially covered by insurance; check to see what your insurance covers.

Difficult decisions may be required at different times during evaluation and treatment. Decisions might include whether to proceed to more complex and expensive tests and therapies, whether to take a break from treatment, or whether to abandon treatment altogether.

Infertility treatment can be stressful, can occupy many hours per week, and requires a substantial commitment to self-care.

Infertility remains unexplained in as many as 20% of couples.

Internet resources for infertility include the Centers for Disease Control and Prevention (www.cdc.gov) and American Society for Reproductive Medicine (www.asrm.org).

MEN

Semen analysis is usually the first test. Several semen specimens are obtained over a period of several weeks to obtain the best evaluation.

Depending on your medical history, physical examination findings, and semen analysis, other diagnostic tests may be done (hormone assay, an ultrasound of your reproductive organs, a biopsy of your testicles, and specialized tests of sperm function).

Corrective measures may include medications, surgery, and methods to reduce the scrotal temperature.

WOMEN

The first evaluation is usually to determine whether you are ovulating each month. An ovulation predictor kit is most often used for this purpose. Self-assessment of your basal body temperature and cervical mucus may also be taught. These assessments are often done at the same time as other tests.

Other common evaluations include an ultrasound examination of your reproductive organs, a laparoscopy or hysteroscopy, and a hysterosalpingogram (x-ray of your uterus and tubes).

For some tests and therapies, an operative procedure is required (e.g., hysteroscopy, laparoscopy, laser surgery, and microsurgery).

Typically, infertility evaluations and treatments require more of the woman's time, energy, physical discomfort, and risk than the man's.

Corrective measures depend on the problem identified. Examples include medications, surgery, and advanced reproductive techniques, such as in vitro fertilization.

32-1 Teaching Women about Fertility Awareness

PURPOSES: To identify whether ovulation occurs and the probable time of ovulation and to monitor therapeutic effects of drugs given to induce ovulation

For additional information about fertility awareness, see the Planned Parenthood website (www.plannedparenthood.org).

BASAL BODY TEMPERATURE

The basal body temperature (BBT) is designed to detect the slight elevation in temperature that accompanies increased progesterone secretion in response to the luteinizing hormone (LH) surge and ovulation.

1. Teach the woman the relationship between her BBT and ovulation:
   a. The BBT is the lowest, or resting, temperature of the body.
   b. During the first half of the woman's menstrual cycle, her temperature is lower than during the second half of the cycle.
   c. The basal temperature often drops slightly just before ovulation. Not all women experience this fall in basal temperature.
   d. Progesterone is secreted during the second half of the cycle, rising just after ovulation. The BBT rises after the slight drop near ovulation and remains higher during the second half of the cycle.
   e. The BBT remains higher if conception occurs and falls about 2 to 4 days before menstruation if conception does not occur.

   This method of fertility awareness requires careful assessment and record keeping by the woman. She is more likely to have an accurate record if she understands the relationship between her basal temperature and ovulation.

2. Explain the occurrences that can interfere with the accuracy of her BBT. Examples include illness, restless or inadequate sleep (fewer than 6 hours), waking later than usual, traveling across time zones (jet lag), alcohol intake the evening before, sleeping under an electric blanket or on a heated waterbed, or performing any activity before taking the temperature. *Temperature changes are very slight at ovulation, and these factors can cause the temperature to rise even if ovulation has not occurred.*

3. Teach the woman how to take her basal temperature:
   a. Show the woman an electronic thermometer that digitally displays tenths of a degree. Determine if she knows how to use it, and answer any questions.
   b. Explain that she should place the thermometer under her tongue as soon as she awakens each morning and before any activity. It should remain in place until the electronic signal sounds.

   The temperature rise is slight (about 0.2° to 0.4° C [0.4° to 0.8° F]) higher than during the first half of the cycle). Understanding thermometer use increases the accuracy of the assessment.

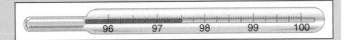

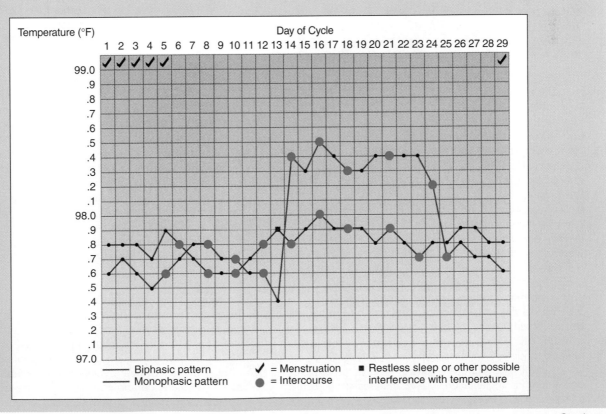

—— Biphasic pattern	✓ = Menstruation	■ Restless sleep or other possible
—— Monophasic pattern	● = Intercourse	interference with temperature

Continued

4. Show the woman the chart for recording her BBT and the symbols for marking relevant events, such as menstrual periods, intercourse, illness, or other occurrences that may alter her BBT. A string of colored beads may also be used, with different colors signifying whether the woman is having her menstrual flow (red), whether pregnancy is unlikely to occur (brown or tan), or if ovulation and fertility are likely (white). *The chart allows a more accurate interpretation of temperature fluctuations.*

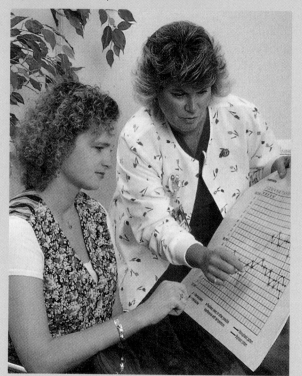

5. Encourage the woman to demonstrate taking her temperature and recording the result. Ask her to list events other than ovulation that can alter the BBT. *Discussion verifies that she has correctly understood the teaching and allows correction of misunderstandings.*
6. As a method to avoid pregnancy: Explain that for the greatest effectiveness, a woman should avoid intercourse from the onset of the menstrual period through the second day of elevated temperature. *The most conservative approach requires a long period of abstinence because the rise in temperature shows that ovulation has already occurred. Also, sperm can remain viable in the woman's reproductive tract for up to 5 days. To reduce the time of abstinence, couples usually combine methods, such as BBT and assessment of the cervical mucus or use a barrier method during the fertile period.*
7. To enhance the chances of conception, this method has limited value because the rise in temperature indicates that ovulation has already occurred. It is helpful as a screening method to identify whether the woman is likely to be ovulating and if progesterone is secreted to prepare the endometrium for implantation. *The woman receiving infertility therapy should understand limitations of the BBT technique.*

Cervical Mucus Assessment

To facilitate survival of the sperm and promote their passage into the woman's uterus, the cervical mucus normally changes just before ovulation.

1. Teach the woman how her cervical mucus changes throughout the menstrual cycle. Spinnbarkeit describes how much the mucus can be stretched between her fingers or between a microscope slide and coverslip. Before and after ovulation the cervical mucus is scant, thick, sticky, and opaque. It stretches less than 6 cm (2.3 inches). Just before and for 2 to 3 days after ovulation, the cervical mucus is thin, slippery, and clear and is similar to raw egg white. It stretches 6 cm or more. When this ovulatory mucus is present, the woman has probably ovulated and could become pregnant. *This method requires careful assessment and record keeping by the woman. She is more likely to perform the assessment and record changes in her cervical mucus accurately if she understands how the changes relate to fertility.*

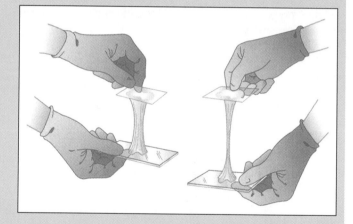

2. Explain common causes of changes in the mucus that are not related to fertility. It may be thicker if she takes antihistamines. Vaginal infections, contraceptive foams or jellies, sexual arousal, and semen can make the mucus thinner even if ovulation has not occurred. Tell her to record these factors. *The women should understand that these factors can interfere with the accuracy of her assessment.*
3. Suggest that the woman simulate stretching mucus using raw egg white at home. *Visual and tactile experiences enhance learning. A return demonstration allows the nurse to determine if the woman understood the teaching.*
4. Teach the woman to wash her hands before and after assessing her mucus. *Handwashing reduces the chance of introducing infection into the reproductive tract and of transferring infectious organisms from the vagina to other areas.*
5. Teach the woman to use a tissue to obtain a small sample of mucus several times a day from just inside her vagina and to note the following:
   a. The general sensation of wetness (around ovulation) or dryness (not near ovulation) on her labia
   b. The appearance and consistency of the mucus: thick, sticky, and whitish; or thin, slippery, and clear or watery

32-1 Teaching Women about Fertility Awareness—cont'd

c. The distance the mucus will stretch between her fingers, usually at least 6 cm (2.3 inches) at the time of ovulation.

This measurement allows the woman to identify cyclic changes in her mucus over the entire duration of her menstrual cycle.

6. Have the woman record the day's mucous characteristics (often combined with the BBT recording). *Recording provides a means of evaluating signs and symptoms associated with ovulation during the entire cycle.*

7. If technique is used as a method of contraception, the woman should avoid intercourse from the time the thin,

stretchy ovulatory mucus appears until 4 days after the end of the slippery mucus. *Avoiding intercourse reduces the chance that sperm are available for fertilization while the ovum is viable.*

8. As a method to enhance conception, the couple should have intercourse every 2 days during the period of ovulatory mucus (approximately days 12 to 16 if the woman has a 28-day cycle). Ovulation predictors available over the counter provide added predictive information that the woman trying to conceive may need. *Timing intercourse with the time of ovulation makes sperm available to fertilize the ovum while it is viable.*

TABLE 32-1 Selected Diagnostic Tests on Infertility

Test and Purpose	Nursing Implications
Male	
Semen Analysis	
Evaluates structure and function of sperm and composition of seminal fluid.	Explain purpose of semen analysis: three or more specimens are usually collected over several weeks' time for accurate analysis.
Semen volume: 2-6 ml	
pH: 7.2-7.8	Explain to the man that he should collect the specimen by masturbation after a 2- to 3-day abstinence; semen may be collected in a condom if masturbation is unacceptable.
Sperm concentration: 20 million/ml or more	
Motility: 50% or more with normal forms	
Morphology: 60% or more with normal forms	Teach the man to note the time the specimen was obtained so the laboratory can evaluate liquefaction of the semen. To maintain warmth, the specimen should be transported near the body and should arrive in the laboratory within 1 hr.
Viability: 50% or more live	
Liquefaction: within 30 min	
Leukocytes (white blood cells): fewer than 1 million/ml	
Fructose: 150-600 mg/dl	
Endocrine Tests	
Evaluate function of hypothalamus, pituitary gland, and the response of the testicles. Assays are made to determine testosterone, estradiol, luteinizing hormone (LH), and follicle-stimulating hormone (FSH) levels.	Teach the man about the relationship between hypothalamic and pituitary function and sperm formation; LH stimulates testosterone production by Leydig cells of the testes, and FSH stimulates Sertoli cells of the testes to produce sperm.
Additional tests may be done based on history and physical findings.	
Ultrasonography	
Evaluates structure of prostate gland, seminal vesicles, and ejaculatory ducts by use of a transrectal probe.	Teach the man that ultrasonography uses sound waves to evaluate these structures; no radiation is involved.
Testicular Biopsy	
An invasive test for obtaining a sample of testicular tissue; identifies pathology and obstructions.	Explain the purpose of the test; a local anesthetic is used, and there should be little discomfort.
Sperm Penetration Assay	
Evaluates fertilizing ability of sperm; assesses ability of sperm to undergo changes that allow penetration of a hamster ovum from which the zona pellucida has been removed.	Explain the purpose of the test; abnormal penetration does not necessarily mean that the sperm cannot fertilize a human ovum.
Female	
Ovulation Prediction	
Identifies the surge of LH, which precedes ovulation by 24 to 36 hr; improves ability to time intercourse to coincide with ovulation, and identifies the absence of ovulation. Common prediction methods include commercial ovulation predictor kits, basal body temperature, and cervical mucus assessment (see Procedure 32-1).	Explain the purpose of the assessments.
	Teach the woman to follow the instructions on commercial ovulation predictor.
	Teach her how to do the basal body temperature and cervical mucus assessment if that is used.
Ultrasonography	
Evaluates structure of pelvic organs. Identifies ovarian follicles and release of ova at ovulation. Evaluates for presence of ectopic or multifetal pregnancy.	Teach the woman that ultrasonography uses sound waves to evaluate these structures; no radiation is involved. Explain preparations needed for specific evaluations.
Postcoital Test	
Evaluates characteristics of cervical mucus and sperm function within that mucus at time of ovulation.	Explain that the test is performed 6 to 12 hours after intercourse; the woman may have to rearrange her personal or work commitments each time this test is done. Use is becoming less frequent, but test remains a valid diagnostic tool.
Ultrasonography ensures proper timing for test.	

Therapies to Facilitate Pregnancy

Evaluation of the couple identifies whether therapy might improve their chances to conceive and complete a pregnancy. A variety of procedures may be used, depending on the couple's initial and ongoing evaluations and their personal choices. Some therapy is simple, such as timing intercourse to better coincide with ovulation. Other procedures may involve considerable expense, discomfort, or unpleasant side effects. Many infertile couples need a combination of treatments to improve their chances of conception.

Identification of appropriate infertility therapy is not always straightforward. Many factors must be considered, including the couple's history, medical evaluations, financial resources, ages and other time constraints, and religious and cultural values. Simple treatments are indicated before more complex ones, but the needs of each couple are considered individually. More aggressive diagnostic testing and therapy may be appropriate if the woman is approaching the end of her reproductive years.

Statistical success rates for various procedures often are difficult for couples to evaluate and vary widely among facilities. Factors that affect a center's success rate for a procedure are numerous. For example, a referral center that is willing to help couples with long-standing infertility may have lower success rates than one that accepts only couples with less severe problems.

Medications

Hormones and other medications may be given to either the man or the woman. A medication may be given to improve semen quality, induce ovulation, prepare the uterine endometrium, or support the pregnancy once it is established. Medications may be given to correct infections. Others may help men for whom erectile dysfunction is the primary problem. Table 32-2 summarizes many of the medications used in infertility therapy.

Ovulation Induction

Medications to induce ovulation may be prescribed for the woman who does not ovulate or who ovulates erratically. Medications also may be given to induce multiple ova if a woman plans to have advanced reproductive techniques such as IVF or gamete intrafallopian transfer (GIFT). Clomiphene citrate is a drug often used to stimulate ovulation in specific types of ovulatory dysfunction. Letrozole, an aromatase inhibitor used in breast cancer treatment, has shown a favorable pregnancy rate and a low multifetal gestation rate when studied as an ovarian stimulant for infertility treatment (Mitwally, Biljan, & Casper, 2005).

TABLE 32-2 Medications Used in Infertility Therapy

Drug	Primary Use
Bromocriptine (Parlodel)	Corrects excess prolactin secretion by anterior pituitary, improving gonadotropin-releasing hormone (GnRH) secretion, in turn normalizing release of follicle-stimulating hormone (FSH) and luteinizing hormone (LH). These drug actions increase ovulation and support early pregnancy by stimulating progesterone secretion by the corpus luteum.
Chorionic gonadotropin, human (hCG; Pregnyl); recombinant deoxyribonucleic acid (DNA) origin (r-hCG; Ovidrel)	Used in conjunction with gonadotropins to stimulate ovulation in the female or sperm formation in the male. Stimulates progesterone production by corpus luteum.
Clomiphene citrate (Clomid)	Induction of ovulation in women who have specific types of ovulatory dysfunction. The drug increases frequency of GnRH secretion from the hypothalamus, thus increasing FSH and LH release, maturing the ovarian follicle, and causing release of the ovum.
FSH, recombinant DNA origin (follitropin [Gonal-F])	Stimulation of ovarian follicle growth; ovulation-induction gonadotropin.
GnRh antagonists (e.g., cetrorelix [Cetrotide], ganirelix [Antagon])	Reduces endometriosis; adjunct to drugs given to stimulate ovulation by suppressing LH and FSH, reducing ovarian hyperstimulation. Depending on drug, doses may be given intranasally, subcutaneously, or intramuscularly.
Gonadotropin-releasing hormone (GnRH) agonists (goserelin [Zoladex], leuprolide [Lupron], nafarelin [Synarel])	Stimulates release of FSH and LH from the pituitary gland in men and women who have deficient GnRH secretion by their hypothalamus. FSH and LH, in turn, stimulate ovulation in the female and stimulate testosterone production and spermatogenesis in the male.
Gonadotropins, human (Bravelle, Humegon, Pergonal, Repronex)	Induction of ovulation with human-derived FSH and LH; brands may differ in the proportions of FSH to LH; recombinant DNA preparations are becoming more common because of their greater purity.
LH, recombinant DNA origin	Replacement of LH; promotes ability of mature ovarian follicle to rupture and luteinize when hCG is secreted; usefulness of drug requires more study.
Progesterone (intramuscular or vaginal preparations)	Luteal phase support; prepares uterine lining and promotes implantation of embryo.
Erectile agents (sildenafil [Viagra], vardenafil [Levitra])	Increase blood flow to the penis, improving erectile function.

Data from Leibowitz, D., & Hoffman, J. (2000). Fertility drug therapies: Past, present, and future. *Journal of Obstetric, Gynecologic, and Neonatal Nursing, 29*(2), 201-210.
Richard-Davis, G. (2002). Ovulation induction for in vitro fertilization: The role of gonadotropin-releasing hormone antagonists. *Infertility and Reproductive Clinics of North America, 13*(3), 437-444.
Thornton, K.L. (2002). Recombinant gonadotropins and IVF. *Infertility and Reproductive Medicine Clinics of North America, 13*(3), 445-458.

DRUG GUIDE

CLOMIPHENE CITRATE (CLOMID, SEROPHENE)

Classification: Ovarian stimulant.

Action: Stimulates pituitary gland to increase secretion of luteinizing hormone (LH) and follicle-stimulating hormone (FSH). LH and FSH stimulate maturation of the ovarian follicle, ovulation, and development of the corpus luteum.

Indications: Female infertility in which estrogen levels are normal.

Dosage and Route: Female sterility: First course: 25 to 50 mg PO daily for 5 days. Second course: Same dose if ovulation occurred with first course. If ovulation did not occur, increase dose to 100 mg daily for 5 days. Some women require up to 250 mg daily. An increased dose is not beneficial if ovulation is triggered.

Absorption: Readily absorbed from the gastrointestinal tract. Time to peak effect is 4 to 10 days after last day of treatment.

Excretion: Excreted in the feces.

Contraindication and Precautions: Pregnancy, liver disease, abnormal bleeding of undetermined origin, ovarian cysts, neoplastic disease. Therapy is ineffective in women with ovarian or pituitary failure.

Adverse Reactions: Ovarian enlargement; symptoms similar to premenstrual syndrome. Ovarian hyperstimulation syndrome. Multiple gestation, if more than one ovum is released. Visual disturbances. Abdominal distention, discomfort, nausea, vomiting. Abnormal uterine bleeding. Breast tenderness. Insomnia, nervousness, headache, depression, fatigue, lightheadedness, dizziness. Hot flashes, increased urination, allergic symptoms, weight gain, reversible alopecia. Dry cervical mucus.

Nursing Considerations: Take the history to determine whether the woman has a history of liver dysfunction or abnormal uterine bleeding. Rule out the possibility of pregnancy. Teach the woman to report abdominal distention, pain in the pelvis or abdomen, and visual disturbances. Teach her to avoid tasks requiring mental alertness or coordination because the drug can cause lightheadedness, dizziness, and visual disturbances. Instruct her to stop taking clomiphene and report to the physician if she suspects she might be pregnant. Teach the woman and her partner that she may notice irritability, mood swings, and other symptoms similar to those in premenstrual syndrome but that these are temporary.

Ovulation induction can increase the chance of multiple births because several ova may be released and fertilized. Another serious complication is ovarian hyperstimulation syndrome, in which marked ovarian enlargement occurs, with exudation of fluid into the woman's peritoneal and pleural cavities. Careful adjustment of medication dose and serial ultrasound examinations prevent most cases of high multifetal pregnancy (triplets or more) and ovarian hyperstimulation syndrome.

Surgical Procedures

Endoscopic procedures may be used to correct obstructions with minimal invasiveness in either the man or the woman. The woman may need a laparotomy to relieve pelvic adhesions and obstructions caused by endometriosis, infection, or previous surgical procedures if these cannot be corrected via laparoscopy. Laser surgical techniques may be used to reduce adhesions because they are minimally invasive, precise, and less likely to cause formation of new adhesions. Correction of a varicocele by ligating or embolizing the dilated vein may improve sperm quality and quantity, although there is not a consensus on its usefulness. Microsurgical techniques may be attempted for correction of obstructions in the fallopian tubes or male tubal structures.

Transcervical balloon tuboplasty is a minimally invasive method to unblock the fallopian tubes. A thin catheter is threaded through the cervix and uterus into the fallopian tube. The balloon is then inflated to clear the blockage.

Therapeutic Insemination

Therapeutic insemination may use either the partner's semen or that of a donor to overcome a low sperm count. Donor insemination also may be used if the woman's partner carries a genetic defect or if a woman wants a biologic child without having a relationship with a male partner. Intrauterine insemination (IUI) is a variation of therapeutic insemination that allows sperm to be placed directly into the uterus, thus bypassing the cervical mucus and reducing some immunologic incompatibilities. This process also removes many of the antibodies that interfere with sperm motility and ability to penetrate the ovum.

The man collects the semen by masturbation after a 3-day abstinence. Sperm that are to be placed directly into the uterus or fallopian tube are prepared by washing and spinning the semen in a centrifuge to remove seminal fluid containing antibodies that interfere with sperm motility and ability to penetrate the ovum. A technique called *sperm swim-up* may be used to concentrate sperm having the best motility. Although the total number of sperm is lower, the remaining ones (those with normal structure and highest motility) are more likely to fertilize the ovum and result in a normal embryo.

If retrograde ejaculation is the man's problem, he takes sodium bicarbonate 2 hours before obtaining the semen to render the urine alkaline. After collecting the semen in a sterile container with a special medium, the sperm are quickly separated from the urine. The sperm are then further prepared for IUI.

Men who donate semen for IUI are screened to reduce the risk of transmitting diseases or genetic defects. They are questioned about their personal and family health history, including genetic disorders and birth defects. Questions about their social habits and personality can disclose high-risk behaviors and also give recipient parents information about traits their child might have. Physical and laboratory examinations are performed to evaluate the man's general health, determine his blood type and Rh factor, and screen for infections such as STDs, hepatitis B, and human immunodeficiency virus (HIV). Carrier testing for specific genetic defects such as sickle cell and Tay-Sachs diseases reduces the risk of passing on these disorders in donors of the racial group at higher risk. Donor semen is frozen and held for 6 months before use to reduce the risk of transmitting diseases that may not be apparent at the initial screening. The man is retested for diseases such as HIV several times during the 6 months.

Inadvertent consanguinity (blood relationship) can occur because half-siblings from two families may not know they were conceived with donor gametes. They may later conceive a child who shares a larger number of genes, both normal and abnormal, than the general population. For this reason, the number of donations may be limited.

Egg Donation

Use of donor oocytes may be an option for some women who do not produce ova because of premature ovarian failure, who do not respond to ovarian stimulation, or whose ova are not successfully fertilized despite apparently normal sperm. It is less successful if used for women who have a birth defect such as Turner's syndrome, in which the ova regress early in life, or for women who have had radiation therapy to the pelvis (Balen & Jacobs, 2003).

As in use of donor semen, egg donation carries with it the risk for infecting the recipient, the fetus, and possibly the male partner of the recipient. Inadvertent consanguinity is a risk with multiple donations, as it is in use of donor semen. In addition to these risks, the procedure carries risks for the donor because she will need medications to stimulate ovulation and an ova retrieval procedure as is done in IVF. Because of the complexity of egg donation, donors are fewer than for sperm donation (ASRM, 2000b; Balen & Jacobs, 2003; Penzias, 2002).

Surrogate Parenting

A surrogate mother may enter the picture if the woman is infertile or cannot carry a fetus to live birth. The surrogate mother may supply her uterus only (gestational surrogate), with the infertile couple supplying the sperm and ovum. Or she may be inseminated with the male partner's sperm and carry the fetus to birth, thus supplying both the genetic component and the gestational component. Surrogacy is different from therapeutic insemination with donor sperm because it is not anonymous. In addition, the woman who carries the child inevitably forms bonds with the fetus during the months of pregnancy. For these reasons, extensive interview and counseling of both the infertile couple and the surrogate mother are required.

Money paid to the surrogate mother can raise ethical issues. Could a poor but fertile woman feel compelled to provide her body for a more well-to-do couple? However, not compensating a woman for the real physical and emotional risks of this undertaking can be construed as coercive as well.

Custody of the resulting child has been the issue in several court cases involving surrogate mothers. In the *Baby M* case, a woman who was inseminated with the man's sperm refused to relinquish the baby as stated in the contract between the birth mother and the infertile couple. Ultimately, custody was awarded to the man providing the sperm and his spouse, but visitation rights were granted to the surrogate mother.

Custody issues when the birth mother is a gestational surrogate are clearer than when she also donates her ovum to the child. Courts have more often recognized the genetic parents as the legal parents and upheld the contracts between them and the gestational surrogate.

Assisted Reproductive Technology

Assisted reproductive technology (ART) uses advanced techniques that bypass many natural obstacles to conception by placing intact gametes together to allow fertilization. These techniques include IVF, GIFT, and zygote intrafallopian transfer (ZIFT). Each procedure begins with ovulation induction to permit retrieval of several ova, thus improving the likelihood of a successful pregnancy. Sperm are prepared and concentrated as they are for therapeutic insemination.

Another class of advanced reproductive techniques involves assisting fertilization with microsurgical techniques. These techniques bypass obstacles to fertilization by penetrating the ovum with tiny needles to allow placement of the sperm within the ovum. The sperm also may be obtained by advanced techniques.

The success rates for ART therapy in carefully selected couples now average approximately 35% (ASRM, 2003; Centers for Disease Control and Prevention [CDC] & ASRM, 2004). Clinics that provide therapy for couples with poorer prognoses for pregnancy may have a lower overall success rate because they may be a "last resort" option for these couples.

IN VITRO FERTILIZATION

The technique of IVF involves bypassing blocked or absent fallopian tubes. The physician removes the ova by laparoscope or ultrasound-guided transvaginal retrieval and mixes them with prepared sperm from the woman's partner or a donor. Fertilized ova are returned to the uterus 1 to 2 days after conception (Figure 32-4). The number of fertilized ova returned is individualized but is approximately 3 or 4. Older women may have more ova transferred than younger women to improve their chances of pregnancy without greatly increasing the risk of having a triplet or higher pregnancy. Supplemental progesterone is given to the woman to promote implantation and support the early pregnancy (luteal phase support). Because of the supplemental progesterone, the woman will not have a menstrual period even if she is not pregnant. Four weeks after implantation, transvaginal ultrasound is used to de-

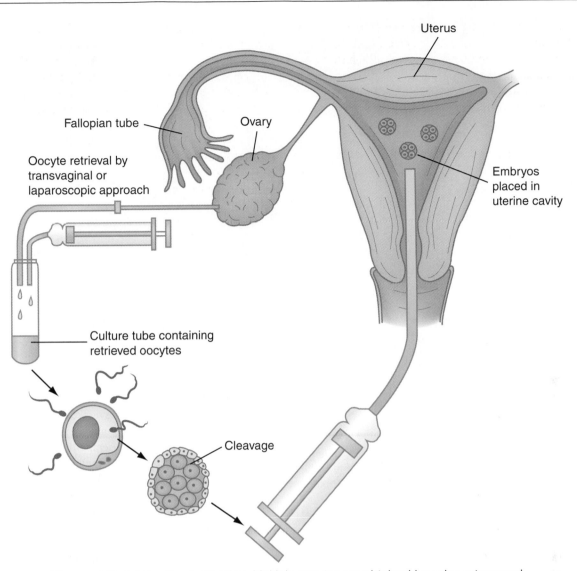

Figure 32-4 ■ In vitro fertilization. Multiple oocytes are obtained by using a transvaginal or laparoscopic approach. The retrieved oocytes are mixed with prepared sperm and incubated 1 to 2 days. Embryos are then transferred to the uterine cavity to allow implantation and continued development.

tect whether one or more gestational sacs are present and to identify if an ectopic (tubal) pregnancy occurred (see Chapter 25).

IVF success rates vary among infertility centers. Bypassing the obstructions does not necessarily result in pregnancy. Not every ovum is successfully fertilized when this technique is used. Embryos transferred to the woman's uterus may not always implant, which is why several are transferred. However, multiple embryos also may implant. Although twins are the most common multifetal pregnancy, triplets or more may occur, raising issues related to the physical and emotional well-being of parents and their babies and possibly raising ethical issues.

GAMETE INTRAFALLOPIAN TRANSFER

The woman must have at least one open fallopian tube for GIFT to take place. The procedure begins in a manner similar to that of IVF, with retrieval of multiple ova and washed sperm. Ova may be retrieved either laparoscopically or transvaginally with ultrasound guidance.

The retrieved ova are drawn into a catheter that also carries prepared sperm. Sperm and up to two ova per tube are injected into each fallopian tube through a laparoscope, in which fertilization may occur. Additional prepared sperm may be injected into the uterus through the cervix to improve the chance of successful fertilization. Progesterone is often given to enhance implantation of any fertilized ova. Progesterone is given as it is in IVF. (See Figure 32-5.)

ZYGOTE INTRAFALLOPIAN TRANSFER

ZIFT, often called *tubal embryo transfer* (TET) is a hybrid of IVF and GIFT. The woman's ova are fertilized outside her body, but the resulting fertilized ova are placed in the fallopian tubes and enter the uterus naturally for implantation. The woman must have at least one patent fallopian tube.

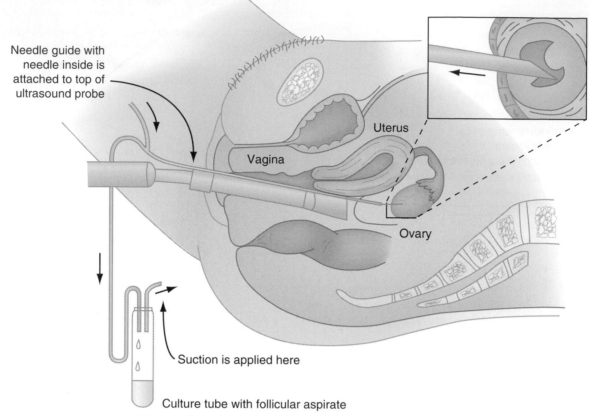

Needle guide with
needle inside is
attached to top of
ultrasound probe

Uterus

Vagina

Ovary

Suction is applied here

Culture tube with follicular aspirate

Figure 32-5 ■ Gamete intrafallopian transfer (GIFT). Multiple ova aspirated from the ovary in this illustration are combined with washed sperm. The mixture of ova and sperm are then transferred directly to a fallopian tube.

COMPARISON OF IN VITRO FERTILIZATION, GAMETE INTRAFALLOPIAN TRANSFER, AND TUBAL EMBRYO TRANSFER

The primary advantage of GIFT and ZIFT over IVF is that people or religious groups may find these procedures more natural and therefore more acceptable than IVF. With IVF or ZIFT there is evidence of fertilization before placement in the uterus or tubes. GIFT and ZIFT have minimally higher success rates than IVF in some clinics, although the success rate for IVF rises with the number of cycles attempted. The GIFT and ZIFT procedures are more invasive, requiring a laparoscopy to place the gametes or fertilized ova in the distal fallopian tube. Tubal pregnancy may result if embryos cannot reach the uterine cavity to implant. For these reasons IVF is used about 98% of the time if a couple requires ART (ASRM, 2004; CDC & ASRM, 2004).

INTRACYTOPLASMIC SPERM INJECTION

Microsurgical techniques are related to IVF but considerably more complex. These techniques now help couples conceive despite severe male factor infertility when standard IVF, GIFT, and ZIFT are unlikely to be successful.

Men who have obstructions to or absence of their epididymis may be able to father children with the use of percutaneous or microsurgical sperm aspiration. The sperm

are retrieved from the epididymis by percutaneous aspiration with a small-gauge needle. Alternately, a microsurgical incision may be made to aspirate the sperm if the percutaneous approach cannot be used. The sperm obtained are then used to fertilize ova by intracytoplasmic sperm injection (ICSI).

PREIMPLANTATION GENETIC TESTING

Preimplantation genetic testing may be offered to couples with higher risks for conceiving an embryo with a diagnosable genetic abnormality. A few cells are withdrawn for analysis before the embryo is implanted. The DNA from the cells allows genetic analysis for some conditions. Because cells are undifferentiated into specialized organ cells at this early stage, their loss is quickly made up. If a genetic defect is identified, the couple has the option of not implanting the embryo.

✓ **CHECK YOUR READING**

12. What elements are included in the history and physical examination for an infertility workup?
13. What medications may be used to induce ovulation?
14. What screening tests are performed if donor sperm is used for therapeutic insemination or GIFT?
15. What are the differences in technique among IVF, GIFT, and ZIFT?

RESPONSES TO INFERTILITY

The desire for children is strong in many people. Even if they delay childbearing, most couples expect to have one or more children before the end of the woman's reproductive years. Those who chose childlessness earlier may reevaluate their decision when they are older. If a couple does not achieve pregnancy or produce a living child as expected, the man and woman often experience psychological distress and a threat to their self-images. Either or both partners may feel like failures. Their marital and family relationships may be stressed, and they may withdraw from relationships with others that they previously found satisfying. Every couple is unique, and many reactions depend on the importance attached to having biologic children. The following discussion describes the ways infertility can alter the lives of those affected.

Assumption of Fertility

Many couples practice contraception for a number of years before they decide to have a baby. They may want to establish a career and financial security, acquire a comfortable home and lifestyle, or perhaps travel and live freely without the responsibility of a child. They usually assume that they are fertile and must take steps to avoid pregnancy until they are ready.

When they do want a child, they discontinue contraception and assume that pregnancy will occur within a few months at most. They may plan conception so that the baby will be born at a certain time of year (such as not during the hottest weather) or to avoid major holidays.

Either or both partners may experiment with the role of parent as they anticipate pregnancy. They develop a heightened awareness of children and parenting. Being with others who are expecting or already have children is exciting because they plan to join their ranks shortly. They may discuss issues like full-time parenting by one partner, child care, and imminent lifestyle changes. The woman often finds that she enjoys shopping in the maternity and children's departments. They may begin acquiring toys and furnishings a child will need. Both partners may develop a fantasy child or a concept of what their baby will be like.

Growing Awareness of a Problem

As the months pass, the couple gradually becomes concerned about the inability to conceive. If the woman is older, they feel the urgency of the limited time before her reproductive years end. The plan to have a baby at a certain time of year is replaced by the desire for a baby any time—and soon.

The couple begins to feel uneasy with child-related activities. Now they are not so sure when they will be parents. They begin to feel hurt when other family members or friends have babies. Events such as baby showers and christenings become melancholy rather than joyful occasions to them. They bypass toy stores and children's departments because of the uncertainty. Family members and friends who are having children may feel guilty when they are around the couple who cannot conceive.

The potential grandparents may feel that their children are waiting too long to start a family or even that they are selfish. If they are aware the couple is trying to conceive, they become even more worried as the months pass without the longed-for announcement of a pregnancy. They are twice saddened—by the lack of a grandchild and the hurt their adult children are enduring.

Seeking Help for Infertility

Eventually, couples must decide whether to seek help to conceive. They may reach this point after only a few menstrual cycles or, at the opposite extreme, may never seek help. Many factors enter into their decision, such as their ages (especially the woman's if menopause is near), how long they have been unable to conceive, how much they want a biologic child, how they regard adoption, and how they feel about a life without children. If they have a biologic child but are unable to conceive another, the couple may consider adoption sooner, including adopting a child from another country.

IDENTIFYING THE IMPORTANCE OF HAVING A BABY

Each partner may place a different priority on having a baby. Conflicts may arise when one partner wants help to conceive sooner than the other. In addition, cultural or religious beliefs influence the way each feels about procreation and whether options such as assisted reproductive procedures or adoption are acceptable. The way in which the couple resolves these differences is crucial to the stability of the relationship.

Men and women often differ in their reactions to infertility. Women may want to talk about their feelings and frustrations, but men often internalize their feelings or feel that they must be strong for their partners. The woman may interpret her partner's stoicism and reluctance to express his feelings as disinterest or lack of concern and care for her.

SHARING INTIMATE INFORMATION

Although the infertility specialist will limit questions to the necessary ones, evaluation and treatment for infertility require that both partners reveal information about their sexual relationship, such as the frequency and timing of intercourse. This is difficult for those who regard this information as intimate. In addition, infertile couples may feel that the evaluation calls their sexual adequacy into question. They may feel defensive if they perceive a threat to their self-image.

CONSIDERING FINANCIAL RESOURCES

Financial concerns enter into the couple's decision about whether to seek treatment and how far to carry it. Techniques such as ovulation predictor kits are inexpensive but have limited usefulness in achieving successful pregnancy. Advanced techniques such as IVF are expensive and may have a low likelihood of success for some couples. Health insurance may not cover infertility treatment at all or may not cover all procedures because the problem is not always seen as a health problem. Treatments that are investigational are usually not covered. The drugs that must be taken to achieve pregnancy are often quite expensive. Expense and restricted coverage limit treatment choices for many low- or middle-income couples. Those who seek and pursue infertility treatment may have greater financial resources than those who do not seek treatment.

COMMITTING TO INVOLVEMENT IN CARE

Infertility evaluation and treatment require a great commitment from the couple in terms of time, emotional and physical energy, and money. Couples can be involved in this process for several years if they do not set a limit on when they want to stop. They participate daily as they do home assessments, take medications, and keep detailed records. The physical effects of drugs that induce ovulation and support conception can result in many side or adverse effects. For infertility diagnosis and therapy to be most effective, couples must consider their ability and desire to be directly involved in the process over what may be a long time.

Reactions during Evaluation and Treatment

Couples undergoing infertility evaluation and treatment have different reactions to the process. While early evaluations often result in simple treatment and quick response, a couple's reactions may change as treatment becomes more complex, demanding, and lengthy.

INFLUENCES ON DECISION MAKING

If their evaluation shows that a treatment or procedure may enable them to conceive, the couple must then decide whether to proceed. The decision-making process begins early and must be repeated during therapy if pregnancy does not occur. A complex array of factors enters into their decisions about beginning and continuing treatment or whether to end their pursuit of pregnancy. Although discussed separately, these factors interact dynamically as the couple makes each decision. The nurse helps them examine each factor and arrive at a decision that is best for them.

SOCIAL, CULTURAL, AND RELIGIOUS VALUES. Some medically appropriate options are not acceptable to every couple within their personal, social, cultural, and religious frameworks. Surrogate parenting, IVF, and therapeutic insemination (especially with donor sperm) are not consistent with the personal or religious beliefs of many people. If a procedure offers the partners hope for a child but is incompatible with their beliefs, their choices are two: use the technology despite their beliefs or be willing to accept childlessness. Adoption may be a third alternative for some couples if the desire for a biologic child is not absolute. As in other decisions, couples must work out conflicting personal values about what therapy is acceptable.

DIFFICULTY OF TREATMENT. The couple must consider how difficult, risky, and uncomfortable therapy

will be. The level of difficulty involves physical, psychological, geographic, and time factors. Employment constraints also may affect treatment decisions.

Several diagnostic tests and treatments for infertility involve invasive procedures or surgery. The person who undergoes the procedure must be the one who ultimately decides whether to do it. That person alone can decide whether the hope for a child is worth the risks and discomfort of the procedure.

Infertility treatment is stressful. Often partners feel or are willing to tolerate different levels of stress. To reduce the stress, they may abandon treatment completely or take a vacation for a few months from the constant preoccupation with conceiving. Women nearing or in their 40s often do not feel they have the luxury of skipping a treatment cycle.

Some couples encounter geographic difficulties if they must travel a long distance for therapy. Time stresses are substantial. The partners, particularly the woman, feel that achieving pregnancy is their new career. One or both partners may spend many hours every week in pursuit of pregnancy.

Employment constraints may be a barrier to infertility therapy because of the time required for treatment. The impact of time is usually greatest on the woman. Time away from work may burden the employer or coworkers. Stopping work may not be an option because the family needs the money and often needs the insurance coverage that comes with employment.

PROBABILITY OF SUCCESS. Couples often have a biased interpretation of their statistical probability of success, especially when they begin treatment with a new procedure. For example, if a procedure has a 20% likelihood of success with each cycle, they tend to expect that they will be in the successful group rather than in the 80% who do not meet with success. As time goes by, however, they must weigh the likelihood of success of any therapy against financial concerns and their own willingness to accept the discomfort and difficulty associated with it. Again, the woman's age imposes an inescapable limit.

FINANCIAL CONCERNS. Some couples, particularly those with ample resources and a strong desire for a biologic child, pursue expensive treatments and do so longer than others of more limited means, despite a low probability of success. Couples with financial limitations find that they must abandon treatment sooner than they want. Other couples go heavily into debt, adding financial strain to the other stresses of treatment in their quest for a biologic child.

PSYCHOLOGICAL REACTIONS

A couple's initial reaction to infertility often is one of shock because the partners are usually healthy and did not expect to have problems conceiving. Their reactions vary according to how easily their infertility is alleviated, their personality and self-image, and the strength of their relationship.

GUILT. A partner having the only identified problem might feel that he or she is depriving the other of children.

This feeling may be compounded if the "normal" partner has children from another relationship. It may be difficult for this person to understand that not all factors affecting fertility are known and what seems like the problem of only one partner is often the couple's problem.

Either partner may feel guilty about past choices that now affect fertility. A woman with adhesions resulting from a sexually transmitted infection may regret her past sexual choices. The man who wanted to delay pregnancy longer than the woman may feel guilty if her age is now reducing her fertility.

ISOLATION. Infertile couples may withdraw from friends and relatives who have children to insulate themselves from painful reminders of their infertility. Some couples develop supportive relationships with others who also are infertile, which somewhat diminishes their sense of isolation.

DEPRESSION. One or both partners may experience depression as their sense of competence and control over their bodies is challenged, especially if therapy is not successful quickly. They often feel as though they are on a roller coaster of hope alternating with despair when the woman has her menstrual period each month. In an attempt to reduce their disappointment, couples with long-term infertility try not to expect too much with each cycle.

The couple may feel envy toward those who conceive easily. They may become judgmental and angry when they see those who seem to "have no business having a baby," such as an adolescent, a woman who abuses drugs, or a poor woman who cannot support an added child.

STRESS ON THE RELATIONSHIP. Because infertility can challenge a person's identity and self-esteem, partners may find less satisfaction in their relationship. They may feel unlovable or unappealing to their mate.

The man may have difficulty performing on demand for semen specimens or postcoital tests, feeling that others will judge his sexual function. The fact that semen samples are best obtained by masturbation is unacceptable to some men. Both partners are stressed when intercourse must be scheduled to coincide with specific evaluations or ovulation. Intercourse can become a chore more than an expression of love. It may come to be associated with failure rather than fulfillment if a child is not forthcoming.

If sperm from an anonymous donor is used for therapeutic insemination or other techniques, the man may feel that his masculinity is further threatened. He does not want to deprive his wife of a child, but he may be ambivalent about use of sperm from a third party. He may have difficulty distinguishing between fatherhood as a biologic achievement and fatherhood as a relationship.

The partners find their relationship strained if they disagree on which treatments are appropriate and how long they should be pursued. One partner may want to keep trying "one more month," and the other may want to abandon treatment. If they are considering adoption, their relationship may be strained if they differ on whether to adopt and what kind of child they are willing to accept.

> ✓ **CHECK YOUR READING**
>
> 16. What factors do couples consider when they are deciding whether to seek help for their infertility?
> 17. What factors must couples consider when they reach decision points during infertility evaluation and treatment?
> 18. What are possible psychological reactions to infertility?

OUTCOMES AFTER INFERTILITY THERAPY

After infertility therapy, three outcomes are possible. The pregnancy may be lost, resulting in mixed emotions of grief and optimism. The couple may become parents, either biologically or through adoption. Infertility therapy may be unsuccessful and the couple must decide whether to pursue adoption or to remain childless.

Pregnancy Loss after Infertility Therapy

Couples who suffer pregnancy loss after infertility therapy may interpret the experience with mixed feelings of loss and gain. Couples undergoing infertility evaluation and treatment often are aware of a pregnancy much earlier than fertile couples. They want to hope yet expect to be disappointed again. If a spontaneous abortion occurs, they may grieve profoundly for what they achieved and then lost.

Yet despite their grief about the pregnancy loss, the partners may be encouraged because they have proved that they can achieve a pregnancy. They may feel that if they succeeded once, they can do it again. A miscarriage may give them the courage to continue treatment. They realize that many pregnancies are lost early, often before most women have any idea that they might be pregnant.

When pregnancy loss has occurred because of an ectopic pregnancy, the woman may lose a fallopian tube, although earlier diagnosis reduces the risks of damage or loss of the affected tube (see p. 627). These couples may have an added threat to their fertility because of the uncertainty of getting pregnant again in addition to the possible loss or blockage of one or both fallopian tubes.

Parenthood after Infertility Therapy

Couples who conceive experience varied emotions. If they have been disappointed before, they may hardly believe the good news. They are thrilled but worry about whether they can complete the pregnancy and take home a baby. Pregnancy after infertility therapy is emotionally tentative for many infertile couples, especially those who have been trying to conceive for a long time or have lost a pregnancy. They may distance themselves from the reality of the pregnancy until much later in gestation than normally fertile couples. The woman has learned to sense and report every symptom and may interpret normal changes of pregnancy as a threat.

The previously infertile couple may find little sympathy from those who do not understand their fear of investing in the pregnancy. Others are annoyed because they expect the couple to be overjoyed at a successful and apparently normal pregnancy. Outsiders may feel that the partners are self-centered and cannot decide what they want. Other infertile couples who have been a source of mutual support may either withdraw from the couple who achieve a pregnancy or rejoice in their success.

The parents' anxiety may be heightened during labor. They are afraid that something will go wrong at the last moment. Even after the birth of a healthy infant, some parents need time to relax and grasp the fact that their baby is really here.

These new parents often need much support as they gain experience with their child. Infertile couples who eventually have biologic or adopted children may have unrealistic expectations about parenting. After investing so many financial, physical, and emotional resources in having a child, they may be reluctant to express any unhappiness or frustration over the difficulties of child-rearing.

Choosing to Adopt

Not every couple who seeks treatment for infertility achieves a "take-home" baby. Some couples discontinue treatment sooner than others, depending on their age and tolerance for the fatigue, stress, and expense. Some couples investigate adoption early in infertility treatment because advanced age may make them ineligible to adopt through many agencies or because a nonbiologic child is acceptable to them. Agencies that coordinate international adoptions are often consulted.

Couples who consider adoption must confront their personal preferences, limitations, and prejudices. As much as they want a child, many couples are not willing to adopt any child. Most couples prefer to adopt a newborn or an infant of their race. Some prefer an infant but also are willing to adopt an older child, one with special needs, one of a mixed or different race, or a group of siblings. Other couples will not consider adopting these children for a variety of reasons.

Some couples fear adopting a child because the woman might become pregnant. Although pregnancy has been their goal for a long time, they may worry that they would love their adopted child differently from their biologic child. If the couple plans to continue trying for a biologic child, they also must come to grips with this issue.

Couples who decide to adopt face further scrutiny of their personal lives. Agencies investigate their home, financial means (which may have been seriously drained), and fitness as parents. Once again, they may feel that their personal competence is questioned. International adoptions often have many additional requirements that the couple does not encounter in their home country.

The couple who decides on adoption may have emotions similar to those who achieve a pregnancy. They may be slow to invest in the process emotionally because they expect disappointment again. In addition, the adopted child often arrives suddenly and unexpectedly. A delay in the adoption process may also occur, bringing further uncertainty to the couple. Although they may have been waiting months for

this happy event, the couple may have little time to adjust to the reality of their new roles as parents.

✔ **CHECK YOUR READING**

19. If the partners become parents, either through birth or adoption, how may they react to parenthood?
20. What are the issues couples must face if they consider adoption?
21. What emotions do couples often experience if they lose a pregnancy after infertility treatment?

Application of the Nursing Process
Care of the Infertile Couple

Nurses may encounter couples facing infertility in many different settings and identify numerous nursing care needs. Regardless of the setting, the nurse often addresses the couple's emotional needs associated with infertility evaluation, treatment, and outcomes of therapy.

Assessment

In many instances, infertile couples previously have had a positive self-image and feelings of competence about themselves. The diagnosis of infertility shakes their positive view. The nurse should be aware that these feelings may be present, regardless of the practice setting in which the couple is encountered.

Determine at what point the couple is in their infertility treatment. Couples who have just discovered that they may have difficulty conceiving may be shocked yet optimistic that therapy will result in a baby. Other couples for whom simple treatments were unsuccessful may face shock again if the more complex treatments such as IVF or ICSI are recommended, particularly if these treatments require them to go into debt. Couples with long-standing infertility may have a deeper sense of failure and a pessimistic outlook. Listen for remarks that are negative, expressing guilt or helplessness.

Evaluate the way infertility has affected the partners' relationship with each other. Are there conflicts or differences in values between the two? Observing their body language, such as eye contact, may provide clues about similarities and differences in their commitment to diagnosis and treatment. Ask them how their relationship has changed. Are they more or less satisfied with their marital relationship than they were before they had problems conceiving? How is each member of the couple adjusting to the situation?

Ask about support systems. Couples suffering from infertility often withdraw from old relationships yet do not form new supportive ones. Do others who are significant in the partners' lives know that they are trying to conceive? Are family members and friends nearby, and are they supportive? Ask whether they have encountered assumptions by others that infertility is the "fault" of one partner or the other. Are they subjected to questions that invade their privacy, such as "When are you two going to have a baby of your own?"

Determine how the couple's culture or religion views infertility and the impact of these values on therapy. Are some therapies unacceptable to one or both partners? The partners may have differing views that can cause conflict during treatment, and they will need help to work these out.

Determine how the couple is coping with the stresses of treatment. How much has infertility cost them in terms of time, money, and discomfort? Identify the successes and failures they have experienced as well as outcomes that have provided them hope or comfort. Their age, especially the woman's, adds another stressor that cannot be ignored in their decisions.

If the woman is pregnant or has given birth recently or the couple has adopted a child recently, observe for high levels of anxiety in either or both parents. Assess them for negative behaviors and comments, such as reluctance to feel joy or a sense that they will "fail" again.

Analysis

A nursing diagnosis commonly encountered is "Situational Low Self-Esteem related to loss of control secondary to the couple's infertility diagnosis and treatment."

Planning

Three expected outcomes are appropriate for this nursing diagnosis, and they may apply to the man, the woman, or both partners. The person(s) will do the following:

- Express feelings about infertility and its evaluation and treatment
- Explore ways to increase control within the situation of infertility
- Identify aspects of self that are positive

Interventions

ASSISTING COMMUNICATION

Therapeutic communication is the primary technique for assessment and intervention related to this nursing diagnosis. Use a variety of communication techniques such as active listening and exploration to encourage the partners to express their feelings honestly. Provide privacy and acceptance of their feelings. Nurses must recognize the validity of the couple's views and emotions, even if they differ from the nurse's own feelings.

Encourage the partners to accept their feelings, both positive and negative. For example, the couple who has finally achieved pregnancy may be living a lie to some extent. The partners may act elated because they believe they should feel happy, yet inside they are cautious and hesitant about becoming attached to their baby. Explain that feelings are not right or wrong but simply exist. Opening the subject of negative feelings (fear of attachment) within a successful situation (pregnancy or birth) may be helpful to reinforce the normality of their emotions. This technique gives them the opportunity to talk about emotional reactions that they or

others feel are inappropriate and might otherwise be reluctant to discuss.

Discuss possible differences in ways the man and the woman communicate. For example, explain that the woman may feel more comfortable than the man in talking about their problem and concerns about treatment. Explain that these differences in communication style can cause misunderstandings because one partner believes that the other does not care as much about their problem. Encourage them to be open with each other for the best mutual support. Support groups provide another means for communication and ventilation of feelings among those who are most likely to understand what an infertile couple is going through.

INCREASING THE COUPLE'S SENSE OF CONTROL

Explore how the couple has dealt with stressors in the past and how these techniques might be used to cope with the present crisis. A couple's pattern of dealing with stress in other parts of life is likely to carry over into infertility diagnosis and treatment and throughout pregnancy and parenthood. Reinforce positive coping skills such as learning more about infertility and the proposed therapy for it.

Couples who experience undue stress may benefit from relaxation techniques such as visualization and moderate exercise. Frequent strenuous exercise may reduce the woman's ability to ovulate. Although a hot tub is relaxing for many people, it should be avoided because the high temperatures may inhibit spermatogenesis. In addition, the woman could become pregnant with any cycle, and high body temperatures may be associated with fetal anomalies.

Discuss behaviors that enhance the ability to handle stress and provide a good environment for a pregnancy that might occur. Reinforce healthy choices such as good nutrition and a balance between exercise and rest. Teach the couple ways to enhance general health if deficiencies are identified.

Explain any procedures and their purpose in language that the couple can understand. Reinforce any medical explanations that may have been given. Encourage questions so that the couple is fully informed. Have the partners restate what was explained to reduce misunderstandings.

Help the couple explore options at each decision point. The couple must decide the best course of action, but the nurse can help identify pros and cons of each choice so that the partners can arrive at a decision appropriate for them. Be nondirective so that the choices are theirs and do not reflect the biases of the nurse or other caregivers.

REDUCING ISOLATION

Because couples often distance themselves from friends and family relationships that they find painful, they may have little social support. Refer them to available support groups to provide emotional outlets, a sense of belonging, and a source of information.

Couples who achieve pregnancy or adopt a child may again find themselves isolated if infertile couples in their circle of support are no longer comfortable with them. Encourage them to take the initiative to reestablish ties with relatives and friends, who can be an important source of aid during pregnancy and child-rearing. Help them identify ways they can improve communication with these significant others. Remind them that they have undergone significant shifts in self-image, which also have affected those around them.

PROMOTING A POSITIVE SELF-IMAGE

Because infertility work often is such a dominant factor in their lives, a continuing inability to conceive erodes the partners' perception of themselves. Explore with them other areas of competence and activities that make them feel good about themselves. Reinforce positive attitudes and self-evaluations. Encourage them to maintain activities such as hobbies, sports, or volunteer work. The career of either partner may be a source of stress that needs relief, or it may be an avenue that fosters a positive self-perception.

Encourage them to avoid activities such as baby showers if these events make them sad. Help them identify the best way to cope with these activities if they do not want to avoid them.

Some people benefit from self-improvement activities such as continuing education courses or enhancement of appearance. Encourage these activities if they help the individuals feel better about themselves. If the activity might impair fertility treatments, such as strict dieting, also inform the person of this fact.

Evaluation

The goals established are achieved if the individual or both partners can:

- Express their feelings about their situation, usually over a period of time
- Explore ways to increase personal control over their lives, as evidenced by expressing feelings of reduced helplessness and dependence
- Identify one or more aspects of self perceived as positive, identifying areas of competence

SUMMARY CONCEPTS

- Nurses may encounter persons having infertility problems in a variety of settings other than infertility clinics, such as maternity and gynecology services, urology services, the perioperative area, and the emergency department. Friends and family members also see the nurse as an information resource about infertility care.
- About 20% of infertile couples have no identified problem that is explained by current evaluation techniques.
- Because many unknown factors in reproduction exist, identification and correction of problems in one or both partners does not necessarily resolve their infertility.
- A variety of structural and functional abnormalities may contribute to a couple's infertility. The man may have abnormalities of the sperm or the seminal fluid or with ejacu-

lation. The woman may have ovulation disorders, anatomic problems such as fallopian tube occlusion, or physiologic disorders such as hormone imbalances.

- A systematic evaluation of both partners, proceeding from simple to more complex, identifies therapy that is most likely to be successful and cost-effective. The couple may decide to stop evaluation or therapy at any point.
- Infertility is a crisis for the couple and often for the extended family. Either or both partners may feel that the inability to conceive represents a personal failure. They may have a variety of psychological reactions.
- Infertile couples must make choices at many points before and during evaluation and therapy. Some major factors that enter into their decisions involve personal, social, cultural, and religious values; difficulty of treatment; probability of success; financial resources; and age, particularly the woman's.
- The possible outcomes after infertility therapy may present new challenges to the couple and their families: unsuccessful therapy and the choice of whether to pursue adoption, pregnancy loss after infertility, and parenthood after infertility.
- Many nursing care needs may be identified as the couple negotiates infertility evaluation and treatment.

REFERENCES & READINGS

Abma, J., Chandra, A., Mosher, W., Peterson, L., & Piccinino, L. (1997). Fertility, family planning, and women's health: New data from the 1995 national survey of family growth. *Vital & Health Statistics, 23*(19). Retrieved March 9, 2005, from www.cdc.gov/nchs/data/series/sr_23/sr23_019.pdf.

Alper, M.M. (2002). Improving and facilitating the delivery of care to patients undergoing in vitro fertilization. *Infertility and Reproductive Medicine Clinics of North America, 13*(3), 431-436.

American Society for Reproductive Medicine. (2000a). *Committee opinion: Effectiveness and treatment for unexplained infertility.* Birmingham, AL: Author.

American Society for Reproductive Medicine. (2000b). *Committee opinion: Repetitive oocyte donation.* Birmingham, AL: Author.

American Society for Reproductive Medicine. (2003). *Assisted reproductive technology.* Birmingham, AL: Author. Retrieved May 4, 2005, from www.asrm.org/Patients/patientbooklets/ART.pdf.

American Society for Reproductive Medicine. (2004). *Frequently-asked questions about infertility.* Retrieved March 9, 2005, from www.asrm.org?patients/faqs.html.

Angard, N.T. (2000). Seeking coverage for infertility: Insurers should offer reasonable services to help couples achieve pregnancy. *AWHONN Lifelines, 4*(3), 22-24.

Balen, A.H., & Jacobs, H.S. (2003). *Infertility in practice* (2nd ed.). Edinburgh: Churchill Livingstone.

Blackburn, S.T. (2003). *Maternal, fetal, and neonatal physiology: A clinical perspective.* Philadelphia: Saunders.

Bowers, N.A. (2000). The multiple birth explosion: Implications for nursing practice. *Journal of Obstetric, Gynecologic, and Neonatal Nursing, 27*(3), 302-310.

Centers for Disease Control and Prevention & American Society for Reproductive Medicine. (2004). *2002 Assisted reproductive technology success rates: National summary and fertility clinic reports.* Atlanta, GA, & Birmingham, AL: Authors. Retrieved March 9, 2005, from www.cdc.gov/reproductivehealth/ART02/download.htm.

Cockey, C.D. (2003). Exploring infertility and endometriosis. *AWHONN Lifelines, 7*(4), 309-310.

Daly, D.C. (2000). Induction of ovulation. In E.J. Quilligan & F.A. Zuspan (Eds.), *Current therapy in obstetrics and gynecology* (5th ed., pp. 80-83). Philadelphia: Saunders.

Devine, K.S. (2003). Caring for the infertile woman. *MCN: American Journal of Maternal/Child Nursing, 28*(2), 100-105.

Gutman, J.N., & Braverman, A.M. (2002). What's in a name? The evolution of gestational surrogacy. *Infertility and Reproductive Medicine Clinics of North America, 13*(3), 595-613.

Guyton, A.C., & Hall, J.E. (2000). *Textbook of medical physiology* (10th ed.). Philadelphia: Saunders.

Hahn, S.J., & Craft-Rosenberg, M. (2002). The disclosure decisions of parents who conceive children using donor eggs. *Journal of Obstetric, Gynecologic, and Neonatal Nursing, 31*(3), 283-293.

Johnson, J. (2003). Infertility. In J.R. Scott, R.S. Gibbs, B.Y. Karlan, & A.F. Haney (Eds.), *Danforth's obstetrics and gynecology* (9th ed., pp. 685-695). Philadelphia: Lippincott Williams & Wilkins.

Jones, E.E., & DeCherney, A.H. (2003a). The female reproductive system. In E.L. Boulpaep & W.F. Boron (Eds.), *Medical physiology* (pp. 1141-1165). Philadelphia: Saunders.

Jones, E.E., & DeCherney, A.H. (2003b). The male reproductive system. In E.L. Boulpaep & W.F. Boron (Eds.), *Medical physiology* (pp. 1122-1140). Philadelphia: Saunders.

Leibowitz, D., & Hoffman, J. (2000). Fertility drug therapies: Past, present, and future. *Journal of Obstetric, Gynecologic, and Neonatal Nursing, 29*(2), 201-210.

Maifeld, M., Hahn, S., Titler, M.G., & Mullen, M. (2003). Decision making regarding multifetal reduction. *Journal of Obstetric, Gynecologic, and Neonatal Nursing, 32*(3), 357-369.

Meldrum, D.R. (2004). Infertility and assisted reproductive technologies. In N.F. Hacker & J.G. Moore (Eds.), *Essentials of obstetrics and gynecology* (4th ed., pp. 413-421). Philadelphia: Saunders.

Mitwally, M.F., Biljan, M.M., & Casper, R.F. (2005). Pregnancy outcome after the use of an aromatase inhibitor for ovarian stimulation. *American Journal of Obstetrics and Gynecology, 192*(2), 381-386.

National Kidney and Urologic Diseases Information Clearinghouse, National Institutes of Health. (2003). *Erectile dysfunction* (NIH Publication No. 04-3923). Retrieved May 4, 2005, from http://www.niddk.nih.gov.

Pagana, K.D., & Pagana, T.J. (2005). *Diagnostic and laboratory test reference.* St. Louis, MO: Elsevier.

Penzias, A.S. (2002). Oocyte donation, 2002. *Infertility and Reproductive Medicine Clinics of North America, 13*(3), 587-594.

Richard-Davis, G. (2002). Ovulation induction for in vitro fertilization: The role of gonadotropin-releasing hormone antagonists. *Infertility and Reproductive Clinics of North America, 13*(3), 437-444.

Richlin, S.S., Shanti, A., & Murphy, A.A. (2003). Assisted reproductive technology. In J.R. Scott, R.S. Gibbs, B.Y. Karlan, & A.F. Haney (Eds.), *Danforth's obstetrics and gynecology* (9th ed., pp. 697-712). Philadelphia: Lippincott Williams & Wilkins.

Wilkinson, E.J. (2003). Benign vulvovaginal disorders. In J.R. Scott, R.S. Gibbs, B.Y. Karlan, & A.F. Haney (Eds.), *Danforth's obstetrics and gynecology* (9th ed., pp. 605-623). Philadelphia: Lippincott Williams & Wilkins.

Women's Health Care

OBJECTIVES

After studying this chapter, you should be able to:

1. Explain examinations and screening procedures recommended to maintain the health of women.
2. Explain benign disorders of the breast, relate them to usual age of onset, and describe the diagnostic procedures used to rule out cancer of the breast.
3. Describe the incidence, risks, pathophysiology, management, and nursing considerations related to malignant breast tumors.
4. Discuss cardiovascular disease in women, including risk factors, signs and symptoms, and prevention measures.
5. Discuss common menstrual cycle disorders.
6. Explain premenstrual syndrome, management options, and nursing considerations.
7. Discuss medical termination of pregnancy in terms of procedures, possible complications, and follow-up care.
8. Describe the physical and psychological changes associated with menopause and options to alleviate uncomfortable changes.
9. Discuss measures to reduce severity of osteoporosis.
10. Describe the major disorders associated with pelvic relaxation in terms of cause, treatment, and nursing considerations.
11. Discuss the most common benign and malignant disorders of the reproductive tract in terms of signs and symptoms, management, and nursing considerations.
12. Describe care of the woman with an infectious disorder of the reproductive tract, including sexually transmissible diseases, pelvic inflammatory disease, and toxic shock syndrome.

Go to your Student CD-ROM for Review Questions keyed to these Objectives.

DEFINITIONS

Adjuvant Therapy Additional treatment that increases or enhances the action of the primary treatment.

Adnexa Accessory parts or organs, such as the fallopian tubes and ovaries associated with the uterus.

Amenorrhea Absence of menstruation. Primary amenorrhea is a delay of the first menstruation. Secondary amenorrhea is cessation of menstruation after its initiation.

Angina Pectoris Myocardial pain usually brought on by physical activity or stress; usually called simply *angina*.

Atrophic Vaginitis Inflammation that occurs when the vagina becomes dry and fragile, usually as a result of estrogen deficit after menopause.

Autogenous Graft Tissue that is moved from one part of the body to another part of the same person's body.

Axillary Tail Wedge of tissue extending from the breast into the axilla (also called the *tail of Spence*).

Carcinoma in Situ Malignant neoplasm in surface tissue that has not extended into deeper tissue.

Climacteric Endocrine, body, and psychic changes occurring at the end of a woman's reproductive cycle. Also informally called *menopause*.

Colposcopy Examination of the vaginal and cervical tissue with a colposcope for magnification of cells.

Condyloma A wartlike growth of the skin seen on the external genitalia, in the vagina, on the cervix, or near the anus; may be caused by human papillomavirus (condyloma acuminatum) or by syphilis (condyloma latum).

DEFINITIONS—cont'd

Cryotherapy Destruction of tissue using extreme cold.

Cystocele Prolapse of the urinary bladder through the anterior vaginal wall.

Dysmenorrhea Painful menstruation.

Dyspareunia Difficult or painful coitus in women.

Dysplasia Abnormal development of tissue.

Dysuria Painful urination often associated with urinary tract infection.

Endometrial Hyperplasia Excessive proliferation of normal cells of the uterine lining; may be caused by administration of estrogen during the postmenopausal period.

Endometriosis Presence of tissue resembling the endometrium outside the uterine cavity.

Laparoscopy Insertion of an illuminated tube into the abdominal cavity to visualize contents, locate bleeding, and perform surgical procedures.

Laparotomy Incision through the abdominal wall to examine the abdominal or pelvic organs or perform other surgical procedures.

Mammogram Study of breast tissue using very-low-dose x-rays; primary tool in the diagnosis of breast tumors.

Menarche Onset of menstruation, usually between 10 and 16 years of age or within 2 years of the start of breast development.

Menometrorrhagia Uterine bleeding that is irregular in frequency and excessive in amount.

Menopause Permanent cessation of menstruation during the climacteric.

Menorrhagia Excessive bleeding at the time of menstruation in number of days' duration, amount of blood lost, or both.

Metrorrhagia Bleeding from the uterus at any time other than during the menstrual period.

Osteoporosis Increased spaces (porosity) in bone; process greatly accelerates after menopause.

Paroxysmal Nocturnal Dyspnea Respiratory distress occurring when lying down; often associated with congestive heart failure.

Peau d'orange Dimpled skin condition in which skin resembles an orange peel; associated with lymphatic edema and often seen over the area of breast cancer.

Phytoestrogen Estrogen substance of plant origin.

Rectocele Herniation (protrusion) of the rectum through the posterior vaginal wall.

Toxic Shock Syndrome Rare, potentially fatal disorder usually caused by toxin produced by *Staphylococcus aureus;* has been associated with improper use of tampons.

This chapter focuses on primary and preventive care of women: routine assessments, screening procedures, and management of specific health concerns. Nurses provide many of the services most valued by women. Some, such as nurse practitioners, provide primary care. Others act as educators and advocates for women. They are responsible for explaining screening and diagnostic procedures and for clarifying options so that women can make informed decisions about care. Finally, nurses traditionally have offered support and comfort to women when they experience disruptions in their health.

NATIONAL EMPHASIS ON WOMEN'S HEALTH

Two national programs have a potential to influence women's health positively. They are the Women's Health Initiative (WHI) of the National Institutes of Health (NIH) and the Healthy People 2010 health promotion and disease prevention agenda coordinated by the U.S. Department of Health and Human Services.

Women's Health Initiative

The WHI is a 15-year health study that began in 1991 and is sponsored by the Heart, Lung, and Blood Institute (NHLBI) within the NIH. The study targets the top causes of death and disability in older women of every race:

- Cardiovascular disease
- Breast cancer
- Colorectal cancer
- Osteoporosis

Long-term studies of these diseases will be done in multiple centers across the United States: (1) a randomized, controlled trial, (2) an observational study, and (3) a community prevention study. The study has now been extended through 2010. For detailed information about the initiative and to determine the status of each study, see the web site at www.nhlbi.nih.gov/whi/index.html.

The randomized, controlled trial will address how hormone replacement therapy (HRT), dietary patterns, and calcium plus vitamin D intake affect these four devastating diseases. This clinical trial has enrolled more than 68,000 women, 50 to 79 years old, in 40 nationwide centers.

The observational study will examine the relationship among lifestyle, health, and risk factors and specific disease outcomes. This study will correlate the medical history and health habits of about 100,000 women over an 8- to 12-year period.

The community prevention study is a collaborative venture between the Centers for Disease Control and Prevention (CDC) and the NIH. Eight community centers will conduct and critically evaluate health programs that encourage women of all races and socioeconomic backgrounds to adopt healthful behaviors. These programs may consist of diet improvement, smoking cessation, exercise, and early detection of treatable health problems.

Healthy People 2010 Goals

The Healthy People 2010 national health promotion and disease prevention initiative has been discussed in other chapters in this text. The Healthy People 2010 home page may be found at http://www.health.gov/healthypeople/default.htm. Several Healthy People 2010 goals also relate to women's health, and many address the goals in the WHI:

- Increase the proportion of adults who are at a healthy weight (body mass index [BMI] of 18.5 to 25) from 42% to 60%
- Reverse the rise in breast cancer deaths from 27.9 per 100,000 women in 1998 to no more than 22.3
- Increase the number of women age 40 or older who have received a mammogram within the preceding 2 years from 67% in 1998 to 70%
- Reduce deaths from cancer of the cervix from 3 per 100,000 women in 1998 to no more than 2
- Increase from 79% in 1998 to 90% the number of women (18 years or older) who received a Pap test for cervical cancer within the last 3 years
- Increase from 35% in 1998 to 50% the number of adults 50 years and older who received a fecal occult blood test within the preceding 2 years
- Reduce the proportion of adults who are hospitalized for vertebral fractures associated with osteoporosis from 17.5 per 10,000 in 1998 to 14 per 10,000
- Reduce the incidence of gonorrhea in women between the ages of 15 and 44 from 123 cases per 100,000 women in 1997 to 19
- Reduce the prevalence of *Chlamydia trachomatis* infections among women under the age of 25 to no more than 3%
- Reduce congenital syphilis from an incidence of 27 per 100,000 live births in 1997 to no more than 1
- Increase the proportion of adolescents in grades 9 through 12 who abstain from sexual intercourse or use condoms if they are sexually active to at least 95%

HEALTH MAINTENANCE

Health maintenance includes measures taken to prevent or detect specific diseases early, when they are most treatable. The most common health maintenance measures include periodic health examinations, immunizations, and screening procedures. Unfortunately, many women do not take advantage of recommended health maintenance measures. Some seek care only when they have a problem. The only regular health care other women receive comes from a gynecologist or nurse practitioner who conducts a gynecologic examination. Therefore those who provide health care for women must be familiar with principles of screening and counseling in areas that are not traditionally associated with gynecology, such as assessing for colon cancer and heart disease.

Health History

The health history identifies risk factors for a variety of conditions and may be obtained from sources such as questionnaires, interviews, and previous records. The focus of a health history depends on the woman's age, but some topics should be discussed with all women. Box 33-1 provides a summary of information to obtain. These topics include dietary intake, physical activity, habits, and sexual practices. Discussions of drugs must include long-term use of prescription and over-the-counter medications. Illicit drugs must also be discussed to provide the safest care for the woman.

Family history identifies many risk factors that cannot be modified. History of hyperlipidemia, heart disease, osteo-

---

BOX 33-1 Health History

Personal History
Demographic data (name, age, marital status or whether living with a partner of either sex)
Reason for seeking medical care (chief complaint)
Current and past state of health, previous surgeries
Height, weight, vital signs
Allergies (drugs, food, environmental allergens)
Medications, usual and reason for taking (over-the-counter; prescribed; illicit)
Use of complementary or alternative therapies, such as herbal or botanical preparations, acupressure
Habits (smoking, use of alcohol, drugs)
Appetite, usual dietary intake
Exercise pattern (type, frequency, duration)
Patterns of elimination (current or chronic problems)
Sleep and rest patterns
Degree of stress and stress management techniques

Menstrual History
Age of menarche
Regularity, duration of menstrual cycle
Menstrual discomfort (time during cycles, intensity, relief measures)
Age at menopause, if applicable

Obstetric History
Gravida, para, length of gestation, weight of infant at birth
Labor experience, medical interventions, and method of delivery

Sexual History
Sexual activity (one partner, multiple partners, age when first sexually active)
Method of contraception (satisfaction with method, adverse reactions, accuracy of use)
Previous sexually transmitted disease
Knowledge and practice of measures for protection from sexually transmitted diseases

Family History
Cardiovascular problems (anemia, hypertension, clotting disorders, stroke, heart attacks)
Cancer (breast, uterine, ovarian, bowel, lung)
Osteoporosis

Psychosocial History
Primary language, additional languages spoken or understood, ability to read
Marital status, employment, occupation, education (relevant to determine financial, social, and emotional support)

COMPLEMENTARY/ALTERNATIVE THERAPY

Many people take herbal or other botanical preparations but do not mention them because they do not consider them drugs. The nurse must specifically ask about use of these preparations or any therapies the woman may use in addition to medically prescribed interventions to obtain the most complete information for the medical history.

porosis, and thyroid disease suggests the best choice of screening tests. A list of family members who had cancer, the type of cancer they had, and their ages when it was discovered provides important information about the woman's risk for cancer, particularly breast and colon cancer.

A family history of heart disease is especially important when the woman is postmenopausal because estrogen, which provides some protection against coronary artery disease (CAD), decreases after menopause, and obesity may increase. If family history, obesity, or other factors increase the woman's risk for heart disease, a baseline electrocardiogram, stress test, and analysis of cholesterol and lipid profiles may identify other risk factors that can be modified.

✓ CHECK YOUR READING

1. How is the WHI expected to affect the health of women?
2. Why is a family history an important part of a health history?
3. What questions should be asked when taking a sexual history?

Physical Assessment

A complete physical examination is essential to detect general health problems. (See a physical assessment text for a full explanation of the process of physical examination.) Blood pressure, temperature, pulse, respirations, and weight are measured at each visit. Height is taken at the initial examination and yearly after that. Loss of height, abnormal curvature of the vertebral column (dorsal kyphosis or scoliosis), and a thickening waistline in the absence of weight gain are important observations in evaluating osteoporosis.

The heart is auscultated to determine rate and rhythm and to detect heart murmurs. Auscultation of the lungs identifies abnormal sounds that may suggest the presence of fluid secondary to heart dysfunction or malignancy. The extremities are observed for varicosities or edema, and pedal pulses are palpated for strength and equality. The abdomen is palpated for tenderness, masses, or distention that may indicate presence of benign or malignant tumors.

Additional assessments are necessary if the woman is in a high-risk group. For instance, if she has a family history of diabetes mellitus, tests such as fasting glucose or a glucose tolerance test may be indicated. If she has a history of multiple sexual partners or a sexual partner with multiple contacts, testing for sexually transmissible diseases (STDs), in-

cluding human immunodeficiency virus (HIV) infection, is indicated.

Preventive Counseling

Physical examination provides an excellent opportunity to counsel women about preventive care. Major preventable problems are overweight and obesity, inactivity, and smoking. Overweight and obesity are associated with numerous health problems such as diabetes, hypertension, and CAD, as well as some cancers of the breast and reproductive organs. Overweight is defined as a BMI of 25 to 29.9. Obesity is defined as a BMI of 30 to 39.9. For both men and women from 20 to 74 years of age, 65% are overweight, including obesity. Of this group, 34% are overweight but not obese, while 31% are obese. Race and ethnic origin show differences among women who are overweight and the percentages within the overweight group who are obese (Figure 33-1) (National Center for Health Statistics, 2004).

- White—57% overweight, 31.3% of this group are obese
- Black—77.5% overweight, 49.5% of this group are obese
- Mexican origin—71.4% overweight, 38.9% of this group are obese

Physical inactivity is linked to overweight and obesity, osteoporosis, high cholesterol levels, and CAD. Women, older adults, and the less affluent are more likely to be inactive. Blacks and Hispanics are less active when compared with whites. Smoking among females is highest in low-income women and those with an education less than high school level (CDC, 2001; National Center for Health Statistics, 2004).

Counseling about diet should be offered, and positive health behaviors, such as adequate physical activity or smoking cessation, should be reinforced. Use of latex con-

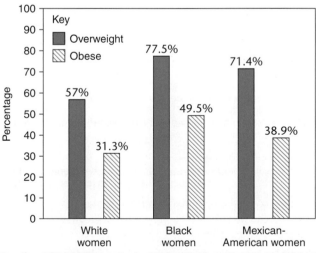

Figure 33-1 ■ The extent of the problem of excess weight in the United States. Overweight is defined as a body mass index (BMI) of 25 to 29.9; obesity is defined as a BMI of 30 to 39.9. The taller bars show the percentage of women who are overweight. The shorter bars for each group show the percentage of women within the overweight group who are obese.

doms should be emphasized for high-risk women with multiple sexual partners or those whose partner has multiple sexual partners. Latex condoms provide some protection against transmission of viruses such as HIV and human papillomavirus (HPV).

The history or physical examination may identify other areas for client counseling. These include the dangers of malignant melanoma with repeated exposure to ultraviolet rays of the sun. In addition, counseling and referral for alcohol and other substance abuse may be needed for some women. Domestic violence may be discovered, requiring counseling for the woman to deal with this complex social problem.

Screening Procedures

The value of screening procedures is based on two assumptions: (1) prevention is better than cure, and (2) early diagnosis allows early treatment while the pathologic process is most curable.

Some screening procedures are recommended for all women of reproductive age, including some screening procedures for early detection of breast cancer as well as vulvar self-examination and screening for cervical cancer. Other screening procedures are recommended for older women or those with higher risk (Box 33-2).

BREAST SELF-EXAMINATION

Breast self-examination (BSE) supplements rather than replaces screening by professional examination and mammography. Although women often discover their abnormalities first, BSE should not be a substitute for clinical breast examination by a clinical professional (ACOG, 2003a). In many parts of the world, however, BSE is the only realistic means of early cancer detection.

BOX 33-2 Risk Factors for Breast Cancer

Female
Age older than 50 years
Early menarche (<10 years of age), late menopause (>50 years of age)
Nulliparity or first pregnancy after 30 years of age
Personal history of breast cancer
Genetic risk factors
Family history in first-degree relative (mother, sister, daughter)
Family history of other cancer
Mutations in the BRCA1 and BRCA2 genes; mutations in the p53 tumor suppressor gene
Mutations in other genes, such as the CHEK-2 gene and the ATM (ataxia-telangiectasia) gene, that have been linked to breast cancer
Previous irradiation of the chest area as a child or young woman as treatment for another cancer (such as Hodgkin's disease or non-Hodgkin's lymphoma)
Previous abnormal breast biopsy results:
    Atypical hyperplasia (increases the risk four to five times)
    Fibrocystic changes without proliferative changes (does not change breast cancer risk)
Long-term hormone replacement therapy with estrogen and progesterone
Physical inactivity

Data from American Cancer Society. (2004). *Detailed guide: Breast Cancer: What are the risk factors for breast cancer?* See www.cancer.org/docroot/home/index.asp.

Most breast cancers are discovered by the woman herself. BSE should be performed monthly by all women after the age of 20 years. Women should perform a BSE about 1 week after the onset of menses, when hormonal influences on the breasts are at a low level. If the woman no longer menstruates, she may choose a day that is easy to remember and perform the examination on that day every month.

CLINICAL BREAST EXAMINATION

Clinical breast examination (CBE) is similar to BSE, but professional examiners may identify questionable areas that the woman misses. It should be routinely performed every 3 years for women ages 20 to 39 years and yearly for those 40 years or older. The American College of Obstetricians and Gynecologists (ACOG) recommends that the CBE be done yearly in all women at the time of the yearly physical examination (ACOG, 2003a; American Cancer Society [ACS], 2004b). Some conditions require more frequent examinations because they are associated with a higher risk for breast cancer than in the general population. The examination includes inspection and palpation and should be part of every gynecologic examination.

INSPECTION

1. While the woman is in an upright position, the examiner inspects the breasts for size, symmetry, color, and skin changes. The nipples and areola are inspected for differences in size and color, unilateral retraction of a nipple, and asymmetric nipple direction, which may indicate an underlying tumor.
2. The woman raises her hands above her head, and the examiner inspects the sides and underneath portions of the breast for asymmetry and differences in color.
3. The woman places her hands on her hips and presses down to reveal skin dimpling or masses.

PALPATION

1. While the woman is in an upright position with her arm relaxed at her side, the axillary, supraclavicular, and suprasternal lymph nodes are palpated for tenderness or enlargement.
2. The woman lies in a supine position for palpation of the breasts. A small pillow or folded towel is placed under the shoulder to stretch the tissue and flatten the breast. The examiner uses the flat part of the first three fingers to palpate the breast, rotating the fingers against the chest wall. Tissue that extends into the axilla, the axillary tail (or tail of Spence), should be palpated. The procedure is repeated on the opposite side. Normal breast tissue is described as firm, lumpy, nodular, tender, and thickened. Abnormal breast tissue is often likened to a raisin, watermelon seed, or grape because a discrete mass can be felt and its size estimated. If a suspicious area is found, follow up by diagnostic mammography, often ultrasonography is recommended.
3. The nipples are compressed to detect the presence of discharge. A sample of any discharge should be collected for culture and examination of cells.

How to Perform Breast Self-Examination

- Lie down. Flatten your right breast by placing a pillow under your right shoulder. If your breasts are large, use your right hand to hold your right breast while you do the examination with your left hand.

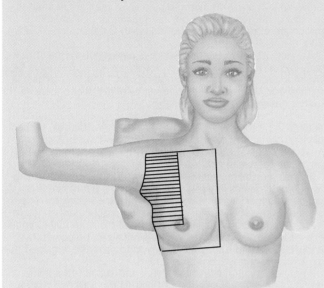

- Use the sensitive pads of the middle three fingers on your left hand and a massaging motion to feel for lumps or changes in the breast tissue.
- Press firmly enough to distinguish different breast textures: light pressure to feel tissues near the skin, medium pressure to feel slightly deeper, and firm pressure to feel tissues near the chest and ribs.
- Completely palpate or feel all parts of the breast and chest area. Be sure to examine the breast tissue that extends toward the shoulder. The amount of time required to completely palpate all the breast tissue depends on the size of the breast. Women with small breasts need at least 2 minutes to examine each breast. Larger breasts take longer.

- Use the same routine or pattern to feel every part of the breast tissue. Any of three patterns can help you make sure you have covered your entire breast: the vertical strip, the circular pattern, and the wedge. Choose the method you find easiest. Evidence suggests the up-and-down pattern is the most effective to avoid missing breast tissue.
- When you have completely examined your right breast, examine the left breast with your right hand using the same method. Compare what you feel in one breast with the other.

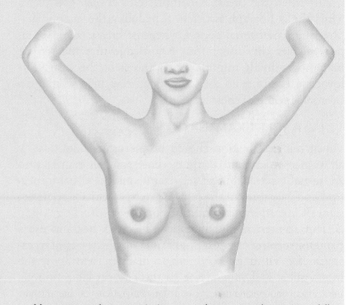

- You may also want to examine your breasts while bathing, when the skin is wet and lumps may be easily palpated.
- You can check your breasts in a mirror by raising your arms and looking for an unusual shape, dimpling of the skin, and any changes in the nipple.
- Examine each underarm, either when sitting or standing, by raising your arm slightly to better feel the area. Raising your arm high will tighten tissues in the area, reducing what you can feel.

Source: American Cancer Society's *How to perform a breast self-exam.* Copyright 2003, American Cancer Society, Inc. www.cancer.org. Reprinted with permission.

MAMMOGRAPHY

Mammography may be used either to screen for cancer or to assist in the diagnosis of a palpable mass in the breast. Mammography is a screening tool that can detect breast lumps well before they are large enough to be palpated. This procedure, often accompanied by ultrasound examination, allows early diagnosis and treatment and thereby increases the chance of long-term survival.

No consensus exists on the frequency of mammography for women in their forties. The ACS (2004b) recommends screening mammography each year for women age 40 and older. ACOG (2003a) recommends that women have a mammogram every 1 to 2 years at age 40 to 49, and yearly after age 50. Women at high risk for breast cancer (see p. 882 for a summary of risk factors) may need earlier or more frequent mammography and should consult their health care providers.

Despite the known value of mammography, many women have never had a mammogram. Reasons for this include lack of a health care professional's recommendation, expense, fear that x-ray exposure will cause cancer, fear of pain, and reluctance to hear "bad news." Nurses provide information and reassurance whenever possible and, in this way, help the woman overcome her objections to the use of this valuable screening tool. Mammography is relatively expensive, but part of its cost is often covered by health insurance, Medicaid, or Medicare. Screening mammograms are frequently offered by community agencies at low cost. The ACS (www.cancer.org) is a source of information about low-cost mammograms. Acknowledge that brief discomfort occurs when the breast is compressed between two plates while the radiograph is taken. Scheduling the mammography after a menstrual period, when the breasts are less tender, reduces the discomfort. Knowledge that the risk of mammography is minimal to nonexistent, because very-low-dose exposure to x-rays is used, may help women to overcome some of their fear.

VULVAR SELF-EXAMINATION

Vulvar self-examination should be performed monthly by all women older than 18 and by those younger than 18 who are sexually active. Vulvar self-examination is visual inspection and palpation of the female external genitalia to detect signs of precancerous conditions or infections.

The woman should sit in a well-lighted area and use a hand mirror to see her external genitalia. She is taught to examine the vulva in a systematic manner, starting at the mons pubis and progressing to the clitoris, labia minora, labia majora, perineum, and anus. Palpation of the vulvar area should accompany visual inspection. She should report new moles, warts or growths of any kind, ulcers, sores, changes in skin color, or areas of inflammation or itching to her health care provider as soon as possible.

PELVIC EXAMINATION

The complete gynecologic assessment includes a pelvic examination. The woman should schedule the examination between menstrual periods and should not douche or have sexual intercourse for at least 48 hours before the examination. She also is advised not to use vaginal medications, sprays, or deodorants that might interfere with interpretation of cytology specimens that are collected.

The procedure is carefully explained before the examination, and the woman empties her bladder. Although pelvic examinations are relatively painless, most women dislike them and welcome sensitive, considerate support. Women who have undergone female genital mutilation (Box 33-3) need extra consideration. The nurse must avoid displaying shock, despite the fact that most nurses in Western countries have an aversion to this often-unfamiliar practice. A pediatric vaginal speculum may be needed for these or other women with a very small vaginal opening. Routine preventive pelvic examinations may be impossible for women who have only a tiny opening left for drainage of urine and menstrual blood.

BOX 33-3 Female Genital Mutilation

Female genital mutilation, sometimes called *female circumcision,* is the ritual disfigurement and the partial or total removal of a girl's external genitalia or other injury to her external genitalia for cultural, religious, or other nontherapeutic reasons.

The practice occurs in Africa and in some areas of the Middle East and Asia. It may be found in immigrant groups in Europe, Australia, New Zealand, Canada, and the United States. Between 100 and 140 million girls and women are estimated to have undergone female genital mutilation, and another 2 million are at risk annually (World Health Organization [WHO], 2000).

The age at which the procedure is performed varies from a few days old to adult. Most are performed when the girl is between 4 and 10 years old, an age at which she cannot give informed consent for a procedure with lifetime consequences for her health.

Female genital mutilation may be done by a village practitioner using crude tools, such as knives, razor blades, broken glass, thorns, or scissors, and without anesthesia. Parents in more developed countries may seek the procedure from a physician to assure pain relief and sterility.

Female genital mutilation is considered a part of the coming-of-age ceremonies in some societies, and a girl may not be considered marriageable unless she has undergone the procedure. Some societies believe that the practice enhances female chastity and increases male sexual pleasure. Other societies consider the external female genitalia to be unsightly and dirty. Therefore they are removed to promote hygiene and the woman's attractiveness.

Female genital mutilation is illegal and subject to criminal prosecution in several countries, including the United States.

Four major types of female genital mutilation exist (WHO, 2000):
- Type I: Excision of the skin surrounding the clitoris (prepuce), with or without excision of all or part of the clitoris
- Type II: Removal of all of the clitoris and part or all of the labia minora. The vaginal opening is visible.
- Type III: Excision of part or all of the external genitalia and stitching or narrowing of the vaginal opening (infibulation).
- Type IV: Various practices of pricking, piercing, and cutting of the clitoris and labia; stretching of the clitoris or labia; cauterization of the clitoris and surrounding tissue.

Other mutilations may include scraping of tissue surrounding the vagina or cutting into the vagina itself, placing corrosive or herbal substances into the vagina to cause bleeding to tighten or narrow the vagina.

Health consequences may include the immediate results of severe pain, shock, hemorrhage, ulceration, urinary retention, and infection. Transmission of human immunodeficiency virus is a concern if unsterile materials are used or if the vaginal opening is so small that anal intercourse is used as an alternative to vaginal intercourse. Infibulation may result in scar formation that causes dyspareunia, difficulty urinating, difficulty with menstruation, recurrent urinary tract infections, and infertility. Painful intercourse and reduced sexual sensitivity may have consequences on psychological health.

Several groups worldwide are working together to target societies and parents where the practice prevails, educating them about its harm to girls and women. The intent is to eradicate the harmful practice through education and legislation.

The adolescent having her first examination also benefits from an understanding nurse who takes the time to explain the equipment and steps of the examination carefully before having the adolescent undress. If she is anxious and fidgeting, she will appreciate a hand to hold and an explanation before each step. Some of the breathing techniques used for birth, such as slow, paced breathing, or use of a focal point (see Chapter 15), may be helpful.

The pelvic examination is done usually with the woman in a lithotomy position, with a pillow under her head. If she wishes, she may be placed in a semi-sitting position and offered a hand mirror so that she can observe the external genitalia and the examination and learn more about her body. She is draped so that only the parts being examined are exposed.

Women who cannot tolerate a lithotomy position, such as a frail elderly woman, may benefit from a side-lying pelvic examination. The pelvic can also be done with the woman in a semi-Fowler's position, with her knees bent and feet on the examination table, rather than using the stirrups and having her hips at the edge of the table. The paraplegic woman, with no control over her lower extremities, usually can be examined with her legs separated in a V shape without her knees being bent.

Necessary equipment to be assembled before the examination begins includes gloves, speculum (several sizes, including pediatric, should be available), slides, cotton swabs, a fixative agent, and a cytobrush and spatula for obtaining material for the cytology specimen, or Pap (Papanicolaou) test (see later in this chapter). A stool specimen may be obtained by the examiner during the rectal examination, and a slide for this specimen also should be available.

EXTERNAL ORGANS. The pelvic examination is conducted systematically and gently. The external organs are inspected for the degree of development or atrophy of the labia, the distribution of hair, and the character of the hymen. Any cysts, tumors, or inflammation of Bartholin's glands is noted. The urinary meatus and Skene's glands are inspected for purulent discharge. Perineal scarring resulting from childbirth is noted.

SPECULUM EXAMINATION. A bivalve speculum of the appropriate size is used to inspect the vagina and cervix. The speculum is warmed with tap water and gently inserted into the vagina. No other lubrication is used because it interferes with accurate cytology results. The size, shape, and color of the cervix are noted. A sample is taken for the Pap test. In addition, a sample of any unusual discharge is obtained for microscopic examination or culture.

BIMANUAL EXAMINATION. The bimanual examination provides information about the uterus, fallopian tubes, and ovaries. The labia are separated, and the gloved, lubricated index finger and middle finger of one hand are inserted into the vaginal introitus.

The cervix is palpated for consistency, size, and tenderness to motion. The uterus is evaluated by placing the other hand on the abdomen with the fingers pressing gently just above the symphysis pubis so that the uterus can be felt between the examining fingers of both hands. The size, configuration, consistency, and mobility of the uterus are evaluated (Figure 33-2).

Feeling the fallopian tubes is usually impossible, although the ovaries may be palpated between the fingers of both hands. Because ovaries atrophy after menopause, palpating the ovaries of a postmenopausal woman is usually not possible.

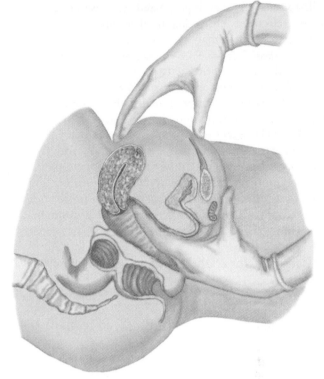

Figure 33-2 ■ Bimanual palpation provides information about the uterus, fallopian tubes, and ovaries.

PAP TEST

PURPOSE. It is known that, in virtually all cases, changes occur in cells of the cervix before cervical cancer develops. These changes have variously been called *cervical intraepithelial neoplasia, dysplasia, squamous intraepithelial lesions (SIL),* and *carcinoma in situ.* Cervical cytology, or the Pap test, is the most useful procedure for detecting precancerous and cancerous cells that may be shed by the cervix. Regular Pap tests can increase the survival for women who develop cervical cancer by identifying it when it is most treatable. Because infection with HPV has been shown to contribute to cervical neoplasms, testing for this virus is often done during the pelvic examination.

PROCEDURE. With the speculum blades open and the cervix in view, samples of the superficial layers of the cervix and endocervix are obtained. Samples are best obtained with a spatula and a cytobrush or with a broom-type sampling device. A sample is taken where most lesions develop, at the squamocolumnar junction (the border where developing squamous tissue meets the immature columnar epithelium). In postmenopausal women the squamocolumnar junction recedes into the endocervix, making cervical specimens obtained by the cytobrush or broom-type device important.

Cervical tissue is placed on slides that are then sprayed with or immersed in a fixative solution before being sent to the laboratory for analysis if the older Pap test technique is used. Specimens obtained with the broom-type device, such as those in the liquid-based Thin-Prep or AutoCyte tests for cervical cancer, are rotated in the liquid that preserves the cells for analysis. The liquid-based tests use image processing to select the slides that need additional reading by a technician for best analysis.

CLASSIFICATION OF CERVICAL CYTOLOGY.
A great deal of variation existed in how cervical cytology findings were reported until recently. The Bethesda system was devised to offer standard terminology and give a narrative, descriptive diagnosis. It consists of three elements: (1) a statement of specimen adequacy, (2) a general categorization (normal or abnormal), and (3) a descriptive diagnosis regarding abnormal cytology. Additional interpretations not related to cancer include presence of infecting organisms (such as *Trichomonas vaginalis*), changes that may be associated with inflammation, radiation, or intrauterine contraceptives), or atrophy of the cervical cells.

Categories for epithelial cell abnormalities include the following:

- Atypical squamous cells of undetermined significance (ASCUS).
- Squamous intraepithelial lesion, which is subdivided into (a) low-grade SIL (including cellular changes of HPV) and (b) high-grade SIL (previously categorized as carcinoma in situ). High-grade SIL is more likely to become cancerous without definitive treatment.
- Squamous cell cancer.

Glandular cell abnormalities are categorized as follows:

- Atypical glandular cells of uncertain significance (AGCUS)
- Adenocarcinoma

The woman's follow-up depends on the nature of the abnormality and whether it is persistent. Pap tests that have persistent ASCUS findings after a 3- to 6-month interval also usually are evaluated by colposcopy. Suspicious lesions are examined with colposcopy and biopsy.

RECTAL EXAMINATION

The anus is inspected for hemorrhoids, inflammation, and lesions. The examiner's lubricated index finger is gently inserted, and sphincter tone is noted. A slide may be prepared to test for the presence of occult blood in stool.

Fecal occult blood testing (FOBT) is a useful yearly screening measure for colorectal cancer beginning at age 50. Special instructions are necessary to prevent false test results when the woman is given materials for FOBT. She should be instructed to do the following:

- Avoid aspirin and nonsteroidal antiinflammatory drugs (NSAIDs) such as ibuprofen or naproxen for at least 7 days before collecting the specimen.
- Avoid red meat, raw fruits and vegetables, horseradish, and vitamin C for 72 hours before testing.
- Collect a specimen from three consecutive stools.
- Return slides as directed within 4 to 6 days after the specimens are collected.

A newer test, the fecal immunochemical test (FIT) may be done, requiring only two samples and having a lower risk of false-positive results (ACS, 2005).

LABORATORY SCREENING TESTS

Additional laboratory tests depend on the age, history, and risk assessment of the woman and might include the following:

- Testing for STDs, such as chlamydial infection, gonorrhea, syphilis, and HIV
- Testing for rubella immunity, which is particularly important in the childbearing years, although the overall incidence of the disease is very low in the United States
- Tuberculosis skin testing or chest x-ray examination
- Cholesterol and other lipid profile testing of women at risk for CAD (particularly important after menopause)
- Fasting glucose testing or other tests to identify development of diabetes, recommended every 3 years after age 45 or earlier if the woman has high-risk factors such as family history or being overweight
- Urinalysis to detect signs of urinary tract infection
- Thyroid function tests, which may be indicated if the woman exhibits signs of thyroid dysfunction, such as heart palpitations and heat intolerance
- Serum testing for genes associated with specific cancers, such as the BRCA1, BRCA2, or p53 genes associated with breast and some other cancers
- Serum testing for CA-125, a tumor marker that may be elevated with ovarian cancer
- Transvaginal ultrasonography, which may be recommended for women who are at increased risk for malignant disorders of the reproductive tract (see Chapter 10)
- A sigmoidoscopy (every 5 years after age 50); a yearly colonoscopy may be recommended if the woman has a family history of colon cancer because the sigmoidoscopy only examines about half the length of the colon
- A colonoscopy every 10 years for more detailed examinations because of personal or family history

See Table 33-1 for a summary of recommended procedures.

✓ CHECK YOUR READING

4. What are the three screening procedures to identify cancer of the breast?
5. Why is vulvar self-examination recommended?
6. What is a Pap test, and why is it performed?
7. Why is fecal occult blood testing important?

Diagnosis of Disorders of the Breast

When a lesion or lump is discovered in the breast, the physician must determine if it is benign or malignant. Ultrasound examination can be used to differentiate fluid-filled cysts from solid tissue, which is more likely to be malignant. Fine needle aspiration (FNA) biopsy can be performed to remove fluid or small tissue fragments for analysis of the cells. Core needle biopsy uses a larger needle to obtain a cylinder of tissue from an area of abnormal breast tissue. Open, or surgical, biopsy is performed to re-

TABLE 33-1 Summary of Screening Procedures

Procedure	Purpose
Breast self-examination (BSE)	For the woman to assess monthly for breast changes or masses that might indicate breast tumors
Clinical breast examination (CBE)	For a health care professional to detect masses that women might miss
Mammography with additional imaging, such as ultrasonography, as needed and yearly in women 40 years or older (routine screening mammography)*	To detect breast lumps before they become palpable, promoting long-term survival; diagnostic mammograms and other imaging may be started at a younger age for women having a higher risk for breast cancer or previous breast cancer or other disorders.
Cholesterol test	To detect blood levels that raise risk for heart disease; often combined with additional tests for high-quality screening, such as triglyceride level, high-density lipoprotein (HDL), and low-density lipoprotein (LDL)
Vulvar self-examination	To detect signs of precancerous conditions or infection
Pelvic examination	To confirm that no disease exists, or for early detection if disease does exist
Pap test	To detect abnormal cervical cytology as early as possible
Rectal examination	To check for hemorrhoids and lesions and to evaluate sphincter control
Fecal occult blood test (FOBT)	To detect blood in stool, an early sign of colon cancer
Urinalysis	To screen for diabetes and urinary infections

Additional Procedures May Be Based on Risk Factors

Procedure	Risk Factors
Sexually transmissible disease (STD) testing	Multiple sexual partners of the woman or her partner, history of STDs
Human immunodeficiency virus (HIV) testing	Seeking treatment for STDs, injection drug use, sexual partner who is HIV-positive or bisexual or injects drugs, recurrent or persistent episodes of STDs such as candidiasis and herpes
Lipid profile	Diabetes, smoking, no estrogen use after menopause, family history of high cholesterol or coronary artery disease, overweight
Fasting glucose test	Overweight, history of gestational diabetes, family history of diabetes
Rubella antibodies	To assess immunity to rubella
Thyroid-stimulating hormone	Signs or strong family history of thyroid disease
Blood tests to evaluate genetic risk for reproductive cancers, such as BRCA1 and BRCA2, CA-125, p53 or other indicated gene evaluation	To determine the degree of higher risk influenced by genetic alterations, improving options for therapy
Transvaginal ultrasound examination	Family history of ovarian cancer
Sigmoidoscopy or colonoscopy	Family history of bowel cancer or age >50 years
Tuberculosis testing	To determine infection in a person at higher risk for tuberculosis

*American Cancer Society. (2004). *Detailed guide: Breast Cancer: What are the risk factors for breast cancer?* Retrieved March 22, 2005, from www.cancer.org/docroot/home/index.asp.

move all or part of the lump of breast tissue if other conditions exist:

- Suspicious mass that persists through a menstrual cycle
- Bloody fluid aspirated from a cyst
- Failure of the mass to disappear completely after fluid aspiration
- Recurrence of the cyst after one or two aspirations
- Solid dominant mass not diagnosed as fibroadenoma
- Serous or serosanguineous nipple discharge
- Nipple ulceration or persistent crusting
- Skin edema and erythema suspicious for inflammatory breast carcinoma
- Suspicious mammography or ultrasound findings

BENIGN DISORDERS OF THE BREAST

Four relatively common benign disorders of the breast tend to occur at different ages.

Fibrocystic Breast Changes

Fibrocystic breast changes are common benign breast changes during the reproductive years before menopause. The early stage is characterized by fibrosis, or thickening of the normal breast tissue, whereas cysts form in the latter

stages and are felt as multiple, smooth, well-delineated nodules, which are usually present bilaterally.

The most common symptom of fibrocystic breast changes is pain and tenderness. The pain is often bilateral and most noticeable during the premenstrual phase of the normal cycle. Women with large breasts may have pain associated with stretching of the breast ligaments. Premenstrual pain is believed to be the result of an imbalanced estrogen-progesterone ratio. Women with fibrocystic breast changes improve dramatically during pregnancy and lactation because of the large amounts of progesterone produced that blocks the excess amounts of estrogens produced when the woman is not pregnant.

The initial therapy varies with the age of the woman and her risk for breast cancer. Aspiration of cysts may relieve pain with follow-up needed only if the cyst disappears and the fluid aspirated is clear. The bilateral nature of the changes and pain suggest that the condition is benign, but definitive studies such as mammogram and ultrasound imaging, FNA of the cysts, or surgical biopsy may be needed to identify malignancy. Fibrocystic breast changes may fall into three categories (Gemignani, 2003; Hacker, 2004a):

- Nonproliferative lesions
- Hyperplasia without atypical cells
- Atypical hyperplasia

Hyperplastic lesions with atypical cellular changes have an increased risk to become malignant, but most women with fibrocystic breast changes do not have a greater risk for breast cancer.

Specific symptom relief for fibrocystic disease has not proven beneficial, but some methods may be worth trying. Avoiding caffeine and other stimulants (coffee, tea, chocolate, and some soft drinks) reduces methylxanthines that may increase discomfort during the last half of the menstrual cycle. Edema may be limited by reducing salt intake, although diuretics are not commonly prescribed.

Fibroadenoma

Fibroadenomas are common benign tumors of the breast, and although they may occur at any age, they are most common during the teenage years and the twenties. Fibroadenomas are composed of both fibrous and glandular tissue. They are firm, freely mobile nodules that may or may not be tender when palpated. Fibroadenomas do not change during the menstrual cycle. They are generally located in the upper, outer quadrant of the breast, and more than one is often present.

Treatment may involve careful observation for a few months to determine if the mass is stable. FNA or core biopsy of the tumor is done if the mass continues to enlarge. The mass may be excised and the specimen analyzed to rule out malignancy if results of other diagnostic tests are not conclusive.

Ductal Ectasia

Ductal ectasia generally occurs as the woman approaches menopause. It is characterized by dilation of the collecting ducts, which become distended and filled with cellular debris. This initiates an inflammatory process resulting in

- A mass that feels firm and irregular
- Enlarged axillary nodes
- Nipple retraction and discharge

These signs are similar to those of breast cancer, and accurate diagnosis is vital. Once an excisional biopsy that removes the mass indicates that the condition is benign mammary duct ectasia, no further treatment is necessary.

Intraductal Papilloma

Intraductal papilloma develops most often just before or during menopause. It occurs when papillomas (small elevations or protuberances) develop in the epithelium of the ducts of the breasts. Most lesions are located under the areola. As the papilloma grows, it causes trauma and erosion within the ducts that result in serous or bloody discharge from the nipple. Ultrasonography and diagnostic mammography aid in the diagnosis of the intraductal papilloma.

Treatment consists of excision of the mass and ductal area, plus analysis of nipple discharge to rule out a malignant tumor. Long-term follow-up is essential to identify any malignancy early.

Nursing Considerations

The nurse must acknowledge the anxiety that all women feel when a breast disorder is discovered. Furthermore, the apprehension continues for most women while they await a final diagnosis. Some women may find it helpful to learn that most breast disorders are benign. However, as discussed, some benign disorders do increase the risk for later occurrence of cancer. For others, the most helpful intervention is to encourage them to express their concerns.

The nurse should explain the diagnostic procedures that are planned, such as ultrasound examination, mammography, needle biopsy, or surgical biopsy. Explanations should include what the procedures entail and how long the woman will have to wait for results to be known. The woman's anxiety may be high, and she will likely need reinforcement of explanations that she has forgotten.

✔ **CHECK YOUR READING**

8. How are fibrocystic breast changes treated?
9. What diagnostic procedures are used to determine whether a breast disorder is benign or malignant?

MALIGNANT TUMORS OF THE BREAST

Incidence

The lifetime risk for a woman to develop breast cancer in the United States is 1 in 7. Although men develop breast cancer, the risk for women is 100 times greater than for men. During 2003 the risk for development of invasive breast cancer was estimated to be approximately 211,300 among women in the United States. Breast cancer is the leading cancer among women of all races. However, in the United States white women have a breast cancer rate that is about 1.2 times higher than the rate for black women and 1.5 times higher than that for Asian and Pacific Islander women. However, African-American women have a higher risk of dying from breast cancer because they are more likely to be diagnosed at a later and more advanced stage. Asian, Hispanic, and Native American women have a lower risk for developing cancer (ACS, 2003a; ACS, 2004b).

Risk Factors

Although the actual cause of breast cancer remains unknown, several factors are known to increase the risk for the development of breast and ovarian cancer or other diseases (see Box 33-2). Mutations in two genes (BRCA1 and BRCA2) thought to be responsible for most cases of familial breast cancer have been identified. Mutation of the CHEK-2 gene has shown higher risk for development of breast cancer in both women and men. Mutation of the p53 tumor suppressor gene has been shown to increase the risk for breast and other cancers. Study of genetic links to many types of cancers and nonmalignant diseases is ongoing. Because research has linked these and other genes to an increased risk for breast or other cancers, testing is offered to the woman having a higher risk or who has developed cancer at a younger age than expected.

Knowing risk factors is important to guide breast cancer screening and treatment processes so that a cancer is diagnosed at the earliest stage possible. It is also important for the nurse to convey to women that many breast cancers develop in women with no known risk factors, whereas other women with one or more risk factors do not develop breast cancer.

Pathophysiology

About 65% to 80% of breast cancers are infiltrating ductal carcinoma, which originates in the epithelial lining of the mammary ducts. The cancer becomes invasive when it is no longer confined to the duct and spreads to surrounding breast tissue. Another 10% to 14% of breast cancers are infiltrating lobular cancer that originates in the milk-secreting pockets of breast tissue. Most breast cancers grow in irregular patterns and invade the lymphatic channels, eventually causing lymphatic edema and the dimpling of the skin that resembles an orange peel (peau d'orange). Several types of breast tumors may be present at the same time (Gemignani, 2003; Hacker, 2004a).

Cancer cells are carried by the lymph channels to the lymph nodes, and 40% to 50% of patients have involvement of axillary lymph nodes at the time of diagnosis. By the time a patient consults a physician, breast cancer may already be a systemic disease rather than being confined to the local tissue. Metastasis occurs when the malignant cells are spread by both blood and lymph systems to distant organs. Distant metastases include the lungs, liver, bones, and brain.

Staging

Although confirmation of malignancy is the first step in evaluating the woman with cancer, staging is necessary to understand the severity of the cancer and plan the best therapy. Staging is based on the TNM (tumor, node, and metastasis) system used to describe the cancer's anatomic extent. Stages of breast cancer progress from stage 1, indicating a small tumor without lymphatic involvement in the local area or metastases, to stage 4, which indicates spread to lymph nodes and metastases to distant organs. The stages are used to guide treatment and help provide a prognosis. The type of cancer cell, the presence of hormone receptors, and the proliferative rate of the breast cancer cells are also important factors in the rate of recurrence and determination of most appropriate treatment.

Management

Many new treatments have emerged over the last decade. A combination of surgical excision of the tumor and locally involved lymph nodes and adjuvant therapy is recom-

mended. The combination of therapies is individualized for each patient. New techniques, medications, and management emerge frequently, and the nurse who cares for women with cancer should stay informed about changes in therapy.

SURGICAL TREATMENT

The surgical procedure depends on the type, stage, and location of the disease. The most common surgeries are the following:

- Breast conservation treatment, which involves wide local excision (lumpectomy) of the tumor to microscopically clean margins for tumors that are small relative to the breast size. Some axillary lymph nodes are removed to determine spread of the disease. Radiation or other adjuvant therapy is indicated to complete the treatment.

- Simple mastectomy, which is removal of the entire breast. Axillary dissection is omitted, although some lymph nodes may be removed for staging purposes. It may be recommended for selected cases in which prophylactic removal of the breast is considered for a woman at high risk for development of breast cancer. Simple mastectomy in the absence of cancer does not eradicate the risk for later breast cancer, however, because a small amount of breast tissue remains.

- Modified radical mastectomy, which involves removal of breast tissue, axillary nodes, and some chest muscles; however, the pectoralis major muscle is preserved. This surgical procedure may be recommended when a single large primary lesion or multiple lesions exist in a relatively small breast because cosmetic results may be less than satisfactory. Other factors include whether the woman can undergo radiation therapy. Radiation therapy after surgery may not be possible if she is pregnant, has had prior breast or chest radiation, or has an autoimmune disease such as systemic lupus erythematosus (Gemignani, 2003).

Sentinel lymph node (SLN) biopsy is a technique to remove a few key lymph nodes to evaluate cancer spread rather than removing most of the nodes in the area (axillary dissection). A radioisotope suspension or a special dye is injected near the tumor site, where it is transported by the lymphatics toward the axillary nodes and trapped by the first one or two lymph nodes, or the "sentinel" nodes. The nodes identified by one or both of these techniques are excised for evaluation. If cancer has not spread to a sentinel node, the surgeon does not have to remove a large number of lymph nodes for staging of the cancer. Reducing the number of lymph nodes removed helps avoid some of the problems caused by lymphedema (see p. 891).

ADJUVANT THERAPY

Adjuvant therapy is supportive or additional therapy that is usually recommended after the surgical procedure. Radiation, chemotherapy, hormone therapy, and immunotherapy are adjuvant therapies that are often recommended. The decision about adjuvant therapy is based on the woman's age, the stage of the disease, the woman's preference, and the hormone receptor status of the lesion. Radiation and chemotherapy are known to improve the chance of long-term survival, and one or both are usually recommended after surgical excision of the tumor. For a more in-depth discussion of cancer treatment, see a medical-surgical nursing text.

RADIATION THERAPY. Radiation uses high-energy rays to destroy cancer cells that remain in the breast, the chest wall, and the underarm area after surgery. The lymph nodes above the clavicle and the internal mammary lymph nodes are also irradiated. Radiation may be used to reduce the size of a large tumor before surgery. A radiation oncologist directs use of radiation in cancer therapy. The skin in the treated area may have a reaction similar to sunburn. Lymphedema is more likely to occur if the axillary lymph nodes are treated. A newer technology to limit the adverse effects of radiation on normal tissues while giving a maximum dose of radiation to the tumor site is intensity-modulated radiation therapy (IMRT).

CHEMOTHERAPY. Chemotherapy drugs are designed to kill the proliferating cancer cells. The specific combination of drugs and number of treatment cycles is individualized for factors such as type of cancer cells, the woman's age, hormone-receptor status of malignant cells, whether she is postmenopausal, and other important factors such as medications she needs for nonmalignant disorders. Depending on the specific drugs, chemotherapeutics often kill normal cells, especially rapidly dividing cells such those in the mucosa, the blood cells, and the platelets. For this reason, the woman often has sore, bleeding gums or other bleeding tendencies and may be more susceptible to infection during treatment. Many chemotherapeutic drugs cause hair loss (head and body hair) or menstrual irregularities during treatment. Anemia, with resulting fatigue, is common because erythrocyte production is impaired.

HORMONAL THERAPY. Estrogen-blocking medications are prescribed because many breast tumors are estrogen receptor–positive, meaning that their growth is stimulated by estrogen. Estrogen receptor–positive tumors may occur in both premenopausal and postmenopausal women. Risks and benefits of proposed estrogen-blocking medications are discussed with the oncologist, particularly in women who have not reached menopause.

Tamoxifen (Nolvadex) blocks estrogen by binding to estrogen receptors, thereby suppressing tumor growth by reducing the effects of estrogen. Hot flashes, vaginal dryness or an increased vaginal discharge, nausea, or anorexia may occur with tamoxifen therapy. Laboratory values for calcium, cholesterol, and triglycerides may be elevated. Anastrozole (Arimidex), exemestane (Aromasin), and letrozole (Femara) are aromatase inhibitors with estrogen-blocking capabilities (they block conversion of androgens to estrogen).

Raloxifene (Evista) is an estrogen modifier to reduce osteoporosis that also blocks the estrogen effects for the breast. Raloxifene also lowers low-density lipoproteins and cholesterol. Because of its estrogen-blocking effects, raloxifene is being studied in the Study of Tamoxifen and Raloxifene (STAR) research backed by National Cancer Institute that is to be completed in the summer of 2006.

IMMUNOTHERAPY. Trastuzumab (Herceptin) is a biologically based therapy that targets cell pathways that promote cancer growth. Some tumors produce excessive amounts of the HER-2 protein, promoting tumor cell growth. Trastuzumab blocks the effect of this protein to inhibit growth of the cancer cells. Research is ongoing into other immunotherapy for breast and other cancers.

BREAST RECONSTRUCTION

TIMING. Breast reconstruction is a standard option in the treatment of breast cancer, and the timing of reconstruction should be discussed with the woman before surgical treatment. Immediate reconstruction has a psychological appeal, but expected therapy after surgery may have aspects which make later reconstruction the best option. The prospect of having a life-threatening breast cancer and simultaneously facing the loss of a breast may be overwhelming for many women. Conversely, delayed reconstruction may give a woman time to learn about the procedure, to heal from the mastectomy, and to consider the extent of the disease and the side effects associated with adjuvant therapy.

METHOD. Several methods of breast reconstruction are available. The tissue expansion method uses an empty silicone prosthesis fitted with a valve that can be accessed by percutaneous needle puncture. The bag is filled with saline in small increments to slowly expand the tissue. When the desired volume is attained, the incision is reopened, the device is removed, and the expander is exchanged for the appropriate implant. In some models, only the valve must be removed and the expander serves as the permanent implant (ACS, 2004a; Resnick & Belcher, 2002).

Tissue flap procedures move autogenous tissue from the back, abdomen, or buttocks to create a breast mound. Although these procedures do not always involve implants of a foreign substance as the tissue expansion method does, they involve at least two incisions: one at the breast and one at the site of the donor tissue. All women are not suitable for muscle flap grafts, particularly those with diabetes or connective tissue disorders and smokers, because these procedures involve altering the blood supply to the transplanted tissue, with the possibility of poor wound healing for these women. Thin women may not have sufficient tissue for transplant to the breast (ACS, 2004a; Gemignani, 2003; Resnick & Belcher, 2002).

Types of tissue flap procedures include the following:

- Transverse rectus abdominis muscle (TRAM) flap, which uses extra abdominal tissue in two common ways, as follows. A pedicle flap allows the tissue to remain attached to its original blood supply while it is tunneled under the skin to its site for breast reconstruction. The *free flap* involves removal of the tissue from its original site for attachment to the breast site. Because blood vessels are disconnected in free flap removal, microsurgery is required to reconnect the vessels and promote tissue-preserving blood flow in the graft.

- Deep inferior epigastric artery perforator (DIEP) flap, which is a newer procedure in which skin and fat tissue are detached from the lower abdominal area. Muscle is not used in creation of the new breast. Microsurgery is also required to connect blood vessels.
- Latissimus dorsi flap, in which muscle and skin tissue are moved from the upper back under the skin to the site of breast reconstruction. Weakness of the back, shoulder, or arm may persist after the surgery.
- Gluteal free flap, in which surgical transfer of skin, fat, muscle, and blood vessels is used to recreate the breast.

Nipple and areola reconstruction improves the natural appearance in the reconstructed breast through a small skin graft. Tissue may be taken from the opposite nipple, from skin that covers the prosthesis mound, or from other body tissue. After the nipple has been reconstructed, tattooing promotes natural coloring to the nipple and areola (Resnick & Belcher, 2002).

Psychosocial Consequences of Breast Cancer

The time from discovery to treatment of breast cancer is the most stressful time for many women. Factors that contribute to presurgery distress include a sense of uncertainty, incomplete information, the need to make difficult treatment decisions, and scheduling problems. Surgery may be preceded by chemotherapy or adjuvant therapy, or these therapies may also follow surgery. Because of the many complexities to be considered for treatment to be most effective, consultations with several specialists, including a surgeon, a radiation oncologist, a plastic surgeon, and a medical oncologist, are needed. Scheduling difficulties arise when women must travel significant distances for treatment. The many appointments with unfamiliar specialists and studies to determine best treatment often result in frustration and confusion for a woman and her family.

Concerns frequently expressed during treatment for breast cancer include fear of death, uncertainty about the quality of life, changes in body image, the effect on sexuality, and side effects of recommended therapy. For most women the knowledge that they will lose their hair as a result of chemotherapy creates one of the most difficult situations in therapy, adding yet another assault on their body image.

Breast cancer has psychological consequences for women and their husbands, significant others, and other family members. Difficulties reported include sleep disturbances, eating disorders, and problems with work responsibilities. Breast cancer can create strain on the marital relationship, primarily in the areas of sexual relations and communication about matters related to the illness. Women and their partners sometimes differ with regard to how much they want to discuss the illness. Some women have a great need to discuss their diagnosis, treatment, and fears of recurrence. Other women and many men view discussion of such fears as negative thinking that delays adjustment.

Nursing Considerations

The woman who is diagnosed with breast cancer depends on the nurse for emotional support and accurate information. The woman needs time to express her feelings, and the nurse must convey a sense of empathetic understanding by quiet presence, touch, and close attention to the woman's concerns. Many women feel that they have lost control and that their lives have been taken over by cancer and the recommended treatment. Some women are concerned about family relationships, and how their sexual partner will respond. Each woman should be allowed to express her fears and worries. In addition to providing time and demonstrating genuine interest in the woman's concerns, use communication techniques, such as clarifying, paraphrasing, and reflecting feelings, so that the woman can participate in decisions about her care.

Most women with a clear understanding of procedures and care experience a reduction in anxiety. Preoperative teaching is often part of the nurse's responsibility, and husbands and significant others should be included as much as possible in the teaching. Many women are relieved to learn that the hospital stay is short after mastectomy, and they may be relieved by knowing exactly what to expect after surgery. For instance, a pressure binder is applied over the wound to prevent bleeding after surgery and maintain a fine surgical scar line. Sutures are not often seen on the skin surface, and the "dressing" over the incision may look more like clear nail polish. Drainage tubes are often placed to prevent accumulation of fluid under the skin flaps. The incision may appear red and raised for the first few weeks. Exercises such as armlifts and pulley exercises may be necessary to promote return to usual flexibility in the surgical areas.

Lymphedema, caused by blocked drainage of the lymphatic system in the arm on the side of the mastectomy, is possible if most axillary lymph nodes must be removed. Lymphedema may not occur for many years and is not anticipated for women who do not require an extensive lymphatic tissue removal in the axilla. Compression armsleeves, similar to thromboembolism deterrent (TED) hose, are an available treatment to control lymphedema if needed.

In addition to self-care of the surgical area, discharge teaching focuses on the need for continued care and treatment. Some areas of concern include how to reduce the risk of wound infection, care of the arm on the affected side, side effects of postoperative medications, and signs and symptoms that should be reported to the physician. If the woman will be discharged with the drains in place, she should be taught how to empty them. Most women also benefit from information about such groups as Reach to Recovery and Encore, which provide support, information, and guidance after mastectomy. Printed information is usually offered because of early discharge.

Relevant nursing diagnoses may include:

- Fear related to uncertain outcome
- Disturbed Body Image related to the loss of breast and temporary loss of hair during chemotherapy
- Interrupted Family Processes related to the illness, inadequate information about the course of the disease, or changes in work and home activities
- Ineffective Sexuality Patterns related to concern about changed body structure or discomfort with intercourse secondary to chemotherapy effects

✔ CHECK YOUR READING

10. What are the major risk factors for breast cancer?
11. Why is staging for breast cancer important?
12. What is meant by *adjuvant therapy,* and why is it used?
13. How and when may breasts be reconstructed after mastectomy?
14. What should preoperative teaching include?
15. What should discharge planning emphasize?

CARDIOVASCULAR DISEASE

Cardiovascular diseases include disorders of the heart and blood vessels, such as myocardial infarction (MI), congenital abnormalities, and stroke. Those discussed here primarily relate to diseases of the blood vessels, particularly CAD. The topic is extensive, and only an overview will be presented in this text. A medical-surgical text should be consulted for more extensive information.

Most women fear dying from cancer, often breast cancer, but cardiovascular disease is the leading cause of death in both men and women in the United States. Almost twice as many U.S. women die of heart disease and stroke as from all forms of cancer, including breast cancer. Most people tend to think of heart and other blood vessel diseases as a male problem, particularly when compared with women before menopause.

Recognition of Coronary Artery Disease

Women are more likely to die from MI than men. In part, this is because they are older and may have other complicating diseases, but it also happens because the MI tends to manifest with atypical, vague symptoms that can delay recognition and treatment. The classic crushing or stabbing chest pain or pressure in the chest is not the usual symptom in women, as it is in men. Women may report having some vague symptoms such as fatigue for several weeks before seeking care that results in diagnosis of an imminent acute MI or one that has already occurred. Some of the symptoms of CAD in women include the following (AWHONN, 2003; Tazbir & Keresztes, 2005):

- Fatigue, weakness
- Angina (chest pain with exertion) or pain at rest
- Dyspnea, sometimes paroxysmal nocturnal dyspnea
- Dizziness, faintness, lightheadedness
- Upper abdominal pain, heartburn, loss of appetite
- Nausea, vomiting, sweating
- Pain in the upper body, but other than the chest (arm, neck, back, jaw, throat, teeth)

Because the pain may be subtle or unlike that which she associates with a heart attack, the woman may not consider MI as a possibility. Caregivers must be aware that the woman's symptoms could be cardiac related. For example, a dentist must consider that a woman with a toothache but no apparent tooth disease could have cardiac ischemia and an MI.

Risk Factors

Many factors increase risk for cardiovascular disease, but common ones include hypertension, inadequate physical activity, overweight and obesity, and a diet of poor nutritional quality. These and other risk factors often contribute to development of other problems that further increase the risk for cardiovascular disease, such as type 2 diabetes. Each risk factor may add to the risk for developing another of the problems listed here.

Risk factors may be fixed, or unmodifiable, or may be factors that can be changed. Aging is a major risk factor, because the woman loses the protection that estrogen, secreted before menopause, exerts on the blood vessels. Estrogen's protective effect delays onset of cardiovascular disease, making most women older at the onset of the disease than men. Other risk factors are listed in Box 33-4 and are similar to those for men. Several risk factors deserve added discussion.

The leading preventable cause of CAD and other diseases in women and men is smoking. Cigarette smoking adds to the burden of heart, blood vessel, and respiratory disorders, cancers, and many other diseases in women. Smoking is often more attractive to a woman if others in her family and friends smoke, she believes that smoking helps control her weight, or she believes that smoking reduces her anxiety.

BOX **33-4** Risk Factors for Coronary Artery Disease in Women

Cigarette smoking
Hypertension (including isolated systolic hypertension)
Serum lipids (dyslipidemia):
    Elevated total cholesterol (normal: ≤199 mg/dl; borderline: 200-239 mg/dl; elevated: ≥240 mg/dl).
    Low levels of high-density lipoprotein (HDL) cholesterol: <35 mg/dl.
    Cholesterol ratio: The ratio of cholesterol to HDL cholesterol is often used instead of total blood cholesterol. The goal is to keep the ratio lower than 5 (total cholesterol):1 (HDL cholesterol), with an optimum ratio of 3.5:1.
Triglyceride levels: >150 mg/dl.
Diabetes mellitus
Overweight and obesity
Sedentary lifestyle
Poor nutrition, especially a diet high in saturated fat and cholesterol but low in fiber and fruit
Age >60
Postmenopausal status
Family history of coronary artery disease

From Association for Women's Health, Obstetric and Neonatal Nurses. (2003). *Cardiovascular health for women: Primary prevention: Evidence-based practice guideline.* Washington, DC: Author; Berra, K. (2003). *Risk reduction in the prevention of cardiovascular disease in women: Lifestyle and medication management.* Washington, DC: Association of Women's Health, Obstetric and Neonatal Nurses; Pagana, K.D., & Pagana, T.J. (2005). *Mosby's diagnostic and test reference* (7th ed.). St. Louis: Mosby; Ralstin, A. (2004). Nursing assessment cardiovascular system. In S.M. Lewis, M.M. Heitkemper, & S.R. Dirksen (Eds.), *Medical-surgical nursing: assessment and management of clinical problems* (6th ed., pp. 799-837). Philadelphia: Mosby.

How to Reduce the Risk for Coronary Artery Disease

- Stop smoking. Your risk begins to decrease within a few months of stopping and reaches the level of a person who has never smoked within 3 to 5 years. Stopping also reduces your risk for lung cancer and many other respiratory diseases.
- Maintain a normal weight. Your risk is much higher if your weight is 30% or more over your ideal weight. See your health care provider about an ideal weight management plan, which usually includes a balanced diet and moderate exercise to lose weight gradually.
- Eat right. A variety of fruits, vegetables, grains, low-fat or nonfat dairy products, fish, legumes, poultry, and lean meats provides a basic healthy eating pattern. Substitute unsaturated fat from vegetables, fish, legumes, and nuts for foods high in saturated fats and cholesterol. Limit salt to less than 6 grams per day.
- Limit alcohol to 1 drink per day if you are a woman. Do not drink when pregnant or trying to become pregnant to avoid fetal alcohol syndrome, and do not drink when breastfeeding.
- Control high blood pressure. Even modest blood pressure elevations can be deadly, causing heart attack and stroke. Measures to reduce your blood pressure include weight reduction, exercise, diet improvement, and stress management. If your physician prescribes drugs to control your blood pressure, take them faithfully, even if you feel fine. Let the doctor know if you are having problems with your drugs for high blood pressure; a change in the drug may be possible.
- Exercise. Aerobic exercise helps reduce your blood pressure, control your weight, and keep your blood glucose levels normal. Resistance and weight-bearing exercise also helps slow osteoporosis. You need at least 30 minutes of moderate-intensity exercise 4 to 6 days each week.
- Control diabetes. Diabetes in a woman cancels many of estrogen's protective benefits, so you must work harder to control your diabetes as well as your cardiovascular risks.
- To learn more about cardiovascular disease and its prevention, visit these websites: American Heart Association, www.americanheart.org, and American Dietetic Association, www.eatright.org.

Both systolic and diastolic blood pressure elevations are associated with CAD and other vascular disorders. Adequate control of hypertension reduces death and disability from MI, stroke, and other blood vessel disorders. The person may not consider hypertension to be a problem because no symptoms are present. Smoking, overweight, and diabetes further contribute to hypertension. Hypertension is more prevalent in African-Americans than in whites.

Inadequate exercise contributes to many of the risk factors listed. Overweight and obesity are more likely when a person is sedentary, and these weight problems increase the likelihood that diabetes and hypertension will occur. Dyslipidemia is more likely in both women and men who do not get adequate exercise, adding further to the risk.

Prevention

Prevention is the key to reducing death and illness from all cardiovascular diseases among women. Although once thought to reduce a woman's risk for cardiovascular disease, estrogen's benefits for this have not proven true when HRT is chosen after natural estrogen declines at menopause (see p. 902).

HYPERTENSION

Lowering hypertension, including isolated systolic hypertension in older women, to levels lower than 140 mm Hg systolic and lower than 90 mm Hg diastolic reduces the risk of CAD and stroke. Even borderline hypertension can be dangerous. Medication should be considered if regular aerobic exercise, weight reduction, improved nutrition, and stress management do not lower the blood pressure adequately (Berry, 2003; Martinez, 2004). The Dietary Approaches to Stop Hypertension (DASH) diet plan from the NHLBI of the NIH is often recommended for people to maintain good control. DASH diet guidelines may be obtained from www.nhlbi.nih.gov/health/public/heart/hbp/dash/.

SMOKING CESSATION

Stopping smoking may cause a woman to gain weight, particularly if she increases food calories or reduces her activity. However, smoking cessation has a positive effect on reducing angina and stopping the progression of CAD. Stopping smoking also reduces the risk for lung cancer, the number one cancer in women. Improvement in other respiratory conditions is likely as well. Medication patches may be prescribed to gradually reduce nicotine intake while stopping and may be helpful for some women.

DIET AND GLUCOSE CONTROL

Women with diabetes have a relatively greater risk for CAD than men, so maintaining weight and glucose within normal limits is especially important. Diet is the primary means to control the lipid profile. Diet recommendations should be individualized, but general guidelines are that fat intake should be a maximum of 30% of daily calories, and saturated fat (found in foods such as meat, butter, cream, and cheese) make up no more than 10% of daily calories. Cholesterol intake maintained lower than 200 mg/day is ideal. Increased evidence shows that fish, especially fatty fish, confers cardiovascular benefits, and at least two servings per week are recommended. Eating a diet high in vegetables, fruits, and low-fat dairy products and limiting salt intake to under 6 g per day and alcohol to a maximum of one drink per day for women has shown to be beneficial at reducing blood pressure (Anderson, 2003; Krauss et al., 2000).

INCREASED ACTIVITY

Aerobic exercise helps control weight, blood pressure, the lipid profile, and glucose. It reduces body fat while increasing muscle mass and improving muscle tone. The Surgeon General has recommended at least 30 minutes of moderate physical activity daily such as a brisk walk or stair climbing. Low- to moderate-intensity exercises also have some benefits.

ASPIRIN

Low-dose aspirin therapy (81 mg or "baby aspirin") each day has shown to be beneficial to inhibit platelet aggregation that can increase clot formation and lead to CAD. Acute chest pain should be treated with a single adult-dose tablet (325 mg, equivalent to 4 baby aspirin tablets) as soon as MI is suspected to reduce clot formation and increase the chances of full recovery. For those unable to tolerate aspirin or who have recent gastrointestinal bleeding, prescription drugs such as clopidogrel (Plavix) may be prescribed. Individual needs are based on age, risk factors, and history.

✔ CHECK YOUR READING

16. What are the symptoms of CAD, such as an MI, in a woman?
17. List appropriate measures to reduce the risk for CAD.

MENSTRUAL CYCLE DISORDERS

The four most common menstrual cycle disorders are absence of menses (amenorrhea), abnormal uterine bleeding, pain associated with the menstrual cycle, and cyclic mood changes, including premenstrual syndrome (PMS). Although most of the disorders are benign, all require comprehensive gynecologic assessment. Nurses must be knowledgeable about underlying processes, diagnostic procedures, and expected treatment in order to fulfill the basic core of nursing activities, which include client advocacy, education, and supportive counseling.

Amenorrhea

Amenorrhea can indicate either normal physiologic processes or pathology in the reproductive system. Amenorrhea before menarche, during pregnancy, during the puerperium and lactation, and after menopause is normal. Amenorrhea at other times is abnormal, and it is called either *primary* or *secondary amenorrhea,* depending on when it occurs.

PRIMARY AMENORRHEA

Menstrual periods should begin within 2 years of breast development, usually between ages 10 and 16. Lack of breast development or other secondary sexual development or a shortened growth spurt in addition to the absence of menstruation provides additional diagnostic clues. Primary amenorrhea is considered if onset of menstrual periods has not occurred, particularly if associated sexual changes have not taken place. Primary amenorrhea may be suspected if the girl is more than 1 year older than the ages at which her mother and sisters had menarche (Jenkins, 2004). The causes for primary amenorrhea may be genetic (ovarian failure) or systemic or may involve anomalies of the reproductive tract.

Ovarian failure may occur in girls who have Turner's syndrome, in which only one of the normal two X chromosomes is present. They have a total of 45 chromosomes, with a single X chromosome. If secondary sex characteristics are present, incomplete development of internal reproductive organs may be the cause of amenorrhea. Other causes may include hormonal imbalances, systemic disease such as cancer with its associated therapy, and abnormalities of the hypothalamic-pituitary axis that result in hormone imbalance.

A common systemic cause of primary amenorrhea is low body weight for height. This may occur in competitive athletes and dancers but also occurs in girls with eating disorders, such as anorexia nervosa, who have a very low body weight. If the girl began sexual development and then restricted calories (or began an intense exercise program), her sexual development may be arrested at the point of the calorie restriction. Other systemic causes of primary amenorrhea include chronic stress, hypothyroidism, abnormal steroid secretion, central nervous system diseases, and drug use (Fritz, 2003).

Abnormalities in the uterus, vagina, or hymen can obstruct the outflow of the menstrual flow. Congenital enzyme abnormalities may disable different aspects of the reproductive cycle.

The condition causes a great deal of concern for the young woman and her family. Amenorrhea is a symptom, not a diagnosis, and they may worry that it indicates a serious disease. Menstruation is a unique function of women, and absence of menstruation may provoke concerns about femininity and the ability to have children. Concern increases if medical treatment is not successful.

Medical management depends on the cause. Counseling for eating disorders, such as anorexia nervosa, and reducing excessive exercise to allow adequate weight gain may prove helpful. Hormone therapy may establish normal menses if the cause is hormone imbalance. However, some conditions cannot be successfully treated. For example, if the cause is reproductive tract or congenital anomalies, normal menses and fertility may not be possible, and psychological support becomes the most important therapy.

SECONDARY AMENORRHEA

Secondary amenorrhea is the cessation of menstruation for a period of at least 6 months in a woman who has established a pattern of menstruation. The most common cause is pregnancy. Other causes include systemic diseases such as diabetes mellitus, tuberculosis, and hypothyroidism. Hormonal imbalances, low weight for height, stress, systemic illness, poor nutrition, use of oral contraceptives or antidepressants, and tumors of the ovary, pituitary, or adrenal gland also may be the cause.

Assessment includes a thorough medical and obstetric history and questions about eating habits, history of dieting, and current exercise pattern. Women are also questioned about their use of drugs, such as oral contraceptives, phenothiazines, and antihypertensives, which can cause secondary amenorrhea.

Medical treatment aims at identifying and correcting the underlying cause after ruling out pregnancy and determining if the woman wants children. Pregnancy testing is done for a sexually active woman, and medications that are potentially teratogenic must be withheld until pregnancy is ruled out. Other treatment may include testing levels of hormones related to the menstrual cycle, therapy to improve timing of the cycle, treatment of anovulation, and identification of other abnormalities that may be related to the disorder. Excess androgen levels may cause polycystic ovary syndrome (PCOS), characterized by acne, excess weight and body hair, as well as the anovulation that results in amenorrhea (Laufer & Patel, 2004).

Dysfunctional Uterine Bleeding

The normal menstrual cycle was described in Chapter 4. Dysfunctional bleeding occurs with abnormal frequency, lasts an abnormal length of time, occurs irregularly, or is excessive in amount. Complications of an unrecognized pregnancy, such as spontaneous abortion, must be considered when making the diagnosis.

ETIOLOGY

The most common causes of abnormal bleeding fall into five basic categories:

1. Pregnancy complications, such as spontaneous abortion
2. Anatomic lesions, either benign or malignant, of the vagina, cervix, or uterus
3. Drug-induced bleeding, such as "breakthrough" bleeding that may occur in women who are taking some oral contraceptives or drugs that mimic or modify natural hormones, such as cancer therapy (London, 2003)
4. Systemic disorders, such as diabetes mellitus, uterine myomas (fibroids), and hypothyroidism
5. Failure to ovulate

MANAGEMENT

Evaluation of abnormal uterine bleeding may include a sensitive pregnancy test, coagulation studies, and tests to determine whether ovulation is occurring. Hormone and liver function tests, plus tests to determine if the woman is anemic, often are done. Ultrasonography or hysteroscopy may be used to look for polyps and check the condition of the uterine lining.

A common hormone treatment is progestin-estrogen combination oral contraceptives that suppress ovulation and allow a more stable endometrial lining to form. Surgical therapy may include dilation and curettage (D&C) to remove polyps or to diagnose endometrial hyperplasia, which may be treated with progesterone to suppress excess uterine lining. Hysterectomy may be performed if the uterus is enlarged as a result of fibroids or adenomyosis (benign invasive growth of the endometrium into the muscular layer of the uterus) and if the woman does not want more children. Laser ablation may be used to permanently remove the endometrial lining without hysterectomy. Treatment of anemia is needed by many women with excessive vaginal bleeding.

NURSING CONSIDERATIONS

Nurses should encourage women to seek medical attention promptly when irregular or prolonged bleeding occurs. Nurses also help the woman keep a record of the bleeding episodes and the amount of blood lost. This involves keeping a calendar and noting any vaginal bleeding (spotting, menses) that occurs in addition to the number of pads and tampons saturated each day.

The nurse teaches the importance of adequate nutrition and discourages rigorous dieting. For women who are concerned about amenorrhea, the nurse should explain that although exercise is beneficial, excessive workouts or aerobic training can cause amenorrhea. In addition, the nurse teaches methods to reduce stress and promote relaxation. Finally, nurses must provide support for women who fear that irregular bleeding indicates a serious disease, such as cancer. Offering false reassurance is unwise, but information about diagnostic procedures, such as pelvic examination, Pap test, and other tests is helpful.

> ✔ **CHECK YOUR READING**
>
> 18. How does primary amenorrhea differ from secondary amenorrhea in terms of onset, cause, and treatment?
> 19. What are possible causes of dysfunctional uterine bleeding, and why should it not be ignored?

Cyclic Pelvic Pain

Cyclic pelvic pain must be distinguished from acute pelvic pain. Acute pelvic pain is sudden in onset and is not experienced with each menstrual cycle. It may indicate a serious disorder, such as ectopic pregnancy or appendicitis. Cyclic pelvic pain occurs repetitively and predictably in a specific phase of the menstrual cycle. The most common causes of cyclic pelvic pain are mittelschmerz, primary dysmenorrhea, and endometriosis.

MITTELSCHMERZ

Mittelschmerz ("middle" pain) is pelvic pain that occurs midway between menstrual periods at the time of ovulation. The pain results from growth of the dominant follicle within the ovary or rupture of the follicle and subsequent spillage of follicular fluid and blood into the peritoneal space. The pain is fairly sharp and is felt on the right or left side of the pelvis. It generally lasts from a few hours to 2 days, and slight vaginal bleeding may accompany the discomfort. Generally, women do not need medical treatment beyond simple explanation of the discomfort or mild analgesics.

PRIMARY DYSMENORRHEA

Primary dysmenorrhea is menstrual pain without identified pathology. Its onset is usually 1 to 3 years after menstruation begins, when ovulatory menstrual cycles are well established, and it is most common in young, nulliparous women. Commonly called "cramps," primary dysmenorrhea causes significant loss of school or work hours. The pain begins within hours of the onset of menses, and it is spasmodic or colicky in nature because of increased prostaglandins secreted at this time. It is felt in the lower abdomen but often radiates to the lower back or down the legs. Nausea, vomiting, loose stools, or dizziness may also occur. The duration of the pain is usually 48 to 72 hours.

Two recommended treatments of primary dysmenorrhea provide marked relief: oral contraceptives and prostaglandin inhibitors. Oral contraceptives decrease the amount of endometrial growth that occurs during the menstrual cycle and thereby reduce the production of endometrial prostaglandin. For women who do not wish to take oral contraceptives, prostaglandin inhibitors offer relief. The most effective prostaglandin inhibitors are NSAIDs such as ibuprofen (Motrin, Advil) and naproxen (Naprosyn, Anaprox). To be effective, the NSAID should be taken around the clock for at least 48 to 72 hours beginning when menstrual flow starts.

Cyclooxygenase (COX)-2 inhibitors such as rofecoxib (Vioxx) and valdecoxib (Bextra) have been effective in relieving dysmenorrhea with less gastric upset. However, recent concerns about cardiovascular problems such as MI or stroke have caused the manufacturer of rofecoxib to withdraw from the market while further U.S. Food and Drug Administration (FDA) studies of these inhibitors continue. The FDA recommended that valdecoxib be withdrawn from the market by its manufacturer in 2005. For updated information on COX-2 inhibitors and other drugs, consult the FDA website—www.fda.gov.

Simple relief measures supplement medical interventions and may be sufficient for a woman. Rest in a comfortable position and application of warmth often provide additional relief.

ENDOMETRIOSIS

PATHOPHYSIOLOGY. Endometriosis is defined as the presence outside the uterus of tissue that resembles the endometrium in both structure and function. The response of this tissue to the stimulation of estrogen and progesterone during the menstrual cycle is identical to that of the endometrial tissue. That is, it grows and proliferates during the follicular and luteal phases of the cycle and then sloughs during menstruation. The menstruation from endometriosis lesions, however, occurs in a closed cavity, which causes pressure and pain on adjacent tissue. In addition, prostaglandins secreted by the endometriosis lesions irritate nerve endings and stimulate uterine contractions that further increase pain. Cyclic bleeding into the pelvic cavity causes chronic inflammatory changes that may make conception and implantation difficult. The most common sites of endometriosis lesions are illustrated in Figure 33-3.

Although endometriosis occurs in 5% to 15% of all women, causes remain unknown. One theory is that reflux of the menstrual flow through the fallopian tubes allows the endometrial cells to attach to nearby structures and proliferate, creating spots of endometrial tissue. Endometrial tissue has been found in distant sites such as the lungs, raising the possibility that the cells are spread by blood circulation. Spread of the endometrial cells by the lymphatics has also been implicated. A genetic predisposition is likely.

Most women with endometriosis are in their 30s and nulliparous, and many have had infertility problems. Most women with endometriosis find that the signs and symptoms regress after menopause, but a few women first develop the symptoms after menopause, even with no estrogen supplementation. Occasionally endometriosis appears in childhood or adolescence, usually related to structural abnormalities of the reproductive organs (Moore & Gambone, 2004b).

SIGNS AND SYMPTOMS. The two major problems associated with endometriosis are pain and infertility. The pain of endometriosis differs from that of primary dysmenorrhea. Endometriosis pain is deep, unilateral or bilateral, and either sharp or dull. It is constant, as opposed to the spasmodic or colicky pain of primary dysmenorrhea. Dyspareunia (painful intercourse) is common, particularly with

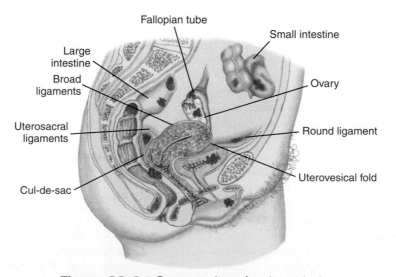

Figure 33-3 ■ Common sites of endometriosis.

deep penetration. Rectal pain is common, especially during defecation. Diarrhea, constipation, and sensations of rectal pressure or urgency are other symptoms of endometriosis. Although causes of infertility may not be known, pelvic adhesions and tubal pathology because of chronic inflammatory changes of endometriosis may be contributing factors.

MANAGEMENT. Treatment may be either medical or surgical, in choosing therapy one must weigh the need for pain relief and the desire to maintain fertility against the side effects that accompany many treatment regimens. Growth of endometriosis tissue depends on adequate production of ovarian hormones during the menstrual cycle. Other factors to be considered include symptom severity, desire for future fertility, the woman's age, and how endometriosis affects nearby organs such as obstructing the urinary or gastrointestinal tracts (Moore & Gambone, 2004b).

Continuous oral contraceptives suppress endometrial tissue proliferation, particularly in a woman who desires pregnancy after medical treatment. Progestins such as medroxyprogesterone acetate (Depo-Provera) or norethindrone (Micronor) directly inhibit growth of the excessive endometrial tissue.

Both the testosterone derivative danazol (Danocrine) and gonadotropin-releasing hormone (GnRH) agonists such as leuprolide acetate (Lupron) and nafarelin (Synarel) interfere with hormones needed for ovulation and the menstrual cycle, creating a "pseudomenopause" while taken. The woman may have hot flashes, vaginal dryness, insomnia, decreased libido, and reduced bone density. In addition, danazol may produce masculinizing effects, such as deepening of the voice, facial and body hair, and weight gain. The woman takes the drug for a varying period of time, often between 3 and 6 months, depending on the drug and the degree of her endometriosis.

Surgical treatment of endometriosis may have different options because of the varied size, number, and location of lesions, the age of the affected woman, and whether endometriosis contributes to her infertility. Laparoscopy may be performed for lysis of adhesions and laser vaporization of the lesions of endometriosis. This procedure is used especially when infertility is a problem. For women with severe pain who no longer wish to have children, a hysterectomy, sometimes including bilateral salpingo-oophorectomy to remove both fallopian tubes and ovaries, and excision of all lesions offer relief. Removal of both ovaries causes loss of their hormone production, resulting in an early menopause. Postoperative HRT may be recommended if endometriosis lesions are removed.

NURSING CONSIDERATIONS

Dysmenorrhea varies from mild "menstrual awareness" to incapacitating pain that affects the quality of life for several days out of each month. Too often the pain is belittled ("It's just cramps"). One of the most important nursing actions is to acknowledge the pain: "I understand this is really uncomfortable, and you are concerned that you have this much pain every month."

COMPLEMENTARY/ALTERNATIVE THERAPY

Women should be instructed in nonpharmacologic measures to relieve pain, such as frequent rest periods, application of heat to the lower abdomen, moderate exercise, and a well-balanced diet. If they want to try an herbal remedy, they should be advised to consult their health care provider about safety and effectiveness, particularly because the possibility of unrecognized pregnancy is always present.

The nurse should advise the woman to schedule stress-provoking situations so that they will not coincide with the menstrual period if possible. If NSAIDs are recommended, these should be taken with foods to reduce gastrointestinal irritation. The woman should be counseled to report unusual side effects, such as headache, dizziness, or unusual fluid retention, to the physician or nurse practitioner.

The nurse must allow time for the woman to express her concerns about the therapy. The woman should be taught expected effects of drugs given for endometriosis and about the drug's precautions and side or adverse effects that may occur. Some women benefit from information about measures that promote sleep and relaxation and, most important, from the knowledge that someone is available to provide support and guidance when needed. A woman may demonstrate emotional distress if she has not had all the children she desires but must decide whether to have a hysterectomy to reduce physical pain that simpler measures have not relieved.

✓ CHECK YOUR READING

20. What causes primary dysmenorrhea, and how may it be treated?
21. How does endometriosis cause dysmenorrhea, and how can it be treated?
22. What are the major side effects of danazol? Of the GnRH agonists?

Premenstrual Syndrome

Many women notice some minor physical and emotional changes related to their menstrual cycles. However, a few women have severe problems associated with these cyclic changes. PMS, also called *premenstrual dysphoric disorder* (PMDD), may affect as many as 10% of women severely enough to cause significant disruption with their daily lives (Pritham, 2002; Reid, 2003). Although PMDD is the official diagnostic name for the diagnostic criteria, PMS is now a term ingrained in lay culture. The following criteria must be met for the condition to be diagnosed as PMS:

- The signs and symptoms must be cyclic and recur in the luteal phase (after ovulation) of the menstrual cycle.
- The woman should be symptom-free during the follicular phase (before ovulation) of the menstrual cycle, and the cycle must include 7 symptom-free days.

- Symptoms must be severe enough to have an impact on work, lifestyle, and relationships.
- Diagnosis should be based on the woman's *prospective* symptom recording, or charting of symptoms as they occur rather than recall of symptoms that occurred in the past (ACOG, 2000).

Some women who have medical or psychiatric disorders have an increased intensity of symptoms during the last half of their cycles, often leading them to assume that they have PMS. Examples of these are depressive disorders, panic disorder, and generalized anxiety disorder. A psychiatric illness such as bipolar disorder may have symptoms unrelated to PMS, but the two disorders may coexist (Laufer & Gambone, 2004b).

BOX 33-5 Symptoms of Premenstrual Syndrome

Physical Symptoms
Headaches, dizziness
Abdominal bloating or swelling; swelling of the extremities
Breast tenderness
Hot flashes
Abdominal cramps
Generalized muscle and joint pain
Fatigue
Appetite changes: binge eating, cravings
Sleep changes: excessive sleep or insomnia
Reduced sexual interest

Behavioral Symptoms
Depressed mood
Feelings of hopelessness
Marked anxiety
Confusion, forgetfulness, poor concentration
Accident proneness
Irritability and anger
Emotional lability: tearfulness or readiness to cry, loneliness, mood instability
Reduced interest in activities of living
Social avoidance
Lethargy or high energy

Numerous symptoms have been ascribed to PMS, but a relatively small number make up the majority of complaints. They can be divided into behavioral and physical symptoms. Box 33-5 lists those that are most common. Several PMS diaries with varied amounts of detail are available for the woman to record her symptoms and their severity, lifestyle impact, and medications (Figure 33-4).

ETIOLOGY

Although the cause of PMS is unknown, several theories or predisposing factors have been proposed. The current theory of PMS etiology is that normal fluctuations in gonadal hormones during a cycle, chiefly estrogen and progesterone, trigger central biochemical responses, specifically serotonin. The premenstrual fall in serotonin levels occurs in most women, but a susceptible woman may show psychiatric symptoms as her estrogen, progesterone, and serotonin levels fall during the luteal phase. Most women show a rapid postmenstrual return to a feeling of well-being.

IMPACT ON FAMILY

PMS puts a consistent strain on family relationships because symptoms recur monthly. The episodes of PMS affect the functioning of the entire family. Clinical descriptions of severe family disruptions include increased family conflict, disrupted communication, and decreased family cohesion. Of particular concern is the group of women who report symptoms of loss of control, child battering, self-injury, and increased accidents. Work and social relationships may suffer.

MANAGEMENT

Treatment of PMS is based on the symptom profile of each woman after ruling out other problems, especially psychiatric diagnoses such as depression. Supportive therapy such as reassuring the woman that PMS is a common problem

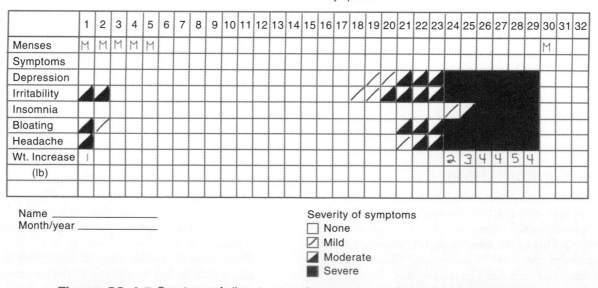

Figure 33-4 ■ One type of diary to record occurrence and severity of premenstrual symptoms.

that has a physiologic basis may reduce her anxiety and should be part of other treatments. Relaxation therapy has shown benefits to women with the more severe PMS symptoms. Exercise has been shown to reduce PMS symptoms and also has many other benefits to a woman's health. Modifying the diet to reduce salty foods, caffeine, chocolate, red meat, dairy products, and alcohol may be helpful. Small and frequent meals may reduce mood swings (ACOG, 2000; Pritham, 2002; Reid, 2003).

Clinical trials have shown that supplementation with calcium (1200 mg/day) has some effectiveness and with magnesium (200 to 400 mg/day) is minimally effective. Carbohydrate-rich food and beverages may improve the mood and reduce food cravings in some women. Reducing caffeine and taking vitamin E (400 international units [IU]/day) during the luteal phase of the cycle may reduce breast pain (mastalgia) in some women. Evening primrose oil also may have some benefit in reducing breast pain (ACOG, 2000; Reid, 2003).

Women with physical, emotional, and cognitive symptoms may be prescribed antidepressant medications, oral contraceptives to suppress ovulation, or both. Estrogen therapy may relieve premenstrual migraines. Danazol taken in low doses relieves mastalgia, but higher doses may be required for the drug to relieve other PMS symptoms. Preferred antidepressants are selective serotonin reuptake inhibitors (SSRIs) such as fluoxetine (Prozac), sertraline (Zoloft), or paroxetine (Paxil), although tricyclic antidepressants may also be useful. Short-acting drugs to reduce anxiety, such as alprazolam (Xanax) or buspirone (BuSpar), have also shown benefit (ACOG, 2000; Pritham, 2002; Reid, 2003).

NURSING CONSIDERATIONS

Many women experience some of the symptoms and diagnose themselves as having PMS. Nurses must discourage this practice, because serious systemic disease can be missed if the criteria for diagnosis are ignored. Instead of self-diagnosis, nurses should recommend that the woman consult with her health care provider so that a complete history and physical examination can be performed to rule out other causes or a problem that may coexist with PMS.

Once the diagnosis of PMS is confirmed, nurses can educate the family about lifestyle changes that may help. Nurses should acknowledge that dietary changes are particularly difficult because many women crave salty or sweet foods, which should be restricted. Women also benefit from education about expected cyclic changes. As they learn to

predict the pattern of symptoms and gain a sense of control over them, the symptoms often diminish.

Education and support must be expanded to include the family. When the woman exhibits symptoms of PMS, family members often respond by withdrawing or confronting the woman. Family members should also be encouraged to express their feelings so that anger and resentment within the family can be diminished.

Nurses must help the woman make concrete arrangements to obtain relief when she feels she is losing control or when she fears that she may harm herself or a child. A neighbor, friend, or family member should be identified to provide immediate relief, without questions or explanations, when the woman feels she is losing control.

> ■ It is more helpful if the family acknowledges feelings they believe the woman is experiencing. For instance saying, "It must be disturbing to feel so irritable. What can I do to help?" provokes a different emotional response than comments that are confrontational or blaming.

The family also should be encouraged to express their feelings so that anger and resentment within the family can be diminished.

Nurses must help the woman make concrete arrangements to obtain relief if she feels she is losing control or if she fears that she may harm herself or a child. A neighbor, friend, or family member should be identified to provide immediate relief, without questions or explanations, when the woman feels she is losing control. The telephone number of this important support person should be posted so that it is easily accessible, and the designated person should be called before symptoms are severe.

MEDICAL TERMINATION OF PREGNANCY

Medical termination of pregnancy, also called *induced abortion*, is a voluntary method of ending a pregnancy. It may be performed to preserve the health of the mother, to prevent the birth of an infant with severe birth defects, or to end a pregnancy caused by rape or incest. A woman may also choose to terminate a pregnancy for economic or social reasons. Termination of pregnancy for the purpose of safeguarding the health of the mother is termed "therapeutic" abortion. Interruption of the pregnancy at the request of the woman but not for reasons of impaired maternal health or fetal disease is often called "elective" abortion. Therapeutic and elective abortions involve many social and ethical issues (see Chapter 3). In 2001 the induced abortion rate was 16 per 1000 women, a decline from the peak of 29.4 per 1000 in 1980 (Strauss et al., 2004).

Methods of Medical Termination of Pregnancy

The technique used to medically terminate pregnancy depends on the length of gestation and may be medical, if only drugs are used to end the pregnancy, or surgical, if a surgical procedure is required. A surgical procedure may sometimes be required to completely evacuate the uterine contents when a medical abortion is done.

COMPLEMENTARY/ALTERNATIVE THERAPY

> Alternative therapy may help some women. Measures include acupuncture, biofeedback, hypnosis, psychotherapy, and stress management. Evening primrose oil may be useful in treating breast tenderness but not other symptoms of PMS (ACOG, 2000).

How to Relieve Symptoms of Premenstrual Syndrome

DIET

- Decrease consumption of caffeine (coffee, tea, colas, chocolate), which increases irritability, insomnia, anxiety, and nervousness.
- Avoid simple sugars (cookies, cake, candy) to prevent high blood glucose followed by a rapid decline and a period of low blood glucose (hypoglycemia).
- Decrease intake of salty foods (chips, pickles) to reduce fluid retention.
- Drink at least 2000 ml (2 quarts) of *water* per day, and do not include other beverages in this total.
- Eat six small meals a day to prevent hypoglycemia. Meals should be well balanced, with emphasis on fresh fruits and vegetables, complex carbohydrates, and non-fat milk products.
- Avoid alcohol, which aggravates depression.

EXERCISE

- Increase physical exercise to relieve tension and to decrease depression. Aerobic activity, such as jogging or walking, several times a week is recommended.

STRESS MANAGEMENT

- During the time when there are no symptoms of PMS, acknowledge the effect of PMS on daily life and make plans to avoid stressful situations during the premenstrual period when symptoms are acute.
- Use guided imagery, conscious relaxation techniques, warm baths, and massage to reduce stress.

SLEEP AND REST

To reduce fatigue and combat insomnia:
- Adhere to a regular schedule for sleep.
- Drink a glass of milk, which is high in tryptophan and is known to promote sleep, before bedtime.
- Schedule exercise in the morning or early afternoon rather than late afternoon.
- Engage in relaxing activities, such as reading, before bedtime, and avoid excitement at this time.

Drugs that may be used in medical abortion regimens include the following:

- Mifepristone (Mifeprex, or RU-486), an antiprogesterone drug, followed by misoprostol (Cytotec), a prostaglandin drug commonly used to reduce gastric acid secretion. Oral or vaginal use of misoprostol in medical abortion is unlabeled by the manufacturer. The woman receives an initial dose of 600 mg of mifepristone orally. Oral or vaginal misoprostol 400 mcg follows in 48 hours to promote expulsion if pregnancy has not ended. The woman usually expels the early pregnancy within 14 days of her first visit. Newer regimens may use a combination of mifepristone 200 mg followed by a client-administered dose of vaginal misoprostol 800 mcg and may be prescribed through 9 weeks of gestation (FDA, 2000; Taylor & Hwang, 2003/2004; Trupin, 2003).
- Methotrexate (Folex, Mexate) is an antimetabolite also used to treat certain types of cancer. Although not FDA-approved for medical abortion, individualized doses have been successfully used for medical pregnancy termination. Misoprostol may be prescribed to enhance expulsion of uterine contents (Taylor & Hwang, 2003/2004; Trupin, 2003).
- Misoprostol (Cytotec), a prostaglandin analog drug normally given to prevent gastric ulcers.

Surgical abortion techniques are needed if the woman has been pregnant for over 7 weeks or if her medical abortion failed and she still desires pregnancy termination. Through 12 weeks' gestation, vacuum aspiration with curettage is the method of choice. The cervix is dilated after locally injecting anesthetic in the area, and a plastic cannula is inserted into the uterine cavity. The contents are aspirated with negative pressure, and the uterine cavity may be scraped with a curet to ensure that the uterus is empty. Cramping may last 20 to 30 minutes after the procedure is completed. Complications may include uterine perforation, hemorrhage, cervical lacerations, and adverse reactions to the anesthetic agent.

For second-trimester abortions, *dilation with removal of the fetus and placenta* is generally performed. The procedure is similar to vacuum curettage but requires greater cervical dilation and a larger aspirator because the products of conception have grown in size and must be removed gradually. Dilation begins with insertion of laminaria, rounded cone-shaped materials that absorb water, into the cervix 24 hours before the procedure. The laminaria draw fluid from the cervical canal and expand, causing the cervix to dilate slowly and with minimal trauma. If needed before aspiration and removal of the products of pregnancy, additional cervical dilation is done.

Medical methods exist for abortion in the second trimester, but these involve labor. Retention of the placenta often occurs, requiring a D&C to fully clean the uterus. Laminaria are inserted about 12 hours before the procedure to start cervical dilation. Prostaglandin E_2, which stimulates contractions, may be given via vaginal suppository or intraamniotic infusion. Oxytocin is not effective at starting labor because of the early gestation, but it may shorten labor after it has been established by other methods. Because of the emotional distress caused by the longer procedure and the increased risks involved, medical termination of pregnancy is not often chosen in the second trimester.

Guidelines for Self-Care after Medical Termination of Pregnancy

Normal activities may be resumed, but strenuous work or exercise should be avoided for a few days.

Bleeding or cramping may occur for a week or two. If either becomes severe, medical advice should be sought. Light "spotting" may occur for about a month.

Sanitary pads should be used instead of tampons for the first week after the abortion to avoid possible infection.

Intercourse should be curtailed for 1 week after the abortion because of the possibility of infection until the uterine lining heals.

Birth control measures should be used if sex is resumed before menstruation begins, because it is possible to become pregnant during this time. Menstruation usually resumes in 4 to 6 weeks.

Temperature should be taken twice a day to detect possible infection; a temperature above 37.8° C (100° F) should be reported to the health care provider.

It is important to keep the follow-up appointment in 2 weeks or as recommended.

Nursing Considerations

The nurse's role in caring for women seeking induced abortion is one of providing physical and emotional support and information. History taking and collection of laboratory data depend on the routine of the health care setting in which the nurse is functioning. Counseling and lending emotional support are nursing responsibilities, although a designated counselor may also perform these services.

Nurses are also responsible for providing information about self-care after an abortion. Self-care is similar to that after spontaneous abortion: observation for excessive bleeding or signs of infection (temperature >37.8° C (100° F, foul-smelling vaginal drainage). Nurses also provide information about follow-up visits and contraception. The Rh-negative woman should receive Rh$_o$(D) immune globulin (RhoGAM).

✓ CHECK YOUR READING

23. What are the criteria for diagnosing PMS?
24. What lifestyle changes can be made to reduce the symptoms of PMS?
25. What drugs can be used in a medical termination of pregnancy?
26. What discharge teaching is appropriate after medical termination of pregnancy?

MENOPAUSE

Menopause means the end of menstruation. However, most people use the term to include the array of endocrine, somatic, and psychic changes that occur at the end of the reproductive period. The entire process, often called the "change of life," is correctly termed the *climacteric*. *Premenopause* refers to the early part of the climacteric, before menstruation ceases but after the woman experiences some of the climacteric symptoms, such as irregular menses. Perimenopause includes premenopause, menopause, and at least 1 year after menopause. *Postmenopause* refers to the phase after menopause, when menstrual periods have ceased.

Unexpected postmenopausal bleeding should be investigated as soon as possible because it suggests endometrial cancer. Conversely, planned or scheduled postmenopausal bleeding is generally not a cause for concern. It occurs when the woman who takes estrogen and progesterone sequentially stops taking the drugs, usually once a month. This allows the uterine lining to be sloughed and prevents endometrial hyperplasia.

Age of Menopause

The average age for natural menopause is 51.5 years (Laufer & Gambone, 2004a). The natural climacteric takes place over 3 to 5 years. Menopause can be induced or created artificially, however, at any age. Surgical removal of the ovaries or destruction of the ovaries by radiation or chemotherapy causes abrupt, permanent cessation of ovarian function, including the production of estrogen. The most common reason for performing these procedures is treatment of cancer or endometriosis. Young women who experience artificial menopause often have more symptoms associated with menopause than do women who go through the process naturally because theirs is not a gradual process as it is for the older woman.

Women can now expect to live another 30 years after menopause. During this period they must deal with physical, psychological, and social changes that often require a reevaluation of their primary roles and restructuring of personal goals.

Physiologic Changes

During the normal reproductive cycle, the ovaries respond to gonadotropins (follicle-stimulating hormone and luteinizing hormone) in a predictable pattern: (1) a follicle matures, (2) the ovary secretes estrogen, (3) ovulation occurs, and (4) the corpus luteum produces progesterone. During the premenopausal period, however, the ovaries are less responsive to gonadotropins, and, although increased amounts of follicle-stimulating hormone are secreted, ovulation is sporadic and menstrual periods are irregular. With progressive aging the ovaries become unresponsive, even to high levels of gonadotropins, and ovulation, menstruation, and the secretion of ovarian hormones (estrogen and progesterone) ceases.

Estrogen is responsible for the secondary sex characteristics of women; when estrogen levels decline, the organs of reproduction undergo regression. The labia become thin and pale. The vaginal mucosa atrophies, and vaginal tissue loses its lubrication and therefore is easily traumatized. Dyspareunia is not uncommon, and bacterial invasion of the epithelium may occur and lead to frequent vaginal infections. This entire process is referred to as *atrophic vaginitis*. Breasts become smaller, and atrophy of the uterus and ovaries occur. However, a concurrent benefit is that uterine myomas (fibroids) and endometriosis lesions also atrophy. Estrogen deficit can also result in atrophic changes in the bladder and urethra that may cause loss of urethral tone and frequent atrophic cystitis.

In addition, absence of estrogen is associated with an adverse change in serum lipids. Serum levels of low-density lipoproteins (LDL), which carry cholesterol to blood vessels, increase. At the same time, levels of high-density lipoproteins (HDL), which are known to carry cholesterol to the liver and to protect against the development of CAD, decrease.

Many menopausal women experience hot flashes or flushes, which are the result of vasomotor instability. The cause of vasomotor instability is not known, but it is closely associated with increased secretion of gonadotropins. Hot flashes are characterized by a sudden feeling of heat or burning of the skin, followed by perspiration. They occur more frequently during the night, and fatigue as a result of interrupted sleep is a major problem for some women. Hot flashes are often more frequent and severe in younger women who undergo the climacteric, particularly if loss of ovarian function was abrupt because of surgery. Many women in the climacteric have few annoyances from the hot flashes, however.

Psychological Responses

It is easy to understand why menopause is called the "change of life." It is accompanied by physical, psychological, and social changes, and individual responses vary widely. Many women are relieved that their childbearing and child-rearing tasks are ending. They see this as an exciting time, when they can pursue personal development. Other women grieve that the possibility of childbearing is past. This may be particularly true for women who have never had a child, whether because of infertility or because of lack of a male partner. However, artificial reproductive techniques have blurred the line that defines the age at which it is and is not possible to bear a child (see Chapter 32).

Menopause requires a woman to come to terms with aging. It may be difficult to accept aging in a society that reveres youth, and many women become extremely concerned with measures that slow the signs of aging. Many women become grandmothers at this time, which also confirms aging and requires a major adjustment in how the woman views herself. A large population of "baby boomers"—those born from 1946 to 1964—are entering menopause. These women are likely to change many of society's ideas about menopause by the sheer size of their group and because they have changed the social fabric of the United States dramatically as they have grown up and matured.

Some symptoms do not have a physiologic explanation, but they are no less real to women who experience them.

Depression, mood swings, irritability, and agitation are common climacteric complaints. Insomnia and fatigue are often mentioned as major problems.

One of the most puzzling aspects of menopause is the wide variation in both physical and psychological symptoms that women experience. For some women, the only changes are mild, infrequent hot flashes and amenorrhea. Other women experience severe, debilitating hot flashes, atrophic vaginitis, and multiple psychological symptoms, such as irritability and prolonged depression.

Therapy for Menopause

Although many women comfortably undergo the age-associated changes of menopause, others seek relief for discomforts such as hot flashes, interrupted sleep, or vaginal dryness. The psychological perception that increasing reproductive hormones would slow the aging process and promote a more youthful appearance has strengthened use of HRT during the climacteric. Additional beneficial effects were thought to be a reduction in cardiovascular disease, colorectal cancer, breast cancer, and osteoporosis, as well as other medical-surgical conditions associated with aging.

As greater research results emerged, including that of the WHI, additional risk factors as well as benefits of hormone therapy emerged. Two groups of perimenopausal women were included in the hormone studies of the WHI research:

- Estrogen and progesterone have been given to women with a uterus. Combining progesterone with estrogen therapy prevents uterine hyperplasia, a precursor to uterine cancer, in this group.
- Estrogen therapy alone has been given to women who have had a hysterectomy, because uterine hyperplasia is not a risk.

The combination of estrogen and progesterone replacement is usually called *hormone replacement therapy*, whereas the estrogen-only replacement therapy may be called *estrogen-replacement therapy* (ERT). It is common to see *HRT* used for either or both therapies, however.

Other hormone replacement research studies were being done as the WHI study continued, and increasing evidence emerged that estrogen plus progesterone therapy significantly increased risks of some disorders, primarily breast cancer and heart disease. Therefore the estrogen-progesterone arm of the study was stopped in 2002. A woman was not obligated to stop taking estrogen-progesterone therapy when this arm of the study was stopped, but they had to make their choices based on both the benefits and the unexpected risks that emerged. Rather than receive estrogen-progesterone supplements through the study, the women received the estrogen-progesterone hormone via prescription from their health care provider. The estrogen-only arm of the study continues, because risk levels in this group have not shown the higher risk levels that the estrogen-progesterone group showed. The WHI hormone study, having a single arm at this time, has continued into 2005, and the study is now scheduled to continue through 2010 to gather health information and identify problems in the women who participate.

RISKS

HRT was not considered safe for all women before the WHI findings. For example, women who have had estrogen- or progesterone-receptor positive breast cancer or blood coagulation disorders do not qualify. A woman who has had breast cancer may take a drug to block effects of estrogen

COMPLEMENTARY/ALTERNATIVE THERAPY

All patients should be asked about their use of complementary and alternative therapy methods, and their response should be documented.

"Natural" should not be assumed to be safe or therapeutic. Errors may be made with natural products because of nonstandardized products, inconsistent quality control, and errors in making a natural product—including misidentifying plant products.

Many biological products should not be used by a woman considering becoming pregnant or during pregnancy and lactation. Natural biological products cannot be assumed to be safe for children.

Botanical products that may be used for hot flashes, although effectiveness is not yet well supported by research, include the following:

- Black cohosh: reduced sweating; suppression of luteinizing hormone; no influence on endometrial thickness, levels of follicle-stimulating hormone, estrogenic or prolactin levels; should not be used with estrogen therapy, anticoagulants, and antihypertensives
- Soy products: Contain phytoestrogens that may serve as weak estrogenic compounds, stimulating estrogen receptors; no convincing evidence that soy products reduce hot flashes more than placebos in some studies; should be avoided in women with estrogen-dependent tumors such as breast, ovarian, or endometrial cancer, because tumor growth may be stimulated; possible interaction between estrogen replacement therapy or the drug tamoxifen; should be avoided in pregnant or lactating women
- Dong Quai: May be used with other herbal products; contains coumarin products that have vasodilation and antispasmodic effects; more study needed to determine effects on hot flashes although it is a traditional Chinese medicine product
- Vitamin E: A fat-soluble vitamin supplement having antioxidant properties; inhibits platelet aggregation and low-density lipoprotein (LDL) oxidation, possibly interfering with therapeutic effects of anticoagulant chemotherapy, or statin drugs designed to normalize lipids; has been associated with gastrointestinal disturbances; recent results have shown an association with heart failure
- Chasteberry: possible reduction in premenstrual symptoms of mood alteration, anger, headache

From American College of Obstetricians and Gynecologists. (2001). *Use of botanicals for management of menopausal symptoms,* Practice Bulletin No. 28. Washington, DC: Author; Gingrich, P.M., & Fogel, C.I. (2003). Herbal therapy use by perimenopausal women. *Journal of Obstetric, Gynecologic, and Neonatal Nursing, 32*(2), 181-189; Phillips, M., Lee, Y.-M., Swanson, B., Keithley, J.K., Zeller, J.M., Hindin, P. (2003). Herbal and dietary supplements for hot flashes: Here's what works—and what doesn't. *AWHONN Lifelines, 7*(5), 414-420; National Institutes of Health: National Center for Complementary and Alternative Medicine. (2005). Consumer advisory: Vitamin E supplements. Retrieved April 2, 2005, from www.nccam.nih.gov.

and reduce the risk of recurrence. Likewise, a woman who has a close family history of breast cancer might not want to take it. Unexplained uterine bleeding or endometrial cancer are contraindications. Smoking, hypertension, diabetes, cardiovascular disease, and renal or liver disease are often contraindications for hormone therapy, whether therapy includes both estrogen and progesterone or estrogen only. Other possible contraindications include seizure disorders, migraines, and gallbladder or pancreatic disease.

Nursing care focuses on helping women understand the physical changes that occur and the psychological responses that may occur during menopause. Nurses must clarify the individual regimen of HRT as well as the risks and benefits of the therapy. For instance, women should be told that although HRT effectively treats atrophic vaginitis and reduces dyspareunia, it may not overcome the loss of libido that some women experience (Box 33-6).

If HRT is contraindicated, nurses are often the primary source of information about alternative measures that mitigate symptoms:

- Using water-soluble lubricants such as K-Y Liquid, K-Y Silk-e, Lubrin, or Replens to relieve vaginal dryness and dyspareunia. Oil-based lubricants should not be used because they adhere to the mucous membrane for long periods of time and provide a medium for bacterial growth.
- Discussing alternatives to estrogen, such as botanical preparations, if the woman does not want ERT. The woman should discuss these with her health care provider, because some have side or adverse effects or interactions with other drugs. Research is often minimal for these therapies. The website for the National Center for Complementary and Alternative Medicine of the NIH, www.nccam.nih.gov, contains updated information.
- Doing Kegel exercises to increase muscle tone around the vagina and urinary meatus and counteract the effects of genital atrophy.
- Drinking at least eight glasses of water a day decreases the concentration of urine, flushes urine from the bladder, and reduces bacterial growth, thereby preventing atrophic cystitis.
- Wiping from front to back after urination and defecation reduces the transfer of bacteria from the anus to the urinary meatus and helps prevent cystitis.

BOX 33-6 Contraindications and Cautions Related to Estrogen Replacement Therapy

Previous episode of breast cancer or other estrogen-dependent tumor
Close family history of breast cancer (first-degree relative)
Uterine cancer
Active thromboembolic disease or prior thromboembolic disorder when on estrogen
Risk for cardiovascular disease
Stroke
Acute or chronic liver disease
Undiagnosed abnormal vaginal bleeding
Gallbladder or pancreatic disease
Diabetes mellitus
Conditions that may be aggravated by fluid retention, such as migraine, epilepsy, cardiac, renal dysfunction, depression

About Hormone Replacement Therapy

Hormone replacement therapy is highly individualized owing to research findings about unfavorable cardiovascular effects of estrogen-progesterone supplementation during the climacteric. However, women may continue using the estrogen-only HRT or the estrogen-progesterone HRT for significant discomforts that are unrelieved by other methods or for beneficial effects such as reduction in osteoporosis. The woman and her caregiver must consider both benefits and risks of HRT to make the decision about whether to use the hormone replacement.

- Take the medication with meals to reduce nausea.
- If you miss a dose, take the medication as soon as you remember, but not immediately before the next scheduled dose. *Do not take double doses.*

- Expect withdrawal bleeding (if your uterus is present) when estrogen and progestin are temporarily discontinued.
- Report unexpected bleeding to your health care provider.
- Stop smoking to reduce the risk of thromboembolism.
- Use sunscreen and protective clothing to prevent increased pigmentation.
- Continue follow-up physical examinations, including blood pressure measurements, Pap tests, and examinations of breasts, abdomen, and pelvis.

✔ CHECK YOUR READING

27. What are the effects of estrogen depletion at menopause (either natural or artificial) on the body?
28. What are the major psychological symptoms associated with menopause?
29. How does hormone replacement affect menopausal and postmenopausal women? What concerns were raised by the WHI research?

Osteoporosis

Osteoporosis is one of the greatest hazards of the postmenopausal years. It is characterized by decreased bone density, leaving the bones porous, fragile, and susceptible to fractures. The vertebrae, wrists, and hips are the most common sites of fractures.

Osteoporosis is a major public health problem that will likely increase as baby boomers age. More than 44 million people in the United States presently have the public health threat of low bone mass or osteoporosis, and 68% of them are women. One in two women over age 50 will have a fracture related to osteoporosis in their lifetime. Osteoporosis causes as many as 300,000 hip fractures, 700,000 vertebral fractures, and 250,000 wrist fractures, in addition to other fractures (NIH, 2003). Hip fractures increase the risk of reduced mobility and death in the elderly.

RISK FACTORS

Small-boned, fair-skinned, white and Asian women are at greatest risk for osteoporosis. Other risk factors include a family history of the disease, early menopause, and a sedentary lifestyle. Women who smoke, drink alcohol, or take corticosteroids or anticonvulsants, as well as those who consume excessive amounts of caffeine, also have an increased risk for osteoporosis (NIH, 2003). Inadequate intake of calcium and vitamin D is a major risk factor because it results in failure to achieve peak bone mass during youth.

SIGNS AND SYMPTOMS

Osteoporosis has been called the "silent thief" because bone mass is lost over many years with no signs or symptoms. The first noticeable evidence is loss of height and back pain that occurs when the vertebrae collapse. Later signs include the "dowager's hump," which occurs when the vertebrae can no longer support the upper body in an upright position. Secondary to this, the waistline disappears and the abdomen protrudes as the rib cage moves closer to the pelvis. Depending on the number of fractures, several inches of height may be lost. Figure 33-5 illustrates progressive changes in posture associated with osteoporosis.

Diagnosis of osteoporosis requires a thorough history, physical examination, and bone mineral analysis. Conventional x-ray examination is of little help, because more than 30% of the bone mass must be lost before changes are apparent. Dual-energy x-ray absorptiometry (DEXA) is a highly accurate, fast, and relatively inexpensive method for measuring bone mineral density. In addition, it involves low exposure to radiation. Single-energy x-ray absorptiometry can be used in mobile units and is good for simple screening at health fairs. Ultrasonography is another method to evaluate bone density of peripheral sites (Curry & Hogstel, 2002; U.S. Preventive Services Task Force, 2002).

PREVENTION AND MEDICAL MANAGEMENT

The main goal of treatment is to prevent the development of osteoporosis and to stabilize remaining bone mass. The major goal of treatment is to prevent or slow osteoporosis and to stabilize remaining bone mass. Although research has upheld estrogen therapy to reduce osteoporosis by inhibition of bone resorption, fewer women are choosing the hormone because of its potential adverse effects.

DRUG THERAPY. Other drug categories to reduce osteoporosis include:

- Calcitonin (Calcimar, Miacalcin), a synthetic thyroid hormone usually prescribed as a daily nasal spray to

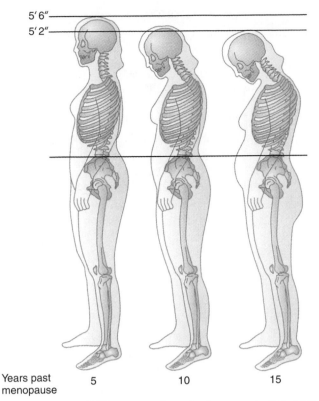

5'6"
5'2"

Years past menopause   5   10   15

Figure 33-5 ■ With progression of osteoporosis, the vertebral column collapses, causing loss of height and back pain. "Dowager's hump" is the term used for this curvature of the upper back.

reduce factors that cause loss of calcium and increase reabsorption of calcium in the gastrointestinal tract.

■ Biophosphonates, which inhibit osteoclasts, reducing bone turnover. Alendronate (Fosamax) has been evaluated extensively, showing significant reduction of osteoporosis-related fractures. Risedronate (Actonel) is a newer drug with similar effects. Alendronate and risedronate may be prescribed in daily or weekly doses. Biophosphonates may be contraindicated for women with ulcers or an inflammatory gastrointestinal disease such as dysphagia or esophagitis. The drugs should be taken at least 30 minutes before eating, drinking fluids other than water, or taking other medicine for improved absorption.

■ Raloxifene (Evista), a selective estrogen receptor modulator, or SERM, that binds to estrogen receptors to reduce bone loss. Because of the combined estrogen agonist and estrogen antagonist effects of SERMs, raloxifene is being studied to see if its effects also improve cardiac health without raising breast or uterine cancer risks.

CALCIUM AND VITAMIN D. Although calcium does not prevent bone loss, other therapies cannot be effective if calcium is deficient. A woman older than 50 years needs 1200 mg of calcium daily, and the woman 65 years or older needs 1500 mg/day. Daily calcium supplements are recommended, because it is difficult to ingest these quantities through food intake only. Vitamin D is necessary for calcium to be absorbed from the intestine. Supplemental vitamin D, 400 to 800 units, is recommended for many women (Cedars & Evans, 2003; Curry & Hogstel, 2002).

EXERCISE. Weight-bearing and resistance exercise has been shown to be beneficial in slowing loss of bone mass to maintain density, if there is adequate calcium and vitamin D intake. Most of the bone mass is acquired by age 18, but muscle-strengthening exercise may continue to build bone into the thirties. High-impact exercise improves bone mineral density but should be avoided in a woman who already has fragile vertebrae from osteoporosis. At least 30 minutes of therapeutic exercise is needed. Other exercises, such as swimming or water-based exercises, often improve cardiovascular and respiratory fitness while managing weight, although their primary use is not to limit bone loss.

NURSING CONSIDERATIONS

Nurses often counsel women about lifestyle factors that contribute to bone loss, such as cigarette smoking, excessive alcohol or caffeine intake, and the importance of following the recommended medical regimen. Adolescents and young women should be counseled about factors that impair as well as promote their ideal amount of peak bone density. Nurses are also concerned about how to prevent falls and thereby reduce the risk of fractures, particularly in older women or those with mobility impairments. A major responsibility is to help the woman make her environment as safe as possible. Lighting should be ample, with switches easily accessible. Loose electrical cords should be kept out of the way, and area rugs should have nonskid backing. The bathtub should have nonskid devices, and grab bars should be installed near toilets and tubs. Stairways should have handrails, and loose items should be kept out of the walking pathways. Consultation with an occupational or physical therapist may be needed if the woman has serious mobility problems.

NURSING DIAGNOSES

A variety of nursing diagnoses may be relevant for the woman with osteoporosis, depending on the severity of the condition. Examples include:

■ Pain related to pressure and inflammation of nerves that exit the vertebral column
■ Activity Intolerance related to discomfort and fear of falling
■ Disturbed Body Image related to postural and functional limitations
■ Self-Care Deficit (specify deficit) related to physical limitations and depression

✓ **CHECK YOUR READING**

30. Why is osteoporosis called the "silent thief"?
31. How can osteoporosis be prevented?
32. What can nurses do to prevent fractures in women with osteoporosis?

PELVIC FLOOR DYSFUNCTION

Pelvic floor dysfunction occurs when muscles, ligaments, and fascia that support the pelvic organs are damaged or weakened. This relaxation of pelvic support allows the pelvic organs to prolapse into, and sometimes out of, the vagina. Pelvic disorders generally occur in the perimenopausal period and may be the delayed result of traumatic childbirth or the effects of aging.

Vaginal Wall Prolapse

The vagina may prolapse at either the anterior or posterior wall. Anterior wall prolapse involves the bladder and urethra and is called *cystocele.* Prolapse of the posterior wall produces enterocele or rectocele.

CYSTOCELE

When the weakened upper anterior wall of the vagina is no longer able to support the weight of urine in the bladder, cystocele develops. The bladder protrudes downward into the vagina, resulting in incomplete emptying of the bladder. Cystitis is likely to occur because of the stagnant urine. Urethral displacement, formerly termed *urethrocele,* may occur when the urethra bulges into the lower anterior vaginal wall, producing stress urinary incontinence (Figure 33-6, *A*).

Stress incontinence is the loss of urine that occurs with a sudden increase in intraabdominal pressure, such as that generated by sneezing, coughing, laughing, lifting, or sudden jarring motions. The two most common causes of stress incontinence are damage to the normal supports of the bladder neck and urethra that occurs during pregnancy and childbirth, and tissue atrophy that occurs after menopause.

ENTEROCELE

Enterocele is prolapse of the upper posterior vaginal wall between the vagina and rectum. This is almost always associated with herniation of the pouch of Douglas (a fold of peritoneum that dips down between the rectum and the uterus) and may contain loops of bowel. Enterocele often accompanies uterine prolapse (Figure 33-6, *B*).

RECTOCELE

Rectocele occurs when the posterior wall of the vagina becomes weakened and thin. Each time the woman strains at defecation, feces are pushed against the thinned wall, causing further stretching, until finally the rectum protrudes into the vagina. Many rectoceles are small and produce few symptoms. If the rectocele is large, the patient may have difficulty emptying the rectum. Some women facilitate bowel elimination by applying digital pressure along the posterior vaginal wall to keep the rectocele from protruding during a bowel movement (Figure 33-6, *C*).

Uterine Prolapse

Uterine prolapse occurs when the cardinal ligaments, which support the uterus and vagina, are unduly stretched during pregnancy and do not return to normal after childbirth. This allows the uterus to sag backward and downward into the

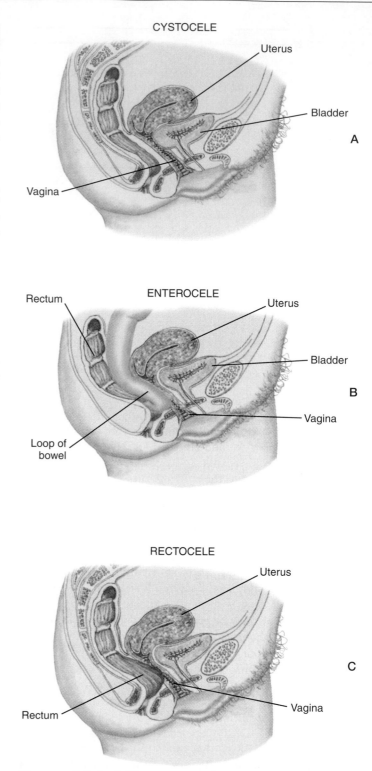

Figure 33-6 ■ Three types of vaginal wall prolapse. **A,** Note bulging of bladder into the vagina. **B,** Note loop of bowel between rectum and uterus. **C,** Note bulging of rectum into vagina.

vagina. Uterine prolapse is less common than in the past, largely because of a reduction in traumatic vaginal deliveries. The condition continues to exist, however, particularly when the woman has had many vaginal deliveries or when the infants were large. Figure 33-7 illustrates three degrees of uterine prolapse from first degree, in which the uterus remains in

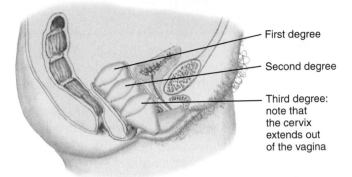

Figure 33-7 ■ Three degrees of uterine prolapse.

the vagina, to third degree, in which the cervix protrudes from the vagina. Detailed staging, from stage 0 through stage IV, provides details about the amount and direction of vaginal wall shape alterations and the descent in specific areas of the vagina (DeLancey & Strohbehn, 2003).

Symptoms

Symptoms of pelvic floor dysfunction generally become obvious during the menopausal period. This is because estrogen diminishes at this time, resulting in atrophic changes in the supporting structures. The most common symptoms of vaginal wall prolapse are feelings of pelvic fullness, a dragging sensation, pelvic pressure, and fatigue. Low backache and a feeling that "everything is falling out" are sometimes described.

Symptoms relate to the structures involved and the level at which support has decreased. For instance, urinary frequency and urgency and urinary incontinence are seen in patients with cystocele because support of the urethra and lower vaginal wall has decreased. Constipation, flatulence, and difficulty defecating are major symptoms of rectocele. Regardless of the location or structure involved, symptoms become worse after prolonged standing, and they are relieved by lying down.

Symptoms of uterine prolapse are produced by the weight of the descending structures and may include sensations of pelvic pressure, backache, and fatigue. Cervical ulceration and bleeding occur if the cervix protrudes from the vaginal introitus.

Management

Treatment of disorders related to pelvic floor dysfunction depends on the woman's age, physical condition, sexual activity, and degree of prolapse. Surgical procedures provide the most satisfactory therapy for women who have significant discomfort. The most common procedures are the anterior and posterior colporrhaphy. The anterior colporrhaphy involves suturing the pubocervical fascia to support the bladder and urethra when a cystocele exists. If a rectocele exists, a posterior colporrhaphy (suturing the fascia and perineal muscles that support the perineum and rectum) is performed. The two colporrhaphy surgeries are often described as an *A and P (anterior and posterior) repair.*

Vaginal hysterectomy, in which the uterus is removed through the vaginal canal rather than through an abdominal incision, is the most common surgery to correct vaginal prolapse. Vaginal hysterectomy often is combined with anterior and posterior repair.

If surgery is contraindicated, a pessary (a device to support pelvic structures) may be inserted into the vagina. The pessary must be inspected and changed frequently by a physician or nurse practitioner to prevent vaginal ulceration, fistula formation, stool impaction, and infection. Vaginal estrogen cream may improve the woman's tolerance of the pessary. Topical or systemic estrogen treatment may be indicated for the woman (Bhatia, 2004; DeLancey & Strohbehn, 2003).

Nursing Considerations

PELVIC EXERCISES

Kegel exercises are known to strengthen the pubococcygeal muscle, which surrounds the urethra, vagina, and rectum and is the main support of the pelvic floor. Before teaching Kegel exercise, determine if the woman can contract the pubococcygeal muscle by asking her to sit with her legs apart while she urinates and to squeeze the muscles to stop the stream of urine. If she can accomplish this, the muscle is contracted and it is possible for her to perform the exercise.

Kegel exercises involve conscious contracting and relaxing of the pelvic muscles. Only the pelvic muscles should be used; the abdomen, thighs, and buttocks should *not* tighten. Women should be taught to exhale and keep the mouth open to avoid bearing down when contracting the pelvic muscles for at least 3 seconds, building to a maximum hold of 10 seconds, and then gradually relaxing the muscle contraction. A minimum of 10 seconds of muscle relaxation should follow the pelvic muscle contractions. Variations exist about how frequently to repeat pelvic muscle contractions each day, but from 24 to 45 daily repetitions are beneficial. To maintain pelvic muscle tone, the woman should continue Kegel exercises for the rest of her life (Newman, 2003b; Sampselle, 2003).

Graduated weight cones may be used as an adjunct to pelvic muscle exercise. Incrementally weighted cones are inserted into the vagina, and the woman attempts to hold the weights in place. As the weight of the cones increases, the resistance against which the pelvic muscles contract increases, thereby strengthening the pelvic muscles.

Measures that help reduce the symptoms of pelvic relaxation may also prove helpful. These include lying down with the legs elevated for a few minutes several times a day. Some women are relieved by assuming a knee-chest position for a few minutes. In addition, teaching may include measures to prevent constipation.

URINARY INCONTINENCE

Evaluation of the characteristics of a woman's urinary incontinence guides treatment. Three major patterns are (Fenner, 2003; Sampselle, 2003):

- Stress incontinence, with urine leakage occurring as the woman increases her intraabdominal pressure. Examples of times when intraabdominal pressure may increase sufficiently include coughing, sneezing, laughter, or physical exertion such as picking up a full shopping bag or heavier load.

- Urge incontinence, characterized by urine leakage that accompanies a woman's strong need to void promptly.
- Mixed incontinence, in which a woman's urine leakage has associated factors from both the stress and urge incontinence patterns.

Overactive bladder (OAB) may occur with both urge and mixed incontinence. OAB is characterized by frequent sensations of urgency and nocturia and may accompany neurologic, anatomic, or structural disorders.

■ Direct questions, such as "Do you have trouble with your bladder?" or "Do you ever unintentionally lose urine?" may encourage women to discuss urine control problems. After the subject is introduced, follow-up questions are asked to determine urinary frequency. For instance, can she sit through a 2-hour movie without emptying her bladder? How many times does she get up to urinate each night? Does she often feel that she must hurry to empty her bladder and that she will lose urine while going to the restroom?

Nursing research has shown that continence can be improved by teaching specific health promotion activities, such as Kegel exercises and bladder training, which involves adhering to a prescribed schedule for emptying the bladder (Sampselle, 2003). Women who cannot execute even a weak pelvic muscle contraction or are unable to implement bladder training may benefit from biofeedback or electrical stimulation provided by a skilled practitioner.

Women often benefit from knowing about some of the commercial products that protect the skin and prevent odor. These products are made of material that traps urine and prevents constant contact with the skin.

Women often restrict fluids, believing that this will decrease urinary incontinence. Restricting fluids may actually make the condition worse because the bladder does not fill to its normal capacity. Furthermore, decreased fluid intake can lead to concentrated urine that can irritate bladder mucous membranes and increase the urge to void. Alcohol and caffeine can also irritate the bladder and worsen incontinence. Obesity is associated with urinary incontinence, increasing the benefits for a woman to achieve her ideal weight range.

Drug treatment may enhance bladder control. Drugs that may be prescribed include (Newman, 2003a):

- Vaginal estrogen using a cream, tablet, or vaginal ring to reduce atrophy of the urinary and vaginal areas
- Anticholinergic drugs, including their long-acting versions, such as oxybutynin or tolterodine

---

✔ CHECK YOUR READING

33. How does cystocele differ from rectocele in terms of location? Symptoms?
34. What causes uterine prolapse, and how is it treated?
35. What are nursing actions to alleviate problems associated with pelvic floor relaxation? Urinary incontinence?

DISORDERS OF THE REPRODUCTIVE TRACT

Benign Disorders

The most common benign conditions of the reproductive tract include cervical polyps, uterine leiomyomas (fibroids), and ovarian cysts.

CERVICAL POLYPS

Polyps are small tumors, usually only a few millimeters in diameter, that are generally on a pedicle (a stalk, or stemlike structure). They are caused by proliferation of cervical mucosa, and often cause intermittent vaginal bleeding.

Cervical polyps are surgically removed in an outpatient setting, and the specimen is sent for pathologic examination to rule out malignancy.

UTERINE LEIOMYOMAS

Leiomyomas, also called *fibroids,* are one of the most common gynecologic conditions encountered. Although the cause is unknown, they develop from uterine smooth muscle cells and are estrogen dependent. As a result, they grow rapidly during the childbearing years, when estrogen is abundant, but shrink during menopause unless growth is maintained by HRT for menopausal symptoms. Fibroids may occur throughout the muscular layer of the uterus and may be prominent near the end of pregnancy as the estrogen levels are high and the uterus is large (Figure 33-8).

Uterine fibroids do not often cause symptoms. Uterine size is sometimes increased, and excessive menstrual bleeding may occur. Excessive bleeding may result in anemia, weakness, and fatigue. Infertility may be related to uterine fibroids. Additional symptoms include feelings of pelvic pressure, bloating, and urinary frequency that occurs when

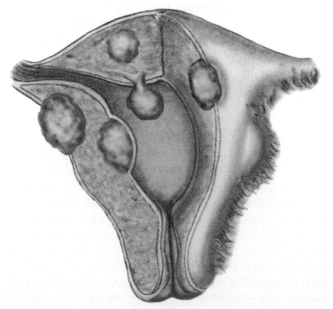

Figure 33-8 ■ Sites within the uterus where fibroids commonly occur.

the tumor applies pressure on the bladder. Pressure on the ureter may cause hydroureter (dilation of the ureter).

Treatment depends on the size of the fibroids and the symptoms experienced. In the absence of symptoms, treatment may consist of observation only. If abnormal bleeding is a problem, surgical intervention may be necessary. The two most common surgeries are myomectomy or removal of the tumor only, and hysterectomy, which is removal of the uterus.

Medical treatment with progesterone-only or combination estrogen-progesterone oral contraceptives may reduce excess menstrual flow. Short courses of GnRH agonists may be effective in reducing the size of myomas and lessen the need for surgical removal of the tumor. GnRH agonists cause hot flashes, vaginal dryness, and other discomforts similar to those of menopause, and therefore are not tolerated well by some women. Loss of bone mineral density is an adverse effect of long-term therapy. Mifepristone (RU-486) is being studied as a drug to reduce fibroid size without loss of bone density (Moore & Nelson, 2004a).

OVARIAN CYSTS

An ovarian cyst may be either follicular or luteal. If the ovarian follicle fails to rupture during ovulation, a follicular cyst may develop. These cysts are usually asymptomatic and may be an incidental finding on an ultrasound. They generally regress during the subsequent menstrual cycle. A lutein cyst may develop if the corpus luteum becomes cystic and fails to regress. A lutein cyst is more likely to cause pain and delay in the next menstrual cycle. Occasionally, an ovarian cyst can rupture or twist on its pedicle and become infarcted, causing pelvic pain and tenderness.

Treatment depends on differentiating a cyst from a solid ovarian tumor that is more likely to indicate cancer. If the woman is in her childbearing years, when the risk of ovarian cancer is less, the physician may wait until after the next menstrual cycle and examine the woman again. Transvaginal ultrasound examination is useful to determine if it is a fluid-filled cyst or a solid tumor. Laparoscopy may be helpful in ruling out endometriosis. Laparotomy may be necessary to remove the cyst from the ovary for examination by a pathologist.

Malignant Disorders

The primary sites for cancer in the female reproductive organs are the uterus, ovaries, and cervix. Cancer of the vagina, vulva, and fallopian tubes is relatively uncommon. Although cancer can occur at any age, the incidence increases with age.

SIGNS AND SYMPTOMS

Cancer of the reproductive organs may not be diagnosed until it is advanced, because few symptoms are experienced in the early stages. When symptoms occur, they are often nonspecific and could be caused by infection or other benign conditions. Cancer of the ovaries is particu-

---

BOX 33-7 Risk Factors for Cancer of the Reproductive Organs

Uterus
African-Americans: higher risk for leiomyosarcoma
Obesity
Nulliparity
Middle-aged and elderly
Late menopause (>52 years old)
Diabetes mellitus
Breast, colon, or ovarian cancer
Estrogen replacement therapy

Cervix
Human papilloma virus (HPV) infection
Sexual risks: Young age at start of intercourse (<20 years), multiple sexual partners, uncircumcised male partners
Many pregnancies
Obesity
Diet low in fruits and vegetables
Smoking
Lower socioeconomic status (may be related to infrequent gynecologic examinations)
History of sexually transmitted diseases, such as chlamydia or human immunodeficiency virus (HIV) infection

Ovaries
Menses started at <12 years of age
No child or first child after 30 years of age
Late menopause (>55 years old)
Infertility; infertility drugs
Family history of ovarian, breast, or colorectal cancer
Personal history of breast cancer

---

larly difficult to diagnose because it may remain "silent" until far advanced, when the chance of long-term survival is greatly reduced.

RISK FACTORS

Risk factors vary according to the site of the cancer. Risk factors for cervical cancer include a history of STDs, particularly condyloma acuminatum, or genital warts caused by HPV. Prolonged use of unopposed ERT (estrogen-only) predisposes to overgrowth (hyperplasia) of endometrial tissue and is a significant risk factor for uterine cancer.

Family history is an important risk factor for ovarian cancer. Other factors such as the use of talcum powder and feminine hygiene products that contain talc have also been implicated, but their role is inconclusive (Berek, 2004). See Box 33-7 for a summary of risk factors for cancer of the reproductive organs.

DIAGNOSIS

Early diagnosis is strongly associated with long-term survival. Many screening and diagnostic tests are useful. Screening tests include periodic pelvic examinations, Pap tests, ultrasonography, and serum tests for tumor markers such as CA-125, which may be increased with ovarian or other cancers. Genes linked to other cancers, such as BRCA1 or BRCA2 (p. 888), may lead to more diagnostic procedures than if the genetic risk is not apparent. Significant family history of specific cancers of the reproductive organs or linked cancers such as breast cancers may alter the risk for a woman's development of cancer. Diagnostic pro-

Symptoms That Should Always Be Investigated

- Irregular vaginal bleeding
- Unexplained postmenopausal bleeding
- Unusual vaginal discharge
- Dyspareunia
- Persistent vulvar or vaginal itching
- Elevated or discolored lesions of the vulva
- Persistent abdominal bloating or constipation
- Persistent anorexia or vomiting
- Blood in stools

cedures such as endometrial biopsy for endometrial cancer and colposcopy can identify patterns of abnormality near the cervical os, where most cancers of the cervix develop.

MANAGEMENT

Treatment of cancer of the reproductive organs is based on location and extent of the disease and the age and desire of the woman to have children. Treatment of one type of cancer may be based on previous cancer treatment in the same or related organs. For instance, treatment of previous breast cancer with the chemotherapy drug adriamycin often means that the woman has reached the maximum lifetime amount that she can take because of the drug's effects on her heart.

CERVICAL CANCER. Testing for HPV often reveals the cervical infection that contributes to cancer. A biopsy of the suspicious area and an endocervical curettage is done for diagnosis if the woman is not pregnant.

Early treatment to destroy abnormal tissue in cervical cancer may consist of cryosurgery, laser, loop electrodiathermy excision (LEEP), electrocoagulation, or surgical conization of the cervix. After treatment, a surveillance schedule should be established because of the risk of recurrent cervical squamous intraepithelial lesion (SIL). See p. 886 for information on the Bethesda system for classifications of cervical cytology.

Surgical staging guides treatment for most advanced cervical cancer to identify the degree of invasive spread. If there is lymphatic or distant spread of cervical cancer, a radical hysterectomy with lymph node dissection is recommended by many gynecologic oncologists. Chemotherapy and radiation therapy may be incorporated into treatment (Hacker, 2004b).

ENDOMETRIAL CANCER. Postmenopausal bleeding is the most common presentation for endometrial cancer. Women who are older, obese, and diabetic are more likely to have endometrial cancer if they have vaginal bleeding after menopause. The highest remission rate is with surgery (hysterectomy and salpingo-oophorectomy), possibly supplemented by radiation therapy. Poor surgical candidates may be treated with radiation therapy alone, and radiation therapy may be given as adjuvant therapy to women at risk for metastatic disease or disease in the upper vagina (vaginal

cuff). Five-year survival rates are less than 50% even if the cancer was found at an early stage (Hacker, 2004c).

OVARIAN CANCER. Surgery, possibly involving removal of the healthy ovary as well as the ovary affected with cancer, is an essential part of therapy and may be curative for women in the earliest stages of ovarian cancer. Chemotherapy may be given to reduce the tumor's size, followed by oophorectomy to remove it. Surgery for more advanced ovarian cancer improves diagnostic information, allows more accurate staging, and permits surgical reduction of the cancer. Chemotherapy is required after surgery for all but the very early cancers, and newer drugs have improved the 5-year survival rate to about 50%. A diagnostic workup identifies the effects of the tumor on adjacent organs in the abdomen and identifies metastases to distant sites. Many patients with advanced tumors relapse or have disease progression despite treatment (Berek, 2004; Cass & Karlan, 2003).

CHECK YOUR READING

36. What are the signs and symptoms of leiomyomas (uterine fibroids), and how are they treated?
37. Why is ultrasonography used to evaluate ovarian cysts?
38. What signs and symptoms are suggestive of cancer of the reproductive organs and should always be investigated?
39. How may cancer of the following reproductive organs be treated: Cervix? Endometrium? Ovary?

INFECTIOUS DISORDERS OF THE REPRODUCTIVE TRACT

Infections of the reproductive tract may cause a variety of problems for women of all ages. Although some, such as candidiasis, are mostly annoying, others, such as the immunodeficiency virus, may be lethal. Some infections are seldom associated with sexual activity, whereas others are almost exclusively spread in this way. Infections may spread silently in the reproductive organs, allowing damage to the organs before the woman has symptoms.

Candidiasis

Candidiasis, also known as *moniliasis* and *yeast infection*, is the most common form of vaginitis. The cause is believed to be related to a change in vaginal pH that allows accelerated growth of *Candida albicans*, a yeastlike fungus commonly found in the digestive tract and on the skin. Some conditions, such as pregnancy, diabetes mellitus, oral contraceptive use, and systemic antibiotic therapy, result in changes in vaginal pH and flora that favor accelerated growth of *C. albicans*. Although not considered an STD, recurrent candidiasis in sexually active women may occur. A small number of male partners may have erythema and itching of their glans penis (balanitis).

The main symptoms for candidiasis are vaginal and perineal itching. Vulvar and vaginal tissues are inflamed, causing burning on urination. Vaginal discharge is white with a typical "cottage cheese" appearance. Diagnosis is made by identifying the spores of *C. albicans.*

Treatment may consist of nonprescription or prescription medications. Medications available without prescription include butoconazole, miconazole, clotrimazole, nystatin, terconazole, and tioconazole by vaginal application. The duration for most of the nonprescription medications for candidiasis ranges from 3 to 7 days, depending on the specific medication. Women should be advised to seek medical attention with the first infection or if the infection persists or recurs frequently. Oral fluconazole is a prescription medication for treatment of uncomplicated candidiasis with a single dose. Patients with a more severe candidiasis may need another dose of diflucan in 4 days. Recurrent yeast infections that resist treatment are associated with diabetes mellitus or HIV infection.

Sexually Transmissible Diseases

Many diseases can be transmitted through sexual activity. For some diseases, such as syphilis, gonorrhea, and chlamydial infection, sexual activity is almost the only method of transmission. For other diseases, such as bacterial vaginosis, sexual activity may or may not be the mode of transmission.

INCIDENCE

STDs are epidemic today, with the highest incidence among adolescents and young adults. Furthermore, the number of untreated infected individuals with no symptoms is most likely immense. For many reasons these diseases remain a major health problem despite advancements in the development of antibiotics. The age of the first sexual experience has been declining steadily, and sexual activity is high among adolescents and young adults. Multiple sexual partners, inadequate knowledge of transmission and prevention, and feelings of invincibility are common among this age group. Because the vagina may have microscopic tears after intercourse that provide favorable conditions for an infection, women are twice as likely as men to have an STD (CDC, 2002).

Methods of contraception have a significant impact on the risk of STDs. Barrier methods, such as condoms and female condoms, offer the best protection from infection. Diaphragms, cervical caps, and spermicidal foams and jellies do not offer the same protection as condoms, although they can decrease the risk of cervical and upper genital tract infections. When counseling teenagers, nurses must emphasize that oral contraceptives prevent pregnancy but do nothing to prevent exposure to STDs.

Major concerns include the following:
- The vulnerability of women to STDs
- The resistance of some organisms to antibiotics
- The relationship between HIV infection and other STDs
- Failure of asymptomatic persons to seek treatment when their sexual partner is infected

See Chapter 26 for the impact of STDs on pregnancy and the fetus.

TYPES OF SEXUALLY TRANSMITTED DISEASES

TRICHOMONIASIS. Trichomoniasis is caused by *T. vaginalis,* an anaerobic protozoon that thrives in an alkaline environment. Most infections are believed to be transmitted by sexual contact. The presenting symptoms include a purulent vaginal discharge that is thin or frothy, malodorous, and yellow green or brownish-gray in color. The pH of the discharge is usually greater than 4.5. Vulvar itching, edema, and redness may also be present. The diagnosis is made by identifying the organism in a wet mount preparation.

If the woman is not pregnant, the treatment of choice is metronidazole (Flagyl, Protostat) 2 g in a single oral dose or 500 mg twice daily for 7 days. Some clinicians prefer to avoid use of metronidazole in the first trimester of pregnancy. Clotrimazole (Gyne-Lotrimin) may provide symptom relief at this time. Metronidazole may be used during the second and third trimesters. Alcohol ingestion when taking metronidazole may result in a disulfiram-like (Antabuse) reaction. Women should be advised to avoid using alcohol during treatment with metronidazole and for 24 hours after treatment is complete.

Sexual partners should refrain from intercourse until a cure is established. Reinfection may result when the woman's partner is not treated. In particular, emphasize that all sexual partners should be treated and that condoms should be used with a new partner.

BACTERIAL VAGINOSIS. This infection, previously referred to as *nonspecific vaginitis,* is associated with organisms that replace normal lactobacilli with *Gardnerella vaginalis* or *Mycoplasma hominis* or with anaerobic bacteria, such as *Prevotella* or *Mobiluncus.* Causes of the bacterial proliferation are not known, although tissue trauma and vaginal intercourse have been identified as contributing factors. Multiple partners, douching, and lack of vaginal lactobacilli are associated with bacterial vaginosis.

Chief signs and symptoms are a thin grayish white vaginal discharge that typically exudes a fishy odor. The diagnosis is made by preparing a saline wet mount and identifying characteristic clue cells (epithelial cells with numerous bacilli clinging to their surface).

Treatment for bacterial vaginosis is directed toward reestablishing the balance of flora in the vagina. Metronidazole has been shown to relieve symptoms and to improve vaginal flora. Clindamycin is an alternative treatment. The woman should refrain from sexual intercourse until cured, or her partner should use a condom. Treatment of her partner has not proved beneficial (CDC, 2002).

CHLAMYDIAL INFECTION. The most common STD in Western countries is caused by the gram-negative bacterium *C. trachomatis.* The incidence is particularly high in sexually active teens and young adults. Chlamydial infection is often asymptomatic in women, which makes diagnosis and control of the disease difficult. It should be suspected when the male sexual partner is treated for nongonococcal urethritis and when the culture results for gonorrhea are negative, yet the woman exhibits symptoms similar to those of gonorrhea, such as a yellowish vaginal discharge and painful urination. Gonorrhea and chlamydial infections often coexist.

Diagnosis of chlamydial infection can be made by isolating the bacterium in tissue culture, by enzyme-linked immunosorbent assay (ELISA), or by direct fluorescent monoclonal antibody. Tissue culture of the organism is most accurate but requires more time.

Untreated, chlamydial infection ascends from the cervix to involve the fallopian tubes, and it is one of the chief causes of tubal scarring that result in pelvic inflammatory disease (PID), infertility, or ectopic pregnancy. Treatment is usually directed to eradicate both chlamydia and gonorrhea, because the two often coexist. Treatment options for chlamydia include azithromycin (Zithromax), doxycycline (Vibramycin), clindamycin (Cleocin), ofloxacin (Floxin), levofloxacin (Levaquin), and erythromycin. Treatment of all sexual partners is essential to prevent recurrence. Use of condoms until a cure is established is essential, as well.

GONORRHEA. Gonorrhea is an infection of the genitourinary tract that is caused by the gonococcus *Neisseria gonorrhoeae*. Gonorrhea may be asymptomatic in women, but when symptoms do occur, they usually include purulent discharge, dysuria, and dyspareunia. Diagnosis is based on a positive culture for the gonococcus. Gonorrhea is associated with PID (which increases the risk of tubal scarring and can result in infertility or ectopic pregnancy), as is chlamydial infection.

Currently, two factors influence the treatment of gonorrhea: the high numbers of organisms that have become resistant to previously used antibiotics, such as penicillin and tetracycline, and the high frequency of chlamydial infections in persons with gonorrhea. Cefixime (Suprax), ceftriaxone (Rocephin), and ciprofloxacin (Cipro) in combination with one of the antibiotics listed for chlamydia, appear to be effective for gonorrhea treatment. All sexual partners should be treated simultaneously, and intercourse should be avoided or the man should use a condom until a cure is confirmed.

SYPHILIS. Syphilis is caused by the spirochete *Treponema pallidum,* and it is divided into primary, secondary, and tertiary stages. The first sign of primary syphilis is a painless chancre that develops on the genitalia, anus, or lips or in the oral cavity. At this time, diagnosis is made by identifying the spirochete on dark-field microscopy in material scraped from the base of the chancre. Serologic test results are generally negative in the primary stage. If untreated the chancre heals in about 6 weeks. The disease is highly infectious at the primary stage.

Although the chancre disappears, the spirochete lives and is carried by the blood to all parts of the body. About 2 months after the initial infection, infected people exhibit symptoms of secondary syphilis, including enlargement of the spleen and liver, headache, anorexia, and a generalized maculopapular skin rash. Skin eruptions, called *condylomata lata,* may develop on the vulva during this time. Condylomata lata resemble warts; they contain numerous spiro-

chetes and are highly contagious. Serologic test results are generally positive at this time.

If untreated the disease enters a latent phase that may last for several years. Tertiary syphilis, which follows the latent phase, may involve the heart, blood vessels, and central nervous system. General paralysis and psychosis may result.

In addition to identification of the spirochete in material scraped from a chancre, diagnosis is also made by serology. The usual screening test is the Venereal Disease Research Laboratory (VDRL) serum test, which is based on the presence of antibodies produced in response to the infection. The rapid plasma reagin (RPR) and fluorescent treponemal antibody absorption (FTA-ABS) tests are more specific and are often done to confirm a positive result of VDRL.

Best treatment of all stages of syphilis is with penicillin. Ceftriaxone and doxycycline can also be useful. Tetracycline is an alternative if the woman is not pregnant. A woman who is allergic to penicillin can be admitted to the hospital for desensitization to penicillin, followed by administration of the drug.

HERPES GENITALIS. Herpes genitalis is an STD caused by the herpes simplex virus (HSV). Two types of HSV have been identified: type 1 and type 2. HSV-2 usually causes genital lesions, and HSV-1 usually causes oral-pharyngeal infection. However, either organism may infect the less-frequent location. Transmission occurs through direct contact with an infected person. A person infected with HSV-1 develops antibodies that may reduce the severity of the first HSV-2 infection. A *primary* HSV-2 infection is one in which the person had no preceding HSV-1 infection, and therefore has no antibodies. Transmission may occur from a partner who is infected but has no visible lesions or symptomatic viral shedding (McGregor, French, & Lench, 2004).

Within 2 to 12 days after the primary infection, vesicles (blisters) appear in a characteristic cluster on the vulva, perineum, or perianal area. The initial lesions may cause severe vulvar pain and tenderness as well as dyspareunia. Lesions may also occur on the cervix or in the vagina. With primary infection, the woman may also experience flulike symptoms, including fever, general malaise, and enlarged lymph nodes. The vesicles rupture within 1 to 7 days and form ulcers that take an average of 7 to 10 days to heal.

When symptoms abate, the virus remains dormant in the nerve ganglia and periodically reactivates, particularly in times of stress, fever, and menses. Recurrent episodes are seldom as extensive or painful as the initial episode, but they are just as contagious. Diagnosis is often based on clinical signs and symptoms and confirmed by viral culture of fluid from the vesicle.

No cure exists, but antiviral drugs reduce or suppress symptoms, shedding, and recurrent episodes. Antiviral drugs include acyclovir (Zovirax), famciclovir (Famvir), and valacyclovir (Valtrex). Women should be advised to abstain from sexual contact while the lesions are present to avoid transmission to their partner. If it is an initial infection, they should

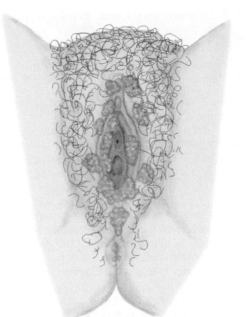

Figure 33-9 ■ Condylomata acuminata, also called *venereal warts,* are caused by the human papillomavirus (HPV).

continue to abstain until they become culture-negative, because prolonged viral shedding may occur in such cases.

CONDYLOMATA ACUMINATA. Condylomata acuminata, also known as *venereal* or *genital warts,* are caused by HPV. The dry, wart-like growths may be small and discrete, or they may cluster and resemble cauliflower (Figure 33-9). Common sites include the vagina, labia, cervix, and perineal area.

Condylomata acuminata are of particular concern because of the association of HPV with cervical cancer. Colposcopy, examination by a magnifying instrument called the colposcope, is generally recommended to evaluate abnormal cervical tissue and to identify HPV. Women with condylomata acuminata should be advised to have Pap tests more frequently to detect cervical dysplasia.

The goal of treatment is to remove the warts, which easily transmit the virus back and forth between sexual partners. Treatment is determined by the site and extent of the warts and the woman's preference. Topical treatment options include podophyllin, trichloroacetic acid (TCA), bichloroacetic acid (BCA), and imiquimod cream. More extensive warts or those that do not respond to topical therapy may require removal by cryotherapy, electrodessication, electrocautery, or laser. Interferon, an antineoplastic drug, is sometimes used to treat condylomata acuminata in women older than 18 years of age who have not responded to conventional therapy.

The woman must understand that none of these treatments eradicate the virus and that she may have recurrences. Furthermore, all sexual partners must be treated. Sexual contact should be avoided until all lesions are healed, and the use of condoms is recommended to reduce transmission.

ACQUIRED IMMUNODEFICIENCY SYNDROME. Acquired immunodeficiency syndrome (AIDS), caused by

HIV, remains the most devastating STD in the world today, although new treatments have improved the outlook considerably. HIV has been isolated from blood, semen, vaginal secretions, urine, saliva, tears, cerebrospinal fluid, amniotic fluid, and breast milk. The primary modes of transmission are intimate contact with infected bodily secretions, exposure to infected blood and blood products, and perinatal transmission from mother to infant.

HIV testing is offered to all pregnant women and to high-risk groups such as those who are poor or who use injectable drugs. However, a woman's risk for infection through a heterosexual relationship has surpassed the risk that her HIV infection stems from injectable drug use. Diagnosis of another STD is an indication to offer HIV testing, as is the presence of infections such as herpesvirus or recurrent candidiasis (CDC, 2002; Minkoff & Gibbs, 2003).

No medications have been shown to cure HIV and AIDS. Researchers continue to examine the benefits and safety of drug regimens that interrupt production of the virus. Zidovudine (a reverse transcriptase inhibitor) is a familiar drug having substantial safety for the fetus during pregnancy. However, combined drug therapy often benefits the HIV-infected woman and may have acceptable safety if she is pregnant. Protease inhibitors, such as indinavir and saquinavir, block the enzyme crucial to one step in the reproductive cycle of HIV. See Chapters 26 and 30 for a discussion of HIV and AIDS management in pregnant women and neonates. Updated guidelines for HIV and AIDS treatment in the pediatric, adult, and perinatal groups may be found at the AIDS Info website, a service of the NIH: http://aidsinfo.nih.gov/guidelines.

NURSING CONSIDERATIONS

As teachers and counselors, nurses can play a major part in preventing the spread of STDs and treating specific infections. Women must often be encouraged regarding ways to avoid acquiring an infection, including HIV infection, from a man who does not want to use condoms as a barrier to infection. To fulfill this role, nurses must be prepared to do the following:

- Teach the signs and symptoms that require medical attention
- Explain diagnostic or screening tests and follow-up testing needed for some infections
- Teach preventive measures and follow-up care to assure a cure for non-HIV infections
- Identify STD preventive measures that are compatible with age, language, male-female relationships in the woman's culture, values for her own well-being, frequency of intercourse, number of partners, and many other factors that may be identified when the woman seeks care
- Refer the woman to support groups and HIV specialists for best treatment options and follow-up if she has HIV infection

CHECK YOUR READING

40. What conditions may change the normal flora of the vagina and result in *C. albicans* vaginitis?
41. How does the vaginal discharge of candidiasis differ from that of trichomoniasis?
42. Why are barrier-type contraceptives recommended to prevent STDs?
43. How do primary and secondary syphilis differ in terms of signs and symptoms and potential for transmitting the disease?
44. How are condylomata acuminata associated with cervical cancer?

Pelvic Inflammatory Disease

PID, infection of the upper genital tract, is a serious health problem in the United States. About 1 million women develop PID each year in the United States and many of them have ectopic pregnancy or infertility as added complications. Women who are more likely to develop PID are under 25 because the cervix is not fully matured, increasing their susceptibility to infectious organisms. Exposure to multiple sexual partners increases the risk of acquiring an infection that causes PID. Douching increases the risk for PID because it changes the natural vaginal flora that helps resist infection and pushes infectious organisms toward the uterine cavity (CDC, 2005; McGregor, French, & Lench, 2004).

ETIOLOGY

About 15% to 30% of PID cases are caused by *C. trachomatis* and *N. gonorrhoeae* infections. The remainder are caused by a mixture of organisms such as *Escherichia coli, G. vaginalis, Streptococcus, Peptostreptococcus, Bacteroides, Prevotella, Mycoplasma, Ureaplasm* and cytomegalovirus (CMV) (CDC, 2002; McGregor, French, & Lench, 2004). These organisms invade the endocervical canal, where they cause cervicitis. Bacteria ascend and infect the endometrium, fallopian tubes, and pelvic cavity. The chronic inflammatory response results in tubal scarring and peritubal adhesions, which interfere with conception or with transport of the fertilized ovum through the obstructed fallopian tubes. Inadequate treatment of a vaginal infection increases the risk that the organisms will ascend into the uterus, infecting deeper reproductive structures and causing PID.

SYMPTOMS

Signs and symptoms of PID vary widely. Some women are asymptomatic or have subtle symptoms, whereas others experience pelvic pain, fever, purulent vaginal discharge, nausea, anorexia, and irregular vaginal bleeding. Findings during physical examination may include abdominal or adnexal tenderness and tenderness of the uterus and cervix when they are moved during bimanual examination (cervical motion tenderness). Laboratory evaluation may reveal a marked leukocytosis and increased sedimentation rate. A urinalysis is needed to rule out urinary tract infection. Cultures for *N. gonorrhoeae, C. trachomatis,* or other suspected infectious organism help diagnose and best treat PID.

MANAGEMENT

Women with serious infection, as manifested by fever, abdominal pain, and leukocytosis, may be admitted to a hospital. They are most often treated with intravenous administration of broad-spectrum antibiotics such as cefoxitin or cefotetan plus doxycycline or clindamycin plus gentamicin. Intravenous antibiotic treatment can usually be changed to oral treatment after 48 hours, and the total duration of antibiotic therapy should be 14 days. Laparoscopy may be required to rule out surgical emergencies such as appendicitis or ectopic pregnancy, which have similar signs and symptoms, and to obtain specimens for culture. Pelvic abscess often requires surgical treatment. Outpatient treatment is appropriate for some women who are not as ill and are able to comply with the recommended regimen (CDC, 2002).

NURSING CONSIDERATIONS

Nurses can play an important role in preventing PID by teaching women how to prevent STDs in themselves and in their partners. Prevention can be thought of as occurring on two levels: primary and secondary. Primary prevention involves avoiding exposure to these diseases or preventing acquisition of infection during exposure. Primary preventive measures include limiting the number of sexual partners and avoiding intercourse with those who have had multiple partners or other high-risk behaviors such as injectable drug use, which is associated with HIV infection. Barrier methods (latex condoms) used consistently and correctly during all sexual activity help prevent STDs.

Secondary prevention involves keeping a lower genital tract infection from ascending to the upper genital tract or from being further transmitted within the community. This involves seeking medical attention promptly after having unprotected sex with someone who is suspected of having an STD and when vaginal discharge or genital lesions are apparent. Periodic medical assessment is necessary if the woman is not in a mutually monogamous relationship, even if she is asymptomatic. Additional measures include taking medication as prescribed and returning for follow-up evaluation. Periodic medical evaluations may be recommended for a woman who is asymptomatic yet engages in sexual activity that increases risk.

Toxic Shock Syndrome

Although toxic shock syndrome is rare, it is a potentially fatal condition caused by toxin-producing strains of *S. aureus.* The toxin alters capillary permeability, which allows intravascular fluid to leak from the blood vessels, leading to hypovolemia, hypotension, and shock. The toxin also causes direct tissue damage to organs and precipitates serious defects in coagulation.

If toxin-producing strains of *S. aureus* inhabit the vagina, certain factors increase the risk that the toxin will gain entry into the bloodstream. These include the use of high-absorbency tampons during menstruation and barrier methods of contraception (cervical cap or diaphragm), both of which may trap and hold bacteria if left in place for a prolonged time. Persons having had nasal surgery or previous *S. aureus* wound infections also have a greater risk.

Symptoms of toxic shock syndrome include a sudden spiking fever and flulike symptoms (headache, sore throat, vomiting, diarrhea), hypotension, a generalized rash resembling sunburn, and skin peeling from the palms of the hands and the soles of the feet 1 and 2 weeks after the onset of the illness.

Treatment consists of fluid replacement, administration of vasopressor drugs, and antimicrobial therapy. Corticosteroids may be used to treat skin changes.

Nurses are often responsible for providing information that may help to prevent toxic shock syndrome. Nurses should instruct women to do the following.

TAMPON USE

- Wash the hands thoroughly to remove bacteria before inserting tampons.
- Change tampons at least every 4 hours to prevent excessive bacterial growth on a tampon that is left in place for a longer time.
- Do not use superabsorbent tampons at any time because they may be left in the vagina for a prolonged period, allowing bacteria to proliferate.
- Use pads rather than tampons during hours of sleep, which usually exceeds 4-hour segments of tampon use.

DIAPHRAGM OR CERVICAL CAP USE

- Wash hands thoroughly before inserting diaphragm or cervical cap.
- Do not use diaphragm or cervical cap during menstrual periods.
- Remove diaphragm or cervical cap within time recommended by health care provider.

✔ **CHECK YOUR READING**

45. What organisms cause PID?
46. How can the risk of toxic shock syndrome be reduced?

SUMMARY CONCEPTS

- *Health maintenance* refers to periodic examinations and screening procedures that provide early detection of specific conditions, such as breast or cervical cancer, and allow for early treatment that increases the chance of long-term survival. Immunizations and routine lab studies recommended according to the woman's age may be included.

- A major role of nurses is to explain screening procedures and to encourage women to have them on a regular basis. The most common screening procedures include breast self-examination, professional breast examination, and mammography or ultrasound studies for breast cancer; vulvar self-examination to detect precancerous conditions or infections; pelvic examination to detect abnormalities of the uterus or ovaries; Pap test for cervical cancer; and screening for fecal occult blood. Additional tests may include transvaginal ultrasonography and serum tests for genes associated with specific cancers.

- Disorders of the breast may be benign, such as fibrocystic changes that occur in relation to the menstrual cycle, or malignant. The discovery of any breast disorder creates anxiety in women, and nurses must be prepared to explain diagnostic procedures, such as mammogram, ultrasound, fine needle aspiration biopsy, core needle biopsy, and surgical biopsy.

- One in seven women in the United States develops breast cancer. Besides gender, the greatest risk factors are advancing age, a prior history of breast cancer, and genetic mutations in the BRCA1 and BRCA2 and p53 genes. Additional factors include family history (mother, sister, daughter) of breast cancer and previous uterine, ovarian, or colon cancer. Lifestyle factors such as a high intake of dietary fat, smoking, and consumption of alcohol are also suspected to increase risk.

- Management of breast cancer includes surgical removal of the tumor plus varying amounts of surrounding tissue and lymph glands. Adjuvant therapy includes radiation, chemotherapy, hormone therapy, and immunotherapy.

- Breast reconstruction is an integral part of the surgical management of breast cancer. Methods include tissue expansion and autogenous grafts. Reconstruction at the time of surgical tumor removal or a later reconstruction are options for many women.

- Nursing care for women with cancer of the breast focuses on providing emotional support and accurate information.

- Cardiovascular disease kills more women than breast cancer. Preventive measures include modifying all risk factors that can be modified, such as maintaining a normal weight and stopping smoking. Added preventive measures include controlling hypertension, diet and glucose control, increasing activity, and, for many women, use of low-dose aspirin on a daily basis.

- Menstrual cycle disorders include amenorrhea, abnormal uterine bleeding, cyclic pelvic pain, and premenstrual syndrome. Some of the disorders, such as premenstrual syndrome, respond to lifestyle alterations such as changes in diet, exercise habits, and stress management.

- Medical termination of pregnancy may be performed by medical or surgical methods, and each method is associated with social and ethical conflicts.

- The climacteric is a combination of endocrine, somatic, and psychic changes that occur at the end of the reproductive cycle. Menopause is the final menstrual period, although most people use the term interchangeably with *climacteric*. Women's responses to menopause vary widely, but all women are in a permanent state of estrogen deficit after menopause that can result in bone loss (osteoporosis), increased risk for coronary artery disease, atrophic vaginitis, and Alzheimer's disease.

- Hormone replacement therapy may be prescribed to manage the symptoms of estrogen deficit, such as hot flashes and atrophic vaginitis, and to decrease bone mineral loss that results in osteoporosis. Greater risk for cardiovascular disease in the estrogen-progesterone arm of the Women's Health Initiative caused cancellation of this part of the study. Each woman and her health care provider must individually evaluate whether hormone replacement therapy is beneficial.

- Hormone replacement therapy has risks and benefits and is contraindicated for women who have thromboembolic disease, undiagnosed vaginal bleeding, previous episodes of breast cancer or untreated uterine cancer, or chronic liver disease. For these women, alternative measures are needed to control the symptoms of menopause.

- Relaxation of pelvic support structures occurs as a delayed result of traumatic childbirth and becomes troublesome when a deficiency in estrogen hastens genital atrophy.

- Many infections of the reproductive tract are transmitted by sexual contact. The incidence of sexually transmitted diseases is reduced by barrier methods of contraception, particularly the condom, which prevents contact between infected skin or mucosal surfaces and prevents potentially infected ejaculate from entering the woman's lower genital tract.

- Pelvic inflammatory disease is often a complication of untreated sexually transmitted diseases, and a large number of cases are caused by chlamydial or gonorrheal infections. Pelvic inflammatory disease can cause infertility or ectopic pregnancy because of scarring of fallopian tubes resulting from inflammatory processes in the pelvic cavity.

- Toxic shock syndrome is a life-threatening condition resulting from infection with toxin-producing strains of *Staphylococcus aureus*. The infection may be related to use of high-absorbency tampons that trap and hold bacteria in nutrient-rich menstrual blood for an extended time. Tampons should be removed every 4 hours, and other items that trap bacteria, such as cervical caps and diaphragms, should be removed as directed by the health care provider.

REFERENCES & READINGS

American Cancer Society. (2003a). *Breast cancer facts and figures 2003-2004.* Atlanta, GA: Author.

American Cancer Society. (2003b). *How to perform a breast self-exam.* Retrieved March 23, 2005, from www.cancer.org.

American Cancer Society. (2004a). *Breast reconstruction after mastectomy.* Retrieved March 26, 2005, from www.cancer.org/docroot/home/index.asp.

American Cancer Society. (2004b). *Detailed guide: Breast Cancer: What are the risk factors for breast cancer?* Retrieved March 22, 2005, from www.cancer.org/docroot/home/index.asp.

American Cancer Society. (2005). *Detailed guide: Colon and rectum cancer: Can colorectal polyps and cancer be detected early.* Retrieved March 25, 2005, from www.cancer.org/docroot/home/index.asp.

American College of Obstetricians and Gynecologists (ACOG). (1999). *Medical management of endometriosis,* Practice Bulletin No. 11. Washington, DC: Author.

American College of Obstetricians and Gynecologists. (2000). *Premenstrual syndrome,* Practice Bulletin No. 15. Washington, DC: Author.

American College of Obstetricians and Gynecologists. (2001). *Use of botanicals for management of menopausal symptoms,* Practice Bulletin No. 28. Washington, DC: Author.

American College of Obstetricians and Gynecologists. (2003a). *Breast cancer screening,* Practice Bulletin No. 42. Washington, DC: Author.

American College of Obstetricians and Gynecologists. (2003b). *Cervical cytology screening,* Practice Bulletin No. 45. Washington, DC: Author.

Anderson, S.L. (2003). Diseases of the heart, blood vessels, and lungs. In S.R. Williams & E.D. Schlenker (Eds.), *Essentials of nutrition and diet therapy* (8th ed., pp. 469-491). St Louis: Mosby.

Association of Women's Health, Obstetric and Gynecologic Nurses (AWHONN). (2003). *Evidence-based clinical practice guideline: Cardiovascular health for women: Primary prevention* (2nd ed.). Washington, DC: Author.

Berek, J.S. (2004). Ovarian cancer. In N.F. Hacker, J.G. Moore, & J.C. Gambone (Eds.), *Essentials of obstetrics and gynecology* (4th ed., pp. 459-468). Philadelphia: Saunders.

Berry, K. (2003). *Risk reduction in the prevention of cardiovascular disease in women: Lifestyle and medication management.* Washington, DC: AWHONN.

Bhatia, N.N. (2004). Genitourinary dysfunction: Pelvic organ prolapse, urinary incontinence, and infections. In N.F. Hacker, J.G. Moore, & J.C. Gambone (Eds.), *Essentials of obstetrics and gynecology* (4th ed., p. 309). Philadelphia: Saunders.

Brucker, M.C., & Youngkin, E.Q. (2002). What's a woman to do? Exploring HRT questions raised by the Women's Health Initiative. *AWHONN Lifelines, 6*(5), 410-417.

Cass, I., & Karlan, B.Y. (2003). Neoplasms of the ovary and fallopian tube. In J.R. Scott, R.S. Gibbs, B.Y. Karlan, & A.F. Haney (Eds.), *Danforth's obstetrics and gynecology* (9th ed., pp. 971-1006). Philadelphia: Lippincott Williams & Wilkins.

Cedars, M.I., & Evans, M. (2003). Menopause. In J.R. Scott, R.S. Gibbs, B.Y. Karlan, & A.F. Haney (Eds.), *Danforth's obstetrics and gynecology* (9th ed., pp. 721-737). Philadelphia: Lippincott Williams & Wilkins.

Centers for Disease Control and Prevention (CDC). (2002). Sexually transmitted diseases treatment guidelines 2002. *MMWR. Morbidity and Mortality Weekly Report, 51*(RR-6), 1-84. Retrieved April 5, 2005, from www.cdc.gov/std/treatment/rr5106.pdf.

Centers for Disease Control & Prevention. (2005). *Fact sheet: Pelvic inflammatory diseases.* Retrieved April 5, 2005, from www.cdc.gov/std/PID/PID.pdf.

Centers for Disease Control and Prevention: National Center for Chronic Disease Prevention and Health Promotion. (2001). *Women and smoking: A report of the surgeon general–2001.* Retrieved May 29, 2005 from www.cdc.gov/tobacco/sgr/sgr_forwomen/index.htm.

Chase, S.K., & Youngkin, E.Q. (2004). Postmenopausal hormone replacement and cardiovascular disease: Incorporating research into practice. *Journal of Obstetric, Gynecologic, and Neonatal Nursing, 33*(5), 648-656.

Curry, L.C., & Hogstel, M.O. (2002). Osteoporosis: Education and awareness can make a difference. *American Journal of Nursing, 102*(1), 26-28.

DeLancey, J.O.L., & Strohbehn, K. (2003). Pelvic organ prolapse. In J.R. Scott, R.S. Gibbs, B.Y. Karlan, & A.F. Haney (Eds.), *Danforth's obstetrics and gynecology* (9th ed., pp. 791-817). Philadelphia: Lippincott Williams & Wilkins.

Fenner, D.E. (2003). Incontinence. In J.R. Scott, R.S. Gibbs, B.Y. Karlan, & A.F. Haney (Eds.), *Danforth's obstetrics and gynecology* (9th ed., pp. 845-867). Philadelphia: Lippincott Williams & Wilkins.

Fontaine, K.L. (2005). *Healing practices: Alternative therapies for nursing* (2nd ed.). Upper Saddle River, NJ: Prentice-Hall.

Fritz, M.A. (2003). Amenorrhea. In J.R. Scott, R.S. Gibbs, B.Y. Karlan, & A.F. Haney (Eds.), *Danforth's obstetrics and gynecology* (9th ed., pp. 625-641). Philadelphia: Lippincott Williams & Wilkins.

Gemignani, M.L. (2003). Disorders of the breast. In J.R. Scott, R.S. Gibbs, B.Y. Karlan, & A.F. Haney (Eds.), *Danforth's obstetrics and gynecology* (9th ed., pp. 889-910). Philadelphia: Lippincott Williams & Wilkins.

Gingrich, P.M., & Fogel, C.I. (2003). Herbal therapy use by perimenopausal women. *Journal of Obstetric, Gynecologic, and Neonatal Nursing, 32*(2), 181-189.

Hacker, N.F. (2004a). Breast disease: A gynecologic perspective. In N.F. Hacker, J.G. Moore, & J.C. Gambone (Eds.), *Essentials of obstetrics and gynecology* (4th ed., pp. 364-371). Philadelphia: Saunders.

Hacker, N.F. (2004b). Cervical dysplasia and cancer. In N.F. Hacker, J.G. Moore, & J.C. Gambone (Eds.), *Essentials of obstetrics and gynecology* (4th ed., pp. 447-458). Philadelphia: Saunders.

Hacker, N.F. (2004c). Uterine corpus cancer. In N.F. Hacker, J.G. Moore, & J.C. Gambone (Eds.), *Essentials of obstetrics and gynecology* (4th ed., pp. 478-485). Philadelphia: Saunders.

Hacker, N.F. (2004d). Vulvar and vaginal cancer. In N.F. Hacker, J.G. Moore, & J.C. Gambone (Eds.), *Essentials of obstetrics and gynecology* (4th ed., pp. 469-477). Philadelphia: Saunders.

Hale, T. (2004). *Medications and mother's milk* (11th ed.). Amarillo, TX: Pharmasoft Publishing.

Jenkins, R.R. (2004). Menstrual problems. In R.E. Behrman, R.M. Kliegman, & H.B. Jenson (Eds.), *Nelson textbook of pediatrics* (17th ed., pp. 663-667). Philadelphia: Saunders.

Kanusky, C. (2003). Health concerns of women in midlife. In E.T. Breslin & V.A. Lucas (Eds.), *Women's health nursing: Toward evidence-based practice* (pp. 628-683). Philadelphia: Saunders.

Kass-Wolff, J.H. (2004). Calcium in women: Healthy bones and much more. *Journal of Obstetric, Gynecologic, and Neonatal Nursing, 33*(1), 21-33.

Kochanek, K., Murphy, S.L., Anderson, R.N., & Scott, C. (2004). Deaths: Final data for 2002. *National Vital Statistics Reports, 53*(5). Hyattsville, MD: National Center for Health Statistics.

Krauss, R.M., Eckel, R.H., Howard, B., Appel, L.J., Daniels, S.R., Deckelbaum, R.J., et al. (2000). AHA Dietary guidelines: Revision 2000: A statement for healthcare professionals from the Nutrition Committee of the American Heart Association. *Circulation, 102*(10), 2296-2311.

Laufer, L.R., & Gambone, J.C. (2004a). Climacteric. In N.F. Hacker, J.G. Moore, & J.C. Gambone (Eds.), *Essentials of obstetrics and gynecology* (4th ed., pp. 422-428). Philadelphia: Saunders.

Laufer, L.R., & Gambone, J.C. (2004b). Menstrual cycle-influenced disorders. In N.F. Hacker, J.G. Moore, & J.C. Gambone (Eds.), *Essentials of obstetrics and gynecology* (4th ed., pp. 429-433). Philadelphia: Saunders.

Laufer, L.R., & Patel, K.S. (2004). Amenorrhea, oligomenorrhea, and hyperandrogenic disorders. In N.F. Hacker, J.G. Moore, & J.C. Gambone (Eds.), *Essentials of obstetrics and gynecology* (4th ed., pp. 422-428). Philadelphia: Saunders.

London, S.N. (2003). Abnormal uterine bleeding. In J.R. Scott, R.S. Gibbs, B.Y. Karlan, & A.F. Haney (Eds.), *Danforth's obstetrics and gynecology* (9th ed., pp. 643-651). Philadelphia: Lippincott Williams & Wilkins.

Martinez, L.G. (2004). Coronary artery disease and acute coronary syndrome. In S.M. Lewis, M.M. Heitkemper, & S.R. Dirksen (Eds.), *Medical-surgical nursing: Assessment and management of clinical problems* (6th ed., pp. 799-837). Philadelphia: Mosby.

McCrink, A. (2004). Evaluating the female pelvic floor: Understanding and treating prolapse, incontinence in women. *AWHONN Lifelines, 7*(6), 516-522.

McEvoy, M., Chang, J., & Coupey, S.M. (2004). Common menstrual disorders in adolescents. *MCN: American Journal of Maternal/Child Nursing, 29*(1), 41-49.

McGregor, J.A., French, J.L., & Lench, J.B. (2004). Pelvic infections: Vulvovaginitis, sexually transmitted infections, and pelvic inflammatory disease. In N.F. Hacker, J.G. Moore, & J.C. Gambone (Eds.), *Essentials of obstetrics and gynecology* (4th ed., pp. 296-308). Philadelphia: Saunders.

Minkoff, H.L., & Gibbs, R.S. (2003). Obstetric and perinatal infections. In J.R. Scott, R.S. Gibbs, B.Y. Karlan, & A.F. Haney (Eds.), *Danforth's obstetrics and gynecology* (9th ed., pp. 339-364). Philadelphia: Lippincott Williams & Wilkins.

Moore, J.G., & Gambone, J.C. (2004a). Dysfunctional uterine bleeding. In N.F. Hacker, J.G. Moore, & J.C. Gambone (Eds.), *Essentials of obstetrics and gynecology* (4th ed., pp. 409-412). Philadelphia: Saunders.

Moore, J.G., & Gambone, J.C. (2004b). Endometriosis and adenomyosis. In N.F. Hacker, J.G. Moore, & J.C. Gambone (Eds.), *Essentials of obstetrics and gynecology* (4th ed., pp. 334-340). Philadelphia: Saunders.

Moore, J.G., & Nelson, A.L. (2004a). Congenital anomalies and benign conditions of the uterine corpus and cervix. In N.F. Hacker, J.G. Moore, & J.C. Gambone (Eds.), *Essentials of obstetrics and gynecology* (4th ed., pp. 268-276). Philadelphia: Saunders.

Moore, J.G., & Nelson, A.L. (2004b). Congenital anomalies and benign conditions of the ovaries and fallopian tubes. In N.F. Hacker, J.G. Moore, & J.C. Gambone (Eds.), *Essentials of obstetrics and gynecology* (4th ed., pp. 277-286). Philadelphia: Saunders.

National Cancer Institute. (2001). Bethesda System 2001. Retrieved March 25, 2005, from http://bethesda2001.cancer.gov/terminology.html.

National Center for Health Statistics. (2004). *Health, United States, 2004, with Chartbook on Trends in the Health of Americans.* Hyattsville, MD: Author.

National Institutes of Health: National Center for Complementary and Alternative Medicine. (2005a). Consumer advisory: Vitamin E supplements. Retrieved April 2, 2005, from nccam.nih.gov.

National Institutes of Health: National Heart, Lung, and Blood Institute. (1998). *Clinical guidelines on the identification, evaluation, and treatment of overweight and obesity in adults. Executive summary.* Retrieved March 22, 2005, from www.nhlbi.nih.gov/guidelines/index.htm.

National Institutes of Health: Osteoporosis and Related Bone Diseases, National Resource Center. (2003). *Facts sheets: Osteoporosis.* Retrieved April 2, 2005, from www.osteo.org/osteolinks.asp.

Nelson, A.L., & Gambone, J.C. (2004). Congenital anomalies and benign conditions of the vulva and vagina. In N.F. Hacker, J.G. Moore, & J.C. Gambone (Eds.), *Essentials of obstetrics and gynecology* (4th ed., pp. 259-267). Philadelphia: Saunders.

Nelson, A.L. (2004). Family planning: Contraception, sterilization, and abortion. In N.F. Hacker, J.G. Moore, & J.C. Gambone (Eds.), *Essentials of obstetrics and gynecology* (4th ed., pp. 341-351). Philadelphia: Saunders.

Newman, D.K. (2003a). Pharmaceutical review: Drugs used to treat incontinence. *American Journal of Nursing, March*(Suppl.), 48.

Newman, D.K. (2003b). Stress urinary incontinence in women. *American Journal of Nursing, 103*(8), 46-55.

Pagana, K.D., & Pagana, T.J. (2005). *Mosby's diagnostic and test reference* (7th ed.). St. Louis: Mosby.

Phillips, M., Lee, Y.-M., Swanson, B., Keithley, J.K., Zeller, J.M., & Hindin, P. (2003). Herbal and dietary supplements for hot flashes: Here's what works—and what doesn't. *AWHONN Lifelines, 7*(5), 412-420.

Pritham, U.A. (2002). Managing PMS and PMDD: Exploring new treatment options. *AWHONN Lifelines, 6*(5), 430-437.

Ralstin, A. (2004). Nursing assessment cardiovascular system. In S.M. Lewis, M.M. Heitkemper, & S.R. Dirksen (Eds.), *Medical-surgical nursing: Assessment and management of clinical problems* (6th ed., pp. 799-837). Philadelphia: Mosby.

Rapkin, A.J., & Gambone, J.C. (2004). Dysmenorrhea and chronic pelvic pain. In N.F. Hacker, J.G. Moore, & J.C. Gambone (Eds.), *Essentials of obstetrics and gynecology* (4th ed., pp. 287-295). Philadelphia: Saunders.

Reid, R.I. (2003). Premenstrual syndrome. In J.R. Scott, R.S. Gibbs, B.Y. Karlan, & A.F. Haney (Eds.), *Danforth's obstetrics and gynecology* (9th ed., pp. 653-662). Philadelphia: Lippincott Williams & Wilkins.

Resnick, B., & Belcher, A.E. (2002). Breast reconstruction: Options, answers, and support for patients making a difficult personal decision. *American Journal of Nursing, 102*(4), 26-33.

Ripkin, A.J., &. Gambone, J.C. (2004). Dysmenorrhea and chronic pelvic pain. In N.F. Hacker, J.G. Moore, & J.C. Gambone (Eds.), *Essentials of obstetrics and gynecology* (4th ed., pp. 287-295). Philadelphia: Saunders.

Sampselle, C.M. (2003). Behavioral interventions in young and middle-aged women. *American Journal of Nursing, March*(Suppl.), 9-19.

Schenken, R.S. (2003). Endometriosis. In J.R. Scott, R.S. Gibbs, B.Y. Karlan, & A.F. Haney (Eds.), *Danforth's obstetrics and gynecology* (9th ed., pp. 713-720). Philadelphia: Lippincott Williams & Wilkins.

Skillman-Hull, L. (2003). Adolescent women's health. In E.T. Breslin & V.A. Lucas (Eds.), *Women's health nursing: Toward evidence-based practice* (pp. 432-552). Philadelphia: Saunders.

Strauss, L.T., Herndon, J., Chang, J., Parker, W.Y., Bowens, S.V., Zane, S.B., & Berg, C.J. (2004). Abortion surveillance—United States 2001. *MMWR. Morbidity and Mortality Weekly Report,* 53(No. SS-9). Retrieved March 30, 2005, from www.cdc.gov/mmwr/PDF/ss/ss5309.pdf.

Taylor, D., & Hwang, A.C. (Dec. 2003/Jan. 2004). Mifepristone for medical abortion: Exploring a new option for nurse practitioners. *AWHONN Lifelines, 7*(5), 524-529.

Tazbir, J., & Keresztes, P.A. (2005). Management of clients with myocardial infarction. In J. M. Black & J.H. Hawks (Eds.)., *Medical-surgical nursing: Clinical management for positive outcomes* (7th ed., pp. 1701-1730). Philadelphia: Saunders.

Teschendorf, M. (2003). Women during the reproductive years. In E.T. Breslin & V.A. Lucas (Eds.), *Women's health nursing: Toward evidence-based practice* (pp. 553-627). Philadelphia: Saunders.

Trupin, S.R. (2003). Induced abortion. In J.R. Scott, R.S. Gibbs, B.Y. Karlan, & A.F. Haney (Eds.), *Danforth's obstetrics and gynecology* (9th ed., pp. 561-580). Philadelphia: Lippincott Williams & Wilkins.

U.S. Department of Health and Human Services. (2005). *Healthy People 2010 Online.* Retrieved March 22, 2005, from www.healthypeople.gov/default.htm.

U.S. Food and Drug Administration. (2000). *FDA approves mifepristone for termination of pregnancy.* Retrieved April 7, 2005, from www.fda.gov.

U.S. Preventive Services Task Force. (2002). Osteoporosis screening. Retrieved April 2, 2005, from www.preventiveservices.ahrq.gov.

World Health Organization (WHO). (2000). *Female genital mutilation: Fact sheet N241.* Retrieved March 25, 2005, from www.who.int/mediacentre/factsheets/fs241/en/.

Wyman, J.F. (2003). Treatment of urinary incontinence in men and women. *American Journal of Nursing, March*(Suppl.), 26-31.

Zaccardi, J.E., & Cox, S.B. (2004). Evaluation and management: Female urinary incontinence. *AWHONN Lifelines, 8*(4), 326-332.

Zangwill, M. (2004). Cervical cancer: The hidden risk of HPV. *Cure, 3*(4), pp. 28-35.

Zawacki, K.L., & Phillips, M. (2002). Cancer genetics and women's health. *Journal of Obstetric, Gynecologic, and Neonatal Nursing, 31*(2), 208-216.

Laboratory Values in Pregnant and Nonpregnant Women and in the Newborn

Laboratory Values in Pregnant and Nonpregnant Women

Value	Nonpregnancy	Pregnancy
Blood volume, total (ml/kg)	55-80	Increases 40%-50%
Plasma volume (ml/kg)	30-45	Increases 50% (1200 to 1300 ml above nonpregnant levels)
Red blood cell volume (ml/kg)	20-35	Increases 25%-33% (average total increase of 250-450 ml)
Red blood cell count (1,000,000/mm^3)	4.2-5.4	Decreases slightly because of hemodilution
Hemoglobin (g/dl)	12-16	At least 11 g/dl during first and third trimesters and at least 10.5 g/dl during second trimester
Hematocrit, packed cell volume (%)	37-47	>33
White blood cell count (1000/mm^3)	5-10	5-12 Rises during labor and early postpartum
Platelets (1000/mm^3)	150-400	150-400 or slightly decreased
Prothrombin time (sec)	11-12.5	Slight decrease but remains within normal limits
Activated partial thromboplastin time (sec)	21-35	Slight decrease but remains within normal limits
D dimer	Negative	Negative
Glucose, blood		
Fasting (mg/dl)	70-105	95 or lower
Postprandial (mg/dl)	<140	<140
Creatinine, serum (mg/dl)	0.5-1.1	0.5
Creatinine clearance, urine (ml/min)	87-107	110-180
Fibrinogen (mg/dl)	200-400	300-600

Data from Blackburn, S.T. (2003). *Maternal, fetal, and neonatal physiology* (2nd ed.). Philadelphia: Saunders; Cunningham, F.G., Leveno, K.J., Bloom, S.L., Hauth, J.C., Gilstrap, L., & Wenstrom, K.D. (2005). *Williams obstetrics* (22nd ed.). New York: McGraw-Hill; Fischbach, F.T. & Dunning, M.B. (2004). *A manual of laboratory and diagnostic tests* (7th ed.). Philadelphia: Lippincott Williams & Wilkins; Gordon, M.C. (2002). Maternal physiology in pregnancy. In S G. Gabbe, J.R. Niebyl, & J.L. Simpson (Eds.). *Obstetrics: Normal and problem pregnancies* (4th ed.). Philadelphia: Churchill Livingstone; Moore, T.R. (2004). Diabetes in pregnancy. In R.K. Creasy & R. Resnik (Eds.). *Maternal-fetal medicine: Principles and practice* (5th ed.). Philadelphia: Saunders; and Pagana, K.D., & Pagana, T.J. (2005). *Mosby's diagnostic and laboratory test reference* (7th ed.). St. Louis: Mosby.

Laboratory Values in the Newborn

Test, Specimen, and Unit of Measurement	Age	Normal Ranges
Red blood cell count, whole blood (1,000,000/mm^3)	Cord	3.9-5.5
	1-3 days	4-6.6
	1 wk	3.9-6.3
	1 mo	3-5.4
Hemoglobin, whole blood (g/dl)	1-3 days (capillary)	14.5-22.5
	2 mo	9-14
Hematocrit, whole blood (%)	1 day (capillary)	48-69
	2 days	48-75
	3 days	44-72
	2 mo	28-42
White blood cell count, whole blood (1000/mm^3)	Birth	9-30
	24 hr	9.4-34
	1 mo	5-19.5
White blood cell differential count, whole blood		
Myelocytes (%)		0
Neutrophils ("bands") (%)		3-5
Neutrophils ("segs") (%)		54-62
Lymphocytes (%)		25-33
Monocytes (%)		3-7
Eosinophils (%)		1-3
Basophils (%)		0-0.75
Platelet count, whole blood (1000/mm^3)	Newborn	84-478
	>1 wk	150-400
Glucose, serum (mg/dl)	Cord	45-96
	1 day	40-60
	Newborn, >1 day	50-90
Calcium, serum (mg/dl)	Cord	9-11.5
	Newborn 3-24 hr	9-10.6
	24-48 hr	7-12
	4-7 days	9-10.9
Magnesium, plasma (mg/dl)	Newborn 0-6 days	1.2-2.6

	Age	Normal Ranges	
		Preterm	Full-Term
Bilirubin, total serum (mg/dl)	Cord	<2	<2
	0-1 day	<8	<6
	1-2 days	<12	<8
	2-5 days	<16	<12
	>5 days	<20	<10
Bilirubin, direct (conjugated) serum (mg/dl)		0-0.2	0-0.2

Adapted from Nicholson, J.F., & Pesce, M.A. (2004). Reference ranges for laboratory tests and procedures. In R.E. Behrman, R.M. Kliegman, & H.B. Jenson (Eds.). *Nelson textbook of pediatrics* (17th ed., pp. 2396-2427). Philadelphia: Saunders.

Use of Drugs and Botanical (Herbal) Preparations during Pregnancy, Breastfeeding, and Women's Health

FDA PREGNANCY RISK CATEGORIES

The U.S. Food and Drug Administration (FDA) has assigned pregnancy risk categories to many drugs on the basis of their known relative safety or danger to the fetus and whether safer alternative drugs exist. Depending on fetal effects or nearness of birth, drugs may carry different risk categories at different points during pregnancy. For many drugs, little is known about the fetal risk. FDA categories are as follows:

A: No evidence of risk to the fetus exists.

B: Animal reproduction studies have not demonstrated a risk to the fetus. No adequate and well-controlled studies have been done in pregnant women.

C: Animal reproduction studies have shown an adverse effect on the fetus, but no adequate, well-controlled studies have been done in humans. Potential benefits may warrant use of the drug in pregnant women despite fetal risks. Or, animal studies show adverse effect on fetus, but human studies with pregnant women have not demonstrated a risk to the fetus in any trimester of pregnancy.

D: There is positive evidence of human fetal risk based on adverse reaction data, but potential benefits may warrant use of the drug in pregnant women despite fetal risks. Essentially, no safer alternatives to the drug are available.

X: There is positive evidence of human fetal risk based on animal or human studies and/or adverse reaction data. The risks of using the drug in pregnant women clearly outweigh potential benefits. Safer alternatives to these drugs may be available.

DRUG USE DURING LACTATION

The effects of many drugs when used during lactation have not been studied. In general, if a drug is safe for use in infants, it is probably safe for the lactating woman to take. Other drugs are known not to be excreted in breast milk or are excreted in an inactive form or very low concentrations. Modifying the time of maternal ingestion may reduce transfer of the drug to the infant. Some drugs are undesirable because they suppress lactation, which is a problem primarily in the earliest stages of breastfeeding.

Maternal use of social and illicit drugs during pregnancy or breastfeeding is discussed in Chapters 24 and 30.

Drug	Use during Pregnancy	Use during Breastfeeding
Amebicides Metronidazole (Flagyl)	*Risk category B.* Previous concern about teratogenic effects on the fetus have not been supported (CDC, 2002). Treatment of choice for trichomoniasis but may also be chosen as part of drug regimen for inflammatory bowel disease or postpartum endometritis.	Breastfeeding may be discontinued for 12-24 hr during single-dose treatment of mother. However, few known adverse infant effects.
Analgesics Aspirin	*Risk category C (D in third trimester).* Has been linked to fetal gastroschisis and small intestine atresia.	Single doses not associated with risk to breastfeeding infant. Greater potential risk if mother requires higher doses for a disorder such as arthritis.

CDC, Centers for Disease Control and Prevention.

Continued

Drug	Use during Pregnancy	Use during Breastfeeding
Analgesics—cont'd		
Acetaminophen (Tylenol, Datril, Tempra)	*Risk category B.* Problems have not been documented, but drug crosses placenta in low concentrations. Maximum dose 4 g/day. Drug often combined with other medications and should be considered when determining the maximum daily dose received.	Safe. Very small amounts secreted into breast milk.
Opiate analgesics: (butorphanol [Stadol], fentanyl [Sublimaze], hydrocodone [Duocet, Lortab, Norco, Vicodin, Zydone], hydromorphone [Dilaudid], meperidine [Demerol], morphine, nalbuphine [Nubain], oxycodone [Percocet, Tylox, Percodan])	*Most are risk category B or C.* Neonatal respiratory depression is the most significant adverse effect when large amounts of opiates are used during labor, making them category D drugs at this time. Neonatal withdrawal may occur if the woman is addicted to an opiate drug.	Most narcotics given briefly and in therapeutic doses are compatible with breastfeeding, including intrathecal (before epidural catheter removal) morphine given postoperatively. Prolonged infant sedation during the early postpartum period may occur with maternal meperidine analgesia.
Nonsteroidal antiinflammatory drugs: (NSAIDs): (fenoprofen [Nalfon], flurbiprofen [Ansaid], ibuprofen [Advil, Motrin, Nuprin], indomethacin [Indocin], ketoprofen [Actron, Orudis], naproxen [Aleve, Anaprox])	*Risk category B or C; category D in third trimester.* May prolong pregnancy or labor because of antiprostaglandin effects. Indomethacin associated with premature closure of ductus arteriosus or oligohydramnios in fetus but may be given in limited doses to stop preterm labor or reduce excess amniotic fluid in hydramnios.	Ibuprofen, indomethacin, and naproxen are AAP approved. All should be used cautiously owing to potential for infant bleeding. Indomethacin has been used for treatment of neonatal patent ductus arteriosus.
COX-2 inhibitors: celecoxib [Celebrex]	*Risk category C.* Associated with oligohydramnios and constriction of the ductus arteriosus. Greater risk of adverse cardiovascular effects has caused two related COX-2 inhibitors (rofecoxib [Vioxx], valdecoxib [Bextra]) to be withdrawn from the market. See www.fda.gov for latest information on COX-2 inhibitors and other drugs.	No adverse effects via milk reported. Observe for infant gastrointestinal (GI) cramping, diarrhea, effects similar to those reported in adults.
Migraine agents: (almotriptan [Axert], frovatriptan [Frova], naratriptan [Amerge], rizatriptan [Maxalt], sumatriptan [Imitrex])	*Risk category C.* Minimal well-controlled studies about fetal safety during pregnancy.	No identified pediatric concerns regarding breast milk, but caution recommended. Pumping and discarding milk for 24 hr after medication administration prevents transfer to infant.
Antiallergics		
Antihistamines (see middle column for drugs)	*Risk category B:* Chlorpheniramine (Chlor-Trimeton), clemastine (Contac, Tavist), diphenhydramine (Benadryl), loratadine (Claritin), meclizine (Antivert, Dramamine). *Risk category C:* astemizole (Hismanal), brompheniramine (Dimetane), phenylephrine (Neo-Synephrine), terfenadine (Seldane), triprolidine (Alleract).	All should be used with caution. Most are safe but may cause infant drowsiness. If these adverse effects occur, a different drug may be tried. Clemastine noted by AAP to be given with caution because of one case of infant irritability, refusal to feed, neurologic symptoms, seizures, and a high-pitched cry.
Antiasthmatics (See also *Decongestants, Hormones, Corticosteroids other than inhalers*)		
Corticosteroid inhalers: (beclomethasone [Beclovent, Vanceril], triamcinolone [Aristocort, Azmacort, Nasacort])	*Risk category C.*	Safety in lactation not fully known, but no reported problems following breast milk ingestion.
NSAID asthma medications: (cromolyn [Intal, NasalCrom, Opticrom], nedocromil [Alocril, Miraze])	*Risk category B.*	Minimal oral absorption. No reported adverse effects via milk.
Epinephrine (Adrenalin, Sus-Phrine, Primatene)	*Risk category C.* To treat bronchospasm in acute asthma attack.	Observe for brief infant stimulation after maternal drug use.
Leukotriene pathway modulators: (montelukast [Singulair], zafirlukast [Accolate], zyleuton [Zyflo])	*Risk category B* (zafirlukast, montelukast) and C (zyleuton).	No reported problems via breast milk; little published experience.
Bronchodilators: (albuterol [Proventil, Ventolin], metaproterenol [Alupent])	*Risk category C.* May inhibit uterine contractions.	Unknown if secreted in milk; use cautiously.

AAP, American Academy of Pediatrics; *COX,* cyclooxygenase.

Drug	Use during Pregnancy	Use during Breastfeeding
Anticoagulants		
Enoxaparin (Lovenox)	*Risk category B.* Not interchangeable with heparin.	Unlikely to produce clinically relevant levels in breast milk because of molecular size.
Heparin	*Risk category C.*	Not excreted in breast milk.
Warfarin (Coumadin)	*Risk category X.* Known teratogen that should be used during pregnancy only if the benefits outweigh risks. Associated with CNS and facial malformations, mental retardation, prenatal growth deficiency, and other fetal defects.	Small amounts secreted in milk. Infant bleeding abnormalities may result. Avoiding breastfeeding during therapy may be recommended.
Anticonvulsants		
Carbamazepine (Tegretol); oxcarbazepine (Trileptal)	*Risk category C.* Associated with craniofacial abnormalities, underdeveloped fingernails, neural tube defects, and developmental delay.	Small amounts secreted in breast milk; accumulation does not seem to occur. Observe infant for sedation.
Clonazepam (Klonopin)	*Risk category D.* No firm evidence that clonazepam is teratogenic. Infant after birth may display mild sedation, hypotonia, poor sucking.	Enters breast milk in a possibly relevant quantity.
Magnesium sulfate	*Risk category A* during early pregnancy. Infants exposed to magnesium sulfate 2 hr before birth may exhibit respiratory depression, hypotonic muscle tone, depressed reflexes, hypocalcemia, or cardiac dysrhythmias. Although infant risks exist when drug used during labor, complications of preeclampsia and eclampsia are greater.	Milk levels return to normal about 24 hr after drug is stopped.
Phenobarbital	*Risk category D.* Fetal addiction with subsequent withdrawal is possible but rare at dose levels used for seizure control. Abnormalities similar to those seen in infants exposed to carbamazepine, phenytoin, and valproic acid have been reported.	Infant serum levels approximately one third of adult levels. Psychomotor delay and sedation possible.
Fosphenytoin (Cerebyx); phenytoin (Dilantin)	*Risk category D.* Few studies of fosphenytoin. Risk for fetal malformations with phenytoin, specifically congenital heart defects and cleft palate, is double that in the general population.	Methemoglobinemia, drowsiness, and poor sucking have been reported. Most studies do not suggest problems.
Primidone (Mysoline)	*Risk category D.*	Drug and its metabolites are secreted into breast milk. Has been associated with neonatal sedation.
Topiramate (Topamax)	*Risk category C.*	No studies available. Use with caution.
Valproic acid (Depakene)	*Risk category D.* Associated with neural tube defects and craniofacial, cardiac, and hand abnormalities.	Secreted in small amounts. May cause drowsiness. Used for treatment of infant seizures.
Antidiabetics		
Insulin	*Risk category B.* Insulin is the drug of choice during pregnancy because it does not cross placenta.	Orally ingested insulin would be destroyed in infant's GI tract.
Oral hypoglycemic agents: (metformin [Glucophage], nateglinide [Starlix], pioglitazone [Actos], repaglinide [Prandin], rosiglitazone [Avandia])	*Risk category B:* Metformin. Risk category C: Remaining drugs.	Safety not established for most oral hypoglycemics. Observe for infant hypoglycemia if used.
Antifungals		
Fluconazole (Diflucan), miconazole (Monistat), nystatin (Mycostatin), terconazole (Terazol)	*Risk category C.*	Fluconazole excreted in breast milk at levels similar to the mother's plasma level. Most considered safe if ingested in breast milk.

CNS, central nervous system.

Continued

Drug	Use during Pregnancy	Use during Breastfeeding
Antihypertensives **(See also *Diuretics*)** *ACE inhibitors:* (benazepril [Lotensin], captopril [Capoten], enalapril [Vasotec], fosinopril [Monopril], lisinopril [Prinivil, Zestril], quinapril [Accupril], ramipril [Altace], trandolapril [Mavik])	*Risk category D* (primarily second and third trimesters). Renal dysplasia leading to oligohydramnios may result in pulmonary hypotension and death after birth.	Observe for infant hypotension. Fewer safety data available for newer agents.
Beta-adrenergic blockers: (acebutolol [Monitan, Sectral], atenolol [Tenormin], betaxolol [Kerlone], labetalol [Normodyne], metoprolol [Lopressor, Toprol], nadolol [Corgard], penbutolol [Levatol], pindolol [Viskin], propranolol [Inderal])	*Risk category B* (pindolol). Possible fetal or neonatal effects include intrauterine growth restriction, neonatal hypotension, bradycardia, transient tachypnea, respiratory depression, and hypoglycemia. *Risk category C* (labetalol, metoprolol, nadolol, penbutolol, propranolol) and D (acebutolol, atenolol).	Acebutalol, labetalol, metoprolol, nadolol, and propranolol considered safe. Less known about other drugs. Observe infant for possible effects listed under "Use during Pregnancy."
Calcium channel blockers: (amlodipine [Norvasc], diltiazem [Cardizem], nicardipine [Cardene], nifedipine [Adalat, Procardia], verapamil [Calan, Isoptin])	*Risk category C.* May benefit fetus by reducing resistance to placental blood flow. Nifedipine and verapamil may be given to reduce preterm contractions, prolonging pregnancy.	Diltiazem, nifedipine, verapamil generally considered safe, although diltiazem levels in breast milk may reach maternal serum levels. Less known about other drugs listed.
Centrally acting antihypertensives: (clonidine [Catapres], guanabenz [Wytensin], guanadrel [Hylorel], guanfacine [Tenex], methyldopa [Aldomet])	*Risk categories B* (guanadrel, guanfacine, methyldopa) and C (clonidine, guanabenz). Methyldopa is an accepted antihypertensive drug during first trimester of pregnancy.	Methyldopa is considered safe. Little information about effects of the other centrally acting antihypertensive drugs on lactation. Observe infant for hypotension.
Vasodilators: (eprosartan [Teveten], hydralazine [Apresoline], minoxidil [Loniten], nitroprusside [Nipride, Nitropress])	*Risk category C;* risk category D in second and third trimesters for eprosartan. Hydralazine is drug of choice for hypertension during pregnancy. Nitroprusside given in carefully titrated doses to control severe hypertension during pregnancy.	Hydralazine considered safe, but less is known about minoxidil use. Nitroprusside is a concern because of drug's conversion to potentially toxic thiocyanate metabolite.
Antimicrobials *Aminoglycosides:* (gentamicin [Garamycin], streptomycin, tobramycin [Tobrex, Nebcin])	*Risk categories C and D.* Associated with hearing loss and renal toxicity. Monitoring of blood levels reduces risk of adverse effects.	Most drugs in this class are considered safe because minimal amounts are secreted in breast milk and drugs are poorly absorbed if orally ingested. Observe for changes in GI flora.
Macrolides: (azithromycin [Zithromax], clarithromycin [Biaxin], erythromycin [EES, Erythrocin, Ilotycin])	*Risk category B.*	Appear to be safe. Drugs available in pediatric preparations.
Cephalosporins (first- through fourth-generation drugs)	*Risk category B.*	Most are considered safe for breastfeeding.
Chloramphenicol (Chloromycetin)	*Risk category D.* Not recommended for use near term because it is associated with neonatal "gray baby syndrome" (rapid respiration, ashen and pale color, poor feeding, abdominal distention, vasomotor collapse, death).	Generally unsafe in breastfeeding mothers because of potential toxicity and "gray baby syndrome" risk for newborns.
Fluoroquinolones: (ciprofloxacin [Cipro], levofloxacin [Levaquin], norfloxacin [Chibroxin], ofloxacin [Floxin])	*Risk category C.* Animal studies have shown skeletal abnormalities.	Potentially hazardous. Ofloxacin and ciprofloxacin reach breast milk concentrations similar to or higher than maternal plasma. Less is known about other drugs. Observe infant for diarrhea.
Nitrofurantoin (Furadantin, Macrodantin)	*Risk category B.* Crosses placenta. Animal studies reassuring, and no evidence suggests drug is teratogenic.	Should avoid if infant is younger than 1 month. Risk for hemolytic anemia if infant has an enzyme (G-6-PD) deficiency.
Penicillins: (amoxicillin [Amoxil], ampicillin [Omnipen, Polycillin], penicillin G)	*Risk category B.* No reported adverse fetal effects. Penicillins combined with beta-lactamase inhibitors (amoxicillin and clavulanate [Augmentin], ticarcillin and clavulanate [Timentin], and ampicillin and sulbactam [Unasyn]) also are risk category B.	Low concentrations of penicillins in breast milk, including those combined with beta-lactamase inhibitors. Observe for infant diarrhea or candidiasis.
Sulfonamides: (sulfadiazine [Coptin], sulfamethoxazole [Gantanol], sulfisoxazole [Gantrisin])	*Risk category C.*	AAP recommends caution in use of breast milk if infant has jaundice or G-6-PD deficiency and in the ill or preterm infant.
Tetracycline	*Risk category D.* Can interfere with tooth enamel formation and cause discolored teeth. Prenatal exposure does not affect permanent teeth.	Thought to be compatible with breastfeeding. Oral ingestion appears to be safe, although few well-controlled studies exist.

Drug	Use during Pregnancy	Use during Breastfeeding
Antimicrobials—cont'd		
Vancomycin (Vancocin)	*Risk category B.* Used for maternal methicillin-resistant *Staphylococcus aureus* infections and prophylaxis to prevent endocarditis.	Thought to be safe because oral absorption by breastfeeding infant is minimal.
Antiretrovirals		
Nucleoside reverse transcriptase inhibitors (NRTIs): (abacavir [ABC, Ziagen], didanosine [ddI, Videx], lamivudine [3TC, Epivir], stavudine [d4T, Zerit], tenofovir DF [Viread, TDF], zalcitabine [ddC, Hivid], zidovudine [ZDV, Retrovir])	*Risk category B* (didanosine) or C (abacavir, lamivudine, stavudine, tenofovir DF, zalcitabine, zidovudine). Zidovudine is recommended for HIV-seropositive women to reduce risk for perinatal transmission of the virus.	Breastfeeding not recommended because of possibility of HIV transmission to infant.
Nonnucleotide reverse transcriptase inhibitors: (NNRTIs) (delavirdine [DLV, Rescriptor], efavirenz [Sustiva, EFV], nevirapine [NVP, Viramune])	*Risk category C.* Efavirenz category C first trimester, category D second and third trimesters.	Breastfeeding not recommended because of possibility of HIV transmission to infant.
Fusion inhibitors: enfuvirtide [Fuzeon, T-20]	*Risk category B.*	Breastfeeding not recommended because of possibility of HIV transmission to infant.
Protease inhibitors (PIs): (amprenavir [Agenerase], indinavir [Crixivan], nelfinavir [Viracept], ritonavir [Norvir], saquinavir [Invirase])	*Risk category B:* Nelfinavir, ritonavir, saquinavir. *Risk category C:* Amprenavir, indinavir.	Breastfeeding not recommended because of possibility of HIV transmission to infant.
Antituberculosis Agents (See also *Antimicrobials*)		
Ethambutol (Myambutol)	*Risk category B.* No evidence of increased abnormalities.	Small amounts of ethambutol are excreted into breast milk.
Isoniazid (INH)	*Risk category C.*	Scant drug levels found in breast milk. Observe infant for hepatitis, vision changes.
Pyrazinamide	*Risk category C.* No adverse experience with this widely prescribed agent.	None reported in breast milk.
Rifampin (Rifadin)	*Risk category C.*	Trace amounts excreted in breast milk.
Antitussives and Expectorants		
Dextromethorphan (Robitussin-DM)	*Risk category C.*	No reported adverse effects.
Guaifenesin (Robitussin)	*Risk category C.* Usefulness as an expectorant is questionable.	No reported adverse effects.
Antiviral Agents		
Genital herpes infection therapy: (acyclovir [Avirax, Zovirax], foscarnet [Foscavir], valacyclovir [Valtrex])	*Risk categories B* (acyclovir) and C (foscarnet, valacyclovir).	Few reported toxicities except foscarnet associated with higher milk levels than other drugs. Wash topical drug from area before nursing, and consult with physician about breastfeeding safety if lesion is present on nipple.
Ribavirin (Virazole)	*Risk category X.* Administered by aerosol, usually to young children only. Women who are pregnant or may become pregnant should avoid exposure.	Drug is most often given to young children hospitalized with respiratory syncytial virus (RSV), so transfer to breast milk is not likely.
Cardiac Medications		
Antiarrhythmics for serious arrhythmias: (amiodarone [Cordarone, Pacerone], bretylium [Bretylol])	*Risk category C* (bretylium) or D (amiodarone). May reduce uterine blood flow. Possible neurotoxic effects of amiodarone.	Used for life-threatening arrhythmias; woman unlikely to be nursing.
Digitoxin (Crystodigin), digoxin (Lanoxin)	*Risk category C.* Has been used to treat fetal cardiac arrhythmias.	Digoxin considered safe, but less known about digitoxin safety.
Lidocaine (used as antiarrhythmic) (Xylocaine)	*Risk category B.*	Lidocaine considered safe for breastfeeding.
Decongestants		
Ephedrine, epinephrine (EpiPen, Sus-Phrine)	*Risk category C.* Ephedrine is also used to support blood pressure during epidural or subarachnoid block during intrapartum period.	Acute, one-time use of ephedrine or epinephrine is likely to be safe. Breastfeeding not recommended if drug regularly used by mother.
Nasal sprays: (oxymetazoline [Afrin, Coricidin, Dristan], phenylephrine [Neo-Synephrine], phenylpropanolamine [Kleer, Propan], fluticasone [Flonase, Flovent])	*Risk category C.* Avoid during third trimester.	Minimal amounts secreted in milk (oxymetazoline and phenylephrine). Less information available about fluticasone and phenylpropanolamine in milk secretion.

HIV, human immunodeficiency virus.

Continued

Drug	Use during Pregnancy	Use during Breastfeeding
Decongestants—cont'd		
Pseudoephedrine (Sufedrine, Sudafed)	*Risk category C.* Avoid during first trimester because fetus may have higher risk for gastroschisis or small intestinal atresia.	Generally considered safe for breastfeeding if used occasionally rather than chronically.
Diuretics		
Carbonic anhydrase inhibitors: (acetazolamide [Diamox], methazolamide [Neptazane])	*Risk category C.*	Acetazolamide is considered safe. Safety of methazolamide unknown.
Loop diuretics: (ethacrynic acid [Edecrin], furosemide [Lasix], torsemide [Demadex])	*Risk category B* (ethacrynic acid) or C (furosemide and torsemide).	Few well-controlled studies; effects probably minimal. Maternal use could suppress lactation.
Potassium-sparing diuretics: (amiloride [Midamor], spironolactone [Aldactone], triamterene [Dyrenium])	*Risk category B* (amiloride, triamterene); category D (spironolactone).	Amiloride concentrated in breast milk. Few studies of triamterene. Spironolactone considered safe by AAP.
Thiazide diuretics: (chlorothiazide [Diuril], hydrochlorothiazide [HydroDIURIL])	*Risk category D.* Decreased intravascular volume may reduce uteroplacental perfusion and result in growth retardation. Metabolic disturbances and thrombocytopenia may occur in mother and fetus.	Considered safe during lactation.
Thiazide-like diuretics: (chlorthalidone [Hygroton], indapamide [Lozide, Lozol], metolazone [Mykrox, Zaroxolyn])	*Risk category B.*	Chlorthalidone considered by AAP to be safe during lactation but may reduce milk supply.
Hormones		
Corticosteroids: (beclomethasone [Vanceril, Beclovent], betamethasone [Celestone], cortisone [Cortone], dexamethasone [Decadron], prednisolone [Delta-Cortef, Prelone], prednisone [Deltasone])	*Risk category C.* Prednisone or prednisolone (category B) is common for asthmatic woman who needs steroids. Betamethasone and dexamethasone are used to accelerate maturation of fetal lungs if preterm delivery is likely.	Prednisone and prednisolone compatible with breastfeeding. Delay nursing 4 hr after dose to reduce transfer to infant. Remove from nipples before nursing if applied topically.
Clomiphene citrate (Clomid)	*Risk category X.* Questionable association with neural tube defects. Drug is discontinued after pregnancy is achieved.	Unlikely to be given during lactation because the drug is for infertility treatment.
Danazol (Danocrine)	*Risk category X.* May cause virilization of female fetus.	Breastfeeding not advised.
Estrogens (Azumon, Conjugen, Ovest, Premarin)	*Risk category X.* No indication for estrogens during pregnancy.	Try to delay drug until breastfeeding is firmly established.
Estradiol (Alora, Climara, Estrace, Estraderm, Estring, FemPatch, Vivelle)	*Risk category X.* Contraceptives; not indicated during pregnancy.	Safe during lactation. Early use sometimes reduces milk volume secreted.
Estrogen-progestin combinations	*Risk category X.* Risks and benefits must be individually evaluated because a higher risk for cardiovascular disease was found in women who take the combination for menopausal symptoms. Doses much higher than those for oral contraceptives and are associated with masculinization of the female fetus' genitalia.	Ideally, avoid until lactation is well established for best quantity and quality of breast milk.
Progesterone (Gesterol 50, Lutolin-S, Progestagect-50, Prometrium, Crinone)	*Risk category D.* Most often given for amenorrhea, hormone replacement therapy, infertility (luteal phase support only during pregnancy).	Generally considered safe for use when breastfeeding.
Psychoactive Drugs		
Benzodiazepines: (alprazolam [Xanax], chlordiazepoxide [Librium, Libritabs], clonazepam [Klonopin], diazepam [Valium], flurazepam [Dalmane], lorazepam [Ativan], midazolam [Versed], oxazepam [Serax], temazepam [Restoril], triazolam [Halcion])	Most are risk category D. Some reports of mild facial abnormalities and developmental delay, but no conclusive studies. Use during the third trimester may slow the infant's neurologic development and result in sedation after birth. Midazolam is primarily used as a brief maternal perioperative sedative. The following sedative-hypnotic drugs in this class are risk category X: flurazepam, temazepam, and triazolam.	Potentially hazardous because of the long half-lives of many drugs in this class and the potential development of dependence. Few reported adverse effects, but observe infant for sedation, poor feeding.
Anxiolytic: (meprobamate [Equanil, Miltown])	*Risk category D.* Has been associated with cardiac malformations.	Concentrations in milk are higher than in maternal serum. Observe for infant sedation.

Drug	Use during Pregnancy	Use during Breastfeeding
Psychoactive Drugs—cont'd		
Antipsychotic: lithium [Eskalith, Lithobid]	*Risk category D.* Slightly increased risk for cardiac abnormalities.	Infant blood concentration of lithium reaches $\frac{1}{2}$ to $\frac{1}{3}$ of the mother's concentration. Infant drug levels should be evaluated. T-wave abnormalities and decreased muscle tone have been noted.
Atypical antidepressants: (bupropion [Wellbutrin], mirtazapine [Remeron], nefazodone [Serzone], trazodone [Desyrel], venlafaxine [Effexor])	*Risk category B* (bupropion); risk category C (mirtazapine; nefazodone; trazodone; venlafaxine).	Trazodone minimally excreted in breast milk. Unknown if other atypical antidepressants are excreted in breast milk.
Phenothiazines: (chlorpromazine [Thorazine], prochlorperazine [Compazine], thioridazine [Mellaril])	*Risk category C.* Risk of malformations is uncertain, but these are probably safe for use in humans. Alcohol may increase CNS depression. Taking other drugs with phenothiazines may alter serum levels of one or more of the drugs taken.	Neonatal hypoglycemia has been reported with chlorpromazine. Less known about breastfeeding effects of maternal prochlorperazine and thioridazine.
Monoamine oxidase inhibitors (MAOIs): (phenelzine [Nardil], tranylcypromine [Parnate])	*Risk category C.* Documented interactions between opioids and MAOIs. Potential risks if taken near the time other drugs were taken. Consult a detailed drug guide. Little documentation of fetal effects.	Few published reports related to entry of these MAOI drugs into breast milk.
Tricyclic antidepressants: (amitriptyline [Elavil], amoxapine [Asendin], clomipramine [Anafranil], desipramine [Norpramin], doxepin [Adepin, Sinequan], imipramine [Tofranil], nortriptyline [Aventyl, Pamelor], protriptyline [Vivactil])	*Risk category C* for most tricyclics. Risk category D for imipramine and nortriptyline, however. Several studies have shown that tricyclic antidepressant use during pregnancy is most likely not teratogenic.	Few contraindications for most tricyclic antidepressants. Infant apnea and drowsiness with maternal doxepin intake have been described.
Selective serotonin reuptake inhibitors (SSRIs): (citalopram [Celexa], escitalopram [Lexapro], fluoxetine [Prozac], fluvoxamine [Luvox], paroxetine [Paxil], sertraline [Zoloft])	*Most risk category C;* sertraline risk category B.	Most considered safe for breastfeeding infant. Citalopram and escitalopram have been associated with excessive somnolence, decreased intake, and infant weight loss.
Other psychoactive drugs: (bupropion [Wellbutrin], mirtazapine, [Remeron], nefazodone [Serzone], trazodone [Desyrel], venlafaxine [Effexor])	*Risk category C* except for bupropion (risk category B).	Few reports on breast milk safety for infants for most drugs. No AAP contraindications for bupropion or trazodone. Observe infant for sedation.
Thyroid Drugs		
Antithyroids: (methimazole [Tapazole], propylthiouracil [PTU])	*Risk category D.* May result in neonatal goiter or hypothyroidism, although uncommon at usual therapeutic doses. Methimazole has possible association with scalp defects. PTU is drug of choice during pregnancy.	Approved by AAP. Neonatal thyroid function apparently unaffected by maternal treatment.
Potassium iodide (SSKI, Thyro-Block)	*Risk category D.* Long-term exposure may produce fetal thyroid enlargement or hypothyroidism.	May cause rash or suppress infant's thyroid function. Dose should not be higher than RDA (recommended daily allowance).
Thyroid replacement hormone: (levothyroxine [Levoxyl, Synthroid])	*Risk category A.* Crosses placenta only to limited extent.	Apparently safe during breastfeeding.
Vitamins and Retinoids		
Retinoids: (isotretinoin [Accutane])	*Risk category X.* Related to vitamin A. Associated with severe fetal malformations (microcephaly, ear abnormalities, cardiac defects, central nervous system abnormalities).	Contraindicated for use during breastfeeding because of severe fetal effects.
Vitamin A	*Risk category A* at doses no higher than 6000 USP units/day. (Risk category X at doses higher than RDA limits [see Table 9-4, pp. 178-179]. Excess intake may lead to abnormalities noted for isotretinoin.	Breast milk usually supplies sufficient vitamin A to infant. Mother should not take more than 6000 international units per day.
Vitamin D	*Risk category A* (risk category D at doses above RDA). Excess intake associated with malformations, including aortic stenosis, facial abnormalities, and mental retardation.	AAP approved. Infant serum level assessment recommended if mother taking a therapeutic dose.

RDA, recommended daily allowance; *USP*, US Pharmacopeia.

Continued

Drug	Use during Pregnancy	Use during Breastfeeding
Miscellaneous Drugs Nicotine gum; nicotine transdermal patch	*Risk category C* (nicotine gum) or D (transdermal nicotine). Risk category X if used in overdose. Stopping nicotine intake by ceasing smoking lowers complications such as preterm birth.	Lactation safe, although drug is passed into breast milk. Infant exposure to passive environmental nicotine smoke is not considered safe, however.

Herbal and Botanical Preparations

Botanical Preparation	Uses	Risks for Use during Pregnancy and Lactation
Black cohosh (baneberry, black snakeroot, bugbane, squaw root, rattle root)	Phytoestrogen effects to reduce symptoms during menopause.	Pregnancy risk category X because of uterine stimulant effects. Unknown lactation effects but may reduce milk production with estrogenic effects.
Blue cohosh (blue ginseng, squaw root, papoose root, yellow ginseng)	Uterine stimulant. Similar to nicotine, resulting in hypertension, gastric stimulation, and coronary vasoconstriction.	Pregnancy risk category X. Has been used short term to stimulate delivery. No data for lactation safety but considered a high-risk herbal supplement.
Capsaicin (Zostrix, Axsain, Capsin, Capzasin-P, No-Pain, Absorbine Jr. Arthritis, Arthricare)	Topical application for pain associated with osteoarthritis, fibromyalgia, peripheral neuropathy, shingles. Avoid eye contact.	Pregnancy category C, little data on risk during lactation. Considered safe for children >2 years of age.
Chamomile (German chamomile, Hungarian chamomile, pinheads, wild chamomile)	Antiinflammatory, antispasmodic, sedative. Treatment of nausea, GI spasms, diarrhea, insomnia. Topical treatment of hemorrhoids. Caution required in those with asthma or allergic to ragweed.	Uterotonic effects with unknown risk. Should be avoided in pregnancy and lactation.
Echinacea (Black Susan, snakeroot, comb flower, red sunflower, scurvy root)	Antiviral, antibiotic effects to reduce cold and flu symptoms, stimulate wound healing. Long-term daily doses may suppress rather than stimulate immune response. Should not be taken by those with autoimmune disease.	Contraindicated in pregnancy. Pregnancy category C because of possible immune suppression. No data on lactation effects.
Evening primrose oil	Treatment of premenstrual syndrome (PMS), menopausal symptoms. Seizure risk increased if combined with antipsychotics.	No pregnancy category assigned. Appears to be safe for use in pregnancy and lactation.
Feverfew (bachelor button, featherfew, midsummer daisy, Santa Maria)	Prevention of migraines. Should not be used with prescription headache drugs. May cause uterine contraction or abortion.	Contraindicated in pregnancy and lactation.
Glucosamine	Treatment of osteoarthritis to reduce pain and improve movement.	Increases blood glucose levels. Avoid use in pregnancy and lactation.
Goldenseal	Antibiotic, antiseptic, antiinflammatory effects. Uses include wound healing, treatment of upper respiratory infections, uterine bleeding, and enhancement of insulin.	Contraindicated in pregnancy and lactation. May cause premature contractions. Short-term use only because product may cause inflammation of mucosa.
Kava (also known as *kava-kava*) (Awa, Kew, Tonga)	Treatment of anxiety, stress, restlessness; sedation or sleep enhancement. Effects similar to alcohol. Mixing with alcohol increases toxicity.	Contraindicated in pregnancy and lactation.
St. John's wort	Treatment of mild to moderate depression. Possible interaction with therapeutic drugs and other herbal preparations: cyclosporine, digoxin, ACE inhibitors, indinavir, ginseng, chamomile, goldenseal, kava, valerian.	Contraindicated in pregnancy and lactation. May cause increased muscle tone of uterus. Pregnancy category C. Infant effects may include colic, drowsiness, lethargy.
Valerian (valerian root)	Sedative for insomnia, sleeping disorders associated with anxiety, restlessness.	Inadequate data to determine effects during pregnancy. Sedative effects discourage use in lactating woman.

ACE, Angiotensin-converting enzyme; *GI,* gastrointestinal.

REFERENCES & READINGS

American Academy of Pediatrics and American College of Obstetricians and Gynecologists. (2002). *Guidelines for perinatal care* (5th ed.). Elk Grove Village, IL, and Washington, DC: Authors.

American Academy of Pediatrics Committee on Drugs. (2000). Use of psychoactive medications during pregnancy and possible effects on the fetus and newborn (RE9866). *Pediatrics, 105*(4), 880-887.

American Academy of Pediatrics Committee on Drugs. (2001). Transfer of drugs and other chemicals into human milk. *Pediatrics, 108*(3), 776-789.

Andrade, S.E., Gurwitz, J.H., Davis, R.L., Chan, K.A., Finkelstein, J.A., Fortman, K., et al. (2004). Prescription drug use in pregnancy. *American Journal of Obstetrics & Gynecology, 191*(2), 398-407.

Andres, R.L. (2004). Effects of therapeutic, diagnostic, and environmental agents and exposure to social and illicit drugs. In R.K. Creasy, R. Resnik, & J.D. Iams (Eds.), *Maternal-fetal medicine: Principles and practice* (5th ed., pp. 281-314). Philadelphia: Saunders.

Blanchard, D.G., & Shabetai, R. (2004). Cardiac diseases. In R.K. Creasy, R. Resnik, & J.D. Iams (Eds.), *Maternal-fetal medicine: Principles and practice* (5th ed., pp. 815-843). Philadelphia: Saunders.

Centers for Disease Control and Prevention. (2002). Sexually transmitted diseases treatment guidelines. *MMWR. Morbidity and Mortality Weekly Report, 51*(RR-6). Atlanta, GA: Author.

Cunningham, F.G., Leveno, K.J., Bloom, S.L., Hauth, J.C., Gilstrap, L.C., & Wenstrom, K.D. (2005). *Williams obstetrics* (22nd ed.). New York: McGraw-Hill.

Fontaine, K.L. (2005). *Complementary and alternative therapies for nursing practice* (2nd ed.). Upper Saddle River, NJ: Prentice-Hall.

Gahart, B.L., & Nazareno, A.R. (2005). *2005 intravenous medications* (21st ed.). St. Louis: Mosby.

Gal, P., & Reed, M.D. (2004). Medications. In R.E. Behrman, R.M. Kliegman, & H.B. Jenson (Eds.), *Nelson's textbook of pediatrics* (17th ed., pp. 2432-2501). Philadelphia: Saunders.

Gibbs, R.S., Sweet, R.L., & Duff, W.P. (2004). Maternal and fetal infectious disorders. In R.K. Creasy, R. Resnik, & J.D. Iams (Eds.), *Maternal-fetal medicine: Principles and practice* (5th ed., pp. 741-801). Philadelphia: Saunders.

Harkness, R., & Bratman, S. (2003). *Mosby's handbook of drug-herb and drug-supplement interactions.* St. Louis: Mosby.

Hale, T.W. (2004). *Medications and mothers' milk* (11th ed.). Amarillo, TX: Pharmasoft Medical Publishing.

Hodgson, B.B. (2005). *Nursing drug handbook 2005.* Philadelphia: Saunders.

Kemper, K.J., & Gardiner, P. (2004). Herbal medicines. In R.E. Behrman, R.M. Kliegman, & H.B. Jenson (Eds.), *Nelson's textbook of pediatrics* (17th ed., pp. 2502-2505). Philadelphia: Saunders.

Lawrence, R.M., & Lawrence, R.A. (2004). The breast and the physiology of lactation. In R.K. Creasy, R. Resnik, & J.D. Iams (Eds.), *Maternal-fetal medicine: Principles and practice* (5th ed., pp. 135-153). Philadelphia: Saunders.

Lawrence, R.M., & Lawrence, R.A. (2005). *Breastfeeding: A guide for the medical profession* (6th ed.). St. Louis: Mosby.

Minkoff, H.L. (2004). Human immunodeficiency virus. In R.K. Creasy, R. Resnik, & J.D. Iams (Eds.), *Maternal-fetal medicine: Principles and practice* (5th ed., pp. 803-814). Philadelphia: Saunders.

Public Health Service Task Force. (2005). *Recommendations for using antiretroviral drugs in pregnant HIV-1 infected women for maternal health and interventions to reduce perinatal HIV-1 transmission in the United States.* Retrieved April 13, 2005, from http://AIDSinfo.nih.gov.

Public Health Service Task Force. (2005). *Safety and toxicity of individual antiretroviral agents in pregnancy.* Retrieved April 13, 2005, from http://AIDSinfo.nih.gov.

Skidmore-Roth, L. (2004). *Mosby's handbook of herbs and natural supplements* (2nd ed.). St. Louis: Mosby.

Skidmore-Roth, L. (2005). *Mosby's nursing drug reference.* St. Louis: Mosby.

Spencer, J.W., & Jacobs, J.J. (2004). *Complementary and alternative medicine: An evidence-based approach* (2nd ed.). St. Louis: Mosby.

U.S. Department of Health and Human Services. (2004). AIDS info: Approved medications to treat HIV infection. Retrieved April 1, 2004, from www.AIDSinfo.nih.gov.

Weiner, C.P,. & Buhimschi, C. (2004). *Drugs for pregnant and lactating women.* New York: Churchill Livingstone.

Keys to Clinical Practice: Components of Daily Care

INTRAPARTUM CARE

Text to Prepare You for Clinical Practice

Chapter 15: Nonpharmacologic techniques (see also Figures 15-5 to 15-8)

Figure 12-4: Pelvic divisions and measurements

Table 13-1: Intrapartum assessment guide

Figure 13-2: Vaginal examination during labor

Figure 13-7: Sequence for delivery

Figure 13-8: Vaginal birth

Table 13-2: Apgar score

Procedure 21-2: Using a bulb syringe

New Terms

Amniotomy
Bloody show
Crowning
Dilation
EDD (also known as *EDB*)
Effacement
Gravida
Lochia
Multipara
Nullipara
Para
Presentation
Primipara
Station
Vaginal birth after cesarean (VBAC)

Equipment and Supplies

Sterile and nonsterile gloves
Lubricant
Urine specimen containers
Amniotic membrane perforator (Amnihook)
Emesis basin
Bedpan
Disposable underpads
Extra linens
Fetal monitoring equipment and related supplies
Electronic fetal monitor and supplies
Doppler transducer
Intravenous (IV) fluids, tubing, venipuncture supplies, IV pumps
Urinary catheters (indwelling and straight)
Oxygen equipment, including water, tubing, and face masks
Emergency cart
"Precip tray" (for emergency birth)
Neonatal warmer
Neonatal oxygen equipment and resuscitation supplies

Normal Assessments

FETUS

GESTATION. 38 to 42 weeks.

FETAL HEART RATE (FHR). Lower limit of 110 to 120 bpm and upper limit of 150 to 160 bpm at term. The rate may slow during contractions but should return to its original level by the end of the contraction.

AMNIOTIC FLUID. Clear (may have particles of white vernix); no foul odor.

WOMAN

TEMPERATURE. Lower than 38° C (100.4° F).

BLOOD PRESSURE. Near baseline levels established during pregnancy. (Report elevations of 140 [systolic]) or 90 [diastolic] or higher.)

PULSE. 60 to 100 beats/minute.

RESPIRATIONS. 12 to 20 breaths/minute.

CONTRACTIONS. No more than 90 to 120 seconds in duration, with at least 30 seconds of uterine relaxation between the end of one contraction and the beginning of the next.

BLOODY SHOW. Dark blood mixed with mucus (has a distinct mucous component). The amount varies but increases as full cervical dilation nears.

LOCHIA (FOURTH STAGE). No more than one saturated pad in 1 hour. (Perineal pads containing cold packs absorb less and are saturated sooner than standard pads.)

FUNDUS (FOURTH STAGE). Firm, between the symphysis and the umbilicus, midline.

Nursing Care

Clinical experiences in the intrapartum setting are primarily observational. The nursing student works with an experienced nurse when caring for the laboring woman. Primary responsibilities of the novice are to promote family attachment, provide comfort and support to the woman and her family, and report maternal or fetal assessments that are not expected.

Personal protective equipment (PPE), such as gloves and water-repellent gowns or aprons, must be worn whenever the possibility of contact with body fluids (amniotic fluid, blood, lochia, colostrum, breast milk, urine, or stool) exists to conform with standard precautions. Protective eyewear also must be worn if splash or spray contamination of the eyes is a possibility.

Assessments

Unless directed otherwise by the experienced nurse, assess the woman and fetus who do not have complications or medications that require special monitoring by using the following guidelines:

1. FHR with continuous electronic fetal monitoring or intermittent auscultation: every hour during the latent phase; every 30 minutes during the active phase; every 15 minutes during the second stage of labor for the low-risk woman.
2. The woman's temperature every 4 hours unless her membranes have ruptured, then every 2 hours.
3. The woman's blood pressure, pulse, and respirations every hour.
4. Contractions: Assess at same time as FHR.
5. If the woman's membranes rupture, assess FHR for at least 1 minute, and observe the color, odor, and amount of fluid. Notify an experienced nurse that the woman's membranes have ruptured.
6. After birth, during the recovery phase, assess the mother's uterine fundus, lochia, blood pressure, pulse, and respirations every 15 minutes for the first hour.

Interventions

1. Assess the woman and the fetus using the guidelines listed previously or according to the facility's policy. Document all assessments, and *report any findings that do not fall within the expected limits.*
2. If no contraindication exists, give the woman ice chips and encourage her to change position as much as she desires. Ask an experienced nurse to be sure.
3. The woman can usually walk to the bathroom if she is not in advanced labor and has not had analgesia or anesthesia that impairs mobility (such as epidural block). Record each time she voids or has a bowel movement.
4. Help the woman cope with labor:
   - A cool, damp washcloth often feels good on her face, arms, and abdomen.
   - If her back hurts, offer to rub it or apply firm pressure in the sacral area. Ask her where and how firmly to press. Encourage her to try alternative positions.
   - Give generous praise and encouragement for her efforts to give birth. Praise the partner's efforts as a coach.
5. Offer a snack to the woman's partner, or encourage the partner to take a break and have a meal.
6. Look at the woman's perineum if she says that the baby is coming or begins making grunting sounds or bearing down. Summon the experienced nurse with the call bell immediately, but *do not leave the woman.*
7. When the infant is born, focus on the respiratory efforts and maintain warmth. Use a bulb syringe to suction excess secretions. Keep the infant under a radiant warmer or wrap in warmed blankets. Do not get between the radiant heat source and the infant.
8. Observe parent-infant attachment behaviors such as making eye contact, talking in soft, high-pitched tones, and making remarks about the infant.
9. In many facilities, the infant remains with the parents during the recovery period, and the same nurse cares for both the mother and the newborn. If this is the case, continue to observe the infant's respiratory effort and maintain the temperature.

POSTPARTUM CARE: PHYSIOLOGIC ASPECTS

Text to Prepare You for Clinical Practice

Procedure 17-1: Assessing the uterine fundus
Procedure 17-2: Assessing the perineum
Figure 17-2: Assessing volume of lochia
Figure 17-7: Clinical pathway for vaginal birth
Figure 17-8: Assessing Homans' sign
Table 17-1: Characteristics of lochia
Table 17-3: Observations of the fundus requiring nursing actions
Critical to Remember: Signs of a distended bladder

New Terms

Afterpains
Atony
Colostrum
Engorgement
Episiotomy
Fundus
Lochia rubra, serosa, alba
Puerperium
REEDA (redness, edema, ecchymosis, drainage, approximation)

Equipment and Supplies

Thermometer
Blood pressure equipment
Watch
Stethoscope
Flashlight

Nonsterile gloves
Peripads
Clean linen
Disposable underpads

Normal Assessments

VITAL SIGNS

TEMPERATURE. Lower than 38° C (100.4° F).

BLOOD PRESSURE. Near the baseline levels established during pregnancy.

PULSE. 60 to 90 beats/minute. 50 to 60 beats/minute may occur. Bradycardia reflects the increased amount of blood returning to the central circulation.

RESPIRATIONS. 12 to 20 breaths/minute. Should be unchanged from preconception levels; the lungs should be free of adventitious breath sounds.

BREASTS

1. First 24 hours: Soft.
2. Days 2 to 3: Firm to very firm, as milk comes in.
3. Nipples: Free of redness, abraded areas, blisters, bruising, and fissures.

GASTROINTESTINAL SYSTEM

1. Mother is hungry and thirsty.
2. Abdomen is soft. Temporary constipation may occur because of dehydration and decreased intake during labor.
3. Bowel sounds usually present within 24 to 36 hours after cesarean birth.
4. Hemorrhoids may be obvious, particularly during the first 24 hours.

GENITOURINARY SYSTEM

1. Fundus should be firm, midline, and located approximately at the umbilicus (±1 cm).
2. Lochia rubra should be scant to moderate with a fleshy, earthy odor.
3. Episiotomy edges should be approximated and without redness or edema.
4. Perineum, labia, or both may be slightly bruised or swollen.
5. Abdominal dressing, if present, should be dry and intact. Follow agency protocol or physician orders for removal. The edges of the surgical incision should be approximated and without signs of infection.
6. Diuresis is normal for the first 2 to 5 days. Mothers often are unaware of the need to urinate.
7. After the woman voids, the bladder should not be palpable and the fundus should remain firm in the midline of the abdomen, and at the level of the umbilicus.

Nursing Care

Preparation before approaching the new mother helps the nurse recognize unusual or abnormal data and initiate the necessary nursing interventions.

Nonsterile gloves must be worn whenever the possibility of contact with body fluids (blood, lochia, colostrum, breast milk, urine, or stool) exists.

The sequence in which postpartum assessments are performed is important because they should progress from areas that are least likely to be contaminated, such as the breasts, to areas that are associated with pathogenic organisms, such as the perineum and anal areas. The following sequence is recommended.

Assessments

1. Explain the purpose of the assessments: "I know we do these assessments several times a day, but they help us determine if everything is progressing as it should. It is also a good time for you to ask any questions you might have."
2. Assess vital signs, usually every 4 to 8 hours, depending on facility protocols and the condition of the mother.
3. Auscultate breath sounds and the ability to breathe deeply and cough if the woman had a cesarean birth, if she smokes, or if she has a history of respiratory disorders.
4. Ask the mother to unfasten her bra or to lower the bra flaps to assess the nipples for redness, fissures, or blisters that may occur with breastfeeding. Note nipple size and shape that may make breastfeeding more difficult (flat, retracted, inverted). Palpate the breasts and ask how well breastfeeding is progressing and whether she has any questions.
5. Lower the top of the bed, and ask the mother to flex her knees for comfort. If the woman had a cesarean birth, auscultate the abdomen for bowel sounds and ask if she is passing flatus. Palpate the abdomen determine if it is soft or distended.
6. If a dressing covers the incision, observe for intactness and drainage. If no dressing is present, observe the cesarean incision for REEDA and note whether a topical skin adhesive, staples, or adhesive strips are in place.
7. Assess for bladder distention (observable or palpable bulge above the symphysis pubis) and time and amount of last voiding (can be validated from the chart before beginning the assessment). If an indwelling catheter is in place, note the color and amount of urine.
8. Palpate the lower extremities for the presence and extent of edema. Press the thumb on the pretibial area and the feet to determine whether pitting edema is present. Note how long it takes for the pit to disappear.
9. Observe and palpate the lower extremities for signs of thrombophlebitis (areas of redness, warmth, tenderness, swelling). Sharply dorsiflex the foot to elicit Homan's sign.
10. Lower the perineal pad(s) and observe flow of lochia while palpating the fundus for firmness and location.
11. Observe the perineal pad(s) for color and amount of lochia and presence of unpleasant or foul odor. Ask how long since the peripad(s) was changed, to determine the amount of flow.
12. Ask the mother to turn onto her side, and assess the episiotomy and perineum for REEDA. Note the number and size of hemorrhoids.
13. Evaluate the mother's ability to ambulate, and elicit information about dizziness, weakness, or lightheaded-

ness during ambulation. Observe her gait for steadiness and balance.

14. Ask the mother about particular problems and concerns. How is her appetite? How much rest is she getting? Does she have discomfort (where, when)? Does she require medication?

Interventions

1. Changes in vital signs may be within expected limits, or they may indicate the beginning of serious problems. Tachycardia or lower-than-expected blood pressure may indicate excessive bleeding and should be reported. Blood pressure that is higher than expected may indicate preeclampsia. The blood pressure should be reassessed with the woman in a left lateral recumbent position. *Temperature above 38° C (100.4° F) suggests infection rather than dehydration and should be reported. Diminished or abnormal breath sounds (wheezes or crackles), as well as difficulty breathing or coughing, should be reported at once.*

2. Nipple trauma provides a portal for entry of pathogenic organisms and creates discomfort during breastfeeding. The new mother often needs information, guidance, and encouragement with breastfeeding.

3. *Intervene at once if you are unable to locate the fundus, if the fundus feels soft (boggy), or if it is above the umbilicus or displaced from the midline.* Massage a boggy fundus and expel clots when the fundus becomes firm. Assist the mother to void, or catheterize her if she is unable to empty her bladder.

4. Report a positive Homan's sign or areas of redness, edema, or tenderness of the legs. Assist the woman to ambulate if her gait is unsteady or she experiences lightheadedness when she ambulates.

5. If necessary, teach self-care measures such as perineal care and sitz bath to reduce perineal discomfort and prevent infection.

6. Provide medication for afterpains or perineal discomfort according to the physician's orders. Reassure the mother that very little of the medication administered for discomfort crosses into the breast milk and the infant should not be affected.

POSTPARTUM CARE: PSYCHOSOCIAL ASPECTS

Text to Prepare You for Clinical Practice

Table 18-1: Assessing maternal adaptation
Table 18-2: Assessing family adaptation
Critical to Remember: Reciprocal attachment behaviors

New Terms

Attachment
Bonding
En face
Engrossment
Entrainment
Fingertipping

Letting-go
Reciprocal bonding behaviors
Taking-hold
Taking-in

Normal Assessments

MATERNAL TOUCH. During the first 24 hours, the mother progresses from the discovery phase, when she "fingertips" the infant, to holding the infant close and demonstrating consoling behaviors.

VERBAL EXPRESSIONS. The mother progresses from referring to the infant as "it" to using "he" or "she" and finally to calling the infant by a given name. Some parents have called the infant by name since an ultrasound during pregnancy.

TAKING-IN PHASE. Mothers are concerned with their own physical needs and the need to recount details of their labor and delivery.

TAKING-HOLD PHASE. Mothers become more independent and focus on learning how to care for themselves and the infant.

FATHERS. Fathers demonstrate intense fascination with the infant and often respond gently to infant signals such as fussing and crying.

FAMILY. Family support is obvious when the grandparents or other relatives call or visit, offer to assist the mother, and demonstrate interest in the newborn.

Nursing Care

To prepare for the psychological assessment, the nurse should review expected maternal behaviors, progression of maternal touch, and verbal interactions.

Assessments

1. Collect data from the woman's chart or Kardex (age, gravida, para, time and type of delivery, sex and weight of infant, unusual characteristics or anomalies of the infant, time the mother was last medicated for discomfort) to identify factors that might affect adjustment.

2. Begin the psychosocial assessment during the physical assessment, and continue to make observations throughout the day.

3. Observe maternal mood, general energy level, and activity.

4. Ask about the mother's comfort, how she slept, and whether she has special concerns.

5. Note the focus of the mother's attention—is it on her own needs or care of the infant? Does she require assistance with hygiene and self-care measures? How much does she talk about the birth experience and what does she say?

6. Observe the mother's interaction with the infant and her readiness to participate in infant care. Note her tone of voice and verbal interaction.

7. Watch how the mother touches the infant and how she responds to infant cues, such as crying and fussing.

8. Note the father's participation in infant care and his comfort in handling the infant.

9. Notice infant behavior (awake, sleepy, gazing, response to parents' voices). Observe how the infant responds to the parents and whether the parents are successful in consoling the infant.
10. Observe visitors, particularly the grandparents and family, who may provide assistance to the parents during the early weeks at home.

Interventions

1. Anticipate the mother's needs, and provide physical care and comfort measures that are particularly important in the early hours after childbirth.
2. Allow time to listen; this is very important in establishing rapport and assisting the mother to integrate the birth experience into her reality system.
3. Promote bonding and attachment by providing long periods of uninterrupted contact between the parents and the infant. Model behaviors such as gently responding when the infant cries and talking to the infant in a high-pitched voice. Point out positive characteristics of the infant to the parents.
4. Prepare to teach basic infant care, including explanations, demonstrations, pamphlets and videos.
5. Answer questions or demonstrate care as the mother indicates a readiness to learn.

THE NEWBORN: INITIAL ASSESSMENTS AND CARE

Text to Prepare You for Clinical Practice

Procedure 20-1: Assessing vital signs in the newborn
Procedure 20-2: Weighing and measuring the newborn
Procedure 20-3: Obtaining blood samples from the newborn by heel puncture
Procedure 21-1: Administering intramuscular injections to newborns
Procedure 21-2: Using a bulb syringe
Figure 21-2: Administration of ophthalmic ointment
Table 20-1: Summary of newborn assessment

New Terms

Acrocyanosis
Caput succedaneum
Cephalhematoma
Hyperbilirubinemia
Lanugo
Milia
Molding
Mongolian spots
Vernix caseosa

Equipment and Supplies

Scale
Radiant warmer
Nonsterile gloves
Stethoscope
Thermometer
Tape measure
Vitamin K, syringe, filter needle, alcohol wipes
Eye medication
Bulb syringe

Normal Assessments

VITAL SIGNS

TEMPERATURE. Axillary 36.5° to 37.5° C (97.7° to 99.5° F).
   HEART RATE. 120 to 160 beats/minute.
   RESPIRATIONS. 30 to 60 breaths/minute.

BLOOD GLUCOSE

Above 40 to 45 mg/dl by screening tests.

MEASUREMENTS

WEIGHT. 2500 to 4000 g (5 lb, 8 oz to 8 lb, 13 oz).
   LENGTH. 48 to 53 cm (19 to 21 inches).
   HEAD CIRCUMFERENCE. 33 to 35.5 cm (13 to 14 inches).
   CHEST CIRCUMFERENCE. 30.5 to 33 cm (12 to 13 inches).

Nursing Care

A typical order in which assessments and care are performed in the labor, delivery, recovery unit or the admission nursery is given here. The elements actually included and the order in which they are performed depend on the facility's routine and the circumstances.

Adhere to standard precautions at all times. Wear nonsterile gloves whenever handling the infant until the bath is given and all blood is removed from the skin. After the bath, wear gloves when soiling with body fluids may occur.

Include family members who are present. They often are very interested in explanations of the assessments and care being given. Promote bonding by encouraging them to touch and talk to the infant.

Assessments

Begin with a quick overall assessment of the infant's general condition. Attend to major problems, such as severe respiratory distress, before continuing the more detailed assessment and routine care. Observe for signs of distress or abnormality in the early hours after birth, when they are most likely to appear. Report and take action, as necessary, for any abnormal findings.

1. Perform a quick general assessment to identify gross abnormalities. *Be constantly alert for signs of respiratory distress.*
2. Assess vital signs. *Report and follow up on abnormalities immediately.*
3. Weigh infant and measure length and head and chest circumferences.
4. Assess blood glucose according to signs of hypoglycemia and agency policy.

5. Perform in-depth assessment (see Table 20-1).

6. Continue monitoring vital signs every 30 minutes until infant has been stable for 2 hours. Assess more often if necessary. Once the infant is stable, vital signs should be checked every 8 hours, or more frequently if abnormal.

Interventions

1. Suction the infant as necessary.

2. Take footprints, if not done previously (according to agency routine).

3. Administer antibiotic ointment to the eyes, and administer vitamin K injection. Note: Do not give vitamin K until after the bath or the leg is well cleaned if the mother is positive for hepatitis B or human immunodeficiency virus (HIV).

4. Allow the infant to rest quietly under a radiant warmer between assessments and care. When the initial assessment and procedures are completed and the temperature is stable, wrap the infant in two blankets, place a hat on the infant's head, and give the infant to the parents to hold.

5. When the temperature is stable, bathe the infant under a radiant warmer to remove blood and excess vernix. Keep the infant warm by drying as quickly as possible and removing wet linens. Dry the hair thoroughly to prevent heat loss.

6. Assist the mother with the initial feeding. If the infant is formula fed, give no more than 1 oz. Burp the infant halfway through the feeding.

7. Watch continuously for circumoral or central cyanosis, or lack of breathing during sucking. Stop the feeding, suction with a bulb syringe, and stimulate the infant by rubbing the back. Continue feeding when the infant has regained color. Place the infant on the right side with a rolled diaper behind the back after feeding, or elevate the head of the bed slightly.

8. Complete a gestational age assessment.

9. Prepare for transfer from the radiant warmer to a crib if all assessments are normal. Place clothing and blankets under the warmer to heat. Take the last set of vital signs, dress the infant, apply a hat, and wrap the infant in two warmed blankets. Complete all charting.

10. Give report if another nurse is taking over care of the infant. Include gravida, para, length of labor, medications and anesthesia used in labor and delivery, time of rupture of membranes, any complications during birth, any problems in the early hours, feeding, voids and stools, and any other pertinent information.

THE NEWBORN: CONTINUED CARE

Text to Prepare You for Clinical Practice

Procedure 21-3: Identifying infants
Box 21-1: Precautions to prevent infant abductions
Parents Want to Know: Caring for the uncircumcised penis
Parents Want to Know: How to care for the circumcision site

New Terms

Erythema toxicum
Hypoglycemia
Nonshivering thermogenesis

Equipment and Supplies

Stethoscope
Thermometer
Alcohol wipes

Normal Assessments

VITAL SIGNS

TEMPERATURE. Axillary 36.5° to 37.5° C (97.7° to 99.5° F).
HEART RATE. 120 to 160 beats/minute.
RESPIRATIONS. 30 to 60 breaths/minute.

BLOOD GLUCOSE

Above 40 to 45 mg/dl by screening tests (according to agency policy).

Nursing Care

Assess and care for infants using the following list as a guide. Keep in mind that the role of the nurse is to continue to observe for abnormalities and complications, as well as to assess progress of mother-infant bonding and the mother's ability to care for the infant.

Assessments

1. *Vital signs.* Assess vital signs once every 8 hours and more often if any abnormalities are present. Before disturbing a sleeping infant, check the respirations and pulse rate. Temperature should be stable after the first day; if not, action is needed. Continue to listen for abnormal heart sounds. Murmurs heard earlier may disappear after the first day as transition to neonatal circulation becomes complete. Note acrocyanosis or central cyanosis. Breath sounds should be clear.

2. *Weight.* Weigh infants daily at the same time of day according to agency routine.

3. *Neurologic.* Note the state of alertness (six stages), movement of extremities, and reflexes (especially Moro, rooting, suck). Observe the eyes for signs of inflammation (redness, drainage); may result from a reaction to eye medication or infection. Cleanse drainage with sterile water from the inner to outer canthus, ensuring that drainage from one eye does not contaminate the other. Watch for signs of hypoglycemia (jitteriness, tremors). Check fontanel with the infant in an upright position. It should be soft and flat. *Report fullness, bulging, depression.*

4. *Skin.* Assess all skin areas to observe for new marks or changes in existing ones. Compare with previous assessments. Expect the skin to be dry and peeling. Look for redness, scratches (keep hands covered), rashes, signs of

skin breakdown, and infection. Erythema toxicum may become more apparent. Resolution of caput succedaneum may occur as early as 12 hours or may take several days. Cephalhematoma resolves in several weeks. Physiologic jaundice may begin to develop after the first 24 hours. Blanch the skin over the nose and bony prominences, and note the color and how far down the body the jaundice extends. Check the cord and base of the cord for redness, foul odor, and serosanguineous or purulent drainage. Note how well the cord is drying. Remove the clamp when the end of the cord is dry and crisp (about 24 hours).

5. *Musculoskeletal.* Note the movement of extremities and muscle tone. The infant should resist when the extremities are extended. Note stiffness, arching of the infant's back, or molding of the infant to the caregiver's body.

6. *Gastrointestinal.* The abdomen should be soft and bowel sounds present. If the mother is giving all feedings, observe at least a part of several feedings. Ask the mother how she feels the feedings are going. Assess for suck and swallow coordination, choking, length of time the feeding lasts, amount taken, and any regurgitation. Note the type and number of stools. Know whether the infant has had a stool during the current shift and when the last stool occurred. (The first stool is generally passed within 12 to 48 hours of birth.)

7. *Genitourinary.* Note the number of voidings and the color of urine on diapers. Know whether the infant has voided on the present shift and when the last voiding occurred. Teach the parents to expect at least two to six wet diapers per day during the first 2 days of life and 6 to 10 wet diapers per day thereafter. (The first voiding should occur within 12 to 24 hours.) Observe the circumcision site for drainage (purulent, serous, sanguineous, frank bleeding, or oozing). Determine whether the infant is voiding after a circumcision is performed.

8. *Bonding.* Observe bonding behaviors in the mother and infant. Note how the mother holds the infant, whether she talks to the infant, calls the infant by name, and so on. Note response of the infant to the mother's care.

9. *Teaching.* Assess in which areas the mother (or the parents) need teaching.

Interventions

The following care of the infant is typical for every shift. In addition, make rounds frequently (at least every hour) to monitor the mother's progress in infant care and determine the need for further interventions.

1. *Cord care.* Care for the cord according to agency policy. Some units apply nothing to the cord or use triple dye or other bactericidal agents once daily. If alcohol is used, apply it to the cord once each shift. Use an alcohol wipe or an applicator dipped in alcohol to cleanse all parts of the cord and the crevices of the umbilicus. Avoid the skin around the cord because alcohol is drying to the skin. Fold the diaper below the cord.

2. *Care of the circumcision site.* Assess the parent's knowledge of care of the circumcision site, and teach as necessary. If a Plastibell was used, no special care is necessary other than observation for complications. If a Gomco clamp was used, instruct parents to squeeze petroleum jelly liberally over the circumcision site (and apply gauze if part of agency routine) at each diaper change for the first 24 hours. Assess the incision throughout the shift for redness, edema, purulent or sanguineous drainage, and odor.

3. *Identification.* If the mother and infant are separated at any time, use the proper identification process each time the infant is reunited with the mother.

4. *Protection.* Maintain vigilance against kidnappers at all times. Follow agency procedures to provide for infant security.

5. *Feedings.* Determine whether the infant is taking feedings adequately (every 2 to 3 hours if breastfed, every 3 to 4 hours if formula fed). Record each feeding including the type, the amount (or how long the infant nursed at each breast), how feedings are taken, and any regurgitation. Teach the parents as necessary.

6. *Elimination.* Record each wet diaper and stool. Note the color, amount, and consistency.

7. *Continue observation.* Observe for problems throughout the shift.

8. *Continue teaching.* Provide additional parent teaching as needed along with the "scheduled" teaching that was planned at the beginning of the shift.

ASSISTING THE INEXPERIENCED BREASTFEEDING MOTHER

Text to Prepare You for Clinical Practice

Table 22-1: The LATCH Scoring Tool
Box 22-2: Hunger cues in infants
Figure 22-3: Cradle hold
Figure 22-4: Football hold
Figure 22-5: Cross-cradle hold
Figure 22-6: Side-lying position
Figure 22-7: C position of hand on breast
Mothers Want to Know: Is my baby getting enough milk?
Mothers Want to Know: Solutions to common breastfeeding problems
Mothers Want to Know: Breastfeeding after the birth of more than one infant

New Terms

Latch-on
Nonnutritive suckling or sucking
Nutritive suckling or sucking

Normal Assessments

1. The infant is positioned facing the breast, and the infant's body is well supported.

2. The mother is comfortable and holds her breast so that the infant can take it into the mouth without interference.

3. The infant's mouth covers the nipple and as much of the areola as possible.
4. Suckling includes audible swallowing.

Nursing Care

This is a summary of information that nurses can use to help the inexperienced mother, especially during the first breastfeeding sessions.

Assessments

1. Assess the mother's knowledge about breastfeeding techniques.
2. Assess the mother's breasts to identify engorgement, flat or inverted nipples, or nipple trauma.
3. Assess the infant's behavior state, sucking reflex, and coordination of sucking and swallowing.

Interventions

1. Plan with the mother when the infant will be fed, and note any questions or concerns that she has about breastfeeding. Be sure that she is comfortable (pain relief needs met) and not in the middle of other care (hygiene, meals). However, if the infant must eat immediately because of concerns about hypoglycemia, meet the mother's needs quickly or postpone her care and help her begin the feeding.
2. Explain that breastfeeding is a learned skill for both the mother and the infant and that practice is required to perfect the skill.
3. Begin the feeding when the infant is awake and showing signs of hunger. Do not wait until the infant is ravenously hungry and upset.
4. Assist the mother to position herself and the infant. Use pillows or blankets for comfort, to protect an abdominal incision, and to raise the infant to nipple level.
   a. *Sitting.* Place the bed in a high Fowler's position. Position pillows behind the mother's back and under her elbow to support her arm.
   b. *Cradle hold.* Place the infant in the mother's arms, with the head at the antecubital space (or at nipple level) and the mother's arm extending along the infant's body. The mother's other hand positions the breast. The infant should be totally on the side facing the breast so that turning of the head is not necessary.
   c. *Cross cradle hold.* The mother holds the infant's head in the hand opposite the breast to be used and supports the infant's body across her lap with the arm. She supports the breast with the hand on the same side as the breast. The infant is turned to the side and facing the breast.
   d. *Football hold.* Place the infant's head in the mother's hand, with the body along her side supported by pillows or blankets.
   e. *Side-lying.* Place pillows behind the mother's back and between her legs. Her lower arm may go under her head or around the infant, while her upper hand positions the breast. Place the infant on the side facing the breast, using pillows to pad the side rails and to maintain the position.
5. Demonstrate the proper hand position, with the hand cupped around the breast, the thumb on top, and the fingers supporting the breast below. Keep the fingers and thumb behind the areola.
6. Elicit latch-on. Brush the nipple against the center of the infant's lips until the infant opens the mouth wide. Bring the infant toward the breast while inserting the nipple and as much of the areola as possible into the infant's mouth.
7. Assess the mouth position. The infant's lips should be 1 to 1½ inches from the base of the nipple with the lips flared. Remove the infant from the breast and start over if the cheeks dimple or clicking or smacking sounds occur.
8. Assess the infant's suck. Nutritive suckling is smooth and continuous with occasional pauses. A swallow follows every one to three sucks and has a "ka" or "ah" sound. Nonnutritive suckling is choppy with no swallowing. Do not jiggle the breast in the infant's mouth to stimulate suckling or the infant may lose the grip and chew on the nipple.
9. When swallowing stops and doesn't resume shortly, remove the infant from the breast and burp the infant, change sides, awaken, or let the infant sleep if the feeding is finished.
10. Demonstrate removal from the breast. Have the mother insert a finger into the corner of the infant's mouth between the gums to release suction. Remove the infant immediately.
11. Instruct the mother to nurse approximately 15 minutes on each breast per feeding. Burp the infant between breasts. Instruct her to nurse every 2 to 3 hours during the day and at least every 4 hours throughout the night to build the milk supply.
12. Observe the mother at intervals after the feeding begins. Help her switch sides to observe for difficulty. Then observe the mother at other feedings to give reinforcement and correct technique as needed. Offer praise generously because feeding the infant may affect the mother's view of her mothering abilities.

Answers to Check Your Reading

CHAPTER 1

1. High rates of maternal and infant mortality among poor women led to federal programs to improve the health of mothers, infants, and young children. Distribution of health care remains inequitable between poor women and more affluent women because many physicians practice in an area in which payment for care is more certain.

2. Family-centered maternity care provides safe, quality care that adapts to both the physical and the psychological needs of the entire family during reproduction and greatly increases the responsibilities of nurses providing care.

3. Birthing centers provide professional care during pregnancy and childbirth in a homelike environment for women with low-risk pregnancies. They are associated with a nearby hospital to which the woman can be transferred in case of unexpected complications. Although the home setting provides comfort and closeness, it may not have adequate equipment or personnel to handle unexpected developments. Family members and friends must assist with care of other children, the mother, and her new infant. LDR and LDRP rooms offer a comfortable setting that promotes family involvement for birth but within the hospital, where emergencies can be handled more easily.

4. Cost-containment strategies have shortened the length of stay in the birth facility for mothers and their infants. This has created concern for nurses, who must provide information for fatigued parents in a very short time. Nurses can also use the demand for cost containment to develop innovative programs for family education.

5. Clinical pathways are guidelines that define expected outcomes for clients, including the length of stay and the time and sequence of interventions that will accomplish the outcomes.

6. A variety of standards guide both agency and community care for perinatal nurses. Standards include agency and organizational standards that spell out the prepara-

tion, responsibilities, and actions of nurses. Legal standards define the scope of practice, and other regulatory bodies such as OSHA, CDC, and FDA provide guidelines. Accrediting agencies such as JCAHO and CHAP give approval when standards reach a certain level.

7. Safety is the major concern with the use of complementary and alternative medicine because these modalities are largely unregulated. Additionally, clients usually refer themselves to practitioners and may either delay care from a conventional health care provider or may not tell the conventional provider about substances they are taking that may be harmful when combined with other medications. Some organic substances have active pharmacologic ingredients of varying strengths.

8. Traditional families are headed by a man and a woman, usually married, who view parenting as the major priority in their lives and whose energies are not depleted by poverty, illness, or substance abuse. Nontraditional families are defined by their unique structure and include single-parent families, blended families, extended families, same-sex parent families, and adoptive families.

9. Families may be identified as high risk if they are below the poverty level; are headed by a single teenage parent; have a preterm, ill, or disabled infant; or have lifestyle problems such as substance abuse or family violence.

10. A healthy family can adapt without undue stress to the changes precipitated by childbirth. Members communicate openly, are flexible in role assignment, agree on the basic principles of parenting, are adaptable to change, and volunteer assistance to aid family members.

11. Factors that interfere with family functioning include lack of family resources, absence of adequate family support, birth of an infant who requires specialized care, unhealthy habits (such as smoking and substance abuse), and the inability to make mature decisions.

12. Nurses should examine their own cultural values and beliefs to determine ways in which their beliefs may

generate conflict with those who hold different cultural beliefs.

13. Differences in language create the greatest difficulty; however, differences in communication style or knowledge about the dominant family member may result in conflicts.

14. Culture is difficult to understand because, like an iceberg, only the tip (the behavior) is visible. Reasons for the behavior (for example, religious beliefs, and moral values) are hidden, much like the submerged part of an iceberg, requiring study.

15. The infant mortality rate is lower today than in the early 1900s because of improved neonatal care, public awareness of preventive measures such as those to prevent SIDS, and availability of prenatal care, including at public clinics.

16. The higher incidence of poverty among African-Americans is associated with inadequate prenatal care and the birth of premature or low-birth-weight infants with short-term or long-term health problems.

17. With regard to infant mortality rate, the United States ranks twenty-eighth among developed nations.

CHAPTER 2

1. Therapeutic communication is purposeful, goal directed, and focused.

2. Major communication techniques include clarifying, paraphrasing, reflecting, silence, structuring, pinpointing, questioning, directing, and summarizing.

3. Major blocks to communication include conveying a lack of interest or haste, displaying a closed posture, interrupting, providing false reassurance, offering inappropriate self-disclosure, giving advice, and failing to acknowledge comments or feelings.

4. Major principles of teaching and learning include readiness to learn, participation, repetition, positive feedback, and acknowledgment of frustration. Effective methods include role modeling, presenting simple tasks before more complex material, and using a variety of teaching methods.

5. Factors that affect learning include developmental level, language, culture, previous experience, physical environment, and the organization and skill of the teacher.

6. Nursing practice based on the best evidence available rather than tradition or intuition is now an expectation for producing the most effective and efficient patient outcomes.

7. The purpose of critical thinking is to identify and overcome habits or impulses that result in poor decisions or inappropriate actions and to make the best clinical judgments.

8. Steps that may be helpful in learning critical thinking can be organized into an "ABCDE" pattern. They include recognizing assumptions, examining possible personal biases, determining the need for closure, developing the ability to collect, organize, and analyze data in an expert manner, and acknowledging how emotions or environmental factors may interfere with the ability to think critically.

9. Reflective skepticism means to suspend judgment to avoid making decisions in haste or with insufficient data.

10. The screening assessment gathers information about all aspects of the client's health. The focused assessment gathers information about an actual health problem or one for which the client appears to have a higher risk. A client's desire to improve health may be identified during both types of assessment.

11. Actual nursing diagnoses reflect health problems that can be validated by the presence of defining characteristics. Risk nursing diagnoses indicate that risk factors are present that make the client vulnerable to the development of a particular problem that has not yet developed.

12. The terms *goals* and *expected outcomes* (outcome criteria) are often used interchangeably to describe desired endpoints of care, but they are different. Broad goals do not have the specific criteria of outcome criteria. Expected outcomes should (1) be stated in terms of the client, (2) be observable and measurable, (3) have a time frame, (4) be realistic, and (5) be worked out with the client and family.

13. Nursing interventions that are not specific and do not spell out exactly what is to be done are difficult to implement. Clearly written interventions that provide detailed, objective instructions correct the problem.

14. Nursing diagnoses describe health problems that nurses can treat independently and for which they are accountable. Collaborative problems are potential complications that nurses do not treat independently but with physicians or advanced practice nurses such as certified nurse-midwives and nurse-practitioners.

15. Client-centered goals or expected outcomes are inappropriate for collaborative problems because they imply accountability for problems that nurses cannot manage independently.

CHAPTER 3

1. Ethics examines conduct and distinctions between right and wrong. Bioethics applies specifically to the ethics of health care.

2. Deontologic theory applies ethical principles to determine what is right. It does not vary the solution according to individual situations. Utilitarian theory analyzes the benefits and burdens to determine a course of action that provides the greatest amount of good in a given situation.

3. Ethical principles may conflict when the application of one principle violates another.

4. Assessment is used to gather data from all concerned persons. Ethical theories and principles are analyzed to determine whether an ethical dilemma exists. Planning involves identifying as many options as possible and choosing a so-

lution. Interventions must be identified to implement the chosen solution, and the results are evaluated.

5. The Supreme Court decision in *Roe v. Wade* declared that abortion was legal anywhere in the United States and that existing state laws prohibiting abortion were unconstitutional because they interfered with a woman's right to privacy.

6. The belief that abortion is a private choice conflicts with the belief that abortion is taking a life.

7. States cannot give a husband veto power over his spouse's decision to have an abortion; states do not have an obligation to pay for abortions, physicians are given broad discretion to determine fetal viability, and states may restrict abortions of viable fetuses. In addition, states may require parental consent for minors to obtain abortion if an alternative (e.g., judge's approval) is available, states may require a woman to wait 24 hours before seeking and obtaining an abortion, and states may not require a married woman to inform her husband before obtaining an abortion.

8. At the time they are employed, nurses must disclose their beliefs about caring for women having an abortion. Nurses must inform a supervisor so that appropriate care can be arranged.

9. Punitive approaches are against the ethical principles of autonomy, bodily integrity, and personal freedom. Although the intended plan may be to protect the fetus, such a plan can have unexpected outcomes, causing the woman to avoid prenatal care or be dishonest with care providers, causing greater harm to her fetus.

10. Problems involved in the use of advanced reproductive techniques include high cost, low success rate, limitation to the affluent, control of unused embryos, and problem or unexpected pregnancy outcomes. Another issue is that the offspring born after menopause are more likely to be orphaned than those of younger mothers.

11. Poverty is the underlying factor that causes problems such as inadequate access to health care. The lack of access to health care is a major reason for the large number of low-birth-weight infants and the high infant mortality rate.

12. The Balanced Budget Act of 1997 has further reduced income from Medicare and Medicaid (a major source of funding for most health care facilities). This requires an even greater conservation of funds. Its emphasis on disease prevention provides a positive challenge for nurses.

13. The focus has long been on treatment and cure of illness, often with expensive technology. However, prevention is less expensive and provides care for greater numbers of people.

14. State boards of nursing administer the individual states' nurse practice acts, which establish what the nurse is allowed and expected to do when practicing nursing in that state.

15. Standards of care and agency policies influence judgment about malpractice because they describe the level of care that can be expected from practitioners.

16. Nursing actions that help defend malpractice claims include securing informed consent appropriately, keeping documentation that provides evidence that the standard of care has been maintained, acting appropriately as a client advocate in terms of taking a problem through the chain of command, and maintaining expertise.

17. Concerns about the use of unlicensed assistive personnel include whether this use compromises the quality of care and the nurse's ability to supervise unlicensed personnel adequately with high workloads.

18. Short lengths of stay lead to concerns about the woman's ability to care for herself and her infant, potential complications that new parents may not identify, and the fact that parents will not have had time to absorb the necessary teaching. Follow-up phone calls help alleviate some concerns and identify some problems that develop after discharge.

19. Facilities that use phone-call triage must have regularly reviewed and updated protocols, good documentation forms, and specific instructions to the client about actions to take if further problems develop.

CHAPTER 4

1. Development of the breasts is the first sign of puberty in girls. In boys, growth of the testes is the first sign, followed by growth of the penis about 1 year later.

2. Usually, Asians and Native Americans have less and finer body hair than either whites or African-Americans. African-Americans usually have body hair that is coarser and curlier than Asians, Native Americans, or whites.

3. The female pelvis has a wide, rounded, basinlike shape that favors efficient passage of the fetus during birth. The male pelvis is heavier and narrower and structurally suited for tasks requiring load bearing.

4. Males generally attain a greater adult height than females because they begin their growth spurt about 1 year later than girls and continue growing for a longer period of time.

5. Female secondary sex characteristics include round hips and breasts and pubic hair, finer skin texture, and a higher-pitched voice. Male secondary sex characteristics include facial and pubic hair, a deeper voice, broader shoulders, and greater muscle mass.

6. The female external reproductive organs are collectively called the *vulva*. The labia majora extend from the mons pubis to the perineum. The labia minora are within and parallel to the labia majora. The clitoris is at the anterior junction of the labia minora. The urinary meatus and vaginal introitus are found within the vestibule (the area enclosed by the labia minora). The hymen partially closes the vaginal opening. The perineum extends from the fourchette (posterior rim of the vaginal opening) to the anus.

7. The three divisions of the uterus are the corpus (body), isthmus, and cervix (neck). The uterine fundus is the

part of the corpus that lies above the entry points of the fallopian tubes.

8. The myometrium is the middle layer of thick uterine muscle between the perimetrium and endometrium. The myometrium includes three types of muscle fibers: (1) longitudinal fibers, mostly in the fundus, to expel the fetus during birth; (2) interlacing figure-eight fibers to compress bleeding blood vessels after birth; and (3) circular fibers to provide constrictions near the fallopian tubes and the internal cervical os, enabling the proper implantation of the fertilized ovum and preventing the reflux of menstrual blood into the fallopian tubes.

9. The fallopian tubes are lined with cells with cilia that beat rhythmically toward the uterine cavity to propel the ovum through the fallopian tube. The fertilized ovum undergoes its early cell divisions in the fallopian tube so that implantation is most likely to occur in the uterine fundus.

10. The two functions of the ovaries are to produce hormones (primarily estrogen and progesterone) and mature an ovum for release during each reproductive cycle.

11. The pelvis is located at the lower end of the spine. The true pelvis is located below the linea terminalis. The true pelvis is the most relevant during birth.

12. Pelvic muscles enclose the lower pelvis and support internal reproductive, urinary, and bowel structures. Ligaments maintain internal reproductive organs and their nerve and blood supplies in the proper positions in the pelvis.

13. The ripening follicle secretes estrogen to form new endometrial epithelium and endometrial glands. After ovulation, the follicle (now called the *corpus luteum*) secretes large amounts of estrogen to continue thickening of the endometrium and progesterone to cause the endometrium to secrete substances to nourish a fertilized ovum.

14. Three ovarian phases of the female reproductive cycle are the follicular (maturation of an ovum), ovulatory (release of the mature ovum), and luteal (secretion of estrogen and progesterone by the corpus luteum). The length of the follicular phase varies more among women than the other two phases.

15. The three phases are the proliferative, secretory, and menstrual phases. The proliferative phase occurs during the first half of the cycle, during which the endometrium thickens in preparation for a fertilized ovum. The secretory phase occurs during the second half of the cycle and is characterized by continued growth of the endometrium, growth of blood vessels and glands, and secretion of substances to nourish a fertilized ovum. If pregnancy does not occur, the endometrium becomes ischemic and necrotic as secretion of estrogen and progesterone from the corpus luteum falls. The old endometrium is shed in the menstrual phase.

16. The cervical mucus becomes thin, clear, and elastic during ovulation to facilitate entrance of sperm from the vagina into the uterus and fallopian tube, thereby enhancing the chances for conception.

17. Montgomery's tubercles secrete a substance during pregnancy and lactation that keeps the nipples soft.

18. A woman's breast size is not related to the amount of milk she can produce. Breast size is influenced by the amount of fatty tissue in the breast.

19. Milk secretion does not occur during pregnancy because estrogen and progesterone produced by the placenta inhibit its production. Estrogen and progesterone stimulate the growth of the alveoli and ductal system during pregnancy.

20. As a urinary organ the penis transports urine from the bladder to outside the body during urination. As a reproductive organ, it carries and deposits semen into the vagina during coitus.

21. The two types of erectile tissue in the penis are the corpus spongiosum that surrounds the urethra and the two columns of corpus cavernosum tissue on each side of the penis. The function of erectile tissue is to facilitate entry of the penis into the female's vagina.

22. The scrotum holds the testes away from the body to keep them cooler than the core body temperature, thus facilitating sperm production.

23. The testes function as endocrine glands to produce testosterone and the male gametes (spermatozoa).

CHAPTER 5

1. DNA is the building block of genes. A varying number of genes makes up each chromosome.

2. Genes are too small to be seen under a microscope. They can be studied by analysis of the products they instruct cells to produce, by direct study of the DNA, or through their close association with another gene that can be studied by one of these other methods.

3. Chromosomes can be seen under a microscope when living nucleated cells are dividing. Cell division during the metaphase is a common time for analysis because each chromosome is compact. Fluorescent *in situ* hybridization (FISH) identifies chromosomal abnormalities in more than one stage of cell division, allowing rapid test results. Spectral karyotyping (SKY) assigns a color to each chromosome to better identify rearrangements and small additions or deletions of chromosomal material that may cause abnormalities.

4. *46,XY* describes the chromosome makeup of a normal human male. *46,XX* describes the chromosomes of a normal human female. Abnormalities are described beginning with the total number of chromosomes, followed by the sex chromosome complement, and followed by the abbreviation that describes the chromosome abnormality.

5. The child of a parent with an autosomal dominant disorder has a 50% chance of having the same disorder.

6. Blood relationship (consanguinity) of parents increases the likelihood that both share some of the same harm-

ful autosomal recessive genes, increasing the chance that their offspring will be affected with a disorder. The closer the parents' blood relationship, the more genes they are likely to share.

7. If both parents carry an abnormal gene for an autosomal recessive disorder, each child has a 25% chance of receiving both copies of the defective gene and having the disorder. Each child also has a 50% chance of receiving only one copy of the defective gene and being a carrier like the parents. Each child also has a 25% chance of receiving the normal gene from each parent, thereby being neither a carrier nor affected and having no chance of passing the gene to future generations.

8. Males are more likely to have X-linked recessive disorders because they do not have a compensating X chromosome with a normal gene. Each son of a female carrier has a 50% chance of having the trait and a 50% chance of being unaffected. Each daughter of the female carrier has a 50% chance of being a carrier and a 50% chance of being unaffected.

9. A trisomy exists when each body cell contains an extra copy of one chromosome. Down syndrome is the most common trisomy and involves three copies of chromosome 21, for a total of 47 chromosomes in each cell.

10. A monosomy exists when each body cell is missing a chromosome. Turner's syndrome (a female with a single X chromosome) is the only monosomy compatible with postnatal life.

11. Genetic material can be lost or duplicated when a chromosome has a structural abnormality. Also, the position of genes on the chromosome may be altered, preventing them from functioning normally.

12. A parent with a balanced chromosomal translocation may have a child with completely normal chromosomes, or the child may have a balanced chromosomal translocation like that of the parent. The offspring may also receive an unbalanced amount of chromosomal material (too much or too little), which often results in spontaneous abortion or birth defects.

13. Multifactorial disorders are typically present and detectable at birth. They are usually isolated defects rather than being present with other unrelated defects. However, sometimes the primary multifactorial defect alters further development and results in other related defects.

14. Factors that may affect the likelihood that a multifactorial disorder will occur or recur include the following: the number of affected close relatives, severity of the defect in those affected, gender of the affected person, geographic location, and seasonal variations.

15. The woman may be able to prevent exposing her fetus to teratogens by being immunized against infections such as rubella at least 28 days (1 month) before pregnancy, eliminating the use of nontherapeutic drugs such as alcohol and illicit drugs, changing therapeutic drugs to those having a lower risk to the fetus, and avoiding radiation exposure when she may be pregnant.

16. A pregnant woman who has phenylketonuria should return to her low-phenylalanine diet when she is pregnant to prevent buildup of toxic products that would damage the developing fetus.

17. Adequate folic acid intake of at least 0.4 mg (400 mcg) has been associated with a lower incidence of neural tube defects. Because the neural tube begins closure at 4 weeks' gestation, the woman should have adequate intake beginning before conception to ensure the best outcome.

CHAPTER 6

1. Meiosis is a type of cell division that halves the number of chromosomes so that only one of each chromosomal pair goes into each gamete. Meiosis also promotes genetic variation by the process of crossing over, or exchange of chromosomal material between each member of the pair of chromosomes. The union of male and female gametes at conception restores the number of chromosomes to 46 in the offspring.

2. Each oogonium produces one mature ovum after two meiotic divisions. The first meiotic division begins in fetal life and is not completed until shortly before that ovum undergoes ovulation. The second meiotic division begins at ovulation but is not completed unless fertilization occurs.

3. Each spermatogonium undergoes two meiotic divisions to result in four mature spermatozoa. Meiosis begins at puberty, and both meiotic divisions are completed before the sperm mature and are ejaculated.

4. Fertilization usually occurs in the distal third of the fallopian tube (the ampulla), near the ovary.

5. Seminal fluid nourishes and protects the sperm from the acidic environment of the woman's vagina.

6. As sperm approach the ovum, they secrete hyaluronidase to digest a pathway through the corona radiata and zona pellucida. When one spermatozoon finally penetrates the ovum, changes in the zona pellucida prevent other spermatozoa from entering. The cell membranes of the ovum and sperm fuse to allow the sperm to penetrate the ovum. The ovum also completes its second meiotic division.

7. Fertilization is complete when the nuclei of the ovum and spermatozoon unite.

8. Implantation begins 6 days after conception and is complete by the tenth day.

9. The upper uterus is the ideal location for implantation for three reasons: (1) it has a rich blood supply for fetal gas exchange and nutrition, (2) the thick uterine lining prevents the placenta from attaching too deeply, and (3) the strong interlacing muscle fibers contract to limit blood loss after birth.

10. Nutritive fluids produced in the thick decidua pass to the conceptus by diffusion before a placental circulation is established. Primary chorionic villi, which will form the fetal side of the placenta, extend from the con-

ceptus into the decidua basalis, which will become the maternal side of the placenta, to tap these nutrients.

11. During the first 8 weeks after conception, all major organ systems develop. The woman may be unaware that she is pregnant and may inadvertently expose the embryo to harmful substances. These substances may damage organs that are developing.

12. At 4 weeks the trachea develops as a bud of the upper digestive tract. After the trachea separates from the upper digestive tract, it branches into the two bronchi, which then divide to form the three lobes of the right lung and the two lobes of the left. Branching continues until terminal air sacs develop.

13. The intestines are contained mostly within the umbilical cord until 10 weeks because they grow more rapidly than the abdominal cavity and the liver and kidneys are relatively large. By 10 weeks after conception, the abdominal cavity has caught up with the growth of its contents and can accommodate them.

14. Gestational age is calculated from the woman's last menstrual period and is about 2 weeks longer than fertilization age. Gestational age is most commonly used because the menstrual period provides a specific marker.

15. The fetus usually assumes a head-down position because this position best fits the egg shape of the uterus. Also, the head is heavier and tends to go downward with gravity in the pool of amniotic fluid.

16. Vernix caseosa protects fetal skin from constant exposure to amniotic fluid. Lanugo helps vernix adhere to the skin. Brown fat helps the infant maintain temperature stability in the cooler external environment. Surfactant keeps the lung alveoli from collapsing with each expiration, thus making breathing easier after birth.

17. The placenta gradually takes over the function of the corpus luteum and secretes estrogen and progesterone.

18. Exchange of oxygen, nutrients, and waste products between the woman and fetus takes place in the intervillous spaces of the placenta.

19. Maternal and fetal blood may be of incompatible blood types and thus should not mix.

20. The fetus can thrive in a relatively low-oxygen environment because of the following:
    a. Fetal hemoglobin carries more oxygen than adult hemoglobin.
    b. The fetus has a higher hemoglobin and hematocrit level than does the newborn or adult.
    c. Rapid diffusion of carbon dioxide into the maternal blood causes the mother to give up oxygen more readily and causes oxygen to combine with fetal blood more readily.

21. Human chorionic gonadotropin (hCG) causes the corpus luteum of the ovary to persist and secrete estrogens and progesterones, which are essential to maintain the uterine lining for implantation. It also facilitates fetal testosterone secretion in the male fetus. Human placental lactogen promotes normal fetal nutrition and growth and maternal breast development. Estrogens cause enlargement of the woman's uterus and genitalia and enlargement and development of the breasts. Progesterone maintains the secretory endometrium and changes the endometrium into the decidua to nourish the conceptus and reduces uterine contractions to prevent spontaneous abortion. Progesterone facilitates growth and development of the mother's breasts and the cells that will secrete milk. Progesterone may allow immune tolerance of the conceptus.

22. The fetal membranes contain the amniotic fluid that cushions the fetus and circulation within the umbilical cord, maintains a stable temperature, and promotes normal prenatal structural development.

23. Oxygenated blood enters the fetus through the umbilical vein. Half the blood goes to the liver, and the rest passes through the ductus venosus to the inferior vena cava. Blood enters the right atrium, where a small amount goes to the right ventricle and the rest goes through the foramen ovale to the left atrium and then to the left ventricle. Some blood from the right ventricle goes to the lungs to nourish their tissue, and the rest goes through the ductus arteriosus, where it joins blood ejected from the left ventricle. After circulation through the body, deoxygenated blood returns to the placenta through the two umbilical arteries.

24. Monozygotic twins are conceived when one spermatozoon fertilizes one ovum and the resulting conceptus later divides into two inner cell masses that will become two fetuses.

25. The placentas and chorions may fuse before birth, making it difficult to determine whether the twins are monozygotic or dizygotic.

26. Dizygotic twins develop from two ova that are each fertilized by a spermatozoon and are like other siblings in a family.

CHAPTER 7

1. By 16 weeks the fundus is midway between the symphysis and the umbilicus. At 20 weeks' gestation, the uterus generally reaches the level of the umbilicus. By 36 weeks, the uterus extends to the xiphoid process, the highest level of uterine growth.

2. In early pregnancy, blood flow in the uterus is mainly to the endometrium and myometrium. As pregnancy progresses, there is an increase in blood flow into intervillous spaces of the placenta to provide oxygen and nutrients to the fetus and remove wastes.

3. The cervical mucus plug blocks ascent of bacteria from the vagina into the uterus, thereby protecting the membranes and the fetus from possible infection.

4. The major purpose of progesterone in early pregnancy is to stop contractions and help prevent fetal tissue rejection.

5. During pregnancy the breasts enlarge and become more vascular; the areolae increase in size and become more

pigmented; the nipples enlarge and become more erect; and Montgomery's tubercles become more prominent.

6. Expanded blood volume is needed for the added maternal tissues of pregnancy, to provide blood flow to the placenta, and to allow for loss of blood at childbirth.

7. Physiologic anemia of pregnancy is caused by a greater increase in plasma volume than in red blood cells, resulting in a dilution but not inadequate hematocrit concentration. Iron deficiency anemia is caused by a true lack of iron that affects hemoglobin levels.

8. It is important to standardize techniques for taking blood pressure because blood pressure in the pregnant woman is affected by position. It is lowest in a lateral recumbent position. If all staff do not use the same Korotkoff's sound, readings from one measurement to another cannot be compared accurately.

9. With the supine position, the weight of the uterus on the vena cava and descending aorta impedes blood flow to and from the lower extremities, resulting in decreased cardiac output and a supine hypotensive syndrome.

10. During pregnancy, increased circulation through the kidneys is needed to remove metabolic wastes generated by the mother and fetus. Increased circulation through the skin is necessary to dissipate heat that is generated by accelerated metabolism.

11. Progesterone causes slight hyperventilation and increases sensitivity of the respiratory center to carbon dioxide leading to a feeling of dyspnea.

12. Flaring of the ribs, widening of the substernal angle, and increased circumference of the chest allow adequate intake of air with each breath.

13. Estrogen causes hyperemia of the gums that may lead to bleeding or gingivitis. Excessive salivation (ptyalism) is a problem for some. Progesterone relaxes smooth muscle in the gastrointestinal tract, which may increase time for nutrient absorption but may lead to heartburn and constipation.

14. Expectant mothers are at increased risk for urinary tract infection because compression of the ureters between the uterus and the pelvic bones causes dilation of the ureters and kidney pelvis and stasis of urine.

15. Softening of pelvic ligaments and joints because of relaxin and progesterone creates instability and results in a wide stance and "waddling" gait. Lordosis occurs when the large uterus causes the woman to lean backward to maintain her balance.

16. The hormones FSH and LH are suppressed during pregnancy to prevent ovulation. Progesterone maintains the endometrium and prevents contractions even though oxytocin is increased.

17. Maternal hormones create increasing resistance of maternal tissues to insulin during the second and third trimesters causing the mother to produce more insulin.

18. Most presumptive signs are subjective, and probable signs are objective; both can be caused by conditions other than pregnancy.

19. Many things such as gas, peristalsis, or pseudocyesis (false pregnancy) can be mistaken by the woman for fetal movement.

20. The most common causes of false-negative pregnancy tests are pregnancy tests performed too soon, urine that is too dilute, impending spontaneous abortion, ectopic pregnancy, and improper use of the test.

21. A preconception visit identifies factors that may cause harm to the fetus or the mother before pregnancy occurs so that steps can be taken to avoid problems.

22. A medical-surgical history and an obstetric history are necessary to identify chronic conditions or past difficulties that might affect the outcome of the pregnancy.

23. A gradual, predictable increase in uterine size occurs as gestation advances. From approximately 16 to 38 weeks, fundal height in centimeters is nearly equal to gestational age in weeks for a single fetus.

24. Major risk factors during pregnancy are age under 16 years, low socioeconomic status, previous problem pregnancies, preexisting medical disorders or infections, and use of substances such as alcohol, tobacco, or illicit drugs.

25. Antepartum visits should begin in the first trimester and continue every 4 weeks until 28 weeks, then every 2 to 3 weeks until 36 weeks, and weekly from 37 weeks to birth.

26. In multifetal pregnancies increased blood volume results in additional work for the heart of the mother. The greatly increased size of the uterus causes greater elevation of the diaphragm and more compression of the large vessels, ureters, and bowel.

27. Increased levels of placental hormones, such as estrogen and hCG, are believed to be responsible for "morning sickness."

28. Correct posture and body mechanics as well as exercises such as pelvic rocking can alleviate backache during pregnancy.

CHAPTER 8

1. The fetus seems vague and unreal during the first trimester. Gradually, physical changes (such as uterine growth, weight gain, quickening) confirm that a fetus is developing, and the expectant mother begins to perceive the fetus as a separate though dependent being.

2. Although sexual responses vary widely during pregnancy, the woman may have increased interest in the first trimester unless she has nausea or fears miscarriage. Interest is often increased in the second trimester because of pelvic vasocongestion and a general feeling of well-being. The discomforts of the third trimester may decrease sexual responsiveness. Some expectant fathers are more interested in sex during pregnancy, but others find the pregnant woman unattractive and fear harming the fetus.

3. The pregnant woman explores the role of mother to develop a sense of herself in the role and selects behaviors that confirm her idea of fulfilling the role.

4. The pregnant woman often experiences a temporary sense of sadness when she realizes she must give up certain aspects of her previous self when she moves into the role of mother.

5. The pregnant woman seeks safe passage for herself and the baby when she seeks the care of a physician or nurse-midwife and follows recommendations about diet, vitamins, rest, and subsequent prenatal care.

6. Experiences that make the child more real serve as reality boosters and include hearing the fetal heart, feeling the fetus move, and seeing the fetus via ultrasound.

7. Nurses can help men gain recognition as parents by focusing on the father as well as the mother, encouraging the father's questions, and including him in the plan of care.

8. Information about infant behavior and care is more relevant and therefore more useful after the infant is born.

9. Some factors that shape the way grandparents respond to a grandchild are their own ages, the number and spacing of other grandchildren, and their perceptions of their role as grandparents.

10. Toddlers do not understand that a birth is expected and should be told shortly before the expected date. Preschoolers may like to be involved and to help prepare for the birth. Adolescents may be embarrassed by evidence of their parents' sexuality.

11. Parents can make any changes in sleeping arrangements several weeks before the infant is born so that other children do not feel displaced by the newborn. They can increase time and attention to older children and reassure them of their love and acceptance.

12. Priorities of low income families often focus primarily on present needs such as food and shelter and focus less on preventive activities such as prenatal care.

13. Some health care workers are unsympathetic to the plights of indigent families, who experience long waits at understaffed health care facilities, hurried examinations, and rudeness.

14. Cultural differences that cause conflict between health care workers and families during pregnancy occur most often in the areas of health care beliefs, communication, and time orientation.

15. Cultural negotiation includes acknowledging that the family may hold different views, being sensitive to special concerns, and providing information in an acceptable manner.

CHAPTER 9

1. Weight gain helps determine fetal growth. Too little weight gain may be associated with low birth weight, and too much gain may be associated with large infants.

2. The average woman should gain 11.5 to 16 kg (25 to 35 lb). Underweight women and those carrying more than one fetus should gain more, and overweight women should gain less.

3. The average woman should gain approximately 1.6 kg (3.5 lb) the first trimester and 0.4 kg (0.88 lb) per week in the second and third trimesters.

4. Although no additional calories are needed during the first trimester, the recommendation for the second and third trimesters is 340 calories and 452 calories.

5. Approximately 71 g of protein per day, an increase of 25 g above prepregnancy needs, is recommended during pregnancy.

6. Vitamins B_6, D, E, and folic acid are likely to be low in the diets of pregnant women.

7. Fat-soluble vitamins (such as A, D, E, K) are stored in the fat and available longer than the water-soluble vitamins (such as B_6, B_{12}, folic acid, thiamin, riboflavin, niacin, C), which must be replenished daily. Excessive intake of fat-soluble vitamins may cause toxicity.

8. If all women consumed 400 mcg of folic acid daily, fewer infants would be born with neural tube defects because women would not be deficient in folic acid during the early weeks of pregnancy, during which time the neural tube is closing.

9. Iron, calcium, zinc, and magnesium are often below the recommended amounts in the diets of pregnant women.

10. Excessive intake of vitamins and minerals may result in toxicity and interfere with absorption of other vitamins and minerals.

11. During pregnancy a woman should drink at least eight 8-oz glasses of fluids (mostly water) daily.

12. During pregnancy the following servings of food are recommended: seven servings of whole grains, 2 cups (five or more servings) of fruits, 2½ cups (five servings) of vegetables, three or more servings of dairy products, servings equal to 7 oz of protein, and 6 teaspoons of saturated fats.

13. The nurse should consider traditional foods from the woman's culture, the degree to which she follows the traditional diet, and her inclusion of nontraditional foods in her diet.

14. Both Southeast Asian and Hispanic women balance yin and yang (cold and hot) foods during pregnancy and may have low intakes of calcium, iron, and vitamin D.

15. The nurse should assess the woman's financial resources for food purchase, need for financial assistance, and education about nutrition.

16. The adolescent may skip meals and vitamin-mineral supplements and eat snacks and fast foods of low nutrient value to be like her peers.

17. The vegan can include nonanimal sources of iron, calcium, and vitamin B_{12} and D and combine incomplete protein foods to ensure intake of all essential amino acids.

18. Lactose-intolerant women can choose calcium-containing foods like leafy green vegetables, broccoli, corn tortillas, tofu, sunflower seeds, nuts, salmon, and sardines.

19. Other conditions presenting nutritional risk factors during pregnancy are excessive nausea and vomiting, anemia, abnormal prepregnancy weight, eating disorders,

pica, grand multiparity, substance abuse, closely spaced pregnancies, and multifetal pregnancy.

20. The lactating woman needs more of most nutrients than the woman who is not pregnant. She needs 330 more calories than her nonpregnant needs during the first 6 months of lactation.

21. The breastfeeding woman should avoid alcohol, caffeine, and foods that seem to cause distress in the infant.

22. The woman who is not breastfeeding should decrease calories to her prepregnant level, continue to eat a well-balanced diet including enough protein and vitamin C, and plan to lose extra weight slowly.

CHAPTER 10

1. Major reasons for ultrasonography during the first trimester are to confirm pregnancy, verify gestational age, locate the fetus, determine multifetal pregnancy and fetal gestation, confirm fetal viability, identify markers that suggest fetal abnormalities, and identify and guide chorionic villus sampling (CVS). Indications during the second and third trimesters are to confirm fetal viability, gestational age, and growth; evaluate fetal anatomy, umbilical cord and vessels, and placenta; evaluate multifetal pregnancies; locate the placenta; determine fetal presentation; evaluate amniotic fluid volume; and guide needle placement for amniocentesis and umbilical cord sampling.

2. Transvaginal ultrasonography is most often performed during the first trimester, when the uterus lies within the pelvis. A transabdominal procedure is more common during the second and third trimesters, when the uterus is above the pelvic brim and the contents are clearly visible.

3. Major advantages of ultrasonography are that it allows clear visualization of the fetus and surrounding structures; it is safe, noninvasive, and relatively comfortable; and the results are available immediately. The major disadvantage is the cost. Also, ultrasonography may reveal findings that might indicate a problem but for which data are inadequate to make a clear diagnosis, thereby requiring further decisions by the woman and her support person.

4. MSAFP must be viewed as the first step in a series of diagnostic procedures offered if abnormal concentrations are found.

5. Elevated MSAFP may be caused by open neural tube defects, esophageal obstruction, open abdominal wall defects, and undetected fetal demise. Additional causes include multifetal gestation, inaccurate fetal age or maternal weight, maternal diabetes, and threatened abortion.

6. Low levels of AFP suggest chromosomal abnormalities or inaccurate gestational age and maternal weight. Gestational trophoblastic disease may also cause low AFP.

7. Multiple marker screening, often called triple marker screening or other names, determines maternal serum levels of AFP, hCG, and unconjugated estriols. Elevation of hCG with low levels of AFP and estriols suggest chromosome abnormalities. Further testing with amniocentesis to positively identify the fetal karyotype will be offered to the woman if triple marker screening is abnormal.

8. CVS is performed slightly sooner than even early amniocentesis, at 10 to 12 weeks' gestation. Obtaining information about fetal anomalies earlier in the pregnancy allows the woman to make a decision about pregnancy termination before the second trimester. CVS is more expensive than amniocentesis and does not provide amniotic fluid for analysis of AFP.

9. Pregnancy loss is slightly higher after CVS than after amniocentesis. The likelihood that chromosome findings will be questionable and lead to additional testing such as amniocentesis is greater.

10. Amniocentesis is most often performed to detect chromosomal abnormalities and other prenatally detectable genetic disorders or to identify if maternal sensitization to Rh-negative blood has affected the fetus. Additional indications include investigating abnormal levels of MSAFP, determining fetal lung maturity, and evaluating the fetus affected by Rh isoimmunization.

11. Fetal lung maturity is confirmed by a 2:1 ratio of lecithin/sphingomyelin and the presence of other lipoproteins such as PG and PI, which comprise pulmonary surfactant. A newer test evaluates the quantity of surfactant phospholipids relative to the quantity of albumin in the amniotic fluid.

12. The degree of bilirubin staining of amniotic fluid reflects the degree of erythrocyte destruction in an Rh-positive fetus whose mother is Rh-sensitized.

13. Early amniocentesis has the same advantage as CVS: information is available early in the pregnancy, allowing parents to make decisions about the pregnancy as early as possible.

14. A nonstress test (so called because the fetus is not challenged or stressed to obtain data) measures acceleration of the fetal heart in response to fetal movement. Acceleration, even without fetal movement felt by the mother, provides reassurance of fetal health.

15. In vibroacoustic stimulation, an artificial larynx is used to stimulate fetal movement and accelerations using sound and vibrations. Fetal accelerations are expected after stimulation. Otherwise, the procedure and interpretation are the same as those in a nonstress test.

16. A contraction stress test indicates fetal response to periodic hypoxia that occurs as a result of uterine contractions. Contractions are initiated by intravenous administration of oxytocin or by breast stimulation. As contractions compress the placental arterioles that supply oxygen to the fetus, a recurrent decrease occurs in fetal oxygen levels.

17. Late decelerations in a CST indicate fetal oxygen reserves are inadequate to tolerate contractions, and fetal acidosis, myocardial depression, or both may result.

18. Loss of fetal tone in a biophysical profile indicates advanced hypoxia and fetal acidosis. Fetal tone develops early in gestation and is one of the parameters of the biophysical profile that is most resistant to the effects of hypoxia.

19. Decreased amniotic fluid volume is associated with prolonged fetal hypoxia, in which blood is shunted away from the fetal lungs and kidneys, which produce amniotic fluid, and toward vital organs such as the fetal heart and brain.

CHAPTER 11

1. The goals of perinatal education are to help women and their support persons become knowledgeable consumers and active participants in pregnancy and childbirth.
2. Couples must choose their health care professional, birth setting, support person(s), and type of education for preparation (if any).
3. Early pregnancy classes emphasize adapting to pregnancy, coping with common discomforts, and learning what to expect in later pregnancy. Later classes discuss preparation for childbirth, the postpartum period, breastfeeding issues, and parenting concerns.
4. The chance that a couple may experience cesarean birth is approximately 26.7%. Therefore all women need to know about cesarean birth.
5. Classes for family members help ease family transition by providing information and opportunities for discussing common feelings.
6. Education, relaxation, and conditioning reduce pain and increase coping ability for childbirth by helping to decrease muscle and mental tension.
7. Cutaneous stimulation and imagery help reduce pain by sending other messages to the brain so that pain messages are not recognized as strongly and perception of pain is reduced.
8. Breathing techniques are used to enhance relaxation during labor.
9. Having a support person during labor increases a woman's satisfaction by helping her deal with stress, focus on her learned techniques, and feel that her experience is being shared.
10. Support roles include active assistance and physical care, verbal encouragement, minimal physical assistance, and presence without active involvement.
11. Specific techniques used by support persons during labor include assistance with relaxation and breathing, encouragement, sacral pressure, massage, and comfort measures.

CHAPTER 12

1. Effacement and dilation of the cervix occur because contractions pull the cervix upward over the fetus and amniotic sac while pushing the fetus and amniotic sac downward against the cervix. The muscle fibers of the upper uterus become shorter to maintain these forces between contractions. In addition, the uterus changes shape and becomes more elongated and narrow to maintain pressure of the fetus and amniotic sac against the cervix.
2. The cervix of the nullipara effaces more before it dilates. The cervix of a multipara is usually thicker than that of a nullipara during the entire labor.
3. Maternal changes occurring during labor include the following:
   a. *Cardiovascular system*—A slight increase in blood pressure and decrease in pulse rate occurs as each contraction temporarily stops blood flow to her uterus. Supine hypotension may occur if she lies on her back because the heavy uterus compresses her inferior vena cava and reduces blood flow to her heart.
   b. *Respiratory system*—The depth and rate of respirations increase.
   c. *Gastrointestinal system*—Although a controversial belief, many authorities think that peristalsis slows during labor.
   d. *Renal system*—The sensation of a full bladder is reduced.
   e. *Hematopoietic system*—Leukocyte counts are as high as 25,000 or more, and levels of clotting factors are elevated.
4. Uterine contractions temporarily stop blood flow to the placenta. If the contractions were sustained, the fetus could not receive freshly oxygenated blood and nutrients and dispose of waste products through the placenta.
5. Labor and vaginal birth benefit the newborn by increasing absorption of fetal lung fluid and compressing the upper airways, causing some lung fluid to be expelled. These effects reduce the amount of lung fluid remaining in the newborn's respiratory tract when breathing begins. Labor also stimulates the fetus to secrete catecholamines, which help speed clearance of the lung fluid after birth, stimulate cardiac contraction and breathing, and aid in temperature regulation.
6. The power of labor during the first stage of labor involves uterine contractions. Powers during the second stage include uterine contractions, augmented by the woman's voluntary pushing efforts.
7. The three divisions of the true pelvis are the inlet, midpelvis, and outlet.
8. The vertex presentation, in which the fetal head is fully flexed forward, allows the smallest diameter of the fetal head to enter the pelvis. It also more effectively dilates the cervix.
9. ROP: The fetal landmark is the occiput, indicating a vertex presentation. It is located in the mother's right posterior pelvic quadrant. OA: The fetal landmark is the occiput, which is located in the mother's anterior pelvis and is not directed toward her left or her right. This is often the presentation just before birth. RSA: The fetal landmark is the sacrum, indicating that the fetus is in a breech presentation. It is located in the mother's right anterior pelvis. LMA: The fetal landmark is the mentum, or chin, indicating that the fetus is in a face presentation. The chin is in the mother's left anterior pelvis.

10. If the fetus is in a face presentation, the occiput is not accessible to the examiner's fingers during vaginal examination. For this reason the fetal chin (mentum) is used to describe the position (such as RMA [right mentum anterior]).

11. The woman may note several changes as labor approaches: increased strength and frequency of Braxton Hicks contractions, lightening, increased vaginal mucus, bloody show, an energy spurt, and a small weight loss.

12. False labor tends to differ from true labor in three major ways. True labor is characterized by contractions that progressively become more frequent, last longer, and are more intense. The discomfort of true labor begins in the lower back and sweeps to the lower abdomen, whereas the discomfort of false labor is more often in the abdomen or groin and is often simply annoying. In true labor, progressive effacement and dilation of the cervix occur, which is the most significant difference from false labor.

13. The transverse diameter of the pelvic inlet is slightly larger than the inlet's anteroposterior diameter. The anteroposterior diameter of the fetal head (in line with the sagittal suture) is slightly larger than the transverse diameter. Therefore the fetal head best fits the pelvis if the sagittal suture is aligned with the pelvic transverse diameter.

14. Because the woman's pelvic outlet is usually slightly larger in its anteroposterior diameter than its transverse diameter, the fetal head turns in the mechanism of internal rotation so that the sagittal suture aligns with the anteroposterior diameter.

15. During the first stage, latent phase, the expectant mother is often sociable, excited, and somewhat anxious. During the first stage, active phase, the woman becomes less sociable and is inwardly focused. During the first stage, transition phase, the woman may become irritable and temporarily lose control. During the second stage, the woman usually concentrates her energy toward pushing her baby out and interacts little with others. She often regains a feeling of control and active participation in the birth during second stage.

16. Contractions vary among women, but the general pattern includes increasing frequency, duration, and intensity throughout labor. In the first stage, latent phase, contractions gradually increase until they are about 5 minutes apart, lasting for 30 to 40 seconds with mild to moderate intensity. In the first stage, active phase, contractions increase to about 2 to 5 minutes apart with a duration of about 40 to 60 seconds and moderate to strong intensity. In the first stage, transition phase, contractions are strong with a frequency of 1.5 to 2 minutes apart and a duration of 60 to 90 seconds. In the second stage, contractions are strong and about 2 to 3 minutes apart and have a duration of about 40 to 60 seconds.

17. Signs that the placenta may have separated include a spherical uterine shape, the rising of the uterus upward in the abdomen, protrusion of the umbilical cord farther outward from the vagina, and a gush of blood.

18. Hemorrhage may occur if the uterus does not remain contracted after birth of the placenta because open blood vessels at the site will not be compressed by the interlacing muscle fibers of the uterus.

CHAPTER 13

1. The nurse should show warmth, concern, and friendliness when the woman and her family enter the hospital or birth center. Determining the woman's and family's expectations about birth, conveying confidence, assigning a primary nurse, and respecting cultural values are specific skills that the nurse can use throughout labor. In addition, a nonjudgmental attitude facilitates communication and shows respect to the woman as an individual.

2. The nurse should try to identify and incorporate beneficial or neutral cultural practices into care during labor and birth by asking about specific practices that are important during birth and facilitating communication by obtaining a fluent interpreter who is acceptable to the woman and her family.

3. The nurse should promptly evaluate the maternal and fetal conditions and the nearness of birth when a woman comes to the hospital or birth center. Prompt assessments should include checking the maternal vital signs, fetal heart rate and patterns, and progress of labor.

4. A lower limit of 110 to 120 bpm and an upper limit of 150 to 160 bpm with a regular rhythm are reassuring. Accelerations and the absence of nonreassuring decelerations from the baseline also are reassuring.

5. Impending birth should be suspected if the woman is grunting, bearing down, sitting on one buttock, or urgently signifying that her baby is about to be born. In that case, the nurse should abbreviate the initial assessment and collect other information after the birth.

6. Two tests assist the nurse, nurse-midwife, or physician to determine whether a woman's membranes have ruptured: the nitrazine test and examination of the amniotic fluid under a microscope for ferning.

7. Hypertonic contractions (too frequent, too long, or an inadequate rest period) reduce blood flow to and from the placenta. This interferes with fetal oxygenation and waste disposal.

8. Routine FHR assessments in uncomplicated labor are documented at least hourly during latent (early) labor, every 30 minutes during active labor, and every 15 minutes during the second stage. The FHR should be assessed after the membranes rupture to detect whether the fetal umbilical cord was displaced with the gush of fluid and is being compressed between the fetal presenting part and maternal pelvis.

9. Greenish amniotic fluid contains meconium, which may have been passed by the fetus in response to transient hypoxia. Cloudy, yellowish, or foul-smelling fluid suggests infection in the amniotic sac.

10. Frequent vaginal examinations may cause infection because microorganisms from the perineal area can be introduced into the uterus.

11. The woman may specifically request other pain management measures including epidural analgesia or other medication, express ineffectiveness of nonpharmacologic measures, show muscle tension during and between contractions, have a tense facial expression, and express an inability to tolerate the pain.

12. Hypotension reduces blood flow to the placenta and therefore reduces fetal oxygenation because it diverts blood away from the uterus to better supply the mother's brain, heart, and kidneys. Hypertension may result in vasospasm that can reduce exchange of oxygen, nutrients, and waste products in the placenta. Fetal hypoxia and acidosis can be the ultimate result of maternal hypotension and hypertension.

13. The supine position allows the heavy uterus to compress the mother's inferior vena cava, reducing blood return to her heart and reducing placental blood supply. A small wedge under her hip, such as a small pillow or rolled towel, is effective to relieve vena cava compression.

14. General physical comfort measures during labor include soft, dim lighting; a comfortable temperature; maintenance of cleanliness; mouth care; observations for a full bladder; positions for comfort; and a warm bath or shower. Caring for the support person includes respect for the couple's wishes about partner involvement in birth. The nurse should provide support that the partner cannot and should consider physical needs for food and rest.

15. Shortly before birth, the woman's perineum bulges and the fetal head becomes visible as the mother pushes. At this time birth can occur suddenly.

CHAPTER 14

1. Fetal oxygenation depends on normal maternal blood flow and volume; normal oxygen saturation of the maternal blood; adequate oxygen-carbon dioxide exchange in the placenta; patent umbilical cord vessels; and normal fetal circulatory and oxygen-carrying function.

2. When the umbilical cord is compressed, the umbilical vein is compressed first, resulting in a slight fetal hypotension and acceleration of the fetal heart rate. Continued compression obstructs the umbilical arteries, resulting in fetal hypertension and slowing of the fetal heart rate. As compression is relieved, these changes are reversed.

3. The fetus increases cardiac output, and therefore oxygenation, primarily by increasing the heart rate. Rates lower than 50 BPM may reduce fetal oxygenation. Rates higher than 200 BPM also may reduce fetal oxygenation because the ventricles do not have time to refill with oxygenated blood.

4. Fetal monitoring should be done more frequently if there are risk factors present. These may include antepartum factors in the woman's history or course of pregnancy. They may also include problems in the woman or fetus that develop intrapartally. Although there are no absolute indications for continuous electronic fetal monitoring, most hospitals use it in both low- and high-risk intrapartum care.

5. Intermittent auscultation promotes the laboring woman's mobility and creates a more natural atmosphere. However, it can assess the fetus for only part of labor, may be distracting for some women, and may require more staff. Continuous electronic fetal monitoring provides more data, is often expected by parents, and can assist the nurse to better observe more than one woman. It allows the nurse to devote more time to coaching the woman and her partner. Its primary drawbacks are reduced maternal mobility, adjustments to the equipment, and its technical atmosphere.

6. The upper grid on the paper strip of the electronic fetal monitor records the constant changes in the fetal heart rate. The lower grid records contractions as a series of bell-shaped curves. Other information that may be printed on the strip includes maternal blood pressure and information charted by the nurse by way of data entry devices. Fetal pulse oximetry data may be recorded on monitors equipped with this technology. The "paper strip" may be on a computer screen rather than printed.

7. The Doppler ultrasound transducer senses fetal heart motion and translates the motion into a heart rate.

8. Four factors may affect the accuracy of the external uterine activity monitor: fetal size, maternal abdominal fat thickness, maternal position, and location of the transducer.

9. The two types of internal uterine activity catheters are the solid and the fluid-filled catheter. The solid catheter tends to record higher intrauterine pressures because it senses fluid pressure above its sensor inside the uterus. The fluid-filled catheter can be affected by its height in relation to the mother's transducer.

10. Fetal heart rate accelerations are a reassuring sign of fetal responsiveness and nonacidosis.

11. In early decelerations, the fetal heart rate slows after the contraction begins and returns to the baseline rate by the end of the contraction. Early decelerations are caused by fetal head compression and are reassuring. Late decelerations are characterized by slowing of the fetal heart rate late in the contraction cycle, often after the peak. They do not return to the baseline until after the contraction has ended. Late decelerations are associated with decreased uteroplacental perfusion and are nonreassuring.

12. Variable decelerations show a fetal heart rate that rises and falls abruptly. They are not consistent in appearance and may not occur at similar times in relation to the contractions. They are caused by compression of the umbilical cord.

13. Fetal scalp stimulation or vibroacoustic stimulation may be done to clarify fetal heart rate patterns as reas-

suring or nonreassuring when they are vague. The reassuring response to stimulation is an increase in the fetal heart rate, peaking 15 BPM above the baseline for at least 15 seconds. This suggests that the fetus has a normal oxygen and acid-base balance.

14. Cord blood gas and pH analysis assesses the newborn's oxygen and acid-base status immediately after birth and identifies if the fetus was adjusting to the stresses of labor.

15. Basic nursing actions for nonreassuring fetal heart rate patterns vary according to the pattern. They include identifying the cause of a nonreassuring pattern by vaginal examination, taking maternal vital signs, reviewing medications, or applying internal monitoring; increasing placental perfusion by reducing excess uterine activity and positioning the woman on her side; giving the mother oxygen; and reducing cord compression by position changes and amnioinfusion.

16. A tocolytic drug reduces the intensity and frequency of uterine contractions, thus allowing more time for the placenta to be supplied with oxygen-rich maternal blood.

17. Amnioinfusion may be used to replace the fluid cushion around the umbilical cord, reducing compression. It may also be used to dilute thick meconium, which might otherwise cause respiratory distress in the newborn.

CHAPTER 15

1. Childbirth pain differs from other painful experiences because it is part of a normal process, the woman has time to prepare for it, it is self-limited and intermittent, and it ends with the birth of the baby.

2. Excessive, unrelieved labor pain may result in a stress response (diverting blood flow from the uterus and compromising fetal oxygenation), maternal acid-base imbalance, and fetal acidosis. It may increase the length of labor. Poor pain relief can lessen the joy of childbirth for the woman and her partner and may have lasting psychological effects

3. Physical and psychological factors interact to alter the ability to tolerate pain. For example, relaxation and working with the forces of labor enhance the chance that the woman who has a large baby and a small pelvis will give birth vaginally.

4. Four sources of pain present in most labors are cervical dilation, uterine ischemia, pressure and pulling on pelvic structures, and distention of the vagina and perineum.

5. Physical factors that influence pain include the following:
   a. A short, intense labor may be more painful because dilation, effacement, and fetal descent occur rapidly.
   b. A cervix that does not efface or dilate easily is likely to be associated with a longer and more uncomfortable labor.
   c. An abnormal fetal position may cause a longer labor as the woman's body maneuvers it into a better position. Back pain is especially noticeable if the fetus is in an occiput posterior position.
   d. Variations in the mother's pelvic size or shape may result in abnormal fetal presentations or positions and in a longer labor because the fetus does not fit through the pelvis easily.
   e. Fatigue reduces the woman's pain tolerance and ability to use coping skills.

6. Psychosocial factors that influence labor pain include culture, anxiety and fear, previous experiences, preparation for childbirth, and the mother's support system.

7. The gate control theory of pain assumes that there is a gating mechanism in the dorsal horn of the spinal cord that controls the transmission of painful impulses to the brain for interpretation. Pain impulses are transmitted through small-diameter fibers, whereas other sensations, such as tactile (massage, heat, cool) are transmitted more quickly through large-diameter fibers. Therefore the impulses transmitted through the large-diameter fibers interfere with or "close the gate" to transmission of pain impulses. Impulses from the brain, such as responses to auditory stimuli (listening to music, for instance), can also impede pain transmission.

8. Nursing actions to promote relaxation include arranging for environmental comfort, maintaining the woman's general comfort, reducing factors that cause anxiety and fear, and using specific relaxation techniques such as helping the woman focus on relaxing specific tense muscles.

9. Accurate information and a focus on the normal aspects of childbirth help reduce anxiety and fear. Avoid referring to the woman as a "patient," because this word is associated with illness. Empowerment of the birthing partners helps them see themselves as competent to give birth successfully.

10. Self-massage might include effleurage, rubbing the hands together, patting or banging the hands on the rail. Massage by others helps relax tense muscles and aids relaxation. Counterpressure, which may include sacral pressure or other variations, is often used to reduce back pain when the fetus is in an occiput posterior position. Warmth relaxes muscles, promoting relaxation. Cool often feels better to the laboring woman who may be hot, or she may want cool only in a local area or ice in her mouth.

11. Hydration must be adequate to offset the diuresis that often occurs with immersion in water. Diuresis could reduce placental perfusion if plasma volume is low. Water temperature must be controlled to prevent hyperthermia or hypothermia, which could raise the mother's metabolic rate, increasing her oxygen and glucose consumption. These changes could reduce oxygen and glucose delivered to the fetus.

12. The more complex breathing techniques are more effective for greater pain, but they are tiring. Advancing

from simpler to more complex breathing techniques too quickly can cause the mother to become fatigued when she most needs to use these methods.

13. The cleansing breath has four purposes: a) to release tension; b) to increase oxygen intake to combat myometrial hypoxia; c) to clear the woman's mind so she can focus on relaxing through the contraction; and d) to signal her labor partner that a contraction has begun.

14. Drugs taken by the mother can affect the fetus directly, such as by decreasing fetal heart rate variability, or indirectly, such as by causing hypotension that reduces placental blood flow and fetal oxygen supply.

15. Aortocaval compression should be offset by placing a wedge under the woman's hip if a supine position is required. Tilting the patient table during surgery reduces compression until the infant is born. The woman is more sensitive to general anesthesia and may have a greater fall in oxygenation when general anesthesia is induced. Reduced peristalsis and tone of the sphincter at the junction of the esophagus and stomach can lead to regurgitation and aspiration of gastric contents, primarily with general anesthesia. Lower doses of anesthetic agents will be needed for epidural or subarachnoid blocks.

16. Drugs (prescribed, over-the-counter, or illicit), botanical preparations, and alcohol may interact with one another. These interactions may be harmful to the woman, the fetus, or both. Knowledge of exactly what drugs she uses allows the safest choices in pharmacologic pain relief methods.

17. Neonatal respiratory depression is the primary drawback to the use of opioid analgesia. This effect can be reduced by timing the dose to reduce the amount transferred to the fetus (which varies according to the drug) and by giving the narcotic in small, frequent, IV doses at the beginning of the contraction. Naloxone (Narcan) is the drug that may be given to reverse opioid-induced respiratory depression in the neonate, with bag-and-mask ventilation being the initial method to oxygenate the infant.

18. Because naloxone's effects are shorter than those of the narcotic, the nurse must observe for a recurrence of respiratory depression.

19. The two major advantages of regional pain management are that the woman can have pain relief and remain alert.

20. Epidural and subarachnoid blocks can cause maternal hypotension. The fall in blood pressure may result in reduced placental blood flow, compromising fetal oxygen supply. Giving the woman IV fluids before the block reduces this effect. Other less serious adverse effects are bladder distention, prolonged second stage of labor (epidural), and postdural puncture headache (usually only subarachnoid block).

21. Epidural or intrathecal opioid analgesics may cause nausea, vomiting, itching, or a combination of these. They may also result in delayed respiratory depression (up to 24 hours), depending on the drug used. Management includes promethazine for nausea and vomiting; diphenhydramine, naloxone, or naltrexone for itching; and pulse oximetry and monitoring of respirations while the opioid is given and up to 24 hours after administration ends, depending on the drug.

22. Maternal regurgitation with aspiration of acidic gastric contents is the major potential adverse effect of general anesthesia. The risk may be reduced by limiting intake to clear fluids, giving drugs to raise the gastric pH, giving drugs to reduce gastric secretions or speed emptying of the stomach, and using cricoid pressure (Sellick's maneuver) to block the esophagus while the endotracheal tube is being inserted. Respiratory depression, primarily in the infant, is minimized by delaying general anesthesia until the surgery team is prepared and by keeping the anesthesia level as light as possible until the umbilical cord is cut.

CHAPTER 16

1. Three major risks of amniotomy are prolapsed umbilical cord, infection, and abruptio placentae.

2. The FHR is assessed before the membranes rupture to identify whether the fetus has a normal rate and pattern and establish a baseline. It is checked after the membranes rupture to identify patterns that suggest umbilical cord compression and other problems.

3. Green amniotic fluid contains meconium, passed from the fetal intestines. It may be seen in postterm gestation or placental insufficiency.

4. Signs of chorioamnionitis include fetal tachycardia (often the first sign), elevated maternal temperature, and amniotic fluid that has a foul or strong odor or a cloudy or yellowish appearance.

5. Five precautions that promote safe oxytocin induction or augmentation of labor include the following:
   a. Dilution of the oxytocin in an isotonic solution
   b. Piggybacking the oxytocin solution into the port of the primary nonadditive (maintenance) IV line that is nearest the venipuncture site
   c. Starting the oxytocin infusion slowly
   d. Increasing the rate of infusion gradually
   e. Monitoring uterine contractions and FHR

6. Labor may be augmented if it stops or contractions become ineffective. The woman whose labor is augmented with oxytocin usually needs less of the drug than the woman whose labor is being induced, because her uterus is more sensitive to its effects.

7. The fetus may have an adverse reaction to oxytocin, manifested by nonreassuring FHR patterns such as bradycardia, tachycardia, late decelerations, or decreased FHR variability.

8. Signs of hypertonic uterine activity include incomplete relaxation of the uterus between contractions or a rest period shorter than 30 seconds or Montevideo units exceeding 400, which may result in inadequate placental

blood flow and a fall in fetal oxygenation. Nonreassuring FHR patterns may occur even if these signs of hypertonic uterine activity are absent.

9. Administration of oxytocin for a prolonged time may lead to postpartum hemorrhage because the fatigued uterus cannot contract properly to compress bleeding vessels at the placenta site (uterine atony).

10. The FHR should be monitored before external version to identify nonreassuring patterns that would preclude the procedure. It should be monitored (by Doppler or real-time ultrasound) as much as possible during and for a short while after external version to detect cord compression that can occur if the umbilical cord becomes entangled during change of the fetal presentation.

11. Uterine activity should be observed after external version for possible onset of labor because this procedure may cause uterine irritability or possible abruptio placentae and is done near term.

12. Forceps and vacuum extraction are used to provide traction to assist the mother in rotation, expulsion, or both, of the fetal head. Special forceps (Piper) can be used to deliver the head of the fetus in a breech presentation, but a vacuum extractor can be used only with a cephalic presentation. Forceps may cause fetal injury such as facial bruising and nerve injury. The vacuum extractor may create an artificial caput called a *chignon*.

13. Catheterization before forceps are used eliminates a full bladder, which would reduce available room in the pelvis. Emptying the bladder also reduces the risk of bladder injury.

14. Use of cold immediately (for the first 12 hours) after episiotomy reduces pain, edema, and formation of hematomas. The nurse should also observe for continuous, bright-red bleeding that suggests a vaginal wall laceration. Warmth after at least 12 hours of cold application promotes resolution of the edema and hematoma.

15. The infant with an asymmetric facial appearance when crying may have facial nerve injury, usually a temporary condition that sometimes occurs when forceps are used to assist birth.

16. The low transverse uterine incision is less likely to rupture during another pregnancy than either of the two vertical incisions. There are, however, valid reasons for the use of vertical incisions.

17. The woman expecting a cesarean birth should be taught the following about the operating room and recovery area:
    a. Preoperative procedures, such as the skin preparation and indwelling catheter.
    b. Personnel who will be present and their functions.
    c. The narrow table, safety strap, and positioning measures.
    d. When her partner or support person can come in.
    e. If a regional anesthetic is planned, that she will be awake and feel pulling and pressure sensations but should not expect pain. If a general anesthetic is planned, that all preparations will be made before she

is put to sleep but that the surgery will not begin before she is asleep and she will not awaken during it.
    f. In the recovery area, use of oxygen, pulse oximeter, and automatic blood pressure cuff for vital signs; checking of her fundus, incision, lochia, and pain relief needs.

18. The woman who has cesarean birth needs care similar to that of the woman who delivers vaginally, in terms of vital signs and fundus and lochia assessments. Additional care includes assessment of oxygen saturation and respiratory status, observation of urine output from the indwelling catheter, pain needs, and respiratory care (turning, coughing, deep breathing). Anesthesia-related care includes level of consciousness (primarily if general anesthesia was used) and return of movement and sensation (primarily if epidural or subarachnoid block was used).

CHAPTER 17

1. The three processes involved in involution are contraction of muscle fibers, catabolism, and regeneration of uterine epithelium.

2. The fundus is expected to descend 1 cm (approximately 1 fingerbreadth) per day so that by 10 days after birth it cannot be palpated.

3. A multipara is expected to experience afterpains because repeated stretching of the uterus makes continuous uterine contraction more difficult. Overdistention of the uterus and breastfeeding also cause afterpains. Afterpains are treated with analgesics. Lying in a prone position also provides relief.

4. Lochia rubra is red, consists mostly of blood, and lasts for 3 days. Lochia serosa is pink to brown-tinged and usually lasts from the fourth to tenth days. Lochia alba is white, cream, or yellowish and may last 3 to 6 weeks.

5. The mother is at risk for urinary retention because she is less sensitive to fluid pressure, decreasing the urge to void even when the bladder is distended. Trauma of childbirth and lingering effects of epidural anesthesia may also make it difficult to void. Urinary tract infection is more likely because stasis of urine allows time for bacteria to multiply. Postpartum hemorrhage may occur because a full bladder displaces the uterus, causing the uterine muscles to relax.

6. Hyperpigmentation decreases because estrogen, progesterone, and melanocyte-stimulating hormone decreases rapidly after childbirth.

7. Breastfeeding delays the return of both ovulation and menstruation.

8. The WBC count is normally elevated to an average of 14,000 to 16,000 mm³ after childbirth. If the woman has a fever or is at increased risk for infection, the nurse should be especially alert for a rising WBC count and other signs of infection.

9. Menses will probably resume about 7 to 9 weeks after childbirth in the woman who is formula feeding her in-

fant. The breastfeeding woman may begin menses between 12 weeks and 18 months after childbirth.

10. Women lose approximately 4.5 to 5.5 kg (10 to 12 lb) during childbirth. They often lose another 2.3 to 3.6 kg (5 to 8 lb) during involution.

11. When tachycardia is noted, assessment of temperature, blood pressure, location and firmness of the uterus, amount of lochia, estimated blood loss at delivery, hemoglobin, and hematocrit values are necessary to help identify the cause. Excitement, fatigue, dehydration, infection, pain, or hypovolemia may cause tachycardia.

12. Orthostatic hypotension, a drop in blood pressure when the mother goes from a supine to a sitting or standing position quickly, results from engorgement of visceral blood vessels from decreased intraabdominal pressure after delivery. Signs and symptoms include a 15- to 20–mm Hg drop in blood pressure, dizziness, lightheadedness, or faintness.

13. Uterine massage is necessary when the uterus is not firmly contracted. The nurse places the nondominant hand above the woman's symphysis pubis to anchor and support the uterus during massage.

14. A cervical or vaginal laceration may cause excessive bleeding even when the uterus is firmly contracted.

15. Frequent respiratory assessments, auscultation of breath sounds and bowel sounds, and inspection of the surgical dressing and wound are necessary for the postcesarean mother.

16. Hypostatic pneumonia can be prevented by frequent turning, coughing, breathing deeply, and ambulating early and frequently.

17. Early ambulation, pelvic lifts, and restriction of carbonated beverages and straws for drinking prevent or minimize abdominal distention.

18. Wearing a snug bra and avoiding nipple stimulation help prevent lactation.

19. Providing adequate information in a short time is a major problem in preparing parents for discharge. Clinical pathways list guidelines for outcomes and a specific time frame for interventions that will help the new mother achieve the stated outcomes.

20. Before discharge the nurse should be sure that the mother has no complications and all assessments are normal. Ambulation and ability to eat and drink should be normal. The mother should indicate understanding of self-care instructions, signs of complications and proper responses, and infant care. She should have adequate support during the early days after discharge.

21. All methods help meet educational needs by answering parents' questions and providing reassurance. Information lines rely on the family to initiate contact and usually deal only with the concern that precipitated the call, whereas telephone interviews allow the nurse to guide the interview. Phone calls are relatively inexpensive, but nurses must rely on observations made by the family. Home visits allow physical examination of the mother, infant, and environment but are expensive because they require the time of a well-prepared nurse. Outpatient clinics are less expensive and allow direct assessment of the mother and infant. Transportation is a problem for some families, however, and not all families will take advantage of clinics.

CHAPTER 18

1. Bonding describes the initial attraction felt by the parents for the infant. Attachment is the development of an enduring, loving relationship between parents and child. It is progressive and requires response from the infant.

2. Maternal touch may progress from fingertipping in the discovery phase to enfolding the infant and then to consoling behaviors.

3. Parents progress from referring to the newborn as "it" to "he" or "she" and then to using the given name. Parents who know the sex of the baby before birth may call the infant by name from birth or before.

4. The mother is focused primarily on her own needs during the taking-in phase. She often is passive and dependent and repeatedly recounts her birth experience. In the taking-hold phase, she becomes more independent, focuses on the infant, and exhibits a heightened readiness to learn.

5. In the letting-go phase, mothers (and fathers) relinquish previous lifestyle patterns to assume the parenting role.

6. The anticipatory stage begins during pregnancy as mothers prepare for the birth of the child. The formal stage begins with birth when parents become acquainted with their child. During the informal stage, parents respond to the unique cues of their child rather than relying on directions from others. The personal stage is attained when the parents feel comfortable with their roles as parents.

7. "Heading toward a new normal" involves appreciating the body, settling in, and becoming a new family.

8. Postpartum blues may be related to emotional letdown, discomfort, and anxiety about parenting and self-image. Nurses can provide reassurance to the mother and teach the family about the condition, the length of time it may last, and the mother's needs at this time.

9. Fathers who are sometimes ignored and not included in infant care may feel left out and unneeded.

10. Siblings may feel jealousy and fear that they will be replaced by the newborn in the affection of the parents.

11. Time must be allowed for the parents to form attachment with each newborn individually. Concerns over the health of the infants and about finances may interfere with attachment.

CHAPTER 19

1. Hypoxia causes decreased PO_2 and pH and increased PCO_2 to affect chemoreceptors that stimulate the respiratory center in the brain. Cool air and handling at birth

cause skin sensors to stimulate the respiratory center. These factors all contribute to the initiation of respirations at birth.

2. Surfactant reduces surface tension in the alveoli and allows them to remain partially open on expiration.

3. Fetal lung fluid begins to move into the interstitial spaces shortly before birth and when air enters the lungs at birth. It is absorbed from the interstitial spaces by the lymphatic and vascular systems. A small part of the fluid is squeezed out during birth.

4. The ductus arteriosus closes as a result of increases in blood oxygen levels and decreased prostaglandins from the placenta. The foramen ovale closes when pressure in the left atrium exceeds that in the right atrium. The ductus venosus closes when the vessels of the cord become occluded.

5. At birth, increasing levels of oxygen cause the pulmonary blood vessels to dilate. In addition, movement of fetal lung fluid into the interstitial tissues allows more room for expansion of the pulmonary blood vessels. The ductus arteriosus constricts because of the increased oxygen level in the blood when the neonate begins to breathe.

6. Newborns have thinner skin with less subcutaneous fat, blood vessels close to the surface, and a larger skin surface area. These all contribute to greater loss of heat than in older children or adults.

7. Newborns respond to low temperatures by increasing activity and flexion, vasoconstriction, and nonshivering thermogenesis. This increases oxygen and glucose consumption and may cause respiratory distress, hypoglycemia, acidosis, and jaundice.

8. Newborns have higher levels of erythrocytes, hemoglobin, and hematocrit than adults because during fetal life, the available oxygen is lower than after birth. More red blood cells are needed to adequately oxygenate the cells.

9. Stools progress from thick, greenish-black meconium to loose greenish-brown transitional stools to milk stools that are frequent, soft, seedy, and mustard-colored if the infant is breastfed, and pale yellow or light brown, firmer, and less frequent if formula fed.

10. Hypoglycemia is a problem for the newborn because glucose is the major source of energy in the brain.

11. Infants have an immature liver and more hemolysis of erythrocytes than adults. Trauma at birth, poor early feeding, and an intestinal enzyme that deconjugates bilirubin also increase jaundice.

12. Physiologic jaundice occurs in normal newborns after the first 24 hours of life as a result of hemolysis of red blood cells and immaturity of the liver. Pathologic jaundice is generally a result of excessive destruction of erythrocytes, causing bilirubin levels to rise faster and higher than in physiologic jaundice. It begins within the first 24 hours and may necessitate phototherapy. Breast milk jaundice lasts longer than physiologic jaundice and may result from enzymes in the milk.

13. The newborn's body is composed of a greater percentage of water, with more located in the extracellular compartment, than the adult's body.

14. Newborns receive passive immunity to infections when IgG crosses the placenta *in utero*. After birth, infants produce IgM and IgA to protect against infection. IgM rises in response to infection. IgA lines the gastrointestinal and respiratory tracts to prevent infection and is present in breast milk.

15. During both periods of reactivity, newborns are active and alert, may be interested in feeding, have elevated pulse and respiratory rates, and may have transient signs of respiratory distress.

16. In the quiet sleep state, the infant is in a deep sleep with regular respirations and little response to outside stimuli. In active sleep, infants move about and may have irregular respirations. The drowsy state is the time between sleep and waking. In the quiet alert state the infant is awake and interested in stimuli. The active alert state is a fussy period that may lead to the crying state if the infant's needs are not met.

CHAPTER 20

1. The early focused assessments of the infant immediately after birth help detect serious abnormalities that need immediate attention. They focus on cardiorespiratory status, thermoregulation, and the presence of anomalies. A more complete assessment follows when the infant is stable.

2. The cardiovascular assessment includes evaluation of history, airway, color, heart sounds, pulses, and blood pressure.

3. Taking a rectal temperature is dangerous because it risks perforation of the rectum, which turns sharply to the right after about 3 cm (1.2 inches).

4. Molding of the head is a change in the shape because of normal temporary overriding of bones during birth. Caput succedaneum is localized swelling from pressure against the cervix, which can cross the suture lines. Cephalhematoma is bleeding between the periosteum and the bone that never crosses suture lines. Molding and caput disappear within a few days, but cephalhematoma may last for several weeks or months.

5. Measurements of the infant help determine if *in utero* growth was adequate for gestational age and if complications are present.

6. Some signs of hypoglycemia are jitteriness, poor muscle tone, respiratory distress (tachypnea, dyspnea, apnea, and cyanosis), high-pitched cry, diaphoresis, low temperature, poor suck, lethargy, irritability, seizures, and coma.

7. Using an incorrect site for heel punctures risks injury to the bone, nerves, or blood vessels of the heel.

8. Newborn reflexes provide information about the status of the neonate's central nervous system.

9. The first feeding allows the nurse to evaluate the newborn's ability to suck, swallow, and breathe in coordi-

nation and assess for signs of a connection between the trachea and esophagus.

10. Newborns usually pass the first stool within 12 to 48 hours of birth. Feeding and taking a rectal temperature may stimulate stool passage.

11. Infants should void within 12 to 24 hours. Infants void at least one to two times during the first 2 days and at least 6 times a day by the fourth day.

12. The nurse documents location, size, color, elevation, and texture of marks on the skin; explains marks to parents; and offers emotional support as needed.

13. The gestational age assessment provides an estimate of the infant's age since conception and alerts the nurse to possible complications related to age and development.

14. The periods of reactivity are important because the infant may need nursing intervention for low temperature, elevated pulse and respirations, and excessive respiratory secretions. During the sleep period, the infant will have relaxed muscle tone and no interest in feeding.

CHAPTER 21

1. All newborns receive vitamin K to prevent vitamin K–dependent bleeding. The eyes are treated with an antibiotic ointment to prevent ophthalmia neonatorum.

2. Nurses can prevent heat loss in newborns by keeping them dry and covered; by keeping them away from cold objects or surfaces, drafts, and outside windows and walls; and by teaching parents.

3. When infants show signs of hypoglycemia, the nurse should check the blood glucose level and temperature, feed the infant, and watch for signs of other complications.

4. Interventions for preventing jaundice include ensuring that the infant is feeding well by working with mothers and infants having difficulty and teaching parents about jaundice and what observations they should make.

5. Nurses can prevent a parent from getting the wrong baby by always checking the infant's identification band against that of the mother or support person every time the two are reunited.

6. Nurses and parents can prevent infant abductions by always being alert for suspicious behavior and stopping anyone who might be taking a baby. Parents must know how to identify hospital staff and should never allow anyone without proper identification to remove their infant from them.

7. Scrupulous handwashing by staff and all who come in contact with newborns is the most important way to prevent infections in newborns.

8. Parents choose circumcision because of the decreased incidence of urinary tract infections, penile cancer, and some sexually transmittable diseases; religious dictates; parental preference; and lack of knowledge about care of the foreskin. Parents decide against circumcision because it causes pain and the risk of bleeding, infection, recurrent phimosis, wound separation, urinary reten-

tion, meatitis, meatal stenosis, chordee, and inclusion cysts. They also question the need for surgery to prevent uncommon conditions.

9. Teach parents not to retract the foreskin on an uncircumcised penis until it begins to separate from the glans later in childhood. They can teach the child to retract it to clean after separation occurs. Teach parents of circumcised infants to watch for bleeding and infection and to apply petroleum jelly as instructed unless a Plastibell was used.

10. Planning parent teaching includes coordinating teaching to include all topics, setting priorities based on parents' needs, using a variety of teaching techniques, modeling behavior, including other family members, and considering culture and language.

11. The first hepatitis B vaccine is given at the birth facility to infants whose mothers are positive for hepatitis B to prevent the infant from being infected. Hepatitis B immune globulin is also given these infants.

12. Newborn screening tests should be performed as close to discharge as possible, as the tests are more sensitive after the first 24 hours of life. If infants are discharged earlier, they should be retested so that any disorders can be diagnosed early.

CHAPTER 22

1. Some infants lose weight after birth because of insufficient intake and normal loss of meconium and extracellular fluid.

2. Colostrum is rich in protein, vitamins, minerals, and immunoglobulins. Transitional milk has less protein and immunoglobulin but more lactose, fat, and calories than colostrum. Mature milk appears less rich than colostrum and transitional milk but supplies all nutrients needed.

3. Breast milk nutrients are in an easily digested form and in proportions required by the newborn. Commercial formulas contain cow's milk adapted to simulate human milk. Infants may develop allergies to modified cow's milk and may need other types of formula, but they are unlikely to be allergic to human milk.

4. Breast milk contains bifidus factor to help establish intestinal flora, leukocytes, lysozymes that are bacteriolytic, lactoferrin to bind iron in bacteria, and immunoglobulins.

5. Commercial formulas include modified cow's milk formula, soy-based or casein hydrolysate formulas, and special formulas for preterm infants or those with special needs.

6. Support from family and friends, cultural influences, employment demands, knowledge about each method, age, and education may influence a woman's choice of feeding method.

7. Suckling causes release of oxytocin from the posterior pituitary, which produces the let-down reflex. Suckling and removal of milk from the breast cause the anterior pituitary to release prolactin to increase milk produc-

tion. Therefore the more frequently the infant breast-feeds, the more milk is produced. Infrequent feedings decrease prolactin output and milk production.

8. During pregnancy, identification of flat and inverted nipples and possible use of breast shells to help correct them are important.

9. The nurse can help the mother establish breastfeeding in the beginning by initiating early feeding, helping position the infant at the breast, and showing the mother ways to position her hands. The nurse also can help the infant latch on to the breast, assess the position of the mouth on the breast, check for swallowing, and remove the infant from the breast properly.

10. The mother should feed the infant every 2 to 3 hours (8 to 12 times each day) for about 10 to 15 minutes on each side or longer if the infant wishes. Length of feedings may vary but should average at least 20 minutes of effective suckling.

11. To wake up a sleepy infant, unwrap the infant's blankets, talk to the infant, change the diaper, rub the infant's back, and express colostrum onto the breast.

12. Sucking from a bottle requires pushing the tongue against the nipple to slow the flow of milk. Suckling from the breast requires drawing the nipple far into the mouth so that the gums compress the areola as the tongue moves over the milk duct in a wave-like motion.

13. To help the mother with engorged breasts, the nurse can encourage nursing frequently, applying heat and cold, massaging, and expressing milk to soften the areola.

14. The nurse should advise the mother with sore nipples to ensure proper positioning of the infant at the breast, vary the position of the infant, apply colostrum or compresses to the nipples, and expose the nipples to air.

15. The mother who plans to work and breastfeed should be taught use of a breast pump, proper storage of milk, and ways to maintain her milk supply.

16. Care available after discharge for the breastfeeding mother includes home visits by nurses, outpatient clinics where nurses assess and teach breastfeeding, telephone access to nurses, and consultation with lactation specialists.

17. A mother might ask about the types of formula available, ways to prepare it correctly, frequency and amount of feedings, and feeding techniques.

18. Propping bottles risks aspiration of milk. Infants who sleep with a propped bottle have more ear infections and may develop cavities when the teeth come in.

CHAPTER 23

1. Parents obtain information about infant care from friends, family, nurses, health care providers, the Internet, child care classes, books, and magazines.

2. Nurses may provide follow-up phone calls, home visits, clinic visits, and child care classes.

3. All equipment should be checked for safety, and parts should be inspected to ensure that they are functioning properly.

4. Car seats must be chosen according to the size of the infant and must be used correctly to maintain safety.

5. Infants are not "spoiled" by prompt attention to their needs. Prompt, consistent response to crying may decrease overall crying later.

6. Nurses can assist parents of crying infants to determine the cause and teach them appropriate techniques for dealing with a crying infant. Nurses can also use therapeutic communication techniques to help parents deal with negative feelings.

7. Signs of teething include drooling, irritability, decreased appetite and sleep, and red, swollen gums.

8. Diaper rash can be prevented by keeping the area clean and dry and avoiding products to which the infant seems sensitive. If rash occurs, parents should expose the area to air and apply creams sparingly.

9. The amount infants eat during the early weeks will vary but will average about $\frac{1}{2}$ to 1 oz per feeding at first and 5 to 6 oz per feeding at 12 weeks.

10. Solid foods cannot be digested completely until age 4 to 6 months and may cause allergies, gastric upsets, and decreased intake of needed nutrients from milk. In addition, the extrusion reflex makes it difficult to feed solids to infants younger than 4 months.

11. Understanding the infant's changing capabilities helps parents assess situations and the home environment to prevent accidents.

12. Well-baby checkups allow the health care provider to assess the infant's growth and development, provide parent teaching, and give immunizations.

13. Immunizations prevent infants from becoming infected with very serious communicable diseases.

14. Immediate help should be obtained if infants have difficulty breathing, are cyanotic, or are hard to arouse from sleep.

15. The cause of sudden infant death syndrome remains unknown, but the risk may be increased with sleeping in a prone position or on soft, loose bedding, overheating, maternal smoking, and sleeping with another person or on an adult bed or sofa. Infants should sleep in a supine position at all times.

CHAPTER 24

1. Pregnancy interrupts developmental tasks such as the achievement of a stable identity, development of a personal value system, completion of educational goals, and achievement of independence from parents.

2. Teenagers experience greater risk for preeclampsia, anemia, nutritional deficiencies, high or low weight gain, abuse, depression, and sexually transmissible diseases. Infants are at greater risk of being born prematurely and weighing less than 2500 g.

3. A variety of teaching methods such as visual aids, videos, group classes, and one-to-one counseling may be effective for teenagers.

4. Infants develop a sense of trust, which is necessary for future development, when their needs are met promptly and gently. Crying indicates a need and does not mean the infant is "spoiled." Physical growth and development proceed slowly from the head downward.

5. Mature primigravidas often have maturity, problem-solving skills, and emotional and financial resources that may be unavailable to younger women.

6. The fetus of a woman older than 35 years is at increased risk for chromosomal anomalies that may be detected by prenatal screening.

7. The older mother may have less energy than younger mothers, and conserving her energy for care of herself and her infant is important.

8. The effects of smoking on the neonate include low birth weight, prematurity, and increased perinatal loss. Later effects include SIDS and delayed neurologic and intellectual development.

9. Fetal alcohol syndrome is characterized by slow growth, central nervous system disorders, and cranial and facial anomalies. Infants with fetal alcohol effects will have fewer and less severe problems than those with fetal alcohol syndrome.

10. Neonates exposed to cocaine have an increased risk of SIDS. Other long-term effects are unclear but may include learning difficulties and slower development of intellectual, language, and motor skills.

11. Pregnant heroin users are placed on methadone to provide a long-acting, steady drug dose to the fetus to avoid the problems of intrauterine overdosage and withdrawal.

12. Prenatal behaviors that suggest substance abuse include prenatal care sought late in pregnancy, failure to keep appointments, inconsistent follow-through with recommended regimens, poor grooming, inadequate weight gain, needle punctures, thrombosed veins, and signs of cellulitis.

13. Signs and symptoms of recent cocaine use include profuse sweating, high blood pressure, irregular respirations, dilated pupils, increased body temperature, sudden onset of severely painful uterine contractions, fetal tachycardia, and excessive fetal activity. Emotional signs include anger, caustic or abusive reactions to the caregiver, emotional lability, and paranoia.

14. Interventions are focused on preventing maternal or fetal injury and may require setting limits in a firm, nonjudgmental manner with a woman who may be abusive and in great pain.

15. Parents experience less anxiety when they are gently told about the condition of the infant and allowed to hold their newborn as soon as possible.

16. Facial, genital, and irreparable defects are likely to affect parenting most.

17. The reaction of parents can be described in terms of a grief response. Initial reactions include shock and disbelief. Denial, anger, and guilt are common.

18. Nurses can promote bonding and attachment by handling the infant gently, emphasizing normal traits, help-

ing parents hold and cuddle the infant, and using communication skills to help parents come to terms with their feelings.

19. Discharge planning for the family of an infant with congenital anomalies should include special feeding and other techniques that the infant may require, follow-up care needed, and referral to agencies and organizations that may be helpful.

20. The way in which the stillborn infant is presented creates memories that the parents will retain. The infant should be washed and taken to the parents while still warm and soft, wrapped in a soft, warm blanket.

21. A memory packet that includes photographs of the baby, handprints, footprints, a birth identification band, and crib card, and if possible, a lock of hair help parents grieve.

22. Mothers see adoption as an act of sacrifice and love when they give up the infant to those who can provide a better life.

23. Adoptive parents must be taught how to care for an infant and what to expect in terms of growth and development.

24. Battering may start or become worse during pregnancy. The abdomen, face, and breasts are frequent targets for battery.

25. Nurses can examine their own biases to determine whether they accept a common myth that blames the victim. In addition, nurses can consciously practice in ways that empower women and make it clear that the woman owns her body and no one deserves to be beaten.

26. The battered woman often appears hesitant, embarrassed, or evasive. She may avoid eye contact and appear ashamed, guilty, or frightened. Signs of present and past injury may be present, such as bruising, swelling, lacerations, scars, and old fractures, as well as genital injuries.

27. Nurses can help establish short-term goals by helping the woman acknowledge the abuse, develop a plan for protecting herself and her children, and identify community resources that provide protection.

CHAPTER 25

1. Bleeding is the most common sign of threatened abortion. It may be accompanied by rhythmic cramping, backache, or feelings of pelvic pressure. Gross rupture of membranes and subsequent uterine contractions and bleeding makes the abortion inevitable.

2. Recurrent spontaneous abortions (also called *miscarriages*) most often occur as a result of genetic or chromosomal abnormalities of the embryo or anomalies of the maternal reproductive tract. Additional causes are believed to be hormonal and immunologic factors or systemic diseases or infections.

3. Nurses can facilitate the grief response by being aware that although many couples grieve over an early pregnancy loss, they often feel a lack of support from fam-

ily, friends, and health care personnel. When nurses demonstrate empathy and unconditional acceptance of the feelings expressed, they facilitate the grief response. Providing information about the grieving and referrals to additional support groups also may be helpful.

4. Disseminated intravascular coagulation is a life-threatening disorder in which procoagulation and anticoagulation factors are activated simultaneously, resulting in profuse bleeding from any vulnerable area. It may occur with missed abortion (primarily if the pregnancy had reached the second trimester when fetal death occurred), abruptio placentae, severe pregnancy-induced hypertension, amniotic fluid embolism, and other conditions such as sepsis.

5. Ectopic pregnancy remains the leading cause of maternal death because of hemorrhage, and it can reduce the woman's chance of subsequent pregnancies because of damage to a fallopian tube. Also, the condition that caused the ectopic pregnancy in the tube may be present in the opposite tube.

6. The increase in incidence of ectopic pregnancy may occur as a result of pelvic inflammatory disease that may complicate untreated sexually transmitted diseases. Scarring of the fallopian tubes that may result from the infection may make it difficult for the fertilized ovum to pass through the obstructed tube. Ectopic pregnancy is also more likely to occur in women who have assisted reproduction for infertility, ovulation disorders, contraceptive devices, and use of progesterone agents. Treatment for ectopic pregnancy may be medical (chemotherapeutic agent) or surgical (salpingostomy or salpingectomy).

7. Hydatidiform mole is a form of gestational trophoblastic disease that involves abnormal development of the placenta as the fetal part of the pregnancy fails to develop. The first phase of treatment is evacuation of the molar pregnancy from the uterus. The second phase is follow-up to detect malignant changes in remaining trophoblastic tissue.

8. Painless vaginal bleeding in the latter half of pregnancy is the classic sign of placenta previa. Strict bed rest, no sexual intercourse, an adult caregiver present at all times, and availability of emergency transportation to the hospital are essential for home care. The woman must also be taught to monitor fetal movement and to report a decrease in movement or increase in vaginal bleeding.

9. The five classic signs of abruptio placentae are (a) bleeding, which may be evident vaginally or concealed behind the placenta; (b) uterine tenderness; (c) excess uterine activity, with poor relaxation between contractions; (d) abdominal pain; and (e) a high uterine resting tone if an intrauterine pressure catheter is being used.

10. Hemorrhagic shock is the major danger of placental abruption for the mother; anoxia, excessive blood loss, or delivery before maturity are major dangers for the fetus.

11. Both morning sickness and hyperemesis gravidarum begin in the first trimester. Morning sickness is self-limiting and causes no serious complications. Hyperemesis is persistent, uncontrollable vomiting that may cause excessive weight loss, dehydration, and electrolyte or acid-base imbalance.

12. Goals of management are to maintain hydration, replace electrolytes and vitamins, maintain nutrition, and provide emotional support.

13. Nurses must use critical thinking to examine biases that may result in lack of comfort and support for women with hyperemesis. Helping the woman identify any reluctance to accept the pregnancy may open the door to solutions that can reduce the intensity of hyperemesis.

14. Persistent vasospasm of uterine arterioles may result in fetal hypoxemia, intrauterine growth restriction, or even fetal death.

15. Classic signs of preeclampsia include hypertension and possibly proteinuria. Although nonspecific, edema that is often severe and generalized is often seen and has recently been considered a classic sign. Headache, hyperreflexia, visual disturbances, and epigastric pain indicate the disease is worsening. Rest, especially in a lateral position, increases cardiac return and circulatory volume, thus improving perfusion of vital organs. Increased renal perfusion decreases angiotensin II levels, thus lowering blood pressure.

16. Vasospasms cause rupture of cerebral capillaries and small cerebral hemorrhages.

17. Magnesium sulfate prevents seizures by reducing central nervous system irritability and decreasing vasoconstriction. The primary adverse effect is central nervous system depression, which includes depression of the respiratory center.

18. Pulmonary edema, circulatory or renal failure, and cerebral hemorrhage are complications of eclampsia. The HELLP syndrome, which demonstrates coagulation and liver function abnormalities, is more likely to occur when a woman has severe preeclampsia or eclampsia. DIC may cause unexpected bleeding as coagulation factors decline.

19. Assessments for the woman with preeclampsia include daily weights, location and degree of edema, vital signs, hourly urinary output, urine for protein, deep tendon reflexes, and subjective signs such as headache, visual disturbances, and epigastric pain. The fetal heart rate should be assessed for nonreassuring patterns. Respiratory rate, oxygen saturation level, consciousness level, and laboratory data such as creatinine, liver enzymes, and magnesium level should be evaluated. Psychosocial assessment should include the reaction of the woman's family and support system. Nursing assessment helps determine whether the condition is responding to medical management or the disease is worsening.

20. To prevent seizures, maintain a quiet environment, reduce environmental stimuli, and maintain a therapeutic level of magnesium. Nurses must remain with the

woman and call for help if a seizure occurs. If time allows, attempt to turn the woman on her side. Note the sequence and time of the seizure. Insert an airway after the seizure and suction the woman's nose and mouth, administer oxygen, administer medications, and prepare for additional medical interventions.

21. To prevent seizure-related injury, the side rails should be padded and raised. The bed should be in the lowest position with the wheels locked. Oxygen and suction should be readily available. Necessary equipment and medications should be kept in the room.

22. Signs of magnesium toxicity include respiratory rate below 12 breaths per minute, hyporeflexia, sweating or flushing, altered sensorium (lethargy, drowsiness, disorientation), and serum magnesium level beyond the therapeutic range. If toxicity occurs, notify the physician so the dose can be altered or the drug discontinued. Calcium gluconate is the antidote for magnesium toxicity.

23. *H,* Hemolysis; *EL,* elevated liver enzymes; *LP,* low platelets. Major symptoms are pain and tenderness in the right upper quadrant. Additional signs and symptoms may include nausea, vomiting, and severe edema. Laboratory data include a low hematocrit, abnormal liver studies, coagulation abnormalities, and often abnormal renal studies. Palpating the liver could cause trauma, including rupture of a subcapsular hematoma.

24. Preeclampsia occurs only during pregnancy and the early postpartum period. Chronic hypertension is present before pregnancy or before the twentieth week of gestation and persists after the postpartum period. Hypertension that remains several weeks postpartum suggests that the woman has chronic hypertension even if her blood pressures were normal when she entered care. Treatment may be similar during pregnancy; however, chronic hypertension is often treated with antihypertensive medications before and during pregnancy. Preeclampsia may further complicate chronic hypertension.

25. Administration of $Rh_o(D)$ immunoglobulin prevents development of maternal anti-Rh antibodies and is recommended after any procedure that includes the possibility of maternal exposure to Rh-positive fetal blood.

26. Maternal anti-Rh antibodies cross the placental barrier and destroy fetal Rh-positive red blood cells. The fetus becomes anemic, bilirubin increases, and in severe cases severe neurologic disease can result.

27. Many women with blood type O have anti-A or anti-B antibodies before they become pregnant, so the first pregnancy can be affected. The effects of ABO incompatibility are milder than Rh sensitization because fewer maternal antibodies cross into fetal blood.

CHAPTER 26

1. The hormones of pregnancy cause resistance of maternal cells to insulin, which increases the availability of glucose for the fetus.

2. The mother is at risk to develop preeclampsia, urinary tract infections, ketoacidosis, and preterm labor. Possible fetal and neonatal effects include congenital malformations; small or large fetal size, depending on the placental vascular supply; fetal hypoxemia; and polycythemia. Neonatal effects include hypoglycemia, hypocalcemia, hyperbilirubinemia, and respiratory distress syndrome.

3. Insulin needs decrease during the first trimester and increase sharply during the second and third trimesters (when placental hormones initiate insulin resistance). During the muscular exertion and reduced oral intake associated with labor, insulin needs must be determined by frequent checks of blood glucose to keep the glucose within normal limits. In the postpartum period insulin needs decrease as placental hormones decline.

4. Glycosylated hemoglobin gives an accurate evaluation of blood glucose for the past 2 to 3 months and is not affected by recent intake of food.

5. Gestational diabetes mellitus is first diagnosed during pregnancy. It is often managed by diet and exercise, although insulin may be needed if fasting or postprandial capillary blood glucose values are persistently high.

6. A glucose challenge test (GCT) is a screening procedure only and requires no fasting before the woman drinks the 50-g glucose solution. A 3-hour oral glucose tolerance test (OGTT) is performed to diagnose diabetes mellitus. The OGTT requires a fasting blood glucose level followed by ingestion of 100 g of glucose solution. Blood glucose levels are drawn hourly after the solution is taken, at 1, 2, and 3 hours.

7. Maternal effects of gestational diabetes mellitus include increased incidence of urinary tract infections, hydramnios (excessive amniotic fluid), premature rupture of membranes, and development of pregnancy-associated hypertension. Fetal effects may include macrosomia, which can result in shoulder dystocia or cesarean birth. The newborn is at risk for hypoglycemia. Preexisting diabetes has similar maternal effects as gestational diabetes, but fetal and infant effects differ. The infant may have IUGR if the woman's diabetes has caused vascular impairment, or macrosomia if her glucose is poorly controlled and no vascular impairment exists. Congenital anomalies are increased in preexisting diabetes, especially if the diabetes is poorly controlled at conception and during early gestation.

8. Increased intravascular volume and increased cardiac output (particularly stroke volume) place an added burden on the heart of a woman who has a cardiac defect.

9. Rheumatic and congenital heart disease are the two major categories of heart disease during pregnancy. Acute problems such as myocardial infarction or conduction disorders may also occur during pregnancy. Functional classification depends on the person's ability to tolerate activity. Class I indicates no limitation on activity. Class II indicates slight restriction if necessary. Class III is associated with marked limitation. Class IV indicates that the person has symptoms such as dyspnea even at rest.

10. Goals of treatment are to prevent anemia so there is an adequate supply of red blood cells to transport oxygen and thus reduce the demands on the heart, limit physical activity so cardiac demand does not exceed the capacity of the heart, and limit weight gain, which would add further demands on the heart.

11. With every contraction, blood is shifted from the uterus and placenta into the central circulation. This can lead to fluid overload if fluids are administered rapidly.

12. An additional 500 ml of blood are added to the central circulation with delivery of the placenta. Also, the compression of the vena cava that characterized much of pregnancy is gone. This increases the load on the heart and can lead to further compromise of the heart.

13. Most women begin pregnancy with marginal iron stores, do not have adequate iron stores to meet the demands of pregnancy, and have difficulty meeting the high iron needs of pregnancy with diet alone.

14. The fetus usually receives adequate iron, even at a cost to the mother. Therefore, neonatal effects of moderate maternal anemia are rare. With very severe maternal anemia, however, the fetus may become hypoxic.

15. The fetal and neonatal effects of folic acid deficiency are increased risk of spontaneous abortion, abruption of the placenta, and fetal anomalies, particularly neural tube defects.

16. Pregnancy may worsen sickle cell disease, and the risk of "sickle cell crisis" is increased.

17. Frequent evaluations of hemoglobin, blood count, serum iron, and iron-binding capacity as well as folate are necessary to determine the degree of anemia. Frequent fetal surveillance and monitoring for signs of sickle cell crisis are also necessary. The nurse must also be aware that the woman's pain could be a pregnancy complication rather than a result of sickle cell crisis.

18. Thalassemia is associated with increased iron absorption and storage, making women with this disorder susceptible to iron overload.

19. The maternal and fetal effects of systemic lupus erythematosus are increased incidence of abortion, fetal death, and preterm delivery. Congenital heart block, often permanent, is a serious complication for the newborn. Pregnancy can exacerbate the disease, and renal complications pose a special risk.

20. There is often marked improvement of rheumatoid arthritis during pregnancy. However, relapse often occurs soon after childbirth.

21. Hypothyroidism in the woman may cause adverse effects on the mental development of the fetus through birth and childhood.

22. Anticonvulsant drugs may be teratogenic. Many have probable or known adverse effects on the fetus. However, generalized seizures may also have adverse fetal effects, so maintaining the anticonvulsant dose as low as possible is important. Newer anticonvulsants have fewer data related to their possible fetal effects.

23. The recommended supportive care for women with Bell's palsy includes eye patching, applying ointment or drops to prevent trauma to the cornea, facial massage, and psychological support. Corticosteroids may be given.

24. A fetus born to a woman who has primary CMV infection during pregnancy has a 40-50% chance of being infected. Five to 10% of these infected newborns are symptomatic at birth and another 5-10% of infants will develop problems within the first 2 years after birth. Problems include enlarged spleen and liver, CNS abnormalities, jaundice, chorioretinitis, hearing loss, and IUGR.

25. The first trimester is the time of organogenesis, when damage can be done to all developing organ systems.

26. A vaccine is available to prevent rubella but it cannot be given during pregnancy. During pregnancy a woman can only avoid situations in which she is likely to contract rubella. Rubella immunization should be given to the woman before discharge after birth, and she should be taught that pregnancy should be avoided for 4 weeks after the immunization.

27. Immunization with varicella-zoster immune globulin is recommended. Infected mothers and infants must be isolated from those who are not immune.

28. Vertical transmission of herpesvirus occurs when organisms ascend after rupture of membranes and during birth when the fetus comes into contact with infectious tissue and secretions.

29. The fetal and neonatal effects of parvovirus B19 infection are failure of red blood cell production, severe fetal anemia, hydrops, and heart failure.

30. Hepatitis B virus is transmitted by contact with infected blood, saliva, vaginal secretions, semen, or breast milk. A newborn whose mother is known to carry the hepatitis B surface antigen should receive hepatitis B immune globulin soon after birth, followed by hepatitis B vaccine. The infant should receive the second and third doses of vaccine at regularly scheduled times.

31. Avoid sexual transmission by abstinence, avoiding intercourse with infected persons, or using recommended barrier methods. Intravenous drug users who refuse rehabilitation must avoid transmission that occurs when needles are shared with those who are infected. Use standard precautions to avoid contact with secretions that may carry the virus.

32. Several combinations of antiretroviral medication regimens may be administered to delay replication of the virus. Medications are also available to prevent *Pneumocystis carinii* pneumonia. Opportunistic diseases are treated. Good hygiene reduces transmission of infectious organisms to the susceptible person, and nutritious meals reduce the risk for opportunistic infection. Zidovudine therapy reduces vertical transmission of HIV to the infant and ideally begins during the second trimester of pregnancy. Additional zidovudine continues after birth for the infant. Maternal therapy often includes additional drugs.

33. Toxoplasmosis can be prevented by cooking meat thoroughly, not touching mucous membranes while han-

dling raw meat, washing kitchen surfaces and hands thoroughly after handling raw meat, avoiding uncooked eggs and unpasteurized milk, washing vegetables and fruit before consumption, and avoiding contact with materials that may be contaminated with cat feces.

34. Risk factors for the mother transmitting GBS to her infant include a prior infant with GBS infection, presence of GBS organisms in the urine in the present pregnancy, preterm birth (before 37 weeks), maternal fever in labor, prolonged membrane rupture ($\geq$18 hours). Intravenous antibacterial therapy is used to prevent colonization.

35. Isoniazid, rifampin, and pyrazinamide given for 9 months are used to treat tuberculosis in the mother. Ethambutol is often added based on drug sensitivity of the organism. Pyridoxine is added to prevent neurotoxicity. The infant is skin tested at birth and may be started on isoniazid therapy until the skin test, which will be repeated, remains negative.

CHAPTER 27

1. Hypotonic labor dysfunction usually occurs during the active phase of first stage labor (4 cm cervical dilation or more), whereas hypertonic dysfunction usually occurs during the latent phase (within the first 3 cm of cervical dilation). Uterine contractions become weaker, shorter, and less frequent in hypotonic dysfunction. In hypertonic dysfunction, contractions are painful but inefficient and the uterine resting tone is high. Hypotonic dysfunction is not painful because the contractions decrease, although the woman may become tired. Hypertonic dysfunction is characterized by a cramping type of pain. Management of both depends on the identified cause. Hypotonic dysfunction often is managed by ensuring adequate intake of fluids and electrolytes, position changes, amniotomy if the membranes are not ruptured, and oxytocin augmentation. Hypertonic dysfunction may be managed by mild sedation or tocolytic drugs to reduce excess uterine activity. Oxytocin in very low doses may be used occasionally to help coordinate uterine activity.

2. Maternal position changes encourage the fetus to rotate from an occiput transverse or occiput posterior position to an occiput anterior position, similar to nesting two spoons together. The convex surface of the rounded fetal back rotates toward the convex surface of the anterior uterus. The squatting position also increases pelvic diameters and straightens the pelvic curve to facilitate both fetal rotation and descent.

3. Other complications are associated with a fetus in a breech presentation that may cause problems, regardless of the method of birth. These include low birth weight, fetal anomalies, and associated pregnancy or labor complications.

4. The staff must be prepared for care of multiple infants. Duplicate staff and equipment should be ready for every infant expected.

5. Bladder distention during labor can consume available room in the woman's pelvis, thus impeding labor progress and fetal descent. In addition, it is a potential source of discomfort.

6. Psychological support reduces stress that otherwise can consume energy the uterus needs, inhibit uterine contractions, reduce placental blood supply, impair the woman's pushing efforts, and increase the woman's pain experience.

7. The average nullipara's cervix dilates about 1.2 cm per hour; minimal fetal descent is 1 cm per hour. The average parous woman's cervix dilates about 1.5 cm per hour, with minimal descent of 2 cm per hour.

8. Nursing care for the woman who has prolonged labor is similar to that for dysfunctional labor. Promoting comfort, energy conservation, position changes, and assessments for related complications such as infection should be done.

9. Trauma is the primary maternal risk of a precipitate labor and may include uterine rupture, cervical lacerations, and hematomas. Fetal risks may include trauma, such as intracranial hemorrhage or nerve damage, and hypoxia. Abruptio placentae may cause maternal hemorrhage and fetal hypoxia because of the premature detachment of the placenta from the uterus.

10. Premature rupture of the membranes (PROM) occurs before true labor any time during pregnancy. Preterm premature rupture of the membranes (PPROM) occurs before 37 weeks of gestation are completed and may be accompanied by contractions. PPROM is more likely to be associated with preterm labor and birth.

11. Infection may be both a cause and result of premature rupture of the membranes, particularly if birth is not desired because of fetal immaturity.

12. Labor is usually induced if a woman with ruptured membranes is near term and has a favorable cervix and if labor does not spontaneously begin within at least 12 to 24 hours. Prostaglandin in the form of Cervidil or Prepidil may be used to soften the cervix if she is at least 36 weeks of gestation. If she is slightly preterm (32 to 35 weeks), the physician will deliver the infant if infection is present, the fetal lungs are mature, or both. If no infection exists and the fetal lungs are not mature, expectant care with periodic tests for fetal lung maturity and fetal well-being are done. Steroids and antibiotics are given to mothers at earlier gestations to speed fetal lung maturation and reduce infections that may have contributed to or be a result of PPROM.

13. The nurse should assess the woman's vital signs and FHR, teach her to avoid insertion of anything into the vagina, avoid breast stimulation, maintain activity restrictions, and note any uterine contractions, and teach her how to observe fetal kick counts.

14. Symptoms of preterm labor often are vague. They include uterine contractions that may often be painless, the fetus "balling up," menstrual-like cramps, backache, pelvic pressure, changed or increased vaginal discharge,

abdominal cramps, thigh pain, and a sense of "feeling bad."

15. Early identification of preterm labor enables management that may delay birth and allow further maturation of the fetus or permit transfer to a facility equipped to care for an immature infant. Corticosteroids may be given to the mother of a fetus between 24 and 34 weeks to accelerate maturation of the lungs before preterm birth.

16. Classifications of drugs to inhibit preterm contractions include beta-adrenergics such as terbutaline, magnesium sulfate, prostaglandin synthesis inhibitors such as indomethacin, and calcium channel blockers such as nifedipine.

17. Corticosteroids are given to the woman who is likely to deliver prematurely to accelerate maturation of the fetal lungs and reduce the incidence of intraventricular hemorrhage. The greatest benefits occur if steroids are in the mother's system at least 24 hours before birth. The newborn who delivers before 24 hours after the mother receives corticosteroids may also benefit.

18. The three potential fetal or newborn risks are reduced placental function and umbilical cord compression before birth and meconium aspiration after birth.

19. If umbilical cord prolapse occurs, the priority of care is to reduce compression of and restore normal blood flow through the cord while giving the mother oxygen to maximize her blood oxygen concentration. At the same time, the nurse should summon help to expedite delivery, usually by cesarean birth.

20. Stimulated contractions are potentially more powerful than natural ones and may cause the pressure in the uterus to exceed the uterine wall's ability to withstand that pressure.

21. Shock and hemorrhage are rapidly developing complications of uterine inversion. They are managed by rapid IV fluid and blood replacement, often using two IV lines. A drug that relaxes the uterus is given to allow uterine replacement, and general anesthesia may be needed. Oxytocin is given *after* the uterus is replaced in the proper position. Hemodynamic monitoring may be required to ensure stabilization.

22. For intrapartum emergencies, nursing considerations include the following: *Prolapsed umbilical cord*—Relieve pressure on the cord to restore adequate blood flow through it until the baby can be delivered. *Uterine rupture*—Attempt to prevent by cautious intrapartum use of uterine stimulants and close monitoring of uterine contractions. *Uterine inversion*—Avoid pressure on the poorly contracted fundus after birth; assess for and correct shock. *Amniotic fluid embolism*—Cardiorespiratory support; hemodynamic monitoring; observe for coagulation deficits.

23. The fetus may suffer direct injury such as skull fracture or intracranial hemorrhage related to maternal injuries such as pelvic fracture, penetrating wounds, or blunt trauma. Fetal injury from indirect causes includes

abruptio placentae and disruption of placental flow because of maternal hemorrhage or shock.

CHAPTER 28

1. The nurse examines a woman's previous records to identify factors that would predispose her to complications such as postpartum hemorrhage.

2. Overdistention of uterine muscles makes their contraction more difficult and excessive bleeding more likely.

3. The nurse cannot be certain that bleeding is controlled because concealed bleeding can occur in soft tissue and produce a hematoma.

4. Initial management of uterine atony focuses on measures to contract the uterus, such as massaging, expressing clots, and emptying the bladder. Pharmacologic measures include fluid replacement and administration of oxytocin, methylergonovine, or other drugs such as carboprost.

5. Large hematomas may require incision and evacuation of clots, as well as ligation of the bleeding vessel. Small hematomas do not require treatment.

6. It may be difficult to recognize hypovolemia because of compensatory mechanisms, such as carotid and aortic baroreceptors, which constrict peripheral blood vessels. This shunts blood to the central circulation, maintains blood pressure, and increases the heart rate.

7. The major signs of subinvolution are prolonged lochial discharge, irregular or excessive uterine bleeding, pelvic pain and heaviness, backache, fatigue, and malaise.

8. Nurses must teach the mother how to palpate the fundus, to estimate fundal height, and to report abnormalities of lochia, a foul odor, or pelvic pain.

9. Venous stasis increases during pregnancy because of compression of the large vessels by the enlarging uterus. At birth, stasis may occur when the woman is in stirrups. Changes in the coagulation and fibrinolytic systems during pregnancy and the postpartum period elevate the factors that favor coagulation and decrease the factors that favor lysis of clots.

10. Signs and symptoms of superficial venous thrombosis include swelling, tenderness, warmth, and redness.

11. Heparin remains the long-term treatment of the pregnant woman with deep venous thrombosis because warfarin (Coumadin) may be teratogenic and predisposes the fetus to hemorrhage. Heparin is changed to warfarin in the postpartum period.

12. Bed rest is prescribed for the woman with deep vein thrombosis to decrease swelling and to promote venous return from the leg.

13. The nurse assesses mothers receiving anticoagulants for unexplained bruising, petechiae, bleeding from the nose, bladder or gums, or increased vaginal bleeding. Signs of hemorrhage, such as tachycardia, falling blood pressure, or other signs of shock, also should be noted.

14. The home care nurse should assess family structure and function that will need to change as a result of prolonged treatment for the mother. The nurse should eval-

uate mother-infant interaction and determine what support system may be available to provide assistance.

15. Cesarean birth or the use of vacuum extraction or forceps may result in trauma that provides a portal of entry for infectious organisms.

16. All parts of the reproductive tract are connected, and organisms can move from the vagina through the cervix, uterus, and fallopian tubes and into the peritoneal cavity. Alkalinity of the vagina during labor, necrosis of the endometrium, and the presence of lochia encourage bacterial growth.

17. When labor is prolonged, organisms have time and opportunity to ascend from the vagina into the uterus, increasing the risk of infection. Also, there may be more vaginal examinations and ruptured membranes for a longer time.

18. Fever, chills, lethargy, malaise, anorexia, abdominal pain and cramping, uterine tenderness, and purulent foul-smelling lochia, tachycardia, and subinvolution are signs and symptoms of metritis. It usually is treated by IV administration of antibiotics, antipyretics, and oxytocics to promote involution.

19. Wound infection most often occurs in cesarean incisions, episiotomies, and lacerations.

20. Incisions and lacerations should be inspected for redness, tenderness, edema, and approximation of the edges of the wound, which may pull apart with infection.

21. To prevent urinary tract infection, the woman should be advised to drink at least 2500 to 3000 ml of fluid each day, empty her bladder every 2 to 3 hours during the day, and practice meticulous hygiene. Cystitis and pyelonephritis may be treated with oral antibiotics on an outpatient basis. Severe pyelonephritis or the infection during pregnancy may require hospitalization and IV antibiotics.

22. Measures to prevent mastitis include correct positioning of the infant, frequent emptying of the breasts, and avoiding nipple trauma and supplemental feedings. In addition, the woman should avoid continuous pressure on the breasts caused by tight bras or infant carriers.

23. The symptoms of postpartum depression differ from those of postpartum "blues" by the number, intensity, and persistence of symptoms. They are present daily for at least 2 weeks. These symptoms include a loss of interest in one's surroundings, a loss of usual emotional responses, and feelings of unworthiness, guilt, and shame.

24. Nurses can demonstrate caring, provide anticipatory guidance, help the mother verbalize her feelings, and make appropriate referrals.

25. Postpartum psychosis usually requires hospitalization, psychotherapy, and appropriate medication.

CHAPTER 29

1. Preterm infants appear frail and weak and are small, with limp extremities, poor muscle tone, red skin, and immature ears, nipples, areolae, and genitals.

2. Factors that increase respiratory problems in preterm infants include lack of surfactant, poor cough reflex, small air passages, and weak muscles.

3. Nursing responsibilities for preterm infants with respiratory problems include working with respiratory therapists to manage equipment, monitoring the infant's changing oxygen needs, positioning infants to promote drainage, and suctioning.

4. Nurses wean infants to the open crib by making gradual changes in the environmental temperature, dressing the infant, and using blankets and a hat when the infant is out of the incubator.

5. To measure intake and output for infants, all fluids (IV and oral), including medications, are measured. Diapers are weighed to calculate urine output, and drainage, regurgitation, and stools are measured.

6. Preterm infants' kidneys do not concentrate or dilute urine well, and they have large insensible water losses. They lack passive antibodies from the mother and have an immature immune system. Pain causes physiologic responses such as vital sign changes and decreases in oxygenation.

7. Nonpharmacologic methods to reduce pain in infants include positioning, swaddling, facilitated tucking, sucking, and sucrose.

8. The nurse can diminish overstimulation by organizing care to provide for rest periods, reducing environmental stimuli, minimizing pain, and discussing the plan of care with others.

9. Feeding tolerance is assessed by checking gastric residual volume before gavage feedings, measuring abdominal girth, testing stools for reducing substances and blood, and observing for regurgitation. During nipple feedings, the nurse watches for signs of respiratory difficulty, decreased oxygenation, and fatigue.

10. When allowed to set the pace of feedings, infants can stop to rest to conserve energy and regulate breathing, and control the flow of milk. Moving the nipple in the infant's mouth may cause fatigue and choking.

11. The nurse can help breastfeeding mothers of preterm infants by teaching them ways to pump and store milk and breastfeeding techniques adapted to the preterm infant's needs and by providing support and encouragement.

12. The nurse can help parents feel comfortable with preterm infants by providing warm support, realistic encouragement, and information about the NICU environment, the infant's condition and characteristics, and the equipment and care. Involving the parents in care also helps.

13. Helping parents take on partial responsibility for care, beginning early in hospitalization, and gradually increasing their responsibility will help them prepare for discharge of their infant. Helping them prepare their home for the infant is also important.

14. Postmature infants may be thin and have loose skin folds, cracked and peeling skin, minimal vernix or lanugo, and meconium staining and may look worried.

15. Postmature infants may have polycythemia, meconium aspiration, hypoglycemia, and poor temperature regulation.

16. In symmetric growth restriction, all body parts are proportionately small. In asymmetric growth restriction, the head is normal in size but seems large for the small body and the length is generally normal.

17. LGA infants may have birth injuries such as fractures, nerve damage, cephalhematoma, hypoglycemia, and polycythemia.

CHAPTER 30

1. Waiting to give an Apgar to an infant who needs resuscitation delays treatment unnecessarily and may make resuscitation more difficult. The Apgar scores can be given during the resuscitation process.

2. The nurse's role in asphyxia is to begin resuscitation promptly, assist the team, and provide follow-up and parental support.

3. Transient tachypnea of the newborn is caused by failure of fetal lung fluid to be absorbed completely in full-term or preterm infants. Respiratory distress syndrome occurs in preterm infants as a result of inadequate surfactant.

4. Meconium staining may be found in normal full-term infants. It is most likely to be present when infants are postterm and have decreased amniotic fluid and cord compression, in SGA infants, and in infants with asphyxia.

5. Infants with PPHN have constriction of the pulmonary blood vessels from inadequate oxygen levels and acidosis. This increases resistance to blood flow into the lungs and causes blood to flow through a patent foramen ovale and ductus arteriosus.

6. Kernicterus can be prevented by identifying women whose infants are at risk for blood incompatibilities, giving Rh-negative mothers Rh immune globulin, recognizing infants with bilirubin levels that are pathological, and instituting phototherapy when it is needed.

7. Nurses can help reduce bilirubin in an infant receiving phototherapy by ensuring that the lights or blankets are functioning and positioned properly; reducing the infant's time out of phototherapy; ensuring adequate intake to increase removal of bilirubin by frequent stools; preventing cold stress or hypoglycemia, which would decrease albumin-binding sites for bilirubin; and turning the infant frequently to expose all areas to the lights.

8. Vertical infection is transmitted from the mother to the infant during pregnancy or birth. Horizontal infection is transmitted from other people to the infant after birth.

9. The role of the nurse in sepsis is to identify early signs, notify the physician, coordinate treatment, observe for change, and support the family.

10. Macrosomia occurs in IDMs because of excessive transfer of glucose, amino acids, and fatty acids from the mother to the fetus. This results in fetal production of insulin and excessive growth in the fetus.

11. IDMs may develop hypoglycemia after birth because they have high levels of insulin even though they no longer receive glucose from the mother. Infants may need early feeding as a result.

12. The nurse can help the drug-exposed infant to rest by minimizing stimulation, swaddling in a flexed position, organizing care to avoid interruptions, and providing a pacifier.

13. The nurse can promote bonding when there has been prenatal drug abuse by helping the mother feel welcome, encouraging her to participate in infant care, teaching her about the infant's behavior and how to respond and about the infant's care, and modeling parenting behaviors.

14. Cyanotic heart defects allow unoxygenated blood flow into the systemic circulation, producing cyanosis. Acyanotic heart defects cause impairment of blood flow or circulation of oxygenated blood into the pulmonary system, usually without cyanosis. Other categories are by blood flow, including increased or decreased pulmonary blood flow, obstruction to blood flow, or mixing of venous and oxygenated blood.

CHAPTER 31

1. Almost all contraceptive methods are used by women, and failure will most affect women.

2. The nurse's role in helping women with contraception is to provide information so that women can choose contraceptives appropriately and use them correctly.

3. Important considerations in choosing contraceptive techniques include safety, protection from sexually transmissible diseases, effectiveness, acceptability, convenience, education needed, benefits, side effects, interference with spontaneity, availability, expense, preference of the woman and her partner, religious beliefs, and culture.

4. Sterilization, hormonal contraceptives, and intrauterine devices may require signed informed consents.

5. Adolescents may have incorrect beliefs, such as that they cannot conceive during first intercourse, without orgasm, or without having menstruated a certain length of time or that douching will prevent pregnancy.

6. Adolescents may not seek contraception because they may fear lack of acceptance, loss of sexual privacy, pelvic examination, or adverse effects of contraception on their health.

7. The nurse can teach adolescents effectively by showing sensitivity to their feelings, being accepting, and providing extensive teaching without hurry, using understandable terms and audiovisual materials.

8. Perimenopausal women who do not smoke and have no other contraindications can use any method of contraception.

9. Important factors to consider when choosing a method of sterilization include time involved, cost, need for hospitalization, and feelings of each partner about a permanent end to the ability to have more children.

10. Hormonal contraceptives alter normal hormone changes, making the cervical mucus unfavorable to sperm, preventing ovulation, and altering the endometrium.

11. Menstrual changes and spotting are the reason some women stop using some hormonal contraceptives.

12. Women using OCs need to know that the pills must be taken consistently and in the right order every day, what to do if pills are missed, common side effects, and signs that may indicate a problem.

13. The first dose of ECP should be taken as soon as possible after unprotected intercourse and within 120 hrs. The second dose can be taken along with the first dose or 12 hours later.

14. Education for women choosing intrauterine devices includes information about side effects, when and how to check the strings, and when to seek medical treatment.

15. Barrier methods kill sperm or prevent them from entering the cervix or both.

16. Natural family planning methods avoid drugs, chemicals, and devices; are inexpensive; and are acceptable to most religions. Couples need extensive education and high motivation, however, and they risk pregnancy if they make an error.

CHAPTER 32

1. Infertility is strictly defined as the inability to conceive after 1 year of unprotected regular intercourse. A more workable definition that considers the age and other individual factors is the inability of a couple to conceive when desired. Primary infertility is that which occurs in couples who have never conceived. Secondary infertility occurs in those who have conceived before and are not able to conceive again.

2. The normal average number of sperm released at ejaculation is 40 to 250 million. Twenty million per milliliter is probably the minimum required for unassisted fertility. At least 30% of the sperm must be living and normal, and half must have normal forward movement. The amount of seminal fluid should be 2 to 6 ml and it should liquefy within 30 minutes. Seminal fluid should have fewer white blood cells than 1 million/ml.

3. Erection problems exist if the man cannot initiate and maintain a penile erection that is sufficient to allow intercourse and deposit of seminal fluid with sperm near the woman's cervix. Ejaculation abnormalities may result from retrograde ejaculation, hypospadias, or abnormal ejaculation response (premature, slow, or absent).

4. Abnormalities of the sperm, ejaculation, or the seminal fluid can result from factors such as abnormal hormone stimulation, systemic illness, infections or abnormalities of the reproductive tract, anatomic abnormalities of the reproductive system, exposure to toxins, therapeutic medications, excessive alcohol intake, illicit drug use, elevated scrotal temperature, obstruction, and immunologic factors.

5. Abnormal ovulation can occur because of hormone disruptions caused by cranial tumors, stress, obesity, anorexia, systemic disease, and abnormalities in the ovaries or other endocrine glands.

6. Hormone abnormalities associated with the ovulation problem interfere with normal buildup and decline of the endometrium. Menstrual periods may be absent, scant, or very heavy.

7. Fallopian tube obstruction may be caused by scarring or adhesions secondary to infections, endometriosis, or pelvic surgery. Congenital anomalies of the reproductive structures also can cause mechanical interference with successful pregnancy.

8. Abnormal cervical mucus can trap sperm and prevent them from entering the uterus and fallopian tube or prevent their preparation (capacitation) for fertilization.

9. Anatomic abnormalities of the woman's reproductive tract may prevent normal fertilization or implantation. They also may prevent normal placental or fetal growth, or they may increase the risk for miscarriage or pre-viable birth.

10. Endocrine abnormalities associated with repeated pregnancy loss include inadequate progesterone secretion, inadequate endometrial response to progesterone, hypothyroidism and hyperthyroidism, and maternal diabetes.

11. Immunologic causes of repeated pregnancy loss include an intolerance of the embryo's foreign tissue and systemic lupus erythematosus.

12. Elements included in the history and physical examination include a reproductive history, past medical history, examination for undiagnosed endocrine disturbances, tumors, chronic disease, and abnormalities of the reproductive organs. Chromosome analysis is sometimes done. Imaging studies are done if structural abnormalities are suspected.

13. Medications used to induce ovulation include clomiphene citrate, chorionic gonadotropins, gonadotropin-releasing hormone, and human gonadotropins. Clomiphene is a common drug for this purpose. Additional drugs may be given to increase the formation and release of ova and to support a pregnancy that results.

14. Screening tests related to use of donor sperm include those for blood type and Rh factor, possible genetic defects, and infection. In addition, the man's history, physical examination, and lifestyle are reviewed for possible problems that might not be revealed by standard tests. Donor sperm are frozen for 6 months to allow identification of infections or other problems that are not evident at the time of collection.

15. *In vitro* fertilization mixes the male and female gametes outside the body and places embryos back into the uterus. Gamete intrafallopian transfer retrieves ova, and then places the ova and sperm into the fallopian tubes, where fertilization takes place. Zygote intrafallopian transfer mixes male and female gametes to allow fertilization and places the fertilized ova into the fallopian tubes.

16. Factors that couples consider when seeking infertility help include their age, the length of their attempt to conceive, their desire for a biologic child, and their feelings about adoption or a child-free life. Financial constraints often are another consideration.

17. When deciding about infertility evaluations and treatments, the couple considers their personal, social, cultural, and religious values; how difficult treatment may be; the probability of success with treatment; and financial concerns.

18. Psychological reactions to infertility may include guilt, isolation, depression, or stress on the relationship.

19. Parenthood after infertility may be marked by anxiety about the pregnancy, loss of support from infertile couples, or unrealistic expectations about parenting abilities.

20. Couples considering adoption must confront their personal preferences, limitations, and prejudices.

21. Couples who lose a pregnancy after a period of infertility often experience grief, but sometimes the grief is mixed with optimism because they were able to achieve pregnancy, even if completion was not possible.

CHAPTER 33

1. The Women's Health Initiative studies the four major diseases that kill women: heart disease, breast cancer, colorectal cancer, and osteoporosis.

2. Family history is an important part of a health history to assess risk factors for conditions such as heart disease, breast and colon cancer, osteoporosis, and other health problems that should be studied.

3. When taking a sexual history, the nurse should ask about sexual activity, number of partners, age when sexual activity began, method of contraception, and knowledge about and measures used for protection from sexually transmitted diseases (STDs).

4. Three screening procedures for cancer of the breast are breast self-examination, clinical breast examination by a professional, and mammography, often with additional ultrasound or other imaging.

5. Vulvar self-examination is recommended to detect signs of precancerous conditions or infections.

6. A Pap test is a cytology specimen of the superficial layers of the cervix and endocervix to detect precancerous and cancerous cells of the cervix.

7. Fecal occult blood testing is important to detect colon or rectal cancer.

8. Medical treatment of fibrocystic breast changes is rare because side effects of the drugs may be more distressing than the breast discomfort. Reducing foods high in caffeine or sodium near the end of the menstrual cycle may reduce pain. Evening primrose oil is a botanical preparation that may help some women.

9. Ultrasound examination, fine needle aspiration biopsy, core needle biopsy, or surgical biopsy is used to determine whether a breast disorder is benign or malignant.

10. Major risk factors for breast cancer are gender (female), age (increases with age), mutations in certain genes (such as BRCA1, BRCA2, CHEK-2, and p53), a history of breast cancer, or first-degree relatives with breast cancer.

11. Staging of breast cancer is important to determine the extent of the breast cancer and to plan appropriate therapy.

12. Adjuvant therapy is supportive or additional therapy recommended after surgery to improve the chance of long-term survival. Adjuvant therapy includes radiation therapy, chemotherapy, hormonal therapy, and immunotherapy.

13. Breasts may be reconstructed during the initial surgery or later. Two major methods are the tissue expansion method and autogenous grafts from another area of the woman's body. Tissue grafting cannot be done in every woman.

14. Preoperative teaching should include a description of the pressure binder, wound suction, wound appearance, and any special exercises that may be recommended.

15. Discharge planning after breast cancer treatment should emphasize the need for continued care, reducing the risk for infection on the affected side, any postoperative medications, and signs and symptoms that should be reported to the physician. Referral to local support groups also may be helpful.

16. Although a woman may have the "classic" crushing chest pain that is associated with a myocardial infarction, she is more likely to have atypical pain that often is confused with other conditions. These symptoms include fatigue or weakness; angina or pain at rest; dyspnea; dizziness or faintness; upper abdominal pain, heartburn, or loss of appetite; nausea, vomiting, or sweating; and pain in the upper body other than the chest (arm, neck, back, jaw, throat, and tooth).

17. Measures to reduce the risk for coronary artery disease include smoking cessation, control of hypertension; diet and glucose control to maintain normal weight and optimum fat and cholesterol intake; increase in activity level; and, for many women, daily aspirin therapy.

18. Primary amenorrhea is menstruation that fails to occur within 2 years of breast development, usually between the ages of 10 and 16 years. Causes include hormonal imbalances, congenital anomalies, chromosomal defects, and systemic diseases as well as rigorous dieting and exercise. Treatment is aimed at identifying and treating the underlying cause. Secondary amenorrhea is cessation of menstruation for a period of at least 6 months in a woman who has an established pattern of menstruation. Pregnancy is the most common cause. Other causes include systemic disorders, hormonal imbalances, low weight for height, stress, poor nutrition, drug therapy for other disorders, and tumors of the ovary, pituitary, or adrenal gland. Once pregnancy is ruled out, treatment may include correction of the underlying cause, hormonal replacement therapy, and ovulation stimulation.

19. Possible causes of dysfunctional uterine bleeding include complications of pregnancy; benign or malignant

lesions of the vagina, cervix, or uterus; drug-induced bleeding; systemic diseases, which require prompt treatment; and failure to ovulate.

20. Primary dysmenorrhea has no identified pathology. High levels of endometrial prostaglandin diffuse into endometrial tissue, causing painful uterine contractions, uterine ischemia, and tissue hypoxia often called "cramps." Effective treatment includes rest, application of warmth, oral contraceptives, and prostaglandin inhibitors.

21. Endometriosis lesions grow and proliferate during the follicular and luteal phases of the menstrual cycle and then slough during menstruation. The menstruation from endometriosis lesions occurs in deeper tissue, causing pressure or pain that is deep, bilateral or unilateral, and dull or sharp. Treatment varies with the woman's age, whether she is nearing menopause, her desire for children, her willingness to take the drugs that inhibit excessive tissue growth, and the problems caused to nearby organs by endometriosis. In addition to delaying pregnancy, drug therapy may induce menopausal symptoms.

22. Side effects of danazol include headache, dizziness, irritability, decreased libido, and masculinizing effects. Most common side effects of GnRH agonists are hot flashes, vaginal dryness, decreased libido, and loss of bone mineral density.

23. Symptoms of PMS must be cyclic and recur in the luteal phase of the menstrual cycle; the woman should be symptom free during the follicular phase; symptoms must be severe enough to alter the work, lifestyle, and relationships of the woman; and the diagnosis must be based on the woman's charting of her symptoms in a diary as they occur rather than by recall.

24. Common nursing education includes planning exercise therapy, dietary measures to reduce fluid retention and other symptoms (such as restricting salty or sweet foods, chocolate, caffeine, and others), educating the family about how to relate to a woman who is very irritable, and helping the woman to make arrangements so that she can avoid harming her child if she becomes very agitated.

25. Mifepristone, methotrexate, and misoprostol may be used for medical termination of pregnancy.

26. The nurse should teach the woman self-care measures: observation for excessive bleeding or signs of infection, information about follow-up visits, and contraception information.

27. Without estrogen, the reproductive organs begin to atrophy and the vagina and labia are thinner and more fragile. The breasts become smaller and atrophy. Bladder changes associated with atrophy make the woman more vulnerable to cystitis. Total cholesterol and low-density lipoproteins ("bad" cholesterol) increase, while high-density lipoproteins ("good" cholesterol) decrease, increasing the woman's risk for coronary artery disease. Hot flashes occur because of vasomotor instability. Bone mineral loss accelerates in the first few years of the

climacteric. Loss of estrogen also appears to increase the risk for Alzheimer's disease.

28. Depression, mood swings, and irritability are common psychological symptoms of menopause as the woman comes to term with aging. A woman may also greet menopause as a freedom from earlier obligations in life as she shifts responsibility to her adult children.

29. Estrogen replacement controls hot flashes, alleviates genital atrophy, and protects against osteoporosis. Estrogen replacement must begin early in the perimenopause to provide significant protection against osteoporosis. If the woman has a uterus, progesterone is given for part of the cycle to prevent excessive buildup of the endometrium. Although once thought to reduce the incidence of cardiovascular disease and breast cancers, estrogen-progesterone replacement showed the opposite effect in the Women's Health Initiative study. At this time a woman must make a careful choice after weighing the benefits and drawbacks of HRT.

30. Osteoporosis is called the "silent thief" because there may be no signs or symptoms until posture changes as the vertebrae collapse or fractures occur.

31. Osteoporosis can be prevented by medications to enhance calcium absorption and inhibit calcium loss, calcium and vitamin D supplementation, and exercise to strengthen muscles and increase weight bearing. HRT also enhances calcium retention, but potential problems with HRT limits its usefulness for many women.

32. Nurses can help women with osteoporosis avoid falls by making their environment as safe as possible and enhancing their exercise programs. Adolescents and young women can also be taught the value of exercise in maintaining long-term bone health.

33. With a cystocele the weakened upper anterior wall of the vagina cannot support the weight of urine, and the bladder protrudes downward into the vagina, resulting in incomplete emptying of the bladder and consequent cystitis and stress incontinence. With a rectocele the rectum protrudes into the vagina as the upper posterior wall of the vagina becomes weakened, which may result in difficulty emptying the rectum.

34. Uterine prolapse is caused when the cardinal ligaments are unduly stretched during pregnancy and do not return to normal. This condition is usually treated surgically according to severity.

35. Pelvic exercises and bladder training may alleviate symptoms of pelvic floor relaxation and urinary incontinence. Additional measures include teaching about the need to maintain hydration and restrict alcohol and caffeine, weight control to reach optimal weight, and use of commercial products to protect the skin and prevent odor. Teaching about any prescribed medications may be indicated.

36. Signs and symptoms of leiomyomas are increased uterine size and excessive vaginal bleeding, which often results in anemia. Other symptoms are pelvic pressure, bloating, and urinary frequency, depending on the size

and location of the fibroids. Treatment depends on size, symptoms, and whether the woman desires more children. Surgical treatment options include removal of the fibroids (myomectomy) or hysterectomy.

37. Ultrasound is used to distinguish a fluid-filled ovarian cyst from a solid tumor, which requires additional evaluation to determine if the solid tumor is malignant.

38. Signs and symptoms that may indicate cancer of the reproductive organs are irregular vaginal bleeding, unexplained postmenopausal bleeding, unusual vaginal discharge, dyspareunia, persistent vaginal itching, elevated or discolored lesions of the vulva, abdominal bloating, persistent constipation, anorexia, or nausea. Reproductive organ cancers such as ovarian cancer may have no symptoms in the early stages.

39. Cervical cancer may be treated by cryosurgery, destruction of tissue by laser, loop electrosurgical excision procedure (LEEP), electrocoagulation surgical conization, or hysterectomy with chemotherapy for more advanced cases. Endometrial cancer is best treated with hysterectomy and bilateral salpingo-oophorectomy plus radiation. Radiation only may be used if the woman is a poor surgical candidate. Ovarian cancer is often treated by chemotherapy to reduce the tumor's size, followed by oophorectomy and more chemotherapy.

40. Pregnancy, diabetes mellitus, oral contraceptive use, and antibiotic therapy may result in vaginitis caused by *Candida albicans.*

41. Candidiasis causes a thick, white discharge, often with "cottage-cheese" characteristics. Trichomoniasis causes a thin or frothy, malodorous, and yellow-green or dirty gray discharge.

42. Barrier methods of contraception (particularly condoms) prevent potentially infected ejaculate from entering the genital tract and prevent contact between the penis and vagina.

43. The major symptom of primary syphilis is a painless chancre that disappears in about 6 weeks; the disease is highly infectious during primary syphilis. Symptoms of secondary syphilis are enlargement of the liver and spleen, headache, anorexia, and skin rash. Condylomata lata that contain numerous spirochetes and are highly contagious may develop.

44. Condylomata acuminata (genital warts) are caused by HPV, which is associated with cervical cancer.

45. *Chlamydia trachomatis* and *Neisseria gonorrhoeae* cause most cases of PID. Other pathogens, including *Escherichia coli, Gardnerella vaginalis, Streptococcus, Peptostreptococcus, Bacteroides, Prevotella, Mycoplasma, Ureaplasm,* and cytomegalovirus may cause PID.

46. The risk of toxic shock syndrome can be reduced by changing tampons at least every 4 hours, avoiding use of superabsorbent tampons, and using pads rather than tampons during hours of sleep. The diaphragm or cervical cap should not be used during menstruation, and the device should be removed within the time limits recommended. Careful handwashing should be done before and after use of tampons, pads, diaphragm, or cervical cap for all women.

Glossary

abortion A pregnancy that ends before 20 weeks' gestation, either spontaneously (miscarriage) or electively. *Miscarriage* is a lay term for spontaneous abortion that is being more frequently used by health professionals.

abruptio placentae Premature separation of a normally implanted placenta.

abstinence syndrome A group of symptoms that occurs when a person who is addicted to a specific drug withdraws or abstains from taking that drug.

acidosis Condition resulting from accumulation of acid (hydrogen ions) or depletion of base (bicarbonate); acid-base balance measured by pH.

acme Peak or period of greatest strength of a uterine contraction.

acrocyanosis Bluish discoloration of the hands and feet because of reduced peripheral circulation.

addiction Physical or psychological dependence on a substance, such as alcohol, tobacco, or drugs, either legal or illicit.

adjuvant therapy Additional treatment that increases or enhances the action of the primary treatment.

adnexa Accessory parts or organs, such as the fallopian tubes and ovaries associated with the uterus.

afterpains Cramping pain after childbirth caused by alternate relaxation and contraction of uterine muscles.

agonist Substance causing a physiologic effect.

alcohol-related birth defects (ARBD) Birth defects that are directly attributed to prenatal exposure to alcohol.

alcohol-related neurodevelopmental disorder (ARND) Neurologic conditions and delayed development resulting from prenatal exposure to alcohol.

alcoholism A chronic, progressive, and potentially fatal disease characterized by tolerance for and physical dependency on alcohol, or by pathologic organ changes resulting from alcohol abuse, or both.

allele An alternate form of a gene.

alpha-fetoprotein Plasma protein produced by the fetus.

ambiguity (ambiguous) Lack of clarity or certainty; having more than one meaning.

ambivalence Simultaneous conflicting emotions, attitudes, ideas, or wishes.

amenorrhea Absence of menstruation. Primary amenorrhea is a delay of the first menstruation and secondary amenorrhea is cessation of menstruation after its initiation.

amniocentesis Transabdominal puncture of the amniotic sac to obtain a sample of amniotic fluid that contains fetal cells and biochemical substances for laboratory examination.

amnioinfusion Infusion of a sterile isotonic solution into the uterine cavity during labor to reduce umbilical cord compression; also done to dilute meconium in amniotic fluid, which reduces the risk that the infant will aspirate thick meconium at birth.

amniotic fluid embolism An embolism in which amniotic fluid with its particulate matter is drawn into the pregnant woman's circulation, lodging in her lungs.

amniotic fluid index (AFI) An ultrasound examination in which the vertical depth of the largest fluid pocket in each of the four quadrants of the uterus is measured and totaled.

amniotomy Artificial rupture of the amniotic sac (fetal membranes).

amphetamines Central nervous system stimulants that create a perception of pleasure unrelated to external stimuli.

analgesic Systemic agent that relieves pain without loss of consciousness.

anaphylactoid syndrome A disorder in which amniotic fluid with its particulate matter enters the pregnant woman's circulation, lodging in her lungs. Previously called amniotic fluid embolism.

anesthesia Loss of sensation, especially to pain, with or without loss of consciousness.

anesthesiologist Physician who specializes in administration of anesthesia.

angina pectoris Myocardial pain usually brought on by physical activity or stress; usually called simply *angina*.

anorexia nervosa Refusal to eat because of a distorted body image and feeling of obesity.

anovulatory (or anovular) Menstrual cycles occurring without ovulation.

antagonist Drug that blocks the action of another drug or of body secretions.

antepartum The time during pregnancy before the onset of labor.

antiphospholipid antibodies Autoimmune antibodies that are directed against phospholipids in cell membranes. It is associated with recurrent spontaneous abortion, fetal loss, and severe preeclampsia.

apneic spells Cessation of breathing for more than 20 seconds or accompanied by cyanosis or bradycardia.

asphyxia Insufficient oxygen and excess carbon dioxide in the blood and tissues.

aspiration pneumonitis Chemical injury to the lungs that may occur with regurgitation and aspiration of acidic gastric secretions.

assisted reproductive techniques (ART) Use of medical, surgical, laboratory, and/or micromanipulation techniques to handle the ovum and sperm to improve chances of conception.

assumptions Beliefs taken for granted without examination.

atony Absence or lack of usual muscle tone.

atrophic vaginitis Inflammation that occurs when the vagina becomes dry and fragile, usually as a result of estrogen deficit after menopause.

attachment Development of strong affectional ties as a result of interaction between an infant and a significant other (such as mother, father, sibling, or caretaker).

attitude Relationship of fetal body parts to one another.

augmentation of labor Artificial stimulation of uterine contractions that have become ineffective.

autogenous graft Tissue that is moved from one part of the body to another part of the same person's body.

autosome Any of the 22 pairs of chromosomes other than the sex chromosomes.

axillary tail Wedge of tissue extending from the breast into the axilla (also called the *tail of Spence*).

azoospermia Absence of sperm in semen.

baroreceptors Cells that are sensitive to blood pressure changes.

basal body temperature Body temperature at rest.

baseline data Information that describes the status of the client before treatment begins.

baseline risk The risk, usually in reference to birth defects or spontaneous abortion, of the general population of pregnant women who have no identified high-risk factors or invasive procedures.

bias A prejudice that sways the mind.

bicornuate (bicornate) uterus Malformed uterus having two horns.

bilirubin Unusable component of hemolyzed erythrocytes.

bilirubin encephalopathy Acute neurological condition resulting from deposits of unconjugated bilirubin in the brain tissue (kernicterus).

bilirubin-induced neurological dysfunction Permanent brain damage resulting from kernicterus.

bioethics Rules or principles that govern right conduct, specifically those that relate to health care.

biophysical profile Method for evaluating fetal status during the antepartum period based on five variables originating with the fetus: fetal heart rate, breathing movements, gross body movements, muscle tone, and amniotic fluid volume.

birth defect An abnormality of structure, function, or body metabolism present at birth that results in physical or mental disability or is fatal.

birth plan A plan describing a couple's preferences for their birth experience (also called a *family preference plan*).

bloody show Mixture of cervical mucus and blood from ruptured capillaries in the cervix; often precedes labor and increases with cervical dilation.

body image Subjective image of one's own physical appearance and capabilities; derived from one's own observations and the evaluation of significant others.

bonding Development of a strong emotional tie of a parent to a newborn; also called *claiming,* or *binding in.*

Braxton Hicks contractions Irregular, usually mild uterine contractions that occur throughout pregnancy and become stronger in the last trimester.

bronchopulmonary dysplasia (BPD) Chronic pulmonary condition in which damage to the infant's lungs requires prolonged dependence on supplemental oxygen.

brown fat (or brown adipose tissue) Highly vascular specialized fat found in the newborn that provides more heat than other fat when metabolized.

bulimia Eating disorder characterized by ingestion of large amounts of food followed by purging behavior, such as induced vomiting or laxative abuse.

café-au-lait spots Light-brown birthmarks.

caput succedaneum Area of edema over the presenting part of the fetus or newborn resulting from pressure against the cervix; often called simply *caput.*

carcinoma in situ Malignant neoplasm in surface tissue that has not extended into deeper tissue.

catabolism Destructive process that converts living cells into simpler compounds; process involved in involution of the uterus after childbirth.

caudal regression syndrome A malformation that results when the sacrum, lumbar spine, and lower extremities fail to develop.

cephalhematoma Bleeding between the periosteum and skull from pressure during birth; does not cross suture lines.

cephalopelvic disproportion Fetal head size that is too large to fit through the maternal pelvis at birth (also called *fetopelvic disproportion*).

cerclage Encircling the cervix with suture to prevent recurrent spontaneous abortion caused by early cervical dilation.

cervical cap A small cuplike device placed over the cervix to prevent sperm from entering, thus preventing pregnancy.

cesarean birth Surgical birth of the fetus through an incision in the abdominal wall and uterus.

Chadwick's sign Bluish purple discoloration of the cervix, vagina, and labia during pregnancy as a result of increased vascular congestion.

chemoreceptors Cells that are sensitive to chemical changes in the blood, specifically changes in oxygen and carbon dioxide levels, and changes in acid-base balance.

chignon Newborn scalp edema created by a vacuum extractor.

choanal atresia Abnormality of the nasal septum that obstructs one or both nasal passages.

chorioamnionitis Inflammation of the amniotic sac (fetal membranes); usually caused by bacterial and viral infections (also called *amnionitis*).

chorionic villus sampling Transcervical or transabdominal procedure to obtain a sample of chorionic villi (projections of the outer fetal membrane) for analysis of fetal cells.

chromosomes Organization of DNA of specific genes into strings within the cell nucleus.

cilia Hairlike processes on the surface of a cell that beat rhythmically to move the cell or to move fluid or other substances over the cell surface.

climacteric Endocrine, body, and psychic changes occurring at the end of a woman's reproductive period. Also informally called *menopause* although this term does not encompass all changes.

coitus Sexual union between a male and a female.

coitus interruptus Withdrawal of the penis from the vagina before ejaculation.

colostrum Breast fluid secreted during pregnancy and the first week after childbirth.

colposcopy Examination of the vaginal and cervical tissue with a colposcope for magnification of cells.

complementary and alternative medicine Nonmainstream or unconventional health care treatments and practices that are generally not used in hospitals and often not reimbursed by insurance companies.

compliance Stretchability or elasticity of the lungs and thorax that allows distention without resistance during respirations.

conceptus Cells and membranes resulting from fertilization of the ovum at any stage of prenatal development.

condom Latex, polyurethane, or natural membrane sheath covering the penis or lining the vagina to prevent sperm from entering the cervix and prevent infection.

condyloma A wartlike growth of the skin seen on the external genitalia, in the vagina, on the cervix, or near the anus; may be caused by human papillomavirus (condyloma acuminatum) or by syphilis (condyloma latum).

congenital Present at birth.

congenital anomaly Abnormal intrauterine development of an organ or structure.

congestive heart failure Condition resulting from failure of the heart to maintain adequate circulation; characterized by weakness, dyspnea, and edema in body parts that are lower than the heart.

containment A method of increasing comfort in infants by swaddling or other means to keep the extremities in a flexed position near the body.

contraception Prevention of pregnancy.

contraceptive vaginal ring Flexible ring releasing small amounts of estrogen and progesterone to prevent pregnancy.

contraction stress test Method for evaluating fetal status during the antepartum period by observing response of the fetal heart to the stress of uterine contractions that may induce recurrent episodes of fetal hypoxia.

corpus luteum Graafian follicle cells remaining after ovulation that produce estrogen and progesterone.

corrected age Gestational age that a preterm infant would be if still in utero. Also may be called *developmental age;* the chronologic age minus the number of weeks the infant was born prematurely.

couvade Pregnancy-related rituals or a cluster of symptoms experienced by some prospective fathers during pregnancy and childbirth.

crack A highly addictive form of cocaine that has been processed to be smoked.

craniosynostosis Premature closure of the sutures of the infant's head.

crowning Appearance of the fetal scalp or presenting part at the vaginal opening.

cryotherapy Destruction of tissue using extreme cold.

cryptorchidism Failure of one or both testes to descend into the scrotum.

culture Sum of values, beliefs, and practices of a group of people that is transmitted from one generation to the next.

cystocele Prolapse of the urinary bladder through the anterior vaginal wall.

decidua Name applied to the endometrium during pregnancy. All except the deepest layer is shed after childbirth.

decrement Period of decreasing strength of a uterine contraction.

Δ **OD$_{450}$** A test used to measure the change in optical density of the amniotic fluid caused by staining with bilirubin.

delegated nursing interventions Physician-prescribed nursing actions that require nursing judgment because nurses are accountable for correct implementation; also called *interdependent nursing interventions.* (See also *independent nursing interventions.*)

deontologic theory Ethical theory holding that the right course of action is the one dictated by ethical principles and moral rules.

developmental task A step in growth and maturation that one must complete before additional growth and maturation are possible.

diabetes mellitus A disorder of carbohydrate metabolism caused by a relative or complete lack of insulin secretion; characterized by glycosuria (glucose in the urine) and hyperglycemia.

diabetogenic Condition such as pregnancy that produces the effects of diabetes mellitus.

diaphragm A latex dome that covers the cervix and prevents entrance of sperm; must be used with a spermicide to be effective.

diastasis recti Separation of the longitudinal muscles of the abdomen (rectus abdominis) during pregnancy.

dietary reference intakes A label for several terms that estimate nutrient needs; includes recommended dietary allowance, adequate intake, tolerable upper intake level, and estimated average requirement.

dilation and curettage (D&C) Stretching of the cervical os to permit suctioning or scraping of the walls of the uterus. The procedure is performed in abortion, to obtain samples of uterine lining tissue for laboratory examination, and during the postpartum period to remove retained fragments of placental tissue.

dilation and evacuation (D&E) Wide cervical dilation followed by mechanical destruction and removal of fetal parts from the uterus. After complete removal of the fetus, a vacuum curet is used to remove the placenta and remaining products of conception.

diploid Having a pair of chromosomes that represents one copy of every chromosome from each parent; the number of chromosomes (46 in humans) normally present in body cells other than gametes.

disturbance in body image Negative feelings about the characteristics, functions, or limits of one's body.

doula A trained labor support person who provides labor or postpartum support.

duration Period from the beginning of a uterine contraction to the end of the same contraction.

dysmenorrhea Painful menstruation.

dyspareunia Difficult or painful coitus in women.

dysplasia Abnormal development of tissue.

dystocia Difficult or prolonged labor; often associated with abnormal uterine activity and cephalopelvic disproportion.

dysuria Painful urination often associated with urinary tract infection.

eclampsia Form of hypertension of pregnancy complicated by generalized (grand mal) seizures.

ectopic pregnancy Implantation of a fertilized ovum in any area other than the uterus; the most common site is the fallopian tube.

EDD Abbreviation for estimated date of delivery; also may be abbreviated *EDB* (estimated date of birth).

effleurage Massage of the abdomen or another body part performed during labor contractions.

egocentrism Interest centered on the self rather than the needs of others.

ejaculation Expulsion of semen from the penis.

emancipated minor An adolescent younger than the age of majority (usually 18 years) who is considered developmentally competent to make certain medical decisions independent of a parent or guardian.

embolus A mass which may be composed of a thrombus (blood clot) or amniotic fluid released into the bloodstream to cause obstruction of pulmonary vessels.

embryo The developing baby from the beginning of the third week through the eighth week after conception.

endometrial hyperplasia Excessive proliferation of normal cells of the uterine lining; may be due to administration of estrogen during the postmenopausal period.

endometriosis Presence of endometrial tissue (uterine lining) outside the uterine cavity.

endometrium Lining of the uterus.

endorphin Substance similar to opioids, which occurs naturally in the central nervous system and modifies pain sensations; related to enkephalins.

en face Position that allows eye-to-eye contact between the newborn and a parent.

engagement Descent of the widest diameter of the fetal presenting part to at least a zero station (the level of the ischial spines in the maternal pelvis).

engorgement Swelling of the breasts resulting from enlarged lymph glands, increased blood flow, and accumulation of milk when milk begins to be produced.

engrossment Intense fascination and close face-to-face observation between the father and newborn.

enkephalin Substance similar to opioids, which occurs naturally in the central nervous system and modifies pain sensations; related to endorphins.

enteral feeding Nutrients supplied to the gastrointestinal tract orally or by feeding tube.

entrainment Newborn movement in rhythm to adult speech, particularly high-pitched tones, which are more easily heard.

epidural space Area outside the dura, between the dura mater and the vertebral canal.

episiotomy Surgical incision of the perineum to enlarge the vaginal opening.

epispadias Abnormal placement of the urinary meatus on the dorsal side of the penis.

erectile dysfunction Consistent inability of a man to achieve or maintain an erection of the penis that is sufficiently rigid to permit successful sexual intercourse. Also called *impotence.*

erythema toxicum Benign rash of unknown cause in newborns, with blotchy red areas that may have white or yellow papules or vesicles in the center.

erythroblastosis fetalis Agglutination and hemolysis of fetal erythrocytes resulting from incompatibility between maternal and fetal blood. In most cases, the fetus is Rh-positive and the mother is Rh-negative.

esophageal atresia Condition in which the esophagus is separated from the stomach and ends in a blind pouch.

essential amino acids Amino acids that cannot be synthesized by the body and must be obtained from foods.

ethical dilemma A situation in which no solution seems completely satisfactory.

ethics Rules or principles that govern right conduct and distinctions between right and wrong.

ethnic Pertaining to religious, racial, national, or cultural group characteristics, especially speech patterns, social customs, and physical characteristics.

ethnicity Condition of belonging to a particular ethnic group; also refers to ethnic pride.

ethnocentrism Opinion that the beliefs and customs of one's own ethnic group are superior.

extremely-low-birth-weight infant An infant weighing 1000 g (2 lb, 3 oz) or less at birth.

extrusion reflex Automatic nervous system response that causes an infant to push anything solid out of the mouth.

familial Presence of a trait or condition in a family more often than would be expected by chance alone.

fantasy Mental images formed to prepare for the birth of a child.

female sterilization Cutting or mechanically occluding the fallopian tubes to prevent passage of ova or sperm, thus preventing pregnancy. May also be called *tubal ligation.*

ferning Microscopic appearance of amniotic fluid resembling fern leaves when the fluid is allowed to dry on a microscope slide; also called *fern test.* Also describes the microscopic, fernlike appearance of dried cervical mucus that is most apparent at the time of ovulation.

fertilization age Prenatal age of the developing baby, calculated from the date of conception. (Also called *postconceptional age.*)

fetal alcohol syndrome A group of physical and mental disorders of the offspring associated with maternal use of alcohol during pregnancy.

fetal lung fluid Fluid that fills the fetal lungs, expanding the alveoli and promoting lung development.

fetus The developing baby from 9 weeks after conception until birth; term used in everyday practice to describe a developing baby during pregnancy, regardless of age.

fingertipping First tactile (touch) experience between the mother and newborn in which the mother explores the infant's body, mainly with her fingertips.

first period of reactivity Period beginning at birth in which newborns are active and alert. It ends when the infant first falls asleep.

fontanel Space at the intersection of sutures connecting fetal or infant skull bones.

foremilk First breast milk received in a feeding.

fornix (pl. fornices) An arch or pouchlike structure at the upper end of the vagina. Also called a *cul-de-sac.*

fourth trimester First 12 weeks after birth; a time of transition for parents and siblings.

frequency Period from the beginning of one uterine contraction to the beginning of the next.

fundus Part of the uterus that is farthest from the cervix, above the openings of the fallopian tubes.

gamete Reproductive cell or germ cell; in the female an ovum and in the male a spermatozoon.

gametogenesis Development and maturation of the sperm and ova.

gastroesophageal reflux Condition in which stomach contents enter the esophagus and may be aspirated into the lungs.

gastroschisis Protrusion of the intestines through a defect in the abdominal wall. The intestines are not covered by a peritoneal sac or skin.

gate control theory A theory about pain based on the premise that a gating mechanism in the dorsal horn of the spinal cord can open or close a "gate" for transmission of pain impulses to the brain.

gene Segment of DNA that directs the production of a specific product needed for body structure or function.

general anesthesia Systemic loss of sensation with loss of consciousness.

genetic Pertaining to the genes or chromosomes.

genetic sex Sex determined at conception by union of two X chromosomes (female) or an X and a Y chromosome (male) (also called *chromosomal sex*).

genotype Genetic makeup of an individual.

gestational age Prenatal age of the developing baby (measured in weeks) calculated from the first day of the woman's last menstrual period; about 2 weeks longer than the fertilization age. (Also called *menstrual age.*)

gestational surrogate A woman who carries the embryo of an infertile couple and relinquishes the child to the couple after birth.

gestational trophoblastic disease Spectrum of diseases that includes both benign hydatidiform mole and gestational trophoblastic tumors, such as invasive moles and choriocarcinoma.

gluconeogenesis Formation of glycogen by the liver from noncarbohydrate sources, such as amino and fatty acids.

gonad Reproductive (sex) gland that produces gametes and sex hormones. The female gonads are ovaries and the male gonads are testes.

gonadotropic hormones Secretions of the anterior pituitary gland that stimulate the gonads, specifically follicle-stimulating hormone and luteinizing hormone. Chorionic gonadotropin is secreted by the placenta during pregnancy.

Goodell's sign Softening of the cervix during pregnancy.

graafian follicle A small sac within the ovary that contains the maturing ovum.

gravida A woman who is or has been pregnant, regardless of the duration or outcome of the pregnancy.

gynecologic age The number of years since menarche (first menstrual period).

habituation Decreased response to a repeated stimulus.

haploid Normal number of chromosomes in male or female gamete; refers to one copy of a chromosome from each pair (23 in humans, or half the diploid number).

Hegar's sign Softening of the lower uterine segment that allows it to be easily compressed by the sixth week of pregnancy.

hematoma Localized collection of blood in a space or tissue.

heme iron Iron obtained from meat, poultry, or fish sources; the form most usable by the body.

heterozygous Having two different alleles for a genetic trait.

hindmilk Breast milk received near the end of a feeding; contains higher fat content than foremilk.

homologous Chromosomes that pair during meiosis, one received from the person's mother and one from the father.

homozygous Having two identical alleles for a genetic trait.

hydatidiform mole Abnormal pregnancy resulting from proliferation of chorionic villi that give rise to multiple cysts and rapid growth of the uterus.

hydramnios Excess volume of amniotic fluid (more than 2000 mL at term). Also called *polyhydramnios.*

hydrops fetalis Heart failure and generalized edema in the fetus secondary to severe anemia resulting from destruction of erythrocytes.

hyperbilirubinemia Excessive amount of bilirubin in the blood.

hypercapnia Excess carbon dioxide in the blood, evidenced by an elevated PCO_2.

hyperemia Excess blood in an area of the body.

hypertonic contractions Uterine contractions that are too long or too frequent, have too short a resting interval, or have an inadequate relaxation period to allow optimal uteroplacental exchange.

hypertonic labor dysfunction Ineffective labor characterized by erratic and poorly coordinated contractions. Uterine resting tone is higher than normal.

hypospadias Abnormal placement of the urinary meatus on the ventral side of the penis.

hypotonic labor dysfunction Ineffective labor characterized by weak, infrequent, and brief but coordinated uterine contractions. Uterine resting tone is normal.

hypovolemia Abnormally decreased volume of circulating fluid in the body.

hypovolemic shock Acute peripheral circulatory failure resulting from loss of circulating blood volume.

hypoxemia Reduced oxygenation of the blood, evidenced by a low PO_2.

hypoxia Reduced availability of oxygen to the body tissues.

iatrogenic An adverse condition resulting from treatment.

impotence See *erectile dysfunction.*

incompetent cervix Inability of the cervix to remain closed long enough during pregnancy for the fetus to reach a maturity sufficient to survive.

incomplete protein food Food that does not contain all the essential amino acids.

increment Period of increasing strength of a uterine contraction.

independent nursing interventions Nurse-prescribed actions used in both nursing diagnoses and collaborative problems. (See also *delegated nursing interventions.*)

induction of labor Artificial initiation of labor.

infant mortality rate Number of deaths per 1000 live births that occurs within the first 12 months of life.

inference The act of drawing a conclusion or making a deduction.

infertility Inability of a couple to conceive after 1 year of regular intercourse (two to three times weekly) without using contraception; also the involuntary inability to conceive and produce viable offspring when the couple chooses. Primary infertility occurs in a couple who has never conceived; secondary infertility occurs in a couple who has conceived at least once before.

intensity Strength of a uterine contraction.

intermittent monitoring Variation of electronic fetal monitoring in which an initial strip is obtained on admission. If patterns are reassuring the woman is remonitored for 15 minutes at regular intervals (such as every 30 to 60 minutes).

interval Period between the end of one uterine contraction and the beginning of the next.

intrapartum The time of labor and childbirth.

intrauterine contraceptive A mechanical device inserted into the uterus to prevent pregnancy; also called intrauterine device (IUD).

intrauterine growth restriction Failure of a fetus to grow as expected for gestational age.

introversion Inward concentration on the self and body.

involution Retrogressive changes that return the reproductive organs, particularly the uterus, to their nonpregnant size and condition.

jaundice Yellow discoloration of the skin and sclera caused by excessive bilirubin in the blood.

judgment An opinion.

karyotype A display of a cell's chromosomes, arranged from largest to smallest pairs.

Kegel exercises Alternate contracting and relaxing of the pelvic muscles. These movements strengthen the pubococcygeal muscle, which surrounds the urinary meatus and vagina.

kernicterus Staining of brain tissue caused by accumulation of unconjugated bilirubin in the brain. Bilirubin encephalopathy is the brain damage that results from these deposits.

ketosis Accumulation of ketone bodies (metabolic products) in the blood; frequently associated with acidosis.

kilocalorie A unit of heat; used to show the energy value in foods (commonly called *calorie*).

lactation Secretion of milk from the breasts; also describes the period of breastfeeding.

lacto-ovovegetarian A vegetarian whose diet includes milk products and eggs.

lactose intolerance Inability to digest most dairy products because of a deficiency of the enzyme lactase.

lactovegetarian A vegetarian whose diet includes milk products.

lanugo Fine, soft hair covering the fetus.

laparoscopy Insertion of an illuminated tube into the abdominal cavity to visualize contents, locate bleeding, and perform surgical procedures.

laparotomy Incision through the abdominal wall to examine the abdominal or pelvic organs or perform other surgical procedures.

large-for-gestational-age infant An infant whose size is above the 90th percentile for gestational age.

latch-on Attachment of the infant to the breast.

late deceleration The slowing of the fetal heart rate after the onset of a uterine contraction and persisting after the contraction ends.

lecithin/sphingomyelin ratio (L/S Ratio) Ratio of two phospholipids in amniotic fluid that is used to determine fetal lung maturity; ratio of 2:1 or greater usually indicates fetal lung maturity.

let-down reflex See *milk-ejection reflex.*

letting-go A phase of maternal adaptation that involves relinquishment of previous roles and assumption of a new role as a parent.

libido Sexual desire.

lie Relationship of the long axis of the fetus to the long axis of the mother.

lightening Descent of the fetus toward the pelvic inlet before labor.

linear salpingostomy Incision along the length of a fallopian tube to remove an ectopic pregnancy and preserve the tube.

lipogenic Substance, such as insulin, that stimulates the production of fat.

lochia Vaginal drainage after birth.

lochia alba White or cream-colored vaginal discharge that follows lochia serosa. Occurs when the amount of blood is decreased and the number of leukocytes is increased.

lochia rubra Reddish vaginal discharge that occurs immediately after childbirth; composed mostly of blood.

lochia serosa Pink or brown-tinged vaginal discharge that follows lochia rubra and precedes lochia alba; consists largely of serous exudate, blood, and leukocytes.

low-birth-weight infant An infant weighing less than 2500 g (5 lb, 8 oz) at birth.

maceration Discoloration and softening of tissues and eventual disintegration of a fetus that is retained in the uterus after its death.

macrosomia Unusually large fetal size; infant birth weight more than 4000 g.

malpractice Negligence by a professional person.

mammogram Study of breast tissue using very-low-dose x-ray; primary tool in the diagnosis of breast tumors.

Marfan syndrome A hereditary condition that involves weakness in connective tissue, bones, and muscles; the vascular system is affected, particularly the aorta.

mastitis Inflammation of the breast usually caused by infection.

maternal mortality rate Number of maternal deaths from births and complications of pregnancy, childbirth, and puerperium (the first 42 days after pregnancy ends) per 100,000 live births.

mature milk Breast milk that appears after the first 2 weeks of lactation.

meconium aspiration syndrome Obstruction and air trapping caused by meconium in the infant's lungs, which may lead to severe respiratory distress.

meiosis Reduction cell division in gametes that halves the number of chromosomes in each cell.

melasma Brownish pigmentation of the face during pregnancy; also called chloasma and "mask of pregnancy."

menarche Onset of menstruation, usually between 10 and 16 years of age or within 2 years from the start of breast development.

meningocele Protrusion of the meninges through a defect in the vertebrae; a form of neural tube defect.

menometrorrhagia Uterine bleeding irregular in frequency and excessive in amount.

menopause Permanent cessation of menstruation during the climacteric.

menorrhagia Excessive bleeding at the time of menstruation in number of days' duration, amount of blood lost, or both.

methadone A synthetic compound with opiate properties; used as an oral substitute for heroin and morphine in the opiate-addicted person.

metrorrhagia Bleeding from the uterus at any time other than during the menstrual period.

milia White cysts, 1 to 2 mm in size, from distended sebaceous glands.

miliaria (prickly heat) Rash caused by heat.

milk-ejection reflex Release of milk from the alveoli into the ducts; also known as the *letdown reflex.*

mimicry Copying the behaviors of other pregnant women or mothers as a method of "trying on" the role of advanced pregnancy or motherhood.

minimal enteral nutrition Very small feedings designed to help the gastrointestinal tract mature. Also called trophic feedings.

mitosis Cell division in body cells other than the gametes.

Mittelschmerz Low abdominal pain that occurs at ovulation.

molding Shaping of the fetal head during movement through the birth canal.

Mongolian spots Bruise-like marks that occur mostly in newborns with dark skin tones.

monosomy Presence of only one of a chromosome pair in every body cell.

Montevideo unit A method to calculate the intensity of uterine contractions in mm Hg as measured with an intrauterine pressure catheter. The baseline intrauterine pressure for each contraction in a 10-minute period is subtracted from the peak pressure. The resulting net pressures (peak minus baseline) are added to calculate Montevideo units, or MVUs.

motor block Loss of voluntary movement caused by regional anesthesia.

multifetal pregnancy A pregnancy in which the woman is carrying two or more fetuses. Also called *multiple gestation.*

multigravida A woman who has been pregnant more than once.

multipara A woman who has given birth after two or more pregnancies of at least 20 weeks' gestation; also informally used to describe a pregnant woman before the birth of her second child.

multiple-marker screening Analysis of maternal serum for abnormal levels of alpha-fetoprotein, human chorionic gonadotropin, and estriols that may predict chromosomal abnormalities of the fetus; often called triple-screen. Addition of tests, such as inhibin A, have improved accuracy of the results, leading to alternate names for the package of tests.

mutation Alteration in DNA sequence in a gene, usually one that adversely affects its function.

mutual recognition model A model of nurse licensure that allows nurses to hold licenses in their states of residence and practice in other states that also recognize the home state's license; also known as a *multistate licensure compact.*

myelomeningocele Protrusion of the meninges and spinal cord through a defect in the vertebrae; a form of neural tube defect.

nadir Lowest point, such as the lowest pulse rate in a series.

narcissism Undue preoccupation with oneself.

natural family planning Method of predicting ovulation based on normal changes in a woman's body.

necrotizing enterocolitis Serious inflammatory condition of the intestines.

negligence Failure to act in the way a reasonable, prudent person of similar background would act in similar circumstances.

neonatal abstinence syndrome A cluster of physical signs exhibited by the newborn exposed in utero to maternal use of substances such as heroin. (See also *abstinence syndrome.*)

neonatal mortality rate Number of deaths per 1000 live births occurring at birth or within the first 28 days of life.

neural tube defect A congenital defect in closure of the bony encasement of the spinal cord or skull. Includes defects such as anencephaly, spina bifida, meningocele, myelomeningocele, and others.

neutral thermal environment Environment in which body temperature is maintained without an increase in metabolic rate or oxygen use.

nevus flammeus Permanent purple birthmark; also called *port wine stain.*

nevus simplex Flat, pink area on the nape of the neck, midforehead, or over the eyelids resulting from dilation of the capillaries; also called *stork bites, salmon patches,* or *telangiectatic nevi.*

nevus vasculosus Rough, red collection of capillaries with a raised surface that disappears with time. Also called strawberry hemangioma.

nidation Implantation of the fertilized ovum (zygote) in the uterine endometrium.

nitrazine paper Paper used to test pH; helps determine whether the amniotic sac has ruptured.

noncompliance Resistance of the lungs and thorax to distention with air during respirations.

nonheme iron Iron obtained from plant and fortified foods.

nonnutritive sucking Sucking during which no milk flow is obtained.

nonshivering thermogenesis Process of heat production, without shivering, by oxidation of brown fat.

nonstress test A method for evaluating fetal status during the antepartum period by observing the response of the fetal heart rate to fetal movement.

nuchal cord Umbilical cord around the fetal neck.

nullipara A woman who has not completed a pregnancy to at least 20 weeks' gestation.

nurse anesthetist A registered nurse who has advanced education and certification in administration of anesthetics; also, certified registered nurse anesthetist (CRNA).

nurse practice acts Laws that determine the scope of nursing practice in each state.

nutrient density The quality and quantity of protein, vitamins, and minerals per 100 calories in foods.

nutritive suckling (sucking) Steady, rhythmic suckling at the breast or sucking at a bottle to obtain milk.

occult prolapse *See prolapsed cord.*

oligohydramnios Abnormally small quantity of amniotic fluid, less than about 500 ml at term.

oligospermia A decreased number of sperm in semen, usually considered to be under 20 million per milliliter.

omphalocele Protrusion of the intestines into the base of the umbilical cord. The intestines are covered by a peritoneal sac.

oogenesis Formation of gametes (ova) in the female.

opiate Any narcotic containing opium or a derivative of opium.

oral contraceptive Drug that inhibits ovulation; contains progestins alone or in combination with estrogen.

osmotic diuresis Secretion and passage of large amounts of urine as a result of increased osmotic pressure that can result from hyperglycemia.

osteoporosis Increased spaces (porosity) in bone; process greatly accelerates after menopause.

ovovegetarian A vegetarian whose diet includes eggs.

ovulation Release of the mature ovum from the ovary.

oxytocin Hormone produced by the posterior pituitary gland that stimulates uterine contractions and the milk-ejection reflex; also prepared synthetically.

pain threshold (or pain perception) The lowest level of stimulus one perceives as painful; relatively constant under different conditions.

pain tolerance Maximum pain one is willing to endure. Pain tolerance may increase or decrease under different conditions.

para A woman who has given birth after a pregnancy of at least 20 weeks' gestation; also designates the number of a woman's pregnancies that have ended after at least 20 weeks' gestation. (A multifetal gestation, such as twins, is considered one birth when calculating parity.)

parenteral nutrition Intravenous infusion of all nutrients known to be needed for metabolism and growth.

paroxysmal nocturnal dyspnea Respiratory distress occurring when lying down, often associated with congestive heart failure.

peau d'orange Dimpled skin condition that resembles an orange peel; associated with lymphatic edema and often seen over the area of breast cancer.

pedigree A graphic representation of a family's medical and hereditary history and the relationships among the family members (also called a *genogram*).

percutaneous umbilical blood sampling (PUBS) Procedure for obtaining fetal blood through ultrasound-guided puncture of an umbilical cord vessel to detect fetal problems, such as inherited blood disorders, acidosis, or infection; also called *cordocentesis.*

perinatologist Physician who specializes in the care of the mother, fetus, and infant during the perinatal period (from about the 20th week of pregnancy to 4 weeks after childbirth).

periodic breathing Cessation of breathing lasting 5 to 10 seconds without changes in color or heart rate.

periventricular-intraventricular hemorrhage Bleeding around and into the ventricles of the brain.

persistent pulmonary hypertension Vasoconstriction of the infant's pulmonary vessels after birth; may result in right-to-left shunting of blood flow through the ductus arteriosus, the foramen ovale, or both.

phenotype The outward expression of a person's genetic makeup; observed characteristics produced by the interaction of genes and environment.

phosphatidylglycerol (PG) A major phospholipid of surfactant whose presence in amniotic fluid indicates fetal lung maturity.

phosphatidylinositol (PI) A phospholipid of surfactant that is produced and secreted in increasing amounts as the fetal lungs mature.

physiologic anemia of pregnancy Decrease in hemoglobin and hematocrit values caused by dilution of erythrocytes by expanded plasma volume rather than by an actual decrease in erythrocytes or hemoglobin.

phytoestrogen Estrogen substance of plant origin.

pica Ingestion of a nonnutritive substance, such as laundry starch, dirt, or ice.

placenta Fetal structure that provides nourishment and removes wastes from the developing baby and secretes hormones necessary for the continuation of pregnancy.

placenta accreta A placenta that is abnormally adherent to the uterus. If the condition is more advanced, it is called *placenta increta* (the placenta extends into the uterine muscle) or *placenta percreta* (the placenta extends through the uterine muscle).

placenta previa Abnormal implantation of the placenta in the lower uterus located at or very near the cervical os.

point of maximum impulse (PMI) Area of the chest in which the heart sounds are loudest when auscultated.

polycythemia Abnormally high number of erythrocytes.

polydactyly More than 10 digits on the hands or feet.

polydipsia Excessive thirst.

polymorphism Alternate form of a gene found in the population at a frequency greater than 1%.

polyphagia Excessive ingestion of food.

polyploidy Having additional full sets of chromosomes, such as 69 (triploidy) or 92 (tetraploidy).

polyuria Excessive excretion of urine.

position Relation of a fixed reference point on the fetus to the quadrants of the maternal pelvis.

postmaturity syndrome Condition in which a postterm infant shows characteristics indicative of poor placental functioning before birth.

postpartum The first 6 weeks after childbirth.

postpartum blues Temporary, self-limited period of tearfulness experienced by many new mothers beginning in the first week after childbirth.

postterm birth One that occurs after the 42nd week of gestation.

postterm infant An infant born after 42 weeks of gestation.

precipitate birth A birth that occurs without a trained attendant present.

precipitate labor An intense, unusually short labor (less than 3 hours).

preeclampsia A hypertensive disorder of pregnancy characterized by hypertension and proteinuria.

premature rupture of the membranes Spontaneous rupture of the membranes before the onset of labor (term, preterm, or postterm gestation).

presentation Fetal part that enters the pelvic inlet, or the presenting part.

preterm birth One that occurs after the 20th week and before the start of the 38th week of gestation.

preterm infant An infant born before the beginning of the 38th week of gestation. Also called *premature infant.*

preterm labor Onset of labor after 20 weeks and before the beginning of the thirty-eighth week of gestation.

primigravida A woman who is pregnant for the first time.

primipara A woman who has given birth after a pregnancy of at least 20 weeks' gestation; also used informally to describe a pregnant woman before the birth of her first child.

progestin Any natural or synthetic form of progesterone.

prolactin Anterior pituitary hormone that promotes growth of breast tissue and stimulates production of milk.

prolapsed cord Displacement of the umbilical cord in front of or beside the fetal presenting part. An occult prolapse is one that is suspected on the basis of fetal heart rate patterns; the umbilical cord cannot be palpated or seen.

prune-belly syndrome An absence of abdominal muscles resulting in a flabby, distended, and creased abdomen that may occur in the infant exposed to cocaine in utero.

pseudomenstruation Vaginal bleeding in the newborn, resulting from withdrawal of placental hormones.

psychoprophylaxis Method of prepared childbirth that emphasizes mental concentration and relaxation to increase pain tolerance.

psychosis Mental state in which a person's ability to recognize reality, communicate, and relate to others is impaired.

puberty Period of sexual maturation accompanied by the development of secondary sex characteristics and the capacity to reproduce.

puerperium Period from the end of childbirth until involution of the reproductive organs is complete; approximately 6 weeks.

pulse oximetry Method of determining the level of blood oxygen saturation by sensors attached to the skin.

reciprocal bonding behaviors Repertoire of infant actions that promotes attachment between the parent and newborn.

recommended dietary allowances Levels of nutrient intake considered to meet the needs of healthy individuals.

rectocele Herniation (protrusion) of the rectum through the posterior vaginal wall.

REEDA Acronym for redness, ecchymosis, edema, discharge, and approximation; useful for assessing wound healing or the presence of inflammation or infection.

reflection Meditation, attentive consideration.

regional anesthesia Anesthesia that blocks pain impulses in a localized area without loss of consciousness.

respiratory distress syndrome Condition caused by insufficient production of surfactant in the lungs; results in atelectasis (collapse of the lung alveoli), hypoxemia (decreased O_2), and hypercapnia (increased CO_2).

retinopathy of prematurity Condition in which damage to blood vessels often associated with oxygen use may cause decreased vision or blindness.

retrograde ejaculation Discharge of semen into the bladder rather than from the end of the penis.

ripening Softening of the cervix as labor nears as the result of an increase in water content and the effects of relaxin on its connective tissue.

role transition Changing from one pattern of behavior and one image of self to another.

ruga (pl. *rugae*) Ridge or fold of tissue, as on the male's scrotum and in the female's vagina.

salpingectomy Surgical removal of a fallopian tube.

seborrheic dermatitis (cradle cap) Yellowish, crusty area of the scalp.

second period of reactivity Period of 4 to 6 hours after the first sleep following birth when the newborn may have an elevated pulse and respiratory rate and excessive mucus.

secondary sex characteristics Physical differences between mature males and females that are not directly related to reproduction.

semen Spermatozoa with their nourishing and protective fluid; discharged at ejaculation.

sensory block Loss of sensation caused by regional anesthesia.

seroconversion Change in a blood test result from negative to positive, indicating the development of antibodies in response to infection or immunization.

sex chromosome The X or Y chromosome. Females have two X chromosomes; males have one X and one Y chromosome.

sexually transmitted (or transmissible) disease (STD) A disease that is passed to others primarily through sexual contact. Also called *sexually transmissible (or transmitted) infection (STI)*.

shoulder dystocia Delayed or difficult birth of the fetal shoulders after the head is born.

sibling rivalry Feelings of jealousy and fear of replacement when a young child must share the attention of the parents with a newborn infant.

skepticism Doubt in the absence of conclusive evidence.

small-for-gestational-age infant An infant whose size is below the 10th percentile for gestational age.

somatic cells Body cells other than the gametes, or germ cells.

somatic sex Gender assignment as male or female on the basis of form and structure of the external genitalia.

spermatogenesis Formation of male gametes (sperm) in the testes.

spermicide A chemical that kills sperm.

spina bifida Defective closure of the bony spine that encloses the spinal cord; a type of neural tube defect.

spinnbarkeit Clear, slippery, stretchy quality of cervical mucus during ovulation.

standard of care Level of care that can be expected of a professional as determined by laws, professional organizations, and health care agencies.

standard procedures Procedures determined by nurses, physicians, and administrators that allow nurses to perform duties usually part of the medical practice.

station Measurement of fetal descent in relation to the ischial spines of the maternal pelvis (see also *engagement*).

sterility Total inability to conceive.

strabismus A turning inward ("crossing") or outward of the eyes because of poor muscle tone in the muscles that control eye movement.

striae gravidarum Irregular reddish streaks on the woman's abdomen, breasts, and thighs resulting from tears in connective tissue.

subarachnoid space Space between the arachnoid mater and the pia mater containing cerebrospinal fluid.

subinvolution A slower-than-expected return of the uterus to its nonpregnancy size after childbirth.

suckling Giving or taking nourishment from the breast. Sometimes used interchangeably with sucking, which refers only to drawing into the mouth with a partial vacuum, as with a bottle or pacifier.

sudden infant death syndrome (SIDS) Sudden death of an infant that is unexplained by history, autopsy, or examination of the scene of death.

surfactant Combination of lipoproteins produced by the lungs of the mature fetus to reduce surface tension in the alveoli, thus promoting lung expansion after birth.

surrogate mother A fertile woman who is inseminated for the purpose of conceiving and relinquishing a child to an infertile couple.

suspend To delay or bring to a stop temporarily.

sutures Narrow areas of flexible tissue that connect fetal skull bones, permitting slight movement during labor.

syndactyly Webbing between fingers or toes.

tachypnea Respiratory rate above 60 breaths per minute in the newborn after the first hour of life.

taking-hold Second phase of maternal adaptation during which the mother assumes control of her own care and initiates care of the infant.

taking-in First phase of maternal adaptation during which the mother passively accepts care, comfort, and details about the newborn.

telemetry Wireless transmission of electronic fetal monitoring data to the bedside or central monitor unit.

teratogen An environmental agent that can cause defects in a developing baby during pregnancy.

term birth One that occurs between the 38th and 42nd weeks of gestation.

thermogenesis Heat production.

thermoregulation Maintenance of body temperature.

thrombus Collection of blood factors, primarily platelets and fibrin that may cause vascular obstruction.

tocolytic Drug that inhibits uterine contractions.

toxic shock syndrome Rare, potentially fatal disorder usually caused by toxin produced by *Staphylococcus aureus;* has been associated with improper use of tampons.

tracheoesophageal fistula Abnormal connection between the esophagus and trachea.

transcutaneous oxygen monitoring Method of continuous noninvasive measurement of oxygen in the blood by transducers attached to the skin.

transdermal contraceptive patch Adhesive patch containing estrogen and progestin, which are absorbed through the skin to prevent pregnancy.

transducer Device that translates one physical quantity to another, such as fetal heart motion into an electrical signal for rate calculation, generation of sound, or a written record.

transient tachypnea of the newborn Condition of rapid respirations caused by inadequate absorption of fetal lung fluid.

transitional milk Breast milk that appears between secretion of colostrum and of mature milk.

translocation Exchange of genetic material between nonhomologous chromosomes.

trimester A division of full term pregnancy into 3 equal parts of 13 weeks each.

trisomy Presence of three copies of a chromosome in each body cell.

ultrasonography Technique for visualizing deep structures of the body by recording the reflections (echoes) of high-frequency sound waves directed into the tissue.

uterine inversion Turning of the uterus inside out after birth of the fetus.

uterine resting tone Degree of uterine muscle tension when the woman is not in labor or during the interval between labor contractions

uterine rupture A tear in the wall of the uterus.

uteroplacental insufficiency Inability of the placenta to exchange oxygen, carbon dioxide, nutrients, and waste products properly between the maternal and fetal circulations.

utilitarian theory Ethical theory stating that the right course of action is the one that produces the greatest good.

vacuum curettage (vacuum aspiration) Removal of the uterine contents by application of a vacuum through a hollow curet or cannula introduced into the uterus.

validate To make certain that the information collected during assessment is accurate.

varicocele Abnormal dilation or varicosity of veins in the spermatic cord.

vasectomy Cutting or occluding the vas deferens to prevent passage of sperm, thus preventing pregnancy.

vasoconstriction Narrowing of the lumen of blood vessels.

VBAC Acronym for *vaginal birth after cesarean.*

vegan A complete vegetarian who does not eat any animal products.

vegetarian An individual whose diet consists wholly or mostly of plant foods and who avoids animal food sources.

vernix caseosa Thick, white substance that protects the skin of the fetus.

version Turning the fetus from one presentation to another before birth, usually from breech to cephalic.

very-low-birth-weight infant An infant weighing 1500 g (3 lb, 5 oz) or less at birth.

vibroacoustic stimulation Use of sound stimulation to elicit fetal movement and acceleration (speeding up) of the fetal heart rate.

withdrawal syndrome See *abstinence syndrome.*

zygote The developing baby from conception through the first week of prenatal life.

Index

Page numbers followed by b indicate boxes; f, figures; t, tables.

A

AAP (American Academy of Pediatrics), 7
Abacavir, risk categories of, 925
ABC. *See* Abacavir.
ABCDEs, of critical thinking, 29-30
Abdomen
  antepartum assessment of, 132
  intrapartum assessment of, 274t
  of newborn, assessment of, 491
  postpartum assessment of, 399
    in cesarean birth, 418
Abdominal breathing exercises, 423f
Abdominal distention, post cesarean, preventing, 419
Abdominal enlargement, as indication of pregnancy, 126
Abdominal exercises, for diastasis recti, 399f
Abdominal wall, in pregnancy, 118
Abduction, infant, preventing, 522-523
ABO incompatibility, 656
Abortion
  in adolescent pregnancy, 591
  complete, 625
  defined, 109, 266, 622
  in early pregnancy, 623-625
  elective, 38-39
  ethical aspects of, 38-39
  history of, 271t
  incomplete, 625
  inevitable, 624
  legal and political aspects of, 39
  medical, 899-901
  nursing considerations in, 626
  spontaneous, 623-625
    recurrent, 625-626
    threatened, 623-624
  surgical techniques of, 900
Abruptio placentae, 634
  in amniotomy, 365
  clinical signs of, 634-635
  concealed hemorrhage in, signs of, 635

Abruptio placentae *(Continued)*
  defined, 364, 622, 697
  and fetal oxygenation, 308
  incidence and etiology of, 634
  nursing considerations in, 635-636
  therapeutic management of, 635
  types of, 635f
Abstinence, 851
Abstinence syndrome, defined, 589
Abused women. *See* Violence, against women.
Acceleration patterns, in fetal heart rate, 319, 319f
Acceptance, of motherhood, securing, 156
Accident prevention. *See* Safety considerations.
Accolate. *See* Zafirlukast.
Accupril. *See* Quinapril.
Accutane. *See* Isotretinoin.
ACE inhibitors, risk category of, 924
Acebutolol, risk category of, 924
Acetaminophen
  postpartum use of, 411t
  risk category of, 922
Acetazolamide, risk category of, 926
ACHES (acronym), 845t
Acidosis, defined, 306
Acme, of contraction, 239
ACOG (American College of Obstetricians and Gynecologists), 7
Acquired immunodeficiency syndrome (AIDS). *See also* HIV (human immunodeficiency virus) infection.
  in pregnancy, 688-690
Acrocyanosis, 475, 493
  defined, 468
Activated partial thromboplastin time values in pregnant and nonpregnant women, 919
Active management, of labor, 369
Actonel. *See* Risedronate.
Actos. *See* Pioglitazone.

Actron. *See* Ketoprofen.
Actual nursing diagnoses, 31t
Acyanotic conditions, of newborn, 823
Acyclovir, risk category of, 925
Adalat. *See* Nifedipine.
Addiction, defined, 589
Adepin. *See* Doxepin.
Adjunctive drugs, and opioid analgesics, 348t, 351
Adjuvant therapy
  in breast cancer, 889-890
  defined, 878
Admission, hospital or birth center, 267-282
  assessments in. *See* Admission assessment(s).
  birth attendant notification in, 275
  communication with families in, 267
  consent forms in, 275
  cultural considerations in, 268-269
  items to bring in, 235b
  nursing responsibilities during, 268-269
  primary nurse assignment in, 268-269
  therapeutic communication in, 268
Admission assessment(s), intrapartum, 270t-274t, 275
  consent forms in, 275
  critical thinking exercises in, 275, 282
  fetal evaluation in, 269, 273t, 280f-281f, 281-282
  focused, 269
  interview in, 270t-272t
  labor status determination in, 269-282, 273t
  maternal evaluation in, 269, 273t-274t, 282-284
Adnexa, defined, 878
Adolescent pregnancy, 160-161, 590-598
  adaptation to, 161, 598